W9-BRC-037

# 1999

# Lippincott's Nursing Drug Guide

# 1999 Lippincott's Nursing Drug Guide

Amy M. Karch, RN, MS

Director of Applied Science/Lecturer
Nazareth College
Rochester, NY

Lippincott
Philadelphia • New York

*Acquisitions Editor:* Margaret Zuccarini
*Assistant Editor:* Sara Lauber
*Project Editor:* Tom Gibbons
*Production Manager:* Helen Ewan
*Production Coordinator:* Michael Carcel
*Design Coordinator:* Doug Smock

Copyright © 1999 by Lippincott-Raven Publishers. All rights reserved. This book is protected by copyright. No part of it may be reproduced, stored in a retrieval system, or transmitted, in any form or by any means—electronic, mechanical, photocopy, recording, or otherwise—without the prior written permission of the publisher, except for brief quotations embodied in critical articles and reviews. Printed in the United States of America. For information write Lippincott-Raven Publishers, 227 East Washington Square, Philadelphia, PA 19106.

ISSN: 1081-857X
ISBN: 0-7817-1731-0
1998 Quick Access Photo Guide to Pills and Capsules—Adapted from Facts and Comparisons, St. Louis, MO

Care has been taken to confirm the accuracy of the information presented and to describe generally accepted practices. However, the authors, editors, and publisher are not responsible for errors or omissions or for any consequences from application of the information in this book and make no warranty, express or implied, with respect to the contents of the publication.

The authors, editors and publisher have exerted every effort to ensure that drug selection and dosage set forth in this text are in accordance with current recommendations and practice at the time of publication. However, in view of ongoing research, changes in government regulations, and the constant flow of information relating to drug therapy and drug reactions, the reader is urged to check the package insert for each drug for any change in indications and dosage and for added warnings and precautions. This is particularly important when the recommended agent is a new or infrequently employed drug.

Some drugs and medical devices presented in this publication have Food and Drug Administration (FDA) clearance for limited use in restricted research settings. It is the responsibility of the health care provider to ascertain the FDA status of each drug or device planned for use in their clinical practice.

9 8 7 6 5 4 3 2 1

# Consultants and Student Reviewers

**Lois Dixon, RN, MSN**
Assistant Professor
Trinity College of Nursing
Moline, Illinois

**Libby Hall**
Nursing Student
University of North Carolina—Chapel Hill
Chapel Hill, North Carolina

**Cynthia Hanson, RN, MSN, CS, CRNP**
Geriatric Nurse Practitioner
Genesis Physician Services
Wayne, Pennsylvania

**Phillis Foster Healy, PhD, RN**
Associate Professor and Graduate Chair
University of Southern Maine
College of Nursing
Portland, Maine

**Mary Regina Jennette, RN, MA, MSN, EdD**
Professor, Director of Nursing Program
West Virginia Northern Community College
Wheeling, West Virginia

**Molly Long**
Nursing Student
University of North Carolina—Chapel Hill
Chapel Hill, North Carolina

**Jane B. Pond, MSN, CRNP**
Director, Ambulatory Care Services
Temple Health Connection
Philadelphia, Pennsylvania

**Sandi Schutte**
Nursing Student
University of Minnesota
Moorhead, Minnesota

**Sharon Staib, RN, MS**
Assistant Professor of Nursing
Ohio University—Zanesville
Zanesville, Ohio

**Deborah Trafton, LPN**
Pediatric Home Health Care
Barnes Jewish Children's Hospital
St. Louis, Missouri

**Dianne R. Wasson, MSN, RN**
Assistant Professor
Trinity College of Nursing
Moline, Illinois

# Consultants to Previous Editions

**Marion J. Anema, RN, PhD**
Professor and Dean, School of Nursing
Tennessee State University
Nashville, Tennessee

**Jeffrey Baldwin, BS (Pharm), PharmD, RPh**
Associate Professor of Pharmacy Practice and (courtesy) Pediatrics
University of Nebraska Medical Center
College of Pharmacy
Omaha, Nebraska

**Nancy Balkon, MS, RN, CS, ANP**
Clinical Assistant Professor
Adult Health Nursing
State University of New York at Stony Brook
Stony Brook, New York

**Jen Bartek, RN, PhD, CARN**
Associate Professor
University of Nebraska Medical Center
Colleges of Nursing and Medicine
Omaha, Nebraska

**Margaret W. Bellak, RN, MN**
Assistant Professor
School of Nursing
Indiana University of Pennsylvania
Indiana, Pennsylvania

**Patricia Brown-Dominguez, RN, MSN**
Assistant Professor
Houston Baptist University
College of Nursing
Houston, Texas

**Brenda L. Burns**
Student Nurse
Clayton State College
Morrow, Georgia

**Sarah Connor, RNCS, BSN, MSN, EdD**
Assistant to Vice President and Dean of Faculty
Armstrong State College
Savannah, Georgia

**Dona M. Sobokta Ely, MPH, BSN, RN, C**
Adjunct Faculty
University of Pennsylvania
Philadelphia, Pennsylvania

**Elizabeth Fisk, RN, MS**
Associate Professor
Nursing Department
Fitchburg State College
Fitchburg, Massachusetts

**Steven S. Golden**
Nursing Student
Rock Island, Illinois

**Barbara Kesler, Registered Pharmacist**
Instruction Coordinator
El Paso Community College
Staff Pharmacist
Thomson General Hospital
El Paso, Texas

**Theresa Moderhack**
Nursing Student
Wauconda, Illinois

**Bette S. Perman, MN, RN, CCRN**
Professor of Nursing
Shoreline Community College
Seattle, Washington

**Rebecca L. Peters**
Nursing Student
Moline, Illinois

**Ann Richardson**
Nursing Student
Moline, Illinois

**Marjorie L. Roark, RN, BSN, MEd**
Nursing Instructor
Angelina College
Lutkin, Texas

**Sally Scavone, RN, BSN, MS**
Assistant Professor
Nursing Department
Erie Community College/City Campus
Erie, New York

**Theresa Schumacher, RN, BSN, MSN**
Area Chairperson, Level 4
School of Nursing
Good Samaritan Hospital
Cincinnati, Ohio

**Robert Stanton, MBA, PharmD**
Clinical Pharmacist
Cabell Huntingdon Hospital
Assistant Professor
Marshall University
Huntingdon, West Virginia

**Vicki M. Stephens, RN, MSN**
Assistant Professor of Nursing
University of Charleston
BSN Program
Charleston, West Virginia

**Majorie Suedekum, MS, RN, CS**
ALT Manager
Department of Nursing and Radiologic Sciences
Mesa State College
Grand Junction, Colorado

**Jessica Twitty**
Nursing Student
Rock Island, Illinois

**Chris Vidman**
Nursing Student
Moline, Illinois

**Patricia Warunek, RN, PhD**
Assistant Vice President for Academic Affairs
Farleigh-Dickinson University
Teaneck, New Jersey

**Laura Zanolla**
Nursing Student
Burbank, Illinois

# Preface

## How To Use This Drug Guide

The number of clinically important drugs increases every year, as does the nurse's responsibility for drug therapy. No nurse can memorize all the drug information needed to provide safe and efficacious drug therapy. The *1999 Lippincott's Nursing Drug Guide* provides the drug information nurses need in a concise, ready-access format and presents nursing considerations related to drug therapy in the format of the nursing process, a framework for applying basic pharmacologic information to patient care. It is intended for both the student nurse who is just learning how to apply pharmacologic data in the clinical situation and the busy practicing professional nurse who needs a quick, easy-to-use guide to the clinical use of drugs. This book provides broad coverage of the drugs commonly encountered by nurses and of drugs whose use commonly involves significant nursing intervention. Commonly used medical abbreviations are found throughout the book and are defined in the list of Commonly Used Medical Abbreviations located on the inside front cover and facing page.

### Part I

The first section of this book provides a concise review of the nursing process and its application to pharmacologic situations, including a concise example of how to use this drug guide to apply the nursing process. A review of selected drug classifications provides a convenient, complete summary of the drug information pertinent to drugs in each class. The Compendium of Adverse Effects includes guidelines for nursing interventions as related to adverse effects.

### Part II

Drug information is presented in monograph form, with the monographs arranged alphabetically by generic name. Each page of the book contains guide words at the top, much like a dictionary, to facilitate easy access to any drug. The right-hand edge of the book contains letter guides, again to facilitate finding a drug as quickly as possible.

## Complete Drug Monographs

Each drug monograph is complete in itself—that is, it includes all of the clinically important information that a nurse needs to know to give the drug safely and effectively. Every monograph begins with the drug's generic (nonproprietary) name; an alphabetical list of the most common brand names, including common brand names found only in Canada (noted by the designation CAN); a notation indicating if the drug is available as an OTC drug; its pregnancy category classification; and its schedule if it is a controlled substance.

- Commonly accepted pronunciation (after *United States Adopted Names [USAN]* and the *United States Pharmacopeia [USP] Dictionary of Drug Names, 1987*) is provided to help the nurse feel more comfortable discussing the drug with other members of the health care team.
- The clinically important drug classes of each drug are indicated to put the drug in appropriate context.
- The therapeutically useful actions of the drug are described, including (when known) the mechanism(s) by which these therapeutic effects are produced; no attempt is made to list *all* of the drug's known actions here.

- Clinical indications for the drug are listed, including important non-FDA approved, or "unlabeled," indications as well as orphan drug uses when appropriate.
- Contraindications to drug use and cautions that should be considered when using the drug are listed.
- The pharmacokinetic profile of the drug is given in table form to allow easy access to such information as half-life, peak levels, and distribution, offering a quick reference to how the drug is handled in the body.
- Dosage information is listed next, including adult, pediatric, geriatric, renal-impaired and hepatic-impaired patients, and dosages for different indications when these differ. Details of drug administration that must not be overlooked for the safe administration of the drug (e.g., "Dilute before infusing," or "Infuse *slowly* over 30 minutes") are included in the dosage section, but other aspects of drug administration (e.g., directions for reconstituting a powder for injection) are presented under "Implementation" in the next section of the monograph. If there is a treatment for the overdose of this drug, that information is indicated in a separate section.
- The **IV Facts** section gives concise, important information that is needed for drugs given IV—preparation guidelines, dilution, flow rate, compatibilities, and monitoring tips—making it unnecessary to have a separate IV handbook.
- Commonly encountered adverse effects are listed by body system, with the most commonly encountered adverse effects appearing in *italics* to make it easier to assess the patient for adverse effects and to teach the patient about what to expect. Potentially life-threatening adverse effects are in **bold** for easy access. Adverse effects that have been reported, but appear less commonly or rarely, are also listed to make the drug information as complete as possible.
- Clinically important interactions are listed separately for easy access—drug–drug, drug–food, and drug–laboratory test interferences to consider when using the drug and any nursing action that is necessary because of this interaction.

### Clinically Focused Nursing Considerations

The remainder of each monograph is concerned with nursing considerations, which are presented in the format of the nursing process. The steps of the nursing process are given slightly different names by different authorities; this drug guide considers assessment (history and physical), implementation, and drug-specific teaching points for each of the drugs presented.

1. ***Assessment:*** Outlines the information that should be collected before administering the drug. This section is further divided into two subsections:
   - *History:* Includes a list of those underlying conditions that constitute contraindications and cautions for use of the drug.
   - *Physical Assessment:* Provides data by organ system that should be collected before beginning drug therapy, both to allow detection of conditions that are contraindications/cautions to the use of the drug and to provide baseline data to allow detection of adverse reactions to the drug and to monitor for therapeutic response.
2. ***Implementation:*** Lists, in chronologic order, those nursing activities that should be undertaken in the course of caring for a patient who is receiving the drug. This includes interventions related to drug preparation and administration, the provision of comfort and safety measures, and drug levels to monitor, as appropriate.
3. ***Drug-Specific Patient Teaching Points:*** Includes specific information that is needed for teaching the patient who is receiving this drug. Proven "what to say advice" can be transferred directly to patient teaching cards and used as a written reminder. (A sample teaching card is provided in the appendices for easy copying.)

Evaluation is usually the last step of the nursing process. In all drug therapy, the patient should be evaluated for the desired effect of the drug, as listed in the *Indications* section;

the occurrence of adverse effects, as listed in the *Adverse Effects* section; and learning following patient teaching, as described in the *Drug-Specific Teaching Points* section. These points are essential. In some cases, evaluation includes monitoring specific therapeutic serum drug levels; these cases are specifically identified under *Implementation*.

## Appendices

The appendices contain information that is useful to nursing practice but may not lend itself to the monograph format—a detailed combination drug reference, biologicals, topical drugs, vitamins, laxatives, ophthalmic preparations, adjuncts to general anesthesia, peripheral vasodilators, general anesthetics, topical corticosteroids, and alternative and complementary therapies—as well as pregnancy categories, schedule of controlled substances, formulas for dosage calculations, pediatric nomograms, list of nursing diagnoses, guide for injection, recommended immunization schedule, equianalgesic dosages for narcotics, common cancer chemotherapy combinations, regimen for endocarditis prophylaxis, guides to drug compatibility and drug compatibility in syringes, the patient teaching guide, important dietary sources for patient teaching, and a list of drugs withdrawn or discontinued since the last edition. A suggested bilbliography follows the appendices.

## Index

An extensive index provides a ready reference to drug information. The **generic** name of each drug is highlighted in bold. If the generic name of a drug is not know, the drug may be found quickly by using *whatever* name is known. *Brand names* are listed in italics; commonly used chemical names, and any commonly used "jargon" names (such as "IDU" for idoxuridine) are in plain print. In addition, the index lists drugs by clinically important classes—pharmacologic and therapeutic. If you know a patient is taking an antianginal drug and don't remember the name, reviewing the list of drugs under **Antianginals** may well help recall the name. Chlorpromazine, for example, is indexed by its generic name, by its brand names, and by classes as an Antipsychotic drug (a therapeutic classification), as a Phenothiazine (a chemical classification), and as a Dopaminergic blocking drug (a classification by postulated mechanism of action). The comprehensive index helps to avoid cross-referencing from within the text, which is time consuming and confusing.

## Plus These Exciting New Features

- More than 50 newly released drugs
- Over 1,000 updates on dosage, indications, precautions, and administration
- Listing of available forms for each drug, making it easier for prescribing or guiding patients
- Simple guide for application of the nursing process, using the monograph format
- More IV facts content
- Expanded section on Alternative and Complimentary Therapies
- Expanded section on Combination Drugs
- Listing of the new standard for endocarditis prophylaxis
- Important dietary sources for patient teaching
- Listing of drugs withdrawn or discontinued since the last edition, to help those looking for a drug they are used to using but can't find
- A 32-page full-color insert presenting nearly 400 of the most commonly prescribed drugs

## Bonus Disk

The free disk has been updated with the most current data on nearly 150 of the most commonly prescribed drugs in the community. Design your own drug cards, create your own study aids, customize patient teaching tools.

### Added Value

With this guide comes a free 1-year subscription to *PharmPhax,* Lippincott's pharmacology newsletter. Get the hottest drug information available, including the latest FDA drug approvals and advances in clinical pharmacology.

This fourth edition incorporates many of the suggestions and requests made by users of earlier editions of the drug guide. It is hoped that the overall organization and concise, straightforward presentation of the material in the *1999 Lippincott's Nursing Drug Guide* will make it a clinically useful reference for the nurse who needs easily accessible information to facilitate drug therapy within the framework of the nursing process. It is further hoped that the thoroughness of the additional sections of the book will make it an invaluable resource that will replace the need for several additional references.

Amy M. Karch, RN, MS

# Acknowledgments

I would like to thank the many people who have helped to make this book possible: My students and colleagues, past and present, who have helped me learn how to make pharmacology usable in different areas of nursing practice and who have so generously shared their experience to make this book even more clinically useful; my editor at Lippincott-Raven Publishers, Margaret Zuccarini, who believed in this project and provided encouragement and humor when it was needed most, and who mastered all of the minute details and kept things in order; Sara Lauber, who kept all of us on our toes and organized; Tom Gibbons, who somehow made it all come together; my husband, Dr. Fred E. Karch, who was able to share his wonderful understanding and knowledge of pharmacology, medicine, and computers, and who offered support and encouragement and tolerated the long nights and late dinners; my children Timothy, Mark, Cortney, and Kathryn for their encouragement and begrudging tolerance; Al and Dorothy Morrison for giving me the potential; and Cider who provided endless hours of company and who always answered all problems and frustrations with a happily wagging tail that kept everything in perspective.

# Contents

A four-color photo guide to pills and capsules is found between pages 594 and 595

# Part 1

# I

# Nursing Process Guidelines Related to Drug Administration

The delivery of medical care today is in a constant state of change and sometimes in crisis. The population is aging, resulting in more chronic disease and more complex care issues. The population is transient, resulting in unstable support systems, fewer at-home care providers and helpers. At the same time, medicine is undergoing a technological boom (eg, CAT scans, NMRIs, experimental drugs). Patients are being discharged earlier from the acute care facility or not being admitted at all for procedures that used to be treated in the hospital with follow-up support and monitoring. Patients are becoming more responsible for their own care and for following complicated medical regimens at home.

Nursing is a unique and complex science and a nurturing and caring art. In the traditional sense, nurses have always been seen as ministering and soothing the sick. In the current state of medical changes, nursing also has become more technical and scientific. Nurses have had to assume increasing responsibilities involved with not only nurturing and caring, but with assessing, diagnosing, and intervening with patients to treat, prevent, and educate to help people cope with various health states.

The nurse deals with the whole person—the physical, emotional, intellectual, and spiritual aspects—considering the ways that a person responds to treatment, disease, and the change in lifestyle that may be required by both. The nurse is the key health care provider in a position to assess the patient—physical, social, and emotional aspects—to administer therapy and medications, teach the patient how best to cope with the therapy to ensure the most effectiveness, and evaluate the effectiveness of therapy. This requires a broad base of knowledge in the basic sciences (anatomy, physiology, nutrition, chemistry, pharmacology), the social sciences (sociology, psychology) and education (learning approaches, evaluation).

Although all nursing theorists do not completely agree on the process that defines the practice of nursing, most include certain key elements in the nursing process. These elements are the basic components of the decision-making or problem-solving process: assessment (gathering of information), diagnosis (defining that information to arrive at some conclusions), intervention (eg, administration, education, comfort measures), and evaluation (determining the effects of the interventions that were performed). The use of this process each time a situation arises ensures a method of coping with the overwhelming scientific and technical information confounding the situation and the unique emotional, social, and physical aspects that each patient brings to the situation. Using the nursing process format in each instance of drug therapy will ensure that the patient receives the best, most efficient, scientifically based holistic care.

## Assessment

The first step of the nursing process is the systematic, organized collection of data about the patient. Because the nurse is responsible for holistic care, these data must include information about physical, intellectual, emotional, social, and environmental factors. They will provide the nurse with information needed to plan discharge, plan educational programs, arrange for appropriate consultations, and monitor physical response to treatment or to disease. In actual clinical practice, this process never ends. The patient is not in a steady state but is dynamic, adjusting to physical, emotional, and environmental influences. Each nurse develops a unique approach to the organization of the assessment, an approach that is functional and useful in the clinical setting and that makes sense to that nurse and that clinical situation.

Drug therapy is a complex, integral, and important part of health care today, and the principles of drug therapy need to be incorporated into every patient assessment plan. The particular information that is needed and that should be assessed will vary with each drug, but the concepts involved are similar and are based on the principles of drug therapy. Two important areas that need to be assessed are history and physical assessment.

### *History*

Past experiences and past illnesses impact the actual effect of a drug.

**Chronic conditions:** These may be contraindications to the use of a drug or may require that caution be used or that drug dosage be adjusted.

**Drug use:** Prescription drugs, OTC drugs, street drugs, alcohol, nicotine, and caffeine all may have an impact on the effect of a drug. Patients often neglect to mention OTC drugs and contraceptives, not considering them actual drugs, and should be asked specifically about OTC drug and contraceptive use.

**Allergies:** Past exposure to a drug or other allergen can predict a future reaction or note a caution for the use of a drug, food, or animal product.

**Level of education:** This information will help to provide a basis for patient education programs and level of explanation.

**Level of understanding of disease and therapy:** This information also will direct the development of educational information.

**Social supports:** Patients are being discharged earlier than ever before and often need assistance at home to provide care and institute and monitor drug therapy.

**Financial supports:** The financial impact of health care and the high cost of medications need to be considered when prescribing drugs and depending on the patient to follow through with drug therapy.

**Pattern of health care:** The way that a patient seeks health care will give the nurse valuable information to include in educational information. Does this patient routinely seek follow-up care or wait for emergency situations?

### *Physical assessment*

**Weight:** Weight is an important factor when determining if the recommended dosage of a drug is appropriate. The recommended dosage is based on the 150-lb adult male. Patients who are much lighter or much heavier will need a dosage adjustment.

**Age:** Patients at the extremes of the age spectrum—pediatric and geriatric—often require dosage adjustments based on the functional level of the liver and kidneys and the responsiveness of other organs.

**Physical parameters related to the disease state or known drug effects:** Assessment of these factors before beginning drug therapy will give a baseline level with which future assessments can be compared to determine the effects of drug therapy. The specific parameters that need to be assessed will depend on the disease process being treated and on the expected therapeutic and adverse effects of the drug therapy. Because the nurse has the greatest direct and continual contact with the patient, the nurse has the best opportunity to detect the minute changes that will determine the course of drug therapy and therapeutic success or discontinuation because of adverse or unacceptable responses.

The monographs in this book include the specific parameters that need to be assessed in relation to the particular drug being discussed (see the sample monograph at the end of this chapter). This assessment provides not only the baseline information needed before giving that drug, but the data needed to evaluate the effects of that drug on the patient. The information given in this area should supplement the overall nursing assessment of the patient, which will include social, intellectual, financial, environmental, and other physical data.

### *Nursing diagnoses*

Once data have been collected, the nurse must organize and analyze that information to arrive at a nursing diagnosis. A nursing diagnosis is simply a statement of the patient's status from a nursing perspective. This statement directs appropriate nursing interventions. A nursing diagnosis will show actual or potential alteration in patient function based on the assessment of the clinical situation. Because drug therapy is only a small part of the overall patient situation, the nursing diagnoses that are related to drug therapy must be incorporated into a total picture of the patient. In many cases the drug therapy will not present a new nursing diagnosis, but the desired effects and adverse effects related to each drug given should be considered in the nursing diagnoses for each patient. The North American Nursing Diagnosis Association (NANDA) list of accepted nursing diagnoses is included as Appendix U.

### *Interventions*

The assessment and diagnosis of the patient's situation will direct specific nursing interventions. Three types of interventions are frequently involved in drug therapy: drug administration, provision of comfort measures, and patient/family teaching.

### *Drug administration*

**Drug:** Ensuring that the drug being administered is the correct dose of the correct drug at the correct time, and is being given to the correct patient, is standard nursing practice.

**Storage:** Some drugs require specific storage environments (eg, refrigeration, protection from light).

**Route:** Determining the best route of administration is often determined by the prescription of the drug. Nurses can often have an impact on modifying the prescribed route to determine the most efficient route and the most comfortable one for the patient based on his or her specific situation. When establishing the prescribed route, it is important to check the proper method of administering a drug by that route.

**Dosage:** Drug dosage may need to be calculated based on available drug form, patient body weight or surface area, or kidney function.

**Preparation:** Some drugs require specific preparation before administration. Oral drugs may need to be shaken, crushed; parenteral drugs may need to be reconstituted or diluted with specific solutions; topical drugs may require specific handling before administration.

**Timing:** Actual administration of a drug may require coordination with the administration of other drugs, foods, or physical parameters. The nurse, as the caregiver most frequently involved in administering a drug, must be aware and juggle all of these factors and educate the patient to do this on his or her own.

**Recording:** Once the nurse has assessed the patient, made the appropriate nursing diagnoses, and delivered the correct drug by the correct route, in the correct dose, and at the correct time, that information needs to be recorded in accordance with the local requirements for recording medication administration.

Each monograph in this book contains pertinent guidelines for storage, dosage, preparation, and administration of the drug being discussed.

### *Comfort measures*

Nurses are in the unique position to help the patient cope with the effects of drug therapy as they impact him or her.

**Placebo effect:** The anticipation that a drug will be helpful (placebo effect) has been proved to have tremendous impact on actual success of drug therapy, so the nurse's attitude and support can be a critical part of drug therapy. A back rub, a kind word, a positive approach may be as beneficial as the drug itself.

**Side effects:** These interventions can be directed at decreasing the impact of the anticipated side effects of the drug and promoting patient safety. Such interventions include environmental control (eg, temperature, lighting), safety measures (eg, avoiding driving, avoiding the sun, using side rails), physical comfort (eg, skin care, laxatives, frequent meals).

**Lifestyle adjustment:** Some drug effects will require that a patient change his or her lifestyle to cope effectively. Diuretic users may have to rearrange the day to be near toilet facilities when the drug works. MAOI users have to adjust their diet to prevent serious drug effects.

Each monograph in this book will include a list of pertinent comfort measures appropriate to that particular drug.

***Education***

With patients becoming more responsible for their own care, it is becoming essential that they have all of the information necessary to ensure safe and effective drug therapy at home. Many states now require that the patient be given written information. Key elements that need to be included in any drug education include the following:

1. Name, dose, and action of drug: With many people seeing more than one health care provider, this information is important for ensuring safe and effective drug therapy.
2. Timing of administration: Patients need to know specifically when to take the drug with regard to frequency, other drugs, and meals.
3. Special storage and preparation instructions: Some drugs require particular handling that the patient will need to have spelled out.
4. Specific OTC drugs to avoid: Many people do not consider OTC drugs to be actual drugs and may inadvertently take them and cause unwanted or even dangerous drug-drug interactions. Spelling out particular problems of which to be aware will help the patient avoid these situations.
5. Special comfort or safety measures that need to be considered: Alerting the patient to ways to cope with anticipated side effects will prevent a great deal of anxiety and noncompliance with drug therapy. The patient also may need to be alerted to the need to return for follow-up tests or evaluation.
6. Safety measures: All patients need to be alerted to keep drugs out of the reach of children. They also need to be reminded to tell any health care provider whom they see that they are taking this drug. This can prevent drug–drug interactions and misdiagnosing based on drug effects.
7. Specific points about drug toxicity: Warning signs of drug toxicity of which the patient should be aware should be listed. He or she can be advised to notify the health care provider if any of these effects occur.
8. Specific warnings about drug discontinuation: Some drugs with a small margin of safety and drugs with particular systemic effects cannot be stopped abruptly without dangerous effects. Patients taking these drugs need to be alerted to the problem and encouraged to call immediately if they cannot take their medication for any reason (eg, illness, financial).

Each drug monograph in this book lists specific teaching points that relate to that particular drug. The appendix presents a basic patient teaching guideline that can be used in conjunction with the drug-specific teaching points to provide the patient with a compact, written drug card.

***Evaluation***

Evaluation is part of the continual process of patient care that leads to changes in assessment, diagnosis, and intervention. The patient is continually evaluated for therapeutic response, the occurrence of drug side effects, and the occurrence of drug–drug or drug–laboratory test interaction. The efficacy of the nursing interventions and the education program must be evaluated. In some situations, the nurse will evaluate the patient simply by reapplying the beginning steps of the nursing process and analyzing for change. In some cases of drug therapy, particular therapeutic drug levels need to be evaluated as well.

Monographs in this book list only specific evaluation criteria, such as therapeutic serum levels, as they apply to each drug. Regular evaluation of drug effects, side effects, and the efficacy of comfort measures and education programs will not be specifically listed but can be deduced from information in the monograph regarding therapeutic effects and adverse effects. See the following example of a nursing care plan using these guidelines.

## NURSING CARE PLAN: PATIENT ON AN NSAID

| Assessment | Nursing Diagnoses | Implementation | Evaluation |
|---|---|---|---|
| ***History*** (contraindications/cautions)<br>Ulcerative GI disease<br>Peptic ulcer<br>Renal dysfunction<br>Hepatic dysfunction<br>Pregnancy<br>Lactation<br>Know allergies to: other NSAIDs, aspirin | Potential sensory-perceptual alteration secondary to CNS effects<br>Potential alteration in comfort related to GI upset, headache<br>Potential ineffective gas exchange related to possible hypersensitivity reaction | Safe and appropriate administration of the drug<br>Provision of safety and comfort and safety measures:<br>Drug given with meals<br>Alleviation of GI upset, headache<br>Safety provisions if dizziness or visual disturbances occur | Monitor for therapeutic effects of the drug: decrease in the signs and symptoms of inflammation<br>Monitor for adverse effects of drug:<br>GI upset<br>Liver function changes<br>CNS effects<br>CHF<br>Renal or urinary tract dysfunction<br>Blood dyscrasias<br>Visual changes<br>Rash<br>Asthma<br>Anaphylactic reactions |
| ***Medication History*** (possible drug–drug interactions)<br>Sulfonamides<br>Hydantoin<br>Probenecid<br>Oral anticoagulants<br>Oral hypoglycemics | Knowledge deficit regarding drug therapy | Patient teaching regarding:<br>Drug<br>Side effects to anticipate<br>Warnings<br>Reactions to report<br>Support and encouragement to cope with disease, therapy, and side effects | |
| ***Physical Assessment*** (screen for contraindications, establish a baseline for effects and adverse effects)<br>CNS: affect, reflexes, peripheral sensation<br>CV: BP, P, peripheral perfusion, auscultation<br>GI: bowel sounds, liver evaluation, stool guaiac<br>Skin: Lesions<br>Blood tests: CBC, liver and renal function tests | | Provision of emergency and life-support measures in cases of acute hypersensitivity | Evaluate effectiveness of patient teaching program: patient can state name of drug, dose of drug, use of drug, adverse effects to expect, reactions to report<br>Evaluate effectiveness of comfort and safety measures<br>Monitor for drug–drug interactions if patient is on an interacting drug<br>Evaluate effectiveness of life-support measures if needed |

Generic name

## anagrelide hydrochloride

Pronunciation guide

*(an* ***agh'*** *rah lide)*

Brand name

Agrylin

FDA pregnancy category

**Pregnancy Category C**

Therapeutic drug class

**Drug classes**

Platelet reducing agent

Action of drug on the body

**Therapeutic actions**

Reduces platelet production by decreasing megakaryocyte hypermaturation; inhibits cyclic AMP and ADP collagen-induced platelet aggregation. At therapeutic doses has no affect on WBC counts or coagulation parameters; may affect RBC parameters.

Uses for the drug

*Evaluation points*—resolution or stabilization of those conditions

**Indications**

- Treatment of essential thrombocytopenia to reduce elevated platelet count and the risk of thrombosis

Conditions limiting use of drug

*Assessment points*—history of these conditions, physical assessment indicating these conditions

**Contraindications/cautions**

- Use caution in the presence of renal or hepatic disorders, pregnancy, lactation, known heart disease, thrombocytopenia.

Forms and dosages available for use

Recommended dose of drug for adults, pediatrics, etc.

**Dosage**

**Available Forms:** Capsules—0.5, 1 mg

*ADULT:* Initially 0.5 mg PO qid or 1 mg PO bid. After 1 wk, reevaluate and adjust the dosage as needed; do not increase by more than 0.5 mg/d each week. Maximum dose 10 mg/d or 2.5 mg as a single dose.

*PEDIATRIC:* Safety and efficacy not established.

Action of body on the drug—*points for assessment* (hepatic function), cautions, and contraindications

**Pharmacokinetics**

| *Route* | *Onset* | *Peak* |
|---|---|---|
| Oral | Rapid | 1 h |

*Metabolism:* Hepatic metabolism; $T_{1/2}$: 3 d

*Distribution:* Crosses placenta; may pass into breast milk

*Excretion:* Urine

Effects of drug on the body—not therapeutic but can be expected

*Assessment points*—baselines for these systems

*Nursing diagnosis*—potential alterations resulting from these effects

*Evaluation*—presence/absence of these effects

**Adverse effects**

- GI: *Diarrhea, nausea, vomiting, abdominal pain,* flatulence, dyspepsia, anorexia, pancreatitis, ulcer, CVA
- Hematological: *Thrombocytopenia*
- CNS: Dizziness, headaches, asthenia, paresthesias

- **CV:** CHF, tachycardia, MI, complete heart block, atrial fibrillation, hypertension, *palpitations*
- **Other:** Rash, purpura

**Clinically important drug-food interactions**

- Reduced availability of anagrelide if taken with food

Anticipated interactions

*Assessment points*—history of use of these drugs, physical response

*Evaluation*—changes from anticipated therapeutic response related to drug interactions

## ■ Nursing Considerations

### Assessment

- ***History:*** Allergy to anagrelide, thrombocytopenia, hemostatic disorders, bleeding ulcer, intracranial bleeding, severe liver disease, lactation, renal disorders, pregnancy, known heart disease
- ***Physical:*** Skin color, lesions; orientation; bowel sounds, normal output; CBC, liver and renal function tests

Points to establish baselines, determine factors contraindicating drug use or requiring caution

### Implementation

- Perform platelet counts q 2 d during the first week of therapy and at least weekly thereafter; if thrombocytopenia occurs, decrease dosage of drug and arrange for supportive therapy.
- Advise patient to use barrier contraceptives while receiving this drug; it may harm the fetus.
- Monitor patient for any sign of excessive bleeding—bruises, dark stools, etc.—and monitor bleeding times.

Nursing actions, in chronologic order, for safe and effective drug therapy

### Drug-specific teaching points

- Take drug on an empty stomach.
- Be aware that it may take longer than normal to stop bleeding while on this drug; avoid contact sports, use electric razors, etc.; apply pressure for extended periods to bleeding sites.
- Avoid pregnancy while on this drug; it could harm the fetus. Use barrier contraceptives.
- Know that upset stomach, nausea, diarrhea, loss of appetite (small, frequent meals may help) may occur.
- Notify any dentist or surgeon that you are on this drug before invasive procedures.
- Report fever, chills, sore throat, skin rash, bruising, bleeding, dark stools or urine, palpitations, chest pain.

Teaching points to include on patient teaching program

*Nursing diagnosis*—knowledge deficit regarding drug therapy

*Evaluation*—points patient should be able to repeat

# II

# Pharmacologic Drug Classification

## Alkylating Agents

### Pregnancy Category D

### Therapeutic actions

Alkylating agents are cytotoxic: they alkylate cellular DNA, interfering with the replication of susceptible cells and causing cell death. Their action is most evident in rapidly dividing cells.

### Indications

- Palliative treatment of chronic lymphocytic leukemia; malignant lymphomas, including lymphosarcoma, giant follicular lymphoma; Hodgkin's disease; multiple myelomas; testicular cancers; brain tumors; pancreatic cancer; ovarian and breast cancers
- Used as part of multiple agent regimens

### Contraindications/cautions

- Contraindications: hypersensitivity to the drugs, concurrent radiation therapy, hematopoietic depression, pregnancy, lactation.

### Adverse effects

- CNS: *Tremors, muscular twitching, confusion,* agitation, ataxia, flaccid paresis, hallucinations, seizures
- GI: Nausea, vomiting, anorexia, **hepatotoxicity**
- Respiratory: Bronchopulmonary dysplasia, pulmonary fibrosis
- Hematologic: *Bone marrow depression,* hyperuricemia
- GU: Sterility
- Dermatologic: Skin rash, urticaria, alopecia, keratitis
- Other: *Cancer, acute leukemia*

### ■ Nursing Considerations

#### Assessment

- *History:* Hypersensitivity to drug, radiation therapy, hematopoietic depression, pregnancy, lactation
- *Physical:* T; weight; skin color, lesions; R, adventitious sounds; liver evaluation; CBC, differential, hemoglobin, uric acid, renal and liver function tests

#### Implementation

- Arrange for blood tests to evaluate hematopoietic function prior to and weekly during therapy.
- Restrict dosage within 4 wk after a full course of radiation therapy or chemotherapy due to risk of severe bone marrow depression.
- Ensure that patient is well hydrated before treatment.
- Arrange for small, frequent meals and dietary consultation to maintain nutrition if GI upset occurs.
- Arrange for skin care for rashes.

#### Drug-specific teaching points

- Possible side effects: nausea, vomiting, loss of appetite (dividing dose may help; small, frequent meals may help; maintain fluid intake and nutrition; drink at least 10–12 glasses of fluid each day); infertility (potentially irreversible and irregular menses to amenorrhea and aspermia; discuss feelings with healthcare provider); this drug can cause severe birth defects; use birth control methods while on this drug.
- Report unusual bleeding or bruising; fever, chills, sore throat; cough, shortness of breath; yellowing of the skin or eyes; flank or stomach pain.

### Representative drugs

busulfan
carboplatin

carmustine
chlorambucil
cisplatin
cyclophosphamide
ifosfamide
lomustine
mechlorethemine
melphalan
streptozocin
thiotepa

## Alpha$_1$-Adrenergic Blockers

### Pregnancy Category C

### Therapeutic actions

Alpha-adrenergic blockers selectively block postsynaptic alpha$_1$-adrenergic receptors, decreasing sympathetic tone on the vasculature, dilating arterioles and veins, and lowering both supine and standing blood pressure; unlike conventional alpha-adrenergic blocking agents (phentolamine), they do not also block alpha$_2$ presynaptic receptors, so they do not cause reflex tachycardia.

### Indications

- Treatment of hypertension (alone or with other agents)
- Treatment of BHP (terazosin, tamsulosin)
- Unlabeled uses: management of refractory CHF and Raynaud's vasospasm; treatment of prostatic outflow obstruction

### Contraindications/cautions

- Contraindications: hypersensitivity to any alpha$_1$-adrenergic blocker, lactation. Use with caution in the presence of CHF, renal failure, pregnancy.

### Adverse effects

- CNS: *Dizziness, headache, drowsiness, lack of energy, weakness,* nervousness, vertigo, depression, paresthesia
- GI: *Nausea,* vomiting, diarrhea, constipation, abdominal discomfort or pain
- CV: *Palpitations,* sodium and water retention, increased plasma volume, edema, dyspnea, syncope, tachycardia, orthostatic hypotension
- GU: Urinary frequency, incontinence, impotence, priapism
- EENT: Blurred vision, reddened sclera, epistaxis, tinnitus, dry mouth, nasal congestion
- Dermatologic: Rash, pruritus, alopecia, lichen planus
- Other: Diaphoresis, lupus erythematosus

### Clinically important drug-drug interactions

- Severity and duration of hypotension following first dose of drug may be greater in patients receiving beta-adrenergic blocking drugs (propranolol), verapamil

## ■ Nursing Considerations

### Assessment

- *History:* Hypersensitivity to alpha$_1$-adrenergic blocker, CHF, renal failure, lactation
- *Physical:* Weight; skin color, lesions; orientation, affect, reflexes; ophthalmologic exam; P, BP, orthostatic BP, supine BP, perfusion, edema, auscultation; R, adventitious sounds, status of nasal mucous membranes; bowel sounds, normal output; voiding pattern, normal output; kidney function tests, urinalysis

### Implementation

- Administer, or have patient take, first dose hs to lessen likelihood of first dose syncope believed due to excessive postural hypotension.
- Have patient lie down, and treat supportively if syncope occurs; condition is self-limiting.
- Monitor patient for orthostatic hypotension: most marked in the morning, accentuated by hot weather, alcohol, exercise.
- Monitor edema, weight in patients with incipient cardiac decompensation, arrange to add a thiazide diuretic to the drug regimen if sodium and fluid retention, signs of impending CHF occur.
- Provide small, frequent meals, frequent mouth care if GI effects occur.

- Establish safety precautions if CNS, hypotensive changes occur (side rails, accompany patient).
- Arrange for analgesic for patients experiencing headache.
- Provide consultations to help patient cope with sexual dysfunction and priapism.

### Drug-specific teaching points

- Take drug exactly as prescribed. Take the first dose at bedtime. Do not drive a car or operate machinery for 4 h after the first dose.
- Avoid OTC drugs (nose drops, cold remedies) while taking this drug. If you feel you need one of these preparations, consult health care provider.
- Possible side effects: dizziness, weakness may occur when changing position, in the early morning, after exercise, in hot weather, and after consuming alcohol; tolerance may occur after taking the drug for awhile, but avoid driving or engaging in tasks that require alertness while experiencing these symptoms; change position slowly, and use caution in climbing stairs; lie down for a while if dizziness persists; GI upset (frequent, small meals may help); impotence (discuss this with health care provider); dry mouth (sucking on sugarless lozenges, ice chips may help); stuffy nose. Most of these effects will gradually disappear with continued therapy.
- Report frequent dizziness or faintness.

### Representative drugs

doxazosin
prazosin
tamsulosin
terazosin

## Aminoglycosides

### Pregnancy Category C

### Therapeutic actions

Aminoglycosides are antibiotics that are bactericidal. They inhibit protein synthesis in susceptible strains of gram-negative bacteria, appear to disrupt the functional integrity of bacterial cell membrane, causing cell death. Oral aminoglycosides are very poorly absorbed and are used for the suppression of GI bacterial flora.

### Indications

- Short-term treatment of serious infections caused by susceptible strains of *Pseudomonas* species, *Escherichia coli,* indole-positive *Proteus* species, *Providencia* species, *Klebsiella-Enterobacter-Serratia* species, *Acinetobacter* species
- Suspected gram-negative infections before results of susceptibility studies are known
- Initial treatment of staphylococcal infections when penicillin is contraindicated or when infection may be caused by mixed organisms
- Neonatal sepsis when other antibiotics cannot be used (used in combination with penicillin-type drug)
- Unlabeled uses: as part of a multidrug regimen for treatment of *Mycobacterium avium* complex (a common infection in AIDS patients) and orally for the treatment of intestinal amebiasis; adjunctive treatment of hepatic coma and for suppression of intestinal bacteria for surgery

### Contraindications/cautions

- Contraindications: allergy to any aminoglycosides, renal disease, hepatic disease, preexisting hearing loss, myasthenia gravis, parkinsonism, infant botulism, lactation. Use caution with elderly patients, patients with diminished hearing, decreased renal function, dehydration, neuromuscular disorders.

### Adverse effects

- CNS: *Ototoxicity;* confusion, disorientation, depression, lethargy, nystagmus, visual disturbances, headache, fever, numbness, tingling, tremor, paresthesias, muscle twitching, convulsions, muscular weakness, neuromuscular blockade, apnea
- GI: *Nausea, vomiting, anorexia, diarrhea,* weight loss, stomatitis, increased salivation, splenomegaly
- CV: Palpitations, hypotension, hypertension

- **Hematologic**: Leukemoid reaction, agranulocytosis, granulocytosis, leukopenia, leukocytosis, thrombocytopenia, eosinophilia, pancytopenia, anemia, hemolytic anemia, increased or decreased reticulocyte count, electrolyte disturbances
- GU: *Nephrotoxicity*
- **Hypersensitivity**: Purpura, rash, urticaria, exfoliative dermatitis, itching
- **Hepatic**: Hepatic toxicity; hepatomegaly
- **Other**: *Superinfections, pain and irritation at IM injection sites*

### Clinically important drug-drug interactions

• Increased ototoxic and nephrotoxic effects if taken with potent diuretics and similarly toxic drugs (cephalosporins) • Increased likelihood of neuromuscular blockade if given shortly after general anesthetics, depolarizing and nondepolarizing neuromuscular junction blockers

## ■ Nursing Considerations

### Assessment

- *History:* Allergy to any aminoglycosides, renal disease, hepatic disease, preexisting hearing loss, myasthenia gravis, parkinsonism, infant botulism, lactation, diminished hearing, decreased renal function, dehydration, neuromuscular disorders.
- *Physical:* Arrange culture and sensitivity tests of infection prior to therapy; check before, during and after renal function, eighth cranial nerve function, and state of hydration, during, and after therapy; hepatic function tests, CBC; skin color, lesions; orientation, affect; reflexes, bilateral grip strength; body weight; bowel sounds

### Implementation

- Arrange for culture and sensitivity testing of infected area prior to treatment.
- Monitor duration of treatment: usual duration is 7–10 d. If no clinical response within 3–5 d, stop therapy. Prolonged treatment leads to increased risk of toxicity. If drug is used longer than 10 d, monitor auditory and renal function daily.
- Give IM dosage by deep injection.
- Ensure that patient is well hydrated before and during therapy.
- Establish safety measures if CNS, vestibular nerve effects occur (use of side rails, assistance with ambulation).
- Provide small, frequent meals if nausea, anorexia occur.
- Provide comfort measures and medication for superinfections.

### Drug-specific teaching points

- Take full course of oral drug; drink plenty of fluids.
- Possible side effects: ringing in the ears, headache, dizziness (reversible; safety measures need to be taken if severe); nausea, vomiting, loss of appetite (small, frequent meals, frequent mouth care may help).
- Report pain at injection site, severe headache, dizziness, loss of hearing, changes in urine pattern, difficulty breathing, rash or skin lesions.

### Representative drugs

amikacin sulfate
gentamicin
kanamycin
neomycin (oral)
netilmicin
tobramycin (parenteral)

# Angiotensin-Converting Enzyme (ACE) Inhibitors

### Pregnancy Category C

### Therapeutic actions

ACE inhibitors block ACE in the lungs from converting angiotensin I, activated when renin is released from the kidneys, to angiotensin II, a powerful vasoconstrictor. Blocking this conversion leads to decreased BP, decreased aldosterone secretion, a small increase in serum potassium levels, and sodium and fluid loss; increased prostaglandin synthesis also may be involved in the antihypertensive action.

**Indications**

- Treatment of hypertension (alone or with thiazide-type diuretics)
- Treatment of CHF in patients who do not respond adequately to conventional therapy (used with diuretics and digitalis)
- Unlabeled uses: management of hypertensive crises; treatment of rheumatoid arthritis; diabetic nephropathy, diagnosis of anatomic renal artery stenosis, hypertension related to scleroderma renal crisis; diagnosis of primary aldosteronism, idiopathic edema; Bartter's syndrome; Raynaud's syndrome; hypertension of Takayasu's disease.

**Contraindications/cautions**

- Contraindications: allergy to the drug, impaired renal function, CHF, salt/volume depletion, or lactation.

**Adverse effects**

- GI: *Gastric irritation, aphthous ulcers, peptic ulcers, dysgeusia,* cholestatic jaundice, hepatocellular injury, anorexia, constipation
- CV: *Tachycardia,* angina pectoris, **myocardial infarction,** Raynaud's syndrome, CHF, hypotension in salt/volume-depleted patients
- Hematologic: Neutropenia, agranulocytosis, thrombocytopenia, hemolytic anemia, **fatal pancytopenia**
- GU: *Proteinuria,* renal insufficiency, renal failure, polyuria, oliguria, urinary frequency
- Dermatologic: *Rash, pruritus,* pemphigoid-like reaction, scalded mouth sensation, exfoliative dermatitis, photosensitivity, alopecia
- Other: *Cough,* malaise, dry mouth, lymphadenopathy

**Clinically important drug-drug interactions**

- Increased risk of hypersensitivity reactions with allopurinal • Decreased antihypertensive effects with indomethacin

**Clinically important drug-food interactions**

- Decreased absorption of selected agents if taken with food

**Drug-lab test interferences**

- False-positive test for urine acetone

## ■ Nursing Considerations

### Assessment

- *History:* Allergy to ACE inhibitors, impaired renal function, CHF, salt/volume depletion, pregnancy, lactation
- *Physical:* Skin color, lesions, turgor; T, P, BP, peripheral perfusion; mucous membranes; bowel sounds; liver evaluation; urinalysis, renal and liver function tests, CBC and differential

### Implementation

- Administer 1 h before or 2 h after meals if affected by food in GI tract.
- Alert surgeon and mark patient's chart that ACE inhibitor is being taken; angiotensin II formation subsequent to compensatory renin release during surgery will be blocked; hypotension may be reversed with volume expansion.
- Monitor patient closely in situations that may lead to a fall in BP due to reduction in fluid volume (excessive perspiration and dehydration, vomiting, diarrhea) because excessive hypotension may occur.
- Arrange for reduced dosage in patients with impaired renal function.
- Arrange for bowel program if constipation occurs.
- Provide small, frequent meals if GI upset is severe.
- Provide for frequent mouth care and oral hygiene if mouth sores, alteration in taste occur.
- Caution patient to change position slowly if orthostatic changes occur.
- Provide skin care as needed.

### Drug-specific teaching points

- Take drug 1 h before or 2 h after meals; do not take with food.
- Do not stop taking the medication without consulting health care provider.

- Possible side effects: GI upset, loss of appetite, change in taste perception (limited effects; if they persist or become a problem, consult health care provider); mouth sores (frequent mouth care may help); skin rash; fast heart rate; dizziness, lightheadedness (passes after a few days of therapy; if it occurs, change position slowly and limit activities requiring alertness and precision).
- Be careful in any situation that may lead to a drop in BP (diarrhea, sweating, vomiting, dehydration); if lightheadedness or dizziness occurs, consult health care provider.
- Avoid OTC medications, especially cough, cold, allergy medications. If you need one of these, consult health care provider.
- Report mouth sores; sore throat, fever, chills; swelling of the hands, feet; irregular heartbeat, chest pains; swelling of the face, eyes, lips, tongue, difficulty in breathing.

### Representative drugs

benazepril
captopril
enalapril
enalaprilat
fosinopril
lisinopril
moexipril
quinapril
ramipril
trandolapril

## Antiarrhythmics

### Pregnancy Category C

### Therapeutic actions

Antiarrhythmics act at specific sites to alter the action potential of cardiac cells and interfere with the electrical excitability of the heart. Most of these drugs may cause new or worsened arrhythmias (proarrhythmic effect) and must be used with caution and with continual cardiac monitoring and patient evaluation.

### Indications

- Treatment of tachycardia when rapid but short-term control of ventricular rate is desirable (patients with atrial fibrillation, flutter, in perioperative or postoperative situations)
- Treatment of noncompensatory tachycardia when heart rate requires specific intervention
- Treatment of atrial arrhythmias

### Contraindications/cautions

- Reserve for emergency situations; there are no contraindications. Use caution during pregnancy or lactation.

### Adverse effects

- CNS: *Lightheadedness, speech disorder, midscapular pain, weakness, rigors,* somnolence, confusion
- GI: *Taste perversion*
- CV: *Hypotension,* pallor
- GU: *Urinary retention*
- Local: *Inflammation,* induration, edema, erythema, burning at the site of infusion
- Other: Fever, rhonchi, flushing

### Clinically important drug-drug interactions

- Monitor patients receiving antiarrhythmics for drug interactions; see specific drug for clinically important interactions.

## ■ Nursing Considerations

### Assessment

- *History:* Cardiac disease, cerebrovascular disease
- *Physical:* P, BP, ECG; orientation, reflexes; R, adventitious sounds; urinary output

### Implementation

- Ensure that more toxic drug is not used in chronic settings when transfer to another agent is anticipated.
- Monitor BP, heart rate, and rhythm closely
- Provide comfort measures for pain, rigors, fever, flushing, if patient is awake.
- Provide supportive measures appropriate to condition being treated.

- Provide support and encouragement to deal with drug effects and discomfort of IV lines.

### Drug-specific teaching points

- Reserved for emergency use. Incorporate any information about drug into the overall teaching program for patient. Patients maintained on oral drug will need specific teaching. See individual monograph for details.

### Representative drugs

*Type I*
moricizine
*Type IA*
disopyramide
procainamide
quinidine
*Type IB*
lidocaine
mexilitine
phenytoin
tocainamide
*Type IC*
flecainide
propafenone
*Type II*
acebutolol
esmolol
propranolol
*Type III*
amiodarone
bretylium
ibutilide
sotalol
*Type IV*
verapamil
*Other*
adenosine
digoxin

## Anticoagulants

### Pregnancy Category D

### Therapeutic actions

Oral anticoagulants interfere with the hepatic synthesis of vitamin K-dependent clotting factors (factors II, prothrombin, VII, IX, and X), resulting in their eventual depletion and prolongation of clotting times; parenteral anticoagulants interfere with the conversion of prothrombin to thrombin, blocking the final step in clot formation but leaving the circulating levels of clotting factors unaffected.

### Indications

- Treatment and prevention of pulmonary embolism and venous thrombosis and its extension
- Treatment of atrial fibrillation with embolization
- Prevention of deep vein thrombosis
- Prophylaxis of systemic emobization after acute MI
- Prevention of thrombi following specific surgical procedures (low-molecular-weight heparins)
- Unlabeled uses: prevention of recurrent transient ischemic attacks, and MI; adjunt to therapy in small-cell carcinoma of the lung.

### Contraindications/cautions

- Contraindications: allergy to the drug; SBE; hemorrhagic disorders; tuberculosis; hepatic diseases; GI ulcers; renal disease; indwelling catheters, spinal puncture; aneurysm; diabetes; visceral carcinoma; uncontrolled hypertension; severe trauma (including recent or contemplated CNS, eye surgery, recent placement of IUD); threatened abortion, menometrorrhagia; pregnancy (oral agents cause fetal damage and death); or lactation (heparin if anticoagulation is required). Use caution in the presence of CHF, diarrhea, fever; thyrotoxicosis; senile, psychotic or depressed patients.

### Adverse effects

- GI: *Nausea,* vomiting, anorexia, abdominal cramping, diarrhea, retroperitoneal hematoma, hepatitis, jaundice, mouth ulcers
- **Hematologic**: Granulocytosis, leukopenia, eosinophilia
- GU: Priapism, nephropathy, red-orange urine
- **Dermatologic**: *Alopecia, urticaria, dermatitis*
- **Bleeding**: *Hemorrhage;* GI or urinary tract bleeding (hematuria, dark stools;

paralytic ileus; intestinal obstruction from hemorrhage into GI tract); petechiae and purpura, bleeding from mucous membranes; hemorrhagic infarction, vasculitis, skin necrosis of female breast; adrenal hemorrhage and resultant adrenal insufficiency; compressive neuropathy secondary to hemorrhage near a nerve
- **Other**: Fever, "purple toes" syndrome

## Clinically important drug-drug interactions

• Increased bleeding tendencies with salicylates, chloral hydrate, phenylbutazone, clofibrate, disulfiram, chloramphenicol, metronidazole, cimetidine, ranitidine, cotrimoxazole, sulfinpyrazone, quinidine, quinine, oxyphenbutazone, thyroid drugs, glucagon, danazol, erythromycin, androgens, amiodarone, cefamandole, cefoperazone, cefotetan, moxalactam, cefazolin, cefoxitin, ceftriaxone, meclofenamate, mefenamic acid, famotidine, nizatidine, nalidixic acid • Possible decreased anticoagulation effect with barbiturates, griseofulvin, rifampin, phenytoin, glutethimide, carbamazepine, vitamin K, vitamin E, cholestyramine, aminoglutethimide, ethchlorvynol • Altered effects of warfarin with methimazole, propylthiouracil • Increased activity and toxicity of phenytoin with oral anticoagulants

## Drug-lab test interferences

- Red-orange discoloration of alkaline urine may interfere with some lab tests.

## ■ Nursing Considerations

### Assessment

- *History:* Allergy to the drug; SBE; hemorrhagic disorders; tuberculosis; hepatic diseases; GI ulcers; renal disease; indwelling catheters, spinal puncture; aneurysm; diabetes; visceral carcinoma; uncontrolled hypertension; severe trauma; threatened abortion, menometrorrhagia; pregnancy; lactation; CHF, diarrhea, fever; thyrotoxicosis; senile, psychotic, or depressed patients.
- *Physical:* Skin lesions, color, T, orientation, reflexes, affect; P, BP, peripheral perfusion, baseline ECG; R, adventitious sounds; liver evaluation, bowel sounds, normal output; CBC, urinalysis, guaiac stools, prothrombin time, renal and hepatic function tests, WBCT, APTT

### Implementation

- Monitor clotting times to adjust dosage.
- Do not change brand names once stabilized; bioavailability problems have been documented.
- Evaluate patient for signs of blood loss (petechiae, bleeding gums, bruises, dark stools, dark urine).
- Establish safety measures to protect patient from injury.
- Do not give patient IM injections. Monitor sites of invasive procedures; ensure prolonged compression of bleeding vessels.
- Double-check other drugs that are ordered for potential interaction: dosage of both drugs may need to be adjusted.
- Use caution when discontinuing other medications; dosage of warfarin may need to be adjusted; carefully monitor PT values.
- Maintain vitamin K on standby in case of overdose of oral agents; maintain protamine sulfate on standby for parenteral drug.
- Arrange for frequent follow-up, including blood tests to evaluate drug effects.
- Evaluate for therapeutic effects: PT, 1.5–2.5 times the control value; WBCT, 2.5–3 times control; APTT, 1.5–2 times normal.

### Drug-specific teaching points

- Many factors may change the body's response to this drug—fever, change of diet, change of environment, other medications. The dosage of the drug may have to be changed. Be sure to write down all changes prescribed.
- Do not change any medication that you are taking (adding or stopping another drug) without consulting health care provider. Other drugs affect the way anticoagulants work; starting or stopping another drug can cause excessive bleeding or interfere with the desired effects of the drug.
- Carry or wear a medical alert tag stating that you are on this drug. This will alert

medical personnel in an emergency that you are taking this drug.
- Avoid situations in which you could be easily injured—contact sports, shaving with a straight razor.
- Possible side effects: stomach bloating, cramps (passes with time; if it becomes too uncomfortable, contact health care provider); loss of hair, skin rash (this is a frustrating and upsetting effect; if it becomes a problem, discuss it with health care provider); orange-red discoloration to the urine (this may be mistaken for blood; add vinegar to urine, the color should disappear).
- Arrange periodic blood tests to check on the action of the drug. It is very important that you have these tests.
- Use contraceptive measures while taking this drug; it is important that you do not become pregnant.
- Report unusual bleeding (when brushing your teeth, excessive bleeding from injuries, excessive bruising), black or bloody stools, cloudy or dark urine, sore throat, fever, chills, severe headaches, dizziness, suspected pregnancy.

### Representative drugs
*Oral*

warfarin sodium

*Parenteral*

heparin

*Low-molecular Weight Heparins*

ardeparin
dalteparin
danaparoid
enoxaparin

## Antidiabetic Agents

### Pregnancy Category C

### Therapeutic actions
Oral antidiabetic agents are called sulfonylureas. They stimulate insulin release from functioning beta cells in the pancreas; may improve binding between insulin and insulin receptors or increase the number of insulin receptors; second-generation sulfonylureas (glipizide and glyburide) are thought to be more potent than first-generation sulfonylureas. New class of agents increases insulin receptor sensitivity (troglitazone).

### Indications
- Adjuncts to diet to lower blood glucose in patients with non–insulin-dependent diabetes mellitus (type II)
- Adjuncts to insulin therapy in the stabilization of certain cases of insulin-dependent maturity-onset diabetes, reducing the insulin requirement and decreasing the chance of hypoglycemic reactions

### Contraindications/cautions
- Contraindications: allergy to sulfonylureas; diabetes complicated by fever, severe infections, severe trauma, major surgery, ketosis, acidosis, coma (insulin is indicated); type I or juvenile diabetes, serious hepatic impairment, serious renal impairment, uremia, thyroid or endocrine impairment, glycosuria, hyperglycemia associated with primary renal disease; labor and delivery (if glipizide is used during pregnancy, discontinue drug at least 1 mo before delivery); lactation, safety not established.

### Adverse effects
- GI: *Anorexia, nausea,* vomiting, *epigastric discomfort, heartburn, diarrhea*
- CV: Increased risk of CV mortality
- **Hematologic**: Leukopenia, thrombocytopenia, anemia
- Hypersensitivity: *Allergic skin reactions,* eczema, pruritus, erythema, urticaria, photosensitivity, fever, eosinophilia, jaundice
- Endocrine: *Hypoglycemia*

### Clinically important drug-drug interactions
• Increased risk of hypoglycemia with sulfonamides, chloramphenicol, fenfluramine, oxyphenbutazone, phenylbutazone, salicylates, clofibrate • Decreased effectiveness of both sulfonylurea and diazoxide if taken concurrently • Increased risk of hyperglycemia with rifampin, thiazides • Risk of hypo-

glycemia and hyperglycemia with ethanol; "disulfiram reaction" also has been reported.

## Nursing Considerations

### Assessment

- *History:* Allergy to sulfonylureas; diabetes complicated by fever, severe infections, severe trauma, major surgery, ketosis, acidosis, coma (insulin is indicated); type I or juvenile diabetes, serious hepatic impairment, serious renal impairment, uremia, thyroid or endocrine impairment, glycosuria, hyperglycemia associated with primary renal disease
- *Physical:* Skin color, lesions; T.; orientation, reflexes, peripheral sensation; R, adventitious sounds; liver evaluation, bowel sounds; urinalysis, BUN, serum creatinine, liver function tests, blood glucose, CBC.

### Implementation

- Administer drug before breakfast; if severe GI upset occurs may be divided and given before meals.
- Monitor urine and serum glucose levels to determine effectiveness of drug and dosage.
- Arrange for transfer to insulin therapy during periods of high stress (infections, surgery, trauma).
- Arrange for use of IV glucose if severe hypoglycemia occurs as a result of overdose.
- Arrange consultation with dietician to establish weight loss program and dietary control as appropriate.
- Arrange thorough diabetic teaching program to include disease, dietary control, exercise, signs and symptoms of hypoglycemia and hyperglycemia, avoidance of infection, hygiene.
- Provide skin care to prevent breakdown.
- Ensure access to bathroom facilities if diarrhea occurs.
- Establish safety precautions if CNS effects occur.

### Drug-specific teaching points

- Do not stop this medication without consulting health care provider.
- Monitor urine or blood for glucose and ketones.
- Do not use this drug during pregnancy.
- Avoid alcohol while on this drug.
- Report fever, sore throat, unusual bleeding or bruising, skin rash, dark urine, light-colored stools, hypoglycemia or hyperglycemic reactions.

### Representative drugs

acarbose
acetohexamide
chlorpropamide
glimepride
glipizide
glyburide
metformin
miglitol
tolazamide
tolbutamide
troglitazone

# Antifungals

### Pregnancy Category C

### Therapeutic actions

Antifungals bind to or impair sterols of fungal cell membranes, allowing increased permeability and leakage of cellular components and causing the death of the fungal cell.

### Indications

- Systemic fungal infections: candidiasis, chronic mucocutaneous candidiasis, oral thrush, candiduria, blastomycosis, coccidioidomycosis, histoplasmosis, chromomycosis, paracoccidioidomycosis, dermatophytosis, ringworm infections of the skin
- Unlabeled uses: treatment of onychomycosis, pityriasis versicolor, vaginal candidiasis; CNS fungal infections (high doses); topical treatment of tinea corporis and tinea cruris caused by *Trichophyton rubrum, Trichophyton mentagrophytes* and *Epidermophyton floccosum;* treatment of tinea versicolor caused by *Malassezia furfur* (topical); and reduction of scaling due to dandruff (shampoo)

### Contraindications/cautions

- Contraindications: allergy to any antifungal, fungal meningitis, pregnancy, or lactation. Use with caution in the presence of hepatocellular failure (increased risk of hepatocellular necrosis).

**Adverse effects**

- CNS: Headache, dizziness, somnolence, photophobia
- GI: Hepatotoxicity, *nausea, vomiting,* abdominal pain
- **Hematologic**: Thrombocytopenia, leukopenia, hemolytic anemia
- GU: Impotence, oligospermia (with very high doses)
- **Hypersensitivity**: Urticaria to anaphylaxis
- General: *Pruritus,* fever, chills, gynecomastia
- Local: *Severe irritation, pruritus, stinging* with topical application.

**Clinically important drug-drug interactions**

• Decreased blood levels with rifampin • Increased blood levels of cyclosporine and risk of toxicity with antifungals • Increased duration of adrenal suppression when methylprednisolone, corticosteroids are taken with antifungals • Risk of cardiac arrhythmias and even death with antihistamines, especially astemizole, terfenadine.

## ■ Nursing Considerations

### Assessment

- *History:* Allergy to antifungals, fungal meningitis, hepatocellular failure, pregnancy, lactation
- *Physical:* Skin color, lesions; orientation, reflexes, affect; bowel sounds, liver evaluation; liver function tests; CBC and differential; culture of area involved

### Implementation

- Arrange for culture before beginning therapy; treatment should begin, prior to lab results.
- Maintain epinephrine on standby in case of severe anaphylaxis after first dose.
- Administer oral drug with food to decrease GI upset.
- Administer until infection is eradicated: candidiasis, 1–2 wk; other systemic mycoses, 6 mo; chronic mucocutaneous candidiasis, often requires maintenance therapy; tinea versicolor, 2 wk of topical application.
- Discontinue treatment and consult physician about diagnosis if no improvement within 2 wk of topical application.
- Discontinue topical applications if sensitivity or chemical reaction occurs.
- Administer shampoo as follows: moisten hair and scalp thoroughly with water; apply sufficient shampoo to produce a lather; gently massage for 1 min; rinse hair with warm water; repeat, leaving on hair for 3 min.
- Provide hygiene measures to control sources of infection or reinfection.
- Provide small, frequent meals if GI upset occurs.
- Provide comfort measures appropriate to site of fungal infection.
- Arrange hepatic function tests prior to therapy and at least monthly during treatment.
- Establish safety precautions if CNS effects occur (siderails, assistance with ambulation).

### Drug-specific teaching points

- Take the full course of therapy. Long-term use of the drug will be needed; beneficial effects may not be seen for several weeks. Take oral drug with meals to decrease GI upset. Apply topical drug to affected area and surrounding area. Shampoo—moisten hair and scalp thoroughly with water; apply to produce a lather; gently massage for 1 min; rinse with warm water; repeat, leaving on for 3 min. Shampoo twice a week for 4 wk with at least 3 d between shampooing.
- Use hygiene measures to prevent reinfection or spread of infection.
- Possible side effects: nausea, vomiting, diarrhea (take drug with food); sedation, dizziness, confusion (avoid driving or performing tasks that require alertness); stinging, irritation (local application).
- Report skin rash, severe nausea, vomiting, diarrhea, fever, sore throat, unusual bleeding or bruising, yellowing of skin or eyes, dark urine or pale stools, severe irritation (local application).

**Representative drugs**

amphotericin B
butenafine
butoconazole
clotrimazole
fluconazole
flucytosine
itraconazole
ketoconazole
miconazole
nystatin

## Antihistamines

**Pregnancy Category C**

**Therapeutic actions**

Antihistamines competitively block the effects of histamine at peripheral $H_1$ receptor sites, have anticholinergic (atropine-like) and antipruritic effects.

**Indications**

- Symptomatic relief of symptoms associated with perennial and seasonal allergic rhinitis, vasomotor rhinitis, allergic conjunctivitis, mild, uncomplicated urticaria and angioedema.
- Amelioration of allergic reactions to blood or plasma
- Treatment of dermatographism
- Adjunctive therapy in anaphylactic reactions
- Unlabeled uses: relief of lower respiratory conditions, such as histamine-induced bronchoconstriction in asthmatics and exercise- and hyperventilation-induced bronchospasm

**Contraindications/cautions**

- Contraindications: allergy to antihistamines, pregnancy, or lactation. Use cautiously with narrow-angle glaucoma, stenosing peptic ulcer, symptomatic prostatic hypertrophy, asthmatic attack, bladder neck obstruction, pyloroduodenal obstruction.

**Adverse effects**

- CNS: *Depression, nightmares,* sedation (terfenadine is less sedating than other antihistamines)
- GI: *Dry mouth, GI upset,* anorexia, increased appetite, nausea, vomiting, diarrhea
- CV: Arrhythmia, increase in QTc intervals
- **Respiratory**: *Bronchospasm, cough, thickening of secretions*
- GU: Galactorrhea, menstrual disorders, dysuria, hesitancy
- **Dermatologic**: *Alopecia,* angioedema, skin eruption and itching
- **Other**: Musculoskeletal pain, mild to moderate transaminase elevations

**Clinically important drug-drug interactions**

• Altered antihistamine metabolism with ketoconazole, troleandomycin • Increased antihistamic anticholinergic effects with MAO Inhibitors • Additive CNS depressant effects with alcohol, CNS depressants • Potentially fatal cardiac arrhythmias if taken with erythromycin, antifungals, astemizole, terfenadine)

### ■ Nursing Considerations

**Assessment**

- *History:* Allergy to any antihistamines, narrow-angle glaucoma, stenosing peptic ulcer, symptomatic prostatic hypertrophy, asthmatic attack, bladder neck obstruction, pyloroduodenal obstruction, pregnancy, lactation
- *Physical:* Skin color, lesions, texture; orientation, reflexes, affect; vision exam; R, adventitious sounds; prostate palpation; serum transaminase levels

**Implementation**

- Administer with food if GI upset occurs.
- Provide mouth care, sugarless lozenges for dry mouth.
- Arrange for humidifier if thickening of secretions, nasal dryness become bothersome; encourage intake of fluids.
- Provide skin care for dermatologic effects.

**Drug-specific teaching points**

- Avoid excessive dosage.
- Take with food if GI upset occurs.
- Possible side effects: dizziness, sedation, drowsiness (use caution driving or perform-

ing tasks that require alertness); dry mouth (mouth care, sucking sugarless lozenges may help); thickening of bronchial secretions, dryness of nasal mucosa (use a humidifier); menstrual irregularities.

- Avoid alcohol; serious sedation could occur.
- Report difficulty breathing, hallucinations, tremors, loss of coordination, unusual bleeding or bruising, visual disturbances, irregular heartbeat.

### Representative drugs

astemizole
azatadine
azelastine
brompheniramine
buclizine
cetirizine
chlorpheniramine
clemastine
cyclizine
cyproheptadine
dechlorpheniramine
dimenhydrinate
diphenhydramine
fexofenadine
hydroxyzine
loratadine
meclizine
methdilazine
promethazine
tripelennamine

## Antimetabolites

### Pregnancy Category D

### Therapeutic actions

Antimetabolites are antineoplastic drugs that inhibit DNA polymerase. They are cell cycle phase specific to S phase (stage of DNA synthesis), causing cell death for cells in the S phase; they also block progression of cells from $G_1$ to S in the cell cycle.

### Indications

- Induction and maintenance of remission in acute myelocytic leukemia (higher response rate in children than in adults), chronic lymphocytic leukemia
- Treatment of acute lymphocytic leukemia, chronic myelocytic leukemia and erythroleukemia, meningeal leukemia, psoriasis and rheumatoid arthritis (methotrexate)
- Palliative treatment of GI adenocarcinoma, carcinoma of the colon, rectum, breast, stomach, pancreas
- Part of combination therapy for the treatment of non-Hodgkin's lymphoma in children

### Contraindications/cautions

- Contraindications: allergy to the drug, pregnancy, lactation, premature infants. Use cautiously with hematopoietic depression secondary to radiation or chemotherapy; impaired liver function.

### Adverse effects

- CNS: Neuritis, neural toxicity
- GI: *Anorexia, nausea, vomiting, diarrhea, oral and anal inflammation or ulceration;* esophageal ulcerations, esophagitis, abdominal pain, *hepatic dysfunction* (jaundice), acute pancreatitis
- **Hematologic**: Bone marrow depression, hyperuricemia
- GU: Renal dysfunction, urinary retention
- **Dermatologic**: Fever, rash, urticaria, freckling, skin ulceration, pruritis, conjunctivitis, alopecia
- **Local**: Thrombophlebitis, cellulitis at injection site
- Other: *Fever, rash*

### Clinically important drug-drug interactions

• Decreased therapeutic action of digoxin with cytarabine • Enhanced toxicity of fluorouracil with leucovorin • Potentially fatal reactions if methotrexate is taken with various NSAIDs

### ■ Nursing Considerations

#### Assessment

- *History:* Allergy to drug, hematopoietic depression, impaired liver function, lactation
- *Physical:* Weight; T; skin lesions, color; hair; orientation, reflexes; R, adventitious

sounds; mucous membranes, liver evaluation, abdominal exam; CBC, differential; renal and liver function tests; urinalysis

### Implementation

- Arrange for tests to evaluate hematopoietic status prior to and during therapy.
- Arrange for discontinuation of drug therapy if platelet count < 50,000/mm$^3$, polymorphonuclear granulocyte count < 1,000/mm$^3$; consult physician for dosage adjustment.
- Monitor injection site for signs of thrombophlebitis, inflammation.
- Provide mouth care for mouth sores.
- Arrange for small, frequent meals and dietary consultation to maintain nutrition when GI effects are severe.
- Establish safety measures if dizziness, CNS effects occur.
- Arrange for patient to obtain a wig or some other suitable head covering if alopecia occurs; ensure that head is covered in extremes of temperature.
- Protect patient from exposure to infections.
- Provide skin care.
- Arrange for comfort measures if anal inflammation, headache, other pain associated with cytarabine syndrome occur.
- Arrange for treatment of fever if it occurs.

### Drug-specific teaching points

- Prepare a calendar of treatment days for the patient.
- Possible side effects: nausea, vomiting, loss of appetite (medication may be ordered; small frequent meals may help; it is important to maintain nutrition); malaise, weakness, lethargy (these are all effects of the drug; consult your health care provider and avoid driving or operating dangerous machinery); mouth sores (frequent mouth care will be needed); diarrhea; loss of hair (you may wish to obtain a wig or other suitable head covering; keep the head covered in extremes of temperature); anal inflammation (consult with health care provider; comfort measures can be ordered).
- Use birth control; this drug may cause birth defects or miscarriages.
- Arrange to have frequent, regular medical follow-up, including frequent blood tests.
- Report black, tarry stools; fever, chills; sore throat; unusual bleeding or bruising; shortness of breath; chest pain; difficulty swallowing.

### Representative drugs

cytarabine
floxuridin
fludarabine
fluorouracil
mercaptopurine
methotrexate
thioguanine

## Antivirals

### Pregnancy Category C

### Therapeutic actions

Antiviral drugs inhibit viral DNA or RNA replication in the virus, preventing replication and leading to viral death.

### Indications

- Initial and recurrent mucosal and cutaneous HSV 1 and 2 infections in immunocompromised patients, encephalitis, herpes zoster
- HIV infections (part of combination therapy)
- CMV retinitis in patients with AIDS
- Severe initial and recurrent genital herpes infections
- Treatment and prevention of influenza A respiratory tract illness
- Treatment of initial HSV genital infections and limited mucocutaneous HSV infections in immunocompromised patients (ointment)
- Unlabeled uses: treatment of herpes zoster, CMV and HSV infection following transplant, herpes simplex infections, infectious mononucleosis, varicella pneumonia, and varicella zoster in immunocompromised patients.

### Contraindications/cautions

- Contraindications: allergy to the drug, seizures, CHF, renal disease, or lactation.

**Adverse effects**

*Systemic Administration*

- CNS: Headache, vertigo, depression, tremors, encephalopathic changes
- GI: *Nausea, vomiting,* diarrhea, anorexia
- GU: Crystalluria with rapid IV administration, hematuria
- Dermatologic: *Inflammation or phlebitis at injection sites,* rash, hair loss

*Topical Administration*

- Skin: *Transient burning at the site of application*

**Clinically important drug-drug interactions**

- Increased drug effects with probenecid
- Increased nephrotoxicity with other nephrotoxic drugs

## ■ Nursing Considerations

### Assessment

- *History:* Allergy to drug, seizures, CHF, renal disease, lactation
- *Physical:* Skin—color, lesions; orientation; BP, P, auscultation, perfusion, edema; R, adventitious sounds; urinary output; BUN, creatinine clearance

### Implementation

*Systemic Administration*

- Ensure that the patient is well hydrated with IV fluids or PO fluids.
- Provide support and encouragement to deal with disease.
- Provide small, frequent meals if systemic therapy causes GI upset.
- Provide skin care, analgesics if necessary for rash.

*Topical Administration*

- Start treatment as soon as possible after onset of signs and symptoms.
- Wear a rubber glove or finger cot when ...lying drug.

### ...cific teaching points

- ... full course of oral therapy, ...ed the prescribed dose.
- ... cure for your disease ... feel better.
- ... vomiting, loss ..., dizziness.
- Avoid sexual intercourse while visible lesions are present.
- Report difficulty urinating, skin rash, increased severity or frequency of recurrences.

*Topical Administration*

- Wear rubber gloves or finger cots when applying the drug to prevent autoinoculation of other sites and transmission of the disease.
- This drug does not cure the disease; application of the drug during symptom-free periods will not prevent recurrences.
- Avoid sexual intercourse while visible lesions are present.
- This drug may cause burning, stinging, itching, rash; notify health care provider if these are pronounced.

**Representative drugs**

acyclovir
acyclovir sodium
amantadine
cidofovir
delaviridine
didanosine
famciclovir
foscarnet
ganciclovir
imiguimod
indinavir
lamivudine
nelfinavir
nevirapine
penciclovir
ribavirin
rimantadine
ritonavir
saguinavir
stavudine
valacyclovir
vidarabine
zalcitabine
zidovudine

## Barbiturates

**Pregnancy Category D**
**C-II controlled substances**

**Therapeutic actions**

Barbiturates act as sedatives, hypnotics, and anticonvulsants. They are general CNS depressants. Barbiturates inhibit impulse conduction in the ascending reticular activating system, depress the cerebral cortex, alter cerebellar function, depress motor output, and can produce excitation, sedation, hypnosis, anesthesia, and deep coma; at anesthetic doses, they have anticonvulsant activity.

### Indications

- Sedatives or hypnotics for short-term treatment of insomnia
- Preanesthetic medications
- Anticonvulsants, in anesthetic doses, for emergency control of certain acute convulsive episodes (eg, status epilepticus, eclampsia, meningitis, tetanus, toxic reactions to strychnine or local anesthetics)

### Contraindications/cautions

- Contraindications: hypersensitivity to barbiturates, manifest or latent porphyria, marked liver impairment, nephritis, severe respiratory distress, respiratory disease with dyspnea, obstruction or cor pulmonale, previous addiction to sedative-hypnotic drugs, pregnancy (causes fetal damage, neonatal withdrawal syndrome), or lactation. Use cautiously with acute or chronic pain (paradoxical excitement or masking of important symptoms could result), seizure disorders (abrupt discontinuation of daily doses of drug can result in status epilepticus), fever, hyperthyroidism, diabetes mellitus, severe anemia, pulmonary or cardiac disease, status asthmaticus, shock, uremia.

### Adverse effects

- CNS: *Somnolence, agitation, confusion, hyperkinesia, ataxia, vertigo, CNS depression, nightmares, lethargy, residual sedation (hangover), paradoxical excitement, nervousness, psychiatric disturbance, hallucinations, insomnia, anxiety, dizziness, thinking abnormality*
- GI: *Nausea, vomiting, constipation, diarrhea, epigastric pain*
- CV: *Bradycardia, hypotension, syncope*
- Respiratory: *Hypoventilation, apnea, respiratory depression,* laryngospasm, bronchospasm, circulatory collapse
- Hypersensitivity: Skin rashes, angioneurotic edema, serum sickness, morbiliform rash, urticaria; rarely, exfoliative dermatitis, **Stevens-Johnson syndrome,** sometimes fatal
- Local: *Pain, tissue necrosis at injection site,* gangrene; arterial spasm with inadvertent intra-arterial injection; thrombophlebitis; permanent neurologic deficit if injected near a nerve
- Other: Tolerance, psychological and physical dependence; **withdrawal syndrome** (sometimes fatal)

### Clinically important drug-drug interactions

• Increased CNS depression with alcohol • Increased nephrotoxicity with methoxyflurane • Decreased effects of the following drugs given with barbiturates: oral anticoagulants, corticosteroids, oral contraceptives and estrogens, beta-adrenergic blockers (especially propranolol, metoprolol), theophylline, metronidazole, doxycycline, griseofulvin, phenylbutazones, quinidine

## ■ Nursing Considerations

### Assessment

- *History:* Hypersensitivity to barbiturates manifest or latent porphyria; marked liver impairment; nephritis; severe respiratory distress; respiratory disease with dyspnea, obstruction, or cor pulmonale; previous addiction to sedative-hypnotic drugs; acute or chronic pain; seizure disorders; pregnancy; lactation; fever, hyperthyroidism; diabetes mellitus; severe anemia; pulmonary or cardiac disease; status asthmaticus; shock; uremia
- *Physical:* Weight; T; skin color, lesions, injection site; orientation, affect, reflexes; P, BP, orthostatic BP; R, adventitious sounds; bowel sounds, normal output, liver evaluation; liver and kidney function tests, blood and urine glucose, BUN

### Implementation

- Do not administer intra-arterially; produce arteriospasm, throm' gangrene.
- Administer IV doses slowly.

- Administer IM doses deep in a muscle mass.
- Do not use parenteral dosage forms if solution is discolored or contains a precipitate.
- Monitor injection sites carefully for irritation, extravasation (IV); solutions are alkaline and very irritating to the tissues.
- Monitor P, BP, R carefully during IV administration.
- Provide resuscitative facilities on standby in case of respiratory depression, hypersensitivity reaction.
- Provide small, frequent meals, frequent mouth care if GI effects occur.
- Use safety precautions if CNS changes occur (side rails, accompany patient).
- Provide skin care if dermatologic effects occur.
- Provide comfort measures, reassurance for patients receiving pentobarbital for tetanus, toxic convulsions.
- Offer support and encouragement to patients receiving this drug for preanesthetic medication.
- Taper dosage gradually after repeated use, especially in epileptic patients.

### Drug-specific teaching points

When giving this drug as preanesthetic, incorporate teaching about the drug into general teaching about the procedure. Include:

- This drug will make you drowsy and less anxious.
- Do not try to get up after you have received this drug (request assistance if you must sit up or move about for any reason).

*Outpatients*

- Take this drug exactly as prescribed. This drug is habit forming; its effectiveness in facilitating sleep disappears after a short time. Do not take this drug longer than 2 wk (for insomnia), and do not increase the dosage without consulting health care provider. If the drug appears to be ineffective, consult health care provider.
- Avoid becoming pregnant while taking this drug. The use of oral contraceptives is not recommended as they lose their effectiveness while you are taking this drug.
- Possible side effects: drowsiness, dizziness, "hangover," impaired thinking (these effects may become less pronounced after a few days; avoid driving a car or engaging in activities that require alertness); GI upset (taking the drug with food may help); dreams, nightmares, difficulty concentrating, fatigue, nervousness (these are effects of the drug that will go away when the drug is discontinued; consult your health care provider if these become bothersome).
- Report severe dizziness, weakness, drowsiness that persists, rash or skin lesions, pregnancy.

### Representative drugs

amobarbital
aprobarbital
butabarbital
mephobarbital
pentobarbital
pentobarbital sodium
phenobarbital
secobarbital

## Benzodiazepines

### Pregnancy Category D
### C-IV controlled substance

### Therapeutic actions

Benzodiazepines are antianxiety agents, anticonvulsants, muscle relaxants, and sedative-hypnotics. Their exact mechanisms of action not understood, but it is known that benzodiazepines potentiate the effects of gamma-aminobutyrate, an inhibitory neurotransmitter.

### Indications

- Management of anxiety disorders, short-term relief of symptoms of anxiety
- Short-term treatment of insomnia
- Alone or as adjunct in treatment of Lennox-Gastaut syndrome (petit mal variant), akinetic and myoclonic seizures
- May be useful in patients with absence (petit mal) seizures who have not responded to succinimides; up to 30% of patients show loss of effectiveness of drug, within 3 mo of therapy (may respond to dosage adjustment)

- Unlabeled use: treatment of panic attacks, periodic leg movements during sleep, hypokinetic dysarthria, acute manic episodes, multifocal tic disorders; adjunct treatment of schizophrenia, neuralgias; treatment of irritable bowel syndrome

### Contraindications/cautions

- Contraindications: hypersensitivity to benzodiazepines, psychoses, acute narrow-angle glaucoma, shock, coma, acute alcoholic intoxication with depression of vital signs, pregnancy (risk of congenital malformations, neonatal withdrawal syndrome), labor and delivery ("floppy infant" syndrome reported), or lactation (infants become lethargic and lose weight). Use cautiously with impaired liver or kidney function, debilitation.

### Adverse effects

- CNS: *Transient, mild drowsiness initially; sedation, depression, lethargy, apathy, fatigue, lightheadedness, disorientation, anger, hostility,* episodes of mania and hypomania, *restlessness, confusion, crying,* delirium, *headache,* slurred speech, dysarthria, stupor, rigidity, tremor, dystonia, vertigo, euphoria, nervousness, difficulty in concentration, vivid dreams, psychomotor retardation, extrapyramidal symptoms; *mild paradoxical excitatory reactions, during first 2 wk of treatment*
- GI: *Constipation, diarrhea, dry mouth,* salivation, *nausea,* anorexia, vomiting, difficulty in swallowing, gastric disorders, hepatic dysfunction, encoporesis
- CV: Bradycardia, tachycardia, CV collapse, hypertension and hypotension, palpitations, edema
- **Hematologic**: Elevations of blood enzymes—LDH, alkaline phosphatase, SGOT, SGPT; blood dyscrasias—agranulocytosis, leukopenia
- GU: Incontinence, urinary retention, changes in libido, menstrual irregularities
- EENT: Visual and auditory disturbances, diplopia, nystagmus, depressed hearing, nasal congestion
- **Dermatologic**: Urticaria, pruritus, skin rash, dermatitis
- **Other**: Hiccups, fever, diaphoresis, paresthesias, muscular disturbances, gynecomastia; *drug dependence with withdrawal syndrome when drug is discontinued; more common with abrupt discontinuation of higher dosage used for longer than 4 mo*

### Clinically important drug-drug interactions

- Increased CNS depression with alcohol
- Increased effect with cimetidine, disulfiram, omeprazole, oral contraceptives
- Decreased effect with theophylline

## ■ Nursing Considerations

### Assessment

- *History:* Hypersensitivity to benzodiazepines, psychoses, acute narrow-angle glaucoma, shock, coma, acute alcoholic intoxication with depression of vital signs, pregnancy, lactation, impaired liver or kidney function, debilitation
- *Physical:* Skin color, lesions; T; orientation, reflexes, affect, ophthalmologic exam; P, BP; R, adventitious sounds; liver evaluation, abdominal exam, bowel sounds, normal output; CBC, liver and renal function tests

### Implementation

- Keep addiction-prone patients under careful surveillance.
- Monitor liver function, blood counts in patients on long-term therapy.
- Ensure ready access to bathroom if GI effects occur; establish bowel program if constipation occurs.
- Provide small, frequent meals, frequent mouth care if GI effects occur.
- Provide measures appropriate to care of urinary problems (protective clothing, bed changing).
- Establish safety precautions if CNS changes occur (eg, side rails, accompany patient).
- Taper dosage gradually after long-term therapy, especially in epileptic patients;

arrange substitution of another antiepileptic drug.
- Monitor patient for therapeutic drug levels; levels vary with drug being used.
- Arrange for patient to wear medical alert identification indicating epilepsy and drug therapy.

### Drug-specific teaching points
- Take drug exactly as prescribed; do not stop taking drug (long-term therapy) without consulting health care provider.
- Avoid alcohol, sleep-inducing, or OTC drugs.
- Possible side effects: drowsiness, dizziness (may become less pronounced after a few days; avoid driving or engaging in other dangerous activities); GI upset (take drug with food); fatigue; depression; dreams; crying; nervousness; depression, emotional changes; bed wetting, urinary incontinence.
- Report severe dizziness, weakness, drowsiness that persists, rash or skin lesions, difficulty voiding, palpitations, swelling in the extremities.

### Representative drugs
alprazolam
chlordiazepoxide
clonazepam
clorazepate
diazepam
estazolam
flurazepam
lorazepam
oxazepam
quazepam
temazepam
triazolam

## Beta-Adrenergic Blockers

### Pregnancy Category C

### Therapeutic actions
Beta-adrenergic blockers are antianginals, antiarrhythmics, and antihypertensives. Beta-blockers competitively block beta-adrenergic receptors in the heart and juxtaglomerular apparatus. They decrease the influence of the sympathetic nervous system on these tissues, the excitability of the heart, cardiac work load and oxygen consumption, the release of renin and lower BP. They have membrane-stabilizing (local anesthetic) effects that contribute to their antiarrhythmic action. They also act in the CNS to reduce sympathetic outflow and vasoconstrictor tone.

### Indications
- Hypertension (alone or with other drugs, especially diuretics)
- Angina pectoris caused by coronary atherosclerosis
- Hypertrophic subaortic stenosis, to manage associated stress-induced angina, palpitations, and syncope; cardiac arrhythmias, especially supraventricular tachycardia, and ventricular tachycardias induced by digitalis or catecholamines; essential tremor, familial or hereditary
- Prevention of reinfarction in clinically stable patients 1–4 wk after MI
- Adjunctive therapy for pheochromocytoma after treatment with an alpha-adrenergic blocker, to manage tachycardia before or during surgery or if the pheochromocytoma is inoperable
- Prophylaxis for migraine headache (propranolol)
- Management of acute situational stress reaction (stage fright) (propranolol)
- Unlabeled uses: treatment of recurrent GI bleeding in cirrhotic patients, schizophrenia, essential tremors, tardive dyskinesia, acute panic symptoms, vaginal contraceptive

### Contraindications/cautions
- Contraindications: allergy to beta-blocking agents, sinus bradycardia, second- or third-degree heart block, cardiogenic shock, CHF, bronchial asthma, bronchospasm, COPD, pregnancy (neonatal bradycardia, hypoglycemia, and apnea have occurred in infants whose mothers received propranolol; low birth weight occurs with chronic maternal use during pregnancy), or lactation. Use cautiously

with hypoglycemia and diabetes, thyrotoxicosis, hepatic dysfunction.

### Adverse effects

- GI: *Gastric pain, flatulence, constipation, diarrhea, nausea, vomiting,* anorexia, ischemic colitis, renal and mesenteric arterial thrombosis, retroperitoneal fibrosis, hepatomegaly, acute pancreatitis
- CV: *Bradycardia, CHF, cardiac arrhythmias, sinoartial or AV nodal block, tachycardia,* peripheral vascular insufficiency, claudication, CVA, pulmonary edema, hypotension
- Respiratory: Bronchospasm, dyspnea, cough, bronchial obstruction, nasal stuffiness, rhinitis, pharyngitis
- Neuro: Dizziness, vertigo, tinnitus, *fatigue,* emotional depression, paresthesias, sleep disturbances, hallucinations, disorientation, memory loss, slurred speech
- GU: *Impotence, decreased libido,* Peyronie's disease, dysuria, nocturia, frequency
- MS: Joint pain, arthralgia, muscle cramp
- EENT: Eye irritation, dry eyes, conjunctivitis, blurred vision
- Dermatologic: Rash, pruritus, sweating, dry skin
- Allergic reactions: Pharyngitis, erythematous rash, fever, sore throat, laryngospasm, respiratory distress
- Other: *Decreased exercise tolerance, development of antinuclear antibodies,* hyperglycemia or hypoglycemia, elevated serum transaminase, alkaline phosphatase, and LDH

### Clinically important drug-drug interactions

• Increased effects with verapamil • Decreased effects with indomethacin, ibuprofen, piroxicam, sulindac, barbiturates • Prolonged hypoglycemic effects of insulin with beta-blockers • Peripheral ishemia possible if combined with ergot alkaloids • Initial hypertensive episode followed by bradycardia with epinephrine • Increased "first-dose response" to prazosin with beta-blockers • Increased serum levels and toxic effects with lidocaine, cimetidine • Increased serum levels of beta-blockers and phenothiazines, hydralazine if the two drugs are taken concurrently • Paradoxical hypertension when clonidine is given with beta-blockers; increased rebound hypertension when clonidine is discontinued • Decreased serum levels and therapeutic effects if taken with methimazole, propylthioracil • Decreased bronchodilator effects of theophyllines • Decreased antihypertensive effects with NSAIDs (eg, ibuprofen, indomethacin, piroxicam, sulindac), rifampin

### Drug-lab test interferences

• Interference with glucose or insulin tolerance tests, glaucoma screening tests

## ■ Nursing Considerations

### Assessment

- *History:* Allergy to beta-blocking agents, sinus bradycardia, second- or third-degree heart block, cardiogenic shock, CHF, bronchial asthma, bronchospasm, COPD, hypoglycemia and diabetes, thyrotoxicosis, hepatic dysfunction, pregnancy, lactation
- *Physical:* Weight, skin color, lesions, edema, T; reflexes, affect, vision, hearing, orientation; BP, P, ECG, peripheral perfusion; R, auscultation; bowel sounds, normal output, liver evaluation; bladder palpation; liver and thyroid function tests, blood and urine glucose

### Implementation

- Do not stop drug abruptly after chronic therapy (hypersensitivity to catecholamines may have developed, causing exacerbation of angina, MI, and ventricular dysrhythmias). Taper drug gradually over 2 wk with monitoring.
- Consult with physician about withdrawing drug if patient is to undergo surgery (controversial).
- Give oral drug with food to facilitate absorption.
- Provide side rails and assistance with walking if CNS, vision changes occur.

- Position patient to decrease effects of edema, respiratory obstruction.
- Space activities, and provide periodic rest periods for patient.
- Provide frequent, small meals if GI effects occur.
- Provide comfort measures to help patient cope with eye, GI, joint, CNS, dermatologic effects.

### Drug-specific teaching points

- Take this drug with meals. Do not stop abruptly; abrupt discontinuation can worsen the disorder for which you are taking the drug.
- Possible side effects: dizziness, drowsiness, lightheadedness, blurred vision (avoid driving or performing hazardous tasks); nausea, loss of appetite (frequent, small meals may help); nightmares, depression (notify your health care provider who may be able to change your medication); sexual impotence (you may want to discuss this with the health care provider).
- Report difficulty breathing, night cough, swelling of extremities, slow pulse, confusion, depression, rash, fever, sore throat.
- For diabetic patients, be aware that the normal signs of hypoglycemia (sweating, tachycardia) may be blocked by this drug; monitor your blood/urine glucose carefully; be sure to eat regular meals, and take your diabetic medication regularly.

### Representative drugs

acebutolol
atenolol
betaxolol
bisoprolol
carteolol
esmolol
labetolol
metoprolol
nadolol
penbutolol
pindolol
propranolol
sotalol
timolol

## Calcium Channel-Blockers

### Pregnancy Category C

### Therapeutic actions

Calcium channel-blockers are antianginal and antihypertensive. They inhibit the movement of calcium ions across the membranes of cardiac and arterial muscle cells; this inhibition of transmembrane calcium flow results in the depression of impulse formation in specialized cardiac pacemaker cells, slowing of the velocity of conduction of the cardiac impulse, depression of myocardial contractility, and dilation of coronary arteries and arterioles and peripheral arterioles; these effects lead to decreased cardiac work, decreased cardiac energy consumption, and increased delivery of oxygen to myocardial cells.

### Indications

- Treatment of angina pectoris due to coronary artery spasm (Prinzmetal's variant angina), chronic stable angina (effort-associated angina), hypertension, arrhythmias (supraventricular, those related to digoxin [verapamil]), subarachnoid hemorrhage (nimodipine)
- Orphan drug use in the treatment of interstitial cystitis, hypertensive emergencies, migraines

### Contraindications/cautions

- Contraindications: allergy to calcium channel-blockers, sick sinus syndrome, heart block, ventricular dysfunction, or pregnancy. Use cautiously during lactation.

### Adverse effects

- CNS: *Dizziness, lightheadedness, headache, asthenia,* fatigue, *nervousness,* sleep disturbances, blurred vision
- GI: *Nausea, diarrhea, constipation,* cramps, flatulence, hepatic injury
- CV: *Peripheral edema, angina,* hypotension, arrhythmias, *bradycardia, AV block,* asystole

- Dermatologic: *Flushing, rash,* dermatitis, pruritus, urticaria
- Other: *Nasal congestion, cough,* fever, chills, shortness of breath, muscle cramps, joint stiffness, sexual difficulties

### Clinically important drug-drug interactions

- Increased effects with cimetidine, ranitidine

## ■ Nursing Considerations

### Assessment

- *History:* Allergy to calcium channel-blockers, sick sinus syndrome, heart block, ventricular dysfunction; pregnancy; lactation
- *Physical:* Skin lesions, color, edema; orientation, reflexes; P, BP, baseline ECG, peripheral perfusion, auscultation; R, adventitious sounds; liver evaluation, normal GI output; liver function tests

### Implementation

- Monitor patient carefully (BP, cardiac rhythm, and output) while drug is being titrated to therapeutic dose; the dosage may be increased more rapidly in hospitalized patients under close supervision.
- Ensure that patients do not chew or divide sustained-release tablets.
- Taper dosage of beta blockers before beginning calcium channel-blocker therapy.
- Protect drug from light and moisture.
- Ensure ready access to bathroom.
- Provide comfort measures for skin rash, headache, nervousness.
- Establish safety precautions if CNS changes occur.
- Position patient to alleviate peripheral edema.
- Provide small, frequent meals if GI upset occurs.

### Drug-specific teaching points

- Do not chew or divide sustained-release tablets. Swallow whole.
- Possible side effects: nausea, vomiting (small, frequent meals may help); dizziness, light headedness, vertigo (avoid driving, operating hazardous machinery; avoid falling); muscle cramps, joint stiffness, sweating, sexual difficulties (should disappear when the drug therapy is stopped; discuss with health care provider if these become too uncomfortable).
- Report irregular heart beat, shortness of breath, swelling of the hands or feet, pronounced dizziness, constipation.

### Representative drugs

amlodipine
bepridil
diltiazem
felodipine
isradipine
mibefradil
nicardipine
nifedipine
nimodipine
nisoldipine
verapamil

# Cephalosporins

### Pregnancy Category B

### Therapeutic actions

Cephalosporins are antibiotics. They are bactericidal, inhibiting synthesis of bacterial cell wall, causing cell death in susceptible bacteria.

### Indications

- Treatment of pharyngitis, tonsillitis caused by *Streptococcus pyogenes;* otitis media caused by *Streptococcus pneumoniae, Haemophilus influenzae, Moraxella catarrhalis, S. pyogenes;* lower respiratory tract infections caused by *S. pneumoniae, Haemophilus parainfluenxae, Staphylococcus aureus, Escherichia coli, Klebsiella, H. influenzae, S. pyogenes;* UTIs caused by *E. coli, Klebsiella pneumoniae;* dermatologic infections caused by *S. aureus, S. pyogenes, E. coli, Klebsiella, Enterobacter;* uncomplicated and disseminated gonorrhea caused by *Neisseria gonorrhoea;* septicemia caused by *S. pneumoniae, S. aureus, E. coli, Klebsiella, H. influenzae;* meningitis caused by *S. pneumoniae, H. influenze, S. aureus, Neisseria meningi-*

*tidis;* bone and joint infections caused by *S. aureus*
- Perioperative prophylaxis

### Contraindications/cautions
- Contraindications: allergy to cephalosporins or penicillins, renal failure, or lactation.

### Adverse effects
- CNS: Headache, dizziness, lethargy, paresthesias
- GI: *Nausea, vomiting, diarrhea, anorexia, abdominal pain, flatulence,* pseudomembranous colitis, liver toxicity
- **Hematologic: Bone marrow depression;** decreased WBC, platelets, Hct
- GU: Nephrotoxicity
- **Hypersensitivity:** *Ranging from rash, fever* to anaphylaxis; serum sickness reaction
- Local: *Pain,* abscess at injection site, *phlebitis,* inflammation at IV site
- Other: *Superinfections, disulfiram-like reaction with alcohol*

### Clinically important drug-drug interactions
• Increased nephrotoxicity with aminoglycosides • Increased bleeding effects with oral anticoagulants • Disulfiram-like reaction may occur if alcohol is taken within 72 h after cephalosporin administration

### Drug-lab test interferences
- Possibility of false results on tests of urine glucose using Benedict's solution, Fehling's solution, Clinitest tablets; urinary 17-keto-steroids; direct Coombs' test.

## ■ Nursing Considerations

### Assessment
- *History:* Allergy to any cephalosporin, liver and kidney dysfunction, lactation, pregnancy
- *Physical:* Skin status, liver and kidney function test, culture of affected area, sensitivity tests

### Implementation
- Culture infected area and arrange for sensitivity tests before beginning drug therapy and during therapy if expected response is not seen.
- Administer oral drug with food to decrease GI upset and enhance absorption.
- Administer liquid drug to children who cannot swallow tablets; crushing the drug results in a bitter, unpleasant taste.
- Have vitamin K available in case hypoprothrombinemia occurs.
- Discontinue drug if hypersensitivity reaction occurs.
- Ensure ready access to bathroom and provide small, frequent meals if GI complications occur.
- Arrange for treatment of superinfections.

### Drug-specific teaching points
*Oral Drug*
- Take full course of therapy.
- This drug is specific to an infection and should not be used to self-treat other problems.
- Swallow tablets whole; do not crush.
- Take the drug with food.
- Avoid drinking alcoholic beverages while taking and for 3 d after stopping this drug because severe reactions often occur (even with parenteral forms).
- Possible side effects: stomach upset or diarrhea.
- Report severe diarrhea with blood, pus, or mucus; rash; difficulty breathing; unusual tiredness, fatigue; unusual bleeding or bruising; unusual itching or irritation, pain at injection site.

### Representative drugs
*First Generation*

cefadroxil
cefazolin
cephalexin
cephalothin
cephapirin
cephradine

*Second Generation*

cefaclor
cefamandole
cefmetazole
cefoxitin
cefonicid
cefotetan

cefprozil
cefpodoxime
cefuroxime
loracarbef

*Third Generation*

cefepime
cefixime
cefoperazone
cefotaxime
ceftazidime
ceftibuten
ceftizoxime
ceftriaxone

## Diuretics

### Pregnancy Category C

### Therapeutic actions

Diuretics are divided into several subgroups. Thiazide and thiazide-related diuretics inhibit reabsorption of sodium and chloride in the distal renal tubule, increasing the excretion of sodium, chloride, and water by the kidney. Loop diuretics inhibit the reabsorption of sodium and chloride in the loop of Henle and in the distal renal tubule; because of this added effect, loop diuretics are more potent. Potassium-sparing diuretics block the effect of aldosterone on the renal tubule, leading to a loss of sodium and water and the retention of potassium; their overall effect is much weaker. Osmotic diuretics pull fluid out of the tissues with a hypertonic effect. Overall effect of diuretics is a loss of water and electrolytes from the body.

### Indications

- Adjunctive therapy in edema associated with CHF, cirrhosis, corticosteroid and estrogen therapy, renal dysfunction.
- Treatment of hypertension, alone or in combination with other antihypertensives
- Unlabeled uses: treatment of diabetes insipidus, especially nephrogenic diabetes insipidus, reduction of incidence of osteoporosis in postmenopausal women

### Contraindications/cautions

- Contraindications: fluid or electrolyte imbalances, renal or liver disease, gout, SLE, glucose tolerance abnormalities, hyperparathyroidism, manic-depressive disorders, or lactation.

### Adverse effects

- CNS: *Dizziness, vertigo,* paresthesias, weakness, headache, drowsiness, fatigue
- GI: *Nausea, anorexia, vomiting, dry mouth, diarrhea, constipation,* jaundice, hepatitis, pancreatitis
- CV: Orthostatic hypotension, venous thrombosis, volume depletion, cardiac arrhythmias, chest pain
- **Hematologic**: Leukopenia, thrombocytopenia, agranulocytosis, aplastic anemia, neutropenia, fluid and electrolyte imbalances
- GU: *Polyuria, nocturia, impotence,* loss of libido
- **Dermatologic**: Photosensitivity, rash, purpura, exfoliative dermatitis
- **Other**: Muscle cramps and muscle spasms, fever, hives, gouty attacks, flushing, weight loss, rhinorrhea, electrolyte imbalance

### Clinically important drug-drug interactions

• Increased thiazide effects and possible acute hyperglycemia with diazoxide • Decreased absorption with cholestyramine, colestipol • Increased risk of cardiac glycoside toxicity if hypokalemia occurs • Increased risk of lithium toxicity • Increased dosage of antidiabetic agents may be needed • Risk of hyperkalemia if potassium-sparing diuretics are given with potassium preparations or ACE inhibitors • Increased risk of ototoxicity it loop diuretics are taken with aminoglycosides or cisplatin

### Drug-lab test interferences

- Monitor for decreased PBI levels without clinical signs of thyroid disturbances

## ■ Nursing Considerations

### Assessment

- *History:* Fluid or electrolyte imbalances, renal or liver disease, gout, SLE, glucose tolerance abnormalities, hyperparathyroidism, manic-depressive disorders, lactation

- *Physical:* Orientation, reflexes, muscle strength; pulses, BP, orthostatic BP, perfusion, edema, baseline ECG; respiratory rate, adventitious sounds; liver evaluation, bowel sounds; CBC, serum electrolytes, blood glucose; liver and renal function tests; serum uric acid, urinalysis

### Implementation

- Administer with food or milk if GI upset occurs.
- Administer early in the day so increased urination will not disturb sleep.
- Ensure ready access to bathroom.
- Establish safety precautions if CNS effects, orthostatic hypotension occur.
- Measure and record regular body weights to monitor fluid changes.
- Provide mouth care, small frequent meals as needed.
- Monitor IV sites for any sign of extravasation.
- Monitor electrolytes frequently with parenteral use, periodically with chronic use.

### Drug-specific teaching points

- Take drug early in the day so sleep will not be disturbed by increased urination.
- Weigh yourself daily, and record weights.
- Protect skin from exposure to the sun or bright lights.
- Avoid foods high in potassium and the use of salt substitutes if taking a potassium-sparing diuretic.
- Take prescribed potassium replacement, and use foods high in potassium if taking a thiazide or loop diuretic.
- Increased urination will occur (stay close to bathroom facilities).
- Use caution if dizziness, drowsiness, feeling faint occur.
- Report rapid weight gain or loss, swelling in ankles or fingers, unusual bleeding or bruising, muscle cramps.

### Representative drugs

*Thiazide and Related Diuretics*

bendroflumethiazide
benzthiazide
chlorothiazide
chlorthalidone
hydrochlorothiazide
hydroflumethiazide
indapamide
methyclothiazide
metolazone
polythiazide
quinethazone
trichlormethiazide

*Loop Diuretics*

bumetanide
ethacrynic acid
furosemide
torsemide

*Potassium-Sparing Diuretics*

amiloride
spironolactone
triamterene

*Osmotic Diuretic*

mannitol

## Fluoroquinolones

### Pregnancy Category C

### Therapeutic actions

Fluoroquinolones are antibacterial. They are bactericidal, interfering with DNA replication in susceptible gram-negative bacteria, preventing cell reproduction and leading to death of bacteria.

### Indications

- Treatment of infections caused by susceptible gram-negative bacteria, including *E. coli, Proteus mirabilis, K. pneumoniae, Enterobacter cloacae, Proteus vulgaris, Providencia rettgeri, Morganella morganii, Pseudomonas aeruginosa, Citrobacter freundii, S. aureus, S. epidermidis,* group D streptococci
- Unlabeled use: treatment of patients with cystic fibrosis who have pulmonary exacerbations

### Contraindications/cautions

- Contraindications: allergy to any fluoroquinolone, pregnancy, or lactation. Use cautiously with renal dysfunction, seizures.

### Adverse effects

- CNS: *Headache,* dizziness, insomnia, fatigue, somnolence, depression, blurred vision
- GI: *Nausea,* vomiting, dry mouth, *diarrhea,* abdominal pain
- Hematologic: Elevated BUN, SGOT, SGPT, serum creatinine and alkaline phosphatase; decreased WBC, neutrophil count, hematocrit
- Other: Fever, rash, **photosensitivity**

### Clinically important drug-drug interactions

• Decreased therapetic effect with iron salts, sucralfate • Decreased absorption with antacids • Increased effects with azlocillin • Increased serum levels and toxic effects of theophyllines with fluoroquinolone

## ■ Nursing Considerations

### Assessment

- *History:* Allergy to fluoroquinolones, renal dysfunction, seizures, lactation
- *Physical:* Skin color, lesions; T; orientation, reflexes, affect; mucous membranes, bowel sounds; renal and liver function tests

### Implementation

- Arrange for culture and sensitivity tests before beginning therapy.
- Continue therapy for 2 d after the signs and symptoms of infection have disappeared.
- Administer oral drug 1 h before or 2 h after meals with a glass of water.
- Ensure that patient is well hydrated during course of drug therapy.
- Administer antacids, if needed, at least 2 h after dosing.
- Monitor clinical response; if no improvement is seen or a relapse occurs, repeat culture and sensitivity.
- Ensure ready access to bathroom if diarrhea occurs.
- Arrange for appropriate bowel training program if constipation occurs.
- Provide small, frequent meals if GI upset occurs.
- Arrange for monitoring of environment (noise, temperature) and analgesics, for headache.
- Establish safety precautions if CNS, visual changes occur.
- Encourage patient to complete full course of therapy.

### Drug-specific teaching points

- Take oral drug on an empty stomach, 1 h before or 2 h after meals. If an antacid is needed, do not take it within 2 h of ciprofloxacin dose.
- Drink plenty of fluids.
- Possible side effects: nausea, vomiting, abdominal pain (small, frequent meals may help); diarrhea or constipation (consult health care provider); drowsiness, blurring of vision, dizziness (observe caution if driving or using hazardous equipment).
- Report rash, visual changes, severe GI problems, weakness, tremors.

### Representative drugs

ciprofloxacin
enoxacin
levofloxacin
lomefloxacin
norfloxacin
ofloxacin
sparfloxacin
trovafloxacin

## Histamine$_2$ ($H_2$) Antagonist

### Pregnancy Category B

### Therapeutic actions

Histamine$_2$ antagonists inhibit the action of histamine at the histamine$_2$ receptors of the stomach, inhibiting gastric acid secretion and reducing total pepsin output; the resultant decrease in acid allows healing of ulcerated areas.

### Indications

- Short-term treatment of active duodenal ulcer and benign gastric ulcer
- Treatment of pathologic hypersecretory conditions (Zollinger-Ellison syndrome) and erosive gastroesophageal reflux

- Prophylaxis of stress-induced ulcers and acute upper GI bleed in critically ill patients

**Contraindications/cautions**
- Contraindications: allergy to $H_2$ blockers, impaired renal or hepatic function, or lactation.

**Adverse effects**
- CNS: *Dizziness, somnolence, headache, confusion, hallucinations,* peripheral neuropathy, symptoms of brain stem dysfunction (dysarthria, ataxia, diplopia)
- GI: *Diarrhea*
- CV: Cardiac arrhythmias, arrest; hypotension (IV use)
- Hematologic: Increases in plasma creatinine, serum transaminase
- Other: *Impotence* (reversible with drug withdrawal), gynecomastia (long-term treatment), rash, vasculitis, pain at IM injection site

**Clinically important drug-drug interactions**
• Increased risk of decreased white blood cell counts with antimetabolites, alkylating agents, other drugs known to cause neutropenia • Increased serum levels and risk of toxicity of warfarin-type anticoagulants, phenytoin, beta-adrenergic blocking agents, alcohol, quinidine, lidocaine, theophylline, chloroquine, certain benzodiazepines (alprazolam, chlordiazepoxide, diazepam, flurazepam, triazolam), nifedipine, pentoxifylline, tricyclic antidepressants, procainamide, carbamazepine when taken with $H_2$ blockers

## ■ Nursing Considerations

### Assessment
- *History:* Allergy to $H_2$ blockers, impaired renal or hepatic function, lactation
- *Physical:* Skin lesions; orientation, affect; pulse, baseline ECG (continuous with IV use); liver evaluation, abdominal exam, normal output; CBC, liver and renal function tests

### Implementation
- Administer drug with meals and hs.
- Decrease doses in renal dysfunction and liver dysfunction.
- Administer IM dose undiluted, deep into large muscle group.
- Ensure ready access to bathroom.
- Provide comfort measures for skin rash, headache.
- Establish safety measures if CNS changes occur (side rails, accompany patient).
- Arrange for regular follow-up, including blood tests to evaluate effects.

### Drug-specific teaching points
- Take drug with meals and at bedtime; therapy may continue for 4–6 wk or longer.
- Take prescribed antacids exactly as prescribed, be careful of the time.
- Inform health care provider about your cigarette smoking habits. Cigarette smoking decreases the effectiveness of this drug.
- Have regular medical follow-up while on this drug to evaluate your response.
- Report sore throat, fever, unusual bruising or bleeding, tarry stools, confusion, hallucinations, dizziness, muscle or joint pain.

**Representative drugs**

cimetidine
famotidine
nizatidine
ranitidine

## HMG CoA Inhibitors

**Pregnancy Category X**

**Therapeutic actions**

HMG CoA inhibitors are antihyperlipidemic. They are a fungal metabolite that inhibits the enzyme that catalyzes the first step in the cholesterol synthesis pathway in humans, resulting in a decrease in serum cholesterol, serum LDLs (associated with increased risk of coronary artery disease) and either an increase or no change in serum HDLs (associated with decreased risk of coronary artery disease).

### Indications
- Adjunct to diet in the treatment of elevated total and LDL cholesterol in patients with primary hypercholesterolemia (types IIa and IIb) whose response to dietary restriction of saturated fat and cholesterol and other nonpharmacologic measures has not been adequate.

### Contraindications/cautions
- Contraindications: allergy to HMG CoA inhibitors, fungal byproducts, pregnancy, or lactation. Use cautiously with impaired hepatic function, cataracts.

### Adverse effects
- CNS: *Headache, blurred vision,* dizziness, insomnia, fatigue, muscle cramps, cataracts
- GI: *Flatulence, abdominal pain, cramps, constipation, nausea, vomiting,* heartburn
- **Hematologic**: Elevations of CPK, alkaline phosphatase, and transaminases

### Clinically important drug-drug interactions
- Monitor patients receiving HMG CoA inhibitors for possible severe myopathy or rhabdomyolysis if taken with cyclosporine, erythromycin, gemfibrozil, niacin

## ■ Nursing Considerations

### Assessment
- *History:* Allergy to HMG CoA inhibitors, fungal byproducts; impaired hepatic function; cataracts; pregnancy; lactation
- *Physical:* Orientation, affect, ophthalmologic exam; liver evaluation; lipid studies, liver function tests

### Implementation
- Administer drug hs; highest rates of cholesterol synthesis are between midnight and 5 AM.
- Consult with dietician regarding low-cholesterol diets.
- Arrange for diet and exercise consultation.
- Arrange for regular follow-up during long-term therapy.
- Provide comfort measures to deal with headache, muscle cramps, nausea.
- Arrange for periodic ophthalmologic exam to check for cataract development.
- Offer support and encouragement to deal with disease, diet, drug therapy, and follow-up.

### Drug-specific teaching points
- Take drug at bedtime.
- Institute appropriate diet changes.
- Possible side effects: nausea (small, frequent meals may help); headache, muscle and joint aches and pains (may lessen with time).
- Have periodic ophthalmic exams while you are on this drug.
- Report severe GI upset, changes in vision, unusual bleeding or bruising, dark urine or light-colored stools.

### Representative drugs
atorvastatin
cerivastatin
fluvastatin
lovastatin
pravastatin
simvastatin

# Macrolide Antibiotics

### Pregnancy Category B

### Therapeutic actions
Macrolides are antibiotics. They are bacteriostatic or bactericidal in susceptible bacteria; they bind to cell membranes and cause changes in protein function, leading to bacteria cell death.

### Indications
- Treatment of acute infections caused by sensitive strains of *S. pneumoniae, Mycoplasma pneumoniae, Listeria monocytogenes, Legionella pneumophila;* URIs, LRIs, skin and soft-tissue infections caused by group A beta-hemolytic streptococci when oral treatment is preferred to injectable benzathine penicillin; PID caused by *N. gonorrhoeae* in patients allergic to penicillin; intestinal amebiasis caused by *Entamoeba histolytica;* infec-

tions in the newborn and in pregnancy that are caused by *Chlamydia trachomatis* and in adult chlamydial infections when tetracycline cannot be used; primary syphilis (*Treponema pallidum*) in penicillin-allergic patients; eliminating *Bordetella pertussis* organisms from the nasopharynx of infected individuals and as prophylaxis in exposed and susceptible individuals; superficial ocular infections caused by susceptible strains of microorganisms; prophylaxis of ophthalmia neonatorum caused by *N. gonorrhoeae* or *C. trachomatis*
- Treatment of acne vulgaris and skin infections caused by sensitive microorganisms
- In conjunction with sulfonamides to treat URIs caused by *H. influenzae*
- Adjunct to antitoxin in infections caused by *Corynebacterium diphtheriae* and *Corynebacterium minutissimum*
- Prophylaxis against alpha-hemolytic streptococcal endocarditis before dental or other procedures in patients allergic to penicillin who have valvular heart disease and against infection in minor skin abrasions
- Unlabeled uses: erythromycin base is used with neomycin before colorectal surgery to reduce wound infection; treatment of severe diarrhea associated with *Campylobacter* enteritis or enterocolitis; treatment of genital, inguinal, or anorectal lymphogranuloma venereum infection; treatment of *Haemophilus ducreyi* (chancroid).

### Contraindications/cautions

- Contraindications: allergy to any macrolide antibiotic. Use cautiously with hepatic dysfunction or lactation (secreted and may be concentrated in breast milk; may modify bowel flora of nursing infant and interfere with fever workups).

### Adverse effects

- CNS: Reversible hearing loss, confusion, uncontrollable emotions, abnormal thinking
- GI: *Abdominal cramping, anorexia, diarrhea, vomiting,* pseudomembranous colitis, hepatotoxicity
- **Dermatologic**: Edema, urticaria, dermatitis, angioneurotic edema
- Hypersensitivity: Allergic reactions ranging from rash to anaphylaxis
- Local: *Irritation, burning, itching* at site of application
- Other: *Superinfections*

### Clinically important drug-drug interactions

• Increased serum levels of digoxin • Increased effects of oral anticoagulants, theophyllines, carbamazepine • Increased therapeutic and toxic effects of corticosteroids • Increased levels of cyclosporine and risk of renal toxicity • Increased irritant effects with peeling, desquamating, or abrasive agents used with dermatologic preparations • Risk of serious CV effects and sudden death in combination with terfenadine; astemizole

### Drug-lab test interferences

• Interferes with fluorometric determination of urinary catecholamines • Decreased urinary estriol levels due to inhibition of hydrolysis of steroids in the gut

## ■ Nursing Considerations

### Assessment

- *History:* Allergy to macrolides, hepatic dysfunction, lactation, viral, fungal, mycobacterial infections of the eye (ophthalmologic)
- *Physical:* Site of infection, skin color, lesions; orientation, affect, hearing tests; R, adventitious sounds; GI output, bowel sounds, liver evaluation; culture and sensitivity tests of infection, urinalysis, liver function tests

### Implementation

- Culture site of infection prior to therapy.
- Administer oral erythromycin base or stearate on an empty stomach, 1 h before or 2–3 h after meals, with a full glass of water (oral erythromycin estolate, ethylsuccinate, and certain enteric-coated tablets; see manufacturer's instructions; may be given without regard to meals).

- Administer drug around the clock to maximize therapeutic effect; scheduling may have to be adjusted to minimize sleep disruption.
- Monitor liver function in patients on prolonged therapy.
- Institute hygiene measures and treatment if superinfections occur.
- If GI upset occurs with oral therapy, some preparations (see above) may be given with meals, or it may be possible to substitute one of these preparations.
- Provide small, frequent meals if GI problems occur.
- Establish safety measures (accompany patient, side rails) if CNS changes occur.
- Give patient support and encouragement to continue with therapy.
- Wash affected area, rinse well, and dry before topical application.

### Drug-specific teaching points

- Take oral drug on an empty stomach, 1 hour before or 2–3 h after meals, with a full glass of water, or, as appropriate, drug may be taken without regard to meals. The drug should be taken around the clock; schedule to minimize sleep disruption. It is important that you finish the *full course* of the drug therapy.
- Possible side effects: stomach cramping, discomfort (taking the drug with meals, if appropriate, may alleviate this problem); uncontrollable emotions, crying, laughing, abnormal thinking (will end when the drug is stopped).
- Report severe or watery diarrhea, severe nausea or vomiting, dark urine, yellowing of the skin or eyes, loss of hearing, skin rash or itching.
- Wash and rinse area and pat it dry before applying topical solution; use fingertips or an applicator; wash hands thoroughly after application.

### Representative drugs

azithromycin
clarithromycin
dirithromycin
erythromycin

## Narcotics

**Pregnancy Category C**
**C-II controlled substance**

### Therapeutic actions

Narcotics act as agonists at specific opioid receptors in the CNS to produce analgesia, euphoria, sedation; the receptors mediating these effects are thought to be the same as those mediating the effects of endogenous opioids (enkephalins, endorphins).

### Indications

- Relief of moderate to severe acute and chronic pain
- Preoperative medication to sedate and allay apprehension, facilitate induction of anesthesia, and reduce anesthetic dosage
- Analgesic adjunct during anesthesia
- A component of most preparations referred to as Brompton's Cocktail or Mixture, an oral alcoholic solution used for chronic severe pain, especially in terminal cancer patients
- Intraspinal use with microinfusion devices for the relief of intractable pain
- Unlabeled use: relief of dyspnea associated with acute left ventricular failure and pulmonary edema

### Contraindications/cautions

- Contraindications: hypersensitivity to narcotics, diarrhea caused by poisoning until toxins are eliminated, during labor or delivery of a premature infant (may cross immature blood-brain barrier more readily), after biliary tract surgery or following surgical anastomosis, pregnancy, or labor (can cause respiratory depression of neonate; may prolong labor). Use cautiously with head injury and increased intracranial pressure; acute asthma, COPD, cor pulmonale, preexisting respiratory depression, hypoxia, hypercapnia (may decrease respiratory drive and increase airway resistance); lactation (may be safer to wait 4–6 h after administration to nurse the baby); acute abdominal conditions; cardiovascular disease, supraventricular tachycardias; myxedema; convulsive disorders; acute alcoholism, delirium tremens; cerebral arteriosclerosis; ulcerative colitis; fever; kyphoscoliosis; Addison's disease; prostatic hypertrophy, urethral stricture; recent GI or GU surgery; toxic psychosis; renal or hepatic dysfunction.

### Adverse effects

- CNS: *Lightheadedness, dizziness, sedation,* euphoria, dysphoria, delirium, insomnia, agitation, anxiety, fear, hallucinations, disorientation, drowsiness, lethargy, impaired mental and physical performance, coma, mood changes, weakness, headache, tremor, convulsions, miosis, visual disturbances, suppression of cough reflex.
- GI: *Nausea, vomiting,* dry mouth, anorexia, constipation, biliary tract spasm; increased colonic motility in patients with chronic ulcerative colitis.
- CV: Facial flushing, peripheral circulatory collapse, tachycardia, bradycardia, arrhythmia, palpitations, chest wall rigidity, hypertension, hypotension, orthostatic hypotension, syncope
- GU: Ureteral spasm, spasm of vesical sphincters, urinary retention or hesitancy, oliguria, antidiuretic effect, reduced libido or potency
- Dermatologic: Pruritus, urticaria, laryngospasm, bronchospasm, edema
- Local: Tissue irritation and induration (SC injection)
- Major hazards: **Respiratory depression, apnea, circulatory depression, respiratory arrest, shock, cardiac arrest**
- Other: *Sweating,* physical tolerance and dependence, psychological dependence

### Clinically important drug-drug interactions

- Increased likelihood of respiratory depression, hypotension, profound sedation, or coma in patients receiving barbiturate general anesthetics.

### Drug-lab test interferences

- Elevated biliary tract pressure (an effect of narcotics) may cause increases in plasma amylase, lipase; determinations of these levels may be unreliable for 24 h

## ■ Nursing Considerations

### Assessment

- *History:* Hypersensitivity to narcotics; diarrhea caused by poisoning; labor or delivery of a premature infant; biliary tract surgery or surgical anastomosis; head injury and increased intracranial pressure; acute asthma, COPD, cor pulmonale, preexisting respiratory depression, hypoxia, hypercapnia; acute abdominal conditions; CV disease, supraventricular tachycardias; myxedema; convulsive disorders; acute alcoholism, delirium tremens; cerebral arteriosclerosis; ulcerative colitis; fever; kyphoscoliosis; Addison's disease; prostatic hypertrophy; urethral stricture; recent GI or GU surgery; toxic psychosis; renal or hepatic dysfunction; pregnancy; lactation
- *Physical:* T; skin color, texture, lesions; orientation, reflexes, bilateral grip strength, affect; P, auscultation, BP, orthostatic BP, perfusion; R, adventious sounds; bowel sounds, normal output; urinary frequency, voiding pattern, normal output; ECG; EEG; thyroid, liver, kidney function tests

### Implementation

- Caution patient not to chew or crush controlled-release preparations.
- Dilute and administer slowly IV to minimize likelihood of adverse effects.
- Direct patient to lie down during IV administration.
- Provide narcotic antagonist, facilities for assisted or controlled respiration on standby during IV administration.
- Use caution when injecting SC or IM into chilled areas or in patients with hypotension or in shock; impaired perfusion may delay absorption; with repeated doses, an excessive amount may be absorbed when circulation is restored.
- Monitor injection sites for irritation, extravasation.

- Instruct postoperative patients in pulmonary toilet; drug suppresses cough reflex.
- Monitor bowel function, and arrange for anthraquinone laxatives for severe constipation.
- Institute safety precautions (side rails, assist walking) if CNS, vision effects occur.
- Provide frequent, small meals if GI upset occurs.
- Provide environmental control if sweating, visual difficulties occur.
- Provide back rubs, positioning, and other nondrug measures to alleviate pain.
- Reassure patient about addiction liability; most patients who receive opiates for medical reasons do not develop dependence syndromes.

### Drug-specific teaching points

When used as preoperative medication, teaching about the drug should be incorporated into the teaching about the procedure.

- Take this drug exactly as prescribed. Avoid alcohol, antihistamines, sedatives, tranquilizers, OTC drugs.
- Possible side effects: nausea, loss of appetite (take the drug with food and lie quietly); constipation (notify health care provider if this is severe; a laxative may help); dizziness, sedation, drowsiness, impaired visual acuity (avoid driving or performing other tasks requiring alertness, visual acuity).
- Do not take any leftover medication for other disorders, and do not let anyone else take your prescription.
- Report severe nausea, vomiting, constipation, shortness of breath or difficulty breathing, skin rash.

### Representative drugs

codeine
fentanyl
hydrocodone
hydromorphone
levomethadyl
levorphanol
meperidine
methadone
morphine sulfate
opium
oxycodone
oxymorphone
propoxyphene
remifentanil
sufentanil

## Nitrates

### Pregnancy Category C

### Therapeutic actions

Nitrates are antianginals. They relax vascular smooth muscle with a resultant decrease in venous return and decrease in arterial blood pressure, which reduces left ventricular workload and decreases myocardial oxygen consumption, relieving the pain of angina.

### Indications

- Treatment of acute angina (sublingual, translingual, inhalant preparations)
- Prophylaxis of angina (oral sustained release, sublingual, topical, transdermal, translingual, transmucosal preparations)
- Treatment of angina unresponsive to recommended doses of organic nitrates or beta-blockers (IV preparations)
- Management of perioperative hypertension, CHF associated with acute myocardial infarction (IV preparations)
- Produce controlled hypertension during surgery (IV preparations)
- Unlabeled uses: reduction of cardiac workload in acute MI and in CHF (sublingual, topical) and adjunctive treatment of Raynaud's disease (topical)

### Contraindications/cautions

- Contraindications: allergy to nitrates, severe anemia, early MI, head trauma, cerebral hemorrhage, hypertrophic, cardiomyopathy, pregnancy, or lactation. Use cautiously with hepatic or renal disease, hypotension or hypovolemia, increased intracranial pressure, constrictive pericarditis, pericardial tamponade, low ventricular filling pressure or low pulmonary capillary wedge pressure (PCWP).

**Adverse effects**

- CNS: Headache, apprehension, restlessness, weakness, vertigo, dizziness, faintness
- GI: Nausea, vomiting, incontinence of urine and feces, abdominal pain
- CV: Tachycardia, retrosternal discomfort, palpitations, **hypotension,** syncope, collapse, postural hypotension, angina
- Dermatologic: Rash, exfoliative dermatitis, cutaneous vasodilation with flushing, pallor, perspiration, cold sweat, contact dermatitis (transdermal preparations), topical allergic reactions (topical nitroglycerin ointment)
- Local: Local burning sensation at the point of dissolution (sublingual)
- Other: Ethanol intoxication with high dose IV use (alcohol in diluent)

**Clinically important drug-drug interactions**

• Increased risk of hypertension and decreased antianginal effect with ergot alkaloids • Decreased pharmacologic effects of heparin

**Drug-lab test interferences**

- False report of decreased serum cholesterol if done by the Zlatkis-Zak color reaction

## ■ Nursing Considerations

### Assessment

- *History:* Allergy to nitrates, severe anemia, early MI, head trauma, cerebral hemorrhage, hypertrophic cardiomyopathy, hepatic or renal disease, hypotension or hypovolemia, increased intracranial pressure, constrictive pericarditis, pericardial tamponade, low ventricular filling pressure or low PCWP, pregnancy, lactation
- *Physical:* Skin color, T, lesions; orientation, reflexes, affect; P, BP, orthostatic BP, baseline ECG, peripheral perfusion; R, adventitious sounds; liver evaluation, normal output; liver function tests (IV); renal function tests (IV); CBC, Hgb

### Implementation

- Administer sublingual preparations under the tongue or in the buccal pouch. Encourage the patient not to swallow. Ask patient if the tablet "fizzles" or burns. Check the expiration date on the bottle; store at room temperature, protected from light. Discard unused drug 6 mo after bottle is opened (conventional tablets); stabilized tablets (Nitrostat) are less subject to loss of potency.
- Administer sustained-release preparations with water; tell the patient not to chew the tablets or capsules; do not crush these preparations.
- Administer topical ointment by applying the ointment over a 6 × 6 in area in a thin, uniform layer using the applicator. Cover area with plastic wrap held in place by adhesive tape. Rotate sites of application to decrease the chance of inflammation and sensitization; close tube tightly when finished.
- Administer transdermal systems to skin site free of hair and not subject to much movement. Shave areas that have a lot of hair. Do not apply to distal extremities. Change sites slightly to decrease the chance of local irritation and sensitization. Remove transdermal system before attempting defibrillation or cardioversion.
- Administer transmucosal tablets by placing them between the lip and gum above the incisors or between the cheek and gum. Encourage patient not to swallow and not to chew the tablet.
- Administer the translingual spray directly onto the oral mucosa; preparation is not to be inhaled.
- Withdraw drug gradually, 4–6 wk recommended period for the transdermal preparations.
- Establish safety measures if CNS effects, hypotension occur.
- Keep environment cool, dim, and quiet.
- Provide periodic rest periods for patient.
- Provide comfort measures and arrange for analgesics if headache occurs.

- Maintain life support equipment on standby if overdose occurs or cardiac condition worsens.
- Provide support and encouragement to deal with disease, therapy, and needed lifestyle changes.

### Drug-specific teaching points

- Place sublingual tablets under your tongue or in your cheek; do not chew or swallow the tablet; the tablet should burn or "fizzle" under the tongue. Take the nitroglycerin before chest pain begins, when you anticipate that your activities or situation may precipitate an attack. Do not buy large quantities; this drug does not store well. Keep the drug in a dark, dry place, in a dark-colored glass bottle with a tight lid; do not combine with other drugs. You may repeat your dose every 5 min for a total of _ tablets; if the pain is still not relieved, go to an emergency room.
- Do not chew or crush the timed-release preparations; take on an empty stomach.
- Spread a thin layer of topical ointment on the skin using the applicator. Do not rub or massage the area. Cover with plastic wrap held in place with adhesive tape. Wash your hands after application. Keep the tube tightly closed. Rotate the sites frequently to prevent local irritation.
- To use transdermal systems, you may need to shave an area for application. Apply to a slightly different area each day. Use care if changing brands; each system has a different concentration.
- Place transmucosal tablets between the lip and gum or between the gum and cheek. Do not chew; try not to swallow.
- Spray translingual spray directly onto oral mucous membranes; do not inhale. Use 5–10 min before activities that you anticipate will precipitate an attack.
- Take drug exactly as directed; do not exceed recommended dosage.
- Possible side effects: dizziness, lightheadedness (this may pass as you adjust to the drug; use care to change positions slowly); headache (lying down in a cool environment and resting may help; OTC preparations may not help); flushing of the neck or face (this usually passes as the drug's effects pass).
- Report blurred vision, persistent or severe headache, skin rash, more frequent or more severe angina attacks, fainting.

### Representative drugs

amyl nitrate
isosorbide dinitrate
nitroglycerin

## Nondepolarizing Neuromuscular Junction Blockers (NMJ Blockers)

### Pregnancy Category C

### Therapeutic actions

NMJ blockers interfere with neuromuscular transmission and cause flaccid paralysis by blocking acetylcholine receptors at the skeletal neuromuscular junction.

### Indications

- Adjuncts to general anesthetics to facilitate endotracheal intubation and relax skeletal muscle, to relax skeletal muscle to facilitate mechanical ventilation.

### Contraindications/cautions

- Contraindications: hypersensitivity to NMJ blockers and the bromide ion. Use cautiously with myasthenia gravis; pregnancy (teratogenic in preclinical studies; may be used in cesarean section, but reversal may be difficult if patient has received magnesium sulfate to manage preeclampsia); renal or hepatic disease, respiratory depression, altered fluid/electrolyte balance; patients in whom an increase in heart rate may be dangerous.

### Adverse effects

- CV: *Increased P*
- Respiratory: *Depressed respiration, apnea,* bronchospasm
- MS: Profound and prolonged muscle paralysis

- **Hypersensitivity:** Hypersensitivity reactions, especially rash

### Clinically important drug-drug interactions

• Increased intensity and duration of neuromuscular block with some anesthetics (isoflurane, enflurane, halothane, diethyl ether, methoxyflurane), some parenteral antibiotics (aminoglycosides, clindamycin, lincomycin, bacitracin, polymyxin B, and sodium colistimethate), ketamine, quinine, quinidine, trimethaphan, calcium channel-blocking drugs (eg, verapamil), $Mg^{2+}$ salts, and in hypokalemia (produced by $K^+$ depleting diuretics) • Decreased intensity of neuromuscular block with acetylcholine, cholinesterase inhibitors, $K^+$ salts, theophyllines, phenytoins, azathioprine, mercaptopurine, carbamazepine

## ■ Nursing Considerations

### Assessment

- *History:* Hypersensitivity to NMJ blockers and the bromide ion, myasthenia gravis, pregnancy, renal or hepatic disease, respiratory depression, altered fluid/electrolyte balance
- *Physical:* Weight, T, skin condition, hydration, reflexes, bilateral grip strength, pulse, BP, respiratory rate and adventitious sounds, liver and kidney function, serum electrolytes

### Implementation

- Drug should be given only by trained personnel (anesthesiologists).
- Arrange to have facilities on standby to maintain airway and provide mechanical ventilation.
- Provide neostigmine, pyridostigmine, or edrophonium (cholinesterase inhibitors) on standby to overcome excessive neuromuscular block.
- Provide atropine or glycopyrrolate on standby to prevent parasympathomimetic effects of cholinesterase inhibitors.
- Provide a peripheral nerve stimulator on standby to assess degree of neuromuscular block, as needed.
- Change patient's position frequently, and provide skin care to prevent decubitus ulcer formation when drug is used for other than brief periods.
- Monitor conscious patient for pain, distress that patient may not be able to communicate.
- Reassure conscious patients frequently.

### Drug-specific teaching points

- Teaching points about what the drug does and how the patient will feel should be incorporated into overall teaching program about the procedure.

### Representative drugs

atracurium
cisatracurium
doxacurium
metocurine
mivacurium
pancuronium
pipecuronium
rocuronium
tubocurarine
vecuronium

## Nonsteroidal Anti-inflammatory Agents (NSAIDs)

### Pregnancy Category B

### Therapeutic actions

NSAIDs have anti-inflammatory, analgesic, and antipyretic activities largely related to inhibition of prostaglandin synthesis; exact mechanisms of action are not known.

### Indications

- Relief of signs and symptoms of rheumatoid arthritis and osteoarthritis
- Relief of mild to moderate pain
- Treatment of primary dysmenorrhea
- Fever reduction
- Unlabeled use: treatment of juvenile rheumatoid arthritis

### Contraindications/cautions

- Contraindications: allergy to salicylates or other NSAIDs (more common in patients with rhinitis, asthma, chronic urticaria, nasal polyps); CV dysfunction, hypertension; peptic ulceration, GI bleeding; pregnancy; or lactation. Use cautiously with impaired hepatic function; impaired renal function.

### Adverse effects

- CNS: *Headache, dizziness, somnolence, insomnia,* fatigue, tiredness, dizziness, tinnitus, ophthalmologic effects
- GI: *Nausea, dyspepsia, GI pain,* diarrhea, vomiting, *constipation,* flatulence
- **Respiratory**: Dyspnea, hemoptysis, pharyngitis, bronchospasm, rhinitis
- **Hematologic**: Bleeding, platelet inhibition with higher doses, neutropenia, eosinophilia, leukopenia, pancytopenia, thrombocytopenia, agranulocytosis, granulocytopenia, aplastic anemia, decreased hemoglobin or hematocrit, bone marrow depression, menorrhagia
- GU: Dysuria, renal impairment
- **Dermatologic**: *Rash,* pruritus, sweating, dry mucous membranes, stomatitis
- **Other**: Peripheral edema, anaphylactoid reactions to fatal anaphylactic shock

### Clinically important drug-drug interactions

• Increased toxic effects of lithium with NSAIDs • Decreased diuretic effect with loop diuretics: bumetanide, furosemide, ethacrynic acid • Potential decrease in antihypertensive effect of beta-adrenergic blocking agents

## ■ Nursing Considerations

### Assessment

- *History:* Allergy to salicylates or other NSAIDs; CV dysfunction, hypertension; peptic ulceration, GI bleeding; impaired hepatic function; impaired renal function; pregnancy; lactation
- *Physical:* Skin color, lesions; T; orientation, reflexes, ophthalmologic evaluation, audiometric evaluation, peripheral sensation; P, BP, edema; R, adventitious sounds; liver evaluation, bowel sounds; CBC, clotting times, urinalysis, renal and liver function tests, serum electrolytes, stool guaiac

### Implementation

- Administer drug with food or after meals if GI upset occurs.
- Establish safety measures if CNS, visual disturbances occur.
- Arrange for periodic ophthalmologic examination during long-term therapy.
- Arrange for discontinuation of drug if eye changes, symptoms of liver dysfunction, renal impairment occur.
- Institute emergency procedures if overdose occurs (gastric lavage, induction of emesis, supportive therapy).
- Provide comfort measures to reduce pain (positioning, environmental control) and to reduce inflammation (warmth, positioning, rest).
- Provide small, frequent meals if GI upset is severe.

### Drug specific teaching points

- Use the drug only as suggested. Do not exceed the prescribed dosage. Take the drug with food or after meals if GI upset occurs.
- Possible side effects: nausea, GI upset, dyspepsia (take with food); diarrhea or constipation; drowsiness, dizziness, vertigo, insomnia (use caution when driving or operating dangerous machinery).
- Avoid OTC drugs while taking this drug. Many of these drugs contain similar medications, and serious overdosage can occur. If you feel that you need one of these preparations, consult with health care provider.
- Report sore throat, fever, rash, itching, weight gain, swelling in ankles or fingers, changes in vision, black or tarry stools.

### Representative drugs

bromfenac
diclofenac
diflunisal
etodolac

fenoprofen
flurbiprofen
ibuprofen
indomethacin
ketoprofen
ketorolac
meclofenamate
mefenamic acid
nabumetone
naproxen
oxaprozin
piroxicam
sulindac
tolmetin

## Penicillins

### Pregnancy Category C

### Therapeutic actions

Penicillins are antibiotics. They are bactericidal, inhibiting the synthesis of cell wall of sensitive organisms, causing cell death in susceptible organisms.

### Indications

- Treatment of moderate to severe infections caused by sensitive organisms: streptococci, pneumococci, staphylococci, *N. gonorrhoeae, T. pallidum,* meningococci, *Actinomyces israelii, Clostridium perfringens, Clostridium tetani, Leptotrichia buccalis* (Vincent's disease), *Spirillium minus* or *Streptobacillus moniliformis, L. monocytogenes, Pasteurella multocida, Erysipelothrix insidiosa, E. coli, Enterobacter aerogenes, Alcaligenes faecalis, Salmonella, Shigella, P. mirabilis, C. diphtheriae, Bacillus anthracis*
- Treatment of syphilis, gonococcal infections
- Unlabeled use: treatment of Lyme disease

### Contraindications/cautions

- Contraindications: allergy to penicillins, cephalosporins, other allergens. Use cautiously with renal disease, pregnancy, lactation (may cause diarrhea or candidiasis in the infant).

### Adverse effects

- CNS: Lethargy, hallucinations, seizures
- GI: *Glossitis, stomatitis, gastritis, sore mouth,* furry tongue, black "hairy" tongue, *nausea, vomiting, diarrhea,* abdominal pain, bloody diarrhea, enterocolitis, pseudomembranous colitis, nonspecific hepatitis
- **Hematologic**: Anemia, thrombocytopenia, leukopenia, neutropenia, prolonged bleeding time
- GU: Nephritis-oliguria, proteinuria, hematuria, casts, azotemia, pyuria
- **Other**: *Superinfections,* sodium overload, leading to CHF
- **Hypersensitivity reactions**: *Rash, fever, wheezing,* anaphylaxis
- **Local**: *Pain, phlebitis,* thrombosis at injection site, Jarisch-Herxheimer reaction when used to treat syphilis

### Clinically important drug-drug interactions

- Decreased effectiveness with tetracyclines
- Inactivation of parenteral aminoglycosides (amikacin, gentamicin, kanamycin, neomycin, netilmicin, streptomycin, tobramycin)

### Drug-lab test interferences

- False-positive Coombs' test (IV)

## ■ Nursing Considerations

### Assessment

- *History:* Allergy to penicillins, cephalosporins, other allergens, renal disease, lactation
- *Physical:* Culture infected area; skin rashes, lesions; R, adventitious sounds; bowel sounds, normal output; CBC, liver function tests, renal function tests, serum electrolytes, hematocrit, urinalysis; skin test with benzylpenicyllolyl-polylysine if hypersensitivity reactions have occurred

### Implementation

- Culture infected area before beginning treatment; reculture area if response is not as expected.
- Use the smallest dose possible for IM injection to avoid pain and discomfort.

- Arrange to continue treatment for 48–72 h beyond the time that the patient becomes asymptomatic.
- Monitor serum electrolytes and cardiac status if penicillin G is given by IV infusion. Na or K preparations have been associated with severe electrolyte imbalances.
- Check IV site carefully for signs of thrombosis or local drug reaction.
- Do not give IM injections repeatedly in the same site; atrophy can occur. Monitor injection sites.
- Explain the reason for parenteral routes of administration; offer support and encouragement to deal with therapy.
- Provide small, frequent meals if GI upset occurs.
- Arrange for comfort and treatment measures for superinfections.
- Provide for frequent mouth care if GI effects occur.
- Ensure that bathroom facilities are readily available if diarrhea occurs.
- Maintain epinephrine, IV fluids, vasopressors, bronchodilators, oxygen, and emergency equipment on standby in case of serious hypersensitivity reaction.
- Arrange for the use of corticosteroids, antihistamines for skin reactions.

### Drug-specific teaching points

- This drug must be given by injection.
- Possible side effects: upset stomach, nausea, vomiting (small, frequent meals may help); sore mouth (frequent mouth care may help); diarrhea; pain or discomfort at the injection site (report this if it becomes too uncomfortable).
- Report unusual bleeding, sore throat, rash, hives, fever, severe diarrhea, difficulty breathing.

### Representative drugs

amoxicillin
ampicillin
bacampicillin
carbenicillin
cloxacillin
dicloxacillin
methicillin
mezlocillin
nafcillin
oxacillin
penicillin G benzathine
penicillin G potassium
penicillin G procaine
penicillin V
piperacillin
ticarcillin

## Phenothiazines

### Pregnancy Category C

### Therapeutic actions

Mechanism of action of phenothiazines is not fully understood. Antipsychotic drugs block postsynaptic dopamine receptors in the brain, but this may not be necessary and sufficient for antipsychotic activity; depresses the RAS, including the parts of the brain involved with wakefulness and emesis; anticholinergic, antihistaminic ($H_1$), and alpha-adrenergic blocking activity also may contribute to some of its therapeutic (and adverse) actions.

### Indications

- Management of manifestations of psychotic disorders
- Control of severe nausea and vomiting, intractable hiccups

### Contraindications/cautions

- Contraindications: coma or severe CNS depression, bone marrow depression, blood dyscrasia, circulatory collapse, subcortical brain damage, Parkinson's disease, liver damage, cerebral arteriosclerosis, coronary disease, severe hypotension or hypertension. Use cautiously with respiratory disorders ("silent pneumonia" may develop); glaucoma, prostatic hypertrophy; epilepsy or history of epilepsy; breast cancer; thyrotoxicosis; peptic ulcer, decreased renal function; myelography within previous 24 h or scheduled within 48 h; exposure to heat or phosphorous insecticides; pregnancy; lactation; children younger than 12 y, especially those with chickenpox, CNS infections (children are especially susceptible to dystonias that may confound the diagnosis of Reye's syndrome).

**Adverse effects**

***Antipsychotic Drugs***

- CNS: *Drowsiness,* insomnia, vertigo, headache, weakness, tremor, ataxia, slurring, cerebral edema, seizures, exacerbation of psychotic symptoms, extrapyramidal syndromes—*pseudoparkinsonism; dystonias; akathisia,* tardive dyskinesias, potentially irreversible (no known treatment), **neuroleptic malignant syndrome**
- CV: Hypotension, orthostatic hypotension, hypertension, tachycardia, bradycardia, cardiac arrest, CHF, cardiomegaly, **refractory arrhythmias,** pulmonary edema
- Respiratory: Bronchospasm, laryngospasm, dyspnea; suppression of cough reflex and potential for aspiration (**sudden death related to asphyxia** or cardiac arrest has been reported)
- Hematologic: Eosinophilia, leukopenia, leukocytosis, anemia; aplastic anemia; hemolytic anemia; thrombocytopenic or nonthrombocytopenic purpura; pancytopenia
- EENT: Glaucoma, *photophobia, blurred vision,* miosis, mydriasis, deposits in the cornea and lens (opacities), pigmentary retinopathy
- Hypersensitivity: Jaundice, urticaria, angioneurotic edema, laryngeal edema, photosensitivity, eczema, asthma, anaphylactoid reactions, exfoliative dermatitis
- Endocrine: Lactation, breast engorgement in females, galactorrhea; syndrome of inappropriate ADH secretion; amenorrhea, menstrual irregularities; gynecomastia in males; changes in libido; hyperglycemia or hypoglycemia; glycosuria; hyponatremia; pituitary tumor with hyperprolactinemia; inhibition of ovulation, infertility, pseudopregnancy; reduced urinary levels of gonadotropins, estrogens, progestins
- Autonomic: Dry mouth, salivation, nasal congestion, nausea, vomiting, anorexia, fever, pallor, flushed facies, sweating, constipation, paralytic ileus, urinary retention, incontinence, polyuria, enuresis, priapism, ejaculation inhibition, male impotence
- Other: *Urine discolored pink to red-brown*

**Clinically important drug-drug interactions**

• Additive CNS depression with alcohol • Additive anticholinergic effects and possibly decreased antipsychotic efficacy with anticholinergic drugs • Increased likelihood of seizures with metrizamide (contrast agent used in myelography) • Increased chance of severe neuromuscular excitation and hypotension if given to patients receiving barbiturate anesthetics (methohexital, thiamylal, phenobarbital, thiopental) • Decreased antihypertensive effect of guanethidine when taken with antipsychotics

**Drug-lab test interferences**

• False-positive pregnancy tests (less likely if serum test is used) • Increase in protein-bound iodine, not attributable to an increase in thyroxine

## ■ Nursing Considerations

### Assessment

- *History:* Coma or severe CNS depression; bone marrow depression; blood dyscrasia; circulatory collapse; subcortical brain damage; Parkinson's disease; liver damage; cerebral arteriosclerosis; coronary disease; severe hypotension or hypertension; respiratory disorders; glaucoma, prostatic hypertrophy; epilepsy or history of epilepsy; breast cancer; thyrotoxicosis; peptic ulcer, decreased renal function; myelography within previous 24 h or myelography scheduled within 48 h; exposure to heat or phosphorous insecticides; pregnancy; children younger than 12 y, especially those with chickenpox, CNS infections
- *Physical:* Weight, T; reflexes, orientation, intraocular pressure; P, BP, orthostatic BP; R, adventitious sounds; bowel sounds and normal output, liver evaluation; urinary output, prostate size; CBC, urinalysis, thyroid, liver and kidney function tests

### Implementation

- Dilute oral concentrate *only* with water, saline, 7-Up, homogenized milk, carbonated orange drink, and pineapple, apricot, prune, orange, V-8, tomato, and grapefruit juices; use 60 ml of diluent for each 16 mg (5 ml) of concentrate.
- Do *not* mix with beverages that contain caffeine (coffee, cola), tannics (tea), or pectinates (apple juice); physical incompatibility may result.
- Give IM injections only to seated or recumbent patients, and observe for adverse effects for a brief period afterward.
- Monitor pulse and BP continuously during IV administration.
- Do not change dosage in chronic therapy more often than weekly; drug requires 4–7 d to achieve steady-state plasma levels.
- Avoid skin contact with oral solution; contact dermatitis has occurred.
- Arrange for discontinuation of drug if serum creatinine, BUN become abnormal or if WBC count is depressed.
- Monitor bowel function, arrange therapy for severe constipation; adynamic ileus with fatal complications has occurred.
- Monitor elderly patients for dehydration, and institute remedial measures promptly; sedation and decreased sensation of thirst related to CNS effects of drug can lead to severe dehydration.
- Consult physician regarding warning of patient or patient's guardian about tardive dyskinesias.
- Consult physician about dosage reduction, use of anticholinergic antiparkinsonian drugs (controversial) if extrapyramidal effects occur.
- Provide safety measures (side rails, assist) if sedation, ataxia, vertigo, orthostatic hypotension, vision changes occur.
- Provide positioning to relieve discomfort of dystonias.
- Provide reassurance to deal with extrapyramidal effect, sexual dysfunction.

### Drug-specific teaching points

- Take drug exactly as prescribed. The full effect may require 6 wk–6 mo of therapy.
- Avoid skin contact with drug solutions.
- Avoid driving or engaging in activities requiring alertness if CNS, vision changes occur.
- Avoid prolonged exposure to sun or use a sunscreen or covering garments if exposure is necessary.
- Maintain fluid intake, and use precautions against heatstroke in hot weather.
- Report sore throat, fever, unusual bleeding or bruising, rash, weakness, tremors, impaired vision, dark urine (pink or reddish brown urine is to be expected), pale stools, yellowing of the skin or eyes.

### Representative drugs

acetophenazine
chlorpromazine
fluphenazine
mesoridazine
methdilazine
methotrimeprazine
perphenazine
prochlorperazine
promazine
promethazine
thioridazine
trifluoperazine
triflupromazine

## Selective Serotonin Reuptake Inhibitors (SSRIs)

### Pregnancy Category B

### Therapeutic actions

The selective serotonin reuptake inhibitors act as antidepressants by inhibiting CNS neuronal uptake of serotonin and blocking uptake of serotonin with little effect on norepinephrine; they are also thought to antagonize muscarinic, histaminergic, and $\alpha_1$-adrenergic receptors. The increase in serotonin levels at neuroreceptors is thought to act as a stimulant, counteracting depression and increasing motivation.

### Indications

- Treatment of depression; most effective in patients with major depressive disorder
- Treatment of obsessive-compulsive disorders
- Unlabeled uses: treatment of obesity, bulemia

### Contraindications/cautions

- Contraindications: hypersensitivity to any SSRI; pregnancy. Use cautiously with impaired hepatic or renal function, diabetes mellitus, lactation

### Adverse effects

- CNS: *Headache, nervousness, insomnia, drowsiness, anxiety, tremor, dizziness, lightheadedness,* agitation, sedation, abnormal gait, convulsions
- GI: *Nausea, vomiting, diarrhea, dry mouth, anorexia, dyspepsia, constipation, taste changes,* flatulence, gastroenteritis, dysphagia, gingivitis
- Dermatologic: *Sweating, rash, pruritus,* acne, alopecia, contact dermatitis
- CV: Hot flashes, palpitations
- Respiratory: *Upper respiratory infections, pharyngitis,* cough, dyspnea, bronchitis, rhinitis
- GU: *Painful menstruation, sexual dysfunction, frequency,* cystitis, impotence, urgency, vaginitis
- Other: *Weight loss, asthenia, fever*

### Clinically important drug-drug interactions

• Increased therapeutic and toxic effects of tricyclic antidepressants with SSRIs • Decreased therapeutic effects with cyproheptadine

## ■ Nursing Considerations

### Assessment

- *History:* Hypersensitivity to any SSRI; impaired hepatic or renal function; diabetes mellitus; lactation; pregnancy
- *Physical:* Weight; T; skin rash, lesions; reflexes, affect; bowel sounds, liver evaluation; P, peripheral perfusion; urinary output, renal function; renal and liver function tests, CBC

### Implementation

- Arrange for lower dose or less frequent administration in elderly patients and patients with hepatic or renal impairment.
- Establish suicide precautions for severely depressed patients. Dispense only a small number of capsules at a time to these patients.
- Administer drug in the morning. If dose of >20 mg/d is needed, administer in divided doses.
- Monitor patient response for up to 4 wk before increasing dose because of lack of therapeutic effect. It frequently takes several weeks to see the desired effect.
- Provide small, frequent meals if GI upset or anorexia occurs. Monitor weight loss; a nutritional consultation may be necessary.
- Provide sugarless lozenges, frequent mouth care if dry mouth is a problem.
- Assure ready access to bathroom facilities if diarrhea occurs. Establish bowel program if constipation is a problem.
- Establish safety precautions (siderails, appropriate lighting, accompanying patient, etc.) if CNS effects occur.
- Provide appropriate comfort measures if CNS effects, insomnia, rash, sweating occur.
- Encourage patient to maintain therapy for treatment of underlying cause of depression.

### Drug-specific teaching points

- It may take up to 4 wk to get a full antidepressant effect from this drug. The drug should be taken in the morning (or in divided doses if necessary).
- The following side effects may occur: dizziness, drowsiness, nervousness, insomnia (avoid driving or performing hazardous tasks); nausea, vomiting, weight loss (small, frequent meals may help; monitor your weight loss—if it becomes marked, consult with your health care provider); sexual dysfunction (drug effect); flulike symptoms (if severe, check with your health care provider for appropriate treatment).
- Do not take this drug during pregnancy. If you think that you are pregnant or you wish to become pregnant, consult with your physician.
- Report rash, mania, seizures, severe weight loss.

### Representative drugs

fluoxetine
fluvoxamine

paroxetine
sertraline
sumatriptan
trazodone

## Sulfonamides

**Pregnancy Category C**
**Pregnancy Category D (at term)**

### Therapeutic actions

Sulfonamides are antibiotics. They are bacteriostatic; competitively antagonize paraaminobenzoic acid, an essential component of folic acid synthesis, in susceptible gram-negative and gram-positive bacteria, causing cell death.

### Indications

- Treatment of ulcerative colitis, otitis media, inclusion conjunctivitis, meningitis, nocardiosis, toxoplasmosis, trachoma, urinary tract infections
- Management of rheumatoid arthritis, collagenous colitis, Crohn's disease

### Contraindications/cautions

- Contraindications: allergy to sulfonamides, sulfonylureas, thiazides; pregnancy (teratogenic in preclinical studies; at term, may bump fetal bilirubin from plasma protein binding sites and cause kernicterus); or lactation (risk of kernicterus, diarrhea, rash). Use cautiously with impaired renal or hepatic function, G-6-PD deficiency, porphyria.

### Adverse effects

- CNS: Headache, peripheral neuropathy, mental depression, convulsions, ataxia, hallucinations, tinnitus, vertigo, insomnia, hearing loss, drowsiness, transient lesions of posterior spinal column, transverse myelitis
- GI: Nausea, emesis, abdominal pains, diarrhea, bloody diarrhea, anorexia, pancreatitis, stomatitis, impaired folic acid absorption, hepatitis, hepatocellular necrosis
- **Hematologic**: Agranulocytosis, aplastic anemia, thrombocytopenia, leukopenia, hemolytic anemia, hypoprothrombinemia, methemoglobinemia, megaloblastic anemia
- GU: Crystalluria, hematuria, proteinuria, nephrotic syndrome, toxic nephrosis with oliguria and anuria, oligospermia, infertility
- **Dermatologic**: Photosensitivity, cyanosis, petechiae, alopecia
- **Hypersensitivity**: Stevens-Johnson syndrome, generalized skin eruptions, epidermal necrolysis, urticaria, serum sickness, pruritus, exfoliative dermatitis, anaphylactoid reactions, periorbital edema, conjunctival and scleral redness, photosensitization, arthralgia, allergic myocarditis, transient pulmonary changes with eosinophilia, decreased pulmonary function
- **Other**: Drug fever, chills, periarteritis nodosum

### Clinically important drug-drug interactions

• Increased risk of hypoglycemia when tolbutamide, tolazamide, glyburide, glipizide, acetohexamide, chlorpropamide are taken concurrently • Increased risk of folate deficiency if taking sulfonamides; monitor patients receiving folic acid carefully for signs of folate deficiency

### Drug-lab test interferences

- Possible false-positive urinary glucose tests using Benedict's method

## ■ Nursing Considerations

### Assessment

- *History:* Allergy to sulfonamides, sulfonylureas, thiazides; pregnancy; lactation; impaired renal or hepatic function; G-6-PD deficiency; porphyria
- *Physical:* T; skin color, lesions; culture of infected site; orientation, reflexes, affect, peripheral sensation; R, adventitious sounds; mucous membranes, bowel sounds, liver evaluation; liver and renal function tests, CBC and differential, urinalysis

### Implementation

- Arrange for culture and sensitivity tests of infected area prior to therapy; repeat cultures if response is not as expected.

- Administer drug after meals or with food to prevent GI upset. Administer the drug around the clock.
- Ensure adequate fluid intake.
- Discontinue drug immediately if hypersensitivity reaction occurs.
- Establish safety precautions if CNS effects occur (side rails, assistance, environmental control).
- Protect patient from exposure to light (use of sunscreen, wear protective clothing) if photosensitivity occurs.
- Provide small, frequent meals if GI upset occurs.
- Provide mouth care for stomatitis.
- Offer support and encouragement to deal with side effects of drug therapy, including changes in sexual function.

### Drug-specific teaching points

- Complete full course of therapy.
- Take the drug with food or meals to decrease GI upset.
- Drink eight glasses of water per day.
- This drug is specific to this disease; do not use to self-treat any other infection.
- Possible side effects: sensitivity to sunlight (use sunscreens; wear protective clothing); dizziness, drowsiness, difficulty walking, loss of sensation (avoid driving or performing tasks that require alertness); nausea, vomiting, diarrhea (ensure ready access to bathroom); loss of fertility; yellow-orange urine.
- Report blood in the urine, rash, ringing in the ears, difficulty breathing, fever, sore throat, chills.

### Representative drugs

sulfadiazine
sulfamethizole
sulfamethoxazole
sulfasalazine
sulfisoxazole

## Tetracyclines

### Pregnancy Category D

### Therapeutic actions

Tetracyclines are antibiotics. They are bacteriostatic; inhibit protein synthesis of susceptible bacteria, preventing cell replication.

### Indications

- Treatment of infections caused by rickettsiae; *M. pneumoniae;* agents of psittacosis, ornithosis, lymphogranuloma venereum, and granuloma inguinale; *Borrelia recurrentis, H. ducreyi, Pasteurella pestis, Pasteurella tularensis, Bartonella bacilliformis, Bacteroides, Vibrio comma, Vibrio fetus, Brucella, E. coli, E. aerogenes, Shigella, Acinetobacter calcoaceticus, H. influenzae, Klebsiella, Diplococcus pneumoniae, S. aureus;* when penicillin is contraindicated, infections caused by *N. gonorrhoeae, T. pallidum, Treponema pertenue, L. monocytogenes, Clostridium, B. anthracis, Fusobacterium fusiforme, Actinomyces, N. meningitidis*
- Adjunct to amebicides in acute intestinal amebiasis
- Treatment of acne
- Treatment of complicated urethral, endocervical or rectal infections in adults caused by *C. trachomatis*
- Treatment of superficial ocular infections due to susceptible strains of microorganisms
- Prophylaxis of ophthalmia neonatorum due to *N. gonorrhoeae* or *C. trachomatis*

### Contraindications/cautions

- Contraindications: allergy to any of the tetracyclines, allergy to tartrazine (in 250-mg tetracycline capsules marketed under brand name *Panmycin*), pregnancy (toxic to the fetus), lactation (causes damage to the teeth of infant). Use cautiously with hepatic or renal dysfunction, presence of ocular viral, mycobacterial, or fungal infections.

### Adverse effects

- GI: *Discoloring and inadequate calcification of primary teeth of fetus if used by pregnant women, discoloring and inadequate calcification of permanent teeth if used during period of dental development,* fatty liver, liver failure, *anorexia, nausea, vomiting, diarrhea, glossitis, dysphagia,* enterocolitis, esophageal ulcers

- **Hematologic**: Hemolytic anemia, thrombocytopenia, neutropenia, eosinophilia, leukocytosis, leukopenia
- **Dermatologic**: *Phototoxic reactions, rash,* exfoliative dermatitis
- **Hypersensitivity**: Reactions from urticaria to anaphylaxis, including intracranial hypertension
- **Local**: *Transient irritation, stinging, itching,* angioneurotic edema, urticaria, dermatitis, superinfections with ophthalmic or dermatologic use
- **Other**: *Superinfections,* local irritation at parenteral injection sites

### Clinically important drug-drug interactions

• Decreased absorption with calcium salts, magnesium salts, zinc salts, aluminum salts, bismuth salts, iron, urinary alkalinizers, food, dairy products, charcoal • Increased digoxin toxicity • Increased nephrotoxicity if taken with methoxyflurane • Decreased effectiveness of oral contraceptives (rare) with a risk of break-through bleeding or pregnancy • Decreased activity of penicillins

## ■ Nursing Considerations

### Assessment

- *History:* Allergy to any of the tetracyclines; allergy to tartrazine; hepatic or renal dysfunction, pregnancy, lactation; ocular viral, mycobacterial or fungal infections
- *Physical:* Site of infection, skin color, lesions; R, adventitious sounds; bowel sounds, output, liver evaluation; urinalysis, BUN, liver function tests, renal function tests

### Implementation

- Administer oral medication on an empty stomach, 1 h before or 2–3 h after meals. Do not give with antacids. If antacids must be used, give them 3 h after the dose of tetracycline.
- Culture infected area prior to drug therapy.
- Do not use outdated drugs; degraded drug is highly nephrotoxic and should not be used.
- Do not give oral drug with meals, antacids, or food.
- Provide frequent hygiene measures if superinfections occur.
- Protect patient from sunlight and bright lights if photosensitivity occurs.
- Arrange for regular renal function tests if long-term therapy is used.
- Use topical preparations of this drug only when clearly indicated. Sensitization from the topical use of this drug may preclude its later use in serious infections. Topical preparations containing antibiotics that are not ordinarily given systemically are preferable.

### Drug-specific teaching points

- Take the drug throughout the day for best results. The drug should be taken on an empty stomach, 1 h before or 2–3 h after meals, with a full glass of water. Do not take the drug with food, dairy products, iron preparations, or antacids.
- Finish your complete prescription; if any is left, discard it immediately. Never take an outdated product.
- There have been reports of pregnancy occurring when taking tetracycline with oral contraceptives. To be absolutely confident of avoiding pregnancy, use an additional type of contraceptive while on this drug.
- Possible side effects: stomach upset, nausea; superinfections in the mouth, vagina (frequent washing may help this problem; if it becomes severe, medication may help); sensitivity of the skin to sunlight (use protective clothing and a sunscreen).
- Report severe cramps, watery diarrhea, rash or itching, difficulty breathing, dark urine or light-colored stools, yellowing of the skin or eyes.
- To give eye drops: lie down or tilt head backward and look at the ceiling. Drop suspension inside lower eyelid while looking up. Close eye, and apply gentle pressure to inner corner of the eye for 1 min.
- Apply ointment inside lower eyelid; close eyes, and roll eyeball in all directions.

- This drug may cause temporary blurring of vision or stinging after application.
- Notify health care provider if stinging or itching becomes severe.
- Take the full course of therapy prescribed; discard any leftover medication.
- Apply dermatologic solution until skin is wet. Avoid eyes, nose, and mouth.
- You may experience transient stinging or burning; this will subside quickly; skin in the treated area may become yellow; this will wash off.
- Use cosmetics as you usually do.
- Wash area before applying (unless contraindicated); this drug may stain clothing.
- Report worsening of condition, rash, irritation.

### Representative drugs

demeclocycline
doxycycline
minocycline
oxytetracyline
tetracycline

## Tricyclic Antidepressants (TCAS)

### Pregnancy Category C

### Therapeutic actions

Mechanism of action is unknown. The TCAs are structurally related to the phenothiazine antipsychotic drugs (eg, chlorpromazine), but in contrast to them, TCAs inhibit the presynaptic reuptake of the neurotransmitters norepinephrine and serotonin; anticholinergic at CNS and peripheral receptors; the relation of these effects to clinical efficacy is unknown.

### Indications

- Relief of symptoms of depression (endogenous depression most responsive; unlike other TCAs, protriptyline is "activating" and may be useful in withdrawn and anergic patients)
- Unlabeled use: treatment of obstructive sleep apnea

### Contraindications/cautions

- Contraindications: hypersensitivity to any tricyclic drug, concomitant therapy with an MAO inhibitor, recent MI, myelography within previous 24 h or scheduled within 48 h, pregnancy (limb reduction abnormalities reported), or lactation. Use cautiously with EST; preexisting CV disorders (severe CHD, progressive heart failure, angina pectoris, paroxysmal tachycardia); angle-closure glaucoma, increased intraocular pressure, urinary retention, ureteral or urethral spasm; seizure disorders (lower seizure threshold); hyperthyroidism (predisposes to CVS toxicity, including cardiac arrhythmias); impaired hepatic, renal function; psychiatric patients; schizophrenic or paranoid may exhibit a worsening of psychosis; manic-depressive disorder may shift to hypomanic or manic phase; elective surgery (discontinue as long as possible before surgery).

### Adverse effects

- CNS: *Sedation and anticholinergic (atropine-like) effects* (dry mouth, blurred vision, disturbance of accommodation for near vision, mydriasis, increased intraocular pressure), *confusion* (especially in elderly), *disturbed concentration,* hallucinations, disorientation, decreased memory, feelings of unreality, delusions, anxiety, nervousness, restlessness, agitation, panic, insomnia, nightmares, hypomania, mania, exacerbation of psychosis, drowsiness, weakness, fatigue, headache, numbness, tingling, paresthesias of extremities, incoordination, motor hyperactivity, akathisia, ataxia, tremors, peripheral neuropathy, extrapyramidal symptoms, *seizures,* speech blockage, dysarthria, tinnitus, altered EEG
- GI: *Dry mouth, constipation,* paralytic ileus, *nausea,* vomiting, anorexia, epigastric distress, diarrhea, flatulence, dysphagia, peculiar taste, increased salivation, stomatitis, glossitis, parotid swelling, abdominal cramps, black tongue
- CV: *Orthostatic hypotension,* hypertension, syncope, tachycardia, palpitations, MI, arrhythmias, heart block, precipitation of CHF, stroke
- **Hematologic**: Bone marrow depression, including agranulocytosis; eosinophila; purpura; thrombocytopenia; leukopenia

- **GU**: Urinary retention, delayed micturition, dilation of the urinary tract, gynecomastia, testicular swelling; breast enlargement, menstrual irregularity and galactorrhea; change in libido; impotence
- **Hypersensitivity**: Skin rash, pruritus, vasculitis, petechiae, photosensitization, edema (generalized, face and tongue), drug fever
- **Endocrine**: Elevated or depressed blood sugar; elevated prolactin levels; inappropriate ADH secretion
- **Withdrawal**: Symptoms with abrupt discontinuation of prolonged therapy; nausea, headache, vertigo, nightmares, malaise
- **Other**: Nasal congestion, excessive appetite, weight change; sweating, alopecia, lacrimation, hyperthermia, flushing, chills

### Clinically important drug-drug interactions

• Increased TCA levels and pharmacologic effects with cimetidine, fluoxetine, ranitidine • Increased half-life and therefore increased bleeding with dicumarol • Altered response, including dysrhythmias and hypertension, with sympathomimetics • Risk of severe hypertension with clonidine • Hyperpyretic crises, severe convulsions, hypertensive episodes, and death with MAO inhibitors • Decreased hypotensive activity of guanethidine

## ■ Nursing Considerations

### Assessment

- *History:* Hypersensitivity to any tricyclic drug; concomitant therapy with an MAO inhibitor; recent MI; myelography within previous 24 h or scheduled within 48 h; pregnancy; lactation; preexisting disorders; angle-closure glaucoma, increased intraocular pressure, urinary retention, ureteral or urethral spasm; seizure disorders; hyperthyroidism; impaired hepatic, renal function; psychiatric, manic-depressive disorder; elective surgery
- *Physical:* Weight; T; skin color, lesions; orientation, affect, reflexes, vision and hearing; P, BP, orthostatic BP, perfusion; bowel sounds, normal output, liver evaluation; urine flow, normal output; usual sexual function, frequency of menses, breast and scrotal examination; liver function tests, urinalysis, CBC, ECG

### Implementation

- Ensure that depressed and potentially suicidal patients have limited access to drug.
- Reduce dosage if minor side effects develop; discontinue drug if serious side effects occur.
- Arrange for CBC if patient develops fever, sore throat, or other sign of infection.
- Ensure ready access to bathroom if GI effects occur; establish bowel program for constipation.
- Provide small, frequent meals, frequent mouth care if GI effects occur; provide sugarless lozenges for dry mouth.
- Establish safety precautions if CNS changes occur (side rails, assist walking).

### Drug-specific teaching points

- Take drug exactly as prescribed; do not stop taking this drug abruptly or without consulting the health care provider.
- Avoid alcohol, sleep-inducing drugs, OTC drugs.
- Avoid prolonged exposure to sunlight or sunlamps; use a sunscreen or protective garments if unavoidable.
- Possible side effects: headache, dizziness, drowsiness, weakness, blurred vision (reversible; safety measures may be needed if severe; avoid driving or performing tasks requiring alertness); nausea, vomiting, loss of appetite, dry mouth (small, frequent meals, mouth care, and sucking sugarless candies may help); nightmares, inability to concentrate, confusion; changes in sexual function.
- Report dry mouth, difficulty in urination, excessive sedation.

### Representative drugs

amitriptyline
amoxapine
clomipramine
desipramine
doxepin
imipramine
nortriptyline
protriptyline
trimipramine

# III

# Compendium of Adverse Effects

All drugs are potentially dangerous. Even though chemicals are carefully screened and tested on animals and in people before they are released as drugs, drug products often cause unexpected or unacceptable reactions when they are given to people in the clinical situation. No drug does just what you want it to do when given to a patient. Drugs are chemicals, and the human body operates by a vast series of chemical reactions. Many effects can be seen when altering just one chemical factor. Today's potent and amazing drugs can cause a great variety of reactions, many of which are more severe than ever seen before.

The nurse, as the caregiver who most frequently administers medications, must be constantly alert for signs of drug reactions of different types. Patients and their families must be taught what to look for when patients are taking drugs at home. Some adverse effects can be countered with specific comfort measures or precautions. Knowing that these effects may occur and what action can be taken to prevent or cope with them may be the critical factor in helping the patient to be compliant with drug therapy and adjust to it successfully.

## Adverse effects

Adverse drug effects can be of several types.

### *Primary actions*

One of the most common occurrences in drug therapy is the development of adverse effects from simple overdosage. The patient suffers from the effects that are merely an extension of the desired effect. For example, a patient taking an anticoagulant must be careful that the drug's actions do not become so effective that excessive and spontaneous bleeding occurs. This type of adverse effect can be avoided by monitoring the patient carefully and adjusting the "recommended dose" to that particular patient. For example, a patient taking an antihypertensive drug may become dizzy, weak, and faint on the "recommended dose" but will be able to adjust to the drug therapy with a reduced dose. This may be because of an individual response to the drug, because of high or low weight, because of age, or even because of underlying pathology that alters the effects of the drug.

### *Secondary actions*

Drugs possess more than just the desired action and can produce a wide variety of effects in addition to the desired pharmacological effect. Sometimes the dose of the drug can be adjusted so that the desired effect can be achieved without producing undesirable secondary reactions. Sometimes this is not possible and the side-effects are almost inevitable. In these cases, the patient must be alerted to the fact that these effects may occur and can be counseled in ways to best cope with the undesired effect. For example, many antihistamines are very effective in drying up secretions and helping breathing, but in doing this they also cause drowsiness. The patient taking these drugs needs to know that driving a car or operating dangerous machinery could be dangerous because of this drowsiness.

### *Hypersusceptibility*

Some patients are excessively responsive to either the primary or the secondary effects of a drug. This can occur because of some pathological condition. For example, many drugs are excreted through the kidneys; if a patient develops kidney problems, the drug may not be excreted and may accumulate in the body, causing toxic effects. This could also occur because the patient has an underlying condition that makes the drug effects especially unpleasant or dangerous: for example, a man with an enlarged prostate who takes an anticholinergic drug may develop urinary retention or even bladder paralysis when the drug's effects block the urinary sphincters. He would need to be taught to empty the bladder before taking the drug, and the dosage may need to be reduced to prevent serious problems due to his underlying condition.

### *Drug allergy*

A drug allergy occurs when a person's body makes antibodies to that particular drug and reacts to it when the person is reexposed to the drug. Many people state that they have a drug allergy because of the effects of a drug. For example, a patient states that she is allergic to the diuretic Lasix. When the nurse further questions her, it is discovered that she is "allergic" because it makes her go to the bathroom—the desired drug effect. Patients who state that they have drug "allergies" should be further questioned as to the nature of the allergy. Many patients do not receive needed treatment because the response to the drug is not understood. Drug allergies fall into four main classifications.

#### Anaphylactic type

This allergy involves an antibody that reacts with specific sites in the body to cause the release of chemicals, including histamine, that give immediate reactions: swelling of the mucous membranes and constricting bronchi, leading to respiratory distress and even respiratory arrest. Reaction is immediate.

**Assessment:** Hives, rash, difficulty breathing, increased BP, dilated pupils, diaphoresis, "panicked" feeling, increased heart rate, respiratory arrest.

**Interventions:** Epinephrine, 0.3 ml of a 1:1000 solution, SC. Massage the site to speed the rate of absorption. Dose may be repeated every 15 to 20 minutes. Notify the prescriber and/or primary care giver. Prevention is the best treatment. Patients with known allergies should wear a Medic-Alert bracelet and may be advised to carry an emergency epinephrine kit.

#### Cytotoxic type

This allergy involves antibodies that are circulating in the blood and that attack antigens (the drug) on cell sites, causing death of that cell. This reaction is not immediate but may be seen over a few days.

**Assessment:** CBC showing damage to blood forming cells—Hct, decreased WBC, decreased platelets; liver function tests showing elevated liver enzymes; renal function test showing decreased renal function.

**Interventions:** Notification of drug prescriber and discontinuation of the drug. The patient may need to be supported to prevent infection and conserve energy until the allergic response is over.

#### Serum-sickness type

This allergy involves antibodies that circulate in the blood and cause damage to various tissues by depositing in blood vessels. This reaction may take up to a week or more after exposure to the drug.

**Assessment:** Itchy rash, high fever, swollen lymph nodes, swollen and painful joints, edema of the face and limbs.

**Interventions:** Discontinue the drug, notify prescriber, provide comfort measures to help the patient cope with the signs and symptoms—cool environment, skin care, positioning, ice to joints, antipyretic or anti-inflammatory agent as appropriate.

#### Delayed allergic reaction

This reaction occurs several hours after exposure and involves antibodies that are bound to specific white cells.

**Assessment:** Rash, hives, swollen joints (similar to the reaction to poison ivy).

**Interventions:** Discontinue drug, notify prescriber, provide skin care and comfort measures that may include antihistamines or topical corticosteroids.

## Drug-induced tissue and organ damage

Drugs can act directly or indirectly to cause many types of adverse effects in various tissues, structures, and organs. Such drug effects account for many of the cautions that are noted before drug administration begins. The possible occurrence of these effects also accounts for the fact that the use of some drugs is contraindicated in patients with a particular history or underlying pathology. These effects occur frequently enough that the nurse should be aware of the presentation of the drug-induced damage and of appropriate interventions should they occur.

***Dermatologic reactions***

**Assessment:** Hives, rashes, lesions. Severe reactions may include **exfoliative dermatitis,** characterized by rash and scaling, fever, enlarged lymph nodes, enlarged liver, and **erythema multiforme exudativum (Stevens-Johnson syndrome),** characterized by dark red papules on the extremities with no pain or itching, often appearing in rings or disk-shaped patches.

**Interventions:** In mild cases or where the benefit of the drug outweighs the discomfort of skin lesion: frequent skin care, avoid rubbing, avoid tight or rough clothing, avoid harsh soaps or perfumed lotions; antihistamines may be suggested. In severe cases, discontinue drug and notify prescriber. In addition to the above, the use of topical corticosteroids, antihistamines, and emollients is frequently recommended.

***Stomatitis (inflammation of the mucous membranes)***

**Assessment:** Swollen gums, inflamed gums (gingivitis), swollen and red tongue (glossitis), difficulty swallowing, bad breath, pain in the mouth and throat.

**Interventions:** Frequent mouth care with a nonirritating solution, nutrition evaluation and development of a tolerated diet usually involving frequent meals; dental consultation may be necessary; antifungal agents and/or local anesthetics are sometimes recommended.

***Superinfections***

**Assessment:** Fever, diarrhea, black-hairy tongue, swollen and red tongue (glossitis), mucous membrane lesions, vaginal discharge and/or itching.

**Interventions:** Supportive therapy as appropriate—frequent mouth care, skin care, access to bathroom facilities, small and frequent meals, antifungal therapy as appropriate. In severe cases the drug may need to be discontinued.

***Blood dyscrasias (bone marrow depression)***

**Assessment:** Fever, chills, sore throat, weakness, back pain, dark urine, decreased Hct (anemia), thrombocytopenia (low platelet count), leukopenia (low WBC count), pancytopenia (a reduction of all cellular elements of the CBC).

**Interventions:** Monitor blood counts, provide supportive measures—rest, protection from exposure to infections, protection from injury, avoidance of activities that might result in injury or bleeding. In severe cases the drug may need to be discontinued or stopped until the bone marrow can recover to a safe level.

***Liver injury***

**Assessment:** Fever, malaise, nausea, vomiting, jaundice, change in color of urine or stools, abdominal pain or colic, elevated liver enzymes (AST [SGOT], ALT [SGPT]), alterations in bilirubin levels, PTT changes.

**Interventions:** Discontinue the drug, notify prescriber, offer supportive measures—small, frequent meals, skin care, cool environment, provision of rest periods.

***Hypoglycemia***

**Assessment:** Fatigue; drowsiness; hunger; anxiety; headache; cold/clammy skin; tremulousness (shaking and lack of coordination); increased heart rate; increased blood pressure; numbness and tingling of the mouth, tongue and/or lips; confusion; rapid and shallow respirations, in severe cases seizures and/or coma may occur.

**Interventions:** Restore glucose (IV or PO if possible); supportive measures including skin care, environmental control of light and temperature, rest; safety measures to prevent injury or falls; reassurance to help patient cope with experience.

***Hyperglycemia***

**Assessment:** Fatigue, increased urination (polyuria), increased thirst (polydipsia), deep respirations (Kussmaul's respirations), restlessness, increased hunger (polyphagia), nausea, hot or flushed skin, fruity odor to breath.

**Interventions:** Insulin therapy to decrease blood glucose, carefully monitor blood glucose levels; support to deal with signs and symptoms, including access to bathroom facilities, controlled environment, reassurance, mouth care.

***Renal injury***

**Assessment:** Elevated BUN, elevated creatinine levels, decreased Hct, electrolyte imbalances, fatigue, malaise, edema, irritability, skin rash.

**Interventions:** Discontinue drug, notify prescriber, offer supportive measures—positioning, diet and fluid restrictions, skin care, electrolyte therapy, rest periods, controlled environment; in severe cases dialysis may be required for survival.

***Hypokalemia***

**Assessment:** Serum potassium ($K^+$) less than 3.5 mEq/l, weakness, numbness and tingling in the extremities, muscle cramps, nausea, vomiting, diarrhea, decreased bowel sounds, irregular pulse, weak pulses, orthostatic hypotension, disorientation. In severe cases paralytic ileus (absent bowel sounds, abdominal distention, acute abdomen) may occur.

**Interventions:** Replacement of serum potassium with careful monitoring of serum levels and patient response; supportive therapy including safety precautions to prevent injury or falls; orient patient; comfort measures for pain and discomfort.

***Hyperkalemia***

**Assessment:** Serum potassium level over 5.0 mEq/l, weakness, muscle cramps, diarrhea, numbness and tingling, slow heart rate, low blood pressure, decreased urine output, difficulty breathing.

**Interventions:** Measures to decrease serum potassium, including use of sodium polystyrene sulfonate; supportive measures to cope with discomfort; safety measures to prevent injury or falls; monitor cardiac effects and be prepared for cardiac emergency; in severe cases dialysis may be needed.

***Ocular toxicity***

**Assessment:** Blurring of vision, color vision changes, corneal damage, blindness.

**Interventions:** Monitor patient's vision carefully when on known ocular-toxic drugs; discontinue drug and notify prescriber; provide supportive measures, especially if vision loss is not reversible; monitor lighting and exposure to sunlight.

***Auditory damage***

**Assessment:** Dizziness, "ringing in the ears," loss of balance, loss of hearing.

**Interventions:** Monitor patient loss or change; provide protective measures to prevent falling or injury; consult with prescriber to decrease dose or discontinue drug; provide supportive measures to cope with drug effects.

***Central nervous system effects***

**Assessment:** Confusion, delirium, insomnia, drowsiness, hyper- or hyporeflexia, bizarre dreams, hallucinations.

**Interventions:** Provide safety measures to prevent injury; caution patient to avoid dangerous situations such as driving a car or operating dangerous machinery; orient patient and provide support; consult with prescriber to decrease drug dose or discontinue drug.

***Atropine-like (cholinergic) effects***

**Assessment:** Dry mouth, altered taste perception, dysphagia, heartburn, constipation, bloating, paralytic ileus, urinary hesitancy and retention, impotence, blurred vision, cycloplegia, photophobia, headache, mental confusion, nasal congestion, palpitations, decreased sweating, dry skin.

**Interventions:** Provide sugarless lozenges, mouth care to help mouth dryness. Arrange for bowel program as appropriate. Have patient void before taking drug to aid voiding. Provide safety measures if vision changes occur. Arrange for appropriate medication for headache, nasal congestion as appropriate. Advise patient to avoid hot environments and to take protective measures if exposed to heat due to decreased sweating.

***Parkinson-like syndrome***

**Assessment:** Lack of activity, akinesia, muscular tremors, drooling, changes in gait, rigidity, akathisia, (extreme restlessness, "jitters"), dyskinesia (spasms).

**Interventions:** Withdrawal of the drug may be necessary; treatment with anticholinergics or antiparkinson drugs may be recommended if benefit outweighs the discomfort of side effects. Provide small, frequent meals if swallowing becomes difficult; provide safety measures if ambulation becomes a problem (dropping things, etc.).

***Neuroleptic malignant syndrome (NMS)***

**Assessment:** Extrapyramidal symptoms, hyperthermia, autonomic disturbances.

**Interventions:** Withdrawal of drug may be necessary; treatment with anticholinergics or antiparkinson drugs may be necessary; supportive care to lower body temperature; safety precautions are necessary.

### *Teratogenicity*

Many drugs that reach the developing fetus or embryo can cause death or congenital defects. The exact effects of a drug on the fetus may not be known. In some cases a predictable syndrome occurs when a drug is given to a pregnant woman. In any situation, a pregnant woman who is given a drug must be advised of the possible side effects on the baby. The actual benefits of any drug should be weighed against the potential risks before administering any drug to a pregnant woman. All pregnant women should be advised not to self-medicate with any medication during the pregnancy.

**Interventions:** Emotional and physical support for dealing with fetal death or birth defects.

### *Poisoning*

Overdoses of some drugs are poisonous. The assessment factors for each drug will vary with the drug being used. The treatment of a drug poisoning will also vary, depending on the agent causing the poisoning. Throughout this book specific antidotes or treatments to poisoning will be identified if known.

# *Part* 2

# abciximab

*(ab **six'** ab mab)*
ReoPro
**Pregnancy Category C**

## Drug classes
Antiplatelet drug

## Therapeutic actions
Interferes with platelet membrane function by inhibiting fibrinogen binding and platelet–platelet interactions; inhibits platelet aggregation and prolongs bleeding time; effect is irreversible for life of the platelet.

## Indications
- Adjunct to percutaneous transluminal coronary angioplasty or atherectomy for the prevention of acute cardiac ischemic complications in patients at high risk for abrupt closure of the treated coronary vessel; intended to be used with heparin and aspirin therapy

## Contraindications/cautions
- Contraindications: allergy to abciximab, neutropenia, thrombocytopenia, hemostatic disorders, bleeding ulcer, intracranial bleeding, major trauma, vasculitis, pregnancy.
- Use cautiously with lactation.

## Dosage
**Available Forms:** Injection—2 mg/ml
*ADULT:* 0.25 mg/kg by IV bolus 10–60 min before therapy, followed by continuous infusion of 10 $\mu$g/min for 12 h.
*PEDIATRIC:* Safety and efficacy not established.

## Pharmacokinetics

| *Route* | *Onset* | *Peak* |
|---|---|---|
| IV | Rapid | 30 min |

*Metabolism:* Hepatic; $T_{1/2}$: <10 min, then 30 min
*Distribution:* Crosses placenta; may enter breast milk
*Excretion:* Urine and feces

## IV facts
**Preparation:** Withdraw the necessary amount through a .2 or 0.22-micron filter for bolus injection. Prepare infusion by withdrawing 4.5 ml through filter into syringe; inject into 250 ml 0.9% Sterile Saline or 5% Dextrose. Do not use any solution that contains visibly opaque particles; discard solution after 12 h. Do not shake; refrigerate solution.
**Infusion:** Give bolus 10–60 min before procedure; give continuous infusion at rate of 10 $\mu$g/min (17 ml/hr solution) for 12 h.
**Compatibilities:** Do not mix in solution with any other medication; give through a separate IV line.

## Adverse effects
- CNS: Dizziness, confusion
- GI: *Nausea, vomiting*
- Hematologic: Thrombocytopenia, **bleeding**
- Respiratory: Pneumonia, pleural effusion
- Local: *Pain, edema*

## ■ Nursing Considerations

### Assessment
- *History:* Allergy to abciximab, neutropenia, thrombocytopenia, hemostatic disorders, bleeding ulcer, intracranial bleeding, severe liver disease, lactation, renal disorders, pregnancy, recent trauma
- *Physical:* Skin color, lesions; orientation; bowel sounds, normal output; CBC, liver and renal function tests

### Implementation
- Monitor CBC count before use and frequently while initiating therapy.
- Arrange for concomitant aspirin and heparin therapy.
- Establish safety precautions to prevent injury and bleeding (electric razor, no contact sports, etc.).
- Provide increased precautions against bleeding during invasive procedures—bleeding will be prolonged.
- Mark chart of any patient receiving abciximab to alert medical personnel to po-

tential for increased bleeding in surgery or dental surgery.

### Drug-specific teaching points

- It may take longer than normal to stop bleeding while on this drug; avoid contact sports, use electrical razors, etc. Apply pressure for extended periods to bleeding sites.
- The following side effects may occur: upset stomach, nausea.
- Report fever, chills, sore throat, skin rash, bruising, bleeding, dark stools or urine.

## acarbose

*(a **kar'** boz)*

Precose, Prandase (CAN)

**Pregnancy Category B**

### Drug classes

Antidiabetic agent

### Therapeutic actions

Alpha-glucosidase inhibitor obtained from the fermentation process of a microorganism; delays the digestion of ingested carbohydrates, leading to a smaller rise in blood glucose following meals and a decrease in glycosylated Hgb; does not enhance insulin secretion, so its effects are additive to those of the sulfonylureas in controlling blood glucose.

### Indications

- Adjunct to diet to lower blood glucose in patients with non–insulin-dependent diabetes mellitus (Type II) whose hyperglycemia cannot be managed by diet alone
- Combination therapy with a sulfonylurea to enhance glycemic control in patients who do not receive adequate control with diet and either drug alone

### Contraindications/cautions

- Contraindications: hypersensitivity to drug; diabetic ketoacidosis; cirrhosis; inflammatory bowel disease; existence of or predisposition to intestinal obstruction; Type I diabetes; conditions that would deteriorate with increased gas in the bowel.
- Use cautiously with renal impairment, pregnancy, lactation.

### Dosage

**Available Forms:** Tablets—50, 100 mg

*ADULT:* Give 3×/d at the start of each meal; maximum dosage 100 mg PO tid. Initial dose of 25 mg PO tid at the start of each meal, increase as needed every 4–8 wk as indicated by 1 h postprandial glucose levels and tolerance.

- ***Combination with sulfonylurea*** Blood glucose may be much lower; monitor closely and adjust dosages of each drug accordingly.

*PEDIATRIC:* Safety and efficacy not established.

### Pharmacokinetics

| *Route* | *Onset* | *Peak* |
|---|---|---|
| Oral | Rapid | 1 h |

*Metabolism:* Intestinal; $T_{1/2}$: 2 h
*Distribution:* Very little
*Excretion:* Feces, small amount in urine

### Adverse effects

- GI: *Abdominal pain, flatulence, diarrhea,* anorexia, nausea, vomiting
- **Hematologic**: Leukopenia, thrombocytopenia, anemia
- **Endocrine**: *Hypoglycemia*

## ■ Nursing Considerations

### Assessment

- ***History:*** Hypersensitivity to drug; diabetic ketoacidosis; cirrhosis; inflammatory bowel disease; existence of or predisposition to intestinal obstruction; Type I diabetes; conditions that would deteriorate with increased gas in bowel; renal impairment; pregnancy; lactation
- ***Physical:*** Skin color, lesions; T; orientation, reflexes, peripheral sensation; R, adventitious sounds; liver evaluation, bowel sounds; urinalysis, BUN, blood glucose, CBC

### Implementation

- Give drug 3×/d with the first bite of each meal.
- Monitor urine and serum glucose levels frequently to determine drug effectivness and dosage.

- Inform patient of likelihood of abdominal pain and flatulence.
- Consult with dietician to establish weight loss program and dietary control.
- Arrange for thorough diabetic teaching program, including disease, dietary control, exercise, signs and symptoms of hypoglycemia and hyperglycemia, avoidance of infection, hygiene.

### Drug-specific teaching points

- Do not discontinue this drug without consulting health care provider.
- Take drug three times a day with first bite of each meal.
- Monitor urine or blood for glucose and ketones as prescribed.
- Continue diet and exercise program established for control of diabetes.
- The following side effects may occur: abdominal pain, flatulence, bloating.
- Report fever, sore throat, unusual bleeding or bruising, severe abdominal pain.

## acebutolol hydrochloride

*(a se **byoo'** toe lole)*

Sectral

**Pregnancy Category B**

### Drug classes

Beta-adrenergic blocking agent ($\beta_1$ selective)
Antiarrhythmic drug
Antihypertensive drug

### Therapeutic actions

Blocks beta-adrenergic receptors of the sympathetic nervous system in the heart and juxtaglomerular apparatus (kidney); decreases excitability of the heart, cardiac output and oxygen consumption, and release of renin from the kidney; and lowers BP.

### Indications

- Hypertension, as a step 1 agent, alone or with other drugs, especially diuretics
- Cardiac arrhythmias, especially ventricular premature beats

### Contraindications/cautions

- Contraindications: sinus bradycardia (HR < 45 beats per minute), second- or third-degree heart block (PR interval > 0.24 sec), cardiogenic shock, CHF, asthma, COPD, lactation.
- Use cautiously with diabetes or thyrotoxicosis, hepatic impairment, renal failure.

### Dosage

**Available Forms:** Capsules—200, 400 mg

*ADULT*

- *Hypertension:* Initially 400 mg/d in one or two doses PO; usual maintenance dosage range is 200–1,200 mg/d given in two divided doses.
- *Ventricular arrhythmias:* 200 mg bid PO; increase dosage gradually until optimum response is achieved (usually at 600–1,200 mg/d); discontinue gradually over 2 wk.

*GERIATRIC:* Because bioavailability doubles, lower doses may be required; maintain at 800 mg/d.

*IMPAIRED RENAL/HEPATIC FUNCTION:* Reduce daily dose by 50% when creatinine clearance is < 50 ml/min; reduce by 75% when creatinine clearance is < 25 ml/min; use caution with hepatic impairment.

*PEDIATRIC:* Safety and efficacy not established.

### Pharmacokinetics

| Route | Onset | Peak | Duration |
|---|---|---|---|
| Oral | Varies | 3–4 h | 6–8 h |

*Metabolism:* Hepatic, $T_{1/2}$: 3–4 h
*Distribution:* Crosses placenta; passes into breast milk
*Excretion:* Urine, bile/feces

### Adverse effects

- CNS: Dizziness, vertigo, tinnitus, fatigue, emotional depression, paresthesias, sleep disturbances, hallucinations, disorientation, memory loss, slurred speech (Because acebutolol is less lipid soluble than propranolol, it is less likely to penetrate the blood–brain barrier and cause CNS effects.)

- GI: *Gastric pain, flatulence, constipation, diarrhea, nausea, vomiting,* anorexia
- CV: *Bradycardia, CHF, cardiac arrhythmias, sinoatrial or AV nodal block, tachycardia,* peripheral vascular insufficiency, claudication, CVA, pulmonary edema, hypotension
- Respiratory: *Bronchospasm*, dyspnea, cough, bronchial obstruction, nasal stuffiness, rhinitis
- GU: *Impotence, decreased libido*, Peyronie's disease, dysuria, nocturia, frequent urination
- MS: Joint pain, arthralgia, muscle cramp
- Derm: Rash, pruritus, sweating, dry skin
- EENT: Eye irritation, dry eyes, conjunctivitis, blurred vision
- Allergic reactions: Pharyngitis, erythematous rash, fever, sore throat, *laryngospasm, respiratory distress*
- Other: *Decreased exercise tolerance, development of antinuclear antibodies*, hyperglycemia or hypoglycemia, elevated serum transaminase

### Clinically important drug-drug interactions

• Increased effects with verapamil • Increased risk of postural hypotension with prazosin • Possible increased BP-lowering effects with aspirin, bismuth subsalicylate, magnesium salicylate, sulfinpyrazone, oral contraceptives • Decreased antihypertensive effects with NSAIDs, clonidine • Possible increased hypoglycemic effect of insulin

### Drug-lab test interferences

• Possible false results with glucose or insulin tolerance tests (oral)

## ■ Nursing Considerations

#### Assessment

- *History:* Sinus bradycardia, second- or third-degree heart block, cardiogenic shock, CHF, asthma, COPD, pregnancy, lactation, diabetes, or thyrotoxicosis
- *Physical:* Weight, skin condition, neurologic status, P, BP, ECG, respiratory status, kidney and thyroid function, blood and urine glucose

#### Implementation

- Give with meals if needed.
- Do not discontinue drug abruptly after chronic therapy. Taper drug gradually over 2 wk with monitoring (abrupt withdrawal may cause serious beta-adrenergic rebound effects).
- Consult with physician about withdrawing drug if patient is to undergo surgery (withdrawal is controversial).
- Provide comfort measures for coping with drug effects.
- Provide safety precautions if CNS effects occur.

#### Drug-specific teaching points

- Take drug with meals.
- Do not stop taking unless so instructed by health care provider.
- Avoid driving or dangerous activities if dizziness, weakness occur.
- The following side effects may occur: dizziness, lightheadedness, loss of appetite, nightmares, depression, sexual impotence.
- Report difficulty breathing, night cough, swelling of extremities, slow pulse, confusion, depression, rash, fever, sore throat.

# acetaminophen

*(a seat a **mee'** noe fen)*

N-acetyl-P-aminophenol

*Suppositories:* Abenol (CAN), Acephen, Feverall, Children's, Feverall, Infants, Neopap

*Oral:* Aceta, Ace-Tabs (CAN), Apacet, Genapap, Genebs, Liquiprin, Mapap, Oraphen (CAN), Panadol, Paraphen (CAN), Robigesic (CAN), Rounox (CAN), Tapanol, Tempra, Tylenol

**Pregnancy Category B**

**Drug classes**
Antipyretic
Analgesic (non-narcotic)

**Therapeutic actions**
Antipyretic: reduces fever by acting directly on the hypothalamic heat-regulating center to cause vasodilation and sweating, which helps dissipate heat
Analgesic: site and mechanism of action unclear

**Indications**
- Analgesic–antipyretic in patients with aspirin allergy, hemostatic disturbances, bleeding diatheses, upper GI disease, gouty arthritis
- Arthritis and rheumatic disorders involving musculoskeletal pain (but lacks clinically significant antirheumatic and anti-inflammatory effects)
- Common cold, "flu," other viral and bacterial infections accompanied by pain and fever
- Unlabeled use: prophylactic for children receiving DPT vaccination to reduce incidence of fever and pain

**Contraindications/cautions**
- Contraindications: allergy to acetaminophen.
- Use cautiously with impaired hepatic function, chronic alcoholism, pregnancy, lactation.

**Dosage**
**Available Forms:** Suppositories—80, 120, 125, 300, 325, 650 mg; chewable tablets—80 mg; tablets—160, 325, 500, 650 mg; caplets—160, 500, 650 mg; gelcaps—650 mg; capsules—500 mg; elixir—120 mg/5 ml, 160 mg/5 ml; liquid—160 mg/5 ml, 500 mg/15 ml; solution—80 mg/1.66 ml, 100 mg/ml
*ADULT:* By suppository, 325–650 mg q4–6h or PO, 1,000 mg 3–4×/d. Do not exceed 4 g/d.
*PEDIATRIC:* Doses may be repeated 4–5×/d; do not exceed five doses in 24 h; give PO or by suppository.

| *Age* | *Dosage (mg)* |
|---|---|
| 0–3 mo | 40 |
| 4–11 mo | 80 |
| 1–2 y | 120 |
| 2–3 y | 160 |
| 4–5 y | 240 |
| 6–8 y | 320 |
| 9–10 y | 400 |
| 11 y | 480 |

**Pharmacokinetics**

| *Route* | *Onset* | *Peak* | *Duration* |
|---|---|---|---|
| Oral | Varies | 0.5–2 h | 3–4 h |

*Metabolism:* $T_{1/2}$: 1–3 h
*Distribution:* Crosses placenta; passes into breast milk
*Excretion:* Urine

**Adverse effects**
- CNS: Headache
- GI: Hepatic toxicity and failure, jaundice
- CV: Chest pain, dyspnea, myocardial damage when doses of 5–8 g/d are ingested daily for several weeks or when doses of 4 g/d are ingested for 1 year
- **Hematologic**: Methemoglobinemia—cyanosis; hemolytic anemia—hematuria, anuria; neutropenia, leukopenia, pancytopenia, thrombocytopenia, hypoglycemia
- GU: Acute kidney failure, renal tubular necrosis
- **Hypersensitivity reactions**: Skin rash, fever
- **Treatment of overdose**: Monitor serum levels regularly, N-acetylcysteine should be available as a specific antidote; basic life support measures may be necessary.

**Clinically important drug-drug interactions**
• Increased toxicity with chronic, excessive ethanol ingestion • Increased hypoprothrombinemic effect of oral anticoagulants • Increased risk of hepatotoxicity and possible decreased therapeutic effects with barbiturates, carbamazepine, hydantoins, rifampin, sulfinpyrazone • Possible delayed or decreased

effectiveness with anticholinergics • Possible reduced absorption of acetaminophen with activated charcoal • Possible decreased effectiveness of zidovudine

### Drug-lab test interferences

• Interference with Chemstrip G, Dextrostix, and Visidex II home blood glucose measurement systems; effects vary

## ■ Nursing Considerations

### Assessment

- *History:* Allergy to acetaminophen, impaired hepatic function, chronic alcoholism, pregnancy, lactation
- *Physical:* Skin color, lesions; T; liver evaluation; CBC, liver and renal function tests

### Implementation

- Do not exceed the recommended dosage.
- Consult physician if needed for children $<$ 3 y; if needed for longer than 10 d; if continued fever, severe or recurrent pain occurs (possible serious illness).
- Avoid using multiple preparations containing acetaminophen. Carefully check all OTC products.
- Give drug with food if GI upset is noted.
- Discontinue drug if hypersensitivity reactions occur.

### Drug-specific teaching points

- Do not exceed recommended dose; do not take for longer than 10 d.
- Take the drug only for complaints indicated; not an anti-inflammatory agent.
- Avoid the use of other OTC preparations. They may contain acetaminophen, and serious overdosage can occur. If you need an OTC preparation, consult your health care provider.
- Report skin rash, unusual bleeding or bruising, yellowing of skin or eyes, changes in voiding patterns.

# acetazolamide

*(a set a **zole'** a mide)*

Apo-Acetazolamide (CAN), Dazamide, Diamox, Diamox Sequels

**Pregnancy Category C**

### Drug classes

Carbonic anhydrase inhibitor
Antiglaucoma agent
Diuretic
Antiepileptic drug
Sulfonamide (nonbacteriostatic)

### Therapeutic actions

Inhibits the enzyme carbonic anhydrase. This action decreases aqueous humor formation in the eye, intraocular pressure, and hydrogen ion secretion by renal tubule cells, and increases sodium, potassium, bicarbonate, and water excretion by the kidney, causing a diuretic effect.

### Indications

- Adjunctive treatment of chronic open-angle glaucoma, secondary glaucoma
- Preoperative use in acute angle-closure glaucoma when delay of surgery is desired to lower intraocular pressure
- Edema caused by CHF, drug-induced edema
- Centrencephalic epilepsy
- Prophylaxis and treatment of acute mountain sickness

### Contraindications/cautions

- Contraindications: allergy to acetazolamide, antibacterial sulfonamides, or thiazides; chronic noncongestive angle-closure glaucoma.
- Use cautiously with fluid or electrolyte imbalance (specifically decreased $Na^+$, decreased $K^+$, hyperchloremic acidosis), renal disease, hepatic disease (risk of hepatic coma if acetazolamide is given), adrenocortical insufficiency, respiratory acidosis, COPD, lactation.

### Dosage

**Available Forms:** Tablets—125, 200 mg; SR capsules—500 mg; powder for injection—500 mg/vial

**ADULT**

- *Open-angle glaucoma:* 250 mg–1 g/d PO, usually in divided doses. Do not exceed 1 g/d.
- *Secondary glaucoma and preoperatively:* 250 mg q4h or 250 mg bid PO, or 500 mg followed by 125–250 mg q4h.

May be given IV for rapid relief of increased intraocular pressure.

- *Diuresis in CHF:* 250–375 mg (5 mg/kg) qd in the morning. Most effective if given on alternate days or for 2 d alternating with a day of rest.
- *Drug-induced edema:* 250–375 mg qd or once daily for 1–2 d followed by a day of rest.
- *Epilepsy:* 8–30 mg/kg per day in divided doses. When given in combination with other antiepileptics, starting dose is 250 mg qd. Sustained-release preparation is not recommended for this use.
- *Acute mountain sickness:* 500 mg–1 g/d in divided doses of tablets or sustained-release capsules. For rapid ascent, the 1-g dose is recommended. When possible, begin dosing 24–48 h before ascent and continue for 48 h or longer as needed while at high altitude.

PEDIATRIC

- *Secondary glaucoma and preoperatively:* 5–10 mg/kg IM or IV q6h, or 10–15 mg/kg per day PO in divided doses q6–8.
- *Epilepsy:* 8–30 mg/kg per day in divided doses. When given with other antiepileptics, starting dose is 250 mg/d.

### Pharmacokinetics

| *Route* | *Onset* | *Peak* | *Duration* |
|---|---|---|---|
| Oral | 1 h | 2–4 h | 6–12 h |
| Sustained release | 2 h | 8–12 h | 18–24 h |
| IV | 1–2 min | 15–18 min | 4–5 h |

*Metabolism:* $T_{1/2}$: 2.5–6 h
*Distribution:* Crosses placenta; passes into breast milk
*Excretion:* Unchanged in the urine

### IV facts

**Preparation:** Reconstitute 500-mg vial with 5 ml of Sterile Water for Injection; stable for 1 week if refrigerated, but use within 24 h is recommended.
**Infusion:** Give over 1 min for single injection, over 4–8 h in solution.
**Compatibility:** Do not mix with diltiazem or in multivitamin infusion.

### Adverse effects

- CNS: Weakness, fatigue, nervousness, sedation, drowsiness, dizziness, depression, tremor, ataxia, headache, paresthesias, convulsions, flaccid paralysis, transient myopia
- GI: *Anorexia, nausea, vomiting, constipation,* melena, hepatic insufficiency
- **Hematologic:** Bone marrow depression
- GU: Hematuria, glycosuria, *urinary frequency,* renal colic, renal calculi, crystalluria, polyuria
- **Dermatologic:** Urticaria, pruritis, rash, photosensitivity, erythema multiforme (Stevens-Johnson syndrome)
- **Other:** Weight loss, fever, acidosis

### Clinically important drug-drug interactions

• Decreased renal excretion of quinidine • Increased excretion of salicylates, lithium • Increased risk of salicylate toxicity due to metabolic acidosis with acetazolamide

### Drug-lab test interferences

• False-positive results of tests for urinary protein

## ■ Nursing Considerations

### Assessment

- *History:* Allergy to acetazolamide, antibacterial sulfonamides, or thiazides; chronic noncongestive angle-closure glaucoma; fluid or electrolyte imbalance; renal or hepatic disease; adrenocortical insufficiency; respiratory acidosis; COPD; lactation
- *Physical:* Skin color, lesions; edema, weight, orientation, reflexes, muscle strength, intraocular pressure; respiratory rate, pattern, adventitious sounds; liver evaluation, bowel sounds, urinary output patterns; CBC, serum electrolytes, liver and renal function tests, urinalysis

### Implementation

- Administer by direct IV if parenteral use is necessary; IM use is painful.
- Give with food or milk if GI upset occurs.

- Use caution if giving with other drugs with excretion inhibited by urine alkalinization.
- Make oral liquid form by crushing tablets and suspending in cherry, chocolate, raspberry, or other sweet syrup, or one tablet may be submerged in 10 ml of hot water with 1 ml of honey or syrup; *do not use alcohol or glycerin* as a vehicle.
- Establish safety precautions if CNS effects occur; protect patient from sun or bright lights if photophobia occurs.
- Obtain regular weight to monitor fluid changes.
- Monitor serum electrolytes and acid–base balance during course of drug therapy.

### Drug-specific teaching points

- Take drug with meals if GI upset occurs.
- Arrange to have intraocular pressure checked periodically.
- Weigh yourself on a regular basis, at the same time of the day and in the same clothing. Record weight on calendar.
- The following side effects may occur: increased volume and frequency of urination; dizziness, feeling faint on arising, drowsiness, fatigue (do not engage in hazardous activities like driving a car); sensitivity to sunlight (use sunglasses, wear protective clothing, or use a sunscreen when out of doors); GI upset (taking the drug with meals, having small frequent meals may help).
- Report weight change of more than 3 lb in 1 day, unusual bleeding or bruising, sore throat, dizziness, trembling, numbness, fatigue, muscle weakness or cramps, flank or loin pain, rash.

## acetohexamide

*(a set oh **hex'** a mide)*
Dimelor (CAN), Dymelor
**Pregnancy Category C**

### Drug classes

Antidiabetic agent
Sulfonylurea—first generation

### Therapeutic actions

Stimulates insulin release from functioning beta cells in the pancreas; may improve binding between insulin and insulin receptors or increase number of insulin receptors and lower blood glucose; has significant uricosuric activity.

### Indications

- Adjunct to diet to lower blood glucose in non–insulin-dependent diabetes mellitus (Type II)
- Adjunct to insulin therapy in the stabilization of certain cases of insulin-dependent, maturity-onset diabetes, reducing the insulin requirement and decreasing the chance of hypoglycemic reactions

### Contraindications/cautions

- Contraindications: allergy to sulfonylureas; conditions in which insulin is indicated to control blood sugar—diabetes complicated by fever, severe infections, severe trauma, major surgery, ketosis, acidosis, coma; Type I or juvenile diabetes; serious hepatic or serious renal impairment; uremia, thyroid, or endocrine impairment; glycosuria; hyperglycemia associated with primary renal disease; pregnancy or lactation.

### Dosage

**Available Forms:** Tablets—250, 500 mg

*ADULT:* 250 mg–1.5 g/d PO. Patients on $<1$ g/d can be controlled with once-daily dosage; if patients are on 1.5 g/d, twice daily dosage, before morning and evening meals is appropriate; do not exceed 1.5 g/d.

*PEDIATRIC:* Safety and efficacy not established.

*GERIATRIC:* Geriatric patients tend to be more sensitive to the drug; start with a lower initial dose, monitor for 24 h, and gradually increase dose as needed.

### Pharmacokinetics

| *Route* | *Onset* | *Peak* | *Duration* |
|---|---|---|---|
| PO | 1 h | 2–4 h | 12–24 h |

*Metabolism:* Hepatic; $T_{1/2}$: 6–8 h
*Distribution:* Enters breast milk
*Excretion:* Renal

### Adverse effects

- GI: *Anorexia, nausea, vomiting, epigastric discomfort, heartburn*
- Hematologic: *Hypoglycemia*, leukopenia, thrombocytopenia, anemia
- Dermatologic: Allergic skin reactions, eczema, pruritus, erythema, urticaria, photosensitivity
- Hypersensitivity: Fever, eosinophilia, jaundice
- Other: Possible increased risk of CV mortality

### Clinically important drug-drug interactions

• Increased risk of hypoglycemia with insulin, sulfonamides, chloramphenicol, fenfluramine, oxyphenbutazone, phenylbutazone, salicylates, probenecid, monoamine oxidase inhibitors, clofibrate • Decreased effect with beta-adrenergic blocking agents (signs of hypoglycemia also may be blocked), rifampin • Decreased effectiveness of acetohexamide and diazoxide if taken concurrently • Increased risk of hyperglycemia with thiazides, other diuretics, phenytoin, nicotinic acid, sympathomimetics • Risk of hypoglycemia and hyperglycemia with ethanol; "disulfiram reaction" also has been reported

## ■ Nursing Considerations

### Assessment

- *History:* Renal, hepatic, endocrine disorders
- *Physical:* Skin color, lesions; T; orientation, reflexes, peripheral sensation; R, adventitious sounds; liver evaluation, bowel sounds; urinalysis, BUN, serum creatinine, liver function tests, blood glucose, CBC

### Implementation

- Give drug before breakfast. If severe GI upset occurs or if dosage is 1.5 g/d, dose may be divided with one dose before breakfast and one before the evening meal.
- Monitor serum glucose levels frequently to determine effectiveness of drug.
- Transfer to insulin therapy during periods of high stress—infections, surgery, trauma, etc.
- Use IV glucose if severe hypoglycemia occurs as a result of overdose.

### Drug-specific teaching points

- Take this drug early in the morning before breakfast. If the drug is to be taken two times a day, take it before breakfast and before the evening meal.
- Do not discontinue this medication without consulting health care provider.
- Do not take this drug during pregnancy; if you think you are pregnant, consult health care provider.
- Monitor urine or blood for glucose and ketones as prescribed.
- Avoid alcohol while on this drug; serious reactions could occur.
- Report fever, sore throat, unusual bleeding or bruising, skin rash, dark urine, light-colored stools, hypoglycemic or hyperglycemic reactions.

## acetohydroxamic acid

*(a see' toe hye drox am ik)*

AHA

Lithostat

**Pregnancy Category A**

### Drug classes

Urinary tract agent

### Therapeutic actions

Inhibits the bacterial enzyme urease, inhibiting the production of ammonia in the urine and lowering the pH of urine infected with urea-splitting organisms. This enhances the effectiveness of antibiotics and increases the cure rate of these infections, which are often accompanied by kidney stone formation.

### Indications

- Adjunctive therapy in chronic urea-splitting urinary tract infections

### Contraindications/cautions

- Allergy to acetohydroxamic acid, physical conditions that are amenable to surgery or antimicrobial treatment, poor renal function, pregnancy (teratogenic–recommend the use of birth control methods while on this drug), lactation.

### Dosage

**Available Forms:** Tablets—250 mg

*ADULT:* 250 mg PO tid to qid for a total dose of 10–15 mg/kg per day; recommended starting dose is 12 mg/kg per day q6–8h; do not exceed 1.5 g/d.

*PEDIATRIC:* Initial dose of 10 mg/kg per day PO; dose titration may be required by hematologic response.

*GERIATRIC OR RENAL IMPAIRED:* Serum creatinine > 1.8 mg/dl: do not exceed 1 g/d with doses at 12-h intervals; do not administer to patients with serum creatinine > 2.5 mg/dl.

### Pharmacokinetics

| *Route* | *Onset* | *Peak* |
|---|---|---|
| PO | 1 h | 15–60 min |

*Metabolism:* Hepatic; $T_{1/2}$: 5–10 h

*Distribution:* Crosses placenta, may enter breast milk

*Excretion:* Unchanged in the urine

### Adverse effects

- CNS: *Headache, depression, anxiety, nervousness, malaise, tremulousness*
- GI: *Nausea, vomiting, anorexia*
- CV: Superficial phlebitis of lower extremities
- Hematologic: **Coombs' negative hemolytic anemia**
- Dermatologic: Nonpruritic, macular skin rash in the upper extremities and face (most common after ingestion of alcohol during long-term use), alopecia

### Clinically important drug-drug interactions

- Rash with alcohol • Absorption of acetohydroxamic acid and iron decreased if both are taken; if needed, space doses at least 2 h apart

## ■ Nursing Considerations

### Assessment

- ***History:*** Allergy to acetohydroxamic acid, physical conditions that are amenable to surgery or antimicrobial treatment, poor renal function, pregnancy, lactation
- ***Physical:*** Skin color, lesions; orientation, affect, reflexes; peripheral perfusion, veins in lower extremities; liver evaluation; CBC, liver and renal function tests

### Implementation

- Arrange for culture and sensitivity tests of urine before beginning therapy; do not administer if urine is infected with non-urease-producing organisms.
- Ensure that patient is not pregnant nor planning to become pregnant. Advise the patient to use birth control.
- Administer on an empty stomach—1 h before or 2 h after meals.
- Arrange for analgesics to relieve headache.

### Drug-specific teaching points

- Take the drug on an empty stomach—1 h before or 2 h after meals.
- The following side effects may occur: headache (analgesics may help); nausea, vomiting, loss of appetite (small, frequent meals may help); skin rash (more common when alcohol is taken with this drug).
- This drug causes birth defects and should not be taken if you are, or are trying to become, pregnant; use of birth control methods is highly recommended; if you think you are pregnant, consult your physician immediately.
- Report unusual bleeding or bruising; malaise, lethargy; leg pain or swelling of

the lower leg; severe nausea and vomiting.

## acetophenazine maleate

*(a set oh **fen'** a zeen)*

Tindal

**Pregnancy Category C**

### Drug classes

Phenothiazine (piperazine)
Dopaminergic blocking drug
Antipsychotic drug

### Therapeutic actions

Mechanism of action not fully understood: antipsychotic drugs block dopamine receptors in the brain, depress the RAS (including those parts of the brain involved with wakefulness and emesis), and are anticholinergic and act as antihistamines.

### Indications

- Management of manifestations of psychotic disorders

### Contraindications/cautions

- Contraindications: coma or severe CNS depression, bone marrow depression, blood dyscrasia, circulatory collapse, subcortical brain damage, Parkinson's disease, liver damage, cerebral arteriosclerosis, coronary disease, severe hypotension or hypertension.
- Use cautiously with respiratory disorders ("silent pneumonia" may develop); glaucoma, prostatic hypertrophy; epilepsy or history of epilepsy; breast cancer; thyrotoxicosis; peptic ulcer, decreased renal function; myelography in prior 24 h or scheduled in next 48 h; exposure to heat or phosphorous insecticides; lactation; children < 12 y, especially those with chickenpox, CNS infections (children are especially susceptible to dystonias that may confound the diagnosis of Reye's syndrome).

### Dosage

**Available Forms:** Tablets—20 mg

Full clinical effects may require 6 wk to 6 mo of therapy.

*ADULT:* 20 mg tid PO; total dosage range is 40–80 mg/d. Hospitalized patients: 80–120 mg/d PO in divided doses (doses as high as 400–600 mg/d have been used).

*PEDIATRIC:* Generally not recommended for children < 12 y.

*GERIATRIC:* Use lower doses, and increase dosage more gradually than in younger patients.

### Pharmacokinetics

| Route | Onset | Peak | Duration |
|---|---|---|---|
| PO | 2–3 h | 2–4 h | 36–48 h |

*Metabolism:* Hepatic; $T_{1/2}$: 10–20 h

*Distribution* : Crosses the placenta; enters breast milk

*Excretion:* 50% renal, 50% enterohepatic

### Adverse effects

- CNS: *Drowsiness*; insomnia; vertigo; headache; weakness; tremor; ataxia; slurring; cerebral edema; seizures; exacerbation of psychotic symptoms; extrapyramidal syndromes—*pseudoparkinsonism, dystonias; akathisia*; tardive dyskinesias potentially irreversible (no known treatment); NMS (rare but 20% fatal)
- CV: Hypotension, orthostatic hypotension, hypertension, tachycardia, bradycardia, **cardiac arrest,** CHF, cardiomegaly, **refractory arrhythmias** (some fatal), pulmonary edema
- Respiratory: Bronchospasm, laryngospasm, dyspnea; suppression of cough reflex and potential for aspiration
- Hematologic: Eosinophilia, leukopenia, leukocytosis, anemia; aplastic anemia; hemolytic anemia; thrombocytopenic or nonthrombocytopenic purpura; pancytopenia
- Hypersensitivity: Jaundice, urticaria, angioneurotic edema, laryngeal edema, photosensitivity, eczema, asthma, anaphylactoid reactions, exfoliative dermatitis
- Endocrine: Lactation, breast engorgement in females, galactorrhea; syndrome

of inappropriate ADH secretion (SIADH); amenorrhea, menstrual irregularities; gynecomastia in males; changes in libido; hyperglycemia or hypoglycemia; glycosuria; hyponatremia; pituitary tumor with hyperprolactinemia; inhibition of ovulation, infertility, pseudopregnancy; reduced urinary levels of gonadotropins, estrogens, progestins
- **Autonomic**: Dry mouth, salivation, nasal congestion, nausea, vomiting, anorexia, fever, pallor, flushed facies, sweating, constipation, paralytic ileus, urinary retention, incontinence, polyuria, enuresis, priapism, ejaculation inhibition, male impotence

### Clinically important drug-drug interactions

• Additive CNS depression with barbiturates, anesthetics, ethanol • Additive anticholinergic effects and possibly decreased antipsychotic efficacy with anticholinergic drugs • Decreased absorption of oral antipsychotic drugs with antidiarrheal mixtures, antacids • Decreased plasma levels of antipsychotic drugs, but severe neurotoxicity with lithium • Increased neurotoxicity of phenytoin • Decreased neuromuscular block with polypeptide antibiotics (bacitracin, capreomycin, colistimethate, polymyxin B) • Increased likelihood of seizures with metrizamide (contrast agent used in myelography) • Decreased antihypertensive effect of guanethidine

### Drug-lab test interferences

• False-positive pregnancy tests (less likely if serum test is used) • Increase in PBI not attributable to an increase in thyroxine

## ■ Nursing Considerations

### Assessment

- *History:* Coma or severe CNS depression; bone marrow depression; blood dyscrasia; circulatory collapse; subcortical brain damage; Parkinson's disease; liver damage; cerebral arteriosclerosis; coronary disease; severe hypotension or hypertension; respiratory disorders; glaucoma, prostatic hypertrophy; history of epilepsy; breast cancer; thyrotoxicosis; peptic ulcer, decreased renal function; myelography within previous 24 h or scheduled within 48 h; exposure to heat or phosphorous insecticides; lactation
- *Physical:* Weight, T; reflexes, orientation, intraocular pressure; P, BP, orthostatic BP; R, adventitious sounds; bowel sounds and normal output, liver evaluation; urinary output, prostate size; CBC, urinalysis; thyroid, liver, and kidney function tests

### Implementation

- Discontinue drug if serum creatinine, BUN become abnormal or if WBC count is depressed.
- Monitor bowel function and arrange therapy for severe constipation; adynamic ileus with fatal complications has occurred.
- Monitor elderly patients for dehydration, and institute remedial measures promptly; sedation and decreased sensation of thirst from CNS effects can lead to dehydration.
- Consult physician regarding warning of patient or patient's guardian about tardive dyskinesias.
- Consult physician about dosage reduction, use of anticholinergic antiparkinsonian drugs (controversial) if extrapyramidal effects occur.

### Drug-specific teaching points

- Take drug exactly as prescribed.
- The following side effects may occur: drowsiness (avoid driving or engaging in other hazardous activities), sensitivity to the sun (avoid prolonged exposure, use a sunscreen or covering garments), pink or reddish brown urine.
- Maintain fluid intake, and use precautions against heatstroke in hot weather; you may not feel thirsty. Urinate before taking your drug; you may experience difficulties urinating if you have prostrate problems.
- Report sore throat, fever, unusual bleeding or bruising, rash, weakness, tremors, impaired vision, dark urine, pale stools, yellowing of the skin or eyes.

## acetylcysteine

*(a se teel **sis'** tay een)*

n-acetylcysteine

Airbron (CAN), Mucomyst, Mucosil, Mucomyst 10 IV

**Pregnancy Category C**

### Drug classes

Mucolytic agent
Antidote

### Therapeutic actions

Mucolytic activity: splits links in the mucoproteins contained in respiratory mucus secretions, decreasing the viscosity of the mucus

Antidote to acetaminophen hepatotoxicity: protects liver cells by maintaining cell function and detoxifying acetaminophen metabolites

### Indications

- Mucolytic adjuvant therapy for abnormal, viscid, or inspissated mucus secretions in acute and chronic bronchopulmonary disease (emphysema with bronchitis, asthmatic bronchitis, tuberculosis, pneumonia), in pulmonary complications of cystic fibrosis, and in tracheostomy care; pulmonary complications associated with surgery, anesthesia, post-traumatic chest conditions; diagnostic bronchial studies
- To prevent or lessen hepatic injury that may occur after ingestion of a potentially hepatotoxic dose of acetaminophen; treatment must start as soon as possible, at least within 24 h of ingestion
- Unlabeled uses: as ophthalmic solution to treat keratoconjunctivitis sicca (dry eye); as an enema to treat bowel obstruction due to meconium ileus or its equivalent

### Contraindications/cautions

- Mucolytic use: contraindicated with hypersensitivity to acetylcysteine; use caution and discontinue immediately if bronchospasm occurs.
- Antidotal use: there are no contraindications; use cautiously with esophageal varices, peptic ulcer.

### Dosage

**Available Forms:** Solution—10%, 20%; injection—orphan drug availability

*Mucolytic use*

- ***Nebulization with face mask, mouthpiece, tracheostomy:*** 1–10 ml of 20% solution or 2–20 ml of 10% solution q2–6h; the dose for most patients is 3–5 ml of the 20% solution or 6–10 ml of the 10% solution tid–qid.
- ***Nebulization with tent, croupette:*** Very large volumes are required, occasionally up to 300 ml, during a treatment period. The dose is the volume or solution that will maintain a very heavy mist in the tent or croupette for the desired period. Administration for intermittent or continuous prolonged periods, including overnight, may be desirable.

*Instillation*

- ***Direct or by tracheostomy:*** 1–2 ml of a 10%–20% solution q1–4h; may be introduced into a particular segment of the bronchopulmonary tree by way of a plastic catheter (inserted under local anesthesia and with direct visualization). Instill 2–5 ml of the 20% solution by a syringe connected to the catheter.
- ***Percutaneous intratracheal catheter:*** 1–2 ml of the 20% solution or 2–4 ml of the 10% solution q1–4h by a syringe connected to the catheter.
- ***Diagnostic bronchogram:*** Before the procedure, give two to three administrations of 1–2 ml of the 20% solution or 2–4 ml of the 10% solution by nebulization or intratracheal instillation.

*Antidotal use:* For acetaminophen overdose, administer acetylcysteine immediately if 24 h or less have elapsed since acetaminophen ingestion, using the following protocol:• Empty the stomach by lavage or by inducing emesis with syrup of ipecac; repeat dose of ipecac if emesis does not occur in 20 min. • If activated charcoal has been administered by lavage, charcoal may adsorb acetylcysteine and reduce its effectiveness. • Draw blood for acetaminophen plasma assay and for baseline SGOT, SGPT, bilirubin, prothrombin time, creatinine, BUN, blood sugar, and electrolytes; if acetaminophen assay cannot be obtained or dose is clearly in the toxic range, give full course of acetylcysteine therapy; monitor hepatic and renal function, fluid and electrolyte balance. • Administer acetylcysteine PO 140 mg/kg loading dose. • Administer 17 maintenance doses of 70 mg/kg q4h, starting 4 h after loading dose; administer full course of doses unless acetaminophen assay reveals a nontoxic level. • If patient vomits loading or maintenance dose within 1 h of administration, repeat that dose. An IV form is being studied as an orphan drug. • If patient persistently vomits the oral dose, administer by duodenal intubation. • Repeat blood chemistry assays in number 3 above daily if acetaminophen plasma level is in toxic range.

### Pharmacokinetics

| Route | Onset | Peak | Duration |
|---|---|---|---|
| Oral | 30–60 min | 1–2 h | |
| Instillation/ inhalation | 1 min | 5–10 min | 2–3 h |

*Metabolism:* Hepatic, $T_{1/2}$: 6.25 h
*Excretion:* Urine (30%)

### Adverse effects

*Lytic Use*

- GI: *Nausea*, stomatitis
- **Respiratory**: Bronchospasm, especially in asthmatics
- **Hypersensitivity**: Urticaria
- Other: *Rhinorrhea*

*Antidotal Use*

- GI: *Nausea, vomiting, other GI symptoms*
- Dermatologic: Rash

## ■ Nursing Considerations

### Assessment

- *History*
  Mucolytic use: Hypersensitivity to acetylcysteine, asthma
  Antidotal use: Esophageal varices, peptic ulcer
- ***Physical:*** Weight, T, skin color, lesions; BP, P; R, adventitious sounds, bowel sounds, liver palpation

### Implementation

*Mucolytic Use*

- Dilute the 20% acetylcysteine solution with either Normal Saline or Sterile Water for Injection; use the 10% solution undiluted. Refrigerate unused, undiluted solution, and use within 96 h. Drug solution in the opened bottle may change color, but this does not alter safety or efficacy.
- Administer the following drugs separately, because they are incompatible with acetylcysteine solutions: tetracyclines, erythromycin lactobionate, amphotericin B, iodized oil, chymotrypsin, trypsin, hydrogen peroxide.
- Use water to remove residual drug solution on the patient's face after administration by face mask.
- Inform patient that nebulization may produce an initial disagreeable odor, but it will soon disappear.
- Monitor nebulizer for buildup of drug from evaporation; dilute with Sterile Water for Injection to prevent concentrate from impeding nebulization and drug delivery.
- Establish routine for pulmonary toilet; have suction equipment on standby.

*Antidotal Use*

- Dilute the 20% acetylcysteine solution with cola drinks or other soft drinks to a final concentration of 5%; if administered by gastric tube or Miller-Abbott tube, water may be used as diluent. Dilution minimizes the risk of vomiting.
- Prepare fresh solutions, and use within 1 h; undiluted solution in opened vials may be kept for 96 h.
- Treat fluid and electrolyte imbalance, hypoglycemia.
- Give vitamin $K_1$ if prothrombin ratio exceeds 1.5; give fresh-frozen plasma if PT ratio exceeds 3.
- Do not administer diuretics.

### Drug-specific teaching points

- The following side effects may occur: increased productive cough, nausea, GI upset.
- Report difficulty breathing or nausea.

## acitretin

*(ass ah* ***tree'*** *tin)*
Soriatane
**Pregnancy Category X**

### Drug classes

Antipsoriatic agent (systemic)
Retinoid

### Therapeutic actions

Related to retinoic acid, vitamin A, a metabolite of etretinate; mechanism of action is not known but improvement seems to be related to a decrease in scale, erythema and thickness of lesions as well as normalization of epidermal differentiation and decreased inflammation in the epidermis and dermis.

### Indications

- Treatment of severe psoriasis in female patients of reproductive potential who are unresponsive to or unable to take other agents

### Contraindications/cautions

- Contraindications: allergy to etretinate, retinoids, pregnancy, lactation, use of alcohol.
- Use cautiously with cardiovascular disease (drug increases triglycerides); diabetes mellitus, obesity, increased alcohol intake, familial history of these conditions (these patients have a tendency to develop hypertriglyceridemia and may be at greater risk of developing this condition in association with etretinate therapy); severe hepatic or renal dysfunction.

### Dosage

**Available Forms:** Capsules—10, 25 mg

*ADULT:* Individualize dosage based on side effects and disease response. Initial dose 25–50 mg PO qd with the main meal. Terminate therapy when lesions resolve. Course may be repeated if relapse occurs.

*PEDIATRIC:* Not recommended.

### Pharmacokinetics

| Route | Onset | Peak | Duration |
|---|---|---|---|
| Oral | Slow | 2–6 h | Wks |

*Metabolism:* Hepatic; $T_{1/2}$: 49 h
*Distribution:* Crosses placenta; may pass into breast milk
*Excretion:* Bile and urine

### Adverse effects

- CNS: *Lethargy, insomnia, fatigue, headache, fever, dizziness, anmesia,* abnormal thinking, pseudotumor cerebri
- CV: *Cardiovascular, thrombotic or obstructive events,* edema, *dyspnea*
- GI: *Cheilitis, chapped lips; dry mouth, thirst; sore mouth and tongue, gingival bleeding/inflammation, nausea,* vomiting, abdominal pain, anorexia, inflammatory bowel disease, **hepatitis** (including fatalities)
- GU: *White cells in the urine, proteinuria, red blood cells in the urine, hematuria,* glycosuria, aceetonuria
- Hematologic: *Elevated mean corpuscular hemoglobin concentration,* reticulocytes, partial thromboplastin time, erythrocyte sedimentation rate; decreased Hgb/Hct, RBC and mean corpuscular volume, increased platelets, *increased or decreased WBC or prothrombin time,* **elevated triglycerides,** AST, ALT, alkaline phosphatase, GGTP, globulin, cholesterol, bilirubin abnormal liver function tests, increased fasting serum glucose, increased BUN and creatinine, increased or decreased potassium
- ENT: Epistaxis, *dry nose, eye irritation, conjunctivitis, corneal opacities, eyeball pain; abnormalities of eyelid, cornea, lens, and retina; decreased visual acuity, double vision;* abnormalities of lacrimation, vision, extraoccular musculature, ocular tension, pupil and vitreous, earache, otitis externa, papilledema
- Musculoskeletal: *Skeletal hyperostosis, arthralgia, muscle cramps,* bone and joint pain and stiffness
- Dermatological: *Skin fragility, dry skin, pruritus, rash, thinning of hair, peeling of palms and soles,* skin infections, nail brittleness, petechiae, sunburn, changes in perspiration

**Clinically important drug-drug interactions**

• Greatly prolonged half-life and toxic effects if taken with alcohol • Possible decreased effectiveness of low estrogen-progesterones used for contraception

## ■ Nursing Considerations

### Assessment

- *History:* Allergy to etretinate, retinoids; cardiovascular disease; diabetes mellitus, obesity, increased alcohol intake, familial history of these conditions; pregnancy, lactation, renal or liver disease
- *Physical:* Body weight; skin color, lesions, turgor, texture; joints—range of motion; orientation, reflexes, affect, ophthalmologic exam; mucous membranes, bowel sounds; hepatic function tests (AST, ALT, LDH), serum triglycerides, cholesterol, HDL, sedimentation rate, CBC and differential, urinalysis, serum electrolytes, pregnancy test

### Implementation

- Ensure that patient is not pregnant before administering; arrange for a pregnancy test 2 wk before beginning therapy. Advise patient to use barrier contraceptive measures during treatment and for an indefinite period after treatment is discontinued (the exact length of time after treatment when pregnancy should be avoided is not known, at least 2–4 months). Patient should receive information in writing and sign informed consent. Repeat pregnancy test and contraceptive teaching periodically during therapy.
- Arrange for patient to have hepatic function tests prior to therapy and at 1 to 2 wk intervals for the first 1–2 mo of therapy, and at intervals of 1–3 mo thereafter.
- Arrange for patient to have blood lipid determinations before therapy and at intervals of 1 or 2 wk until the lipid response is established (usually within 4–8 wk). If elevations occur, institute other measures to lower serum triglycerides: weight reduction, reduction in dietary fat, exercise, increased intake of insoluble fiber, decreased alcohol consumption.
- Administer drug with main meal of the day; do not crush capsules.
- Discontinue drug if signs of papilledema occur and arrange for patient to consult a neurologist for further care.
- Discontinue drug if visual disturbances occur and arrange for an ophthalmologic exam.
- Discontinue drug if abdominal pain, rectal bleeding or severe diarrhea occurs and consult with physician.
- Do not allow blood donation from patients taking acitretin due to the teratogenic effects of the drug; do not donate blood for 3 years after treatment is finished.
- Protect patient from exposure to the sun—use sunscreen, protective clothing, avoid the use of sunlamps.

### Drug-specific teaching points

- Take drug with main meal of the day. Do not crush capsules.
- This drug has been associated with severe birth defects and miscarriages; it is contraindicated in pregnant women. It is important to use barrier contraceptive measures during treatment and for 1 month after treatment is discontinued. If you think that you have become pregnant, consult with your physician immediately. Oral contraceptives may not be effective while on this drug; barrier measures are needed.
- Do not take vitamin A supplements while you are taking this drug.
- Do not use alcohol while on this drug and for 2 months after treatment is finished; it makes the drug's effects stronger and the toxic reactions more severe.
- You will not be permitted to donate blood while on this drug and for 3 years after treatment is finished because of its possible effects on the fetus of a blood recipient.
- The following side effects may occur: exacerbation of psoriasis during initial therapy; dizziness, lethargy, headache, visual changes (avoid driving or performing tasks that require alertness if these oc-

cur); sensitivity to the sun (avoid sunlamps, exposure to the sun; use sunscreens, protective clothing if sun cannot be avoided); diarrhea, abdominal pain, loss of appetite (taking the drug with meals may help); dry mouth (sucking sugarless lozenges is often helpful); eye irritation and redness, inability to wear contact lenses; dry skin, itching, redness.
- Report headache with nausea and vomiting, yellowing of the skin or eyes, pale-colored stools, visual difficulties.

## acyclovir

*(ay sye' kloe ver)*
acycloguanosine
Zovirax
**Pregnancy Category C**

### Drug classes
Antiviral

### Therapeutic actions
Antiviral activity; inhibits viral DNA replication

### Indications
- Initial and recurrent mucosal and cutaneous herpes simplex virus (HSV) 1 and 2 infections in immunocompromised patients
- Severe initial and recurrent genital herpes infections in selected patients
- Herpes simplex encephalitis in patients >6 mo
- Ointment: initial HSV genital infections; limited mucocutaneous HSV infections in immunocompromised patients
- Unlabeled uses: treatment of herpes zoster, cytomegalovirus and HSV infection following transplant, herpes simplex infections, infectious mononucleosis, varicella pneumonia, disseminated primary eczema herpeticum

### Contraindications/cautions
- Contraindications: allergy to acyclovir, seizures, CHF, renal disease, lactation.

### Dosage
**Available Forms:** Tablets—400, 800 mg; capsules—200 mg; suspension—200 mg/5 ml; powder for injection—500 mg/vial, 1,000 mg/vial; ointment: 50 mg/g

ADULT
- ***Parenteral:*** 5–10 mg/kg infused IV over 1 h, q8h (15 mg/kg/d) for 7 d.
- ***Oral***
  - *Initial genital herpes:* 200 mg q4h while awake (1000 mg/d) for 10 d.
  - *Chronic suppressive therapy:* 400 mg bid for up to 12 mo.

PEDIATRIC
- ***Parenteral:*** <12 y: 250–500 mg/m$^2$ infused IV over 1 h, q8h (750 mg/m$^2$/d) for 7 d. >12 y: adult dosage.
- ***Oral:*** Safety not established.

GERIATRIC OR RENAL IMPAIRED
- ***Oral:*** Creatinine clearance <10 ml/min: 200 mg q12h.
- ***IV:***

| Creatinine Clearance (ml/min) | Dosage (IV) |
|---|---|
| >50 | 5 mg/kg q8h |
| 25–50 | 5 mg/kg q12h |
| 10–25 | 5 mg/kg qd |
| 0–10 | 2.5 mg/kg qd |

***Topical***
- *Ointment (all ages):* Apply sufficient quantity to cover all lesions 6×/d for 7 d; 1.25 cm (1/2 in) ribbon of ointment covers 2.5 cm$^2$ (4 in$^2$) surface area q3h.

### Pharmacokinetics

| Route | Onset | Peak | Duration |
|---|---|---|---|
| Oral | Varies | 1.5–2 h | |
| IV | Immediate | 1 h | 8 h |

*Metabolism:* $T_{1/2}$: 2.5–5 h
*Distribution:* Crosses placenta; enters breast milk
*Excretion:* Unchanged in urine

### IV facts
**Preparation:** Reconstitute drug in 10 ml Sterile Water for Injection or Bacteriostatic Water for Injection containing benzyl alcohol; concentration will be 50 mg/ml. Do *not* dilute drug with bacteriostatic water containing parabens. Use reconstituted solution within 12 h; dilute

IV solution to concentration of 7 mg/ml or less. Do not use biologic or colloidal fluids such as blood products or protein solutions. Warm drug to room temperature to dissolve precipitates formed during refrigeration.

**Infusion:** Administer by slow IV infusion of parenteral solutions; avoid bolus or rapid injection. Infuse over 1 h to avoid renal damage.

**Incompatibilities:** Do not mix with diltiazem, dobutamine, dopamine, fludarabine, foscarnet, idarubicin, meperidine, morphine, ondansetron, piperacillin, sagramostim, vinorelbine.

### Adverse effects

*Systemic Administration*

- CNS: Headache, vertigo, depression, tremors, encephalopathic changes
- GI: *Nausea, vomiting,* diarrhea, anorexia
- GU: Crystalluria with rapid IV administration, hematuria
- Dermatologic: *Inflammation or phlebitis at injection sites,* rash, hair loss

*Topical Administration*

- Dermatologic: *Transient burning at site of application*

### Clinically important drug-drug interactions

*Systemic Administration*

• Increased effects with probenecid • Increased nephrotoxicity with other nephrotoxic drugs • Extreme drowsiness with zidovudine

## ■ Nursing Considerations

### Assessment

- *History:* Allergy to acyclovir, seizures, CHF, renal disease, lactation
- *Physical:* Skin color, lesions; orientation; BP, P, auscultation, perfusion, edema; R, adventitious sounds; urinary output; BUN, creatinine clearance

### Implementation

*Systemic Administration*

- Ensure that the patient is well hydrated.

*Topical Administration*

- Start treatment as soon as possible after onset of signs and symptoms.
- Wear a rubber glove or finger cot when applying drug.

### Drug-specific teaching points

*Systemic Administration*

- Complete the full course of oral therapy, and do *not* exceed the prescribed dose.
- Oral acyclovir is *not* a cure for your disease but should make you feel better.
- The following side effects may occur: nausea, vomiting, loss of appetite, diarrhea; headache, dizziness.
- Avoid sexual intercourse while visible lesions are present.
- Report difficulty urinating, skin rash, increased severity or frequency of recurrences.

*Topical Administration*

- Wear rubber gloves or finger cots when applying the drug to prevent autoinnoculation of other sites and transmission to others.
- This drug does not cure the disease; application during symptom-free periods will not prevent recurrences.
- Avoid sexual intercourse while visible lesions are present.
- This drug may cause burning, stinging, itching, rash; notify your physician if these are pronounced.

## adenosine

*(a **den'** oh seen)*

Adenocard, Adenoscan

**Pregnancy Category C**

### Drug classes

Antiarrhythmic

### Therapeutic actions

Slows conduction through the AV node; can interrupt the reentry pathways through the AV node and restore sinus rhythm in patients with paroxysmal supraventricular tachycardias

a

### Indications

- Conversion to sinus rhythm of paroxysmal supraventricular tachycardia, including that associated with accessory bypass tracts (Wolff-Parkinson-White Syndrome), after attempting vagal maneuvers when appropriate (Adenocard)
- Assessment of patients with suspected CAD in conjuction with thallium tomography (Adenoscan)
- Orphan drug use: treatment of brain tumors in conjunction with BCNU

### Contraindications/cautions

- Contraindications: hypersensitivity to adenosine; second- or third-degree AV heart block, sick sinus syndrome (unless artificial pacemake in place); atrial flutter, atrial fibrillation, ventricular tachycardia.
- Use cautiously with asthma (could produce bronchospasm in asthma patients).

### Dosage

**Available Forms:** Injection—3 mg/ml
For rapid bolus IV use only.

**ADULT**

- *Conversion of arrhythmia:*
  - *Initial dose:* 6 mg as a rapid IV bolus administered over 1–2 sec.
  - *Repeat administration:* 12 mg as a rapid IV bolus if initial dose does not produce elimination of the supraventricular tachycardia within 1–2 min. 12-mg bolus may be repeated a second time if needed. Doses > 12 mg are not recommended.
- *Assessment of suspected CAD:* 140 mcg/kg/min IV infused over 6 min. Inject thallium at 3 min.

**PEDIATRIC:** Not recommended.

### Pharmacokinetics

| *Route* | *Onset* | *Peak* | *Duration* |
|---|---|---|---|
| IV | Immediate | 10 sec | 20–30 sec |

*Metabolism:* Hepatic; $T_{1/2}$: > 10 sec
*Distribution:* Rapidly picked up by red blood cells

### IV facts

**Preparation:** Store drug at room temperature; do not refrigerate. Solution must be clear at time of use; discard any unused portion of vial.

**Infusion:** By rapid IV bolus only, given over 1–2 sec; administer directly into a vein or as proximal as possible; follow with a rapid saline flush.

### Adverse effects

- CNS: *Headache, lightheadness,* dizziness, tingling in arms, numbness, apprehension, blurred vision, burning sensation, heaviness in arms, neck and back pain
- GI: *Nausea,* metallic taste, tightness in throat, pressure in groin
- CV: *Facial flushing, arrhythmias,* sweating, palpitations, chest pain, hypotension
- Respiratory: *Shortness of breath/dyspnea, chest pressure,* hyperventilation

### Clinically important drug-drug interactions

• Increased degree of heart block with carbamazepine • Increased effects of adenosine with dipyridamole • Decreased effects with methylxanthines (caffeine, theophylline), which antagonize adenosine's activity

## ■ Nursing Considerations

### Assessment

- *History:* Hypersensitivity to adenosine, second- or third-degree AV heart block, sick sinus syndrome, atrial flutter, atrial fibrillation, ventricular tachycardia, asthma (use caution), adenosine
- *Physical:* Orientation; BP, P, auscultation, ECG; R, adventitious sounds

### Implementation

- Assess asthma patients carefully for signs of exacerbation of asthma.
- Monitor patient's ECG continually during administration. Be alert for the possibility of arrhythmias. These usually last only a few seconds.
- Maintain emergency equipment on standby at time of administration.

- Have methlyxanthines available as antagonists if problems occur.

**Drug-specific teaching points**

- The following side effects may occur: rapid or irregular heartbeat (usually passes quickly), facial flushing, headache, lightheadedness, dizziness, nausea, shortness of breath.
- Report chest pain, difficulty breathing, numbness, tingling so appropriate measures can be taken.

## albendazole

*(al **ben'** da zole)*

Albenza

**Pregnancy Category C**

### Drug classes
Anthelmintic

### Therapeutic actions
Inhibitory effect on tubulin polymerization resulting in loss of cytoplasmic microtubules and death of susceptible larva.

### Indications
- Treatment of parenchymal neurocysticercosis due to active lesions caused by larval forms of pork tapeworm *T. solium*
- Treatment of cystic hydatid disease of the liver, lung, and peritoneum caused by larval form of dog tapeworm *E. granulosus* (surgery is the optimal treatment with albendazole given in pre- and post-surgical settings; 3 treatment courses most effective)

### Contraindications/cautions
- Contraindications: hypersensitivity to benzimidazole compounds; pregnancy (embryotoxic and teratogenic in preclinical studies; avoid use in pregnancy, do not become pregnant for at least 1 mo after therapy).
- Use cautiously with hepatic impairment, lactation.

### Dosage
**Available Forms:** Tablets—200 mg

ADULT
- *Hydatid disease:* >60 kg: 400 mg PO bid with meals for 28 d followed by 14 d with no abendazole, repeat for total of 3 cycles; <60 kg: 15 mg/kg/d PO in divided doses bid with meals for 28 d followed by 14 d with no abendazole, repeat for a total of 3 cycles.
- *Neurocysticercosis:* >60 kg: 400 mg PO bid with meals for 8–30 d; < 60 kg: 15 mg/kg/d PO in divided doses bid with meals for 8–30 d.

PEDIATRIC: Safety and efficacy for use in children <6 y not established.

### Pharmacokinetics

| Route | Onset | Peak |
|---|---|---|
| Oral | Slow | 2–5 h |

*Metabolism:* Hepatic; $T_{1/2}$: 8–12 h
*Distribution:* Crosses placenta; may pass into breast milk
*Excretion:* Feces and urine

### Adverse effects
- CNS: Headache, dizziness, vertigo
- GI: *Abnormal liver function tests; abdominal pain,* nausea, vomiting
- Hematologic: Neutropenia, leukopenia, **bone marrow depression**
- Renal: **Acute renal failure**
- Other: Fever, rash, reversible alopecia

### Clinically important drug-drug interactions
- Increased effects with dexamethasone, praziquantel, cimetidine; monitor for increased adverse effects

## ■ Nursing Considerations

### Assessment
- *History:* Allergy to benzimidazole compounds; pregnancy, hepatic impairment, lactation
- *Physical:* T; orientation; skin color, lesions; CBC, liver and renal function tests

### Implementation
- Give drug with food.
- Arrange for 3 courses of treatment for hydatid disease.

- Assure that patients with neurocysticercosis also receive appropriate steroid and anticonvulsant therapy as required.
- Alert patient to risk of fetal harm with drug; suggest use of barrier contraceptives during and for 1 mo after therapy.

**Drug-specific teaching points**

- Take this drug with food. Follow the cycle days carefully if taking drug for hydatid disease; mark calendar with drug and drug-free days.
- This drug can cause serious fetal harm; do not take while you are pregnant. Use of a barrier contraceptive is recommended during and for 1 mo after therapy.
- The following side effects may occur: nausea, vomiting (small, frequent meals may help); headache (use analgesics); dizziness (avoid driving or operating dangerous machinery).
- Report fever, bruising, infections, pregnancy.

## albumin, human

*(al* ***byoo'*** *min)*

normal serum albumin

*5%:* Albuminar-5, Albutein 5%, Buminate 5%, Plasbumin-5

*25%:* Albuminar-25, Albutein 25%, Buminate 25%, Plasbumin-25

**Pregnancy Category C**

**Drug classes**

Blood product
Plasma protein

**Therapeutic actions**

Normal blood protein; maintains plasma osmotic pressure and is important in maintaining normal blood volume

**Indications**

- Supportive treatment of shock due to burns, trauma, surgery, and infections
- Burns: albumin 5% used to prevent hemoconcentration and water and protein losses in conjunction with adequate infusions of crystalloid
- Hypoproteinemia in nephrotic syndrome, hepatic cirrhosis, toxemia of pregnancy, postoperative patients, tuberculous patients, premature infants
- Adult respiratory distress syndrome: albumin 25% with a diuretic may be helpful.
- Cardiopulmonary bypass: preoperative blood dilution with 25% albumin
- Acute liver failure
- Sequestration of protein-rich fluids
- Erythrocyte resuspension: albumin 25% may be added to the isotonic suspension of washed red cells immediately before transfusion.
- Acute nephrosis: albumin 25% and loop diuretic may help to control edema.
- Renal dialysis: albumin 25% may be useful in treatment of shock and hypotension
- Hyperbilirubinemia and erythroblastosis fetalis: adjunct in exchange transfusions

**Contraindications/cautions**

- Contraindications: allergy to albumin; severe anemia, cardiac failure, normal or increased intravascular volume, current use of cardiopulmonary bypass.
- Use cautiously with hepatic or renal failure.

**Dosage**

**Available Forms:** Injection—5%, 25%

Administer by IV infusion only; contains 130–160 mEq sodium/L.

**ADULT**

- *Hypovolemic shock:* 5% albumin: Initial dose of 500 ml given as rapidly as possible; additional 500 ml may be given in 30 min. Base therapy on clinical response if more than 1,000 ml is required; consider the need for whole blood. In patients with low blood volume, administer at rate of 2–4 ml/min. 25% albumin: Base therapy on clinical response. Administer as rapidly as tolerated; 1 ml/min may be given to patients with low blood volume.
- *Hypoproteinemia:* 5% albumin may be given for acute replacement of protein; if edema is present, use 25% albumin 50–75 g/d. Do not exceed 2 ml/min. Adjust the rate of infusion based on patient response.

- *Burns:* 5% or 25% albumin can be helpful in maintaining colloid osmotic pressure; suggested regimen has not been established.
- *Hepatic cirrhosis:* 25% may be effective in temporary restoration of plasma protein levels.
- *Nephrosis:* Initial dose of 100–200 ml of 25% albumin may be repeated at intervals of 1–2 d; effects are not sustained because of the underlying problem.

PEDIATRIC

- *Hypovolemic shock:* 50 ml of 5% albumin; base dosage on clinical response.
- *Hypoproteinemia:* 25 g/d of 25% albumin.
- *Hyperbilirubinemia and erythroblastosis fetalis:* 1 g/kg 1–2 h before transfusion, or 50 ml of albumin may be substituted for 50 ml of plasma in the blood to be transfused.

### Pharmacokinetics

*Metabolism:* Tissue, $T_{1/2}$: unknown
*Distribution:* Crosses placenta; passes into breast milk
*Excretion:* Urine

### IV facts

**Preparation:** Swab stopper top with antiseptic immediately before removing seal and entering the vial. Inspect for particulate matter and discoloration. Store at room temperature; do not freeze. Do not dilute 5% albumin; 25% albumin may be undiluted or diluted in Normal Saline.

**Infusion:** Give by IV infusion slowly enough to prevent rapid plasma volume expansion. Give in combination with or through the same administration set as solutions of saline or carbohydrates. Do not use with alcohol or protein hydrolysates—precipitates may form.

### Adverse effects

- CV: Hypotension, CHF, **pulmonary edema after rapid infusion**
- Hypersensitivity reactions: Fever, chills, *changes in blood pressure,* flushing, nausea, vomiting, changes in respiration, rashes

## ■ Nursing Considerations

### Assessment

- *History:* Allergy to albumin, severe anemia, CHF, current use of cardiopulmonary bypass, hepatic failure, renal failure
- *Physical:* Skin color, lesions; T; P, BP, peripheral perfusion; R, adventitious sounds; liver and renal function tests, Hct, serum electrolytes

### Implementation

- Give to all blood groups or types.
- Consider using whole blood; infusion provides only symptomatic relief of hypoproteinemia.
- Monitor BP; discontinue infusion if hypotension occurs.
- Stop infusion if headache, flushing, fever, changes in BP occur; treat reaction with antihistamines. If a plasma protein is still needed, try material from a different lot number.
- Monitor patient's clinical response, and adjust infusion rate accordingly.

### Drug-specific teaching points

- Report headache; nausea, vomiting; difficulty breathing; back pain.

## albuterol

*(al* ***byoo'*** *ter ole)*

albuterol sulfate

Salbutamol (CAN), Novo-Salmol (CAN), Proventil, Ventodisk (CAN), Ventolin, Volmax

**Pregnancy Category C**

### Drug classes

Sympathomimetic drug
Beta-2 selective adrenergic agonist
Bronchodilator
Antiasthmatic drug

### Therapeutic actions

In low doses, acts relatively selectively at $\beta_2$-adrenergic receptors to cause bronchodilation and vasodilation; at higher doses, $\beta_2$-selectivity is lost, and the drug acts at

$\beta_1$ receptors to cause typical sympathomimetic cardiac effects.

**Indications**

- Relief of bronchospasm in patients with reversible obstructive airway disease
- Prevention of exercise-induced bronchospasm
- Unlabeled use: adjunct in treating serious hyperkalemia in dialysis patients; seems to lower potassium concentrations when inhaled by patients on hemodialysis

**Contraindications/cautions**

- Contraindications: hypersensitivity to albuterol; tachyarrhythmias, tachycardia caused by digitalis intoxication; general anesthesia with halogenated hydrocarbons or cyclopropane (these sensitize the myocardium to catecholamines); unstable vasomotor system disorders; hypertension; coronary insufficiency, CAD; history of stroke; COPD patients with degenerative heart disease.
- Use cautiously with diabetes mellitus (large IV doses can aggravate diabetes and ketoacidosis); hyperthyroidism; history of seizure disorders; psychoneurotic individuals; labor and delivery (oral use has delayed second stage of labor; parenteral use of $\beta_2$-adrenergic agonists can accelerate fetal heart beat and cause hypoglycemia, hypokalemia, pulmonary edema in the mother and hypoglycemia in the neonate); lactation.

**Dosage**

**Available Forms:** Tablets—2, 4 mg; SR tablets—4 mg; syrup—2 mg/5 ml; aerosol—90 μg/actuation; solution for injection—0.083%, 0.5%; capsules for inhalation—200 μg

ADULT

- ***Oral:*** Initially, 2 or 4 mg (1–2 tsp syrup) tid–qid PO; may cautiously increase dosage if necessary to 4 or 8 mg qid, not to exceed 32 mg/d.
- ***Inhalation:*** Each actuation of aerosol dispenser delivers 90 μg albuterol. 2 inhalations q4–6h; some patients may require only 1 inhalation q4h; more frequent administration or larger number of inhalations not recommended.
  - ***Prevention of exercise-induced bronchospasm:*** 2 inhalations 15 min prior to exercise.

PEDIATRIC

- ***Oral, tablets***
  - ***12 years or older:*** Same as adult.
- ***Oral, syrup***
  - ***> 14 y:*** Same as adult.
  - ***6–14 y:*** 2 mg (1 tsp) tid–qid; if necessary, cautiously increase dosage. Do not exceed 24 mg/d in divided doses.
  - ***2–6 y:*** Initially, 0.1 mg/kg tid, not to exceed 2 mg (1 tsp) tid; if necessary, cautiously increase stepwise to 0.2 mg/kg tid. Do not exceed 4 mg (2 tsp) tid.
  - ***< 2 y:*** Safety and efficacy not established.
- ***Inhalation***
  - ***12 y or older:*** Same as adult.
  - ***< 12 y:*** Safety and efficacy not established.

GERIATRIC AND PATIENTS SENSITIVE TO BETA-ADRENERGIC STIMULATION: Restrict initial dose to 2 mg tid–qid; individualize dosage thereafter. Patients > 60 y are more likely to develop adverse effects.

**Pharmacokinetics**

| Route | Onset | Peak | Duration |
|---|---|---|---|
| Oral | 30 min | 2–2 1/2 h | 4–8 h |
| Inhalation | 5 min | 1 1/2–2 h | 3–8 h |

*Metabolism:* Hepatic, $T_{1/2}$: 2–4 h
*Distribution:* Crosses placenta; passes into breast milk
*Excretion:* Urine

**Adverse effects**

- CNS: *Restlessness, apprehension, anxiety, fear, CNS stimulation*, hyperkinesia, insomnia, tremor, drowsiness, irritability, weakness, vertigo, headache
- GI: *Nausea*, vomiting, heartburn, unusual or bad taste
- CV: *Cardiac arrhythmias,* tachycardia, palpitations, PVCs (rare), anginal pain
- **Respiratory**: Respiratory difficulties, pulmonary edema, coughing, bronchospasm, paradoxical airway resistance with

repeated, excessive use of inhalation preparations
- GU: Increased incidence of leiomyomas of uterus when given in higher than human doses in preclinical studies
- Dermatologic: *Sweating, pallor, flushing*

**Clinically important drug-drug interactions**
• Increased sympathomimetic effects with other sympathomimetic drugs • Increased risk of toxicity, especially cardiac, when used with theophylline, aminophylline, oxtriphylline • Decreased bronchodilating effects with beta-adrenergic blockers (eg, propranolol) • Decreased effectiveness of insulin, oral hypoglycemic drugs • Decreased serum levels and therapeutic effects of digoxin

## ■ Nursing Considerations

### Assessment
- *History:* Hypersensitivity to albuterol; tachyarrhythmias, tachycardia caused by digitalis intoxication; general anesthesia with halogenated hydrocarbons or cyclopropane; unstable vasomotor system disorders; hypertension; coronary insufficiency, CAD; history of stroke; COPD patients who have developed degenerative heart disease; diabetes mellitus; hyperthyroidism; history of seizure disorders; psychoneurotic individuals; lactation.
- *Physical:* Weight; skin color, temperature, turgor; orientation, reflexes, affect; P, BP; R, adventitious sounds; blood and urine glucose, serum electrolytes, thyroid function tests, ECG

### Implementation
- Use minimal doses for minimal periods; drug tolerance can occur with prolonged use.
- Maintain a beta-adrenergic blocker (cardioselective beta-blocker, such as atenolol, should be used with respiratory distress) on standby in case cardiac arrhythmias occur.
- Do not exceed recommended dosage; administer pressurized inhalation drug forms during second half of inspiration, because the airways are open wider, and the aerosol distribution is more extensive.

### Drug-specific teaching points
- Do not exceed recommended dosage; adverse effects or loss of effectiveness may result. Read the instructions that come with respiratory inhalant.
- The following may occur: dizzines, drowsiness, fatigue, headache (use caution if driving or performing tasks that require alertness); nausea, vomiting, change in taste (small, frequent meals may help); rapid heart rate, anxiety, sweating, flushing.
- Report chest pain, dizziness, insomnia, weakness, tremors or irregular heart beat, difficulty breathing, productive cough, failure to respond to usual dosage.

## aldesleukin

*(al des **loo'** ken)*

Interleukin-2, IL-2

Proleukin

**Pregnancy Category C**

**Drug classes**
Antineoplastic

**Therapeutic actions**
Human interleukin produced by *Escherichia coli* bacteria; activates human cellular immunity and inhibits tumor growth through increases in lymphocytes, platelets, and cytokines (tumor necrosis factor and interferon)

**Indications**
- Metastatic renal cell carcinoma in adults
- Treatment of adult patients with metastatic melanoma
- Unlabeled uses: treatment of Kaposi's sarcoma with zidovudine; treatment of metastatic melanoma with cyclophosphamide; treatment of non-Hodgkin's lymphoma with lymphokine-actived killer cells; treatment of phase I AIDS, advanced ARC with zidovudine

## Contraindications/cautions

- Contraindications: hypersensitivity to aldesleukin; abnormal thallium stress test; abnormal pulmonary function test; organ allografts; lactation.
- Use cautiously with renal, liver, or CNS impairment.

## Dosage

**Available Forms:** Powder for injection—22 X $10^6$ IU/vial

*ADULT:* Administer by 15 min IV infusion q8h.

- ***Metastatic renal cell carcinoma:*** Each course of treatment consists of two 5-d cycles of 600,000 IU/kg q8h IV over 15 min, separated by a rest, for a total of 14 doses, then 9 d of rest followed by 14 more doses. Treatment may be stopped because of toxicity.

*PEDIATRIC:* Safety not established.

## Pharmacokinetics

| *Route* | *Onset* | *Peak* | *Duration* |
|---|---|---|---|
| IV | 5 min | 13 min | 180–240 min |

*Metabolism:* Renal, $T_{1/2}$: 85 min
*Distribution:* Crosses placenta; passes into breast milk
*Excretion:* Urine

## IV facts

**Preparation:** Reconstitute each vial (22 million IU) with 1.2 ml Sterile Water for Injection, USP; direct the Sterile Water at the side of the vial, and swirl contents gently to avoid excess foaming; do not shake. Resultant liquid should be clear, colorless to yellow, and contain 18 million IU/ml. Use plastic, not glass, containers, and avoid in-filters while administering. Dilute in 50 ml of 5% Dextrose Injection, USP. Avoid dilution in bacteriostatic water or 0.9% Sodium Chloride Injection; aggregation can occur. Do not dilute with albumin; do not mix with any other drugs. Store vials in refrigerator before and after reconstitution; do not freeze. Administer within 48 h after reconstitution; discard any unused portions.

**Infusion:** Bring solution to room temperature before use; infuse over 15 min.
**Incompatibility:** Do not mix with other drugs.

## Adverse effects

- CNS: *Mental status changes, dizziness,* sensory dysfunction, syncope, headache, conjunctivitis
- GI: *Nausea, vomiting, diarrhea, stomatitis, anorexia,* **GI bleed**
- CV: **Capillary leak syndrome**—third spacing of fluids and severe hypotension, which may proceed to shock and death; *hypotension, sinus tachycardia, arrhythmias*
- Respiratory: *Respiratory difficulties, dyspnea,* pulmonary edema, coughing, bronchospasm
- Hematologic: *Anemia, thrombocytopenia, leukopenia,* coagulation disorders
- GU: *Oliguria/anuria,* proteinuria, hematuria
- Dermatologic: *Pruritus, erythema, rash,* dry skin, exudative dermatitis
- General: *Fever, chills, pain, fatigue, weakness, malaise, edema, infection*

## Clinically important drug-drug interactions

• Increased hypotensive effects with antihypertensives • Decreased effectiveness with corticosteroids • Increased toxicity of cardiotoxic, hepatotoxic, myelotoxic, and nephrotoxic agents: doxorubicin, methotrexate, asparaginase, aminoglycosides, indomethacin

## ■ Nursing Considerations

### Assessment

- ***History:*** Hypersensitivity to aldesleukin; abnormal thallium stress test, pulmonary function test; organ allografts; lactation; renal, liver, or CNS impairment
- ***Physical:*** Weight; skin color, temperature, turgor; orientation, reflexes, affect; P, BP; R, adventitious sounds; bowel sounds; CBC, serum electrolytes, thyroid, liver and renal function tests; ECG, stress test, pulmonary function tests

### Implementation

- Give only in intensive care settings with emergency life support available.
- Ensure that patient has normal thallium stress test and normal pulmonary function tests, including baseline blood gases, before giving drug.
- Monitor patient, watching vital signs, weight, cardiac monitoring (if BP falls), respiratory sounds, and pulse oximetry; cardiac sounds and perfusion evaluation; orientation.
- Caution patient to use birth control methods during drug use; nursing patients should select another method of feeding baby.
- Monitor patient for signs of infection; advise patient to avoid exposure to many people or to contagious diseases.
- Stop drug if patient becomes disoriented, somnolent or very lethargic; continued use could result in a coma.
- Stop drug if severe side effects occur (arrhythmias, hypotension, chest pain, oliguria, liver failure, bullous dermatitis); drug may be restarted if a period of rest returns affected systems to normal.

### Drug-specific teaching points

- This drug is given in 5-d cycles with a period of rest (9 wk) to allow the body to recover. This drug can only be given IV, and you will need to be closely monitored while it is given.
- You will need to have many tests to evaluate the effects of this drug and the advisability of continuing treatment.
- Avoid exposure to any infections or contagious diseases (eg, crowds); you will be more susceptible to infection.
- The following side effects may occur: fever, chills, rash, fluid retention, difficulty breathing, nausea, vomiting, diarrhea.
- Report chest pain, dizziness, weakness, irregular heart beat, difficulty breathing, swelling, fever, malaise, fatigue, changes in stool or urine color.

## alendronate sodium

*(ah **len'** dro nate)*

Fosamax

**Pregnancy Category C**

### Drug classes

Calcium regulator

### Therapeutic actions

Slows normal and abnormal bone resorption without inhibiting bone formation and mineralization.

### Indications

- Treatment of osteoporosis in postmenopausal women
- Treatment of Paget's disease of bone in patients with alkaline phosphatase at least two times upper limit of normal, those who are symptomatic, those at risk for future complications

### Contraindications/cautions

- Contraindications: allergy to biphosphonates; hypocalcemia, pregnancy, lactation.
- Use cautiously with renal dysfunction, upper GI disease.

### Dosage

**Available Forms:** Tablets—10, 40 mg

*ADULT*

- ***Postmenopausal osteoporosis:*** 10 mg/d PO in AM with full glass of water, at least 30 min before other beverage, food, or medication.
- ***Paget's disease:*** 40 mg/d PO in AM with full glass of water, at least 30 min before other beverage, food, or medication for 6 mo; may retreat after 6-mo treatment-free period.
- ***Unlabeled Use:*** Prevention of osteoporosis in premenopausal women, 5 mg PO qd.

*PEDIATRIC:* Safety and efficacy not established.

*RENAL IMPAIRED:* Dosage adjustment not necessary for Ccr 35–60 ml/min; not recommended if Ccr <35 ml/min.

### Pharmacokinetics

| Route | Onset | Duration |
|---|---|---|
| PO | Slow | Days |

*Metabolism:* Not metabolized

*Distribution:* Crosses placenta; may enter breast milk

*Excretion:* Urine

**Adverse effects**
- CNS: *Headache*
- GI: *Nausea, diarrhea*
- Skeletal: *Increased or recurrent bone pain,* focal osteomalacia

**Clinically important drug-drug interactions**
- Increased risk of GI distress with aspirin
- Decreased absorption if taken with antacids, calcium, iron, multivalent cations; separate dosing by at least 30 min

**Clinically important drug-food interactions**
- Significantly decreased absorption and serum levels if taken with food; separate dosing from food and beverage by at least 30 min

## ■ Nursing Considerations

### Assessment
- *History:* Allergy to biphosphonates, renal failure, upper GI disease, lactation
- *Physical:* Muscle tone, bone pain; bowel sounds; urinalysis, serum calcium

### Implementation
- Give in AM with full glass of water at least 30 min before any beverage, food, or medication.
- Monitor serum calcium levels before, during, and after therapy.
- Recommend concomitant hormone replacement therapy in treatment of osteoporosis.
- Ensure 6-mo rest period after treatment for Paget's disease if retreatment is required.
- Ensure adequate vitamin D and calcium intake.
- Provide comfort measures if bone pain returns.

### Drug-specific teaching points
- Take drug in morning with a full glass of plain water (not mineral water), at least 30 min before any beverage, food, or medication.
- The following side effects may occur: nausea, diarrhea; bone pain, headache (analgesic may help).
- Report twitching, muscle spasms, dark-colored urine, severe diarrhea.

## alglucerase

*(al **gloo'** sir ace)*
Ceredase
**Pregnancy Category C**

**Drug classes**
Enzyme

**Therapeutic actions**
Modified form of a naturally occurring human enzyme that is essential for the breakdown of glucocerebroside, a breakdown product of membrane lipids.

**Indications**
- Long-term enzyme replacement therapy for patients with type 1 Gaucher's disease who have moderate-to-severe anemia, thrombocytopenia, bone disease, hepatomegaly, splenomegaly

**Contraindications/cautions**
- Contraindicated in the presence of hypersensitivity to alglucerase.
- Use caution during lactation.

### Dosage
**Available Forms:** Injection—10 U/ml$^2$, 80 U/ml$^2$
*ADULT:* Administer by IV infusion over 1–2 h. Initial dosage of 60 U/kg per infusion, repeated every 2–4 wk depending on response. Dosage may be lowered every 3–6 mo.
*PEDIATRIC:* Safety and efficacy not established.

**Pharmacokinetics**

| *Route* | *Onset* | *Peak* | *Duration* |
|---|---|---|---|
| IV | 3–5 min | 10–15 min | 60 min |

*Metabolism:* $T_{1/2}$: 3–10 min

**IV facts**
**Preparation:** Dilute dose with Normal Saline to a final volume not to exceed 100 ml. Do not shake; shaking may render the drug inactive. Refrigerate; do not

use any bottle with particulate matter or discoloration or after expiration date. Discard any unused portion.
**Infusion:** Infuse over 1–2 h; use an in-line particulate filter.

### Adverse effects

- CNS: Fever, chills
- GI: Nausea, vomiting, abdominal discomfort
- **Local**: Discomfort, swelling, burning and swelling at venipuncture site

## ■ Nursing Considerations

### Assessment

- *History:* Sensitivity to alglucerase, lactation
- *Physical:* Venipuncture site, abdominal exam, CBC, bone density evaluation

### Implementation

- Explain risk of viral infection when using blood products. Assure patient that side effects are usually transient.
- Monitor response to establish most convenient and effective treatment schedule.
- Monitor IV site for signs of irritation.

### Drug-specific teaching points

- Drug must be given IV, and the schedule will be determined by your response and convenience; drug replaces an enzyme that is missing in your body and will need to be taken long-term.
- The following side effects may occur: abdominal discomfort, nausea, vomiting, discomfort at injection site.
- Report swelling, burning at injection site.

# allopurinol

*(al oh **pure'** i nole)*
Lopurin, Purinol (CAN), Zyloprim
**Pregnancy Category C**

### Drug classes

Antigout drug

### Therapeutic actions

Inhibits the enzyme responsible for the conversion of purines to uric acid, thus reducing the production of uric acid with a decrease in serum and sometimes in urinary uric acid levels, relieving the signs and symptoms of gout

### Indications

- Management of the signs and symptoms of primary and secondary gout
- Management of patients with malignancies that result in elevations of serum and urinary uric acid
- Management of patients with recurrent calcium oxalate calculi whose daily uric acid excretion exceeds 800 mg/d (males) or 750 mg/d (females)
- Orphan drug use: treatment of Chagas' disease; cutaneous and visceral leishmaniasis

### Contraindications/cautions

- Contraindications: allergy to allopurinol, blood dyscrasias.
- Use cautiously with liver disease, renal failure, lactation, pregnancy.

### Dosage

**Available Forms:** Tablets—100, 300 mg

**ADULT**

- *Gout and hyperuricemia:* 100–800 mg/d PO in divided doses, depending on the severity of the disease (200–300 mg/d is usual dose). *Maintenance:* Establish dose that maintains serum uric acid levels within normal limits.
- *Prevention of acute gouty attacks:* 100 mg/d PO; increase the dose by 100 mg at weekly intervals until uric acid levels are within normal limits.
- *Prevention of uric acid nephropathy in certain malignancies:* 600–800 mg/d for 2–3 d; maintenance dose should then be established as above.
- *Recurrent calcium oxalate stones:* 200–300 mg/d PO; adjust dose up or down based on 24-h urinary urate determinations.

**PEDIATRIC**

- *Secondary hyperuricemia associated with various malignancies: 6–10 y:* 300 mg/d PO. *<6 y:* 150 mg/d; adjust dosage after 48 h of treatment based on serum uric acid levels.

*GERIATRIC OR RENAL IMPAIRED:* Geriatric or renal-impaired creatine clearance 10–20 ml/min–200 mg/d; CCr <10 ml/min–100 mg/d; CCr <3 ml/min–intervals between doses will need to be extended, based on patient's serum uric acid levels.

### Adverse effects

- CNS: *Headache, drowsiness,* peripheral neuropathy, neuritis, paresthesias
- GI: *Nausea, vomiting, diarrhea,* abdominal pain, gastritis, hepatomegaly, hyperbilirubinemia, cholestatic jaundice
- Hematologic: Anemia, leukopenia, agranulocytosis, thrombocytopenia, aplastic anemia, bone marrow depression
- GU: Exacerbation of gout and renal calculi, renal failure
- Dermatologic: **Rashes—*maculopapular*, scaly or exfoliative—sometimes fatal**

### Clinically important drug-drug interactions

• Increased risk of hypersensitivity reaction with ACE inhibitors • Increased toxicity with thiazide diuretics • Increased risk of skin rash with ampicillin • Increased risk of bone marrow suppression with cyclophosphamide, other cytotoxic agents • Increased half-life of oral anticoagulants • Increased serum levels of theophylline, 6-MP (azathioprine dose and dose of 6-MP should be reduced to one-third to one-fourth the usual dose)

## ■ Nursing Considerations

### Assessment

- *History:* Allergy to allopurinol, blood dyscrasias, liver disease, renal failure, lactation
- *Physical:* Skin lesions, color; orientation, reflexes; liver evaluation, normal urinary output; normal output; CBC, renal and liver function tests, urinalysis

### Implementation

- Administer drug following meals.
- Force fluids—2.5 to 3.0 L/d to decrease the risk of renal stone development.
- Check urine alkalinity—urates crystallize in acid urine; sodium bicarbonate or potassium citrate may be ordered to alkalinize urine.
- Arrange for regular medical follow-up and blood tests.

### Drug-specific teaching points

- Take the drug following meals.
- The following side effects may occur: exacerbation of gouty attack or renal stones (drink plenty of fluids while on this drug, 2.5–3 L/d); nausea, vomiting, loss of appetite (take after meals or eat small frequent meals); drowsiness (use caution while driving or performing hazardous tasks).
- Avoid OTC medications. Many of these preparations contain vitamin C or other agents that might increase the likelihood of kidney stone formation. If you need an OTC preparation, check with your health care provider.
- Report skin rash; unusual bleeding or bruising; fever, chills; gout attack; numbness or tingling; flank pain.

# alpha$_1$-proteinase inhibitor (human)

Prolastin

**Pregnancy Category C**

### Drug classes

Blood product

### Therapeutic actions

A human enzyme that inhibits neutrophil elastase, an enzyme that degrades the elastin tissue essential for maintaining lung integrity; failure to replace the enzyme in deficient patients results in slowly progressive, severe, panacinar emphysema.

### Indications

- Congenital alpha$_1$-antitrypsin deficiency; chronic replacement in adults with early evidence of panacinar emphysema.

### Contraindications/cautions

- CHF (risk of circulatory overload), hepatitis

### Dosage

**Available Forms:** Injection—20 mg/ml

*ADULT:* 60 mg/kg IV once a week to increase and maintain a level of functional alpha$_1$-proteinase inhibitor in the lower respiratory tract.

*PEDIATRIC:* Safety and efficacy not established.

### Pharmacokinetics

| *Route* | *Onset* | *Duration* |
|---|---|---|
| IV | Slow | Weeks |

*Metabolism:* Intravascular, $T_{1/2}$: 4.5–5.2 d

*Distribution:* Crosses placenta; enters breast milk

#### IV facts

**Preparation:** Reconstitute with provided solution; administer within 3 h of reconstitution; refrigerate, avoid freezing; do not refrigerate after reconstitution; may reconstitute with Normal Saline if necessary.

**Infusion:** Administer alone; do not mix with other agents or diluting solutions. May be given at rate of 0.08 ml/kg/min or greater.

| *Body weight (lb/kg)* | *Dosage (mg)* | *IV rate (ml/min)* |
|---|---|---|
| 75/34 | 2040 | 2.7 |
| 90/41 | 2460 | 3.3 |
| 105/48 | 2880 | 3.8 |
| 120/55 | 3300 | 4.4 |
| 135/61 | 3660 | 4.9 |
| 150/68 | 4080 | 5.5 |
| 165/75 | 4500 | 6.0 |
| 180/82 | 4920 | 6.5 |
| 195/89 | 5340 | 7.1 |
| 210/96 | 5760 | 7.6 |
| 225/102 | 6120 | 8.2 |
| 240/109 | 6540 | 8.7 |

### Adverse effects

- CNS: Lightheadedness, dizziness
- GI: **Hepatitis** (prepared from pools of human blood products)
- CV: *Circulatory overload*, CHF, hypertension, palpitations
- Other: Fever, usually within first 24 h of treatment

## ■ Nursing Considerations

### Assessment

- ***History:*** CHF, hepatitis
- ***Physical:*** T; P, BP, perfusion; R, adventitious sounds; liver evaluation; liver function tests, HBsAg, respiratory function tests, HIV antibody screen

### Implementation

- Arrange for immunization against hepatitis B using a hepatitis B vaccine before treatment.
- Arrange for administration of single dose of hepatitis B immune globulin, 0.06 ml/kg IM, with initial dose of hepatitis B vaccine if alpha$_1$-proteinase inhibitor is needed before the required waiting time for full immunization with hepatitis B vaccine.
- Monitor T for first few hours of treatment; monitor for signs of circulatory overload: tachycardia, $S_3$, edema, rapid respirations, elevated JVP.
- Arrange for periodic screening for liver function, hepatitis B, and HIV exposure.

### Drug-specific teaching points

- Drug must be given IV. Weekly treatment will be needed to maintain drug level in lung.
- There is a risk of hepatitis and AIDS when receiving blood products. Blood products are carefully screened but some risk remains. Immunization with hepatitis B vaccine is required to eliminate some risk.
- The following side effects may occur: fever (this usually passes within a few hours); lightheadedness, dizziness
- Report shortness of breath, palpitations or irregular heart beats, fever, chills, sore throat, unusual bleeding or bruising.

## alprazolam

*(al **pray'** zoe lam)*

Apo-Alpraz (CAN), Novo-Alprazol (CAN), Nu-Alpraz (CAN), Xanax

**Pregnancy Category D**
**C-IV controlled substance**

**Drug classes**
Benzodiazepine
Antianxiety drug

**Therapeutic actions**
Exact mechanisms of action not understood; main sites of action may be the limbic system and reticular formation; increases the effects of gamma-aminobutyrate, an inhibitory neurotransmitter; anxiety blocking effects occur at doses well below those necessary to cause sedation, ataxia.

**Indications**
- Management of anxiety disorders, short-term relief of symptoms of anxiety; anxiety associated with depression.
- Treatment of panic attacks with or without agoraphobia
- Unlabeled uses: social phobia, premenstrual syndrome, depression

**Contraindications/cautions**
- Contraindications: hypersensitivity to benzodiazepines, psychoses, acute narrow-angle glaucoma, shock, coma, acute alcoholic intoxication with depression of vital signs, pregnancy (crosses the placenta; risk of congenital malformations, neonatal withdrawal syndrome), labor and delivery ("floppy infant" syndrome), lactation (secreted in breast milk; infants become lethargic and lose weight).
- Use cautiously with impaired liver or kidney function, debilitation.

**Dosage**
**Available Forms:** Tablets—0.25, 0.5, 1, 2 mg
Individualize dosage; increase dosage gradually to avoid adverse effects.

ADULT
- *Anxiety disorders:* Initially, 0.25–0.5 mg PO tid; titrate to maximum daily dose of 4 mg/d in divided doses.
- *Panic disorder:* Initially 0.5 mg PO tid; increase dose at 3- to 4-d intervals in increments of no more than 1 mg/d; ranges of 1–10 mg/d have been needed.
- *Social phobia:* 2–8 mg/d PO.
- *Premenstrual syndrome:* 0.25 mg PO tid.

GERIATRIC PATIENTS OR THOSE WITH DEBILITATING DISEASE: Initially 0.25 mg bid–tid; gradually increase if needed and tolerated.

**Pharmacokinetics**

| *Route* | *Onset* | *Peak* | *Duration* |
|---|---|---|---|
| Oral | 30 min | 1–2 h | 4–6 h |

*Metabolism:* Hepatic, $T_{1/2}$: 6.3–26.9 h
*Distribution:* Crosses placenta; passes into breast milk
*Excretion:* Urine

**Adverse effects**
- CNS: *Transient, mild drowsiness initially; sedation, depression, lethargy, apathy, fatigue, lightheadedness, disorientation, anger, hostility,* episodes of mania and hypomania, *restlessness, confusion, crying,* delirium, *headache,* slurred speech, dysarthria, stupor, rigidity, tremor, dystonia, vertigo, euphoria, nervousness, difficulty in concentration, vivid dreams, psychomotor retardation, extrapyramidal symptoms; *mild paradoxical excitatory reactions, during first 2 weeks of treatment*
- GI: *Constipation, diarrhea, dry mouth,* salivation, *nausea,* anorexia, vomiting, difficulty in swallowing, gastric disorders, hepatic dysfunction
- CV: Bradycardia, tachycardia, cardiovascular collapse, hypertension, hypotension, palpitations, edema
- **Hematologic**: Elevations of blood enzymes—LDH, alkaline phosphatase, SGOT, SGPT; blood dyscrasias—agranulocytosis, leukopenia
- GU: Incontinence, urinary retention, changes in libido, menstrual irregularities
- **Dermatologic**: Urticaria, pruritus, skin rash, dermatitis
- **EENT**: Visual and auditory disturbances, diplopia, nystagmus, depressed hearing, nasal congestion

- **Other**: Hiccups, fever, diaphoresis, paresthesias, muscular disturbances, gynecomastia. *Drug dependence with withdrawal syndrome when drug is discontinued; more common with abrupt discontinuation of higher dosage used for longer than 4 mo.*

**Clinically important drug-drug interactions**

• Increased CNS depression with alcohol, other CNS depressants, propoxyphene • Increased effect with cimetidine, disulfiram, omeprazole, isoniazid, oral contraceptives, valproic acid • Decreased effect with carbamazepine, rifampin, theophylline • Possible increased risk of digitalis toxicity with digoxin • Decreased antiparkinson effectiveness of levodopa with benzodiazepines • Contraindicated with ketoconazole, itraconazole; serious toxicity can occur

## ■ Nursing Considerations

### Assessment

- *History:* Hypersensitivity to benzodiazepines; psychoses; acute narrow-angle glaucoma; shock; coma; acute alcoholic intoxication with depression of vital signs; labor and delivery; lactation; impaired liver or kidney function; debilitation.
- *Physical:* Skin color, lesions; T; orientation, reflexes, affect, ophthalmologic exam; P, BP; liver evaluation, abdominal exam, bowel sounds, normal output; CBC, liver and renal function tests

### Implementation

- Arrange to taper dosage gradually after long-term therapy, especially in epileptic patients.

### Drug-specific teaching points

- Take this drug exactly as prescribed.
- Do not stop taking drug (long-term therapy) without consulting health care provider.
- Avoid alcohol, sleep-inducing, or OTC drugs.
- The following side effects may occur: drowsiness, dizziness (less pronounced after a few days, avoid driving a car or engaging in other dangerous activities if these occur); GI upset (take drug with food); fatigue; depression; dreams; crying; nervousness.
- Report severe dizziness, weakness, drowsiness that persists, rash or skin lesions, difficulty voiding, palpitations, swelling in the extremities.

## alprostadil

*(al **pross'** ta dil)*

PGE$_1$

*IV:* Prostin VR Pediatric

*Intracavernous:* Caverject, Edex, MUSE

**Pregnancy Category (not applicable)**

**Drug classes**

Prostaglandin

**Therapeutic actions**

Relaxes vascular smooth muscle; the smooth muscle of the ductus arteriosus is especially sensitive to this action and will relax and stay open; this is beneficial in infants who have congenital defects that restrict pulmonary or systemic blood flow and who depend on a patent ductus arteriosus for adequate blood oxygenation and lower body perfusion. Treatment of erectile dysfunction due to neurogenic, vasculogenic, psychogenic, or mixed etiology.

**Indications**

- Palliative therapy to temporarily maintain the patency of the ductus arteriosus until corrective or palliative surgery can be performed in neonates with congenital heart defects who depend on a patent ductus (eg, pulmonary atresia or stenosis, tetralogy of Fallot, coarctation of the aorta)
- Treatment of erectile dysfunction (intracavernous injection)

**Contraindications/cautions**

- Contraindications: respiratory distress syndrome; conditions that might predispose to priapism, deformation of the penis, penile implants (intracavernous injection).

- Use caution in the presence of bleeding tendencies (drug inhibits platelet aggregation).

## Dosage

**Available Forms:** Powder for injection—6.15, 11.9, 23.2 μg; pellets—125, 250, 500, 1000 μg; injection (IV)—500 μg/ml; injection (penile)—5, 10, 20, 40 μg/vial

Preferred administration is through a continuous IV infusion into a large vein; may be administered through an umbilical artery catheter placed at the ductal opening. Begin infusion with 0.1 μg/kg per minute. After an increase in $Po_2$ or in systemic BP and blood pH is achieved, reduce infusion to the lowest possible dosage that maintains the response (often achieved by reducing dosage from 0.1–0.05 to 0.025–0.01 μg/kg per minute). Up to 0.4 μg/kg per minute may be used for maintenance if required; higher dosage rates are not more effective.

- ***Intracavernous injection:*** 0.2–140 μg by intracavernous injection using 1/2-in 27–30 gauge needle; may be repeated up to 3× weekly. Self injection over 6-mo period has been successful. Reduce dose if erection lasts > 1 h.

## Pharmacokinetics

| *Route* | *Onset* | *Peak* |
|---|---|---|
| IV | 5–25 min | — |
| Intracavernous | 10 min | 30–60 min |

*Metabolism:* Lungs, $T_{1/2}$: 5–10 min
*Excretion:* Urine

## IV facts

**Preparation:** Prepare solution by diluting 500 μg alprostadil with Sodium Chloride Injection or Dextrose Injection; dilute to volumes required for pump delivery system. Discard and prepare fresh infusion solutions q24h; refrigerate drug ampules.

**Infusion:**

| *Add 500 mg Alprostadil to* | *Approx. Concentration of Resulting Solution* | *Infusion Rate (ml/min/kg)* |
|---|---|---|
| 250 ml | 2 mcg/ml | 0.05 |
| 100 ml | 5 mcg/ml | 0.02 |
| 50 ml | 10 mcg/ml | 0.01 |
| 25 ml | 20 mcg/ml | 0.005 |

## Adverse effects

- CNS: *Seizures,* cerebral bleeding, hypothermia, jitteriness, lethargy, stiffness
- GI: Diarrhea
- CV: *Bradycardia, flushing, tachycardia, hypotension,* cardiac arrest, heart block, CHF
- **Respiratory:** *Apnea,* respiratory distress
- **Hematologic:** Inhibited platelet aggregation, bleeding, anemia, disseminated intravascular coagulation, hypokalemia
- **Other:** Cortical proliferation of the long bones (with prolonged use, regresses after treatment is stopped), sepsis
- GU (with intracavernous injection): Penile pain, rash, **fibrosis,** erection, priapism.

## ■ Nursing Considerations

### Assessment

- *History:* Respiratory distress, bleeding tendencies
- *Physical:* T; cyanosis; skeletal development, reflexes, state of agitation, arterial pressure (using auscultation or Doppler), P, auscultation, peripheral perfusion; R, adventitious sounds, bleeding times, arterial blood gases, blood pH

### Implementation

*IV*

- Constantly monitor arterial pressure; decrease infusion rate immediately if any fall in arterial pressure occurs.
- Regularly monitor arterial blood gases to determine efficacy of alprostadil ($PO_2$ in infants with restricted pulmonary flow; pH and systemic blood pressure in infants with restricted systemic flow).

*Intracavernous*

- Reconstitute vial with 1 ml diluent. I ml of solution will contain 10.5–20.5 μg of alprostadil.
- Use solution immediately after reconstitution; do not store or freeze.
- Inject along dorsal-lateral aspect of proximal third of penis using sterile technique.

## Drug-specific teaching points

*IV*

Teaching about this drug should be incorporated into a total teaching program for the parent(s) of the infant with a cyanotic congential heart defect; specifics about the drug that they will need to know include:

- Your infant will be continually monitored and have frequent blood tests to follow the effects of the drug.
- The baby may look better, breathe easier, become fussy, and so forth, but the drug treatment is only a temporary solution, and the baby will require corrective surgery.

*Intracavernous*

- Learn and repeat self-injection technique. Do not self-inject >3×/wk; wait at least 24 hr between injections.
- Return for regular medical follow-up and evaluation.
- The following side effects may occur: penile pain, swelling, rash.
- Report prolonged erection, swelling, or pain.

# alteplase, recombinant (tissue-type plasminogen activator)

*(al ti **plaze'**)*

rt-PA (recombinant tissue plasminogen activator), TPA

Activase

**Pregnancy Category C**

## Drug classes

Thrombolytic enzyme

## Therapeutic actions

Human tissue enzyme produced by recombinant DNA techniques; converts plasminogen to the enzyme plasmin (fibrinolysin), which degrades fibrin clots; lyses thrombi and emboli; is most active at the site of the clot and causes little systemic fibrinolysis.

## Indications

- Treatment of coronary artery thrombosis associated with acute MI
- Treatment of acute, massive pulmonary embolism in adults
- Treatment of acute ischemic stroke
- Unlabeled use: treatment of unstable angina

## Contraindications/cautions

- Contraindications: allergy to TPA; active internal bleeding,; recent (within 2 mo) CVA; intracranial or intraspinal surgery or neoplasm; recent major surgery, obstetric delivery, organ biopsy, or rupture of a noncompressible blood vessel; recent serious GI bleed; recent serious trauma, including CPR; SBE; hemostatic defects; cerebrovascular disease; early-onset, insulin-dependent diabetes; septic thrombosis; severe uncontrolled hypertension.
- Use cautiously with liver disease, old age (> 75 y—risk of bleeding may be increased).

## Dosage

**Available Forms:** Powder for injection—50, 100 mg

Careful patient assessment and evaluation are needed to determine the appropriate dose of this drug. Because experience is limited with this drug, careful monitoring is essential.

### ADULT

- *Acute MI:* Total dose of 100 mg IV given as follows: 60 mg the first hour, with an initial bolus of 6–10 mg given over 1–2 min and the rest infused slowly over the rest of the hour; then 20 mg infused slowly over the second hour and 20 mg more infused slowly over the third hour. For patients weighing less than 65 kg, decrease total dose to 1.25 mg/kg. **Do not use a total dose of 150 mg because of the increased risk of intracranial bleeding.**
- *Pulmonary embolism:* 100 mg administered by IV infusion over 2 h, followed immediately by heparin therapy.
- *Acute ischemic stroke:* 0.9 mg/kg infused over 60 mm with 10% given as an IV bolus over the first 1 min

### Pharmacokinetics

| Route | Onset | Peak | Duration |
|---|---|---|---|
| IV | Immediate | 5–10 min | 2 1/2–3 h |

*Metabolism:* $T_{1/2}$: 26 min
*Distribution:* Crosses placenta
*Excretion:* Cleared by the liver

#### IV facts

**Preparation:** Do not use if vacuum is not present; add volume of the Sterile Water for Injection provided with vial using a large bore needle and directing stream into the cake; slight foaming may occur but will dissipate after standing undisturbed for several minutes; reconstitute immediately before use. Refrigerate reconstituted solution and use within 3 h. Do not use Bacteriostatic Water for Injection. Reconstituted solution should be colorless or pale yellow and transparent; contains 1 mg/ml with a pH of 7.3.

**Infusion:** Administer as reconstituted or further dilute with an equal volume of 0.9% Sodium Chloride Injection or 5% Dextrose Injection to yield 0.5 mg/ml; stable for up to 8 h in these solutions. Avoid excessive agitation; mix by gentle swirling or slow inversion. Discard unused solution.

**Compatibilities:** Do not add other medications to infusion solution; use 0.9% Sodium Chloride Injection or 5% Dextrose Injection and no other solutions.

### Adverse effects

- CV: Cardiac arrhythmias with coronary reperfusion, hypotension
- Hematologic: *Bleeding*—particularly at venous or arterial access sites, GI bleeding, intracranial hemorrhage
- Other: Urticaria, nausea, vomiting, fever

### Clinically important drug-drug interactions

- Increased risk of hemorrhage if used with heparin or oral anticoagulants, aspirin, dipyridamole

## ■ Nursing Considerations

### Assessment

- *History:* Allergy to TPA; active internal bleeding; recent (within 2 mo) obstetric delivery, organ biopsy, or rupture of a noncompressible blood vessel; recent serious GI bleed; recent serious trauma, including CPR; SBE; hemostatic defects; cerebrovascular disease; early-onset insulin-dependent diabetes; septic thrombosis; severe uncontrolled hypertension; liver disease
- *Physical:* Skin color, temperature, lesions; orientation, reflexes; P, BP, peripheral perfusion, baseline ECG; R, adventitous sounds; liver evaluation, Hct, platelet count, TT, APTT, PT

### Implementation

- Discontinue heparin and alteplase if serious bleeding occurs.
- Monitor coagulation studies; PT or APPT should be less than 2X control.
- Apply pressure or pressure dressings to control superficial bleeding (at invaded or disturbed areas).
- Avoid arterial invasive procedures.
- Type and cross-match blood in case serious blood loss occurs and whole blood transfusions are required.
- Institute treatment within 6 h of onset of symptoms for evolving myocardial infarction, within 3 h of onset of stroke.

### Drug-specific teaching points

- This drug can only be given IV. You will be closely monitored during drug treatment.
- Report difficulty breathing, dizziness, disorientation, headache, numbness, tingling.

## altretamine

*(al **tret'** a meen)*
hexamethylmelamine
Hexalen
**Pregnancy Category D**

**Drug classes**
Antineoplastic

**Therapeutic actions**
Cytotoxic; mechanisms by which it is able to cause cell death are not known.

**Indications**
- Single agent in the palliative treatment of persistent or recurrent ovarian cancer following first-line therapy with a cisplatin or alkylating agent-based combination

**Contraindications/cautions**
- Hypersensitivity to altretamine, bone marrow depression, severe neurologic toxicity, lactation.

**Dosage**
**Available Forms:** Capsules—50 mg
*ADULT:* Dosage is determined by body surface area.
260 mg/m$^2$ per day PO given for 14 or 21 consecutive days in a 28-d cycle. Total daily dose is given as divided doses after meals and hs.
Temporarily discontinue altretamine for > 14 days if GI intolerance, WBC < 2,000/mm$^3$ or granuloctyes < 1,000/mm$^3$, platelet count < 75,000/mm$^3$, or progressive neuropathy occurs; restart with 200 mg/m$^2$ per day.

**Pharmacokinetics**

| Route | Onset | Peak |
|---|---|---|
| Oral | Rapid | 1/2–3 h |

*Metabolism:* Hepatic, $T_{1/2}$: 4.7–10 h
*Distribution:* Crosses placenta; passes into breast milk
*Excretion:* Urine

**Adverse effects**
- CNS: **Peripheral sensory neuropathy** (mild to severe); fatigue, seizures
- GI: *Nausea, vomiting*, increased alkaline phosphatase, anorexia
- GU: Increased BUN
- Hematologic: **Bone marrow depression**
- Other: Carcinogenesis, impairment of fertility, mutagenesis

**Clinically important drug-drug interactions**
- Increased effects with cimetidine • Increased risk of postural hypotension with MAO inhibitors

## ■ Nursing Considerations

### Assessment
- *History:* Hypersensitivity to altretamine; bone marrow depression; severe neurologic toxicity; lactation
- *Physical:* Neurologic status, T, abdominal exam, kidney and liver function tests, CBC

### Implementation
- Give drug with meals and at bedtime.
- Discontinue drug if GI effects are intractable; severe neuropathy occurs; bone marrow depression becomes dangerous. Reevaluate patient, and consider restarting drug after up to 14 d of rest.
- Arrange for blood counts before and at least monthly during treatment.
- Monitor neurologic status frequently.
- Consider antiemetics or decreased dose if nausea and vomiting are severe.

### Drug-specific teaching points
- Take drug with meals and at bedtime.
- Arrange to have regular blood tests and neurologic exams while on drug.
- The following side effects may occur: nausea and vomiting (this may be severe; antiemetics may help and can be ordered for you; small, frequent meals also may help); weakness, lethargy (frequent rest periods may help); increased susceptibility to infection (avoid crowds and situations that might involve exposure to many people or diseases); numbness and tingling in the fingers or toes (use care to avoid injury to these areas; use care if trying to perform tasks that require precision).
- Report severe nausea and vomiting; fever, chills, sore throat; unusual bleeding or

bruising; numbness or tingling in your fingers or toes.

## Aluminum preparations

### aluminum carbonate gel, basic

*(a loo' mi num)*

Basaljel

### aluminum hydroxide gel

ALternaGEL, Alu-Cap, Alu-Tab, Amphojel

**Pregnancy Category C**

#### Drug classes

Antacid

#### Therapeutic actions

Neutralizes or reduces gastric acidity, resulting in an increase in the pH of the stomach and duodenal bulb and inhibiting the proteolytic activity of pepsin, which protects the lining of the stomach and duodenum; binds with phosphate ions in the intestine to form insoluble aluminum-phosphate complexes, lowering phosphate in hyperphosphatemia and chronic renal failure but may cause hypophosphatemia in other states.

#### Indications

- Symptomatic relief of upset stomach associated with hyperacidity
- Hyperacidity associated with peptic ulcer, gastritis, peptic esophagitis, gastric hyperacidity, hiatal hernia
- Treatment, control, or management of hyperphosphatemia — aluminum carbonate
- Prevention of formation of phosphate urinary stones, used in conjunction with a low-phosphate diet — aluminum carbonate
- Unlabeled use for aluminum hydroxide: prophylaxis of GI bleeding, stress ulcer; reduction of phosphate absorption in hyperphosphatemia in patients with chronic renal failure

#### Contraindications/cautions

- Allergy to aluminum products, gastric outlet destruction, hypertension, CHF, hypophosphatemia, lactation

#### Dosage

**Available Forms:** Aluminum carbonate gel: Tablets—500 mg; suspension—400 mg/5 ml; aluminum hydroxide gel: Tablets—300, 500, 600 mg; capsules—400, 500 mg; suspension—450 mg/5 ml, 675 mg/5 ml; liquid—600 mg/5 ml

ADULT

**Aluminum hydroxide gel:** 500–1,800 mg 3–6×/d PO between meals and hs.

**Aluminum carbonate gel:** Antacid: 2 capsules or tablets, 10 ml of regular suspension or 5 ml of extra strength suspension as often as q2h, up to 12 times per day PO

- *Prevention of phosphate stones:* Administer PO 1 h after meals and hs.
- *Capsules or tablets:* 2 to 6;
- *Suspension:* 10 to 30 ml;
- *Extra strength suspension:* 5 to 15 ml in water or fruit juice.
- *Hyperphosphatemia:* Administer PO tid–qid with meals.
- *Capsules, tablets:* take 2;
- *Suspension:* take 12 ml;
- *Extra strength suspension:* take 5 ml.

PEDIATRIC

**Aluminum hydroxide gel**

- *Hyperphosphatemia:* 50–150 mg/kg every 24 h PO in divided doses q4–6h; titrate dose to normal serum phosphorus.
- *General guidelines:* 5–15 ml PO q3–6h or 1–3h after meals and hs.
- *Prophylaxis of GI bleeding in critically ill infants:* 2–5 ml/dose q1–2h PO.
- *Prophylaxis of GI bleeding in critically ill children:* 5–15 ml/dose q1–2h PO.

#### Pharmacokinetics

| Route | Onset |
|---|---|
| Oral | Varies |

*Metabolism:* Hepatic
*Distribution:* hronic use, small amounts may be absorbed systemically and cross the placenta and enter breast milk
*Excretion:* GI bound in the feces

### Adverse effects

- GI: *Constipation;* intestinal obstruction, decreased absorption of fluoride, accumulation of aluminum in serum, bone, and CNS
- MS: Osteomalacia and chronic phosphate deficiency with bone pain, malaise, muscular weakness

### Clinically important drug-drug interactions

• Do not administer *other oral drugs* within 1–2 h of antacid; change in gastric pH may interfere with absorption of oral drugs. • Decreased pharmacologic effect of corticosteroids, diflunisal, digoxin, iron, isoniazid, penicillamine, phenothiazines, ranitidine, tetracyclines. • Increased pharmacologic effect of benzodiazepines.

## ■ Nursing Considerations

### Assessment

- ***History:*** Allergy to aluminum products; gastric outlet obstruction; hypertension, CHF; hypophosphatemia; lactation
- ***Physical:*** Bone strength, muscle strength; P, auscultation, BP, peripheral edema; abdominal exam, bowel sounds; serum phosphorous, serum fluoride; bone x-ray is appropriate

### Implementation

- Give hourly for first 2 wk when used for acute peptic ulcer; during the healing stage, give 1–3 h after meals and hs.
- Do not administer oral drugs within 1–2 h of antacid administration.
- Have patient chew tablets thoroughly; follow with a glass of water.
- Monitor serum phosphorus levels periodically during long-term therapy.

### Drug-specific teaching points

- Take this drug between meals and at bedtime; ulcer patients need to strictly follow prescribed dosage pattern. If tablets are being used, chew thoroughly before swallowing, and follow with a glass of water.
- Do not take maximum dosage of antacids for more than 2 weeks except under medical supervision.
- Do not take this drug with any other oral medications; absorption of those medications can be inhibited. Take other oral medications at least 1–2 h after aluminum salt.
- Constipation may occur.
- Report constipation; bone pain, muscle weakness; coffee ground vomitus, black tarry stools; no relief from symptoms being treated.

## amantadine HCl

*(a **man'** ta deen)*

Symmetrel

**Pregnancy Category C**

### Drug classes

Antiviral drug
Antiparkinsonism drug

### Therapeutic actions

May inhibit penetration of influenza A virus into the host cell; may increase dopamine release in the nigostriatal pathway of parkinsonism patients, relieving their symptoms.

### Indications

- Prevention and treatment of influenza A virus respiratory infection, especially in high-risk patients
- Adjunct to late vaccination against influenza A virus, to provide interim coverage; supplement to vaccination in immunodeficient patients; prophylaxis when vaccination is contraindicated
- Parkinson's disease and drug-induced extrapyramidal reactions

### Contraindications/cautions

- Allergy to drug product, seizures, liver disease, eczematoid rash, psychoses, CHF, renal disease, lactation.

### Dosage

**Available Forms:** Capsules—100 mg; syrup—50 mg/5 ml

*Influenza A Virus*

- ADULT
  - ***Prophylaxis:*** 200 mg/d PO or 100 mg bid PO for 10 d after exposure, for up to

90 d if vaccination is impossible and exposure is repeated.

– *Treatment:* Same dose as above; start treatment as soon after exposure as possible, continuing for 24–48 h after symptoms are gone.

***Patients with seizure disorders:***
100 mg/d.

***Patients with renal disease:***

| *Creatinine Clearance (ml/min)* | *Dosage* |
|---|---|
| 10–19 | Alternate 200 mg/100 mg q7d |
| 20–29 | 100 mg three/week |
| 30–39 | 200 mg two/week |
| 40–59 | 100 mg/d |
| 60–79 | 200 mg/100 mg on alternate days |
| 80 and over | 100 mg bid |

- *PEDIATRIC:* Not recommended for children > 1 y.

*Prophylaxis: 1–9 y:* 2–4 mg/lb per d PO in two to three divided doses, not to exceed 150 mg/lb per d. *9–12 y:* 100 mg PO bid. *Treatment:* As above; start as soon after exposure as possible, continuing for 24–48 h after symptoms are gone.

*Parkinsonism Treatment*

- *ADULT:* 100 mg bid (up to 400 mg/d) PO when used alone; reduce in patients receiving other antiparkinsonism drugs.
- *GERIATRIC: > 65 years with no recognized renal disease:* 100 mg once daily PO in parkinsonism treatment; 100 mg bid (up to 400 mg/d) when used alone; reduce dosage in patients receiving other antiparkinsonian drugs.

***Patients With Renal Disease:***

| *Creatinine Clearance (ml/min)* | *Dosage* |
|---|---|
| 10–19 | Alternate 200 mg/100 mg q7d |
| 20–29 | 100 mg three/week |
| 30–39 | 200 mg two/week |
| 40–59 | 100 mg/d |
| 60–79 | 200 mg/100 mg on alternate days |
| 80 and over | 100 mg bid |

*Drug-induced Extrapyramidal Reactions*

- *ADULT:* 100 mg bid PO, up to 300 mg/d in divided doses has been used.

**Pharmacokinetics**

| *Route* | *Onset* | *Peak* |
|---|---|---|
| Oral | 36–48 h | 4 h |

*Metabolism:* $T_{1/2}$: 15–24 h
*Distribution:* Crosses placenta; passes into breast milk
*Excretion:* Unchanged in the urine

**Adverse effects**

- CNS: *Lightheadedness, dizziness, insomnia,* confusion, irritability, ataxia, psychosis, depression, hallucinations
- GI: *Nausea,* anorexia, constipation, dry mouth
- CV: CHF, orthostatic hypotension, dyspnea
- GU: Urinary retention

**Clinically important drug-drug interactions**

• Increased atropine-like side effects with anticholinergic drugs • Increased amantadine effects with hydrochlorothiazide, triamterene

## ■ Nursing Considerations

### Assessment

- *History:* Allergy to drug product, seizures, liver disease, eczematoid rash, psychoses, CHF, renal disease, lactation
- *Physical:* Orientation, vision, speech, reflexes; BP, orthostatic BP, P, auscultation, perfusion, edema; R, adventitious sounds; urinary output; BUN, creatinine clearance

### Implementation

- Do not discontinue abruptly when treating parkinsonism syndrome; parkinsonian crisis may occur.

### Drug-specific teaching points

- Mark your calendar if you are on alternating dosage schedules; it is very important to take the full course of the drug.
- The following may occur: drowsiness, blurred vision (use caution when driving

or using dangerous equipment); dizziness, light-headedness (avoid sudden position changes); irritability or mood changes (common effect; if severe, drug may be changed).

- Report swelling of the fingers or ankles; shortness of breath; difficulty urinating, walking; tremors, slurred speech.

## ambenonium chloride

*(am be **noe'** nee um)*

Mytelase

**Pregnancy Category C**

### Drug classes

Cholinesterase inhibitor
Parasympathomimetic drug (indirectly acting)
Antimyasthenic drug

### Therapeutic actions

Increases the concentration of acetylcholine at the sites of cholinergic transmission (parasympathetic neurons and skeletal muscles) and prolongs and exaggerates the effects of acetylcholine by inhibiting the enzyme acetylcholinesterase; this causes parasympathomimetic effects and facilitates transmission at the skeletal neuromuscular junction. Also has direct stimulating effects on skeletal muscle and has a longer duration of effect and fewer side effects than other agents.

### Indications

- Symptomatic control of myasthenia gravis

### Contraindications/cautions

- Contraindications: hypersensitivity to anticholinesterases; intestinal or urogenital tract obstruction; peritonitis; lactation.
- Use cautiously with asthma, peptic ulcer, bradycardia, cardiac arrhythmias, recent coronary occlusion, vagotonia, hyperthyroidism, epilepsy.

### Dosage

**Available Forms:** Tablets—10 mg

*ADULT:* 5–25 mg PO tid–qid (5–75 mg per dose has been used). Start dosage with 5 mg, and gradually increase to determine optimum dosage based on optimal muscle strength and no GI disturbances; increase dose every 1–2 d. Dosage above 200 mg/d requires close supervision to avoid overdose.

*PEDIATRIC:* Safety and efficacy not established.

### Pharmacokinetics

| Route | Onset | Peak |
|---|---|---|
| Oral | 20–30 min | 3–8 h |

*Metabolism:* $T_{1/2}$: Unknown
*Distribution:* Crosses placenta; passes into breast milk
*Excretion:* Unknown

### Adverse effects

*Parasympathomimetic Effects*

- GI: *Salivation, dysphagia, nausea, vomiting, increased peristalsis, abdominal cramps,* flatulence, diarrhea
- CV: *Bradycardia, cardiac arrhythmias,* AV block and nodal rhythm, cardiac arrest; decreased cardiac output, leading to hypotension, syncope
- **Respiratory**: *Increased pharyngeal and tracheobronchial secretions*, laryngospasm, bronchospasm, bronchiolar constriction, dyspnea
- GU: *Urinary frequency and incontinence*, urinary urgency
- EENT: *Lacrimation, miosis,* spasm of accommodation, diplopia, conjunctival hyperemia
- Dermatologic: Diaphoresis, flushing

*Skeletal Muscle Effects*

- CNS: Convulsions, dysarthria, dysphonia, drowsiness, dizziness, headache, loss of consciousness
- **Peripheral**: Skeletal muscle weakness, fasciculations, muscle cramps, arthralgia
- **Respiratory**: Respiratory muscle paralysis, central respiratory paralysis

### Clinically important drug-drug interactions

• Decreased neuromuscular blockade of succinylcholine • Decreased effects of ambenonium and possible muscular depression with corticosteroids

a

## ■ Nursing Considerations

### Assessment

- *History:* Hypersensitivity to anticholinesterases, intestinal or urogenital tract obstruction, peritonitis, asthma, peptic ulcer, bradycardia, cardiac arrhythmias, recent coronary occlusion, vagotonia, hyperthyroidism, epilepsy, lactation
- *Physical:* Skin color, texture, lesions; reflexes, bilateral grip strength; P, auscultation, BP; R, adventious sounds; salivation, bowel sounds, normal output; frequency, voiding pattern, normal urinary output; EEG, thyroid tests

### Implementation

- Overdosage can cause muscle weakness (cholinergic crisis) that is difficult to differentiate from myasthenic weakness (use of edrophonium for differential diagnosis is recommended). The administration of atropine may mask the parasympathetic effects of anticholinesterase overdose and further confound the diagnosis.
- Maintain atropine sulfate on standby as an antidote and antagonist in case of cholinergic crisis or hypersensitivity reaction.
- Monitor patient response carefully if increasing dosage.
- Discontinue drug and consult physician if excessive salivation, emesis, frequent urination, or diarrhea occurs.
- Arrange for decreased dosage of drug if excessive sweating, nausea, or GI upset occur.

### Drug-specific teaching points

- Take this drug exactly as prescribed; does not need to be taken at night. Patient and significant other need to know about the effects of the drug, the signs and symptoms of myasthenia gravis, the fact that muscle weakness may be related to drug overdosage and to exacerbation of the disease, and that it is important to report muscle weakness promptly to the nurse or physician so that proper evaluation can be made.
- The following side effects may occur: blurred vision, difficulty with far vision, difficulty with dark adaptation (use caution while driving, especially at night, or performing hazardous tasks in reduced light); increased urinary frequency, abdominal cramps (if these become a problem, notify your health care provider); sweating (avoid hot or excessively humid environments).
- Report muscle weakness, nausea, vomiting, diarrhea, severe abdominal pain, excessive sweating, excessive salivation, frequent urination, urinary urgency, irregular heartbeat, difficulty in breathing.

## ☆ amifostine

*(am ah fohs' teen)*
Ethyol
**Pregnancy Category C**

### Drug classes

Cytoprotective agent

### Therapeutic actions

Metabolized to a thiol metabolite that protects healthy cells from toxic effects of cisplatin; thought to react to normal pH and vascularity of nontumor cells; may also act as a scavenger of free radicals that may be generated after exposure of tissues to cisplatin.

### Indications

- Reduction of renal toxicity associated with repeated administration of cisplatin in patients with advanced ovarian cancer
- Unlabeled use: Protection of lung fibroblasts from damaging effects of paclitaxel

### Contraindications/cautions

- Contraindications: hypersensitivity to mannitol or aminothiol compounds
- Use cautiously with hypocalcemia, pregnancy, lactation, CV or CNS disease

### Dosage

**Available Forms:** Powder for injection—500 mg

*ADULT:* 910 mg/m$^2$ IV qid as 15-min infusion given within 30 min of starting chemotherapy

*GERIATRIC:* No data available for use in patients >70 y.

### Pharmacokinetics

| *Route* | *Onset* | *Duration* |
|---|---|---|
| IV | Immediate | 6–8 min |

*Metabolism:* $T_{1/2}$: 8 min
*Distribution:* Crosses placenta; may enter breast milk
*Excretion:* Urine

#### IV facts

**Preparation:** Reconstitute with 9.5 ml 0.9% Sodium Chloride; refrigerate vial; stable for 5 h at room temperature after reconstitution or 24 h if refrigerated.
**Infusion:** Infuse slowly over 15 min.

### Adverse effects

- CNS: *Somnolence,* loss of consciousness
- GI: *Severe nausea, vomiting, hiccoughs*
- CV: **Hypotension**
- Hematologic: Hypocalcemia
- Other: *Flushing, feeling of warmth, chills/fever,* skin rash

### Clinically important drug-drug interactions

- Possibility of severe hypotension with antihypertensives or any drug regimen that lowers blood pressure

## ■ Nursing Considerations

#### Assessment

- *History:* Hypersensitivity to mannitol or aminothiol compounds; hypocalcemia; pregnancy; lactation; CV or CNS disease
- *Physical:* T; skin color, texture, lesions; orientation; BP, P, perfusion; abdominal exam; serum calcium, renal function tests

#### Implementation

- Arrange for antiemetic medication before and in conjunction with amifostine (dexamethasone, 20 mg IV and any serotonin antagonist are recommended); further antiemetic therapy may be needed with cisplatin regimen; monitor fluid balance carefully.
- Monitor BP continuously during infusion; interrupt if systolic BP falls 20 points (if baseline <100 mm Hg) to 50 points (if baseline >180 mm Hg). If BP returns to baseline within 5 min after infusion is stopped, full dose may be resumed. If full dose cannot be tolerated, start next dose at 740 mg/m$^2$.
- Monitor serium calcium levels, especially for patients at risk (eg, nephrotic syndrome). Arrange for calcium supplements as required.

#### Drug-specific teaching points

- This drug will be given IV to help prevent some of the side effects of your chemoapy.
- The following side effecs may occur: nausea and vomiting (medication will be given); flushing, dizziness, feeling of warmth or chills.
- Report severe dizziness, weakness, hiccoughs, shaking.

## amikacin sulfate

*(am i **kay'** sin)*
Amikacin, Amikin
**Pregnancy Category C**

### Drug classes

Aminoglycoside antibiotic

### Therapeutic actions

Bactericidal: inhibits protein synthesis in susceptible strains of gram-negative bacteria, and the functional integrity of bacterial cell membrane appears to be disrupted, causing cell death.

### Indications

- Short-term treatment of serious infections caused by susceptible strains of *Pseudomonas* species, *E. coli,* indole-positive *Proteus* species, *Providencia* species, *Klebsiella, Enterobacter, and Serratia* species, *Acinetobacter* species
- Suspected gram-negative infections before results of susceptibility studies are known (effective in infections caused by

gentamicin- or tobramycin-resistant strains of gram-negative organisms)
- Initial treatment of staphylococcal infections when penicillin is contraindicated or infection may be caused by mixed organisms
- Neonatal sepsis when other antibiotics cannot be used (often used in combination with penicillin-type drug)
- Unlabeled uses: intrathecal/intraventricular administration at 8 mg/24 h; part of a multidrug regimen for treatment of *Mycobacterium avium* complex, a common infection in AIDS patients

## Contraindications/cautions

- Contraindications: allergy to any aminoglycosides, renal or hepatic disease, preexisting hearing loss, myasthenia gravis, parkinsonism, infant botulism, lactation.
- Use cautiously with elderly patients, any patient with diminished hearing, decreased renal function, dehydration, neuromuscular disorders.

## Dosage

**Available Forms:** Injection—50 mg/ml, 250 mg/ml

IM or IV (dosage is the same)

*ADULT AND PEDIATRIC:* 15 mg/kg per day divided into two to three equal doses at equal intervals, not to exceed 1.5 g/d.

- *UTIs:* 250 mg bid; treatment is usually required for 7–10 d. If treatment is required for longer, carefully monitor serum levels and renal and neurologic function.

*NEONATAL:* Loading dose of 10 mg/kg then 7.5 mg/kg q12h.

*GERIATRIC OR RENAL FAILURE PATIENTS:* Reduce dosage, and carefully monitor serum drug levels and renal function tests throughout treatment; regulate dosage based on these values. If CCr is not available and patient condition is stable, calculate a dosage interval in hours for the normal dose by multiplying patient's serum creatinine by 9. Dosage guide if CCr is known: Maintenance dose q12h observed CCr ÷ normal CCr × calculated loading dose (mg).

## Pharmacokinetics

| Route | Onset | Peak |
|---|---|---|
| IV | Immediate | 30 min |
| IM | Varies | 45–120 min |

*Metabolism:* $T_{1/2}$: 2–3 hours

*Distribution:* Crosses placenta; passes into breast milk

*Excretion:* Unchanged in the urine

## IV facts

**Preparation:** Prepare IV solution by adding the contents of a 500-mg vial to 100 or 200 ml of sterile diluent. Do not physically mix with other drugs. Administer amikacin separately. Prepared solution is stable in concentrations of 0.25 and 5 mg/ml for 24 h at room temperature.

**Infusion:** Administer to adults or pediatric patients over 30–60 min; infuse to infants over 1–2 h.

**Compatibilities:** Amikacin is stable in 5% Dextrose Injection; 5% Dextrose and 0.2%, 0.45%, or 0.9% Sodium Chloride Injection; Lactated Ringer's Injection; Normosol M in 5% Dextrose Injection; Normosol R in 5% Dextrose Injection; Plasma-Lyte 56 or 148 Injection in 5% Dextrose in Water.

## Adverse effects

- CNS: *Ototoxicity*, confusion, disorientation, depression, lethargy, nystagmus, visual disturbances, headache, fever, numbness, tingling, tremor, paresthesias, muscle twitching, convulsions, muscular weakness, neuromuscular blockade, apnea
- GI: *Nausea, vomiting, anorexia, diarrhea*, weight loss, stomatitis, increased salivation, splenomegaly
- CV: Palpitations, hypotension, hypertension
- **Hematologic**: Leukemoid reaction, agranulocytosis, granulocytosis, leukopenia, leukocytosis, thrombocytopenia, eosinophilia, pancytopenia, anemia, he-

molytic anemia, increased or decreased reticulocyte count, electrolyte disturbances
- GU: *Nephrotoxicity*
- **Hepatic**: Hepatic toxicity; hepatomegaly
- **Hypersensitivity**: Purpura, rash, urticaria, exfoliative dermatitis, itching
- **Other**: *Superinfections, pain and irritation at IM injection sites*

### Clinically important drug-drug interactions

• Increased ototoxic and nephrotoxic effects with potent diuretics and other similarly toxic drugs (eg, cephalosporins). • Risk of inactivation if mixed parenterally with penicillins. • Increased likelihood of neuromuscular blockade if given shortly after general anesthetics, depolarizing and nondepolarizing neuromuscular junction blockers.

## ■ Nursing Considerations

### Assessment

- *History:* Allergy to any aminoglycosides, renal or hepatic disease, preexisting hearing loss, myasthenia gravis, parkinsonism, infant botulism, lactation, diminished hearing, decreased renal function, dehydration, neuromuscular disorders
- *Physical:* Arrange culture and sensitivity tests on infection prior to therapy; renal function, eighth cranial nerve function and state of hydration prior to, during, and after therapy; hepatic function tests, CBC, skin color and lesions, orientation and affect, reflexes, bilateral grip strength, weight, bowel sounds.

### Implementation

- Arrange for culture and sensitivity testing of infected area before treatment.
- Monitor duration of treatment: usually 7–10 d. If clinical response does not occur within 3-5 days, stop therapy. Prolonged treatment leads to increased risk of toxicity. If drug is used longer than 10 d, monitor auditory and renal function daily.
- Give IM dosage by deep injection.
- Ensure that patient is well hydrated before and during therapy.

### Drug-specific teaching points

- This drug is only available for IM or IV use.
- The following side effects may occur: ringing in the ears, headache, dizziness (reversible; safety measures may need to be taken if severe); nausea, vomiting, loss of appetite (small frequent meals, frequent mouth care may help).
- Report pain at injection site, severe headache, dizziness, loss of hearing, changes in urine pattern, difficulty breathing, rash or skin lesions.

# amiloride hydrochloride

(*a* ***mill'*** *oh ride*)

Midamor

**Pregnancy Category B**

### Drug classes

Potassium-sparing diuretic

### Therapeutic actions

Inhibits sodium reabsorption in the renal distal tubule, causing loss of sodium and water and retention of potassium.

### Indications

- Adjunctive therapy with thiazide or loop diuretics in edema associated with CHF and in hypertension to treat hypokalemia or to prevent hypokalemia in patients who would be at high risk if hypokalemia occurred (digitalized patients, patients with cardiac arrhythmias)
- Unlabeled uses: inhalation in the treatment of cystic fibrosis; reduction of lithium-induced polyuria without increasing lithium levels

### Contraindications/cautions

- Allergy to amiloride, hyperkalemia, renal or liver disease, diabetes mellitus, metabolic or respiratory acidosis, lactation.

### Dosage

**Available Forms:** Tablets—5, 10 mg

*ADULT:* Add 5 mg/d to usual antihypertensive or dosage of kaluretic diuretic; if necessary, increase dose to 10 mg/d or to 15–20 mg/d with careful monitoring of electrolytes.

- *Single-drug therapy:* Start with 5 mg/d; if necessary, increase to 10 mg/d or to 15–20 mg/d with careful monitoring of electrolytes.

*PEDIATRIC:* Safety and efficacy not established.

### Pharmacokinetics

| Route | Onset | Peak | Duration |
|---|---|---|---|
| Oral | 2 h | 6–10 h | 24 h |

*Metabolism:* $T_{1/2}$: 6–9 h
*Distribution:* Crosses placenta; passes into breast milk
*Excretion:* Unchanged in the urine

### Adverse effects

- CNS: *Headache*, dizziness, drowsiness, fatigue, paresthesias, tremors, confusion, encephalopathy
- GI: *Nausea, anorexia, vomiting, diarrhea*, dry mouth, constipation, jaundice, gas pain, GI bleeding
- Respiratory: Cough, dyspnea
- GU: *Hyperkalemia*, polyuria, dysuria, *impotence*, loss of libido
- MS: *Weakness, fatigue, muscle cramps* and muscle spasms, joint pain
- Other: Rash, pruritus, itching, alopecia

### Clinically important drug-drug interactions

• Increased hyperkalemia with triamterene, spironolactone, potassium supplements, diets rich in potassium, captopril, enalapril, lisinopril • Reduced effectiveness of digoxin with amiloride.

## ■ Nursing Considerations

### Assessment

- *History:* Allergy to amiloride, hyperkalemia, renal or liver disease, diabetes mellitus, metabolic or respiratory acidosis, lactation
- *Physical:* Skin color, lesions, edema; orientation, reflexes, muscle strength; pulses, baseline ECG, BP; respiratory rate, pattern, adventitious sounds; liver evaluation, bowel sounds, urinary output patterns; CBC, serum electrolytes, blood sugar, liver and renal function tests, urinalysis

### Implementation

- Administer with food or milk to prevent GI upset.
- Administer early in the day so increased urination does not disturb sleep.
- Measure and record weights to monitor mobilization of edema fluid.
- Avoid foods and salt substitutes high in potassium.
- Provide frequent mouth care, sugarless lozenges to suck.
- Arrange for regular evaluation of serum electrolytes.

### Drug-specific teaching points

- Take single dose early in the day so increased urination will not disturb sleep.
- Take the drug with food or meals to prevent GI upset.
- Avoid foods that are high in potassium and any flavoring that contains potassium (eg, salt substitute).
- Weigh yourself on a regular basis at the same time and in the same clothing, and record the weight on your calendar.
- The following side effects may occur: increased volume and frequency of urination; dizziness, feeling faint on arising, drowsiness (avoid rapid position changes, hazardous activities like driving, and the use of alcohol which may intensify these problems); decrease in sexual function; increased thirst (sucking on sugarless lozenges may help; frequent mouth care also may help); avoid foods that are rich in potassium (eg, fruits, Sanka).
- Report loss or gain of more than 3 lb in one day; swelling in your ankles or fingers; dizziness, trembling, numbness, fatigue; muscle weakness or cramps.

# amino acids

*(a mee' noe)*

Aminess, Aminosyn, BranchAmin, FreAmine, HepatAmine, NephrAmine, Novamine, ProcalAmine, RenAmin, Travasol, TrophAmine

**Pregnancy Category C**

## Drug classes
Protein substrate
Caloric agent

## Therapeutic actions
Essential and nonessential amino acids provided in various combinations to supply calories and proteins and provide a protein-building and a protein-sparing effect for the body (a positive nitrogen balance).

## Indications
- Provide nutrition to patients who are in a negative nitrogen balance when GI tract cannot absorb protein; when protein needs exceed the ability to absorb protein (burns, trauma, infections); when bowel rest is needed; when tube feeding cannot supply adequate nutrition; when health can be improved or restored by replacing lost amino acids
- Treatment of hepatic encephalopathy in patients with cirrhosis or hepatitis
- Nutritional support of uremic patients when oral nutrition is not feasible

## Contraindications/cautions
- Contraindications: hypersensitivity to any component of the solution; severe electrolyte or acid–base imbalance; inborn errors in amino acid metabolism; decreased circulating blood volume; severe kidney or liver disease; hyperammonemia; bleeding abnormalities.
- Use cautiously with liver or renal impairment; diabetes mellitus; CHF; hypertension.

## Dosage
**Available Forms:** Many forms available for IV injections

Dosage must be individualized with careful observation of cardiac status and BUN and evaluation of metabolic needs.

*ADULT:* 1–1.7 g/kg per day amino acid injection IV into a peripheral vein; 250–500 ml/d amino acid injection IV mixed with appropriate dextrose, vitamins, and electrolytes as part of a TPN solution.

*PEDIATRIC:* 2–3 g/kg per day amino acid IV mixed with dextrose as appropriate.

## Pharmacokinetics

| Route | Onset |
|---|---|
| IV | Immediate |

*Metabolism:* Part of normal anabolic processes
*Distribution:* Crosses placenta; passes into breast milk
*Excretion:* Urine as urea nitrogen

### IV Facts
**Preparation:** Strict aseptic technique is required in mixing solution; use of a laminar flow hood in the pharmacy is recommended. A 0.22-$\mu$m filter should be used to block any particulate matter and bacteria. Use mixed solution immediately. If not used within 1 h, refrigerate solution. Mixed solutions must be used within 24 h. Use strict aseptic technique when changing bottles, catheter, tubing, and so forth. Replace all IV apparatus every 24 h. Change dressing every 24 h to assess insertion site.

**Infusion:** Use a volumetric infusion pump. Infuse only if solution is absolutely clear and without particulate matter. Infuse slowly. If infusion falls behind, do not try to speed up infusion rate; serious overload could occur. Infusion rates of 20–30 ml/h up to a maximum of 60–100 ml/h have been used.

**Compatibilities:** Do not mix with amphotericin B, ampicillin, carbenicillin, cephradine, gentamicin, metronidazole, tetracycline, ticarcillin.

## Adverse effects
- CNS: *Headache, dizziness*, mental confusion, **loss of consciousness**
- GI: *Nausea, vomiting,* abdominal pain, liver impairment, fatty liver

- CV: Hypertension, CHF, **pulmonary edema**, tachycardia, *generalized flushing*
- Endocrine: Hypoglycemia, hyperglycemia, fatty acid deficiency, azotemia, hyperammonemia
- Local: *Pain, infection,* phlebitis, venous thrombosis, tissue sloughing at injection site
- Hypersensitivity: Fever, chills, rash, papular eruptions

### Clinically important drug-drug interactions

- Reduced protein-sparing effects of amino acids if taken with tetracyclines

## ■ Nursing Considerations

### Assessment

- *History:* Hypersensitivity to any component of the solution; severe electrolyte or acid–base imbalance; inborn errors in amino acid metabolism; decreased circulating blood volume; kidney or liver disease; hyperammonemia; bleeding abnormalities, diabetes mellitus; congestive heart failure; hypertension
- *Physical:* T, weight, height; orientation, reflexes; P, BP, edema; R, lung auscultation; abdominal exam; urinary output; CBC, platelet count, PT, electrolytes, BUN, blood glucose, uric acid, bilirubin, creatinine, plasma proteins, renal and liver function tests; urine glucose, osmolarity

### Implementation

- Assess nutritional status before and frequently during treatment; weigh patient daily to monitor fluid load and nutritional status.
- Monitor vital signs frequently during infusion; monitor I&O continually during treatment.
- Observe infusion site at least daily for infection, phlebitis; change dressing using strict aseptic technique at least q24h.
- Arrange to give $D_5W$ or $D_{10}W$ for injection by a peripheral line to avoid hypoglycemia rebound if TPN infusion needs to be stopped.
- Monitor urine glucose, acetone, and specific gravity q6h during initial infusion period, at least bid when the infusion has stabilized; stop solution at any sign of renal failure.
- Monitor patient for vascular overload or hepatic impairment; decrease rate of infusion or discontinue.

### Drug-specific teaching points

- This drug can be given only through an intravenous or central line.
- This drug will help you to build new proteins and regain your strength and healing power.
- The following side effects may occur: headache, dizziness (medication may be ordered to help); nausea, vomiting; pain at infusion site.
- Report fever, chills, severe pain at infusion site, changes in color of urine or stool, severe headache, rash.

# aminocaproic acid

*(a mee noe ka **proe'** ik)*

Amicar

**Pregnancy Category C**

### Drug classes

Systemic hemostatic agent

### Therapeutic actions

Inhibits fibrinolysis by inhibiting plasminogen activator substances and by antiplasmin activity; this action prevents the breakdown of clots.

### Indications

- Treatment of excessive bleeding resulting from systemic hyperfibrinolysis and urinary fibrinolysis.
- Unlabeled uses: prevention of recurrence of subarachnoid hemorrhage; management of amegakaryocytic thrombocytopenia; to decrease the need for platelet administration; to abort and treat attacks of hereditary angioneurotic edema

### Contraindications/cautions

- Allergy to aminocaproic acid, active intravascular clotting (DIC), cardiac disease, renal dysfunction, hematuria of upper urinary tract origin, hepatic dysfunction, lactation.

### Dosage

**Available Forms:** Tablets—500 mg; syrup—250 mg/ml; injection—250 mg/ml

*ADULT:* Initial dose of 5 g PO or IV followed by 1–1.25 g/h to produce and sustain plasma levels of 0.13 mg/ml; do not administer more than 30 g/d.

- *Acute bleeding:* 4–5 g IV in 250 ml of diluent during the first hour of infusion; then continuous infusion of 1 g/h in 50 ml of diluent. Continue for 8 h or until bleeding stops.
- *Prevention of recurrence of subarachnoid hemorrhage:* 36 g/d in six divided doses, PO or IV.
- *Amegakaryocytic thrombocytopenia:* 8–24 g/d for 3 d to 13 mo.

*PEDIATRIC:* 100 mg/kg PO or IV during the first hour; then 33.3 mg/kg per hour for a maximum of 18g/m$^2$ per day.

### Pharmacokinetics

| *Route* | *Onset* | *Peak* | *Duration* |
|---|---|---|---|
| Oral | Rapid | 2 h | |
| IV | Immediate | Minutes | 2–3 h |

*Distribution:* Crosses placenta; passes into breast milk

*Excretion:* Unchanged in the urine

### IV facts

**Preparation:** Dilute in compatible IV fluid. Rapid IV infusion undiluted is not recommended. Dilute 4 ml (1 g) of solution with 50 ml of diluent. For acute bleed, dilute 4–5 g in 250 ml diluent and give over 1 h; then a continuous infusion of 1–1.25 g/h given in 50 ml diluent. Store at room temperature.

**Infusion:** Infuse at 4–5 g the first hour of treatment, then 1 g/h by continuous infusion; administer slowly to avoid hypotension, bradycardia, arrhythmias.

**Compatibilities:** Compatible with Sterile Water for Injection, Normal Saline, 5% Dextrose, Ringer's Solution.

### Adverse effects

- CNS: *Dizziness, tinnitus, headache,* delirium, hallucinations, psychotic reactions, weakness, conjunctivial suffusion, nasal stuffiness
- GI: *Nausea, cramps, diarrhea*
- CV: Hypotension, cardiac myopathy
- **Hematologic**: *Elevated serum CPK,* aldolase, SGOT, elevated serum potassium
- GU: Intrarenal obstruction, renal failure, *fertility problems*
- MS: *Malaise,* myopathy, symptomatic weakness, fatigue
- **Other**: Skin rash, thrombophlebitis

### Clinically important drug-drug interactions

- Risk of hypercoagulable state with oral contraceptives, estrogens.

### Drug-lab test interferences

- Elevation of serum $K^+$ levels, especially with impaired renal function

## ■ Nursing Considerations

### Assessment

- *History:* Allergy to aminocaproic acid, active intravascular clotting, cardiac disease, renal dysfunction; hematuria of upper urinary tract origin, hepatic dysfunction, lactation
- *Physical:* Skin color, lesions; muscular strength; orientation, reflexes, affect; BP, P, baseine ECG, peripheral perfusion; liver evaluation, bowel sounds, output; clotting studies, CPK, urinalysis, liver and kidney function tests

### Implementation

- Patient on oral therapy may have to take up to 10 tablets the first hour of treatment and tablets around the clock during treatment.
- Orient patient, and offer support if hallucinations, delirium, psychoses occur.
- Monitor patient for signs of clotting.

**Drug-specific teaching points**

- The following side effects may occur: dizziness, weakness, headache, hallucinations (avoid driving or the use of dangerous machinery; take special precautions to avoid injury); nausea, diarrhea, cramps (small, frequent meals may help); infertility problems (menstrual irregularities, dry ejaculation—should go away when the drug is stopped); weakness, malaise (plan activities, take rest periods as needed).
- Report severe headache, restlessness, muscle pain and weakness, blood in the urine.

## aminoglutethemide

*(a meen oh gloo* ***teth'*** *i mide)*

Cytadren

**Pregnancy Category D**

**Drug classes**

Antineoplastic
Hormone antagonist

**Therapeutic actions**

Inhibits the conversion of cholesterol to the steroid base necessary for producing adrenal glucocorticoids, mineralocorticoids, estrogens, and androgens.

**Indications**

- Suppression of adrenal function in selected patients with Cushing's syndrome—those awaiting surgery or in whom other treatment is not appropriate
- Unlabeled use: to produce medical adrenalectomy in patients with advanced breast cancer and in patients with metastatic prostate carcinoma

**Contraindications/cautions**

- Hypersensitivity to glutethemide or to aminoglutethemide; hypotension; hypothyroidism; pregnancy (causes fetal harm); lactation.

**Dosage**

**Available Forms:** Tablets—250 mg

*ADULT*

- *Cushing's Disease:* 250 mg PO q6h; may be increased in increments of 250 mg/d at intervals of 1–2 wk to a total daily dose of 2 g.
- *Cancer:* 250 mg PO bid with hydrocortisone 60 mg hs, 20 mg on arising, and 20 mg at 2 PM for 2 weeks; then 250 mg PO qid and hydrocortisone 20 mg hs, 10 mg on arising, and 10 mg at 2 PM.

*PEDIATRIC:* Safety and efficacy not established.

**Pharmacokinetics**

| *Route* | *Onset* | *Peak* |
|---|---|---|
| Oral | 3–5 d | 36–72 h |

*Metabolism:* $T_{1/2}$: 11–16 h
*Distribution:* Crosses placenta; passes into breast milk
*Excretion:* Urine

**Adverse effects**

- CNS: *Drowsiness,* dizziness, headache
- GI: *Nausea, anorexia*
- CV: *Hypotension*, tachycardia
- Dermatologic: *Morbiliform rash*, pruritus, urticaria
- Endocrine: Adrenal insufficiency, **hypothyroidism**, masculinization, and hirsutism
- Other: Myalgia, fever

**Clinically important drug-drug interactions**

• Decreased therapeutic effects of warfarin, anisindione, dicumarol • Possible decreased effectiveness of aminophylline, oxtriphylline, theophylline, medroxyprogesterone • Decreased effectiveness with dexamethasone, hydrocortisone

### ■ Nursing Considerations

**Assessment**

- *History:* Hypersensitivity to glutethemide or to aminoglutethemide; hypotension; hypothyroidism; pregnancy, lactation
- *Physical:* Weight, skin condition, fever, neurologic status, reflexes, P, BP, thyroid function, renal and liver function tests, cortisol levels

**Implementation**

- Begin therapy in a hospital setting until response has stabilized.

- Monitor patient carefully; if extreme drowsiness, severe skin rash, or excessively low cortisol levels occur, reduce dose or discontinue.
- Monitor patient for signs of hypothyroidism (slow pulse, lethargy, dry skin, thick tongue), and arrange for appropriate replacement therapy.
- Discontinue drug if skin rash persists for longer than 5–8 d or becomes severe; it may be possible to restart therapy at a lower dose once the rash has disappeared.
- Caution patient to avoid pregnancy if taking this drug; recommend birth control.

### Drug-specific teaching points

- Avoid driving or dangerous activities if dizziness, weakness occur.
- The following side effects may occur: dizziness, lightheadedness (change position slowly, avoid dangerous situations); loss of appetite, nausea (maintain nutrition); headache (if severe, medication may be ordered).
- A Medic-Alert system may help notify medical workers in an emergency situation that you are on this drug.
- Avoid pregnancy while taking this drug; discuss contraceptive methods.
- Report skin rash, severe drowsiness or dizziness, headache, severe nausea.

## aminophylline

*(am in off' i lin)*

theophylline ethylenediamine

Phyllocontin, Truphylline

**Pregnancy Category C**

### Drug classes

Bronchodilator
Xanthine

### Therapeutic actions

Relaxes bronchial smooth muscle, causing bronchodilation and increasing vital capacity, which has been impaired by bronchospasm and air trapping; in higher concentrations, it also inhibits the release of slow-reacting substance of anaphylaxis (SRS-A) and histamine.

### Indications

- Symptomatic relief or prevention of bronchial asthma and reversible bronchospasm associated with chronic bronchitis and emphysema
- Unlabeled uses: respiratory stimulant in Cheyne-Stokes respiration; treatment of apnea and bradycardia in premature babies

### Contraindications/cautions

- Contraindications: hypersensitivity to any xanthine or to ethylenediamine, peptic ulcer, active gastritis; rectal or colonic irritation or infection (use rectal preparations).
- Use cautiously with cardiac arrhythmias, acute myocardial injury, CHF, cor pulmonale, severe hypertension, severe hypoxemia, renal or hepatic disease, hyperthyroidism, alcoholism, labor, lactation.

### Dosage

**Available Forms:** Tablets—100, 200 mg; CR tablets—225 mg; liquid—105 mg/5 ml; injection—250 mg/10 ml; suppositories—250, 500 mg

Individualize dosage, base adjustments on clinical responses; monitor serum theophylline levels; maintain therapeutic range of 10–20 μg/ml; base dosage on lean body mass; 127 mg aminophylline dihydrate 100 mg theophylline anhydrous.

ADULT

- ***Acute symptoms requiring rapid theophyllinization in patients not receiving theophylline:*** An initial loading dose is required, as indicated below:

| *Patient Group* | *Oral Loading* | *Followed by* | *Maintenance* |
|---|---|---|---|
| Young adult smokers | 7.6 mg/kg | 3.8 mg/kg q4h × 3 doses | 3.8 mg/kg q6h |
| Non-smoking adults who are otherwise healthy | 7.6 mg/kg | 3.8 mg/kg q6h × 2 doses | 3.8 mg/kg q8h |

- *Chronic therapy:* Usual range is 600–1,600 mg/d PO in three to four divided doses.

– ***Rectal:*** 500 mg q6–8h by rectal suppository or retention enema.

PEDIATRIC: Use in children <6 mo not recommended; use of timed-release products in children >6 y not recommended. Children are very sensitive to CNS stimulant action of theophylline; use caution in younger children who cannot complain of minor side effects.

- *Acute therapy:* For acute symptoms requiring rapid theophyllinization in patients not receiving theophylline, a loading dose is required. Dosage recommendations are as follows:

| Patient Group | Oral Loading | Followed by | Maintenance |
|---|---|---|---|
| Children 6 mo–6 y | 7.6 mg/kg | 5.1 mg/kg q4h × 3 doses | 5.1 mg/kg q6h |
| Children 9–16 y | 7.6 mg/kg | 3.8 mg/kg q4h × 3 doses | 3.8 mg/kg q6h |

- *Chronic therapy:* 12 mg/kg per 24 h PO; slow clinical titration of the oral preparations is preferred; monitor clinical response and serum theophylline levels. In the absence of serum levels, titrate up to the maximum dosage shown below, providing the dosage is tolerated.

| Age | Maximum Daily Dose |
|---|---|
| <9 y | 30.4 mg/kg/d |
| 9–12 y | 25.3 mg/kg/d |
| 12–16 y | 22.8 mg/kg/d |
| >16 y | 16.5 mg/kg/d or 1100 mg, whichever is less |

GERIATRIC OR IMPAIRED ADULT: Use caution, especially in elderly men and in patients with cor pulmonale, CHF, liver disease (half-life of aminophylline may be markedly prolonged in CHF, liver disease). For acute symptoms requiring rapid theophyllinization in patients not receiving theophylline, a loading dose is necessary as follows

| Patient Group | Oral Loading | Followed by | Maintenance |
|---|---|---|---|
| Older patients and cor pulmonale | 7.6 mg/kg | 2.5 mg/kg q6h × 2 doses | 2.5 mg/kg q8h |
| CHF | 7.6 mg/kg | 2.5 mg/kg q8h × 2 doses | 1.3–2.5 mg/kg q12h |

**Pharmacokinetics**

| Route | Onset | Peak | Duration |
|---|---|---|---|
| Oral | 1–6 h | 4–6 h | 6–8 h |
| IV | Immediate | 30 min | 4–8 h |

*Metabolism:* Hepatic, $T_{1/2}$: 3–15 h
*Distribution:* Crosses placenta; passes into breast milk
*Excretion:* Urine

## IV facts

**Preparation:** May be infused in 100–200 ml of 5% Dextrose Injection or 0.9% Sodium Chloride Injection.

**Infusion:** Do not exceed 25 mg/min infusion rate. Substitute oral therapy or IV therapy as soon as possible; administer maintenance infusions in a large volume to deliver the desired amount of drug each hour.

*Adult:* 6 mg/kg. For acute symptoms requiring rapid theophyllinization in patients receiving theophylline: a loading dose is required. Each 0.6 mg/kg IV administered as a loading dose will result in about a 1 μg/ml increase in serum theophylline. Ideally, defer loading dose until serum theophylline determination is made; otherwise, base loading dose on clinical judgment and the knowledge that 3.2 mg/kg aminophylline will increase serum theophylline levels by about 5 μg/ml and is unlikely to cause dangerous adverse effects if the patient is not experiencing theophylline toxicity before this dose. Aminophylline IV maintenance infusion rates (mg/kg per h) are given below:

| *Patient Group* | *First 12 h* | *Beyond 12 h* |
|---|---|---|
| Young adult smokers | 1 | 0.8 |
| Nonsmoking adults, otherwise healthy | 0.7 | 0.5 |

***Pediatric:*** After an IV loading dose, the following maintenance rates (mg/kg per h) are recommended:

| *Patient Group* | *First 12 h* | *Beyond 12 h* |
|---|---|---|
| Children 6 mo–6 y | 1.2 | 1 |
| Children 9–16 y | 1 | 0.8 |

***Geriatric:*** After a loading dose, the following maintenance infusion rates (mg/kg per hour) are recommended:

| *Patient Group* | *First 12 h* | *Beyond 12 h* |
|---|---|---|
| Other patients, cor pulmonale | 0.6 | 0.3 |
| CHF, liver disease | 0.5 | 0.1–0.2 |

**Compatibility:** Aminophylline is compatible with most IV solutions, but do not mix in solution with other drugs, including vitamins.

## Adverse effects

- **Serum theophylline levels < 20 μg/ml**: adverse effects uncommon
- **Serum theophylline levels > 20–25 μg/ml**: nausea, vomiting, diarrhea, headache, insomnia, irritability (75% of patients)
- **Serum theophylline levels > 30–35 μg/ml**: hyperglycemia, hypotension, cardiac arrhythmias, tachycardia (> 10 μg/ml in premature newborns); **seizures, brain damage, death**
- CNS: Irritability (especially children); restlessness, dizziness, muscle twitching, convulsions, severe depression, stammering speech; abnormal behavior characterized by withdrawal, mutism and unresponsiveness alternating with hyperactive periods
- GI: Loss of appetite, hematemesis, epigastric pain, gastroesophageal reflux during sleep, increased SGOT
- CV: Palpitations, sinus tachycardia, ventricular tachycardia, life-threatening ventricular arrhythmias, circulatory failure
- **Respiratory**: Tachypnea, respiratory arrest
- GU: Proteinuria, increased excretion of renal tubular cells & RBCs; diuresis (dehydration), urinary retention in men with prostate enlargement
- **Other**: Fever, flushing, hyperglycemia, SIADH, rash

## Clinically important drug-drug interactions

• Increased effects with cimetidine, erythromycin, troleandomycin, clindamycin, lincomycin, influenza virus vaccine, oral contraceptives • Possibly increased effects with thiabendazole, rifampin, allopurinol • Increased cardiac toxicity with halothane; increased likelihood of seizures when given with ketamine; increased likelihood of adverse GI effects when given with tetracyclines • Increased or decreased effects with furosemide, dextrothyroxine, levothyroxine, liothyronine, liotrix, thyroglobulin, thyroid • Decreased effects in patients who are cigarette smokers (1–2 packs per day); theophylline dosage may eed to be increased 50%–100% • Decreased effects with phenobarbital, aminoglutethimide • Increased effects, toxicity of sympathomimetics (especially ephedrine) with theophylline preparations • Decreased effects of phenytoin and theophylline preparations when given concomitantly • Decreased effects of lithium carbonate, nondepolarizing neuromuscular blockers given with theophylline preparations • Mutually antagonistic effects of beta-blockers and theophylline preparations

## Clinically important drug-food interactions

• Elimination is increased by a low-carbohydrate, high-protein diet and by charcoal broiled beef • Elimination is decreased by a high-carbohydrate, low-protein diet • Food may alter bioavailability and absorption of timed-release theophylline preparations, causing toxicity. These forms should by taken on an empty stomach.

**Drug-lab test interferences**

• Interference with spectrophotometric determinations of serum theophylline levels by furosemide, phenylbutazone, probenecid, theobromine; coffee, tea, cola beverages, chocolate, acetaminophen cause falsely high values • Alteration in assays of uric acid, urinary catecholamines, plasma free fatty acids by theophylline preparations

## ■ Nursing Considerations

### Assessment

- ***History:*** Hypersensitivity to any xanthine or to ethylenediamine, peptic ulcer, active gastritis, cardiac arrhythmias, acute myocardial injury, CHF, cor pulmonale, severe hypertension, severe hypoxemia, renal or hepatic disease, hyperthyroidism, alcoholism, labor, lactation, rectal or colonic irritation or infection (aminophylline rectal preparations).
- ***Physical:*** Bowel sounds, normal output; P, auscultation, BP, perfusion, ECG; R, adventitious sounds; frequency of urination, voiding, normal output pattern, urinalysis, renal function tests; liver palpation, liver function tests; thyroid function tests; skin color, texture, lesions; reflexes, bilateral grip strength, affect, EEG

### Implementation

- Administer to pregnant patients only when clearly needed—neonatal tachycardia, jitteriness, and withdrawal apnea observed when mothers received xanthines up until delivery.
- Caution patient not to chew or crush enteric-coated timed-release forms.
- Give immediate-release, liquid dosage forms with food if GI effects occur.
- Do not give timed-release forms with food; these should be given on an empty stomach 1 h before or 2 h after meals.
- Maintain adequate hydration.
- Monitor results of serum theophylline levels carefully, and arrange for reduced dosage if serum levels exceed therapeutic range of 10–20 μg/ml.
- Take serum samples to determine peak theophylline concentration drawn 15–30 min after an IV loading dose.
- Monitor for clinical signs of adverse effects, particularly if serum theophylline levels are not available.
- Maintain diazepam on standby to treat seizures.

### Drug-specific teaching points

- Take this drug exactly as prescribed; if a timed-release product is prescribed, take this drug on an empty stomach, 1 h before or 2 h after meals.
- Do not to chew or crush timed-release preparations.
- Administer rectal solution or suppositories after emptying the rectum.
- It may be necessary to take this drug around the clock for adequate control of asthma attacks.
- Avoid excessive intake of coffee, tea, cocoa, cola beverages, chocolate.
- Smoking cigarettes or other tobacco products impacts the drug's effectiveness. Try not to smoke. Notify the care provider if smoking habits change while taking this drug.
- Be aware that frequent blood tests may be necessary to monitor the effect of this drug and to ensure safe and effective dosage; keep all appointments for blood tests and other monitoring.
- The following side effects may occur: nausea, loss of appetite (taking this drug with food may help if taking the immediate-release or liquid dosage forms); difficulty sleeping, depression, emotional lability (reversible).
- Report nausea, vomiting, severe GI pain, restlessness, convulsions, irregular heartbeat.

# amiodarone hydrochloride

*(a mee o' da rone)*

Cordarone, Cordarone IV

**Pregnancy Category C**

### Drug classes
Antiarrhythmic
Adrenergic blocker (not used as sympatholytic agent)

### Therapeutic actions
Type III antiarrhythmic: acts directly on cardiac cell membrane; prolongs repolarization and refractory period; increases ventricular fibrillation threshold; acts on peripheral smooth muscle to decrease peripheral resistance

### Indications
- Only for treatment of the following documented life-threatening recurrent ventricular arrhythmias that do not respond to other antiarrhythmics or when alternative agents are not tolerated: recurrent ventricular fibrillation, recurrent hemodynamically unstable ventricular tachycardia. Serious and even fatal toxicity has been reported with this drug; use alternative agents first; very closely monitor patient receiving this drug.
- Unlabeled uses: treatment of refractory sustained or paroxysmal atrial fibrillation and paroxysmal supraventricular tachycardia; treatment of symptomatic atrial flutter; may produce benefit in left ventricular ejection fraction, exercise tolerance, and ventricular arrhythmias in patients with CHF

### Contraindications/cautions
- Hypersensitivity to amiodarone, sinus node dysfunction, heart block, severe bradycardia, hypokalemia, lactation.

### Dosage
**Available Forms:** Tablets—200 mg; injection—50 mg/ml

Careful patient assessment and evaluation with continual monitoring of cardiac response are necessary for titrating the dosage. Therapy should begin in the hospital with continual monitoring and emergency equipment on standby. The following is a guide to usual dosage.

ADULT
- ***PO:*** *Loading dose:* 800–1,600 mg/d PO in divided doses, for 1–3 wk; reduce dose to 600–800 mg/d in divided doses for 1 mo; if rhythm is stable, reduce dose to 400 mg/d in one to two divided doses for maintenance dose. Titrate to the lowest possible dose to limit side effects.
- ***IV:*** 1000 mg IV over 24 h—150 mg loading dose over 10 min, followed by 360 mg over 6 h at rate of 1 mg/min; maintenance infusion: 540 mg at 0.5 mg/min over 18 h. May be continued up to 96 h or until rhythm is stable. Switch to oral form as soon as possible.

PEDIATRIC: Safety and efficacy not established.

### Pharmacokinetics
| Route | Onset | Peak | Duration |
|---|---|---|---|
| Oral | 2–3 d | 3–7 h | 6–8 h |
| IV | Immediate | 10 min | Infusion |

*Metabolism:* Hepatic, $T_{1/2}$: 2.5–10 d, then 40–55 d
*Distribution:* Crosses placenta; passes into breast milk
*Excretion:* Bile and feces

### IV facts
**Preparation:** Do not use PVC container. Dilute 150 mg in 100 ml $D_5W$ for rapid loading dose (1.5 mg/ml). Dilute 900 mg in 500 ml $D_5W$ for slow infusions (1.8 mg/ml). Store at room temperature and use within 24 h.
**Infusion:** Infuse loading dose over 10 min. Immediately follow with slow infusion of 1 mg/min or 33.3 ml/hr. Maintenance infusion of 0.5 mg/min or 16.6 ml/hr can be continued up to 96 h. Use of an infusion pump is advised.
**Compatibility:** Do not mix in solution with other drugs.

### Adverse effects
- CNS: *Malaise, fatigue, dizziness, tremors, ataxia,* paresthesias, lack of coordination
- GI: *Nausea, vomiting, anorexia, constipation, abnormal liver function tests,* ***liver toxicity***
- CV: **Cardiac arrhythmias**, congestive heart failure, **cardiac arrest**

- Respiratory: *Pulmonary toxicity*—pneumonitis, infitrates (shortness of breath, cough, rales, wheezes)
- Endocrine: *Hypothyroidism* or *hyperthyroidism*
- EENT: *Corneal microdeposits* (photophobia, dry eyes, halos, blurred vision); **Ophthalmic abnormalities** including permanent blindness
- Other: *Photosensitivity*, angioedema

### Clinically important drug-drug interactions

• Increased digitalis toxicity with digoxin • Increased quinidine toxicity with quinidine • Increased procainamide toxicity with procainamide • Increased flecainide toxicity with amiodarone • Increased phenytoin toxicity with phenytoin, ethotoin, mephenytoin • Increased bleeding tendencies with warfarin • Potential sinus arrest and heart block with $\beta$-blockers, calcium channel-blockers

### Drug-lab test interferences

• Increased $T_4$ levels, increased serum reverse $T_3$ levels

## ■ Nursing Considerations

### Assessment

- ***History:*** Hypersensitivity to amiodarone, sinus node dysfunction, heart block, severe bradycardia, hypokalemia, lactation
- ***Physical:*** Skin color, lesions; reflexes, gait, eye exam; P, BP, auscultation, continuous ECG monitoring; R, adventitious sounds, baseline chest x-ray; liver evaluation; liver function tests, serum electrolytes, $T_4$ and $T_3$

### Implementation

- Monitor cardiac rhythm continuously.
- Monitor for an extended period when dosage adjustments are made.
- Monitor for safe and effective serum levels (0.5–2.5 $\mu$g/ml).
- Doses of digoxin, quinidine, procainamide, phenytoin, and warfarin may need to be reduced one-third to one-half when amiodarone is started.
- Give drug with meals to decrease GI problems.
- Arrange for ophthalmologic exams; reevaluate at any sign of optic neuropathy.
- Arrange for periodic chest x-ray to evaluate pulmonary status (every 3–6 mo).
- Arrange for regular periodic blood tests for liver enzymes, thyroid hormone levels.

### Drug-specific teaching points

- Drug dosage will be changed in relation to response of arrhythmias; you will need to be hospitalized during initiation of drug therapy; you will be closely monitored when dosage is changed.
- The following side effects may occur: changes in vision (halos, dry eyes, sensitivity to light; wear sunglasses, monitor light exposure); nausea, vomiting, loss of appetite (take with meals; small, frequent meals may help); sensitivity to the sun (use a sunscreen or protective clothing when outdoors); constipation (a laxative may be ordered); tremors, twitching, dizziness, loss of coordination (do not drive, operate dangerous machinery, or undertake tasks that require coordination until drug effects stabilize and your body adjusts to it).
- Have regular medical follow-up, monitoring of cardiac rhythm, chest x-ray, eye exam, blood tests.
- Report unusual bleeding or bruising; fever, chills; intolerance to heat or cold; shortness of breath, difficulty breathing, cough; swelling of ankles or fingers; palpitations; difficulty with vision.

## ☆ amitriptyline hydrochloride

*(a mee **trip'** ti leen)*

Elavil, Levate (CAN), Meravil (CAN), Novotriptyn (CAN)

**Pregnancy Category C**

### Drug classes

Tricyclic antidepressant (TCA; tertiary amine)

### Therapeutic actions

Mechanism of action unknown; TCAs act to inhibit the reuptake of the neurotransmitters norepinephrine and serotonin, leading to an increase in their effects; anticholinergic at CNS and peripheral receptors; sedative.

### Indications

- Relief of symptoms of depression (endogenous most responsive); sedative effects may help when depression is associated with anxiety and sleep disturbance.
- Unlabeled uses: control of chronic pain (eg, intractable pain of cancer, peripheral neuropathies, postherpetic neuralgia, tic douloureux, central pain syndromes); prevention of onset of cluster and migraine headaches; treatment of pathologic weeping and laughing secondary to forebrain disease (due to multiple sclerosis)

### Contraindications/cautions

- Contraindications: hypersensitivity to any tricyclic drug; concomitant therapy with an MAO inhibitor; recent MI; myelography within previous 24 h or scheduled within 48 h; lactation.
- Use cautiously with electroshock therapy; preexisting CV disorders (severe coronary heart disease, progressive heart failure, angina pectoris, paroxysmal tachycardia); angle-closure glaucoma, increased intraocular pressure, urinary retention, ureteral or urethral spasm; seizure disorders; hyperthyroidism; impaired hepatic, renal function; psychiatric patients (schizophrenic or paranoid patients may exhibit a worsening of psychosis with TCA therapy); manic-depressive patients; elective surgery (discontinue as long as possible before surgery).

### Dosage

**Available Forms:** Injection—10 mg/ml; tablets—10, 25, 50, 75, 100, 150 mg

**ADULT**

- ***Depression, hospitalized patients:*** Initially, 100 mg/d PO in divided doses: gradually increase to 200–300 mg/d as required. May be given IM 20–30 mg qid, initially only in patients unable or unwilling to take drug PO. Replace with oral medication as soon as possible.
- ***Outpatients:*** Initially, 75 mg/d PO, in divided doses; may increase to 150 mg/d. Increases should be made in late afternoon or hs. Total daily dosage may be administered hs. Initiate single daily dose therapy with 50–100 mg hs; increase by 25–50 mg as necessary to a total of 150 mg/d. Maintenance dose is 40–100 mg/d, which may be given as a single bedtime dose. After satisfactory response, reduce to lowest effective dosage. Continue therapy for 3 mo or longer to lessen possibility of relapse.
- ***Chronic pain:*** 75–150 mg/d PO
- ***Prevention of cluster/migraine headaches:*** 50–150 mg/d PO.
- ***Prevention of weeping in MS patients with forebrain disease:*** 25–75 mg PO.

**PEDIATRIC:** Not recommended in children < 12 y.

### Pharmacokinetics

| *Route* | *Onset* | *Peak* | *Duration* |
|---|---|---|---|
| Oral | Varies | 2–4 h | 20–4 wk |

*Metabolism:* Hepatic, $T_{1/2}$: 10–50 h
*Distribution:* Crosses placenta; passes into breast milk
*Excretion:* Urine

### Adverse effects

- CNS: *Sedation and anticholinergic (atropine-like) effects*; *confusion* (especially in elderly), *disturbed concentration*, hallucinations, disorientation, decreased memory, feelings of unreality, delusions, anxiety, nervousness, restlessness, agitation, panic, insomnia, nightmares, hypomania, mania, exacerbation of psychosis, drowsiness, weakness, fatigue, headache, numbness, tingling, paresthesias of extremities, incoordination, motor hyperactivity, akathisia, ataxia, tremors, peripheral neuropathy, extrapyramidal symptoms, seizures, speech blockage, dysarthria, tinnitus, altered EEG
- GI: *Dry mouth, constipation*, paralytic ileus, *nausea*, vomiting, anorexia, epi-

gastric distress, diarrhea, flatulence, dysphagia, peculiar taste, increased salivation, stomatitis, glossitis, parotid swelling, abdominal cramps, black tongue, hepatitis, jaundice (rare), elevated transaminase, altered alkaline phosphatase

- CV: *Orthostatic hypotension*, hypertension, syncope, tachycardia, palpitations, MI, arrhythmias, heart block, precipitation of CHF, stroke
- **Hematologic**: Bone marrow depression, including agranulocytosis; eosinophila, purpura, thrombocytopenia, leukopenia
- GU: Urinary retention, delayed micturition, dilation of the urinary tract, gynecomastia, testicular swelling; breast enlargement, menstrual irregularity and galactorrhea; increased or decreased libido; impotence
- **Endocrine**: Elevated or depressed blood sugar, elevated prolactin levels, inappropriate ADH secretion
- **Hypersensitivity**: Skin rash, pruritus, vasculitis, petechiae, photosensitization, edema (generalized, face, tongue), drug fever
- **Withdrawal**: Symptoms on abrupt discontinuation of prolonged therapy: nausea, headache, vertigo, nightmares, malaise
- **Other**: Nasal congestion, excessive appetite, weight change; sweating, alopecia, lacrimation, hyperthermia, flushing, chills

**Clinically important drug-drug interactions**

• Increased TCA levels and pharmacologic (especially anticholinergic) effects with cimetidine, fluoxetine • Increased TCA levels with methylphenidate, phenothiazines, oral contraceptives, disulfiram • Hyperpyretic crises, severe convulsions, hypertensive episodes and deaths with MAO inhibitors, furazolidone • Increased antidepressant response and cardiac arrhythmias with thyroid medication. • Increased or decreased effects with estrogens • Delirium with disulfiram • Sympathetic hyperactivity, sinus tachycardia, hypertension, agitation with levodopa • Increased biotransformation of TCAs in patients who smoke cigarettes • Increased sympathomimetic (especially $\alpha$-adrenergic) effects of direct-acting sympathomimetic drugs (norepinephrine, epinephrine) • Increased anticholinergic effects of anticholinergic drugs (including anticholinergic antiparkisonism drugs) • Increased response (especially CNS depression) to barbiturates • Increased effects of dicumarol • Decreased antihypertensive effect of guanethidine, clonidine, other antihypertensives • Decreased effects of indirect-acting sympathomimetic drugs (ephedrine)

## ■ Nursing Considerations

### Assessment

- ***History:*** Hypersensitivity to any tricyclic drug; concomitant therapy with an MAO inhibitor; recent MI; myelography within previous 24 h or scheduled within 48 h; lactation; EST; preexisting CV disorders; angle-closure glaucoma, increased intraocular pressure, urinary retention, ureteral or urethral spasm; seizure disorders; hyperthyroidism; impaired hepatic, renal function; psychiatric patients; manic-depressive patients; elective surgery
- ***Physical:*** Weight; T; skin color, lesions; orientation, affect, reflexes, vision and hearing; P, BP, orthostatic BP, perfusion; bowel sounds, normal output, liver evaluation; urine flow, normal output; usual sexual function, frequency of menses, breast and scrotal exam; liver function tests, urinalysis, CBC, ECG

### Implementation

- Restrict drug access for depressed and potentially suicidal patients.
- Give IM only when oral therapy is impossible.
- Do not administer IV.
- Administer major portion of dose at bedtime if drowsiness, severe anticholinergic effects occur (note that the elderly may not tolerate single daily dose therapy).

- Reduce dosage if minor side effects develop; discontinue if serious side effects occur.
- Arrange for CBC if patient develops fever, sore throat, or other sign of infection.

### Drug-specific teaching points

- Take drug exactly as prescribed; do not stop abruptly or without consulting health care provider.
- Avoid using alcohol, other sleep-inducing drugs, OTC drugs.
- Avoid prolonged exposure to sunlight or sunlamps; use a sunscreen or protective garments.
- The following side effects may occur: headache, dizziness, drowsiness, weakness, blurred vision (reversible; if severe, avoid driving and tasks requiring alertness while these persist); nausea, vomiting, loss of appetite, dry mouth (small frequent meals, frequent mouth care and sucking sugarless candies may help); nightmares, inability to concentrate, confusion; changes in sexual function.
- Report dry mouth, difficulty in urination, excessive sedation.

## amlodipine

*(am **loe'** di peen)*

Norvasc

**Pregnancy Category C**

### Drug classes

Calcium channel-blocker
Antianginal drug
Antihypertensive

### Therapeutic actions

Inhibits the movement of calcium ions across the membranes of cardiac and arterial muscle cells; inhibits transmembrane calcium flow, which results in the depression of impulse formation in specialized cardiac pacemaker cells, slowing of the velocity of conduction of the cardiac impulse, depression of myocardial contractility, and dilation of coronary arteries and arterioles and peripheral arterioles; these effects lead to decreased cardiac work, decreased cardiac oxygen consumption, and in patients with vasospastic (Prinzmetal's) angina, increased delivery of oxygen to cardiac cells.

### Indications

- Angina pectoris due to coronary artery spasm (Prinzmetal's variant angina)
- Chronic stable angina, alone or in combination with other agents
- Essential hypertension, alone or in combination with other antihypertensives

### Contraindications/cautions

- Contraindications: allergy to diltiazem, impaired hepatic or renal function, sick sinus syndrome, heart block (second or third degree), lactation
- Use cautiously with CHF

### Dosage

**Available Forms:** Tablets—2.5, 5, 10 mg

*ADULT:* Initially 5 mg PO qd; dosage may be gradually increased over 10–14 d to a maximum dose of 10 mg PO qd.

*PEDIATRIC:* Safety and efficacy not established.

*GERIATRIC OR HEPATIC IMPAIRMENT:* Initially, 2.5 mg PO qd; dosage may be gradually titrated over 7–14 d based on clinical assessment

### Pharmacokinetics

| Route | Onset | Peak |
|---|---|---|
| Oral | Unknown | 6–12 h |

*Metabolism:* Hepatic, $T_{1/2}$: 30–50 h

*Distribution:* Crosses placenta; passes into breast milk

*Excretion:* Urine

### Adverse effects

- CNS: *Dizziness, lightheadedness, headache*, asthenia, *fatigue, lethargy*
- GI: *Nausea*, abdominal discomfort
- CV: *Peripheral edema*, arrhythmias
- Dermatologic: *Flushing*, rash

### Clinically important drug-drug interactions

- Possible increased serum levels and toxicity of cyclosporine if taken concurrently

a

## Nursing Considerations

### Assessment
- *History:* Allergy to amlodipine, impaired hepatic or renal function, sick sinus syndrome, heart block, lactation, CHF
- *Physical:* Skin lesions, color, edema; P, BP, baseline ECG, peripheral perfusion, auscultation; R, adventitious sounds; liver evaluation, GI normal output; liver and renal function tests, urinalysis

### Implementation
- Monitor patient carefully (BP, cardiac rhythm, and output) while titrating drug to therapeutic dose; use special caution if patient has CHF.
- Monitor BP very carefully if patient is also on nitrates.
- Monitor cardiac rhythm regularly during stabilization of dosage and periodically during long-term therapy.
- Administer drug without regard to meals.

### Drug-specific teaching points
- Take with meals if upset stomach occurs.
- The following side effects may occur: nausea, vomiting (small, frequent meals may help); headache (adjust lighting, noise, and temperature; medication may be ordered).
- Report irregular heart beat, shortness of breath, swelling of the hands or feet, pronounced dizziness, constipation.

# ammonia spirit, aromatic

*(ah **mo'** nee a)*

**Pregnancy Category C**

### Drug classes
Respiratory and circulatory stimulant

### Therapeutic actions
Stimulates the respiratory and CV centers of the medulla by causing irritation of the sensory receptors in nasal membranes, esophageal mucosa, and fundus of the stomach.

### Indications
- Prevention and treatment of fainting (smelling salts)

### Contraindications/cautions
- Contraindications: severe hypertension, lactation.

### Dosage
**Available Forms:** Vials

Inhale vapors as required.

### Pharmacokinetics
*Metabolism:* Lung and liver, $T_{1/2}$: unknown

*Distribution:* Crosses placenta; may pass into breast milk

*Excretion:* Unknown

### Adverse effects
- CV: Hypertension, tachycardia
- Local: Nasal irritation
- GI: Nausea, vomiting

## Nursing Considerations

### Assessment
- *History:* Blood dyscrasias, recent infection
- *Physical:* Status of mucous membranes; BP, P

### Implementation
- Wrap glass vial in gauze or cloth; break between fingers.
- Store vials in dark in tightly closed container.
- Evaluate patient if frequent fainting spells occur; refer to appropriate medical consultation.

### Drug-specific teaching points
- Nausea, nasal irritation, headache may occur.
- Report frequent use of drug, frequent fainting spells, severe headache.

# ammonium chloride

*(ah **mo'** nee um)*

**Pregnancy Category C**

### Drug classes
Electrolyte

Urinary acidifier

### Therapeutic actions
Converted to urea in the liver; liberated hydrogen and chloride ions in blood and ex-

tracellular fluid lower the pH and correct alkalosis; lowers the urinary pH, producing an acidic urine that changes the excretion rate of many metabolites and drugs.

### Indications

- Treatment of hypochloremic states and metabolic alkalosis
- Acidification of urine

### Contraindications/cautions

- Renal function impairment; hepatic impairment; metabolic alkalosis due to vomiting of hydrochloric acid when it is accompanied by loss of sodium

### Dosage

**Available Forms:** Injection—26.75% (5 μg/ml); tablets—500 mg; coated tablets—486 mg

**ADULT/PEDIATRIC**

- ***IV:*** Dosage is determined by patient's condition and tolerance; monitor dosage rate and amount by repeated serum bicarbonate determinations.

**ADULT**

- ***PO:*** 4–12 g/d PO divided q4–6h for no longer than 6 d

**PEDIATRIC**

- ***PO:*** 75 mg/kg per day PO in four divided doses for no longer than 6 d

### Pharmacokinetics

| *Route* | *Onset* | *Peak* |
|---|---|---|
| IV | Rapid | 1–3 h |
| PO | Varies | 3–6 h |

*Metabolism:* Hepatic
*Distribution:* Crosses placenta; passes into breast milk
*Excretion:* Urine

### IV facts

**Preparation:** Add contents of one or two vials (100–200 mEq) to 500 or 1,000 ml isotonic (0.9%) Sodium Chloride Injection. Concentration should not exceed 1%–2% ammonium chloride. Avoid excessive heat; protect from freezing. If crystals do appear, warm the solution to room temperature in a water bath prior to use.

**Infusion:** Do not exceed rate of 5 ml/min in adults (1,000 ml infused over 3 h). Infuse slowly. Reduce rate in infants and children.

**Compatibilities:** Do not mix with codeine, levorphanol, methadone, nitrofurantoin, warfarin.

### Adverse effects

- GI: *Nausea*, vomiting, gastric irritation (oral); **severe hepatic impairment**
- **Metabolic**: Metabolic acidosis, hypervolemia, ammonia toxicity—pallor, sweating, irregular breathing, retching, bradycarida, arrhythmias, twitching, convulsion, coma
- **Local**: *Pain or irritation at injection site*, fever, venous thrombosis, phlebitis, extravasation (IV)

### Clinically important drug-drug interactions

- Decreased therapeutic levels due to increased elimination of amphetamine, methamphetamine, dextroamphetamine, ephedrine, pseudoephedrine, methadone, mexiletine when taken with ammonium chloride • Increased effects of chlorpropamide with ammonium chloride

## ■ Nursing Considerations

### Assessment

- ***History:*** Renal or hepatic impairment; metabolic alkalosis due to vomiting of hydrochloric acid when it is accompanied by loss of sodium
- ***Physical:*** P, BP; skin color, texture; T; injection site evaluation; liver evaluation; renal and liver function tests, serum bicarbonate, urinalysis

### Implementation

- Infuse by IV route slowly to avoid irritation; check infusion site frequently to monitor for reaction.
- Monitor IV doses for possible fluid overload.
- Monitor for acidosis (increased R, restlessness, sweating, increased blood pH); decrease infusion as appropriate. Maintain sodium bicarbonate or sodium lactate on standby for overdose situations.

**Drug-specific teaching points**

- Do not take oral drug for longer than 6 d.
- Frequent monitoring of blood tests is needed when receiving IV drugs to determine dosage and rate of drug.
- Report pain or irritation at IV site; confusion, restlessness, sweating, headache; severe GI upset, fever, chills, changes in stool or urine color (oral drug)

## amobarbital

*(am oh **bar'** bi tal)*

amobarbital sodium, amylobarbitone

Amytal Sodium, Novamobarb (CAN)

**Pregnancy Category D**
**C-II controlled substance**

### Drug classes

Barbiturate (intermediate acting)
Sedative
Hypnotic
Anticonvulsant

### Therapeutic actions

General CNS depressant; barbiturates act on the ascending RAS, depress the cerebral cortex, alter cerebellar function, depress motor output, and can produce excitation, sedation, hypnosis, anesthesia and deep coma; at anesthetic doses, has anticonvulsant activity.

### Indications

- Oral: sedation and relief of anxiety; hypnotic effects; preanesthetic medication; control of convulsions
- Parenteral: management of catatonic and negativistic reactions, manic reactions and epileptiform seizures; useful in narcoanalysis and narcotherapy; diagnostic aid in schizophrenia; control of convulsive seizures due to chorea, eclampsia, meningitis, tetanus, procaine or cocaine reactions, poisoning from drugs, such as strychnine or picrotoxin.

### Contraindications/cautions

- Contraindications: hypersensitivity to barbiturates; manifest or latent porphyria; marked liver impairment; nephritis; severe respiratory distress, respiratory disease with dyspnea, obstruction, or cor pulmonale; previous addiction to sedative-hypnotic drugs; pregnancy.
- Use cautiously with acute or chronic pain (drug may cause paradoxical excitement or mask important symptoms); seizure disorders (abrupt discontinuation of daily doses can result in status epilepticus); lactation; fever, hyperthyroidism, diabetes mellitus, severe anemia, pulmonary or cardiac disease, status asthmaticus, shock, uremia; impaired liver or kidney function, debilitation.

### Dosage

**Available Forms:** Tablets—30, 50, 100 mg; capsules—65, 200 mg; powder for injection: 250, 500 mg/vial

**ADULT**

- ***Oral:*** Dosage range: 15–120 mg bid–qid
  - *Daytime sedation:* 30–50 mg bid–tid PO
  - *Hypnotic:* 100–200 mg PO
  - *Insomnia:* 65–200 mg (as sodium) hs, PO
- ***IM:*** Usual dose is 65–500 mg; maximum dose should not exceed 500 mg. Do not give more than 5 ml concentration in one injection; solutions of 20% can be used to minimize volume.
  - *Preanesthetic sedation:* 200 mg (as sodium) 1–2 h before surgery, IM
  - *Labor:* Initial dose is 200–400 mg (as sodium); additional doses: 200–400 mg at 1- to 3-h intervals for a total dose of not more than 1 g, IM
- ***IV:*** Same dose as IM. Do not exceed a rate of 1 ml/min. Use of the 10% solution may cause serious respiratory depression.

**PEDIATRIC:** Use caution. Barbiturates may produce irritability, excitability, inappropriate tearfulness, and aggression. Base dosage on weight, age, and response. Because of higher metabolic rates, children tolerate comparatively higher doses; ordinarily, 65–500 mg may be given to a child 6-12 y old. Administer by slow IV injection, and monitor response carefully.

GERIATRIC PATIENTS OR THOSE WITH DEBILITATING DISEASE: Reduce dosage and monitor closely; may produce excitement, depression, confusion.

### Pharmacokinetics

| Route | Onset | Peak | Duration |
|---|---|---|---|
| Oral | 45–60 min | | 6–8 h |
| IV | 5 min | 15 min | 3–6 h |

*Metabolism:* Hepatic, $T_{1/2}$: 16–40 h
*Distribution:* Crosses placenta; passes into breast milk
*Excretion:* Urine

**IV facts**

**Preparation:** Add Sterile Water for Injection to the vial, then rotate it to dissolve the powder. Do not shake the vial. Use only a solution that is absolutely clear after 5 min. Inject contents within 30 min of opening the vial. Amobarbital is unstable on exposure to air.
**Infusion:** Infuse slowly. Do not give intra-arterially; can cause severe spasm. Do not exceed rate of 1 ml/min. Monitor patient continually during infusion.
**Compatibilities:** Incompatible with many other drugs in solution; **do not mix in solution with any drugs.**

### Adverse effects

- CNS: *Somnolence, agitation, confusion, hyperkinesia, ataxia, vertigo, CNS depression, nightmares, lethargy, residual sedation (hangover),* paradoxical excitement, nervousness, psychiatric disturbance, hallucinations, insomnia, anxiety, dizziness, thinking abnormality
- GI: *Nausea, vomiting, constipation, diarrhea,* epigastric pain
- CV: Bradycardia, hypotension, syncope
- Respiratory: *Hypoventilation*, **apnea, respiratory depression**, laryngospasm, bronchospasm, circulatory collapse
- Hypersensitivity: Skin rashes, angioneurotic edema, serum sickness, morbiliform rash, urticaria; rarely, exfoliative dermatitis, **Stevens-Johnson syndrome, sometimes fatal**
- Injection site: *Local pain*, tissue necrosis, gangrene; arterial spasm with inadvertent intra-arterial injection; thrombophlebitis; permanent neurologic deficit if injected near a nerve
- Other: *Tolerance, psychological and physical dependence*; withdrawal syndrome, sometimes fatal

### Clinically important drug-drug interactions

• Increased CNS depression with alcohol, other CNS depressants, phenothiazines, antihistamines, tranquilizers • Increased blood levels and pharmacologic effects of barbiturates with MAO inhibitors • Increased renal toxicity if taken with methoxyflurane • Decreased effects of the following: oral anticoagulants, digitoxin, tricyclic antidepressants, corticosteroids, oral contraceptives and estrogens, acetaminophen, metronidazole, phenmetrazine, carbamazepine, beta blockers, griseofulvin, phenylbutazones, theophyllines, quinidine, doxycycline • Altered effectiveness of phenytoin with barbiturates

## ■ Nursing Considerations

### Assessment

- *History:* Hypersensitivity to barbiturates; manifest or latent porphyria; marked liver impairment; nephritis; severe respiratory distress, respiratory disease with dyspnea, obstruction or cor pulmonale; previous addiction to sedative-hypnotic drugs; acute or chronic pain; seizure disorders; lactation; fever, hyperthyroidism, diabetes mellitus, severe anemia, pulmonary or cardiac disease, status asthmaticus, shock, uremia; debilitation.
- *Physical:* Weight; T; skin color, lesions; orientation, affect, reflexes; P, BP, orthostatic BP; R, adventitious sounds; bowel sounds, normal output, liver evaluation; liver and kidney function tests, blood and urine glucose, BUN.

### Implementation

- Monitor patient responses, blood levels if any of the above interacting drugs are given with amobarbital; suggest alterna-

tive contraceptives to oral ones if amobarbital is used.
- Do not give intra-arterially (may produce arteriospasm, thrombosis, gangrene).
- Give IM doses deep in a muscle mass.
- Monitor sites carefully for irritation, extravasation with IV use (alkaline solutions are irritating to tissues).
- Monitor P, BP, respiration carefully during IV administration.
- Have resuscitative facilities on standby in case of respiratory depression, hypersensitivity reaction.
- Taper dosage gradually after repeated use, especially in epileptic patients.

### Drug-specific teaching points

Incorporate teaching about the drug with the general teaching about the procedure for patients receiving this drug as preanesthetic medication or during labor; include the following:
- This drug will make you drowsy and less anxious.
- Do not try to get up after you have received this drug (request assistance if you feel you must sit up or move around).

*Oral Use*
- This drug is habit forming; its effectiveness in facilitating sleep disappears after a short time.
- Do not take this drug longer than 2 wk (for insomnia), and do not increase the dosage without consulting health care provider.
- Consult health care provider if drug appears to be ineffective; do not increase the dose.
- Avoid alcohol, sleep-inducing, or OTC drugs while on this drug because these could be dangerous.
- Use contraception other than oral contraceptives. Avoid becoming pregnant while taking this drug.
- The following side effects may occur: drowsiness, dizziness, "hangover," impaired thinking (these effects may become less pronounced after a few days; avoid driving or dangerous activities); GI upset (taking the drug with food may help); dreams, nightmares, difficulty concentrating, fatigue, nervousness (reversible; will go away when drug is discontinued).
- Report severe dizziness, weakness, drowsiness that persists; rash or skin lesions; pregnancy.

## amoxapine

*(a **mox'** a peen)*

Asendin

**Pregnancy Category C**

### Drug classes

Tricyclic antidepressant (TCA)
Antianxiety drug

### Therapeutic actions

Mechanism of action unknown; TCAs inhibit the reuptake of the neurotransmitters norepinephrine and serotonin, leading to an increase in their effects; anticholinergic at CNS and peripheral receptors; sedative.

### Indications

- Relief of symptoms of depression (endogenous depression most responsive)
- Antianxiety drug

### Contraindications/cautions

- Contraindications: hypersensitivity to any tricyclic drug; concomitant therapy with an MAO inhibitor; recent MI; myelography within previous 24 h or scheduled within 48 h; lactation.
- Use cautiously with EST; preexisting CV disorders (severe coronary heart disease, progressive heart failure, angina pectoris, paroxysmal tachycardia); angle-closure glaucoma, increased intraocular pressure, urinary retention, ureteral or urethral spasm; seizure disorders; hyperthyroidism; impaired hepatic, renal function; psychiatric patients (schizophrenic or paranoid patients may exhibit a worsening of psychosis); manic-depressive patients; elective surgery (discontinue as soon as possible before surgery).

### Dosage

**Available Forms:** Tablets—25, 50 mg

*ADULT:* Initially 50 mg PO bid–tid; gradually increase to 100 mg bid–tid by end of first week if tolerated; increase above 300 mg/d only if this dosage ineffective for at least 2 wk. Hospitalized patients refractory to antidepressant therapy and with no history of convulsive seizures may be given up to 600 mg/d in divided doses; after effective dosage is established, drug may be given in single hs dose (up to 300 mg).

*PEDIATRIC:* Not recommended in children < 16 y.

*GERIATRIC:* Initially, 25 mg bid–tid; if tolerated, dosage may be increased by end of first week to 50 mg bid–tid. For many elderly patients, 100–150 mg/d may be adequate; some may require up to 300 mg/d.

### Pharmacokinetics

| *Route* | *Onset* | *Peak* | *Duration* |
|---|---|---|---|
| Oral | Varies | 2–4 h | 2–4 wk |

*Metabolism:* Hepatic, $T_{1/2}$: 8–30 h
*Distribution:* Crosses placenta; passes into breast milk
*Excretion:* Urine

### Adverse effects

- CNS: *Sedation and anticholinergic (atropine-like) effects*; *confusion* (especially in elderly), *disturbed concentration*, hallucinations, disorientation, decreased memory, feelings of unreality, delusions, anxiety, nervousness, restlessness, agitation, panic, insomnia, nightmares, hypomania, mania, exacerbation of psychosis, drowsiness, weakness, fatigue, headache, numbness, tingling, paresthesias of extremities, incoordination, motor hyperactivity, akathisia, ataxia, tremors, peripheral neuropathy, extrapyramidal symptoms, seizures, speech blockage, dysarthria, tinnitus, altered EEG
- GI: *Dry mouth, constipation*, paralytic ileus, *nausea*, vomiting, anorexia, epigastric distress, diarrhea, flatulence, dysphagia, peculiar taste, increased salivation, stomatitis, glossitis, parotid swelling, abdominal cramps, black tongue, hepatitis, jaundice (rare); elevated transaminase, altered alkaline phosphatase
- CV: *Orthostatic hypotension*, hypertension, syncope, tachycardia, palpitations, MI, arrhythmias, heart block, precipitation of CHF, stroke
- **Hematologic**: Bone marrow depression
- GU: Urinary retention, delayed micturition, dilation of the urinary tract, gynecomastia, testicular swelling in men; breast enlargement, menstrual irregularity, and galactorrhea in women; changes in libido; impotence
- **Endocrine**: Elevated or depressed blood sugar, elevated prolactin levels, inappropriate ADH secretion
- **Hypersensitivity**: Skin rash, pruritus, vasculitis, petechiae, photosensitization, edema (generalized, facial, tongue), drug fever
- **Withdrawal**: Symptoms on abrupt discontinuation of prolonged therapy; nausea, headache, vertigo, nightmares, malaise
- **Other**: Nasal congestion, excessive appetite, weight gain or loss, sweating, alopecia, lacrimation, hyperthermia, flushing, chills

### Clinically important drug-drug interactions

• Increased TCA levels and pharmacologic (especially anticholinergic) effects with cimetidine, fluoxetine • Increased TCA levels with methylphenidate, phenothiazines, oral contraceptives, disulfiram, cimetidine, ranitidine • Hyperpyretic crises, severe convulsions, hypertensive episodes, and deaths with MAO inhibitors, furazolidone • Increased antidepressant response and cardiac arrhythmias with thyroid medication. • Increased or decreased effects with estrogens • Delirium with disulfiram • Sympathetic hyperactivity, sinus tachycardia, hypertension, agitation with levodopa • Increased biotransformation of TCAs in patients who smoke cigarettes • Increased sympathomimetic (especially $\alpha$-adrenergic) effects of direct-acting sympathomimetic drugs (norepinephrine, epinephrine) • Increased anticholinergic effects of anticholinergic drugs (including anticholinergic antiparkisonism drugs) • Increased response (especially CNS depression) to barbiturates

• Increased effects of dicumarol • Decreased antihypertensive effect of guanethidine, clonidine, other antihypertensives • Decreased effects of indirect-acting sympathomimetic drugs (ephedrine)

## ■ Nursing Considerations

### Assessment

- *History:* Hypersensitivity to any tricyclic drug; concomitant therapy with an MAO inhibitor; recent MI; myelography within previous 24 h or scheduled within 48 h; lactation; EST; preexisting CV disorders; angle-closure glaucoma, increased intraocular pressure; urinary retention, ureteral or urethral spasm; seizure disorders; hyperthyroidism; impaired hepatic, renal function; psychiatric patients; manic-depressive patients; elective surgery
- *Physical:* Weight; T; skin color, lesions; orientation, affect, reflexes, vision and hearing; P, BP, orthostatic BP, perfusion; bowel sounds, normal output, liver evaluation; urine flow, normal output; usual sexual function, frequency of menses, breast and scrotal exam; liver function tests, urinalysis, CBC, ECG

### Implementation

- Restrict drug access for depressed and potentially suicidal patients.
- Give major portion of dose hs if drowsiness, severe anticholinergic effects occur (the elderly may not tolerate single daily dose).
- Reduce dosage if minor side effects develop; discontinue if serious side effects occur.
- Arrange for CBC if patient develops fever, sore throat, or other sign of infection.
- Encourage elderly men or men with prostate problems to void before taking drug.

### Drug-specific teaching points

- Do not stop taking this drug abruptly or without consulting health care provider.
- Avoid using alcohol, other sleep-inducing drugs, OTC drugs.
- Avoid prolonged exposure to sunlight or sunlamps; use a sunscreen or protective garments.
- The following side effects may occur: headache, dizziness, drowsiness, weakness, blurred vision (reversible; safety measures may need to be taken if severe; avoid driving or tasks requiring alertness); nausea, vomiting, loss of appetite, dry mouth (small frequent meals, frequent mouth care and sucking sugarless candies may help); nightmares, inability to concentrate, confusion; changes in sexual function.
- Report dry mouth, difficulty in urination, excessive sedation.

## amoxicillin

*(a mox i **sill'** in)*

Amoxil, Apo-Amoxi (CAN), Biomox, Novamoxin (CAN), Nu-Amoxi (CAN), Polymox, Trimox, Wymox

**Pregnancy Category B**

### Drug classes

Antibiotic, penicillin–ampicillin type

### Therapeutic actions

Bactericidal: inhibits synthesis of cell wall of sensitive organisms, causing cell death.

### Indications

- Infections due to susceptible strains of *Haemophilus influenzae, E. coli, Proteus mirabilis, Neisseria gonorrhoeae, Streptococcus pneumoniae*, streptococci, nonpencillinase-producing staphylococci
- Unlabeled use: *Chlamydia trachomatis* in pregnancy

### Contraindications/cautions

- Contraindications: allergies to penicillins, cephalosporins, or other allergens.
- Use cautiously with renal disorders, lactation.

### Dosage

**Available Forms:** Chewable tablets—125, 250 mg; capsules—250, 500 mg; powder for oral suspension—50 mg/ml; 125 mg/5 ml, 250 mg/5 ml

Available in oral preparations only.

**ADULTS AND CHILDREN > *20 KG***

- ***URIs, GU infections, skin and soft-tissue infections:*** 250–500 mg PO q8h.

- *Lower respiratory infections:* 500 mg PO q8h.
- *Uncomplicated gonococcal infections:* 3 g amoxicillin with 1 g probenecid PO.
- *C. trachomatis* in pregnancy: 500 mg PO tid for 7 d.
- *Prevention of SBE: Dental, oral, or upper respiratory procedures:* 3 g 1 h before procedure, then 1.5 g 6 h after initial dose.
- *GI or GU procedures:* 2 g ampicillin plus 1.5 mg/kg gentamicin IM or IV one-half hour before procedure, followed by 1.5 g amoxicillin; for low-risk patients, 3 g 1 h before procedure, then 1.5 g 6 h after initial dose.

PEDIATRIC < 20 KG

- *URIs, GU infections, skin, and soft-tissue infections:* 20 mg/kg per day PO in divided doses q8h.
- *Lower respiratory infections:* 40 mg/kg per day PO in divided doses q8h.
- *Prevention of SBE: Dental, oral, or upper respiratory procedures:* 3 g 1 h before procedure, then 1.5 g 6 h after initial dose.
- *GI or GU procedures:* 50 mg/kg ampicillin plus 2 mg/kg gentamicin IM or IV one-half hour before procedure followed by 25 mg/kg amoxicillin. For low-risk patients, 3 g 1 h before procedure, then 1.5 g 6 hours after initial dose

### Pharmacokinetics

| *Route* | *Onset* | *Peak* | *Duration* |
|---|---|---|---|
| Oral | Varies | 1 h | 6–8 h |

*Metabolism:* $T_{1/2}$: 1–1.4 h
*Distribution:* Crosses placenta; passes into breast milk
*Excretion:* Unchanged in the urine

### Adverse effects

- CNS: Lethargy, hallucinations, seizures
- GI: *Glossitis, stomatitis, gastritis, sore mouth*, furry tongue, black "hairy" tongue, *nausea, vomiting, diarrhea, abdominal pain*, bloody diarrhea, enterocolitis, pseudomembranous colitis, nonspecific hepatitis
- Hematologic: Anemia, thrombocytopenia, leukopenia, neutropenia, prolonged bleeding time
- GU: Nephritis
- Hypersensitivity reactions: *Rash, fever, wheezing,* ***anaphylaxis***
- Other: *Superinfections*—oral and rectal moniliasis, vaginitis

### Clinically important drug-drug interactions

• Increased effect with probenecid • Decreased effectiveness with tetracyclines, chloramphenicol • Decreased efficacy of oral contraceptives

### Clinically important drug-food interactions

• Delayed or reduced GI absorption with food

## ■ Nursing Considerations

### Assessment

- *History:* Allergies to penicillins, cephalosporins, or other allergens; renal disorders; lactation
- *Physical:* Culture infected area; skin color, lesion; R, adventitious sounds; bowel sounds; CBC, liver and renal function tests, serum electrolytes, Hct, urinalysis

### Implementation

- Culture infected area prior to treatment; reculture area if response is not as expected.
- Give in oral preparations only; absorption may be affected by presence of food; drug should be taken 1 h before or 2 h after meals.
- Continue therapy for at least 2 d after signs of infection have disappeared; continuation for 10 full days is recommended.
- Use corticosteroids, antihistamines for skin reactions.

### Drug-specific teaching points

- Take this drug around the clock. The drug should be taken on an empty stomach, 1 h before or 2 h after meals.
- Take the full course of therapy; do not stop because you feel better.

- This antibiotic is specific for this problem and should not be used to self-treat other infections.
- The following side effects may occur: nausea, vomiting, GI upset (small frequent meals may help); diarrhea; sore mouth (frequent mouth care may help).
- Report unusual bleeding or bruising, sore throat, fever, rash, hives, severe diarrhea, difficulty breathing.

## amphotericin B

*(am foe **ter'** i sin)*

Fungizone, Fungizone Intravenous, Abelcet, Amphotec, AmBisome

**Pregnancy Category B**

### Drug classes

Antifungal antibiotic

### Therapeutic actions

Binds to sterols in the fungal cell membrane with a resultant change in membrane permeability, an effect that can destroy fungal cells and prevent their reproduction; fungicidal or fungistatic depending on concentration and organism.

### Indications

- Reserve use for patients with progressive, potentially fatal infections: cryptococcosis; North American blastomycosis; disseminated moniliasis; coccidioidomycosis and histoplasmosis; mucormycosis caused by species of *Mucor, Rhizopus, Absidia, Entomophthora, Basidiobolus;* sporotrichosis; aspergillosis.
- Adjunct treatment of American mucocutaneous leishmaniasis (not choice in primary therapy).
- Treatment of aspergillosis in patients refractory to conventional therapy (Abelcet, Amphotec)
- Treatment of cutaneous and mucocutaneous mycotic infections caused by *Candida* species (topical application)
- Treatment of invasive aspergillosis where renal toxicity precludes use of conventional amphotericin B (Amphotec)
- Treatment of presumed fungal infections in febrile, neutropenic patients (AmBisome)
- Treatment of *Aspergillis, Candida or Cryptococcus* infections in patients intolerant to or refractory to Funjizone (AmBisome)
- Treatment of any type of progressive fungal infection that does not respond to conventional therapy
- Unlabeled use: prophylactic use to prevent fungal infections in bone marrow transplants

### Contraindications/cautions

- Allergy to amphotericin B, renal dysfunction, lactation (except when life-threatening and treatable only with this drug).

### Dosage

**Available Forms:** Injection—50 mg; suspension for injection—100 mg/20 ml; powder for injection—50, 100 mg; powder for infusion 50 mg/vial

**ADULT AND PEDIATRIC:** For test dose, give 1 mg slowly IV to determine patient tolerance. Administer by slow IV infusion over 6 h at a concentration of 0.1 mg/ml. Increase daily dose based on patient tolerance and response. Usual dose is 0.25 mg/kg per day; do not exceed 1.5 mg/kg per day.

- ***Fungizone***
  - ***Sporotrichosis:*** 20 mg per injection; therapy may extend for 9 mo.
  - ***Aspergillosis:*** Treat up to 11 mo, with a total dose of 3.6 g.
  - ***Rhinocerebral phycomycosis:*** Control diabetes; amphotericin B cumulative dose of 3 g; disease is usually rapidly fatal; treatment must be aggressive.
  - ***Bladder irrigation (adults):*** 50 mg/1,000 ml sterile water instilled intermittently or continuously
  - ***For topical application:*** Liberally apply to candidal lesions 2–4×/d; treatment ranges from 2–4 wk based on response.
- ***Abelcet***
  - ***Aspergillosis:*** 5 mg/kg/d given as a single infusion at 2.5 mg/kg/h.
- ***Amphotec***
  - ***Aspergillosis:*** Initially 3–4 mg/kg/d, may increase to 6 mg/kg/d IV. Infuse at 1 mg/kg/h over at least 2 h.

- *AmBisome*
– *Aspergillosis:* 3–5 mg/kg/d IV, give over > 2 h.

**Pharmacokinetics**

| *Route* | *Onset* | *Peak* | *Duration* |
|---|---|---|---|
| IV | 20–30 min | 1–2 h | 20–24 h |

*Metabolism:* $T_{1/2}$: 24 h initially and then 15 d; 173.4 h (Abelcet)
*Distribution:* Crosses placenta; may pass into breast milk
*Excretion:* Urine

**IV facts**

**Preparation:** Fungizone: 5 mg/ml: rapidly inject 10 ml Sterile Water for Injection without a bacteriostatic agent directly into the lyophilized cake using a sterile needle (minimum diameter, 20 gauge); shake vial until clear; 0.1 mg/ml solution is obtained by further dilution with 5% Dextrose Injection of pH above 4.2; use strict aseptic technique. Do not dilute with saline; do not use if any precipitation is found. Refrigerate vials and protect from exposure to light; store in dark at room temperature for 24 h or refrigerated for 1 wk. Discard any unused material. Use solutions prepared for IV infusion promptly.
Abelcet: shake vial gently until no yellow sediment is seen. Withdraw dose, replace needle with a 5$\mu$ filter needle. Inject into bag containing 5% Dextrose Injection to a concentration of 1 mg/ml. May be further diluted. Store vials in refrigerator; stable for 15 h once prepared if refrigerated, for 6 h at room temperature.
Amphotec: Reconstitute with sterile water for injection. 10 ml to 50 mg/vial or 20 ml to 100 mg/vial. Dilute to 0.06 mg/ml. Refrigerate after reconstitution; use within 24 h.

**Infusion:** Fungizone: protect from exposure to light if not infused within 8 h of preparation. Infuse slowly over 6 h. Abelcet: infuse at rate of 2.5 mg/kg/h. If infusion takes >2 h, remix bag by shaking.
Amphotec: Infuse at 1 mg/kg/min over at least 2 h; do *not* use an in-line filter. AmBisome: Infuse over > 2 h if tolerated; stop immediately at any sign of anaphylactic reaction.

**Compatibilities:** Do not mix with saline-containing solution, parenteral nutrional solutions, aminoglycosides, penicillins, phenothiazines, calcium preparations, cimetidine, metaraminol, methyldopa, polymyxin, potassium chloride, ranitidine, verapamil, clindamycin, cotrimoxazole, dopamine, dobutamine, tetracycline, vitamins, lidocaine, procaine or heparin. **If line must be flushed, do not use heparin or saline; use D5W.**

**Adverse effects**

*Systemic Administration*

- CNS: *Fever (often with shaking chills), headache, malaise,* generalized pain
- GI: *Nausea, vomiting, dyspepsia, diarrhea,* cramping, epigastric pain, anorexia
- **Hematologic:** Normochromic, normocytic anemia
- GU: Hypokalemia, azotemia, hyposthenuria, renal tubular acidosis, nephrocalcinosis
- **Local:** *Pain at the injection site* with phlebitis and thrombophlebitis
- **Other:** Weight loss

*Topical Application*

- Skin: *Drying effect on skin, local irritation* (cream); *pruritus,* allergic contact dermatitis (lotion); *local irritation* (ointment)

**Clinically important drug-drug interactions**

• Do not administer with corticosteroids unless these are needed to control symptoms. • Increased risk of nephrotoxicity with other nephrotoxic antibiotics, antineoplastics. • Increased effects and risk of toxicity of digitalis, skeletal muscle relaxants, flucytosine. • Increased nephrotoxic effects with cyclosporine.

## ■ Nursing Considerations

### Assessment

- *History:* Allergy to amphotericin B, renal dysfunction, lactation

- *Physical:* Skin color, lesions; T; weight; injection site; orientation, reflexes, affect; bowel sounds, liver evaluation; renal function tests; CBC and differential; culture of area involved

### Implementation

- Arrange for immediate culture of infection but begin treatment before lab results are returned.
- Monitor injection sites and veins for signs of phlebitis.
- Cleanse affected lesions before applying topical drug; apply liberally to lesions and rub in gently; do not cover with plastic wrap.
- Use soap and water to wash hands, fabrics, skin areas that may discolor as a result of topical application.
- Provide aspirin, antihistamines, antiemetics, maintain sodium balance to ease drug discomfort. Minimal use of IV corticosteroids may decrease febrile reactions. Meperidine has been used to relieve chills and fever.
- Monitor renal function tests weekly; discontinue or decrease dosage of drug at any sign of increased renal toxicity.
- Continue topical adminstration for long-term therapy until infection is eradicated, usually 2–4 wk.
- Discontinue topical application if hypersensitivity reaction occurs.

### Drug-specific teaching points

- Be aware that long-term use of this drug will be needed; beneficial effects may not be seen for several weeks; the systemic form of the drug can only be given IV.
- For topical application, apply topical drug liberally to affected area after first cleansing area.
- Use hygiene measures to prevent reinfection or spread of infection.
- Know that the following side effects may occur: nausea, vomiting, diarrhea (small, frequent meals may help); discoloring, drying of the skin, staining of fabric (washing with soap and water or cleaning fabric with standard cleaning fluid should remove stain; topical); stinging, irritation with local application; fever, chills, muscle aches and pains, headache (medications may be ordered to help you to deal with these discomforts of the drug).
- Report pain, irritation at injection site; GI upset, nausea, loss of appetite; difficulty breathing; local irritation, burning (topical application).

# Ampicillins

## ampicillin

*(am pi **sill' in**)*

*Oral:* Ampicin (CAN), Apo-Ampi (CAN), D-Amp, Novo-Ampicillin (CAN), Nu-Ampi (CAN), Omnipen, Penbritin (CAN), Polycillin, Principen, Totacillin

## ampicillin sodium

*Parenteral:* Omnipen-N, Polycillin-N, Totacillin-N

**Pregnancy Category B**

### Drug classes

Antibiotic
Penicillin

### Therapeutic actions

Bactericidal action against sensitive organisms; inhibits synthesis of bacterial cell wall, causing cell death.

### Indications

- Treatment of infections caused by susceptible strains of *Shigella, Salmonella, E. coli, H. influenzae, P. mirabilis, N. gonorrhoeae,* enterococci, gram-positive organisms (penicillin G-sensitive staphylococci, streptococci, pneumococci).
- Meningitis caused by *Neisseria meningitidis.*
- Unlabeled use: prophylaxis in cesarean section in certain high-risk patients

### Contraindications/cautions

- Contraindications: allergies to penicillins, cephalosporins, or other allergens.
- Use cautiously with renal disorders.

### Dosage

**Available Forms:** Capsules—250, 500 mg; powder for oral suspension—100 mg/ml, 125 mg/5 ml, 250 mg/5 ml, 500 mg/

5 ml; powder for injection—125, 250, 500 mg, 1, 2, 10 g
Maximum recommended dosage: 8 mg/d; may be given IV, IM, or PO. Use parenteral routes for severe infections, and switch to oral route as soon as possible.
***Respiratory and soft-tissue infections:*** *Patients weighing 40 kg or more:* 250–500 mg IV or IM q6h. *Patients weighing <40 kg:* 25–50 mg/kg per day IM or IV in equally divided doses at 6–8h intervals. *Patients weighing >20 kg:* 250 mg PO q6h. *Patients weighing < 20 kg:* 50 mg/kg per day PO in equally divided doses q6–8h.
***GI and GU infections, including women with N. gonorrhoeae:*** *Patients weighing >40 kg:* 500 mg IM or IV q6h. *Patients weighing <40 kg:* 50 mg/kg per day IM or IV in equally divided doses q6–8h. *Patients weighing >20 kg:* 500 mg PO q6h. *Patients weighing <20 kg:* 100 mg/kg per day PO in equallly divided doses q6–8h.
***Gonococcal infections:*** 1 g q6h for penicillin-sensitive organism.
***Bacterial meningitis (adult and pediatric):*** 150–200 mg/kg per day by continuous IV drip and then IM injections in equally divided doses q3–4h.
***Prevention of bacterial endocarditis for GI or GU surgery or instrumentation:***

- *ADULT:* 2 g ampicillin IM or IV plus 1.5 mg/kg gentamicin IM or IV. First dose 1/2–1 h before the procedure, followed by 1.5 mg amoxicillin 6 h after initial dose, or repeat parenteral dose 8 h after initial dose.
- *PEDIATRIC:* 50 mg/kg ampicillin plus 2 mg/kg gentamicin at the same dosage schedule as adults.

***Prevention of bacterial endocarditis for dental, oral, or upper respiratory procedures***

- *ADULT:* 1–2 g ampicillin IM or IV plus 1.5 mg/kg gentamicin IM or IV. First dose 1/2–1 h before the procedure, followed by 1.5 mg amoxicillin 6 h after initial dose, or repeat parenteral dose 8 h after initial dose.
- *PEDIATRIC:* 50 mg/kg ampicillin plus 1.5 mg/kg gentamicin at the same dosage schedule as adults.

***Septicemia (adult and pediatric):*** 150–200 mg/kg per day IV for at least 3 days, then IM q3–4h.
***Sexually transmitted diseases (adult):*** Rape victims: Prophylaxis against infection. Pregnant women and patients allergic to tetracycline: 3.5g ampicillin PO with 1 g probenecid. Prophylaxis in cesarean section: Single IV or IM dose of 25–100 mg/kg immediately after cord is clamped.

### Pharmacokinetics

| *Route* | *Onset* | *Peak* | *Duration* |
|---|---|---|---|
| Oral | 30 min | 2 h | 6–8 h |
| IM | 15 min | 1 h | 6–8 h |
| IV | Immediate | 5 min | 6–8 h |

*Metabolism:* $T_{1/2}$: 1–2 h
*Distribution:* Crosses placenta; passes into breast milk
*Excretion:* Unchanged in the urine

### IV facts

**Preparation:** Reconstitute with Sterile or Bacteriostatic Water for Injection; piggyback vials may be reconstituted with Sodium Chloride Injection; use reconstituted solution within 1 h. Do not mix in the same IV solution as other antibiotics. Use within 1 h after preparation because potency may decrease significantly after that.
**Infusion:** Direct IV administration; give slowly over 3–5 min. *Rapid administration can lead to convulsions.* ***IV drip****: dilute as above before further dilution.* ***IV piggyback:*** *administer alone or further dilute with compatible solution.*
**Compatibility:** Ampicillin is compatible with 0.9% Sodium Chloride, 5% Dextrose in Water, or 0.45% Sodium Chloride Solution, 10% Invert Sugar Water, M/6 Sodium Lactate Solution, Lactated Ringer's Solution, Sterile Water for Injection. Diluted solutions are stable for 2–8 h; check manufacturer's inserts for specifics. Discard solution after allotted time period.
**Incompatibility:** Do not mix with lidocaine, verapamil, other antibiotics, dextrose solutions

a

**Adverse effects**
- CNS: Lethargy, hallucinations, seizures
- GI: *Glossitis, stomatitis, gastritis, sore mouth*, furry tongue, black "hairy" tongue, *nausea, vomiting, diarrhea*, abdominal pain, bloody diarrhea, enterocolitis, pseudomembranous colitis, nonspecific hepatitis
- CV: CHF
- Hematologic: Anemia, thrombocytopenia, leukopenia, neutropenia, prolonged bleeding time
- GU: **Nephritis**
- Local: *Pain, phlebitis,* thrombosis at injection site (parenteral)
- Hypersensitivity reactions: *Rash, fever, wheezing,* ***anaphylaxis***
- Other: *Superinfections*—oral and rectal moniliasis, vaginitis

**Clinically important drug-drug interactions**

• Increased ampicillin effect with probenecid • Increased risk of skin rash with allopurinol • Increased bleeding effect with heparin, oral anticoagulants • Decreased effectiveness with tetracyclines, chloramphenicol • Decreased efficacy of oral contraceptives, atenolol with ampicillin

**Clinically important drug-food interactions**

• Oral ampicillin may be less effective with food; take on an empty stomach

**Drug-lab test interferences**

• False-positive Coombs' test if given IV. • Decrease in plasma estrogen concentrations in pregnant women. • False-positive urine glucose tests if Clinitest, Benedict's solution, or Fehling's solution is used; enzymatic glucose oxidase methods (Clinistix, Tes-Tape) should be used to check urine glucose.

## ■ Nursing Considerations

### Assessment
- *History:* Allergies to penicillins, cephalosporins, or other allergens; renal disorders; lactation
- *Physical:* Culture infected area; skin color, lesion; R, adventitious sounds; bowel sounds; CBC, liver and renal function tests, serum electrolytes, hematocrit, urinalysis.

### Implementation
- Culture infected area before treatment; reculture area if response is not as expected.
- Check IV site carefully for signs of thrombosis or drug reaction.
- Do not give IM injections in the same site; atrophy can occur. Monitor injection sites.
- Administer oral drug on an empty stomach, 1 h before or 2 h after meals with a full glass of water—no fruit juice or soft drinks.

### Drug-specific teaching points
- Take this drug around the clock.
- Take the full course of therapy; do not stop taking the drug if you feel better.
- Take the oral drug on an empty stomach, 1 h before or 2 h after meals; the oral solution is stable for 7 d at room temperature.
- This antibiotic is specific to your problem and should not be used to self-treat other infections.
- The following side effects may occur: nausea, vomiting, GI upset (small frequent meals may help), diarrhea.
- Report pain or discomfort at sites, unusual bleeding or bruising, mouth sores, rash, hives, fever, itching, severe diarrhea, difficulty breathing.

# amrinone lactate

*(am' ri none)*
Inocor
**Pregnancy Category C**

**Drug classes**
Cardiotonic drug

**Therapeutic actions**
Increases force of contraction of ventricles (positive inotropic effect); causes vasodilation by a direct relaxant effect on vascular smooth muscle.

### Indications
- CHF: short time management of patients who have not responded to digitalis, diuretics, or vasodilators

### Contraindications/cautions
- Allergy to amrinone or bisulfites, severe aortic or pulmonic valvular disease, acute MI, decreased fluid volume, lactation

### Dosage
**Available Forms:** Injection—5 mg/ml

*ADULT*
- *Initial dose:* 0.75 mg/kg IV bolus, given over 2–3 min. A supplemental IV bolus of 0.75 mg/kg may be given after 30 min if needed.
- *Maintenance infusion:* 5–10 μg/kg per minute. Do not exceed a total of 10 mg/kg per day.

*PEDIATRIC:* Not recommended.

### Pharmacokinetics

| Route | Onset | Peak | Duration |
|---|---|---|---|
| IV | Immediate | 10 min | 2 h |

*Metabolism:* Hepatic, $T_{1/2}$: 3.6–5.8 h
*Distribution:* Crosses placenta; may pass into breast milk
*Excretion:* Urine (63%) and feces (18%)

### IV facts
**Preparation:** Give as supplied or dilute in normal or one-half normal saline solution to a concentration of 1–3 mg/ml. Use diluted solution within 24 h. Protect ampules from exposure to light.
**Infusion:** Administer IV bolus slowly over 2–3 min. Maintenance infusion should not exceed 5–10 μg/kg per minute. Monitor doses; do not exceed a daily dose of 10 mg/kg.
**Compatibilities:** Do not mix directly with dextrose-containing solutions; may be injected into a Y-connector or into tubing when a dextose solution is running. Do not mix with furosemide.

### Adverse effects
- GI: Nausea, vomiting, abdominal pain, anorexia, hepatoxicity
- CV: *Arrhythmias*, hypotension
- Hematologic: *Thrombocytopenia*
- **Hypersensitivity**: Pericarditis, pleuritis, ascites, vasculitis
- **Other**: Fever, chest pain, burning at injection site

### Clinically important drug-drug interactions
- Precipitate formation in solution if given in the same IV line with furosemide

## ■ Nursing Considerations

### Assessment
- *History:* Allergy to amrinone or bisulfites, severe aortic or pulmonic valvular disease, acute MI, decreased fluid volume, lactation
- *Physical:* Weight, orientation, P, BP, cardiac auscultation, peripheral pulses, peripheral perfusion; R, adventitious sounds; bowel sounds, liver evaluation; urinary output; serum electrolyte levels, platelet count, liver enzymes

### Implementation
- Protect drug vial from light.
- Monitor BP and P, and reduce dose if marked decreases occur.
- Monitor I&O and electrolyte levels; record daily weights.
- Monitor platelet counts if patient is on prolonged therapy. Reduce dose if platelet levels fall.

### Drug-specific teaching points
- You will need frequent BP and P monitoring.
- You may experience increased voiding while on this drug.
- Report pain at IV injection site; dizziness; weakness, fatigue; numbness or tingling.

## ☆ amyl nitrite

*(am' il)*

**Pregnancy Category C**

### Drug classes
Antianginal drug
Nitrate

### Therapeutic actions

Relaxes vascular smooth muscle, which results in a decrease in venous return and arterial blood pressure; this reduces left ventricular workload and decreases myocardial oxygen consumption.

### Indications

- Relief of angina pectoris

### Contraindications/cautions

- Allergy to nitrates, severe anemia, head trauma, cerebral hemorrhage, hypertrophic cardiomyopathy, lactation.

### Dosage

**Available Forms:** Inhalation—0.3 ml

*ADULT:* 0.18 or 0.3 ml by inhalation of vapor from crushed capsule; may repeat in 3–5 min for relief of angina. 1–6 inhalations are usually sufficient to produce desired effect.

*PEDIATRIC:* Safety and efficacy not established.

### Pharmacokinetics

| *Route* | *Onset* | *Peak* | *Duration* |
|---|---|---|---|
| Inhalation | 30 sec | 3 min | 3–5 min |

*Metabolism:* Hepatic metabolism, $T_{1/2}$: 1–4 min

*Distribution:* Crosses placenta; may passes into breast milk

*Excretion:* Urine

### Adverse effects

- CNS: *Headache, apprehension, restlessness, weakness*, vertigo, dizziness, faintness, euphoria
- GI: *Nausea,* vomiting, incontinence of urine and feces, abdominal pain
- CV: *Tachycardia*, retrosternal discomfort, palpitations, *hypotension*, syncope, collapse, postural hypotension, angina
- **Dermatologic:** Rash, exfoliative dermatitis, *cutaneous vasodilation with flushing*
- **Drug abuse:** Abused for sexual stimulation and euphoria, effects of inhalation are instantaneous
- **Other:** Muscle twitching, pallor, perspiration, cold sweat

### Clinically important drug-drug interactions

• Increased risk of severe hypotension and CV collapse if used with alcohol • Increased risk of hypotension with antihypertensive drugs, beta-adrenergic blockers, phenothiazines

### Drug-lab test interferences

• False report of decreased serum cholesterol if done by the Zlatkis-Zak color reaction

## ■ Nursing Considerations

### Assessment

- *History:* Allergy to nitrates, severe anemia, head trauma, cerebral hemorrhage, hypertrophic cardiomyopathy, lactation
- *Physical:* Skin color, temperature, lesions; orientation, reflexes, affect; P, BP, orthostatic BP, baseline ECG, peripheral perfusion; R, adventitious sounds; liver evaluation; normal urinary output; CBC, hemoglobin

### Implementation

- Crush the capsule and wave under the patient's nose; 2–6 inhalations are usually sufficient; may repeat every 3–5 min.
- Protect the drug from light; store in a cool place.
- Gradually reduce dose if anginal treatment is being terminated; rapid discontinuation can cause withdrawal.

### Drug-specific teaching points

- Crush the capsule, and inhale 2–6× by waving under your nose; repeat in 3–5 min if necessary.
- Do not use where vapors may ignite; vapors are highly flammable.
- Protect the drug from light; store in a cool place.
- Avoid alcohol while on amyl nitrite.
- The following side effects may occur: dizziness, lightheadedness (transient; use care to change positions slowly; lie or sit down when taking dose); headache (lie down and rest in a cool environment; OTC preparations may not help); flushing of the neck or face (transient).

- Report blurred vision, persistent or severe headache, skin rash, more frequent or more severe angina attacks, fainting.

## anagrelide hydrochloride

*(an* ***agh'*** *rah lide)*
Agrylin
**Pregnancy Category C**

### Drug classes
Antiplatelet agent

### Therapeutic actions
Reduces platelet production by decreasing megakaryocyte hypermaturation; inhibits cyclic AMP and ADP collagen-induced platelet aggregation. At therapeutic doses has no affect on WBC counts or coagulation parameters; may affect RBC parameters.

### Indications
- Treatment of essential thrombocytopenia to reduce elevated platelet count and the risk of thrombosis

### Contraindications/cautions
- Use cautiously with renal or hepatic disorders, pregnancy, lactation, known heart disease, thrombocytopenia.

### Dosage
**Available Forms:** Capsules—0.5, 1 mg

**ADULT:** Initially 0.5 mg PO qid or 1 mg PO bid. After 1 wk, reevaluate and adjust the dosage as needed; do not increase by more than 0.5 mg/d each week. Maximum dose 10 mg/d or 2.5 mg as a single dose.

**PEDIATRIC:** Safety and efficacy not established.

### Pharmacokinetics

| *Route* | *Onset* | *Peak* |
|---|---|---|
| Oral | Rapid | 1 h |

*Metabolism:* Hepatic metabolism; $T_{1/2}$: 3 d
*Distribution:* Crosses placenta; may pass into breast milk
*Excretion:* Urine

### Adverse effects
- CNS: Dizziness, headaches, asthenia, paresthesias
- CV: CHF, tachycardia, MI, complete heart block, atrial fibrillation, hypertension, *palpitations*
- GI: *Diarrhea, nausea, vomiting, abdominal pain,* flatulence, dyspepsia, anorexia, pancreatitis, ulcer, CVA
- Hematologic: *Thrombocytopenia*
- Other: Rash, purpura

### Clinically important drug-food interactions
- Reduced availability of anagrelide if taken with food

## ■ Nursing Considerations

### Assessment
- *History:* Allergy to anagrelide, thrombocytopenia, hemostatic disorders, bleeding ulcer, intracranial bleeding, severe liver disease, lactation, renal disorders, pregnancy, known heart disease
- *Physical:* Skin color, lesions; orientation; bowel sounds, normal output; CBC, liver and renal function tests

### Implementation
- Perform platelet counts q 2 d during the first week of therapy and at least weekly thereafter; if thrombocytopenia occurs, decrease dosage of drug and arrange for supportive therapy.
- Administer drug on an empty stomach if at all tolerated.
- Establish safety precautions to prevent injury and bleeding (electric razor, no contact sports, etc.).
- Advise patient to use barrier contraceptives while receiving this drug; it may harm the fetus.
- Monitor patient for any sign of excessive bleeding—bruises, dark stools, etc.—and monitor bleeding times.
- Mark chart of any patient receiving anagrelide to alert medical personnel of potential for increased bleeding in cases of surgery or dental surgery, invasive procedures.

### Drug-specific teaching points

- Take drug on an empty stomach.
- You will require frequent and regular blood tests to monitor your response to this drug.
- It may take longer than normal to stop bleeding while on this drug; avoid contact sports, use electric razors, etc.; apply pressure for extended periods to bleeding sites.
- Avoid pregnancy while on this drug; it could harm the fetus.
- The following side effects may occur: upset stomach, nausea, diarrhea, loss of appetite (small, frequent meals may help).
- Notify any dentist or surgeon that you are on this drug before invasive procedures.
- Report fever, chills, sore throat, skin rash, bruising, bleeding, dark stools or urine, palpitations, chest pain.

## anastrazole

*(an abs' troh zol)*

Arimidex

**Pregnancy Category D**

### Drug classes

Antiestrogen

### Therapeutic actions

Selective nonsteroidal aromatase inhibitor that significantly reduces serum estradiol levels with no significant effect on adrenocortical steroids or aldosterone.

### Indications

- Treatment of advanced breast cancer in postmenopausal women with disease progression following tamoxifen therapy

### Contraindications/cautions

- Contraindications: allergy to anastrazole, pregnancy, lactation.
- Use cautiously with hepatic or renal impairment, high cholesterol states.

### Dosage

**Available Forms:** Tablets for injection—1 mg

*ADULT:* 1 mg PO qd.

*PEDIATRIC:* Not recommended.

*HEPATIC/RENAL IMPAIRMENT:* No change in dosage is recommended.

### Pharmacokinetics

| *Route* | *Onset* | *Peak* |
|---|---|---|
| Oral | Varies | 10–12 h |

*Metabolism:* Hepatic; $T_{1/2}$: 50 h

*Distribution:* Crosses placenta; enters breast milk

*Excretion:* Feces and urine

### Adverse effects

- CNS: Depression, lightheadedness, dizziness, asthenia
- GI: *Nausea, vomiting,* food distaste, dry mouth, *pharyngitis*
- GU: Vaginal bleeding, vaginal pain, UTIs
- **Dermatologic**: *Hot flashes, skin rash*
- **Other**: Peripheral edema, *bone pain, back pain*

## ■ Nursing Considerations

### Assessment

- *History:* Allergy to anastrazole, hepatic or renal dysfunction, pregnancy, lactation, treatment profile for breast cancer, hypercholesterolemia
- *Physical:* Skin lesions, color, turgor; pelvic exam; orientation, affect, reflexes; peripheral pulses, edema; liver and renal function tests

### Implementation

- Administer once daily without regard to meals.
- Arrange for periodic lipid profiles during therapy.
- Arrange for appropriate analgesic measures if pain and discomfort become severe.

### Drug-specific teaching points

- Take the drug once a day without regard to meals.
- The following side effects may occur: bone pain; hot flashes (staying in cool temperatures may help); nausea, vomiting (small, frequent meals may help); dizziness, headache, lightheadedness (use caution if driving or performing tasks that require alertness).

- Report changes in color of stool or urine, severe vomiting, or inability to eat.

# anistreplase

*(an is tre **plaze'**)*

anisoylated plasminogen streptokinase activator complex, APSAC

Eminase

**Pregnancy Category C**

## Drug classes
Thrombolytic enzyme

## Therapeutic actions
A complex of streptokinase with human plasminogen, which is activated to plasmin in the body; plasmin lyses formed thrombi.

## Indications
- Management of acute MI for the lysis of thrombi obstructing coronary arteries, the reduction of infarct size, the improvement of ventricular function following acute MI, and the reduction of mortality associated with acute MI.

## Contraindications/cautions
- Allergic reactions to anistreplase or streptokinase, active internal bleeding, CVA within 2 mo, intracranial or intraspinal surgery or neoplasm, arteriovenous malformation, aneurysm, recent major surgery, obstetric delivery, organ biopsy, rupture of a noncompressible blood vessel, recent serious GI bleed, recent serious trauma, including CPR, hemostatic defects, cerebrovascular disease, SBE, severe uncontrolled hypertension, liver disease, old age (> 75 y), lactation

## Dosage
**Available Forms:** Powder for injection—30 U/vial

Give as soon as possible after the onset of symptoms.

*ADULT:* 30 U given only by IV injection over 2–5 min into an IV line or directly into vein.

## Pharmacokinetics

| *Route* | *Onset* | *Peak* | *Duration* |
|---|---|---|---|
| IV | Immediate | 45 min | 4–6 h |

*Metabolism:* Plasma, $T_{1/2}$: 2 h

*Distribution:* Crosses placenta; may pass into breast milk

### IV facts
**Preparation:** Reconstitute by slowly adding 5 ml of Sterile Water for Injection to the vial. Gently roll the vial, mixing the dry powder and fluid; reconstituted solution should be colorless to a pale yellow transparent solution. Withdraw the entire contents of the vial. Reconstitute immediately before use. Must be used within 30 min of reconstitution. Discard any unused solution. Avoid excess agitation during dilution. Swirl gently to mix. *Do not shake.* Minimize foaming.

**Infusion:** Give as soon as possible after onset of symptoms. Administer over 2–5 min into an IV line or directly into a vein.

**Compatibilities:** Do not further dilute before administration; do not add to any infusion fluids. Do not add any other medications to the vial or to the syringe.

## Adverse effects
- CV: **Cardiac arrhythmias with coronary reperfusion, *hypotension***
- Hematologic: *Bleeding*, particularly at venous or arterial access sites, gastrointestinal bleeding, intracranial hemorrhage
- Hypersensitivity: Anaphylactic and anaphylactoid reactions, bronchospasm, itching, flushing, rash
- Other: Urticaria, nausea, vomiting, fever, chills, headache

## Clinically important drug-drug interactions
- Increased risk of hemorrhage if used with heparin or oral anticoagulants, aspirin, dipyridamole

## Drug-lab test interferences
- Decrease in plasminogen and fibrinogen results in increases in thrombin time, APTT, PT, tests may be unreliable

## ■ Nursing Considerations

### Assessment

- *History:* Allergic reactions to anistreplase or streptokinase, active internal bleeding, CVA within 2 mo, intracranial or intraspinal surgery or neoplasm, arteriovenous malformation, aneurysm, recent major surgery, obstetric delivery, organ biopsy, rupture of a noncompressible blood vessel, recent serious GI bleed, recent serious trauma, including CPR, hemostatic defects, cerebrovascular disease, SBE, severe uncontrolled hypertension, liver disease, old age (> 75 y), lactation
- *Physical:* Skin color, temperature, lesions; orientation, reflexes; P, BP, peripheral perfusion, baseline ECG; R, adventitous sounds; liver evaluation; Hct, platelet count, TT, APTT, PT

### Implementation

- Discontinue heparin and alteplase if serious bleeding occurs.
- Regularly monitor coagulation studies.
- Apply pressure or pressure dressings to control superficial bleeding.
- Avoid any arterial invasive procedures during therapy.
- Arrange for typing and cross-matching of blood in case serious blood loss occurs and whole blood transfusions are required.
- Institute treatment as soon as possible after onset of symptoms for evolving MI.

### Drug-specific teaching points

- Report difficulty breathing, dizziness, disorientation, headache, numbness, tingling.

## antihemophilic factor

*(an tee hee moe **fill'** ik)*

AHF, Factor VIII

Alphanate, Bioclate, Helixate, Hemofil M, Humate-P, Koate-HP, Kogenate, Monoclate-P, Recombinate

**Pregnancy Category C**

### Drug classes

Antihemophilic agent

### Therapeutic actions

A normal plasma protein that is needed for the transformation of prothrombin to thrombin, the final step of the intrinsic clotting pathway.

### Indications

- Treatment of classical hemophilia (Hemophilia A), in which there is a demonstrated deficiency of Factor VIII; provides a temporary replacement of clotting factors to correct or prevent bleeding episodes or to allow necessary surgery.

### Contraindications/cautions

- Antibodies to mouse protein.

### Dosage

**Available Forms:** IV injection—250, 500, 1,000, 1,500 U/vial in numerous preparations

Administer IV using a plastic syringe; dose depends on weight, severity of deficiency, and severity of bleeding. Follow treatment carefully with Factor VIII level assays.

Formulas used as a guide for dosage are:

$$\text{Expected Factor VHI increase (\% of normal)} = \frac{\text{AHF/IU given} \times 2.0}{\text{weight in kg}}$$

$$\text{AHF/IU required} = \text{weight (kg)} \times \text{desired Factor VIII increase (\% normal)} \times 0.5$$

*Prophylaxis of spontaneous hemorrhage:* Level of Factor VIII required to prevent spontaneous hemorrhage is 5% of normal; 30% of normal is the minimum required for hemostasis following trauma or surgery; smaller doses may be needed if treated early.

*Mild hemorrhage:* Do not repeat therapy unless further bleeding occurs.

*Moderate hemorrage or minor surgery:* 30%–50% of normal is desired for Factor VIII levels; initial dose of 15–25 AHF/IU/kg with maintenance dose of 10–15 AHF/IU/kg is usually sufficient.

*Severe hemorrhage:* Factor VIII level of 80%–100% normal is desired; initial dose of 40–50 AHF/IU/kg and a maintenance dose of 20–25 AHF/IU/kg is given q8–12 h.

*Major surgery:* Dose of AHF to achieve Factor VIII levels of 80%–100% of normal given an hour before surgery; second dose of half the size about 5 h later. Maintain Factor VIII levels at at least 30% normal for a healing period of 10–14 d.

**Pharmacokinetics**

| Route | Onset |
|---|---|
| IV | Immediate |

*Metabolism:* $T_{1/2}$: 12 h
*Distribution:* Does not readily cross placenta
*Excretion:* Cleared from the body by normal metabolism

**IV facts**

**Preparation:** Reconstitute using solution provided. Refrigerate unreconstituted preparations. Before reconstitution, warm diluent and dried concentrate to room temperature. Add diluent and rotate vial, or shake gently, until completely dissolved. Do not refrigerate reconstituted preparations; give within 3 h of reconstitution.

**Infusion:** Give by IV only; use a plastic syringe; solutions may stick to glass. Give preparations containing 34 or more U/ml at a maximum rate of 2 ml/min; give preparations containing $< 34$ AHF U/ml at a rate of 10–20 ml over 3 min.

**Adverse effects**
- Hematologic: Hemolysis with large or frequently repeated doses
- Allergic reactions: Erythema, hives, fever, backache, bronchospasm, urticaria, chills, nausea, *stinging at the infusion site*, vomiting, headache
- Other: **Hepatitis, AIDS**—risks associated with repeated use of blood products

## ■ Nursing Considerations

### Assessment
- *History:* Antibodies to mouse protein
- *Physical:* Skin color, lesions; P, peripheral perfusion; R, adventitious sounds; factor VIII levels, Hct, direct Coombs' test, HIV screening, hepatitis screening

### Implementation
- Monitor pulse during administration; if a significant increase occurs, reduce the rate or discontinue and consult physician.
- Monitor patient's clinical response and factor VIII levels regularly; if no response is noted with large doses, consider the presence of factor VIII inhibitors and need for anti-inhibitor complex therapy.

### Drug-specific teaching points
- Dosage is highly variable. All known safety precautions are taken to ensure that this blood product is pure and the risk of AIDS and hepatitis is as minimal as possible.
- Wear or carry a medical alert ID tag to alert medical emergency personnel that you require this treatment.
- Report headache; rash, itching; backache; difficulty breathing.

## antithrombin

***(an' tee throm bin)***
ATnativ, Kybernin, Thrombate III
**Pregnancy Category C**

**Drug classes**
Coagulation inhibitor

**Therapeutic actions**
A normal plasma factor identical to heparin cofactor I, necessary for heparin to exert its anticoagulant effect.

**Indications**
- Treatment of patients with hereditary antithrombin III (AT III) deficiency in connection with surgical or obstetric procedures or when they suffer from thromboembolism
- Replacement therapy in congenital AT III deficiency

**Contraindications/cautions**
- Use caution in neonates of parents with AT III deficiency and in pregnancy.

### Dosage
**Available Forms:** Powder for injection—500 IU

Administer IV only; dosage is based on the amount of drug needed to replace each individual patient's deficiency. Once appropriate AT III levels are achieved, maintain that level for 2–8 d depending on the situation involved.

Formulas used as a guide for dosage are:

$$\text{Dosage Units} = \frac{[\text{desired AT-III level } (\%) - \text{baseline AT-III } (\%)] \times \text{body weight}}{1\%/(\text{IU/kg})}$$

*PEDIATRIC:* Safety and efficacy not established.

### Pharmacokinetics

| Route | Onset |
|---|---|
| IV | Immediate |

*Metabolism:* $T_{1/2}$: 3 d
*Distribution:* May cross placenta
*Excretion:* Cleared from the body by normal metabolism

### IV facts

**Preparation:** Dissolve the powder in 10 ml Sterile Water for Injection, USP. Gently swirl the vial to dissolve the powder. Do not shake. Bring the solution to room temperature, and administer within 3 h following reconstitution. May be reconstituted with 0.9% Sodium Chloride Injection or 5% Dextrose Injection. After reconstitution, may be further diluted with the same diluent.

**Infusion:** Administer by IV route only; infuse over 5–10 min. Recommended rate is 50 IU/ min (1 ml/min); do not exceed 100 IU/min (2 ml/min). Avoid rapid infusion.

### Adverse effects

- Immunologic: Hepatitis, AIDS—risks associated with repeated use of blood products
- **Other**: Diuretic and vasodilatory effects in patients with severe DIC

### Clinically important drug-drug interactions

- Increased effects of heparin if given with antithrombin III

## ■ Nursing Considerations

### Assessment

- *History:* Clear history of AT III deficiency based on family history of venous thrombosis, decreased plasma AT III level, and exclusion of an acquired deficiency
- *Physical:* Skin color, lesions; P, peripheral perfusion; R, adventitious sounds; AT III levels, HIV screening, hepatitis screening

### Implementation

- Monitor AT III levels before, 30 min after the first dose, and periodically during therapy; the first dose should increase the AT III levels to about 120% of normal. Maintenance doses, q24h, should keep that level at > 80% normal for therapeutic effect.
- Decrease heparin doses during treatment with AT III to avoid excessive bleeding.

### Drug-specific teaching points

- Dosage varies greatly. Frequent blood tests will evaluate the effectiveness of drug therapy. All known safety precautions are taken to ensure that this blood product is pure and the risk of AIDS and hepatitis is as minimal as possible.
- Wear or carry a medical alert ID tag so that medical emergency personnel will know that you require this treatment.
- Report pain or discomfort at IV site.

## aprobarbital

*(a pro **bar'** bi tal)*
Alurate

**Pregnancy Category D**
**C-III controlled substance**

### Drug classes

Barbiturate (short acting)
Sedative
Hypnotic

### Therapeutic actions

General central nervous system depressant; barbiturates act on the ascending RAS, depress the cerebral cortex, alter cerebellar function, depress motor output, and can produce excitation, sedation, hypnosis, anesthesia, and deep coma.

### Indications

- Short-term sedation and sleep induction

### Contraindications/cautions

- Contraindications: hypersensitivity to barbiturates; manifest or latent porphyria; marked liver impairment; nephritis; severe respiratory distress, respiratory disease with dyspnea, obstruction or cor pulmonale; previous addiction to sedative-hypnotic drugs; pregnancy.
- Use cautiously with acute or chronic pain (drug may cause paradoxical excitement or mask important symptoms); seizure disorders (abrupt discontinuation of daily doses can result in status epilepticus); lactation; fever, hyperthyroidism, diabetes mellitus, severe anemia, pulmonary or cardiac disease, status asthmaticus, shock, uremia; impaired liver or kidney function, debilitation.

### Dosage

**Available Forms:** Elixir—40 mg/5 ml

ADULT

- *Sedation:* 40 mg tid, PO.
- *Mild insomnia:* 40–80 mg at bedtime, PO.
- *Pronounced insomnia:* 80–160 mg at bedtime, PO.

PEDIATRIC: Safety and efficacy not established.

GERIATRIC PATIENTS OR THOSE WITH DEBILITATING DISEASE: Reduce dosage and monitor closely; may produce excitement, depression, confusion.

### Pharmacokinetics

| *Route* | *Onset* | *Duration* |
|---|---|---|
| Oral | 45–60 min | 6–8 h |

*Metabolism:* Hepatic, $T_{1/2}$: 14–34 h
*Distribution:* Crosses placenta; passes into breast milk
*Excretion:* Urine

### Adverse effects

- CNS: *Somnolence, agitation, confusion, hyperkinesia, ataxia, vertigo, CNS depression, nightmares, lethargy, residual sedation (hangover),* paradoxical excitement, nervousness, psychiatric disturbance, hallucinations, insomnia, anxiety, dizziness, thinking abnormality
- GI: *Nausea, vomiting, constipation, diarrhea,* epigastric pain
- CV: Bradycardia, hypotension, syncope
- Respiratory: *Hypoventilation,* **apnea, respiratory depression**, laryngospasm, bronchospasm, circulatory collapse
- Hypersensitivity: Skin rashes, angioneurotic edema, serum sickness, morbiliform rash, urticaria, rarely exfoliative dermatitis, **Stevens-Johnson syndrome, sometimes fatal**
- Other: *Tolerance, psychological and physical dependence,* withdrawal syndrome, sometimes fatal

### Clinically important drug-drug interactions

• Increased CNS depression with alcohol, other CNS depressants, phenothiazines, antihistamines, tranquilizers • Increased blood levels and pharmacologic effects of barbiturates with MAO inhibitors • Increased renal toxicity with methoxyflurane • Decreased effects of the following: oral anticoagulants, digitoxin, tricyclic antidepressants, corticosteroids, oral contraceptives and estrogens, acetaminophen, metronidazole, phenmetrazine, carbamazepine, beta-blockers, griseofulvin, phenylbutazones, theophyllines, quinidine, doxycycline • Altered effectiveness of phenytoin barbiturates

## ■ Nursing Considerations

### Assessment

- *History:* Hypersensitivity to barbiturates; manifest or latent porphyria; marked liver impairment; nephritis; severe respiratory distress, respiratory disease with dyspnea, obstruction, or cor pulmonale; previous addiction to sedative-hypnotic drugs; acute or chronic pain; seizure disorders; lactation; fever, hyperthyroidism, diabetes mellitus, severe anemia, cardiac disease, status asthmaticus, shock, uremia; debilitation.

- *Physical:* Weight; T; skin color, lesions; orientation, affect, reflexes; P, BP, orthostatic BP; R, adventitious sounds; bowel sounds, normal output, liver evaluation; liver and kidney function tests, blood and urine glucose, BUN.

### Implementation

- Monitor patient responses, blood levels if interacting drugs are given with aprobarbital; suggest alternative contraceptives to oral ones if aprobarbital is used.
- Taper dosage gradually after repeated use, especially in epileptic patients.

### Drug-specific teaching points

- This drug is habit forming; its ability to facilitate sleep disappears in a short time.
- Do not take this drug longer than 2 wk (for insomnia), and do not increase the dosage without consulting the physician.
- Consult care provider if the drug appears to be ineffective; do not increase the dose.
- Avoid alcohol, sleep-inducing, or OTC drugs while on this drug because these could be dangerous.
- Use a means of contraception other than oral contraceptives. Avoid becoming pregnant.
- The following side effects may occur: drowsiness, dizziness, "hangover," impaired thinking (may be reduced in time; avoid driving or engaging in dangerous activities); GI upset (take drug with food); dreams, nightmares, difficulty concentrating, fatigue, nervousness (reversible).
- Report severe dizziness, weakness, drowsiness that persists; rash or skin lesions; pregnancy.

## aprotinin

(*ah **pro'** tin in*)

Trasylol

**Pregnancy Category B**

### Drug classes

Systemic hemostatic

### Therapeutic actions

Derived from bovine lung, aprotinin forms complexes with plasmin, kallikreins, and other factors to block activation of the kinin and fibrinolytic systems.

### Indications

- Prophylactic use: to reduce blood loss and the need for transfusion in patients undergoing cardiopulmonary bypass in the course of repeat coronary artery bypass graft surgery
- Prophylactic use: to reduce blood loss in select first-time coronary bypass surgery when the patient is at special risk for bleeding

### Contraindications/cautions

- Contraindictations: allergy to aprotinin, first time CABG surgery (except in rare cases).
- Use cautiously with pregnancy, lactation

### Dosage

**Available Forms:** Injection—10,000 kIU/ml

Provided in a solution containing 1.4 mg/ml or 10,000 KIU/ml.

*Adult:* Test dose of 1 ml IV 10 min before loading dose. 1–2 million KIU IV loading dose, 1–2 million KIU into pump prime, 250,000–500,000 KIU/h of operation as continuous IV infusion.

### Pharmacokinetics

| Route | Peak |
|---|---|
| IV | Immediately |

*Metabolism:* $T_{1/2}$: 150 min

*Distribution* : Crosses placenta; passes into breast milk

*Excretion* : Urine

### IV facts

**Preparation:** No further preparation is required.

**Infusion:** Give loading dose over 20–30 min, then continuous infusion of 25–50 ml/h.

**Compatibilities:** Do not give in solution with corticosteroids, heparin, tetracyclines, fat emulsions, amino acids. Give other drugs through a separate line.

**Adverse effects**

- CV: *Atrial fibrillation, MI,* CHF, atrial flutter, ventricular tachycardia, heart block, shock, hypotension
- Respiratory: Asthma, dyspnea, respiratory distress
- Other: Anaphylactic reactions

**Clinically important drug-drug interactions**

• Increased bleeding tendencies with heparin • Blocked antihypertensive effect with cimetidine

## ■ Nursing Considerations

### Assessment

- *History:* Allergy to aprotinin, first time CABG surgery , pregnancy
- *Physical:* Skin lesions, color, temperature; P, BP, peripheral perfusion, baseline ECG; R, adventitious sounds; prothrombin time, renal and hepatic function tests

### Implementation

- Give test dose of 10 ml before any administration.
- Give loading dose slowly with patient in the supine position; sudden drops in BP may occur.
- Evaluate patient regularly for signs of CV effects.

### Drug-specific teaching points

- Patients receiving this drug will be unaware of its effects; information about this drug can be incorporated into the general teaching about coronary artery bypass surgery.

## ardeparin sodium

*(are **da'** pear in)*

Normiflo

**Pregnancy Category C**

**Drug classes**

Antithrombotic
Low-molecular-weight heparin

**Therapeutic actions**

Low-molecular-weight heparin that inhibits thrombus and clot formation by blocking Factor Xa and Factor IIa, accelerating the activity of antithrombin III, and inhibiting the binding of heparin cofactor II. Ardeparin is derived from porcine heparin.

**Indications**

- Prevention of deep vein thrombosis, which may lead to pulmonary embolism, following knee replacement surgery

**Contraindications/cautions**

- Contraindications: hypersensitivity to ardeparin, heparin or pork products; severe thrombocytopenia; uncontrolled bleeding.
- Use cautiously with pregnancy or lactation, severe liver or renal disease, recent brain surgery, retinopathy, asthma, history of GI bleed.

### Dosage

Available Forms: Injection—5,000 anti-Xa U/0.5 ml, 10,000 anti-Xa U/0.5 ml

*Adult:* 50 anti-Xa U SC q12h with the initial dose given the evening before surgery and continue for up to 14 days or until the patient is fully ambulatory.

*Pediatric:* Safety and efficacy not established.

**Pharmacokinetics**

| *Route* | *Onset* | *Peak* | *Duration* |
|---|---|---|---|
| SC | 20–60 min | 3–5 h | 12 h |

*Metabolism:* $T_{1/2}$: 4 hours
*Distribution:* May cross placenta
*Excretion:* Urine

**Adverse effects**

- CV: Chest pain, dizziness, CVA
- Hematological: **Hemorrhage,** *bruising,* thrombocytopenia, elevated SGOT, SGPT levels, hyperkalemia
- Hypersensitivity: Chills, fever, urticaria, asthma
- Other: Fever, pain, local irritation, hematoma, erythema at site of injection
- Treatment of Overdose: Protamin sulfate (1% solution). Each mg of protamine neutralizes 100 anti-Xa U ardeparin. Give very slowly IV over 10 min.

**Clinically important drug-drug interactions**
- Increased bleeding tendencies with drugs that affect hemostasis (anticoagulants, platelet inhibitors, etc.)

## ■ Nursing Considerations

### Assessment
- *History:* Recent surgery or injury; sensitivity to heparin, pork products, ardeparin; lactation; renal or liver disease; retinopathy; history of GI bleed.
- *Physical:* Peripheral perfusion, R, stool guaiac test, partial thromboplastin time (PTT) or other tests of blood coagulation; platelet count, kidney and liver function tests

### Implementation
- Arrange to give drug the evening before knee replacement surgery and q12 h after that.
- Give deep subcutaneous injection; *do not* give ardeparin by IM injection.
- Administer by deep SC injection; patient should be lying down; alternate administration between the abdomen, outer aspect of the upper arm and anterior aspect of the thigh. Introduce the whole length of the needle into a skin fold held between the thumb and forefinger; hold the skin fold throughout the injection.
- Apply pressure to all injection sites after needle is withdrawn; inspect injection sites for signs of hematoma.
- Do not massage injection sites.
- Provide for safety measures (electric razors, soft toothbrush) to prevent injury to patient who is at risk for bleeding.
- Check patient for signs of bleeding, monitor blood tests.
- Alert all health care providers that patient is on ardeparin.
- Have protamine sulfate (ardeparin antidote) on standby in case of overdose.

### Drug-specific teaching points
- This drug must be given by a parenteral route (cannot be taken orally).
- Periodic blood tests will be needed to monitor response to this drug.
- Avoid injury while on this drug: use electric razor, avoid activities that might lead to injury.
- Report nose bleed, bleeding gums, unusual bruising, black or tarry stools, cloudy or dark urine, abdominal/lower back pain, severe headache.

# asparaginase

*(a* ***spare'*** *a gi nase)*

colaspase

Elspar, Kidrolase (CAN)

**Pregnancy Category C**

**Drug classes**

Antineoplastic agent

**Therapeutic actions**

Asparaginase is an enzyme that hydrolyzes the amino acid asparagine, which is needed by some malignant cells (but not normal cells) for protein synthesis; it inhibits malignant cell proliferation by interruption of protein synthesis; maximal effect in G1 phase of the cell cycle.

**Indications**
- Acute lymphocytic leukemia as part of combination therapy to induce remissions in children
- Unlabeled uses: other leukemias, lymphosarcoma

**Contraindications/cautions**
- Allergy to asparaginase, pancreatitis or history of pancreatitis, impaired hepatic function, bone marrow depression, lactation.

### Dosage
**Available Forms:** Powder for injection—10,000 IU

PEDIATRIC
- ***Induction regimen I:*** Prednisone 40 mg/m² per day PO in three divided doses for 15 d, followed by tapering of dosage as follows: 20 mg/m² for 2 d, 10 mg/m² for 2 d, 5 mg/m² for 2 d, 2.5 mg/m² for 2 d, and then discontinue. Vincristine sulfate 2 mg/m² IV once weekly on days 1, 8, 15; maximum dose should not ex-

ceed 2 mg. Asparaginase 1,000 IU/kg per day IV for 10 successive days beginning on day 22.

- *Induction regimen II:* Prednisone 40 mg/m$^2$ per day PO in three divided doses for 28 d, then gradually discontinue over 14 d. Vincristine sulfate 1.5 mg/m$^2$ IV weekly for four doses on days 1, 8, 15, 22; maximum dose should not exceed 2 mg. Asparaginase 6,000 IU/m$^2$ IM on days 4, 7, 10, 13, 16, 19, 22, 25, 28.
- *Maintenance:* When remission is obtained, institute maintenance therapy; do not use asparaginase in maintenance regimen.
- *Single-agent induction therapy:* Used only when combined therapy is inappropriate or when other therapies fail; 200 IU/kg per day IV for 28 d (children or adults).

### Pharmacokinetics

| *Route* | *Onset* |
|---|---|
| IM | Varies |
| IV | 30–40 min |

*Metabolism:* $T_{1/2}$: 8–30 h
*Distribution:* Crosses placenta; may pass into breast milk
*Excretion:* Urine

### IV facts

**Preparation:** Reconstitute vial with 5 ml of Sterile Water for Injection or Sodium Chloride Injection. Ordinary shaking does not inactivate the drug. May be used for direct IV injection or further diluted with Sodium Chloride Injection or 5% Dextrose Injection. Stable for 8 h once reconstituted; use only when clear. Discard any cloudy solution.
**Infusion:** Infuse over not less than 30 min into an already running IV infusion of Sodium Chloride Injection or 5% Dextrose Injection.

### Adverse effects

- Hypersensitivity: *Skin rashes, urticaria, arthralgia,* respiratory distress to anaphylaxis
- CNS: CNS depression
- GI: *Hepatotoxicity, nausea, vomiting, anorexia,* abdominal cramps, pancreatitis
- Hematologic: Bleeding problems, **bone marrow depression**
- GU: Uric acid nephropathy, **renal toxicity**
- Endocrine: Hyperglycemia—glucosuria, polyuria
- Other: Chills, fever, weight loss; **fatal hyperthermia**

### Clinically important drug-drug interactions

- Increased toxicity if given IV with or immediately before vincristine or prednisone
- Diminished or decreased effect of methotrexate on malignant cells if given with or immediately after asparaginase

### Drug-lab test interferences

- Inaccurate interpretation of thyroid-function tests because of decreased serum levels of thyroxine-binding globulin; levels usually return to pretreatment levels within 4 wk of the last dose of asparaginase.

## ■ Nursing Considerations

### Assessment

- *History:* Allergy to asparaginase, pancreatitis or history of pancreatitis, impaired hepatic function, bone marrow depression, lactation
- *Physical:* Weight; T; skin color, lesions; orientation, reflexes; liver evaluation, abdominal exam; CBC, blood sugar, liver and renal function tests, serum amylase, clotting time, urinalysis, serum uric acid levels

### Implementation

- Perform an intradermal skin test prior to initial administration and if there is a week or more between doses because of risk of severe hypersensitivity reactions. Prepare skin test solution as follows: reconstitute 10,000-IU vial with 5 ml of diluent; withdraw 0.1 ml (200 IU/ ml), and inject it into a vial containing 9.9 ml of diluent, giving a solution of 20 IU/ ml. Use 0.1 ml of this solution (2 IU) for the skin test. Observe site for 1 h for a wheal or erythema that indicates allergic reaction.

- Arrange for desensitization to hypersensitivity reaction. Check manufacturer's literature for desensitization dosages, or arrange for patient to receive *Erwinia* asparaginase (available from the National Cancer Institute).
- Arrange for lab tests (CBC, serum amylase, blood glucose, liver function tests, uric acid) prior to therapy and frequently during therapy.
- For IM administration, reconstitute by adding 2 ml of Sodium Chloride Injection to the 10,000-U vial. Stable for 8 h once reconstituted; use only if clear. Limit injections at each site to 2 ml; if more is required use two injection sites.
- Monitor for signs of hypersensitivity (eg, rash, difficulty breathing). If any occur, discontinue drug and consult with physician.
- Monitor for pancreatitis; if serum amylase levels rise, discontinue drug and consult with physician.
- Monitor for hyperglycemia—reaction may resemble hyperosmolar, nonketotic hyperglycemia. If present, discontinue drug and be ready to use IV fluids and insulin.

### Drug-specific teaching points

- Prepare a calendar for patients who must return for specific treatments and additional therapy. Drug can be given only in the hospital under the direct supervision of physician.
- The following side effects may occur: loss of appetite, nausea, vomiting (frequent mouth care, small frequent meals may help; good nutrition is important; dietary services are available; antiemetic may be ordered); fatigue, confusion, agitation, hallucinations, depression (reversible; use special precautions to avoid injury).
- Have regular blood tests to monitor the drug's effects.
- Report fever, chills, sore throat; unusual bleeding or bruising; yellow skin or eyes; light-colored stools, dark urine; thirst, frequent urination.

## aspirin

*(as' pir in)*

Apo-ASA (CAN), Aspergum, Bayer, Easprin, Ecotrin, Empirin, Entrophen (CAN), Genprin, Norwich, Novasen (CAN), PMS-ASA (CAN), ZORprin

*Buffered aspirin products:*
Alka-Seltzer, Ascriptin, Bufferin, Buffex, Wesprin Buffered

**Pregnancy Category D**

### Drug classes

Antipyretic
Analgesic (non-narcotic)
Anti-inflammatory
Antirheumatic
Antiplatelet
Salicylate
NSAID

### Therapeutic actions

Analgesic and antirheumatic effects are attributable to aspirin's ability to inhibit the synthesis of prostaglandins, important mediators of inflammation. Antipyretic effects are not fully understood, but aspirin probably acts in the thermoregulatory center of the hypothalamus to block effects of endogenous pyrogen by inhibiting synthesis of the prostaglandin intermediary. Inhibition of platelet aggregation is attributable to the inhibition of platelet synthesis of thromboxane $A_2$, a potent vasoconstrictor and inducer of platelet aggregation. This effect occurs at low doses and lasts for the life of the platelet (8 d). Higher doses inhibit the synthesis of prostacyclin, a potent vasodilator and inhibitor of platelet aggregation.

### Indications

- Mild to moderate pain
- Fever
- Inflammatory conditions—rheumatic fever, rheumatoid arthritis, osteoarthritis
- Reduction of risk of recurrent TIAs or stroke in males with history of TIA due to fibrin platelet emboli
- Reduction of risk of death or nonfatal MI in patients with history of infarction or unstable angina pectoris

- Unlabeled use: prophylaxis against cataract formation with long-term use

## Contraindications/cautions

- Allergy to salicylates or NSAIDs (more common with nasal polyps, asthma, chronic urticaria); allergy to tartrazine (cross-sensitivity to aspirin is common); hemophilia, bleeding ulcers, hemmorhagic states, blood coagulation defects, hypoprothrombinemia, vitamin K deficiency (increased risk of bleeding); impaired or renal function; chickenpox, influenza (risk of Reye's syndrome in children and teenagers); children with fever accompanied by dehydration; surgery scheduled within 1 wk; pregnancy (maternal anemia, antepartal and postpartal hemorrhage, prolonged gestation, and prolonged labor have been reported; readily crosses the placenta; possibly teratogenic; maternal ingestion of aspirin during late pregnancy has been associated with the following adverse fetal effects: low birth weight, increased intracranial hemorrhage, stillbirths, neonatal death); lactation.

## Dosage

**Available Forms:** Tablets—325, 500, 650, 975 mg; SR tablets—650, 800 mg; suppositories: 120, 200, 300, 600 mg

Available in oral and suppository forms. Also available as chewable tablets, gum; enteric coated, sustained release, and buffered preparations (sustained-release aspirin is not recommended for antipyresis, short-term analgesia, or children < 12 y).

### ADULT

- *Minor aches and pains:* 325–650 mg q4h.
- *Arthritis and rheumatic conditions:* 3.2–6.0 g/d in divided doses.
- *Acute rheumatic fever:* 5–8 g/d; modify to maintain serum salicylate level of 15–30 mg/dl.
- *TIAs in men:* 1,300 mg/d in divided doses (650 mg bid or 325 mg qid).
- *MI:* 300–325 mg/d.

### PEDIATRIC

- *Analgesic and antipyretic:* 65 mg/kg per 24 h in four to six divided doses, not to exceed 3.6 g/d. Dosage recommendations by age follow:

| Age (years) | Dosage (mg q4h) |
|---|---|
| 2–3 | 162 |
| 4–5 | 243 |
| 6–8 | 324 |
| 9–10 | 405 |
| 11 | 486 |
| 12 and older | 648 |

- *Juvenile rheumatoid arthritis:* 60–110 mg/kg per 24 h in divided doses at 4- to 6-h intervals. Maintain a serum level of 200–300 μg/ml.
- *Acute rheumatic fever:* 100 mg/kg/d initially, then decrease to 75 mg/kg/d for 4–6 wk. Therapeutic serum salicylate level is 15–30 mg/dl.
- *Kawasaki disease:* 80–180 mg/kg per day; very high doses may be needed during acute febrile period; after fever resolves, dosage may be adjusted to 10 mg/kg per day.

## Pharmacokinetics

| Route | Onset | Peak | Duration |
|---|---|---|---|
| Oral | 5–30 min | 0.25–2 h | 3–6 h |
| Rectal | 1–2 h | 4–5 h | 6–8 h |

*Metabolism:* Hepatic (salicylate), $T_{1/2}$: 15 min–12 h

*Distribution:* Crosses placenta; passes into breast milk

*Excretion:* Urine

## Adverse effects

*NSAIDs*

- GI: *Nausea, dyspepsia, heartburn, epigastric discomfort*, anorexia, hepatotoxicity
- Hematologic: *Occult blood loss, hemostatic defects*
- **Hypersensitivity**: Anaphylactoid reactions to fatal anaphylactic shock
- **Aspirin intolerance**: Exacerbation of bronchospasm, rhinitis (with nasal polyps, asthma, rhinitis)

- Salicylism: *Dizziness, tinnitus, difficulty hearing, nausea*, vomiting, diarrhea, mental confusion, lassitude (dose related)
- Acute aspirin toxicity: Respiratory alkalosis, hyperpnea, tachypnea, hemorrhage, excitement, confusion, asterixis, pulmonary edema, convulsions, tetany, metabolic acidosis, **fever, coma, cardiovascular collapse**, renal and respiratory failure (dose related 20–25 g in adults, 4 g in children)

### Clinically important drug-drug interactions

• Increased risk of bleeding with oral anticoagulants, heparin • Increased risk of GI ulceration with steroids, phenylbutazone, alcohol, NSAIDs • Increased serum salicylate levels due to decreased salicylate excretion with urine acidifiers (ammonium chloride, ascorbic acid, methionine) • Increased risk of salicylate toxicity with carbonic anhydrase inhibitors, furosemide • Decreased serum salicylate levels with corticosteroids • Decreased serum salicylate levels due to increased renal excretion of salicylates with acetazolamide, methazolamide, certain antacids, alkalinizers • Decreased absorption of aspirin with nonabsorbable antacids • Increased methotrexate levels and toxicity with aspirin • Increased effects of valproic acid secondary to displacement from plasma protein sites • Greater glucose lowering effect of sulfonylureas, insulin with large doses (> 2 g/d) of aspirin • Decreased antihypertensive effect of captopril, beta-adrenergic blockers with salicylates; consider discontinuation of aspirin • Decreased uricosuric effect of probenecid, sulfinpyrazone • Possible decreased diuretic effects of spironolactone, furosemide (in patients with compromised renal function) • Unexpected hypotension may occur with nitroglycerin

### Drug-lab test interferences

• Decreased serum protein bound iodine (PBI) due to competition for binding sites • False-negative readings for urine glucose by glucose oxidase method and copper reduction method with moderate to large doses of aspirin • Interference with urine 5-HIAA determinations by fluorescent methods but not by nitrosonaphthol colorimetric method • Interference with urinary ketone determination by the ferric chloride method • Falsely elevated urine VMA levels with most tests; a false decrease in VMA using the Pisano method

## ■ Nursing Considerations

### Assessment

- *History:* Allergy to salicylates or NSAIDs; allergy to tartrazine; hemophilia, bleeding ulcers, hemmorhagic states, blood coagulation defects, hypoprothrombinemia, vitamin K deficiency; impaired hepatic function; impaired renal function; chickenpox, influenza; children with fever accompanied by dehydration; surgery scheduled within 1 wk; pregnancy; lactation
- *Physical:* Skin color, lesions; temperature; eighth cranial nerve function, orientation, reflexes, affect; P, BP, perfusion; R, adventitious sounds; liver evaluation, bowel sounds; CBC, clotting times, urinalysis, stool guaiac, renal and liver function tests

### Implementation

- Give drug with food or after meals if GI upset occurs.
- Give drug with full glass of water to reduce risk of tablet or capsule lodging in the esophagus.
- Do not crush, and ensure that patient does not chew sustained-release preparations.
- Do not use aspirin that has a strong vinegar-like odor.
- Institute emergency procedures if overdose occurs: gastric lavage, induction of emesis, activated charcoal, supportive therapy.

### Drug-specific teaching points

- OTC aspirins are equivalent. Price does not reflect effectiveness.

- Use the drug only as suggested; avoid overdose. Take the drug with food or after meals if GI upset occurs.
- The following side effects may occur: nausea, GI upset, heartburn (take drug with food); easy bruising, gum bleeding (related to aspirin's effects on blood clotting)
- Avoid the use of other OTC drugs while taking this drug. Many of these drugs contain aspirin, and serious overdosage can occur.
- Report ringing in the ears; dizziness, confusion; abdominal pain; rapid or difficult breathing; nausea, vomiting.
- Take extra precautions to keep this drug out of the reach of children; this drug can be very dangerous for children.

## astemizole

*(a **stem'** mi zole)*

Hismanal

**Pregnancy Category C**

### Drug classes
Antihistamine (nonsedating type)

### Therapeutic actions
Competitively blocks the effects of histamine at peripheral $H_1$ receptor sites; has anticholinergic (atropine-like) and antipruritic effects.

### Indications
- Relief of symptoms associated with perennial and seasonal allergic rhinitis; vasomotor rhinitis; allergic conjunctivitis; mild, uncomplicated urticaria and angioedema
- Amelioraton of allergic reactions to blood or plasma
- Dermatographism
- Adjunctive therapy in anaphylactic reactions

### Contraindications/cautions
- Allergy to any antihistamines; narrow-angle glaucoma, stenosing peptic ulcer, symptomatic prostatic hypertrophy, asthmatic attack, bladder neck obstruction, pyloroduodenal obstruction; lactation

### Dosage
**Available Forms:** Tablets—10 mg

**ADULT AND PEDIATRIC > 12 Y:** 10 mg PO bid; to achieve the optimal dose, 30 mg may be given the first day, 20 mg the second day, and 10 mg daily thereafter.

**PEDIATRIC < 12 Y:** Safety and efficacy not established.

**GERIATRIC OR HEPATIC IMPAIRMENT:** More likely to cause dizziness, sedation, syncope, toxic confusional states, and hypotension; use with caution.

### Pharmacokinetics

| *Route* | *Onset* | *Peak* | *Duration* |
|---|---|---|---|
| Oral | 1–2 h | 2–4 h | 4–6 h |

*Metabolism:* Hepatic, $T_{1/2}$: 20 h first phase, 7–11 d second phase

*Distribution:* Crosses placenta; passes into breast milk

*Excretion:* Urine and feces

### Adverse effects
- CNS: *Headache, nervousness, dizziness*, depression
- GI: *Appetite increase*, nausea, diarrhea, abdominal pain
- CV: Palpitation, edema
- **Respiratory**: Bronchospasm, pharyngitis
- **General**: *Weight gain*
- **Other**: Fever, photosensitivity, rash, myalgia, arthralgia, angioedema

### Clinically important drug-drug interactions
• Additive CNS depressant effects with alcohol, other CNS depressants • Increased and prolonged anticholinergic (drying) effects with MAO inhibitors; avoid this combination • Risk of sudden cardiac death in combination with macrolide antibiotics (indinavir, ritonavir, saquinavir, nelfinavir, fluoxetine, fluvoxamine, sertraline, nefazodone, paroxetine, zileuton)

### Drug-lab test interferences
• False skin testing procedures if done while patient is on antihistamines

## ■ Nursing Considerations

### Assessment

- *History:* Allergy to antihistamines; narrow-angle glaucoma, stenosing peptic ulcer, symptomatic prostatic hypertrophy, asthmatic attack, bladder neck obstruction, pyloroduodenal obstruction; lactation
- *Physical:* Skin color, lesions, texture; orientation, reflexes, affect; vision exam; R, adventitious sounds; prostate palpation; serum transaminase levels.

### Implementation

- Administer on an empty stomach, 1 h before or 2 h after meals.

### Drug-specific teaching points

- Take this drug on an empty stomach, 1 h before or 2 h after meals or food.
- The following side effects may occur: dizziness, sedation, drowsiness (use caution driving or performing tasks that require alertness); headache (consult with health care provider for treatment); thickening of bronchial secretions, dryness of nasal mucosa (humidifier may help).
- Avoid alcohol; serious sedation could occur.
- Report difficulty breathing, hallucinations, tremors, loss of coordination, irregular heartbeat.

## atenolol

*(a ten' o lole)*

Apo-Atenol (CAN), Novo-Atenol (CAN), Tenormin

**Pregnancy Category C**

### Drug classes

Beta-adrenergic blocking agent ($\beta_1$ selective)
Antihypertensive drug

### Therapeutic actions

Blocks beta-adrenergic receptors of the sympathetic nervous system in the heart and juxtaglomerular apparatus (kidney), thus decreasing the excitability of the heart, decreasing cardiac output and oxygen consumption, decreasing the release of renin from the kidney, and lowering blood pressure.

### Indications

- Treatment of angina pectoris due to coronary atherosclerosis
- Hypertension, as a step 1 agent, alone or with other drugs, especially diuretics
- Treatment of myocardial infarction
- Unlabeled uses: prevention of migraine headaches; alcohol withdrawal syndrome, treatment of ventricular arrhythmias

### Contraindications/cautions

- Contraindications: sinus bradycardia, second- or third-degree heart block, cardiogenic shock, CHF.
- Use cautiously with renal failure, diabetes or thyrotoxicosis (atenolol can mask the usual cardiac signs of hypoglycemia and thyrotoxicosis), lactation.

### Dosage

**Available Forms:** Tablets—25, 50, 100 mg; injection—5 mg/10 ml

ADULT

- *Hypertension:* Initially 50 mg PO once a day; after 1–2 wk, dose may be increased to 100 mg
- *Angina pectoris:* Initially 50 mg PO qd. If optimal response is not achieved in 1 wk, increase to 100 mg qd; up to 200 mg/d may be needed.
- *Acute MI:* Initially 5 mg IV given over 5 min as soon as possible after diagnosis; follow with IV injection of 5 mg 10 min later. Switch to 50 mg PO 10 min after the last IV dose; follow with 50 mg PO 12 h later. Thereafter, administer 100 mg PO qd or 50 mg PO bid for 6–9 d or until discharge from the hospital.

GERIATRIC OR RENAL IMPAIRED: Dosage reduction is required because atenolol is excreted through the kidneys. The following dosage is suggested:

| *Creatinine Clearance (ml/min/1.73m²* | *Half-life (h)* | *Maximum Dosage* |
|---|---|---|
| 15–35 | 16–27 | 50 mg/d |
| <14 | >27 | 50 mg qod |

*HEMODIALYSIS PATIENTS:* 50 mg after each dialysis; give only in hospital setting; severe hypotension can occur.
*PEDIATRIC:* Safety and efficacy not established.

**Pharmacokinetics**

| *Route* | *Onset* | *Peak* | *Duration* |
|---|---|---|---|
| Oral | Varies | 2–4 h | 24 h |
| IV | Immediate | 5 min | 24 h |

*Metabolism:* $T_{1/2}$: 6–7 h
*Distribution:* Crosses placenta; passes into breast milk
*Excretion:* Urine (40%–50%) and bile/feces (50%–60%)

**IV facts**
**Preparation:** May be diluted in Dextrose Injection, Sodium Chloride Injection, or Sodium Chloride and Dextrose Injection. Stable for 48 h after mixing.
**Infusion:** Initiate treatment as soon as possible after admission to the hospital; inject 5 mg over 5 min; follow with another 5-mg IV injection 10 min later.

**Adverse effects**
- CNS: Dizziness, vertigo, tinnitus, fatigue, emotional depression, paresthesias, sleep disturbances, hallucinations, disorientation, memory loss, slurred speech
- GI: *Gastric pain, flatulence, constipation, diarrhea, nausea, vomiting,* anorexia, ischemic colitis, renal and mesenteric arterial thrombosis, retroperitoneal fibrosis, hepatomegaly, acute pancreatitis
- CV: *Bradycardia, CHF, cardiac arrhythmias, sinoartial or AV nodal block, tachycardia,* peripheral vascular insufficiency, claudication, CVA, pulmonary edema, hypotension
- **Respiratory**: Bronchospasm, dyspnea, cough, bronchial obstruction, nasal stuffiness, rhinitis, pharyngitis (less likely than with propranolol)
- GU: *Impotence, decreased libido*, Peyronie's disease, dysuria, nocturia, frequent urination
- MS: Joint pain, arthralgia, muscle cramp
- EENT: Eye irritation, dry eyes, conjunctivitis, blurred vision
- **Dermatologic**: Rash, pruritus, sweating, dry skin
- **Allergic reactions**: Pharyngitis, erythematous rash, fever, sore throat, laryngospasm, respiratory distress
- **Other**: *Decreased exercise tolerance, development of antinuclear antibodies*, hyperglycemia or hypoglycemia, elevated serum transaminase, alkaline phosphatase, and LDH

**Clinically important drug-drug interactions**
• Increased effects with verapamil, anticholinergics, quinidine • Increased risk of postural hypotension with prazosin • Increased risk of lidocaine toxicity with atenolol • Possible increased blood pressure-lowering effects with aspirin, bismuth subsalicylate, magnesium salicylate, sulfinpyrazone, oral contraceptives • Decreased antihypertensive effects with NSAIDs, clonidine • Decreased antihypertensive and antianginal effects of atenolol with ampicillin, calcium salts • Possible increased hypoglycemic effect of insulin

**Drug-lab test interferences**
• Possible false results with glucose or insulin tolerance tests

## ■ Nursing Considerations

### Assessment
- *History:* Sinus bradycardia, second- or third-degree heart block, cardiogenic shock, CHF, renal failure, diabetes or thyrotoxicosis, lactation
- *Physical:* Baseline weight, skin condition, neurologic status, P, BP, ECG, respiratory status, kidney and thyroid function, blood and urine glucose

### Implementation
- Do not discontinue drug abruptly after chronic therapy (hypersensitivity to catecholamines may have developed, causing exacerbation of angina, MI, and ventricular dysrhythmias). Taper drug gradually over 2 wk with monitoring.

- Consult physician about withdrawing drug if patient is to undergo surgery (withdrawal is controversial).

#### Drug-specific teaching points

- Take drug with meals if GI upset occurs.
- Do not stop taking this drug unless told to by a health care provider.
- Avoid driving or dangerous activities if dizziness, weakness occur.
- The following side effects may occur: dizziness, lightheadedness, loss of appetite, nightmares, depression, sexual impotence.
- Report difficulty breathing, night cough, swelling of extremities, slow pulse, confusion, depression, rash, fever, sore throat.

## atorvastatin calcium

*(ah **tor'** va stah tin)*
Lipitor
**Pregnancy Category X**

### Drug classes

Antihyperlipidemic
HMG CoA inhibitor

### Therapeutic actions

Inhibits HMG co-enzyme A, the enzyme that catalyzes the first step in cholesterol synthesis pathway, resulting in a decrease in serum cholesterol, serum LDLs (associated with increased risk of CAD), and increases serum HDLs (associated with decreased risk of CAD); increases hepatic LDL recapture sites, enhances reuptake and catabolism of LDL; lowers triglyceride levels.

### Indications

- Adjunct to diet in treatment of elevated total cholesterol and LDL cholesterol in patients with primary hypercholesterolemia (types IIa and IIb) and mixed dyslipidemia, and homozygous familial hypercholesterolemia whose response to dietary restriction of saturated fat and cholesterol and other nonpharmacologic measures has not been adequate

### Contraindications/cautions

- Contraindications: allergy to atorvastatin, fungal byproducts, active liver disease or unexplained and persistent elevations of transaminase levels, pregnancy, lactation
- Use cautiously with impaired endocrine function

### Dosage

**Available Forms:** Tablets—10, 20, 40 mg

*ADULT:* Initial: 10 mg PO qd once daily without regard to meals; maintenance: 10–80 mg PO qd. May be combined with bile acid binding resin.

*PEDIATRIC:* Safety and efficacy not established.

### Pharmacokinetics

| *Route* | *Onset* | *Peak* |
|---|---|---|
| Oral | Slow | 1–2 h |

*Metabolism:* Hepatic and cellular; $T_{1/2}$: 14 h
*Distribution:* Crosses placenta; passes into breast milk
*Excretion:* Bile

### Adverse effects

- CNS: *Headache,* asthenia
- GI: *Flatulence, abdominal pain, cramps, constipation, nausea,* dyspepsia, heartburn, **liver failure**
- Respiratory: Sinusitis, pharyngitis
- Other: **Rhabdomyolysis with acute renal failure,** arthralgia, myalgia

### Clinically important drug-drug interactions

• Possible severe myopathy or rhabdomyolysis with erythromycin, cyclosporine, niacin, antifungals • Increased digoxin levels with possible toxicity if taken together; monitor digoxin levels • Increased estrogen levels with oral contraceptives; monitor patients on this combination

### ■ Nursing Considerations

#### Assessment

- *History:* Allergy to atorvastatin, fungal byproducts; active hepatic disease; acute serious illness; pregnancy, lactation

- *Physical:* Orientation, affect, muscle strength; liver evaluation, abdominal exam; lipid studies, liver and renal function tests

## Implementation

- Obtain liver function tests as a baseline and periodically during therapy; discontinue drug if AST or ALT levels increase to 3 X normal levels.
- Withhold atorvastatin in any acute, serious condition (severe infection, hypotension, major surgery, trauma, severe metabolic or endocrine disorder, seizures) that may suggest myopathy or serve as risk factor for development of renal failure.
- Ensure that patient has tried cholesterol-lowering diet regimen for 3–6 mo before beginning therapy.
- Administer drug without regard to food, but at same time each day.
- Consult dietician regarding low-cholesterol diets.
- Ensure that patient is not pregnant and has appropriate contraceptives available during therapy; serious fetal damage has been associated with drug.

## Drug-specific teaching points

- Take this drug once a day, at about the same time each day; may be taken with food.
- Institute appropriate dietary changes that need to be made.
- The following side effects may occur: nausea (eat small, frequent meals); headache, muscle and joint aches and pains (may lessen over time).
- Arrange to have periodic blood tests while you are on this drug.
- Alert any health care provider that you are on this drug; it will need to be discontinued if acute injury or illness occurs.
- Do not become pregnant while you are on this drug; use barrier contraceptives. If you wish to become pregnant or think you are pregnant, consult your health care provider.
- Report muscle pain, weakness, tenderness; malaise; fever; changes in color of urine or stool; swelling.

# atovaquone

*(a **toe'** va kwon)*
Mepron
**Pregnancy Category C**

## Drug classes
Antiprotozoal

## Therapeutic actions
Directly inhibits enzymes required for nucleic acid and ATP synthesis in protozoa; effective against *Pneumocystis carinii.*

## Indications
- Acute oral treatment of mild to moderate *P. carinii* pneumonia (PCP) in patients who are intolerant to trimethoprim-sulfamethoxazole.

## Contraindications/cautions
- Contraindications: development or history of potentially life-threatening allergic reactions to any of the components of the drug.
- Use cautiously with severe PCP infections, the elderly, lactation.

## Dosage
**Available Forms:** Suspension—750 mg/5 ml

*ADULT:* 750 mg PO tid administered with food for 21 d.

*PEDIATRIC:* Safety and efficacy not established.

*GERIATRIC:* Use caution, and evaluate patient response regularly.

## Pharmacokinetics

| Route | Onset | Peak | Duration |
|---|---|---|---|
| Oral | Varies | 1–8 h | 3–5 d |

*Metabolism:* $T_{1/2}$: 2.2–2.9 d
*Distribution:* Crosses placenta; may pass into breast milk
*Excretion:* Feces

## Adverse effects
- CNS: Dizziness, *insomnia*, *headache*
- GI: Constipation, *diarrhea, nausea, vomiting,* anorexia, abdominal pain, oral monilia infections
- **Dermatologic**: *Rash*, pruritus, sweating, dry skin

- Other: *Fever*, elevated liver enzymes, hyponatremia

**Clinically important drug-drug interactions**

- Decreased effects of other highly protein-bound drugs

**Clinically important drug-food interactions**

- Markedly increased absorption of atovaquone when taken with food

## ■ Nursing Considerations

### Assessment

- *History:* History of potentially life-threatening allergic reactions to any components of the drug, severe PCP infections, elderly, lactation
- *Physical:* T, skin condition, neurologic status, abdominal evaluation, serum electrolytes, liver function tests

### Implementation

- Give drug with meals.
- Ensure that this drug is taken for 21 d.

### Drug-specific teaching points

- Take drug with food; food increases the absorption of the drug.
- The following side effects may occur: dizziness, insomnia, headache (medication may be ordered); nausea, vomiting (small frequent meals may help); diarrhea or constipation (consult your health care provider for appropriate treatment); superinfections (therapy may be ordered); rash (good skin care may help).
- Report fever, mouth infection, severe headache, severe nausea or vomiting, rash.

## atropine sulfate

*(a' troe peen)*

*Parenteral and oral preparations:* Minims (CAN)

*Ophthalmic solution:* Atropine Sulfate S.O.P., Atropisol (CAN), Dioptic's Atropine (CAN), Isopto-Atropine Ophthalmic, R.O. Atropine (CAN)

**Pregnancy Category C**

**Drug classes**

Anticholinergic
Antimuscarinic
Parasympatholytic
Antiparkinsonism drug
Antidote
Diagnostic agent (ophthalmic preparations)
Belladonna alkaloid

**Therapeutic actions**

Competitively blocks the effects of acetylcholine at muscarinic cholinergic receptors that mediate the effects of parasympathetic postganglionic impulses, depressing salivary and bronchial secretions, dilating the bronchi, inhibiting vagal influences on the heart, relaxing the GI and GU tracts, inhibiting gastric acid secretion (high doses), relaxing the pupil of the eye (mydriatic effect), and preventing accommodation for near vision (cycloplegic effect); also blocks the effects of acetylcholine in the CNS.

**Indications**

*Systemic Administration*

- Antisialogogue for preanesthetic medication to prevent or reduce respiratory tract secretions
- Treatment of parkinsonism; relieves tremor and rigidity
- Restoration of cardiac rate and arterial pressure during anesthesia when vagal stimulation produced by intra-abdominal traction causes a decrease in pulse rate, lessening the degree of AV block when increased vagal tone is a factor (eg, some cases due to digitalis)
- Relief of bradycardia and syncope due to hyperactive carotid sinus reflex
- Relief of pylorospasm, hypertonicity of the small intestine, and hypermotility of the colon
- Relaxation of the spasm of biliary and ureteral colic and bronchospasm
- Relaxation of the tone of the detrusor muscle of the urinary bladder in the treatment of urinary tract disorders
- Control of crying and laughing episodes in patients with brain lesions

- Treatment of closed head injuries that cause acetylcholine release into CSF, EEG abnormalities, stupor, neurologic signs
- Relaxation of uterine hypertonicity
- Management of peptic ulcer
- Control of rhinorrhea of acute rhinitis or hay fever
- Antidote (with external cardiac massage) for CV collapse from overdose of parasympathomimetic (cholinergic) drugs (choline esters, pilocarpine), or cholinesterase inhibitors (eg, physostigmine, isoflurophate, organophosphorus insecticides)
- Antidote for poisoning by certain species of mushroom (eg, *Amanita muscaria)*
- **Ophthalmic preparations:** diagnostically to produce mydriasis and cycloplegiapupillary dilation in acute inflammatory conditions of the iris and uveal tract

## Contraindications/cautions

- Contraindications: hypersensitivity to anticholinergic drugs.
- Systemic administration: Contraindicated in the presence of glaucoma, adhesions between iris and lens, stenosing peptic ulcer, pyloroduodenal obstruction, paralytic ileus, intestinal atony, severe ulcerative colitis, toxic megacolon, symptomatic prostatic hypertrophy, bladder neck obstruction, bronchial asthma, COPD, cardiac arrhythmias, tachycardia, myocardial ischemia, impaired metabolic, liver or kidney function, myasthenia gravis.
- Use cautiously with Down's syndrome, brain damage, spasticity, hypertension, hyperthyroidism, lactation.
- Ophthalmic solution: Contraindicated with glaucoma or tendency to glaucoma.

## Dosage

**Available Forms:** Tablets—0.4 mg; injection—0.05, 0.1, 0.3, 0.4, 0.5, 0.8, 1 mg/ml; ophthalmic ointment—1%; ophthalmic solution—0.5%, 1%, 2%

ADULT

- *Systemic administration:* 0.4–0.6 mg IM, SC, IV
- *Hypotonic radiography:* 1 mg IM.
- *Surgery:* 0.5 mg (0.4–0.6 mg) IM (or SC, IV) prior to induction of anesthesia; during surgery, give IV; reduce dose to < 0.4 mg with cyclopropane anesthesia.
- *Bradyarrhythmias:* 0.4–1 mg (up to 2 mg) IV every 1–2 h as needed.
- *Antidote:* For poisoning due to cholinesterase inhibitor insecticides, give large doses of at least 2–3 mg parenterally, and repeat until signs of atropine intoxication appear; for "rapid" type of mushroom poisoning, give in doses sufficient to control parasympathetic signs before coma and CV collapse intervene.
- ***Ophthalmic solution***
- *For refraction:* Instill 1–2 drops into eye(s) 1 h before refracting.
- *For uveitis:* Instill 1–2 drops into eye(s) four times daily.

PEDIATRIC

- ***Systemic administration:*** Refer to the following chart:

| *Weight* | *Dose (mg)* |
|---|---|
| 7–16 lb (3,2–7.3 kg) | 0.1 |
| 16–24 lb (7.3–10.9 kg) | 1.15 |
| 24–40 lb (10.9–18.1 kg) | 0.2 |
| 40–65 lb (18.1–29.5 kg) | 0.3 |
| 65–90 lb (29.5–40.8 kg) | 0.4 |
| >90 lb (>40.8 kg) | 0.4–0.6 |

- *Surgery:* 0.1 mg (newborn) to 0.6 mg (12 y) injected SC 30 min before surgery.

GERIATRIC: More likely to cause serious adverse reactions, especially CNS reactions, in elderly patients; use with caution.

## Pharmacokinetics

| *Route* | *Onset* | *Peak* | *Duration* |
|---|---|---|---|
| IM | 10–15 min | 30 min | 4 h |
| IV | Immediate | 2–4 min | 4 h |
| SC | Varies | 1–2 h | 4 h |
| Topical | 5–10 min | 30–40 min | 7–14 d |

*Metabolism:* Hepatic, $T_{1/2}$: 2.5 h

*Distribution:* Crosses placenta; passes into breast milk

*Excretion:* Urine

## IV facts

**Preparation:** Give undiluted or dilute in 10 ml sterile water.

**Infusion:** Give direct IV; administer 1 mg or less over 1 min

### Adverse effects

*Systemic Administration*

- CNS: *Blurred vision, mydriasis, cycloplegia, photophobia*, increased intraocular pressure, headache, flushing, nervousness, weakness, dizziness, insomnia, mental confusion or excitement (after even small doses in the elderly), nasal congestion
- GI: *Dry mouth, altered taste perception, nausea*, vomiting, dysphagia, heartburn, constipation, bloated feeling, **paralytic ileus**, gastroesophageal reflux
- CV: *Palpitations, bradycardia* (low doses), *tachycardia* (higher doses)
- GU: *Urinary hesitancy and retention*; impotence
- Other: *Decreased sweating and predisposition to heat prostration*, suppression of lactation

*Ophthalmic Preparations*

- Local: *Transient stinging*
- Systemic: Systemic adverse effects, depending on amount absorbed

### Clinically important drug-drug interactions

• Increased anticholinergic effects with other drugs that have anticholinergic activity: certain antihistamines, certain antiparkinson drugs, TCAs, MAO inhibitors. • Decreased antipsychotic effectiveness of haloperidol with atropine • Decreased effectiveness of phenothiazines, but increased incidence of paralytic ileus

## ■ Nursing Considerations

### Assessment

- *History:* Hypersensitivity to anticholinergic drugs; glaucoma; adhesions between iris and lens; stenosing peptic ulcer, pyloroduodenal obstruction, paralytic ileus, intestinal atony, severe ulcerative colitis, toxic megacolon, symptomatic prostatic hypertrophy, bladder neck obstruction, bronchial asthma, COPD, cardiac arrhythmias, myocardial ischemia, impaired metabolic, liver or kidney function, myasthenia gravis, Down syndrome, brain damage, spasticity, hypertension, hyperthyroidism, lactation
- *Physical:* Skin color, lesions, texture; T; orientation, reflexes, bilateral grip strength; affect; ophthalmic exam; P, BP; R, adventitious sounds; bowel sounds, normal GI output; normal urinary output, prostate palpation; liver and kidney function tests, ECG

### Implementation

- Ensure adequate hydration; provide environmental control (temperature) to prevent hyperpyrexia.
- Have patient void before taking medication if urinary retention is a problem.

### Drug-specific teaching points

When used preoperatively or in other acute situations, incorporate teaching about the drug with teaching about the procedure; the ophthalmic solution is used mainly acutely and will not be self-administered by the patient; the following apply to oral medication for outpatients:

- Take as prescribed, 30 min before meals; avoid excessive dosage.
- Avoid hot environments; you will be heat intolerant, and dangerous reactions may occur.
- The following side effects may occur: dizziness, confusion (use caution driving or performing hazardous tasks); constipation (ensure adequate fluid intake, proper diet); dry mouth (sugarless lozenges, frequent mouth care may help; may be transient); blurred vision, sensitivity to light (reversible; avoid tasks that require acute vision; wear sunglasses in bright light); impotence (reversible); difficulty in urination (empty the bladder prior to taking drug).
- Report skin rash; flushing; eye pain; difficulty breathing; tremors, loss of coordination; irregular heartbeat, palpitations; headache; abdominal distention; hallucinations; severe or persistent dry mouth; difficulty swallowing; difficulty in urination; constipation; sensitivity to light.

# auranofin

*(au rane' oh fin)*
Ridaura
**Pregnancy Category C**

## Drug classes
Antirheumatic agent
Gold compound

## Therapeutic actions
Suppresses and prevents arthritis and synovitis—taken up by macrophages with resultant inhibition of phagocytosis and inhibition of activities of lysosomal enzymes; decreases concentrations of rheumatoid factor and immunoglobulins; mechanisms not known; no substantial evidence of remission induction.

## Indications
- Management of adults with active classic or definite rheumatoid arthritis who have insufficient response or are intolerant to NSAIDs (given only orally)
- Unlabeled use: alternative or adjuvant to corticosteroids in treatment of pemphigus, SLE; for psoriatic arthritis in patients who do not tolerate or respond to NSAIDs

## Contraindications/cautions
- Contraindications: allergy to gold preparations; history of gold-induced disorders, necrotizing entercolitis, pulmonary fibrosis, exfoliative dermatitis, bone marrow aplasia, severe hematologic disorders, lactation.
- Use cautiously with diabetes mellitus, CHF, hypertension, compromised liver or renal function, compromised cerebral or CV circulation, inflammatory bowel disease, blood dyscrasias.

## Dosage
**Available Forms:** Capsules—3 mg
Contains approximately 29% gold

**ADULT:** 6 mg/d PO, either as 3 mg bid or 6 mg qd. If response is not adequate after 6 mo, dosage may be increased to 9 mg/d (3 mg tid). If response is not adequate after another 3 mo, discontinue drug; do not exceed 9 mg/d.
- *Transfer from injectable gold:* Discontinue injectable agent, and start auranofin 6 mg/d PO.

**PEDIATRIC:** 0.1 mg/kg/d PO initially; titrate up to 0.15 mg/kg/d; do not exceed 0.2 mg/kg/d.

**GERIATRIC:** Monitor patients carefully; tolerance to gold decreases with age.

## Pharmacokinetics

| *Route* | *Onset* | *Peak* |
|---|---|---|
| Oral | Varies | 1–2 h |

*Metabolism:* $T_{1/2}$: 26 d
*Distribution:* Crosses placenta; passes into breast milk
*Excretion:* Urine and feces

## Adverse effects
- GI: *Nausea, vomiting, anorexia, abdominal cramps, diarrhea, stomatitis, glossitis,* gingivitis, metallic taste, pharyngitis, gastritis, colitis, conjunctivitis, hepatitis with jaundice
- Respiratory: Gold bronchitis, **interstitial pneumonitis and fibrosis**, cough, shortness of breath, tracheitis
- Hematologic: *Anemias*, granulocytopenia, thromobocytopenia, leukopenia, eosinophilia
- GU: Nephrotic syndrome or glomerulitis with proteinuria and hematuria; **acute tubular necrosis and renal failure,** vaginitis
- Dermatologic: *Dermatitis; pruritis, erythema,* exfoliative dermatitis, chrysiasis (gray-blue color to the skin due to gold deposition)
- Allergic reactions: Nitroid reactions: flushing, fainting, dizziness, sweating, nausea, vomiting, malaise, weakness

## Clinically important drug-drug interactions
- Do not use with penicillamine, antimalarials, cytotoxic drugs, immunosuppressive agents other than low doses of corticosteroids

## ■ Nursing Considerations

### Assessment
- *History:* Allergy to gold preparations, history of gold-induced disorders, diabe-

tes mellitus, CHF, hypertension, compromised liver or renal function, compromised cerebral or CV circulation, inflammatory bowel disease, blood dyscrasias, lactation

- *Physical:* Skin color, lesions; T; edema; R, adventitious sounds; GI mucous membranes, bowel sounds, liver evaluation; CBC, renal and liver function tests, chest x-ray

### Implementation

- Do not give to patients with idiosyncratic or severe reactions to gold therapy.
- Monitor hematologic status, liver and kidney function, respiratory status regularly during the course of drug therapy.
- Discontinue at first sign of toxic reaction.
- Use low-dose systemic corticosteroids for treatment of severe stomatitis, dermatitis, renal, hematologic, pulmonary, enterocolitic complications.
- Protect from sunlight or ultraviolet light to decrease risk of chrysiasis.

### Drug-specific teaching points

- Take this drug as prescribed; do not take more. Drug's effects are not seen immediately; several months of therapy are needed.
- This drug does not cure the disease but stops its effects.
- The following side effects may occur: diarrhea; mouth sores, metallic taste (frequent mouth care will help); rash, gray-blue color to the skin (avoid exposure to the sun or ultraviolet light); nausea, loss of appetite (small, frequent meals may help).
- Avoid pregnancy while using this drug; if you decide to become pregnant, consult with physician about discontinuing drug.
- Report unusual bleeding or bruising; sore throat, fever; severe diarrhea; skin rash; mouth sores.

## aurothioglucose

*(aur oh thye oh **gloo'** kose)*

Solganal

**Pregnancy Category C**

### Drug classes

Antirheumatic agent
Gold compound

### Therapeutic actions

Suppresses and prevents arthritis and synovitis; taken up by macrophages with resultant inhibition of phagocytosis and inhibition of activities of lysosomal enzymes; decreases concentrations of rheumatoid factor and immunoglobulins; no substantial evidence of remission induction.

### Indications

- Treatment of selected cases of adult and juvenile rheumatoid arthritis; most effective early in disease; later, when damage has occurred, gold only prevents further damage.

### Contraindications/cautions

- Allergy to gold preparations; history of gold-induced disorders—necrotizing entercolitis, pulmonary fibrosis, exfoliative dermatitis, bone marrow aplasia, severe hematologic disorders; uncontrolled diabetes mellitus; CHF; SLE; marked hypertension, compromised liver or renal function, compromised cerebral or CV circulation, inflammatory bowel disease, blood dyscrasias, recent radiation treatments; lactation.

### Dosage

**Available Forms:** Injection suspension—50 mg/ml

Contains approximately 50% gold. Give by IM injection only, preferably intragluteally.

*ADULT*

- **Weekly injections**: First: 10 mg IM; second and third: 25 mg IM; fourth and subsequent: 50 mg IM until 0.8–1 g has been given. If patient improves without toxicity, continue 50-mg dose at 3- to 4-wk intervals.

*PEDIATRIC*

- **6–12 years**: Administer one-fourth the adult dose governed by body weight; do not exceed 25 mg/dose.

*GERIATRIC:* Monitor patients carefully; tolerance to gold decreases with age.

**Pharmacokinetics**

| Route | Onset | Peak |
|---|---|---|
| IM | Slow | 4–6 h |

*Metabolism:* $T_{1/2}$: 3–7 d
*Distribution:* Crosses placenta; passes into breast milk
*Excretion:* Urine and feces

**Adverse effects**

- GI: *Nausea, vomiting, anorexia*, abdominal cramps, diarrhea, *stomatitis, glossitis,* gingivitis, metallic taste, pharyngitis, gastritis, colitis, conjunctivitis, hepatitis with jaundice
- Respiratory: Gold bronchitis, **interstitial pneumonitis and fibrosis**, cough, shortness of breath, tracheitis
- Hematologic: *Anemias*, granulocytopenia, thromobocytopenia, leukopenia, eosinophilia
- GU: Nephrotic syndrome or glomerulitis with proteinuria and hematuria, **acute tubular necrosis** and renal failure, vaginitis
- Dermatologic: *Dermatitis; pruritis, erythema,* exfoliative dermatitis, chrysiasis (gray-blue color to the skin due to gold deposition)
- Immediate postinjection effects: **Anaphylactic shock**, syncope, bradycardia, thickening of the tongue, dysphagia, dyspnea, angioneurotic edema
- Nonvasomotor postinjection reaction: Arthralgia for 1–2 d after the injection; usually subsides after the first few injections
- Allergic reactions: Nitroid reactions: flushing, fainting, dizziness, sweating, nausea, vomiting, malaise, weakness

**Clinically important drug-drug interactions**

- Do not use with penicillamine, antimalarials, cytotoxic drugs, immunosuppressive agents other than low doses of corticosteroids

## ■ Nursing Considerations

### Assessment

- *History:* Allergy to gold preparations; history of gold-induced disorders; uncontrolled diabetes mellitus; CHF; SLE; marked hypertension; compromised liver or renal function; compromised cerebral or CV circulation; inflammatory bowel disease; blood dyscrasias; recent radiation treatments; lactation
- *Physical:* Skin color, lesions; T; edema; P, BP; R, adventitious sounds; GI mucous membranes, bowel sounds, liver evaluation; CBC, renal and liver function tests, chest x-ray

### Implementation

- Do not give drug to patients with history of idosyncratic or severe reactions to gold therapy.
- Monitor hematologic status, liver and kidney function, respiratory status regularly.
- Give by intragluteal IM injection.
- Monitor patient carefully at time of injection for possible postinjection reaction.
- Discontinue drug at first sign of toxic reaction.
- Use low-dose systemic corticosteroids for treatment of severe stomatitis, dermatitis, renal, hematologic, pulmonary, enterocolitic complications.
- Protect patient from exposure to sun or ultraviolet light to decrease risk of chrysiasis.

### Drug-specific teaching points

- Prepare a calendar of projected injection dates. Drug's effects are not seen immediately; several months of therapy are needed.
- The following side effects may occur: increased joint pain for 1–2 d after injection (usually subsides after the first few injections); diarrhea; mouth sores, metallic taste (frequent mouth care will help); rash, gray-blue color to the skin (avoid exposure to sun or ultraviolet light); nausea, loss of appetite (small, frequent meals may help).
- Avoid pregnancy while on this drug. If you decide to become pregnant, consult with physician about discontinuing drug.
- Report unusual bleeding or bruising; sore throat, fever; severe diarrhea; skin rash; mouth sores.

# azatadine maleate

*(a za' te deen)*
Optimine
**Pregnancy Category C**

## Drug classes
Antihistamine (piperidine type)

## Therapeutic actions
Competitively blocks the effects of histamine at $H_1$ receptor sites; has anticholinergic (atropine-like), antiserotonin, antipruritic, sedative, and appetite-stimulating effects.

## Indications
- Relief of symptoms associated with perennial and seasonal allergic rhinitis; vasomotor rhinitis; allergic conjunctivitis; mild, uncomplicated urticaria and angioedema; amelioraton of allergic reactions to blood or plasma; dermatographism; adjunctive therapy in anaphylactic reactions
- Treatment of cold urticaria
- Unlabeled uses: stimulation of appetite in underweight patients and those with anorexia nervosa; treatment of vascular cluster headaches

## Contraindications/cautions
- Contraindications: allergy to any antihistamines, lactation, third trimester of pregnancy.
- Use cautiously with narrow-angle glaucoma, stenosing peptic ulcer, symptomatic prostatic hypertrophy, asthmatic attack, bladder neck obstruction, pyloroduodenal obstruction.

## Dosage
**Available Forms:** Tablets—1 mg
*ADULT:* 1–2 mg PO bid.
*PEDIATRIC:* Safety and efficacy not established in children < 12 y.
*GERIATRIC:* More likely to cause dizziness, sedation, syncope, toxic confusional states, and hypotension in elderly patients; use with caution.

## Pharmacokinetics

| Route | Onset | Peak |
|---|---|---|
| Oral | Varies | 4 h |

*Metabolism:* Hepatic, $T_{1/2}$: 12 h
*Distribution:* Crosses placenta; passes into breast milk
*Excretion:* Urine

## Adverse effects
- CNS: *Drowsiness, sedation, dizziness, disturbed coordination*, fatigue, confusion, restlessness, excitation, nervousness, tremor, headache, blurred vision, diplopia, vertigo, tinnitus, acute labryinthitis, hysteria, tingling, heaviness and weakness of the hands
- GI: *Epigastric distress,* anorexia, increased appetite and weight gain, nausea, vomiting, diarrhea or constipation
- CV: Hypotension, palpitations, bradycardia, tachycardia, extrasystoles
- Respiratory: *Thickening of bronchial secretions*, chest tightness, wheezing, nasal stuffiness, dry mouth, dry nose, dry throat, sore throat
- Hematologic: Hemolytic anemia, hypoplastic anemia, thrombocytopenia, leukopenia, agranulocytosis, pancytopenia
- GU: Urinary frequency, dysuria, urinary retention, early menses, decreased libido, impotence
- Other: Urticaria, rash, **anaphylactic shock**, photosensitivity, excessive perspiration

## Clinically important drug-drug interactions
- Increased and prolonged anticholinergic (drying) effects with MAO inhibitors

## Drug-lab test interferences
- Increase in PBI not attributable to an increase in thyroxine • False-positive pregnancy test (less likely if serum test is used)

## ■ Nursing Considerations

### Assessment
- *History:* Allergy to antihistamines; narrow-angle glaucoma, stenosing peptic

ulcer, symptomatic prostatic hypertrophy, asthmatic attack, bladder neck obstruction, pyloroduodenal obstruction; lactation
- *Physical:* Skin color, lesions, texture; orientation, reflexes, affect; vision exam; P, BP; R, adventitious sounds; bowel sounds; prostate palpation; CBC with differential

### Implementation
- Administer with food if GI upset occurs.
- Monitor patient response. Maintain at lowest possible effective dosage.

### Drug-specific teaching points
- Take as prescribed; avoid excessive dosage.
- Take with food if GI upset occurs.
- The following side effects may occur: dizziness, sedation, drowsiness (use caution driving or performing tasks that require alertness); epigastric distress, diarrhea or constipation (take drug with meals; consult health care provider about diarrhea or constipation); dry mouth (use frequent mouth care, suck sugarless lozenges); thickening of bronchial secretions, dryness of nasal mucosa (use humidifier).
- Avoid alcohol; serious sedation could occur.
- Report difficulty breathing, hallucinations, tremors, loss of coordination, unusual bleeding or bruising, visual disturbances, irregular heartbeat.

## azathioprine

*(ay za **thye'** oh preen)*

Imuran

**Pregnancy Category D**

### Drug classes
Immunosuppressive

### Therapeutic actions
Suppresses cell-mediated hypersensitivities and alters antibody production; exact mechanisms of action in increasing homograft survival and affecting autoimmune diseases not clearly understood.

### Indications
- Renal homotransplantation: adjunct for prevention of rejection
- Rheumatoid arthritis: use only with adults meeting criteria for classic rheumatoid arthritis and not responding to conventional management
- Unlabeled use: treatment of chronic ulcerative colitis, myasthenia gravis, Behçet's syndrome, Crohn's disease

### Contraindications/cautions
- Allergy to azathioprine; rheumatoid arthritis patients previously treated with alkylating agents, increasing their risk for neoplasia; pregnancy.

### Dosage
**Available Forms:** Tablets—50 mg; injection—100 mg/vial

**ADULT**
- ***Renal homotransplantation:*** Initial dose of 3–5 mg/kg per day PO or IV as a single dose on the day of transplant; maintenance levels are 1–3 mg/kg per day PO. Do not increase dose to decrease risk of rejection.
- ***Rheumatoid arthritis:*** Usually given daily; initial dose of 1 mg/kg PO given as a single dose or bid. Dose may be increased at 6–8 wk and thereafter by steps at 4-wk intervals. Dose increments should be 0.5 mg/kg per day up to a maximum dose of 2.5 mg/kg per day. Once patient is stabilized, dose should be decreased to lowest effective dose; decrease in 0.5-mg/kg increments. Patients who do not respond in 12 wk are probably refractory.

**PEDIATRIC**
- ***Renal homotransplantation:*** Initial dose of 3–5 mg/kg per day IV or PO followed by a maintenance dose of 1–3 mg/kg per day.

**GERIATRIC OR RENAL IMPAIRED:** Lower doses may be required because of decreased rate of excretion and increased sensitivity to the drug.

### Pharmacokinetics

| *Route* | *Onset* | *Peak* |
|---|---|---|
| Oral | Varies | 1–2 h |
| IV | Immediate | 30–45 min |

*Metabolism:* Hepatic, $T_{1/2}$: 5 h
*Distribution:* Crosses placenta; may pass into breast milk
*Excretion:* Urine

### IV facts

**Preparation:** Add 10 ml Sterile Water for Injection and swirl until a clear solution results; use within 24 h. Further dilution into sterile saline or dextrose is usually made for infusion.

**Infusion:** Infuse over 30–60 min; ranges from 5 min to 8 h for the daily dose are possible.

### Adverse effects

- GI: *Nausea, vomiting*, hepatotoxicity (especially in homograft patients)
- Hematologic: *Leukopenia, thrombocytopenia, macrocytic anemia*
- Other: **Serious infections** (fungal, bacterial, protozoal infections secondary to immuosuppression; may be fatal), *carcinogenesis* (increased risk of neoplasia, especially in homograft patients)

### Clinically important drug-drug interactions

• Increased effects with allopurinol; reduce azathioprine to one-third to one-fourth the usual dose • Reversal of the neuromuscular blockade of nondepolarizing neuromuscular junction blockers (atracurium, gallamine, pancuronium, tubocurarine, vecuronium) with azathioprine

## ■ Nursing Considerations

### Assessment

- *History:* Allergy to azathioprine; rheumatoid arthritis patients previously treated with alkylating agents; pregnancy or male partners of women trying to become pregnant; lactation
- *Physical:* T; skin color, lesions; liver evaluation, bowel sounds; renal and liver function tests, CBC

### Implementation

- Give drug IV if oral administration is not possible; switch to oral route as soon as possible.
- Administer in divided daily doses or with food if GI upset occurs.
- Monitor blood counts regularly; severe hematologic effects may require the discontinuation of therapy.

### Drug-specific teaching points

- Take drug in divided doses with food if GI upset occurs.
- Avoid infections; avoid crowds or people who have infections. Notify your physician at once if injured.
- Notify your physician if you think you are pregnant or if you wish to become pregnant (also applies to men whose sexual partners wish to become pregnant).
- The following side effects may occur: nausea, vomiting (take drug in divided doses or with food); diarrhea; skin rash.
- Report unusual bleeding or bruising; fever, sore throat, mouth sores; signs of infection; abdominal pain; severe diarrhea; darkened urine or pale stools; severe nausea and vomiting.

## azelastine hydrochloride

*(az ah **las'** teen)*

Astlein

**Pregnancy Category C**

### Drug classes

Antihistamine

### Therapeutic actions

Competitively blocks the effects of histamine at peripheral $H_1$ receptor sites, has no effects on cardiac repolarization, may cause drowsiness.

### Indications

- Relief of symptoms associated with seasonal allergic rhinitis in adults and children > 12 y

### Contraindications/cautions

- Contraindications: allergy to any antihistamines, pregnancy, lactation.
- Use cautiously with COPD.

### Dosage

**Available Forms:** Nasal spray—137 μg/actuation

**ADULT AND CHILDREN > 12 YRS:** 2 sprays per nostril bid.

**PEDIATRIC < 12 Y:** Not recommended.

**Pharmacokinetics**

| *Route* | *Onset* | *Peak* |
|---|---|---|
| Nasal | Rapid | 2–3 h |

*Metabolism:* Hepatic metabolism; $T_{1/2}$: 22 h
*Distribution:* Crosses placenta; may pass into breast milk
*Excretion:* Feces and urine

**Adverse effects**
- CNS: Fatigue, drowsiness, headache, somnolence
- GI: Nausea, dyspepsia, bitter taste, dry mouth
- Other: Nasal burning, sneezing, rhinitis

**Clinically important drug-drug interactions**
• Increased sedative effects with CNS depressants, alcohol • Increased level of azelastine if taken with cimetidine

## ■ Nursing Considerations

### Assessment
- *History:* Allergy to any antihistamines, renal or hepatic impairment, pregnancy, lactation
- *Physical:* Mucous membranes, oropharnyx, R, adventitious sounds; orientation, affect; renal and liver function tests

### Implementation
- Arrange for use of humidifier if thickening of secretions, nasal dryness become bothersome; encourage adequate intake of fluids.
- Teach patient proper use of the nasal spray, including priming before initial use and if not used for > 3 d.
- Advise patient not to use this drug during pregnancy and to use barrier contraceptives as appropriate

### Drug-specific teaching points
- Avoid excessive dosage; take only the dosage prescribed. Read the manufacturer's insert to assure proper delivery of the medication.
- Avoid the use of alcohol while on this drug; serious sedation could occur; do not use OTC antihistamines without consulting health care provider.
- The following side effects may occur: dizziness, sedation, drowsiness (use caution if driving or performing tasks that require alertness); thickening of bronchial secretions, dryness of nasal mucosa (use of humidifier may help); dry mouth, bitter taste, nausea (frequent mouth care, sucking sugarless lozenges may help).
- Report difficulty breathing, severe nausea, nasal pain or continued rhinitis.

# azithromycin

*(ay zi thro **my'** sin)*
Zithromax
**Pregnancy Category B**

**Drug classes**
Macrolide antibiotic

**Therapeutic actions**
Bacteriostatic or bactericidal in susceptible bacteria.

**Indications**
- Treatment of lower respiratory tract infections: acute bacterial exacerbations of COPD due to *H. influenzae, Moraxella catarrhalis, S. pneumoniae;* community-acquired pneumonia due to *S. pneumoniae, H. influenzae*
- Treatment of lower respiratory tract infections: streptococcal pharyngitis/tonsillitis due to *Streptococcus pyogenes* in those who cannot take penicillins
- Treatment of uncomplicated skin infections due to *Staphylococcus aureus, S. pyogenes, Streptococcus agalactiae*
- Treatment of nongonococcal urethritis and cervicitis due to *C. trachomatis*; treatment of PID
- Treatment of otitis media caused by *H. influenzae, M. catarrhalis, S. pneumoniae* in children >6 mo
- Treatment of pharyngitis/tonsillitis in children >2 y who cannot use first-line therapy
- Prevention of disseminated *Mycobacterium avium* complex (MAC) in patients with advanced AIDS

a

**Contraindications/cautions**

- Contraindications: hypersensitivity to azithromycin, erythromycin, or any macrolide antibiotic.
- Use cautiously with gonorrhea or syphilis, pseudomembranous colitis, hepatic or renal impairment, lactation.

**Dosage**

**Available Forms:** Tablets—250, 600 mg; powder for injection—500 mg; powder for oral suspension—100 mg/5 ml, 200 mg/5 ml, 1 g/packet

**ADULT**

- *Mild to moderate acute bacterial exacerbations of COPD, pneumonia, pharyngitis/tonsillitis (as second-line:* 500 mg PO single dose on first day, followed by 250 mg PO qd on days 2–5 for a total dose of 1.5 g.
- *Nongonococcal urethritis and cervicitis due to C. trachomatis*: A single 1-g PO dose.

**PEDIATRIC**

- *Otitis media:* Initially 10 mg/kg PO as a single dose, then 5 mg/kg on days 2–5.
- *Pharyngitis/tonsillitis:* 12 mg/kg/d PO on days 1–5.

**Pharmacokinetics**

| Route | Onset | Peak | Duration |
|---|---|---|---|
| Oral | Varies | 2.5–3.2 h | 24 h |

*Metabolism:* $T_{1/2}$: 11–48 h

*Distribution:* Crosses placenta; passes into breast milk

*Excretion:* Unchanged in biliary excretion and urine

**Adverse effects**

- CNS: Dizziness, headache, vertigo, somnolence, fatigue
- GI: *Diarrhea, abdominal pain, nausea,* dyspepsia, flatulence, vomiting, melena, pseudomembranous colitis
- Other: *Superinfections,* **angioedema,** rash, photosensitivity, vaginitis

**Clinically important drug-drug interactions**

• Decreased serum levels and effectiveness of azithromycin with aluminum and magnesium-containing antacids • Possible decreased effects of theophylline • Possible increased anticoagulant effects of warfarin

**Clinically important drug-food interactions**

• Food greatly decreases the absorption of azithromycin

## ■ Nursing Considerations

**Assessment**

- *History:* Hypersensitivity to azithromycin, erythromycin, or any macrolide antibiotic; gonorrhea or syphilis, pseudomembranous colitis, hepatic or renal impairment, lactation
- *Physical:* Site of infection; skin color, lesions; orientation, GI output, bowel sounds, liver evaluation; culture and sensitivity tests of infection, urinalysis, liver and renal function tests

**Implementation**

- Culture site of infection before therapy.
- Administer on an empty stomach—1 h before or 2–3 h after meals. Food affects the absorption of this drug.
- Counsel patients being treated for STDs about appropriate precautions and additional therapy.

**Drug-specific teaching points**

- Take this drug on an empty stomach—1 h before or 2–3 h after meals; it should never be taken with food. Take the full course prescribed. Do not take with antacids.
- The following side effects may occur: stomach cramping, discomfort, diarrhea; fatigue, headache (medication may help); additional infections in the mouth or vagina (consult with health care provider for treatment).
- Report severe or watery diarrhea, severe nausea or vomiting, skin rash or itching, mouth sores, vaginal sores.

## aztreonam

*(az' tree oh nam)*

Azactam

**Pregnancy Category B**

### Drug classes
Monobactam antibiotic

### Therapeutic actions
Bactericidal: interferes with bacterial cell wall synthesis, causing cell death in susceptible gram-negative bacteria, ineffective against gram-positive and anaerobic bacteria.

### Indications
- Treatment of urinary tract infections, lower respiratory tract infections, skin and skin-structure infections, septicemia, intra-abdominal infections and gynecologic infections caused by suseptible strains of *E. coli, Enterobacter, Serratia, Proteus, Salmonella, Providencia, Pseudomonas, Citrobacter, Haemophilus, Neisseria, Klebsiella*

### Contraindications/cautions
- Contraindications: allergy to aztreonam.
- Use cautiously with immediate hypersensitivity reaction to penicillins or cephalosporins, renal and hepatic disorders, lactation.

## Dosage
**Available Forms:** Powder for injection—500 mg, 1 g, 2 g

Available for IV and IM use only; maximum recommended dose, 8 g/d.

**ADULT**
- *UTIs:* 500 mg–1 g q8–12h.
- ***Moderately severe systemic infection:*** 1–2 g q8–12h.
- ***Severe systemic infection:*** 2 g q6–8h.

*PEDIATRIC:* Safety and efficacy not established.

*GERIATRIC OR IMPAIRED RENAL FUNCTION:* Reduce dosage by one-half in patients with estimated creatinine clearances between 10 and 30 ml/min/1.73m$^2$ after an initial loading dose of 1 or 2 g. *Patients on hemodialysis:* give 500 mg, 1 g, or 2 g initially; maintenance dose should be one-fourth the usual initial dose at fixed intervals of 6, 8, or 12 h.

### Pharmacokinetics

| Route | Onset | Peak | Duration |
|---|---|---|---|
| IM | Varies | 1–1.5 h | 6–8 h |
| IV | Immediate | 30 min | 6–8 h |

*Metabolism:* $T_{1/2}$: 1.5–2 h

*Distribution:* Crosses placenta; passes into breast milk

*Excretion:* Urine

## IV facts
**Preparation:** After adding diluent to container, shake immediatley and vigorously. Constituted solutions are not for multiple-dose use; discard any unused solution. Solution should be colorless to light straw yellow, which may develop a slight pink tint on standing. **IV injection:** reconstitute contents of 15-ml vial with 6–10 ml Sterile Water for Injection. **IV infusion:** Reconstitute contents of 100-ml bottle to make a final concentration not > 2% w/v (add *with* at least 50 ml/g *azetreonam* of one of the following solutions per gram of aztreonam): 0.9% Sodium Chloride Injection, Ringer's Injection, Lactated Ringer's Injection, 5% or 10% Dextrose Injection, 5% Dextrose and 0.2%, 0.45%, or 0.09% Sodium Chloride, Sodium Lactate Injection, Ionosol B with 5% Dextrose, Isolyte E, Isolyte E with 5% Dextrose, Isolyte M with 5% Dextrose, Normosol-R, Normosol-R and 5% Dextrose, Normosol-M and 5% Dextrose, 5% and 10% Mannitol Injection, Lactated Ringer's and 5% Dextrose Injection, Plasma-Lyte M and 5% Dextrose, 10% Travert Injection, 10% Travert and Electrolyte no. 1, 2, or 3 Injection. Use reconstituted solutions promptly after preparation; those prepared with Sterile Water for Injection or Sodium Chloride Injection should be used within 48 h if stored at room temperature and within 7 d if refrigerated.

**Infusion: IV injection:** Inject slowly over 3–5 min directly into vein or into IV tubing of compatible IV infusion. **IV infusion:** Administer over 20–60 min. If giving into IV tubing that is used to administer other drugs, flush tubing with delivery solution before and after aztreonam administration.

**Compatabilities:** Do not mix with nafcillin sodium, cephradine, metronidazole; other admixtures are not recommended because data are not available.

**Adverse effects**
- GI: *Nausea, vomiting, diarrhea*, transient elevation of SGOT, SGPT, LDH
- Dermatologic: *Rash, pruritus*
- Local: *Local phlebitis/thrombophlebitis* at IV injection site, *swelling/discomfort* at IM injection site
- Hypersensitivity: **Anaphylaxis**
- Other: Superinfections

**Clinically important drug-drug interactions**
- Incompatible in solution with nafcillin sodium, cephradine, metronidazole

## ■ Nursing Considerations

### Assessment
- *History:* Allergy to aztreonam, immediate hypersensitivity reaction to penicillins or cephalosporins, renal and hepatic disorders, lactation
- *Physical:* Skin color, lesions; injection sites; T; GI mucous membranes, bowel sounds, liver evaluation; GU mucous membranes; culture and sensitivity tests of infected area; liver and renal function tests

### Implementation
- Arrange for culture and sensitivity tests of infected area before therapy. In acutely ill patients, therapy may begin before test results are known. If therapeutic effects are not noted, reculture area.
- **IM administration:** Reconstitute contents of 15-ml vial with at least 3 ml of diluent per gram of aztreonam. Appropriate diluents are Sterile Water for Injection, Bacteriostatic Water for Injection, 0.9% Sodium Chloride Injection, Bacteriostatic Sodium Chloride Injection. Inject deeply into a large muscle mass. Do not mix with any local anesthetic.
- Discontinue drug and provide supportive measures if hypersensitivity reaction, anaphylaxis occurs.
- Monitor injection sites and provide comfort measures.
- Provide treatment and comfort measures if superinfections occur.
- Monitor patient's nutritional status, and provide small, frequent meals, mouth care if GI effects, superinfections interfere with nutrition.

### Drug-specific teaching points
- This drug can only be given IM or IV.
- The following side effects may occur: nausea, vomiting, diarrhea.
- Report pain, soreness at injection site; difficulty breathing; mouth sores.

# bacampicillin hydrochloride

*(ba kam pi **sill'** in)*

Spectrobid, Penglobe (CAN)

**Pregnancy Category A**

**Drug classes**

Antibiotic

Penicillin, ampicillin-type

**Therapeutic actions**

Metabolized to ampicillin during absorption; bactericidal—inhibits synthesis of cell wall of sensitive organisms causing cell death.

**Indications**
- Upper and lower respiratory tract infections caused by *beta-hemolytic streptococci, Streptococcus pyogenes, Streptococcus pneumoniae, Haemophilus influenzae,* nonpenicillinase-producing staphylococci
- UTIs caused by *Escherichia coli, Proteus mirabilis, Streptococcus faecalis*
- Skin and surface-structure infections due to streptococci and susceptible staphylococci
- Gonorrhea due to *Neisseria gonorrhoeae*

**Contraindications/cautions**
- Contraindications: allergies to penicillins, cephalosporins, or other allergens.
- Use cautiously with renal disorders, lactation.

### Dosage
**Available Forms:** Tablets—400 mg

ADULT (BODY WEIGHT > 25 KG)

- *Upper respiratory infections, UTIs, skin and soft-structure infections:* 400 mg PO q12h.
- *Severe infections caused by less susceptible organisms:* 800 mg PO q12h.
- *Lower respiratory tract infections:* 800 mg PO q12h.
- *Gonorrhea:* 1.6 g bacampicillin plus 1 g probenecid.

PEDIATRIC

- *Upper respiratory infections, UTIs, skin and soft-structure infections:* 25 mg/kg per day PO in two equally divided doses q12h.
- *Severe infections caused by less susceptible organisms:* 50 mg/kg per day PO in two equally divided doses q12h.
- *Lower respiratory tract infections:* 50 mg/kg per day PO in two equally divided doses q12h.

### Pharmacokinetics

| *Route* | *Onset* | *Peak* |
|---|---|---|
| Oral | Varies | 1 h |

*Metabolism:* Hepatic, $T_{1/2}$: 1.5 h
*Distribution:* Crosses placenta; passes into breast milk
*Excretion:* Urine

### Adverse effects

- CNS: Lethargy, hallucinations, seizures
- GI: *Glossitis, stomatitis, gastritis, sore mouth*, furry tongue, black "hairy" tongue, *nausea, vomiting, diarrhea,* abdominal pain, bloody diarrhea, enterocolitis, **pseudomembranous colitis**, nonspecific hepatitis
- CV: CHF (sodium overload with sodium preparations)
- Hematologic: Anemia, thrombocytopenia, leukopenia, neutropenia, prolonged bleeding time
- GU: Nephritis, oliguria, proteinuria, hematuria, casts, azotemia, pyuria
- Hypersensitivity reactions: *Rash, fever, wheezing,* ***anaphylaxis***
- Local: *Pain, phlebitis,* thrombosis at injection site (parenteral)
- Other: *Superinfections*—oral and rectal moniliasis, vaginitis

### Clinically important drug-drug interactions

• Increased effect with probenecid • Decreased effectiveness with tetracyclines, chloramphenicol • Decreased efficacy of oral contraceptives • Do not administer to a patient who is taking disulfiram.

### Clinically important drug-food interactions

• Decreased absorption and effectiveness of bcampicillin if taken with food

## ■ Nursing Considerations

### Assessment

- *History:* Allergies to penicillins, cephalosporins, or other allergens; renal disorders; lactation
- *Physical:* Skin color, lesion; R, adventitious sounds; bowel sounds; CBC, liver and renal function tests, serum electrolytes, Hct, urinalysis

### Implementation

- Culture infected area before treatment; reculture area if response is not as expected.
- Administer drug without regard to meals; may be given with food.

### Drug-specific teaching points

- Take this drug around the clock as prescribed.
- Take the full course of therapy; do not stop taking the drug when you feel better.
- This drug can be taken with food or meals.
- This antibiotic is specific for the current problem and should not be used to self-treat other infections.
- The following side effects may occur: nausea, diarrhea, GI upset (small frequent meals may help); mouth sores (try frequent mouth care).
- Report unusual bleeding or bruising; rash, hives, fever, severe diarrhea; difficulty breathing.

# bacitracin

*(bass i **tray'** sin)*

*Powder for Injection:* Baci-IM

*Ophthalmic:* AK-Tracin

*Topical ointment:* Baciguent, Bacitin (CAN)

**Pregnancy Category C**

## Drug classes

Antibiotic

## Therapeutic actions

Antibacterial: inhibits cell wall synthesis of susceptible bacteria, primarily staphylococci, causing cell death.

## Indications

- IM: Pneumonia and empyema caused by susceptible strains of staphylococci in infants
- Ophthalmic preparations: Infections of the eye caused by susceptible strains of staphylococci
- Topical ointment: Prophylaxis of minor skin abrasions; treatment of superficial infections of the skin caused by susceptible staphylococci
- Unlabeled use (oral preparation): Antibiotic-associated pseudomembranous enterocolitis

## Contraindications/cautions

- Allergy to bacitracin, renal disease, lactation

## Dosage

**Available Forms:** Powder for injection—50,000 U; ophthalmic ointment—500 U/g; topical ointment—500 U/g

***IM use***

- *INFANTS* $<$ *2.5 KG:* 900 U/kg per day IM or IV in two to three divided doses.
- *INFANTS* $>$ *2.5 KG:* 1,000 U/kg per day IM or IV in two to three divided doses.

***Ophthalmic use:*** Half-inch ribbon in the infected eye bid to q3–4h as needed.

***Topical use:*** Apply to affected area one to five times per day; cover with sterile bandage if needed.

## Pharmacokinetics

| *Route* | *Onset* | *Peak* | *Duration* |
|---|---|---|---|
| IM | Rapid | 1–2 h | 12–14 h |

*Metabolism:* $T_{1/2}$: 6 h

*Distribution:* Crosses placenta; passes into breast milk

*Excretion:* Urine

## Adverse effects

- GI: Nausea, vomiting
- GU: *Nephrotoxicity*
- **Local:** *Pain at IM injection site* (IM); *contact dermatitis* (topical ointment); *irritation, burning, stinging, itching, blurring of vision* (ophthalmic preparations)
- Other: Superinfections

## Clinically important drug-drug interactions

• Increased neuromuscular blockade and muscular paralysis with anesthetics, nondepolarizing neuromuscular blocking drugs, drugs with neuromuscular blocking activity • Increased risk of respiratory paralysis and renal failure with aminoglycosides

## ■ Nursing Considerations

### Assessment

- ***History:*** Allergy to bacitracin, renal disease, lactation
- ***Physical:*** Site of infection; skin color, lesions; normal urinary output; urinalysis, serum creatinine, renal function tests

### Implementation

- For IM use: Reconstitute 50,000-U vial with 9.8 ml Sodium Chloride Injection with 2% procaine hydrochloride; reconstitute the 10,000-U vial with 2.0 ml of diluent (resulting concentration of 5,000 U/ml). Refrigerate unreconstituted vials. Reconstituted solutions are stable for 1 wk, refrigerated.
- Topical application: Cleanse the area before applying new ointment.
- Culture infected area before therapy.
- Ensure adequate hydration to prevent renal toxicity.

- Monitor renal function tests daily during therapy (IM use).

### Drug-specific teaching points

- Give ophthalmic preparation as follows: tilt head back; place medication into eyelid and close eyes; gently hold the inner corner of the eye for 1 min. Do not touch tube to eye. For topical application, cleanse area being treated before applying new ointment; cover with sterile bandage (if possible).
- The following side effects may occur: superinfections (frequent hygiene measures, medications may help); burning, stinging, blurring of vision with ophthalmic use (transient).
- Report rash or skin lesions; change in urinary voiding patterns; changes in vision, severe stinging, or itching (ophthalmic).

## baclofen

*(bak' loe fen)*

Alpha-Baclofen (CAN), Lioresal

**Pregnancy Category C**

### Drug classes

Centrally acting skeletal muscle relaxant

### Therapeutic actions

Precise mechanism not known; GABA analog but does not appear to produce clinical effects by actions on GABA minergic systems; inhibits both monosynaptic and polysynaptic spinal reflexes; CNS depressant.

### Indications

- Alleviation of signs and symptoms of spasticity resulting from multiple sclerosis, particularly for the relief of flexor spasms and concomitant pain, clonus, muscular rigidity (for patients with reversible spasticity to aid in restoring residual function); treatment of central spasticity (via SynchroMed pump)
- Spinal cord injuries and other spinal cord diseases—may be of some value
- Unlabeled uses: trigeminal neuralgia (tic douloureux); may be beneficial in reducing spasticity in cerebral palsy in children (intrathecal use)

### Contraindications/cautions

- Contraindications: hypersensitivity to baclofen; skeletal muscle spasm resulting from rheumatic disorders.
- Use cautiously with stroke, cerebral palsy, Parkinson's disease, seizure disorders, lactation.

### Dosage

**Available Forms:** Tablets—10, 20 mg; intrathecal—10 mg/20 ml, 10 mg/5 ml

**ADULT**

- ***Oral:*** Individualize dosage; start at low dosage and increase gradually until optimum effect is achieved (usually 40–80 mg/d). The following dosage schedule is suggested: 5 mg PO tid for 3 d; 10 mg tid for 3 d; 15 mg tid for 3 d; 20 mg tid for 3 d. Thereafter, additional increases may be needed, but do not exceed 80 mg/d (20 mg qid); use lowest effective dose. If benefits are not evident after a reasonable trial period, gradually withdraw the drug.
- ***Intrathecal:*** Refer to manufacturer's instructions on pump implantation and intiation of chronic infusion. Testing is usually done with 50 μg/ml injected into intrathecal space over 1 min. Patient is observed for 24 h, then dose of 75 μg/1.5 ml is given; final screening bolus of 100 μg/2 ml is given 24 h later. Patients who do not respond to this dose are not candidates for the implant. Maintenance dose is determined by monitoring patient response and ranges from 12–1,500 μg/d. Smallest dose possible to achieve muscle tone without adverse effects is desired.

**PEDIATRIC:** Safety for use in children < 12 y not established; orphan drug use to decrease spasticity in children with cerebral palsy is being studied.

**GERIATRIC OR RENAL IMPAIRED:** Dosage reduction may be necessary; monitor closely (drug is excreted largely unchanged by the kidneys).

### Pharmacokinetics

| *Route* | *Onset* | *Peak* | *Duration* |
|---|---|---|---|
| Oral | 1 h | 2 h | 4–8 h |
| Intrathecal | 1/2–1 h | 4 h | 4–8 h |

*Metabolism:* $T_{1/2}$: 3–4 h
*Distribution:* Crosses placenta; passes into breast milk
*Excretion:* Urine

**Adverse effects**

- CNS: *Transient drowsiness, dizziness, weakness, fatigue, confusion, headache, insomnia*
- GI: *Nausea, constipation*
- CV: *Hypotension,* palpitations
- GU: *Urinary frequency,* dysuria, enuresis, impotence
- Other: Rash, pruritus, ankle edema, excessive perspiration, weight gain, nasal congestion, increased SGOT, elevated alkaline phosphatase, elevated blood sugar

**Clinically important drug-drug interactions**

- Increased CNS depression with alcohol, other CNS depressants

## ■ Nursing Considerations

### Assessment

- ***History:*** Hypersensitivity to baclofen, skeletal muscle spasm resulting from rheumatic disorders, stroke, cerebral palsy, Parkinson's disease, seizure disorders, lactation
- ***Physical:*** Weight; T; skin color, lesions; orientation, affect, reflexes, bilateral grip strength, visual exam; P, BP; bowel sounds, normal GI output, liver evaluation; normal urinary output; liver and kidney function tests, blood and urine glucose

### Implementation

- Patients given implantable device for intrathecal delivery need to learn about the programmable delivery system, frequent checks; how to adjust dose and programming.
- Give with caution to patients whose spasticity contributes to upright posture or balance in locomotion or whenever spasticity is used to increase function.
- Taper dosage gradually to prevent hallucinations, possible psychosis.

### Drug-specific teaching points

- Take this drug exactly as prescribed. Do not stop taking this drug without consulting the care provider; abrupt discontinuation may cause hallucinations.
- Avoid alcohol, sleep-inducing, or OTC drugs because these could cause dangerous effects.
- The following side effects may occur: drowsiness, dizziness, confusion (avoid driving or engaging in activities that require alertness); nausea (frequent small meals may help); insomnia, headache, painful or frequent urination (effects reversible; will go away when the drug is discontinued).
- Do not take this drug during pregnancy. If you decide to become pregnant or find that you are pregnant, consult your physician.
- Report frequent or painful urination, constipation, nausea, headache, insomnia, confusion that persist or are severe.

# beclomethasone dipropionate

*(be **kloe meth'** a sone)*

Beclodisk (CAN), Becloforte Inhaler (CAN), Beclovent, Beclovent Rotocaps (CAN), Beconase Inhalation, Beconase AQ Nasal Spray, Vancenase Nasal Inhaler, Vancenase AQ Nasal, Vanceril, Vanceril Double Strength

**Pregnancy Category C**

**Drug classes**

Corticosteroid
Glucocorticoid
Hormonal agent

**Therapeutic actions**

Anti-inflammatory effects; local administration into lower respiratory tract or nasal passages maximizes beneficial effects on these tissues while decreasing the likelihood of adverse corticosteroid effects from systemic absorption.

### Indications

- Respiratory inhalant use: Control of bronchial asthma that requires corticosteroids along with other therapy
- Intranasal use: Relief of symptoms of seasonal or perennial rhinitis that respond poorly to other treatments

### Contraindications/cautions

- Respiratory inhalant therapy: Acute asthmatic attack, status asthmaticus, systemic fungal infections (may cause excerbations), allergy to any ingredient, lactation
- Intranasal therapy: Untreated local infections (may cause exacerbations); nasal septal ulcers, recurrent epistaxis, nasal surgery or trauma (interferes with healing); lactation

### Dosage

**Available Forms:** Aerosol—42 μg/actuation; nasal spray—0.042%

***Respiratory inhalant use:*** 50 μg released at the valve delivers 42 μg to the patient.

- *ADULT:* Two inhalations (84 μg) tid or qid. In severe asthma, start with 12 to 16 inhalations per day, and adjust dosage downward. Do not exceed 20 inhalations (840 μg/d).
- *PEDIATRIC (6–12 Y):* 1 or 2 inhalations tid or qid, not to exceed 10 inhalations (420 μg/d). Do not use in children < 6 y.

***Intranasal therapy:*** Each actuation of the inhaler delivers 42 μg. Discontinue therapy after 3 wk in the absence of significant symptomatic improvement.

- *ADULT:* One inhalation (42 μg) in each nostril bid–qid (total dose 168–336 μg/d).
- *PEDIATRIC (> 12 Y):* One inhalation in each nostril bid–qid; not recommended for children < 12 y.

### Pharmacokinetics

| Route | Onset | Peak |
|---|---|---|
| Inhalation | Rapid | 1–2 wk |

*Metabolism:* Lungs, GI, and liver, $T_{1/2}$: 3–15 h

*Distribution:* Crosses placenta; may pass into breast milk

*Excretion:* Feces

### Adverse effects

*Respiratory Inhalant Use*

- **Endocrine:** Cushing's syndrome with overdosage, suppression of hypothalamic-pituitary-adrenal (HPA) function due to systemic absorption
- Local: *Oral, laryngeal, pharyngeal irritation*, fungal infections

*Intranasal Use*

- Respiratory: *Epistaxis, rebound congestion*, perforation of the nasal septum, anosmia
- Local: *Nasal irritation*, fungal infections
- Other: *Headache, nausea*, urticaria

## ■ Nursing Considerations

### Assessment

- *History:* Acute asthmatic attack, status asthmaticus; systemic fungal infections; allergy to any ingredient; lactation; untreated local infections, nasal septal ulcers, recurrent epistaxis, nasal surgery or trauma
- *Physical:* Weight, T; P, BP, auscultation; R, adventitious sounds; chest x-ray before respiratory inhalant therapy; exam of nares before intranasal therapy

### Implementation

- Taper systemic steroids carefully during transfer to inhalational steroids; deaths resulting from adrenal insufficiency have occurred during and after transfer from systemic to aerosol steroids.
- Use decongestant nose drops to facilitate penetration of intranasal steroids if edema, excessive secretions are present.

### Drug-specific teaching points

- This respiratory inhalant has been prescribed to prevent asthmatic attacks, not for use during an attack.
- Allow at least 1 min between puffs (respiratory inhalant); if you also are using an inhalational bronchodilator (isoproterenol,

metaproterenol, epinephrine), use it several minutes before using the steroid aerosol.
- Rinse your mouth after using the respiratory inhalant aerosol.
- Use a decongestant before the intranasal steroid, and clear your nose of all secretions if nasal passages are blocked; intranasal steroids may take several days to produce full benefit.
- Use this product exactly as prescribed; do not take more than prescribed, and do not stop taking the drug without consulting your health care provider. The drug must not be stopped abruptly but must be slowly tapered.
- The following side effects may occur: local irritation (use the device correctly), headache (consult your health care provider for treatment).
- Report sore throat or sore mouth.

## benazepril hydrochloride

*(ben a' za pril)*

Lotensin

**Pregnancy Category C**

### Drug classes
Antihypertensive
Angiotensin-converting enzyme (ACE) inhibitor

### Therapeutic actions
Blocks ACE from converting angiotensin I to angiotensin II, a potent vasoconstrictor, leading to decreased BP, decreased aldosterone secretion, a small increase in serum potassium levels, and sodium and fluid loss; increased prostaglandin synthesis also may be involved in the antihypertensive action.

### Indications
- Treatment of hypertension alone or in combination with thiazide-type diuretics

### Contraindications/cautions
- Contraindications: allergy to benazepril or other ACE inhibitors.
- Use cautiously with impaired renal function, CHF, salt/volume depletion, lactation.

### Dosage
**Available Forms:** Tablets—5, 10, 20, 40 mg

**ADULT:** Initial dose 10 mg PO qd. Maintenance dose: 20–40 mg/day PO: single or two divided doses. Patients using diuretics should discontinue them 2–3 d prior to benazepril therapy. If BP is not controlled, add diuretic slowly. If diuretic cannot be discontinued, begin benazepril therapy with 5 mg.

**PEDIATRIC:** Safety and efficacy not established.

**GERIATRIC AND RENAL IMPAIRED:** Ccr $< 30$ ml/min/1.73 $m^2$ (serum creatinine $> 3$ mg/dl): 5 mg PO qd. Dosage may be titrated upward until blood pressure is controlled up to a maximum of 40 mg/d.

### Pharmacokinetics

| *Route* | *Onset* | *Peak* | *Duration* |
|---|---|---|---|
| Oral | 0.5–1 h | 3–4 h | 24 h |

*Metabolism:* Hepatic, $T_{1/2}$: 10–11 h
*Distribution:* Crosses placenta; passes into breast milk
*Excretion:* Urine

### Adverse effects
- GI: *Nausea*, abdominal pain, vomiting, constipation
- CV: Angina pectoris, hypotension in salt/volume depleted patients, palpitations
- Respiratory: *Cough,* asthma, bronchitis, dyspnea, sinusitis
- Dermatologic: Rash, pruritus, diaphoresis, flushing
- Other: Angioedema, impotence, decreased libido, asthenia, myalgia, arthralgia

### Clinically important drug-drug interactions
• Increased risk of hypersensitivity reactions with allopurinal • Increased coughing with capsaicin • Decreased antihypertensive effects with indomethacin • Increased lithium levels and neurotoxicity may occur

## ■ Nursing Considerations

### Assessment
- *History:* Allergy to benazepril other ACE inhibitors, impaired renal function, CHF, salt/volume depletion, lactation

- *Physical:* Skin color, lesions, turgor; T; P, BP, peripheral perfusion; mucous membranes, bowel sounds, liver evaluation; urinalysis, renal and liver function tests, CBC and differential

### Implementation

- Alert surgeon: Note use of benazepril on patient's chart; the angiotensin II formation subsequent to compensatory renin release during surgery will be blocked; hypotension may be reversed with volume expansion.
- Monitor patient for possible fall in BP secondary to reduction in fluid volume (excessive perspiration and dehydration, vomiting, diarrhea) because excessive hypotension may occur.
- Reduce dosage in patients with impaired renal function.

### Drug-specific teaching points

- Do not stop taking the medication without consulting your physician.
- The following side effects may occur: GI upset, loss of appetite (transient effects, if persistent consult healthcare provider); lightheadedness (transient; change position slowly, and limit activities to those that do not require alertness and precision); dry cough (irritating but not harmful; consult health care provider).
- Be careful in any situation that may lead to a drop in blood pressure (diarrhea, sweating, vomiting, dehydration); if lightheadedness or dizziness occurs, consult your health care provider.
- Report mouth sores; sore throat, fever, chills; swelling of the hands, feet; irregular heartbeat, chest pains; swelling of the face, eyes, lips, tongue, difficulty in breathing, persistent cough.

## bendroflumethiazide

*(ben droe floo me **thye'** a zide)*

Naturetin

**Pregnancy Category C**

### Drug classes

Thiazide diuretic

### Therapeutic actions

Inhibits reabsorption of sodium and chloride in distal renal tubule, increasing the excretion of sodium, chloride, and water by the kidney.

### Indications

- Adjunctive therapy in edema associated with CHF
- Hypertension, as sole therapy or in combination with other antihypertensives
- Unlabeled uses: calcium nephrolithiasis alone or with amiloride or allopurinal to prevent recurrences in hypercalciuric or normal calciuric patients; diabetes insipidus, especially nephrogenic diabetes insipidus

### Contraindications/cautions

- Contraindications: allergy to thiazides, sulfonamides; fluid or electrolyte imbalance; renal disease (risk of azotemia with thiazides); liver disease (thiazide-induced alterations in fluid and electrolyte balance may precipitate hepatic coma); gout (risk of precipitation of attack).
- Use cautiously with SLE; glucose tolerance abnormalities, diabetes mellitus; hyperparathyroidism; manic-depressive disorders aggravated by hypercalcemia; lactation.

### Dosage

**Available Forms:** Tablets—5, 10 mg

ADULT

- *Edema:* 5 mg PO qd, best in the morning. Up to 20 mg once a day or divided into two doses. **Maintenance:** 2.5–5 mg PO qd. Intermittent therapy may be best for some patients; every other day or a 3- to 5-d/wk schedule.
- *Hypertension:* Initial: 5–20 mg/d PO. **Maintenance:** 2.5–15 mg/d PO.

PEDIATRIC: Safety and efficacy not established.

### Pharmacokinetics

| *Route* | *Onset* | *Peak* | *Duration* |
|---|---|---|---|
| Oral | 2 h | 4 h | 6–12 h |

*Metabolism:* $T_{1/2}$: 3–4 h
*Distribution:* Crosses placenta; passes into breast milk
*Excretion:* Unchanged in the urine

**Adverse effects**

- CNS: *Dizziness, vertigo,* paresthesias, weakness, headache, blurred vision
- GI: *Nausea, anorexia, vomiting, dry mouth*, diarrhea, constipation, jaundice, hepatitis, pancreatitis
- CV: Orthostatic hypotension
- GU: Impotence, loss of libido
- **Dermatologic**: Photosensitivity, rash, purpura, exfoliative dermatitis, hives
- **Endocrine**: Hyperglycemia, hyperurecemia, glycosuria
- **Other**: Muscle cramps and muscle spasms, fever, gouty attacks, flushing, weight loss, rhinorrhea

**Clinically important drug-drug interactions**

• Increased thiazide effects with diazoxide • Decreased absorption with cholestyramine, colestipol • Increased risk of cardiac glycoside toxicity if hypokalemia occurs • Increased risk of lithium toxicity • Decreased effectiveness of antidiabetic agents with bendroflumethiazide

**Drug-lab test interferences**

• Decreased PBI levels without clinical signs of thyroid disturbance • Increased creatinine, BUN

## ■ Nursing Considerations

### Assessment

- *History:* Allergy to thiazides, sulfonamides; fluid or electrolyte imbalance, renal or liver disease; gout; SLE; glucose tolerance abnormalities, diabetes mellitus; hyperparathyroidism; manic-depressive disorders; lactation
- *Physical:* Skin color, lesions, edema; orientation, reflexes, muscle strength; pulses, baseline ECG, BP, orthostatic BP, perfusion; R, pattern, adventitious sounds; liver evaluation, bowel sounds; urinary output patterns; CBC, serum electrolytes, blood glucose, liver and renal function tests, serum uric acid, urinalysis

### Implementation

- Give with food or milk for GI upset.
- Mark calendars or use other reminders of drug days if every other day or 3–5 d/wk therapy is best for treating edema.
- Reduce dosage of other antihypertensive drugs by at least 50% if given with thiazides; readjust dosages gradually as BP responds.
- Give early in the day so increased urination will not disturb sleep; monitor weight.

### Drug-specific teaching points

- Record dates on a calendar or dated envelopes for use as intermittent therapy.
- Take the drug early in the day so increased urination will not disturb sleep. Take with food or meals if GI upset occurs.
- Weigh yourself on a regular basis at the same time of the day and in the same clothing, and record the weight on your calendar.
- The following side effects may occur: increased volume and frequency of urination; dizziness, feeling faint on arising, drowsiness (avoid rapid position changes, hazardous activities: driving a car and using alcohol); sensitivity to sunlight (use sunglasses, wear protective clothing, or use a sunscreen); decrease in sexual function; increased thirst (sucking on sugarless lozenges, frequent mouth care may help).
- Report change of more than 3 lb in one day, swelling in your ankles or fingers, unusual bleeding or bruising, dizziness, trembling, numbness, fatigue, muscle weakness or cramps.

# benzalkonium chloride

*(benz al **koe'** nee um)*

BAC, Benza, Zephiran

**Pregnancy Category C**

**Drug classes**

Antibiotic
Antiinfective
Surface active agent

### Therapeutic actions

Exact mechanism is not known; bacteriostatic or bactericidal depending on concentration; may work by enzyme inactivation; known to have deodorant, wetting, detergent, keratolytic, and emulsifying action, possibly also due to enzyme activation.

### Indications

- **Aqueous solutions:** antisepsis of skin, mucous membranes, and wounds; preoperative preparation of skin, surgeon's hands; treatment of wounds; preservation of ophthalmic solutions; irrigations of eye and body cavities, bladder, and urethra; vaginal douching
- **Tinctures and sprays:** preoperative treatment of skin; treatment of minor skin wounds and abrasions

### Contraindications/cautions

- Use in occlusive dressings, casts, anal or vaginal packs (irritation and chemical burns may result)

### Dosage

Available Forms: Concentrate—17%; solution—1:750; disinfectant—17%; tincture—1:750; tincture spray—1:750; tissue—1:750

ADULT AND PEDIATRIC: Recommended dilutions for specific administration sites:

- *Bladder retention lavage:* 1:20,000–1:40,000 aqueous solution
- *Bladder and urethral irrigation:* 1:5,000–1:20,000 aqueous solution
- *Breast/nipple hygiene:* 1:1,000–1:2,000 aqueous solution
- *Catheters and other adsorbent articles:* 1:500 aqueous solution
- *Deep infected wounds:* 1:3,000–1:20,000 aqueous solution
- *Denuded skin and mucous membranes:* 1:5,000–1:10,000 aqueous solution
- *Eye irrigation:* 1:5,000–1:10,000 aqueous solution
- *Hospital disinfections:* 1:750 aqueous solution
- *Minor wounds, lacerations:* 1:750 tincture or spray
- *Oozing and open infections:* 1:2,000–1:5,000 aqueous solution
- *Postepisiotomy care:* 1:5,000–1:10,000 aqueous solution
- *Preoperative disinfection of skin:* 1:750 tincture, spray, or aqueous solution
- *Preservation of ophthalmic solution:* 1:5,000–1:7,500 aqueous solution
- *Surgeon's hands and arms:* 1:750 aqueous solution
- *Vaginal douche/irrigation:* 1:2,000–1:5,000 aqueous solution
- *Wet dressings:* 1:5,000 or less aqueous solution
- *Preoperative prep:* Perform preoperative periorbital skin or head prep only before the patient or eye is anesthesized

### Pharmacokinetics

Not absorbed systemically.

### Adverse effects

- Allergic reactions: hypersensitivity reaction
- Local: Stinging, burning, erythema

### Clinically important drug-drug interactions

- Incompatible in solution with iodine, silver nitrate, fluorescein, nitrates, peroxide, lanolin, potassium permanganate, aluminum, caramel, kaolin, pine oil, zinc sulfate, zinc oxide, yellow oxide of mercury

## ■ Nursing Considerations

### Assessment

- *History:* Hypersensitivity to benzalkonium
- *Physical:* Skin condition

### Implementation

- Use Sterile Water for Injection as a diluent for aqueous solutions intended for deep wounds or irrigation of body cavities; otherwise, freshly distilled water may be used. Tap water contains metallic ions or organic matter that may reduce antibacterial potency.

- Do not use a cork stopper to close BAC solution container; do not store cotton, wool, rayon, or other materials in solution; use sterile gauze sponges to apply solution; dip into solution immediately before application.
- Rinse area thoroughly if soap and anionic detergents have been used; these agents may inactivate BAC.
- Avoid prolonged contact of solution with patient's skin; avoid pooling on operating table.
- Do not use tinted tincture or spray near an open flame or cautery; these contain flammable organic solvents.
- Irrigate eye immediately and repeatedly with water if solution stronger than 1:5,000 enters the eye.
- Further dilute solution if area for application is inflamed or irritated.

### Drug-specific teaching points

- Teaching should be incorporated into that about the procedures being performed.

## benzonatate

*(ben **zoe'** na tate)*

Tessalon Perles

**Pregnancy Category C**

### Drug classes

Antitussive (nonnarcotic)

### Therapeutic actions

Related to the local anesthetic tetracaine; anesthesizes the stretch receptors in the respiratory passages, lungs, and pleura, dampering their activity and reducing the cough reflex at its source.

### Indications

- Symptomatic relief of nonproductive cough

### Contraindications/cautions

- Allergy to benzonatate or related compounds (tetracaine); lactation

### Dosage

**Available Forms:** Capsules—100 mg

*ADULT AND PEDIATRIC (> 10 Y):* 100 mg PO tid; up to 600 mg/d may be used.

### Pharmacokinetics

| *Route* | *Onset* | *Duration* |
|---|---|---|
| Oral | 15–20 min | 3–8 h |

*Metabolism:* Hepatic

*Distribution:* Crosses placenta; may pass into breast milk

*Excretion:* Urine

### Adverse effects

- CNS: *Sedation, headache, mild dizziness*, nasal congestion, sensation of burning in the eyes
- GI: *Constipation, nausea*, GI upset
- **Dermatologic**: Pruritus, skin eruptions
- **Other**: Vague "chilly" feeling, numbness in the chest

### ■ Nursing Considerations

#### Assessment

- ***History:*** Allergy to benzonatate or related compounds (tetracaine); lactation
- ***Physical:*** Nasal mucous membranes; skin color, lesions; orientation, affect; adventitious sounds

#### Implementation

- Administer orally; caution patient not to chew or break capsules but to swallow them whole.

#### Drug-specific teaching points

- Swallow the capsules whole; do not chew or break capsules because numbness of the throat and mouth could occur, and swallowing could become difficult.
- The following side effects may occur: rash, itching (skin care may help); constipation, nausea, GI upset; sedation, dizziness (avoid driving or tasks that require alertness).
- Report restlessness, tremor, difficulty breathing, constipation, rash.

## benzquinamide hydrochloride

*(benz **kwin'** a mide)*

**Pregnancy Category C**

### Drug classes

Antiemetic

### Therapeutic actions
Mechanism in humans is not known; antiemetic, antihistaminic, anticholinergic, and sedative activity seen in animals.

### Indications
- Prevention and treatment of nausea and vomiting associated with anesthesia and surgery. Prophylactic use should be reserved for patients in whom emesis would endanger the surgical outcome or result in harm to the patient.

### Contraindications/cautions
- Hypersensitivity to benzquinamide; CV disease, hypertension, lactation.

### Dosage
**Available Forms:** Injection—50 mg/vial

*ADULT*
- ***IM:*** 50 mg (0.5–1 mg/kg). Repeat in 1 h, then q3–4 hours as necessary. Prophylactic use, give 15 min prior to emergence from anesthesia.
- ***IV:*** 25 mg (0.2–0.4 mg/kg) as a single dose slowly (1 ml/0.5–1 min). All subsequent doses should be IM.

*PEDIATRIC:* Safety and efficacy not established.

*GERIATRIC:* Administer with caution; if given IV, give smaller dose over longer period, and monitor patient carefully.

### Pharmacokinetics

| Route | Onset | Peak | Duration |
|---|---|---|---|
| IM, IV | 15 min | 30 min | 3–4 h |

*Metabolism:* Hepatic, $T_{1/2}$: 40 min
*Distribution:* Crosses placenta
*Excretion:* Urine

### IV facts
**Preparation:** Reconstitute initially with 2.2 ml Sterile Water or Bacteriostatic Water for Injection with benzyl alcohol or with methylparabens and propylparabens. This yields 2 ml of a solution equivalent to 25 mg benzquinamide/ml. Potent for 14 d. Store at room temperature.

**Infusion:** Infuse slowly; 1 ml every 30–60 sec. Do not use IV route with patients with CV disease or on CV drugs.

### Adverse effects
- CNS: *Drowsiness,* dizziness, vertigo, tinnitus, fatigue, restlessness, headache, *dry mouth*, shivering, sweating, hiccoughs, fever, chills
- GI: Nausea, anorexia
- CV: *Hypertension*, hypotension, atrial arrhythmias
- MS: Twitching, shaking, weakness
- Dermatologic: Rash, pruritus, sweating

## ■ Nursing Considerations

### Assessment
- ***History:*** Hypertension, hypotension, CV disease, lactation
- ***Physical:*** Weight, skin condition, neurologic status, orientation,P,BP

### Implementation
- Give drug to prevent postoperative nausea and vomiting 15 min prior to emergence from anesthesia.
- Do not give IV to patients with CV disease; sudden increase or decrease in BP could be dangerous.
- Give with caution to elderly or debilitated patients; use lower range of dose, and monitor closely.

### Drug-specific teaching points
- Dry mouth may occur: use mouth care, sugarless lozenges.
- Report headache, anxiety, lack of relief from nausea.

## benzthiazide

*(benz **thye'** a zide)*

Exna

**Pregnancy Category C**

### Drug classes
Thiazide diuretic

### Therapeutic actions
Inhibits reabsorption of sodium and chloride in distal renal tubule, increasing ex-

cretion of sodium, chloride, and water by the kidney.

**Indications**

- Adjunctive therapy in edema associated with CHF, cirrhosis, corticosteroid and estrogen therapy, renal dysfunction
- Hypertension: alone or with other antihypertensives
- Unlabeled use: diabetes insipidus, especially nephrogenic diabetes insipidus

**Contraindications/cautions**

- Contraindications: allergy to thiazides, sulfonamides; fluid or electrolyte imbalance; renal disease (risk of azotemia with thiazides); liver disease (thiazide-induced alterations in fluid and electrolyte balance may precipitate hepatic coma); gout (risk of attack).
- Use cautiously with SLE; glucose tolerance abnormalities, diabetes mellitus; hyperparathyroidism; manic-depressive disorders aggravated by hypercalcemia; lactation.

**Dosage**

**Available Forms:** Tablets—50 mg

*ADULT*

- *Edema:* Initially 50–200 mg PO qd for several days. Administer dosages > 100 mg/d in two divided doses. **Maintenance:** 50–150 mg qd.
- *Hypertension:* Initially: 50–100 mg PO qd in two doses of 25 or 50 mg each after breakfast and after lunch. **Maintenance:** individualize to patient's response; maximum dose of 200 mg/d.

**Pharmacokinetics**

| *Route* | *Onset* | *Peak* | *Duration* |
|---|---|---|---|
| Oral | 2 h | 4–6 h | 6–18 h |

*Metabolism:* $T_{1/2}$: unknown

*Distribution:* Crosses placenta; passes into breast milk

*Excretion:* Urine

**Adverse effects**

- CNS: *Dizziness, vertigo,* paresthesias, weakness, headache, blurred vision
- GI: *Nausea, anorexia, vomiting, dry mouth,* diarrhea, constipation, jaundice, hepatitis, pancreatitis
- CV: Orthostatic hypotension
- GU: Impotence, loss of libido
- **Dermatologic:** Photosensitivity, rash, purpura, exfoliative dermatitis, hives
- **Endocrine:** Hyperglycemia, hyperuremia, glycosuria
- **Other:** Muscle cramps and muscle spasms, fever, gouty attacks, flushing, weight loss, rhinorrhea

**Clinically important drug-drug interactions**

• Increased thiazide effects if taken with diazoxide • Decreased absorption with cholestyramine, colestipol • Increased risk of cardiac glycoside toxicity if hypokalemia occurs • Increased risk of lithium toxicity • Decreased effectiveness of antidiabetic agents when taken concurrently with bendroflumethiazide

**Drug-lab test interferences**

• Decreased PBI levels without clinical signs of thyroid disturbance • Increased creatinine, BUN

## ■ Nursing Considerations

**Assessment**

- *History:* Allergy to thiazides, sulfonamides; fluid or electrolyte imbalance, renal or liver disease; gout; SLE; glucose tolerance abnormalities, diabetes mellitus; hyperparathyroidism; manic-depressive disorders; lactation
- *Physical:* Skin color, lesions, edema; orientation, reflexes, muscle strength; pulses, baseline ECG, BP, orthostatic BP, perfusion; R, pattern, adventitious sounds; liver evaluation, bowel sounds; urinary output patterns; CBC, serum electrolytes, blood glucose, liver and renal function tests, serum uric acid, urinalysis

**Implementation**

- Administer early in the day so increased urination will not disturb sleep; administer with food or milk if GI upset occurs.

**Drug-specific teaching points**

- Take the drug early in the day so increased urination will not disturb sleep.

May be taken with food or meals if GI upset occurs.

- Weigh yourself on a regular basis, at the same time and in the same clothing, and record the weight on calendar.
- The following side effects may occur: increased volume and frequency of urination; dizziness, feeling faint on arising, drowsiness (avoid rapid position changes; hazardous activities, such as driving and alcohol); sensitivity to sunlight (use sunglasses, wear protective clothing, or use a sunscreen); decrease in sexual function; increased thirst (suck sugarless lozenges, use frequent mouth care).
- Report weight change of more than 3 lb in one day, swelling in ankles or fingers, unusual bleeding or bruising, dizziness, trembling, numbness, fatigue, muscle weakness or cramps.

## benztropine mesylate

***(benz' troe peen)***

Apo-Benztropine (CAN), Cogentin, PMS Benztropine (CAN)

**Pregnancy Category C**

### Drug classes

Antiparkinsonism drug (anticholinergic type)

### Therapeutic actions

Has anticholinergic activity in the CNS that is believed to help normalize the hypothesized imbalance of cholinergic/dopaminergic neurotransmission in the basal ganglia of the brain of a parkinsonism patient. Reduces severity of rigidity and to a lesser extent, akinesia and tremor; less effective overall than levodopa; peripheral anticholinergic effects suppress secondary symptoms of parkinsonism, such as drooling.

### Indications

- Adjunct in the therapy of parkinsonism (postencephalitic, arteriosclerotic, and idiopathic types)
- Control of extrapyramidal disorders (except tardive dyskinesia) due to neuroleptic drugs (phenothiazines)

### Contraindications/cautions

- Contraindications: hypersensitivity to benztropine; glaucoma, especially angle-closure glaucoma; pyloric or duodenal obstruction, stenosing peptic ulcers, achalasia (megaesophagus); prostatic hypertrophy or bladder neck obstructions; myasthenia gravis.
- Use cautiously with tachycardia, cardiac arrhythmias, hypertension, hypotension, hepatic or renal dysfunction, alcoholism, chronic illness, work in hot environments; hot weather; lactation.

### Dosage

**Available Forms:** Tablets—0.5, 1, 2 mg; injection—1 mg/ml

*ADULT*

- *Parkinsonism:* Initially 0.5–1 mg PO hs; a total daily dose of 0.5–6 mg given hs or in two to four divided doses is usual. Increase initial dose in 0.5-mg increments at 5- to 6-d intervals to the smallest amount necessary for optimal relief. Maximum daily dose is 6 mg. May be given IM or IV in same dosage as oral. When used with other drugs, gradually substitute benztropine for all or part of them and gradually reduce dosage of the other drug.
- *Drug-induced extrapyramidal symptoms:* Acute dystonic reactions: Initially 1–2 mg IM (preferred) or IV to control condition; may repeat if parkinsonian effect begins to return. After that, 1–2 mg PO bid to prevent recurrences.
- *Extrapyramidal disorders occurring early in neuroleptic treatment:* 1–2 mg PO bid–tid. Withdraw drug after 1 or 2 wk to determine its continued need; reinstitute if disorder reappears.

*PEDIATRIC:* Safety and efficacy not established.

*GERIATRIC:* Strict dosage regulation may be necessary; patients > 60 y often develop increased sensitivity to the CNS effects of anticholinergic drugs.

### Pharmacokinetics

| Route | Onset | Duration |
|---|---|---|
| Oral | 1 h | 6–10 h |
| IM/IV | 15 min | 6–10 h |

*Metabolism:* Hepatic
*Distribution:* Crosses placenta; passes into breast milk

**IV facts**
**Preparation:** Give undiluted. Store in tightly covered, light-resistant container. Store at room temparature.
**Infusion:** Administer direct IV at a rate of 1 mg over 1 min.

### Adverse effects

*Peripheral Anticholinergic Effects*
- GI: *Dry mouth, constipation,* dilation of the colon, paralytic ileus, *nausea,* vomiting, epigastric distress
- CV: Tachycardia, palpitations, hypotension, orthostatic hypotension
- GU: *Urinary retention, urinary hesitancy,* dysuria, difficulty achieving or maintaining an erection
- EENT: *Blurred vision,* mydriasis, diplopia, increased intraocular tension, angle-closure glaucoma
- Dermatologic: Skin rash, urticaria, other dermatoses
- Other: Flushing, decreased sweating, elevated temperature

*CNS Effects, Some Characteristic of Centrally Acting Anticholinergic Drugs*
- CNS: *Disorientation, confusion,* memory loss, hallucinations, psychoses, agitation, nervousness, delusions, delirium, paranoia, euphoria, excitement, lightheadedness, dizziness, depression, drowsiness, weakness, giddiness, paresthesia, heaviness of the limbs
- Other: Muscular weakness, muscular cramping; inability to move certain muscle groups (high doses), numbness of fingers

### Clinically important drug-drug interactions

• Paralytic ileus, sometimes fatal, when given with other anticholinergic drugs, or drugs that have anticholinergic properties (phenothiazines,TCAs) • Additive adverse CNS effects (toxic psychosis) with other drugs that have CNS anticholinergic properties (TCAs, phenothiazines) • Possible masking of the development of persistent extrapyramidal symptoms, tardive dyskinesia, in patients on long-term therapy with antipsychotic drugs (phenothiazines, haloperidol) • Decreased therapeutic efficacy of antipsychotic drugs (phenothiazines, haloperidol), possibly due to central antagonism

## ■ Nursing Considerations

### Assessment

- ***History:*** Hypersensitivity to benztropine; glaucoma; pyloric or duodenal obstruction, stenosing peptic ulcers, achalasia; prostatic hypertrophy or bladder neck obstructions; myasthenia gravis; cardiac arrhythmias, hypertension, hypotension; hepatic or renal dysfunction; alcoholism, chronic illness, people who work in hot environment; lactation
- ***Physical:*** Weight; T; skin color, lesions; orientation, affect, reflexes, bilateral grip strength, visual exam including tonometry; P, BP, orthostatic BP; adventitious sounds; bowel sounds, normal output, liver evaluation; normal urinary output, voiding pattern, prostate palpation; liver and kidney function tests

### Implementation

- Decrease dosage or discontinue temporarily if dry mouth makes swallowing or speaking difficult.
- Give with caution and reduce dosage in hot weather. Drug interferes with sweating and body's ability to maintain heat equilibrium; provide sugarless lozenges, ice chips to suck for dry mouth.
- Give with meals if GI upset occurs; give before meals for dry mouth; give after meals if drooling or nausea occur.
- Ensure patient voids before receiving each dose if urinary retention is a problem.

### Drug-specific teaching points

- Take this drug exactly as prescribed.
- Avoid alcohol, sedatives, and OTC drugs (could cause dangerous effects).
- The following side effects may occur: drowsiness, dizziness, confusion, blurred vision (avoid driving engaging in activi-

ties that require alertness and visual acuity); nausea (try frequent small meals); dry mouth (suck sugarless lozenges or ice chips); painful or difficult urination (empty bladder immediately before each dose); constipation (maintain adequate fluid intake and exercise regularly); use caution in hot weather (you are susceptible to heat prostration).
- Report difficult or painful urination; constipation; rapid or pounding heartbeat; confusion, eye pain, or rash.

## bepridil hydrochloride

*(be' pri dil)*
Vascor
**Pregnancy Category C**

### Drug classes
Calcium channel-blocker
Antianginal drug

### Therapeutic actions
Inhibits the movement of calcium ions across the membranes of cardiac and arterial muscle cells; inhibition of transmembrane calcium flow results in the depression of impulse formation in specialized cardiac pacemaker cells, slowing of the velocity of conduction of the cardiac impulse, depression of myocardial contractility, and dilation of coronary arteries and arterioles and peripheral arterioles; these effects lead to decreased cardiac work, decreased cardiac energy consumption, and in patients with vasospastic (Prinzmetal's) angina, increased delivery of oxygen to cardiac cells.

### Indications
- Chronic stable angina in those unresponsive to or intolerant of other antianginals; can cause serious arrhythmias and agranulocytosis

### Contraindications/cautions
- Allergy to bepridil, sick sinus syndrome, heart block (second or third degree), hypotension, history of serious ventricular arrhythmias, uncompensated CHF, congenital QT interval prolongation, lactation.

### Dosage
**Available Forms:** Tablets—200, 300, 400 mg

*ADULT:* Individualize dosage. Initially 200 mg/d PO. After 10 d, dosage may be adjusted upward. *Maintenance:* 300 mg/d PO. Maximum daily dose is 400 mg.

*PEDIATRIC:* Safety and efficacy not established.

*GERIATRIC:* Same starting dose as adult dosage; monitor more closely for adverse effects.

### Pharmacokinetics

| Route | Onset | Peak |
|---|---|---|
| Oral | 60 min | 2–3 h |

*Metabolism:* Hepatic, $T_{1/2}$: 24 h
*Distribution:* Crosses placenta; passes into breast milk
*Excretion:* Urine

### Adverse effects
- CNS: *Dizziness, lightheadedness, nervousness, headache, asthenia,* fatigue
- GI: *Nausea*, hepatic injury, *constipation*
- CV: *Peripheral edema*, hypotension, arrhythmias, *bradycardia, AV block,* ***ventricular tachycardia, asystole***
- Hematologic: **Agranulocytosis**
- Dermatologic: *Rash*

### Clinically important drug-drug interactions
- Cumulative negative chronotropic effects and decreased heart rate with digoxin

## ■ Nursing Considerations

### Assessment
- *History:* Allergy to bepridil, sick sinus syndrome, heart block, hypotension, history of serious ventricular arrhythmias, uncompensated CHF, congenital QT interval prolongation, lactation
- *Physical:* Skin lesions, color, edema; P, BP, baseline ECG, peripheral perfusion, auscultation, R, adventitious sounds; liver

evaluation, GI normal output; liver and renal function tests, CBC

### Implementation

- Give only if unresponsive to or intolerant of other antianginal drugs.
- Monitor patient carefully (BP, cardiac rhythm, and output) during titration to therapeutic dose; dosage may be increased more rapidly in hospital under close supervision.
- Monitor BP carefully if patient is also on nitrates.
- Monitor cardiac rhythm and CBC regularly during stabilization of dosage and periodically during long-term therapy.

### Drug-specific teaching points

- Take this drug exactly as prescribed.
- The following side effects may occur: nausea, vomiting (small, frequent meals may help); headache (adjust lighting, noise, and temperature; medication may be ordered if this becomes severe); dizziness, shakiness (avoid driving or operating dangerous machinery).
- Report irregular heart beat, shortness of breath, swelling of the hands or feet, pronounced dizziness, constipation, unusual bleeding or bruising.

## beractant

*(ber ak' tant)*

DDPC, natural lung surfactant

Survanta

### Drug classes

Lung surfactant

### Therapeutic actions

A natural bovine compound containing lipids and apoproteins that reduce surface tension and allow expansion of the alveoli; replaces the surfactant missing in the lungs of neonates suffering from respiratory distress syndrome (RDS).

### Indications

- Prophylactic treatment of infants at risk of developing RDS; infants with birth weights < 1,350 g or infants with birth weights > 1,350 gm who have evidence of pulmonary immaturity
- Rescue treatment of infants who have developed RDS

### Contraindications/cautions

- Because beractant is used as an emergency drug in acute respiratory situations, the benefits usually outweigh any possible risks.

### Dosage

**Available Forms:** Suspension—25 mg suspended in 0.9% sodium chloride injection

Accurate determination of birth weight is essential for correct dosage. Beractant is instilled into the trachea using a catheter inserted into the endotracheal tube.

***Prophylactic treatment:*** Give first dose of 100 mg phospholipids/kg birth weight (4 ml/kg) soon after birth. Four doses can be administered in the first 48 h of life. Give no more frequently than q6h.

***Rescue treatment:*** Administer 100 mg phospholipids/kg birth weight (4 ml/kg) intratracheally. Administer the first dose as soon as possible after the diagnosis of RDS is made and patient is on the ventilator. Repeat doses can be given based on clinical improvement and blood gases. Administer subsequent doses no sooner than q6h.

### Pharmacokinetics

| *Route* | *Onset* | *Peak* |
|---|---|---|
| Intratracheal | Immediate | Hrs |

*Metabolism:* Normal surfactant metabolic pathways, $T_{1/2}$: unknown

*Distribution:* Lung tissue

### Adverse effects

- CNS: Seizures
- CV: *Patent ductus arteriosus,* ***intraventricular hemorrhage, hypotension, bradycardia***
- Respiratory: **Pneumothorax,** ***pulmonary air leak,*** **pulmonary hemorrhage (more often seen with infants > 700 g),** apnea, pneumomediastinum, emphysema

- **Hematologic:** *Hyperbilirubinemia, thrombocytopenia*
- **Other:** *Sepsis, nonpulmonary infections*

## ■ Nursing Considerations

### Assessment

- ***History:*** Time of birth, exact birth weight
- ***Physical:*** Skin temperature, color; R, adventitious sounds, oximeter, endotracheal tube position and patency, chest movement; ECG, P, BP, peripheral perfusion, arterial pressure (desirable); oxygen saturation, blood gases, CBC; muscular activity, facial expression, reflexes

### Implementation

- Monitor ECG and transcutaneous oxygen saturation continually during administration.
- Ensure that endotracheal tube is in the correct position, with bilateral chest movement and lung sounds.
- Have staff view manufacturer's teaching video before regular use to cover all the technical aspects of administration.
- Suction the infant immediately before administration, but do not suction for 2 h after administration unless clinically necessary.
- Check vial of off-white to brown liquid for settling; gentle mixing should be attempted. Warm to room temperature before using—20 min or 8 min by hand. Do not use other warming methods.
- Store drug in refrigerator. Protect from light. Enter drug vial only once. Discard remaining drug after use.
- Insert 5 French catheter into the endotracheal tube; do not instill into the mainstream bronchus.
- Instill dose slowly; inject one-fourth dose over 2–3 sec; remove catheter and reattach infant to ventilator for at least 30 sec or until stable; repeat procedure administering one-fourth dose at a time.
- Do not suction infant for 1 h after completion of full dose; do not flush catheter.
- Continually monitor patient's color, lung sounds, ECG, oximeter, and blood gas readings during administration and for at least 30 min after.

### Drug-specific teaching points

- Details of drug effects and administration are best incorporated into parents' comprehensive teaching program.

# betaine anhydrous

***beh' tayne)***
Cystadane
**Pregnancy Category C**

### Drug classes
Homocysteine reducer

### Therapeutic actions
Methyl group donor in the remethylation of homocysteine to methionine in patients with homocystinuria; reduces the toxic blood levels of homocysteine that can lead to cardiovascular thrombosis, osteoporosis, skeletal abnormalities and optic lens dislocation.

### Indications
- Treatment of homocystinuria to decrease elevated homocysteine levels

### Contraindications/cautions
- Use cautiously with pregnancy, lactation.

### Dosage
**Available Forms:** Powder—1 g/1.7 ml

*ADULT AND PEDIATRIC:* 6 g/d PO in divided doses of 3 g bid. Up to 20 g/d may be required to decrease homocysteine levels.

### Pharmacokinetics

| *Route* | *Onset* | *Duration* |
|---|---|---|
| Oral | Days | Wks |

*Metabolism:* Hepatic metabolism; $T_{1/2}$: weeks
*Distribution:* Crosses placenta; may pass into breast milk
*Excretion:* Urine

### Adverse effects
- CNS: Psychological changes
- GI: Nausea, GI distress, nausea, diarrhea

• **Other:** Body odor changes, powder aspiration

## ■ Nursing Considerations

### Assessment

• *History:* Pregnancy, lactation
• *Physical:* GI evaluation; homocysteine levels

### Implementation

• Obtain baseline homocysteine levels and then regular levels during treatment.
• Shake bottle lightly before removing cap; measure with scoop provided (one level scoop equals 1 g of betaine); dissolve powder in 4–6 oz water for immediate use; store powder at room temperature.

### Drug-specific teaching points

• Shake bottle lightly before removing cap; measure with scoop provided (one level scoop equals 1 g of betaine); dissolve powder in 4–6 oz water for immediate use; store powder at room temperature.
• Regular blood tests required to monitor homocysteine levels.
• The following side effects may occur: nausea, diarrhea, GI distress (taking the drug with meals may help).
• Report chest pain, difficulty breathing, visual changes, severe GI upset.

# Betamethasone

## betamethasone

*(bay ta **meth'** a sone)*

*Oral:* Celestone

## betamethasone benzoate

*Topical dermatologic ointment, cream, lotion, gel:* Bepen (CAN), Uticort

## betamethasone dipropionate

*Topical dermatologic ointment, cream, lotion, aerosol:* Alphatrex, Diprolene, Diprosone, Maxivate, Occlucort (CAN), Rhoprosone (CAN), Taro-Sone (CAN)

## betamethasone sodium phosphate

*Systemic, including IV and local injection:* Betnesol (CAN), Celestone phosphate, Ced-U-Jec

## betamethasone sodium phosphate and acetate

*Systemic, IM, and local intra-articular, intralesional, intradermal injection:* Celestone Soluspan

## betamethasone valerate

*Topical dermatologic ointment, cream, lotion:* Betacort (CAN), Betaderm (CAN), Betatrex, Beta-Val, Betnovate (CAN), Celestoderm (CAN), Prevex B (CAN), Rholosone (CAN), Valisone

**Pregnancy Category C**

### Drug classes

Corticosteroid (long acting)
Glucocorticoid
Hormonal agent

### Therapeutic actions

Binds to intracellular corticosteroid receptors, thereby initiating many natural complex reactions that are responsible for its anti-inflammatory and immunosuppressive effects.

### Indications

- **Systemic administration:** Hypercalcemia associated with cancer
- Short-term management of inflammatory and allergic disorders, such as rheumatoid arthritis, collagen diseases (SLE), dermatologic diseases (pemphigus), status asthmaticus, and autoimmune disorders
- Hematologic disorders: thrombocytopenia purpura, erythroblastopenia
- Ulcerative colitis, acute exacerbations of mutiple sclerosis, and palliation in some leukemias and lymphomas
- Trichinosis with neurologic or myocardial involvement
- Unlabeled use: Prevention of respiratory distress syndrome in premature neonates
- **Intra-articular or soft-tissue administration:** Arthritis, psoriatic plaques, and so forth
- **Dermatologic preparations:** Relief of inflammatory and pruritic manifestations of steroid-responsive dermatoses.

### Contraindications/cautions

- Systemic (oral and parenteral) administration: Contraindications: infections, especially tuberculosis, fungal infections, amebiasis, vaccinia and varicella, and antibiotic-resistant infections, lactation.
- Use cautiously with kidney or liver disease, hypothyroidism, ulcerative colitis with impending perforation, diverticulitis, active or latent peptic ulcer, inflammatory bowel disease, CHF, hypertension, thromboembolic disorders, osteoporosis, convulsive disorders, diabetes mellitus.

### Dosage

**Available Forms:** Tablets—0.6 mg; syrup—0.6 mg/5 ml; injection—4 mg, 3 mg betamethasone sodium phosphate with 3 mg betamethasone acetate; ointment—0.1%; cream—0.01%, 0.1%; lotion—0.1%

**ADULT**

- *Systemic administration:* Individualize dosage, based on severity and response. Give daily dose before 9 AM to minimize adrenal suppression. Reduce initial dose in small increments until the lowest dose that maintains satisfactory clinical response is reached. If long-term therapy is needed, alternate-day therapy with a short-acting corticosteroid should be considered. After long-term therapy, withdraw drug slowly to prevent adrenal insufficiency.
  - ***Oral (betamethasone):*** Initial dosage 0.6–7.2 mg/d
  - ***IV (betamethasone sodium phosphate):*** Initial dosage up to 9 mg/d.
  - ***IM (betamethasone sodium phosphate; betamethasone sodium phosphate and acetate):*** Initial dosage 0.5–9.0 mg/d. Dosage range: 1/3—1/2 oral dose given q12h. In life-threatening situations, dose can be in multiples of the oral dose.
  - ***Intabursal, intra-articular, intradermal, intralesional (betamethasone sodium phosphate and acetate):*** 0.25–2.0 ml intra-articular, depending on joint size; 0.2 ml/$cm^3$ intradermally, not to exceed 1 ml/wk; 0.25–1.0 ml at 3- to 7-d intervals for disorders of the foot.
  - ***Topical dermatologic cream, ointment (betamethasone dipropionate):*** Apply sparingly to affected area bid–qid.

**PEDIATRIC:** Individualize dosage on the basis of severity and response rather than by formulae that correct adult doses for age or weight. Carefully observe growth and development in infants and children on prolonged therapy.

### Pharmacokinetics

| *Route* | *Onset* | *Duration* |
|---|---|---|
| Systemic | Varies | 3 d |

*Metabolism:* Hepatic, $T_{1/2}$: 36–54 h

*Distribution:* Crosses placenta; passes into breast milk

*Excretion:* Unchanged in the urine

### IV facts

**Preparation:** No further preparation needed.

**Infusion:** Infuse by direct IV injection over 1 min or into the tubing of running IV of dextrose or saline solutions.

### Adverse effects

- CNS: *Vertigo, headache*, paresthesias, insomnia, convulsions, psychosis, cataracts, increased intraocular pressure, glaucoma (long-term therapy)
- GI: Peptic or esophageal ulcer, pancreatitis, abdominal distention, nausea, vomiting, *increased appetite, weight gain (long-term therapy)*
- CV: Hypotension, shock, hypertension, and CHF secondary to fluid retention, thromboembolism, thrombophlebitis, fat embolism, cardiac arrhythmias
- MS: Muscle weakness, steroid myopathy, loss of muscle mass, osteoporosis, spontaneous fractures (long-term therapy)
- **Endocrine**: Amenorrhea, irregular menses, growth retardation, decreased carbohydrate tolerance, diabetes mellitus, cushingoid state (long-term effect), increased blood sugar, increased serum cholesterol, decreased $T_3$ and $T_4$ levels, hypothalamic-pituitary-adrenal (HPA) suppression with systemic therapy longer than 5 d
- **Electrolyte imbalance**: *$Na^+$ and fluid retention*, hypokalemia, hypocalcemia
- **Other**: *Immunosuppression, aggravation, or masking of infections; impaired wound healing*; thin, fragile skin; petechiae, ecchymoses, purpura, striae; subcutaneous fat atrophy; hypersensitivity or anaphylactoid reactions

The following effects are related to various local routes of steroid administration:

- **Intra-articular**: Osteonecrosis, tendon rupture, infection
- **Intralesional therapy**: Blindness, face and head
- **Topical dermatologic ointments, creams, sprays**: *Local burning, irritation*, acneiform lesions, striae, skin atrophy

### Clinically important drug-drug interactions

• Risk of severe deterioration of muscle strength in myasthenia gravis patients receiving ambenonium, edrophonium, neostigmine, pyridostigmine • Decreased steroid blood levels with barbiturates, phenytoin, rifampin • Decreased effectiveness of salicylates with betamethasone

### Drug-lab test interferences

• False-negative nitroblue-tetrazolium test for bacterial infection • Suppression of skin test reactions.

## ■ Nursing Considerations

### Assessment

- ***History (Systemic administration):*** Infections, fungal infectons, amebiasis, vaccinia and varicella, and antibiotic-resistant infections; kidney or liver disease; hypothyroidism; ulcerative colitis with impending perforation; diverticulitis; active or latent peptic ulcer; inflammatory bowel disease; CHF; hypertension; thromboembolic disorders; osteoporosis; convulsive disorders; diabetes mellitus; lactation
- ***Physical:*** Baseline weight, T, reflexes and grip strength, affect and orientation, P, BP, peripheral perfusion, peripheral perfusion, prominence of superficial veins, R and adventitious sounds, serum electrolytes, blood glucose

### Implementation

*Systemic Use*

- Give daily dose before 9 AM to mimic normal peak corticosteroid blood levels.
- Increase dosage when patient is subject to stress.
- Taper doses when discontinuing high-dose or long-term therapy.
- Do not give live virus vaccines with immunosuppressive doses of corticosteroids.

*Topical Dermatologic Preparations*

- Examine area for infections, skin integrity before application.
- Administer cautiously to pregnant patients; topical corticosteroids have caused teratogenic effects and can be absorbed from systemic site.
- Use caution when occlusive dressings, tight diapers cover affected area; these can increase systemic absorption of the drug.

- Avoid prolonged use near eyes, in genital and rectal areas, and in skin creases.

## Drug-specific teaching points

*Systemic Use*

- Do not to stop taking the drug (oral) without consulting health care provider.
- Take single-dose or alternate day doses before 9 AM.
- Avoid exposure to infections; ability to fight infections is reduced.
- Wear a medical alert tag so emergency care providers will know that you are on this medication.
- The following side effects may occur: increase in appetite, weight gain (counting calories may help); heartburn, indigestion (try small, frequent meals, antacids); poor wound healing (consult with your care provider); muscle weakness, fatigue (frequent rest periods will help).
- Report unusual weight gain, swelling of the extremities, muscle weakness, black or tarry stools, fever, prolonged sore throat, colds or other infections, worsening of original disorder.

***Intrabursal, Intra-articular Therapy***

- Do not overuse joint after therapy, even if pain is gone.

*Topical Dermatologic Preparations*

- Apply sparingly; do not cover with tight dressings.
- Avoid contact with the eyes.
- Report irritation or infection at the site of application.

# betaxolol hydrochloride

(be ***tax'*** oh lol)

Ophthalmic: Betoptic, Betoptic S

Oral: Kerlone

**Pregnancy Category C**

## Drug classes

Beta-adrenergic blocking agent ($\beta_1$ selective)
Antihypertensive
Antiglaucoma agent

## Therapeutic actions

Blocks beta-adrenergic receptors of the sympathetic nervous system in the heart and juxtaglomerular apparatus (kidney), decreasing the excitability of the heart, decreasing cardiac output and oxygen consumption, decreasing the release of renin from the kidney, and lowering blood pressure.
Decreases intraocular pressure by decreasing the secretion of aqueous humor.

## Indications

- Hypertension, used alone or with other antihypertensive agents, particularly thiazide-type diuretics (oral)
- Treatment of ocular hypertension and open-angle glaucoma (ophthalmic)

## Contraindications/cautions

- Contraindications: sinus bradycardia, second or third-degree heart block, cardiogenic shock, CHF.
- Use cautiously with renal failure, diabetes or thyrotoxicosis (betaxolol masks the cardiac signs of hypoglycemia and thyrotoxicosis), lactation.

## Dosage

**Available Forms:** Tablets—10, 20 mg; ophthalmic solution—5.6 mg/ml; ophthalmic suspension—2.8 mg/ml

ADULT

- ***Oral:*** Initially 10 mg PO qd, alone or added to diuretic therapy. Full antihypertensive effect is usually seen in 7–14 d. If desired response if not achieved, dose may be doubled.
- ***Ophthalmic:*** One drop bid to affected eye(s).

PEDIATRIC: Safety and efficacy not established.

GERIATRIC:

- ***Oral:*** Consider reducing initial dose to 5 mg PO qd.

## Pharmacokinetics

| Route | Onset | Peak | Duration |
|---|---|---|---|
| Oral | 30–60 min | 2 h | 12–15 h |

*Metabolism:* Hepatic; $T_{1/2}$: 14–22 h
*Distribution:* Crosses placenta; passes into breast milk
*Excretion:* Urine

### Adverse effects

- CNS: Dizziness, vertigo, tinnitus, fatigue, emotional depression, paresthesias, sleep disturbances, hallucinations, disorientation, memory loss, slurred speech
- GI: *Gastric pain, flatulence, constipation, diarrhea, nausea, vomiting,* anorexia, ischemic colitis, renal and mesenteric arterial thrombosis, retroperitoneal fibrosis, hepatomegaly, acute pancreatitis
- CV: *Bradycardia, CHF, cardiac arrhythmias, sinoartial or AV nodal block, tachycardia,* peripheral vascular insufficiency, claudication, CVA, pulmonary edema, hypotension
- **Respiratory**: Bronchospasm, dyspnea, cough, bronchial obstruction, nasal stuffiness, rhinitis, pharyngitis (less likely than with propranolol)
- GU: *Impotence, decreased libido*, Peyronie's disease, dysuria, nocturia, frequent urination
- **MS**: Joint pain, arthralgia, muscle cramp
- **EENT**: Eye irritation, dry eyes, conjunctivitis, blurred vision
- **Dermatologic**: Rash, pruritus, sweating, dry skin
- **Allergic reactions**: Pharyngitis, erythematous rash, fever, sore throat, laryngospasm, respiratory distress
- **Other**: *Decreased exercise tolerance, development of antinuclear antibodies (ANA)*, hyperglycemia or hypoglycemia, elevated serum transaminase, alkaline phosphatase, and LDH

*Specifically Documented for Betaxolol Ophthalmic Solution*

- CNS: Insomnia, depressive neurosis
- **Local**: *Brief ocular discomfort, occasional tearing, itching, decreased corneal sensitivity*, corneal staining, keratitis, photophobia

### Clinically important drug-drug interactions

• Increased effects with verapamil, anticholinergics • Increased risk of postural hypotension with prazosin • Possible increased antihypertensive effects with aspirin, bismuth subsalicylate, magnesium salicylate, sulfinpyrazone, oral contraceptives • Decreased antihypertensive effects with NSAIDs • Possible increased hypoglycemic effect of insulin with betaxolol

### Drug-lab test interferences

• Possible false results with glucose or insulin tolerance tests

## ■ Nursing Considerations

### Assessment

- *History:* Sinus bradycardia, second or third-degree heart block, cardiogenic shock, CHF, renal failure, diabetes or thyrotoxicosis, lactation
- *Physical:* Baseline weight, skin condition, neurologic status, P, BP, ECG, R, kidney and thyroid function tests, blood and urine glucose

### Implementation

- Do not discontinue drug abruptly after chronic therapy (hypersensitivity to catecholamines may develop, exacerbating angina, MI, and ventricular dysrhythmias). Taper drug gradually over 2 wk with monitoring.
- Consult with physician about withdrawing drug if patient is to undergo surgery (withdrawal is controversial).
- Protect eye from injury if corneal sensitivity is lost (ophthalmic).

### Drug-specific teaching points

- Administer eye drops to minimize systemic absorption of the drug.
- Do not stop taking unless told to do so by a health care provider.
- Avoid driving or dangerous activities if dizziness, weakness occur.
- The following side effects may occur: dizziness, lightheadedness, loss of appetite, nightmares, depression, sexual impotence.
- Report difficulty breathing, night cough, swelling of extremities, slow pulse, confusion, depression, rash, fever, sore throat, eye pain or irritation (ophthalmic).

# bethanechol chloride

*(be than' e kole)*

Duvoid, Myotonachol, PMS-Bethanechol Chloride (CAN), Urecholine

**Pregnancy Category C**

## Drug classes
Parasympathomimetic drug

## Therapeutic actions
Acts at cholinergic receptors in the urinary bladder (and GI tract) to mimic the effects of acetylcholine and parasympathetic stimulation; increases the tone of the detrusor muscle and causes the emptying of the urinary bladder; not destroyed by the enzyme acetylcholinesterase, so effects are more prolonged than those of acetylcholine.

## Indications
- Acute postoperative and postpartum nonobstructive urinary retention and neurogenic atony of the urinary bladder with retention
- Unlabeled use: reflux esophagitis, gastroesophageal reflux

## Contraindications/cautions
- Contraindication: unusual sensitivity to bethanechol, hyperthyroidism, peptic ulcer, latent or active asthma, bradycardia, vasomotor instability, coronary artery disease, epilepsy, parkinsonism, hypotension, obstructive uropathies or intestinal obstruction, recent surgery on GI tract or bladder.
- Use caution when lactating.

## Dosage
**Available Forms:** Tablets—5, 10, 25, 50 mg; injection—5 mg/ml

Determine and use the minimum effective dose; larger doses may increase side effects.

ADULT
- ***Oral:*** 10–50 mg bid–qid. Initial dose of 5–10 mg with gradual increases hourly until desired effect is seen; do not exceed single dose of 50 mg. Alternatively, give 10 mg initially, then 25 and 50 mg at 6-h intervals.
- ***SC:*** 2.5–5 mg initially; repeat dose at 15- to 30-min intervals up to a maximum of 4 doses unless adverse effects intervene. Minimum effective dose may be repeated tid–qid.

PEDIATRIC: Safety and efficacy not established for children < 8 y.

## Pharmacokinetics

| Route | Onset | Peak | Duration |
|---|---|---|---|
| Oral | 30–90 min | 60–90 min | 1–6 h |
| SC | 5–15 min | 15–30 min | 1–3 h |

*Metabolism:* Unknown

*Distribution:* Crosses placenta; may pass into breast milk

## Adverse effects
- GI: *Abdominal discomfort, salivation, nausea, vomiting,* involuntary defecation, abdominal cramps, diarrhea, belching
- CV: **Transient heart block, transient cardiac arrest**, dyspnea, orthostatic hypotension (with large doses)
- GU: Urinary urgency
- Other: Malaise, headache, *sweating, flushing*

## Clinically important drug-drug interactions
- Increased cholinergic effects with other cholinergic drugs, cholinesterase inhibitors
- Critical fall in BP may occur if taken with ganglionic blockers

## ■ Nursing Considerations

### Assessment
- *History:* Unusual sensitivity to bethanechol, hyperthyroidism, peptic ulcer, latent or active asthma, bradycardia, vasomotor instability, CAD, epilepsy, parkinsonism, hypotension, obstructive uropathies or intestinal obstruction, recent surgery on GI tract or bladder, lactation
- *Physical:* Skin color, lesions; T; P, rhythm, BP; bowel sounds, urinary bladder palpation; bladder tone evaluation, urinalysis

### Implementation
- Administer on an empty stomach to avoid nausea and vomiting

- Do not administer IM or IV, serious reactions may occur; administer parenteral preparations by SC route only.
- Monitor response to establish minimum effective dose.
- Have atropine on standby to reverse overdosage or severe response.
- Monitor bowel function, especially in elderly patients who may become impacted or develop serious intestinal problems.

### Drug-specific teaching points

- Take this drug on an empty stomach to avoid nausea and vomiting.
- Dizziness, lightheadedness, fainting may occur when getting up from sitting or lying position.
- The following side effects may occur: increased salivation, sweating, flushing, abdominal discomfort.
- Report diarrhea, headache, belching, substernal pressure or pain, dizziness.

## bicalutamide

*(bye cal* ***loo'*** *ta mide)*

Casodex

**Pregnancy Category X**

### Drug classes

Antiandrogen

### Therapeutic actions

A nonsteroidal agent, exerts potent antiandrogenic activity by inhibiting androgen uptake or by inhibiting cytosol binding of androgen in target tissues.

### Indications

- Treatment of advanced prostatic carcinoma in combination with LHRH analogue

### Contraindications/cautions

- Contraindications: hypersensitivity to bicalutamide or any component of the preparation; pregnancy; lactation.
- Use cautiously with moderate to severe hepatic impairment.

### Dosage

**Available Forms:** Tablets—50 mg

*ADULT:* 50 mg PO qd at the same time each day.

*PEDIATRIC:* Safety and efficacy not established.

### Pharmacokinetics

| *Route* | *Onset* | *Peak* | *Duration* |
|---|---|---|---|
| Oral | slow | 31.3 hours | days |

*Metabolism:* Hepatic; $T_{1/2}$: 5.8 days

*Distribution:* Crosses placenta; passes into breast milk

*Excretion:* Urine

### Adverse effects

- CNS: drowsiness, confusion, depression, anxiety, nervousness
- **GI:** *nausea, vomiting, diarrhea, GI disturbances*, jaundice, hepatitis, hepatic necrosis
- **GU:** *impotence, loss of libido*
- **Endocrine:** *gynecomastia and breast pain, hot flashes*
- **Hematologic:** *anemia, leukopenia*, thrombocytopenia, elevated AST, ALT
- **Dermatologic:** *rash*, photosensitivity
- **Other:** carcinogenesis, mutagenesis

## ■ Nursing Considerations

### Assessment

- *History:* Hypersensitivity to bicalutamide or any component of the preparation; pregnancy; lactation, hepatic impairment
- *Physical:* Skin color, lesions; reflexes, affect; urinary output; bowel sounds, liver evaluation; CBC, Hct, electrolytes, liver function tests

### Implementation

- Administer bicalutamide concomitantly with an LHRH analogue.
- Arrange for periodic monitoring of liver function tests and Prostate Specific Antigen levels regularly during therapy.
- Provide small, frequent meals if GI upset occurs; monitor nutritional status and arrange for appropriate consults if necessary.
- Offer support and encouragement to deal with diagnosis, change in self-concept and alteration in sexual functioning.

**Drug-specific teaching points**

- Take this drug concomitantly with other drugs to treat your problem. Do not interrupt dosing or stop taking these medications without consulting your health care provider.
- Arrange for periodic blood tests to monitor drug effects. It is important that you keep appointments for these tests.
- The following side effects may occur: dizziness, drowsiness (avoid driving or performing hazardous tasks); nausea, vomiting, diarrhea (proper nutrition is important, consult with your dietitian to maintain nutrition); impotence, loss of libido.
- Report: change in stool or urine color, yellow skin, difficulty breathing, malaise.

# Biperiden

## biperiden hydrochloride (oral)

*(bye **per'** i den)*

## biperiden lactate (injection)

Akineton

**Pregnancy Category C**

### Drug classes

Antiparkinsonism drug (anticholinergic type)

### Therapeutic actions

Anticholinergic activity in the CNS that is believed to help normalize the hypothesized imbalance of cholinergic/dopaminergic neurotransmission in the basal ganglia in the brain of a parkinsonism patient. Reduces severity of rigidity, and to a lesser extent akinesia and tremor characterizing parkinsonism; less effective overall than levodopa; peripheral anticholinergic effects suppress secondary symptoms of parkinsonism, such as drooling.

### Indications

- Adjunct in the therapy of parkinsonism (postencephalitic, arteriosclerotic, and idiopathic types)
- Relief of symptoms of extrapyramidal disorders that accompany phenothiazine and reserpine therapy

### Contraindications/cautions

- Contraindications: hypersensitivity to benztropine; glaucoma, especially angle-closure glaucoma; pyloric or duodenal obstruction, stenosing peptic ulcers, achalasia (megaesophagus); prostatic hypertrophy or bladder neck obstructions; myasthenia gravis.
- Use cautiously with tachycardia, cardiac arrhythmias, hypertension, hypotension, hepatic or renal dysfunction, alcoholism, chronic illness, people who work in hot environment; hot weather; lactation.

### Dosage

**Available Forms:** Tablets—2 mg; injection— 5 mg/ml

**ADULT**

- *Parkinsonism:* 2 mg PO tid–qid; individualize dosage with a maximum dose of 16 mg/d.
- ***Drug-induced extrapyramidal disorders***

– ***Oral:*** 2 mg PO qid–tid.

– ***Parenteral:*** 2 mg IM or IV; repeat q1/2h until symptoms are resolved, do not give more than 4 consecutive doses per 24 h.

**PEDIATRIC:** Safety and efficacy not established.

**GERIATRIC:** Strict dosage regulation may be necessary; patients > 60 y often develop increased sensitivity to the CNS effects of anticholinergic drugs.

### Pharmacokinetics

| Route | Onset | Peak |
|---|---|---|
| Oral | 1 h | 1–1.5 h |
| IM | 15 min | Unknown |

*Metabolism:* Hepatic, $T_{1/2}$: 18.4–24.3 h

*Distribution:* Crosses placenta; passes into breast milk

### IV facts

**Preparation:** Give undiluted. Store in tightly covered, light-resistant container. Store at room temparature.

**Infusion:** Administer direct IV at a rate of 1 mg over 1 min; do not give more than four consecutive doses per 24 h.

### Adverse effects

- CNS: Some are characteristic of centrally acting anticholinergic drugs: *disorientation, confusion*, memory loss, hallucinations, psychoses, agitation, *nervousness,* delusions, delirium, paranoia, euphoria, excitement, *lightheadedness, dizziness*, depression, drowsiness, weakness, giddiness, paresthesia, heaviness of the limbs

*Peripheral Anticholinergic Effects*

- GI: *Dry mouth, constipation,* dilation of the colon, paralytic ileus, acute suppurative parotitis, nausea, vomiting, epigastric distress
- CV: Tachycardia, palpitations, hypotension, orthostatic hypotension
- GU: *Urinary retention, urinary hesitancy*, dysuria, difficulty achieving or maintaining an erection
- EENT: *Blurred vision, mydriasis,* diplopia, increased intraocular tension, angle-closure glaucoma
- **Dermatologic**: Skin rash, urticaria, other dermatoses
- **Other**: *Flushing, decreased sweating*, elevated temperature, muscular weakness, muscular cramping

### Clinically important drug-drug interactions

• Paralytic ileus, sometimes fatal, with other anticholinergic drugs, with drugs that have anticholinergic properties (phenothiazines, tricyclic antidepressants) • Additive adverse CNS effects (toxic psychosis) with drugs that have CNS anticholinergic properties (TCAs, phenothiazines) • Possible masking of extrapyramidal symptoms, tardive dyskinesia, in long-term therapy with antipsychotic drugs (phenothiazines, haloperidol) • Decreased therapeutic efficacy of antipsychotic drugs (phenothiazines, haloperidol), possibly due to central antagonism

## ■ Nursing Considerations

### Assessment

- *History:* Hypersensitivity to benztropine; glaucoma; pyloric or duodenal obstruction, stenosing peptic ulcers, achalasia; prostatic hypertrophy or bladder neck obstructions; myasthenia gravis; cardiac arrhythmias, hypertension, hypotension; hepatic or renal dysfunction; alcoholism, chronic illness, work in hot environment; lactation
- *Physical:* Body weight; T; skin color, lesions; orientation, affect, reflexes, bilateral grip strength, visual exam, including tonometry; P, BP, orthostatic BP; adventitious sounds; bowel sounds, normal output, liver evaluation; normal urinary output, voiding pattern, prostate palpation; liver and kidney function tests

### Implementation

- Decrease dosage or discontinue temporarily if dry mouth makes swallowing or speaking difficult.
- Give with caution, and reduce dosage in hot weather. Drug interferes with sweating and ability of body to maintain heat equilibrium; anhidrosis and fatal hyperthermia have occurred.
- Give with meals if GI upset occurs; give before meals to patients with dry mouth; give after meals if drooling or nausea occurs.
- Ensure that patient voids just before receiving each dose of drug if urinary retention is a problem.

### Drug-specific teaching points

- Take this drug exactly as prescribed.
- Avoid the use of alcohol, sedative, and OTC drugs (can cause dangerous effects).
- The following side effects may occur: drowsiness, dizziness, confusion, blurred vision (avoid driving or engaging in activities that require alertness and visual acuity); nausea (try frequent small meals); dry mouth (suck sugarless lozenges or ice chips); painful or difficult urination (empty the bladder immedi-

ately before each dose); constipation (maintain adequate fluid intake and exercise regularly); use caution in hot weather (you are susceptible to heat prostration).
- Report difficult or painful urination; constipation; rapid or pounding heartbeat; confusion, eye pain, or rash.

## bismuth subsalicylate

*(bis' mith)*

Bismatrol, Bismatrol Extra Strength, Pepto-Bismol, Pepto-Bismol Maximum Strength, Pepto-Diarrhea Control

**Pregnancy Category C**

### Drug classes
Antidiarrheal agent

### Therapeutic actions
Adsorbent actions remove irritants from the intestine; forms a protective coating over the mucosa and soothes the irritated bowel lining.

### Indications
- Indigestion, nausea, and control of diarrhea within 24 h
- Relief of gas pains and abdominal cramps
- Unlabeled use: prevention and treatment of traveler's diarrhea

### Contraindications/cautions
- Allergy to any components

### Dosage
**Available Forms:** Tablets—262 mg; liquid—262 mg/15 ml, 524 mg/15 ml

**ADULT:** 2 tablets or 30 ml PO, q30 min–1 h as needed, up to eight doses/24 h.
- *Traveler's diarrhea:* 60 ml PO qid.

**PEDIATRIC**
- *9–12 y:* 1 tablet or 15 ml PO.
- *6–9 y:* 2/3 tablet or 10 ml PO.
- *3–6 y:* 1/3 tablet or 5 ml PO.
- *< 3 y:* Dosage not established.

### Pharmacokinetics

| Route | Onset |
|---|---|
| Oral | Varies |

*Metabolism:* Hepatic
*Distribution:* Crosses placenta
*Excretion:* Urine

### Adverse effects
- GI: *Darkening of the stool,* impaction in infants, debilitated patients
- Salicylate toxicity: Ringing in the ears, rapid respirations

### Clinically important drug-drug interactions
• Increased risk of salicylate toxicity with aspirin-containing products • Increased toxic effects of methotrexate, valproic acid if taken concurrently with salicylates • Use caution with drugs used for diabetes • Decreased effectiveness with corticosteroids • Decreased absorption of oral tetracyclines • Decreased effectiveness of sulfinpyrazone with salicylates

### Drug-lab test interferences
• May interfere with radiologic exams of GI tract; bismuth is radiopaque

## ■ Nursing Considerations

### Assessment
- *History:* Allergy to any components
- *Physical:* T; orientation, reflexes; R and depth of respirations; abdominal exam, bowel sounds; serum electrolytes; acid–base levels

### Implementation
- Shake liquid well before administration; have patient chew tablets thoroughly or dissolve in mouth; do not swallow whole.
- Discontinue drug if any sign of salicylate toxicity occurs (ringing in the ears).

### Drug-specific teaching points
- Take this drug as prescribed; do not exceed prescribed dosage. Shake liquid well before using. Chew tablets thoroughly or dissolve in your mouth; do not swallow whole.

- Darkened stools may occur.
- Do not take this drug with other drugs containing aspirin or aspirin products; serious overdosage can occur.
- Report fever, diarrhea that does not stop after 2 d, ringing in the ears, rapid respirations.

## bisoprolol fumarate

*(bis **oh'** pro lole)*
Zebeta
**Pregnancy Category C**

### Drug classes
Beta-adrenergic blocking agent ($\beta$1 selective)
Antihypertensive

### Therapeutic actions
Blocks beta-adrenergic receptors of the sympathetic nervous system in the heart and juxtaglomerular apparatus (kidney), thus decreasing the excitability of the heart, decreasing cardiac output and oxygen consumption, decreasing the release of renin from the kidney, and lowering blood pressure.

### Indications
- Management of hypertension, used alone or with other antihypertensive agents

### Contraindications/cautions
- Contraindications: sinus bradycardia, second or third-degree heart block, cardiogenic shock, CHF.
- Use cautiously with renal failure, diabetes or thyrotoxicosis (bisoprolol can mask the usual cardiac signs of hypoglycemia and thyrotoxicosis), lactation.

### Dosage
**Available Forms:** Tablets—5, 10 mg
*ADULT:* Initially 5 mg PO qid, alone or added to diuretic therapy; 2.5 mg may be added; up to 20 mg PO qid has been used.
*PEDIATRIC:* Safety and efficacy not established.
*RENAL OR HEPATIC IMPAIRMENT:* Initially 2.5 mg PO; titrate, and use extreme caution.

### Pharmacokinetics

| Route | Onset | Peak | Duration |
|---|---|---|---|
| Oral | 30–60 min | 2 h | 12–15 h |

*Metabolism:* Hepatic; $T_{1/2}$: 9–12 h
*Distribution:* Crosses placenta; passes into breast milk
*Excretion:* Urine

### Adverse effects
- CNS: Dizziness, vertigo, tinnitus, fatigue, emotional depression, paresthesias, sleep disturbances, hallucinations, disorientation, memory loss, slurred speech
- GI: *Gastric pain, flatulence, constipation, diarrhea, nausea, vomiting,* anorexia, ischemic colitis, renal and mesenteric arterial thrombosis, retroperitoneal fibrosis, hepatomegaly, acute pancreatitis
- CV: *Bradycardia, CHF, cardiac arrhythmias, sinoartial or AV nodal block, tachycardia,* peripheral vascular insufficiency, claudication, CVA, pulmonary edema, hypotension
- **Respiratory**: Bronchospasm, dyspnea, cough, bronchial obstruction, nasal stuffiness, rhinitis, pharyngitis (less likely than with propranolol)
- GU: *Impotence, decreased libido*, Peyronie's disease, dysuria, nocturia, frequent urination
- MS: Joint pain, arthralgia, muscle cramp
- EENT: Eye irritation, dry eyes, conjunctivitis, blurred vision
- Dermatologic: Rash, pruritus, sweating, dry skin
- **Allergic reactions**: Pharyngitis, erythematous rash, fever, sore throat, laryngospasm, respiratory distress
- Other: *Decreased exercise tolerance, development of antinuclear antibodies,* hyperglycemia or hypoglycemia, elevated serum transaminase, alkaline phosphatase, and LDH

### Clinically important drug-drug interactions

• Increased effects with verapamil, anticholinergics • Increased risk of postural hypotension with prazosin • Possible increased BP-lowering effects with aspirin, bismuth subsalicylate, magnesium salicylate, sulfinpyrazone, oral contraceptives • Decreased antihypertensive effects with NSAIDs • Possible increased hypoglycemic effect of insulin

### Drug-lab test interferences

• Possible false results with glucose or insulin tolerance tests

## ■ Nursing Considerations

### Assessment

- ***History:*** Sinus bradycardia, cardiac arrhythmias, cardiogenic shock, CHF, renal failure, diabetes or thyrotoxicosis, lactation
- ***Physical:*** Baseline weight, skin condition, neurologic status, P, BP, ECG, R, kidney and liver function tests, blood and urine glucose

### Implementation

- Do not discontinue drug abruptly after chronic therapy (hypersensitivity to catecholamines may have developed, causing exacerbation of angina, MI, and ventricular dysrhythmias). Taper drug gradually over 2 wk with monitoring.
- Consult with physician about withdrawing drug if patient is to undergo surgery (withdrawal is controversial).

### Drug-specific teaching points

- Do not stop taking this drug unless instructed to do so by a health care provider.
- Avoid OTC medications.
- Avoid driving or dangerous activities if dizziness, weakness occur.
- The following side effects may occur: dizziness, lightheadedness, loss of appetite, nightmares, depression, sexual impotence.
- Report difficulty breathing, night cough, swelling of extremities, slow pulse, confusion, depression, rash, fever, sore throat.

# bitolterol mesylate

*(bye **tole'** ter ole)*

Tornalate

**Pregnancy Category C**

### Drug classes

Sympathomimetic drug
$\beta_2$-selective adrenergic agonist
Bronchodilator
Antiasthmatic drug

### Therapeutic actions

Prodrug that is converted by tissue and blood enzymes to active metabolite (colterol); in low doses, acts relatively selectively at $\beta_2$ adrenergic receptors to cause bronchodilation (and vasodilation); at higher doses, $\beta_2$ selectivity is lost,and the drug acts at $\beta_1$ receptors to cause typical sympathomimetic cardiac effects.

### Indications

- Prophylaxis and treatment of bronchial asthma and reversible bronchospasm

### Contraindications/cautions

- Hypersensitivity to bitolterol; tachyarrhythmias, tachycardia caused by digitalis intoxication; general anesthesia with halogenated hydrocarbons or cyclopropane, which sensitize the myocardium to catecholamines; unstable vasomotor system disorders; hypertension; coronary insufficiency, CAD; history of stroke; COPD patients with degenerative heart disease; hyperthyroidism; history of seizure disorders; psychoneurotic individuals; labor and delivery (parenteral use of $\beta_2$-adrenergic agonists can accelerate fetal heart beat; cause hypoglycemia, hypokalemia, pulmonary edema in the mother, and hypoglycemia in the neonate; systemic absorption after inhalation may be less than with systemic administration, but use only if potential benefit to mother justifies risk to mother and fetus); lactation

### Dosage

**Available Forms:** Aerosal—0.37 mg/ actuation

*ADULT:*

- *Treatment of bronchospasm:* 2 inhalations at intervals of at least 1–3 min, followed by a 3rd inhalation if needed.
- *Prevention of bronchospasm:* 2 inhalations q8h; do not exceed 3 inhalations q6h or 2 inhalations q4h.

*PEDIATRIC*

- *> 12 y:* Same as adult
- *< 12 y:* Safety and efficacy not established.

*GERIATRIC:*

Patients > 60 y more risk of adverse effects; use extreme caution.

### Pharmacokinetics

| *Route* | *Onset* | *Peak* | *Duration* |
|---|---|---|---|
| Inhalation | 3–4 min | 1/2–2 h | 5–8 h |

*Metabolism:* $T_{1/2}$: 3 h
*Distribution:* Crosses placenta; may pass into breast milk
*Excretion:* Lungs

### Adverse effects

- CNS: *Restlessness, apprehension*, anxiety, fear, CNS stimulation, hyperkinesia, *insomnia,* tremor, drowsiness, *irritability,* weakness, vertigo, headache
- CV: **Cardiac arrhythmias**, tachycardia, palpitations, PVCs (rare), anginal pain (less likely with bronchodilator doses than with bronchodilator doses of a nonselective beta-agonist ie, isoproterenol), changes in BP, sweating, pallor, flushing
- Hypersensitivity: Immediate hypersensitivity (allergic) reactions
- Respiratory: Respiratory difficulties, **pulmonary edema**, coughing, bronchospasm, paradoxical airway resistance with repeated use of inhalation preparations
- GI: *Nausea,* vomiting, heartburn, unusual or bad taste

### Clinically important drug-drug interactions

• Increased sympathomimetic effects with other sympathomimetic drugs • Enhanced toxicity, especially cardiotoxicity, with aminophylline, oxtriphylline, theophylline

## ■ Nursing Considerations

### Assessment

- *History:* Hypersensitivity to bitolterol; tachyarrhythmias; general anesthesia with halogenated hydrocarbons or cyclopropane; unstable vasomotor system disorders; hypertension; coronary insufficiency; history of stroke; COPD patients with degenerative heart disease; hyperthyroidism; history of seizure disorders; psychoneurotic individuals; labor or delivery; lactation
- *Physical:* Weight, skin color, temperature, turgor; orientation, reflexes, affect; P, BP; R, adventitious sounds; blood and urine glucose, serum electrolytes, thyroid function tests, ECG, CBC, liver function tests (SGOT)

### Implementation

- Use minimal doses for minimum time; drug tolerance can occur with prolonged use.
- Maintain a beta-adrenergic blocker (a cardioselective beta-blocker, such as atenolol should be used for respiratory distress) on standby in case cardiac arrhythmias occur.
- Do not exceed recommended dosage; give during second half of inspiration, because airways open wider, and aerosol distribution is more extensive.

### Drug-specific teaching points

- Do not exceed recommended dosage; adverse effects or loss of effectiveness may result. Read product instructions, and ask health care provider or pharmacist any questions.
- The following side effects may occur: drowsiness, dizziness, fatigue, apprehension (use caution if driving or performing tasks that require alertness); nausea, heartburn, change in taste (small, frequent meals may help); sweating, flushing, rapid heart rate.
- Avoid OTC drugs; they can interfere with or cause serious side effects when used with this drug. If you need one of these products, consult health care provider.

- Report chest pain, dizziness, insomnia, weakness, tremor or irregular heart beat, difficulty breathing, productive cough, failure to respond to usual dosage.

## bleomycin sulfate

*(blee oh **mye'** sin)*

BLM, Blenoxane

**Pregnancy Category D**

### Drug classes

Antibiotic
Antineoplastic agent

### Therapeutic actions

Inhibits DNA, RNA, and protein synthesis in susceptible cells, preventing cell division; cell cycle phase-specific agent with major effects in G2 and M phases.

### Indications

- Palliative treatment of squamous cell carcinoma, lymphomas, testicular carcinoma, alone or with other drugs
- Treatment of malignant pleural effusion

### Contraindications/cautions

- Allergy to bleomycin sulfate; lactation

### Dosage

**Available Forms:** Powder for injection—15, 30 units

*ADULT:* Treat lymphoma patients with 2 U or less for the first two doses; if no acute anaphylactoid reaction occurs, use the regular dosage schedule:

- *Squamous cell carcinoma, lymphosarcoma, reticulum cell sarcoma, testicular carcinoma:* 0.25–0.50 U/kg IV, IM, or SC, once or twice weekly.
- *Hodgkin's disease:* 0.25–0.50 U/kg IV, IM, or SC once or twice weekly. After a 50% response, give maintenance dose of 1 U/d or 5 U/wk, IV or IM. Response should be seen within 2 wk (Hodgkin's disease, testicular tumors) or 3 wk (squamous cell cancers). If no improvement is seen by then, it is unlikely to occur.

### Pharmacokinetics

| Route | Onset | Peak |
|---|---|---|
| IV | Immediate | 10–20 min |
| IM, SC | 15–20 min | 30–60 min |

*Metabolism:* $T_{1/2}$: 2 h
*Distribution:* May cross placenta; may pass into breast milk
*Excretion:* Urine

### IV facts

**Preparation:** Dissolve contents of 15- or 30-unit vial with 5 or 10 ml physiologic saline or glucose; stable for 24 h at room temperature in NaCl, 5% Dextrose solutions, and 5% Dextrose containing heparin 100 or 1,000 U/ml; powder should be refrigerated.
**Infusion:** Infuse slowly over 10 min.
**Compatabilities:** Incompatible in solution with aminophylline, ascorbic acid, carbenicillin, diazepam, hydrocortisone, methotrexate, mitomycin, naficillin, penicillin G, terbutaline.

### Adverse effects

- GI: Hepatic toxicity, *stomatitis, vomiting,* anorexia, weight loss
- Respiratory: *Dyspnea, rales, pneumonitis,* ***pulmonary fibrosis***
- GU: Renal toxicity
- Dermatologic: *Rash, striae, vesiculation, hyperpigmentation, skin tenderness, hyperkeratosis, nail changes, alopecia, pruritus*
- Hypersensitivity: Idiosyncratic reaction similar to anaphylaxis: hypotension, mental confusion, fever, chills, wheezing (lymphoma patients, 1% occurrence)
- Other: *Fever, chills*

### Clinically important drug-drug interactions

- Decreased serum levels and effectiveness of digoxin and phenytoin

## ■ Nursing Considerations

### Assessment

- *History:* Allergy to bleomycin sulfate, pregnancy, lactation
- *Physical:* T; skin color, lesions; weight; R, adventitious sounds; liver evaluation,

abdominal status; pulmonary function tests, urinalysis, liver and renal function tests, chest x-ray

### Implementation

- Reconstitute for IM, SC use by dissolving contents of 15-unit vial in 1–5 ml 30-unit vial with 5–10ml of Sterile Water for Injection, Sodium Chloride for Injection, 5% Dextrose Injection, Bacteriostatic Water for Injection.
- Label drug solution with date and hour of preparation; check label before use. Stable at room temperature for 24 h in Sodium Chloride, 5% Dextrose Solution, 5% Dextrose containing heparin 100 or 1,000 U/ml; discard after that time.
- Monitor pulmonary function regularly and chest x-ray weekly or biweekly to monitor onset of pulmonary toxicity; consult physician immediately if changes occur.
- Arrange for periodic monitoring of renal and liver function tests.

### Drug-specific teaching points

- This drug has to be given by injection. Mark calendar with dates for injection.
- The following side effects may occur: rash, skin lesions, loss of hair, changes in nails (you may want to invest in a wig, skin care may help); loss of appetite, nausea, mouth sores (try frequent mouth care, small frequent meals may help; maintain good nutrition).
- Report difficulty breathing, cough, yellowing of skin or eyes, severe GI upset, fever, chills.

## bretylium tosylate

*(bre til' ee um)*

Bretylate (CAN)

**Pregnancy Category C**

### Drug classes

Antiarrhythmic

Adrenergic neuron blocker (not used as sympatholytic agent)

### Therapeutic actions

Type III antiarrhythmic: prolongs repolarization, prolongs refractory period, and increases ventricular fibrillation threshold.

b

### Indications

- Prevention and treatment of ventricular fibrillation
- Treatment of ventricular arrhythmias that are resistant to other antiarrhythmic agents
- Unlabeled use: second-line agent for advanced cardiac life support during CPR

### Contraindications/cautions

- Because bretylium is used in life-threatening situations, the benefits usually outweigh any possible risks of therapy.
- Use caution in the presence of hypotension, shock; aortic stenosis; pulmonary hypertension; renal disease; lactation.

### Dosage

**Available Forms:** Injection—50 mg/ml

Drug is for short-term use only. Careful patient assessment and evaluation are needed to determine the dose. Continual monitoring of cardiac response is necessary to establish the correct dosage. The following is a guide to usual dosage.

ADULT

- *Emergency use:* Undiluted 5 mg/kg by rapid IV bolus: increase dose to 10 mg/kg, and repeat if arrhythmia persists. **Maintenance:** continuously infuse diluted solution IV at 1–2 mg/min, or infuse intermittently at 5–10 mg/kg over 10–30 min, q6h.
- *Other arrhythmias:* Infuse diluted solution at 5–10 mg/kg over > 8 min, and repeat q1–2h. **Maintenance:** same dose at 6-h intervals or continuous infusion of 1–2 mg/min.
  - ***IM:*** 5–10 mg/kg undiluted, repeated at 1- to 2-h intervals if arrhythmia persists. **Maintenance:** same dose at 6- to 8-h intervals.

PEDIATRIC

- *Acute ventricular fibrillation:* 5 mg/kg per dose IV followed by 10 mg/kg at 15- to 30-min intervals; maximum total dose 30 mg/kg. **Maintenance:** 5–10 mg/kg per dose q6h.

- *Other ventricular arrhythmias:* 5–10 mg/kg per dose q6h.

**Pharmacokinetics**

| Route | Onset | Peak | Duration |
|---|---|---|---|
| IM | Varies | 6–9 h | 24 h |
| IV | Minutes | 1–4 h | 24 h |

*Metabolism:* $T_{1/2}$: 6.9–8.1 h
*Distribution:* Crosses placenta; may pass into breast milk
*Excretion:* Urine

### IV facts

**Preparation:** Dilute 1 ampule (10 ml containing 500 mg bretylium) to a minimum of 50 ml with 5% Dextrose Injection or Sodium Chloride Injection.
**Infusion:** Administer undiluted by rapid IV injection for emergency. Administer at a constant infusion of 1–2 mg/min using the following chart.

| *Amount Bretylium* | *Volume IV Fluid* | *Dose mg/min* | *Microdrips/ min & ml/h* |
|---|---|---|---|
| 500 mg | 50 ml | 1 | 7 |
| | | 1.5 | 11 |
| | | 2 | 14 |
| 2 g | 500 ml | 1 | 16 |
| 1 g | 250 | 1.5 | 24 |
| | | 2 | 32 |
| 1 g | 500 | 1 | 32 |
| 500 g | 250 | 1.5 | 47 |
| | | 2 | 63 |

**Compatibilities:** Bretylium is compatible with 5% Dextrose Injection, 5% Dextrose in 0.45% Sodium Chloride, 5% Dextrose in 0.9% Sodium Chloride, 5% Dextrose in Lactated Ringer's, 0.9% Sodium Chloride, 5% Sodium Bicarbonate, 20% Mannitol, 1/6 M Sodium Lactate, Lactated Ringer's, Calcium Chloride in 5% Dextrose, Potassium Chloride in 5% Dextrose.

**Adverse effects**

- CNS: Dizziness/lightheadedness, syncope
- GI: *Nausea, vomiting*
- CV: *Hypotension, orthostatic hypotension,* transient hypertension, cardiac arrhythmias, congestive heart failure
- Local: *Pain, burning* at injection site; tissue necrosis with extravasation

**Clinically important drug-drug interactions**

• Increased digitalis toxicity if taken with digitalis glycosides • Increased pressor effects of dopamine, norepinephrine, catecholamines when given with bretylium

## ■ Nursing Considerations

### Assessment

- *History:* Hypotension, shock; aortic stenosis; pulmonary hypertension; renal disease; lactation
- *Physical:* Orientation, speech, reflexes; P, BP, auscultation, continuous ECG monitoring; R, adventitious sounds; renal function tests

### Implementation

- Monitor cardiac rhythm and BP continuously.
- Keep patient supine until tolerance of orthostatic hypotension develops.
- Increase dosage interval in patients with renal failure.
- Do not give more than 5 ml in any one IM injection site.
- Monitor for safe and effective serum drug levels (0.5–1.5 μg/ml).

### Drug-specific teaching points

- Drug dosage is changed frequently in response to cardiac arrhythmia on monitor, and you will need frequent monitoring of cardiac rhythm and BP.
- Blood pressure will fall during drug therapy; because of this, it is important for you to remain lying down. Ask for assistance to move or sit up. You may feel lightheaded or dizzy even while lying down. Most people adjust to the blood pressure changes in a few days. Continue to change position slowly.
- Report chest pain, pain at IV site or IM injection site.

## bromfenac sodium

***(brom' fen ak)***

Duract

**Pregnancy Category C**

b

### Drug classes
Analgesic (non-narcotic)
Nonsteroidal anti-inflammatory drug (NSAID)

### Therapeutic actions
Inhibits prostaglandin synthetase to cause a peripheral anti-inflammatory effect; the exact mechanism of action is not known.

### Indications
- Short term treatment of pain (less than 10 days)

### Contraindications/cautions
- Contraindications: allergy to aspirin, significant liver impairment, preganancy, lactation.
- Use cautiously with hepatic or renal impairment, asthma, hypertension, CHF, history of GI bleed, coagulation disorders.

### Dosage
**Available Forms:** Capsules—25 mg

*ADULT:* 25 mg PO q 6–8 h as needed; maximum dose 150 mg/d.

*PEDIATRIC:* Safety and efficacy not established.

### Pharmacokinetics

| Route | Onset | Peak | Duration |
|---|---|---|---|
| Oral | 30 min | 2–3 h | 6–7 h |

*Metabolism:* Hepatic metabolism; $T_{1/2}$: 30–54 min

*Distribution:* Crosses placenta; passes into breast milk

*Excretion:* Urine

### Adverse effects
- CNS: *Headache, dizziness,* somnolence, insomia, fatigue, tiredness, asthenia
- GI: *Nausea, dyspepsia, GI pain, diarrhea,* vomiting, *constipation,* flatulence, liver enzyme changes, **fulminant hepatitis, liver failure**

### Clinically important drug-drug interactions
• Increased serum levels and increased risk of lithium toxicity if taken with bromfenac • Cimetidine levels may be increased in used in combination • May increase serum levels and toxicity of anticoagulants

## ■ Nursing Considerations

### Assessment
- *History:* Allergy to aspirin, liver impairment, pregnancy, lactation; renal impairment, asthma, hypertension, CHF, history of GI bleed, coagulation disorders
- *Physical:* Skin color and lesions; orientation, reflexes, liver evaluation; CBC, renal and liver function tests

### Implementation
- Administer drug with food or after meals if GI upset occurs.
- Provide further comfort measures to reduce pain (positioning, environmental control, etc.).
- Administer for short term (up to 10 days) only.

### Drug-specific teaching points
- Take drug with food or meals if GI upset occurs.
- Take only the prescribed dosage for a short time (not more than 10 d).
- The following side effects may occur: dizziness, drowsiness (avoid driving or the use of dangerous machinery while on this drug).
- Report sore throat, fever, rash, changes in vision, black or tarry stools, yellowing of eyes.

# bromocriptine mesylate

*(broe moe **krip'** teen)*

Parlodel

**Pregnancy Category C**

### Drug classes
Antiparkinsonism drug
Dopamine receptor agonist
Semisynthetic ergot derivative

### Therapeutic actions
**Parkinsonism:** Acts as an agonist directly on postsynaptic dopamine receptors of neurons in the brain, mimicking the effects of the neurotransmitter, dopamine, which is

deficient in parkinsonism. Unlike levodopa, bromocriptine does not require biotransformation by the nigral neurons that are deficient in parkinsonism patients; thus, bromocriptine may be effective when levodopa has begun to lose its efficacy.

**Hyperprolactinemia:** Acts directly on postsynaptic dopamine receptors of the prolactin-secreting cells in the anterior pituitary, mimicking the effects of prolactin inhibitory factor, inhibiting the release of prolactin and galactorrhea. Also restores normal ovulatory menstrual cycles in patients with amenorrhea or galactorrhea, and inhibits the release of growth hormone in patients with acromegaly.

## Indications

- Treatment of postencephalitic or idiopathic Parkinson's disease; may provide additional benefit in patients currently maintained on optimal dosages of levodopa with or without carbidopa, beginning to deteriorate or develop tolerance to levodopa, and experiencing "end of dose failure" on levodopa therapy; may allow reduction of levodopa dosage and decrease the dyskinesias and "on-off" phenomenon associated with long-term levodopa therapy
- Short-term treatment of amenorrhea or galactorrhea associated with hyperprolactinemia due to various etiologies, excluding demonstrable pituitary tumors
- Treatment of hyperprolactinemia associated with pituitary adenomas to reduce elevated prolactin levels, cause shrinkage of macroprolactinomas; may be used to reduce the tumor mass before surgery
- Female infertility associated with hyperprolactinemia in the absence of a demonstrable pituitary tumor
- Prevention of physiologic lactation (secretion, congestion, and engorgement) 'after parturition when the mother does not breastfeed or after stillbith or abortion
- Acromegaly: used alone or with pituitary irradiation or surgery to reduce serum growth hormone level

## Contraindications/cautions

- Contraindications: hypersensitivity to bromocriptine or any ergot alkaloid; severe ischemic heart disease or peripheral vascular disease; pregnancy, lactation.
- Use cautiously with history of MI with residual arrhythmias (atrial, nodal, or ventricular); renal, hepatic disease; history of peptic ulcer (fatal bleeding ulcers have occurred in patients with acromegaly treated with bromocriptine).

## Dosage

**Available Forms:** Capsules—5 mg; tablets—2.5 mg

**ADULT:** Give drug with food; individualize dosage; increase dosage gradually to minimize side effects; titrate dosage carefully to optimize benefits and minimize side effects.

- *Hyperprolactinemia:* Initially, one-half to one 2.5-mg tablet PO daily; an additional 2.5-mg tablet may be added as tolerated q3–7d until optimal response is achieved; usual dosage is 5–7.5 mg/d; range is 2.5–15 mg/d. Treatment should not exceed 6 mo.
- *Physiologic lactation:* Start therapy only after vital signs have stabilized and no sooner than 4 h after delivery; 2.5 mg PO bid; usual dosage is 2.5 mg qid–tid. Continue therapy for 14 d or up to 21 d if necessary.
- *Acromegaly:* Initially, 1.25–2.5 mg PO for 3 d when going to sleep; add 1.25–2.5 mg as tolerated q3–7d until optimal response is achieved. Evaluate patient monthly, and adjust dosage based on growth hormone levels. Usual dosage range is 20–30 mg/d; do not exceed 100 mg/d; withdraw patients treated with pituitary irradiation for a yearly 4- to 8-wk reassessment period.
- *Parkinson's disease:* 1.25 mg PO bid; assess every 2 wk, and titrate dosage carefully to ensure lowest dosage producing optimal response. If needed, increase dosage by increments of 2.5 mg/d q14–28d; do not exceed 100 mg/d. Efficacy for > 2 y not established.

**PEDIATRIC:** Safety for use in children < 15 y not established.

## Pharmacokinetics

| *Route* | *Onset* | *Peak* | *Duration* |
|---|---|---|---|
| Oral | Varies | 1–3 h | 14 h |

*Metabolism:* Hepatic; $T_{1/2}$: 3 h initial phase, 45–50 h terminal phase
*Excretion:* Bile

**Adverse effects**

*Hyperprolactinemic Indications*
- CNS: *Dizziness, fatigue, lightheadedness, nasal congestion, drowsiness,* cerebrospinal fluid rhinorrhea in patients who have had transsphenoidal surgery, pituitary radiation
- GI: *Nausea, vomiting, abdominal cramps, constipation, diarrhea, headache*
- CV: Hypotension

*Physiologic Lactation*
- CNS: *Headache, dizziness, nausea, vomiting,* fatigue, syncope
- GI: Diarrhea, cramps
- CV: Hypotension

*Acromegaly*
- CNS: Nasal congestion, digital vasospasm, drowsiness
- GI: *Nausea, constipation, anorexia,* indigestion, dry mouth, vomiting, GI bleeding
- CV: Exacerbation of Raynaud's syndrome, *postural hypotension*

*Parkinson's Disease*
- CNS: *Abnormal involuntary movements, hallucinations, confusion, "on-off" phenomenon, dizziness, drowsiness, faintness, asthenia, visual disturbance, ataxia, insomnia, depression, vertigo*
- GI: *Nausea, vomiting, abdominal discomfort, constipation*
- CV: *Hypotension, shortness of breath*

**Clinically important drug-drug interactions**

• Increased serum bromocriptine levels and increased pharmacologic and toxic effects with erythromycin • Decreased effectiveness with phenothiazines for treatment of prolactin-secreting tumors

## ■ Nursing Considerations

### Assessment
- ***History:*** Hypersensitivity to bromocriptine or any ergot alkaloid; severe ischemic heart disease or peripheral vascular disease; pregnancy; history of MI with residual arrhythmias; renal, hepatic disease; history of peptic ulcer, lactation
- ***Physical:*** Skin temperature (especially fingers), color, lesions; nasal mucous membranes; orientation, affect, reflexes, bilateral grip strength, vision exam, including visual fields; P, BP, orthostatic BP, auscultation; R, depth, adventitious sounds; bowel sounds, normal output, liver evaluation; liver and kidney function tests, CBC with differential

### Implementation
- Evaluate patients with amenorrhea or galactorrhea before drug therapy begins; syndrome may result from pituitary adenoma that requires surgical or radiation procedures.
- Arrange to administer drug with food.
- Taper dosage in patients with Parkinson's disease if drug must be discontinued.
- Monitor BP carefully for several days in patients receiving drug to inhibit postpartum lactation.
- Monitor hepatic, renal, hematopoietic function periodically during therapy.

### Drug-specific teaching points
- Take drug exactly as prescribed with food; take the first dose at bedtime while lying down.
- Do not discontinue drug without consulting health care provider (patients with macroadenoma may experience rapid growth of tumor and recurrence of original symptoms).
- Use mechanical contraceptives while taking this drug (amenorrhea or galactorrhea); pregnancy may occur before menses, and the drug is contraindicated in pregnancy (estrogen contraceptives may stimulate a prolactinoma).
- The following side effects may occur: drowsiness, dizziness, confusion (avoid driving or engaging in activities that require alertness); nausea (take the drug with meals, eat frequent small meals); dizziness or faintness when getting up (change position slowly, be careful climb-

ing stairs); headache, nasal stuffiness (medication may help).

- Report fainting; lightheadedness; dizziness; uncontrollable movements of the face, eyelids, mouth, tongue, neck, arms, hands, or legs; mental changes; irregular heartbeat or palpitations; severe or persistent nausea or vomiting; coffee-ground vomitus; black tarry stools; vision changes (macroadenoma); any persistent watery nasal discharge (hyperprolactinemic).

## brompheniramine maleate

*(brome fen **ir'** a meen)*

parabromdylamine maleate

Bromphen, Cophene-B, Diamine T.D., Dimetane Extentabs, Nasahist B, ND-Stat

**Pregnancy Category C**

### Drug classes

Antihistamine (alkylamine type)

### Therapeutic actions

Competitively blocks the effects of histamine at $H_1$ receptor sites; has anticholinergic (atropine-like), antipruritic, and sedative effects.

### Indications

- **Oral preparations:** Symptomatic relief of symptoms associated with perennial and seasonal allergic rhinitis; vasomotor rhinitis; allergic conjunctivitis; mild, uncomplicated urticaria and angioedema; amelioraton of allergic reactions to blood or plasma; dermatographism; adjunctive therapy in anaphylactic reactions
- **Parenteral preparations:** Amelioration of allergic reactions to blood or plasma; in anaphylaxis as an adjunct to epinephrine and other measures; other uncomplicated allergic conditions when oral therapy is not possible

### Contraindications/cautions

- Contraindications: allergy to any antihistamines, third trimester of pregnancy (newborn or premature infants may have severe reactions).
- Use cautiously with narrow-angle glaucoma, stenosing peptic ulcer, symptomatic prostatic hypertrophy, asthmatic attack, bladder neck obstruction, pyloroduodenal obstruction, lactation.

### Dosage

**Available Forms:** Tablets—4, 8, 12 mg; TR tablets—8, 12 mg; injection—10 mg/ml

ADULT AND CHILDREN > 12 Y

- ***Oral:*** 4 mg PO q4–6h; do not exceed 24 mg in 24 h.
- ***Sustained-release forms:*** 8–12 mg PO q8–12h; do not exceed 24 mg in 24 h.
- ***Parenteral:*** 10 mg/ml injection is intended for IM, or SC administration undiluted; give IV either undiluted or 1:10 with Sterile Saline for Injection. 100 mg/ml injection is intended for IM or SC use only; use undiluted or diluted 1:10 in saline. **Usual dose:** 5–20 mg bid; maximum dose is 40 mg/24 h.

PEDIATRIC

- ***Oral***
  - ***6–12 y:*** 2 mg q4–6h; do not exceed 12 mg in 24 h.
  - ***< 6 y:*** Standard dosage not developed.
- ***Sustained-release forms***
  - *6–12 y:* Use only as directed by physician.
  - *< 6 y:* Not recommended.
- ***Parenteral***
  - *< 12 y:* 0.5 mg/kg per day or 15 mg/$m^2$ per day in 3—4 divided doses.

GERIATRIC: More likely to cause dizziness, sedation, syncope, toxic confusional states, and hypotension in elderly patients; use with caution.

### Pharmacokinetics

| *Route* | *Onset* | *Peak* | *Duration* |
|---|---|---|---|
| Oral | 15–30 min | 1–2 h | 4–6 h |
| IM | 20 min | 1–2 h | 8–12 h |
| IV | Immediate | 30–60 min | 8–12 h |

*Metabolism:* Hepatic; $T_{1/2}$: 12–35 h

*Distribution:* Crosses placenta; passes into breast milk

*Excretion:* Urine

### IV facts

**Preparation:** May be diluted 1:10 with Sterile Saline for Injection. May be added to Normal Saline, 5% glucose, or whole blood.

**Infusion:** May give IV dosage undiluted. Administer slowly, monitoring patient response.

### Adverse effects

- CNS: *Drowsiness, sedation, dizziness, faintness, disturbed coordination*, fatigue, confusion, restlessness, excitation, nervousness, tremor, headache, blurred vision, diplopia, vertigo, tinnitus, acute labryinthitis, hysteria, tingling, heaviness and weakness of the hands
- GI: *Epigastric distress*, anorexia, increased appetite and weight gain, nausea, vomiting, diarrhea or constipation
- CV: Hypotension, palpitations, bradycardia, tachycardia, extrasystoles
- Respiratory: *Thickening of bronchial secretions*, chest tightness, wheezing, nasal stuffiness, dry mouth, dry nose, dry throat, sore throat
- **Hematologic**: Hemolytic anemia, hypoplastic anemia, thrombocytopenia, leukopenia, agranulocytosis, pancytopenia
- GU: Urinary frequency, dysuria, urinary retention, early menses, decreased libido, impotence
- **Hypersensitivity**: Urticaria, rash, anaphylactic shock, photosensitivity

### Clinically important drug-drug interactions

• Increased depressant with alcohol, other CNS depressants • Increased and prolonged anticholinergic (drying) effects with MAO inhibitors.

## ■ Nursing Considerations

### Assessment

- *History:* Allergy to any antihistamines, narrow-angle glaucoma, stenosing peptic ulcer, symptomatic prostatic hypertrophy, asthmatic attack, bladder neck obstruction, pyloroduodenal obstruction, third trimester of pregnancy, lactation
- *Physical:* Skin color, lesions, texture; orientation, reflexes, affect; vision exam; P, BP; R, adventitious sounds; bowel sounds; prostate palpation; CBC with differential

### Implementation

- Give orally with food if GI upset occurs; caution patient not to crush or chew sustained-release forms.
- Administer 10 mg/ml injection IM or SC undiluted.
- Provide supportive measures when allergic reactions require parenteral administration.
- Maintain epinephrine 1:1,000 readily available when using parenteral preparations; hypersensitivity reactions, including anaphylaxis, have occurred.

### Drug-specific teaching points

- Take as prescribed; avoid excessive dosage; take with food if GI upset occurs.
- Do not crush or chew the sustained-release preparations.
- The following side effects may occur: dizziness, sedation, drowsiness (use caution if driving or performing tasks that require alertness); epigastric distress, diarrhea or constipation (take with meals); dry mouth (frequent mouth care, sucking sugarless lozenges may help); thickening of bronchial secretions, dryness of nasal mucosa (try a humidifier).
- Avoid alcohol while on this drug; serious sedation could occur.
- Report difficulty breathing, hallucinations, tremors, loss of coordination, unusual bleeding or bruising, visual disturbances, irregular heartbeat.

## buclizine hydrochloride

***(byoo' kli zeen)***

Bucladin-S Softabs

**Pregnancy Category C**

### Drug classes

Antiemetic
Anti-motion sickness drug

Antihistamine
Anticholinergic drug

### Therapeutic actions

Reduces sensitivity of the labyrinthine apparatus; probably acts partly by blocking cholinergic synapses in the vomiting center, which receives input from the chemoreceptor trigger zone and from peripheral nerve pathways; peripheral anticholinergic effects may contribute to efficacy; mechanism not totally understood.

### Indications

- Control of nausea, vomiting, and dizziness of motion sickness

### Contraindications/cautions

- Contraindications: allergy to buclizine; allergy to tartrazine (more common in patients who are allergic to aspirin); lactation.
- Use caution with narrow-angle glaucoma, stenosing peptic ulcer, symptomatic prostatic hypertrophy, bronchial asthma, bladder neck obstruction, pyloroduodenal obstruction, cardiac arrhythmias (conditions that may be aggravated by anticholinergic therapy).

### Dosage

**Available Forms:** Tablets—50 mg

*ADULT:* 50 mg PO usually alleviates nausea. Up to 150 mg/d may be used. 50 mg PO at least 1/2 h before travel; for extended travel, a second tablet may be taken in 4–6 h. Usual maintenance dose is 50 mg bid; up to 150 mg/d may be given.

*PEDIATRIC:* Safety and efficacy not established.

*GERIATRIC:* More likely to cause dizziness, sedation in elderly patients; use with caution.

### Pharmacokinetics

| Route | Onset | Duration |
|---|---|---|
| Oral | 1 h | 4–6 h |

*Metabolism:* Hepatic
*Distribution:* Crosses placenta; passes into breast milk
*Excretion:* Urine

### Adverse effects

- CNS: *Drowsiness, dry mouth, headache, jitteriness*

## ■ Nursing Considerations

### Assessment

- ***History:*** Allergy to buclizine; allergy to tartrazine; lactation; narrow-angle glaucoma, stenosing peptic ulcer, symptomatic prostatic hypertrophy, bronchial asthma, bladder neck obstruction, pyloroduodenal obstruction, cardiac arrhythmias
- ***Physical:*** Orientation, reflexes, affect; vision exam; P, BP; R, adventitious sounds; bowel sounds, normal GI output; prostate palpation, normal urinary output

### Implementation

- Arrange for analgesics if needed for headache.

### Drug-specific teaching points

- Take this drug as prescribed. Tablets can be taken without water; place tablet in mouth, and dissolve, chew, or swallow whole. Avoid excessive dosage.
- Works best if used before motion sickness occurs.
- The following side effects may occur: dizziness, sedation, drowsiness (use caution if driving or performing tasks that require alertness); dry mouth (use frequent mouth care, suck sugarless lozenges); headache (consult health care provider for analgesic); jitteriness (reversible, will stop when you discontinue the drug).
- Avoid OTC drugs; many of them contain ingredients that cause serious reactions with this drug.
- Avoid alcohol; serious sedation could occur.
- Report difficulty breathing; hallucinations, tremors, loss of coordination; visual disturbances; irregular heartbeat.

# budesonide

*(bue **des'** oh nide)*

Pulmicort Turbuhaler, Rhinocort

**Pregnancy Category C**

## Drug classes

Corticosteroid

## Therapeutic actions

Anti-inflammatory effect; local administration into nasal passages maximizes beneficial effects on these tissues, while decreasing the likelihood of adverse effects from systemic absorption.

## Indications

- Management of symptoms of seasonal or perennial allergic rhinitis in adults and children; nonallergic perennial rhinitis in adults

## Contraindications/cautions

- Presence of untreated local nasal infections, nasal trauma, septal ulcers, recent nasal surgery, lactation.

## Dosage

**Available Forms:** Aerosal—32 μg/actuation; dry powder for inhalation—200 μg/inhalation

***Adult and Children > 6 Y:*** Initial dose 256 μg/day given as 2 sprays in each nostril morning and evening or 4 sprays in each nostril in the morning. After desired clinical effect is achieved, reduce dose to the smallest dose possible to maintain the control of symptoms. Generally takes 3–7 d to achieve maximum clinical effect. *Pulmicort Turbuhaler:* previously on inhaled corticosteroids—initially 200–400 μg twice daily, maximum dose 800μg bid (4 inhalations), 200 μg bid for children > 6y; previously on bronchodilators alone—200–400 μg bid, 200 μg bid for children > 6y; previously on oral corticosteroids—400–800 μg bid, 400 μg bid for children > 6y.

***Pediatric < 6 Y:*** Not recommemded.

## Pharmacokinetics

| *Route* | *Onset* | *Peak* | *Duration* |
|---|---|---|---|
| Intranasal | Immediate | Rapid | 8–12 h |

*Metabolism:* Hepatic; $T_{1/2}$: unknown

*Distribution* : Crosses placenta; may pass into breast milk

*Excretion* : Urine

## Adverse effects

- GI: Nausea, dyspepsia, dry mouth
- **Respiratory**: Epistaxis, rebound congestion, *pharyngitis, cough*
- **Dermatologic**: Rash, edema, pruritis, alopecia
- **Endocrine**: HPA suppression, Cushing's syndrome with overdosage and systemic absorption
- **Local**: *Nasal irritation,* fungal infection

## ■ Nursing Considerations

### Assessment

- *History:* Untreated local nasal infections, nasal trauma, septal ulcers, recent nasal surgery, lactation
- *Physical:* BP, P, auscultation; R, adventitious sounds; exam of nares

### Implementation

- Taper systemic steroids carefully during transfer to inhalational steroids; deaths from adrenal insufficiency have occurred.
- Arrange for use of decongestant nose drops to facilitate penetration if edema, excessive secretions are present.
- Prime unit before use for Pulmicort Turbuhaler; have patient rinse mouth after each use

### Drug-specific teaching points

- Do not use more often than prescribed; do not stop without consulting your health care provider.
- It may take several days to achieve good effects; do not stop if effects are not immediate.
- Use decongestant nose drops first if nasal passages are blocked.

- The following side effects can occur: local irritation (use your device correctly), dry mouth (suck sugarless lozenges).
- Prime unit before use for Pulmicort Turbuhaler; rinse mouth after each use.
- Report sore mouth, sore throat, worsening of symptoms, severe sneezing, exposure to chickenpox or measles, eye infections.

## bumetanide

*(byoo **met'** a nide)*
Bumex
**Pregnancy Category C**

### Drug classes
Loop (high ceiling) diuretic

### Therapeutic actions
Inhibits the reabsorption of sodium and chloride from the proximal and distal renal tubules and the loop of Henle, leading to a natriuretic diuresis.

### Indications
- Edema associated with CHF, cirrhosis, renal disease
- Acute pulmonary edema (IV)
- Unlabeled use: treatment of adult nocturia

### Contraindications/cautions
- Allergy to bumetanide; electrolyte depletion; anuria, severe renal failure; hepatic coma; SLE; gout; diabetes mellitus; lactation.

### Dosage
**Available Forms:** Tablets—0.5, 1, 2 mg; injection—0.25 mg/ml

**ADULT:** 0.5–2.0 mg/d PO in a single dose; may repeat at 4- to 5-h intervals up to a maximum daily dose of 10 mg. Intermittent dosage schedule of drug and rest days: 3–4 on/1–2 off is most effective with edema.

- ***Parenteral therapy:*** 0.5–1.0 mg IV or IM. Give over 1–2 min. Dose may be repeated at intervals of 2–3 h. *Do not exceed 10 mg/d.*

**PEDIATRIC:** Not recommended for children < 18 y.

**GERIATRIC OR RENAL IMPAIRED:** A continuous infusion of 12 mg over 12 h may be more effective and less toxic than intermittent bolus therapy.

### Pharmacokinetics

| Route | Onset | Peak | Duration |
|---|---|---|---|
| Oral | 30–60 min | 60–120 min | 4–6 h |
| IV | Minutes | 15–30 min | 1/2–1 h |

*Metabolism:* $T_{1/2}$: 60–90 min
*Distribution:* Crosses placenta; may pass into breast milk
*Excretion:* Urine

### IV facts
**Preparation:** May be given direct IV or diluted in solution with 5% Dextrose in Water, 0.9% Sodium Chloride, Lactated Ringer's Solution. Discard unused solution after 24 h.
**Infusion:** Give by direct injection slowly, over 1–2 min. Further diluted in solution; give slowly; do not exceed 10 mg/d.

### Adverse effects
- CNS: *Asterixis, dizziness*, vertigo, paresthesias, confusion, fatigue, nystagmus, *weakness, headache, drowsiness*, fatigue, blurred vision, tinnitus, irreversible hearing loss
- GI: *Nausea, anorexia, vomiting, diarrhea*, gastric irritation and pain, dry mouth, acute pancreatitis, jaundice
- CV: *Orthostatic hypotension*, volume depletion, cardiac arrhythmias, thrombophlebitis
- **Hematologic:** *Hypokalemia*, leukopenia, anemia, thrombocytopenia
- GU: *Polyuria, nocturia*, glycosuria, renal failure
- Local: *Pain, phlebitis at injection site*
- Other: Muscle cramps and muscle spasms, weakness, arthritic pain, fatigue, hives, photosensitivity, rash, pruritus, sweating, nipple tenderness

**Clinically important drug-drug interactions**

• Decreased diuresis and natriuresis with NSAIDs • Increased risk of cardiac glycoside toxicity (secondary to hypokalemia) • Increased risk of ototoxicity if taken with aminoglycoside antibiotics, cisplatin

## ■ Nursing Considerations

### Assessment

- *History:* Allergy to bumetanide, electrolyte depletion, anuria, severe renal failure, hepatic coma, SLE, gout, diabetes mellitus, lactation
- *Physical:* Skin—color, lesions; edema; orientation, reflexes, hearing; pulses, baseline ECG, BP, orthostatic BP, perfusion; R, pattern, adventitious sounds; liver evaluation, bowel sounds; urinary output patterns; CBC, serum electrolytes (including calcium), blood sugar, liver and renal function tests, uric acid, urinalysis

### Implementation

- Give with food or milk to prevent GI upset.
- Mark calendars or use reminders if intermittent therapy is best for treating edema.
- Give single dose early in day so increased urination will not disturb sleep.
- Avoid IV use if oral use is possible.
- Arrange to monitor serum electrolytes, hydration, liver function during long-term therapy.
- Provide diet rich in potassium or supplemental potassium.

### Drug-specific teaching points

- Record alternate day or intermittent therapy on a calendar or dated envelopes.
- Take the drug early in day so increased urination will not disturb sleep; take with food or meals to prevent GI upset.
- Weigh yourself on a regular basis, at the same time, and in the same clothing; record the weight on your calendar.
- The following side effects may occur: increased volume and frequency of urination; dizziness, feeling faint on arising, drowsiness (avoid rapid position changes; hazardous activities, such as driving; and alcohol consumption); sensitivity to sunlight (use sunglasses, sunscreen, wear protective clothing); increased thirst (suck sugarless lozenges; use frequent mouth care); loss of body potassium (a potassium-rich diet, or supplement will be needed).
- Report weight change of more than 3 lb in one day; swelling in ankles or fingers; unusual bleeding or bruising; nausea, dizziness, trembling, numbness, fatigue; muscle weakness or cramps.

# buprenorphine hydrochloride

*(byoo pre **nor'** feen)*

Buprenex

**Pregnancy Category C**
**C-V controlled substance**

**Drug classes**

Narcotic agonist-antagonist analgesic

**Therapeutic actions**

Acts as an agonist at specific opioid receptors in the CNS to produce analgesia; also acts as an opioid antagonist; exact mechanism of action not understood.

**Indications**

- Relief of moderate-to-severe pain

**Contraindications/cautions**

- Contraindications: hypersensitivity to buprenorphine.
- Use caution with physical dependence on narcotic analgesics (withdrawal syndrome may occur); compromised respiratory function; increased intracranial pressure (buprenorphine may elevate CSF pressure; may cause miosis and coma, which could interfere with patient evaluation), myxedema, Addison's disease, toxic psychosis, prostatic hypertrophy or urethral stricture, acute alcoholism, delirium tremens, kyphoscoliosis, biliary tract dysfunction (may cause spasm of the sphincter of Oddi), hepatic or renal dysfunction, lactation.

### Dosage

**Available Forms:** Injection—0.324 mg/ml

*ADULT:* 0.3 mg IM or by slow (over 2 min) IV injection. May repeat once, 30–60 min

after first dose. If necessary, nonrisk patients may be given up to 0.6 mg by deep IM injection.
*PEDIATRIC (< 13 Y):* Safety and efficacy not established.
*GERIATRIC OR DEBILITATED:* Reduce dosage to one-half usual adult dose.

### Pharmacokinetics

| Route | Onset | Peak | Duration |
|---|---|---|---|
| IM | 15 min | 1 h | 6 h |
| IV | 10 min | 30–45 min | 6 h |

*Metabolism:* Hepatic; $T_{1/2}$: 2–3 h
*Distribution:* Crosses placenta; may pass into breast milk
*Excretion:* Feces

#### IV facts

**Preparation:** May be diluted with Isotonic Saline, Lactated Ringer's Solution, 5% Dextrose and 0.9% Saline, 5% Dextrose. Protect from light and excessive heat.
**Infusion:** Administer slowly over 2 min.
**Compatibilities:** Compatible IV with scopolamine HBr, haloperidol, glycopyrrolate, droperidol and hydroxyzine HCl; incompatible IV with diazepam and lorazepam.

### Adverse effects

- CNS: *Sedation, dizziness/vertigo, headache*, confusion, dreaming, psychosis, euphoria, weakness/fatigue, nervousness, slurred speech, paresthesia, depression, malaise, hallucinations, depersonalization, coma, tremor, dysphoria/agitation, convulsions, tinnitus
- GI: *Nausea, vomiting*, dry mouth, constipation, flatulence
- CV: *Hypotension,* hypertension, tachycardia, bradycardia, Wenckebach's block
- Respiratory: *Hypoventilation*, dyspnea, cyanosis, apnea
- EENT: *Miosis*, blurred vision, diplopia, conjunctivitis, visual abnormalities, amblyopia
- Dermatologic: *Sweating*, pruritus, rash, pallor, urticaria
- Local: Injection site reaction

### Clinically important drug-drug interactions

- Potentiation of effects of buprenorphine with other narcotic analgesics, phenothiazines, tranquilizers, barbiturates, general anesthetics

## ■ Nursing Considerations

### Assessment

- *History:* Hypersensitivity to buprenorphine, physical dependence on narcotic analgesics, compromised respiratory function, increased intracranial pressure, myxedema, Addison's disease, toxic psychosis, prostatic hypertrophy or urethral stricture, acute alcoholism, delirium tremens, kyphoscoliosis, biliary tract dysfunction, hepatic or renal dysfunction, lactation
- *Physical:* Skin color, texture, lesions; orientation, reflexes, bilateral grip strength, affect; pupil size, vision; pulse, auscultation, BP; R, adventitious sounds; bowel sounds, normal output, liver palpation; prostate palpation, normal urine output; liver, kidney, thyroid, adrenal function tests

### Implementation

- Provide narcotic antagonist, facilities for assisted or controlled respiration on standby in case respiratory depression occurs.

### Drug-specific teaching points

- The following side effects may occur: dizziness, sedation, drowsiness, impaired visual acuity (avoid driving, performing other tasks that require alertness); nausea, loss of appetite (lying quietly, eating frequent small meals may help).
- Report severe nausea, vomiting, palpitations, shortness of breath or difficulty breathing, urinary difficulty.

## bupropion HCl

*(byoo* ***proe'*** *pee on)*
Wellbutrin, Wellbutrin SR, Zyban
**Pregnancy Category B**

**Drug classes**
Antidepressant
Smoking Deterrent

**Therapeutic actions**
The neurochemical mechanism of the antidepressant effect of bupropion is not understood; it is chemically unrelated to other antidepressant agents; it is a weak blocker of neuronal uptake of serotonin and norepinephrine and inhibits the reuptake of dopamine to some extent.

**Indications**
- Treatment of depression (effectiveness if used > 6 wk is unknown)
- Aid to smoking cessation treatment (Zyban)

**Contraindications/cautions**
- Contraindications: hypersensitivity to bupropion; history of seizure disorder, bulimia or anorexia, head trauma, CNS tumor (increased risk of seizures); lactation.
- Use caution with treatment with MAO inhibitor; renal or liver disease; heart disease, history of MI.

**Dosage**
**Available Forms:** Tablets—75,100 mg; SR tablets—100 mg, 150 mg (Zyban)
*ADULT:* Depression: 300 mg PO given as 100 mg tid; begin treatment with 100 mg PO bid; if clinical response warrants, increase 3 d after beginning treatment. If 4 wk after treatment, no clinical improvement is seen, dose may be increased to 150 mg PO tid (450 mg/d). Do not exceed 150 mg in any one dose. Discontinue drug if no improvement occurs at the 450 mg/d level.
Smoking Cessation: 150 mg PO qd for 3 days, then increase to 300 mg/d in 2 divided doses at least 8h apart. Treat for 7–12 weeks.
*PEDIATRIC:* Safety and efficacy in children < 18 y not established.
*GERIATRIC:* Bupropion is excreted through the kidneys; use with caution, and monitor older patients carefully.

**Pharmacokinetics**

| Route | Onset | Peak | Duration |
|---|---|---|---|
| Oral | Varies | 2 h | 8–12 h |

*Metabolism:* Hepatic; $T_{1/2}$: 8–24 h
*Distribution:* May cross placenta; may pass into breast milk
*Excretion:* Urine and feces

**Adverse effects**
- CNS: *Agitation, insomnia, headache/migraine, tremor*, ataxia, incoordination, seizures, mania, increased libido, hallucinations, visual disturbances
- GI: *Dry mouth, constipation,* nausea, vomiting, stomatitis
- CV: *Dizziness, tachycardia*, edema, ECG abnormalities, chest pain, shortness of breath
- GU: Nocturia, vaginal irritation, testicular swelling
- Dermatologic: Rash, alopecia, dry skin
- Other: *Weight loss*, flulike symptoms

**Clinically important drug-drug interactions**
• Increased risk of adverse effects with levodopa • Increased risk of toxicity with MAO inhibitors • Increased risk of seizures with drugs that lower seizure threshold

## ■ Nursing Considerations

**Assessment**
- *History:* Hypersensitivity to bupropion, history of seizure disorder, bulimia or anorexia, head trauma, CNS tumor, treatment with MAO inhibitor, renal or liver disease, heart disease, lactation
- *Physical:* Skin, weight; orientation, affect, vision, coordination; P, rhythm, auscultation; R, adventitious sounds; bowel sounds, condition of mouth

**Implementation**
- Administer drug 3 ×d for depression; do not administer more than 150 mg in any one dose.
- Increase dosage slowly to reduce the risk of seizures.
- Administer 100-mg tablets 4 ×d for depression, with at least 4 h between doses,

if patient is receiving > 300 mg/d; use combinations of 75-mg tablets to avoid giving > 150 mg in any single dose.
- Arrange for patient evaluation after 6 wk; effects of drug after 6 wk are not known.
- Discontinue MAO inhibitor therapy for at least 14 d before beginning bupropion.
- Monitor liver and renal function tests in patients with a history of liver or renal impairment.
- Have patient quit smoking within first 2wk of treatment for smoking cessation; may be used with transdermal nicotine.
- Monitor response and behavior; suicide is a risk in depressed patients.

### Drug-specific teaching points

- Take this drug in equally divided doses 3—4 ×d as prescribed for depression. Do not combine doses or make up missed doses. Take once a day, or divided into 2 doses at least 8h apart for smoking cessation.
- The following side effects may occur: dizziness, lack of coordination, tremor (avoid driving or performing tasks that require alertness); dry mouth (use frequent mouth care, suck sugarless lozenges); headache, insomnia (consult with care provider if these become a problem; do not self-medicate); nausea, vomiting, weight loss (small, frequent meals may help).
- Avoid or limit the use of alcohol while on this drug. Seizures can occur if these are combined.
- May be used with transdermal nicotine; most effective for smoking cessation if combined with behavioral support program.
- Report dark urine, light-colored stools; rapid or irregular heart beat; hallucinations; severe headache or insomnia; fever, chills, sore throat.

## buspirone hydrochloride

*(byoo **spye'** rone)*

BuSpar

**Pregnancy Category B**

### Drug classes

Antianxiety agent

### Therapeutic actions

Mechanism of action not known; lacks anticonvulsant, sedative, or muscle relaxant properties; binds serotonin receptors, but the clinical significance unclear.

### Indications

- Management of anxiety disorders or short-term relief of symptoms of anxiety
- Unlabeled use: decreasing the symptoms (aches, pains, fatigue, cramps, irritability) of PMS

### Contraindications/cautions

- Hypersensitivity to buspirone; marked liver or renal impairment; lactation.

### Dosage

**Available Forms:** Tablets—5, 10 mg

*ADULT:* Initially 15 mg/d PO (5 mg tid). Increase dosage 5 mg/d at intervals of 2–3 d to achieve optimal therapeutic response. Do not exceed 60 mg/d. Divided doses of 20–30 mg/d have been used.

*PEDIATRIC:* Safety and efficacy for children < 18 y not established.

### Pharmacokinetics

| *Route* | *Onset* | *Peak* |
|---|---|---|
| Oral | 7–10 d | 40–90 min |

*Metabolism:* Hepatic; $T_{1/2}$: 3–11 h
*Distribution:* May pass into breast milk
*Excretion:* Urine

### Adverse effects

- CNS: *Dizziness, headache, nervousness, insomnia, lightheadedness,* excitement, dream disturbances, drowsiness, decreased concentration, anger, hostility, confusion, depression, tinnitus, blurred vision, numbness, paresthesia, incoordination, tremor, depersonalization, dysphoria, noise intolerance, euphoria, akathisia, fearfulness, loss of interest, disassociative reaction, hallucinations, suicidal ideation, seizures, altered taste and smell, involuntary movements, slowed reaction time
- GI: *Nausea, dry mouth, vomiting, abdominal/gastric distress, diarrhea,* con-

stipation, flatulence, anorexia, increased appetite, salivation, irritable colon and rectal bleeding
- CV: Nonspecific chest pain, tachycardia/palpitations, syncope, hypotension, hypertension
- **Respiratory**: Hyperventilation, shortness of breath, chest congestion
- GU: Urinary frequency, urinary hesitancy, dysuria, increased or decreased libido, menstrual irregularity, spotting
- **Other**: Musculoskeletal aches and pains, sweating, clamminess, sore throat, nasal congestion

### Clinically important drug-drug interactions
• Give with caution to patients taking alcohol, other CNS depressants • Decreased effects with fluoxetine

## ■ Nursing Considerations

### Assessment
- *History:* Hypersensitivity to buspirone, marked liver or renal impairment, lactation
- *Physical:* Weight; T; skin color, lesions; mucous membranes, throat color, lesions, orientation, affect, reflexes, vision exam; P, BP; R, adventitious sounds; bowel sounds, normal GI output, liver evaluation; normal urinary output, voiding pattern; liver and kidney function tests, urinalysis, CBC and differential

### Implementation
- Provide sugarless lozenges, ice chips, if dry mouth, altered taste occur.
- Arrange for analgesic for headache, musculoskeletal aches.

### Drug-specific teaching points
- Take this drug exactly as prescribed.
- Avoid the use of alcohol, sleep-inducing, or OTC drugs; these could cause dangerous effects.
- The following side effects may occur: drowsiness, dizziness, lightheadedness (avoid driving or operating complex machinery); GI upset (frequent small meals may help); dry mouth (suck ice chips or sugarless candies); dreams, nightmares, difficulty concentrating or sleeping, confusion, excitement (reversible; will stop when the drug is discontinued).
- Report abnormal involuntary movements of facial or neck muscles, motor restlessness; sore or cramped muscles; abnormal posture; yellowing of the skin or eyes.

## busulfan

*(byoo **sul'** fan)*
Myleran
**Pregnancy Category D**

### Drug classes
Alkylating agent
Antineoplastic drug

### Therapeutic actions
Cytotoxic: interacts with cellular thiol groups causing cell death; cell cycle nonspecific.

### Indications
- Palliative treatment of chronic myelogenous leukemia; less effective in patients without the Philadelphia chromosome (Ph1); ineffective in the blastic stage

### Contraindications/cautions
- Allergy to busulfan, history of resistance to busulfan, chronic lymphocyctic leukemia, acute leukemia, blastic phase of chronic myelogenous leukemia, hematopoietic depression, pregnancy, lactation.

### Dosage
Available Forms: Tablets—2 mg

ADULT
- *Remission induction:* 4–8 mg total dose PO daily. Continue until WBC has dropped to 15,000/mm$^3$; WBC may continue to fall for 1 mo after drug is discontinued. Normal WBC count is usually achieved in approximately 12–20 wk in most cases.
- *Maintenance therapy:* Resume treatment with induction dosage when WBC reaches 50,000/mm$^3$. If remission is shorter than 3 mo, maintenance therapy

of 1–3 mg PO qid is advised to keep hematologic status under control.

**Pharmacokinetics**

| *Route* | *Onset* | *Peak* | *Duration* |
|---|---|---|---|
| Oral | 0.5–2 h | 2–3 h | 4 h |

*Metabolism:* Hepatic; $T_{1/2}$: unknown
*Distribution:* Crosses placenta; passes into breast milk
*Excretion:* Urine

**Adverse effects**
- GI: Dryness of the oral mucous membranes and cheilosis
- Respiratory: **Pulmonary fibrosis,** bronchopulmonary dysplasia
- Hematologic: *Leukopenia, thrombocytopenia, anemia, pancytopenia* (prolonged)
- GU: Hyperuricemia
- EENT: Cataracts (with prolonged use)
- Dermatologic: *Hyperpigmentation*, urticaria, Stevens-Johnson syndrome, erythema nodosum, alopecia, porphyria cutanea tarda, excessive dryness and fragility of the skin with anhidrosis
- Endocrine: *Amenorrhea, ovarian suppression, menopausal symptoms*; interference with spermatogenesis, testicular atrophy, syndrome resembling adrenal insufficiency (weakness, fatigue, anorexia, weight loss, nausea, vomiting, melanoderma)
- Other: Cancer

## ■ Nursing Considerations

### Assessment
- *History:* Allergy to or history of resistance to busulfan, chronic lymphocyctic leukemia, acute leukemia, blastic phase of chronic myelogenous leukemia, hematopoietic depression, pregnancy, lactation
- *Physical:* Weight; skin color, lesions, turgor; earlobe tophi; eye exam; bilateral hand grip; R, adventitious sounds; mucous membranes; CBC, differential; urinalysis; serum uric acid; pulmonary function tests; bone marrow exam if indicated

### Implementation
- Arrange for blood tests to evaluate bone marrow function prior to, weekly during, and for at least 3 wk after therapy has ended.
- Arrange for respiratory function tests before beginning therapy, periodically during therapy, and periodically after busulfan therapy has ended.
- Reduce dosage in cases of bone marrow depression.
- Give at the same time each day.
- Suggest contraceptive use during therapy.
- Ensure patient is hydrated before and during therapy; alkalinization of the urine or allopurinol may be needed to prevent adverse effects of hyperuricemia.
- Monitor patient for cataracts.

### Drug-specific teaching points
- Take drug at the same time each day.
- Drink 10–12 glasses of fluid each day.
- The following side effects may occur: darkening of the skin, rash, dry and fragile skin (skin care suggestions will be outlined for you to help to prevent skin breakdown); weakness, fatigue (consult with care provider if pronounced); loss of appetite, nausea, vomiting, weight loss (try small frequent meals); amenorrhea in women, change in sperm production in men (may effect fertility).
- Have regular medical follow up, including blood tests, to monitor effects of the drug.
- Consider using contraceptives. This drug has been known to cause fetal damage.
- Report unusual bleeding or bruising; fever, chills, sore throat; stomach, flank, or joint pain; cough, shortness of breath.

## butabarbital sodium

*(byoo ta **bar'** bi tal)*
secbutabarbital
secbutobarbitone
Butisol Sodium
**Pregnancy Category D**
**C-III controlled substance**

b

**Drug classes**

Barbiturate (intermediate acting)
Sedative
Hypnotic

**Therapeutic actions**

General CNS depressant; barbiturates inhibit impulse conduction in the ascending reticular activating system, depress the cerebral cortex, alter cerebellar function, depress motor output, and can produce excitation (especially with subanesthetic doses in the presence of pain), sedation, hypnosis, anesthesia, deep coma.

**Indications**

- Short-term use as a sedative and hypnotic

**Contraindications/cautions**

- Contraindications: hypersensitivity to barbiturates, tartrazine (in 30-, 50-mg tablets, and elixir marketed as *Butisol Sodium*); manifest or latent porphyria; marked liver impairment; nephritis; severe respiratory distress, respiratory disease with dyspnea, obstruction, or cor pulmonale; previous addiction to sedative-hypnotic drugs; pregnancy.
- Use cautiously with acute or chronic pain (may cause paradoxical excitement or mask important symptoms); seizure disorders (abrupt discontinuation of daily doses can result in status epilepticus); lactation (can cause drowsiness in nursing infants); fever, hyperthyroidism, diabetes mellitus, severe anemia, pulmonary or cardiac disease, status asthmaticus, shock, uremia; impaired liver or kidney function, debilitation.

**Dosage**

**Available Forms:** Tablets—15, 30, 50, 100 mg; elixir—30 mg/5 ml

ADULT

- *Daytime sedation:* 15–30 mg PO tid–qid.
- *Hypnotic:* 50–100 mg PO at hs. Drug loses effectiveness within 2 wk and should not be used longer than that.
- *Preanesthetic sedation:* 50–100 mg PO 60–90 min before surgery. *Note:* It is not considered safe to administer oral medication when a patient is NPO for surgery or anesthesia.

PEDIATRIC: Use caution: barbiturates may produce irritability, excitability, inappropriate tearfulness, and aggression.

- *Daytime sedation:* 7.5–30 mg PO, depending on age, weight, and sedation desired. (For methods to calculate pediatric dosage based on age and weight, see Appendix C).
- *Hypnotic:* Dosage based on age and weight.
- *Preanesthetic sedation:* 2–6 mg/kg; maximum dose 100 mg (see note above).

GERIATRIC PATIENTS OR THOSE WITH DEBILITATING DISEASE: Reduce dosage and monitor closely; may produce excitement, depression, confusion.

**Pharmacokinetics**

| Route | Onset | Peak | Duration |
|---|---|---|---|
| Oral | 45–60 min | 3–4 h | 6–8 h |

*Metabolism:* Hepatic; $T_{1/2}$: 50–100 h
*Distribution:* Crosses placenta; passes into breast milk
*Excretion:* Urine

**Adverse effects**

- CNS: *Somnolence, agitation, confusion, hyperkinesia, ataxia, vertigo, CNS depression, nightmares, lethargy, residual sedation (hangover), paradoxical excitement, nervousness, psychiatric disturbance, hallucinations, insomnia, anxiety, dizziness, thinking abnormality*
- GI: *Nausea, vomiting, constipation, diarrhea, epigastric pain*
- CV: *Bradycardia, hypotension, syncope*
- Respiratory: *Hypoventilation, apnea, respiratory depression,* laryngospasm, bronchospasm, **circulatory collapse**
- Hypersensitivity: Skin rashes, angioneurotic edema, serum sickness, morbiliform rash, urticaria; rarely, exfoliative dermatitis, **Stevens-Johnson syndrome, sometimes fatal**

- **Other:** Tolerance, psychological and physical dependence; withdrawal syndrome (sometimes fatal)

### Clinically important drug-drug interactions

• Increased CNS depression with alcohol • Increased risk of nephrotoxicity with methoxyflurane • Decreased effects of: theophyllines, oral anticoagulants, beta-blockers, doxycycline, griseofulvin corticosteroids, oral contraceptives and estrogens, metronidazole, phenylbutazones, quinidine, carbamazepine

## ■ Nursing Considerations

### Assessment

- *History:* Hypersensitivity to barbiturates, tartrazine, manifest or latent porphyria; marked liver impairment, nephritis, respiratory disease; previous addiction to sedative-hypnotic drugs, acute or chronic pain, seizure disorders, fever, hyperthyroidism, diabetes mellitus, severe anemia, cardiac disease, shock, uremia, debilitation, pregnancy, lactation
- *Physical:* Weight; T; skin color, lesions; orientation, affect, reflexes; P, BP, orthostatic BP; R, adventitious sounds; bowel sounds, normal output, liver evaluation; liver and kidney function tests, blood and urine glucose, BUN

### Implementation

- Monitor responses, blood levels if any of the above interacting drugs are given with butabarbital; suggest alternatives to oral contraceptives.
- Provide resuscitative facilities on standby in case of respiratory depression, hypersensitivity reaction.
- Taper dosage gradually after repeated use, especially in epileptic patients.

### Drug-specific teaching points

- This drug will make you drowsy and less anxious.
- Try not to get up after you have received this drug (request assistance to sit up or move about).

*Outpatients Taking This Drug*

- Take this drug exactly as prescribed.
- This drug is habit-forming; its effectiveness in facilitating sleep disappears after a short time. Do not take this drug longer than 2 wk (for insomnia), and do not increase the dosage without consulting the physician.
- Consult the care provider if the drug appears to be ineffective.
- Avoid alcohol, sleep-inducing, or OTC drugs; they could cause dangerous effects.
- Use an alternative to oral contraceptives; avoid becoming pregnant while taking this drug.
- The following side effects may occur: drowsiness, dizziness, "hangover," impaired thinking (less pronounced after a few days; avoid driving or engaging in dangerous activities); GI upset (take the drug with food); dreams, nightmares, difficulty concentrating, fatigue, nervousness (reversible, will go away when the drug is discontinued).
- Report severe dizziness, weakness, drowsiness that persists, rash or skin lesions, pregnancy.

# butoconazole nitrate

(*byoo toe* ***koe'*** *na zole*)

Femstat, Femstat One

**Pregnancy Category C**

### Drug classes

Antifungal

### Therapeutic actions

Fungicidal and fungistatic: binds to the cell membrane of the fungus with a resultant change in membrane permeability, allowing leakage of intracellular components and cell death.

### Indications

- Local treatment of vulvovaginal candidiasis (moniliasis)

### Contraindications/cautions

- Allergy to butoconazole or components used in preparation; lactation.

### Dosage

**Available Forms:** Vaginal cream—2%

*Pregnant patients (second and third trimesters only):* 1 applicator (5 g) intravaginally hs for 6 d.

*Nonpregnant patients:* 1 applicator (5 g) intravaginally hs for 3 d (may be extended to 6 d).

### Pharmacokinetics

| Route | Onset |
|---|---|
| Vaginal | Immediate |

*Metabolism:* Hepatic; $T_{1/2}$: 21–24 h

*Distribution:* Crosses placenta; may pass into breast milk

*Excretion:* Urine and feces

### Adverse effects

- Local: *Vulvovaginal burning,* vulvar itching; discharge, soreness, swelling, itchy fingers

## ■ Nursing Considerations

### Assessment

- *History:* Allergy to butoconazole or components used in preparation, pregnancy, lactation
- *Physical:* Pelvic exam, exam of mucous membranes and vulvar area; culture of area involved; KOH smear to confirm diagnosis of candidiasis

### Implementation

- Culture fungus prior to therapy.
- Administer vaginal cream high into vagina using the applicator supplied with the product. Administer for 3–6 consecutive nights, even during menstrual period.
- Monitor response to drug therapy; if no response is noted, arrange for further cultures to determine causative organism.
- Ensure that patient receives the full course of therapy to eradicate the fungus and prevent recurrence.
- Discontinue administration if rash or sensitivity occurs.

### Drug-specific teaching points

- Take the full course of drug therapy, even if symptoms improve. Continue during menstrual period if vaginal route is being used. Vaginal cream should be inserted high into the vagina using the applicator provided.
- Use hygiene measures to prevent reinfection or spread of infection; refrain from sexual intercourse, or advise partner to use a condom to avoid reinfection.
- This drug is specific for the fungus being treated; do not self-medicate other problems with this drug.
- Use a sanitary napkin to prevent staining of clothing.
- The following side effects may occur: local irritation, burning, stinging.
- Report worsening of the condition being treated, local irritation, burning.

## butorphanol tartrate

*(byoo* ***tor'*** *fa nole)*

Stadol, Stadol NS

**Pregnancy Category C during pregnancy**

**Pregnancy Category D during labor/delivery**

### Drug classes

Narcotic agonist-antagonist analgesic

### Therapeutic actions

Acts as an agonist at opioid receptors in the CNS to produce analgesia, sedation (therapeutic effects), but also acts to cause hallucinations (adverse effect); has low abuse potential; not in any schedule of the Federal Controlled Substances Act.

### Indications

- Relief of moderate to severe pain
- Relief of migraine headache pain (nasal spray)
- For preoperative or preanesthetic medication, to supplement balanced anesthesia, and to relieve prepartum pain

### Contraindications/cautions

- Contraindications: hypersensitivity to butorphanol, physical dependence on a narcotic analgesic, pregnancy, lactation.
- Use cautiously with bronchial asthma, COPD, respiratory depression, anoxia, in-

creased intracranial pressure, acute MI, ventricular failure, coronary insufficiency, hypertension, biliary tract surgery, renal or hepatic dysfunction.

## Dosage

**Available Forms:** Injection—1 mg/ml, 2 mg/ml; nasal spray 10 mg/ml

*ADULT*

- ***IM:*** Usual single dose is 2 mg q3–4h. Dosage range is 1–4 mg q3–4h; single doses should not exceed 4 mg.
- ***IV:*** Usual single dose is 1 mg q3–4h. Dosage range is 0.5–2 mg q3–4h.
  - ***Preoperative:*** 2 mg IM, 60–90 min before surgery.
  - ***Balanced anesthesia:*** 2 mg IV shortly before induction or 0.5–1 mg IV in increments during anesthesia.
  - ***Labor:*** 1–2 mg IV or IM at full term during early labor; repeat q4h.
- ***Nasal:*** 1 mg (1 spray per nostril). May repeat in 60–90 min if adequate relief is not achieved. May repeat two-dose sequence q3–4h.

*PEDIATRIC (< 18 Y):* Not recommended.

*GERIATRIC OR RENAL OR HEPATIC IMPAIRMENT*

- ***Parenteral:*** Use one-half the usual dose at twice the usual interval. Monitor patient response.
- ***Nasal:*** 1 mg initially. Allow 90–120 min to elapse before a second dose is given.

## Pharmacokinetics

| *Route* | *Onset* | *Peak* | *Duration* |
|---|---|---|---|
| IV | Rapid | 0.5–1 h | 3–4 h |
| IM | 10–15 min | 0.5–1 h | 3–4 h |
| Nasal | 15 min | 1–2 h | 4–5 h |

*Metabolism:* Hepatic; $T_{1/2}$:2.1–9.2 h

*Distribution:* Crosses placenta; passes into breast milk

*Excretion:* Urine and feces

### IV facts

**Preparation:** May be given undiluted. Store at room temperature. Protect from light.

**Infusion:** Administer direct IV at rate of 2 mg every 3–5 min.

**Compatibilities:** Do not mix in solution with dimenhydrinate, pentobarbital.

## Adverse effects

- CNS: *Sedation, clamminess, sweating, headache, vertigo, floating feeling, dizziness, lethary, confusion, lightheadedness,* nervousness, unusual dreams, agitation, euphoria, hallucinations
- GI: *Nausea,* dry mouth
- CV: Palpitation, increase or decrease in blood pressure
- **Respiratory**: Slow, shallow respiration
- **EENT**: Diplopia, blurred vision
- **Dermatologic**: Rash, hives, pruritus, flushing, warmth, sensitivity to cold

## Clinically important drug-drug interactions

- Potentiation of effects of butorphanol when given with barbiturate anesthetics

## ■ Nursing Considerations

### Assessment

- ***History:*** Hypersensitivity to butorphanol, physical dependence on a narcotic analgesic, pregnancy, lactation, bronchial asthma, COPD, increased intracranial pressure, acute MI, ventricular failure, coronary insufficiency, hypertension, biliary tract surgery, renal or hepatic dysfunction
- ***Physical:*** Orientation, reflexes, bilateral grip strength, affect; pupil size, vision; pulse, auscultation, BP; R, adventitious sounds; bowel sounds, normal output; liver, kidney function tests

### Implementation

- Provide narcotic antagonist, facilities for assisted or controlled respiration on standby during parenteral administration.

### Drug-specific teaching points

- The following side effects may occur: dizziness, sedation, drowsiness, impaired visual acuity (avoid driving, performing other tasks that require alertness); nausea, loss of appetite (lying quietly, eating frequent small meals may help).
- Report severe nausea, vomiting, palpitations, shortness of breath or difficulty breathing, nasal lesions or discomfort (nasal spray).

# cabergoline

*(ca **ber'** go lyne)*

Dostinex

**Pregnancy Category B**

## Drug classes

Dopamine receptor agonist

## Therapeutic actions

Synthetic argot derivative; long-acting dopamine receptor agonist with a high affinity for $D_2$ receptors that cause a decrease in prolactin levels in the anterior pituitary; it is thought that the secretion of prolactin from the anterior pituitary may be suppressed by dopamine from the hypothalamus.

## Indications

- Treatment of hyperprolactinemia disorders, idiopathic or due to pituitary tumors
- Unlabeled uses: Treatment of Parkinson's disease; normalization of androgen levels and improvement of menstrual cycling in polycystic ovary system

## Contraindications/cautions

- Contraindications: allergy to ergot products, fungal byproducts, uncontrolled hypertension, pregnancy-induced hypertension, postpartum lactation.
- Use cautiously with impaired liver function, pregnancy, lactation.

## Dosage

**Available Forms:** Tablets—0.5 mg

*ADULT:* Initial dose 0.25 mg PO 2 X/wk; increase based on prolactin levels by 0.25 mg 2 X/wk, maximum dose 1 mg 2 X/wk; do not increase dose more often than every 4 wk.

*PEDIATRIC:* Safety and efficacy not established.

## Pharmacokinetics

| Route | Onset | Peak | Duration |
|---|---|---|---|
| Oral | Slow | 2–3 h | Days–weeks |

*Metabolism:* Hepatic and renal; $T_{1/2}$: 63–69 h

*Distribution:* Crosses placenta; may pass into breast milk

*Excretion:* Urine

## Adverse effects

- CNS: *Headache, dizziness,* somnolence, vertigo, paresthesias, depression, nervousness, fatigue, asthenia
- GI: *Nausea, constipation,* abdominal pain, dyspepsia, vomiting, dry mouth, flatulence
- CV: Hypotension, orthostatic hypotension
- Other: Breast pain, dysmenorrhea, nasal stuffiness, acne

## Clinically important drug-drug interactions

- Additive hypotensive effects with antihypertensive agents; adjust dosage of antihypertensives accordingly • Decreased effectiveness with dopamine antagonists

## ■ Nursing Considerations

### Assessment

- ***History:*** Allergy to ergot products, fungal byproducts, uncontrolled hypeertension, pregnancy-induced hypertension, postpartum lactation, impaired liver function, pregnancy, lactation
- ***Physical:*** Orientation, strength, affect; BP, orthostatic BP; liver evaluation, abdominal exam; serum prolactin level

### Implementation

- Obtain serum prolactin levels before and periodically during drug therapy. Continue therapy until a normal prolactin level has been achieved for 6 mo ($<$20 $\mu$g/L for women, $<$15 $\mu$g/L for men); then periodically check prolactin levels to determine if cabergoline therapy should be restarted.
- Ensure that patient is not pregnant and has appropriate contraceptives available during therapy; serious fetal damage could occur.
- Monitor patient for orthostatic BP changes; if dizziness occurs with position change, provide safety precautions and encourage patient to move slowly.

### Drug-specific teaching points

- This drug is taken twice a week; mark calendar with drug days to ensure that you get the drug as prescribed.

- Arrange to have regular blood tests, which will be needed to adjust drug dose and evaluate its effects on your prolactin level.
- The following side effects may occur: dizziness, drowsiness (avoid driving or operating dangerous machinery, change position slowly); nausea (small, frequent meals may help); constipation (consult with your health care provider if this becomes a problem); headache (analgesics may be available).
- Do not become pregnant while on this drug; use a barrier contraceptive. If you wish to become pregnant or think you are pregnant, consult with your health care provider.
- Report nasal stuffiness, hallucinations, fainting, severe headache.

## caffeine

*(kaf **een'**)*

Caffedrine, NoDoz, Quick Pep, Tirend, Vivarin

**Pregnancy Category C**

### Drug classes
Analeptic
Xanthine

### Therapeutic actions
Increases calcium permeability in sarcoplasmic reticulum, promotes the accumulation of cAMP, and blocks adenosine receptors; stimulates the CNS, cardiac activity, gastric acid secretion, and diuresis.

### Indications
- An aid in staying awake and restoring mental awareness
- Adjunct to analgesic formulations
- Possibly an analeptic in conjunction with supportive measures to treat respiratory depression associated with overdosage with CNS depressants (IM)
- Unlabeled uses: neonatal apnea, headache, alcoholism, asthma, orthostatic hypotension

### Contraindications/cautions
- Depression, duodenal ulcers, diabetes mellitus, lactation

### Dosage
**Available Forms:** Tablets—100, 150, 200 mg; TR tablets—200 mg; TR capsules—200 mg; injection—250 mg/ml

*ADULT:* 100–200 mg PO q3–4h as needed; timed-release preparation, 200 mg PO q3–4h.

- ***Respiratory depression:*** 500 mg–1 g caffeine and sodium benzoate (250–500 mg caffeine) IM; do not exceed 2.5 g/d; may be given IV in severe emergency situation.

*PEDIATRIC:* Safety and efficacy not established.

### Pharmacokinetics

| *Route* | *Onset* | *Peak* |
| --- | --- | --- |
| Oral | 15 min | 15–45 min |

*Metabolism:* Hepatic; $T_{1/2}$: 3–7.5 h
*Distribution:* Crosses placenta; passes into breast milk
*Excretion:* Urine

### IV facts
**Preparation:** Dissolve 10 g caffeine citrate powder in 250 ml Sterile Water for Injection USP qs to 500 ml; filter and autoclave. Final concentration is 10 mg/ml caffeine base (20 mg/ml caffeine citrate). Stable for 3 mo. Or dissolve 10 mg caffeine powder and 10.94 citric acid powder in Bacteriostatic Water for Injection, USP qs to 1 L. Sterilize by filtration.
**Infusion:** IV single dose of 500 mg caffeine may be given slowly over 2 min in emergency situations; not recommended.

### Adverse effects
- CNS: *Insomnia, restlessness, excitement*, nervousness, tinnitus, muscular tremor, headaches, lightheadedness
- CV: *Tachycardia*, extrasystoles, palpitations
- GI: Nausea, vomiting, diarrhea, stomach pain
- GU: *Diuresis*

- **Other:** Withdrawal syndrome: headache, anxiety, muscle tension

**Clinically important drug-drug interactions**
• Increased CNS effects of caffeine with cimetidine, oral contraceptives, disulfiram, ciprofloxacin, enoxacin, phenylpropanolamine • Decreased effects of caffeine while smoking

**Clinically important drug-food interactions**
• Decreased absorption of iron if taken with or 1 h after coffee or tea

**Drug-lab test interferences**
• Possible false elevations of serum urate, urine VMA, resulting in false-positive diagnosis of pheochromocytoma or neuroblastoma

## ■ Nursing Considerations

### Assessment

- *History:* Depression, duodenal ulcer, diabetes mellitus, lactation
- *Physical:* Neurologic status, P, BP, ECG, normal urinary output, abdominal exam, blood glucose

### Implementation

- Do not stop the drug abruptly after long-term use.
- Monitor diet for presence of caffeine-containing foods that may contribute to overdose.

### Drug-specific teaching points

- Do not stop taking this drug abruptly; withdrawal symptoms may occur.
- Avoid foods high in caffeine (coffee, tea, cola, chocolate), which may cause symptoms of overdose.
- Avoid driving or dangerous activities if dizziness, tremors, restlessness occur.
- Consult with your health care provider if fatigue continues.
- The following side effects may occur: diuresis, restlessness, insomnia, muscular tremors, lightheadedness; nausea, abdominal pain.
- Report abnormal heart rate, dizziness, palpitations.

# Calcitonin

C

## calcitonin, human

*(kal si* ***toe'*** *nin)*

Cibacalcin

## calcitonin, salmon

Calcimar, Miacalcin, Miacalcin Nasal Spray, Osteocalcin, Salmonine

**Pregnancy Category B (salmon)**

**Pregnancy Category C (human)**

**Drug classes**
Hormonal agent
Calcium regulator

**Therapeutic actions**
The calcitonins are polypeptide hormones secreted by the thyroid; human calcitonin is a synthetic product; salmon calcitonin appears to be a chemically identical polypeptide but with greater potency per milligram and longer duration; inhibits bone resorption; lowers elevated serum calcium in children and patients with Paget's disease; increases the excretion of filtered phosphate, calcium, and sodium by the kidney.

**Indications**

- Paget's disease (human and salmon calcitonin)
- Postmenopausal osteoporosis in conjunction with adequate calcium and vitamin D intake to prevent loss of bone mass (salmon calcitonin)
- Hypercalcemia, emergency treatment (salmon calcitonin)

**Contraindications/cautions**

- Contraindications: allergy to salmon calcitonin or fish products, lactation.
- Use cautiously with renal insufficiency, osteoporosis, pernicious anemia.

## Dosage

**Available Forms:** Injection (human)—1 mg/ml; injection (salmon)—200 IU/ml; nasal spray (salmon)—200 IU/actuation

ADULT

- ***Calcitonin, human***
  - ***Paget's disease*** Starting dose of 0.5 mg/d SC; some patients may respond to 0.5 mg two to three times per week or 0.25 mg/d. Severe cases may require up to 1 mg/d for 6 mo. Discontinue therapy when symptoms are relieved.
- ***Calcitonin, salmon***
  - ***Skin testing:*** 0.1 ml of a 10 IU/ml solution injected SC.
  - ***Paget's disease:*** Initial dose 100 IU/d SC or IM. *Maintenance dose:* 50 IU/d or every other day. Actual dose should be determined by patient response.
  - ***Postmenopausal osteoporosis:*** 100 IU/d SC or IM, with supplemental calcium (calcium carbonate, 1.5 g/d) and vitamin D (400 U/d) or 200 IU intranasally qd.
  - ***Hypercalcemia:*** Initial dose: 4 IU/kg q12h SC or IM. If response is not satisfactory after 1–2 d, increase to 8 IU/kg q12h; if response remains unsatisfactory after 2 more d, increase to 8 IU/kg q6h.

PEDIATRIC: Safety and efficacy not established.

## Pharmacokinetics

| *Route* | *Onset* | *Peak* | *Duration* |
|---|---|---|---|
| IM, SC | 15 min | 3–4 h | 8–24 h |

*Metabolism:* Renal; $T_{1/2}$: 1.2 h (salmon) 1 h (human)
*Distribution:* May pass into breast milk
*Excretion:* Urine

## Adverse effects

- GI: *Nausea, vomiting*
- Dermatologic: *Flushing of face or hands*, skin rash
- GU: *Urinary frequency* (calcitonin-human)
- Local: *Local inflammatory reactions at injection site* (salmon), nasal irritation (nasal spray)

## ■ Nursing Considerations

### Assessment

- ***History:*** Allergy to salmon calcitonin or fish products, lactation, osteoporosis, pernicious anemia, renal disease
- ***Physical:*** Skin lesions, color, temperature; muscle tone; urinalysis, serum calcium, serum alkaline phosphatase and urinary hydroxyproline excretion

### Implementation

- Give skin test to patients with any history of allergies; salmon calcitonin is a protein, and risk of allergy is significant. Prepare solution for skin test as follows: withdraw 0.05 ml of the 200 IU/ml solution or 0.1 ml of the 100 IU/ml solution into a tuberculin syringe. Fill to 1 ml with Sodium Chloride Injection. Mix well. Discard 0.9 ml, and inject 0.1 ml (approximately 1 IU) SC into the inner aspect of the forearm. Observe after 15 min; the presence of a wheal or more than mild erythema indicates a positive response. Risk of allergy is less in patients being treated with human calcitonin.
- Use reconstituted human calcitonin within 6h.
- Maintain parenteral calcium on standby in case of development of hypocalcemic tetany.
- Monitor serum alkaline phosphatase and urinary hydroxyproline excretion prior to therapy and during first 3 mo and q3–6 mo during long-term therapy.
- Inject doses of more than 2 ml IM, not SC; use multiple injection sites.

### Drug-specific teaching points

- This drug is given SC or IM; you or a significant other must learn how to do this at home. Refrigerate the drug vials.
- For intranasal use, alternate nostrils daily; notify health care provider if significant nasal irritation occurs.
- The following side effects may occur: nausea, vomiting (this passes); irritation at injection site (rotate sites); flushing of the face or hands, skin rash.

- Report twitching, muscle spasms; dark urine; hives, skin rash; difficulty breathing.

## calcitriol

*(kal si **trye'** ole)*

1,25-dihydroxycholecalciferol

1,252-D3

Calcijex, Rocaltrol

**Pregnancy Category C**

### Drug classes
Vitamin
Calcium regulator

### Therapeutic actions
Fat-soluble vitamin; helps to regulate calcium homeostasis, bone growth, and maintenance; increases serum calcium levels and decreases alkaline phosphatase, parathyroid hormone levels.

### Indications
- Management of hypocalcemia in patients on chronic renal dialysis
- Reduction of elevated parathyroid hormone levels in some patients; possibly effective
- Unlabeled use: used orally and topically for 6 mo to decrease the severity of psoriatic lesions in patients with psoriasis vulgaris

### Contraindications/cautions
- Contraindications: allergy to vitamin D, hypercalcemia, vitamin D toxicity, hypervitaminosis D, pregnancy (teratogenic in preclinical studies).
- Use cautiously with renal stones, lactation.

### Dosage
**Available Forms:** Capsules—0.25, 0.50 μg; injection—1 μg/ml, 2 μg/ml

*ADULT:* 0.25 μg/d PO; if satisfactory response is not observed, dosage may be increased by 0.25 μg/d at 4- to 8-wk intervals. Most patients respond to 0.5–1 μg/d. 0.5 μg IV 3×/wk at the end of dialysis; may need up to 3 μg IV 3×/wk.

*PEDIATRIC*
- *>6 y:* 0.5 – 2 μg/d PO.
- *1–5 y:* 0.25–0.75 μg/d.

### Pharmacokinetics

| *Route* | *Onset* | *Peak* | *Duration* |
|---|---|---|---|
| Oral, IV | 2–6 h | 10–12 h | 3–5 d |

*Metabolism:* Renal; $T_{1/2}$: 3–6 h
*Distribution:* May cross placenta; passes into breast milk
*Excretion:* Bile

### IV facts
**Preparation:** No further preparation is needed.
**Infusion:** Administer undiluted, direct IV over 30–60 sec.

### Adverse effects
- CNS: *Weakness, headache, somnolence,* irritability
- GI: *Nausea, vomiting, dry mouth, constipation, metallic taste,* anorexia, pancreatitis, elevated liver function tests
- GU: Polyuria, polydipsia, nocturia, decreased libido, elevated renal function tests
- CV: Hypertension, cardiac arrhythmias
- Other: Muscle pain, bone pain, weight loss, photophobia, rhinorrhea, pruritus, hyperthermia

### Clinically important drug-drug interactions
• Risk of hypermagnesemia with magnesium-containing antacids • Reduced intestinal absorption of fat-soluble vitamins with cholestyramine, mineral oil • Possible risk of hypercalcemia if given with thiazide diuretics

## ■ Nursing Considerations

### Assessment
- *History:* Allergy to vitamin D; hypercalcemia, vitamin D toxicity, hypervitaminosis D; renal stones; lactation
- *Physical:* Skin color, lesions; T; weight; orientation, strength, taste; liver evaluation, mucous membranes; serum calcium, phosphorus, magnesium, alkaline

phosphatase; renal and hepatic function tests; x-rays of bones

### Implementation

- Monitor serum calcium prior to therapy and at least weekly during therapy; if hypercalcemia occurs, discontinue until calcium levels return to normal.
- Provide supportive measures to aid with GI, CNS effects of drug (eg, pain medication, relief of constipation, help with ADLs).
- Arrange for nutritional consultation if GI problems become severe.

### Drug-specific teaching points

- The following side effects may occur: weakness, bone and muscle pain, somnolence (rest often, avoid tasks that are taxing or require alertness); nausea, vomiting, constipation (consult with health care provider for corrective measures).
- Do not use mineral oil, antacids, or laxatives containing magnesium.
- Have blood tests twice-weekly at start and weekly thereafter to monitor your blood calcium levels.
- Report weakness, lethargy; loss of appetite, weight loss, nausea, vomiting; abdominal cramps, constipation, diarrhea; dizziness; excessive urine output, excessive thirst, dry mouth; muscle or bone pain.

## Calcium salts

**calcium carbonate**

Calciday, Caltrate, Chooz, Dicarbosil, Equilet, Os-Cal, Oyst-Cal, Oystercal, Tums

**calcium chloride**

**calcium gluceptate**

**calcium gluconate**

**calcium lactate**

**Pregnancy Category C**

### Drug classes

Electrolyte
Antacid

### Therapeutic actions

Essential element of the body; helps maintain the functional integrity of the nervous and muscular systems; helps maintain cardiac function, blood coagulation; is an enzyme cofactor and affects the secretory activity of endocrine and exocrine glands; neutralizes or reduces gastric acidity (oral use).

### Indications

- Dietary supplement when calcium intake is inadequate
- Treatment of calcium deficiency in tetany of the newborn, acute and chronic hypoparathyroidism, pseudohypoparathyroidism, postmenopausal and senile osteoporosis, rickets, osteomalacia
- Prevention of hypocalcemia during exchange transfusions
- Adjunctive therapy for insect bites or stings, such as black widow spider bites; sensitivity reactions, particularly when characterized by urticaria; depression due to overdosage of magnesium sulfate; acute symptoms of lead colic
- Combats the effects of hyperkalemia as measured by ECG, pending correction of increased potassium in the extracellular fluid (calcium chloride)
- Improves weak or ineffective myocardial contractions when epinephrine fails in cardiac resuscitation, particularly after open heart surgery
- Symptomatic relief of upset stomach associated with hyperacidity; hyperacidity associated with peptic ulcer, gastritis, peptic esophagitis, gastric hyperacidity, hiatal hernia (calcium carbonate)
- Prophylaxis of GI bleeding, stress ulcers, and aspiration pneumonia; possibly useful (calcium carbonate)
- Unlabeled use: treatment of hypertension in some patients with indices suggesting calcium "deficiency"

### Contraindications/cautions

- Allergy to calcium; renal calculi; hypercalcemia; ventricular fibrillation during cardiac resuscitation and patients with the risk of existing digitalis toxicity.

## Dosage

**Available Forms:** Tablets—500, 650, 975 mg, 1 g, 1.25 g, 1.5 g; powder—1250 mg; injection—10%, 1.1 g/5 ml

ADULT

- *Calcium carbonate or lactate*
  - *RDA:* 800 mg.
  - *Dietary supplement:* 500 mg–2 g PO, bid–qid.
  - *Antacid:* 0.5–2.0 g PO calcium carbonate as needed.
- *Calcium chloride:* For IV use only: 1 g contains 272 mg (13.6 mEq) calcium.
  - *Hypocalcemic disorders:* 500 mg–1 g at intervals of 1–3 d.
  - *Magnesium intoxication:* 500 mg promptly. Observe patient for signs of recovery before giving another dose.
  - *Hyperkalemic ECG disturbances of cardiac function:* Adjust dose according to ECG response.
  - *Cardiac resuscitation:* 500 mg–1 g IV or 200–800 mg into the ventricular cavity.
- *Calcium gluconate:* IV infusion preferred: 1 g contains 90 mg (4.5 mEq) calcium. 0.5–2.0 g as required; daily dose 1–15 g.
- *Calcium gluceptate:* IM or IV use: 1.1 g contains 90 mg (4.5 mEq) calcium; solution for injection contains 1.1 g/5 ml. 2–5 ml IM; 5–20 ml IV.

PEDIATRIC

- *Calcium gluconate:* 500 mg/kg per day IV given in divided doses.
- *Calcium gluceptate:* Exchange transfusions in newborns: 0.5 ml after every 100 ml of blood exchanged.

## Pharmacokinetics

| *Route* | *Onset* | *Peak* |
|---|---|---|
| Oral | 3–5 min | |
| IV | Immediate | 3–5 min |

*Metabolism:* Hepatic; $T_{1/2}$: 1–3 h
*Distribution:* Crosses placenta; passes into breast milk
*Excretion:* Feces, urine

## IV facts

**Preparation:** Warm solutions to body temperature; use a small needle inserted into a large vein to decrease irritation.
**Infusion:** Infuse slowly, 0.5–2 ml/min. Stop infusion if patient complains of discomfort; resume when symptoms disappear. Repeated injections are often necessary.
**Compatibilities:** Avoid mixing calcium salts with carbonates, phosphates, sulfates, tartrates.

C

## Adverse effects

- CV: *Slowed heart rate, tingling, "heat waves"* (rapid IV administration); *peripheral vasodilation, local burning,* fall in blood pressure (calcium chloride injection)
- Metabolic: Hypercalcemia (*anorexia, nausea, vomiting, constipation*, abdominal pain, dry mouth, thirst, polyuria), *rebound hyperacidity* and milk-alkali syndrome (hypercalcemia, alkalosis, renal damage with calcium carbonate used as an antacid)
- Local: *Local irritation*, severe necrosis, sloughing and abscess formation (IM, SC use of calcium chloride)

## Clinically important drug-drug interactions

• Decreased serum levels of oral tetracyclines, salicylates, iron salts with oral calcium salts. Give these drugs at least 1 h apart. • Increased serum levels of quinidine and possible toxicity with calcium salts • Antagonism of effects of verapamil with calcium.

## Clinically important drug-food interactions

• Decreased absorption if oral calcium when taken concurrently with oxalic acid (found in rhubarb and spinach), phytic acid (bran and whole cereals), phosphorus (milk and dairy products).

## Drug-lab test interferences

• False-negative values for serum and urinary magnesium

## ■ Nursing Considerations

### Assessment

- *History:* Allergy to calcium; renal calculi; hypercalcemia; ventricular fibrillation during cardiac resuscitation; digitalis toxicity
- *Physical:* Injection site; P, auscultation, BP, peripheral perfusion, ECG; abdominal exam, bowel sounds, mucous membranes; serum electrolytes, urinalysis

### Implementation

- Give drug hourly for first 2 wk when treating acute peptic ulcer. During healing stage, administer 1–3 h after meals and hs.
- Do not administer oral drugs within 1–2 h of antacid administration.
- Have patient chew antacid tablets thoroughly before swallowing; follow with a glass of water or milk.
- Give calcium carbonate antacid 1 and 3 h after meals and hs.
- Avoid extravasation of IV injection; it irritates the tissues and can cause necrosis and sloughing. Use a small needle in a large vein.
- Have patient remain recumbent for a short time after IV injection.
- Administer into ventricular cavity during cardiac resuscitation, not into myocardium.
- Warm calcium gluconate if crystallization has occurred.
- Monitor serum phosphorus levels periodically during long-term oral therapy.
- Monitor cardiac response closely during parenteral treatment with calcium.

### Drug-specific teaching points

*Parenteral Calcium*

- Report any pain or discomfort at the injection site as soon as possible.

*Oral Calcium*

- Take drug between meals and at bedtime. Ulcer patients must take drug as prescribed. Chew tablets thoroughly before swallowing, and follow with a glass of water or milk.
- Do not take with other oral drugs. Absorption of those medications can be blocked; take other oral medications at least 1–2 h after calcium carbonate.
- The following side effects may occur: constipation (can be medicated), nausea, GI upset, loss of appetite (special dietary consultation may be necessary).
- Report loss of appetite; nausea, vomiting, abdominal pain, constipation; dry mouth, thirst, increased voiding.

## capreomycin sulfate

*(kap ree oh **mye'** sin)*

Capastat Sulfate

**Pregnancy Category C**

### Drug classes

Antituberculous drug ("third line")
Antibiotic

### Therapeutic actions

Polypeptide antibiotic; mechanism of action against *Mycobacterium tuberculosis* unknown.

### Indications

- Treatment of pulmonary tuberculosis that is not responsive to first-line antituberculosis agents but is sensitive to capreomycin in conjunction with other antituberculosis agents

### Contraindications/cautions

- Contraindications: allergy to capreomycin; renal insufficiency; preexisting auditory impairment.
- Use caution if lactating.

### Dosage

**Available Forms:** Powder for injection—1 g/10 ml

Always give in combination with other antituberculosis drugs.

**Adult:** 1 g daily (not to exceed 20 mg/kg per day) IM for 60–120 d, followed by 1 g IM two to three times weekly for 18–24 mo.

**Pediatric:** 15 mg/kg/d (maximum 1 g) has been recommended.

GERIATRIC OR RENAL IMPAIRED

| Creatinine Clearance (ml/min) | Dose (mg/kg) at the following intervals 24h | 48h | 72h |
|---|---|---|---|
| 0 | 1.29 | 2.58 | 3.87 |
| 10 | 2.43 | 4.87 | 7.3 |
| 20 | 3.58 | 7.16 | 10.7 |
| 30 | 4.72 | 9.45 | 14.2 |
| 40 | 5.87 | 11.7 | |
| 50 | 7.01 | 14 | |
| 60 | 8.16 | | |
| 80 | 10.4 | | |
| 100 | 12.7 | | |
| 110 | 13.9 | | |

### Pharmacokinetics

| Route | Onset | Peak | Duration |
|---|---|---|---|
| IM | 20–30 min | 1–2 h | 8–12 h |

*Metabolism:* $T_{1/2}$: 4–6 h
*Distribution:* Crosses placenta; may pass into breast milk
*Excretion:* Urine

### Adverse effects

- CNS: *Ototoxicity*
- GI: Hepatic dysfunction
- Hematologic: Leukocytosis, leukopenia, eosinophilia, hypokalemia
- GU: *Nephrotoxicity*
- Hypersensitivity: Urticaria, skin rashes, fever
- Local: Pain, induration at injection sites, sterile abscesses

### Clinically important drug-drug interactions

• Increased nephrotoxicity and ototoxicity if used with similarly toxic drugs • Increased risk of peripheral neuromuscular blocking action with nondepolarizing muscle relaxants (atracurium, gallamine, metocurine iodide, pancuronium, tubocurarine, vecuronium)

## ■ Nursing Considerations

### Assessment

- *History:* Allergy to capreomycin; renal insufficiency; auditory impairment; lactation
- *Physical:* Skin color, lesions; T; orientation, reflexes, affect, audiometric measurement, vestibular function tests; liver evaluation; liver and renal function tests, CBC, serum $K^+$

### Implementation

- Arrange for culture and sensitivity studies before use.
- Administer this drug only when other forms of therapy have failed.
- Administer only in conjunction with other antituberculous agents to which the mycobacteria are susceptible.
- Prepare solution by dissolving in 2 ml of 0.9% Sodium Chloride Injection or Sterile Water for Injection; allow 2–3 min for dissolution. To administer 1 g, use entire vial—if less than 1 g is needed, see the manufacturer's instructions for dilution. Reconstituted solution may be stored for 48 h at room temperature or 14 d refrigerated. Solution may acquire a straw color and darken with time; this is not associated with loss of potency.
- Administer by deep IM injection into a large muscle mass.
- Arrange for audiometric testing and assessment of vestibular function, renal function tests, and serum potassium before and at regular intervals during therapy.

### Drug-specific teaching points

- This drug must be given by IM injection.
- Take this drug regularly; avoid missing doses. *Do not* discontinue this drug without first consulting your physician.
- The following side effects may occur: dizziness, vertigo, loss of hearing (avoid injury).
- Arrange to have regular, periodic medical checkups, including blood.
- Report skin rash, loss of hearing, decreased urine output, palpitations.

## captopril

***(kap' toe pril)***

Apo-Capto (CAN), Capoten, Novo-Captopril (CAN), Nu-Capto (CAN), Syn-Captopril (CAN)

**Pregnancy Category C**

### Drug classes
Antihypertensive
Angiotensin-converting enzyme (ACE) inhibitor

### Therapeutic actions
Blocks ACE from converting angiotensin I to angiotensin II, a powerful vasoconstrictor, leading to decreased blood pressure, decreased aldosterone secretion, a small increase in serum potassium levels, and sodium and fluid loss; increased prostaglandin synthesis also may be involved in the antihypertensive action.

### Indications
- Treatment of hypertension alone or in combination with thiazide-type diuretics
- Treatment of CHF in patients unresponsive to conventional therapy; used with diuretics and digitalis
- Treatment of diabetic nephropathy
- Treatment of left ventricular dysfunction after MI
- Unlabeled uses: management of hypertensive crises; treatment of rheumatoid arthritis; diabetic nephropathy, diagnosis of anatomic renal artery stenosis, hypertension related to scleroderma renal crisis; diagnosis of primary aldosteronism, idiopathic edema; Bartter's syndrome; Raynaud's syndrome; hypertension of Takayasu's disease

### Contraindications/cautions
- Allergy to captopril; impaired renal function; CHF; salt/volume depletion, lactation.

### Dosage
**Available Forms:** Tablets—12.5, 25, 50, 100 mg

**ADULT**

- *Hypertension:* 25 mg PO bid or tid; if satisfactory response is not noted within 1–2 wk, increase dosage to 50 mg bid–tid; usual range is 25–150 mg bid–tid PO with a mild thiazide diuretic. Do not exceed 450 mg/d.
- *CHF:* 6.25–12.5 mg PO tid in patients who may be salt/volume depleted. Usual initial dose is 25 mg PO tid; maintenance dose of 50–100 mg PO tid. Do not exceed 450 mg/d. Use in conjuction with diuretic and digitalis therapy.
- *Left ventricular dysfunction after MI:* 50 mg PO tid, starting as early as 3 days post MI. Initial dose of 6.25 mg, then 12.5 mg tid, increasing slowly to 50 mg tid.
- *Diabetic nephropathy:* 25 mg PO tid.

**PEDIATRIC:** Safety and efficacy not established.

**GERIATRIC AND RENAL IMPAIRED:** Excretion is reduced in renal failure; use smaller initial dose; titrate at smaller doses with 1- to 2-wk intervals between increases; slowly titrate to smallest effective dose. Use a loop diuretic with renal dysfunction.

### Pharmacokinetics

| Route | Onset | Peak |
|---|---|---|
| Oral | 15 min | 1/2–1 1/2 h |

*Metabolism:* $T_{1/2}$: 2 h
*Distribution:* Crosses placenta; passes into breast milk
*Excretion:* Urine

### Adverse effects
- CV: *Tachycardia*, angina pectoris, **MI**, Raynaud's syndrome, CHF, hypotension in salt/volume depleted patients
- GI: *Gastric irritation*, *aphthous ulcers, peptic ulcers, dysgeusia*, cholestatic jaundice, hepatocellular injury, anorexia, constipation
- Hematologic: Neutropenia, agranulocytosis, thrombocytopenia, hemolytic anemia, **fatal pancytopenia**
- GU: *Proteinuria*, renal insufficiency, renal failure, polyuria, oliguria, urinary frequency
- Dermatologic: *Rash, pruritus,* pemphigoid-like reaction, scalded mouth sensation, exfoliative dermatitis, photosensitivity, alopecia
- Other: *Cough,* malaise, dry mouth, lymphadenopathy

### Clinically important drug-drug interactions
• Increased risk of hypersensitivity reactions with allopurinal • Decreased antihypertensive effects with indomethacin

### Clinically important drug-food interactions
• Decreased absorption of captopril with food

### Drug-lab test interferences
• False-positive test for *urine acetone*

## ■ Nursing Considerations

### Assessment
• *History:* Allergy to captopril, impaired renal function, CHF, salt/volume depletion, pregnancy, lactation
• *Physical:* Skin color, lesions, turgor; T; P, BP, peripheral perfusion; mucous membranes, bowel sounds, liver evaluation; urinalysis, renal and liver function tests, CBC and differential

### Implementation
• Administer 1 h before or 2 h after meals.
• Alert surgeon and mark patient's chart with notice that captopril is being taken; the angiotensin II formation subsequent to compensatory renin release during surgery will be blocked; hypotension may be reversed with volume expansion.
• Monitor patient closely for fall in BP secondary to reduction in fluid volume (excessive perspiration and dehydration, vomiting, diarrhea); excessive hypotension may occur.
• Reduce dosage in patients with impaired renal function.

### Drug-specific teaching points
• Take drug 1 h before or 2 h after meals; do not take with food. Do not stop without consulting your physician.
• The following side effects may occur: GI upset, loss of appetite, change in taste perception (limited effects, will pass); mouth sores (frequent mouth care may help); skin rash; fast heart rate; dizziness, lightheadedness (usually passes after the first few days; change position slowly, and limit your activities to those that do not require alertness and precision).
• Be careful of drop in blood pressure (occurs most often with diarrhea, sweating, vomiting, dehydration); if lightheadedness or dizziness occurs, consult your care provider.
• Avoid OTC medications, especially cough, cold, allergy medications that may contain ingredients that will interact with it.
• Report mouth sores; sore throat, fever, chills; swelling of the hands, feet; irregular heartbeat, chest pains; swelling of the face, eyes, lips, tongue, difficulty breathing.

C

## carbamazepine

*(kar ba **maz'** e peen)*

Apo-Carbamazepine (CAN), Atretol, Carbatrol, Epitol, Novo-Carbamaz (CAN), Tegretol, Tegretol-XR

**Pregnancy Category C**

### Drug classes
Antiepileptic agent

### Therapeutic actions
Mechanism of action not understood; antiepileptic activity may be related to its ability to inhibit polysynaptic responses and block post-tetanic potentiation. Drug is chemically related to the tricyclic antidepressants (TCAs).

### Indications
• Refractory seizure disorders: partial seizures with complex symptoms (psychomotor, temporal lobe epilepsy), generalized tonic-clonic (grand mal) seizures, mixed seizure patterns or other partial or generalized seizures. Reserve for patients unresponsive to other agents with seizures difficult to control or who are experiencing marked side effects, such as excessive sedation
• Trigeminal neuralgia (tic douloureux): treatment of pain associated with true trigeminal neuralgia; also beneficial in glossopharyngeal neuralgia
• Unlabeled uses: neurogenic diabetes insipidus; certain psychiatric disorders, including bipolar disorders, schizoaffective illness, resistant schizophrenia, and dyscontrol syndrome associated with limbic system dysfunction; alcohol withdrawal

## Contraindications/cautions

- Contraindications: hypersensitivity to carbamazepine or TCAs; history of bone marrow depression; concomitant use of MAOIs, lactation.
- Use cautiously with history of adverse hematologic reaction to any drug (increased risk of severe hematologic toxicity); glaucoma or increased intraocular pressure; history of cardiac, hepatic, or renal damage; psychiatric patients (may activate latent psychosis).

## Dosage

**Available Forms:** Tablets—200 mg; chewable tablets—100 mg; ER tablets—100, 200, 400 mg; ER capsule; suspension—100 mg/5 ml

Individualize dosage; a low initial dosage with gradual increase is advised.

### Adult

- *Epilepsy:* Initial dose of 200 mg PO bid on the first day; increase gradually by up to 200 mg/d in divided doses q6–8h, until best response is achieved. Do not exceed 1200 mg/d in patients >15 y; doses up to 1600 mg/d have been used in adults (rare). *Maintenance:* adjust to minimum effective level, usually 800–1200 mg/d.
- *Trigeminal neuralgia:* Initial dose of 100 mg PO bid on the first day; may increase by up to 200 mg/d, using 100-mg increments q12h as needed. Do not exceed 1200 mg/d. **Maintenance:** control of pain can usually be maintained with 400–800 mg/d (range 200–1200 mg/d). Attempt to reduce the dose to the minimum effective level or to discotinue the drug at least once every 3 mo.
- *Combination therapy:* When added to existing antiepileptic therapy, do so gradually while other antiepileptics are maintained or discontinued.

### Pediatric

- *Children >12 y:* Use adult dosage. Do not exceed 1000 mg/d in patients 12–15 y; 1200 mg/d in patients >15 y.
- *Children 6–12 y:* Initial dose is 100 mg PO bid on the first day. Increase gradually by adding 100 mg/d at 6- to 8-h intervals until best response is achieved. Do not exceed 1000 mg/d. Dosage also may be calculated on the basis of 20–30 mg/kg per day in divided doses tid–qid.
- *Children <6 y:* Safety and efficacy not established.

**Geriatric:** Use caution; drug may cause confusion, agitation.

## Pharmacokinetics

| Route | Onset | Peak |
|---|---|---|
| Oral | Slow | 4–5 h |

*Metabolism:* Hepatic; $T_{1/2}$: 25–65 h, then 12–17 h

*Distribution:* Crosses placenta; passes into breast milk

*Excretion:* Urine and feces

## Adverse effects

- CNS: *Dizziness, drowsiness, unsteadiness,* disturbance of coordination, confusion, headache, fatigue, visual hallucinations, depression with agitation, behavioral changes in children, talkativeness, speech disturbances, abnormal involuntary movements, paralysis and other symptoms of cerebral arterial insufficiency, peripheral neuritis and paresthesias, tinnitus, hyperacusis, blurred vision, transient diplopia and oculomotor disturbances, nystagmus, scattered punctate cortical lens opacities, conjunctivitis, ophthalmoplegia, fever, chills; syndrome of inappropriate antidiuretic hormone (SIADH)
- GI: *Nausea, vomiting,* gastric distress, abdominal pain, diarrhea, constipation, anorexia, dryness of mouth or pharynx, glossitis, stomatitis; abnormal liver function tests, cholestatic and hepatocellular jaundice, **fatal hepatitis, fatal massive hepatic cellular necrosis with total loss of intact liver tissue**
- CV: CHF, aggravation of hypertension, hypotension, syncope and collapse, edema, primary thrombophlebitis, recurrence of thrombophlebitis, aggravation of

CAD, arrhythmias and AV block; **fatal CV complications**

- Respiratory: Pulmonary hypersensitivity characterized by fever, dyspnea, pneumonitis or pneumonia
- Hematologic: **Potentially fatal hematologic disorders**
- GU: Urinary frequency, acute urinary retention, oliguria with hypertension, renal failure, azotemia, impotence, proteinuria, glycosuria, elevated BUN, microscopic deposits in urine
- Dermatologic: Pruritic and erythematous rashes, urticaria, Stevens-Johnson syndrome, photosensitivity reactions, alterations in pigmentation, exfoliative dermatitis, alopecia, diaphoresis, erythema multiforme and nodosum, purpura, aggravation of lupus erythematosus

### Clinically important drug-drug interactions

• Increased serum levels and manifestations of toxicity with erythromycin, troleandomycin, cimetidine, danazol, isoniazid, propoxyphene, verapamil; dosage of carbamazepine may need to be reduced (reductions of about 50% recommended with erythromycin) • Increased CNS toxicity with lithium • Increased risk of hepatotoxicity with isoniazid (MAOI); because of the chemical similarity of carbamazepine to the TCAs and because of the serious adverse interaction of TCAs and MAOIs, discontinue MAOIs for minimum of 14 d before carbamazepine administration • Decreased absorption with charcoal • Decreased serum levels and decreased effects of carbamazepine with barbiturates • Increased metabolism but no loss of seizure control with phenytoin, primidone • Increased metabolism of phenytoin, valproic acid • Decreased anticoagulant effect of warfarin, oral anticoagulants; dosage of warfarin may need to be increased during concomitant therapy but decreased if carbamazepine is withdrawn • Decreased effects of nondepolarizing muscle relaxants, haloperidol • Decreased antimicrobial effects of doxycycline

## ■ Nursing Considerations

### Assessment

- ***History:*** Hypersensitivity to carbamazepine or TCAs; history of bone marrow depression; concomitant use of MAOIs; history of adverse hematologic reaction to any drug; glaucoma or increased intraocular pressure; history of cardiac, hepatic, or renal damage; pychiatric history; lactation
- ***Physical:*** Weight; T; skin color, lesions; palpation of lymph glands; orientation, affect, reflexes; ophthalmologic exam (including tonometry, funduscopy, slit lamp exam); P, BP, perfusion; auscultation; peripheral vascular exam; R, adventitious sounds; bowel sounds, normal output; oral mucous membranes; normal urinary output, voiding pattern; CBC including platelet, reticulocyte counts and serum iron; hepatic function tests, urinalysis, BUN, thyroid function tests, EEG

### Implementation

- Use only for classifications listed. Do not use as a general analgesic. Use only for epileptic seizures that are refractory to other safer agents.
- Give drug with food to prevent GI upset.
- Reduce dosage, discontinue, or substitute other antiepileptic medication gradually. Abrupt discontinuation of all antiepileptic medication may precipitate status epilepticus.
- Arrange for frequent liver function tests; discontinue drug immediately if hepatic dysfunction occurs.
- Arrange for patient to have CBC, including platelet, reticulocyte counts, and serum iron determination, before initiating therapy; repeat weekly for the first 3 mo of therapy and monthly thereafter for at least 2–3 y. Discontinue drug if there is evidence of marrow suppression, as follows:

| | |
|---|---|
| Erythrocytes | $<4$ million/mm$^3$ |
| Hematocrit | $<32\%$ |
| Hemoglobin | $<11$ g/100 ml |
| Leukocytes | $<4000$/mm$^3$ |
| Platelets | $<100{,}000$/mm$^3$ |
| Reticulocytes | $<0.3\%$ (20,000/mm$^3$) |
| Serum iron | 150 g/100 ml |

- Arrange for frequent eye exams, urinalysis, and BUN determinations.
- Arrange for frequent monitoring of serum levels of carbamazepine and other antiepileptic drugs given concomitantly, especially during the first few weeks of therapy. Adjust dosage on basis of data and clinical response.
- Counsel women who wish to become pregnant.
- Evaluate for therapeutic serum levels (usually 4–12 $\mu$g/ml).

### Drug-specific teaching points

- Take drug with food as prescribed.
- Do not discontinue this drug abruptly or change dosage, except on the advice of your physician.
- Avoid alcohol, sleep-inducing, or OTC drugs; these could cause dangerous effects.
- Arrange for frequent checkups, including blood tests, to monitor your response to this drug. Keep all appointments for checkups.
- Use contraceptive techniques at all times; if you wish to become pregnant, you should consult your physician.
- The following side effects may occur: drowsiness, dizziness, blurred vision (avoid driving or performing other tasks requiring alertness or visual acuity); GI upset (take the drug with food or milk, eat frequent small meals).
- Wear a medical alert tag at all times so that any emergency medical personnel will know that you are an epileptic taking antiepileptic medication.
- Report bruising, unusual bleeding, abdominal pain, yellowing of the skin or eyes, pale feces, darkened urine, impotence, CNS disturbances, edema, fever, chills, sore throat, mouth ulcers, skin rash, pregnancy.

## carbenicillin indanyl sodium

*(kar ben i **sill'** in)*

Geocillin, Geopen Oral (CAN)

**Pregnancy Category B**

### Drug classes

Antibiotic

Penicillin with extended spectrum

### Therapeutic actions

Bactericidal: inhibits synthesis of cell wall of sensitive organisms, causing cell death.

### Indications

- UTIs caused by susceptible strains of *Escherichia coli, Proteus mirabilis, Morganella morganii, Providencia rettgeri, Proteus vulgaris, Pseudomonas, Enterobacter*, and enterococci
- Treatment of prostatitis due to susceptible strains of *E. coli, Streptococcus faecalis, P. mirabilis, Clostridium Enterobacter*

### Contraindications/cautions

- Contraindications: allergies to penicillins, cephalosporins, or other allergens.
- Use cautiously with renal disorders, lactation (may cause diarrhea or candidiasis in the infant).

### Dosage

ADULT

- ***UTIs caused by E. coli, Proteus, Enterobacter***: 382–764 mg PO qid.
- ***UTIs caused by Pseudomonas, Enterococci***: 764 mg qid PO.

PEDIATRIC: Safety and efficacy not established.

### Pharmacokinetics

| *Route* | *Onset* | *Peak* |
|---|---|---|
| Oral | Varies | 1 h |

*Metabolism:* $T_{1/2}$: 60–70 min

*Distribution:* Crosses placenta; passes into breast milk

*Excretion:* Urine

### Adverse effects

- CNS: Lethargy, hallucinations, seizures, decreased reflexes
- GI: *Glossitis, stomatitis, gastritis, sore mouth*, furry tongue, black "hairy" tongue, *nausea, vomiting, diarrhea*, abdominal pain, bloody diarrhea, enterocolitis, pseudomembranous colitis, nonspecific hepatitis

- **Hematologic**: Anemia, thrombocytopenia, leukopenia, neutropenia, prolonged bleeding time, hemorrhagic episodes at high doses
- GU: Nephritis: oliguria, proteinuria, hematuria, casts, azotemia, pyuria
- **Hypersensitivity reactions:** *Rash, fever, wheezing,* anaphylaxis
- Other: *Superinfections*: oral and rectal moniliasis, vaginitis

**Clinically important drug-drug interactions**

• Increased bleeding effects if taken in high doses with heparin, oral anticoagulants • Decreased effectiveness with tetracyclines • Decreased activity of gentamicin, tobramycin, kanamycin, neomycin, amikacin, netilimicin, streptomycin • Decreased efficacy of oral contraceptives is possible

**Clinically important drug-food interactions**

• Decreased absorption and decreased serum levels with food

## ■ Nursing Considerations

### Assessment

- *History:* Allergies to penicillins, cephalosporins, or other allergens; renal disorders; lactation
- *Physical:* Culture infected area; skin color, lesion; R, adventitious sounds; bowel sounds; CBC, liver and renal function tests, serum electrolytes, hematocrit, urinalysis

### Implementation

- Give on an empty stomach, 1 h before or 2 h after meals, with a full glass of water. Do not give with fruit juice or soft drinks.
- Continue treatment for 10 d.

### Drug-specific teaching points

- Take drug around the clock as prescribed; take the full course of therapy, usually 10 d.
- Take the drug on an empty stomach, 1 h before or 2 h after meals, with a full glass of water.
- This antibiotic is specific for this infection and should not be used to self-treat other infections.
- The following side effects may occur: stomach upset, nausea, diarrhea, mouth sores.
- Report unusual bleeding or bruising, fever, chills, sore throat, hives, rash, severe diarrhea, difficulty breathing.

## carboplatin

***(kar' boe pla tin)***

Paraplatin

**Pregnancy Category D**

**Drug classes**

Alkylating agent
Antineoplastic

**Therapeutic actions**

Cytotoxic: heavy metal that produces cross-links within and between strands of DNA, thus preventing cell replication; cell cycle nonspecific.

**Indications**

- Palliative treatment of patients with ovarian carcinoma recurrent after prior chemotherapy, including patients who have been treated with cisplatin
- Unlabeled uses: alone or with other agents to treat small-cell lung cancer, squamous cell cancer of the head and neck, endometrial cancer, relapsed or refractory acute leukemia, seminoma of testicular cancer

**Contraindications/cautions**

- Contraindications: history of severe allergic reactions to carboplatin, cisplatin, platinum compounds, mannitol; severe bone marrow depression; pregnancy, lactation.
- Use caution in renal impairment.

### Dosage

**Available Forms:** Powder for injection—50, 150, 450 mg

ADULT

- *As a single agent:* 360 mg/$m^2$ IV on day 1 every 4 wk. Do not repeat single doses of carboplatin until the neutrophil count is at least 2,000/$mm^3$ and the platelet count is at least 100,000/mm$^3$. The following adjustment of dosage can be used: platelets > 100,00 and neutrophils > 2,000—dosage 125% prior course; platelets 100,000 and neutrophils 2,000—no adjustment in dosage; platelets < 50,000 and neutophils < 500—dosage 75% of previous course. Doses > 125% are not recommended.

*PEDIATRIC:* Safety and efficacy not established.

*GERIATRIC AND RENAL IMPAIRED:* Increased risk of bone marrow depression with renal impairment. Use caution.

| *Creatinine Clearance (ml/min)* | *Dose (mg/m$^2$ on day 1)* |
|---|---|
| 41–59 | 250 |
| 16–40 | 200 |
| ≥14 | No data available |

### Pharmacokinetics

| *Route* | *Onset* | *Duration* |
|---|---|---|
| IV | Rapid | 48–96 h |

*Metabolism:* $T_{1/2}$: 1.2–2 h, then 2.6–5.9 h
*Distribution:* Crosses placenta; may pass into breast milk
*Excretion:* Urine

### IV facts

**Preparation:** Immediately before use, reconstitute the content of each vial with Sterile Water for Injection, 5% Dextrose in Water, or Sodium Chloride Injection. For a concentration of 10 mg/ml, combine 50-mg vial with 5 ml of diluent, 150-mg vial with 15 ml of diluent, or 450-mg vial with 45 ml of diluent. Carboplatin can be further diluted using 5% Dextrose in Water or Sodium Chloride Injection. Store unopened vials at room temperature. Protect from exposure to light. Reconstituted solution is stable for 8 h at room temperature. Discard after 8 h. Do not use needles of IV administration sets that contain aluminum; carboplatin cam precipitate and lose effectiveness when in contact with aluminum.

**Infusion:** Administer by slow infusion lasting >15 min.

### Adverse effects

- CNS: *Peripheral neuropathies*, ototoxicity, visual disturbances, change in taste perception
- GI: *Vomiting, nausea, abdominal pain, diarrhea, constipation*
- Hematologic: **Bone marrow depression**, *decreased serum sodium, magnesium, calcium, potassium*
- GU: *Increased BUN* or *serum creatinine*
- Hypersensitivity: *Anaphylactic-like reaction,* rash, urticaria, erythema, pruritis, brochospasm
- Other: *Pain, alopecia, asthenia,* cancer

### Clinically important drug-drug interactions

- Decreased potency of carboplatin and precipitate formation in solution using needles or administration sets containing aluminum

## ■ Nursing Considerations

### Assessment

- *History:* Severe allergic reactions to carboplatin, cisplatin, platinum compounds, mannitol; severe bone marrow depression; renal impairment; pregnancy, lactation
- *Physical:* Weight, skin, and hair evaluation; eighth cranial nerve evaluation; reflexes; sensation; CBC, differential; renal function tests; serum electrolytes; serum uric acid; audiogram

### Implementation

- Evaluate bone marrow function before and periodically during therapy. Do not give next dose if bone marrow depression is marked. Consult physician for dosage.
- Maintain epinephrine, corticosteroids, and antihistamines on standby in case of anaphylatic-like reactions, which may occur with minutes of administration.
- Arrange for an antiemetic if nausea and vomiting are severe.

### Drug-specific teaching points

- This drug can only be given IV. Prepare a calendar of treatment days.
- The following side effects may occur: nausea, vomiting (medication may be ordered; small, frequent meals also may help); numbness, tingling, loss of taste, ringing in ears, dizziness, loss of hearing; rash, loss of hair (obtain a wig).
- Use birth control while on this drug. This drug may cause birth defects or miscarriages.
- Have frequent, regular medical follow-up, including frequent blood tests to monitor drug effects.
- Report loss of hearing, dizziness; unusual bleeding or bruising; fever, chills, sore throat; leg cramps, muscle twitching; changes in voiding patterns; difficulty breathing.

## carboprost tromethamine

*(kar' boe prost)*
Hemabate
**Pregnancy Category C**

### Drug classes

Prostaglandin
Abortifacient

### Therapeutic actions

Stimulates the myometrium of the gravid uterus to contract in a manner that is similar to the contractions of the uterus during labor, thus evacuating the contents of the gravid uterus.

### Indications

- Termination of pregnancy 13–20 wk from the first day of the last menstrual period
- Evacuation of the uterus in instance of missed abortion or intrauterine fetal death in the second trimester
- Postpartum hemmorhage due to uterine atony unresponsive to conventional methods

### Contraindications/cautions

- Contraindications: allergy to prostaglandin preparations; acute PID; active cardiac, hepatic, pulmonary, renal disease.
- Use cautiously with history of asthma; hypotension; hypertension; cardiovascular, adrenal, renal, or hepatic disease; anemia; jaundice; diabetes; epilepsy; scarred uterus; cervicitis, infected endocervical lesions; acute vaginitis.

### Dosage

**Available Forms:** Injection—250 μg/ml

ADULT

- ***Abortion:*** 250 μg (1 ml) IM; give 250 μg IM at 1 1/2- to 3 1/2-h intervals, depending on uterine response; may be increased to 500 μg if uterine contractility is inadequate after several 250-μg doses; do not exceed 12 mg total dose or continuous administration over 2 d.
- ***Refractory postpartum uterine bleeding:*** 250 μg IM as one dose; in some cases, multiple doses at 15- to 90-min intervals may be used; do not exceed a total dose of 2 mg (8 doses)

### Pharmacokinetics

| Route | Onset | Peak |
|---|---|---|
| IM | 15 min | 2 h |

*Metabolism:* Hepatic and lung; $T_{1/2}$: 8 h
*Distribution:* Crosses placenta; passes into breast milk
*Excretion:* Urine

### Adverse effects

- CNS: Headache, paresthesias, *flushing*, anxiety, weakness, syncope, dizziness
- GI: Vomiting, diarrhea, *nausea*
- CV: *Hypotension*, arrhythmias, chest pain
- **Respiratory**: Coughing, dyspnea
- GU: Endometritis, perforated uterus, uterine rupture, uterine/vaginal pain, incomplete abortion
- **Other**: Chills, diaphoresis, backache, breast tenderness, eye pain, skin rash, pyrexia

## ■ Nursing Considerations

### Assessment

- ***History:*** Allergy to prostaglandin preparations; acute PID; active cardiac, he-

patic, pulmonary, renal disease; history of asthma; hypotension; hypertension; anemia; jaundice; diabetes; epilepsy; scarred uterus; cervicitis, infected endocervical lesions; acute vaginitis
- *Physical:* T; BP, P, auscultation; R, adventitious sounds; bowel sounds, liver evaluation; vaginal discharge, pelvic exam, uterine tone; liver and renal function tests, WBC, urinalysis, CBC

### Implementation
- Refrigerate unopened vials. Stable at room temperature for 9 d.
- Administer a test dose of 100 μg (0.4 ml) prior to abortion if indicated.
- Administer by deep IM injection.
- Arrange for pretreatment or concurrent treatment with antiemetic and antidiarrheal drugs to decrease the incidence of GI side effects.
- Ensure that abortion is complete or that other measures are used to complete the abortion if drug effects are not sufficient.
- Monitor T, using care to differentiate prostaglandin-induced pyrexia from postabortion endometritis pyrexia.
- Monitor uterine tone and vaginal discharge during procedure and several days after to assess drug effects and recovery.
- Ensure adequate hydration throughout procedure.

### Drug-specific teaching points
- Several IM injections may be required to achieve desired effect.
- The following side effects may occur: nausea, vomiting, diarrhea, uterine/vaginal pain, fever, headache, weakness, dizziness.
- Report severe pain, difficulty breathing, palpitations, eye pain, rash.

## carisoprodol

*(kar eye soe **proe'** dol)*

isomeprobamate

Soma

**Pregnancy Category C**

### Drug classes
Centrally acting skeletal muscle relaxant

### Therapeutic actions
Precise mechanism not known; chemically related to meprobamate, an antianxiety drug; has sedative properties; also found in animal studies to inhibit interneuronal activity in descending reticular formation and spinal cord; does not directly relax tense skeletal muscles.

### Indications
- Relief of discomfort associated with acute, painful musculoskeletal conditions as an adjunct to rest, physical therapy, and other measures

### Contraindications/cautions
- Allergic or idiosyncratic reactions to carisoprodol, meprobamate (reported cross-reactions with meprobamate); acute intermittent porphyria, suspected porphyria, lactation.

### Dosage
**Available Forms:** Tablets—350 mg

*ADULT:* 350 mg PO tid–qid; take last dose hs.

*PEDIATRIC:* Not recommended for children <12 y.

*GERIATRIC PATIENTS OR THOSE WITH HEPATIC OR RENAL IMPAIRMENT:* Dosage reduction may be necessary; monitor closely.

### Pharmacokinetics

| *Route* | *Onset* | *Peak* | *Duration* |
|---|---|---|---|
| Oral | 30 min | 1–2 h | 4–6 h |

*Metabolism:* Hepatic; $T_{1/2}$: 8 h

*Distribution:* Crosses placenta; passes into breast milk

*Excretion:* Urine

### Adverse effects
- CNS: *Dizziness, drowsiness, vertigo, ataxia, tremor, agitation, irritability*
- GI: Nausea, vomiting, hiccups, epigastric distress
- CV: Tachycardia, postural hypotension, facial flushing

- Hypersensitivity: **Allergic or idiosyncratic reactions** (seen with first to fourth dose in patients new to drug): skin rash, erythema multiforme, pruritus, eosinophila, fixed drug eruption; asthmatic episodes, fever, weakness, dizziness, angioneurotic edema, smarting eyes, hypotension, anaphylactoid shock

## ■ Nursing Considerations

### Assessment

- *History:* Allergic or idiosyncratic reactions to carisoprodol, meprobamate; acute intermittent porphyria, suspected porphyria; lactation
- *Physical:* T; skin color, lesions; orientation, affect; P, BP, orthostatic BP; bowel sounds, liver evaluation; liver and kidney function tests, CBC

### Implementation

- Reduce dose with liver dysfunction.

### Drug-specific teaching points

- Take this drug exactly as prescribed; do not take a higher dosage.
- Avoid alcohol, sleep-inducing, or OTC drugs; these could cause dangerous effects; if you feel you need one of these preparations, consult your health care provider.
- The following side effects may occur: drowsiness, dizziness, vertigo (avoid driving or activities that require alertness); dizziness when you get up or climb stairs (avoid sudden changes in position, use caution climbing stairs); nausea (take drug with food, eat frequent small meals); insomnia, headache, depression (transient effects).
- Report skin rash, severe nausea, dizziness, insomnia, fever, difficulty breathing.

## carmustine

*(car **mus'** teen)*

BCNU

BiCNU, Gliadel, Gliadel

**Pregnancy Category D**

### Drug classes

Alkylating agent, nitrosourea

Antineoplastic

### Therapeutic actions

Cytotoxic: alkylates DNA and RNA and inhibits several enzymatic processes, leading to cell death.

### Indications

Palliative therapy alone or with other agents for the following:

- Brain tumors: glioblastomas, brainstem glioma, medullablastoma, astrocytoma, ependymoma, metastatic brain tumors
- Hodgkin's disease and non-Hodgkin's lymphomas (as secondary therapy)
- Multiple myeloma (with prednisolone)
- Treatment of recurrent glioblastoma as implantable wafer after removal of tumor (Gliadel)
- Unlabeled use: Treatment of mycosis fungoides

### Contraindications/cautions

- Allergy to carmustine; radiation therapy; chemotherapy; hematopoietic depression; impaired renal or hepatic function; pregnancy (teratogenic, and embryotoxic); lactation.

### Dosage

**Available Forms:** Powder for injection—100 mg; wafer (Gliadel)—7.7 mg

Do not give doses more often than every 6 wk because of delayed bone marrow toxicity.

**ADULT AND PEDIATRIC:** As single agent in untreated patients: 150–200 mg/m² IV every 6 wk as a single dose or in divided daily injections (75–100 mg/m² on 2 successive d). Do not repeat dose until platelets > 100,000/mm³, leukocytes > 4,000/mm³, adjust dosage after initial dose based on hematologic response, as follows:

| *Leukocytes* | *Platelets* | *Percentage of Prior Dose to Give* |
|---|---|---|
| >4000 | >100,000 | 100% |
| 3000–3999 | 75,000–99,999 | 100% |
| 2000–2999 | 25,000–74,999 | 70% |
| <2000 | <25,000 | 50% |

### Pharmacokinetics

| Route | Onset | Peak |
|---|---|---|
| IV | Immediate | 15 min |

*Metabolism:* Hepatic; $T_{1/2}$: 15–30 min
*Distribution:* Crosses placenta; passes into breast milk
*Excretion:* Urine and lungs (10%)

### IV facts

**Preparation:** Reconstitute with 3 ml of supplied sterile diluent, then add 27 ml of Sterile Water for Injection to the alcohol solution; resulting solution contains 3.3 mg/ml of carmustine in 10% ethanol, pH is 5.6–6.0; may be further diluted with Sodium Chloride Injection or 5% Dextrose Injection. Refrigerate unopened vials. Protect reconstituted solution from light; lacking preservatives, solution decomposes with time. Check vials before use for absence of oil film residue; if present, discard vial.

**Infusion:** Administer reconstituted solution by IV drip over 1–2 h; shorter infusion time may cause intense pain and burning.

### Adverse effects

- CNS: Ocular toxicity: nerve fiber-layer infarcts, retinal hemorrhage
- GI: *Nausea, vomiting, stomatitis,* hepatotoxicity
- **Respiratory:** *Pulmonary infiltrates,* fibrosis
- **Hematologic:** *Myelosuppression, leukopenia, thrombocytopenia, anemia* (delayed for 4–6 wk)
- GU: Renal toxicity: decreased renal size, azotemia, renal failure
- **Other:** *Local burning at site of injection*; intense flushing of the skin, suffusion of the conjunctiva with rapid IV infusion; cancer

### Clinically important drug-drug interactions

• Increased toxicity and myelosuppression with cimetidine • Decreased serum levels of digoxin, phenytoin

## ■ Nursing Considerations

### Assessment

- ***History:*** Allergy to carmustine; radiation therapy; chemotherapy; hematopoietic depression; impaired renal or hepatic function; pregnancy; lactation
- ***Physical:*** T; weight; ophthamologic exam; R, adventitious sounds; mucous membranes, liver evaluation; CBC, differential; urinalysis, liver and renal function tests; pulmonary function tests

### Implementation

- Evaluate hematopoietic function before therapy and weekly during and for at least 6 wk after therapy.
- Do not give full dosage within 2–3 wk after a full course of radiation therapy or chemotherapy because of the risk of severe bone marrow depression; reduced dosage may be needed.
- Reduce dosage in patients with depressed bone marrow function.
- Arrange for pretherapy medicating with antiemetic to decrease the severity of nausea and vomiting.
- Monitor injection site for any adverse reaction; accidental contact of carmustine with the skin can cause burning and hyperpigmentation of the area.
- Monitoring ophthalmologic status.
- Monitor urine output for volume and any sign of renal failure.
- Monitor liver, renal, and pulmonary function tests.

### Drug-specific teaching points

- This drug can only be given IV.
- The following side effects may occur: nausea, vomiting, loss of appetite (an antiemetic may be ordered; eat small frequent meals); increased susceptibility to infection (avoid exposure to infection by avoiding crowded places, avoid injury).
- Maintain your fluid intake and nutrition.
- Use birth control; this drug can cause severe birth defects.
- Report unusual bleeding or bruising; fever, chills, sore throat; stomach or flank pain; changes in vision; difficulty

breathing, shortness of breath; burning or pain at IV injection site.

## carteolol hydrochloride

*(**kar'** tee oh lole)*

Cartrol

**Pregnancy Category C**

### Drug classes

Beta adrenergic blocker
Antihypertensive

### Therapeutic actions

Blocks beta-adrenergic receptors of the sympathetic nervous system in the heart and juxtaglomerular apparatus (kidney), thus decreasing the excitability of the heart, decreasing cardiac output and oxygen consumption, decreasing the release of renin from the kidney, and lowering blood pressure.

### Indications

- Management of hypertension, alone as a Step 1 agent, or with other drugs, particularly a thiazide diuretic.
- Unlabeled use: prophylaxis for angina attacks

### Contraindications/cautions

- Contraindications: sinus bradycardia (HR > 45 beats per minute), second- or third-degree heart block (PR interval > 0.24 sec), cardiogenic shock, CHF, asthma, COPD, lactation.
- Use cautiously with diabetes or thyrotoxicosis, hepatic impairment, renal failure.

### Dosage

**Available Forms:** Tablets—2.5, 5 mg

**ADULT:** Initially 2.5 mg as a single daily oral dose, alone or with a diuretic. If inadequate, gradually increase to 5–10 mg as a single daily dose. Doses > 10 mg are not likely to produce further benefit and may decrease response. *Maintenance:* 2.5–5 mg PO qd.

**PEDIATRIC:** Safety and efficacy not established.

**GERIATRIC OR IMPAIRED RENAL FUNCTION:** Because bioavailability increases twofold, lower doses may be required. Creatinine clearance of > 60 ml/min, administer q24h; creatinine clearance of 20–60 ml/min, administer q48h; creatinine clearance of < 30 ml/min, administer q72h.

C

### Pharmacokinetics

| *Route* | *Onset* | *Peak* | *Duration* |
|---|---|---|---|
| Oral | Varies | 1–3 h | 24–48 h |

*Metabolism:* Hepatic; $T_{1/2}$: 6 h
*Distribution:* Crosses placenta; passes into breast milk
*Excretion:* Urine

### Adverse effects

- CNS: Dizziness, vertigo, tinnitus, fatigue, emotional depression, paresthesias, sleep disturbances, hallucinations, disorientation, memory loss, slurred speech (carteolol is less lipid-soluble than propranolol; it is less likely to penetrate the blood–brain barrier and cause CNS effects)
- GI: *Gastric pain, flatulence, constipation, diarrhea, nausea, vomiting,* anorexia,
- CV: *Bradycardia, CHF, cardiac arrhythmias, sinoartial or AV nodal block, tachycardia,* peripheral vascular insufficiency, claudication, CVA, pulmonary edema, hypotension
- Respiratory: **Bronchospasm,** dyspnea, cough, bronchial obstruction, nasal stuffiness, rhinitis
- GU: *Impotence, decreased libido,* Peyronie's disease, dysuria, nocturia, frequent urination
- MS: Joint pain, arthralgia, muscle cramp
- EENT: Eye irritation, dry eyes, conjunctivitis, blurred vision
- Dermatologic: Rash, pruritus, sweating, dry skin
- Allergic: Pharyngitis, erythematous rash, fever, sore throat, **laryngospasm, respiratory distress**
- Other: *Decreased exercise tolerance, development of antinuclear antibodies,* hyperglycemia or hypoglycemia, elevated serum transaminase

**Clinically important drug-drug interactions**

• Increased effects with verapamil • Decreased effects of theophyllines and carteolol if taken concurrently • Increased risk of postural hypotension with prazosin • Possible increased blood pressure-lowering effects with aspirin, bismuth subsalicylate, magnesium salicylate, sulfinpyrazone • Decreased antihypertensive effects with NSAIDs, clonidine • Possible increased hypoglycemic effect of insulin • Initial hypertensive episode followed by bradycardia if combined with epinephrine • Peripheral ischemia and possible gangrene if combined with ergot alkaloids

**Drug-lab test interferences**

• Monitor for possible false results with glucose or insulin tolerance tests.

## ■ Nursing Considerations

### Assessment

- *History:* Arrhythmias, cardiogenic shock, CHF, asthma, COPD, pregnancy, lactation, diabetes or thyrotoxicosis
- *Physical:* Weight, skin condition, neurologic status, P, BP, ECG, respiratory status, kidney and thyroid function, blood and urine glucose

### Implementation

- Give carteolol once a day. Monitor response and maintain at lowest possible dose.
- Do not discontinue drug abruptly after chronic therapy (hypersensitivity to catecholamines may have developed, causing exacerbation of angina, MI, and ventricular dysrhythmias); taper drug gradually over 2 wk with monitoring).
- Consult with physician about withdrawing drug if patient is to undergo surgery (withdrawal is controversial).

### Drug-specific teaching points

- Take drug with meals.
- Do not stop taking this drug unless told to by a health care provider.
- Avoid driving or dangerous activities if dizziness, weakness occur.
- The following side effects may occur: dizziness, lightheadedness, loss of appetite, nightmares, depression, sexual impotence.
- Report difficulty breathing, night cough, swelling of extremities, slow pulse, confusion, depression, rash, fever, sore throat.

## carvedilol

*(kar vah' da lol)*

Coreg

**Pregnancy Category C**

**Drug classes**

Alpha/Beta adrenergic blocker
Antihypertensive

**Therapeutic actions**

Competitively blocks $\alpha_1$ and $\beta_1$- and $\beta_2$-adrenergic receptors, and has some sympathomimetic activity at $\beta_2$-receptors. Both alpha and beta blocking actions contribute to the BP-lowering effect; beta blockade prevents the reflex tachycardia seen with most alpha-blocking drugs and decreases plasma renin activity. Significantly reduces plasma renin activity.

**Indications**

- Hypertension, alone or with other oral drugs, especially diuretics
- Treatment of mild to moderate CHF of ischemic or cardiomyopathic origin with digitalis, diuretics, ACE inhibitors
- Unlabeled uses: angina, idiopathic cardiomyopathy

**Contraindications/cautions**

- Contraindications: decompensated CHF, bronchial asthma, heart block, cardiogenic shock, hypersensitivity to carvedilol, pregnancy, lactation.
- Use cautiously with hepatic impairment, peripheral vascular disease, thyrotoxicosis, diabetes, anesthesia or major surgery.

### Dosage

**Available Forms:** Tablets—3.125, 6.25, 12.5, 25 mg

**ADULT**

- *Hypertension:* 6.25 mg PO bid; maintain for 7–14 d, then increase to 12.5 mg PO bid if needed to control BP. Do not exceed 50 mg/d.
- *CHF:* Monitor patient very closely, individualize dose based on patient response.

Initial dose: 3.125 mg PO bid for 2 wk, may then be increased to 6.25 mg PO bid. Maximum dose: 25 mg PO bid in patients <85 kg or 50 mg PO bid in patients >85 kg.

PEDIATRIC: Safety and efficacy not established.

HEPATIC IMPAIRMENT: Do not administer to any patient with severe hepatic impairment.

### Pharmacokinetics

| *Route* | *Onset* | *Peak* | *Duration* |
|---|---|---|---|
| Oral | Rapid | 30 min | 8–10 h |

*Metabolism:* Hepatic; $T_{1/2}$: 7–10 h
*Distribution:* Crosses placenta; enters breast milk
*Excretion:* Bile, feces

### Adverse effects

- CNS: *Dizziness, vertigo, tinnitus, fatigue,* emotional depression, paresthesias, sleep disturbances
- GI: *Gastric pain, flatulence, constipation, diarrhea,* **hepatic failure**
- CV: *Bradycardia, orthostatic hypertension,* CHF, cardiac arrhythmias, pulmonary edema, hypotension
- Respiratory: *Rhinitis,* pharyngitis, dyspnea
- Other: *Fatigue,* back pain, infections

### Clinically important drug-drug interactions

• Increased effectiveness of antidiabetic agents; monitor blood glucose and adjust dosages appropriately • Increased effectiveness of clonidine; monitor patient for potential severe bradycardia and hypotension • Increased serum levels of digoxin; monitor serum levels and adjust dose accordingly • Increased plasma levels of carvedilol with rifampin • Potential for dangerous conduction system disturbances with verapamil or diltiazem; if this combination is used, closely monitor ECG and BP

### Clinically important drug-food interactions

• Slowed rate of absorption, but not decreased effectiveness with food

## ■ Nursing Considerations

### Assessment

- *History:* CHF, bronchial asthma, heart block, cardiogenic shock, hypersensitivity to carvedilol, pregnancy, lactation, hepatic impairment, peripheral vascular disease, thyrotoxicosis, diabetes, anesthesia or major surgery
- *Physical:* Baseline weight, skin condition, neurologic status, P, BP, ECG, respiratory status, kidney and thyroid function, blood and urine glucose, liver function tests

### Implementation

- Do not discontinue drug abruptly after chronic therapy (hypersensitivity to catecholamines may have developed, causing exacerbation of angina, MI and ventricular dysrhythmias); taper drug gradually over 2 wk with monitoring.
- Consult with physician about withdrawing drug if patient is to undergo surgery (withdrawal is controversial).
- Give with food to decrease orthostatic hypotension and adverse effects.
- Monitor for orthostatic hypotension and provide safety precautions.
- Monitor patient for any sign of liver dysfunction (pruritus, dark urine or stools, anorexia, jaundice, pain); arrange for liver function tests and discontinue drug if tests indicate liver injury. Do not restart carvedilol.

### Drug-specific teaching points

- Take drug with meals.
- Do not stop taking drug unless instructed to do so by a health care provider.
- Avoid use of OTC medications.
- The following side effects may occur: dizziness, lightheadedness, depression (avoid driving or performing dangerous activities; getting up and changing positions slowly may help ease dizziness).
- Report difficulty breathing, swelling of extremities, changes in color of stool or urine, very slow heart rate, continued dizziness.

# cefaclor

*(sef' a klor)*
Ceclor, Ceclor CD
**Pregnancy Category B**

## Drug classes
Antibiotic
Cephalosporin (first generation)

## Therapeutic actions
Bactericidal: inhibits synthesis of bacterial cell wall, causing cell death.

## Indications
- Lower respiratory tract infections caused by *Streptococcus pneumoniae, Haemophilus influenzae, S. pyogenes*
- Upper respiratory infections caused by *S. pyogenes*
- Dermatologic infections caused by *Staphylococcus aureus, S. pyogenes*
- UTIs caused by *E. coli, P. mirabilis, Klebsiella,* coagulase-negative staphylococci
- Otitis media caused by *S. pneumoniae, H. influenzae, S. pyogenes,* staphylococci
- Unlabeled use: acute uncomplicated UTI in select patients, single 2-g dose

## Contraindications/cautions
- Allergy to cephalosporins or penicillins; renal failure; lactation

## Dosage
**Available Forms:** Capsules—250, 500 mg; ER tablets—375, 500 mg; powder for suspension—125 mg/5 ml, 187 mg/5 ml, 250 mg/5 ml, 375 mg/5 ml

*Adult:* 250 mg PO q8h; dosage may be doubled in severe cases. **Do not exceed 4 g/d.**

*Pediatric:* 20 mg/kg per day PO in divided doses q8h; in severe cases 40 mg/kg per day may be given. **Do not exceed 1 mg/d.**

- ***Otitis media and pharyngitis:*** Total daily dosage may be divided and administered q12h.

## Pharmacokinetics

| Route | Peak | Duration |
|---|---|---|
| PO | 30–60 min | 8–10h |

*Metabolism:* $T_{1/2}$: 30–60 min
*Distribution:* Crosses the placenta; enters breast milk
*Excretion:* Renal, unchanged

## Adverse effects
- CNS: Headache, dizziness, lethargy, paresthesias
- GI: *Nausea, vomiting, diarrhea, anorexia, abdominal pain, flatulence, pseudomembranous colitis*, liver toxicity
- **Hematologic: Bone marrow depression**
- GU: Nephrotoxicity
- **Hypersensitivity:** *Ranging from rash, fever* to *anaphylaxis*; serum sickness reaction
- Other: *Superinfections*

## Clinically important drug-drug interactions
• Increased nephrotoxicity with aminoglycosides • Increased bleeding effects with oral anticoagulants • Disulfiram-like reaction may occur if alcohol is taken within 72 h after cefaclor administration.

## Drug-lab test interferences
• Possibility of false results on tests of urine glucose using Benedict's solution, Fehling's solution, Clinitest tablets; urinary 17-ketosteroids; direct Coombs' test.

## ■ Nursing Considerations

### Assessment
- ***History:*** Penicillin or cephalosporin allergy, pregnancy or lactation
- ***Physical:*** Kidney function, respiratory status, skin status, culture and sensitivity tests of infected area

### Implementation
- Culture infection before drug therapy.
- Give drug with meals or food to decrease GI discomfort.
- Refrigerate suspension after reconstitution, and discard after 14 d.
- Discontinue drug if hypersensitivy reaction occurs.

- Give patient yogurt or buttermilk in case of diarrhea.
- Arrange for oral vancomycin for serious colitis that fails to respond to discontinuation of drug.

### Drug-specific teaching points

- Take this drug with meals or food.
- Complete the full course of this drug, even if you feel better.
- This drug is prescribed for this particular infection; do not self-treat any other infection.
- The following side effects may occur: stomach upset, loss of appetite, nausea (take drug with food); diarrhea; headache, dizziness.
- Report severe diarrhea with blood, pus, or mucus; rash or hives; difficulty breathing; unusual tiredness, fatigue; unusual bleeding or bruising.

## cefadroxil

*(sef a **drox'** ill)*
Duricef
**Pregnancy Category B**

### Drug classes

Antibiotic
Cephalosporin (first generation)

### Therapeutic actions

Bactericidal: inhibits the formation of bacterial cell wall, causing the cell's death.

### Indications

- UTIs caused by *E. coli, P. mirabilis, Klebsiella*
- Pharyngitis, tonsillitis caused by group A $\beta$-hemolytic streptococci
- Dermatologic infections caused by staphylococci, streptococci

### Contraindications/cautions

- Allergy to cephalosporins or penicillins, renal failure, lactation

### Dosage

**Available Forms:** Capsules—500 mg; tablets—1 g; oral suspension—125, 250, 500 mg/5 ml

ADULT

- *UTIs:* 1–2 g/d PO in single or two divided doses for uncomplicated lower UTIs. For all other UTIs, 2 g/d in two divided doses.
- *Dermatologic infections:* 1 g/d PO in single or two divided doses.
- *Pharyngitis, tonsillitis caused by group A $\beta$-hemolytic streptococci:* 1 g/d PO in single or two divided doses for 10 d.

PEDIATRIC

- *UTIs, dermatologic infections:* 30 mg/kg per day PO in divided doses q12h.
- *Pharyngitis, tonsillitis caused by group A $\beta$ -hemolytic streptococci:* 30 mg/kg per day in single or two divided doses, continue for 10 d.

GERIATRIC OR IMPAIRED RENAL FUNCTION: 1 g PO loading dose, followed by 500 mg PO at the following intervals:

| Creatinine Clearance (ml/min) | Interval (hours) |
|---|---|
| 0–10 | 36 |
| 10–25 | 24 |
| 25–50 | 12 |
| >50 | Usual adult dosage |

### Pharmacokinetics

| Route | Peak | Duration |
|---|---|---|
| PO | 1.5–2 h | 20–22 h |

*Metabolism:* $T_{1/2}$: 78–96 min
*Distribution:* Crosses the placenta; enters breast milk
*Excretion:* Renal

### Adverse effects

- CNS: Headache, dizziness, lethargy, paresthesias
- GI: *Nausea, vomiting, diarrhea, anorexia, abdominal pain, flatulence,* **pseudomembranous colitis**, liver toxicity
- Hematologic: Bone marrow depression
- GU: Nephrotoxicity
- Hypersensitivity: *Ranging from rash* to *fever* to **anaphylaxis**; serum sickness reaction
- Other: *Superinfections*

### Clinically important drug-drug interactions

• Decreased bactericidal activity if used with bacteriostatic agents • Increased serum levels of cephalosporins if used with probenecid

### Drug-lab test interferences

• False-positive urine glucose using Benedict's solution, Fehling's solution, Clinitest tablets • False-positive direct Coombs' test • Falsely elevated urinary 17-ketosteroids

## ■ Nursing Considerations

### Assessment

- ***History:*** Penicillin or cephalosporin allergy, pregnancy or lactation
- ***Physical:*** Kidney function, respiratory status, skin status, culture and sensitivity tests of infected area

### Implementation

- Culture infection before drug therapy.
- Give drug with meals or food to decrease GI discomfort.
- Refrigerate suspension after reconstitution, and discard after 14 d; shake refrigerated suspension well before using.
- Discontinue if hypersensitivy reaction occurs.
- Give the patient yogurt or buttermilk in case of diarrhea.
- Arrange for oral vancomycin for serious colitis that fails to respond to discontinuation of drug.

### Drug-specific teaching points

- Take this drug only for this infection; do not use to self-treat other problems.
- Refrigerate the suspension, and discard unused portion after 14 d; shake suspension well before each use.
- The following side effects may occur: stomach upset, loss of appetite, nausea (take drug with food), diarrhea, headache, dizziness.
- Report severe diarrhea with blood, pus, or mucus; skin rash; difficulty breathing; unusual tiredness, fatigue; unusual bleeding or bruising.

# cefamandole nafate

*(sef a **man'** dole)*

Mandole

**Pregnancy Category B**

### Drug classes

Antibiotic

Cephalosporin (second generation)

### Therapeutic actions

Bactericidal: inhibits synthesis of bacterial cell wall and causes cell death.

### Indications

- Lower respiratory tract infections caused by *S. pneumoniae, S. aureus,* group A $\beta$-hemolytic streptococci, *Klebsiella, H. influenzae, P. mirabilis*
- Dermatologic infections caused by *S. aureus, S. pyogenes, E. coli, P. mirabilis, H. influenzae, Enterobacter* species
- UTIs caused by *E. coli, Proteus* species, *Klebsiella, Enterobacter* species, *S. epidermidis,* group D streptococci
- Septicemia caused by *S. pneumoniae, S. aureus,* group A $\beta$-hemolytic streptocci, *E. coli, H. infuenzae*
- Peritonitis caused by *E. coli, Enterobacter* species
- Bone and joint infections caused by *S. aureus*
- Mixed infections with many organisms isolated
- Perioperative prophylaxis

### Contraindications/cautions

- Allergy to cephalosporins or penicillins, renal failure, pregnancy, lactation.

### Dosage

**Available Forms:** Powder for injection—1 g

*ADULT:* 500 mg–1 g IM or IV q4–8h, depending on severity of infection.

- ***Acute UTI:*** 500 mg q8h to 1 g q8h, IM or IV.
- ***Severe infections:*** 1 g q4–6h, up to 2 g q4h, IM or IV.
- ***Perioperative prophylaxis:*** 1–2 g IM or IV 1/2–1 h prior to initial incision; 1–2 g q6h for 24 h after surgery.
- ***Prosthetic arthroplasty:*** Continue above doses for 72 h.

- *Cesarean section:* Give first dose just prior to clamping or after cord is clamped.

PEDIATRIC: 50–100 mg/kg per day IM or IV in equally divided doses q4–8h. Up to 150 mg/kg per day in severe infections.

- *Perioperative prophylaxis:* 50–100 mg/kg per day IM or IV in equally divided doses, starting 1/2–1 h before initial incision and continuing for 24 h after surgery.

GERIATRIC OR IMPAIRED RENAL FUNCTION: IM loading dose of 1–2 g. Maintenance dosages are as follows:

| Creatinine Clearance (ml/min) | Severe Infection | Less Severe Infection |
|---|---|---|
| >80 | 2 g q4h | 1.2 g q6h |
| 50–80 | 1.4 g q4h or 2 g q6h | 0.75–1.5 g q6h |
| 25–50 | 1.5 g q6h or 2 g q8h | 0.75–1.5 g q8h |
| 10–25 | 1 g q6h or 1.25 g q8h | 0.5–1 g q8h |
| 2–10 | 0.67 g q8h or 1 g q12h | 0.5–0.75 g q12h |
| <2 | 0.5 g q8h or 0.75 g q12h | 0.25–0.5 g q12h |

### Pharmacokinetics

| Route | Peak | Duration |
|---|---|---|
| IM | 30–120 min | 6–8 h |
| IV | 10 min | 6–8 hs |

*Metabolism:* $T_{1/2}$: 30–60 min

*Distribution* : Crosses the placenta; enters breast milk

*Excretion:* Renal

### IV facts

**Preparation:** Dilute each gram of drug with 10 ml of Sterile Water for Injection, 5% Dextrose Injection, or 0.9% Sodium Chloride Injection, or add drug to IV solutions of 5% Dextrose Injection; 5% or 10% Dextrose and 0.2%, 0.45%, or 0.9% Sodium Chloride Injection; or Sodium Lactate Injection (M/6). To give by continuous IV infusion, dilute each gram with 10 ml Sterile Water for Injection; may be added to IV container of above solutions. Stable for 96 h if refrigerated, 24 h at room temperature.

**Infusion:** By intermittent IV injections, inject slowly over 3–5 min. If using a piggy-back IV setup, discontinue the other solution while cefamandole is being given. If given as part of combination therapy with aminoglycosides, give each antibiotic at a different site.

**Incompatibilities:** Do not mix aminoglycosides and cefamandole in the same IV solution.

C

### Adverse effects

- CNS: Headache, dizziness, lethargy, paresthesias
- GI: *Nausea, vomiting, diarrhea, anorexia, abdominal pain, flatulence,* **pseudomembranous colitis**, liver toxicity
- Hematologic: Bone marrow depression
- GU: Nephrotoxicity
- Hypersensitivity: *Ranging from rash* to *fever* to **anaphylaxis;** serum sickness reaction
- Other: *Superinfections, pain*, abscess (redness, tenderness, heat, tissue sloughing), inflammation at injection site, *phlebitis, disulfiram-like reaction with alcohol*

### Clinically important drug-drug interactions

• Increased nephrotoxicity with aminoglycosides • Increased bleeding effects with oral anticoagulants • Disulfiram-like reaction may occur if alcohol is taken within 72 h after cefamandole administration.

### Drug-lab test interferences

• False results of urine glucose using Benedict's solution, Fehling's solution, Clinitest tablets; urinary 17-ketosteroids; direct Coombs' test.

## ■ Nursing Considerations

### Assessment

- *History:* Penicillin or cephalosporin allergy, pregnancy or lactation

- *Physical:* Kidney function, respiratory status, skin status, culture and sensitivity tests of infected area, injection site

### Implementation

- Culture infection, arrange for sensitivity tests before drug therapy.
- Dilute each gram with 3 ml Sterile Water for Injection, Bacteriostatic Water for Injection, 0.9% Sodium Chloride Injection, or Bacteriostatic Sodium Chloride Injection for IM use. Shake well until dissolved.
- Reconstituted solution is stable for 24 h at room temperature or 4 d if refrigerated.
- Discontinue if hypersensitivy reaction occurs.
- Have vitamin K available in case hypoprothrombinemia occurs.

### Drug-specific teaching points

- Do not use alcohol while on this drug and for 3 d after, because severe reactions often occur.
- The following side effects may occur: stomach upset, loss of appetite, nausea (take drug with food); diarrhea; headache, dizziness.
- Report severe diarrhea, difficulty breathing, unusual tiredness or fatigue, pain at injection site.

## cefazolin sodium

*(sef a' zoe lin)*

Ancef (CAN), Gen-Cefazolin (CAN), Kefzol, Zolicef

**Pregnancy Category B**

### Drug classes

Antibiotic

Cephalosporin (first generation)

### Therapeutic actions

Bactericidal: inhibits synthesis of bacterial cell wall and causes cell death.

### Indications

- Respiratory tract infections caused by *S. pneumoniae, S. aureus*, group A $\beta$-hemolytic streptococci, *Klebsiella, H. influenzae*
- Dermatologic infections caused by *S. aureus*, group A $\beta$-hemolytic streptococci, other strains of streptococci
- GU infections caused by *E. coli, P. mirabilis, Klebsiella,* sensitive strains of *Enterobacter*, and enterococci
- Biliary tract infections caused by *E. coli*, streptococci, *P. mirabilis, Klebsiella, S. aureus*
- Septicemia caused by *S. pneumoniae, S. aureus, E. coli, P. mirabilis, Klebsiella*
- Bone and joint infections caused by *S. aureus*
- Endocarditis caused by *S. aureus,* group A $\beta$-hemolytic streptococci
- Perioperative prophylaxis

### Contraindications/cautions

- Allergy to cephalosporins or penicillins, renal failure, lactation

### Dosage

**Available Forms:** Powder for injection—250, 500 mg; 1, 5, 10, 20 g

*ADULT:* 250–500 mg IM or IV q4–8h.

- ***Moderate to severe infection:*** 500 mg–1 g IM or IV q6–8h.
- ***Life-threatening infections:*** 1–1.5 g IM or IV q6h.
- ***Acute UTI:*** 1 g IM or IV q12h.
- ***Perioperative prophylaxis:*** 1 g IV 1/2–1 h prior to initial incision; 0.5–1 g IV or IM during surgery at appropriate intervals; 0.5–1 g IV or IM q6–8h for 24 h after surgery. Prophylactic treatment may be continued for 3–5 d.

*PEDIATRIC*

- ***Mild infections:*** 25–50 mg/kg per day IM or IV in three to four equally divided doses.
- ***Severe infections:*** Increase total daily dose to 100 mg/kg IM or IV. Adjust dosage for impaired renal function (see package insert for details).
- ***Premature infants and infants <1 mo:*** Safety and efficacy not established.
- ***Perioperative prophylaxis:*** Adjust dose according to body weight or age (see Appendix III for formulas).

*GERIATRIC OR IMPAIRED RENAL FUNCTION:* IV or IM loading dose of 500 mg; maximum maintenance dosages are as follows:

| *Creatinine Clearance (ml/min)* | *Mild to Moderate Infection* | *Severe Infection* |
|---|---|---|
| ≥55 | 250–500 mg q6–8h | 500–1000 mg q6–8h |
| 35–54 | 250–500 mg q8h | 500–1000 mg q12h |
| 11–34 | 125–250 mg q12h | 250–500 mg q12h |
| ≤10 | 125–250 mg q18–24h | 250–800 mg q18–24h |

**Pharmacokinetics**

| *Route* | *Onset* | *Peak* | *Duration* |
|---|---|---|---|
| IM | 30 min | 1.5–2 h | 6–8 h |
| IV | Immediate | 5 min | 6–8 h |

*Metabolism:* $T_{1/2}$: 90–120 min
*Distribution:* Crosses the placenta; enters breast milk
*Excretion:* Renal, unchanged

**IV facts**

**Preparation:** Use a volume control set or separate piggy-back container. Dilute reconstituted 500 mg–1 g of cefazolin in 50–100 ml of 0.9% Sodium Chloride Injection; 5% or 10% Dextrose Injection; 5% Dextrose in Lactated Ringer's Injection; 5% Dextrose and 0.2%, 0.45%, or 0.9% Sodium Chloride Injection; Lactated Ringer's Injection; 5% or 10% Invert Sugar in Sterile Water for Injection; 5% Sodium Bicarbonate in Sterile Water for Injection; Ringer's Injection; Normosol-M in D5-W; Ionosol B with Dextrose 5%; Plasma-Lyte with 5% Dextrose. For direct IV injection as follows: dilute reconstituted 500 mg–1 g cefazolin with at least 10 ml of Sterile Water for Injection. Shake well until dissolved. Stable for 24 h at room temperature.

**Infusion:** By direct IV injection, inject slowly over 3–5 min; by infusion give each g over at least 5 min.

**Incompatibilities:** If given as part of combination therapy with aminoglycosides, give each antibiotic at a different site. **Do not mix aminoglycosides and cefazolin in the same IV solution.**

**Adverse effects**

- CNS: Headache, dizziness, lethargy, paresthesias
- GI: *Nausea, vomiting, diarrhea, anorexia, abdominal pain, flatulence,* **pseudomembranous colitis**, liver toxicity
- Hematologic: Bone marrow depression
- GU: Nephrotoxicity
- Hypersensitivity: *Ranging from rash* to *fever* to **anaphylaxis;** serum sickness reaction
- Other: *Superinfections, pain,* abscess (redness, tenderness, heat, tissue sloughing), inflammation at injection site, *phlebitis, disulfiram-like reaction with alcohol*

**Clinically important drug-drug interactions**

• Increased nephrotoxicity with aminoglycosides • Increased bleeding effects with oral anticoagulants • Disulfiram-like reaction may occur if alcohol is taken within 72 h of cefazolin administration.

**Drug-lab test interferences**

• False results of urine glucose using Benedict's solution, Fehling's solution, Clinitest tablets; urinary 17-ketosteroids; direct Coombs' test.

## ■ Nursing Considerations

### Assessment

- *History::* Penicillin or cephalosporin allergy, pregnancy or lactation
- *Physical::* Kidney function, respiratory status, skin status; culture and sensitivity tests of infected area, injection site

### Implementation

- Culture infection, arrange for sensitivity tests before drug therapy.
- Reconstitute for IM use using Sterile Water for Injection, Bacteriostatic Water for Injection, or 0.9% Sodium Chloride Injection as follows:

| Vial Size | Diluent to Add | Available Volume | Concentration |
|---|---|---|---|
| 250 mg | 2 ml | 2 ml | 125 mg/ml |
| 500 mg | 2 ml | 2.2 ml | 225 mg/ml |
| 1 g | 2.5 ml | 3 ml | 330 mg/ml |

- Inject IM doses deeply into large muscle group.
- Solution is stable for 24 h at room temperature or 4 d if refrigerated; redissolve by warming to room temperature and agitating slightly.
- Have vitamin K available in case hypoprothrombinemia occurs.

### Drug-specific teaching points

- Do not use alcohol while on this drug and for 3 d after because severe reactions often occur.
- The following side effects may occur: stomach upset, loss of appetite, nausea (take drug with food); diarrhea; headache, dizziness.
- Report severe diarrhea, difficulty breathing, unusual tiredness or fatigue, pain at injection site.

## cefepime hydrochloride

*(sef' ah pime)*

Maxipime

**Pregnancy Category B**

### Drug classes

Antibiotic

Cephalosporin (third generation)

### Therapeutic actions

Bactericidal: inhibits synthesis of bacterial cell wall, causing cell death.

### Indications

- Urinary tract infections caused by *E. coli, P. mirabilis, Klebsiella, K. pneumoniae*
- Pneumonia caused by *S. pneumoniae, Pseudomonas aeruginosa, K. pneumoniae, Enterobacter*
- Dermatologic infections caused by *S. aureus,* group or *S. pyogenes*

### Contraindications/cautions

- Contraindications: allergy to cephalosporins or penicillins; renal failure; lactation

### Dosage

**Available Forms:** Powder for injection—500 mg; 1, 2 g

ADULT: 0.5–2 g IV or IM q12h.

- ***Mild to moderate UTI:*** 0.5–1 g IM or IV q12h for 7–10 d.
- ***Severe UTI:*** 2 g IV q12h for 10 d.
- ***Moderate to severe pneumonia:*** 1–2 g IV q12h for 10 d.
- ***Moderate to severe skin infections:*** 2 g IV q12h for 10 d.

PEDIATRIC: Not recommended.

GERIATRIC OR IMPAIRED RENAL FUNCTION: Recommended starting dose as adult, then maintenance dose as follows:

| CCr (ml/min) | Mild infection | Moderate infection | Severe infection |
|---|---|---|---|
| >60 | 500 mg q12h | 1 g q12h | 2 g q12h |
| 30–60 | 500 mg q24h | 1 g q24h | 2 g q24h |
| 11–29 | 500 mg q24h | 500 mg q24h | 1 g q24h |
| <10 | 250 mg q24h | 250 mg q24h | 500 mg q24h |

### Pharmacokinetics

| Route | Onset | Peak | Duration |
|---|---|---|---|
| IM | 30 min | 1.5–2 h | 10–12 h |
| IV | Immediate | 5 min | 10–12 h |

*Metabolism:* $T_{1/2}$: 102–138 min

*Distribution:* Crosses placenta; enters breast milk

*Excretion:* Renal—unchanged

### IV facts

**Preparation:** Dilute with 50–100 ml 0.9% Sodium Chloride, 5% and 10% Dextrose Injection, M/6 Sodium Lactate Injection, 5% Dextrose and 0.9% Sodium Chloride Injection, Lactated Ringer's and 5% Dextrose Injection, *Normosol-R, Normosol-M* in 5% Dextrose Injection. Diluted solution is stable for 24 h at room temperature or up to 7 d if refrigerated. Protect from light.

**Infusion:** Infuse slowly over 30 min.
**Incompatibilities:** Do not mix with ampicillin, metronidazole, vancomycin, gentamicin, tobramycin, netilmicin, or aminophylline. If concurrent therapy is needed, administer each drug separately. If possible, do not give any other drug in same solution as cefepime.

### Adverse effects

- CNS: Headache, dizziness, lethargy, paresthesias
- GI: *Nausea, vomiting, diarrhea, anorexia, abdominal pain, flatulence,* **pseudomembranous colitis,** liver toxicity
- Hematologic: Bone marrow depression
- GU: Nephrotoxicity
- Hypersensitivity: Ranging from *rash, fever* to **anaphylaxis**; serum sickness reaction
- Other: *Superinfections, pain,* abscess (redness, tenderness, heat, tissue sloughing), inflammation at injection site, *phlebitis, disulfiram-like reaction with alcohol*

### Clinically important drug-drug interactions

• Increased nephrotoxicity with aminoglycosides; monitor renal function tests • Increased bleeding effects with oral anticoagulants; reduced dosage may be needed • Disulfiram-like reaction may occur with alcohol if taken within 72 h of cefepime administration

### Drug-lab test interferences

• False reports of urine glucose using Benedict's solution, Fehling's solution, Clinitest tablets; urinary 17-ketosteroids; direct Coombs' test

## ■ Nursing Considerations

### Assessment

- *History:* Penicillin or cephalosporin allergy; pregnancy, lactation
- *Physical:* Kidney function, respiratory status, skin status; culture and sensitivity tests of infection area, injection site

### Implementation

- Culture infected area and arrange for sensitivity tests before beginning therapy.
- Reconstitute for IM use with 0.9% Sodium Chloride, 5% Dextrose Injection, 0.5% or 1% lidocaine HCl or bacteriostatic water with parabens or benzyl alcohol. Reserve IM use for mild to moderate UTIs due to *E. coli.*
- Have vitamin K available in case hypoprothrombinemia occurs.

### Drug-specific teaching points

- Do not use alcohol while on this drug and for 3 d after drug has been stopped; severe reactions may occur.
- The following side effects may occur: stomach upset, loss of appetite, nausea (take drug with food); diarrhea (stay near bathroom); headache, dizziness.
- Report severe diarrhea, difficulty breathing, unusual tiredness or fatigue, pain at injection site.

## cefixime

*(sef* ***icks'*** *ime)*
Suprax
**Pregnancy Category B**

### Drug classes

Antibiotic
Cephalosporin (third generation)

### Therapeutic actions

Bactericidal: inhibits synthesis of bacterial cell wall, causing cell death.

### Indications

- Uncomplicated UTIs caused by *E. coli, P. mirabilis*
- Otitis media caused by *H. influenzae* (beta-lactamase positive and negative strains), *Moraxella catarrhalis, S. pyogenes*
- Pharyngitis, tonsillitis caused by *S. pyogenes*
- Acute bronchitis and acute exacerbations of chronic bronchitis caused by *S. pneumoniae, H. influenzae* (beta-lactamase positive and negative strains)

- Uncomplicated gonorrhea caused by *Neisseria gonorrhoeae*

**Contraindications/cautions**

- Allergy to cephalosporins or penicillins; renal failure; lactation

**Dosage**

**Available Forms:** Tablets—200, 400 mg; powder for oral suspension—100 mg/5 ml

*ADULT AND CHILDREN > 50 KG OR > 12 Y:* 400 mg/d PO as a single 400-mg tablet or as 200 mg q12h. For *S. pyogenes* infections, administer cefixime for at least 10 d.

*PEDIATRIC:* 8 mg/kg per day suspension as a single daily dose or as 4 mg/kg q12h. Treat otitis media with suspension; in clinical studies, the suspension resulted in higher blood levels than tablets.

*GERIATRIC OR IMPAIRED RENAL FUNCTION:*

| *Creatinine Clearance (ml/min)* | *Dosage* |
|---|---|
| >60 | Standard |
| 21–60 or on hemodialysis | 75% of standard |
| ≤20 or on continuous peritoneal dialysis | 50% of standard |

**Pharmacokinetics**

| *Route* | *Peak* |
|---|---|
| PO | 2–6 h |

*Metabolism:* $T_{1/2}$: 3–4 h
*Distribution* : Crosses the placenta; enters breast milk
*Excretion:* Renal and bile

**Adverse effects**

- CNS: Headache, dizziness, lethargy, paresthesias
- GI: *Nausea, vomiting, diarrhea, anorexia, abdominal pain, flatulence,* **pseudomembranous colitis**, liver toxicity
- Hematologic: Bone marrow depression
- GU: Nephrotoxicity
- Hypersensitivity: *Ranging from rash to fever* to **anaphylaxis**; serum sickness reaction
- Other: *Superinfections*

**Clinically important drug-drug interactions**

- Decreased bactericidal activity with bacteriostatic agents • Increased serum levels of cephalosporins with probenecid

**Drug-lab test interferences**

- False-positive urine glucose using Benedict's solution, Fehling's solution, Clinitest tablets • False-positive direct Coombs' test • Falsely elevated urinary 17-ketosteroids

## ■ Nursing Considerations

**Assessment**

- ***History:*** Penicillin or cephalosporin allergy, pregnancy or lactation
- ***Physical:*** Kidney function, respiratory status, skin status, culture and sensitivity tests of infected area

**Implementation**

- Culture infection before drug therapy.
- Shake refrigerated suspension well before using.
- Give drug with meals or food to decrease GI discomfort.
- Refrigerate suspension after reconstitution, and discard after 14 d.
- Discontinue if hypersensitivy reaction occurs.
- Give the patient yogurt or buttermilk in case of diarrhea.
- Arrange for oral vancomycin for serious colitis that fails to respond to discontinuation of drug.

**Drug-specific teaching points**

- Take this drug only for this specific infection; do not use to self-treat other problems.
- Refrigerate suspension, and discard unused portion after 14 d; shake suspension well before each use.
- The following side effects may occur: stomach upset, loss of appetite, nausea (take drug with food); diarrhea; headache, dizziness.
- Report severe diarrhea with blood, pus, or mucus; skin rash; difficulty breathing; unusual tiredness, fatigue; unusual bleeding or bruising.

## cefmetazole sodium

*(sef **met'** a zol)*
Zefazone
**Pregnancy Category B**

### Drug classes
Antibiotic
Cephalosporin (second generation)

### Therapeutic actions
Bactericidal: inhibits the formation of bacterial cell wall, causing cell death.

### Indications
- UTIs caused by *E. coli*
- Lower respiratory tract infections caused by *S. aureus, S. pneumoniae, E. coli, H. influenzae*
- Dermatologic infections caused by *S. aureus, S. epidermidis, S. pyogenes, Streptococcus agalactiae, E. coli, P. mirabilis, P. vulgaris, M. morganii, Proteus stuartii, Klebsiella pneumoniae, Klebsiella oxytoca, Bacteroides fragilis, Bacteroides melaninogenicus*
- Intra-abdominal infections caused by *E. coli, K. pneumoniae, K. oxytoca, B. fragilis, Clostridium perfringens*
- Perioperative prophylaxis for cesarean section, abdominal or vaginal hysterectomy, cholecystectomy, colorectal surgery

### Contraindications/cautions
- Allergy to cephalosporins or penicillins, renal failure, lactation

### Dosage
**Available Forms:** Powder for injection—1, 2 g

*ADULT:* 2 g IV q6–12h for 5–14 d.
- ***Perioperative prophylaxis:***
- *Vaginal hysterectomy:* 2-g single dose 30–90 min before surgery or 1-g doses 30–90 min before surgery and repeated 8 and 16 h later.
- *Abdominal hysterectomy:* 1-g doses 30–90 min before surgery and repeated 8 and 16 h later.
- *Cesarean section:* 2-g single dose after clamping cord or 1-g doses after clamping cord; repeated at 8 and 16 h later.
- *Colorectal surgery:* 2-g single dose 30–90 min before surgery or 2-g doses 30–90 min before surgery and repeated 8 and 16 h later.
- *Cholecystectomy (high risk):* 1-g doses 30–90 min before surgery and repeated 8 and 16 h later.

*PEDIATRIC:* Safety and efficacy not established.

*GERIATRIC OR IMPAIRED RENAL FUNCTION:*

| *Creatinine Clearance (ml/min)* | *Dose (g)* | *Frequency* |
|---|---|---|
| 50–90 | 1–2 | q12h |
| 30–49 | 1–2 | q16h |
| 10–29 | 1–2 | q24h |
| <10 | 1–2 | q48h |

### Pharmacokinetics

| *Route* | *Onset* | *Peak* |
|---|---|---|
| IV | Rapid | End of infusion |

*Metabolism:* $T_{1/2}$: 1.2 h
*Distribution:* Enters breast milk
*Excretion* : Urine

### IV facts
**Preparation:** Use Sterile Water for Injection, Bacteriostatic Water for Injection, or 0.9% Sodium Chloride Injection. Dilute 1 g with 3.7 ml to yield 250 mg/ml or 1 g with 10 ml to yield 100 mg/ml; 2 g diluted with 7 ml will yield 250 mg/ml, or 2 g with 15 ml yields 125 mg/ml. Primary solutions may be further diluted to concentrations of 1–20 mg/ml in 0.9% Sodium Chloride Injection, 5% Dextrose Injection, or Lactated Ringer's Injection. Stable for 24 h at room temperature, 7 d if refrigerated, or 6 wk if frozen. Do not refreeze thawed solutions; discard any unused solution.

**Infusion:** If using a piggy-back IV setup, discontinue the other solution while cefmetazole is being given. If given as part of combination therapy with aminoglycosides, give each antibiotic at a different site. Do not mix aminoglycosides and cefmetazole in the same IV solution. Direct IV infusion over 3–5 min; slow infusion over 10–60 min.

**Incompatibilites:** Do not mix in solution with aminoglycosides.

### Adverse effects

- CNS: Headache, dizziness, lethargy, paresthesias
- GI: *Nausea, vomiting, diarrhea, anorexia, abdominal pain, flatulence,* pseudomembranous colitis, liver toxicity
- **Hematologic**: bone marrow depression: decreased WBC, decreased platelets, decreased Hct
- GU: Nephrotoxicity
- **Hypersensitivity**: *Ranging from rash* to *fever* to anaphylaxis, serum sickness reaction
- **Local**: *Pain,* abscess at injection site, *phlebitis*, inflammation at IV site
- **Other**: *Superinfections, disulfiram-like reaction with alcohol*

### Clinically important drug-drug interactions

• Increased nephrotoxicity with aminoglycosides • Increased bleeding effects with oral anticoagulants • Disulfiram-like reaction may occur if alcohol is taken within 72 h after cefmetazole administration.

### Drug-lab test interferences

• Possibility of false results on tests of urine glucose using Benedict's solution, Fehling's solution, Clinitest tablets; urinary 17-ketosteroids; direct Coombs' test.

## ■ Nursing Considerations

### Assessment

- *History:* Liver and kidney dysfunction, lactation, pregnancy
- *Physical:* Skin status, liver and kidney function test, culture of affected area, sensitivity tests

### Implementation

- Have vitamin K available in case hypoprothrombinemia occurs.
- Discontinue drug if hypersensitivy reaction occurs.

### Drug-specific teaching points

- The following side effects may occur: stomach upset, diarrhea.
- Avoid alcohol while on this drug and for 3 d after because severe reactions often occur.
- Report severe diarrhea, difficulty breathing, unusual tiredness or fatigue, pain at injection site.

## cefonicid

*(se **fon'** i sid)*

Monocid

**Pregnancy Category B**

### Drug classes

Antibiotic

Cephalosporin (second generation)

### Therapeutic actions

Bactericidal: inhibits synthesis of bacterial cell wall, causing cell death.

### Indications

- Lower respiratory tract infections caused by *S. pneumoniae, K. pneumoniae, H. influenzae, E. coli*
- UTIs caused by *E. coli, Proteus* species, *K. pneumoniae*
- Dermatologic infections caused by *S. aureus, S. pyogenes, S. epidermidis, S. agalactiae*
- Septicemia caused by *S. pneumoniae, E. coli*
- Bone and joint infections caused by *S. aureus*
- Perioperative prophylaxis

### Contraindications/cautions

- Allergy to cephalosporins or penicillins, renal failure, lactation.

### Dosage

**Available Forms:** Powder for injection—500 mg; 1, 10 g (bulk vials)

**ADULT:** 1 g/d IM or IV. Up to 2 g/d may be tolerated.

- *Perioperative prophylaxis:* 1 g IV 1 h prior to initial incision; 1 g/d for 24 h after surgery.
- *Cesarean section:* Give *after* the cord is clamped.

**GERIATRIC (OR IMPAIRED RENAL FUNCTION):** Initial dose of 7.5 mg/kg IV or IM followed by:

| *Creatinine Clearance (ml/min)* | *Moderate Infections* | *Severe Infections* |
|---|---|---|
| 60–79 | 10 mg/kg q24h | 25 mg/kg q24h |
| 40–59 | 8 mg/kg q24h | 20 mg/kg q24h |
| 20–39 | 4 mg/kg q24h | 15 mg/kg q24h |
| 10–19 | 4 mg/kg q48h | 15 mg/kg q48h |
| 5–9 | 4 mg/kg q 3–5 d | 15 mg/kg q 3–5d |
| <5 | 3 mg/kg q 3–5 d | 4 mg/kg q 3–5 d |

### Pharmacokinetics

| *Route* | *Onset* | *Peak* | *Duration* |
|---|---|---|---|
| IV | Immediate | 5 min | 24 h |
| IM | 1 h | 1 h | 24 h |

*Metabolism:* $T_{1/2}$: 4.5–5.8 h
*Distribution:* Enters breast milk
*Excretion* : Urine

### IV facts

**Preparation:** Reconstitute single-dose vials as follows: 500-mg vial, add 2 ml Sterile Water for Injection (220 mg/ml concentration); 1-g vial, add 2.5 ml Sterile Water for Injection (325 mg/ml concentration). For IV infusion, add reconstituted solution to 50–100 ml of one of the following: 0.9% Sodium Chloride; 5% or 10% Dextrose Injection; 5% Dextrose and 0.2%, 0.45%, or 0.9% Sodium Chloride Injection; Ringer's Injection; Lactated Ringer's Injection; 5% Dextrose and Lactated Ringer's Injection; 10% Invert Sugar in Sterile Water for Injection; 5% Dextrose and 0.15% Potassium Chloride Injection; Sodium Lactate Injection. Reconstituted or diluted solution is stable for up to 24 h at room temperature, 72 h if refrigerated; discard unused solutions within the allotted time period.

**Infusion:** Give bolus injections slowly over 3–5 min into vein or IV tubing; for infusion, give over 30 min. If given as part of combination therapy with aminoglycosides, give each antibiotic at a different site: do not mix aminoglycosides and cefonicid in the same IV solution.

**Incompatibilities:** Incompatible in solution with aminoglycosides.

### Adverse effects

- CNS: Headache, dizziness, lethargy, paresthesias
- GI: *Nausea, vomiting, diarrhea, anorexia, abdominal pain, flatulence,* pseudomembranous colitis, liver toxicity
- **Hematologic: Bone marrow depression:** decreased WBC, decreased platelets, decreased Hct
- GU: Nephrotoxicity
- **Hypersensitivity:** *Ranging from rash* to *fever* to anaphylaxis; serum sickness reaction
- **Local:** *Pain,* abscess at injection site, *phlebitis*, inflammation at IV site
- **Other:** *Superinfections, disulfiram-like reaction with alcohol*

### Clinically important drug-drug interactions

• Increased nephrotoxicity with aminoglycosides • Increased bleeding effects with oral anticoagulants • Disulfiram-like reaction may occur if alcohol is taken within 72 h after cefonicid administration.

### Drug-lab test interferences

• Possibility of false results on tests of urine glucose using Benedict's solution, Fehling's solution, Clinitest tablets; urinary 17-ketosteroids; direct Coombs' test.

## ■ Nursing Considerations

### Assessment

- *History:* Liver and kidney dysfunction, lactation, pregnancy
- *Physical:* Skin status, liver and kidney function test, culture of affected area, sensitivity tests

### Implementation

- Culture infection, arrange for sensitivity tests before and during therapy if expected response is not seen.
- Divide IM doses of 2 g once daily and give as two equal doses deeply into two different large muscles.

- Have vitamin K available in case hypoprothrombinemia occurs.
- Discontinue drug if hypersensitivy reaction occurs.

### Drug-specific teaching points

- The following side effects may occur: stomach upset, diarrhea.
- Avoid alcohol while on this drug and for 3 d after because severe reactions often occur.
- Report severe diarrhea, difficulty breathing, unusual tiredness or fatigue, pain at injection site.

## cefoperazone sodium

*(sef oh **per'** a zone)*

Cefobid

**Pregnancy Category B**

### Drug classes

Antibiotic

Cephalosporin (third generation)

### Therapeutic actions

Bactericidal: inhibits synthesis of bacterial cell wall, causing cell death.

### Indications

- Respiratory tract infections caused by *S. pneumoniae, S. aureus, S. pyogenes, Pseudomonas aeruginosa, K. pneumoniae, H. influenzae, E. coli, Proteus, Enterobacter*
- Dermatologic infections caused by *S. aureus, S. pyogenes, P. aeruginosa*
- UTIs caused by *E. coli, P. aeruginosa*
- Septicemia caused by *S. pneumoniae, S. aureus, S. agalactiae,* enterococci, *H. influenzae, P. aeruginosa, E. coli, Klebsiella, Proteus, Clostridium,* anaerobic gram-positive cocci
- Peritonitis and intra-abdominal infections caused by *E. coli, P. aeruginosa,* anaerobic gram-positive cocci, anaerobic gram-positive and gram-negative bacilli
- Pelvic inflammatory disease, endometritis caused by *N. gonorrhoeae, S. epidermidis, S. agalactiae, E. coli, Clostridium, Bacteroides,* and anaerobic gram-positive cocci

### Contraindications/cautions

- Allergy to cephalosporins or penicillins, hepatic failure, lactation.

### Dosage

**Available Forms:** Powder for injection—1, 2 g; injection—1, 2 g

**ADULT:** 2–4 g/d IM or IV in equal divided doses q12h; up to 6–12 g/d if severe.

**PEDIATRIC:** Safety and efficacy not established.

**HEPATIC IMPAIRED:** Total daily dose of 4 g. Monitor patient carefully.

### Pharmacokinetics

| *Route* | *Onset* | *Peak* | *Duration* |
|---|---|---|---|
| IV | 5–10 min | 15–20 min | 6–12 h |
| IM | 1 h | 1–2 h | 6–12 h |

*Metabolism:* $T_{1/2}$: 1.75–2.5 h

*Distribution:* Enters breast milk

*Excretion* : Bile

### IV facts

**Preparation:** For IV infusion; concentrations of 2–50 mg/ml are recommended. Reconstitute powder for IV use in 5% or 10% Dextrose Injection; 5% Dextrose and 0.2% or 0.9% Sodium Chloride Injection; 5% Dextrose and Lactated Ringer's Injection; Lactated Ringer's Injection; 0.9% Sodium Chloride Injection; Normosol M and 5% Dextrose Injection; Normosol R. After reconstituting, allow to stand until all foaming is gone; vigorous agitation may be necessary. Reconstituted solution is stable for 24 h at room temperature or up to 5 d if refrigerated.

| *Vial Dose* | *Desired Concentration* | *Diluent to Add* | *Resulting Volume* |
|---|---|---|---|
| 1 g | 333 mg/ml | 2.6 ml | 3 ml |
| | 250 mg/ml | 3.8 ml | 4 ml |
| 2 g | 333 mg/ml | 5 ml | 6 ml |
| | 250 mg/ml | 7.2 ml | 8 ml |

**Infusion:** Administer single dose over 15–30 min, continuous infusion over 6–24 h. If using a piggy-back IV setup, discontinue the other solution while cefoperazone is being given. If given with aminoglycosides, give each at a different site.

**Incompatibilities:** Do not mix aminoglycosides and cefoperazonein the same IV solution.

**Adverse effects**

- CNS: Headache, dizziness, lethargy, paresthesias
- GI: *Nausea, vomiting, diarrhea, anorexia, abdominal pain, flatulence,* pseudomembranous colitis, liver toxicity
- **Hematologic**: Bone marrow depression: decreased WBC, decreased platelets, decreased Hct
- GU: Nephrotoxicity
- **Hypersensitivity**: *Ranging from rash* to *fever* to anaphylaxis; serum sickness reaction
- Local: *Pain,* abscess at injection site; *phlebitis,* inflammation at IV site
- Other: *Superinfections, disulfiram-like reaction with alcohol*

**Clinically important drug-drug interactions**

• Increased nephrotoxicity with aminoglycosides • Increased bleeding effects with oral anticoagulants • Disulfiram-like reaction may occur if alcohol is taken within 72 h after cefoperazone administration.

**Drug-lab test interferences**

• Possibility of false results on tests of urine glucose using Benedict's solution, Fehling's solution, Clinitest tablets; urinary 17-ketosteroids; direct Coombs' test.

## ■ Nursing Considerations

### Assessment

- *History:* Liver and kidney dysfunction, lactation, pregnancy
- *Physical:* Skin status, liver and kidney function test, culture of affected area, sensitivity tests

### Implementation

- Culture infection, arrange for sensitivity tests before and during therapy if expected response is not seen.
- Keep dosage under 4 g/d, or monitor serum concentrations in patients with liver disease or biliary obstruction.
- To prepare drug for IM use: reconstitute powder in Bacteriostatic Water for Injection, Sterile Water for Injection, or 0.5% Lidocaine HCl Injection (concentrations >250 mg/ml).
- Maintain vitamin K on standby in case hypoprothrombinemia occurs.
- Discontinue drug if hypersensitivy reaction occurs.

### Drug-specific teaching points

- The following side effects may occur: stomach upset, diarrhea.
- Avoid alcohol while on this drug and for 3 days after because severe reactions often occur.
- Report severe diarrhea, difficulty breathing, unusual tiredness or fatigue, pain at injection site.

## cefotaxime sodium

*(sef oh* ***taks'*** *eem)*

Claforan

**Pregnancy Category B**

**Drug classes**

Antibiotic

Cephalosporin (third generation)

**Therapeutic actions**

Bactericidal: inhibits synthesis of bacterial cell wall, causing cell death.

**Indications**

- Lower respiratory tract infections caused by *S. pneumoniae, S. aureus, Klebsiella, H. influenzae, E. coli, P. mirabilis, Enterobacter, Serratia marcescens, S. pyogenes*
- UTIs caused by *Enterococcus, S. epidermidis, S. aureus, Citrobacter, Enterobacter, E. coli, Klebsiella, P. mirabilis, Proteus, S. marcescens*
- Gyn infections caused by *S. epidermidis, Enterococcus, E. coli, P. mirabilis, Bacteroides, Clostridium, Peptococcus, Peptostreptococcus,* streptococci; and uncomplicated gonorrhea caused by *N. gonorrhoeae*
- Dermatologic infections caused by *S. aureus, E. coli, Serratia, Proteus, Klebsiella, Enterobacter, Pseudomonas, S. marcescens, Bacteroides, Peptococcus, Peptostreptococcus, P. mirabilis, S. epidermidis, S. pyogenes, Enterococcus*

- Septicemia caused by *E. coli, Klebsiella, S. marcescens*
- Peritonitis and intra-abdominal infections caused by *E. coli, Peptostreptococcus, Bacteroides, Peptococcus, Klebsiella*
- CNS infections caused by *E. coli, H. influenzae, Neisseria meningitidis, S. pneumoniae, K. pneumoniae*
- Bone and joint infections caused by *S. aureus*
- Perioperative prophylaxis

### Contraindications/cautions

- Allergy to cephalosporins or penicillins, renal failure, lactation.

### Dosage

**Available Forms:** Powder for injection—1, 2 g; injection—1, 2 g

ADULT: 2–8 g/d IM or IV in equally divided doses q6–8h. Do not exceed 12 g/d.

- ***Gonorrhea:*** 1 g IM in a single injection.
- ***Disseminated infection:*** 500 mg IV qid for 7 d.
- ***Gonococcal ophthalmia:*** 500 mg IV qid.
- ***Perioperative prophylaxis:*** 1 g IV or IM 30–90 min before surgery.
- ***Cesarean section:*** 1 g IV after cord is clamped and then 1 g IV or IM at 6 and 12 h.

PEDIATRIC

- ***0–1 wk:*** 50 mg/kg IV q12h.
- ***1–4 wk:*** 50 mg/kg IV q8h.
- ***1 mo–12 y (<50 kg):*** 50–180 mg/kg per day IV or IM in four to six divided doses.

GERIATRIC (OR REDUCED RENAL FUNCTION): If creatinine clearance is < 20 ml/min, reduce dosage by half.

### Pharmacokinetics

| *Route* | *Onset* | *Peak* | *Duration* |
|---|---|---|---|
| IV | Immediate | 5 min | 18–24 h |
| IM | 5–10 min | 30 min | 18–24 h |

*Metabolism:* $T_{1/2}$: 1 h

*Distribution:* Crosses the placenta; enters breast milk

*Excretion* : Urine

### IV facts

**Preparation:** Reconstitute for intermittent IV injection with 1 or 2 g with 10 ml Sterile Water for Injection. Reconstitute vials for IV infusion with 10 ml of Sterile Water for Injection. Reconstitute infusion bottles with 50 or 100 ml of 0.9% Sodium Chloride Injection or 5% Dextrose Injection. Drug solution may be further diluted with 50–100 ml of 5% or 10% Dextrose Injection; 5% Dextrose and 0.2%, 0.45%, or 0.9% Sodium Chloride Injection; Lactated Ringer's Solution; 0.9% Sodium Chloride Injection; Sodium Lactate Injection (M/6); 10% Invert Sugar. Reconstituted solution is stable for 24 h at room temperature or 5 d if refrigerated. Powder and reconstituted solution darken with storage.

**Infusion:** Inject slowly into vein over 3–5 min or over a longer time through IV tubing; give continuous infusion over 6–24 h. If administered with aminoglycosides, administer at different sites.

**Incompatibilities: Do not mix in solutions with aminoglycoside solutions.**

### Adverse effects

- CNS: Headache, dizziness, lethargy, paresthesias
- GI: *Nausea, vomiting, diarrhea, anorexia, abdominal pain, flatulence,* pseudomembranous colitis, liver toxicity
- Hematologic: Bone marrow depression: decreased WBC, decreased platelets, decreased Hct
- GU: Nephrotoxicity
- Hypersensitivity: *Ranging from rash* to *fever* to anaphylaxis; serum sickness reaction
- Local: *Pain,* abscess at injection site, *phlebitis*, inflammation at IV site
- Other: *Superinfections, disulfiram-like reaction with alcohol*

### Clinically important drug-drug interactions

• Increased nephrotoxicity with aminoglycosides • Increased bleeding effects with oral anticoagulants • Disulfiram-like reaction may occur if alcohol is used within 72 h after cefotaxime is given.

**Drug-lab test interferences**

• Possibility of false results on tests of urine glucose using Benedict's solution, Fehling's solution, Clinitest tablets; urinary 17-ketosteroids; direct Coombs' test.

## ■ Nursing Considerations

### Assessment

- *History:* Liver and kidney dysfunction, lactation, pregnancy
- *Physical:* Skin status, liver and kidney function test, culture of affected area, sensitivity tests

### Implementation

- Culture infection, arrange for sensitivity tests before and during therapy if expected response is not seen.
- Reconstitution of drug varies by size of package; see manufacturer's directions for details.
- Reconstitute drug for IM use with Sterile Water or Bacteriostatic Water for Injection; divide doses of 2 g and administer at two different sites by deep IM injection.
- Discontinue if hypersensitivy reaction occurs.

### Drug-specific teaching points

- The following side effects may occur: stomach upset, diarrhea.
- Avoid alcohol while on this drug and for 3 days after because severe reactions often occur.
- Report severe diarrhea, difficulty breathing, unusual tiredness or fatigue, pain at injection site.

## cefotetan disodium

*(sef' oh tee tan)*

Cefotan

**Pregnancy Category B**

**Drug classes**

Antibiotic

Cephalosporin (third generation)

**Therapeutic actions**

Bactericidal: inhibits synthesis of bacterial cell wall, causing cell death.

**Indications**

- Lower respiratory tract infections caused by *S. pneumoniae, S. aureus, Klebsiella, H. influenzae, E. coli*
- UTIs caused by *E. coli, Klebsiella, P. vulgaris, P. mirabilis, Morganella morganii, Providencia rettgeri*
- Intra-abdominal infections caused by *E. coli, K. pneumoniae Klebsiella, Streptococcus* (excluding enterococci), *Bacteroides*
- Gynecologic infections caused by *S. aureus, S. epidermidis, Streptococcus* (excluding enterococci), *E. coli, P. mirabilis, N. gonorrhoeae, Bacteroides, Fusobacterium, Peptococcus, Peptostreptococcus*
- Dermatologic infections caused by *S. aureus, S. pyogenes, S. epidermidis, Streptococcus* (excluding enterococci), *E. coli*
- Bone and joint infections caused by *S. aureus*
- Perioperative prophylaxis

**Contraindications/cautions**

- Allergy to cephalosporins or penicillins, renal failure, lactation.

### Dosage

**Available Forms:** Powder for injection—1, 2, 10 g

*ADULT:* 1–2 g/d IM or IV in equally divided doses q12h for 5–10 d. Do not exceed 6 g/d.

- *UTI:* 1–4 g/d given as 500 mg q12h IV, IM or 1–2 g q24h IV or IM, or 1–2 g q12h IV or IM.
- *Other infections:* 2–4 g/d given as 1–2 g q12h IV or IM.
- *Severe infections:* 4 g/d given as 2 g q12h IV.
- *Life-threatening infections:* 6 g/d given as 3 g q12h IV.
- *Perioperative prophylaxis:* 1–2 g IV 1/2–1 h before surgery.
- *Cesarean section:* Administer 1–2 g IV after the cord is clamped.

### Geriatric (or Impaired Renal Function)

| Creatinine Clearance (ml/min) | Dosage |
|---|---|
| >30 | 1–2 g q12h |
| 10–30 | 1–2 g q24h |
| <10 | 1–2 g q48h |

### Pharmacokinetics

| Route | Onset | Peak | Duration |
|---|---|---|---|
| IV | 15–20 min | 30 min | 18–24 h |
| IM | 30–60 min | 1 1/2–3 h | 18–24 h |

*Metabolism:* $T_{1/2}$: 3–4.5 h
*Distribution:* Crosses the placents; enters breast milk
*Excretion* : Urine, bile

### IV facts

**Preparation:** Reconstitute for IV use with Sterile Water for Injection. **1-g vial**: add 10 ml diluent; withdraw 10.5 ml; concentration is 95 mg/ml. **2-g vial**: add 10–20 ml diluent; withdraw 11–21 ml; concentration is 182–195 mg/ml. Reconstituted solution is stable for 24 h at room temperature or 4 d if refrigerated. Protect drug from light.
**Infusion:** Inject slowly over 3–5 min into vein or over a longer time into IV tubing. Discontinue infusion of other solutions temporarily while cefotetan is running. If given with aminoglycosides, give each antibiotic at a different site.
**Incompatibilities:** Do not mix aminoglycosides and cefonicid in the same IV solution.

### Adverse effects

- CNS: Headache, dizziness, lethargy, paresthesias
- GI: *Nausea, vomiting, diarrhea, anorexia, abdominal pain, flatulence,* pseudomembranous colitis, liver toxicity
- **Hematologic**: Bone marrow depression: decreased WBC, decreased platelets, decreased Hct
- GU: Nephrotoxicity
- **Hypersensitivity**: *Ranging from rash to fever* to anaphylaxis, serum sickness reaction
- Local: *Pain,* abscess at injection site; *phlebitis*, inflammation at IV site
- Other: *Superinfection, disulfiram-like reaction with alcohol*

### Clinically important drug-drug interactions

• Increased nephrotoxicity with aminoglycosides • Increased bleeding effects with oral anticoagulants • Disulfiram-like reaction may occur if alcohol is used within 72 h after cefotetan administration.

### Drug-lab test interferences

• Possibility of false results on tests of urine glucose using Benedict's solution, Fehling's solution, Clinitest tablets; urinary 17-ketosteroids; direct Coombs' test.

## ■ Nursing Considerations

### Assessment

- *History:* Liver and kidney dysfunction, lactation, pregnancy
- *Physical:* Skin status, liver and kidney function test, culture of affected area, sensitivity tests

### Implementation

- Culture infection, arrange for sensitivity tests before and during therapy if expected response is not seen.
- Reconstitute for IM use with Sterile Water for Injection, 0.9% Sodium Chloride Solution, Bacteriostatic Water for Injection, 0.5% or 1% lidocaine HCl; inject deeply into large muscle group.
- Protect drug from light.
- Have vitamin K available in case hypoprothrombinemia occurs.
- Discontinue if hypersensitivy reaction occurs.

### Drug-specific teaching points

- The following side effects may occur: stomach upset, diarrhea.
- Avoid alcohol while on this drug and for 3 days after because severe reactions often occur.

- Report severe diarrhea, difficulty breathing, unusual tiredness or fatigue, pain at injection site.

## cefoxitin sodium

*(se **fox'** i tin)*
Mefoxin
**Pregnancy Category B**

### Drug classes
Antibiotic
Cephalosporin (second generation)

### Therapeutic actions
Bactericidal: inhibits synthesis of bacterial cell wall, causing cell death.

### Indications
- Lower respiratory tract infections caused by *S. pneumoniae, S. aureus*, streptococci, *E. coli, Klebsiella, H. influenzae, Bacteroides*
- Dermatologic infections caused by *S. aureus, S. epidermidis*, streptococci, *E. coli, P. mirabilis, Klebsiella, Bacteroides, Clostridium, Peptococcus, Peptostreptococcus*
- UTIs caused by *E. coli, P. mirabilis, Klebsiella, M. morganii, P. rettgeri, P. vulgaris, Providencia*, uncomplicated gonorrhea caused by *N. gonorrhoeae*
- Intra-abdominal infections caused by *E. coli, Klebsiella, Bacteroides, Clostridium*
- Gynecologic infections caused by *E. coli, N. gonorrhoeae, Bacteroides, Clostridium, Peptococcus, Peptostreptococcus*, group B streptococci
- Septicemia caused by *S. pneumoniae, S. aureus, E. coli, Klebsiella, Bacteroides*
- Bone and joint infections caused by *S. aureus*
- Perioperative prophylaxis
- Treatment of oral bacterial *Eikenella corrodens*

### Contraindications/cautions
- Allergy to cephalosporins or penicillins, renal failure, lactation.

### Dosage
**Available Forms:** Powder for injection—1, 2 g; injection—1, 2 g in 5% Dextrose in water

ADULT: 1–2 g IM or IV q6–8h, depending on the severity of the infection.
- ***Uncomplicated gonorrhea:*** 2 g IM with 1 g oral probenecid.
- ***Perioperative prophylaxis:*** 2 g IV or IM 1/2–1 h prior to initial incision and q6h for 24 h after surgery.
- ***Cesarean section:*** 2 g IV as soon as the umbilical cord is clamped, followed by 2 g IM or IV at 4 and 8 h, then q6h for up to 24 h.
- ***Transurethral prostatectomy:*** 1 g prior to surgery and then 1 g q8h for up to 5 d.

PEDIATRIC
- ***>3 mo:*** 80–160 mg/kg per day IM or IV in divided doses q4–6h. Do not exceed 12 g/d.
- ***Prophylactic use:*** 30–40 mg/kg per dose IV or IM q6h.

GERIATRIC OR IMPAIRED RENAL FUNCTION: IV loading dose of 1–2 g:. Maintenance dosages are as follows:

| *Creatinine Clearance (ml/min)* | *Maintenance Dosage* |
|---|---|
| 30–50 | 1–2 g q8–12h |
| 10–29 | 1–2 g q12–24h |
| 5–9 | 0.5–1 g q12–24h |
| <5 | 0.5–1 g q24–48h |

### Pharmacokinetics

| *Route* | *Onset* | *Peak* | *Duration* |
|---|---|---|---|
| IV | Immediate | 5 min | 6–8 h |
| IM | 5–10 min | 20–30 min | 6–8 h |

*Metabolism:* $T_{1/2}$: 45–60 min
*Distribution:* Crosses the placents; enters breast milk
*Excretion* : Urine

### IV facts
**Preparation:** For IV intermittent administration, reconstitute 1 or 2 g with 10–20 ml Sterile Water for Injection. For continuous IV infusion, add reconstituted solution to 5% Dextrose Injection, 0.9% Sodium Chloride Injection, 5% Dextrose and 0.9% Sodium Chloride Injection, or

5% Dextrose Injection with 0.02% Sodium Bicarbonate Solution. Store dry powder in cool, dry area. Powder and reconstituted solution darkens with storage. Stable for 24 h at room temperature.
**Infusion:** *Intermittent administration:* Slowly inject over 3–5 min, or give over longer time through IV tubing; discontinue other solutions temporarily. If given with aminoglycosides, give each at a different site.
**Incompatibilities:** Do not mix aminoglycosides and cefonicid in the same IV solution.

### Adverse effects

- CNS: Headache, dizziness, lethargy, paresthesias
- GI: *Nausea, vomiting, diarrhea, anorexia, abdominal pain, flatulence,* pseudomembranous colitis, liver toxicity
- **Hematologic:** Bone marrow depression: decreased WBC, decreased platelets, decreased Hct
- GU: Nephrotoxicity
- **Hypersensitivity:** *Ranging from rash to fever* to anaphylaxis, serum sickness reaction
- Local: *Pain,* abscess at injection site, *phlebitis,* inflammation at IV site
- Other: *Superinfections, disulfiram-like reaction with alcohol*

### Clinically important drug-drug interactions

• Increased nephrotoxicity with aminoglycosides • Increased bleeding effects with oral anticoagulants • Disulfiram-like reaction may occur if alcohol is taken within 72 h after cefoxitin administration

### Drug-lab test interferences

• Possibility of false results on tests of urine glucose using Benedict's solution, Fehling's solution, Clinitest tablets; urinary 17-ketosteroids; direct Coombs' test.

## ■ Nursing Considerations

### Assessment

- *History:* Liver and kidney dysfunction, lactation, pregnancy
- *Physical:* Skin status, liver and kidney function test, culture of affected area, sensitivity tests

### Implementation

- Culture infection, arrange for sensitivity tests before and during therapy if expected response is not seen.
- Reconstitute each gram for IM use with 2 ml Sterile Water for Injection or with 2 ml of 0.5% Lidocaine HCl Solution (without epinephrine) to decrease pain at injection site. Inject deeply into large muscle group.
- Dry powder and reconstituted solutions darken slightly at room temperature.
- Have vitamin K available in case hypoprothrombinemia occurs.
- Discontinue if hypersensitivity reaction occurs.

### Drug-specific teaching points

- The following side effects may occur: stomach upset or diarrhea.
- Avoid alcohol while on this drug and for 3 days after because severe reactions often occur.
- Report severe diarrhea, difficulty breathing, unusual tiredness or fatigue, pain at injection site.

## cefpodoxime proxetil

*(sef poe **docks'** eem)*
Vantin
**Pregnancy Category B**

### Drug classes

Antibiotic
Cephalosporin (second generation)

### Therapeutic actions

Bactericidal: inhibits synthesis of bacterial cell wall, causing cell death.

### Indications

- Lower respiratory tract infections caused by *S. pneumoniae, H. influenzae*
- Upper respiratory infections caused by *S. pyogenes, H. influenzae, Moraxella catharrhalis*

- Dermatologic infections caused by *S. aureus, S. pyogenes*
- UTIs caused by *E. coli, P. mirabilis, Klebsiella, Staphylococcus saprophyticus*
- Otitis media caused by *S. pneumoniae, H. influenzae, M. catarrhalis*
- Sexually transmitted disease caused by *N. gonorrhoeae*

### Contraindications/cautions

- Allergy to cephalosporins or penicillins, renal failure, lactation.

### Dosage

**Available Forms:** Tablets—100, 200 mg; granules for suspension—50, 100 mg/5 ml

*ADULT:* 100–400 mg q12h PO depending on severity of infection; continue for 7–14 d

*PEDIATRIC:* 5 mg/kg per dose PO q12h; do not exceed 100–200 mg per dose; continue for 10 d

- *Acute otitis media:* 10 mg/kg/d PO; do not exceed 400-mg dose; continue for 10 d.

*GERIATRIC OR RENAL IMPAIRED:* Creatinine clearance < 30 ml/min: increase dosing interval to q24h.

### Pharmacokinetics

| Route | Peak | Duration |
|---|---|---|
| PO | 30–60 min | 16–18 h |

*Metabolism:* $T_{1/2}$: 120–180 min
*Distribution:* Crosses the placenta; enters breast milk;
*Excretion:* Renal, unchanged

### Adverse effects

- CNS: Headache, dizziness, lethargy, paresthesias
- GI: *Nausea, vomiting, diarrhea, anorexia, abdominal pain, flatulence, pseudomembranous colitis*, liver toxicity
- **Hematologic: Bone marrow depression**
- GU: Nephrotoxicity
- **Hypersensitivity:** *Ranging from rash* to *fever* to *anaphylaxis*; serum sickness reaction
- Other: *Superinfections*

### Clinically important drug-drug interactions

- Increased nephrotoxicity with aminoglycosides • Increased bleeding effects with oral anticoagulants • Disulfiram-like reaction if alcohol is used within 72 h after cefpodoxime administration

### Clinically important drug-food interactions

- Increased absorption and increased effects of cefpodoxime if taken with food

### Drug-lab test interferences

- Possibility of false results on tests of urine glucose using Benedict's solution, Fehling's solution, Clinitest tablets; urinary 17-ketosteroids; direct Coombs' test.

## ■ Nursing Considerations

### Assessment

- *History:* Penicillin or cephalosporin allergy, pregnancy or lactation
- *Physical:* Kidney function, respiratory status, skin status; culture and sensitivity tests of infected area

### Implementation

- Culture infection before drug therapy.
- Give drug with meals or food to enhance absorption.
- Prepare suspension as follows: suspend 50 mg/5 ml strength in a total of 58 ml distilled water. Gently tap the bottle to loosen the powder. Add 25 ml distilled water and shake vigorously for 15 seconds. Add 33 ml distilled water, and shake vigorously for 3 min or until all particles are suspended. Suspend 100 mg/5 ml strength in a total of 57 ml distilled water. Proceed as above, adding 25 ml distilled water and 32 ml distilled water, respectively.
- Refrigerate suspension after reconstitution; shake vigorously before use, and discard after 14 d.
- Discontinue drug if hypersensitivity reaction occurs.
- Give the patient yogurt or buttermilk in case of diarrhea.
- Arrange for oral vancomycin for serious colitis that fails to respond to discontinuation

### Drug-specific teaching points

- Take this drug with food.
- Complete the full course of this drug even if you feel better.

- This drug is prescribed for this particular infection; do not self-treat any other infection.
- The following side effects may occur: stomach upset, loss of appetite, nausea (take drug with food); diarrhea; headache, dizziness.
- Report severe diarrhea with blood, pus, or mucus; rash or hives; difficulty breathing; unusual tiredness, fatigue; unusual bleeding or bruising.

# cefprozil monohydrate

*(sef* ***pro'*** *zil)*

Cefzil

**Pregnancy Category B**

## Drug classes
Antibiotic
Cephalosporin (second generation)

## Therapeutic actions
Bactericidal: inhibits synthesis of bacterial cell wall, causing cell death.

## Indications
- Pharyngitis/tonsillitis caused by *S. pyogenes*
- Secondary bacterial infection of acute bronchitis and exacerbation of chronic bronchitis caused by *S. pneumoniae, H. influenzae, M. catarrhalis*
- Dermatologic infections caused by *S. aureus, S. pyogenes*
- Otitis media caused by *S. pneumoniae, H. influenzae, M. catarrhalis*
- Acute sinusitis caused by *S. pneumoniae, S. aureus, H. influenzae, M. catarrhalis*

## Contraindications/cautions
- Allergy to cephalosporins or penicillins, renal failure, lactation.

## Dosage
**Available Forms:** Tablets—250, 500 mg; powder for suspension—125, 250 mg/5 ml

*ADULT:* 250–500 mg PO q12h. Continue treatment for 10 d.

*PEDIATRIC:* 2–12 y: 7.5–15 mg/kg PO q12h; continue treatment for 10 d. 6 mo–2 y: 15 mg/kg PO q12h for 10 d for otitis media.

*GERIATRIC OR RENAL IMPAIRED:* Creatinine clearance 30–120 ml/min, use standard dose; creatinine clearance 0–30 ml/min, use 50% of standard dose.

## Pharmacokinetics

| *Route* | *Peak* | *Duration* |
|---|---|---|
| PO | 6–10 h | 24–28 h |

*Metabolism:* $T_{1/2}$: 78 min
*Distribution:* Crosses the placenta, enters breast milk
*Excretion:* Renal, unchanged

## Adverse effects
- CNS: Headache, dizziness, lethargy, paresthesias
- GI: *Nausea, vomiting, diarrhea, anrexia, abdominal pain, flatulence, pseudomembranous colitis*, liver toxicity
- **Hematologic: Bone marrow depression**
- GU: Nephrotoxicity
- Hypersensitivity: *Ranging from rash to fever to anaphylaxis*; serum sickness reaction
- Other: *Superinfections*

## Clinically important drug-drug interactions
• Increased nephrotoxicity with aminoglycosides • Increased bleeding effects if taken with oral anticoagulants • Disulfiram-like reaction if alcohol is taken within 72 h after cefprozil administration

## Drug-lab test interferences
• Possibility of false results on tests of urine glucose using Benedict's solution, Fehling's solution, Clinitest tablets; urinary 17-ketosteroids; direct Coombs' test.

## ■ Nursing Considerations

### Assessment
- *History:* Penicillin or cephalosporin allergy, pregnancy or lactation
- *Physical:* Kidney function, respiratory status, skin status, culture and sensitivity tests of infected area

### Implementation

- Culture infection before drug therapy.
- Give drug with food to decrease GI discomfort.
- Refrigerate suspension after reconstitution, and discard after 14 d.
- Discontinue if hypersensitivy reaction occurs.
- Give the patient yogurt or buttermilk in case of diarrhea.
- Arrange for oral vancomycin for serious colitis that fails to respond to discontinuation

### Drug-specific teaching points

- Take this drug with food.
- Complete the full course of this drug, even if you feel better.
- This drug is prescribed for this particular infection; do not self-treat any other infection.
- The following side effects may occur: stomach upset, loss of appetite, nausea (take drug with food); diarrhea; headache, dizziness.
- Report severe diarrhea with blood, pus, or mucus; rash or hives; difficulty breathing; unusual tiredness, fatigue; unusual bleeding or bruising.

## ceftazidime

***(sef' tay zi deem)***

Ceptaz, Fortaz, Tazicef, Tazidime

**Pregnancy Category B**

### Drug classes

Antibiotic
Cephalosporin (third generation)

### Therapeutic actions

Bactericidal: inhibits synthesis of bacterial cell wall, causing cell death.

### Indications

- Lower respiratory tract infections caused by *P. aeruginosa,* other *Pseudomonas, S. pneumoniae, S. aureus, Klebsiella, H. influenzae, P. mirabilis, E. coli, Enteroter, Serratia, Citrobacter*
- UTIs caused by *P. aeruginosa, Enterobacter, E. coli, Klebsiella, P. mirabilis, Proteus*
- Gynecologic infections caused by *E. coli*
- Dermatologic infections caused by *P. aeruginosa, S. aureus, E. coli, Serratia, Proteus, Klebsiella, Enterobacter, S. pyogenes*
- Septicemia caused by *P. aeruginosa, E. coli, Klebsiella, H. influenzae, Serratia, S. pneumoniae, S. aureus*
- Intra-abdominal infections caused by *E. coli, S. aureus, Bacteroides, Klebsiella*
- CNS infections caused by *H. influenzae, N. meningitidis*
- Bone and joint infections caused by *P. aeruginosa, Klebsiella, Enterobacter, S. aureus*

### Contraindications/cautions

- Allergy to cephalosporins or penicillins, renal failure, lactation.

### Dosage

**Available Forms:** Powder for injection—500 mg, 1, 2, 6, 10 g; injection—1, 2 g

*ADULT:* Usual dose: 1 g (range 250 mg–2 g) q8–12h IM or IV. Do not exceed 6 g/d. Dosage will vary with infection.

- *UTI:* 250–500 mg IV or IM q8–12h.
- ***Pneumonia, dermatologic infections:*** 500 mg–1 g IV or IM q8h.
- ***Bone and joint infections:*** 2 g IV q12h.
- ***Gynecologic, intra-abdominal, life-threatening infections, meningitis:*** 2 g IV q8h.

*PEDIATRIC*

- ***0–4 wk:*** 30 mg/kg IV q12h.
- ***1 mo–12 y:*** 30 mg/kg IV q8h. Do not exceed 6 g/d.

*GERIATRIC OR REDUCED RENAL FUNCTION:* Loading dose of 1 g IV, followed by:

| *Creatinine Clearance (ml/min)* | *Dosage* |
|---|---|
| 50–31 | 1 g q12h |
| 30–16 | 1 g q24h |
| 15–6 | 500 mg q24h |
| <5 | 500 mg q48h |

### Pharmacokinetics

| *Route* | *Onset* | *Peak* | *Duration* |
|---|---|---|---|
| IV | Rapid | 1 h | 24–28 h |
| IM | 30 min | 1 h | 24–28 h |

*Metabolism:* $T_{1/2}$: 114–120 min
*Distribution:* Crosses the placents; enters breast milk
*Excretion* : Urine

### IV facts

**Preparation:** Reconstitute drug for direct IV injection with Sterile Water for Injection. Reconstituted solution is stable for 18 h at room temperature or 7 d if refrigerated. **500-mg vial**: mix with 5 ml diluent; resulting concentration, 11 mg/ml. **1-g vial:** mix with 5 (10) ml diluent; resulting concentration, 180 (100) mg/ml. **2-g vial** mix with 10 ml diluent; resulting concentration, 170–180 mg/ml.

**Infusion:** For IV, reconstitute 1- or 2-g infusion pack with 100 ml Sterile Water for Injection; infuse slowly. Direct injection: slowly over 3–5 min. Infusion: over 30 min. If patient is also receiving aminoglycosides, administer at seperate sites.

**Incompatibilities:** Sodium Bicarbonate Injection and aminoglycoside solutions.

### Adverse effects

- CNS: Headache, dizziness, lethargy, paresthesias
- GI: *Nausea, vomiting, diarrhea, anorexia, abdominal pain, flatulence*, pseudomembranous colitis, liver toxicity
- Hematologic: Bone marrow depression: decreased WBC, decreased platelets, decreased Hct
- GU: Nephrotoxicity
- Hypersensitivity: *Ranging from rash* to *fever* to anaphylaxis; serum sickness reaction
- Local: *Pain,* abscess at injection site; *phlebitis*, inflammation at IV site
- Other: *Superinfections, disulfiram-like reaction with alcohol*

### Clinically important drug-drug interactions

• Increased nephrotoxicity with aminoosides • Increased bleeding effects with oral anticoagulants • Disulfiram-like reaction may occur if alcohol is used within 72 h after ceftazidime administration.

### Drug-lab test interferences

• Possibility of false results on tests of urine glucose using Benedict's solution, Fehling's solution, Clinitest tablets; urinary 17-ketosteroids; direct Coombs' test.

## ■ Nursing Considerations

### Assessment

- ***History:*** Liver and kidney dysfunction, lactation, pregnancy
- ***Physical:*** Skin status, liver and kidney function test, culture of affected area, sensitivity tests

### Implementation

- Culture infection, arrange for sensitivity tests before and during therapy if expected response is not seen.
- Reconstitute drug for IM use with Sterile Water or Bacteriostatic Water for Injection or with 0.5% or 1% Lidocaine HCl Injection to reduce pain; inject deeply into large muscle group.
- Do *not* mix with aminoglycoside solutions. Administer these drugs seperately.
- Powder and reconstituted solution darken with storage.
- Have vitamin K available in case hypoprothrombinemia occurs.
- Discontinue if hypersensitivity reaction occurs.

### Drug-specific teaching points

- The following side effects may occur stomach upset or diarrhea.
- Avoid alcohol while on this drug and for 3 days after because severe reactions often occur.
- Report severe diarrhea, difficulty breathing, unusual tiredness or fatigue, pain at injection site.

## ceftibuten hydrochloride

*(sef ta **byoo'** ten)*
Cedax
**Pregnancy Category B**

C

**Drug classes**
Antibiotic
Cephalosporin (third generation)

**Therapeutic actions**
Bactericidal: inhibits synthesis of bacterial cell wall, causing cell death.

**Indications**
- Acute bacterial exacerbations of chronic bronchitis due to *Haemophilus influenzae, Moraxella catarrhalis, Streptococcus pneumoniae*
- Acute bacterial otitis media due to *H. influenzae, M. catarrhalis, Streptococcus pyogenes*
- Pharyngitis and tonsillitis due to *S. pyogenes*

**Contraindications/cautions**
- Allergy to cephalosporins or penicillins; renal failure; lactation.

**Dosage**
**Available Forms:** Capsules—400 mg; oral suspension—90, 180 mg/5 ml
*ADULT:* 400 mg PO qd for 10 d.
*PEDIATRIC:* 9 mg/kg/d PO for 10 d to a maximum daily dose of 400 mg/d.
*RENAL IMPAIRED*

| *Creatinine Clearance (ml/min)* | *Dose* |
|---|---|
| >50 | 9 mg/kg or 400 mg PO in 24 h |
| 30–49 | 4.5 mg/kg or 200 mg PO in 24 h |
| 5–29 | 2.25 mg/kg or 100 mg PO in 24 h |

**Pharmacokinetics**

| *Route* | *Peak* | *Duration* |
|---|---|---|
| PO | 30–60 min | 8–10 h |

*Metabolism:* $T_{1/2}$: 30–60 min
*Distribution:* Crosses placenta; enters breast milk
*Excretion:* Renal—unchanged

**Adverse effects**
- CNS: Headache, dizziness, lethargy, paresthesias
- GI: *Nausea, vomiting, diarrhea, anorexia, abdominal pain, flatulence,* **pseudomembranous colitis,** liver toxicity
- GU: Nephrotoxicity
- Hematologic: Bone marrow depression
- Hypersensitivity: Ranging from *rash, fever* to **anaphylaxis**; serum sickness reaction
- Other: *Superinfections*

**Clinically important drug-drug interactions**
• Increased nephrotoxicity with aminoglycosides • Increased bleeding effects with oral anticoagulants • Disulfiram-like reaction may occur if alcohol is taken within 72 h after administration

**Drug-lab test interferences**
• Possibility of false results on tests of urine glucose using Benedict's solution, Fehling's solution, Clinitest tablets; urinary 17-ketosteroids; direct Coombs' test

## ■ Nursing Considerations

### Assessment
- *History:* Allergy to penicllin or cephalosporin; pregnancy, lactation
- *Physical:* Kidney function, respiratory status, skin status; culture and sensitivity tests of infection

### Implementation
- Culture infection before beginning drug therapy.
- Give capsules with meals to decrease GI discomfort; suspension must be given on an empty stomach at least 2 h before or 1 h after meals.
- Refrigerate suspension after reconstitution; shake vigorously before use and discard after 14 d.
- Discontinue drug if hypersensitivity reaction occurs.
- Give patient yogurt or buttermilk in case of diarrhea.
- Arrange for treatment of superinfections.
- Reculture infection if patient fails to respond.

### Drug-specific teaching points
- Take capsules with meals or food; suspension must be taken on an empty

stomach, at least 2 hours before or 1 hour after meals.
- Refrigerate suspension; shake vigorously after use and discard after 14 days.
- Complete the full course of this drug, even if you feel better before the course of treatment is over.
- This drug is prescribed for this particular infection; do not use it to self-treat any other infection.
- The following side effects may occur: stomach upset, loss of appetite, nausea (take drug with food); diarrhea; headache, dizziness.
- Report severe diarrhea with blood, pus or mucus; rash or hives; difficulty breathing; unusual tiredness, fatigue; unusual bleeding or bruising.

## ceftizoxime sodium

*(sef ti **zox'** eem)*

Cefizox

**Pregnancy Category B**

### Drug classes
Antibiotic
Cephalosporin (third generation)

### Therapeutic actions
Bactericidal: inhibits synthesis of bacterial cell wall, causing cell death.

### Indications
- Lower respiratory tract infections caused by *S. pneumoniae, S. aureus, Klebsiella, H. influenzae, E. coli, P. mirabilis, Enterobacter, Serratia, Bacteroides*
- UTIs caused by *S. aureus, Citrobacter, Enterobacter, E. coli, Klebsiella, P. aeruginosa, P. vulgaris, P. rettgeri, P. mirabilis, M. morganii, S. marcescens, Enterobacter*
- Uncomplicated cervical and urethral gonorhea caused by *N. gonorrhoeae*
- PID caused by *N. gonnorrhoeae, E. coli, S. agalactiae*
- Intra-abdominal infections caused by *E. coli, S. epidermidis, Streptococcus* (except enterococci), *Enterobacter, Klebsiella, Bacteroides, Peptococcus, Peptostreptococcus*
- Dermatologic infections caused by *S. aureus, E. coli, Klebsiella, Enterobacter, Bacteroides, Peptococcus, Peptostreptococcus, P. mirabilis, S. epidermidis, S. pyogenes*
- Septicemia caused by *E. coli, Klebsiella, S. pneumoniae, S. aureus, Bacteroides, Serratia*
- Bone and joint infections caused by *S. aureus, Streptococci* (excluding enterococci), *P. mirabilis, Bacteroides, Peptococcus, Peptostreptococcus*
- Meningitis caused by *H. influenzae*, some cases caused by *S. pneumoniae*

### Contraindications/cautions
- Allergy to cephalosporins or penicillins, renal failure, lactation

### Dosage
**Available Forms:** Powder for injection—500 mg, 1, 2, 10 g; injection in D-5-W—1, 2 g

**ADULT:** Usual dose: 1–2 g (range 1–4 g) IM or IV q8–12h. Do not exceed 12 g/d. Dosage will vary with infection.
- ***Gonorrhea:*** Single 1-gm IM dose.
- ***Uncomplicated UTIs:*** 500 mg q12h IM or IV
- ***PID:*** 2 g q8h IV

**PEDIATRIC**
- ***>6 mo:*** 50 mg/kg q6–8h; up to 200 mg/kg per day in severe infections

**GERIATRIC OR REDUCED RENAL FUNCTION:** Initial dose of 500 mg–1 g IM or IV followed by:

| Creatinine Clearance (ml/min) | Usual Dosage | Maximum Dosage |
|---|---|---|
| 79–80 | 500 mg q8h | 0.75–1.5 g q8h |
| 49–5 | 250–500 mg q12h | 0.5–1 g q12h |
| 4–0 | 500 mg q48h or 250 mg q24h | 0.5–1 g q48h or 0.5 g q24h |

### Pharmacokinetics

| Route | Onset | Peak | Duration |
|---|---|---|---|
| IV | Rapid | 1 h | 18–24 h |
| IM | 30 min | 1 h | 18–24 h |

*Metabolism:* $T_{1/2}$: 84–114 min
*Distribution:* Crosses the placenta; enters breast milk
*Excretion* : Urine

### IV facts

**Preparation:** Dilute reconstituted solution for IV infusion with 50–100 ml of 5% or 10% Dextrose Injection; 5% Dextrose and 0.2%, 0.45%, or 0.9% Sodium Chloride Injection; Lactated Ringer's Injection; Ringer's Injection; 0.9% Sodium Chloride Injection; Invert Sugar 10% in Sterile Water for Injection; 5% Sodium Bicarbonate in Sterile Water for Injection; or 5% Dextrose in Lactated Ringer's Injection if reconstituted with 4% Sodium Bicarbonate Injection.

| *Package Size* | *Diluent to Add* | *Resulting Volume* | *Concentration* |
|---|---|---|---|
| 1-g vial | 10 ml | 10.7 ml | 95 mg/ml |
| 2-g vial | 20 ml | 21.4 ml | 95 mg/ml |
| 10-g vial | 30 ml | 37 ml | 1 g/3.5 ml |
| | 45 ml | 51 ml | 1 g/5 ml |

Piggy-back vials should be reconstituted with 50–100 ml of any of the above solutions. Shake well, and administer as a single dose with primary IV fluids. Reconstituted solution is stable for 24 h at room temperature or 4 d if refrigerated; discard solution after allotted time.

**Infusion:** If given with aminoglycosides, give each antibiotic at a different site. Direct injection: administer slowly over 3–5 min directly or through tubing. Infusion: over 30 min.

**Incompatibilities:** Do not mix aminoglycosides and ceftizoxime in the same IV solution.

### Adverse effects

- CNS: Headache, dizziness, lethargy, paresthesias
- GI: *Nausea, vomiting, diarrhea, anorexia, abdominal pain, flatulence,* pseudomembranous colitis, liver toxicity
- **Hematologic**: Bone marrow depression: decreased WBC, decreased platelets, decreased Hct
- GU: Nephrotoxicity
- **Hypersensitivity**: *Ranging from rash* to *fever* to anaphylaxis; serum sickness reaction
- Local: *Pain,* abscess at injection site; *phlebitis*, inflammation at IV site
- Other: *Superinfections, disulfiram-like reaction with alcohol*

### Clinically important drug-drug interactions

• Increased nephrotoxicity with aminoglycosides • Increased bleeding effects with oral anticoagulants • Disulfiram-like reaction may occur if alcohol is taken within 72 h after ceftizoxime administration.

### Drug-lab test interferences

• Possibility of false results on tests of urine glucose using Benedict's solution, Fehling's solution, Clinitest tablets; urinary 17-ketosteroids; direct Coombs' test.

## ■ Nursing Considerations

### Assessment

- *History:* Liver and kidney dysfunction, lactation, pregnancy
- *Physical:* Skin status, liver and kidney function test, culture of affected area, sensitivity tests

### Implementation

- Culture infection, arrange for sensitivity tests before and during therapy if expected response is not seen.
- Divide and administer IM doses of 2 g at two different sites by deep IM injection.
- Give each antibiotic at a different site, if given as part of combination therapy with aminoglycosides.
- Discontinue if hypersensitivy reaction occurs.
- Have vitamin K available in case hypoprothrombinemia occurs.

### Drug-specific teaching points

- The following side effects may occur: stomach upset or diarrhea.
- Avoid alcohol while on this drug and for 3 days after because severe reactions often occur.

- Report severe diarrhea, difficulty breathing, unusual tiredness or fatigue, pain at injection site.

## ceftriaxone sodium

*(sef try **ax'** one)*

Rocephin

**Pregnancy Category B**

### Drug classes
Antibiotic
Cephalosporin (third generation)

### Therapeutic actions
Bactericidal: inhibits synthesis of bacterial cell wall, causing cell death.

### Indications
- Lower respiratory tract infections caused by *S. pneumoniae, S. aureus, Klebsiella, H. influenzae, E. coli, P. mirabilis, E. aerogens, Serratia maecescens, Haemophilus parainfluenzae,* Streptococus (excluding enterococci)
- UTIs caused by *E. coli, Klebsiella, P. vulgaris, P. mirabilis, M. morganii*
- Gonorrhea caused by *N. gonorrhoeae*
- Intra-abdominal infections caused by *E. coli, K. pneumoniae*
- PID caused by *N. gonorrhoeae*
- Dermatologic infections caused by *S. aureus, Klebsiella, Enterobacter cloacae, P. mirabilis, S. epidermidis, P. aeruginosa, Streptococcus* (excluding enterococci)
- Septicemia caused by *E. coli, S. pneumoniae, H. influenzae, S. aureus, K. pneumoniae*
- Bone and joint infections caused by *S. aureus, Streptococci* (excluding enterococci), *P. mirabilis, S. pneumoniae, E. coli, K. pneumoniae, Enterobacter*
- Meningitis caused by *H. influenzae, S. pneumoniae, N. meningitidis*
- Perioperative prophylaxis for patients undergoing coronary artery bypass surgery
- Unlabeled use: treatment of Lyme disease in doses of 2 g IV bid for 14 d

### Contraindications/cautions
- Allergy to cephalosporins or penicillins, renal failure, lactation

### Dosage
**Available Forms:** Powder for injection—250, 500 mg, 1, 2, 10 g; injection—1, 2 g

**ADULT:** 1–2 g/d IM or IV qid or in equal divided doses bid. Do not exceed 4 g/d.
- *Gonorrhea:* Single 250 mg IM dose.
- *Meningitis:* 100 mg/kg per day IV or IM in divided doses q12h. Do not exceed 4 g/d.
- *Perioperative prophylaxis:* 1 g IV 1/2–1 h before surgery.

**PEDIATRIC:** 50–75 mg/kg per day IV or IM in divided doses q12h. Do not exceed 2 g/d.
- *Meningitis:* 100 mg/kg per day IV or IM in divided doses q12h, with or without a loading dose of 75 mg/kg

### Pharmacokinetics

| Route | Onset | Peak | Duration |
|---|---|---|---|
| IV | Rapid | Immediate | 15–18 h |
| IM | 30 min | 1.5–4 h | 15–18 h |

*Metabolism:* $T_{1/2}$: 5–10 h
*Distribution:* Crosses the placents; enters breast milk
*Excretion* : Urine and bile

### IV facts
**Preparation:** Dilute reconstituted solution for IV infusion with 50–100 ml of 5% or 10% Dextrose Injection, 5% Dextrose and 0.45% or 0.9% Sodium Chloride Injection, 0.9% Sodium Chloride Injection, 10% Invert Sugar, 5% Sodium Bicarbonate, FreAmine 111, Normosol-M in 5% Dextrose, Ionosol-B in 5% Dextrose, 5% or 10% Mannitol, Sodium Lactate.

| Package Size | Diluent to Add | Resulting Concentration |
|---|---|---|
| 250-mg vial | 2.4 ml | 100 mg/ml |
| 5000-g vial | 4.8 ml | 100 mg/ml |
| 1-g vial | 9.6 ml | 100 mg/ml |
| 2-g vial | 19.2 ml | 100 mg/ml |
| Piggyback 1 g | 10 ml | |
| Piggyback 2 g | 20 ml | |

Stability of reconstituted and diluted solution depends on diluent, concentration and type of container (eg, glass, PVC); check manufacturer's inserts for specific details. Protect drug from light.

**Infusion:** Administer by intermittent infusion over 15–30 min. Do not mix ceftriaxone with any other antimicrobial drug.

**Incompatibilities:** Do not mix aminoglycosides and ceftriaxone in the same IV solution.

### Adverse effects

- CNS: Headache, dizziness, lethargy, paresthesias
- GI: *Nausea, vomiting, diarrhea, anorexia, abdominal pain, flatulence,* pseudomembranous colitis, liver toxicity
- Hematologic: **Bone marrow depression:** decreased WBC, decreased platelets, decreased Hct
- GU: Nephrotoxicity
- Hypersensitivity: *Ranging from rash to fever* to anaphylaxis; serum sickness reaction
- Local: *Pain,* abscess at injection site; *phlebitis,* inflammation at IV site
- Other: *Superinfections, disulfiram-like reaction with alcohol*

### Clinically important drug-drug interactions

• Increased nephrotoxicity with aminoglycosides • Increased bleeding effects with oral anticoagulants • Disulfiram-like reaction may occur if alcohol is taken within 72 h after ceftriaxone administration.

### Drug-lab test interferences

• Possibility of false results on tests of urine glucose using Benedict's solution, Fehling's solution, Clinitest tablets; urinary 17-ketosteroids; direct Coombs' test.

## ■ Nursing Considerations

### Assessment

- *History:* Liver and kidney dysfunction, lactation, pregnancy
- *Physical:* Skin status, liver and kidney function test, culture of affected area, sensitivity tests

### Implementation

- Culture infection, arrange for sensitivity tests before and during therapy if expected response is not seen.
- Reconstitute for IM use with Sterile Water for Injection, 0.9% Sodium Chloride Solution, 5% Dextrose Solution, Bacteriostatic Water with 0.9% Benzyl Alcohol, or 1% Lidocaine Solution (without epinephrine); inject deeply into a large muscle group.
- Check manufacturer's inserts for specific details. Stability of reconstituted and diluted solution depends on diluent, concentration and type of container (eg, glass, PVC).
- Protect drug from light.
- Do not mix ceftriaxone with any other antimicrobial drug.
- Monitor ceftriaxone blood levels in patients with severe renal impairment and in patients with renal and hepatic impairment.
- Have vitamin K available in case hypoprothrombinemia occurs.
- Discontinue if hypersensitivy reaction occurs.

### Drug-specific teaching points

- The following side effects may occur: stomach upset or diarrhea.
- Avoid alcohol while on this drug and for 3 days after because severe reactions often occur.
- Report severe diarrhea, difficulty breathing, unusual tiredness or fatigue, pain at injection site.

# Cefuroxime

## cefuroxime axetil

*(se fyoor ox' em)*

Ceftin

## cefuroxime sodium

Kefurox, Zinacef

**Pregnancy Category B**

### Drug classes

Antibiotic

Cephalosporin (second generation)

### Therapeutic actions

Bactericidal: inhibits synthesis of bacterial cell wall, causing cell death.

## Indications

*Oral (Cefuroxime Axetil)*

- Pharyngitis, tonsilitis caused by *S. pyogenes*
- Otitis media caused by *S. pneumoniae, H. influenzae, M. catarrhalis, S. pyogenes*
- Lower respiratory tract infections caused by *S. pneumoniae, H. parainfluenxae, H. influenzae*
- UTIs caused by *E. coli, K. pneumoniae*
- Dermatologic infections, including impetigo caused by *S. aureus, S. pyogenes*
- Treatment of early Lyme disease

*Parenteral (Cefuroxime Sodium)*

- Lower respiratory tract infections caused by *S. pneumoniae, S. aureus, E. coli, Klebsiella, H. influenzae, S. pyogenes*
- Dermatologic infections caused by *S. aureus, S. pyogenes, E. coli, Klebsiella, Enterobacter*
- UTIs caused by *E. coli, Klebsiella*
- Uncomplicated and disseminated gonorrhea caused by *N. gonorrhoea*
- Septicemia caused by *S. pneumoniae, S. aureus, E. coli, Klebsiella, H. influenzae*
- Meningitis caused by *S. pneumoniae, H. influenzae, S. aureus, N. meningitidis*
- Bone and joint infections caused by *S. aureus*
- Perioperative prophylaxis

## Contraindications/cautions

- Allergy to cephalosporins or penicillins, renal failure, lactation

## Dosage

**Available Forms:** Tablets—125, 250, 500 mg; suspension—125 mg/5 ml; powder for injection—750 mg, 1.5, 7.5 g; injection—750 mg, 1.5 g

*Oral*

ADULT AND CHILDREN > 12 Y: 250 mg bid. For severe infections, may be increased to 500 mg bid.

- *Uncomplicated UTIs:* 125 mg bid. Increase to 250 mg bid in severe cases.

PEDIATRIC < 12 Y: 125 mg bid.

- *Otitis media:* **<2 y:** 125 mg bid. **>2 y**: 250 mg bid.

*Parenteral*

ADULT: 750 mg–1.5 g IM or IV q8h, depending on severity of infection.

- *Uncomplicated gonorrhea:* 1.5 g IM (at two different sites) with 1 g of oral probenecid.
- *Perioperative prophylaxis:* 1.5 g IV 1/2–1 h prior to initial incision; then 750 mg IV or IM q8h for 24 h after surgery.

PEDIATRIC

- *>3 Mo:* 50–100 mg/kg per day IM or IV in divided doses q6–8h.
- *Bacterial meningitis:* 200–240 mg/kg per day IV in divided doses q6–8h.
- *Impaired renal function:* Adjust adult dosage for renal impairment by weight or age of child

GERIATRIC OR ADULT IMPAIRED RENAL FUNCTION:

| Creatinine Clearance (ml/min) | Dosage |
|---|---|
| >20 | 750 mg–1.5 g q8h |
| 10–20 | 750 mg q12h |
| <10 | 750 mg q24h |

## Pharmacokinetics

| Route | Onset | Peak | Duration |
|---|---|---|---|
| IV | Rapid | Immediate | 18–24 h |
| IM | 20 min | 30 min | 18–24 h |
| PO | Varies | 2 h | 18–24 h |

*Metabolism:* $T_{1/2}$: 1–2 h

*Distribution:* Crosses the placenta; enters breast milk

*Excretion* : Urine

### IV facts

**Preparation:** Preparation of parenteral drug solutions and suspensions differs for different starting preparations and different brand names; check the manufacturer's directions carefully. Reconstitute parenteral drug with Sterile Water for Injection, 5% Dextrose in Water, 0.9% Sodium Chloride, or any of the following, which also may be used for further dilution: 0.9% Sodium Chloride, 5% or 10% Dextrose Injection, 5% Dextrose and 0.45% or 0.9% Sodium Chloride Injection, or M/6 Sodium Lactate Injection. Stability of solutions depends on diluent and concentration: Check manufacturer's specifications. **Do not mix** with IV solutions containing aminoglycosides. Powder form, solutions, and suspensions darken during storage.

**Infusion:** Inject slowly over 3–5 minutes directly into vein for IV administration, or infuse over 30 min, 6–24 h if by continuous infusion. Give aminoglycosides and cefuroxime at different sites.

**Incompatibilities:** Do not mix aminoglycosides and cefuroxime in the same IV solution.

### Adverse effects

- CNS: Headache, dizziness, lethargy, paresthesias
- GI: *Nausea, vomiting, diarrhea, anorexia, abdominal pain, flatulence,* pseudomembranous colitis, liver toxicity
- Hematologic: Bone marrow depression: decreased WBC, decreased platelets, decreased Hct
- GU: Nephrotoxicity
- Hypersensitivity: *Ranging from rash* to *fever* to anaphylaxis, serum sickness reaction
- Local: *Pain,* abscess at injection site; *phlebitis,* inflammation at IV site
- Other: *Superinfections, disulfiram-like reaction with alcohol*

### Clinically important drug-drug interactions

• Increased nephrotoxicity with aminoglycosides • Increased bleeding effects with oral anticoagulants • Disulfiram-like reaction may occur if alcohol is taken within 72 h after cefuroxime administration.

### Drug-lab test interferences

• Possibility of false results on tests of urine glucose using Benedict's solution, Fehling's solution, Clinitest tablets; urinary 17-ketosteroids; direct Coombs' test.

## ■ Nursing Considerations

### Assessment

- *History:* Liver and kidney dysfunction, lactation, pregnancy
- *Physical:* Skin status, liver and kidney function test, culture of affected area, sensitivity tests

### Implementation

- Culture infection, arrange for sensitivity tests before and during therapy if expected response is not seen.
- Give oral drug with food to decrease GI upset and enhance absorption.
- Give oral drug to children who can swallow tablets; crushing the drug results in a bitter, unpleasant taste.
- Have vitamin K available in case hypoprothrombinemia occurs.
- Discontinue if hypersensitivy reaction occurs.

### Drug-specific teaching points

*Parenteral Drug*

- The following side effects may occur: stomach upset or diarrhea.
- Avoid alcohol while on this drug and for 3 days after because severe reactions often occur.
- Report severe diarrhea, difficulty breathing, unusual tiredness or fatigue, pain at injection site.

*Oral Drug*

- Take full course of therapy.
- This drug is specific for this infection and should not be used to self-treat other problems.
- Swallow tablets whole; do not crush. Take the drug with food.
- The following side effects may occur: stomach upset or diarrhea.
- Report severe diarrhea with blood, pus, or mucus; rash; difficulty breathing; unusual tiredness, fatigue; unusual bleeding or bruising; unusual itching or irritation.

## cellulose sodium phosphate

***(sell' u loos)***

CSP

Calcibind, Calcisorb (CAN)

**Pregnancy Category C**

**Drug classes**
Antilithic agent
Resin exchange agent
Cation

**Therapeutic actions**
Binds calcium and magnesium in the bowel; promotes the excretion of calcium and reduces serum calcium levels, decreasing the formation of renal calculi.

**Indications**
- Absorptive hypercalciuria Type I (recurrent passage or formation of calcium oxalate or calcium phosphate renal stones not eliminated by diet)

**Contraindications/cautions**
- Contraindications: primary or secondary hyperparathyroidism; high fasting urinary calcium or hypophosphatemia; pregnancy; children.
- Use cautiously with CHF, ascites, nephrotic syndrome.

**Dosage**
**Available Forms:** Powder—300 g bulk
ADULT: Initial dose of 15 g/d PO (5 g with each meal) in patients with urinary calcium > 300 mg/d; when urinary calcium declines to < 150 mg/d, reduce to 10 g/d (5 g with supper and 2.5 g with two other meals). Patients with urinary calcium < 300 mg/d but > 200 mg/d, 10 g/d.
PEDIATRIC: Safety and efficacy not established.

**Pharmacokinetics**
Not absorbed systemically.

**Adverse effects**
- GI: *Bad taste, loose stools, diarrhea, dyspepsia*
- Other: *Decreased magnesium levels*

## ■ Nursing Considerations

**Assessment**
- *History:* Primary or secondary hyperparathyroidism; high fasting urinary calcium or hypophosphatemia; lactation; CHF, ascites, nephrotic syndrome
- *Physical:* Weight, skin condition, neurologic status, abdominal exam, urinary calcium, serum electrolytes

**Implementation**
- Give drug with meals.
- Arrange for supplemental magnesium gluconate with this drug. Those receiving 15 g CSP/d should receive 1.5 g magnesium gluconate before breakfast and again hs. Those receiving 10 g CSP/d should receive 1 g magnesium gluconate twice a day. Give magnesium 1 h before or 2 h after CSP to prevent binding.
- Suspend each dose of CSP powder in a glass of water, soft drink, or fruit juice. Give 1 h before meal.
- Monitor 24-h urinary calcium levels periodically during therapy; adjust dosage accordingly.
- Arrange for dietary consultation to help patient moderate calcium and dietary oxalate intake.
- Increase fluid intake each day.

**Drug-specific teaching points**
- Take drug 1 h before meals as ordered. Take magnesium supplement 1 h before the CSP; suspend each dose in a glass of water, soft drink, or juice.
- Avoid vitamin C supplements.
- Drink as much fluid as tolerable.
- Moderate your calcium intake (dairy products), oxalate intake (spinach, rhubarb, chocolate, brewed tea), salt intake.
- The following side effects may occur: bad taste, loose stools, diarrhea, indigestion.
- Report swelling of extremities, tremors, palpitations.

# Cephalexin

## cephalexin
*(sef a* ***lex'*** *in)*

Apo-Cephalex (CAN), Keflex, Novo-Lexin (CAN), Nu-Cephalex (CAN)

## cephalexin hydrochloride monohydrate

Biocef, Cefanex, Keftab

**Pregnancy Category B**

**Drug classes**
Antibiotic
Cephalosporin (first generation)

**Therapeutic actions**
Bactericidal: inhibits synthesis of bacterial cell wall, causing cell death.

**Indications**
- Respiratory tract infections caused by *S. pneumoniae,* group A $\beta$-hemolytic streptococci
- Dermatologic infections caused by staphylococci, streptococci
- Otitis media caused by *S. pneumoniae, H. influenzae,* streptococci, staphylococci, *M. catarrhalis*
- Bone infections caused by staphylococci, *P. mirabilis*
- GU infections caused by *E. coli, P. mirabilis, Klebsiella*

**Contraindications/cautions**
- Allergy to cephalosporins or penicillins; renal failure; lactation

**Dosage**
**Available Forms:** Capsules—250, 500 mg, 1 g; oral suspension—125, 250 mg/5 ml

*ADULT:* 1–4 g/d in divided dose; 250 mg PO q6h usual dose.
- ***Skin and skin-structure infections:*** 500 mg PO q12h. Larger doses may be needed in severe cases; *do not exceed* 4 g/d.

*PEDIATRIC:* 25–50 mg/kg per day PO in divided doses.
- ***Skin and skin-structure infections:*** Divide total daily dose, and give q12h. Dosage may be doubled in severe cases.
- ***Otitis media:*** 75–100 mg/kg per day PO in four divided doses.

**Pharmacokinetics**

| *Route* | *Peak* | *Duration* |
|---|---|---|
| PO | 60 min | 8–10 h |

*Metabolism:* $T_{1/2}$: 50–80 min
*Distribution* : Crosses the placenta, enters breast milk
*Excretion:* Renal

**Adverse effects**
- CNS: Headache, dizziness, lethargy, paresthesias
- GI: *Nausea, vomiting, diarrhea, anorexia, abdominal pain, flatulence,* **pseudomembranous colitis**, liver toxicity
- Hematologic: Bone marrow depression
- GU: Nephrotoxicity
- Hypersensitivity: *Ranging from rash* to *fever* to **anaphylaxis**; serum sickness reaction
- Other: *Superinfections*

**Clinically important drug-drug interactions**
• Increased nephrotoxicity with aminoglycosides • Increased bleeding effects with oral anticoagulants • Disulfiram-like reaction may occur if alcohol is taken within 72 h after cephalexin administration.

**Drug-lab test interferences**
• Possibility of false results on tests of urine glucose using Benedict's solution, Fehling's solution, Clinitest tablets; urinary 17-ketosteroids; direct Coombs' test.

## ■ Nursing Considerations

**Assessment**
- *History:* Penicillin or cephalosporin allergy, pregnancy or lactation
- *Physical:* Kidney function, respiratory status, skin status; culture and sensitivity tests of infected area

**Implementation**
- Arrange for culture and sensitivity tests of infection before and during therapy if infection does not resolve.
- Give drug with meals; arrange for small, frequent meals if GI complications occur.
- Refrigerate suspension, discard after 14 d.

**Drug-specific teaching points**
- Take this drug with food. Refrigerate suspension; discard any drug after 14 d.
- Complete the full course of this drug even if you feel better.
- This drug is prescribed for this particular infection; do not self-treat any other infection.

- The following side effects may occur: stomach upset, loss of appetite, nausea (take drug with food); diarrhea; headache, dizziness.
- Report severe diarrhea with blood, pus, or mucus; rash or hives; difficulty breathing; unusual tiredness, fatigue; unusual bleeding or bruising.

## cephalothin sodium

*(sef a' loe thin)*

**Pregnancy Category B**

### Drug classes

Antibiotic
Cephalosporin (first generation)

### Therapeutic actions

Bactericidal: inhibits synthesis of bacterial cell wall, causing cell death.

### Indications

- Respiratory tract infections caused by *S. pneumoniae,* staphylococci, group A $\beta$-hemolytic streptococci, *Klebsiella, H. influenzae*
- Dermatologic infections caused by staphylococci, group A $\beta$-hemolytic streptococci, *E. coli, P. mirabilis,, Klebsiella*
- GU infections caused by *E. coli, P. mirabilis, Klebsiella*
- Septicemia caused by *S. pneumoniae,* staphylococci, group A $\beta$-hemolytic streptococci, *S. viridans, E. coli, P. mirabilis, Klebsiella*
- GI infections caused by *Salmonella, Shigella*
- Meningitis caused by *S. pneumoniae,* group A $\beta$-hemolytic streptococci, staphylococci
- Bone and joint infections caused by staphylococci
- Perioperative prophylaxis

### Contraindications/cautions

- Allergy to cephalosporins or penicillins, renal failure, lactation

### Dosage

**Available Forms:** Powder for injection—1, 2 g

*ADULT:* 500 mg–1 g IM or IV q4–6h, depending on severity of infection (up to 2 g q4h in life-threatening infections).

- ***Perioperative prophylaxis:*** 1–2 g 1/2–1 h before initial incision; 1–2 g during surgery; 1–2 g q6h for 24 h after surgery.

*PEDIATRIC:* Usual dose 100 mg/kg per day (range 80–160 mg/kg per day) IM or IV in divided doses.

- ***Perioperative prophylaxis:*** 20–30 mg/kg 1/2–1 h before initial incision; 20–30 mg/kg during surgery; 20–30 mg/kg q6h for 24 h after surgery.

*GERIATRIC OR IMPAIRED RENAL FUNCTION:* IV loading dose of 1–2 g. Maximum maintenance dosages are:

| *Creatinine Clearance (ml/min)* | *Maximum Dosage* |
|---|---|
| 50–80 | 2 g q6h |
| 25–50 | 1.5 g q6h |
| 10–25 | 1 g q6h |
| 2–10 | 0.5 g q6h |
| <2 | 0.5 g q8h |

### Pharmacokinetics

| *Route* | *Onset* | *Peak* | *Duration* |
|---|---|---|---|
| IV | Rapid | 15 min | 18–24 h |
| IM | 20 min | 30 min | 18–24 h |

*Metabolism:* $T_{1/2}$: 30–50 min
*Distribution:* Crosses the placenta; enters breast milk
*Excretion* : Urine

### IV facts

**Preparation:** Dilute 1–2 g with at least 10 ml of Sterile Water for Injection and add to Acetated Ringer's Injection, 5% Dextrose Injection, 5% Dextrose in Lactated Ringer's Injection, Ionosol B in D5W, Isolyte M with 5% Dextrose, Lactated Ringer's Injection, Normosol-M in D5-W, Plasma-Lyte Injection, Plasma-Lyte-M in 5% Dextrose, Ringer's Injection, or 0.9% Sodium Chloride Injection. Concentrated solutions darken slightly at room temperature. Use IV infusions within 12 h, and complete use within 24 h. Discard solution after 24 h; solution is stable for 4 d if refrigerated. Redissolve

prepared solution by warming to room temperature and agitating slightly.
**Infusion:** Administer intermittent IV by slowly injecting a solution of 1 g in 10 ml diluent directly into the vein over 3–5 min or inject into IV tubing.
**Incompatibilities:** Do not mix aminoglycosides and cephalothin in the same IV solution.

### Adverse effects

- CNS: Headache, dizziness, lethargy, paresthesias
- GI: *Nausea, vomiting, diarrhea, anorexia, abdominal pain, flatulence,* pseudomembranous colitis, liver toxicity
- **Hematologic**: Bone marrow depression: decreased WBC, decreased platelets, decreased Hct
- GU: Nephrotoxicity
- **Hypersensitivity**: *Ranging from rash* to *fever* to anaphylaxis; serum sickness reaction
- Local: *Pain,* abscess at injection site; *phlebitis,* inflammation at IV site
- Other: *Superinfections, disulfiram-like reaction with alcohol*

### Clinically important drug-drug interactions

• Increased nephrotoxicity with aminoglycosides • Increased bleeding effects with oral anticoagulants • Disulfiram-like reaction may occur if alcohol is taken within 72 h after cephalothin administration.

### Drug-lab test interferences

• Possibility of false results on tests of urine glucose using Benedict's solution, Fehling's solution, Clinitest tablets; urinary 17-ketosteroids; direct Coombs' test, creatinine levels.

## ■ Nursing Considerations

### Assessment

- *History:* Liver and kidney dysfunction, lactation, pregnancy
- *Physical:* Skin status, liver and kidney function test, culture of affected area, sensitivity tests

### Implementation

- Culture infection, arrange for sensitivity tests before and during therapy if expected response is not seen.
- Add 6 mg/100 ml cephalothin to peritoneal dialysis solution, and instill into the peritoneum if necessary.
- Prepare IM injection as follows: Reconstitute each gram with 4 ml Sterile Water; if contents do not dissolve, add 0.2–0.4 ml diluent, and warm gently; use within 12 h.
- Give IM injections deeply into large muscle mass.
- Give patient yogurt or buttermilk if diarrhea occurs.
- Arrange for oral vancomycin for severe colitis that does not respond to discontinuation of drug.
- Arrange for prophylactic dose for 3–5 d if postoperative site is infected; do culture and sensitivity tests and arrange for change of antibiotic as needed.

### Drug-specific teaching points

- The following side effects may occur: stomach upset or diarrhea, headache, dizziness.
- Avoid alcohol while on this drug and for 3 days after because severe reactions often occur.
- Report severe diarrhea, difficulty breathing, unusual tiredness or fatigue, pain at injection site.

## cephapirin sodium

*(sef a **pye'** rin)*
Cefadyl
**Pregnancy Category B**

### Drug classes

Antibiotic
Cephalosporin (first generation)

### Therapeutic actions

Bactericidal: inhibits synthesis of bacterial cell wall, causing cell death.

### Indications

- Respiratory tract infections caused by *S. pneumoniae, S. aureus*, group A $\beta$-hemolytic streptococci, *Klebsiella, H. influenzae*
- Dermatologic infections caused by *S. aureus*, group A $\beta$-hemolytic streptococci, *E. coli, P. mirabilis, Klebsiella, S. epidermidis*
- GU infections caused by *S. aureus, E. coli, P. mirabilis, Klebsiella*
- Septicemia caused by *S. aureus*, group A $\beta$-hemolytic streptocci, *S. viridans, E. coli, Klebsiella*
- Endocarditis caused by *S. viridans, S. aureus*
- Osteomyelitis caused by *S. aureus, Klebsiella, P. mirabilis*, group A $\beta$-hemolytic streptococci
- Perioperative prophylaxis

### Contraindications/cautions

- Allergy to cephalosporins or penicillins, renal failure, lactation.

### Dosage

**Available Forms:** Powder for injection—500 mg, 1, 2, 4, 20 g

*ADULT:* 500 mg–1 g IM or IV q4–6h, depending on severity of infection; up to 12 g daily in severe cases.

- *Perioperative prophylaxis:* 1–2 g 1/2–1 h before initial incision; 1–2 g during surgery; 1–2 g q6h for 24 h after surgery or up to 3–5 d.

*PEDIATRIC:* 40–80 mg/kg per day IM or IV in four divided doses. **Do not use in infants <3 mo.**

- *Perioperative prophylaxis:* Reduce adult dose according to weight or age (see Appendix III for formulas).

*GERIATRIC OR RENAL IMPAIRED:* Serum creatinine > 5 mg/100 ml, 7.5–15 mg/kg q12h.

### Pharmacokinetics

| *Route* | *Onset* | *Peak* | *Duration* |
|---|---|---|---|
| IV | Rapid | 5 min | 6–8 h |
| IM | 10 min | 30 min | 6–8 h |

*Metabolism:* $T_{1/2}$: 24–36 min

*Distribution:* Crosses the placenta; enters breast milk

*Excretion* : Urine

### IV facts

**Preparation:** Prepare IV intermittent doses, reconstituting 500 mg or 1- to 2-g vial with 10 ml diluent. Stability of diluted IV solutions varies: See manufacturer's inserts. Prepare IV doses with compatible solutions: Sodium Chloride Injection; 5% Sodium Chloride in Water; 5%, 10%, 20% Dextrose in Water; Sodium Lactate Injection; 10% Invert Sugar in Normal Saline or Water; 5% Lactated Ringer's Injection; Lactated Ringer's with 5% Dextrose; Ringer's Injection; Sterile Water for Injection; 5% Dextrose in Ringer's Injection; Normosol R; Normosol R in 5% Dextrose Injection; Ionosol D-CM; Ionosol G in 10% Dextrose Injection.

**Infusion:** Inject intermittent dose slowly over 3–5 min. If giving cephapirin IV piggyback, stop other infusion while cephapirin is being infused; infuse 1 g over 5 min or longer. Give aminoglycosides and cephapirin at different sites.

**Incompatibilities:** Do not mix aminoglycosides and cephapirin in the same IV solution.

### Adverse effects

- CNS: Headache, dizziness, lethargy, paresthesias
- GI: *Nausea, vomiting, diarrhea, anorexia, abdominal pain, flatulence*, pseudomembranous colitis, liver toxicity
- **Hematologic**: Bone marrow depression: decreased WBC, decreased platelets, decreased Hct
- GU: Nephrotoxicity
- **Hypersensitivity**: *Ranging from rash to fever* to anaphylaxis; serum sickness reaction
- Local: *Pain*, abscess at injection site; *phlebitis*, inflammation at IV site
- **Other**: *Superinfections, disulfiram-like reaction with alcohol*

**Clinically important drug-drug interactions**
• Increased nephrotoxicity with aminoglycosides • Increased bleeding effects with oral anticoagulants • Disulfiram-like reaction if alcohol is taken within 72 h after cephapirin administration

**Drug-lab test interferences**
• Possibility of false results on tests of urine glucose using Benedict's solution, Fehling's solution, Clinitest tablets; urinary 17-ketosteroids; direct Coombs' test.

## ■ Nursing Considerations

### Assessment

- ***History:*** Liver and kidney dysfunction, lactation, pregnancy
- ***Physical:*** Skin status, liver and kidney function test, culture of affected area, sensitivity tests

### Implementation

- Culture infection, arrange for sensitivity tests before and during therapy if expected response is not seen.
- Prepare IM solution as follows: reconstitute 500-mg vials with 1 ml of Sterile Water for Injection or Bacteriostatic Water for Injection; reconstitute 1-g vials with 2 ml of diluent; each 1.2 ml contains 500 mg cephapirin.
- Give IM injections deeply into large muscle mass.
- Have vitamin K available in case hypoprothrombinemia occurs.
- Discontinue if hypersensitivy reaction occurs.

### Drug-specific teaching points

- The following side effects may occur: stomach upset or diarrhea.
- Avoid alcohol while on this drug and for 3 days after because severe reactions often occur.
- Report severe diarrhea, difficulty breathing, unusual tiredness or fatigue, pain at injection site.

## cephradine

*(sef' ra deen)*
Velosef
**Pregnancy Category B**

**Drug classes**
Antibiotic
Cephalosporin (first generation)

**Therapeutic actions**
Bactericidal: inhibits synthesis of bacterial cell wall, causing cell death.

**Indications**
*Oral Use*

- Respiratory tract infections caused by group A β-hemolytic streptococci, *S. pneumoniae*
- Otitis media caused by group A β-hemolytic streptococci, *S. pneumoniae, H. influenzae,* and staphylococci
- Dermatologic infections caused by staphylococci and β-hemolytic streptococci
- UTIs caused by *E. coli, P. mirabilis, Klebsiella,* enterococci

*Parenteral Use*

- Respiratory tract infections caused by *S. pneumoniae, Klebsiella, H. influenzae, S. aureus,* and group A β-hemolytic streptococci
- UTIs caused by *E. coli, P. mirabilis, Klebsiella*
- Dermatologic infections caused by *S. aureus,* group A β-hemolytic streptococci
- Bone infections caused by *S. aureus*
- Septicemia caused by *S. pneumoniae, S. aureus, P. mirabilis, E. coli*
- Perioperative prophylaxis

**Contraindications/cautions**

- Allergy to cephalosporins or penicillins, renal failure, lactation

### Dosage

**Available Forms:** Capsules—250, 500 mg; oral suspension—125, 500 mg/5 ml; powder for injection—250, 500 mg, 1, 2 g

**ADULT:** 250–500 mg PO q6–12h (dose depends on the severity of infection); 2–4 g/d IV or IM in equal divided doses qid.

- ***Perioperative prophylaxis:*** 1 g IV or IM 30–90 min before surgery; then 1 g q4–6h for up to 24 h.
- ***Cesarean section:*** 1 g IV as soon as cord is clamped; then 1 g IM or IV at 6 and 12 h.

**PEDIATRIC**

- *>9 mo:* 25–50 mg/kg/d in equally divided doses PO q6–12h.

- *Otitis media:* 75–100 mg/kg/d PO in equal divided doses q6–12h. **Do not exceed 4 g/d.** 50–100 mg/kg/d day IV or IM in four equally divided doses.

GERIATRIC OR REDUCED RENAL FUNCTION: Loading dose of 1 g and then maintenance dosage as follows:

| *Creatinine Clearance (ml/min)* | *Dosage* |
|---|---|
| >20 | 500 mg q6h |
| 5–20 | 250 mg q6h |
| <5 | 250 mg q12h |

### Pharmacokinetics

| *Route* | *Onset* | *Peak* | *Duration* |
|---|---|---|---|
| IV | Rapid | 5 min | 6–8 h |
| IM | 20 min | 1–2 h | 6–8 h |
| PO | Varies | 1 h | 6–8 h |

*Metabolism:* $T_{1/2}$: 48–80 min
*Distribution:* Crosses the placenta; enters breast milk
*Excretion* : Urine

### IV facts

**Preparation:** Prepare for direct IV injections by diluting drug with Sterile Water for Injection, 5% Dextrose Injection, or Sodium Chloride Injection using 5 ml with the 250- to 500-mg vials, 10 ml with the 1-g vial, or 20 ml with the 2-g vial. Prepare for IV infusion as follows: add 10, 20, or 40 ml Sterile Water for Injection to 1-, 2-, or 4-g preparations; withdraw and dilute further with 5% or 10% Dextrose Injection, Sodium Chloride Injection, M/6 Sodium Lactate, Dextrose and Sodium Chloride Injection, 10% Invert Sugar in Water, Normosol-R, or Ionosol B with 5% Dextrose. Use direct IV solutions within 2 h at room temperature. IV infusion solution is stable for 10 h at room temperature or 48 h if refrigerated; for prolonged infusions replace solution every 10 h. Protect solutions from light or direct sunlight.

**Infusion:** Inject direct IV slowly over 3–5 min, or give through IV tubing; infuse 1 g over 5 min or longer.

**Incompatibilities:** Do not mix cephradine with any other antibiotic. Do not use with Lactated Ringer's Injection.

### Adverse effects

- CNS: Headache, dizziness, lethargy, paresthesias
- GI: *Nausea, vomiting, diarrhea, anorexia, abdominal pain, flatulence*, pseudomembranous colitis, liver toxicity
- **Hematologic**: Bone marrow depression: decreased WBC, decreased platelets, decreased Hct
- GU: Nephrotoxicity
- **Hypersensitivity**: *Ranging from rash* to *fever* to anaphylaxis; serum sickness reaction
- **Local**: *Pain,* abscess at injection site; *phlebitis*, inflammation at IV site
- **Other**: *Superinfections, disulfiram-like reaction with alcohol*

### Clinically important drug-drug interactions

• Increased nephrotoxicity with aminoglycosides • Increased bleeding effects with oral anticoagulants • Disulfiram-like reaction may occur if alcohol is taken within 72 h after cephradine administration.

### Drug-lab test interferences

• Possibility of false results on tests of urine glucose using Benedict's solution, Fehling's solution, Clinitest tablets; urinary 17-ketosteroids; direct Coombs' test.

## ■ Nursing Considerations

### Assessment

- *History:* Liver and kidney dysfunction, lactation, pregnancy
- *Physical:* Skin status, liver and kidney function test, culture of affected area, sensitivity tests

### Implementation

- Culture infection, arrange for sensitivity tests before and during therapy if expected response is not seen.
- Prepare for IM use by reconstituting drug with Sterile Water or Bacteriostatic Water for Injection; inject deeply into large muscle group.

- Use IM solution within 2 h if stored at room temperature.
- Protect solutions from light or direct sunlight.
- Do not mix cephradine with any other antibiotic.
- Give oral drug with meals.
- Have vitamin K available in case hypoprothrombinemia occurs.
- Discontinue if hypersensitivy reaction occurs.

### Drug-specific teaching points

*Parenteral Drug*

- The following side effects may occur: stomach upset or diarrhea.
- Avoid alcohol while on this drug and for 3 days after because severe reactions often occur.
- Report severe diarrhea, difficulty breathing, unusual tiredness or fatigue, pain at injection site.

*Oral Drug*

- Take full course of therapy.
- This drug is specific for this infection and should not be used to self-treat other problems.
- Take drug with food.
- Avoid alcohol while on this drug and for 3 days after because severe reactions often occur.
- The following side effects may occur: stomach upset or diarrhea.
- Report severe diarrhea with blood, pus, or mucus; rash; difficulty breathing; unusual tiredness, fatigue; unusual bleeding or bruising; unusual itching or irritation.

## cerivastatin sodium

*(sar ah va* ***stah'*** *tin)*

Baycol

**Pregnancy Category X**

### Drug classes

Antihyperlipidemic
HMG CoA inhibitor

### Therapeutic actions

Inhibits HMG CoA, the enzyme that catalyzes the first step in the cholesterol synthesis pathway, resulting in a decrease in serum cholesterol, serum LDLs (associated with increased risk of CAD) and either an increase or no change in serum HDLs (associated with decreased risk of CAD); increases hepatic LDL recapture sites, enhances reuptake and catabolism of LDL; lowers triglyceride levels and increases HDL levels.

### Indications

- As an adjunct to diet in the treatment of elevated total cholesterol and LDL cholesterol in patients with primary hypercholesterolemia (types IIa and IIb) and mixed dyslipidemia, and homozygous familial hypercholesterolemia whose response to dietary restriction of saturated fat and cholesterol and other nonpharmacologic measures has not been adequate

### Contraindications/cautions

- Contraindications: allergy to cerivastatin, fungal byproducts; active liver disease or unexplained and persistent eleveations of transaminase levels; pregnancy, lactation.
- Use cautiously with impaired endocrine function.

### Dosage

**Available Forms:** Tablets—0.2, 0.3 mg

*ADULT:* 0.3 mg PO qd in the evening; effectiveness is increased if combined with a bile acid–binding resin—give cerivastatin >2 h after the resin.

*PEDIATRIC:* Safety and efficacy not established.

*RENAL IMPAIRMENT:* Mild renal impairment—no adjustment needed; moderate renal impairment (Ccr 60 ml/min)—use starting dose of 0.2 mg.

### Pharmacokinetics

| *Route* | *Onset* | *Peak* |
|---|---|---|
| Oral | Slow | 2.5 h |

*Metabolism:* Hepatic and cellular; $T_{1/2}$: hours
*Distribution:* Crosses placenta; passes into breast milk
*Excretion:* Bile

### Adverse effects

- CNS: *Headache,* asthenia
- GI: *Flatulence, abdominal pain, cramps, constipation, nausea,* dyspepsia, heartburn, **liver failure**

- Other: **Rhabdomyolysis with acute renal failure,** arthralgia, myalgia

### Clinically important drug-drug interactions

• Possible severe myopathy or rhabdomyolysis with erythromycin, cyclosporin, niacin, antifungals • Increased digoxin levels with possible toxicity if taken together; monitor digoxin levels • Increased estrogen levels when taken with oral contraceptives; monitor patients on this combination • Increased effectiveness with bile acid–binding resin

## ■ Nursing Considerations

### Assessment

- *History:* Allergy to cerivastatin, fungal byproducts; active hepatic disease; acute, serious illness; pregnancy, lactation
- *Physical:* Orientation, affect, muscle strength; liver evaluation, abdominal exam; lipid studies, liver and renal function tests

### Implementation

- Obtain liver function tests as a baseline and periodically during therapy; discontinue drug if AST or ALT levels increase to three times normal levels.
- Withhold cerivastatin in any acute, serious condition (severe infection, hypotension, major surgery, trauma, severe metabolic or endocrine disorder, seizures) that may suggest a myopathy or serve as a risk factor for development of renal failure.
- Ensure that patient has tried a cholesterol-lowering diet regimen for 3–6 mo before beginning therapy.
- Administer drug without regard to food, in the evening.
- Consult with dietitian regarding low-cholesterol diets.
- Ensure that patient is not pregnant and has appropriate contraceptives available during therapy; serious fetal damage could occur.

### Drug-specific teaching points

- Take this drug once a day, in the evening; may be taken with food.
- Institute appropriate diet changes that need to be made.
- The following side effects may occur: nausea (small, frequent meals may help); headache, muscle and joint aches and pains (may lessen over time).
- Arrange to have periodic blood tests while you are on this drug.
- Alert any health care provider that you are on this drug; it will need to be discontinued if acute injury or illness occurs.
- Do not become pregnant while on this drug; use barrier contraceptives. If you wish to become pregnant or think you are pregnant, consult with your health care provider.
- Report muscle pain, weakness, tenderness; malaise; fever; change in color of urine or stool; swelling.

# cetirizine

*(se **tear'** i zeen)*

Zyrtec

**Pregnancy Category C**

### Drug classes

Antihistamine

### Therapeutic actions

Potent histamine ($H_1$) receptor antagonist; inhibits histamine release and eosinophil chemotaxis during inflammation, leading to reduced swelling and decreased inflammatory response

### Indications

- Management of seasonal and perennial allergic rhinitis
- Treatment of chronic, idiopathic urticaria

### Contraindications/cautions

- Contraindications: allergy to any antihistamines; narrow-angle glaucoma, stenosing peptic ulcer, symptomatic prostatic hypertrophy, asthmatic attack, bladder neck obstruction, pyloroduodenal obstruction (avoid use or use with caution as condition may be exacerbated by drug effects); lactation

### Dosage

**Available Forms:** Tablets—5, 10 mg; syrup—5 mg/5 ml

*ADULT AND PEDIATRIC > 12 Y:* 5–10 mg qd PO; maximum dose 20 mg/d.

*HEPATIC OR RENAL IMPAIRED:* 5 mg PO qd.

### Pharmacokinetics

| Route | Onset | Peak | Duration |
|---|---|---|---|
| Oral | Rapid | 1 h | 24 h |

*Metabolism:* Hepatic; $T_{1/2}$: 7–10 h

*Distribution:* Crosses placenta; enters breast milk

*Excretion:* Urine and feces

### Adverse effects

- CNS: *Somnolence, sedation*
- GI: Nausea, diarrhea, abdominal pain, constipation
- CV: Palpitation, edema
- Respiratory: Bronchospasm, pharyngitis
- Other: Fever, photosensitivity, rash, myalgia, arthralgia, angioedema

## ■ Nursing Considerations

### Assessment

- ***History:*** Allergy to any antihistamines; narrow-angle glaucoma, stenosing peptic ulcer, symptomatic prostatic hypertrophy, asthmatic attack, bladder neck obstruction, pyloroduodenal obstruction; lactation
- ***Physical:*** Skin color, lesions, texture; orientation, reflexes, affect; vision exam; R, adventitious sounds; prostate palpation; renal function tests

### Implementation

- Give without regard to meals.
- Provide syrup form for pediatric use if needed.
- Arrange for use of humidifier if thickening of secretions, nasal dryness become bothersome; encourage adequate intake of fluids.
- Provide skin care for urticaria.

### Drug-specific teaching points

- Take this drug without regard to meals.
- The following side effects may occur: dizziness, sedation, drowsiness (use caution if driving or performing tasks that require alertness); thickening of bronchial secretions, dryness of nasal mucosa (humidifier may help).
- Report difficulty breathing, hallucinations, tremors, loss of coordination, irregular heartbeat.

C

## charcoal, activated

***(char' kole)***

*OTC:* Actidose-Aqua, Actidose with Sorbitol, Charcoaid, Charcodote (Can), Liqui-Char

**Pregnancy Category C**

### Drug classes

Antidote

### Therapeutic actions

Adsorbs toxic substances swallowed into the GI tract, inhibiting GI absorption; maximum amount of toxin absorbed is 100–1,000 mg/g charcoal.

### Indications

- Emergency treatment in poisoning by most drugs and chemicals

### Contraindications/cautions

- Poisoning or overdosage of cyanide, mineral acids, alkalies, ethanol, methanol, and iron salts

### Dosage

**Available Forms:** Powder—15, 30, 40, 120, 240 g; liquid—208 mg/ml; suspension—15, 30 g

*ADULT:* 30–100 g or 1 g/kg PO or approximately 5–10 times the amount of poison ingested, as an oral suspension; administer as soon as possible after poisoning.

- *Gastric dialysis:* 20–40 g q6h for 1–2 d for severe poisonings; for optimum effect, administer within 30 min of poisoning.

### Pharmacokinetics

Not absorbed systemically. Excreted in the feces.

### Adverse effects
- GI: *Vomiting* (related to rapid ingestion of high doses), *constipation, diarrhea*, black stools

### Clinically important drug-drug interactions
- Adsorption and inactivation of syrup of ipecac, laxatives with activated charcoal
- Decreased effectiveness of other medications because of adsorption by activated charcoal

## ■ Nursing Considerations

### Assessment
- *History:* Poisoning or overdosage of cyanide, mineral acids, alkalies, ethanol, methanol, and iron salts
- *Physical:* Stools, bowel sounds

### Implementation
- Induce emesis before giving activated charcoal.
- Give drug to conscious patients only.
- Give drug as soon after poisoning as possible; most effective results are seen if given within 30 min.
- Prepare suspension of powder in 6–8 oz of water; taste may be gritty and disagreeable. Sorbitol is added to some preparations to improve taste; diarrhea more likely with these preparations.
- Store in closed containers; activated charcoal adsorbs gases from the air and will lose its effectiveness with prolonged exposure to air.
- Maintain life-support equipment on standby for poisoning and overdose.

### Drug-specific teaching points
- The following side effects may occur: black stools, diarrhea or constipation.

## chenodiol

*(kee noe **dye'** ole)*

chenodeoxycholic acid

Chenix

**Pregnancy Category X**

### Drug classes
Gallstone solubilizing agent

### Therapeutic actions
Suppresses hepatic synthesis of cholesterol and cholic acid, leading to cholesterol in the bile and dissolution of cholesterol gallstones.

### Indications
- Treatment of selected patients with radiolucent gallstones in well-opacifying gallbladders when elective surgery is contraindicated

### Contraindications/cautions
- Allergy to chenodiol, hepatic dysfunction, bile ductal abnormalities, pregnancy, lactation

### Dosage
**Available Forms:** Tablets—250 mg

**ADULT:** 13–16 mg/kg per day PO in two divided doses, morning and night. Start with 250 mg bid for 2 wk, and increase by 250 mg/d each week thereafter until the recommended dose is reached.

**PEDIATRIC:** Safety and efficacy not established.

### Pharmacokinetics

| Route | Onset | Peak | Duration |
|---|---|---|---|
| Oral | Varies | 15–14 min | 2–4 h |

*Metabolism:* Hepatic; $T_{1/2}$: 3.1 min, then 16 1/2 min

*Distribution:* Crosses placenta; may pass into breast milk

*Excretion:* Feces

### Adverse effects
- GI: Increased incidence of intrahepatic cholestasis; *hepatitis; elevated SGPT, diarrhea, cramps,* heartburn, constipation, nausea, vomiting, anorexia, epigastric distress, dyspepsia, flatulence, abdominal pain
- Hematologic: *Elevated serum total cholesterol, LDL;* decreased serum triglycerides; decreased WBC count
- Other: **Colon cancer**

**Clinically important drug-drug interactions**

• Decreased absorption with bile acid sequestering agents (cholestyramine, colestipol) • Reduced absorption of acetaminophen, barbiturates, carbamazepine, digitoxin, digoxin, furosemide, glutethimide, hydantoins, methotrexate, nizatidine, phenothiazines, phenylbutazones, propoxyphene, salicylates, sulfones, sulfonylureas, tetracyclines, theophyllines, tricyclic antidepressants, valproic acid

## ■ Nursing Considerations

### Assessment

- ***History:*** Allergy to chenodiol, hepatic dysfunction, bile ductal abnormalities, pregnancy, lactation
- ***Physical:*** Liver evaluation, abdominal exam; liver function tests, serum lipids, WBC, serum aminotransferase, serum cholesterol; hepatic and biliary radiologic studies

### Implementation

- Give drug twice a day, in the morning and at night.
- Arrange for periodic, regular monitoring of serum aminotransferase levels, serum cholesterol.
- Arrange for patient to be scheduled for periodic oral cholecystograms or ultrasonograms to evaluate drug effectiveness.
- Advise patient to use birth control; drug can cause serious problems for the fetus.

### Drug-specific teaching points

- Take this drug in the morning and at night. Take the drug as long as prescribed.
- This drug may dissolve your gallstones; it does not "cure" the problem that caused the stones in the first place, and the stones can recur; medical follow-up is important.
- Use birth control. This drug must not be taken by pregnant women. If you think you may be pregnant, consult with your physician immediately.
- Receive periodic x-rays or ultrasound tests of your gallbladder. Periodic blood tests are needed to evaluate your response to this drug. Keep follow-up appointments.
- The following side effects may occur: diarrhea (request adjusted dosage); nausea, GI upset, flatulence (small, frequent meals may help).
- Report gallstone attacks (abdominal pain, nausea, vomiting); yellowing of the skin or eyes.



# chloral hydrate

***(klor' al bye' drate)***

Aquachloral Supprettes

**Pregnancy Category C**
**C-IV controlled substance**

**Drug classes**

Sedative/hypnotic (nonbarbiturate)

**Therapeutic actions**

Mechanism by which CNS is affected is not known; hypnotic dosage produces mild cerebral depression and quiet, deep sleep; does not depress REM sleep, produces less "hangover" than most barbiturates and benzodiazepines.

**Indications**

- Nocturnal sedation
- Preoperative sedation to lessen anxiety and induce sleep without depressing respiration or cough reflex
- Adjunct to opiates and analgesics in postoperative care and control of pain

**Contraindications/cautions**

- Contraindications: hypersensitivity to chloral derivatives; allergy to tartrazine (in 324-mg suppositories marketed as Aquachloral Supprettes); severe cardiac disease, gastritis; hepatic or renal impairment; lactation.
- Use cautiously with acute intermittent porphyria (may precipitate attacks).

### Dosage

**Available Forms:** Capsules—500 mg; syrup—250, 500 mg/5 ml; suppositories—324, 500, 648 mg

*ADULT:* Single doses or daily dosage should not exceed 2 g.

- ***Hypnotic:*** 500 mg–1 g PO or rectally 15–30 min before bedtime or 30 min before surgery (*Note:* it is not usually considered safe practice to give oral medication to patients who are NPO for anesthesia or surgery).

- *Sedative:* 250 mg PO or rectally tid after meals.

PEDIATRIC

- *Hypnotic:* 50 mg/kg per day PO up to 1 g per single dose; may be given in divided doses.
- *Sedative:* 25 mg/kg per day PO up to 500 mg per single dose; may be given in divided doses.

### Pharmacokinetics

| *Route* | *Onset* | *Peak* | *Duration* |
|---|---|---|---|
| Oral/PR | 30–60 min | 1–3 h | 4–8 h |

*Metabolism:* Hepatic; $T_{1/2}$: 7–10 h
*Distribution:* Crosses placenta; passes into breast milk
*Excretion:* Urine and bile

### Adverse effects

- CNS: *Somnambulism, disorientation, incoherence, paranoid behavior,* excitement, delirium, drowsiness, staggering gait, ataxia, lightheadedness, vertigo, nightmares, malaise, mental confusion, headache, hallucinations
- GI: *Gastric irritation, nausea, vomiting,* **gastric necrosis** (following intoxicating doses), flatulence, diarrhea, unpleasant taste
- Hematologic: *Leukopenia, eosinophilia*
- Dermatologic: *Skin irritation;* allergic skin rashes including hives, erythema, eczematoid dermatitis, urticaria
- Other: Physical, psychological dependence; tolerance; withdrawal reaction

### Clinically important drug-drug interactions

• Additive CNS depression with alcohol, other CNS depressants • Mutual inhibition of metabolism with alcohol (possible vasodilation reaction characterized by tachycardia, palpitations, and facial flushing) • Complex effects on oral (coumarin) anticoagulants given with chloral hydrate (monitor prothrombin levels and adjust coumarin dosage whenever chloral hydrate is instituted or withdrawn from drug regimen)

### Drug-lab test interferences

• Interference with the copper sulfate test for glycosuria, fluorometric tests for urine catecholamines, and urinary 17-hydroxycorticosteroid determinations (when using the Reddy, Jenkins, and Thorn procedure)

## ■ Nursing Considerations

### Assessment

- *History:* Hypersensitivity to chloral derivatives, allergy to tartrazine, severe cardiac disease, gastritis, hepatic or renal impairment, acute intermittent porphyria, lactation
- *Physical:* Skin color, lesions; orientation, affect, reflexes; P, BP, perfusion; bowel sounds, normal output, liver evaluation; liver and kidney function tests, CBC and differential, stool guaiac test

### Implementation

- Give capsules with a full glass of liquid; ensure that patient swallows capsules whole; give syrup in half glass of water, fruit juice, or ginger ale.
- Supervise dose and amount of drug prescribed for patients who are addiction prone or alcoholic; give least amount feasible to patients who are depressed or suicidal.
- Withdraw gradually over 2 wk if patient has been maintained on high doses for weeks or months; if patient has built up high tolerance, withdrawal should occur in a hospital, using supportive therapy similar to that for barbiturate withdrawal; fatal withdrawal reactions have occurred.
- Reevaluate patients with prolonged insomnia; therapy for the underlying cause (eg, pain, depression) is preferable to prolonged use of sedative–hypnotic drugs.

### Drug-specific teaching points

- Take this drug exactly as prescribed: Swallow capsules whole with a full glass of liquid (take syrup in half glass of water, fruit juice, or ginger ale).

- Do not discontinue the drug abruptly. Consult your care provider if you wish to discontinue the drug.
- Avoid alcohol, sleep-inducing, or OTC drugs; these could cause dangerous effects.
- The following side effects may occur: drowsiness, dizziness, lightheadedness (avoid driving or performing tasks requiring alertness); GI upset (frequent small meals may help); sleep-walking, nightmares, confusion (use caution: close doors, keep medications out of reach so inadvertent overdose does not occur while confused).
- Report skin rash, coffee ground vomitus, black or tarry stools, severe GI upset, fever, sore throat.

## chlorambucil

*(klor* ***am'*** *byoo sil)*

Leukeran

**Pregnancy Category D**

### Drug classes

Alkylating agent, nitrogen mustard
Antineoplastic

### Therapeutic actions

Cytotoxic: alkylates cellular DNA, interfering with the replication of susceptible cells.

### Indications

- Palliative treatment of chronic lymphocytic leukemia; malignant lymphomas, including lymphosarcoma; giant follicular lymphoma; and Hodgkin's disease
- Unlabeled uses: treatment of uveitis and meningoencephalitis associated with Behçet's disease; treatment of idiopathic membranous nephropathy; treatment of rheumatoid arthritis

### Contraindications/cautions

- Allergy to chlorambucil; cross-sensitization with melphalen; radiation therapy, chemotherapy; hematopoietic depression; pregnancy, lactation.

### Dosage

**Available Forms:** Tablets—2 mg

Individualize dosage based on hematologic profile and response.

**ADULT**

- *Initial dose and short course therapy:* 0.1–0.2 mg/kg per day PO for 3–6 wk; single daily dose may be given.
- *Chronic lymphocytic leukemia (alternate regimen):* 0.4 mg/kg PO q2 wk, increasing by 0.1 mg/kg with each dose until therapeutic or toxic effect occurs.
- *Maintenance dose:* 0.03–0.1 mg/kg PO per day. Do not exceed 0.1 mg/kg per day. Short courses of therapy are safer than continuous maintenance therapy; base dosage and duration on patient response and bone marrow status.

**PEDIATRIC:** Safety and efficacy not established.

### Pharmacokinetics

| *Route* | *Onset* | *Peak* | *Duration* |
|---|---|---|---|
| Oral | Varies | 1 h | 15–20 h |

*Metabolism:* Hepatic; $T_{1/2}$: 60–90 min
*Distribution:* Crosses placenta; passes into breast milk
*Excretion:* Urine

### Adverse effects

- CNS: *Tremors, muscular twitching, confusion,* agitation, ataxia, flaccid paresis, hallucinations, seizures
- GI: Nausea, vomiting, anorexia, **hepatotoxicity**, jaundice (rare)
- Respiratory: Bronchopulmonary dysplasia, pulmonary fibrosis
- Hematologic: **Bone marrow depression**, hyperuricemia
- GU: *Sterility* (especially in prepubertal or pubertal males and adult men; amenorrhea can occur in females)
- Dermatologic: Skin rash, urticaria, alopecia, keratitis
- Other: *Cancer, acute leukemia*

## ■ Nursing Considerations

### Assessment

- *History:* Allergy to chlorambucil, cross-sensitization with melphalen (skin rash), radiation therapy, chemotherapy, hematopoietic depression, pregnancy, lactation

- *Physical:* T; weight; skin color, lesions; R, adventitious sounds; liver evaluation; CBC, differential, hemoglobin, uric acid, liver function tests

### Implementation

- Arrange for blood tests to evaluate hematopoietic function before and weekly during therapy.
- Do not give full dosage within 4 wk after a full course of radiation therapy or chemotherapy because of risk of severe bone marrow depression.
- Ensure that patient is well hydrated before treatment.
- Monitor uric acid levels; ensure adequate fluid intake, and prepare for appropriate treatment of hyperuricemia if it occurs.
- Divide single daily dose if nausea and vomiting occur with large single dose.

#### Drug-specific teaching points

- Take this drug once a day. If nausea and vomiting occur, consult health care provider about dividing the dose.
- The following side effects may occur: nausea, vomiting, loss of appetite (dividing dose, small frequent meals also may help; maintain your fluid intake and nutrition; drink at least 10–12 glassses of fluid each day); infertility (from irregular menses to complete amenorrhea; men may stop producing sperm—may be irreversible; discuss with health care provider); severe birth defects—use birth control.
- Report unusual bleeding or bruising; fever, chills, sore throat; cough, shortness of breath; yellow color of the skin or eyes; flank or stomach pain.

## Chloramphenicol

### chloramphenicol

*(klor am **fen'** i kole)*

*Ophthalmic solution:* Chloromycetin Ophthalmic, Chloroptic Ophthalmic

*Otic solution:* Chloromycetin Otic

### chloramphenical sodium succinate

**Pregnancy Category C**

### Drug classes

Antibiotic

### Therapeutic actions

Bacteriostatic effect against susceptible bacteria; prevents cell replication.

### Indications

*Systemic*

- Serious infections for which no other antibiotic is effective
- Acute infections caused by *Salmonella typhi*
- Serious infections caused by *Salmonella, H. influenzae*, rickettsiae, lymphogranuloma—psittacosis group
- Cystic fibrosis regimen

*Ophthalmic Preparations*

- Treatment of superficial ocular infections caused by susceptible microorganisms

*Otic Solution*

- Treatment of superficial infections of the external auditory canal (inner ear infections should be treated with systemic antibiotics)

### Contraindications/cautions

- Allergy to chloramphenical, renal failure, hepatic failure, G-6-PD deficiency, intermittent porphyria, pregnancy (may cause gray syndrome), lactation

### Dosage

**Available Forms:** Capsules—250 mg; powder for injection—100 mg/ml; ophthalmic solution—5 mg/5 ml; ophthalmic ointment—10 mg/g; ophthalmic powder for solution—25 mg vial; otic solution—0.5%

*SYSTEMIC:* Severe and sometimes fatal blood dyscrasias (adults) and severe and sometimes fatal gray syndromes (in newborns and premature infants) may occur. Use should be restricted to situations in which no other antibiotic is effective. Serum levels should be monitored at least weekly to minimize risk of toxicity (therapeutic concentrations: peak, 10–20 μg/ml; trough, 5–10 μg/ml).

*ADULT AND PEDIATRIC:* 50 mg/kg per day PO or IV in divided doses q6h up to 100 mg/kg per day in severe cases.

- *Newborns:* 25 mg/kg PO or IV per day in four doses q6h; after 2 weeks of age, full-term infants usually tolerate 50 mg/kg per day in four doses q6h (dosage should be monitored using serum concentrations of the drug as a guide).

- ***Infants and children with immature metabolic processes:*** 25 mg/kg per day PO or IV (monitor serum concentration carefully).

*GERIATRIC OR RENAL OR HEPATIC FAILURE:* Use serum concentration of the drug to adjust dosage.

*Otic:* Instill 2–3 drops into the ear tid.

*Ophthalmic:* Instill ointment or solution as prescribed.

**Pharmacokinetics**

| *Route* | *Onset* | *Peak* | *Duration* |
|---|---|---|---|
| Oral | Varies | 1–3 h | 48–72 h |
| IV | 20–30 min | 1 h | 48–72 h |

*Metabolism:* Hepatic; $T_{1/2}$: 1.5–4 h
*Distribution:* Crosses placenta; passes into breast milk
*Excretion:* Urine

**IV facts**

**Preparation:** Dilute with 10 ml of Water for Injection, or 5% Dextrose Injection.
**Infusion:** Administer as a 10% solution over 3–5 min, single-dose infusion over 30–60 min. Substitute oral dosage as soon as possible.

**Adverse effects**

*Systemic*

- CNS: *Headache,* mild depression, mental confusion, delirium
- GI: *Nausea, vomiting, glossitis, stomatitis, diarrhea*
- Hematologic: *Blood dyscrasias*
- Other: Fever, macular rashes, urticaria, anaphylaxis; **gray syndrome** (seen in neonates and premature babies: abdominal distension, pallid cyanosis, vasomotor collapse, irregular respirations; may lead to death), superinfections

*Ophthalmic Solution, Otic Solution, Dermatologic Cream*

- Hematologic: **Bone marrow hypoplasia, aplastic anemia,** and **death** with prolonged or frequent intermittent ocular use
- Hypersensitivity: *Irritation, burning, itching,* angioneurotic edema, urticaria, dermatitis
- Other: Superinfections

**Clinically important drug-drug interactions**

• Increased serum levels and drug effects of dicumarol, anisindione, warfarin, phenytoins, tolbutamide, acetohexamide, glipizide, glyburide, tolazamide with chloramphenicol • Decreased hematologic response to iron salts, vitamin $B_{12}$ with chloramphenicol

## ■ Nursing Considerations

### Assessment

- *History:* Allergy to chloramphenicol, renal or hepatic failure, G-6-PD deficiency, intermittent porphyria, lactation
- *Physical:* Culture infection; orientation, reflexes, sensation; R, adventitious sounds; bowel sounds, output, liver function; urinalysis, BUN, CBC, liver function tests, renal function tests

### Implementation

*Systemic Administration*

- Culture infection before beginning therapy.
- Give drug on an empty stomach, 1 h before or 2 h after meals. If severe GI upset occurs, give drug with meals.
- **Do not** give this drug IM because it is ineffective.
- Monitor hematologic data carefully, especially with long-term therapy by any route of administration.
- Reduce dosage in patients with renal or hepatic disease.
- Monitor serum levels periodically as indicated in dosage section.

*Ophthalmic and Otic Solution*

- Topical preparations of the drug should be used only when necessary. Sensitization from the topical use of this drug may preclude its later use in serious infections. Topical preparations that contain antibiotics that are not ordinarily given systemically are preferable.

### Drug-specific teaching points

- **Never** use any leftover medication to self-treat any other infection.

*Oral Therapy*

- Take this drug q6h around the clock; schedule doses to minimize sleep disruption. Take drug on an empty stomach, 1 h before or 2 h after meals. Take the full course of this medication.
- The following side effects may occur: nausea, vomiting (if this becomes severe, the drug can be taken with food); diarrhea (reversible); headache (request medication); confusion (avoid driving or operating delicate machinery); superinfections (frequent hygiene measures may help; medications are available if severe).
- Report sore throat, tiredness; unusual bleeding or bruising (even as late as several weeks after you finish the drug); numbness, tingling, pain in the extremities; pregnancy.

*Ophthalmic Solution*

- Give eye drops as follows: lie down or tilt head backward, and look at ceiling. Drop solution inside lower eyelid while looking up. After instilling eye drops, close eyes, and apply gentle pressure to the inside corner of the eye for 1 min.
- The following side effects may occur: temporary stinging or blurring of vision after administration (notify health care provider if pronounced).

*Otic Solution*

- Give as follows: lie on side or tilt head so that ear to be treated is uppermost. Grasp ear and gently pull up and back (adults) or down and back (children); drop medication into the ear canal. Stay in this position for 2–3 min. Solution should be warmed to near body temperature before use; **do not** use cold or hot solutions.

## chlordiazepoxide hydrochloride

*(klor dye az e **pox'** ide)*

metaminodiazepoxide hydrochloride

Apo-Chlorodiazepoxide (CAN), Librium, Libritabs, Mitran, Reposans-10, Solium (CAN)

**Pregnancy Category D**
**C-IV controlled substance**

### Drug classes

Benzodiazepine
Antianxiety agent

### Therapeutic actions

Exact mechanisms of action not understood; acts mainly at subcortical levels of the CNS; main sites of action may be the limbic system and reticular formation; potentiates the effects of gamma-aminobutyric acid (GABA).

### Indications

- Management of anxiety disorders or for short-term relief of symptoms of anxiety
- Acute alcohol withdrawal; may be useful in symptomatic relief of acute agitation, tremor, delirium tremens, hallucinosis
- Preoperative relief of anxiety and tension

### Contraindications/cautions

- Contraindications: hypersensitivity to benzodiazepines, psychoses, acute narrow-angle glaucoma, shock, coma, acute alcoholic intoxication with depression of vital signs, pregnancy (increased risk of congenital malformations, neonatal withdrawal syndrome), labor and delivery ("floppy infant" syndrome reported), lactation (infants may become lethargic and lose weight).
- Use cautiously with impaired liver or kidney function, debilitation.

### Dosage

**Available Forms:** Capsules—5, 10, 25 mg; tablets—10, 25 mg; powder for injection—100 mg/amp

Individualize dosage; increase dosage cautiously to avoid adverse effects.

ADULT

– ***Oral***

- *Anxiety disorders:* 5 or 10 mg, up to 20 or 25 mg, tid–qid, depending on severity of symptoms.
- *Preoperative apprehension:* 5–10 mg tid–qid on days preceding surgery.
- *Alcohol withdrawal:* Parenteral form usually used initially. If given orally, initial dose is 50–100 mg, followed by repeated doses as needed up to 300 mg/d; then reduce to maintenance levels.

– ***Parenteral***
- *Severe anxiety:* 50–100 mg IM or IV initially; then 25–50 mg tid–qid if necessary, or switch to oral dosage form.
- *Preoperative apprehension:* 50–100 mg IM 1 h prior to surgery.
- *Alcohol withdrawal:* 50–100 mg IM or IV initially; repeat in 2–4 h if necessary. Up to 300 mg may be given in 6 h; do not exceed 300 mg/24 h.

PEDIATRIC

– ***Oral***
- *>6 Y:* 5 mg bid–qid initially; may be increased in some children to 10 mg bid–tid.
- *<6 Y:* Not recommended.

– ***Parenteral, older children:*** 25–50 mg IM or IV.

GERIATRIC PATIENTS OR THOSE WITH DEBILITATING DISEASE: 5 mg PO bid–qid; 25–50 mg IM or IV.

### Pharmacokinetics

| Route | Onset | Peak | Duration |
|---|---|---|---|
| Oral | Varies | 1–4 h | 48–72 h |
| IM | 10–15 min | 15–30 min | 48–72 h |
| IV | Immediate | 3–30 min | 48–72 h |

*Metabolism:* Hepatic; $T_{1/2}$: 5–30 h
*Distribution:* Crosses placenta; passes into breast milk
*Excretion:* Urine

### IV facts

**Preparation:** Add 5 ml sterile physiologic saline or Sterile Water for Injection to contents of ampule; agitate gently until drug is dissolved.

**Infusion:** Administer IV doses slowly over 1 min. Change patients on IV therapy to oral therapy as soon as possible.

### Adverse effects

- CNS: *Transient, mild drowsiness initially; sedation, depression, lethargy, apathy, fatigue, lightheadedness, disorientation, restlessness, confusion,* crying, delirium, headache, slurred speech, dysarthria, stupor, rigidity, tremor, psychomotor retardation, extrapyramidal symptoms; *mild paradoxical excitatory reactions, during first 2 wk of treatment* (especially in psychiatric patients, aggressive children, and those with high dosage), visual and auditory disturbances, diplopia, nystagmus, depressed hearing, nasal congestion
- GI: *Constipation, diarrhea,* dry mouth, salivation, nausea, anorexia, vomiting, difficulty in swallowing, gastric disorders, hepatic dysfunction, jaundice
- CV: *Bradycardia, tachycardia,* CV collapse, hypertension and hypotension, palpitations, edema
- **Hematologic**: Decreased hematocrit, blood dyscrasias
- GU: *Incontinence, urinary retention, changes in libido,* menstrual irregularities
- **Dermatologic**: Urticaria, pruritus, skin rash, dermatitis
- **Dependence**: *Drug dependence with withdrawal syndrome* when drug is discontinued (more common with abrupt discontinuation of higher dosage used for longer than 4 mo)
- **Other**: Phlebitis and thrombosis at IV injection sites, hiccups, fever, diaphoresis, paresthesias, muscular disturbances, gynecomastia, pain, burning, and redness after IM injection

### Clinically important drug-drug interactions

• Increased CNS depression with alcohol, omeprazole • Increased pharmacologic effects with cimetidine, disulfiram, oral contraceptives • Decreased sedative effects with theophylline, aminophylline, dyphylline, oxitriphylline

## ■ Nursing Considerations

### Assessment

- *History:* Hypersensitivity to benzodiazepines; psychoses; acute narrow-angle glaucoma; shock; coma; acute alcoholic intoxication; pregnancy; lactation; impaired liver or kidney function, debilitation.
- *Physical:* Skin color, lesions; T; orientation, reflexes, affect, ophthalmologic exam; P, BP; R, adventitious sounds; liver

evaluation, abdominal exam, bowel sounds, normal output; CBC, liver and renal function tests.

### Implementation

- Do not administer intra-arterially; arteriospasm, gangrene may result.
- Reconstitute solutions for IM injection only with special diluent provided; do not use diluent if it is opalescent or hazy; prepare injection immediately before use, and discard any unused solution.
- Do not use drug solutions made with physiologic saline or Sterile Water for Injection for IM injections because of pain.
- Give IM injection slowly into upper outer quadrant of the gluteus muscle; monitor injection sites.
- Do not use small veins (dorsum of hand or wrist) for IV injection.
- Monitor P, BP, R carefully during IV administration.
- Keep patients receiving parenteral benzodiazepines in bed for 3 h; do not permit ambulatory patients to drive following an injection.
- Reduce dosage of narcotic analgesics in patients receiving IV benzodiazepines; doses should be reduced by at least one-third or totally eliminated.
- Monitor liver and kidney function, CBC at intervals during long-term therapy.
- Taper dosage gradually after long-term therapy, especially in epileptic patients.

### Drug-specific teaching points

- Take drug exactly as prescribed.
- Do not stop taking this drug (long-term therapy) without consulting health care provider. Avoid alcohol, sleep-inducing, or OTC drugs.
- The following side effects may occur: drowsiness, dizziness (transient; avoid driving or engaging in other dangerous activities); GI upset (take drug with water); depression, dreams, emotional upset, crying.
- Report severe dizziness, weakness, drowsiness that persists, rash or skin lesions, palpitations, swelling of the extremities, visual changes, difficulty voiding.

# Chloroquine

## chloroquine hydrochloride

***(klo' ro kwin)***

*IM:* Aralen HCl

## chloroquine phosphate

*Oral:* Aralen Phosphate

**Pregnancy Category C**

### Drug classes

Amebicide
Antimalarial
4-aminoquinoline

### Therapeutic actions

Inhibits protozoal reproduction and protein synthesis. Mechanism of anti-inflammatory action in rheumatoid arthritis is not known.

### Indications

- Treatment of extraintestinal amebiasis
- Prophylaxis and treatment of acute attacks of malaria caused by susceptible strains of *Plasmodia*
- Unlabeled use: treatment of rheumatoid arthritis and discoid lupus erythematosus

### Contraindications/cautions

- Allergy to chloroquine and other 4-aminoquinolines, porphyria, psoriasis, retinal disease, hepatic disease, G-6-PD deficiency, alcoholism, lactation.

### Dosage

**Available Forms:** Tablets—250, 500 mg; injection—50 mg/ml

ADULT

- *Amebicide:* **Oral**: 1 g (600 mg base)/d for 2 d; then 500 mg (300 mg base)/d for 2–3 wk. **IM:** 200–250 mg (160–200 mg base)/d for 10–12 d.
- *Antimalarial:* **Suppression:** 300 mg base PO once a week on the same day for 2 wk before exposure and continuing until 6–8 wk after exposure. **Acute attack:** 600 mg base PO initially; then 300 mg 6 h later and on days 2 and 3; or 160–200 mg base IM initially and 6 h later if needed. Do not exceed 800 mg

base/day. **Antirheumatoid:** 200 mg (160 mg base) PO qid or bid.

*PEDIATRIC*

- *Amebicide:* Not recommended.
- *Antimalarial:* **Suppression:** 5 mg base/kg PO once a week on the same day for 2 wk before exposure and continuing until 6–8 wk after exposure. **Acute attack:** 10 mg base/kg PO initially; then 5 mg base/kg 6 h later and on days 2 and 3; or 5 mg base/kg IM initially and 6 h later if needed. Do not exceed 10 mg base/kg per day.

### Pharmacokinetics

| *Route* | *Onset* | *Peak* | *Duration* |
|---|---|---|---|
| Oral | Varies | 1–2 h | wk |
| IM | Rapid | 45–60 min | wk |

*Metabolism:* Hepatic; $T_{1/2}$: 70–120 h
*Distribution:* Crosses placenta; passes into breast milk
*Excretion:* Urine

### Adverse effects

- CNS: *Visual disturbances*, retinal changes (blurring of vision, difficulty in focusing), ototoxicity, muscle weakness
- GI: *Nausea, vomiting, diarrhea*, loss of appetite, abdominal pain
- CV: *Hypotension, ECG changes*
- Hematologic: Blood dyscrasias, hemolysis in patients with G-6-PD deficiency

### Clinically important drug-drug interactions

• Increased effects of chloroquine with cimetidine • Decreased GI absorption of both drugs with magnesium trisilicate

## ■ Nursing Considerations

### Assessment

- *History:* Allergy to chloroquine and other 4-aminoquinolines, porphyria, psoriasis, retinal disease, hepatic disease, G-6-PD deficiency, alcoholism, lactation
- *Physical:* Reflexes, muscle strength, auditory and ophthalmologic screening; BP, ECG; liver palpation; CBC, G-6-PD in deficient patients, liver function tests

### Implementation

- Administer with meals if GI upset occurs.
- Schedule weekly, same-day therapy on a calendar.
- Double check pediatric doses; children are very susceptible to overdosage.
- Arrange for ophthalmologic exams during long-term therapy.

### Drug-specific teaching points

- Take full course of drug therapy. Take drug with meals if GI upset occurs. Mark your calendar with the drug days for malarial prophylaxis.
- The following side effects may occur: stomach pain, loss of appetite, nausea, vomiting, or diarrhea.
- Arrange to have regular ophthalmologic exams if long-term use is indicated.
- Report blurring of vision, loss of hearing, ringing in the ears, muscle weakness, fever.

# Chlorothiazide

## chlorothiazide

*(klor oh **thye'** a zide)*

Diurigen, Diuril

## chlorothiazide sodium

Diuril Sodium

**Pregnancy Category C**

### Drug classes

Thiazide diuretic

### Therapeutic actions

Inhibits reabsorption of sodium and chloride in distal renal tubule, increasing the excretion of sodium, chloride, and water by the kidney.

### Indications

- Adjunctive therapy in edema associated with CHF, cirrhosis, corticosteroid, and estrogen therapy, renal dysfunction
- Treatment of hypertension, alone or with other antihypertensives
- Unlabeled uses: treatment of diabetes insipidus, especially nephrogenic diabetes

insipidus; reduction of incidence of osteoporosis in postmenopausal women

### Contraindications/cautions

- Fluid or electrolyte imbalances, renal or liver disease, gout, SLE, glucose tolerance abnormalities, hyperparathyroidism, manic-depressive disorders, lactation

## Dosage

**Available Forms:** Tablets—250, 500 mg; oral suspension—250 mg/5 ml; powder for injection—500 mg

**ADULT**

- *Edema:* 0.5–2 g PO or IV (if patient unable to take PO) qid or bid.
- *Hypertension:* 0.5–2 g/d PO as a single or divided dose; adjust dose to BP response, giving up to 2 g/d in divided doses. IV use is not recommended.

**PEDIATRIC:** 22 mg/kg per day PO in two doses.

- *Infants <6 mo:* Up to 33 mg/kg per day in two doses. IV use not recommended.

### Pharmacokinetics

| *Route* | *Onset* | *Peak* | *Duration* |
|---|---|---|---|
| Oral | 2 h | 3–6 h | 6–12 h |
| IV | 15 min | 30 min | 2 h |

*Metabolism:* $T_{1/2}$: 45–120 min
*Distribution:* Crosses placenta; passes into breast milk
*Excretion:* Urine

#### IV facts

**Preparation:** Dilute vial for parenteral solution with 18 ml Sterile Water for Injection. Never add less than 18 ml. Discard diluted solution after 24 h.
**Infusion:** Administer slowly, 0.5 g over 5 min. Switch to oral drug as soon as possible.
**Incompatibilities:** Compatible with dextrose and sodium chloride solutions. Do not give parenteral solution with whole blood or blood products.

### Adverse effects

- CNS: *Dizziness, vertigo,* paresthesias, weakness, headache, drowsiness, fatigue
- GI: *Nausea, anorexia, vomiting, dry mouth, diarrhea, constipation*, jaundice, hepatitis, pancreatitis
- CV: Orthostatic hypotension, venous thrombosis, volume depletion, cardiac arrhythmias, chest pain
- Hematologic: **Leukopenia, thrombocytopenia, agranulocytosis, aplastic anemia, neutropenia,** fluid and electrolyte imbalances
- GU: *Polyuria, nocturia, impotence*, loss of libido
- Dermatologic: Photosensitivity, rash, purpura, exfoliative dermatitis
- Other: Muscle cramps and muscle spasms, fever, hives, gouty attacks, flushing, weight loss, rhinorrhea

### Clinically important drug-drug interactions

• Increased thiazide effects and chance of acute hyperglycemia with diazoxide • Decreased absorption with cholestyramine • Increased risk of cardiac glycoside toxicity if hypokalemia occurs • Increased risk of lithium toxicity • Increased dosage of antidiabetic agents may needed

### Drug-lab test interferences

• Monitor for decreased PBI levels without clinical signs of thyroid disturbances.

## ■ Nursing Considerations

### Assessment

- *History:* Fluid or electrolyte imbalances, renal or liver disease, gout, SLE, glucose tolerance abnormalities, hyperparathyroidism, manic-depressive disorders, lactation
- *Physical:* Orientation, reflexes, muscle strength; pulses, BP, orthostatic BP, perfusion, edema, baseline ECG; R, adventitious sounds; liver evaluation, bowel sounds; CBC, serum electrolytes, blood glucose, liver and renal function tests, serum uric acid, urinalysis

### Implementation

- Administer with food or milk if GI upset occurs.
- Administer early in the day, so increased urination will not disturb sleep.

- Measure and record weight to monitor fluid changes.

### Drug-specific teaching points

- Take drug early in the day, so sleep will not be disturbed by increased urination.
- Weigh yourself daily, and record weights.
- Protect skin from exposure to the sun or bright lights.
- Increased urination will occur.
- Use caution if dizziness, drowsiness, feeling faint occur.
- Report rapid weight change, swelling in ankles or fingers, unusual bleeding or bruising, muscle cramps.

## chlorotrianisene

*(klor oh trye **an'** i seen)*

Tace

**Pregnancy Category X**

### Drug classes

Hormone
Estrogen

### Therapeutic actions

Estrogens are endogenous female sex hormones; important in the development of the female reproductive system and secondary sex characteristics; cause capillary dilatation, fluid retention, protein anabolism, and thin cervical mucus; conserve calcium and phosphorus and encourage bone formation; inhibit ovulation and prevent postpartum breast discomfort.

### Indications

- Palliation of moderate to severe vasomotor symptoms, atrophic vaginitis, kraurosis vulvae associated with menopause
- Treatment of female hypogonadism
- Palliation in prostatic carcinoma (inoperable and progressing)

### Contraindications/cautions

- Contraindications: allergy to estrogens, breast cancer, estrogen-dependent neoplasm; undiagnosed abnormal genital bleeding, active thrombophlebitis or thromboembolic disorders or history of such from previous estrogen use, pregnancy, lactation.
- Use cautiously with metabolic bone disease, renal insufficiency, CHF.

### Dosage

**Available Forms:** Capsules—12, 25 mg

Administer PO; give cyclically (3 wk of therapy followed by 1 wk of rest), and use for short term unless otherwise indicated.

ADULT

- *Moderate to severe vasomotor symptoms associated with menopause:* 12–25 mg/d PO given cyclically for 30 d; one or more courses may be used.
- *Atrophic vaginitis and kraurosis vulvae:* 12–25 mg/d PO given cyclically for 30–60 d.
- *Female hypogonadism:* 12–25 mg/d PO given cyclically for 21 d; may follow immediately by 100 mg progesterone IM or by oral progestin during the last 5 d of therapy. Next course may begin on the fifth day of induced uterine bleeding.
- *Prostatic carcinoma:* 12–25 mg/d PO given chronically.

PEDIATRIC: Not recommended due to effect on the growth of the long bones.

### Pharmacokinetics

| Route | Onset |
|---|---|
| Oral | 14 d |

*Metabolism:* Hepatic
*Distribution:* Crosses placenta; passes into breast milk

### Adverse effects

- CNS: *Steepening of the corneal curvature with a resultant change in visual acuity and intolerance to contact lenses, headache,* migraine, dizziness, mental depression, chorea, convulsions
- GI: *Gallbladder disease, nausea, vomiting, abdominal cramps, bloating,* cholestatic jaundice, colitis, acute pancreatitis, **hepatic adenoma**
- CV: *Increased blood pressure,* **thromboembolic and thrombotic disease**, peripheral edema

- GU: *Increased risk of endometrial cancer* in postmenopausal women, *breakthrough bleeding, change in menstrual flow, dysmenorrhea, premenstrual-like syndrome, amenorrhea*, vaginal candidiasis, cystitis-like syndrome, endometrial cystic hyperplasia, changes in libido
- Dermatologic: Photosensitivity, chloasma, erythema nodosum or multiforme, hemorrhagic eruption, loss of scalp hair, hirsutism, urticaria, dermatitis
- Other: Decreased glucose tolerance, *weight changes*, aggravation of porphyria, *breast tenderness*

### Clinically important drug-drug interactions

• Increased therapeutic and toxic effects of corticosteroids with chlorotrianisene • Risk of breakthrough bleeding, pregnancy, spotting with barbiturates, hydantoins, rifampin

### Drug-lab test interferences

• Increased sulfobromophthalein retention • Increased prothrombin and factors VII, VIII, IX, and X • Decreased antithrombin III • Increased thyroid binding globulin with increased PBI, $T_4$, increased uptake of free $T_3$ resin (free $T_4$ is unaltered) • Impaired glucose tolerance • Decreased pregnanediol excretion • Reduced response to metyrapone test • Reduced serum folate concentration • Increased serum triglycerides and phospholipid concentration

## ■ Nursing Considerations

### Assessment

- *History:* Allergy to estrogens, breast cancer, estrogen-dependent neoplasm, undiagnosed abnormal genital bleeding, active thrombophlebitis or thromboembolic disorders or history of such from previous estrogen use, metabolic bone disease, renal insufficiency, CHF, pregnancy, lactation
- *Physical:* Skin color, lesions, edema; breast exam; orientation, affect, reflexes; P, auscultation, BP, peripheral perfusion; R, adventitious sounds; bowel sounds, liver evaluation, abdominal exam; pelvic exam; serum calcium, phosphorus; liver and renal function tests; Pap smear; glucose tolerance test

### Implementation

- Arrange for pretreatment and periodic (at least annual) history and physical, which should include BP, breasts, abdomen, pelvic organs, and a Pap smear.
- Caution patient before beginning therapy of the risks involved with estrogen use, the need to prevent pregnancy during treatment, the need for frequent medical followup, the need for periodic rests from treatment.
- Give cyclically for short-term or cyclic use only when treating postmenopausal conditions because of the risk of endometrial neoplasm; taper to the lowest effective dose, and provide a drug-free week each month if possible.
- Arrange for progestin therapy during chronic estrogen therapy in women; this will mimic normal physiologic cycling and allow for cyclic uterine bleeding, which may decrease the risk of endometrial cancer.
- Protect patient from exposure to sun or ultraviolet light if photosensitivity occurs.

### Drug-specific teaching points

- Use drug in cycles or for short periods.
- Prepare a calendar of drug days, rest days, and drug-free period.
- Many potentially serious problems have occurred with the use of this drug, including development of cancers, blood clots, liver problems; this drug cannot be given to pregnant women because of serious fetal toxic effects.
- Have periodic medical exams throughout therapy.
- The following side effects may occur: nausea, vomiting, bloating; headache, dizziness, mental depression (use caution if driving or performing tasks that require alertness); sensitivity to sunlight (use a sunscreen and wear protective clothing); skin rash, loss of scalp hair, darkening of the skin on the face; changes in menstrual patterns.

- Report pain in the groin or calves, chest pain or sudden shortness of breath, abnormal vaginal bleeding, lumps in the breast, sudden severe headache, dizziness or fainting, changes in vision or speech, weakness or numbness in the arm or leg, severe abdominal pain, yellowing of the skin or eyes, severe mental depression.

## chlorphenesin carbamate

*(klor **fen'** e sin)*

Maolate

**Pregnancy Category C**

### Drug classes

Skeletal muscle relaxant, centrally acting

### Therapeutic actions

Precise mechanism not known; has sedative properties; does not directly relax tense skeletal muscles; does not directly affect the motor endplate or motor nerves.

### Indications

- Relief of discomfort from acute, painful musculoskeletal conditions
- Adjunct to rest, physical therapy, and other measures

### Contraindications/cautions

- Allergic or idiosyncratic reactions to chlorphenesin, tartrazine; lactation.

### Dosage

**Available Forms:** Tablets—400 mg

**ADULT:** Initially, 800 mg PO tid until desired effect is obtained; reduce maintenance dosage to 400 mg qid or less.

**PEDIATRIC:** Safety and efficacy not established for children < 12 y.

**GERIATRIC PATIENTS OR THOSE WITH HEPATIC IMPAIRMENT:** Dosage reduction may be necessary; monitor closely.

### Pharmacokinetics

| *Route* | *Onset* | *Peak* | *Duration* |
|---|---|---|---|
| Oral | Varies | 1–3 h | 8–12 h |

*Metabolism:* Hepatic; $T_{1/2}$: 3.5 h

*Distribution:* Crosses placenta; may pass into breast milk

*Excretion:* Urine

### Adverse effects

- CNS: *Dizziness, drowsiness, confusion,* paradoxical stimulation, insomnia, headache
- GI: *Nausea, epigastric distress*
- Hematologic: Leukopenia, thrombocytopenia, agranulocytosis, pancytopenia
- Hypersensitivity: **Anaphylactoid reactions,** drug fever

### ■ Nursing Considerations

#### Assessment

- *History:* Allergic or idiosyncratic reactions to chlorphenesin, tartrazine, lactation
- *Physical:* Skin color, lesions; orientation, affect; liver evaluation; liver function tests, CBC with differential

#### Implementation

- Reduce dosage with liver dysfunction.

#### Drug-specific teaching points

- Take this drug exactly as prescribed; do not take a higher dosage.
- Avoid alcohol, sleep-inducing, or OTC drugs; these could cause dangerous effects.
- The following side effects may occur: drowsiness, dizziness, confusion (avoid driving or engaging in activities that require alertness); nausea (take with food and eat frequent small meals); insomnia, headache (reversible).
- Report skin rash, severe nausea, dizziness, insomnia, fever, difficulty breathing.

## chlorpheniramine maleate

*(klor fen **ir'** a meen)*

Aller-Chlor, Chlo-Amine, Chlorate, Chlorphen (CAN), Chlor-Pro, Chlor-Trimeton, Chlor-Tripolon (CAN), Novopheniram (CAN), Telachlor, Telachlor

**Pregnancy Category B**

**Drug classes**
Antihistamine (alkylamine type)

**Therapeutic actions**
Competitively blocks the effects of histamine at $H_1$ receptor sites; has atropine-like, antipruritic, and sedative effects.

**Indications**
- Oral preparations: symptomatic relief of symptoms associated with perennial and seasonal allergic rhinitis; vasomotor rhinitis; allergic conjunctivitis; mild, uncomplicated urticaria and angioedema; amelioraton of allergic reactions to blood or plasma; dermatographism; adjunctive therapy in anaphylactic reactions.
- Parenteral preparations: amelioration of allergic reactions to blood or plasma; in anaphylaxis as adjunct to epinephrine and other measures; other uncomplicated allergic conditions when oral therapy is not possible.

**Contraindications/cautions**
- Contraindications: allergy to any antihistamines, narrow-angle glaucoma, stenosing peptic ulcer, symptomatic prostatic hypertrophy, asthmatic attack, bladder neck obstruction, pyloroduodenal obstruction, third trimester of pregnancy, lactation.
- Use caution in pregnancy.

**Dosage**
**Available Forms:** Chewable tablets—2 mg; tablets—4, 8, 12 mg; ER tablets—8, 12 mg; ER capsules—8 mg

*ADULT AND CHILDREN > 12 Y*
- *Tablets or syrup:* 4 mg PO q4–6h; do not exceed 24 mg in 24 h.
- *Sustained-release forms:* 8–12 mg PO hs or q8–12h during the day; do not exceed 24 mg in 24 h.
- *Parenteral:* 10 mg/ml injection is used for IV, IM, or SC administration; 100 mg/ml injection is used for IM or SC use only.
  - *Allergic reactions to blood or plasma:* 10–20 mg IM, IV, or SC, single dose; maximum dose is 40 mg in 24 h.
  - *Anaphylaxis:* 10–20 mg IV as a single dose.
  - *Uncomplicated allergic conditions:* 5–20 mg IM, IV, or SC, as a single dose.

*PEDIATRIC*
- *Tablets or syrup: 6–12 y:* 2 mg q4–6h PO; do not exceed 12 mg in 24 h. *2–5 y:* 1 mg q4–6h PO; do not exceed 4 mg in 24 h.
- *Sustained-release forms: 6–12 y:* 8 mg PO hs or during the day. *< 6 y:* Not recommended.

*GERIATRIC:* More likely to cause dizziness, sedation, syncope, toxic confusional states, and hypotension in elderly patients; use with caution.

**Pharmacokinetics**

| Route | Onset | Peak |
|---|---|---|
| Oral | 1/2–6 h | 2–6 h |

*Metabolism:* Hepatic, $T_{1/2}$: 12–15 h
*Distribution:* Crosses placenta; enters breast milk
*Excretion:* Urine

**IV facts**
**Preparation:** No preparation necessary.
**Infusion:** Administer slowly, 10 mg over 1 min, by direct injection or into tubing of running line.

**Adverse effects**
- CNS: *Drowsiness, sedation, dizziness, disturbed coordination*, fatigue, confusion, restlessness, excitation, nervousness, tremor, headache, blurred vision, diplopia, vertigo, tinnitus, acute labryinthitis, hysteria, tingling, heaviness and weakness of the hands
- GI: *Epigastric distress,* anorexia, increased appetite and weight gain, nausea, vomiting, diarrhea or constipation
- CV: Hypotension, palpitations, bradycardia, tachycardia, extrasystoles
- **Respiratory**: *Thickening of bronchial secretions*, chest tightness, wheezing, nasal stuffiness, dry mouth, dry nose, dry throat, sore throat

- **Hematologic**: Hemolytic anemia, hypoplastic anemia, thrombocytopenia, leukopenia, agranulocytosis, pancytopenia
- **GU**: Urinary frequency, dysuria, urinary retention, early menses, decreased libido, impotence
- **Other**: Urticaria, rash, anaphylactic shock, photosensitivity, excessive perspiration, chills

**Clinically important drug-drug interactions**

• Increased depressant effects with alcohol, other CNS depressants

## ■ Nursing Considerations

### Assessment

- *History:* Allergy to any antihistamines; narrow-angle glaucoma, stenosing peptic ulcer, symptomatic prostatic hypertrophy, asthmatic attack, bladder neck obstruction, pyloroduodenal obstruction, pregnancy, lactation
- *Physical:* Skin color, lesions, texture; orientation, reflexes, affect; vision exam; P, BP ; R, adventitious sounds; bowel sounds; prostate palpation; CBC with differential

### Implementation

- Administer oral preparations with food if GI upset occurs.
- Caution patient not to crush or chew sustained-release preparations.
- Administer 10 mg/ml injection IV, IM, or SC; give 100 mg/ml injection IM or SC.
- Maintain epinephrine 1:1000 readily available when using parenteral preparations; hypersensitivity reactions, including anaphylaxis, have occurred.
- Arrange for periodic blood tests during prolonged therapy.

### Drug-specific teaching points

- Take as prescribed; avoid excessive dosage. Take with food if GI upset occurs; do not crush or chew the sustained-release preparations.
- The following side effects may occur: dizziness, sedation, drowsiness (use caution driving or performing tasks that require alertness); epigastric distress, diarrhea, or constipation (take with meals; consult care provider if severe); dry mouth (frequent mouth care, sucking sugarless lozenges may help); thickening of bronchial secretions, dryness of nasal mucosa (use a humidifier).
- Avoid OTC drugs; many contain ingredients that could cause serious reactions if taken with this antihistamine.
- Avoid alcohol; serious sedation may occur.
- Report difficulty breathing; hallucinations, tremors, loss of coordination; unusual bleeding or bruising; visual disturbances; irregular heartbeat.

# chlorpromazine hydrochloride

*(klor **proe'** ma zeen)*

Largactil (CAN), Ormazine, Thorazine

**Pregnancy Category C**

**Drug classes**

Phenothiazine
Dopaminergic blocking agent
Antipsychotic
Antiemetic
Antianxiety agent

**Therapeutic actions**

Mechanism not fully understood; antipsychotic drugs block postsynaptic dopamine receptors in the brain; depresses those parts of the brain involved with wakefulness and emesis; anticholinergic, antihistaminic ($H_1$), and alpha-adrenergic blocking.

**Indications**

- Management of manifestations of psychotic disorders; control manic phase of manic-depressive illness
- Relief of preoperative restlessness and apprehension
- Adjunct in treatment of tetanus
- Acute intermittent porphyria therapy
- Severe behavioral problems in children: therapy for combativeness, hyperactivity

- Control of nausea and vomiting and intractable hiccups
- Possibly effective in the treatment of nonpsychotic anxiety (not drug of choice)

**Contraindications/cautions**

- Allergy to chlorpromazine; comatose or severely depressed states; bone marrow depression; circulatory collapse; subcortical brain damage, Parkinson's disease; liver damage; cerebral or coronary arteriosclerosis; severe hypotension or hypertension; respiratory disorders; glaucoma; epilepsy or history of epilepsy; peptic ulcer or history of peptic ulcer; decreased renal function; prostate hypertrophy; breast cancer; thyrotoxicosis; myelography within 24 h or scheduled within 48 h; lactation; exposure to heat, phosphorous insecticides; children with chickenpox, CNS infections (makes children more susceptible to dystonias, confounding the diagnosis of Reye's syndrome or other encephalopathy; antiemetic effects of drug may mask symptoms of Reye's syndrome, encephalopathies)

**Dosage**

**Available Forms:** Tablets—10, 25, 50, 100, 200 mg; SR capsules—30, 75, 150, 200, 300 mg; syrup—10 mg/5 ml; concentrate—30, 100 mg/ml; suppositories—25, 100 mg; injection—25 mg/ml

Full clinical antipsychotic effects may require 6 wk to 6 mo of therapy.

ADULT

- ***Excessive anxiety, agitation in psychiatric patients:*** 25 mg IM; may repeat in 1 h. Increase dosage gradually in inpatients, up to 400 mg q4–6h. Switch to oral dosage as soon as possible: 25–50 mg PO tid for outpatients; up to 2,000 mg/d PO for inpatients. Initial oral dosage: 10 mg tid–qid PO or 25 mg PO bid–tid; increase daily dosage by 20–50 mg semiweekly until optimum dosage is reached (maximum response may require months); doses of 200–800 mg/d PO are not uncommon in discharged mental patients.
- ***Surgery:*** Preoperatively, 25–50 mg PO 2–3 h before surgery or 12.5–25.0 mg IM 1–2 h before surgery; intraoperatively, 12.5 mg IM, repeated in 1/2 h or 2 mg IV repeated q 2 min up to 25 mg total to control vomiting (if no hypotension occurs); postoperatively, 10–25 mg PO q4–6h or 12.5–25.0 mg IM repeated in 1 h (if not, hypotension occurs).
- ***Acute intermittent porphyria:*** 25–50 mg PO or 25 mg IM tid–qid.
- ***Tetanus:*** 25–50 mg IM tid–qid, usually with barbiturates, or 25–50 mg IV diluted and infused at rate of 1 mg/min.
- ***Antiemetic:*** 10–25 mg PO q4–6h; 50–100 mg rectally q6–8h; 25 mg IM. If no hypotension, give 25–50 mg q3–4h. Switch to oral dose when vomiting ends.
- ***Intractable hiccups:*** 25–50 mg PO tid–qid. If symptoms persist for 2–3 d, give 25–50 mg IM; if inadequate response, give 25–50 mg IV in 500–1,000 ml of saline with BP monitoring.

PEDIATRIC: Generally not used in children < 6 mo.

- ***Psychiatric outpatients:*** 0.5 mg/kg PO q4–6h; 1 mg/kg rectally q6–8h; 0.5 mg/kg IM q6–8h, not to exceed 40 mg/d (up to 5 y) or 75 mg/d (5–12 y).
- ***Surgery:*** Preoperatively, 0.5 mg/kg PO 2–3 h before surgery or 0.5 mg/kg IM 1–2 h before surgery; intraoperatively, 0.25 mg/kg IM or 1 mg (diluted) IV, repeated at 2-min intervals up to total IM dose; postoperatively, 0.5 mg/kg PO q4–6h or 0.5 mg/kg IM, repeated in 1 h if no hypotension.
- ***Psychiatric inpatients:*** 50–100 mg/d PO; maximum of 40 mg/d IM for children up to 5 y; maximum of 75 mg/d IM for children 5–12 y.
- ***Tetanus:*** 0.5 mg/kg IM q6–8h or 0.5 mg/min IV, not to exceed 40 mg/d for children up to 23 kg; 75 mg/d for children 23–45 kg.
- ***Antiemetic:*** 0.55 mg/kg PO q4–6h; 1.1 mg/kg rectally q6–8h or 0.55 mg/kg IM q6–8h. Maximum IM dosage 40 mg/d for children up to 5 y or 75 mg/d for children 5–12 y.

GERIATRIC: Start dosage at one-fourth to one-third that given in younger adults and increase more gradually.

**Pharmacokinetics**

| Route | Onset | Peak | Duration |
|---|---|---|---|
| Oral | 30–60 min | 2–4 h | 4–6 h |
| IM | 10–15 min | 15–20 min | 4–6 h |

*Metabolism:* Hepatic, $T_{1/2}$: 2 h, then 30 h
*Distribution:* Crosses placenta; enters breast milk
*Excretion:* Urine

**IV facts**
**Preparation:** Dilute drug for IV injection to a concentration of 1 mg/ml or less.
**Infusion:** Reserve IV injections for hiccups, tetanus, or use during surgery. Administer at a rate of 1 mg/2 min.
**Incompatibilities:** Precipitate or discoloration may occur when mixed with morphine, meperidine, cresols.

**Adverse effects**

- CNS: *Drowsiness, insomnia, vertigo,* headache, weakness, tremors, ataxia, slurring, cerebral edema, seizures, exacerbation of psychotic symptoms, *extrapyramidal syndromes*, neuroleptic malignant syndrome
- GI: *Dry mouth, salivation, nausea, vomiting, anorexia, constipation*, paralytic ileus, incontinence
- CV: *Hypotension, otrhostatic hypotension,* hypertension, tachycardia, bradycardia, cardiac arrest, CHF, cardiomegaly, refractory arrhythmias, pulmonary edema
- Respiratory: Bronchospasm, laryngospasm, dyspnea, suppression of cough reflex and potential aspiration
- Hematologic: **Eosinophilia, leukopenia, leukocytosis, *anemia*, aplastic anemia, hemolytic anemia, thrombocytopenic or nonthrombocytopenic purpura, pancytopenia, elevated serum cholesterol**
- GU: *Urinary retention,* polyuria, incontinence, priapism, ejaculation inhibition, male impotence, urine discolored pink to red-brown
- EENT: Nasal congestion, glaucoma, *photophobia, blurred vision*, miosis, mydriasis, deposits in the cornea and lens, pigmentary retinopathy
- Hypersensitivity: Jaundice, *urticaria*, angioneurotic edema, laryngeal edema, photosensitivity, eczema, asthma, anaphylactoid reactions, exfoliative dermatitis, contact dermatitis
- Endocrine: Lactation, breast engorgement in females, galactorrhea, syndrome of inappropriate ADH secretion, amenorrhea, menstrual irregularities, gynecomastia, changes in libido, hyperglycemia, inhibition of ovulation, infertility, pseudopregnancy, reduced urinary levels of gonadotropins, estrogens and progestins
- Other: Fever, heat stroke, pallor, flushed facies, sweating, *photosensitivity*

**Clinically important drug-drug interactions**

• Additive anticholinergic effects and possibly decreased antipsychotic efficacy with anticholinergic drugs • Additive CNS depression, hypotension if given preoperatively with barbiturate anesthetics, alcohol, meperidine • Additive effects of both drugs if concurrently with beta-blockers • Increased risk of tachycardia, hypotension with epinephrine, norepinephrine • Increased risk of seizure with metrizamide • Decreased hypotension effect with guanethidine

**Drug-lab test interferences**

• False-positive pregnancy tests (less likely if serum test is used) • Increase in protein-bound iodine, not attributable to an increase in thyroxine

## ■ Nursing Considerations

### Assessment

- *History:* Allergy to chlorpromazine; comatose or severely depressed states; bone marrow depression; circulatory collapse; subcortical brain damage, Parkinson's disease; liver damage; cerebral or coronary arteriosclerosis; severe hypotension or hypertension; respiratory disorders;

glaucoma; epilepsy or history of epilepsy; peptic ulcer or history of peptic ulcer; decreased renal function; prostate hypertrophy; breast cancer; thyrotoxicosis; myelography within 24 h or scheduled within 48 h; lactation; exposure to heat, phosphorous insecticides; children with chickenpox; CNS infections

- *Physical:* T, weight; skin color, turgor; reflexes, orientation, intraocular pressure, ophthalmologic exam; P, BP, orthostatic BP, ECG; R, adventitious sounds; bowel sounds, normal output, liver evaluation; prostate palpation, normal urine output; CBC; urinalysis; thyroid, liver, and kidney function tests; EEG

### Implementation

- Do not change brand names of oral dosage forms or rectal suppositories; bioavailability differs.
- Dilute the oral concentrate just before administration in 60 ml or more of tomato or fruit juice, milk, simple syrup, orange syrup, carbonated beverage, coffee, tea, or water, or in semisolid foods (soup, puddings).
- Protect oral concentrate from light.
- Do not allow the patient to crush or chew the sustained-release capsules.
- Do not give by SC injection; give slowly by deep IM injection into upper outer quadrant of buttock.
- Keep recumbent for 1/2 h after injection to avoid orthostatic hypotension.
- Avoid skin contact with oral concentrates and parenteral drug solutions due to possible contact dermatitis.
- Patient or the patient's guardian should be advised about the possibility of tardive dyskinesias.
- Be alert to potential for aspiration because of suppressed cough reflex.
- Monitor renal function tests, discontinue if serum creatinine, BUN become abnormal.
- Monitor CBC, discontinue if WBC count is depressed.
- Consult with physician about dosage reduction or use of anticholinergic antiparkinsonian drugs (controversial) if extrapyramidal effects occur.
- Withdraw drug gradually after high-dose therapy; possible gastritis, nausea, dizziness, headache, tachycardia, insomnia after abrupt withdrawal.
- Monitor elderly patients for dehydration; sedation and decreased sensation of thirst; CNS effects can lead to dehydration, hemoconcentration, and reduced pulmonary ventilation; promptly institute remedial measures.
- Avoid epinephrine as vasopressor if drug-induced hypotension occurs.

### Drug-specific teaching points

- Take drug exactly as prescribed. Avoid OTC drugs and alcohol unless you have consulted your health care provider.
- Do not change brand names without consulting your health care provider.
- Learn how to dilute oral drug concentrate; how to use rectal suppository.
- Do not get oral concentrate on your skin or clothes; contact dermatitis can occur.
- The following side effects may occur: drowsiness (avoid driving or operating dangerous machinery; avoid alcohol, increases drowsiness); sensitivity to the sun (avoid prolonged sun exposure, wear protective garments or use a sunscreen); pink or reddish-brown urine (expected effect); faintness, dizziness (change position slowly; use caution climbing stairs; usually transient).
- Use caution in hot weather; risk of heat stroke; keep up fluid intake, and do not overexercise in a hot climate.
- Report sore throat, fever, unusual bleeding or bruising, rash, weakness, tremors, impaired vision, dark urine, pale stools, yellowing of the skin and eyes.

## chlorpropamide

*(klor **proe'** pa mide)*

Apo-Chlorpropamide (CAN), Diabinese

**Pregnancy Category C**

### Drug classes

Antidiabetic agent
Sulfonylurea, first generation

**Therapeutic actions**

Stimulates insulin release from functioning beta cells in the pancreas; may improve binding between insulin and insulin receptors or increase the number of insulin receptors; can increase the effect of ADH (antidiuretic hormone).

**Indications**

- Adjunct to diet to lower blood glucose in patients with non–insulin-dependent diabetes mellitus (type II)
- Unlabeled uses: treatment of neurogenic diabetes insipidus at doses of 200–500 mg/d; temporary adjunct to insulin therapy in type II diabetes to improve diabetic control

**Contraindications/cautions**

- Allergy to sulfonylureas; diabetes complicated by fever, severe infections, severe trauma, major surgery, ketosis, acidosis, coma; type I or juvenile diabetes, serious hepatic impairment, serious renal impairment, uremia, thyroid or endocrine impairment, glycosuria, hyperglycemia associated with primary renal disease; pregnancy, lactation

**Dosage**

**Available Forms:** Tablets—100, 250 mg

ADULT

- *Initial therapy:* 250 mg/d PO. *Maintenance therapy:* 100–250 mg/d PO. Up to 500 mg/d may be needed; do not exceed 750 mg/d.

PEDIATRIC: Safety and efficacy not established.

GERIATRIC: Greater sensitivity to drug; start with initial dose of 100–125 mg/d PO; monitor for 24 h, and gradually increase as needed.

**Pharmacokinetics**

| *Route* | *Onset* | *Peak* | *Duration* |
|---|---|---|---|
| Oral | 1 h | 3–4 h | 60 h |

*Metabolism:* Hepatic, $T_{1/2}$: 36 h
*Distribution:* Crosses placenta; enters breast milk
*Excretion:* Urine and bile

**Adverse effects**

- GI: *Anorexia, nausea, vomiting, epigastric discomfort, heartburn*
- CV: Possible increased risk of CV mortality
- Hematologic: ***Hypoglycemia***, leukopenia, thrombocytopenia, anemia
- Hypersensitivity: Allergic skin reactions, eczema, pruritus, erythema, urticaria, photosensitivity, fever, jaundice
- Endocrine: SIADH

**Clinically important drug-drug interactions**

• Increased risk of hypoglycemia if chlorpropamide with sulfonamides, urine acidifiers, chloramphenicol, fenfluramine, oxyphenbutazone, phenylbutazone, salicylates, monoamine oxidase inhibitors, clofibrate, dicumarol, rifampin • Decreased effectiveness of chlorpropamide and diazoxide if taken concurrently • Increased risk of hyperglycemia if chlorpropamide with urine alkalinizers, thiazides, other diuretics • Risk of hypoglycemia and hyperglycemia if chlorpropamide with ethanol; "disulfiram reaction" also has been reported

## ■ Nursing Considerations

**Assessment**

- *History:* Allergy to sulfonylureas; diabetes complicated by fever, severe infections, severe trauma, major surgery, ketosis, acidosis, coma; type I or juvenile diabetes, serious hepatic or renal impairment, uremia, thyroid or endocrine impairment, glycosuria, hyperglycemia associated with primary renal disease; pregnancy, lactation
- *Physical:* Skin color, lesions; T; orientation, reflexes, peripheral sensation; R, adventitious sounds; liver evaluation, bowel sounds; urinalysis, BUN, serum creatinine, liver function tests, blood glucose, CBC

**Implementation**

- Give drug before breakfast; if severe GI upset occurs, divide dose—one before breakfast and one before evening meal.
- Monitor urine and serum glucose levels often to determine efficacy and dosage.

- Transfer to insulin therapy during periods of high stress (infections, surgery, trauma).
- Use IV glucose if severe hypoglycemia occurs due to overdose; support and monitoring may be prolonged for 3–5 d because of the long half-life of chlorpropamide.

### Drug-specific teaching points
- Do not discontinue this medication without consulting physician.
- Monitor urine or blood for glucose and ketones.
- Do not use this drug during pregnancy.
- Avoid OTC drugs and alcohol.
- Report fever, sore throat, unusual bleeding or bruising, skin rash, dark urine, light-colored stools, hypoglycemic or hyperglycemic reactions.

## chlorthalidone

*(klor **thal'** i done)*

Apo-Chlorthalidone (CAN), Hygroton, Thalitone

**Pregnancy Category C**

### Drug classes
Thiazide-like diuretic

### Therapeutic actions
Inhibits reabsorption of sodium and chloride in distal renal tubule, increasing excretion of sodium, chloride, and water by the kidney.

### Indications
- Adjunctive therapy in edema associated with CHF, cirrhosis, corticosteroid and estrogen therapy, renal dysfunction
- Hypertension, alone or with other antihypertensives

### Contraindications/cautions
- Fluid or electrolyte imbalances, renal or liver disease, gout, SLE, glucose tolerance abnormalities, hyperparathyroidism, manic-depressive disorders, lactation

### Dosage
**Available Forms:** Tablets—15, 25, 50, 100 mg

ADULT
- *Edema:* 50–100 mg/d PO or 100 mg every other day: up to 200 mg/d.
- *Hypertension:* 25–100 mg/d PO based on patient response (doses > 25 mg/d are likely to increase $K^+$ excretion, but provide no further increase in $Na^+$ excretion or decrease in BP).

PEDIATRIC: Safety and efficacy not established.

### Pharmacokinetics

| Route | Onset | Peak | Duration |
|---|---|---|---|
| Oral | 2 h | 3–6 h | 24–72 h |

*Metabolism:* Hepatic, $T_{1/2}$: 54 h
*Distribution:* Crosses placenta; enters breast milk
*Excretion:* Urine

### Adverse effects
- CNS: *Dizziness, vertigo,* paresthesias, weakness, headache, drowsiness, fatigue
- GI: *Nausea, anorexia, vomiting, dry mouth, diarrhea, constipation*, jaundice, hepatitis, pancreatitis
- GU: *Polyuria, nocturia, impotence*, loss of libido
- **Hematologic**: Leukopenia, thrombocytopenia, agranulocytosis, aplastic anemia, neutropenia, fluid and electrolyte imbalances
- CV: Orthostatic hypotension, venous thrombosis, volume depletion, cardiac arrhythmias, chest pain
- **Dermatologic**: Photosensitivity, rash, purpura, exfoliative dermatitis
- **Other**: Muscle cramps and muscle spasms, fever, hives, gouty attacks, flushing, weight loss

### Clinically important drug-drug interactions
• Increased thiazide effects and chance of acute hyperglycemia with diazoxide • Decreased absorption with cholestyramine, colestipol • Increased risk of cardiac glycoside toxicity if hypokalemia occurs • Increased risk of lithium toxicity • Increased dosage of antidiabetic agents may be needed

**Drug-lab test interferences**
• Decreased PBI levels without clinical signs of thyroid disturbances.

## ■ Nursing Considerations

### Assessment
- *History:* Fluid or electrolyte imbalances, renal or liver disease, gout, SLE, glucose tolerance abnormalities, hyperparathyroidism, manic-depressive disorders, lactation
- *Physical:* Skin color and lesions; orientation, reflexes, muscle strength; pulses, BP, orthostatic BP, perfusion, edema, baseline ECG; R, adventitious sounds; liver evaluation, bowel sounds; CBC, serum electrolytes, blood glucose, liver and renal function tests, serum uric acid, urinalysis

### Implementation
- Give with food or milk if GI upset occurs.
- Administer early in the day, so increased urination will not disturb sleep.
- Mark calendars or other reminders of drug days for outpatients on every other day or 3- to 5-d/wk therapy.
- Measure and record weight to monitor fluid changes.

### Drug-specific teaching points
- Take drug early in the day, so sleep will not be disturbed by increased urination.
- Weigh yourself daily, and record weights.
- Protect skin from exposure to the sun or bright lights.
- Increased urination will occur.
- Use caution if dizziness, drowsiness, feeling faint occur.
- Report rapid weight change, swelling in ankles or fingers, unusual bleeding or bruising, muscle cramps.

## chlorzoxazone

*(klor **zox'** a zone)*

Paraflex, Parafon Forte DSC, Remular-S

**Pregnancy Category C**

**Drug classes**
Skeletal muscle relaxant, centrally acting

**Therapeutic actions**
Precise mechanism not known; has sedative properties; acts at spinal and supraspinal levels of the CNS to depress reflex arcs involved in producing and maintaining skeletal muscle spasm.

**Indications**
- Relief of discomfort associated with acute, painful musculoskeletal conditions, adjunct to rest, physical therapy, and other measures

**Contraindications/cautions**
- Contraindicated with allergic or idiosyncratic reactions to chlorzoxazone.
- Use caution in the presence of history of allergies or allergic drug reactions, lactation.

### Dosage
**Available Forms:** Tablets—250, 500 mg; capsules—250, 500 mg

**ADULT:** Initially, 500 mg PO tid–qid; may increase to 750 mg tid–qid; reduce dosage as improvement occurs.

**PEDIATRIC:** Safety and efficacy not established.

**Pharmacokinetics**

| Route | Onset | Peak | Duration |
|---|---|---|---|
| Oral | 30–60 min | 1–2 h | 3–4 h |

*Metabolism:* Hepatic, $T_{1/2}$: 60 min
*Distribution:* Crosses placenta; may enter breast milk
*Excretion:* Urine

**Adverse effects**
- CNS: *Dizziness, drowsiness, lightheadedness,* malaise, overstimulation
- GI: *GI disturbances*; GI bleeding (rare)
- GU: Urine discoloration—orange to purple-red
- Hypersensitivity: skin rashes, petechiae, ecchymoses, angioneurotic edema, **anaphylaxis** (rare)

**Clinically important drug-drug interactions**
• Additive CNS effects with alcohol, other CNS depressants

## ■ Nursing Considerations

### Assessment
- *History:* Allergic or idiosyncratic reactions to chlorzoxazone; history of allergies or allergic drug reactions; lactation
- *Physical:* Skin color, lesions; orientation; liver evaluation; liver function tests

### Implementation
- Discontinue if signs or symptoms of liver dysfunction or allergic reaction (urticaria, redness, or itching) occur.

### Drug-specific teaching points
- Take this drug exactly as prescribed; do not take a higher dosage.
- Avoid alcohol, sleep-inducing, or OTC drugs; these could cause dangerous effects.
- The following side effects may occur: drowsiness, dizziness, lightheadedness (avoid driving or engaging in activities that require alertness); nausea (take with food and eat frequent small meals); discolored urine (expected effect).
- Report skin rash, severe nausea, coffee-ground vomitus, black or tarry stools, pale stools, yellow skin or eyes, difficulty breathing.

# cholestyramine

*(koe **less'** tir a meen)*

Questran, Questron Light, Prevalite

**Pregnancy Category C**

### Drug classes
Antihyperlipidemic agent
Bile acid sequestrant

### Therapeutic actions
Binds bile acids in the intestine, allowing excretion in the feces; as a result, cholesterol is oxidized in the liver to replace the bile acids lost; serum cholesterol and LDL are lowered.

### Indications
- Adjunctive therapy: reduction of elevated serum cholesterol in patients with primary hypercholesterolemia (elevated LDL)
- Pruritus associated with partial biliary obstruction
- Unlabeled uses: antibiotic-induced pseudomembranous colitis; bile salt-mediated diarrhea, postvagotomy diarrhea; chlordecone *(Kepone)* pesticide poisoning to bind the poison in the intestine

### Contraindications/cautions
- Allergy to bile acid sequestrants, tartrazine (tartrazine sensitivity occurs often with allergies to aspirin); complete biliary obstruction; abnormal intestinal function; pregnancy; lactation.

### Dosage
*ADULT:* 4 g one to six times per day PO. Individualize dose based on response.

*PEDIATRIC:* Safety and efficacy not established.

### Pharmacokinetics
Not absorbed systemically; excreted in the feces.

### Adverse effects
- CNS: Headache, anxiety, vertigo, dizziness, fatigue, syncope, drowsiness
- GI: *Constipation to fecal impaction, exacerbation of hemorrhoids,* abdominal cramps, pain, flatulence, anorexia, heartburn, nausea, vomiting, steatorrhea
- Hematologic: *Increased bleeding tendencies related to vitamin K malabsorption,* vitamins A and D deficiencies, reduced serum and red cell folate, hyperchloremic acidosis
- GU: Hematuria, dysuria, diuresis
- Dermatologic: Rash and irritation of skin, tongue, perianal area
- Other: Osteoporosis, backache, muscle and joint pain, arthritis, fever

### Clinically important drug-drug interactions
- Decreased or delayed absorption with warfarin, dicumarol, thiazide diuretics, digitalis preparations, thyroid, corticosteroids
- Malabsorption of fat-soluble vitamins with cholestyramine

## ■ Nursing Considerations

### Assessment
- *History:* allergy to bile acid sequestrants, tartrazine; complete biliary obstruction; abnormal intestinal function; lactation

- *Physical:* Skin lesions, color, temperature; orientation, affect, reflexes; P, auscultation, baseline ECG, peripheral perfusion; liver evaluation, bowel sounds; lipid studies, liver function tests, clotting profile

### Implementation

- Mix contents of one packet or one level scoop of powder with 4–6 fluid oz of beverage (water, milk, fruit juices, noncarbonates), highly fluid soup, pulpy fruits (applesauce, pineapple); do not give drug in dry form.
- Administer drug before meals.
- Monitor intake of other oral drugs due to risk of binding in the intestine and delayed or decreased absorption, give oral medications 1 h before or 4–6 h after the cholestyramine.
- Alert patient and concerned others about high cost of drug.

### Drug-specific teaching points

- Take drug before meals; do not take the powder in the dry form; mix one packet or one scoop with 4–6 oz of fluid—water, milk, juice, noncarbonates, highly fluid soups, cereals, pulpy fruits.
- Take other medications 1 h before or 4–6 h after cholestyramine.
- The following side effects may occur: constipation (consult about measures that may help); nausea, heartburn, loss of appetite (small, frequent meals may help); dizziness, drowsiness, vertigo, fainting (avoid driving and operating dangerous machinery); headache, muscle and joint aches and pains (may lessen with time).
- Report unusual bleeding or bruising, severe constipation, severe GI upset, chest pain, difficulty breathing, rash, fever.

## choline magnesium trisalicylate

*(**ko'** leen mag **nee'** see um tri **sal'** i ci late)*

Tricosal, Trilisate

**Pregnancy Category C**

### Drug classes

Nonsteroidal anti-inflammatory drug (NSAID)
Salicylate
Analgesic–antipyretic

### Therapeutic actions

Inhibits prostaglandin synthesis; action lowers fever, decreases inflammation.

### Indications

- Treatment of osteoarthritis, rheumatoid arthritis
- Relief of moderate pain, fever

### Contraindications/cautions

- Contraindications: allergy to salicylates, NSAIDs.
- Use cautiously with chronic renal failure, peptic ulcer, hepatic failure, children with chickenpox or CNS symptoms, lactation.

### Dosage

**Available Forms:** 750, 1000 mg

ADULT

- *Arthritis:* 1.5–2.5 g/d PO in 1 to 3 divided doses. Do not exceed 4.5 g/d.
- *Pain, fever:* 2–3 g/d PO in 2 divided doses.

PEDIATRIC

- *Pain, fever:* 50 mg/kg per day PO in two divided doses.

### Pharmacokinetics

| Route | Onset | Peak |
|---|---|---|
| Oral | 30 min | 1–3 h |

*Metabolism:* Hepatic, $T_{1/2}$: 2–3 h
*Distribution:* Crosses placenta; passes into breast milk
*Excretion:* Urine

### Adverse effects

- CNS: Dizziness, vertigo, confusion, drowsiness, headache, tinnitus
- GI: *Diarrhea, nausea,* GI lesion, GI bleed

### Clinically important drug-drug interactions

- Increased risk of salicylate toxicity with aminosalicylic acid, ammonium chloride, acidifying agents, carbonic anhydrase inhibitors • Increased risk of bleeding with oral anticoagulants • Increased risk of toxicity of methotrexate with choline magnesium trisalicylate • Decreased effectiveness of probenecid, sulfinpyrazone

## ■ Nursing Considerations

### Assessment

- *History:* Allergy to salicylates or NSAIDs, peptic ulcer disease, hepatic failure, chronic renal failure, lactation
- *Physical:* Skin condition, T, neurologic status, abdominal exam, kidney and liver function tests, urinalysis, bleeding times

### Implementation

- Give with meals to decrease GI effects.

### Drug-specific teaching points

- Take drug with meals; use the drug only as prescribed.
- Know that the following side effects may occur: dizziness, lightheadedness, drowsiness (avoid driving or operating dangerous machinery it this occurs); nausea, diarrhea.
- Report sore throat, fever, rash, itching, black or tarry stools.

## choline salicylate

***(ko' leen sal' i ci late)***

*OTC:* Arthropan

**Pregnancy Category C**

### Drug classes

Nonsteroidal anti-inflammatory drug (NSAID)
Salicylate
Analgesic–antipyretic

### Therapeutic actions

Inhibits prostaglandin synthesis, which lowers fever, decreases inflammation.

### Indications

- Treatment of osteoarthritis, rheumatoid arthritis
- Relief of moderate pain, fever

### Contraindications/cautions

- Contraindications: allergy to salicylates, NSAIDs.
- Use cautiously with chronic renal failure, peptic ulcer, hepatic failure, children with chickenpox or CNS symptoms, lactation.

### Dosage

**Available Forms:** Liquid—870 mg/5 ml

*ADULT AND CHILDREN > 12 Y:* 870 mg PO q3–4h; do not exceed 6 doses per day. Patients with rheumatoid arthritis may start with 5–10 ml, up to qid.

*PEDIATRIC:* 2 g/m$^2$ per day PO in 4 to 6 divided doses.

### Pharmacokinetics

| *Route* | *Onset* | *Peak* |
|---|---|---|
| Oral | 5–10 min | 10–30 min |

*Metabolism:* Hepatic, $T_{1/2}$: 2–3 h
*Distribution:* Crosses placenta; enters breast milk
*Excretion:* Urine

### Adverse effects

- CNS: Dizziness, vertigo, confusion, drowsiness, headache, tinnitus, sweating
- GI: *Diarrhea, nausea,* hepatotoxicity

### Clinically important drug-drug interactions

- Increased risk of salicylate toxicity with aminosalicylic acid, ammonium chloride, acidifying agents, carbonic anhydrase inhibitors • Increased risk of bleeding with oral anticoagulants • Increased risk of toxicity of methotrexate with choline magnesium trisalicylate • Decreased effectiveness of probenecid, sulfinpyrazone

## ■ Nursing Considerations

### Assessment

- *History:* Allergy to salicylates or NSAIDs, peptic ulcer disease, hepatic or chronic renal failure, lactation
- *Physical:* Skin condition, T, neurologic status, abdominal exam, kidney and liver function tests, urinalysis, bleeding times

### Implementation

- Give with meals to decrease GI effects; may be mixed with fruit juice or carbonated beverage to improve taste.

### Drug-specific teaching points

- Take drug with meals; use as prescribed. May take with fruit juice, carbonated beverages to improve taste. Store drug at room temperature.
- The following side effects may occur: dizziness, lightheadedness, drowsiness (avoid driving or operating dangerous machinery); nausea, diarrhea.
- Report sore throat, fever, rash, itching, black or tarry stools.

## chorionic gonadotropin

*(goe **nad'** oh troe pin)*

human chorionic gonadotropin (HCG)

A.P.L., Chorex, Choron 10, Gonic, Pregnyl, Profasi

**Pregnancy Category C**

### Drug classes

Hormone

### Therapeutic actions

A human placental hormone with actions identical to pituitary leutenizing hormone (LH); stimulates production of testosterone and progesterone.

### Indications

- Prepubertal cryptorchidism not due to anatomic obstruction
- Treatment of selected cases of hypogonadotropic hypogonadism in males
- Induction of ovulation in the anovulatory, infertile woman in whom the cause of anovulation is secondary and not due to primary ovarian failure and who has been pretreated with human menotropins

### Contraindications/cautions

- Contraindications: known sensitivity to chorionic gonadotropin, precocious puberty, prostatic carcinoma or androgen-dependent neoplasm.
- Use cautiously with epilepsy, migraine, asthma, cardiac or renal disease, lactation.

### Dosage

**Available Forms:** Powder for injection—5,000, 10,000, 20,000 U/vial with 10 ml diluent

For IM use only; individualize dosage; the following dosage regimens are suggested:

***Prepubertal cryptorchidism not due to anatomic obstruction:*** 4,000 USP U IM, 3× per week for 3 wk; 5,000 USP U IM, every second day for 4 injections; 15 injections of 500–1,000 USP U over 6 wk; 500 USP U 3× per week for 4–6 wk; if not successful, start another course 1 mo later, giving 1,000 USP U/injection.

***Hypogonadotropic hypogonadism in males:*** 500–1,000 USP U, IM 3× per week for 3 wk; followed by the same dose twice a week for 3 wk; 1,000–2,000 USP U IM 3× per week; 4,000 USP U 3× per week for 6–9 mo; reduce dosage to 2,000 USP Units 3× per week for an additional 3 mo.

***Use with menotropins to stimulate spermatogenesis:*** 5,000 IU IM three times per week for 4–6 mo; with the beginning of menotropins therapy, HCG dose is continued at 2,000 IU twice a week.

***Induction of ovulation and pregnancy:*** 5,000–10,000 IU IM, 1 d following the last dose of menotropins.

### Pharmacokinetics

| Route | Onset | Peak |
|---|---|---|
| IM | 2 h | 6 h |

*Metabolism:* Hepatic, $T_{1/2}$: 23 h

*Distribution:* Crosses placenta; may enter breast milk

*Excretion:* Urine

### Adverse effects

- CNS: *Headache, irritablilty, restlessness,* depression, fatigue
- CV: Edema, arterial thromboembolism
- Endocrine: *Precocious puberty, gynecomastia*, ovarian hyperstimulation (sudden ovarian enlargement, ascites, rupture of ovarian cysts, multiple births)
- Other: *Pain at injection site*

## ■ Nursing Considerations

### Assessment

- *History:* Sensitivity to chorionic gonadotropin, precocious puberty, prostatic carcinoma or androgen-dependent neoplasm, epilepsy, migraine, asthma, cardiac or renal disease, lactation
- *Physical:* Skin texture, edema; prostate exam; injection site; sexual development; orientation, affect, reflexes; R, adventitious sounds; P, auscultation, BP, peripheral edema; liver evaluation; renal function tests

### Implementation

- Prepare solution for injection using manufacturers' instructions; brand and concentrations vary.
- Discontinue at any sign of ovarian overstimulation, and have patient admitted to the hospital for observation and supportive measures.
- Provide comfort measures for CNS effects, pain at injection site.

### Drug-specific teaching points

- This drug can only be given IM. Prepare a calendar with treatment schedule.
- The following side effects may occur: headache, irritability, restlessness, depression, fatigue (reversible; if uncomfortable, consult health care provider).
- Report pain at injection site, severe headache, restlessness, swelling of ankles or fingers, difficulty breathing, severe abdominal pain.

# chymopapain

*(kye' moe pa pane)*

Chymodiactin

**Pregnancy Category C**

### Drug classes

Enzyme

### Therapeutic actions

A protein-dissolving enzyme, which hydrolyzes the polypeptides and proteins that maintain the structure of the chondromucoproteins when injected into the lumbar intervertebral disk. This decreases the pressure and relieves compression symptoms in that area.

### Indications

- Treatment of herniated lumbar intervertebral disks unresponsive to conservative therapy.

### Contraindications/cautions

- Allergy to chymopapain, papaya; severe spondyloisthesis; spinal stenosis; paralysis; spinal cord tumor; previous injection of chymopapain; use in any spinal region other than the lumbar area

### Dosage

**Available Forms:** Powder for injection—4 nKat U/vial

ADULT: 2–4 nKat U/disk injected; usually 3 nKat U/disk, or a volume of injection of 1–2 ml. Maximum dose in patient with multiple herniations is 8 nKat U injected.

PEDIATRIC: Safety and efficacy not established.

### Pharmacokinetics

| *Route* | *Onset* | *Duration* |
|---|---|---|
| Intradiscal | 30 min | 24 h |

*Metabolism:* Plasma, $T_{1/2}$: 18–20 h
*Distribution:* May cross placenta
*Excretion:* Urine

### Adverse effects

- CNS: Paraplegia, paralysis, CNS hemorrhage, myelopathy, paraparesis, headache, dizziness, hypalegesia, leg weakness, calf cramping, foot drop, tingling and numbness in toes and legs
- GI: Nausea, paralytic ileus
- GU: Urinary retention
- MS: *Back pain, stiffness, soreness; back spasm;* ***discitis***
- Allergic: Erythema, pilomotor erection, rash, pruritic urticaria, conjunctivitis, vasomotor rhinitis, angioedema, **anaphylaxis**

## ■ Nursing Considerations

### Assessment

- *History:* Lumbar spine lesion, allergy to papaya or chymopapain, previous injection with chymopapain, spinal tumor, paralysis, spinal stenosis

- *Physical:* Weight, neurologic status, skin evaluation, abdominal exam, urinary output

### Implementation

- Pretreat patient with histamine receptor agonists to lessen severity of allergic reaction. Cimetidine 300 mg PO q6h and diphenhydramine 50 mg PO q6h for 24 h before procedure.
- Prepare solution: cleanse vial stopper with alcohol; allow to air dry before inserting needle (alcohol deactivates the enzyme); reconstitute with 5 ml Sterile Water for Injection. Do not use Bacteriostatic Water for Injection. Store refrigerated. Use within 2 h of reconstitution. Discard drug after that time.
- Provide comfort measures for pain of injection, back spasm, and back pain (which may persist for several weeks).

### Drug-specific teaching points

- This drug will be injected directly into the lumbar spine.
- The following side effects may occur: back spasm, back pain, back soreness, numbness and tingling.
- Report difficulty breathing, rash, itchy or runny eyes, running nose, swelling, vomiting, loss of movement and feeling in the extremities.

## cidofovir

*(si doh' foh ver)*

Vistide

**Pregnancy Category C**

### Drug classes

Antiviral

### Therapeutic actions

Antiviral activity; selectively inhibits CMV replication by inhibition of viral DNA synthesis.

### Indications

- Treatment of CMV retinitis in AIDS patients

### Contraindications/cautions

- Contraindications: allergy to cidofovir, probenecid, or sulfa; pregnancy, lactation
- Use cautiously with renal impairment and in elderly

### Dosage

**Available Forms:** Injection—75 mg/ml

*ADULT:* 5 mg/kg IV infused over 1 hr once per wk for 2 consecutive wk during induction; 5 mg/kg IV once every 2 wk for maintenance. Probenecid must be administered orally with each dose, 2 g PO 3 h before cidofovir and 1 g at 2 h and 8 h after completion of infusion.

*PEDIATRIC:* Safety and efficacy not established in children <12 y.

*RENAL IMPAIRMENT*

| CCr (ml/min) | Induction dose | Maintenance dose |
|---|---|---|
| 41–44 | 2 mg/kg IV once per wk for 2 wk | 2 mg/kg IV once every 2 wk |
| 30–40 | 1.5 mg/kg IV once per wk for 2 wk | 1.5 mg/kg IV once every 2 wk |
| 20–29 | 1 mg/kg IV once per wk for 2 wk | 1 mg/kg IV once every 2 wk |
| <19 | 0.5 mg/kg IV once per wk for 2 wk | 0.5 mg/kg IV once every 2 wk |

### Pharmacokinetics

| Route | Onset | Peak |
|---|---|---|
| IV | Rapid | 15 min |

*Metabolism:* $T_{1/2}$: 1 h

*Distribution:* Crosses placenta; may enter breast milk

*Excretion:* Renal

### IV facts

**Preparation:** Patient should receive 2 g probenecid before starting infusion and 1 g 2 and 8 h after infusion; patient should be hydrated with 1 L normal saline before each dose and 2 L after dose, if tolerated. Dilute in 100 ml 0.9% Saline Solution before administration. Store at room temperature; mixtures may be stored up to 24 h refrigerated; warm to room temperature before using.

**Infusion:** Infuse over 1 h.

**Compatibilities:** Do not mix in solution with other drugs.

### Adverse effects

- CNS: *Headache,* ocular hypotony, asthenia
- GI: *Nausea, vomiting, diarrhea,* anorexia, dry mouth
- CV: Palpitations
- Respiratory: Dyspnea, sinusitis
- Hematologic: **Neutropenia,** metabolic acidosis, elevated serum creatinine
- GU: **Nephrotoxicity,** proteinuria
- Dermatologic: Alopecia, rash
- Other: Infection, chills, fever

### Clinically important drug-drug interactions

• Avoid other nephrotoxic drugs (amphotericin B, aminoglycosides, foscarnet, IV pentamidine) • Risk of increased serum levels of zidovudine when probenecid (required pretreatment with cidofovir) is given concurrently; reduce dosage of zidovudine by up to 50% on day of cidofovir therapy or discontinue for that day

## ■ Nursing Considerations

### Assessment

- *History:* Allergy to cidofovir, probenecid, sulfa drugs; renal dysfunction, pregnancy, lactation
- *Physical:* T; orientation, reflexes; BP, P, peripheral perfusion; R, adventitious sounds; bowel sounds; urinary output; skin color, perfusion, hydration; renal function tests

### Implementation

- Medicate patient with 2 g probenecid PO 3 h before starting cidofovir infusion and 1 g 2 and 8 h after infusion; patient should be hydrated with 1 L normal saline before each dose and 2 L after dose, if tolerated.
- Monitor renal function carefully before and during therapy; dosage must be adjusted based on renal function; for serum creatinine increase of 0.3–0.4 mg/dL, reduce dose from 5 mg/kg to 3 mg/kg. Discontinue drug and notify physician if serum creatinine >0.5 mg/dL or $3^+$ proteinuria.
- Monitor hydration carefully; increase fluids as tolerated.

### Drug-specific teaching points

- This drug can only be given IV. You will need to receive normal saline IV before drug is given. Mark calendar with dates to return for subsequent doses.
- This drug does not cure your CMV retinitis; other AIDS therapy should be continued. If on zidovudine, dosage adjustments will be needed when probenecid is taken.
- Return for medical follow-up, including blood tests to monitor kidney function; decreases in kidney function may require discontinuation of this drug.
- The following side effects may occur: nausea, vomiting, loss of appetite, diarrhea, abdominal pain; headache, dizziness, insomnia.
- Report severe diarrhea, severe nausea, flank pain, discomfort at IV site.

## cimetidine

*(sye met' i deen)*

Novo-Cimetine (CAN), Nu-Cimet (CAN), Peptol (CAN), Tagamet, Tagamet HB

**Pregnancy Category B**

### Drug classes

Histamine 2 (H2) antagonist

### Therapeutic actions

Inhibits the action of histamine at the histamine$_2$ ($H_2$) receptors of the stomach, inhibiting gastric acid secretion and reducing total pepsin output.

### Indications

- Short-term treatment of active duodenal ulcer
- Short-term treatment of benign gastric ulcer
- Treatment of pathologic hypersecretory conditions (Zollinger-Ellison syndrome)
- Prophylaxis of stress-induced ulcers and acute upper GI bleeding in critical patients

- Treatment of erosive gastroesophageal reflux
  Relief of symptoms of heartburn, acid indigestion, sour stomach (OTC use)
- Relief of symptoms of heartburn, acid indigestion, sour stomach, (OTC use)

## Contraindications/cautions

- Allergy to cimetidine, impaired renal or hepatic function, lactation.

## Dosage

**Available Forms:** Tablets—100, 200, 300, 400, 800 mg; liquid—300 mg/5 ml; injection—300 mg/2 ml

*ADULT*

- *Active duodenal ulcer:* 800 mg PO at bedtime or 300 mg PO qid at meals and hs or 400 mg PO bid; continue for 4–6 wk. For intractable ulcers, 300 mg IM or IV q6–8h.
- *Maintenance therapy for duodenal ulcer:* 400 mg PO at bedtime.
- *Active gastric ulcer:* 300 mg PO qid at meals and hs.
- *Pathologic hypersecretory syndrome:* 300 mg PO qid at meals and hs, or 300 mg IV or IM q6h. Individualize doses as needed; **do not exceed 2,400 mg/d**.
- *Erosive gastroesophageal reflux disease:* 1,600 mg PO qd for 12 wk.
- *Prevention of upper GI bleeding:* Continuous IV infusion of 50 mg/h. Do not treat beyond 7 d.
- *Heartburn, acid indigestion:* Heartburn, acid indigestion: 200mg as symptoms occur: up to 4 tablets/24h

*PEDIATRIC:* Not recommended for children < 16 y.

*GERIATRIC OR IMPAIRED RENAL FUNCTION:* Accumulation may occur. Use lowest dose possible: 300 mg PO or IV q12h; may be increased to q8h if patient tolerates it, and levels are monitored.

## Pharmacokinetics

| Route | Onset | Peak |
|---|---|---|
| Oral | Varies | 1–1.5 h |
| IV/IM | Rapid | 1–1.5 h |

*Metabolism:* Hepatic, $T_{1/2}$: 2 h
*Distribution:* Crosses placenta; enters breast milk
*Excretion:* Urine

### IV facts

**Preparation:** *IV injections:* Dilute in 0.9% Sodium Chloride Injection, 5% or 10% Dextrose Injection, Lactated Ringer's Solution, 5% Sodium Bicarbonate Injection to a volume of 20 ml. Solution is stable for 48 h at room temperature. *IV infusions*: Dilute 300 mg in 100 ml of 5% Dextrose Injection or one of above listed solutions.

**Infusion:** Inject by direct injection over not less than 2 min; by infusion, slowly over 15–20 min.

**Incompatibilities:** Incompatible with aminophylline, barbiturate in IV solutions; pentobarbital sodium and pentobarbital sodium/atropine in the same syringe.

## Adverse effects

- CNS: *Dizziness, somnolence, headache, confusion, hallucinations*, peripheral neuropathy; symptoms of brain stem dysfunction (dysarthria, ataxia, diplopia)
- GI: *Diarrhea*
- CV: Cardiac arrhythmias, arrest; hypotension (IV use)
- **Hematologic**: Increases in plasma creatinine, serum transaminase
- Other: *Impotence* (reversible), gynecomastia (in long-term treatment), rash, vasculitis, pain at IM injection site

## Clinically important drug-drug interactions

• Increased risk of decreased white blood cell counts with antimetabolites, alkylating agents, other drugs known to cause neutropenia • Increased serum levels and risk of toxicity of warfarin-type anticoagulants, phenytoin, beta-adrenergic blocking agents, alcohol, quinidine, lidocaine, theophylline, chloroquine, certain benzodiazepines (alprazolam, chlordiazepoxide, diazepam, flurazepam, triazolam), nifedipine, pentoxifylline, tricyclic antidepressants, procainamide, carbamazepine when taken with cimetidine

## ■ Nursing Considerations

### Assessment

- *History:* Allergy to cimetidine, impaired renal or hepatic function, lactation
- *Physical:* Skin lesions; orientation, affect; pulse, baseline ECG (continuous with IV use); liver evaluation, abdominal exam, normal output; CBC, liver and renal function tests

### Implementation

- Give drug with meals and at hs.
- Decrease doses in renal and liver dysfunction.
- Administer IM dose undiluted deep into large muscle group.
- Arrange for regular followup, including blood tests to evaluate effects.

### Drug-specific teaching points

- Take drug with meals and at bedtime; therapy may continue for 4–6 wk or longer.
- Take antacids as prescribed, and at recommended times.
- Inform your health care provider about your cigarette smoking habits. Cigarette smoking decreases drug efficacy.
- Have regular medical followups to evaluate your response to drug.
- Report sore throat, fever, unusual bruising or bleeding, tarry stools, confusion, hallucinations, dizziness, muscle or joint pain.

## cinoxacin

*(sin **ox'** a sin)*
Cinobac Pulvules
**Pregnancy Category B**

### Drug classes

Urinary tract anti-infective
Antibacterial

### Therapeutic actions

Bactericidal; interferes with DNA replication in susceptible gram-negative bacteria, preventing cell division.

### Indications

- Urinary tract infections caused by susceptible gram-negative bacteria, including *E. coli, P. mirabilis, P. vulgaris, K. pneumoniae, Klebsiella* species, *Enterobacter* species

### Contraindications/cautions

- Allergy to cinoxacin; renal dysfunction (do not use with anuric patients); liver dysfunction; pregnancy, lactation

### Dosage

**Available Forms:** Capsules—250, 500 mg

*ADULT:* 1 g/d in two to four divided doses PO for 7–14 d.

*PEDIATRIC:* Not recommended for < 12 y.

*GERIATRIC OR IMPAIRED RENAL FUNCTION:* Initial dose of 500 mg PO, then the following maintenance schedule is suggested:

| *Creatinine Clearance (ml/min)* | *Dosage* |
|---|---|
| >80 | 500 mg bid |
| 80–50 | 250 mg tid |
| 50–20 | 250 mg bid |
| <20 | 250 mg/d |

### Pharmacokinetics

| *Route* | *Onset* | *Peak* | *Duration* |
|---|---|---|---|
| Oral | 2 h | 2–4 h | 10–12 h |

*Metabolism:* Hepatic, $T_{1/2}$: 1–1.5 h
*Distribution:* Crosses placenta; enters breast milk
*Excretion:* Urine

### Adverse effects

- CNS: *Headache, dizziness,* insomnia, nervousness, confusion
- GI: *Nausea*, abdominal cramps, vomiting, dairrhea, anorexia, perineal burning
- Hematologic: Elevated BUN, SGOT, SGPT, serum creatinine, alkaline phosphatase

- Hypersensitivity: *Rash, urticaria, pruritis*, edema

### Clinically important drug-drug interactions

- Lowered urine concentrations of cinoxacin if pretreated with **probenecid**

## ■ Nursing Considerations

### Assessment

- *History:* Allergy to cinoxacin, renal or liver dysfunction, pregnancy, lactation
- *Physical:* Skin—color, lesions; orientation, reflexes; liver and renal function tests

### Implementation

- Arrange for culture and sensitivity tests.
- Administer drug with food if GI upset occurs.
- Arrange for periodic renal and liver function tests during prolonged therapy.
- Monitor clinical response; if no improvement is seen or a relapse occurs, send urine for repeat culture and sensitivity.
- Encourage patient to complete full course of therapy.

### Drug-specific teaching points

- Take drug with food. Complete full course of therapy.
- Know that the following side effects may occur: nausea, vomiting, abdominal pain (try small, frequent meals); diarrhea; drowsiness, blurring of vision, dizziness (use caution driving or using dangerous equipment).
- Report rash, visual changes, severe GI problems, weakness, tremors.

## ciprofloxacin hydrochloride

*(si proe **flox'** a sin)*

Ciloxin (CAN), Cipro, Cipro I.V.

**Pregnancy Category C**

### Drug classes

Antibacterial

### Therapeutic actions

Bactericidal; interferes with DNA replication in susceptible gram-negative bacteria preventing cell reproduction.

### Indications

- For the treatment of infections caused by susceptible gram-negative bacteria, including *E. coli, P. mirabilis, K. pneumoniae, Enterobacter cloacae, P. vulgaris, P. rettgeri, M. morganii, P. aeruginosa, Citrobacter freundii, S. aureus, S. epidermidis,* group D streptococci
- Treatment of chronic bacterial prostatitis
- Unlabeled use: effective in patients with cystic fibrosis who have pulmonary exacerbations

### Contraindications/cautions

- Contraindications: allergy to ciprofloxacin, norfloxacin, pregnancy, lactation.
- Use cautiously with renal dysfunction, seizures.

### Dosage

**Available Forms:** Tablets—250, 500, 750 mg; injection—200, 400 mg; ophthalmic solution—3.5 mg/ml

**ADULT**

- ***Uncomplicated urinary tract infections:*** 250 mg q12h PO for 7–14 d or 200 mg IV q12h.
- ***Complicated urinary tract infections:*** 500 mg bid PO for 10–21 d or 400 mg IV.
- ***Respiratory, bone, joint infections:*** 500 mg q12h PO for 4–6 wk or 400 mg IV.
- ***Severe skin infections:*** 750 mg q12h PO for 4–6 wk.
- ***Infectious diarrhea:*** 500 mg q12h PO for 5–7 d.
- ***Ophthalmic infections caused by susceptible organisms not responsive to other therapy:*** 1-2 gtt/eye qd–bid.

**PEDIATRIC:** Not recommended; produced lesions of joint cartilage in immature experimental animals.

*GERIATRIC OR IMPAIRED RENAL FUNCTION*

- *Creatinine clearance > 50 (oral), > 30 (IV):* **Usual dosage (30–50)**: 250–500 mg q12h; **5–29:** 250–500 mg q18h (oral), 200–400 mg q18–24h (IV); **hemodialysis:** 250–500 mg q24h, after dialysis.

### Pharmacokinetics

| *Route* | *Onset* | *Peak* | *Duration* |
|---|---|---|---|
| Oral | Varies | 1–1 1/2 h | 4–5 h |
| IV | 10 min | 30 min | 4–5 h |

*Metabolism:* Hepatic, $T_{1/2}$: 3 1/2–4 h
*Distribution:* Crosses placenta; enters breast milk
*Excretion:* Urine and bile

### IV facts

*Preparation:* Dilute to a final concentration of 1–2 mg/ml with 0.9% NaCl Injection or 5% Dextrose Injection. Stable up to 14 d refrigerated or at room temperature.
**Infusion:** Administer slowly over 60 min.
**Incompatibilities:** Discontinue the administration of any other solutions during ciprofloxacin infusion.

### Adverse effects

- CNS: *Headache*, dizziness, insomnia, fatigue, somnolence, depression, blurred vision
- GI: *Nausea*, vomiting, dry mouth, *diarrhea*, abdominal pain
- Hematologic: Elevated BUN, SGOT, SGPT, serum creatinine and alkaline phosphatase; decreased WBC, neutrophil count, Hct
- Other: Fever, rash

### Clinically important drug-drug interactions

• Decreased therapeutic effect with iron salts, sulcrafate • Decreased absorption antacids • Increased effects with azlocillin • Increased serum levels and toxic effects of theophyllines if taken concurrently with ciprofloxacin

## ■ Nursing Considerations

### Assessment

- *History:* Allergy to ciprofloxacin, norfloxacin; renal dysfunction; seizures; lactation
- *Physical:* Skin color, lesions; T; orientation, reflexes, affect; mucous membranes, bowel sounds; renal and liver function tests

### Implementation

- Arrange for culture and sensitivity tests before beginning therapy.
- Continue therapy for 2 d after signs and symptoms of infection are gone.
- Give oral drug 1 h before or 2 h after meals with a glass of water.
- Ensure that patient is well hydrated.
- Give antacids at least 2 h after dosing.
- Monitor clinical response; if no improvement is seen or a relapse occurs, repeat culture and sensitivity.
- Encourage patient to complete full course of therapy.

### Drug-specific teaching points

- Take oral drug on an empty stomach—1 h before or 2 h after meals. If an antacid is needed take it at least 2 h before or after dose.
- Drink plenty of fluids while you are on this drug.
- Know that the following side effects may occur: nausea, vomiting, abdominal pain (small, frequent meals may help); diarrhea or constipation; drowsiness, blurring of vision, dizziness (observe caution if driving or using dangerous equipment).
- Report rash, visual changes, severe GI problems, weakness, tremors.

## cisapride

*(sis' a pride)*
Propulsid, Propulsid Quicksolv
**Pregnancy Category C**

### Drug classes

Prokinetic agent
GI drug

### Therapeutic actions
Increases the release of acetylcholine in the myenteric plexus; thus, improves GI motility with little to no dopaminergic action.

### Indications
- Symptomatic treatment of nocturnal heartburn due to gastroesophageal reflux disease

### Contraindications/cautions
- Allergy to cisapride, gallbladder disease, GI hemorrhage, GI obstruction, pregnancy, lactation, prolonged Q-T interval.

### Dosage
**Available Forms:** Tablets—10, 20 mg; suspension—1 mg/ml

*ADULT:* 5–20 mg PO tid; usual dose, 10 mg qid. Administer drug at least 15 min before meals and at hs.

*PEDIATRIC:* Safety and efficacy not established.

### Pharmacokinetics

| Route | Onset | Peak | Duration |
|---|---|---|---|
| Oral | Rapid | 1–1 1/2 h | 8–10 h |

*Metabolism:* Hepatic, $T_{1/2}$: 6–12 h

*Distribution:* Crosses placenta; enters breast milk

*Excretion:* Urine and feces

### Adverse effects
- CNS: *Headache,* fatigue, somnolence
- GI: *Abdominal pain, diarrhea, constipation, nausea, vomiting,* borborygamus, bloating
- CV: **Serious cardiac arrhythmias** when used in combination drug regimens
- Respiratory: *Rhinitis,* sinusitis, coughing, upper respiratory infections

### Clinically important drug-drug interactions
• Increased sedative effects with alcohol, benzodiazepines • Increased coagulation times with oral anticoagulants • Risk of serious ventricular arrhythmias with ketoconazole, itraconazol, miconazole IV, troleandomycin • Increased cisapride absorption and increased H2 antagonist activity when taken in combination

## ■ Nursing Considerations

### Assessment
- *History:* Severe gallbladder disease, GI bleeding, GI obstruction, pregnancy, lactation
- *Physical:* Neurologic status, abdominal exam, R, adventitious sounds, ECG including Q-T interval

### Implementation
- Administer at least 15 min before each meal and at hs.

### Drug-specific teaching points
- Take drug at least 15 min before meals and at bedtime.
- Avoid alcohol; serious sedation could occur.
- The following side effects may occur: headache (consult with your health care provider for correctives), stomach rumbling, diarrhea, abdominal pain, nausea, vomiting, constipation.
- Report severe abdominal pain, prolonged diarrhea, weight loss, extreme fatigue.

## cisplatin

*(sis' pla tin)*

CDDP, Platinol-AQ

**Pregnancy Category D**

### Drug classes
Alkylating agent

Antineoplastic

### Therapeutic actions
Cytotoxic: heavy metal that inhibits cell replication; cell cycle nonspecific.

### Indications
- **Metastatic testicular tumors:** combination therapy with bleomycin sulfate and vinblastine sulfate after surgery or radiotherapy
- **Metastatic ovarian tumors:** as single therapy in resistant patients or in combination therapy with doxorubicin after surgery or radiotherapy
- **Advanced bladder cancer:** single agent for transitional cell bladder cancer

no longer amenable to surgery or radiotherapy

## Contraindications/cautions

- Allergy to cisplatin, platinum-containing products; hematopoietic depression; impaired renal function; hearing impairment; pregnancy; lactation

## Dosage

**Available Forms:** Injection—1 mg/ml

*ADULT*

- *Metastatic testicular tumors:*
  - *Remission induction*
    - **Cisplatin:** 20 mg/m² per day IV for 5 consecutive d (days 1–5) every 3 wk for three courses of therapy. Bleomycin: 30 U IV weekly (day 2 of each week) for 12 consecutive doses. Vinblastine: 0.15–0.2 mg/kg IV twice weekly (days 1 and 2) every 3 wk for four courses.
  - *Maintenance:* Vinblastine: 0.3 mg/kg IV every 4 wk for 2 y.
- *Metastatic ovarian tumors*
  - **Combination therapy:** Administer cisplatin and doxorubicin sequentially.
    - **Cisplatin:** 50 mg/m² IV once every 3 wk (day 1). Doxorubicin: 50 mg/m² IV once every 3 wk (day 1). As a single agent: 100 mg/m² IV every 4 wk.
- *Advanced bladder cancer:* 50–70 mg/m² IV once every 3–4 wk; in heavily pretreated (radiotherapy or chemotherapy) patients, give an initial dose of 50 mg/m² repeated every 4 wk. Do not give repeated courses until serum creatinine is $< 1.5$ mg/100 ml or BUN is $> 25$ mg/100 ml or until platelets $> 100{,}000$/mm³ and WBC $> 4{,}000$/mm³. Do not give subsequent doses until audiometry indicates hearing is within normal range.

## Pharmacokinetics

| *Route* | *Onset* | *Peak* | *Duration* |
|---|---|---|---|
| IV | 8–10 h | 18–23 d | 30–35 d |

*Metabolism:* Hepatic, $T_{1/2}$: 25–49 min, then 58–73 h

*Distribution:* Crosses placenta; enters breast milk

*Excretion:* Urine

## IV facts

**Preparation:** Dissolve the powder in the 10-mg and 50-mg vials with 10 or 50 ml of Sterile Water for Injection respectively; resulting solution contains 1 mg/ml cisplatin; stable for 20 h at room temperature—do not refrigerate. Dilute reconstituted drug in 1–2 L of 5% Dextrose in One-Half or One-Third Normal Saline containing 37.5 g mannitol.

**Infusion:** Hydrate patient with 1–2 L of fluid infused for 8–12 h before drug therapy; infuse dilute drug over 6–8 h.

## Adverse effects

- CNS: *Ototoxicity*, peripheral neuropathies, seizures, loss of taste
- GI: *Nausea, vomiting, anorexia*
- **Hematologic:** *Leukopenia, thrombocytopenia, anemia*, hypomagnesemia, hypocalcemia, hypokalemia, hypophosphatemia, hyperuricemia
- GU: *Nephrotoxicity*, dose limiting
- **Hypersensitivity:** Anaphylactic-like reactions, facial edema, bronchoconstriction, tachycardia, hypotension (treat with epinephrine, corticosteroids, antihistamines)

## Clinically important drug-drug interactions

- Additive ototoxicity with furosemide, bumetanide, ethacrynic acid • Decreased serum levels of phenytoins with cisplatin

## ■ Nursing Considerations

### Assessment

- *History:* Allergy to cisplatin, platinum-containing products; hematopoietic depression; impaired renal function; hearing impairment; pregnancy, lactation
- *Physical:* Weight; eighth cranial nerve evaluation; reflexes; sensation; CBC, differential; renal function tests; serum electrolytes; serum uric acid; audiogram

### Implementation

- Arrange for tests to evaluate serum creatinine, BUN, creatinine clearance, magnesium, calcium, potassium levels before initiating therapy and before each subsequent course of therapy. Do not give if there is evidence of nephrotoxicity.

- Arrange for audiometric testing before beginning therapy and prior to subsequent doses. Do not give dose if audiometric acuity is outside normal limits.
- Do not use needles of IV sets containing aluminum parts; can cause precipitate and loss of drug potency. Use gloves while preparing drug to prevent contact with the skin or mucosa; contact can cause skin reactions. If contact occurs, wash area immediately with soap and water.
- Maintain adequate hydration and urinary output for the 24 h following drug therapy.
- Use an antiemetic if nausea and vomiting are severe; (metoclopramide).
- Monitor uric acid levels; if markedly increased, allopurinol may be ordered.
- Monitor electrolytes and maintain by supplements.

### Drug-specific teaching points

- This drug can only be given IV. Prepare a calendar of treatment days.
- The following side effects may occur: nausea, vomiting (medication may be ordered; small frequent meals also may help); numbness, tingling, loss of taste, ringing in the ears, dizziness, loss of hearing (reversible).
- Use birth control; drug may cause birth defects or miscarriages.
- Have frequent, regular medical follow-up, including frequent blood tests to monitor drug effects.
- Report loss of hearing, dizziness; unusual bleeding or bruising, fever, chills, sore throat, leg cramps, muscle twitching, changes in voiding patterns.

## cladribine

***(kla' dri been)***

CdA, 2-chlorodeoxyadenosine

Leustatin

**Pregnancy Category D**

### Drug classes

Antineoplastic

### Therapeutic actions

Blocks DNA synthesis and repair, causing cell death in active and resting lymphocytes and monocytes.

### Indications

- Treatment of active hairy cell leukemia
- Unlabeled uses: advanced cutaneous T-cell lymphomas, chronic lymphocytic leukemia, non-Hodgkin's lymphomas, acute myeloid leukemia, autoimmune hemolytic anemia, mycosis fungoides, Sezary syndrome

### Contraindications/cautions

- Contraindications: hypersensitivity to cladribine or any components, pregnancy, lactation.
- Use cautiously with active infection, myelosuppression, debilitating illness, renal or hepatic impairment.

### Dosage

**Available Forms:** Solution—1 mg/ml

*ADULT:* Single course given by continuous IV infusion of 0.09 mg/kg per day for 7 d.

*PEDIATRIC:* Safety and efficacy not established.

### Pharmacokinetics

| *Route* | *Onset* | *Duration* |
|---|---|---|
| IV | Rapid | 8–10 h |

*Metabolism:* Hepatic, $T_{1/2}$: 5.4 h

*Distribution:* Crosses placenta; may enter breast milk

*Excretion:* Urine

### IV facts

**Preparation:** Prepare daily dose by adding calculated dose to 500-ml bag of 0.9% Sodium Chloride Injection. Stable for 24 h at room temperature. Prepare 7-d infusion using aseptic technique, and add calculated dose to 100 ml Bacteriostatic, 0.9% Sodium Chloride Injection (0.9% benzyl alcohol preserved) through a sterile 0.22-$\mu$m filter. Store unopened vials in refrigerator, and protect from light. Vials are single-use only, discard after use.

**Infusion:** Infuse daily dose slowly over 24 h. 7-d dose should be infused continuously over the 7-d period.

**Incompatibilities:** Do not mix with any other solutions, drugs, or additives. Do not infuse through IV line with any other drug or additive.

### Adverse effects

- GI: *Nausea, anorexia, vomiting, diarrhea,* constipation, abdominal pain
- CNS: *Fatigue, headache,* dizziness, insomnia, **neurotoxicity**
- CV: Tachycardia, edema
- Respiratory: *Cough, abnormal breath sounds*, shortness of breath
- Hematologic: *Neutropenia,* ***myelosuppression***
- Dermatologic: *Rash*, pruritus, pain, erythema, petechiae, purpura
- Local: *Injection site redness, swelling, pain;* thrombosis, phlebitis
- Other: *Fever, chills*, asthenia, diaphoresis, myalgia, arthralgia, **infection**, cancer

## ■ Nursing Considerations

### Assessment

- ***History:*** Allergy to cladribine or any component, renal or hepatic impairment, myelosuppression, infection, pregnancy, lactation
- ***Physical:*** Weight, skin condition, neurologic status, abdominal exam, P, respiratory status, kidney and liver function tests, CBC, uric acid levels

### Implementation

- Use disposable gloves and protective garments when handling cladribine. If drug contacts skin or mucous membranes, wash immediately with copious amounts of water.
- Ensure continuous infusion of drug over 7 d.
- Alert childbearing age patients to drug's severe efects on fetus; advise using birth control during and for several weeks after treatment.
- Monitor complete hematologic profile, renal and liver function tests before and frequently during treatment. Consult with physician at first sign of toxicity; consider delaying or discontinuing dose if neurotoxicity or renal toxicity occur.

### Drug-specific teaching points

- This drug must be given continuously for 7 d.
- Frequent monitoring of blood tests are needed during the treatment and for several weeks thereafter to assess the drug's effect.
- The following side effects may occur: fever, headache, rash, nausea, vomiting, fatigue, pain at injection site.
- Report numbness or tingling, severe headache, nausea, rash, extreme fatigue, edema, pain or swelling at injection site.

# clarithromycin

*(klar* ***ith'*** *ro my sin)*

Biaxin Filmtabs

**Pregnancy Category C**

### Drug classes

Macrolide antibiotic

### Therapeutic actions

Inhibits protein synthesis in susceptible bacteria, causing cell death.

### Indications

- Treatment of upper respiratory infections caused by *S. pyogenes, S. pneumoniae*
- Treatment of lower respiratory infections caused by *Mycoplasma pneumoniae, S. pneumoniae, H. influenzae, M. catarrhalis*
- Treatment of skin and structure infections caused by *S. aureus, S. pyogenes*
- Treatment of disseminated mycobacterial infections due to *M. avium* and *M. intracellulare*
- Treatment of active duodenal ulcer with *H. pylori* in combination with omeprazole
- Treatment of acute otitis media due to *H. influenzae, M. cararrhalis, S. pneumoniae*

### Contraindications/cautions

- Contraindications: hypersensitivity to clarithromycin, erythromycin, or any macrolide antibiotic.
- Use cautiously with colitis, hepatic or renal impairment, pregnancy, lactation.

### Dosage

**Available Forms:** Tablets—250, 500 mg; granules for suspension—125, 250 mg/5 ml

ADULT

- *Pharyngitis, tonsilitis; pneumonia due to S. pneumoniae, M. pneumoniae;* skin or skin-structure infections; lower respiratory infections due to *S. pneumoniae, M. catawhalis*: 250 mg PO q12h for 7–14 d.
- *Acute maxillary sinusitis, lower respiratory infection caused by H. influenzae*: 500 mg PO q12h for 7–14 d.
- *Mycobacterial infections:* 500 mg PO bid.

PEDIATRIC: Usual dosage 15 mg/kg/d PO q12h for 10 d.

- *Mycobacterial infections:* 7.5 mg/kg PO bid.

GERIATRIC OR IMPAIRED RENAL FUNCTION: Decrease dosage or prolong dosing intervals as appropriate.

### Pharmacokinetics

| Route | Onset | Peak |
|---|---|---|
| Oral | Varies | 2 h |

*Metabolism:* Hepatic, $T_{1/2}$: 3–7 h
*Distribution:* Crosses placenta; enters breast milk
*Excretion:* Urine

### Adverse effects

- CNS: Dizziness, headache, vertigo, somnolence, fatigue
- GI: *Diarrhea, abdominal pain, nausea,* dyspepsia, flatulence, vomiting, melena, **pseudomembranous colitis**
- Other: *Superinfections*

### Clinically important drug-drug interactions

- Increased serum levels and effects of carbamazepine, theophylline, lovastatin, phenytoin

### Clinically important drug-food interactions

- Food decreases the rate of absorption of clarithromycin but does not alter effectiveness

## ■ Nursing Considerations

### Assessment

- *History:* Hypersensitivity to clarithromycin, erythromycin, or any macrolide antibiotic; pseudomembranous colitis, hepatic or renal impairment, lactation
- *Physical:* Site of infection, Skin color, lesions; orientation, GI output, bowel sounds, liver evaluation; culture and sensitivity tests of infection, urinalysis, liver and renal function tests

### Implementation

- Culture infection before therapy.
- Monitor patient for anticipated response.
- Administer without regard to meals; administer with food if GI effects occur.

### Drug-specific teaching points

- Take drug with food if GI effects occur. Take the full course of therapy.
- Shake suspension before use; do not refrigerate.
- The following side effects may occur: stomach cramping, discomfort, diarrhea; fatigue, headache (medication may be ordered); additional infections in the mouth or vagina (consult with care provider for treatment).
- Report severe or watery diarrhea, severe nausea or vomiting, skin rash or itching, mouth sores, vaginal sores.

## clemastine fumarate

***(klem' as teen)***

Tavist, Tavist-1

**Pregnancy Category B**

### Drug classes

Antihistamine

### Therapeutic actions

Blocks the effects of histamine at $H_1$ receptor sites; has atropine-like, antipruritic, and sedative effects.

### Indications

- Symptomatic relief of symptoms associated with perennial and seasonal allergic rhinitis; vasomotor rhinitis; allergic conjunctivitis; mild, uncomplicated urticaria and angioedema; amelioraton of allergic reactions to blood or plasma; dermatographism; adjunctive therapy in anaphylactic reactions.
- Treatment of the common cold

### Contraindications/cautions

- Contraindications: allergy to any antihistamines, third trimester of pregnancy, lactation.
- Use caution in the presence of narrow-angle glaucoma, stenosing peptic ulcer, symptomatic prostatic hypertrophy, asthmatic attack, bladder neck obstruction, pyloroduodenal obstruction.

### Dosage

**Available Forms:** Tablets—1.34, 2.68 mg; syrup—0.65 mg/5 ml

*ADULT AND PEDIATRIC > 12 Y:* 1.34 mg PO bid to 2.68 mg PO tid. Do not exceed 8.04 mg/d. For dermatologic conditions, use 2.68 mg tid only.

*PEDIATRIC < 12 Y:* Safety and efficacy not established.

*GERIATRIC:* More likely to cause dizziness, sedation, syncope, toxic confusional states, and hypotension in elderly patients; use with caution.

### Pharmacokinetics

| Route | Onset | Peak | Duration |
|---|---|---|---|
| Oral | 15–30 min | 1–2 h | 4–6 h |

*Metabolism:* Hepatic, $T_{1/2}$: 3–4 h
*Distribution:* Crosses placenta; enters breast milk
*Excretion:* Urine

### Adverse effects

- CNS: *Drowsiness, sedation, dizziness, disturbed coordination*, fatigue, confusion, restlessness, excitation, nervousness, tremor, headache, blurred vision, diplopia, vertigo, tinnitus, acute labryinthitis, hysteria, tingling, heaviness and weakness of the hands
- GI: *Epigastric distress,* anorexia, increased appetite and weight gain, nausea, vomiting, diarrhea or constipation
- CV: Hypotension, palpitations, bradycardia, tachycardia, extrasystoles
- Respiratory: *Thickening of bronchial secretions,* chest tightness, wheezing, nasal stuffiness, dry mouth, dry nose, dry throat, sore throat
- Hematologic: Hemolytic anemia, hypoplastic anemia, thrombocytopenia, leukopenia, agranulocytosis, pancytopenia
- GU: Urinary frequency, dysuria, urinary retention, early menses, decreased libido, impotence
- Other: Urticaria, rash, anaphylactic shock, photosensitivity, excessive perspiration, chills

### Clinically important drug-drug interactions

• Increased depressant effects with alcohol, other CNS depressants • Increased and prolonged anticholinergic (drying) effects with MAO inhibitors.

## ■ Nursing Considerations

### Assessment

- *History:* Allergy to any antihistamines; narrow-angle glaucoma, stenosing peptic ulcer, symptomatic prostatic hypertrophy, asthmatic attack, bladder neck obstruction, pyloroduodenal obstruction; lactation
- *Physical:* Skin color, lesions, texture; orientation, reflexes, affect; vision exam; P, BP; R, adventitious sounds; bowel sounds; prostate palpation; CBC with differential

### Implementation

- Administer with food if GI upset occurs.
- Administer syrup form if patient is unable to take tablets.
- Monitor patient response, adjust to lowest possible effective dose.

### Drug-specific teaching points

- Take drug as prescribed; avoid excessive dosage.
- Take with food if GI upset occurs.
- The following side effects may occur: dizziness, sedation, drowsiness (use caution

if driving or performing tasks that require alertness); epigastric distress, diarrhea, or constipation (take with meals; consult care provider); dry mouth (frequent mouth care, sucking sugarless lozenges may help); thickening of bronchial secretions, dryness of nasal mucosa (use a humidifier).

- Avoid alcohol; serious sedation could occur.
- Report difficulty breathing, hallucinations, tremors, loss of coordination, unusual bleeding or bruising, visual disturbances, irregular heartbeat.

## Clindamycin

### clindamycin hydrochloride

*(klin da **mye'** sin)*

*Oral:* Cleocin

### clindamycin palmitate hydrochloride

*Oral:* Cleocin Pediatric

### clindamycin phosphate

*Oral, parenteral, topical dermatologic solution for acne, vaginal preparation:* Cleocin Phosphate, Cleocin T, Dalacin C (CAN)

**Pregnancy Category B**

### Drug classes

Lincosamide antibiotic

### Therapeutic actions

Inhibits protein synthesis in susceptible bacteria, causing cell death.

### Indications

- **Systemic administration:** serious infections caused by susceptible strains of anaerobes, streptococci, staphylococci, pneumococci; reserve use for penicillin-allergic patients or when penicillin is inappropriate; less toxic antibiotics (erythromycin) should be considered
- **Parenteral form:** treatment of speticemia caused by staphylococci, streptococci; acute hematogenous osteomyelitis; adjunct to surgical treatment of chronic bone and joint infections due to susceptible organisms
- **Topical dermatologic solution:** Treatment of acne vulgaris
- **Vaginal preparation:** Treatment of bacterial vaginosis; do not use to treat meningitis; does not cross the blood–brain barrier.

### Contraindications/cautions

- **Systemic administration:** allergy to clindamycin, history of asthma or other allergies, tartrazine (in 75- and 150-mg capsules); hepatic or renal dysfunction; lactation.
- **Topical dermatologic solution, vaginal preparation:** allergy to clindamycin or lincomycin; history of regional enteritis or ulcerative colitis; history of antibiotic-associated colitis.

## Dosage

**Available Forms:** Capsules—75, 150, 300 mg; granules for oral solution—75 mg/5 ml; injection—150 mg/ml; topical gel—10 mg; topical lotion—10 mg; topical solution—10 mg; vaginal cream—2%

*ADULT:*

- ***Oral:*** 150–300 mg q6h, up to 300–450 mg q6h in more severe infections.
- ***Parenteral:*** 600–2,700 mg/d in 2 to 4 equal doses; up to 4.8 g/d IV or IM may be used for life-threatening situations.
- ***Vaginal preparation:*** One applicator (100 mg clindamycin phosphate) intravaginally, preferably at hs, for 7 consecutive d.

*PEDIATRIC*

- ***Oral***

**Clindamycin HCl:** 8–20 mg/kg per day in 3 to 4 equal doses.

**Clindamycin palmitate HCl:** 8–25 mg/kg/d in 3–4 equal doses; children weighing <10 kg–37.5 mg tid as the minimum dose.

- ***Parenteral (> 1 mo):*** 15–40 mg/kg per day in three to four equal doses;

in severe infections, give 300 mg/d regardless of weight.

GERIATRIC OR RENAL FAILURE PATIENTS: Reduce dose, and monitor patient's serum levels carefully.

*Topical dermatologic solution:* Apply a thin film to affected area bid.

### Pharmacokinetics

| *Route* | *Onset* | *Peak* | *Duration* |
|---|---|---|---|
| Oral | Varies | 1–2 h | 8–12 h |
| IM | 20–30 min | 1–3 h | 8–12 h |
| IV | Immediate | Minutes | 8–12 h |
| Topical | Minimally absorbed systemically | | |

*Metabolism:* Hepatic, $T_{1/2}$: 2–3 h

*Distribution:* Crosses placenta; enters breast milk

*Excretion:* Urine and feces

### IV facts

**Preparation:** Store unreconstituted product at room temperature. Reconstitute by adding 75 ml of water to 100-ml bottle of palmitate in two portions. Shake well; do *not* refrigerate reconstituted solution. Reconstituted solution is stable for 2 wk at room temperature. Dilute reconstituted solution to a concentration of 300 mg/50 ml or more of diluent using 0.9% Sodium Chloride Injection, 5% Dextrose Injection, or Lactated Ringer's solution. Solution is stable for 16 d at room temperature.

**Infusion:** Do not administer more than 1,200 mg in a single 1-h infusion. Infusion rates: 300 mg in 50 ml diluent, 10 min; 600 mg in 50 ml diluent, 20 min; 900 mg in 50–100 ml diluent, 30 min; 1,200 mg in 100 ml diluent, 40 min.

**Incompatibilities:** Calcium gluconate, ampicillin, phenytoin, barbiturates, aminophylline, and magnesium sulfate. May be mixed with sodium chloride, dextrose, calcium, potassium, vitamin B complex, cephalothin, kanamycin, gentamicin, penicillin, carbencillin.

### Adverse effects

*Systemic Administration*

- GI: Severe colitis, including **pseudomembranous colitis**, *nausea, vomiting, diarrhea, abdominal pain, esophagitis, anorexia*, jaundice, liver function changes
- Hematologic: Neutropenia, leukopenia, agranulocytosis, eosinophilia
- Hypersensitivity: *Skin rashes*, urticaria to anaphylactoid reactions
- Local: *Pain following injection*, induration and sterile abscess after IM injection, thrombophlebitis after IV use

*Topical Dermatologic Solution*

- CNS: *Fatigue, headache*
- GI: Pseudomembranous colitis, diarrhea, bloody diarrhea; abdominal pain, sore throat
- GU: Urinary frequency
- Dermatologic: *Contact dermatitis, dryness*, gram-negative folliculitis

*Vaginal Preparation*

- GU: *Cervicitis, vaginitis*, vulvar irritation

### Clinically important drug-drug interactions

- *Systemic Administration*

Increased neuromuscular blockade with neuromuscular blocking agents • Decreased GI absorption with kaolin, aluminum salts

## ■ Nursing Considerations

### Assessment

- *History:* Allergy to clindamycin, history of asthma or other allergies, allergy to tartrazine (in 75- and 150-mg capsules); hepatic or renal dysfunction; lactation; history of regional enteritis or ulcerative colitis; history of antibiotic associated colitis
- *Physical:* Site of infection or acne; Skin color, lesions; BP; R, adventitious sounds; bowel sounds, output, liver evaluation; complete blood count, renal and liver function tests

### Implementation

*Systemic Administration*

- Administer oral drug with a full glass of water or with food to prevent esophageal irritation.

- Do not give IM injections of more than 600 mg; inject deep into large muscle to avoid serious problems.
- Culture infection before therapy.
- Do not use for minor bacterial or viral infections.
- Monitor renal and liver function tests, and blood counts with prolonged therapy.

*Topical Dermatologic Administration*

- Keep solution away from eyes, mouth and abraded skin or mucous membranes; alcohol base will cause stinging.
- Keep cool tap water available to bathe eye, mucous membranes, abraded skin inadvertently contacted by drug solution.

*Vaginal Preparation*

- Give intravaginally, preferably at hs.

### Drug-specific teaching points

- Take oral drug with a full glass of water or with food. Apply thin film of acne solution to affected area twice daily, being careful to avoid eyes, mucous membranes, abraded skin; if solution contacts one of these areas, flush with copious amounts of cool water. Use vaginal prepartion for 7 consecutive d, preferably at betime.
- Take full prescribed course of drug (oral). Do not stop taking without notifying health care provider.

*Vaginal Preparation*

- Refrain from sexual intercourse during treatment with this product.
- The following side effects may occur: nausea, vomiting (small frequent meals may help); superinfections in the mouth, vagina (use frequent hygiene measures, request treatment if severe).
- Report with oral therapy, severe or watery diarrhea, abdominal pain, inflamed mouth or vagina, skin rash or lesions. With acne solution, abdominal pain, diarrhea. With vaginal preparation: vaginal irritation, itching; diarrhea, no improvement in complaint being treated.

## clofazimine

*(kloe fa' zi meen)*
Lamprene
**Pregnancy Category C**

### Drug classes
Leprostatic agent

### Therapeutic actions
Inhibits growth of *Mycobacterium leprae,* leading to cell death; has anti-inflammatory effects in controlling erythema nodosum leprosum reactions.

### Indications
- Treatment of lepromatous leprosy, including dapsone-resistant lepromatous leprosy and lepromatous leprosy complicated by erythema nodosum leprosum
- Part of combination therapy in the initial treatment of multibacillary leprosy to prevent the development of drug resistance

### Contraindications/cautions
- Contraindication: allergy to clofazimine.
- Use cautiously with GI problems, diarrhea, pregnancy (infant may be born with pigmented skin), lactation.

### Dosage
**Available Forms:** Capsules—50 mg

**ADULT**

- *Dapsone-resistant leprosy:* 100 mg/d PO with one or more other antileprosy drugs for 3 y, then 100 mg/d as single agent.
- *Dapsone-sensitive multibacillary leprosy:* Give triple-drug regimen for at least 2 y, and continue until negative skin smears are obtained; then monotherapy with the appropriate agent.
- *Erythema nodosum leprosum:* 100 mg/d PO. If nerve injury or skin ulceration is threatened, give corticosteroids. If prolonged corticosteroid therapy is needed, give 100–200 mg clofazimine/d for up to 3 mo; do not exceed 200 mg/d, and taper to 100 mg/d a soon as possible. Keep patient under medical surveillance.

**PEDIATRIC:** Safety and efficacy not established.

### Pharmacokinetics

| Route | Onset | Duration |
|---|---|---|
| Oral | Varies | Months |

*Metabolism:* Hepatic, $T_{1/2}$: 70 d
*Distribution:* Crosses placenta; enters breast milk
*Excretion:* Urine, bile, sputum, sweat

### Adverse effects

- CNS: Depression, suicidal tendencies
- GI: *Abdominal, epigastric pain; diarrhea; nausea; vomiting; GI intolerance*; splenic infarction
- **Hematologic**: Elevated blood sugar, elevated sedimentation rate
- GU: *Discolored urine or feces, sputum, sweat*
- EENT: Conjunctival and corneal pigmentation due to crystal deposits, dryness, burning, itching, irritation
- **Dermatologic**: *Pink to brownish-black pigmentation of skin; ichthyosis and dryness; rash and pruritus*

## ■ Nursing Considerations

### Assessment

- ***History:*** Allergy to clofazimine, GI problems, diarrhea, lactation
- ***Physical:*** Skin lesions, color, turgor texture; ocular exam; bowel sounds, feces color; culture of lesions

### Implementation

- Assess patient, and consult with physician if leprosy reactional episodes occur (worsening of leprosy activity related to therapy). Use of other leprostatics, analgesics, corticosteroids, or surgery may be necessary.
- Protect drug from exposure to moisture, heat.
- Administer drug with meals.
- Provide skin care for dermatologic reactions. Apply oil if dryness and ichthyosis occur.
- Arrange for treatment with corticosteroids if needed with erythema nodosum leprosum; monitor closely.
- Reduce dosage if abdominal pain, diarrhea, colic occur. Monitor patient for possible severe abdominal symptoms.
- Tears, sweat, sputum, urine, feces may be discolored as a result of therapy.
- Offer support and encouragement to deal with skin pigmentation; assure patient that it is usually reversible but may take several months to years to disappear. Suicides have been reported due to severe depression due to pigmentation effects.
- Contact support groups to help the patient to cope with disease and drug therapy: National Hansen's Disease Center; Carville, LA 70721; telephone: (504) 642-7771.

### Drug-specific teaching points

- Follow the prescription, do not exceed the prescribed dose. Take the drug with meals. To be effective, this drug will be needed for a prolonged period.
- Have regular medical followups.
- The following side effects may occur: nausea, loss of appetite, vomiting, diarrhea (take with meals); discoloring of the tears, sweat, sputum, urine, feces, whites of the eyes, pigmentation of the skin from pink to brownish-black (reversible; return to normal color may take several months or years); dryness of the skin (apply oil).
- Report worsening of Hansen's disease symptoms, severe GI upset, colicky pain, severe depression.

## clofibrate

*(kloe fye' brate)*
Atromid S
**Pregnancy Category C**

### Drug classes

Antihyperlipidemic

### Therapeutic actions

Stimulates the liver to increase breakdown of VLDL to LDL; decreases liver synthesis of VLDL; inhibits cholesterol formation, lowering serum lipid levels; has antiplatelet effect.

### Indications

- Primary dysbetalipoproteinemia (type III hyperlipidemia) that does not respond to diet

- Very high serum triglycerides (type IV and V hyperlipidemia) with abdominal pain and pancreatitis that does not respond to diet

### Contraindications/cautions

- Allergy to clofibrate, hepatic or renal dysfunction, primary biliary cirrhosis, peptic ulcer, pregnancy, lactation.

### Dosage

**Available Forms:** Capsules—500 mg

*ADULT:* 2 g/d PO in divided doses. **Caution:** use this drug only if strongly indicated, and lipid studies show a definite response; hepatic tumorigenicity occurs in lab animals.

*PEDIATRIC:* Safety and efficacy not established.

### Pharmacokinetics

| Route | Onset | Peak | Duration |
|---|---|---|---|
| Oral | Varies | 3–6 h | Weeks |

*Metabolism:* Hepatic, $T_{1/2}$: 15 h
*Distribution:* Crosses placenta; enters breast milk
*Excretion:* Urine

### Adverse effects

- GI: *Nausea*, vomiting, diarrhea, dyspepsia, flatulence, bloating, stomatitis, gastritis, gallstones (with long-term therapy), peptic ulcer, GI hemorrhage
- CV: Angina, arrhythmias, swelling, phlebitis, thrombophlebitis, pulmonary emboli
- Hematologic: Leukopenia, anemia, eosinophilia, increased SGOT and SGPT, increased thymol turbidity, increased CPK, BSP retention
- GU: *Impotence, decreased libido*, dysuria, hematuria, proteinuria, decreased urine output
- Dermatologic: *Skin rash*, alopecia, dry skin, dry and brittle hair, pruritus, urticaria
- Other: *Myalgia, "flu-like" syndromes*, arthralgia, weight gain, polyphagia, increased perspiration, systemic lupus erythematosus, blurred vision, gynecomastia

### Clinically important drug-drug interactions

• Increased bleeding tendencies if oral anticoagulants are also given; reduce dosage of anticoagulant, usually by 50% • Increased pharmacologic effects of sulfonylureas, insulin, with resultant increased risk of hypoglycemia

## ■ Nursing Considerations

### Assessment

- *History:* Allergy to clofibrate, hepatic or renal dysfunction, primary biliary cirrhosis, peptic ulcer, lactation
- *Physical:* Skin lesions, color, T; P, BP, auscultation, baseline ECG, peripheral perfusion, edema; bowel sounds, normal output, liver evaluation; normal output; lipid studies, CBC, clotting profile, liver and renal function tests, urinalysis

### Implementation

- Administer drug with meals or milk if GI upset occurs.
- Arrange for regular follow-up including blood tests for lipids, liver function, CBC during long-term therapy.
- Monitor urine output.

### Drug-specific teaching points

- Take the drug with meals or with milk if GI upset occurs.
- The following side effects may occur: diarrhea, loss of appetite (eat small frequent meals); dry skin, dry and brittle hair, excessive sweating (frequent skin care, use of nonabrasive lotion may help); loss of libido, impotence.
- Have regular follow-ups for blood tests.
- Report chest pain, shortness of breath, palpitations, severe stomach pain with nausea and vomiting, fever and chills or sore throat, blood in the urine, little urine output, swelling of the ankles or legs, unusual weight gain.

## clomiphene citrate

***(kloe' mi feen)***

Clomid, Milophene, Serophene

**Pregnancy Category X**

### Drug classes
Hormone
Fertility drug

### Therapeutic actions
Binds to estrogen receptors, decreasing the number of available estrogen receptors, which gives the hypothalamus the false signal to increase in FSH and LH secretion, resulting in ovarian stimulation.

### Indications
- Treatment of ovarian failure in patients with normal liver function and normal endogenous estrogen levels, whose partners are fertile and potent
- Unlabeled use: treatment of male infertility

### Contraindications/cautions
- Known sensitivity to clomiphene, liver disease, abnormal bleeding of undetermined origin, ovarian cyst, lactation.

### Dosage
**Available Forms:** Tablets—50 mg

*Treatment of ovarian failure*
- *Initial therapy:* 50 mg/day PO for 5 d started anytime there has been no recent uterine bleeding or about the fifth day of the cycle if uterine bleeding does occur.
- *Second course:* If ovulation does not occur after the first course, administer 100 mg/d PO for 5 d; start this course as early as 30 d after the previous one.
- *Third course:* Repeat second course regimen; if patient does not respond to three courses of treatment, further treatment is not recommended.

*Male sterility:* 50–400 mg/d PO for 2–12 mo.

### Pharmacokinetics

| *Route* | *Onset* | *Duration* |
|---|---|---|
| Oral | 5–8 d | 6 wk |

*Metabolism:* Hepatic, $T_{1/2}$: 5 d
*Distribution:* Crosses placenta
*Excretion:* Feces

### Adverse effects
- CNS: Visual symptoms (blurring, spots, flashes), nervousness, insomnia, dizziness, light headedness
- GI: *Abdominal discomfort, distention, bloating, nausea, vomiting*
- CV: *Vasomotor flushing*
- GU: Uterine bleeding, *ovarian enlargement*, ovarian overstimulation, birth defects in resulting pregnancies
- Other: *Breast tenderness*

### Drug-lab test interferences
- Increased levels of serum thyroxine, thyroxine-binding globulin

## ■ Nursing Considerations

### Assessment
- ***History:*** Sensitivity to clomiphene, liver disease, abnormal bleeding of undetermined origin, ovarian cyst, pregnancy
- ***Physical:*** Skin color, T; affect, orientation, ophthalmologic exam; abdominal exam, pelvic exam, liver evaluation; urinary estrogens and estriol levels (women); liver function tests

### Implementation
- Complete a pelvic exam before each treatment to rule out ovarian enlargement, pregnancy, other uterine difficulties.
- Check urine estrogen and estriol levels before therapy; normal levels indicate appropriate patient selection.
- Refer for complete ophthalmic exam; if visual symptoms occur, discontinue drug.
- Discontinue drug at any sign of ovarian overstimulation, admit patient to hospital for observation and supportive measures.
- Provide women with calendar of treatment days and explanations about signs of estrogen and progesterone activity; caution patient that 24-h urine collections will be needed periodically; timing of intercourse is important for achieving pregnancy.
- Alert to risks and hazards of multiple births.
- Explain failure to respond after 3 courses of therapy, probably means drug will not help, and treatment will be discontinued.

### Drug-specific teaching points
- Prepare a calendar showing the treatment schedule, plotting ovulation.

- The following side effects may occur: abdominal distention; flushing; breast tenderness; dizziness, drowsiness, lightheadedness, visual disturbances (use caution driving or performing tasks that require alertness).
- There is an increased incidence of multiple births in women using this drug.
- Report bloating, stomach pain, blurred vision, yellow skin or eyes, unusual bleeding or bruising, fever, chills, visual changes or blurring.

## clomipramine hydrochloride

*(kloe **mi'** pra meen)*

Anafranil

**Pregnancy Category C**

### Drug classes

Tricyclic antidepressant (TCA) (tertiary amine)

### Therapeutic actions

Mechanism unknown; inhibits the presynaptic reuptake of the neurotransmitters norepinephrine and serotonin; anticholinergic at CNS and peripheral receptors; sedative.

### Indications

- Treatment of obsessions and compulsions in patients with obsessive-compulsive disorder (OCD), whose obsessions or compulsions cause marked distress, are time-consuming, or interfere with social or occupational functioning.

### Contraindications/cautions

- Contraindications: hypersensitivity to any tricyclic drug, concomitant therapy with an MAO inhibitor, recent MI, myelography within previous 24 h or scheduled within 48 h, lactation.
- Use cautiously with EST, preexisting CV disorders (eg, severe coronary heart disease, progressive heart failure, angina pectoris, paroxysmal tachycardia); angle-closure glaucoma, increased intraocular pressure, urinary retention, ureteral or urethral spasm; seizure disorders; hyperthyroidism; impaired hepatic, renal function; psychiatric patients (schizophrenic or paranoid patients may exhibit a worsening of psychosis with TCA therapy); manic-depressive patients; elective surgery.

### Dosage

**Available Forms:** Capsules—25, 50, 75 mg

#### ADULT

- *Initial:* 25 mg PO qid; gradually increase as tolerated to approximately 100 mg during the first 2 wk. Then increase gradually over the next several weeks to a maximum dose of 250 mg/d. At maximum dose, give once a day at hs to minimize sedation.
- *Maintenance:* Adjust to maintain the lowest effective dosage, and periodically assess need for treatment. Effectiveness after 10 wk has not been documented.

#### PEDIATRIC

- *Initial:* 25 mg PO qid; gradually increase as tolerated during the first 2 wk to a maximum of 3 mg/kg or 100 mg, whichever is smaller. Then increase dosage to a daily maximum of 3 mg/kg or 200 mg, whichever is smaller. At maximum give once a day hs to minimize sedation.
- *Maintenance:* Adjust dosage to maintain lowest effective dosage, and periodically assess patient to determine the need for treatment. Effectiveness after 10 wk has not been documented.

### Pharmacokinetics

| *Route* | *Onset* | *Duration* |
|---|---|---|
| Oral | slow | 1–6wk |

*Metabolism:* Hepatic, $T_{1/2}$: 21–31 h
*Distribution:* Crosses placenta; enters breast milk
*Excretion:* Bile/feces

### Adverse effects

- CNS: *Sedation and anticholinergic (atropine-like) effects; confusion* (especially in elderly), *disturbed concentration*, hallucinations, disorientation, decreased memory, feelings of unreality, delusions, anxiety, nervousness, restlessness, agitation, panic, insomnia, nightmares, hypomania, mania, *asthenia, aggressive reaction*
- GI: *Dry mouth, constipation*, paralytic ileus, *nausea*, vomiting, anorexia, epi-

gastric distress, diarrhea, flatulence, dysphagia, peculiar taste, increased salivation, stomatitis, parotid swelling, abdominal cramps, black tongue, *eructation*

- CV: *Orthostatic hypotension*, hypertension, syncope, tachycardia, palpitations, MI, arrhythmias, heart block, precipitation of CHF, stroke
- Hematologic: Bone marrow depression, including agranulocytosis; eosinophila, purpura, thrombocytopenia, leukopenia, *anemia*
- GU: Urinary retention, delayed micturition, dilation of the urinary tract, gynecomastia, testicular swelling; breast enlargement, *menstrual irregularity* and galactorrhea in women; increased or decreased libido; *impotence*
- Endocrine: Elevated or depressed blood sugar; elevated prolactin levels; SIADH secretion
- Hypersensitivity: Skin rash, pruritus, vasculitis, petechiae, photosensitization, edema (generalized, facial, tongue), drug fever
- Withdrawal: Symptoms on abrupt discontinuation of prolonged therapy: nausea, headache, vertigo, nightmares, malaise
- Other: *Nasal congestion*, *laryngitis*, excessive appetite, weight change; sweating hyperthermia, flushing, chills

### Clinically important drug-drug interactions

• Increased TCA levels and pharmacologic effects with cimetidine • Increased TCA levels with fluoxetine, methylphenidate, phenothiazines, oral contraceptives, disulfiram • Hyperpyretic crises, severe convulsions, hypertensive episodes and deaths when MAO inhibitors, furazolidone are given with TCAs • Increased antidepressant response and cardiac arrhythmias when given with thyroid medication • Increased anticholinergic effects of anticholinergic drugs when given with TCAs • Increased response to alcohol, barbiturates, benzodiazepines, other CNS depressants with TCAs • Decreased effects of indirect-acting sympathomimetic drugs (ephedrine) with TCAs

## ■ Nursing Considerations

### Assessment

- ***History:*** Hypersensitivity to any tricyclic drug; concomitant therapy with an MAO inhibitor; recent MI; myelography within previous 24 h or scheduled within 48 h; lactation; EST; preexisting CV disorders; angle-closure glaucoma, increased intraocular pressure, urinary retention, ureteral or urethral spasm; seizure disorders ; hyperthyroidism, impaired hepatic, renal function; psychiatric patients; elective surgery.
- ***Physical:*** Weight; T; skin color, lesions; orientation, affect, reflexes, vision and hearing; P, BP, orthostatic BP, perfusion; bowel sounds, normal output, liver evaluation; urine flow, normal output; usual sexual function, frequency of menses, breast and scrotal exam; liver function tests, urinalysis, CBC, ECG.

### Implementation

- Limit depressed and potentially suicidal patients' access to drug.
- Administer in divided doses with meals to reduce GI side effects while increasing dosage to therapeutic levels.
- Give maintenance dose once-daily at hs to decrease daytime sedation.
- Reduce dose if minor side effects develop; discontinue drug if serious side effects occur.
- Arrange for CBC if patient develops fever, sore throat, or other sign of infection.

### Drug-specific teaching points

- Take this drug as prescribed; do not to stop taking abruptly or without consulting health care provider.
- Avoid alcohol, sleep-inducing drugs, OTC drugs.
- Avoid prolonged exposure to sun or sunlamps; use a sunscreen or protective garments if exposure to sun is unavoidable.
- The following side effects may occur: headache, dizziness, drowsiness, weakness,

blurred vision (reversible; take safety measures if severe; avoid driving or performing tasks that require alertness); nausea, vomiting, loss of appetite, dry mouth (small, frequent meals; frequent mouth care; and sucking sugarless candies may help); nightmares, inability to concentrate, confusion; changes in sexual function.
- Report dry mouth, difficulty urinating, excessive sedation.

## clonazepam

*(kloe **na'** ze pam)*

Klonopin, Rivotril (CAN)

**Pregnancy Category D**
**C-IV controlled substance**

### Drug classes
Benzodiazepine
Antiepileptic agent

### Therapeutic actions
Exact mechanisms not understood; benzodiazepines potentiate the effects of GABA, an inhibitory neurotransmitter.

### Indications
- Used alone or as adjunct in treatment of Lennox-Gastaut syndrome (petit mal variant), akinetic and myoclonic seizures; may be useful in patients with absence (petit mal) seizures who have not responded to succinimides; up to 30% of patients show loss of effectiveness of drug, often within 3 mo of therapy (may respond to dosage adjustment).
- Unlabeled uses: treatment of panic attacks, periodic leg movements during sleep, hypokinetic dysarthria, acute manic episodes, multifocal tic disorders, adjunct treatment of schizophrenia, neuralgias

### Contraindications/cautions
- Contraindications: hypersensitivity to benzodiazepines, psychoses, acute narrow-angle glaucoma, shock, coma, acute alcoholic intoxication with depression of vital signs; pregnancy (risk of congenital malformations, neonatal withdrawal syndrome), labor and delivery ("floppy infant" syndrome), lactation (infants become lethargic and lose weight).
- Use caution in the presence of impaired liver or kidney function, debilitation.

### Dosage
**Available Forms:** Tablets—0.5, 1, 2 mg

Individualize dosage; increase dosage gradually to avoid adverse effects; drug is available only in oral dosage forms.

*ADULT:* Initial dose should not exceed 1.5 mg/d PO divided into 3 doses; increase in increment of 0.5–1 mg PO every 3 days until seizures are adequately controlled or until side effects preclude further increases. Maximum recommended dosage is 20 mg/d.

*PEDIATRIC:* Infants and children up to 10 y or 30 kg: 0.01–0.03 mg/kg per day PO initially; do not exceed 0.05 mg/kg per day PO, given in 2 to 3 doses. Increase dosage by not more than 0.25–0.5 mg every third day until a daily maintenance dose of 0.1–0.2 mg/kg has been reached, unless seizures are controlled by lower dosage or side effects preclude increases. Whenever possible, divide daily dose into three equal doses, or give largest dose at hs.

### Pharmacokinetics

| *Route* | *Onset* | *Peak* | *Duration* |
|---|---|---|---|
| Oral | Varies | 1–2 h | weeks |

*Metabolism:* Hepatic, $T_{1/2}$: 18–50 h
*Distribution:* Crosses placenta; enters breast milk
*Excretion:* Urine

### Adverse effects
- CNS: *Transient, mild drowsiness initially; sedation, depression, lethargy, apathy, fatigue, lightheadedness, disorientation, anger, hostility,* episodes of mania and hypomania, *restlessness, confusion, crying,* delirium, *headache*, slurred speech, dysarthria, stupor, rigidity, tremor, dystonia, vertigo, euphoria, nervousness, difficulty in concentration, vivid dreams, psychomotor retardation, extrapyramidal symptoms; *mild paradoxical excitatory reactions, during first two weeks of treatment*
- GI: *Constipation, diarrhea, dry mouth,* salivation, *nausea*, anorexia, vomiting,

difficulty in swallowing, gastric disorders, hepatic dysfunction, encoporesis
- **CV**: Bradycardia, tachycardia, CV collapse, hypertension and hypotension, palpitations, edema
- **Hematologic**: Elevations of blood enzymes: LDH, alkaline phosphatase, SGOT, SGPT; blood dyscrasias: agranulocytosis, leukopenia
- **GU**: Incontinence, urinary retention, changes in libido, menstrual irregularities
- **EENT**: Visual and auditory disturbances, diplopia, nystagmus, depressed hearing, nasal congestion
- **Dermatologic**: Urticaria, pruritus, skin rash, dermatitis
- **Other**: Hiccups, fever, diaphoresis, paresthesias, muscular disturbances, gynecomastia. Drug dependence with withdrawal syndrome when drug is discontinued; more common with abrupt discontinuation of higher dosage used for longer than 4 mo.

### Clinically important drug-drug interactions
- Increased CNS depression with alcohol
- Increased effect with cimetidine, disulfiram, omeprazole, oral contraceptives
- Decreased effect with theophylline

## ■ Nursing Considerations

### Assessment
- *History:* Hypersensitivity to benzodiazepines; psychoses; acute narrow-angle glaucoma; shock; coma; acute alcoholic intoxication; pregnancy; lactation; impaired liver or kidney function, debilitation.
- *Physical:* Skin color, lesions; T; orientation, reflexes, affect, ophthalmologic exam; P, BP; R, adventitious sounds; liver evaluation, abdominal exam, bowel sounds, normal output; CBC, liver and renal function tests.

### Implementation
- Monitor addiction-prone patients carefully because of their predisposition to habituation and drug dependence.
- Monitor liver function, blood counts periodically in patients on long-term therapy.
- Taper dosage gradually after long-term therapy, especially in epileptic patients; substitute another antielipetic drug.
- Monitor patient for therapeutic drug levels: 20–80 ng/ml.
- Arrange for patient to wear medical alert ID indicating epilepsy and drug therapy.

### Drug-specific teaching points
- Take drug exactly as prescribed; do not stop taking drug (long-term therapy) without consulting health care provider.
- Avoid alcohol, sleep-inducing, or OTC drugs.
- The following side effects may occur: drowsiness, dizziness (may become less pronounced; avoid driving or engaging in other dangerous activities); GI upset (take drug with food); fatigue; dreams; crying; nervousness; depression, emotional changes; bed-wetting, urinary incontinence.
- Report severe dizziness, weakness, drowsiness that persists, rash or skin lesions, difficulty voiding, palpitations, swelling in the extremities.

# clonidine hydrochloride

*(**kloe'** ni deen)*

*Antihypertensives:* Apo-Clonidine (CAN), Catapres, Catapres-TTS (transdermal preparation), Dixarit (CAN), Nu-Clonidine (CAN)

*Analgesic:* Duraclon

**Pregnancy Category C**

### Drug classes
Antihypertensive
Sympatholytic, centrally acting
Central analgesic

### Therapeutic actions
Stimulates CNS alpha$_2$-adrenergic receptors, inhibits sympathetic cardioaccelerator and

vasoconstrictor centers, and decreases sympathetic outflow from the CNS.

### Indications

- Hypertension (stepped-care approach, clonidine is a step 2 drug)
- Treatment of severe pain in cancer patients in combination with opiates; epidural more effective with neuropathic pain (Duraclon)
- Unlabeled uses: Gilles de la Tourette's syndrome; migraine, decreases severity and frequency; menopausal flushing, decreases severity and frequency of episodes; chronic methadone detoxification; rapid opiate detoxification (in doses up to 17 $\mu$g/kg per day); alcohol and benzodiazepine withdrawal treatment; management of hypertensive "urgencies" (oral clonidine "loading" is used; initial dose of 0.2 mg then 0.1 mg every hour until a dose of 0.7 mg is reached or until BP is controlled)

### Contraindications/cautions

- Contraindications: hypersensitivity to clonidine or any adhesive layer components of the transdermal system.
- Use cautiously with severe coronary insufficiency, recent MI, cerebrovascular disease; chronic renal failure; pregnancy, lactation.

### Dosage

**Available Forms:** Tablets—0.1, 0.2, 0.3 mg; transdermal—0.1, 0.2, 0.3 mg/24 hr; epidural injection—100 $\mu$g/ml

ADULT:

- ***Oral therapy:*** Individualize dosage. Initial dose: 0.1 mg bid; maintenance dose: increase in increments of 0.1 or 0.2 to reach desired response. Common range is 0.2–0.8 mg/d, in divided doses; maximum dose is 2.4 mg/d. Minimize sedation by slowly increasing daily dosage; giving majority of daily dose at hs.
- ***Transdermal system:*** Apply to a hairless area of intact skin of upper arm or torso once every 7 d. Change skin site for each application. If system loosens while wearing, apply adhesive overlay directly over the system to ensure adhesion. Start with the 0.1-mg system (releases 0.1 mg/24 h); if, after 1–2 wk, desired BP reduction is not achieved, add another 0.1-mg system, or use a larger system. Dosage of more than two 0.3-mg systems does not improve efficacy. Antihypertensive effect may only begin 2–3 d after application; therefore, when substituting transdermal systems, a gradual reduction of prior dosage is advised. Previous antihypertensive medication may have to be continued, particularly with severe hypertension.
- ***Pain management:*** 30 $\mu$g/h by continuous epidural infusion.

PEDIATRIC: Safety and efficacy not established.

### Pharmacokinetics

| Route | Onset | Peak | Duration |
|---|---|---|---|
| Oral | 30–60 min | 3–5 h | 24 h |
| Transdermal | Slow | 2–3 d | 7 d |
| Epidural | Rapid | 19 min | |

*Metabolism:* Hepatic, $T_{1/2}$: 12–16 h, 19 h (transdermal system); 48 h (epidural)

*Distribution:* Crosses placenta; enters breast milk

*Excretion:* Urine

### Adverse effects

- CNS: *Drowsiness, sedation, dizziness,* headache, fatigue that tend to diminish within 4–6 wk, dreams, nightmares, insomnia, hallucinations, delirium, nervousness, restlessness, anxiety, depression, retinal degeneration
- GI: *Dry mouth, constipation,* anorexia, malaise, nausea, vomiting, parotid pain, parotitis, mild transient abnormalitities in liver function tests
- CV: CHF, orthostatic hypotension, palpitations, tachycardia, bradycardia, Raynaud's phenomenon, ECG abnormalities manifested as Wenckebach period or ventricular trigeminy
- GU: Impotence, decreased sexual activity, loss of libido, nocturia, difficulty in micturition, urinary retention

- **Dermatologic**: Rash, angioneurotic edema, hives, urticaria, hair thinning and alopecia, pruritus, dryness, itching or burning of the eyes, pallor
- **Other**: Weight gain, transient elevation of blood glucose or serum creatine phosphokinase, gynecomastia, weakness, muscle or joint pain, cramps of the lower limbs, dryness of the nasal mucosa, fever

*Transdermal System*

- CNS: *Drowsiness*, fatigue, headache, lethargy, sedation, insomnia, nervousness
- GI: *Dry mouth*, constipation, nausea, change in taste, dry throat
- GU: Impotence, sexual dysfunction
- Local: *Transient localized skin reactions*, pruritus, erythema, allergic contact sensitization and contact dermatitis, localized vesiculation, hyperpigmentation, edema, excoriation, burning, papules, throbbing, blanching, generalized macular rash

### Clinically important drug-drug interactions

• Decreased antihypertensive effects with TCAs (imipramine) • Paradoxical hypertension with propranolol; also greater withdrawal hypertension when abruptly discontinued and patient is taking beta-adrenergic blocking agents

## ■ Nursing Considerations

### Assessment

- *History:* Hypersensitivity to clonidine or adhesive layer components of the transdermal system; severe coronary insufficiency, recent MI, cerebrovascular disease; chronic renal failure; lactation
- *Physical:* Body weight; body temperature; skin color, lesions, temperature; mucous membranes—color, lesion; breast exam; orientation, affect, reflexes; ophthalmologic exam; P, BP, orthostatic BP, perfusion, edema, auscultation; bowel sounds, normal output, liver evaluation, palpation of salivary glands; normal urinary output, voiding pattern; liver function tests, ECG

### Implementation

- Do not discontinue abruptly; discontinue therapy by reducing the dosage gradually over 2–4 d to avoid rebound hypertension, tachycardia, flushing, nausea, vomiting, cardiac arrhythmias (hypertensive encephalopathy and death have occurred after abrupt cessation of clonidine).
- Do not discontinue prior to surgery; monitor BP carefully during surgery; have other BP-controlling drugs on standby.
- Reevaluate therapy if clonidine tolerance occurs; giving concomitant diuretic increases the antihypertensive efficacy of clonidine.
- Monitor BP carefully when discontinuing clonidine; hypertension usually returns within 48 h.
- Assess compliance with drug regimen in a supportive manner; pill counts, or other methods.

### Drug-specific teaching points

- Take this drug exactly as prescribed. Do not miss doses. Do not discontinue the drug unless so instructed. Do not discontinue abruptly; life-threatening adverse effects may occur. If you travel, take an adequate supply of drug.
- Store epidural injection at room temperature; discard any unused portions.
- Use the transdermal system as prescribed; refer to directions in package insert, or contact your health care provider with questions.
- Attempt lifestyle changes that will reduce your BP: stop smoking and alcohol use; lose weight; restrict intake of sodium (salt); exercise regularly.
- Use caution with alcohol. Your sensitiviity may increase while using this drug.
- The following side effects may occur: drowsiness, dizziness, lightheadedness, headache, weakness (often transient; observe caution driving or performing other tasks that require alertness or physical dexterity); dry mouth (sucking on sugarless lozenges or ice chips may help); GI upset (eat frequent small meals); dreams, nightmares (reversible); dizziness, lightheadedness when you

change position (get up slowly; use caution climbing stairs); impotence, other sexual dysfunction, decreased libido (discuss with care providers); breast enlargement, sore breasts; palpitations.
- Report urinary retention, changes in vision, blanching of fingers, skin rash.

## clopidogrel

*(cloe **pid'** oh grel)*
Plavix
**Pregnancy Category B**

### Drug classes
Adenosine diphosphate (ADP) receptor antagonist
Antiplatelet agent

### Therapeutic actions
Inhibits platelet aggregation by blocking ADP receptors.

### Indications
- Treatment of patients at risk for ischemic events—history of MI, ischemic stroke, peripheral artery disease

### Contraindications/cautions
- Contraindications: allergy to clopidogrel, pregnancy, lactation
- Use cautiously with bleeding disorders, recent surgery, closed head injury

### Dosage
**Available Forms:** Tablets—75 mg
*ADULT:* 75 mg PO qd.

### Pharmacokinetics

| *Route* | *Onset* | *Peak* | *Duration* |
|---|---|---|---|
| Oral | Varies | 75 min | 3–4 h |

*Metabolism:* Hepatic; $T_{1/2}$: 8 h
*Distribution:* Crosses placenta; passes into breast milk
*Excretion:* Bile and urine

### Adverse effects
- CNS: *Headache, dizziness,* weakness, syncope, flushing
- GI: Nausea, GI distress, constipation, diarrhea
- Dermatologic: *Skin rash,* pruritus

### ■ Nursing Considerations

#### Assessment
- *History:* Allergy to clopidogrel, pregnancy, lactation, bleeding disorders, recent surgery, closed head injury
- *Physical:* Skin color, temperature, lesions; orientation, reflexes, affect; P, BP, orthostatic BP, baseline ECG, peripheral perfusion; R, adventitious sounds

#### Implementation
- Provide small, frequent meals if GI upset occurs (not as common as with aspirin).
- Provide comfort measures and arrange for analgesics if headache occurs.

#### Drug-specific teaching points
- Take daily as prescribed.
- The following side effects may occur: dizziness, lightheadedness (this may pass as you adjust to the drug); headache (lie down in a cool environment and rest; OTC preparations may help); nausea, gastric distress (eat small, frequent meals).
- Report skin rash, chest pain, fainting, severe headache.

## clorazepate dipotassium

*(klor **az'** e pate)*
Apo-Clorazepate (CAN), Gen-Xene, Novo-Clopate (CAN), Tranxene, Tranxene-SD
**Pregnancy Category D**
**C-IV controlled substance**

### Drug classes
Benzodiazepine
Antianxiety agent
Antiepileptic agent

### Therapeutic actions
Exact mechanisms not understood; benzodiazepines potentiate the effects of GABA, an inhibitory neurotransmitter; anxiolytic effects occur at doses well below those necessary to cause sedation, ataxia.

## Indications

- Management of anxiety disorders or for short-term relief of symptoms of anxiety
- Symptomatic relief of acute alcohol withdrawal
- Adjunctive therapy for partial seizures

## Contraindications/cautions

- Contraindications: hypersensitivity to benzodiazepines; psychoses; acute narrow-angle glaucoma; shock; coma; acute alcoholic intoxication with depression of vital signs; pregnancy (risk of congenital malformations, neonatal withdrawal syndrome); labor and delivery (''floppy infant'' syndrome); lactation (infants tend to become lethargic and lose weight).
- Use cautiously with impaired liver or kidney function, debilitation.

## Dosage

**Available Forms:** Tablets—3.75, 7, 15 mg; single-dose tablets—11.25, 22.5 mg

Individualize dosage; increase dosage gradually to avoid adverse effects. Drug is available only in oral forms.

### Adult

- *Anxiety:* Usual dose is 30 mg/d PO in divided doses tid; adjust gradually within the range of 15–60 mg/d; also may be given as a single daily dose at hs; start with a dose of 15 mg. *Maintenance:* give the 22.5-mg PO tablet in a single daily dose as an alternate form for patients stabilized on 7.5 mg PO tid; do not use to initiate therapy; the 11.5-mg tablet may be given as a single daily dose.
- ***Adjunct to antiepileptic medication:*** Maximum initial dose is 7.5 mg PO tid. Increase dosage by no more than 7.5 mg every wk, do not exceed 90 mg/d.
- ***Acute alcohol withdrawal:*** *Day 1:* 30 mg PO initially, then 30–60 mg in divided doses. *Day 2:* 45–90 mg PO in divided doses. *Day 3:* 22.5–45 mg PO in divided doses. *Day 4:* 15–30 mg PO in divided doses. Thereafter, gradually reduce dose to 7.5–15 mg/d PO, and stop as soon as condition is stable.

### Pediatric:

- ***Adjunct to antiepileptic medication***
  - *>12 y:* Same as adult.
  - *9–12 y:* Maximum initial dose is 7.5 mg PO bid; increase dosage by no more than 7.5 mg every wk, and do not exceed 60 mg/d.
  - *<9 y:* Not recommended.

### Geriatric Patients or Those With Debilitating Disease

- *Anxiety:* Initially, 7.5–15 mg/d PO in divided doses. Adjust as needed and tolerated.

## Pharmacokinetics

| *Route* | *Onset* | *Peak* | *Duration* |
|---|---|---|---|
| Oral | Fast | 1–2 h | Days |

*Metabolism:* Hepatic, $T_{1/2}$: 30–100 h

*Distribution:* Crosses placenta; enters breast milk

*Excretion:* Urine

## Adverse effects

- CNS: *Transient, mild drowsiness initially; sedation, depression, lethargy, apathy, fatigue, lightheadedness, disorientation, anger, hostility,* episodes of mania and hypomania, *restlessness, confusion, crying,* delirium, *headache,* slurred speech, dysarthria, stupor, rigidity, tremor, dystonia, vertigo, euphoria, nervousness, difficulty in concentration, vivid dreams, psychomotor retardation, extrapyramidal symptoms; *mild paradoxical excitatory reactions, during first 2 wk of treatment*
- GI: *Constipation, diarrhea, dry mouth,* salivation, *nausea,* anorexia, vomiting, difficulty in swallowing, gastric disorders, hepatic dysfunction, encoporesis
- CV: Bradycardia, tachycardia, CV collapse, hypertension and hypotension, palpitations, edema
- Hematologic: Elevations of blood enzymes—LDH, alkaline phosphatase, SGOT, SGPT; blood dyscrasias—agranulocytosis, leukopenia

- **GU**: Incontinence, urinary retention, changes in libido, menstrual irregularities
- **EENT**: Visual and auditory disturbances, diplopia, nystagmus, depressed hearing, nasal congestion
- **Dermatologic**: Urticaria, pruritus, skin rash, dermatitis
- **Other**: Hiccups, fever, diaphoresis, paresthesias, muscular disturbances, gynecomastia. Drug dependence with withdrawal syndrome is common with abrupt discontinuation of higher dosage used for longer than 4 mo.

### Clinically important drug-drug interactions

- Increased CNS depression with alcohol
- Increased effect with cimetidine, disulfiram, omeprazole, oral contraceptives
- Decreased effect with theophylline

## ■ Nursing Considerations

### Assessment

- *History:* Hypersensitivity to benzodiazepines; psychoses; acute narrow-angle glaucoma; shock; coma; acute alcoholic intoxication; pregnancy; lactation; impaired liver or kidney function; debilitation
- *Physical:* Skin color, lesions; T; orientation, reflexes, affect, ophthalmologic exam; P, BP; R, adventitious sounds; liver evaluation, abdominal exam, bowel sounds, normal output; CBC, liver and renal function tests

### Implementation

- Taper dosage gradually after long-term therapy, especially in epileptics.
- Arrange for epileptics to wear medical alert ID, indicating disease and medication usage.

### Drug-specific teaching points

- Take drug exactly as prescribed; do not stop taking drug (long-term therapy) without consulting health care provider.
- Avoid alcohol, sleep-inducing, or OTC drugs.
- The following side effects may occur: drowsiness, dizziness (may be transient; avoid driving a car or engaging in other dangerous activities); GI upset (take with food); fatigue; depression; dreams; crying; nervousness; depression, emotional changes; bed-wetting, urinary incontinence.
- Report severe dizziness, weakness, drowsiness that persists, rash or skin lesions, difficulty voiding, palpitations, swelling in the extremities.

## clotrimazole

*(kloe **trim'** a zole)*

*Troche preparation:* Canesten (CAN), Mycelex

*Vaginal preparations:* Gyne-Lotrimin, Mycelex-G, Mycelex-7, Myclo (CAN)

*Topical preparations:* Clotrimaderm (CAN), Lotrimin, Mycelex, Mycelex

**Pregnancy Category C (troche)**

**Pregnancy Category B (topical, vaginal)**

### Drug classes

Antifungal

### Therapeutic actions

Fungicidal and fungistatic: binds to fungal cell membrane with a resultant change in membrane permeability, allowing leakage of intracellular components, causing cell death.

### Indications

- Treatment of oropharyngeal candidiasis (troche)
- Local treatment of vulvovaginal candidiasis (moniliasis; vaginal preparations)
- Topical treatment of tinea pedia, tinea cruris, tinea corporis due to *Trichophyton rubrum, Trichophyton mentagrophytes, Epidermophyton floccosum, Microsporum canis*; candidiasis due to *Candida albicans*; tinea versicolor due to *Microsporum furfur* (topical preparations)

### Contraindications/cautions

- Allergy to clotrimazole or components used in preparation

### Dosage

**Available Forms:** Troche—10 mg; vaginal cream, solution, lotion—1% ; topical cream, solution, lotion—1%

***Troche:*** Administer 1 troche five times a day for 14 consecutive d.

***Vaginal preparation, tablet:*** Insert one 100-mg tablet intravaginally hs for 7 nights or two 100-mg tablets intravaginally hs for 3 nights, or insert one 500-mg tablet intravaginally one time only.

***Vaginal preparation, cream:*** One applicator (5 g/d), preferably hs for 7–14 consecutive d; 14-d treatments have a higher success rate.

***Topical:*** Gently massage into affected and surrounding skin areas bid in the morning and evening for 1–4 wk. With no improvement in 4 wk, reevaluate diagnosis.

### Pharmacokinetics

Action is primarily local; pharmacokinetics are not known.

### Adverse effects

*Troche*

- GI: *Nausea, vomiting, abnormal liver function tests*

*Vaginal*

- GI: *Lower abdominal cramps,* bloating
- GU: *Slight urinary frequency; burning or irritation in the sexual partner*
- Dermatologic: Skin rash

*Topical*

- Local: *Erythema, stinging,* blistering, peeling, edema, pruritus, urticaria, general skin irritation

## ■ Nursing Considerations

### Assessment

- *History:* Allergy to clotrimazole or components used in preparation
- *Physical:* Skin color, lesions, area around lesions; bowel sounds; culture of area involved, liver function tests

### Implementation

- Culture fungus involved before therapy.
- Have patient dissolve troche slowly in mouth.
- Insert vaginal tablets high into the vagina; use hs; if this is not possible, have patient remain recumbent for 10–15 min after insertion. Provide sanitary napkin to protect clothing from stains.
- Administer vaginal cream high into vagina using the applicator supplied with the product. Administer for 7–14 consecutive nights, even during menstrual period.
- Cleanse affected area before topical application. Do not apply to eyes or eye areas.
- Monitor response to drug therapy. If no response is noted, arrange for more cultures to determine causative organism.
- Ensure that patient receives full course of therapy to eradicate the fungus and prevent recurrence.
- Discontinue topical or vaginal administration if rash or sensitivity occurs.

### Drug-specific teaching points

- Take the full course of drug therapy, even if symptoms improve. Continue during menstrual period if vaginal route is being used. Long-term use of the drug may be needed; beneficial effects may not be seen for several weeks. Vaginal tablets and creams should be inserted high into the vagina. Troche preparation should be allowed to dissolve slowly in the mouth. Apply topical preparation with a gently massage into the affected area.
- Use hygiene measures to prevent reinfection or spread of infection.
- Vaginal use: Refrain from sexual intercourse, or advise partner to use a condom to avoid reinfection. Use a sanitary napkin to prevent staining of clothing.
- The following side effects may occur: nausea, vomiting, diarrhea (oral use); irritation, burning, stinging (local).
- Report worsening of the condition being treated, local irritation, burning (topical),

rash, irritation, pelvic pain (vaginal), nausea, GI distress (oral administration).

## cloxacillin sodium

*(klox a **sill'** in)*

Apo-Cloxi (CAN), Cloxapen, Novo-Cloxin (CAN), Nu-Cloxi (CAN), Orbenin (CAN), Tegopen

**Pregnancy Category B**

### Drug classes

Antibiotic
Penicillinase-resistant pencillin

### Therapeutic actions

Bactericidal: inhibits cell wall synthesis of sensitive organisms, causing cell death.

### Indications

- Infections due to penicillinase-producing staphylococci

### Contraindications/cautions

- Contraindications: allergies to penicillins, cephalosporins, or other allergens.
- Use cautiously with renal disorders, lactation (causes diarrhea or candidiasis in infants).

### Dosage

**Available Forms:** Capsules—250, 500 mg; powder for solution—125 mg/5 ml
*ADULT:* 250 mg q6h PO; up to 500 mg q6h PO in severe infections.
*PEDIATRIC <20 KG:* 50 mg/kg/day PO in equally divided doses q6h; up to 100 mg/kg per day PO in equally divided doses q6h in severe infections.

### Pharmacokinetics

| Route | Onset | Peak |
|---|---|---|
| Oral | Varies | 1 h |

*Metabolism:* $T_{1/2}$: 30–90 min
*Distribution:* Crosses placenta; enters breast milk
*Excretion:* Urine

### Adverse effects

- CNS: Lethargy, hallucinations, seizures, decreased reflexes
- GI: *Glossitis, stomatitis, gastritis, sore mouth,* furry tongue, black "hairy" tongue, *nausea, vomiting, diarrhea,* abdominal pain, bloody diarrhea, enterocolitis, pseudomembranous colitis, nonspecific hepatitis
- **Hematologic**: Anemia, thrombocytopenia, leukopenia, neutropenia, prolonged bleeding time, hemorrhagic episodes at high doses
- GU: Nephritis—oliguria, proteinuria, hematuria, casts, azotemia, pyuria
- **Hypersensitivity**: *Rash, fever, wheezing,* anaphylaxis
- Other: *Superinfections*—oral and rectal moniliasis, vaginitis

### Clinically important drug-drug interactions

- Decreased effectiveness with tetracyclines
- Decreased efficacy of oral contraceptives is possible

### Clinically important drug-food interactions

- Decreased absorption and decreased serum levels if taken with food

## ■ Nursing Considerations

### Assessment

- *History:* Allergies to penicillins, cephalosporins, or other allergens; renal disorders, lactation
- *Physical:* Culture infected area; skin color, lesion; R, adventitious sounds; bowel sounds; CBC, liver and renal function tests, serum electrolytes, Hct, urinalysis

### Implementation

- Administer on an empty stomach, 1 h before or 2 h after meals, with a full glass of water. Do not give with fruit juice or soft drinks.
- Continue treatment for 10 full days.

### Drug-specific teaching points

- Take around the clock; take the full course of therapy, usually 10 d. Take on an empty stomach, 1 h before or 2 h after meals, with a full glass of water.
- This antibiotic is for this infection and should not be used to self-treat other infections.

- The following side effects may occur: stomach upset, nausea, diarrhea, mouth sores (if severe, consult health care provider for treatment).
- Report unusual bleeding or bruising, fever, chills, sore throat, hives, rash, severe diarrhea, difficulty breathing.

## clozapine

*(kloe ' za peen)*

Clozaril

**Pregnancy Category B**

### Drug classes

Antipsychotic

Dopaminergic blocking agent

### Therapeutic actions

Mechanism not fully understood: blocks dopamine receptors in the brain, depresses the RAS; anticholinergic, antihistaminic ($H_1$), and alpha-adrenergic blocking activity may contribute to some of its therapeutic (and adverse) actions. Clozapine produces fewer extrapyramidal effects than other antipsychotics.

### Indications

- For severely ill schizophrenics who are unresponsive to standard antipsychotic drugs.

### Contraindications/cautions

- Contraindications: allergy to clozapine, myeloproliferative disorders, history of clozapine-induced agranulocytosis or severe granulocytopenia, severe CNS depression, comatose states, history or seizure disorders, lactation.
- Use cautiously with CV disease, prostate enlargement, narrow-angle glaucoma, pregnancy.

### Dosage

**Available Forms:** Tablets—25, 100 mg

ADULT

- *Initial:* 25 mg PO qid or bid; then gradually increase with daily increments of 25–50 mg/d, if tolerated, to a dose of 300–450 mg/d by the end of second week. Adjust later dosage no more often than twice weekly in increments < 100 mg. Do not exceed 900 mg/d.
- *Maintenance:* Maintain at the lowest effective dose for remission of symptoms.
- *Discontinuation:* Gradual reduction over a 2-wk period is preferred. If abrupt discontinuation is required, carefully monitor patient for signs of acute psychotic symptoms.
- *Reinitiation of treatment:* Follow initial dosage guidelines, use extreme care; increased risk of severe adverse effects with reexposure.

PEDIATRIC: Safety and efficacy in children < 16 y not established.

### Pharmacokinetics

| Route | Onset | Peak | Duration |
|---|---|---|---|
| Oral | Varies | 1–6 h | Weeks |

*Metabolism:* Hepatic, $T_{1/2}$: 4–12 h

*Distribution:* Crosses placenta; enters breast milk

*Excretion:* Urine and feces

### Adverse effects

- CNS: *Drowsiness, sedation, seizures, dizziness, syncope, headache,* tremor, distubed sleep, nightmares, restlessness, agitation, increased salivation, sweating
- GI: *Nausea, vomiting, constipation,* abdominal discomfort, dry mouth
- CV: *Tachycardia, hypotension,* ECG changes, hypertension
- **Hematologic**: Leukopenia, granulocytopenia, agranulocytopenia
- GU: Urinary abnormalities
- **Other**: *Fever,* weight gain, rash

### Clinically important drug-drug interactions

• Increased therapeutic and toxic effects with cimetidine • Decreased therapeutic effect with phenytoin, mephenytoin, ethotoin

## ■ Nursing Considerations

### Assessment

- *History:* Allergy to clozapine, myeloproliferative disorders, history of clozapine-induced agranulocytosis or severe gran-

ulocytopenia, severe CNS depression, comatose states, history or seizure disorders, CV disease, prostate enlargement, narrow-angle glaucoma, lactation
- *Physical:* T, weight; reflexes, orientation, intraocular pressure, ophthalmologic exam; P, BP, orthostatic BP, ECG; R, adventitious sounds; bowel sounds, normal output, liver evaluation; prostate palpation, normal urine output; CBC, urinalysis, liver and kidney function tests, EEG.

### Implementation
- Use only when unresponsive to conventional antipsychotic drugs.
- Obtain clozapine through the Clozaril Patient Management System.
- Dispense only 1 wk supply at a time.
- Monitor WBC carefully prior to first dose.
- Weekly monitoring of WBC during treatment and for 4 wk thereafter.
- Monitor T. If fever occurs, rule out underlying infection, and consult physician for comfort measures.
- Monitor elderly patients for dehydration. Institute remedial measures promptly; sedation and decreased thirst related to CNS effects can lead to dehydration.
- Encourage voiding before taking drug to decrease anticholinergic effects of urinary retention.
- Follow guidelines for discontinuation or reinstitution of the drug.

### Drug-specific teaching points
- Weekly blood tests will be taken to determine safe dosage; dosage will be increased gradually to achieve most effective dose. Only 1 wk of medication can be dispensed at a time. Do not take more than your prescribed dosage. Do not make up missed doses, instead contact care provider. Do not stop taking this drug suddenly; gradual reduction of dosage is needed to prevent side effects.
- The following effects may occur as a result of drug therapy: drowsiness, dizziness, sedation, seizures (avoid driving, operating machinery, or performing tasks that require concentration); dizziness, faintness on arising (change positions slowly); increased salivation (reversible); constipation (consult care provider for correctives); fast heart rate (rest, take your time).
- This drug cannot be taken during pregnancy. If you think you are pregnant or wish to become pregnant, contact your care provider.
- Report lethargy, weakness, fever, sore throat, malaise, mouth ulcers, and "flu-like" symptoms.

## codeine phosphate

*(koe' deen)*
**Pregnancy Category C during pregnancy**
**Pregnancy Category D during labor**
**C-II controlled substance**

### Drug classes
Narcotic agonist analgesic
Antitussive

### Therapeutic actions
Acts at opioid receptors in the CNS to produce analgesia, euphoria, sedation; acts in medullary cough center to depress cough reflex.

### Indications
- Relief of mild to moderate pain in adults and children
- Coughing induced by chemical or mechanical irritation of the respiratory system

### Contraindications/cautions
- Contraindications: hypersensitivity to narcotics, physical dependence on a narcotic analgesic (drug may precipitate withdrawal).
- Use cautiously with pregnancy, labor, lactation, bronchial asthma, COPD, respiratory depression, anoxia, increased intracranial pressure, acute MI, ventricular failure, coronary insufficiency, hypertension, biliary tract surgery, renal or hepatic dysfunction.

### Dosage
**Available Forms:** Tablets—15, 30, 60 mg; injection—30, 60 mg; soluble tablets—30, 60 mg

ADULT
- *Analgesic:* 15–60 mg PO, IM, IV or SC q4–6h; do not exceed 120 mg/24 h.
- *Antitussive:* 10–20 mg PO q4–6h; do not exceed 120 mg/24 h.

PEDIATRIC: Contraindicated in premature infants.
- *Analgesic*
  – *1 y OR OLDER:* 0.5 mg/kg SC, IM or PO q4–6h.
- *Antitussive*
  – *6–12 y:* 5–10 mg PO q4–6h; do not exceed 60 mg/24 h.
  – *2–6 y:* 2.5–5 mg PO q4–6h; do not exceed 30 mg/24 h.

GERIATRIC OR IMPAIRED ADULT: Use caution; respiratory depression may occur in elderly, the very ill, those with respiratory problems. Reduced dosage may be necessary.

### Pharmacokinetics

| Route | Onset | Peak | Duration |
|---|---|---|---|
| Oral/IM/IV | 10–30 min | 30–60 min | 4–6 h |

*Metabolism:* Hepatic, $T_{1/2}$: 2.5–4 h
*Distribution:* Crosses placenta; enters breast milk
*Excretion:* Urine

### IV facts
**Preparation:** Protect vials from light.
**Infusion:** Administer slowly over 5 min by direct injection or into running IV tubing.

### Adverse effects
- CNS: *Sedation, clamminess, sweating, headache, vertigo, floating feeling, dizziness, lethargy, confusion, lightheadedness,* nervousness, unusual dreams, agitation, euphoria, hallucinations, delirium, insomnia, anxiety, fear, disorientation, impaired mental and physical performance, coma, mood changes, weakness, headache, tremor, convulsions
- GI: *Nausea, vomiting,* dry mouth, anorexia, constipation, biliary tract spasm
- CV: Palpitation, increase or decrease in BP, circulatory depression, **cardiac arrest**, **shock**, tachycardia, bradycardia, arrhythmia, palpitations
- Respiratory: Slow, shallow respiration; apnea; suppression of cough reflex; laryngospasm; bronchospasm
- GU: Ureteral spasm, spasm of vesical sphincters, urinary retention or hesitancy, oliguria, antidiuretic effect, reduced libido or potency
- EENT: Diplopia, blurred vision
- Dermatologic: Rash, hives, pruritus, flushing, warmth, sensitivity to cold
- Local: Phlebitis following IV injection, pain at injection site; tissue irritation and induration (SC injection)
- Other: Physical tolerance and dependence, psychological dependence

### Clinically important drug-drug interactions
- Potentiation of effects of codeine with barbiturate anesthetics; decrease dose of codeine when coadministering.

### Drug-lab test interferences
- Elevated biliary tract pressure may cause increases in plasma amylase, lipase; determinations of these levels may be unreliable for 24 h after administration of narcotics.

## ■ Nursing Considerations

### Assessment
- *History:* Hypersensitivity to codeine, physical dependence on a narcotic analgesic, pregnancy, labor, lactation, bronchial asthma, COPD, increased intracranial pressure, acute MI, ventricular failure, coronary insufficiency, hypertension, biliary tract surgery, renal or hepatic dysfunction
- *Physical:* Orientation, reflexes, bilateral grip strength, affect; pupil size, vision; pulse, auscultation, BP; R, adventitious sounds; bowel sounds, normal output; liver and kidney function tests

### Implementation
- Give to nursing women 4–6 h before scheduled feeding to minimize drug in milk.

- Provide narcotic antagonist, facilities for assisted or controlled R on standby during parenteral administration.
- Use caution when injecting SC into chilled body areas or in patients with hypotension or in shock; impaired perfusion may delay absorption; with repeated doses, an excessive amount may be absorbed when circulation is restored.
- Instruct postoperative patients in pulmonary toilet; drug suppresses cough reflex.
- Monitor bowel function, arrange for laxatives (especially senna compounds—approximate dose of 187 mg senna concentrate per 120 mg codeine equivalent), bowel training program if severe constipation occurs.

### Drug-specific teaching points

- Take drug exactly as prescribed.
- The following side effects may occur: dizziness, sedation, drowsiness, impaired visual acuity (avoid driving and performing other tasks that require alertness); nausea, loss of appetite (lie quietly, eat frequent, small meals); constipation (use a laxative).
- Do not to take any leftover medication for other disorders, and do not to let anyone else take the prescription.
- Report severe nausea, vomiting, palpitations, shortness of breath or difficulty breathing.

## colchicine

*(kol chi seen)*

**Pregnancy Category C**

**Pregnancy Category D (parenteral)**

### Drug classes

Antigout drug

### Therapeutic actions

Exact mechanism unknown; decreases deposition of uric acid; inhibits kinin formation and phagocytosis, and decreases inflammatory reaction to urate crystal deposition.

### Indications

- Pain relief of acute gout attack; also used between attacks as prophylaxis; IV use reserved for rapid response or when GI side effects interfere with use
- Orphan drug use: arrest progression of neurologic disability caused by chronic progressive multiple sclerosis
- Unlabeled uses: hepatic cirrhosis, familial Mediterranean fever, skin manifestations of scleroderma, psoriasis, dermatitis herpetiformis, treatment of Behçet's disease

### Contraindications/cautions

- Allergy to colchicine, blood dyscrasias, serious GI disorders, liver, renal or cardiac disorders, pregnancy, lactation

### Dosage

**Available Forms:** Tablets—0.5, 0.6 mg; injection—1 mg

ADULT

- *Acute gouty arthritis:* 0.5–1.2 mg PO followed by 0.5–1.2 mg q1–2h until pain is relieved or nausea, vomiting, or diarrhea occurs. IV dose: 2 mg followed by 0.5 mg q6h until desired effect is achieved; *do not exceed 4 g/24 h.*
- *Prophylaxis in intercritical periods:* Less than one attack per year: 0.5–0.6 mg/d PO for 3–4 d/wk. More frequent attacks (> 1/y): 0.5–0.6 mg/d; up to 1.8 mg/d PO may be needed in severe cases. *IV dose:* 0.5–1 mg qid or bid; change to oral therapy as soon as possible.
- *Prophylaxis for patients undergoing surgery:* 0.5–0.6 mg tid PO for 3 d before and 3 d after the procedure.

PEDIATRIC: Safety and efficacy not established.

GERIATRIC OR RENAL IMPAIRED: Use with caution; reduce dosage if weakness, anorexia, nausea, vomiting, or diarrhea occurs.

### Pharmacokinetics

| Route | Onset | Peak |
|---|---|---|
| Oral | 0.5–2 h | 12 h |
| IV | 30–50 min | 6–12 h |

*Metabolism:* Hepatic, $T_{1/2}$: 20–60 min

*Distribution:* Crosses placenta; enters breast milk

*Excretion:* Urine and bile

### IV facts

**Preparation:** Use undiluted or diluted in 0.9% Sodium Chloride Injection, that does not have a bacteriostatic agent. Do not dilute with 5% Dextrose in Water. Do not use solutions that have become turbid.

**Infusion:** Infuse slowly over 2–5 min by direct injection or into tubing of running IV.

### Adverse effects

- CNS: Peripheral neuritis, purpura, myopathy
- GI: *Diarrhea, vomiting*, abdominal pain, nausea
- **Hematologic**: Bone marrow depression, elevated alkaline phosphatase, SGOT levels
- GU: Azoospermia (reversible)
- **Dermatologic**: Dermatoses, loss of hair
- **Local**: Thrombophlebitis at IV sites

### Clinically important drug-drug interactions

• Decreased absorption of vitamin $B_{12}$ when taken with colchicine

### Drug-lab test interferences

• False-positive results for urine RBC, urine hemoglobin • Decreased thrombocyte levels

## ■ Nursing Considerations

### Assessment

- *History:* Allergy to colchicine, blood dyscrasias, serious GI, liver, renal or cardiac disorders, pregnancy, lactation
- *Physical:* Skin lesions, color; orientation, reflexes; P, cardiac auscultation, BP; liver evaluation, normal bowel output; normal urinary output; CBC, renal and liver function tests, urinalysis

### Implementation

- Monitor for relief of pain, signs and symptoms of gout attack; usually abate within 12 h and are gone within 24–48 h.
- Parenteral drug is to be used IV only; SC or IM use causes severe irritation.
- Arrange for opiate antidiarrheal medication if diarrhea is severe.
- Discuss the dosage regimen with patients who have been using colchicine; these patients know when to stop the medication before GI side effects occur.
- Administration should begin at the first sign of an acute attack; delay can decrease drug's effectiveness in alleviating symptoms of gout.
- Have regular medical follow-ups and blood tests.

### Drug-specific teaching points

- Take this drug at the first warning of an acute attack; delay will impair the drug's effectiveness in relieving your symptoms. Stop drug at the first sign of nausea, vomiting, stomach pain, or diarrhea.
- The following side effects may occur: nausea, vomiting, loss of appetite (take drug following meals or eat small, frequent meals); loss of fertility (reversible); loss of hair (reversible).
- Report severe diarrhea, skin rash, sore throat, fever, unusual bleeding or bruising, fever, chills, sore throat, persistence of gout attack, numbness or tingling, tiredness, weakness.

## colestipol hydrochloride

*(koe **les'** ti pole)*

Colestid

**Pregnancy Category C**

### Drug classes

Antihyperlipidemic
Bile acid sequestrant

### Therapeutic actions

Binds bile acids in the intestine to form a complex that is excreted in the feces; as a result, cholesterol is lost, oxidized in the liver, and serum cholesterol and LDL are lowered.

### Indications

- Reduction of elevated serum cholesterol in patients with primary hypercholesterolemia (elevated LDL) (adjunctive therapy)

### Contraindications/cautions

- Allergy to bile acid sequestrants, complete biliary obstruction, abnormal intestinal function, pregnancy, lactation

### Dosage

**Available Forms:** Tablets—1 g; granules—5 g/7.5 g powder

*ADULT:* 5–30 g/d PO in divided doses 2–4 ×/d. Start with 5 g qid or bid PO, and increase in 5-g/d increments at 1- to 2-mo intervals; tablets: 2–16 g/d.

*PEDIATRIC:* Safety and efficacy not established.

### Pharmacokinetics

Not absorbed systemically. Eliminated in the feces.

### Adverse effects

- CNS: *Headache*, anxiety, vertigo, dizziness, fatigue, syncope, drowsiness
- GI: *Constipation* to fecal impaction, *exacerbation of hemorrhoids*, abdominal cramps, *abdominal pain,* flatulence, anorexia, heartburn, nausea, vomiting, steatorrhea
- **Hematologic**: Increased bleeding tendencies related to vitamin K malabsorption, vitamin A and D deficiencies, hyperchloremic acidosis
- GU: Hematuria, dysuria, diuresis
- **Dermatologic**: Rash and irritation of skin, tongue, perianal area
- **Other**: Osteoporosis, chest pain, backache, muscle and joint pain, arthritis, fever

### Clinically important drug-drug interactions

• Decreased serum levels or delayed absorption of thiazide diuretics, digitalis preparations • Malabsorption of fat-soluble vitamins

## ■ Nursing Considerations

### Assessment

- *History:* Allergy to bile acid sequestrant, complete biliary obstruction, abnormal intestinal function, pregnancy, lactation
- *Physical:* Skin lesions, color, temperature; orientation, affect, reflexes; P, auscultation, baseline ECG, peripheral perfusion; liver evaluation, bowel sounds; lipid studies, liver function tests, clotting profile

### Implementation

- Do not administer drug in dry form. Mix in liquids, soups, cereals, or pulpy fruits; add the prescribed amount to a glassful (90 ml) of liquid; stir until completely mixed. The granules will not dissolve. May be mixed with carbonated beverages, slowly stirred in a large glass. Rinse the glass with a small amount of additional beverage to ensure all of the dose has been taken.
- Ensure that patient swallows tablets whole; do not cut, crush, or chew. Tablets should be taken with plenty of fluids.
- Administer drug before meals.
- Monitor administration of other oral drugs for binding in the intestine and delayed or decreased absorption. Give them 1 h before or 4–6 h after the colestipol.
- Arrange for regular follow-up during long-term therapy.
- Alert patient and concerned others about the high cost of drug.

### Drug-specific teaching points

- Take drug before meals. Do not take the powder in the dry form. Mix in liquids, soups, cereals, or pulpy fruit; add the prescribed amount to a glassful of the liquid; stir until completely mixed. The granules will not dissolve; rinse the glass with a small amount of additional liquid to ensure that you receive the entire dose of the drug; carbonated beverages may be used; mix by slowly stirring in a large glass. If taking tablet form, swallow whole with plenty of fluids; do not cut, crush, or chew.
- This drug may interfere with the absorption of other oral medications. Take other oral medications 1 h before or 4–6 h after colestipol.

- The following side effects may occur: constipation (transient, if it persists, request correctives); nausea, heartburn, loss of appetite (small, frequent meals may help); dizziness, drowsiness, vertigo, fainting (avoid driving and operating dangerous machinery); headache, muscle and joint aches and pains (may lessen in time).
- Report unusual bleeding or bruising, severe constipation, severe GI upset, chest pain, difficulty breathing, rash, fever.

## colfosceril palmitate

*(kole **fos'** seer el)*

synthetic lung surfactant, dipalmitoylphosphatidylcholine, DPPC

Exosurf Neonatal

### Drug classes

Lung surfactant

### Therapeutic actions

A natural compound that reduces surface tension in the alveoli, allowing expansion of the alveoli; replaces the surfactant missing in the lungs of neonates suffering from RDS.

### Indications

- Prophylactic treatment of infants at risk of developing RDS; infants with birth weights < 1,350 g or infants with birth weights > 1,350 g who have evidence of pulmonary immaturity
- Rescue treatment for infants with RDS

### Contraindications/cautions

- Colfosceril is used as an emergency drug in acute respiratory situations; benefits outweigh any potential risks of therapy.

### Dosage

**Available Forms:** Powder for injection—108 mg

Accurate birth weight is necessary for determing correct dosage. Colfosceril is instilled into the trachea using the endotracheal tube adapter that comes with the product.

**PROPHYLACTIC TREATMENT:** Give drug in a single 5-ml/kg intratracheal dose as soon as possible after birth. Give second (12 h) and third (24 h) doses to all infants who remain on mechanical ventilation.

**RESCUE TREATMENT:** Administer in two 5-ml/kg doses. Give first dose as soon as possible after the diagnosis of RDS is made. The second dose should be given in 12 h, if the infant remains on mechanical ventilation. Data on safety and efficacy of rescue treatment with more than two doses are not available.

### Pharmacokinetics

| Route | Onset | Duration |
|---|---|---|
| Intratracheal | Rapid | 12 h |

*Metabolism:* Lung, $T_{1/2}$: 12 h

*Excretion:* Respiratory

### Adverse effects

- CNS: **Seizures**
- CV: *Patent ductus arteriosus, intraventricular hemorrhage, hypotension*
- Respiratory: *Pneumothorax, pulmonary air leak,* ***pulmonary hemorrhage****, apnea,* pneumomediastinum, emphysema
- Hematologic: *Hyperbilirubinemia, thrombocytopenia*
- Other: *Sepsis, nonpulmonary infections*

## ■ Nursing Considerations

### Assessment

- *History:* Time of birth, history of gestation
- *Physical:* T, color; R, adventitious sounds, oximeter, endotracheal tube position and patency, chest movement; ECG, P, BP, peripheral perfusion, arterial pressure (desirable); oxygen saturation, blood gases, CBC; motor activity, facial expression, reflexes

### Implementation

- Monitor ECG and transcutaneous oxygen saturation continually during administration.

- Ensure that endotracheal tube is in the correct position, with bilateral chest movement and lung sounds.
- Arrange for staff to preview teaching videotape, available from the manufacturer, before regular use to cover all the technical aspects of administration.
- Suction the infant immediately before administration; do not suction for 2 h after administration unless clinically necessary.
- Reconstitute immediately before use with the 8 ml of diluent that comes with the product; **do not use** Bacteriostatic Water for Injection. Reconstitute using the manufacturer's directions to ensure proper mixing and dilution.
- Check reconstituted vial, it should appear as a milky liquid; if flakes or precipitates appear, attempt gentle mixing. If precipitate remains, do not use.
- Insert correct size endotracheal adapter into the endotracheal tube; attach the breathing circuit to the adapter; remove cap from the sideport of the adapter; attach syringe containing the drug into the sideport and administer correct dose.
- Instill dose slowly over 1–2 min, 30–50 ventilations, moving infant after each half dose to ensure adequate instillation into both lungs.
- Continually monitor color, lung sounds, ECG, oximeter, and blood gas readings during administration and for at least 30 min following administration.

### Drug-specific teaching points

- Parents of the critically ill infant will need a comprehensive teaching and support program, including details of drug effects.

## corticotropin

*(kor ti koe **troe'** pin)*

ACTH, adenocorticotropin, corticotrophin

*Injection:* Acthar

*Repository injection:* H.P. Achthar Gel, ACTH-80

**Pregnancy Category C**

### Drug classes

Anterior pituitary hormone
Diagnostic agent

### Therapeutic actions

Stimulates the adrenal cortex to synthesize and secrete adrenocortical hormones.

### Indications

- Diagnostic tests of adrenal function
- Therapy of some glucocorticoid-sensitive disorders
- Nonsuppurative thyroiditis
- Hypercalcemia associated with cancer
- Acute exacerbations of multiple sclerosis
- Tuberculous meningitis with subarachnoid block
- Trichinosis with neurologic or myocardial involvement
- Rheumatic, collagen, dermatologic, allergic, ophthalmologic, respiratory, hematologic, edematous, and GI diseases
- Unlabeled use: treatment of infantile spasms

### Contraindications/cautions

- Adrenocortical insufficiency or hyperfunction; infections, especially systemic fungal infections, ocular herpes simplex; scleroderma, osteoporosis; recent surgery; CHF, hypertension; allergy to pork or pork products (corticotropin is isolated from porcine pituitaries); liver disease; ulcerative colitis with impending perforation; diverticulitis; recent GI surgery; active or latent peptic ulcer; inflammatory bowel disease; diabetes mellitus; hypothyroidism; pregnancy, lactation

### Dosage

**Available Forms:** Powder for injection—25, 40 U/vial; repository injection—40, 80 U/ml

ADULT

- *Diagnostic tests:* 10–25 U dissolved in 500 ml of 5% dextrose injection infused IV over 8 h.
- *Therapy:* 20 U IM or SC qid; when indicated, gradually reduce dosage by increasing intervals between injections or decreasing the dose injected, or both.
- *Acute exacerbations of multiple sclerosis:* 80–120 U/d IM for 2–3 wk.

- *Repository injection:* 40–80 U IM or SC q24–72h.

*PEDIATRIC:* Use only if necessary, and only intermittently and with careful observation. Prolonged use will inhibit skeletal growth.

- *Infantile spasms:* 20–40 U/d or 80 U every other day IM for 3 mo or 1 mo after cessation of seizures.

### Pharmacokinetics

| *Route* | *Onset* | *Peak* | *Duration* |
|---|---|---|---|
| IM/IV | Rapid | 1 h | 2–4 h |

*Metabolism:* $T_{1/2}$: 15 min
*Distribution:* Does not cross placenta; may enter breast milk

### IV facts

**Preparation:** Reconstitute powder by dissolving in Sterile Water for Injection or Sodium Chloride Injection. Refrigerate reconstituted solution. Stable for 24 h.
**Infusion:** 10–25 U dissolved in 500 ml of 5% Dextrose Injection infused over 8 h.

### Adverse effects

- CNS: Convulsions, vertigo, *headaches*, pseudotumor cerebri, *euphoria, insomnia, mood swings, depression*, psychosis, intracerebral hemorrhage, reversible cerebral atrophy in infants, cataracts, increased intraocular pressure, glaucoma
- GI: Peptic or esophageal ulcer, pancreatitis, abdominal distention
- CV: *Hypertension*, CHF, necrotizing angiitis
- Hematologic: *Fluid and electrolyte disturbances*, negative nitrogen balance
- GU: *Amenorrhea, irregular menses*
- MS: *Muscle weakness*, steroid myopathy, loss of muscle mass, osteoporosis, spontaneous fractures
- Endocrine: Growth retardation, decreased carbohydrate tolerance, diabetes mellitus, cushingoid state, *secondary adrenocortical and pituitary unresponsiveness*
- Hypersensitivity: **Anaphylactoid** or hypersensitivity reactions
- Other: *Impaired wound healing, petechiae, ecchymoses, increased sweating, thin and fragile skin, acne, immunosuppression and masking of signs of infection,* activation of latent infections, including tuberculosis, fungal, and viral eye infections, pneumonia, abscess, septic infection, GI and GU infections

### Clinically important drug-drug interactions

• Decreased effects with barbiturates • Decreased effects of anticholinesterases with corticotropin; profound muscular depression is possible

### Drug-lab test interferences

• Suppression of skin test reactions

## ■ Nursing Considerations

### Assessment

- *History:* Adrenocortical insufficiency or hyperfunction; infections, ocular herpes simplex; scleroderma, osteoporosis; recent surgery; CHF, hypertension; allergy to pork or pork products; liver disease: cirrhosis; ulcerative colitis; diverticulitis; active or latent peptic ulcer; inflammatory bowel disease, lactation; diabetes mellitus; hypothyroidism
- *Physical:* Weight, T; skin color, integrity; reflexes, bilateral grip strength, ophthalmologic exam, affect, orientation; P, BP, auscultation, peripheral perfusion, status of veins; R, adventitious sounds, chest x-ray; upper GI x-ray (peptic ulcer symptoms), liver palpation; CBC, serum electrolytes, 2-h postprandial blood glucose, thyroid function tests, urinalysis

### Implementation

- Verify adrenal responsiveness (increased urinary and plasma corticosteroid levels) to corticotropin before therapy, use the administrative route proposed for treatment.
- Administer corticotropin repository injection only by IM or SC injection.
- Administer IV injections only for diagnostic purposes or to treat thrombocytopenic purpura.
- Prepare solutions for IM and SC injections: Reconstitute powder by dissolving in Sterile Water for Injection or Sodium

Chloride Injection so that the individual dose will be contained in 1–2 ml of solution. Refrigerate reconstituted solutions, and use within 24 h.

- Use minimal doses for minimal duration to minimize adverse effects.
- Taper doses when discontinuing high-dose or long-term therapy.
- Administer a rapidly acting corticosteroid before, during, and after stress when patients are on long-term therapy.
- Do not give patients receiving corticotropins live virus vaccines.

### Drug-specific teaching points

- Avoid immunizations with live vaccines.
- Diabetics may require an increased dosage of insulin or oral hypoglycemic drug; consult your health care provider.
- Take antacids between meals to reduce "heartburn."
- Avoid exposure to people and contagious diseases. This drug masks signs of infection and decreases resistance to infection; wash hands carefully after touching contaminated surfaces.
- Report unusual weight gain, swelling of lower extremities, muscle weakness, abdominal pain, seizures, headache, fever, prolonged sore throat, cold or other infection, worsening of symptoms for which drug is being taken.

## cortisone acetate

***(kor' ti sone)***

Cortone Acetate

**Pregnancy Category C**

### Drug classes

Adrenal cortical hormone
Corticosteroid, short acting
Hormone

### Therapeutic actions

Enters target cells where it has anti-inflammatory and immunosuppressive (glucocorticoid) and salt-retaining (mineralocorticoid) effects.

### Indications

- Replacement therapy in adrenal cortical insufficiency
- Hypercalcemia associated with cancer
- Short-term management of various inflammatory and allergic disorders: rheumatoid arthritis, collagen diseases (SLE), dermatologic diseases (pemphigus), status asthmaticus, and autoimmune disorders
- Hematologic disorders: thrombocytopenic purpura, erythroblastopenia
- Trichinosis with neurologic or myocardial involvement
- Ulcerative colitis, acute exacerbations of multiple sclerosis, and palliation in some leukemias and lymphomas

### Contraindications/cautions

- Contraindications: infections, especially tuberculosis, fungal infections, amebiasis, vaccinia and varicella, and antibiotic-resistant infections, pregnancy, lactation.
- Use cautiously with renal or hepatic disease; hypothyroidism, ulcerative colitis with impending perforation; diverticulitis; active or latent peptic ulcer; inflammatory bowel disease; CHF, hypertension, thromboembolic disorders; osteoporosis; convulsive disorders; diabetes mellitus.

### Dosage

Available Forms: Tablets—5, 10, 25 mg; injection—50 mg/ml

**Physiologic replacement:** 0.5–0.75 mg/kg per day PO or 25 mg/m$^2$ per day PO divided into equal doses q8h; 0.25–0.35 mg/kg per day or 12–15 mg/m$^2$ per day IM.

ADULT: Individualize dosage based on severity and response. In long-term therapy, alternate-day therapy should be considered. After long-term therapy, withdraw drug slowly to avoid adrenal insufficiency.

- *Initial:* 25–300 mg/d PO; 20–330 mg/d IM.
- *Maintenance:* Reduce dose in small increments at intervals until the lowest dose that maintains satisfactory clinical response is reached.

PEDIATRIC: Individualize dosage on the basis of severity and response, rather than by adherence to formulas that correct adult doses for age or weight. Carefully observe growth and development in infants and children on prolonged therapy.

### Pharmacokinetics

| *Route* | *Onset* | *Peak* | *Duration* |
|---|---|---|---|
| Oral | Rapid | 2 h | 1–1.5 d |
| IM | Slow | 20–40 h | 1–1.5 d |

*Metabolism:* Hepatic, $T_{1/2}$: 30 min
*Distribution:* Crosses placenta; enters breast milk
*Excretion:* Urine

### Adverse effects

- CNS: Convulsions, *vertigo, headaches,* pseudotumor cerebri, *euphoria, insomnia, mood swings, depression,* psychosis, **intracerebral hemorrhage**, reversible cerebral atrophy in infants, cataracts, increased intraocular pressure, glaucoma
- GI: Peptic or esophageal ulcer, pancreatitis, abdominal distention
- CV: *Hypertension,* CHF, necrotizing angiitis
- Hematologic: *Fluid and electrolyte disturbances*, negative nitrogen balance, increased blood sugar, glycosuria, increased serum cholesterol, decreased serum $T_3$ and $T_4$ levels
- GU: *Amenorrhea, irregular menses*
- MS: *Muscle weakness*, steroid myopathy, loss of muscle mass, osteoporosis, spontaneous fractures
- Endocrine: Growth retardation, decreased carbohydrate tolerance, diabetes mellitus, cushingoid state, *secondary adrenocortical and pituitary unresponsiveness*
- Hypersensitivity: Anaphylactoid or hypersensitivity reactions
- Other: *Impaired wound healing, petechiae, ecchymoses, increased sweating, thin and fragile skin, acne, immunosuppression and masking of signs of infection,* activation of latent infections including tuberculosis, fungal and viral eye infections, pneumonia, abscess, septic infection, GI and GU infections

### Clinically important drug-drug interactions

• Increased therapeutic and toxic effects of cortisone if taken concurrently with troleandomycin • Decreased effects of anticholinesterases if taken concurrently with corticotropin; profound muscular depression is possible • Decreased steroid blood levels if taken concurrently with phenytoin, phenobarbital, rifampin • Decreased serum levels of salicylates if taken concurrently with cortisone.

### Drug-lab test interferences

• False-negative nitroblue-tetrazolium test for bacterial infection • Suppression of skin test reactions

## ■ Nursing Considerations

### Assessment

- ***History:*** Infections, hypothyroidism, ulcerative colitis; diverticulitis; active or latent peptic ulcer; inflammatory bowel disease; CHF, hypertension, thromboembolic disorders; osteoporosis; convulsive disorders; diabetes mellitus, lactation
- ***Physical:*** Baseline body weight, T; reflexes, and grip strength, affect, and orientation; P, BP, peripheral perfusion, prominence of superficial veins; R and adventitious sounds; serum electrolytes, blood glucose

### Implementation

- Give daily doses before 9 AM to mimic peak corticosteroid blood levels.
- Increase dosage when patient is subject to stress.
- Taper doses when discontinuing high-dose or long-term therapy.
- Do not give live virus vaccines with immunosuppressive doses of corticosteroids.

### Drug-specific teaching points

- Do not to stop taking the drug (oral) without consulting health care provider.
- Avoid exposure to infection.
- Report unusual weight gain, swelling of the extremities, muscle weakness, black or tarry stools, fever, prolonged sore throat, colds or other infections, worsening of this disorder.

## cosyntropin

*(koe sin **troe'** pin)*

Cortrosyn, Synacthen Depot (CAN)

**Pregnancy Category C**

### Drug classes
Diagnostic agent

### Therapeutic actions
Stimulates the adrenal cortex to synthesize and secrete adrenocortical hormones.

### Indications
- Diagnostic tests of adrenal function

### Contraindications/cautions
- Adrenocortical insufficiency or hyperfunction; infections, especially systemic fungal infections, ocular herpes simplex; scleroderma, osteoporosis; recent surgery; CHF, hypertension; liver disease; ulcerative colitis with impending perforation; diverticulitis; recent GI surgery; active or latent peptic ulcer; inflammatory bowel disease; diabetes mellitus; hypothyroidism; pregnancy, lactation.

### Dosage
**Available Forms:** Injection—0.25 mg

*ADULT:* 0.25–0.075 mg IM or IV; 0.25 mg IM is suggested starting point.

*PEDIATRIC < 2 Y:* 0.125 mg IM or IV.

### Pharmacokinetics

| *Route* | *Onset* | *Peak* | *Duration* |
|---|---|---|---|
| IM/IV | Rapid | 1 h | 2–4 h |

*Metabolism:* $T_{1/2}$: 15 min

*Distribution:* Does not cross placenta; may enter breast milk

### IV facts
**Preparation:** Add 0.25 mg to dextrose or saline solution.

**Infusion:** Infuse at a rate of 0.04 mg/h over 4–8 h.

### Adverse effects
- CNS: **Convulsions**, vertigo, *headaches*, pseudotumor cerebri, *euphoria, insomnia, mood swings, depression,* psychosis, intracerebral hemorrhage, reversible cerebral atrophy in infants
- GI: Peptic or esophageal ulcer, pancreatitis, abdominal distention
- CV: *Hypertension,* CHF, necrotizing angiitis
- Hematologic: *Fluid and electrolyte disturbances*, negative nitrogen balance
- GU: *Amenorrhea, irregular menses*
- MS: *Muscle weakness*, steroid myopathy, loss of muscle mass, osteoporosis, spontaneous fractures
- Endocrine: *Secondary adrenocortical and pituitary unresponsiveness*
- Hypersensitivity: **Anaphylactoid** or hypersensitivity reactions
- Other: *Impaired wound healing, petechiae, ecchymoses, increased sweating, thin and fragile skin, acne, immunosuppression and masking of signs of infection,* activation of latent infections including tuberculosis, fungal and viral eye infections, pneumonia, abscess, septic infection, GI and GU infections

### Clinically important drug-drug interactions
• Decreased effects with barbiturates • Decreased effects of anticholinesterases with corticotropin; profound muscular depression is possible

### Drug-lab test interferences
• Suppression of skin test reactions

## ■ Nursing Considerations

### Assessment
- *History:* Adrenocortical insufficiency or hyperfunction; infections; scleroderma, osteoporosis; recent surgery; CHF, hypertension; liver disease; ulcerative colitis; diverticulitis; active or latent peptic ulcer; inflammatory bowel disease; lactation; diabetes mellitus; hypothyroidism
- *Physical:* Weight, T; skin color, integrity; reflexes, bilateral grip strength, ophthalmologic exam, affect, orientation; P, BP, auscultation, peripheral perfusion, status of veins; R, adventitious sounds, chest x-ray; upper GI x-ray (peptic ulcer symptoms), liver palpation; CBC, serum elec-

trolytes, 2-h postprandial blood glucose, thyroid function tests, urinalysis

### Implementation

- Verify adrenal responsiveness (increase in urinary and plasma corticosteroid levels) to corticotropin before therapy, using the administrative route proposed for treatment.
- Prepare solutions for IM injections by dissolving suggested dose in Sterile Saline.
- Do not give patients live virus vaccines.

### Drug-specific teaching points

- Diabetics may require an increased dosage of insulin or oral hypoglycemic drug; your health care provider will give you details.
- Know that this drug may mask signs of infection and decrease your resistance to infection; wash your hands carefully after touching contaminated surfaces. Avoid exposure to people and contagious diseases.
- Report unusual weight gain, swelling of lower extremities, muscle weakness, abdominal pain, seizures, headache, fever, prolonged sore throat, cold or other infection, pain at injection site.

## cromolyn sodium

*(kroe' moe lin)*

disodium cromoglycate, cromoglicic acid, cromoglycic acid

Gastrocrom

*Respiratory inhalant, nasal solution, ophthalmic solution:*
Intal, Nasalcrom, Opticrom 4%, Rynacrom (CAN)

**Pregnancy Category B**

### Drug classes

Antiasthmatic drug (prophylactic)
Antiallergic agent

### Therapeutic actions

Inhibits the allergen-triggered release of histamine and slow-releasing substance of anaphylaxis, leukotriene, from mast cells; decreases the overall allergic response.

### Indications

- **Respiratory inhalant:** Prophylaxis of severe bronchial asthma; prevention of exercise-induced bronchospasm
- **Nasal preparations:** Prevention and treatment of allergic rhinitis
- **Ophthalmic solution:** Treatment of allergic disorders (vernal keratoconjunctivitis and conjunctivitis, giant papillary conjunctivitis, vernal keratitis, allergic keratoconjunctivitis)
- **Oral use:** orphan drug use—mastocytosis
- **Unlabeled uses**: prevention of GI and systemic reactions to food allergies; treatment of eczema, dermatitis, ulcerations, urticaria pigmentosa, chronic urticaria, hay fever, postexercise bronchospasm

### Contraindications/cautions

- Allergy to cromolyn, pregnancy, lactation.
- Respiratory inhalant and nasal products: Impaired renal or hepatic function.

### Dosage

Available Forms: Nebulizer solution—20 mg/amp; aerosol spray—800 μg/actuation; nasal solution—5.2 mg/actuation; capsules—100 mg; ophthalmic solution—4%

***Respiratory Inhalant Product Used in Spinhaler:***

- *Adult and Children > 5 Y:* Initially 20 mg (contents of 1 capsule) inhaled qid at regular intervals.
- *Children < 5 Y:* Safety and efficacy not established; use of capsule product not recommended.

***Nebulizer Solution for Oral Inhalation:***

- *Adults and children > 2 y:* Initially 20 mg qid at regular intervals, administered from a power-operated nebulizer with an adequate flow rate and equipped with a suitable face mask; do not use a hand-operated nebulizer.
- *Children <2 Y:* Safety and efficacy not established.
- *Children < 2 Y: Prevention of exercise-induced bronchospasm:* Inhale 20 mg no more than 1 h before anticipated exercise; during prolonged exercise, repeat as needed for protection.

***Nasal Solution Used With Nasalmatic Metered-Spray Device:***

- *ADULTS AND CHILDREN > 6 Y:* 1 spray in each nostril three to six times per day at regular intervals.
- *CHILDREN < 6 Y:* Safety and efficacy not established.
- *Seasonal (pollenotic) rhinitis and prevention of rhinitis caused by exposure to other specific inhalant allergens:* Begin use before exposure, and continue during exposure.

***Ophthalmic solution:***

- *ADULTS AND CHILDREN > 4 Y:* 1–2 drops in each eye from four to six times per day at regular intervals.
- *CHILDREN < 4 Y:* Safety and efficacy not established.

***Oral:***

- *ADULTS:* 2 capsules qid PO, 1/2 h before meals and at hs.
- *PEDIATRIC*
- *Premature to term infants:* Not recommended.
- *Term to 2 y:* 20 mg/kg PO per day in four divided doses.
- *2–12 y:* One capsule PO qid 1/2 h before meals and at hs. Dosage may be increased if satisfactory results are seen within 2–3 wk. Do not exceed 40 mg/kg per day (30 mg/kg per day in children 6 mo–2 y).

## Pharmacokinetics

| *Route* | *Onset* | *Peak* | *Duration* |
|---|---|---|---|
| All | 1 wk | 15 min | 6–8 h |

*Metabolism:* Hepatic, $T_{1/2}$: 80 min
*Distribution:* Crosses placenta; may enter breast milk
*Excretion:* Urine and bile; respiratory (inhalation)

## Adverse effects

*Respiratory Inhalant Product*

- CNS: *Dizziness, headache,* lacrimation
- GI: *Nausea, dry and irritated throat,* swollen parotid glands
- GU: Dysuria, frequency
- Dermatologic: Urticaria, rash, angioedema, joint swelling and pain

*Nebulizer Solution*

- GI: Abdominal pain
- Respiratory: *Cough, nasal congestion, wheezing, sneezing,* nasal itching, epistaxis, nose burning

*Nasal Solution*

- CNS: *Headaches*
- GI: Bad taste in mouth
- Respiratory: *Sneezing, nasal stinging or burning, nasal irritation,* epistaxis, postnasal drip
- Dermatologic: Rash

*Ophthalmic Solution*

- Local: *Transient ocular stinging or burning on instillation*

*Oral*

- CNS: *Dizziness, fatigue, paresthesia, headache,* migraine, psychosis, anxiety, depression, insomnia, behavior change, hallucinations, lethargy
- GI: *Taste perversion, diarrhea,* esophagospasm, flatulence, dysphagia, hepatic function tests abnormality, burning in the mouth and throat
- Dermatologic: *Flushing,* urticaria, angioedema, skin erythema and burning

## ■ Nursing Considerations

### Assessment

- *History:* Allergy to cromolyn, impaired renal or hepatic function, lactation
- *Physical:* Skin color, lesions; palpation of parotid glands; joint size, overlying color and T; orientation; R, auscultation, patency of nasal passages (with respiratory inhalant and nasal products); liver evaluation; normal output; renal and liver function tests, urinalysis

### Implementation

*Respiratory Inhalant Products*

- Do not use during acute asthma attack; begin therapy when acute episode is over and patient can inhale.
- Arrange for continuation of treatment with bronchdilators and corticosteroids during initial cromolyn therapy, tapering

corticosteroids or reinstituting them based on patient stress.

- Use caution if cough or bronchospasm occurs after inhalation; this may (rarely) preclude continuation of treatment.
- Discontinue therapy if eosinophilic pneumonia occurs.
- Taper cromolyn if withdrawal is desired.
- Mix cromolyn solution only with compatible solutions: compatible with metaproterenol sulfate, isoproterenol HCl, 0.25% isoetharine HCl, epinephrine HCl, terbutaline sulfate, and 20% acetylcysteine solution for at least 1 h after their admixture.
- Store nebulizer solution below 30°C; protect from light.

*Nasal Solution*

- Have patient clear nasal passages before use.
- Have patient inhale through nose during administration.
- Observable response to treatment may require 2–4 wk (perennial allergic rhinitis); continued use of antihistamines and nasal decongestants may be necessary.
- Replace Nasalmatic pump device every 6 mo.

*Ophthalmic Solution*

- Instruct patients not to wear soft contact lenses.
- Although symptomatic response is usually evident within a few days, up to 6 wk of treatment may be needed.

*All*

- Give corticosteroids as needed.
- Carefully teach patients how to use the specialized Spinhaler, Nasalmatic, or power nebulizer devices.

*Oral*

- Give drug 1/2 h before meals and at hs.
- Prepare solution for patients who cannot take capsules: open capsule, and pour contents into half glass of hot water; stir until completely dissolved; add equal quantity of cold water. Do not mix with fruit juice, milk, or foods. Drink all of the liquid.
- Do not give oral capsules for inhalation.

### Drug-specific teaching points

- Take drug at regular intervals. When drug is used to prevent sprecific allergen exposure reactions or to prevent exercise-induced bronchospasm, instruct patient about the best time to take drug.
- Take drug as follows: *Respiratory inhalant and nasal solution:* See manufacturer's insert; do not swallow capsule used in *Spinhaler*. *Ophthalmic solution:* Lie down or tilt head back, and look at ceiling; drop solution inside lower eyelid while looking up. After instilling eye drops, close eyes; apply gentle pressure to inside corner of eye for 1 min.
- Do not discontinue abruptly except on advice of your health care provider (respiratory inhalant and nasal products).
- Do not wear soft contact lenses while using cromolyn eye drops.
- Be aware that you may experience transient stinging or burning in your eyes on instillation of the eye drops.
- The following side effects may occur (oral): dizziness, drowsiness, fatigue. If this occurs, avoid driving or operating dangerous machinery.
- Report coughing, wheezing (respiratory products); change in vision (ophthalmic products); swelling, difficulty swallowing, depression (oral product).

## cyanocobalamin, nasal

***(sigh' an oh coh ball' a meen)***

Nascobal

**Pregnancy Category C**

### Drug classes

Vitamin

### Therapeutic actions

Intranasal gel that allows absorption of vitamin $B_{12}$, which is essential to cell growth and reproduction, hematopoiesis, and nucleoprotein and myelin synthesis, and has been associated with fat and carbohydrate metabolism and protein synthesis.

### Indications

- Maintenance of patients in hematologic remission after IM vitamin $B_{12}$ therapy for pernicious anemia, inadequate secretion of intrinsic factor, dietary deficiency, malabsorption, competition by intestinal bacteria or parasites, or inadequate utilization of vitamin $B_{12}$

**Contraindications/cautions**

- Use cautiously with pregnancy or lactation, Leber's disease, nasal lesions, or upper respiratory infections.

## Dosage

**Available Forms:** Intranasal gel—500 $\mu$g/0.1 ml

*ADULT:* One spray (500 $\mu$g) in one nostril, once/wk.

*PEDIATRIC:* Safety and efficacy not established.

**Pharmacokinetics**

| *Route* | *Onset* | *Peak* |
|---|---|---|
| Nasal | Slow | 1–2 h |

*Metabolism:* $T_{1/2}$: unknown
*Distribution:* May cross placenta, may enter breast milk
*Excretion:* Urine

**Adverse effects**

- CNS: *Headache*
- Hematologic: Bone marrow suppression
- Local: *Rhinitis, nasal congestion*
- Other: Fever, pain, local irritation

**Clinically important drug-drug interactions**

- Decreased effectiveness may be seen with antibiotics, methotrexate, pyrimethamine

## ■ Nursing Considerations

### Assessment

- *History:* Pregnancy or lactation, Leber's disease, nasal lesions or upper respiratory infections; history of pernicious anemia, vitamin $B_{12}$ deficiency, dates of IM cyanocobalamin therapy
- *Physical:* State of nasal mucous membranes; serum vitamin $B_{12}$ levels, CBC, potassium level

### Implementation

- Confirm diagnosis before administering; ensure that patient is hemodynamically stable after IM therapy.
- Teach patient proper technique for administering nasal gel.
- Monitor serum vitamin $B_{12}$ levels before starting, 1 mo after starting, and every 3–6 mo during therapy.
- Do not administer if nasal congesion, rhinitis, or upper respiratory infection is present.
- Evaluate patient response and consider need for folate or iron replacement.

### Drug-specific teaching points

- Learn the proper technique for administering nasal gel. Mark calendar with date for weekly dose.
- Periodic blood tests will be needed to monitor your response to this drug.
- Do not administer if you have nasal congestion, rhinitis, or upper respiratory infection; consult with your health care provider.
- The following side effects may occur: headache (analgesics may help), nausea (take small, frequent meals).
- Report nasal pain, nasal sores, fatigue, weakness, easy bruising.

# cyclizine hydrochloride

*(sye' kli zeen)*

Marezine

**Pregnancy Category B**

**Drug classes**

Antiemetic
Anti-motion sickness agent
Antihistamine
Anticholinergic

**Therapeutic actions**

Reduces sensitivity of the labyrinthine apparatus; peripheral anticholinergic effects may contribute to efficacy.

**Indications**

- Prevention and treatment of nausea, vomiting, motion sickness

### Contraindications/cautions

- Contraindication: allergy to cyclizine.
- Use cautiously with pregnancy, lactation, narrow-angle glaucoma, stenosing peptic ulcer, symptomatic prostatic hypertrophy, bronchial asthma, bladder neck obstruction, pyloroduodenal obstruction, cardiac arrhythmias; postoperative patients (hypotensive effects may be confusing and dangerous).

### Dosage

**Available Forms:** Tablets—50 mg

*ADULT:* 50 mg PO 1/2 h before exposure to motion; repeat q4–6h. Do not exceed 200 mg in 24 h.

*PEDIATRIC (6–12 Y):* 25 mg PO up to three times a day.

*GERIATRIC:* More likely to cause dizziness, sedation, syncope, toxic confusional states, and hypotension in elderly patients; use with caution.

### Pharmacokinetics

| *Route* | *Onset* | *Peak* | *Duration* |
|---|---|---|---|
| Oral | 30–60 min | 1–1 1/2 h | 4–6 h |

*Metabolism:* Hepatic, $T_{1/2}$: 2–3 h

*Distribution:* Crosses placenta; enters breast milk

*Excretion:* Unknown

### Adverse effects

- CNS: *Drowsiness, confusion,* euphoria, nervousness, restlessness, insomnia and excitement, convulsions, vertigo, tinnitus, blurred vision, diplopia, auditory and visual hallucinations
- GI: *Dry mouth, anorexia, nausea*, vomiting, diarrhea or constipation, cholestatic jaundice
- CV: Hypotension, palpitations, tachycardia
- **Respiratory:** Respiratory depression, death, dry nose and throat
- GU: *Urinary frequency, difficult urination*, urinary retention
- Dermatologic: Urticaria, drug rash

### Clinically important drug-drug interactions

- Increased depressant effects with alcohol, other CNS depressants

## ■ Nursing Considerations

### Assessment

- *History:* Allergy to cyclizine, narrow-angle glaucoma, stenosing peptic ulcer, symptomatic prostatic hypertrophy, bronchial asthma, bladder neck obstruction, pyloroduodenal obstruction, cardiac arrhythmias, recent surgery, lactation
- *Physical:* Skin color, lesions, texture; orientation, reflexes, affect; vision exam; P, BP; R, adventitious sounds; bowel sounds; prostate palpation; CBC

### Implementation

Monitor elderly patients carefully for adverse effects.

### Drug-specific teaching points

- Take drug as prescribed; avoid excessive dosage.
- Use before motion sickness occurs; antimotion sickness drugs work best if used prophylactically.
- The following side effects may occur: dizziness, sedation, drowsiness (use caution driving or performing tasks that require alertness); epigastric distress, diarrhea or constipation (take drug with food); dry mouth (use frequent mouth care, suck sugarless lozenges); thickening of bronchial secretions, dryness of nasal mucosa (consider another type of motion sickness remedy).
- Avoid alcohol; serious sedation could occur.
- Report difficulty breathing, hallucinations, tremors, loss of coordination, unusual bleeding or bruising, visual disturbances, irregular heartbeat.

## cyclobenzaprine hydrochloride

*(sye kloe **ben'** za preen)*

Flexeril

**Pregnancy Category B**

### Drug classes

Skeletal muscle relaxant, centrally acting

**Therapeutic actions**
Precise mechanism not known; does not directly relax tense skeletal muscles but appears to act mainly at brain stem levels or in the spinal cord.

**Indications**
- Relief of discomfort associated with acute, painful musculoskeletal conditions, as adjunct to rest, physical therapy
- Unlabeled use: adjunct in the management of fibrositis syndrome

**Contraindications/cautions**
- Contraindications: hypersensitivity to cyclobenzaprine, acute recovery phase of MI, arrhythmias, heart block or conduction disturbances, CHF, hyperthyroidism.
- Use cautiously with urinary retention, angle-closure glaucoma, increased intraocular pressure, lactation.

**Dosage**
**Available Forms:** Tablets—10 mg
*ADULT:* 10 mg PO tid (range 20–40 mg/d in divided doses); do not exceed 60 mg/d; do not use longer than 2 or 3 wk.
*PEDIATRIC:* Safety and efficacy in children < 15 y not established.

**Pharmacokinetics**

| *Route* | *Onset* | *Peak* | *Duration* |
|---|---|---|---|
| Oral | 1 h | 4–6 h | 12–24 h |

*Metabolism:* Hepatic, $T_{1/2}$: 1–3 d
*Distribution:* Crosses placenta; may enter breast milk
*Excretion:* Urine

**Adverse effects**
- CNS: *Drowsiness, dizziness,* fatigue, tiredness, asthenia, blurred vision, headache, nervousness, confusion
- GI: *Dry mouth*, nausea, constipation, dyspepsia, unpleasant taste, liver toxicity

**Clinically important drug-drug interactions**
- Additive CNS effects with alcohol, barbiturates, other CNS depressants

■ **Nursing Considerations**

**Assessment**
- ***History:*** Hypersensitivity to cyclobenzaprine, acute recovery phase of MI, arrhythmias, CHF, hyperthyroidism, urinary retention, angle-closure glaucoma, increased intraocular pressure, lactation
- ***Physical:*** Orientation, affect, ophthalmic exam (tonometry); bowel sounds, normal GI output; prostate palpation, normal voiding pattern; thyroid function tests

**Implementation**
- Arrange for analgesics if headache occurs (possible adjunct for relief of muscle spasm).

**Drug-specific teaching points**
- Take this drug exactly as prescribed. Do not take a higher dosage.
- Avoid alcohol, sleep-inducing, or OTC drugs; these may cause dangerous effects.
- The following side effects may occur: drowsiness, dizziness, blurred vision (avoid driving or engaging in activities that require alertness); dyspepsia (take drug with food, eat frequent small meals); dry mouth (suck sugarless lozenges or ice chips).
- Report urinary retention or difficulty voiding, pale stools, yellow skin or eyes.

## cyclophosphamide

***(sye kloe foss' fa mide)***
Cytoxan, Neosar, Procytox (CAN)
**Pregnancy Category D**

**Drug classes**
Alkylating agent
Nitrogen mustard
Antineoplastic

**Therapeutic actions**
Cytotoxic: interferes with the replication of susceptible cells. Immunosuppressive: lymphocytes are especially sensitive to drug effects.

### Indications

- Treatment of malignant lymphomas, multiple myeloma, leukemias, mycosis fungoides, neuroblastoma, adenocarcinoma of the ovary, retinoblastoma, carcinoma of the breast; used concurrently or sequentially with other antineoplastic drugs
- Unlabeled uses: severe rheumatologic conditions, Wegener's granulomatosis, steroid-resistant vasculidites, SLE

### Contraindications/cautions

- Contraindications: allergy to cyclophosphamide, allergy to tartrazine (in tablets marketed as Cytoxan), pregnancy, lactation.
- Use cautiously with radiation therapy; chemotherapy; tumor cell infiltration of the bone marrow; adrenalectomy with steroid therapy; infections, especially varicella-zoster; hematopoietic depression, impaired hepatic or renal function.

### Dosage

**Available Forms:** Tablets—25, 50 mg; powder for injection—75 mg mannitol/100 mg cyclophosphamide, 82 mg sodium bicarbonate/100 mg cyclophosphamide

Individualize dosage based on hematologic profile and response.

**ADULT**

- *Induction therapy:* 40–50 mg/kg IV given in divided doses over 2–5 d or 1–5 mg/kg per day PO.
- *Maintenance therapy:* 1–5 mg/kg per day PO, 10–15 mg/kg IV every 7–10 d, or 3–5 mg/kg IV twice weekly.

*Hepatic dysfunction:* Bilirubin of 3.1–5.0 mg% or SGOT > 180: reduce dose by 25%. Bilirubin > 5 mg%: omit dose.

*Renal dysfunction:* Glomerular filtration rate < 10 ml/min: decrease dose by 50%.

### Pharmacokinetics

| Route | Onset | Peak |
|---|---|---|
| Oral | Varies | 1 h |
| IV | Rapid | 15–30 min |

*Metabolism:* Hepatic, $T_{1/2}$: 3–12 h

*Distribution:* Crosses placenta; enters breast milk

*Excretion:* Urine

### IV facts

**Preparation:** Add Sterile Water for Injection or Bacteriostatic Water for Injection to the vial, and shake gently. Use 5 ml for 100-mg vial, 10 ml for 200-mg vial, 25 ml for 500-mg vial, 50 ml for 1-g vial. Prepared solutions may be injected IV, IM, intraperitoneally, intrapleurally. Use within 24 h if stored at room temperature or within 6 d if refrigerated.

**Infusion:** Infuse in 5% Dextrose Injection, 5% Dextrose and 0.9% Sodium Chloride Injection; each 100 mg infused over 15 min.

### Adverse effects

- GI: *Anorexia, nausea, vomiting, diarrhea*, stomatitis
- CV: Cardiotoxicity
- Respiratory: Interstitial pulmonary fibrosis
- Hematologic: *Leukopenia*, thrombocytopenia, anemia (rare), increased serum uric acid levels
- GU: *Hemorrhagic cystitis*, bladder fibrosis, hematuria to potentially fatal **hemorrhagic cystitis**, increased urine uric acid levels, gonadal suppression
- Dermatologic: *Alopecia*, darkening of skin and fingernails
- Other: SIADH, immunosuppression secondary neoplasia

### Clinically important drug-drug interactions

• Prolonged apnea with succinylcholine: metabolism is inhibited by cyclophosphamide • Decreased serum levels and therapeutic acitivity of digoxin

## ■ Nursing Considerations

### Assessment

- *History:* Allergy to cyclophosphamide, allergy to tartrazine, radiation therapy, chemotherapy, tumor cell infiltration of

the bone marrow, adrenalectomy with steroid therapy, infections, hematopoietic depression, impaired hepatic or renal function, pregnancy, lactation
- *Physical:* T; weight; skin color, lesions; hair; P, auscultation, baseline ECG; R, adventitious sounds; mucous membranes, liver evaluation; CBC, differential; urinalysis; liver and renal function tests

### Implementation
- Arrange for blood tests to evaluate hematopoietic function before therapy and weekly during therapy.
- Do not give full dosage within 4 wk after a full course of radiation therapy or chemotherapy due to the risk of severe bone marrow depression; reduced dosage may be needed.
- Arrange for reduced dosage in patients with impaired renal or hepatic function.
- Ensure that patient is well hydrated before treatment to decrease risk of cystitis.
- Prepare oral solution by dissolving injectable cyclophosphamide in aromatic elixir. Refrigerate and use within 14 d.
- Give tablets on an empty stomach. If severe GI upset occurs, tablet may be given with food.
- Counsel male patients not to father a child during or immediately after therapy; infant cardiac and limb abnormalities have occurred.

### Drug-specific teaching points
- Take drug on an empty stomach. If severe GI upset occurs, the tablet may be taken with food.
- The following side effects may occur: nausea, vomiting, loss of appetite (take drug with food, eat small frequent meals); darkening of the skin and fingernails; loss of hair (obtain a wig or other head covering prior to hair loss; head must be covered in extremes of temperature).
- Try to maintain your fluid intake and nutrition (drink at least 10–12 glassses of fluid each day).
- Use birth control during drug use and for a time thereafter (male and female); this drug can cause severe birth defects.
- Report unusual bleeding or bruising, fever, chills, sore throat, cough, shortness of breath, blood in the urine, painful urination, rapid heart beat, swelling of the feet or hands, stomach or flank pain.

C

## cycloserine

*(sye kloe ser' een)*
Seromycin Pulvules
**Pregnancy Category C**

### Drug classes
Antituberculous drug ("third line")
Antibiotic

### Therapeutic actions
Inhibits cell wall synthesis in susceptible strains of gram-positive and gram-negative bacteria and in *Mycobacterium tuberculosis*, causing cell death.

### Indications
- Treatment of active pulmonary and extrapulmonary (including renal) tuberculosis that is not responsive to first-line antituberculous drugs in conjunction with other antituberculous drugs
- UTIs caused by susceptible bacteria

### Contraindications/cautions
- Allergy to cycloserine, epilepsy, depression, severe anxiety or psychosis, severe renal insufficiency, excessive concurrent use of alcohol, lactation.

### Dosage
**Available Forms:** Capsules—250 mg

ADULT
- *Initial dose:* 250 mg bid PO at 12-h intervals for first 2 wk; monitor serum levels (above 30 μg/ml is generally toxic).
- *Maintenance dose:* 500 mg–1 g/d PO in divided doses.

PEDIATRIC: Safety and dosage not established.

### Pharmacokinetics

| Route | Onset | Peak | Duration |
|---|---|---|---|
| Oral | Varies | 3–4 h | 48–72 h |

*Metabolism:* $T_{1/2}$: 10 h
*Distribution:* Crosses placenta; enters breast milk
*Excretion:* Urine and feces

**Adverse effects**

- CNS: *Convulsions, drowsiness, somnolence, headache, tremor, vertigo, confusion*, disorientation, loss of memory, **psychoses** (possibly with suicidal tendencies), hyperirritability, aggression, paresis, hyperreflexia, paresthesias, seizures, coma
- Hematologic: Elevated serum transaminase levels
- Dermatologic: Skin rash

## ■ Nursing Considerations

### Assessment

- *History:* Allergy to cycloserine, epilepsy, depression, severe anxiety or psychosis, severe renal insufficiency, excessive concurrent use of alcohol, lactation
- *Physical:* Skin color, lesions; orientation, reflexes, affect, EEG; liver evaluation; liver function tests

### Implementation

- Arrange for culture and sensitivity studies before use.
- Give this drug only when other therapy has failed, and only in conjunction with other antituberculosis agents when treating tuberculosis.
- Arrange for follow-up of liver and renal function tests, hematologic tests, and serum drug levels.
- Consult with physician regarding the use of anticonvulsants, sedatives, or pyridoxine if CNS effects become severe.
- Discontinue drug, and notify physician if skin rash, severe CNS reactions occur.

### Drug-specific teaching points

- Avoid excessive alcohol consumption.
- Take this drug regularly; avoid missing doses. *Do not* discontinue this drug without first consulting your physician.
- The following side effects may occur: drowsiness, tremor, disorientation (use caution operating a car or dangerous machinery); depression, personality change, numbness and tingling.
- Have regular, periodic medical checkups, that include blood tests to evaluate the drug effects.
- Report skin rash, headache, tremors, shaking, confusion, dizziness.

# cyclosporine

*(sye' kloe spor een)*
cyclosporin A
Sandimmune
**Pregnancy Category C**

**Drug classes**
Immunosuppressant

**Therapeutic actions**
Exact mechanism of immunosuppressant is not known; specifically and reversibly inhibits immunocompetent lymphocytes in the $G_0$ or $G_1$ phase of the cell cycle; inhibits T-helper and T-suppressor cells, lymphokine production, and release of interleukin-2 and T-cell growth factor.

**Indications**

- Prophylaxis for organ rejection in kidney, liver, and heart transplants in conjunction with adrenal corticosteroids
- Treatment of chronic rejection in patients previously treated with other immunosuppressive agents
- Unlabeled use: limited but successful use in other procedures, including pancreas, bone marrow, heart and lung transplants

**Contraindications/cautions**

- Contraindications: allergy to cyclosporine or polyoxyethylated castor oil (oral preparation), pregnancy, lactation.
- Use caution in the presence of impaired renal function, malabsorption.

### Dosage

**Available Forms:** Capsules—25, 50, 100 mg; oral solution—100 mg/ml; IV solution—50 mg/ml

ADULT, PEDIATRIC

- *Oral:* 15 mg/kg per day PO initially given 4–12 h prior to transplantation; continue dose postoperatively for 1–2 wk, then taper by 5%/wk to a maintainence level of 5–10 mg/kg per day.
- ***Parenteral:*** Patients unable to take oral solution preoperatively or postoperatively may be given IV infusion at one-third the oral dose (ie, 5–6 mg/kg per day given 4–12 h prior to transplantation, administered as a slow infusion over 2–6 h). Continue this daily dose postoperatively. Switch to oral drug as soon as possible.

### Pharmacokinetics

| *Route* | *Onset* | *Peak* |
|---|---|---|
| Oral | Varies | 3 1/2 h |
| IV | Rapid | 1–2 h |

*Metabolism:* Hepatic, $T_{1/2}$: 19–27 h
*Distribution:* Crosses placenta; enters breast milk
*Excretion:* Bile and urine

### IV facts

**Preparation:** Dilute IV solution immediately before use. Dilute 1 ml concentrate in 20–100 ml of 0.9% Sodium Chloride Injection or 5% Dextrose Injection. Protect from exposure to light.
**Infusion:** Give in a slow IV infusion over 2–6 h.

### Adverse effects

- CNS: *Tremor*, convulsions, headache, paresthesias
- GI: **Hepatotoxicity**, *gum hyperplasia*, *diarrhea*, nausea, vomiting
- CV: *Hypertension*
- Hematologic: Leukopenia
- GU: *Renal dysfunction*, nephrotoxicity
- Other: *Hirsuitism*, *acne*, lymphomas, infections

### Clinically important drug-drug interactions

• Increased risk of nephrotoxicity with other nephrotoxic agents (erythromycin) • Increased risk of digoxin toxicity • Risk of severe myopathy or rhabdomyolysis with lovastatin • Increased risk of toxicity if taken with diltiazem, metoclopramide, nicardipine • Increased plasma concentration of cyclosporine with ketoconazole • Decreased therapeutic effect with hydantoins, rifampin, sulfonamides

## ■ Nursing Considerations

### Assessment

- *History:* Allergy to cyclosporine or polyoxyethylated castor oil, impaired renal function, malabsorption, lactation
- *Physical:* T; skin color, lesions; BP, peripheral perfusion; liver evaluation, bowel sounds, gum evaluation; renal and liver function tests, CBC

### Implementation

- Mix oral solution with milk, chocolate milk or orange juice at room temperature. Stir well, and administer at once. Do not allow mixture to stand before drinking. Use a glass container, and rinse with more diluent to ensure that the total dose is taken.
- Use parenteral administration only if patient is unable to take the oral solution; transfer to oral solution as soon as possible.
- Do not refrigerate oral solution; store at room temperature and use within 2 mo after opening.
- Monitor renal and liver function tests prior to and during therapy; marked decreases in function may require dosage adjustment or discontinuation.
- Monitor BP; heart transplant patients may require concomitant antihypertensive therapy.

### Drug-specific teaching points

- Dilute solution with milk, chocolate milk or orange juice at room temperature; drink immediately after mixing. Rinse the glass with the solution to ensure that all the dose is taken. Store solution at room temperature. Use solution within 2 mo of opening the bottle.
- Avoid infection; avoid crowds or people who have infections. Notify your physician at once if you injure yourself.
- The following side effects may occur: nausea, vomiting (take the drug with

food); diarrhea; skin rash; mouth sores (frequent mouth care may help).
- This drug should not be taken during pregnancy. If you think that you are pregnant or you want to become pregnant, discuss this with your physician.
- Have periodic blood tests to monitor your response to drug effects.
- Do not discontinue this medication without your physician's advice.
- Report unusual bleeding or bruising, fever, sore throat, mouth sores, tiredness.

# cyproheptadine hydrochloride

*(si proe **hep'** ta deen)*

Periactin, PMS-Cyproheptadine (CAN)

**Pregnancy Category B**

## Drug classes
Antihistamine (piperidine type)

## Therapeutic actions
Blocks the effects of histamine at $H_1$ receptor sites; has atropine-like, antiserotonin, antipruritic, sedative, and appetite-stimulating effects.

## Indications
- Relief of symptoms associated with perennial and seasonal allergic rhinitis; vasomotor rhinitis; allergic conjunctivitis; mild, uncomplicated urticaria and angioedema; amelioraton of allergic reactions to blood or plasma; dermatographism; adjunctive therapy in anaphylactic reactions
- Treatment of cold urticaria
- Unlabeled uses: stimulation of appetite in underweight patients and those with anorexia nervosa; treatment of vascular cluster headaches

## Contraindications/cautions
- Contraindications: allergy to any antihistamines, third trimester of pregnancy.
- Use cautiously with narrow-angle glaucoma, stenosing peptic ulcer, symptomatic prostatic hypertrophy, asthmatic attack, bladder neck obstruction, pyloroduodenal obstruction, lactation.

## Dosage
**Available Forms:** Tablets—4 mg; syrup—2 mg/5 ml

ADULT
- ***Initial therapy***: 4 mg tid PO.
- ***Maintenance therapy***: 4–20 mg/d PO; do not exceed 0.5 mg/kg per day.

PEDIATRIC: 0.25 mg/kg per day PO or 8 $mg/m^2$.
- *7–14 y:* 4 mg PO bid or tid; do not exceed 16 mg/d.
- *2–6 y:* 2 mg PO bid or tid; do not exceed 12 mg/d.

GERIATRIC: More likely to cause dizziness, sedation, syncope, toxic confusional states, and hypotension in elderly patients; use with caution.

## Pharmacokinetics

| *Route* | *Onset* | *Peak* | *Duration* |
|---|---|---|---|
| Oral | 15–30 min | 1–2 h | 4–6 h |

*Metabolism:* Hepatic, $T_{1/2}$: 3–4 h
*Distribution:* Crosses placenta; enters breast milk
*Excretion:* Urine

## Adverse effects
- CNS: *Drowsiness, sedation, dizziness, disturbed coordination*, fatigue, confusion, restlessness, excitation, nervousness, tremor, headache, blurred vision, diplopia, vertigo, tinnitus, acute labryinthitis, hysteria, tingling, heaviness and weakness of the hands
- GI: *Epigastric distress,* anorexia, increased appetite and weight gain, nausea, vomiting, diarrhea or constipation
- CV: Hypotension, palpitations, bradycardia, tachycardia, extrasystoles
- Respiratory: *Thickening of bronchial secretions*, chest tightness, wheezing, nasal stuffiness, dry mouth, dry nose, dry throat, sore throat
- **Hematologic**: Hemolytic anemia, hypoplastic anemia, thrombocytopenia, leukopenia, agranulocytosis, pancytopenia

- GU: Urinary frequency, dysuria, urinary retention, early menses, decreased libido, impotence
- Other: Urticaria, rash, **anaphylactic shock**, photosensitivity, excessive perspiration, chills

**Clinically important drug-drug interactions**

• Subnormal pituitary-adrenal response to metyrapone • Decreased effects of fluoxetine • Increased and prolonged anticholinergic (drying) effects if taken with MAO inhibitors

## ■ Nursing Considerations

### Assessment

- *History:* Allergy to any antihistamines; narrow-angle glaucoma, stenosing peptic ulcer, symptomatic prostatic hypertrophy, asthmatic attack, bladder neck obstruction, pyloroduodenal obstruction; lactation
- *Physical:* Skin color, lesions, texture; orientation, reflexes, affect; vision exam; P, BP; R, adventitious sounds; bowel sounds; prostate palpation; CBC with differential

### Implementation

- Administer with food if GI upset occurs.
- Give syrup form if unable to take tablets.
- Monitor patient response, and adjust dosage to lowest possible effective dose.

### Drug-specific teaching points

- Take as prescribed; avoid excessive dosage.
- Take drug with food if GI upset occurs.
- The following side effects may occur: dizziness, sedation, drowsiness (use caution if driving or performing tasks that require alertness); epigastric distress, diarrhea, or constipation (take drug with meals); dry mouth (use frequent mouth care, suck sugarless lozenges); thickening of bronchial secretions, dryness of nasal mucosa (use humidifier).
- Avoid alcohol, serious sedation could occur.
- Report difficulty breathing, hallucinations, tremors, loss of coordination, unusual bleeding or bruising, visual disturbances, irregular heartbeat.

# cysteamine bitartrate

*(sis **tee'** ah meen)*

Cystagon

**Pregnancy Category C**

C

**Drug classes**

Urinary tract agent

**Therapeutic actions**

Depletes cystine in the cells of patients with cystinosis, an inherited defect of lysosomal transport by participating with the lysosomes in an interchange reaction which allows cystine byproducts to exit the lysosome.

**Indications**

- Management of adults and children with nephropathic cystinosis

**Contraindications/cautions**

- Allergy to cysteamine or penicillamine, pregnancy, lactation.

### Dosage

**Available Forms:** Capsules—50, 150 mg

Maintenance dosage should be reached over a 5–6 wk period with slow incrementation based on leukocyte cystine measurement.

*ADULT AND CHILDREN > 12 Y:* 2 g/d PO divided into 4 doses.

*PEDIATRIC < 12 Y:* 1.3 $g/m^2/d$ of free base divided into 4 doses. Do not give intact capsules to children < 6 y; open capsule and sprinkle over food.

**Pharmacokinetics**

| *Route* | *Onset* | *Peak* |
|---|---|---|
| Oral | Slow | 5–6 h |

*Metabolism:* $T_{1/2}$: unknown

*Distribution* : Crosses placenta; may pass into breast milk

*Excretion* : Urine

**Adverse effects**

- CNS: Nervousness, abnormal thinking, depression, emotional lability, hallucinations, nightmares, *headache,* ataxia, confusion, **seizures**
- GI: *Nausea, vomiting, bad breath, abdominal pain,* dyspepsia, constipation, gastroenteritis, duodenitis, duodenal ulcer

- **Hematologic:** Abnormal liver function tests, leukopenia, anemia
- **Other:** *Rash, fever*

## ■ Nursing Considerations

### Assessment

- ***History:*** Allergy to cysteamine or penicillamine, pregnancy, lactation.
- ***Physical:*** Skin color, lesions, turgor; T; mucous membranes, bowel sounds, liver evaluation; urinalysis, renal and liver function tests, CBC and differential; leukocyte cystine measurement

### Implementation

- Obtain leukocyte cystine measurements 5–6 h after first dose; at 3 wk intervals with any dosage change; every 3 mo during maintenance treatment.
- Temporarily discontinue if initial therapy is poorly tolerated due to GI symptoms or rash; drug may be reinstituted at a lower dose with gradual increases.

### Drug-specific teaching points

- Do not stop taking the medication without consulting your physician.
- Have regular blood tests during treatment.
- The following side effects may occur: GI upset, loss of appetite (transient effects), skin rash, dizziness, loss of sleep, abnormal thinking (avoid driving or performing tasks that require alertness).
- Report fever, rash, severe GI complaints, changes in gait, concentration

## cytarabine

*(sye **tare'** a been)*

cytosine arabinoside

Ara-C, Cytosar-U

**Pregnancy Category D**

### Drug classes

Antimetabolite
Antineoplastic

### Therapeutic actions

Inhibits DNA polymerase; cell cycle phase specific—S phase (stage of DNA synthesis); also blocks progression of cells from $G_1$ to S.

### Indications

- Induction and maintenance of remission in acute myelocytic leukemia (higher response rate in children than in adults)
- Treatment of acute lymphocytic leukemia in adults and children; treatment of chronic myelocytic leukemia and erythroleukemia
- Treatment of meningeal leukemia (intrathecal use)
- Treatment of non-Hodgkin's lymphoma in children (in combination therapy)

### Contraindications/cautions

- Contraindications: allergy to cytarabine, pregnancy, lactation, premature infants.
- Use cautiously with hematopoietic depression secondary to radiation or chemotherapy; impaired liver function.

### Dosage

**Available Forms:** Powder for injection—100, 500 mg, 1, 2 g

Given by IV infusion or injection or SC.

**ADULT**

- ***Acute myelocytic leukemia (AML) induction of remission:*** 200 mg/m² per day by continuous infusion for 5 d for a total dose of 1000 mg/m²; repeat every 2 wk. Individualize dosage based on hematologic response.
- ***Maintenance of AML:*** Use same dosage and schedule as induction; often a longer rest period is allowed.
- ***Acute lymphocytic leukemia (ALL):*** Dosage similar to AML.
- ***Intrathecal use for meningeal leukemia:*** 5 mg/m² to 75 mg/m² once daily for 4 d or once every 4 d. Most common dose is 30 mg/m² every 4 d until CSF is normal, followed by one more treatment.

**PEDIATRIC**

- ***Remission induction and maintenance of AML:*** Calculate dose by body weight or surface area.
- ***ALL:*** Same dosage as AML.

- ***Intrathecal use (has been used as treatment of meningeal leukemia and prophylaxis in newly diagnosed patients):*** Cytarabine, 30 mg/m$^2$; hydrocortisone sodium succinate, 15 mg/m$^2$; methotrexate, 15 mg/m$^2$.
- **Combination therapies:** For persistent leukemias—give at 2- to 4-wk intervals.
- **Combination therapy**
- ► **Cytarabine:** 100 mg/m$^2$/d by continuous IV infusion, days 1–10. **Doxorubicin:** 30 mg/m$^2$/d by IV infusion over 30 min, days 1–3.
- ► **Cytarabine** 100 mg/m$^2$/d by IV infusion over 30 min q12h, days 1–7. **Thioguanine:** 100 mg/m$^2$ PO q12h, days 1–7. **Daunorubicin:** 60 mg/m$^2$/d by IV infusion, days 5–7.
- ► **Cytarabine:** 100 mg/m$^2$/d by continuous infusion, days 1–7. **Doxorubicin:** 30 mg/m$^2$/d by IV infusion, days 1–3. **Vincristine:** 1.5 mg/m$^2$/d by IV infusion, days 1 and 5. **Prednisone:** 40 mg/m$^2$/d by IV infusion q12h, days 1–5.
- ► **Cytarabine:** 100 mg/m$^2$/d IV q12h, days 1–7. **Daunorubicin:** 70 mg/m$^2$/d by infusion, days 1–3. **Thioguanine:** 100 mg/m$^2$/d PO q12h, days 1–7. **Prednisone:** 40 mg/m$^2$/d PO, days 1–7.**Vincristine:** 1 mg/m$^2$/d by IV infusion, days 1 and 7.
- ► **Cytarabine:** 100 mg/m$^2$/d by continuous infusion, days 1–7. **Daunorubicin:** 45 mg/m$^2$/d by IV push, days 1–3.

### Pharmacokinetics

| *Route* | *Onset* | *Peak* | *Duration* |
|---|---|---|---|
| IV | Rapid | 20–60 min | 12–18 h |

*Metabolism:* Hepatic, $T_{1/2}$: 1–3 h
*Distribution:* Crosses placenta; enters breast milk
*Excretion:* Urine

### IV facts

**Preparation:** Reconstitute 100-mg vial with 5 ml of Bacteriostatic Water for Injection with benzyl alcohol 0.9%; resultant solution contains 20 mg/ml cytarabine. Reconstitute 500-mg vial with 10 ml of the above; resultant solution contains 50 mg/ml cytarabine. Store at room temperature for up to 48 h. Discard solution if a slight haze appears. Can be further diluted with Water for Injection, 5% Dextrose in Water, or Sodium Chloride Injection; stable for 8 d.

**Infusion:** Administer by IV infusion over at least 30 min, IV injection over 1–3 min for each 100 mg, or SC; patients can usually tolerate higher doses when given by rapid IV injection. There is no clinical advantage to any particular route.

### Adverse effects

- CNS: Neuritis, neural toxicity
- GI: *Anorexia, nausea, vomiting, diarrhea, oral and anal inflammation or ulceration*; esophageal ulcerations, esophagitis, abdominal pain, *hepatic dysfunction* (jaundice), acute pancreatitis
- **Hematologic**: Bone marrow depression, hyperuricemia
- GU: Renal dysfunction, urinary retention
- **Dermatologic**: Fever, rash, urticaria, freckling, skin ulceration, pruritus, conjunctivitis, alopecia
- **Local**: Thrombophlebitis, cellulitis at injection site
- **Other**: Cytarabine syndrome (fever, myalgia, bone pain, occasional chest pain, maculopapular rash, conjunctivitis, malaise, which is sometimes responsive to corticosteroids), *fever, rash*

### Clinically important drug-drug interactions

- Decreased therapeutic action of digoxin if taken with cytarabine

## ■ Nursing Considerations

### Assessment

- *History:* Allergy to cytarabine, hematopoietic depression, impaired liver function, lactation
- *Physical:* Weight; T; skin lesions, color; hair; orientation, reflexes; R, adventitious sounds; mucous membranes, liver evaluation, abdominal exam; CBC, differen-

tial; renal and liver function tests; urinalysis

### Implementation

- Evaluate hematopoietic status before and frequently during therapy.
- Discontinue drug therapy if platelet count < 50,000/$mm^3$, polymorphonuclear granuloctye count < 1,000/$mm^3$; consult physician for dosage adjustment.
- Use Elliott's B solution for diluent, similar to CSF, for intrathecal use.
- Give comfort measures for anal inflammation, headache, other pain associated with cytarabine syndrome.

### Drug-specific teaching points

- Prepare a calendar of treatment days. Drug must be given IV or SC.
- The following side effects may occur: nausea, vomiting, loss of appetite (medication may be ordered; eat small frequent meals; maintain nutrition); malaise, weakness, lethargy (reversible; avoid driving or operating dangerous machinery); mouth sores (use frequent mouth care); diarrhea; loss of hair (obtain a wig or other head covering; keep the head covered in extreme temperatures); anal inflammation (use comfort measures).
- Use birth control; this drug may cause birth defects or miscarriages.
- Have frequent, regular medical follow-ups, including blood tests to assess drug effects.
- Report black, tarry stools, fever, chills, sore throat, unusual bleeding or bruising, shortness of breath, chest pain, difficulty swallowing.

## dacarbazine

*(da **kar'** ba zeen)*

DTIC, imidazole carboxamide

DTIC-Dome

**Pregnancy Category C**

### Drug classes

Antineoplastic

### Therapeutic actions

Cytotoxic: exact mechanism of action unknown; inhibits DNA and RNA synthesis, causing cell death; cell cycle nonspecific.

### Indications

- Metastatic malignant melanoma
- Hodgkin's disease—second-line therapy in combination with other drugs

### Contraindications/cautions

- Contraindications: allergy to dacarbazine, pregnancy, lactation.
- Use cautiously with impaired hepatic function, bone marrow depression.

### Dosage

**Available Forms:** Injection—10 mg/ml

***Adult and pediatric malignant melanoma:*** 2–4.5 mg/kg per day IV for 10 d, repeated at 4-wk intervals or 250 mg/$m^2$ per day IV for 5 d, repeated every 3 wk.

***Hodgkin's disease:*** 150 mg/$m^2$ per day for 5 d with other drugs, repeated every 4 wk or 375 mg/$m^2$ on day 1 with other drugs, repeated every 15 d.

### Pharmacokinetics

| Route | Onset | Duration |
|---|---|---|
| IV | 15–20 min | 6–8 h |

*Metabolism:* Hepatic; $T_{1/2}$: 19 min then 5 h
*Distribution:* Crosses placenta; enters breast milk
*Excretion:* Urine

### IV facts

**Preparation:** Reconstitute 100-mg vials with 9.9 ml and the 200-mg vials with 19.7 ml of Sterile Water for Injection; the resulting solution contains 10 mg/ml of dacarbazine. Reconstituted solution may be further diluted with 5% Dextrose Injection or Sodium Chloride Injection and administered as an IV infusion. Reconstituted solution is stable for 72 h if refrigerated, 8 h at room temperature. If further diluted, solution is stable for 24 h if refrigerated or 8 h at room temperature.

**Infusion:** Infuse slowly over 30–60 min; avoid extravasation.

**Adverse effects**

- **GI:** *Anorexia, nausea, vomiting,* hepatotoxicity, hepatic necrosis
- **Hematologic:** *Hemopoietic depression*
- **Dermatologic:** *Photosensitivity,* erythematous and urticarial rashes, alopecia
- **Hypersensitivity:** Anaphylaxis
- **Local:** *Local tissue damage and pain if extravasation occurs*
- **Other:** Facial paresthesias, flulike syndrome, cancer

## ■ Nursing Considerations

### Assessment

- ***History:*** Allergy to dacarbazine, impaired hepatic function, bone marrow depression, lactation
- ***Physical:*** Weight; temperature; skin—color, lesions; hair; mucous membranes, liver evaluation; CBC, liver function tests

### Implementation

- Arrange for lab tests (WBC, RBC, platelets) before and frequently during therapy.
- Give IV only; avoid extravasation into the subcutaneous tissues during administration because tissue damage and severe pain may occur.
- Apply hot packs to relieve pain locally if extravasation occurs.
- Restrict oral intake of fluid and foods for 4–6 h before therapy to alleviate nausea and vomiting.
- Consult with physician for antiemetic if severe nausea and vomiting occur. Phenobarbital and prochloperazine may be used. Assure patient that nausea usually subsides after 1–2 d.

### Drug-specific teaching points

- Prepare a calendar for treatment days and additional therapy.
- The following side effects may occur: loss of appetite, nausea, vomiting (frequent mouth care, small frequent meals may help; maintain good nutrition; consult dietician; antiemetic available); rash; loss of hair (reversible; obtain a wig or other suitable head covering; keep head covered in extreme temperature); sensitivity to ultraviolet light (use a sunscreen and protective clothing).
- Have regular blood tests to monitor drug's effects.
- Report fever, chills, sore throat, unusual bleeding or bruising, yellow skin or eyes, light-colored stools, dark urine, pain or burning at IV injection site.



## dactinomycin

*(dak ti noe* ***mye'*** *sin)*
actinomycin D, ACT
Cosmegan
**Pregnancy Category C**

**Drug classes**
Antibiotic
Antineoplastic

**Therapeutic actions**
Cytotoxic: inhibits synthesis of messenger RNA, causing cell death; cell cycle nonspecific.

**Indications**

- Wilms' tumor, rhabdomyosarcoma, metastatic and nonmetastatic choriocarcinoma, Ewing's sarcoma, sarcoma botryoides, in combination therapy.
- Nonseminomatous testicular carcinoma
- Potentiation of effects of radiation therapy

**Contraindications/cautions**

- Contraindications: allergy to dactinomycin; chickenpox, herpes zoster (severe, generalized disease and death could result); pregnancy; lactation.
- Use cautiously with bone marrow suppression, radiation therapy.

### Dosage

**Available Forms:** Powder for injection—0.5 mg

Individualize dosage. Toxic reactions are frequent, limiting the amount of the drug that can be given. Give drug in short courses.

**ADULT**

- ***IV:*** 0.5 mg/d for up to 5 d. Give a second course after at least 3 wk. Do not exceed

15 μg/kg per day for 5 d. Calculate dosage for obese or edematous patients on the basis of surface area as an attempt to relate dosage to lean body mass. Do not exceed 400–600 μg/$m^2$ per day.

– ***Isolation-perfusion technique:*** 0.05 mg/kg for lower extremity or pelvis; 0.035 mg/kg for upper extremity. Use lower dose for obese patients or when previous therapy has been used.

*PEDIATRIC:* Do not give to children < 6–12 mo.

- ***IV:*** 0.015 mg/kg per day for 5 d or a total dose of 2.5 mg/$m^2$ over 1 wk; give a second course after at least 3 wk.

### Pharmacokinetics

| *Route* | *Onset* | *Duration* |
|---|---|---|
| IV | Rapid | 9 d |

*Metabolism* : Hepatic; $T_{1/2}$: 36 h
*Distribution:* Crosses placenta; enters breast milk
*Excretion:* Urine and bile

### IV facts

**Preparation:** Reconstitute by adding 1.1 ml of Sterile Water for Injection (*without preservatives)* to vial, creating a 0.5 mg/ml concentration solution. Discard any unused portion.

**Infusion:** Add to IV infusions of 5% Dextrose or to Sodium Chloride, or inject into IV tubing of a running IV infusion. Direct drug injection without infusion requires 2 needles, one sterile needle to remove drug from vial and another for the direct IV injection. Do not inject into IV lines with cellulose ester membrane filters; drug may be partially removed by filter. Inject over 2–3 min; infuse slowly over 20–30 min.

### Adverse effects

- GI: *Cheilitis, dysphagia, esophagitis*, ulcerative stomatitis, pharyngitis, *anorexia, abdominal pain, diarrhea*, GI ulceration, proctitis, nausea, vomiting, hepatic abnormalities
- **Hematologic:** *Anemia, aplastic anemia, agranulocytosis, leukopenia, thrombocytopenia, pancytopenia, reticulopenia*
- **Dermatologic:** *Alopecia, skin eruptions*, acne, erythema, increased pigmentation of GU renal abnormalities
- **Local:** *Tissue necrosis at sites of extravasation*
- **Other:** *Malaise, fever, fatigue, lethargy, myalgia*, hypocalcemia, death, increased incidence of second primary tumors with radiation

### Drug-lab test interferences

- Inaccurate bioassay procedure results for determination of antibacterial drug levels

## ■ Nursing Considerations

### Assessment

- ***History:*** Allergy to dactinomycin; chickenpox, herpes zoster; bone marrow suppression, radiation therapy; pregnancy, lactation
- ***Physical:*** Temperature; skin color, lesions; weight; hair; local injection site; mucous membranes, abdominal exam; CBC, hepatic and renal function tests, urinalysis

### Implementation

- Do not give IM or SC; severe local reaction and tissue necrosis occur; IV use only.
- Monitor injection site for extravasation, burning, or stinging. Discontinue infusion immediately, apply cold compresses to the area, and restart in another vein. Local infiltration with injectable corticosteroid and flushing with saline may lessen reaction.
- Monitor response, including CBC, often at start of therapy; adverse effects may require a decrease in dose or discontinuation of the drug; consult physician.
- Adverse effects may not occur immediately, may be maximal 1–2 wk after therapy.

### Drug-specific teaching points

- Prepare a calendar for therapy days.
- The following side effects may occur: rash, skin lesions, loss of hair (obtain a wig; use skin care); loss of appetite, nausea, mouth sores (frequent mouth care,

small frequent meals may help; maintain good nutrition; consult a dietician; antiemetic may be ordered).
- Adverse effects of the drug may not occur immediately; may be 1–2 wk after therapy before maximal effects.
- Have regular medical followup, including blood tests to monitor the drug's effects.
- Report severe GI upset, diarrhea, vomiting, burning or pain at injection site, unusual bleeding or bruising, severe mouth sores, GI lesions.

## dalteparin

*(dahl' tep ah rin)*

Fragmin

**Pregnancy Category B**

### Drug classes

Antiplatelet agent
Low-molecular-weight heparin

### Therapeutic actions

Low molecular weight heparin that inhibits thrombus and clot formation by blocking factor Xa, factor IIa, preventing the formation of clots.

### Indications

- Prevention of deep vein thrombosis, which may lead to pulmonary embolism, following abdominal surgery.

### Contraindications/cautions

- Contraindications: hypersensitivity to dalteparin, heparin, pork products; severe thrombocytopenia; uncontrolled bleeding.
- Use cautiously with pregnancy or lactation, history of GI bleed.

### Dosage

**Available Forms:** Solution—16 mg/0.2ml, 32 mg/0.2ml

**ADULT:** 2500 IU SC each day starting 1–2 h before surgery and repeating once daily for 5–10 d post-op.

**PEDIATRIC:** Safety and efficacy not established

### Pharmacokinetics

| *Route* | *Onset* | *Peak* | *Duration* |
|---|---|---|---|
| SC | 20–60 min | 3–5 h | 12 h |

*Metabolism:* $T_{1/2}$: 4.5 h; distribution: may cross placenta, may enter breast milk

*Excretion:* Urine

### Adverse effects

- Hematologic: **Hemorrhage** ; *bruising*; thrombocytopenia; elevated SGOT, SGPT levels; hyperkalemia
- Hypersensitivity: Chills, fever, urticaria, asthma
- Other: Fever; pain; local irritation, hematoma, erythema at site of injection
- Treatment of overdose: Protamine sulfate (1% solution). Each mg of protamine neutralizes 1 mg dalteparin. Give very slowly IV over 10 min.

### Clinically important drug-drug interactions

- Increased bleeding tendencies with oral anticoagulants, salicylates, penicillins, cephalosporins

### Drug-lab test interferences

- Increased AST, ALT levels

## ■ Nursing Considerations

### Assessment

- *History:* Recent surgery or injury; sensitivity to heparin, pork products, enoxaparin; lactation; history of GI bleed.
- *Physical:* Peripheral perfusion, R, stool guaiac test, PTT or other tests of blood coagulation, platelet count, kidney function tests

### Implementation

- Give 1–2 h before abdominal surgery.
- Give deep subcutaneous injections; **do not** give dalteparin by IM injection.
- Administer by deep SC injection; patient should be lying down; alternate administration between the left and right anterolateral and left and right posterolateral abdominal wall. Introduce the whole length of the needle into a skin fold held between the thumb and forefinger; hold the skin fold througout the injection.

- Apply pressure to all injection sites after needle is withdrawn; inspect injection sites for signs of hematoma.
- Do not massage injection sites.
- Do not mix with other injections or infusions.
- Store at room temperature; fluid should be clear, colorless to pale yellow.
- Alert all health care providers that patient is on dalteparin.
- If thromboembolic episode should occur despite therapy, discontinue and initiate appropriate therapy.
- Have protamine sulfate (dalteparin antidote) on standby in case of overdose.

### Drug-specific teaching points

- This drug must be given by a parenteral route (not orally).
- Periodic blood tests are needed to monitor response.
- Avoid injury while on this drug: use an electric razor, avoid potentially injurious activities.
- Report nose bleed, bleeding of the gums, unusual bruising, black or tarry stools, cloudy or dark urine, abdominal or lower back pain, severe headache.

## danaparoid sodium

*(dah **nap'** a royed)*
Orgaran
**Pregnancy Category B**

### Drug classes

Antithrombotic
Low-molecular-weight heparin

### Therapeutic actions

Low-molecular-weight heparin that inhibits thrombus and clot formation by blocking Factor Xa and Factor IIa, accelerating the activity of antithrombin III, and inhibiting the binding of heparin cofactor II. Danaparoid is derived from porcine intestinal mucosa.

### Indications

- Prevention of deep vein thrombosis, which may lead to pulmonary embolism, following elective hip replacement surgery

### Contraindications/cautions

- Contraindications: hypersensitivity to danaparoid, heparin or pork products; severe thrombocytopenia; uncontrolled bleeding.
- Use cautiously with pregnancy or lactation, severe liver or renal disease, recent brain surgery, retinopathy, asthma, history of GI bleed.

### Dosage

**Available Forms:** Injection—750 anti-Xa U/0.6 ml

*ADULT:* 750 anti-Xa U SC bid with the initial dose give 1–4 h before surgery and then no sooner than 2 h after surgery. Continue for at least 7–10 d; up to 14 d may be necessary.

*PEDIATRIC:* Safety and efficacy not established.

### Pharmacokinetics

| *Route* | *Onset* | *Peak* | *Duration* |
|---|---|---|---|
| SC | 20–60 min | 2–5 h | 12 h |

*Metabolism:* $T_{1/2}$: 24 h
*Distribution:* May cross placenta, may enter breast milk
*Excretion:* Urine

### Adverse effects

- CV: Chest pain, dizziness, CVA
- Hematological: **Hemorrhage;** *bruising;* thromobocytopenia; elevated SGOT, SGPT levels; hyperkalemia
- Hypersensitivity: Chills, fever, urticaria, asthma
- Other: Fever, pain, local irritation, hematoma, erythema at site of injection
- Treatment of overdose: No known agent is effective for the treatment of overdose; protamine sulfate may have some effect. If overdose occurs, discontinue danaparoid and administer whole blood or blood products.

**Clinically important drug-drug interactions**

- Increased bleeding tendencies with drugs that affect hemostasis (anticoagulants, platelet inhibitors, etc.)

## ■ Nursing Considerations

### Assessment

- *History:* Recent surgery or injury; sensitivity to heparin, pork products, danaparoid; lactation; renal or liver disease; retinopathy; history of GI bleed
- *Physical:* Peripheral perfusion, R, stool guaic test, partial thromboplastin time (PTT) or other tests of blood coagulation, platelet count, kidney and liver function tests

### Implementation

- Arrange to give drug 1–4 h before surgery and no sooner than 2 h post-op.
- Give deep subcutaneous injection; *do not* give danaparoid by IM injection.
- Administer by deep SC injection; patient should be lying down; alternate administration between the left and right anterolateral and the left and right posterolateral abdomen. Introduce the whole length of the needle into a skin fold held between the thumb and forefinger; hold the skin fold throughout the injection.
- Apply pressure to all injection sites after needle is withdrawn; inspect injection sites for signs of hematoma.
- Do not massage injection sites.
- Provide for safety measures (electric razor, soft toothbrush) to prevent injury to patient who is at risk for bleeding.
- Check patient for signs of bleeding; monitor blood tests.
- Alert all health care providers that patient is on danaparoid.

### Drug-specific teaching points

- This drug must be given by subcutaneous injection into your abdomen.
- Periodic blood tests will be needed to monitor your response to this drug.
- Be careful to avoid injury while you are on this drug; use an electric razor, avoid activities that might lead to injury.
- Report nose bleed, bleeding of the gums, unusual bruising, black or tarry stools, cloudy or dark urine, abdominal or lower back pain, severe headache.

## danazol

*(da na zole)*
Cyclomen (CAN), Danocrine
**Pregnancy Category C**

**Drug classes**

Androgen
Hormone

**Therapeutic actions**

Synthetic androgen that suppresses the release of the pituitary gonadotropins FSH and LH, which inhibits ovulation and decreases estrogen and progesterone levels; inhibits sex steroid synthesis and binds to steroid receptors in cells of target tissues. Therapeutic effects in hereditary angioedema are probably due to drug effects in the liver; danazol partially or completely corrects the primary defect in this disorder.

**Indications**

- Treatment of endometriosis amenable to hormonal management
- Treatment of fibrocystic breast disease; decreases nodularity, pain, and tenderness; symptoms return after therapy
- Prevention of attacks of hereditary angioedema
- Unlabeled uses: treatment of precocious puberty, gynecomastia, menorrhagia

**Contraindications/cautions**

- Known sensitivity to danazol; undiagnosed abnormal genital bleeding; impaired hepatic, renal, or cardiac function; pregnancy; lactation.

### Dosage

**Available Forms:** Capsules—50, 100, 200 mg

ADULT

- *Endometriosis:* Begin during menstruation, or ensure patient is not pregnant; 800 mg/d PO, in two divided doses; downward titration to a dose sufficient to maintain amenorrhea may be considered. For mild cases, give 200–400 mg PO, in 2 divided doses. Continue for 3–

6 mo or up to 9 mo. Reinstitute if symptoms recur after termination.
- *Fibrocystic breast disease:* Begin therapy during menstruation, or ensure that patient is not pregnant; 100–400 mg/d PO in two divided doses; 2–6 mo of therapy may be required to alleviate all signs and symptoms.
- *Hereditary angioedema:* Individualize dosage; starting dose of 200 mg PO bid or tid. After favorable response, decrease dose by 50% or less at 1- to 3-mo intervals. If an attack occurs, increase dose to 200 mg/d; monitor response closely during adjustment of dose.

### Pharmacokinetics

| *Route* | *Peak* | *Duration* |
|---|---|---|
| Oral | 6–8 wk | 3–6 mo |

*Metabolism* : Hepatic; $T_{1/2}$: 4 1/2 h
*Distribution:* Crosses placenta; enters breast milk
*Excretion:* Unknown

### Adverse effects

- CNS: Dizziness, headache, sleep disorders, fatigue, tremor
- GI: Hepatic dysfunction
- GU: Fluid retention
- **Endocrine**: *Androgenic effects* (acne, edema, mild hirsutism, decrease in breast size, deepening of the voice, oily skin or hair, weight gain, clitoral hypertrophy or testicular atrophy), *hypoestrogenic effects* (flushing, sweating, vaginitis, nervousness, emotional lability)

### Clinically important drug-drug interactions

• Prolongation of PT in patients stabilized on oral anticoagulants • Increased carbamazepine toxicity

## ■ Nursing Considerations

### Assessment

- *History:* Known sensitivity to danazol; undiagnosed abnormal genital bleeding; impaired hepatic, renal or cardiac function; pregnancy; lactation
- *Physical:* Weight; hair distribution pattern; skin color, texture, lesions; breast exam; orientation, affect, reflexes; P, auscultation, BP, peripheral edema; liver evaluation; liver and renal function tests, semen and sperm evaluation

### Implementation

- Ensure patient is not pregnant before therapy; begin therapy for endometriosis and fibrocystic breast disease during menstruation.
- Ensure there is no carcinoma of the breast before therapy for fibrocystic breast disease; rule out carcinoma if nodule persists or enlarges.
- Alert patient that androgenic effects may not be reversible.
- Arrange for periodic liver function tests during therapy; hepatic dysfunction occurs with long-term use.
- Periodic tests of semen and sperm, especially in adolescents; marked changes may indicate need to discontinue therapy.

### Drug-specific teaching points

- The following side effects may occur: masculinizing effects (acne, hair growth, deepening of voice, oily skin or hair; may not be reversible), low-estrogen effects (flushing, sweating, vaginal irritation, mood changes, nervousness).
- Use a nonhormonal form of birth control during therapy. If you become pregnant, discontinue the drug, and consult with your physician immediately. This drug is contraindicated during pregnancy.
- Report abnormal growth of facial hair, deepening of the voice, unusual bleeding or bruising, fever, chills, sore throat, vaginal itching or irritation.

## dantrolene sodium

***(dan' troe leen)***

Dantrium, Dantrium Intravenous

**Pregnancy Category C**

### Drug classes

Skeletal muscle relaxant, direct acting

**Therapeutic actions**

Relaxes skeletal muscle within the skeletal muscle fiber, probably by interfering with the release of calcium from the sarcoplasmic reticulum; does not interfere with neuromuscular transmission or affect the surface membrane of skeletal muscle.

**Indications**

- Oral: Control of clinical spasticity resulting from upper motor neuron disorders, such as spinal cord injury, stroke, cerebral palsy, or multiple sclerosis; not indicated for relief of skeletal muscle spasm resulting from rheumatic disorders; continued long-term administration is justified if use significantly reduces painful or disabling spasticity, (clonus); significantly reduces the intensity or degree of nursing care required; rids the patient of problematic manifestation of spasticity.
- Preoperatively to prevent or attenuate the development of malignant hyperthermia in susceptible patients who must undergo surgery or anesthesia; after a malignant hyperthermia crisis to prevent recurrence
- Unlabeled use: exercise-induced muscle pain
- Parenteral (IV): management of the fulminant hypermetabolism of skeletal muscle characteristic of malignant hyperthermia crisis; preoperative prevention of malignant hyperthermia

**Contraindications/cautions**

- See discussion above on chronic use of drug; malignant hyperthermia is a medical emergency that would override contraindications and cautions.
- Contraindications: active hepatic disease; spasticity used to sustain upright posture, balance in locomotion or to gain or retain increased function; lactation.
- Use cautiously with female patients and patients > 35 y (increased risk for potentially fatal, hepatocellular disease); impaired pulmonary function; severely impaired cardiac function due to myocardial disease; history of previous liver disease or dysfunction.

**Dosage**

**Available Forms:** Capsules—25, 50, 100 mg; powder for injection—20 mg/vial

ADULT

- *Oral*
  - *Chronic spasticity:* Titrate and individualize dosage; establish a therapeutic goal before therapy, and increase dosage until maximum performance compatible with the dysfunction is achieved. Initially, 25 mg qd; increase to 25 mg bid–qid; then increase in increments of 25 mg up to as high as 100 mg bid–qid if necessary. Most patients will respond to 400 mg/d or less; maintain each dosage level for 4–7 d to evaluate response. Discontinue drug after 45 d if benefits are not evident.
  - *Preoperative prophylaxis of malignant hyperthermia:* 4–8 mg/kg per d PO in three to four divided doses for 1–2 d prior to surgery; give last dose about 3–4 h before scheduled surgery with a minimum of water. Adjust dosage to the recommended range to prevent incapacitation due to drowsiness and excessive GI irritation.
  - *Postcrisis follow-up:* 4–8 mg/kg per d PO in four divided doses for 1–3 d to prevent recurrence.
- *Parenteral*
  - *Treatment of malignant hyperthermia:* Discontinue all anesthetics as soon as problem is recognized. Give dantrolene by continuous rapid IV push beginning at a minimum dose of 1 mg/kg and continuing until symptoms subside or a maximum cumulative dose of 10 mg/kg has been given. If physiologic and metabolic abnormalities reappear, repeat regimen. Give continuously until symptoms subside.
  - *Preoperative prophylaxis of malignant hyperthermia:* 2.5 mg/kg IV 1 h before surgery infused over 1 h.

PEDIATRIC: Safety for use in children < 5 y not established. Since adverse effects may appear only after many years, weigh benefits and risks of long-term use carefully.

- ***Oral***
  - *Chronic spasticity:* Use an approach similar to that described above for the adult. Initially, 0.5 mg/kg bid PO. Increase to 0.5 mg/kg tid–qid; then increase by increments of 0.5 mg/kg up to

d

3 mg/kg, bid–qid if necessary. Do not exceed dosage of 100 mg qid.
– *Malignant hyperthermia:* Dosage orally and IV is same as adult.

**Pharmacokinetics**

| *Route* | *Onset* | *Peak* | *Duration* |
|---|---|---|---|
| Oral | Slow | 4–6 h | 8–10 h |
| IV | Rapid | 5 h | 6–8 h |

*Metabolism:* Hepatic; $T_{1/2}$: 9 h (oral) 4–8 h (IV)
*Distribution:* Crosses placenta; enters breast milk
*Excretion:* Urine

**IV facts**

**Preparation:** Add 60 ml of Sterile Water for Injection (without bacteriostatic agents); shake until solution is clear. Protect from light, and use within 6 h. Store at room temperature, protected from light.
**Infusion:** Administer by rapid continuous IV push. Administer continuously until symptoms subside; prophylactic doses infused over 1 h.

**Adverse effects**

*Oral*

- CNS: *Drowsiness, dizziness, weakness, general malaise, fatigue*, speech disturbance, seizure, headache, lightheadedness, visual disturbance, diplopia, alteration of taste, insomnia, mental depression, mental confusion, increased nervousness
- GI: *Diarrhea*, constipation, GI bleeding, anorexia, dysphagia, gastric irritation, abdominal cramps, **hepatitis**
- CV: Tachycardia, erratic BP, phlebitis, effusion with pericarditis
- GU: Increased urinary frequency, hematuria, crystalluria, difficult erection, urinary incontinence, nocturia, dysuria, urinary retention
- Dermatologic: Abnormal hair growth, acnelike rash, pruritus, urticaria, eczematoid eruption, sweating, photosensitivity
- Other: Myalgia, backache, chills and fever, feeling of suffocation

*Parenteral*

- None of the above reactions with short-term IV therapy for malignant hyperthermia

## ■ Nursing Considerations

### Assessment

- *History:* Active hepatic disease; spasticity used to sustain upright posture and balance in locomotion or to gain and retain increased function; female patient and patients > 35 y; impaired pulmonary function; severely impaired cardiac function; history of previous liver disease; lactation
- *Physical:* T; skin color, lesions; orientation, affect, reflexes, bilateral grip strength, vision; P, BP, auscultation; adventitious sounds; bowel sounds, normal GI output; prostate palpation, normal output, voiding pattern; urinalysis, liver function tests (SGOT, SGPT, alkaline phosphatase, total bilirubin)

### Implementation

- Monitor IV injection sites, and ensure that extravasation does not occur—drug is very alkaline and irritating to tissues.
- Ensure that other measures are used to treat malignant hyperthermia: discontinuation of triggering agents, monitoring and providing for increased oxygen requirements, managing metabolic acidosis and electrolyte imbalance, cooling if necessary.
- Establish a therapeutic goal before beginning chronic oral therapy to gain or enhance ability to engage in therapeutic exercise program, use of braces, transfer maneuvers.
- Withdraw drug for 2–4 d to confirm therapeutic benefits; clinical impression of exacerbation of spasticity would justify use of this potentially dangerous drug.
- Discontinue if diarrhea is severe; it may be possible to reinstitute it at a lower dose.

- Monitor liver function tests periodically; arrange to discontinue at first sign of abnormality; early detection of liver abnormalities may permit reversion to normal function.

### Drug-specific teaching points

*Preoperative Prophylaxis of Malignant Hyperthermia*

- Call for assistance if you wish to get up; do not move about alone; this drug can cause drowsiness.
- Report GI upset; a dosage change is possible; eat small frequent meals.

*Chronic Oral Therapy for Spasticity*

- Take this drug exactly as prescribed; do not take a higher dosage.
- Avoid alcohol, sleep-inducing, or OTC drugs; these could cause dangerous effects.
- The following side effects may occur: drowsiness, dizziness, blurred vision (avoid driving or engaging in activities that require alertness); diarrhea; nausea (take with food, eat frequent small meals); difficulty urinating, increased urinary frequency, urinary incontinence (empty bladder just before taking medication); headache, malaise (an analgesic may be allowed); photosensitivity (avoid sun and ultraviolet light or use sunscreens, protective clothing).
- Report skin rash, itching, bloody or black tarry stools, pale stools, yellowish discoloration of the skin or eyes, severe diarrhea.

## dapsone

*(dap' sone)*

DDS, diaphenylsulfone

Avlosulfan (CAN)

**Pregnancy Category A**

### Drug classes

Leprostatic agent

### Therapeutic actions

Bactericidal and bacteriostatic against *Mycobacterium leprae*; mechanism of action in dermatitis herpetiformis is not established.

### Indications

- Hansen's disease (leprosy—all forms)
- Dermatitis herpetiformis
- Unlabeled uses: Relapsing polychondritis, prophylaxis of malaria, alone or in combination with trimethoprim for treatment of *Pneumocystis carinii* pneumonia; brown recluse spider bites; SLE

### Contraindications/cautions

- Contraindications: allergy to dapsone or its derivatives, lactation.
- Use cautiously with anemia, severe cardiopulmonary disease, G-6-PD deficiency, methemoglobin reductase deficiency, hemoglobin M, hepatic dysfunction, pregnancy.

### Dosage

**Available Forms:** Tablets—25, 100 mg

ADULT

- ***Dermatitis herpetiformis:*** 50 mg daily PO; individualize dosage to 50–300 mg daily. Maintenance dosage may be reduced after 6 mo on a gluten-free diet.
- ***Leprosy:*** 6–10 mg/kg per week PO (50–100 mg daily).
- ***Bacteriologically negative tuberculoid and indeterminate type leprosy:*** 50 mg/d PO. Continue therapy for at least 3 y after clinical control is established.
- ***Lepromatous and borderline patients:*** 50 mg/d PO for *at least 10 y* after patient is bacteriologically negative, usually for life.

PEDIATRIC: Use correspondingly smaller doses than with adults.

### Pharmacokinetics

| Route | Onset | Peak | Duration |
|---|---|---|---|
| Oral | 8 d | 4–8 h | 3 wk |

*Metabolism:* Hepatic; $T_{1/2}$: 28 h

*Distribution:* May cross placenta; enters breast milk

*Excretion:* Urine

### Adverse effects

- CNS: Peripheral neuropathy in nonleprosy patients, headache, psychosis, insomnia, vertigo, paresthesias, blurred vision, tinnitus
- GI: *Nausea, vomiting*, abdominal pain, anorexia, toxic hepatits, cholestatic jaundice
- **Hematologic**: *Hemolysis, including hemolytic anemia,* aplastic anemia, agranulocytosis; methemoglobinemia, hypoalbuminemia
- GU: Albuminuria, nephrotic syndrome, renal papillary necrosis, male infertility
- **Dermatologic**: Hyperpigmented macules, drug-induced lupus erythematosus, phototoxicity
- Other: Fever, carcinogenic in small animals

### Clinically important drug-drug interactions

- Decreased dapsone levels with rifampin

Increased dapsone levels due to decreased excretion with probenecid

## ■ Nursing Considerations

### Assessment

- ***History:*** Allergy to dapsone or its derivatives, anemia, severe cardiopulmonary disease, G-6-PD deficiency, methemoglobin reductase deficiency, hemoglobin M, hepatic dysfunction, lactation
- ***Physical:*** Skin lesions, color; temperature; orientation, affect, reflexes, vision; P, auscultation, BP, edema; R, auscultation; bowel sounds, liver evaluation; CBC, liver and renal function tests

### Implementation

- Monitor patient closely during administration; fatalities have been reported from agranulocytosis, aplastic anemia, and other blood dyscrasias.
- Arrange for regular blood counts during therapy: weekly for first month, monthly for 6 mo, and then every 6 mo. Discontinue, and consult with physician if significant leukopenia, thrombocytopenia, or decreased hematopoiesis occurs.
- Discontinue, and consult with physician if any sign of hypersensitivity occurs (dermatologic reactions).
- Monitor liver function tests; discontinue and consult with physician if any abnormality occurs.
- Assess patient and consult with physician if leprosy reactional episodes occur (worsening of leprosy activity related to therapy); use of other leprostatics, analgesics, steroids, or surgery may be necessary.
- Give drug with meals if GI upset occurs.
- Suspect secondary dapsone resistance when a lepromatous or borderline lepromatous patient relapses clinically and bacteriologically. Arrange for clinical confirmation of dapsone resistance, and change drugs as ordered.
- Contact support groups to help the patient to cope with disease and drug therapy: National Hansen's Disease Center; Carville, LA, 70721; telephone, (504) 642-7771.

### Drug-specific teaching points

- Take with food if GI upset occurs. Follow the prescription carefully: efficacy depends on prolonged use.
- Arrange regular medical follow-up, including blood tests.
- The following side effects may occur: nausea, loss of appetite, vomiting (take drug with meals); sensitivity to sunlight (wear protective clothing; use a sunscreen); numbness, tingling, weakness (use caution to avoid injury).
- Report worsening of Hansen's disease symptoms, severe GI upset, unusual bleeding or bruising, sore throat, fever, chills, yellowing of skin or eyes.

## daunorubicin citrate liposomal

*(daw noe **roo'** bi sin)*

DNR

DaunoXome

**Pregnancy Category D**

**Drug classes**
Antibiotic
Antineoplastic

**Therapeutic actions**
Cytotoxic, antimiotic, immunosuppressive: binds to DNA and inhibits DNA synthesis, causing cell death; encapsulated in lipid to increase selectivity to tumor cells.

**Indications**
- First-line treatment for advanced HIV-associated Kaposi's sarcoma

**Contraindications/cautions**
- Contraindications: allergy to daunorubicin; systemic infections; myelosuppression; cardiac disease; pregnancy; lactation.
- Use cautiously with impaired hepatic or renal function

**Dosage**
**Available Forms:** Injection—2 mg/ml
*ADULT:* 40 $mg/m^2$ IV infused over 1 h; repeat q 2 wk.
*PEDIATRIC:* Safety and efficacy not established.
*IMPAIRED HEPATIC OR RENAL FUNCTION:*

| *Serum Bilirubin (mg/dl)* | *Serum Creatinine (mg/dl)* | *Dose* |
|---|---|---|
| 1.2–3.0 | | 3/4 normal dose |
| >3 | >3 | 1/2 normal dose |

**Pharmacokinetics**

| *Route* | *Onset* |
|---|---|
| IV | Slow |

*Metabolism:* Hepatic; $T_{1/2}$: 4.4 h
*Distribution:* Crosses placenta; enters breast milk
*Excretion:* Bile and urine

**IV facts**
**Preparation:** Dilute 1:1 with 5% Dextrose Injection before administration. Do not use an in-line filter. Refrigerate. Store reconstituted solution up to 6 h. Protect from light.
**Infusion:** Infuse over 1 h.
**Incompatibilities:** Do not mix with other drugs or heparin.

**Adverse effects**
- GI: *Nausea, vomiting,* mucositis, diarrhea
- CV: Cardiac toxicity, CHF
- **Hematologic**: ***Myelosuppression***
- GU: *Hyperuricemia* due to cell lysis, *red urine*
- **Dermatologic**: *Complete but reversible alopecia*, skin rash
- **Local**: *Local tissue necrosis if extravasation occurs*
- **Other**: Fever, chills, cancer

## ■ Nursing Considerations

### Assessment
- ***History:*** Allergy to daunorubicin; systemic infections; myelosuppression; cardiac disease; impaired hepatic or renal function; lactation.
- ***Physical:*** T; skin color, lesions; weight; hair; local injection site; auscultation, peripheral perfusion, pulses, ECG; R, adventitious sounds; liver evaluation, mucus membranes; CBC, liver and renal function tests, serum uric acid

### Implementation
- Do not give IM or SC; severe local reaction and tissue necrosis occurs.
- Monitor injection site for extravasation: reports of burning or stinging. Discontinue infusion immediately, and restart in another vein. Local SC extravasation: local infiltration with corticosteroid may be ordered, flood area with normal saline; apply cold compress to area. If ulceration begins, arrange consultation with plastic surgeon.
- Monitor patient's response, frequently at beginning of therapy: serum uric acid level, cardiac output (listen for $S_3$), ECG, CBC. Changes may require a decrease in dose; consult physician. Drug therapy for hyperuricemia, CHF may be advisable.

### Drug-specific teaching points
- Prepare a calendar of dates for therapy.
- The following side effects may occur: rash, skin lesions, oss of hair, changes in

nails (obtain a wig; use good skin care); loss of appetite, nausea, mouth sores (frequent mouth care, small frequent meals may help; maintain good nutrition; consult a dietician; antiemetics may be helpful).

- Have regular medical followups, including blood tests to monitor effects.
- Report difficulty breathing, sudden weight gain, swelling, burning or pain at injection site, unusual bleeding or bruising.

## deferoxamine mesylate

*(de fer* ***ox'*** *a meen)*

Desferal

**Pregnancy Category C**

### Drug classes

Chelating agent
Coumarin derivative

### Therapeutic actions

Binds with iron and prevents it from entering into chemical reactions.

### Indications

- Acute iron toxicity
- Treatment of chronic iron overload
- Unlabeled use: management of aluminum accumulation in bone in renal failure and aluminum-induced dialysis encephalopathy

### Dosage

**Available Forms:** Powder for injection—500 mg

ADULT

- *Acute iron toxicity:* 1 g IM, then 0.5 g IM q4h. Subsequently give 0.5 g q4–12h based on response. Do not exceed 6 g/d. Or 15 mg/kg per hour IV; switch to IM as soon as possible.
- *Chronic overload:* 0.5–1 g IM qid. Give 2 g IV with each unit of blood. Do not exceed 15 mg/kg per day. Or 1–2 g/d (20–40 mg/kg per day) SC over 8–24 h with a continuous infusion pump.

PEDIATRIC: 50 mg/kg per dose IM or IV q6h or up to 15 mg/kg per hour by continuous IV infusion. Do not exceed 6 g/24 h or 2 g/dose.

### Pharmacokinetics

| Route | Onset |
|---|---|
| IV, IM | Rapid |

*Metabolism:* Plasma; $T_{1/2}$: 1 h
*Distribution:* Crosses placenta; enters breast milk
*Excretion:* Urine

### IV facts

**Preparation:** Add 2 ml Sterile Water for Injection to each vial. Add to saline, glucose in water, or Ringer's Lactate Solution for infusion. Protect from light. Do not store reconstituted solution longer than 1 wk.

**Infusion:** Infuse slowly; do not exceed 15 mg/kg/h; use of an unfusion pump is preferable.

### Adverse effects

- GI: Diarrhea, abdominal discomfort
- CNS: Blurred vision, cataracts (long-term), auditory disturbances, loss of hearing
- Local: *Pain, induration at injection site*, skin irritation and swelling
- Hypersensitivity: Generalized itching, rash, anaphylactic reaction
- Other: Tachycardia, fever

## ■ Nursing Considerations

### Assessment

- *History:* Severe renal disease, anuria, primary hemochromatosis, lactation
- *Physical:* Skin condition, neurologic exam, including vision and hearing, eye exam, abdominal exam, CBC, serum iron levels

### Implementation

- Administer IM, by continuous SC infusion, or by slow IV infusion.
- Monitor patient response to drug, including evaluation for cataracts, skin reaction, local injection site.

### Drug-specific teaching points

- This drug is given IM, SC, or IV. Its effects will be monitored carefully.
- The following side effects may occur: discomfort at injection site, skin rash, vision changes (use caution if vision becomes impaired).
- Report loss of hearing, vision changes, skin rash with itching, difficulty breathing, fever, pain at injection site.

## delavirdine mesylate

*(dell ah* ***vur'*** *den)*

Rescriptor

**Pregnancy Category C**

### Drug classes

Antiviral

### Therapeutic actions

Non-nucleoeside inhibitor of HIV reverse transcriptase; binds directly to HIV's reverse transcriptase and blocks RNA-dependent and DNA-dependent DNA polymerase activities.

### Indications

- Treatment of HIV-1 infection in combination with other appropriate retroviral agents when therapy is warranted; not intended as a monotherapy—resistant virus ermerges rapidly

### Contraindications/cautions

- Contraindications: life-threatening allergy to any component, pregnancy, lactation.
- Use cautiously with compromised impaired liver function.

### Dosage

**Available Forms:** Tablets—100 mg

**ADULTS AND CHILDREN > 16 Y:** 400 mg PO tid used in combination with appropriate agents.

**PEDIATRIC:** Not recommended <16 y.

### Pharmacokinetics

| *Route* | *Onset* | *Peak* |
|---|---|---|
| Oral | Rapid | 1 h |

*Metabolism:* Hepatic; $T_{1/2}$: 2–11 h

*Distribution:* Crosses placenta; passes into breast milk

*Excretion:* Urine

### Adverse effects

- CNS: *Headache,* insomnia, myalgia, *asthenia,* malaise, dizziness, paresthesia, somnolence, fatigue
- GI: *Nausea,* GI pain, *diarrhea,* anorexia, vomiting, dyspepsia, increased liver enzymes
- Skin: *Rash,* pruritus, maculopapular rash, nodules, urticaria
- Other: Anemia, arthralgia, breast enlargement.

### Clinically important drug-drug interactions

- Potentially serious or life-threatening adverse effects may occur in combination with terfenadine, astemizole, clarithromycin, dapsone, rifabutin, benzodiazepines, cisapride, calcium channel blockers, ergot derivatives, indinavir, saquinavir, quinidine or warfarin; avoid these combinations if at all possible; if the combination cannot be avoided, monitor patient very closely and decrease dosage as appropriate

## ■ Nursing Considerations

### Assessment

- ***History:*** Life-threatening allergy to any component, impaired liver function, pregnancy, lactation
- ***Physical:*** Skin rashes, lesions, texture; T; affect, reflexes, peripheral sensation; bowel sounds, liver function tests, CBC and differential

### Implementation

- Arrange to monitor hematologic indices and liver function periodically during therapy.
- Monitor patient for signs of opportunistic infections that will need to be treated appropriately.
- Administer the drug concurrently with appropriate antiretroviral agents.
- Offer support and encouragement to the patient to deal with the diagnosis; explain

that this drug must be taken in combination with other agents and that the long-term effects of the use of this drug are not known.

### Drug-specific teaching points

- Take drug as prescribed; take concurrently with other prescribed drugs; do not change dose or alter routine without checking with your health care provider.
- These drugs are not a cure for AIDS or ARC; opportunistic infections may occur and regular medical care should be sought to deal with the disease.
- Frequent blood tests are needed during the course of treatment; results of blood counts may indicate a need for decreased dosage or discontinuation of the drug for a period of time.
- This drug may interact with several other drugs; alert any health care provider that you are on this drug. If you are taking antacids, take them at least 1 h apart from delavirdine.
- The following side effects may occur: nausea, loss of appetite, change in taste (small, frequent meals may help); headache, fever, muscle aches (an analgesic may help; consult with your care provider); rash (skin care will be important).
- Delavirdine does not reduce the risk of transmission of HIV to others by sexual contact or blood contamination; use appropriate precautions.
- Report skin rash, severe headache, severe nausea, vomiting, changes in color of urine or stool, fatigue.

## demeclocycline hydrochloride

*(dem e kloe sye' kleen)*

demethylchlortetracycline hydrochloride

Declomycin

**Pregnancy Category D**

### Drug classes

Antibiotic
Tetracycline antibiotic

### Therapeutic actions

Bacteriostatic: inhibits protein synthesis of susceptible bacteria, preventing cell reproduction.

### Indications

- Infections caused by rickettsiae; *Mycoplasma pneumoniae;* agents of psittacosis, ornithosis, lymphogranuloma venereum, and granuloma inguinale; *Borrelia recurrentis; Haemophilus ducreyi; Pasteurellia pestis; Pasteurellia tularensis; Bartonella bacilliformis; Bacteroides; Vibrio comma; Vibrio fetus; Brucella; Escherichia coli; Enterobacter aerogenes; Shigella; Acinetobacter calcoaceticus; Haemophilus influenzae; Klebsiella; Diplococcus pneumoniae; Staphylococcus aureus*
- When penicillin is contraindicated, infections caused by *Neisseria gonorrhoeae, Treponema pallidum, Treponema pertenue, Listeria monocytogenes, Clostridium, Bacillus anthracis, Fusobacterium fusiforme, Actinomyces, Neisseria meningitidis*
- As an adjunct to amebicides in acute intestinal amebiasis
- Treatment of acne, uncomplicated urethral, endocervical or rectal infections in adults caused by *Chlamydia trachomatis*
- Unlabeled use: management of the chronic form of the syndrome of inappropriate antidiuretic hormone secretion (SIADH)

### Contraindications/cautions

- Allergy to tetracyclines, renal or hepatic dysfunction, pregnancy, lactation.

### Dosage

**Available Forms:** Capsules—150 mg; tablets—150, 300 mg

*ADULT:* 150 mg qid PO or 300 mg bid PO

- *Gonococcal infection:* 600 mg PO then 300 mg q12h for 4 d to a total of 3 g.

*PEDIATRIC (>8 Y):* 6–12 mg/kg per day PO in two to four divided doses. Not recommended for children < 8 y.

### Pharmacokinetics

| Route | Onset | Peak | Duration |
|---|---|---|---|
| Oral | Varies | 3–4 h | 18–20 h |

*Metabolism:* Hepatic; $T_{1/2}$: 12–16 h
*Distribution:* Crosses placenta; enters breast milk
*Excretion:* Urine and feces

### Adverse effects

- GI: Fatty liver, liver failure, *anorexia, nausea, vomiting, diarrhea, glossitis,* dysphagia, enterocolitis, esophageal ulcer
- **Hematologic**: Hemolytic anemia, thrombocytopenia, neutropenia, eosinophilia, leukocytosis, leukopenia
- **Dermatologic**: *Phototoxic reactions, rash,* exfoliative dermatitis (especially frequent and severe with this tetracycline)
- **Dental**: *Discoloring and inadequate calcification of primary teeth of fetus if used by pregnant women, discoloring and inadequate calcification of permanent teeth if used during period of dental development*
- **Other**: Superinfections, nephrogenic diabetes insipidus syndrome (polyuria, polydipsia, weakness) in patients being treated for SIADH

### Clinically important drug-drug interactions

• Decreased absorption with antacids, iron, alkali • Increased digoxin toxicity • Increased nephrotoxicity with methoxyflurane • Decreased activity of penicillin.

### Clinically important drug-food interactions

• Decreased effectiveness of demeclocycline if taken with food, dairy products

### Drug-lab test interferences

• Interference with culture studies for several days following therapy

## ■ Nursing Considerations

### Assessment

- *History:* Allergy to tetracyclines, renal or hepatic dysfunction, pregnancy, lactation.
- *Physical:* Skin status, R and sounds, GI function and liver evaluation, urinary output and concentration, urinalysis and BUN, liver and renal function tests; culture infected area before beginning therapy.

### Implementation

- Give oral form on an empty stomach; if severe GI upset occurs, give with food.
- Discontinue drug if diabetes insipidus occurs in SIADH patients.

### Drug-specific teaching points

- Take drug throughout the day for best results; take on an empty stomach, 1 h before or 1 h after meals, unless GI upset occurs; then it can be taken with food.
- The following side effects may occur: sensitivity to sunlight (use protective clothing and sunscreen), diarrhea.
- Report rash, itching; difficulty breathing; dark urine or light-colored stools; severe cramps; increased thirst, increased urination, weakness (SIADH patients).

d

# desipramine hydrochloride

*(dess **ip'** ra meen)*
Norpramin, Pertofrane
**Pregnancy Category C**

### Drug classes

Tricyclic antidepressant (TCA) (secondary amine)

### Therapeutic actions

Mechanism of action unknown; inhibits the presynaptic reuptake of the neurotransmitters norepinephrine and serotonin; anticholinergic at CNS and peripheral receptors; sedating.

### Indications

- Relief of symptoms of depression (endogenous depression most responsive)
- Unlabeled uses: facilitation of cocaine withdrawal (50–200 mg/d), treatment of eating disorders

### Contraindications/cautions

- Contraindications: hypersensitivity to any tricyclic drug, concomitant therapy with an MAO inhibitor, recent MI, myelography within previous 24 h or scheduled within 48 h, lactation.

- Use cautiously with EST; preexisting CV disorders (eg, severe coronary heart disease, progressive heart failure, angina pectoris, paroxysmal tachycardia; possibly increased risk of serious CVS toxicity with TCAs); angle-closure glaucoma, increased intraocular pressure, urinary retention, ureteral or urethral spasm (anticholinergic effects of TCAs may exacerbate these conditions); seizure disorders (TCAs lower the seizure threshold); hyperthyroidism (predisposes to CVS toxicity, including cardiac arrhythmias); impaired hepatic, renal function; psychiatric patients (schizophrenic or paranoid patients may exhibit a worsening of psychosis with TCA therapy); manic-depressive patients (may shift to hypomanic or manic phase); elective surgery (TCAs should be discontinued as long as possible before surgery).

## Dosage

**Available Forms:** Tablets—10, 25, 50, 75, 100, 150 mg

**ADULT**

- *Depression:* 100–200 mg/d PO as single dose or in divided doses initially. May gradually increase to 300 mg/d. Do not exceed 300 mg/d. Patients requiring 300 mg/d should generally have treatment initiated in a hospital. Continue a reduced maintenance dosage for at least 2 mo after a satisfactory response has been achieved.

*PEDIATRIC:* Not recommended in children < 12 y.

*GERIATRIC:* Initially 25–100 mg/d PO; dosages more than 150 mg are not recommended.

## Pharmacokinetics

| *Route* | *Onset* | *Peak* | *Duration* |
|---|---|---|---|
| Oral | Varies | 2–4 h | 3–4 d |

*Metabolism:* Hepatic; $T_{1/2}$: 12–24 h

*Distribution:* Crosses placenta; enters breast milk

*Excretion:* Urine

## Adverse effects

- CNS: *Sedation and anticholinergic effects, confusion* (especially in elderly), *disturbed concentration*, hallucinations, disorientation, decreased memory, feelings of unreality, delusions, anxiety, nervousness, restlessness, agitation, panic, insomnia, nightmares, hypomania, mania, exacerbation of psychosis, drowsiness, weakness, fatigue, headache, numbness, tingling, paresthesias of extremities, incoordination, motor hyperactivity, akathisia, ataxia, tremors, peripheral neuropathy, extrapyramidal symptoms, *seizures*, speech blockage, dysarthria, tinnitus, altered EEG
- GI: *Dry mouth, constipation*, paralytic ileus, *nausea*, vomiting, anorexia, epigastric distress, diarrhea, flatulence, dysphagia, peculiar taste, increased salivation, stomatitis, glossitis, parotid swelling, abdominal cramps, black tongue
- CV: *Orthostatic hypotension*, hypertension, syncope, tachycardia, palpitations, MI, arrhythmias, heart block, precipitation of CHF, stroke
- **Hematologic**: Bone marrow depression
- GU: Urinary retention, delayed micturition, dilation of the urinary tract, gynecomastia, testicular swelling in men; breast enlargement, menstrual irregularity and galactorrhea in women; increased or decreased libido; impotence
- **Endocrine**: Elevated or depressed blood sugar; elevated prolactin levels; SIADH secretion
- **Hypersensitivity**: Skin rash, pruritus, vasculitis, petechiae, photosensitization, edema (generalized or of face and tongue), drug fever
- **Withdrawal**: Symptoms on abrupt discontinuation of prolonged therapy: nausea, headache, vertigo, nightmares, malaise
- **Other**: Nasal congestion, excessive appetite, weight gain or loss; sweating (paradoxical effect in a drug with prominent anticholinergic effects), alopecia, lacrimation, hyperthermia, flushing, chills

**Clinically important drug-drug interactions**

• Increased TCA levels and pharmacologic (especially anticholinergic) effects with cimetidine, fluoxetine, ranitidine • Increased serum levels and risk of bleeding with oral anticoagulants. • Altered response, including dysrhythmias and hypertension with sympathomimetics • Risk of severe hypertension with clonidine • Hyperpyretic crises, severe convulsions, hypertensive episodes, and deaths when MAO inhibitors are given with TCAs • Decreased hypotensive activity of guanethidine.

## ■ Nursing Considerations

### Assessment

- *History:* Hypersensitivity to any tricyclic drug; concomitant therapy with an MAO inhibitor; recent MI; myelography within previous 24 h or scheduled within 48 h; lactation; EST; preexisting CV disorders; angle-closure glaucoma, increased intraocular pressure, urinary retention, ureteral or urethral spasm; seizure disorders; hyperthyroidism; impaired hepatic, renal function; psychiatric patients; elective surgery.
- *Physical:* Body weight; temperature; skin color, lesions; orientation, affect, reflexes, vision and hearing; P, BP, orthostatic BP, perfusion; bowel sounds, normal output, liver evaluation; urine flow, normal output; usual sexual function, frequency of menses, breast and scrotal exam; liver function tests, urinalysis, CBC, ECG.

### Implementation

- Limit access of depressed and potentially suicidal patients to drug.
- Give major portion of dose hs if drowsiness, severe anticholinergic effects occur.
- Reduce dosage if minor side effects develop; discontinue if serious side effects occur.
- Arrange for CBC if patient develops fever, sore throat, or other sign of infection.

### Drug-specific teaching points

- Take drug exactly as prescribed; do not to stop taking this drug abruptly or without consulting the healthcare provider.
- Avoid alcohol, other sleep-inducing drugs, OTC drugs while on this drug.
- Avoid prolonged exposure to sunlight or sunlamps; use a sunscreen or protective garments with prolonged exposure to sunlight.
- The following side effects may occur: headache, dizziness, drowsiness, weakness, blurred vision (reversible; if severe, avoid driving or performing tasks that require alertness); nausea, vomiting, loss of appetite, dry mouth (small frequent meals, frequent mouth care, and sucking sugarless candies may help); nightmares, inability to concentrate, confusion; changes in sexual function.
- Report dry mouth, difficulty in urination, excessive sedation.

d

# desmopressin acetate

*(des moe **press'** in)*

1-deamino-8-D-arginine vasopressin

DDAVP, Stimate

**Pregnancy Category B**

**Drug classes**

Hormone

**Therapeutic actions**

Synthetic analog of human ADH; promotes resorption of water in the renal tubule; increases levels of clotting factor VIII.

**Indications**

- DDAVP: neurogenic diabetes insipidus (not nephrogenic in origin; intranasal and parenteral); hemophilia A (with factor VIII levels >5%; parenteral); von Willebrand's disease (type I; parenteral); primary nocturnal enuresis (intranasal)
- Stimate: treatment of hemophilia A, von Willebrand's disease
- Unlabeled use: treatment of chronic autonomic failure (intranasal)

**Contraindications/cautions**

- Contraindications: allergy to desmopressin acetate; type II von Willebrand's disease.

- Use cautiously with vascular disease or hypertension, lactation, water intoxication, fluid and electrolyte imbalance.

## Dosage

**Available Forms:** Tablets—0.1, 0.2 mg; nasal solution—0.1 mg/ml DDAVP, 1.5 mg/ml Stimate; injection—4 μg/ml

ADULT

- ***Diabetes insipidus:*** 0.1–0.4 ml/d intranasally as a single dose or divided into two to three doses; 1 spray/nostril for total of 300 mg. 0.5–1.0 ml/d SC or IV, divided into two doses, adjusted to achieve a diurnal water turnover pattern, or 0.05 mg PO bid—adjust according to water turnover pattern.
- ***Hemophilia A or von Willebrand's disease:*** 0.3 μg/kg diluted in 50 ml sterile physiologic saline; infuse IV slowly over 15–30 min. If needed preoperatively, infuse 30 min before the procedure. Determine need for repeated administration based on patient reponse.

ADULT AND CHILDREN >6 Y

- ***Primary nocturnal enuresis:*** 20 μg (0.2 ml) intranasal hs. Up to 40 μg may be needed.

PEDIATRIC

- ***Diabetes insipidus (3 mo–12 y):*** 0.05–0.3 ml/d intranasally as a single dose or divided into two doses; 1 spray/nostril for total of 300 mg; or 0.05 mg PO qd—adjust according to water turnover pattern..
- ***Hemophilia A or von Willebrand's disease (10 kg or less):*** 0.3 μg/kg diluted in 10 ml of sterile physiologic saline. Infuse IV slowly over 15–30 min.

## Pharmacokinetics

| *Route* | *Onset* | *Peak* | *Duration* |
|---|---|---|---|
| Oral | 1 h | 1–1.5 h | 7 h |
| IV/SC | 30 min | 90–120 min | |
| Nasal | 15–60 min | 1–5 h | 5–21 h |

*Metabolism:* $T_{1/2}$: 7.8 min then 75.5 min
*Distribution:* Crosses placenta; enters breast milk

## IV facts

**Preparation:** Use drug as provided; refrigerate vial.
**Infusion:** Administer by direct IV injection over 1 min; infuse for hemophilia A or von Willebrand's disease over 15–30 min.

## Adverse effects

- CNS: Transient headache
- GI: Nausea, mild abdominal cramps
- CV: Slight elevation of BP, facial flushing (with high doses)
- GU: Vulval pain, fluid retention, water intoxication, hyponatremia (high doses)
- Local: *Local erythema, swelling, burning pain* (parenteral injection)

# ■ Nursing Considerations

## Assessment

- *History:* Allergy to desmopressin acetate; type II von Willebrand's disease; vascular disease or hypertension; lactation
- *Physical:* Nasal mucous membranes; skin color; P, BP, edema; R, adventitous sounds; bowel sounds, abdominal exam; urine volume and osmolality, plasma osmolality; factor VIII coagulant activity, skin bleeding times, factor VIII coagulant levels, factor VIII antigen and ristocetin cofactor levels (as appropriate)

## Implementation

- Refrigerate nasal solution and injection.
- Administer intranasally by drawing solution into the rhinyle or flexible calibrated plastic tube supplied with preparation. Insert one end of tube into nostril; blow on the other end to deposit solution deep into nasal cavity. Administer to infants, young children, or obtunded adults by using an air-filled syringe attached to the plastic tube. Spray form also available (1 spray/nostril).
- Monitor condition of nasal passages during long-term therapy; inappropriate administration can lead to nasal ulcerations.

- Monitor patients with CV diseases very carefully for cardiac reactions.
- Arrange to individualize dosage to establish a diurnal pattern of water turnover; estimate response by adequate duration of sleep and adequate, not excessive, water turnover.
- Monitor P and BP during infusion for hemophilia A or von Willebrand's disease. Monitor clinical response and lab reports to determine effectiveness of therapy and need for more desmopression or use of blood products.

### Drug-specific teaching points

- Administer intranasally by drawing solution into the rhinyle or flexible calibrated plastic tube supplied with preparation. Insert one end of tube into nostril; blow on the other end to deposit soluton deep into nasal cavity. Review proper administration technique for nasal use.
- The following side effects may occur: GI cramping, facial flushing, headache, nasal irritation (proper administration may decrease these problems).
- Report drowsiness, listlessness, headache, shortness of breath, heartburn, abdominal cramps, vulval pain, severe nasal congestion or irritation.

# Dexamethasone

## dexamethasone

*(dex a* ***meth'*** *a sone)*

*Oral, topical dermatologic aerosol and gel, ophthalmic suspension:* Aeroseb-Dex, Decadron, Dexasone (CAN), Dexone, Hexadrol, Maxidex Ophthalmic

## dexamethasone acetate

*IM, intra-articular, or soft-tissue injection:* Dalalone, Decadron-LA, Decaject-L.A., Desxasone-L.A., Dexone L.A., Solurex L.A.

## dexamethasone sodium phosphate

*IV, IM, intra-articular, intrlesional injection; respiratory inhalant; intranasal steroid; ophthalmic solution and ointment; topical dermatologic cream:* AK-Dex, Dalalone, Decadron Phosphate, Decadron Phosphate Ophthalmic, Decadron Phosphate Respihaler, Decaject, Dexasone, Dexone, Hexadrol Phosphate, Maxidex Ophthalmic, Solurex, Turbinaire Decadron Phosphate

**Pregnancy Category C**

### Drug classes

Corticosteroid
Glucocorticoid
Hormone

### Therapeutic actions

Enters target cells and binds to specific receptors, initiating many complex reactions that are responsible for its antiinflammatory and immunosuppressive effects.

### Indications

- Hypercalcemia associated with cancer
- Short-term management of various inflammatory and allergic disorders, such as rheumatoid arthritis, collagen diseases (SLE), dermatologic diseases (pemphigus), status asthmaticus, and autoimmune disorders
- Hematologic disorders: thrombocytopenic purpura, erythroblastopenia
- Trichinosis with neurologic or myocardial involvement
- Ulcerative colitis, acute exacerbations of multiple sclerosis, and palliation in some leukemias and lymphomas
- Cerebral edema associated with brain tumor, craniotomy, or head injury
- Testing adrenocortical hyperfunction
- Unlabeled uses: Antiemetic for cisplatin-induced vomiting, diagnosis of depression
- **Intra-articular or soft-tissue administration:** Arthritis, psoriatic plaques
- **Respiratory inhalant:** Control of bronchial asthma requiring corticosteroids in conjunction with other therapy

- **Intranasal:** Relief of symptoms of seasonal or perennial rhinitis that responds poorly to other treatments
- **Dermatologic preparations:** Relief of inflammatory and pruritic manifestations of dermatoses that are steroid-responsive
- **Ophthalmic preparations:** Inflammation of the lid, conjunctiva, cornea, and globe

## Contraindications/cautions

- Contraindications: infections, especially tuberculosis, fungal infections, amebiasis, vaccinia and varicella, and antibiotic-resistant infections.
- Use cautiously with renal or hepatic disease; hypothyroidism, ulcerative colitis with impending perforation; diverticulitis; active or latent peptic ulcer; inflammatory bowel disease; CHF, hypertension, thromboembolic disorders; osteoporosis; convulsive disorders; diabetes mellitus; lactation.

## Dosage

**Available Forms:** Tablets—0.25, 0.5, 0.75, 1, 1.5, 2, 4, 6 mg; elixir—0.5 mg/5ml; oral solution—0.5 mg/5ml; injection—8 mg/ml, 16 mg/ml, 4 mg/ml, 10 mg/ml, 20 mg/ml, 24 mg/ml; aerosol—84 μg/actuation; ophthalmic solution—0.1%; ophthalmic suspension—0.1%; ophthalmic ointment—0.05%; topical ointment—0.05%; topical cream 0.05%, 0.1%; topical aerosol—0.01%, 0.04%

***Systemic Administration***

- ADULT: Individualize dosage, based on severity of condition and response. Give daily dose before 9 AM to minimize adrenal suppression. If long-term therapy is needed, alternate-day therapy with a short-acting steroid should be considered. After long-term therapy, withdraw drug slowly to avoid adrenal insufficiency. For maintenance therapy, reduce initial dose in small increments at intervals until the lowest clinically satisfactory dose is reached.
- PEDIATRIC: Individualize dosage, based on severity of condition and response, rather than by strict adherence to formulas that correct adult doses for age or body weight. Carefully observe growth and development in infants and children on long-term therapy.

***Oral (dexamethasone, oral):*** 0.75–9.0 mg/d.

- *Suppression tests: For Cushing's syndrome:* 1 mg at 11 PM; assay plasma cortisol at 8 PM the next day. For greater accuracy, give 0.5 mg q6h for 48 h, and collect 24-h urine to determine 17-OH-corticosteroid excretion. *Test to distinguish Cushing's syndrome due to ACTH excess from that resulting from other causes:* 2 mg q6h for 48 h. Collect 24-h urine to determine 17-OH-corticosteroid excretion.

***IM (dexamethasone acetate):*** 8–16 mg; may repeat in 1–3 wk. Dexamethasone phosphate: 0.5–0.9 mg/d; usual dose range is one-third to one-half the oral dose.

***IV (dexamethasone sodium phosphate):*** 0.5–9.0 mg/d.

- *Cerebral edema:* 10 mg IV and then 4 mg IM q6h; change to oral therapy, 1–3 mg tid, as soon as possible and taper over 5–7 d.
- PEDIATRIC
  - *Unresponsive shock:* 1–6 mg/kg as a single IV injection (as much as 40 mg initially followed by repeated injections q2–6h has been reported).
  - *Dexamethasone acetate:* 4–16 mg intra-articular, soft tissue; 0.8–1.6 mg intralesional.
  - *Dexamethasone sodium phosphate:* 0.4–6.0 mg (depending on joint or soft-tissue injection site).

***Respiratory Inhalant (Dexamethasone Sodium Phosphate) (84 μg released with each actuation).***

- ADULT: 3 inhalations tid–qid, not to exceed 12 inhalations/d.
- PEDIATRIC: 2 inhalations tid–qid, not to exceed 8 inhalations/d.

***Intranasal (Dexamethasone Sodium Phosphate) (Each spray delivers 84 μg dexamethasone).***

- ADULT: 2 sprays (168 μg) into each nostril bid–tid, not to exceed 12 sprays (1,008 μg)/d.

- *PEDIATRIC:* 1 or 2 sprays (84–168 μg) into each nostril bid, depending on age, not to exceed 8 sprays (672 μg). Arrange to reduce dose and discontinue therapy as soon as possible.

***Topical Dermatologic Preparations:*** Apply sparingly to affected area bid–qid.

***Ophthalmic Solutions/Suspensions:*** Instill 1–2 drops into the conjunctival sac q1h during the day and q2h during the night; after a favorable response, reduce dose to 1 drop q4h and then 1 drop tid–qid.

***Ophthalmic Ointment:*** Apply a thin coating in the lower conjunctival sac tid–qid; reduce dosage to bid and then qid after improvement.

## Pharmacokinetics

| *Route* | *Onset* | *Peak* | *Duration* |
|---|---|---|---|
| Oral | Slow | 1–2 h | 2–3 d |
| IM | Rapid | 30–60 min | 2–3 d |
| IV | Rapid | 30–60 min | 2–3 d |

*Metabolism:* Hepatic; $T_{1/2}$: 110–210 min
*Distribution:* Crosses placenta; enters breast milk
*Excretion:* Urine

## IV facts

**Preparation:** No preparation required.
**Infusion:** Administer by slow, direct IV injection over 1 min.

## Adverse effects

Adverse effects depend on dose, route, and duration of therapy. The first list is primarily associated with absorption; the list following is related to specific routes of administration.

- CNS: Convulsions, *vertigo*, *headaches*, pseudotumor cerebri, *euphoria*, *insomnia*, *mood swings*, *depression*, psychosis, intracerebral hemorrhage, reversible cerebral atrophy in infants, cataracts, increased intraocular pressure, glaucoma
- GI: Peptic or esophageal ulcer, pancreatitis, abdominal distention
- CV: *Hypertension*, CHF, necrotizing angiitis
- Hematologic: *Fluid and electrolyte disturbances*, negative nitrogen balance, increased blood sugar, glycosuria, increased serum cholesterol, decreased serum $T_3$ and $T_4$ levels
- GU: *Amenorrhea*, *irregular menses*
- MS: *Muscle weakness*, steroid myopathy, loss of muscle mass, osteoporosis, spontaneous fractures
- Endocrine: Growth retardation, decreased carbohydrate tolerance, diabetes mellitus, cushingoid state, *secondary adrenocortical and pituitary unresponsiveness*
- Hypersensitivity: Anaphylactoid or hypersensitivity reactions
- Other: *Impaired wound healing; petechiae; ecchymoses; increased sweating; thin and fragile skin; acne; immunosuppression and masking of signs of infection*; activation of latent infections, including tuberculosis, fungal, and viral eye infections; pneumonia; abscess; septic infection; GI and GU infections

*Intra-articular*

- Musculoskeletal: Osteonecrosis, tendon rupture, infection

*Intralesional Therapy*

- CNS: Blindness (when used on face and head—rare)

*Respiratory Inhalant*

- Respiratory: Oral, laryngeal, pahryngeal irritation
- Endocrine: Suppression of HPA function due to systemic absorption
- Other: Fungal infections

*Intranasal*

- CNS: Headache
- GI: Nausea
- Respiratory: Nasal irritation, fungal infections, epistaxis, rebound congestion, perforation of the nasal septum, anosmia
- Dermatologic: Urticaria
- Endocrine: suppression of HPA function due to systemic absorption

*Topical Dermatologic Ointments, Creams, Sprays*

- Local: Local burning, irritation, acneiform lesions, striae, skin atrophy

- **Endocrine**: Suppression of HPA function due to systemic absorption, growth retardation in children (children may be at special risk for systemic absorption because of their large skin surface area to body weight ratio)

*Ophthalmic Preparations*

- **Local**: Infections, especially fungal; glaucoma, cataracts with long-term use
- **Endocrine**: Suppression of HPA function due to systemic absorption; more common with long-term use

## Clinically important drug-drug interactions

• Increased therapeutic and toxic effects of cortisone with troleandomycin • Decreased effects of anticholinesterases with corticotropin; profound muscular depression is possible • Decreased steroid blood levels with phenytoin, phenobarbital, rifampin • Decreased serum levels of salicylates with cortisone.

## Drug-lab test interferences

• False-negative nitroblue-tetrazolium test for bacterial infection • Suppression of skin test reactions

# ■ Nursing Considerations

### Assessment

- ***History for systemic administration***: Active infections; renal or hepatic disease; hypothyroidism, ulcerative colitis; diverticulitis; active or latent peptic ulcer; inflammatory bowel disease; CHF, hypertension, thromboembolic disorders; osteoporosis; convulsive disorders; diabetes mellitus; lactation.
- ***For ophthalmic preparations:*** Acute superficial herpes simplex keratitis, fungal infections of ocular structures; vaccinia, varicella, and other viral diseases of the cornea and conjunctiva; ocular tuberculosis.
- ***Physical for systemic administration***: Baseline body weight, temperature; reflexes, and grip strength, affect, and orientation; P, BP, peripheral perfusion, prominence of superficial veins; R and adventitious sounds; serum electrolytes, blood glucose. *For topical dermatologic preparations:* Affected area for infections, skin injury

### Implementation

- *For systemic administration:* Do not give drug to nursing mothers; drug is secreted in breast milk.
- Give daily doses before 9 AM to mimic normal peak corticosteroid blood levels.
- Increase dosage when patient is subject to stress.
- Taper doses when discontinuing high-dose or long-term therapy.
- Do not give live virus vaccines with immunosuppressive doses of corticosteroids.
- *For respiratory inhalant, intranasal preparation:* Do not use respiratory inhalant during an acute asthmatic attack or to manage status asthmaticus.
- Do not use intranasal product with untreated local nasal infections, epistaxis, nasal trauma, septal ulcers, or recent nasal surgery.
- Taper systemic steroids carefully during transfer to inhalational steroids; adrenal insufficiency deaths have occurred.
- *For topical dermatologic preparations:* Use caution when occlusive dressings, tight diapers; cover affected area; these can increase systemic absorption.
- Avoid prolonged use near the eyes, in genital and rectal areas, and in skin creases.

### Drug-specific teaching points

- *For systemic administration:* Do not stop taking the drug (oral) without consulting health care provider.
- Avoid exposure to infection.
- Report unusual weight gain, swelling of the extremities, muscle weakness, black or tarry stools, fever, prolonged sore throat, colds or other infections, worsening of this disorder.
- *For intra-articular administration:* Do not overuse joint after therapy, even if pain is gone.
- *For respiratory inhalant, intranasal preparation:* Do not use more often than prescribed.
- Do not stop using this drug without consulting health care provider.

- Use the inhalational bronchodilator drug before using the oral inhalant product when using both.
- Administer decongestant nose drops first if nasal passages are blocked.
- *For topical dermatologic preparations:* Apply the drug sparingly.
- Avoid contact with eyes.
- Report any irritation or infection at the site of application.
- *For ophthalmic preparations:* Administer as follows: Lie down or tilt head backward and look at ceiling. Warm tube of ointment in hand for several minutes. Apply 1/4–1/2 inch of ointment, or drop suspension inside lower eyelid while looking up. After applying ointment, close eyelids and roll eyeball in all directions. After instilling eye drops, release lower lid, but do not blink for at least 30 sec; apply gentle pressure to the inside corner of the eye for 1 min. Do not close eyes tightly, and try not to blink more often than usual; do not touch ointment tube or dropper to eye, fingers, or any surface.
- Wait at least 10 min before using any other eye preparations.
- Eyes will become more sensitive to light (use sunglasses).
- Report worsening of the condition, pain, itching, swelling of the eye, failure of the condition to improve after 1 wk.

## dexchlorpheniramine maleate

*(dex klor fen ir' a meen)*

Dexchlor, Poladex, Polaramine

**Pregnancy Category B**

### Drug classes
Antihistamine (alkylamine type)

### Therapeutic actions
Blocks the effects of histamine at $H_1$ receptor sites, has atropine-like, antipruritic, and sedative effects.

### Indications
- Relief of symptoms associated with perennial and seasonal allergic rhinitis; vasomotor rhinitis; allergic conjunctivitis; mild, uncomplicated urticaria and angioedema; amelioraton of allergic reactions to blood or plasma; dermatographism; adjunctive therapy in anaphylactic reactions

### Contraindications/cautions
- Contraindications: allergy to any antihistamines, narrow-angle glaucoma, stenosing peptic ulcer, symptomatic prostatic hypertrophy, asthmatic attack, bladder neck obstruction, pyloroduodenal obstruction, third trimester of pregnancy, lactation.
- Use cautiously with pregnancy.

### Dosage
**Available Forms:** Tablets—2 mg; TR tablets—4, 6 mg; syrup—2 mg/5ml

**ADULT AND PEDIATRIC > 12 Y:** 2 mg q4–6h PO, or 4–6 mg repeat-action tablets at bedtime PO or q8–10h PO during the day.

**PEDIATRIC**

- *6–11 y:* 1 mg q4–6h PO or 4 mg repeat-action tablet once daily at hs; 2–5 y: 0.5 mg q4–6h PO; do not use repeat-action tablets.

**GERIATRIC:** More likely to cause dizziness, sedation, syncope, toxic confusional states, and hypotension in elderly patients; use with caution.

### Pharmacokinetics

| *Route* | *Onset* | *Peak* |
|---|---|---|
| Oral | 15–30 min | 3 h |

*Metabolism:* Hepatic; $T_{1/2}$: 12–15 h

*Distribution:* Crosses placenta; enters breast milk

*Excretion:* Urine

### Adverse effects
- CNS: *Drowsiness, sedation, dizziness, disturbed coordination*, fatigue, confusion, restlessness, excitation, nervousness, tremor, headache, blurred vision, diplopia, vertigo, tinnitus, acute labryinthitis, hysteria, tingling, heaviness and weakness of the hands

- GI: *Epigastric distress,* anorexia, increased appetite and weight gain, nausea, vomiting, diarrhea or constipation
- CV: Hypotension, palpitations, bradycardia, tachycardia, extrasystoles
- **Respiratory:** *Thickening of bronchial secretions,* chest tightness, wheezing, nasal stuffiness, dry mouth, dry nose, dry throat, sore throat
- **Hematologic:** Hemolytic anemia, hypoplastic anemia, thrombocytopenia, leukopenia, agranulocytosis, pancytopenia
- GU: Urinary frequency, dysuria, urinary retention, early menses, decreased libido
- **Other:** Urticaria, rash, anaphylactic shock, photosensitivity, excessive perspiration

### Clinically important drug-drug interactions

- Increased depressant effects with alcohol, other CNS depressants

## ■ Nursing Considerations

### Assessment

- ***History:*** Allergy to any antihistamines; narrow-angle glaucoma, stenosing peptic ulcer, symptomatic prostatic hypertrophy, asthmatic attack, bladder neck obstruction, pyloroduodenal obstruction, pregnancy, lactation
- ***Physical:*** Skin color, lesions, texture; orientation, reflexes, affect; vision exam; P, BP; R, adventitious sounds; bowel sounds; prostate palpation; CBC with differential

### Implementation

- Administer with food if GI upset occurs.
- Administer syrup form if patient is unable to take tablets.
- Monitor patient response, and adjust dosage to lowest possible effective dose.

### Drug-specific teaching points

- Take as prescribed; avoid excessive dosage. Take with food if GI upset occurs; do not crush or chew the sustained-release preparations.
- The following side effects may occur: dizziness, sedation, drowsiness (use caution driving or performing tasks that require alertness); epigastric distress, diarrhea, or constipation (take with meals); dry mouth (frequent mouth care, sucking sugarless lozenges may help); thickening of bronchial secretions, dryness of nasal mucosa (use a humidifier).
- Avoid alcohol; serious sedation can occur.
- Report difficulty breathing; hallucinations, tremors, loss of coordination; unusual bleeding or bruising; visual disturbances; irregular heartbeat.

## dexpanthenol

*(dex **pan'** the nole)*

dextropantothenyl alcohol

Ilopan

**Pregnancy Category C**

### Drug classes

GI stimulant

### Therapeutic actions

Mechanism is unknown; is the alcohol analog of pantothenic acid, a cofactor in the synthesis of the neurotransmitter acetylcholine; acetylcholine is the transmitter released by parasympathetic postganglionic nerves; the parasympathetic nervous system provides stimulation to maintain intestinal function.

### Indications

- Prophylactic use immediately after major abdominal surgery to minimize paralytic ileus, intestinal atony causing abdominal distention.
- Treatment of intestinal atony causing abdominal distention; postoperative or postpartum retention of flatus; postoperative delay in resumption of intestinal motility; paralytic ileus

### Contraindications/cautions

- Allergy to dexpanthenol, hemophilia, ileus due to mechanical obstruction, lactation.

### Dosage

**Available Forms:** Injection—250 mg/ml

*ADULT*

- ***Prevention of postoperative adynamic ileus:*** 250–500 mg IM; repeat in 2 h, then q6h until danger of adynamic ileus has passed.
- ***Treatment of adynamic ileus:*** 500 mg IM; repeat in 2 h, then q6h as needed.
  - ***IV administration:*** 500 mg diluted in IV solutions.

*PEDIATRIC:* Safety and efficacy not established.

**Pharmacokinetics**

| *Route* | *Onset* | *Peak* |
|---|---|---|
| IM | Rapid | 4 h |

*Metabolism:* Hepatic; $T_{1/2}$: unknown
*Distribution:* Crosses placenta; enters breast milk
*Excretion:* Urine and feces

**IV facts**

**Preparation:** Dilute with bulk solutions of glucose or Lactated Ringer's.
**Infusion:** Infuse slowly over 3–6 h. Do not administer by direct IV injection.

**Adverse effects**

- GI: *Intestinal colic* (1/2 h after administration), *nausea, vomiting; diarrhea*
- CV: *slight drop in blood pressure*
- Respiratory: Dyspnea
- Dermatologic: Itching, tingling, red patches of skin, generalized dermatitis, urticaria

## ■ Nursing Considerations

### Assessment

- *History:* Allergy to dexpanthenol, hemophilia, ileus due to mechanical obstruction, lactation.
- *Physical:* Skin color, lesions, texture; P, BP; bowel sounds, normal output

### Implementation

- Monitor BP carefully during IV administration.

### Drug-specific teaching points

Teaching about this drug should be incorporated into the overall postoperative or postpartum teaching. Intestinal colic may occur within 1/2 h of administration.

- The following side effects may occur: nausea, vomiting, diarrhea, itching, skin rash.
- Report difficulty breathing, severe itching, or rash.

d

# dextran, high molecular weight

*(dex' tran)*

Dextran 70, Dextran 75, Gendex 75, Gentran 70, Macrodex

**Pregnancy Category C**

**Drug classes**

Plasma volume expander
nonbacteriostatic

**Therapeutic actions**

Synthetic polysaccharide used to approximate the colloidal properties of albumin.

**Indications**

- Adjunctive therapy for treatment of shock or impending shock due to hemorrhage, burns, surgery, or trauma; to be used only in emergency situations when blood or blood products are not available

**Contraindications/cautions**

- Allergy to dextran (dextran 1 can be used prophylactically in patients known to be allergic to clinical dextran); marked hemostatic defects (risk for increased bleeding effects); severe cardiac congestion; renal failure or anuria.

### Dosage

**Available Forms:** Injection—6% dextran 75 in 0.9% sodium chloride, 6% dextran 70 in 0.9% sodium chloride, 6% dextran 75 in 5% dextrose, 6% dextran 70 in 5% dextrose

*ADULT:* 500 ml, given at a rate of 24–40 ml/min IV as an emergency procedure. Do not exceed 20 ml/kg the first 24 h of treatment.

*PEDIATRIC:* Determine dosage by body weight or surface area of the patient. Do not exceed 20 ml/kg IV.

**Pharmacokinetics**

| *Route* | *Onset* | *Peak* | *Duration* |
|---|---|---|---|
| IV | Minutes | Minutes | 12 h |

*Metabolism:* Hepatic; $T_{1/2}$: 24 h
*Distribution:* Crosses placenta; enters breast milk
*Excretion:* Urine

**IV facts**

**Preparation:** Administer in unit provided. Discard any partially used containers. Do not use unless the solution is clear.
**Infusion:** Infuse at rate of 20–40 ml/min.

**Adverse effects**

- GI: Nausea, vomiting
- Hematologic: *Hypervolemia, coagulation problems*
- Hypersensitivity: Urticaria, nasal congestion, wheezing, tightness of chest, mild hypotension (antihistamines may be helpful in relieving these symptoms)
- Local: Infection at injection site, extravasation
- Other: Fever, joint pains

**Drug-lab test interferences**

• Falsely elevated blood glucose assays • Interference with bilirubin assays in which alcohol is used, with total protein assays using biuret reagent • Blood typing and cross-matching procedures using enzyme techniques may give unreliable readings; draw blood samples before giving infusion of dextran

## ■ Nursing Considerations

### Assessment

- *History:* Allergy to dextran; marked hemostatic defects; severe cardiac congestion; renal failure or anuria
- *Physical:* T; skin color, lesions; P, BP, adventitious sounds, peripheral edema; R, adventitious sounds; urinalysis, renal and liver function tests, clotting times, PT, PTT, Hgb, Hct, urine output

### Implementation

- Administer by IV infusion only; monitor rates based on patient response.
- Do not give more than recommended dose.
- Use only clear solutions. Discard partially used containers; solution contains no bacteriostat.
- Monitor patients carefully for any sign of hypervolemia or the development of CHF; supportive measures may be needed.

### Drug-specific teaching points

- Report difficulty breathing, skin rash, unusual bleeding or bruising, pain at IV site.

# dextran, low molecular weight

***(dex' tran)***

Dextran 40, Gentran 40, 10% LMD, Rheomacrodex

**Pregnancy Category C**

**Drug classes**

Plasma volume expander nonbacteriostatic

**Therapeutic actions**

Synthetic polysaccharide used to approximate the colloidal properties of albumin.

**Indications**

- Adjunctive therapy for treatment of shock or impending shock due to hemorrhage, burns, surgery or trauma
- Priming fluid in pump oxygenators during extracorporeal circulation
- Prophylaxis against deep vein thrombosis (DVT) and pulmonary emboli (PE) in patients undergoing procedures known to be associated with a high incidence of thromboembolic complications, such as hip surgery

**Contraindications/cautions**

- Allergy to dextran (dextran 1 can be used prophylactically in patients known to be allergic to clinical dextran); marked hemostatic defects; severe cardiac congestion; renal failure or anuria.

### Dosage

**Available Forms:** Injection—10% dextran 40 in 0.9% sodium chloride, 10% dextran 40 in 5% dextrose

ADULT

- ***Adjunctive therapy in shock:*** Total dosage of 20 ml/kg IV in first 24 h. The first 10 ml/kg should be infused rapidly, the remaining dose administered slowly. Beyond 24 h, total daily dosage should not exceed 10 ml/kg. Do not continue therapy for more than 5 d.
- ***Hemodiluent in extracorporeal circulation:*** Generally 10–20 ml/kg are added to perfusion circuit. Do not exceed a total dosage of 20 ml/kg.
- ***Prophylaxis therapy for DVT, PE:*** 500–1,000 ml IV on day of surgery, continue treatment at dose of 500 ml/d for an additional 2–3 d. Thereafter, based on procedure and risk, 500 ml may be administered every second to third day for up to 2 wk.

### Pharmacokinetics

| *Route* | *Onset* | *Peak* | *Duration* |
|---|---|---|---|
| IV | Immediate | Minutes | 12 h |

*Metabolism:* Hepatic; $T_{1/2}$: 3 h
*Distribution:* Crosses placenta; enters breast milk
*Excretion:* Urine

### IV facts

**Preparation:** Protect from freezing. Use in bottles provided, no further preparation necessary.
**Infusion:** Administer first 10 ml rapidly, remainder of solution slowly over 8–24 h, monitoring patient response.

### Adverse effects

- GI: Nausea, vomiting
- CV: Hypotension, anaphylactoid shock, *hypervolemia*
- Hypersensitivity: Ranging from mild cutaneous eruptions to generalized urticaria
- Local: Infection at site of injection, extravasation, venous thrombosis or phlebitis
- Other: Headache, fever, wheezing

### Drug-lab test interferences

- Falsely elevated blood glucose assays
- Interference with bilirubin assays in which alcohol is used, with total protein assays using biuret reagent • Blood typing and cross-matching procedures using enzyme techniques may give unreliable readings; draw blood samples before giving infusion of dextran

## ■ Nursing Considerations

### Assessment

- ***History:*** Allergy to dextran; marked hemostatic defects; severe cardiac congestion; renal failure or anuria; lactation
- ***Physical:*** T; skin color, lesions; P, BP, adventitious sounds, peripheral edema; R, adventitious sounds; urinalysis, renal and liver function tests, clotting times, PT, PTT, Hgb, Hct, urine output

### Implementation

- Administer by IV infusion only; monitor rates based on patient response.
- Do not administer more than recommended dose.
- Monitor urinary output carefully; if no increase in output is noted after 500 ml of dextran, discontinue drug until diuresis can be induced by other means.
- Monitor patients carefully for signs of hypervolemia or development of CHF; slow rate or discontinue drug if rapid CVP increase occurs.

### Drug-specific teaching points

- Report difficulty breathing, skin rash, unusual bleeding or bruising, pain at IV site.

## dextroamphetamine sulfate

*(dex troe am* ***fet'*** *a meen)*
Dexedrine
**Pregnancy Category C**
**C-II controlled substance**

## Drug classes
Amphetamine
Anorexiant
Central nervous system stimulant

## Therapeutic actions
Acts in the CNS to release norepinephrine from nerve terminals; in higher doses also releases dopamine; suppressess appetite; increases alertness, elevates mood; often improves physical performance, especially when fatigue and sleep-deprivation have caused impairment; efficacy in hyperkinetic syndrome, attention-deficit disorders in children appears paradoxical and is not understood.

## Indications
- Narcolepsy
- Adjunct therapy for abnormal behavioral syndrome in children (attention-deficit disorder, hyperkinetic syndrome) that includes psychological, social, educational measures
- Exogenous obesity, short-term adjunct to caloric restriction in patients refractory to alternative therapy

## Contraindications/cautions
- Hypersensitivity to sympathomimetic amines, tartrazine (Dexedrine); advanced arteriosclerosis, symptomatic CV disease, moderate to severe hypertension, hyperthyroidism, glaucoma, agitated states, history of drug abuse; pregnancy; lactation.

## Dosage
**Available Forms:** Tablets—5, 10 mg; SR capsules—5, 10, 15 mg

### ADULT
- *Narcolepsy:* Start with 10 mg/d PO in divided doses; increase in increments of 10 mg/d at weekly intervals. If insomnia, anorexia occur, reduce dose. Usual dosage is 5–60 mg/d PO in divided doses. Give first dose on awakening, additional doses (1 or 2) q4–6h; long-acting forms can be given once a day.
- *Exogenous obesity:* 5–30 mg/d PO in divided doses of 5–10 mg, 30–60 min before meals. *Long-acting form:* 10–15 mg in the morning.

### PEDIATRIC
- *Narcolepsy*
  - *6–12 Y:* Condition is rare in children < 12 y; when it does occur, initial dose is 5 mg/d PO. Increase in increments of 5 mg at weekly intervals until optimal response is obtained.
  - *12 Y OR OLDER:* Use adult dosage.
- *Attention-deficit disorder*
  - *<3 Y:* Not recommended.
  - *3–5 Y:* 2.5 mg/d PO. Increase in increments of 2.5 mg/d at weekly intervals until optimal response is obtained.
  - *6 Y OR OLDER:* 5 mg PO qd–bid. Increase in increments of 5 mg/d at weekly intervals until optimal response is obtained. Dosage will rarely exceed 40 mg/d. Give first dose on awakening, additional doses (1 or 2) q4–6h. Long-acting forms may be used once a day.
- *Obesity:* Not recommended for children < 12 y.

## Pharmacokinetics

| *Route* | *Onset* | *Peak* | *Duration* |
|---|---|---|---|
| Oral | Rapid | 1–5 h | 8–10 h |

*Metabolism:* Hepatic; $T_{1/2}$: 10–30 h
*Distribution:* Crosses placenta; enters breast milk
*Excretion:* Urine

## Adverse effects
- CNS: *Overstimulation, restlessness, dizziness, insomnia*, dyskinesia, euphoria, dysphoria, tremor, headache, psychotic episodes
- GI: *Dry mouth, unpleasant taste, diarrhea*, constipation, anorexia and weight loss
- CV: *Palpitations, tachycardia, hypertension*
- GU: Impotence, changes in libido
- **Dermatologic**: Urticaria
- **Endocrine**: Reversible elevations in serum thyroxine with heavy use
- **Other**: Tolerance, psychological dependence, social disability with abuse

**Clinically important drug-drug interactions**

• Hypertensive crisis and increased CNS effects if given within 14 d of monoamine oxidase inhibitors (MAOIs); DO NOT GIVE DEXTROAMPHETAMINE to patients who are taking or who have recently taken MAOIs • Increased duration of effects if taken with urinary alkalinizers, (acetazolamide, sodium bicarbonate), furazolidone • Decreased effects if taken with urinary acidifiers • Decreased efficacy of antihypertensive drugs (guanethidine) given with amphetamines

## ■ Nursing Considerations

### Assessment

- *History:* Hypersensitivity to sympathomimetic amines, tartrazine; advanced arteriosclerosis, symptomatic CV disease, moderate to severe hypertension, hyperthyroidism, glaucoma, agitated states, history of drug abuse; lactation.
- *Physical:* Weight; T; skin color, lesions; orientation, affect, ophthalmic exam (tonometry); P, BP, auscultation; R, adventitious sounds; bowel sounds, normal output; thyroid function tests, blood and urine glucose, baseline ECG

### Implementation

- Ensure proper diagnosis before administering to children for behavioral syndromes: drug should not be used until other causes (learning disability, EEG abnormalities, neurologic deficits) are ruled out.
- Interrupt drug dosage periodically in children being treated for behavioral disorders to determine if symptomatic response still validates drug therapy.
- Monitor growth of children on long-term amphetamine therapy.
- Discontinue use of amphetamines as anorexiants if tolerance develops; do not increase dosage.
- Dispense the lowest feasible dose to minimize risk of overdosage.
- Give drug early in the day to prevent insomnia.
- Monitor BP frequently early in therapy.
- Monitor obese diabetics taking amphetamines closely, adjust insulin dosage.

### Drug-specific teaching points

- Take this drug exactly as prescribed. This drug has short-term efficacy for weight loss. Do not increase the dosage without consulting your physician. If the drug appears ineffective, consult your health care provider.
- Do not crush or chew sustained-release or long-acting tablets.
- Take drug early in the day (especially sustained-release preparations) to avoid insomnia.
- Avoid pregnancy while on this drug. This drug can cause harm to the fetus.
- The following side effects may occur: nervousness, restlessness, dizziness, insomnia, impaired thinking (may diminish in a few days; avoid driving or engaging in activities that require alertness); headache, loss of appetite, dry mouth.
- Report nervousness, insomnia, dizziness, palpitations, anorexia (except in patients taking drug for this effect), GI disturbances.

d

## dextromethorphan hydrobromide

*(dex troe meth or' fan)*

Benylin DM, Delsym, Demo-Cineal (CAN), Hold, Koffex (CAN), Pedia Care, Pertussin, Robidex (CAN), Scot Tussin Cough, St. Joseph Cough, Sedatuss (CAN), Sucrets Cough Control

**Pregnancy Category C**

### Drug classes

Nonnarcotic antitussive

### Therapeutic actions

Lacks analgesic and addictive properties; controls cough spasms by depressing the cough center in the medulla; analog of codeine.

### Indications

- Control of nonproductive cough

### Contraindications/cautions

- Hypersensitivity to any component (check label of products for flavorings, vehicles); sensitivity to bromides; cough that persists for more than 1 wk, tends to recur, is accompanied by excessive secretions, high fever, rash, nausea, vomiting, or persistent headache (dextromethorphan should not be used; patient should consult a physician); lactation

### Dosage

**Available Forms:** Lozenges—2.5, 5, 7.5 mg; liquid—3.5, 7.5, 15 mg/5 ml; syrup—10 mg/5 ml; sustained action liquid—30 mg/5 ml

ADULT

- *Lozenges, syrup and chewy squares:* 10–30 mg q4–8h PO. Do not exceed 120 mg/24 h.
- *Sustained action liquid:* 60 mg bid PO.

PEDIATRIC

- *CHILDREN >12 Y:* As for adults.
- *Lozenges, syrup, and chewy squares*
  - *CHILDREN 6–12 Y:* 5–10 mg q4h PO or 15 mg q6–8h. Do not exceed 60 mg/24 h.
- *Sustained-action liquid:* 30 mg bid PO.
- *Syrup and chewy squares*
  - *CHILDREN 2–6 Y:* 2.5–7.5 mg q4–8h PO. Do not exceed 30 mg/24 h. Do not give lozenges to this age group.
- *Sustained-action liquid:* 15 mg bid PO.
  - *CHILDREN < 2 Y:* Use only as directed by a physician.

### Pharmacokinetics

| *Route* | *Onset* | *Peak* | *Duration* |
|---|---|---|---|
| Oral | 15–30 min | 2 h | 3–6 h |

*Metabolism:* Hepatic; $T_{1/2}$: 2–4 h
*Distribution:* Crosses placenta; enters breast milk
*Excretion:* Urine

### Adverse effects

- Respiratory: **Respiratory depression (with overdose)**

## ■ Nursing Considerations

### Assessment

- ***History:*** Hypersensitivity to any component; sensitivity to bromides; cough that persists for more than 1 wk or is accompanied by excessive secretions, high fever, rash, nausea, vomiting, or persistent headache; lactation
- ***Physical:*** T; R, adventitious sounds

### Implementation

- Ensure drug is used only as recommended. Coughs may be symptomatic of a serious underlying disorder that should be diagnosed and properly treated; drug may mask symptoms of serious disease.

### Drug-specific teaching points

- Take this drug exactly as prescribed. Do not take more than or for longer than recommended.
- Report continued or recurring cough, cough accompanied by fever, rash, persistent headache, nausea, vomiting.

## dextrothyroxine sodium

*(dex troe thye **rox'** een)*

Choloxin

**Pregnancy Category C**

### Drug classes

Antihyperlipidemic

### Therapeutic actions

Stimulates the liver to increase the breakdown and excretion of cholesterol into the bile and feces; lowers the serum cholesterol and LDLs.

### Indications

- Adjunct to diet and other measures to reduce elevated serum cholesterol in euthyroid patients with no known CV disease

### Contraindications/cautions

- Contraindications: history of organic heart disease, cardiac arrhythmias, rheu-

matic heart disease, CHF, hypertension, advanced liver or renal disease, pregnancy, lactation, allergy to tartrazine.
- Use cautiously with impaired renal or hepatic function; pending surgery (discontinue at least 2 wk before surgery).

### Dosage

**Available Forms:** Tablets—2, 4 mg

*ADULT:* 1–2 mg/d PO; increase by 1–2 mg at intervals of not less than 1 mo to a maximum of 4–8 mg/d.

- *Maintenance:* 4–8 mg/d PO.

*PEDIATRIC:* 0.05 mg/kg per day PO; increase in up to 0.05 mg/kg per day increments at monthly intervals to a maximum of 0.4 mg/kg per day or 4 mg/d. *Maintenance:* 0.1 mg/kg per day.

### Pharmacokinetics

| Route | Onset |
|---|---|
| Oral | Gradual |

*Metabolism:* Hepatic; $T_{1/2}$: 18 h

*Distribution:* Crosses placenta; enters breast milk

*Excretion:* Urine and feces

### Adverse effects

- CNS: Insomnia, nervousness, tremors, headache, tinnitis, dizziness, visual disturbances, exophthalmos, retinopathy, lid lag
- GI: Dyspepsia, nausea, vomiting, constipation, diarrhea, anorexia, weight loss
- CV: Angina, arrhythmias, ischemic myocardial changes, *MI*
- Dermatologic: Hair loss, skin rash, itching
- Other: sweating, flushing, hyperthermia, changes in libido, edema

### Clinically important drug-drug interactions

• Increased bleeding effects with oral anticoagulants • Increased effects and accumulation of theophyllines with dextrothyroxine • Alteration in serum levels of digitalis glycosides • Increased CNS stimulation when taken with TCAs • Risk of increased drug effects if taken with thyroid hormones

## ■ Nursing Considerations

### Assessment

- ***History:*** Allergy to tartrazine, history of organic heart disease, cardiac arrhythmias, rheumatic heart disease, CHF, hypertension, liver or renal disease, pregnancy, lactation, scheduled surgery.
- ***Physical:*** Weight; T; skin color, lesions, hair; reflexes, orientation, eye exam; cardiac evaluation, ECG, liver evaluation; liver and renal function tests, serum cholesterol, LDLs

### Implementation

- Arrange for lab tests of serum cholesterol and fractionated lipids before beginning therapy and frequently during therapy.
- Discontinue drug at least 2 wk before scheduled surgery; notify surgeon of drug therapy in emergency surgery.
- Discontinue drug and notify physician if any signs of cardiac disease develop.

### Drug-specific teaching points

- Take drug as prescribed; monthly blood tests will be needed to monitor your response and adjust dosage.
- The following side effects may occur: loss of appetite, nausea, vomiting (eat small, frequent meals); rash, loss of hair (reversible); dizziness, nervousness, tremors, visual disturbances (use caution driving or operating dangerous machinery).
- Report chest pain, palpitations, edema, skin rash, diarrhea, headache.

# dezocine

***(dez' oh seen)***

Dalgan

**Pregnancy Category C**

**Pregnancy Category D (labor & delivery)**

### Drug classes

Narcotic agonist-antagonist analgesic

### Therapeutic actions

Acts as an agonist at specific opioid receptors in the CNS to produce analgesia, sedation, but also acts to cause hallucinations; seems to have low abuse potential; not in any schedule of the Federal Controlled Substances Act.

### Indications

- Relief of moderate to severe pain when opiate analgesic is appropriate
- For preoperative or preanesthetic medication to supplement balanced anesthesia and relieve prepartum pain

### Contraindications/cautions

- Contraindications: hypersensitivity to dezocine, physical dependence on a narcotic analgesic (may precipitate withdrawal); pregnancy, lactation.
- Use cautiously with bronchial asthma, COPD, respiratory depression, anoxia, increased intracranial pressure, acute MI, ventricular failure, coronary insufficiency, hypertension, biliary tract surgery, renal or hepatic dysfunction.

### Dosage

**Available Forms:** Injection—5, 10, 15 mg/ml

ADULT

- ***IM single dose:*** 5–20 mg (usual, 10 mg). Adjust dosage according to patient's weight, age, severity of pain, physical status, and other medications. May be repeated q3–6h as needed. Do not exceed 20 mg/dose. Upper limit is 120 mg/d.
- ***IV:*** 2.5–10 mg repeated q2–4h. Initial dose is usually 5 mg.
- ***SC:*** Not recommended. Repeated injections lead to irritation, inflammation, thrombophlebitis.

PEDIATRIC (< 18 Y): Not recommended.

### Pharmacokinetics

| *Route* | *Onset* | *Peak* |
|---|---|---|
| IV | 5 min | 5–15 min |
| IM | 10–15 min | 10–90 min |

*Metabolism:* Hepatic; $T_{1/2}$: 2.4 h
*Distribution:* Crosses placenta; enters breast milk
*Excretion:* Urine

### IV facts

**Preparation:** Administer as provided. Store at room temperature; protect from light. Do not use if solution contains precipitate.
**Infusion:** Infuse slowly, each 5 mg over 2–3 min.

### Adverse effects

- CNS: *Sedation, clamminess, sweating, headache, vertigo, floating feeling, dizziness, lethargy, confusion, lightheadedness,* nervousness, unusual dreams, agitation, euphoria, hallucinations
- GI: *Nausea, vomiting,* dry mouth
- CV: Palpitation, changed BP
- **Respiratory**: Slow, shallow respiration
- **Dermatologic**: Rash, hives, pruritus, flushing, warmth, sensitivity to cold
- EENT: Diplopia, blurred vision
- Local: *Injection site reactions*

### Clinically important drug-drug interactions

- Increased CNS depression with general anesthetics, sedatives, tranquilizers, hypnotics, other opioid analgesics.

## ■ Nursing Considerations

### Assessment

- *History:* Hypersensitivity to dezocine, physical dependence on a narcotic analgesic; bronchial asthma, COPD, respiratory depression, anoxia, increased intracranial pressure, acute MI, ventricular failure, coronary insufficiency, hypertension, biliary tract surgery, renal or hepatic dysfunction; lactation.
- *Physical:* Orientation, reflexes, bilateral grip strength, affect; pupil size, vision; pulse, auscultation, BP; R, adventitious sounds; bowel sounds, normal output; liver, kidney function tests.

### Implementation

- Provide narcotic antagonist, facilities for assisted or controlled respiration on standby during parenteral administration.

**Drug-specific teaching points**

Incorporate teaching about drug into preoperative teaching when used in the acute setting. For other patients:

- The following side effects may occur: dizziness, sedation, drowsiness, impaired visual acuity (avoid driving, performing other tasks that require alertness); nausea, loss of appetite (lying quietly, eating frequent small meals may help).
- Report severe nausea, vomiting, palpitations, shortness of breath or difficulty breathing, pain at injection site.

## diazepam

*(dye az' e pam)*

Apo-Diazepam (CAN), Diastat, Diazemuls (CAN), Valium, Vivol (CAN)

**Pregnancy Category D**
**C-IV controlled substance**

### Drug classes

Benzodiazepine
Antianxiety agent
Antiepileptic agent
Skeletal muscle relaxant, centrally acting

### Therapeutic actions

Exact mechanisms of action not understood; acts mainly at the limbic system and reticular formation; may act in spinal cord and at supraspinal sites to produce skeletal muscle relaxation; potentiates the effects of GABA, an inhibitory neurotransmitter; anxiolytic effects occur at doses well below those necessary to cause sedation, ataxia; has little effect on cortical function.

### Indications

- Management of anxiety disorders or for short-term relief of symptoms of anxiety
- Acute alcohol withdrawal; may be useful in symptomatic relief of acute agitation, tremor, delirium tremens, hallucinosis
- Muscle relaxant: adjunct for relief of reflex skeletal muscle spasm due to local pathology (inflammation of muscles or joints) or secondary to trauma; spasticity caused by upper motoneuron disorders (cerebral palsy and paraplegia); athetosis, stiff-man syndrome
- Treatment of tetanus (parenteral)
- Antiepileptic: adjunct in status epilepticus and severe recurrent convulsive seizures (parenteral); adjunct in convulsive disorders (oral)
- Preoperative: relief of anxiety and tension and to lessen recall in patients prior to surgical procedures, cardioversion, and endoscopic procedures (parenteral)
- Management of selected, refractory patients with epilepsy who require intermittent use to control bouts of increased seizure activity (rectal)
- Unlabeled use: treatment of panic attacks

### Contraindications/cautions

- Contraindications: hypersensitivity to benzodiazepines; psychoses, acute narrow-angle glaucoma, shock, coma, acute alcoholic intoxication; pregnancy (cleft lip or palate, inguinal hernia, cardiac defects, microcephaly, pyloric stenosis when used in first trimester; neonatal withdrawal syndrome reported in babies); lactation.
- Use cautiously with elderly or debilitated patients; impaired liver or kidney function.

### Dosage

**Available Forms:** Tablets—2, 5, 10 mg; SR capsule—15 mg; oral solution—5 mg/5 ml; rectal pediatric tip—2.5, 5, 10 mg; rectal adult tip—10, 15, 20 mg; injection 5 mg/ml

Individualize dosage; incease dosage cautiously to avoid adverse effects.

**ADULT**

- ***Oral***
  - *Anxiety disorders, skeletal muscle spasm, convulsive disorders:* 2–10 mg bid–qid.
  - *Alcohol withdrawal:* 10 mg tid–qid first 24 h; reduce to 5 mg tid–qid, as needed.
- ***Oral sustained release***
  - *Anxiety disorders:* 15–30 mg/d.
  - *Alcohol withdrawal:* 30 mg first 24 h; reduce to 15 mg/d as needed.

- ***Rectal:*** 0.2 mg/kg PR; treat no more than one episode q 5 days. May be given a second dose in 4–12 h.
- ***Parenteral:*** Usual dose is 2–20 mg IM or IV. Larger doses may be required for some indications (tetanus). Injection may be repeated in 1 h.
  - *Anxiety:* 2–10 mg IM or IV; repeat in 3–4 h if necessary.
  - *Alcohol withdrawal:* 10 mg IM or IV initially, then 5–10 mg in 3–4 h if necessary.
  - *Endoscopic procedures:* 10 mg or less, up to 20 mg IV just before procedure or 5–10 mg IM 30 min prior to procedure. Reduce or omit dosage of narcotics.
  - *Muscle spasm:* 5–10 mg IM or IV initially, then 5–10 mg in 3–4 h if necessary.
  - *Status epilepticus:* 5–10 mg, preferably by slow IV. May repeat q 5–10 min up to total dose of 30 mg. If necessary, repeat therapy in 2–4 h; other drugs are preferable for long-term control.
  - *Preoperative:* 10 mg IM.
  - *Cardioversion:* 5–15 mg IV 5–10 min before procedure.

PEDIATRIC

- *Oral*
  - *> 6 Mo:* 1–2.5 mg PO tid–qid initially. Gradually increase as needed and tolerated. Can be given rectally if needed.
- ***Rectal:*** 2 y—not recommended; 2–5 y—0.5 mg/kg; 6–11 y—0.3 mg/kg; >12 adult dose; may give a second dose in 4–12 h.
- ***Parenteral:*** Maximum dose of 0.25 mg/kg IV administered over 3 min; may repeat after 15–30 min. If no relief of symptoms after 3 doses, adjunctive therapy is recommended.
  - *Tetanus (> 30 d):* 1–2 mg IM or IV slowly q3–4h as necessary.
  - *Tetanus (5 y or older):* 5–10 mg q 3–4 h.
  - *Status epilepticus (> 30 d but < 5 y):* 0.2–0.5 mg slowly IV q 2–5 min up to a maximum of 5 mg.
  - *Status epilepticus (5 y or older):* 1 mg IV q 2–5 min up to a maximum of 10 mg; repeat in 2–4 h if necessary.

GERIATRIC PATIENTS OR THOSE WITH DEBILITATING DISEASE: 2–2.5 mg PO qd–bid or 2–5 mg parenteral initially; reduce rectal dose. Gradually increase as needed and tolerated.

## Pharmacokinetics

| *Route* | *Onset* | *Peak* | *Duration* |
|---|---|---|---|
| Oral | 30–60 min | 1–2 h | 3 h |
| IM | 15–30 min | 30–45 min | 3 h |
| IV | 1–5 min | 30 min | 15–60 min |
| Rectal | Rapid | 1.5 h | 3 h |

*Metabolism:* Hepatic; $T_{1/2}$: 20–50 h
*Distribution:* Crosses placenta; enters breast milk
*Excretion:* Urine

### IV facts

**Preparation:** Do not mix with other solutions; do not mix in plastic bags or tubing.
**Infusion:** Inject slowly into large vein, 1 ml/min at most; for children do not exceed 3 min; do not inject intrarterially; if injected into IV tubing, inject as close to vein insertion as possible.
**Incompatibilities:** Do not mix with other solutions; do not mix with any other drugs.

## Adverse effects

- CNS: *Transient, mild drowsiness initially*; *sedation, depression, lethargy, apathy, fatigue, lightheadedness, disorientation, restlessness, confusion*, crying, delirium, headache, slurred speech, dysarthria, stupor, rigidity, tremor, dystonia, vertigo, euphoria, nervousness, difficulty in concentration, vivid dreams, psychomotor retardation, extrapyramidal symptoms; *mild paradoxical excitatory reactions, during first 2 wk of treatment*, visual and auditory disturbances, diplopia, nystagmus, depressed hearing, nasal congestion
- GI: *Constipation; diarrhea*; dry mouth; salivation; nausea; anorexia; vomiting;

difficulty in swallowing; gastric disorders; elevations of blood enzymes—LDH, alkaline phosphatase, SGOT, SGPT; hepatic dysfunction; jaundice
- CV: *Bradycardia, tachycardia*, CV collapse, hypertension and hypotension, palpitations, edema
- **Hematologic**: Decreased hematocrit, blood dyscrasias
- GU: *Incontinence, urinary retention, changes in libido*, menstrual irregularities
- **Dermatologic**: Urticaria, pruritus, skin rash, dermatitis
- **Dependence**: *Drug dependence with withdrawal syndrome* when drug is discontinued (common with abrupt discontinuation of higher dosage used for longer than 4 mo); IV diazepam: 1.7% incidence of fatalities; oral benzodiazepines ingested alone; no well-documented fatal overdoses
- **Other**: Phlebitis and thrombosis at IV injection sites, hiccups, fever, diaphoresis, paresthesias, muscular disturbances, gynecomastia; pain, burning, and redness after IM injection

### Clinically important drug-drug interactions

• Increased CNS depression with alcohol, omeprazole • Increased pharmacologic effects of diazepam cimetidine, disulfiram, oral contraceptives • Decreased effects of diazepam with theophyllines, ranitidine

## ■ Nursing Considerations

### Assessment

- *History:* Hypersensitivity to benzodiazepines; psychoses, acute narrow-angle glaucoma, shock, coma, acute alcoholic intoxication; elderly or debilitated patients; impaired liver or kidney function; pregnancy, lactation.
- *Physical:* Weight; skin color, lesions; orientation, affect, reflexes, sensory nerve function, ophthalmologic exam; P, BP; R, adventitious sounds; bowel sounds, normal output, liver evaluation; normal output; liver and kidney function tests, CBC

### Implementation

- Do not administer intra-arterially; may produce arteriospasm, gangrene.
- Change from IV therapy to oral therapy as soon as possible.
- Do not use small veins (dorsum of hand or wrist) for IV injection.
- Reduce dose of narcotic analgesics with IV diazepam; dose should be reduced by at least one-third or eliminated.
- Carefully monitor P, BP, respiration during IV administration.
- Maintain patients receiving parenteral benzodiazepines in bed for 3 h; do not permit ambulatory patients to operate a vehicle following an injection.
- Monitor EEG in patients treated for status epilepticus; seizures may recur after initial control, presumably because of short duration of drug effect.
- Monitor liver and kidney function, CBC during long-term therapy.
- Taper dosage gradually after long-term therapy, especially in epileptic patients.
- Arrange for epileptic patients to wear medical alert ID indicating that they are epileptics taking this medication.

### Drug-specific teaching points

- Take this drug exactly as prescribed. Do not stop taking this drug (long-term therapy, antiepileptic therapy) without consulting your health care provider.
- Care-giver should learn to assess seizures, administer rectal form and monitor patient
- The following side effects may occur: drowsiness, dizziness (may lessen; avoid driving or engaging in other dangerous activities); GI upset (take drug with food); dreams, difficulty concentrating, fatigue, nervousness, crying (reversible).
- Report severe dizziness, weakness, drowsiness that persists, rash or skin lesions, palpitations, swelling of the ankles, visual or hearing disturbances, difficulty voiding.

# diazoxide

*(di az* ***ok'*** *sid)*

*Oral:* Proglycem

*Parenteral:* Hyperstat

**Pregnancy Category C**

**Drug classes**
Glucose-elevating agent (oral)
Antihypertensive
Thiazide diuretic

**Therapeutic actions**
Increases blood glucose by decreasing insulin release and decreasing glucose.
Decreases BP by relaxing arteriolar smooth muscle.

**Indications**
- Oral: management of hypoglycemia due to hyperinsulinism in infants and children and to inoperable pancreatic islet cell malignancies
- Parenteral: short-term use in malignant and nonmalignant hypertension, used primarily in hospital

**Contraindications/cautions**
- Contraindications: allergy to thiazides or other sulfonamide derivatives; pregnancy, lactation.
- Use extreme caution with functional hypoglycemia, decreased cardiac reserve, decreased renal function, gout or hyperuricemia when using oral diazoxide; compensatory hypertension, dissecting aortic aneurysm, pheochromocytoma, decreased cerebral or cardiac circulation, labor and delivery (IV use may stop uterine contractions and cause neonatal hyperbilirubinemia, thrombocytopenia) when using parenteral diazoxide.

**Dosage**
**Available Forms:** Capsules—50 mg; oral suspension—50 mg/ml; injection—15 mg/ml

***Oral Diazoxide***
- *ADULT:* 3–8 mg/kg per day PO in 2–3 doses q8–12 h. *Starting dose:* 3 mg/kg per day in 3 equal doses q8h.
- *PEDIATRIC:* 3–8 mg/kg per day PO in 2–3 doses q8–12 h. *Starting dose:* 3 mg/kg per day in 3 equal doses q8h.
- *INFANTS AND NEWBORNS:* 8–15 mg/kg per day PO in 2–3 doses q8–12 h. *Starting dose:* 10 mg/kg per day in 3 equal doses q8h.

***Parenteral Diazoxide***
- *ADULT:* 1–3 mg/kg (maximum dose 150 mg) undiluted and rapidly by IV injection in a bolus dose within 30 sec; repeat bolus doses q 5–15 min until desired decrease in BP is achieved. Repeat doses q4–24h until oral antihypertensive medications can be started. Treatment is seldom needed for longer than 4–5 d and should not be continued for more than 10 d.

**Pharmacokinetics**

| *Route* | *Onset* | *Peak* | *Duration* |
|---|---|---|---|
| Oral | 1 h | 8 h | |
| IV | 30–60 min | 5 min | 2–12 h |

*Metabolism:* Hepatic; $T_{1/2}$: 21–45 h
*Distribution:* Crosses placenta; enters breast milk
*Excretion:* Urine

**IV facts**
**Preparation:** Do not mix or dilute solution. Protect from light.
**Infusion:** Inject directly as rapid bolus, 30 sec or less; maximum of 150 mg in one injection.

**Adverse effects**
- CNS: Cerebral ischemia, headache, hearing loss, blurred vision, apprehension, cerebral infarction, coma, convulsions, paralysis, *dizziness, weakness*, altered taste sensation
- GI: *Nausea, vomiting*, hepatotoxicity, anorexia, parotid swelling, constipation, diarrhea, acute pancreatitis
- CV: *Hypotension* (managed by Trendelenburg position or sympathomimetics), occasional hypertension, angina, MI, cardiac arrhythmias, palpitations, *CHF secondary to fluid and sodium retention*
- **Respiratory**: Dyspnea, choking sensation
- **Hematologic**: Thrombocytopenia, decreased Hgb, decreased Hct, hyperuricemia
- GU: Renal toxicity
- **Dermatologic**: Hirsutism, rash
- **Metabolic**: Hyperglycemia, glycosuria, ketoacidosis, and nonketotic hyperosmolar coma
- **Local**: Pain at IV injection site

**Clinically important drug-drug interactions**

• Increased therapeutic and toxic effects of diazoxide if taken concurrently with thiazides • Increased risk of hyperglycemia if taken concurrently with acetohexamide, chlorpropamide, glipizide, glyburide, tolazamide, tolbutamide • Decreased serum levels and effectiveness of hydantoins taken concurrently with diazoxide

**Drug-lab test interferences**

• Hyperglycemic and hyperuricemic effects of diazoxide prevent testing for disorders of glucose and xanthine metabolism • False-negative insulin response to glucagon

## ■ Nursing Considerations

### Assessment

- *History:* Allergy to thiazides or other sulfonamide derivatives; pregnancy; lactation; functional hypoglycemia, decreased cardiac reserve, decreased renal function, gout or hyperurecemia; compensatory hypertension, dissecting aortic aneurysm, pheochromocytoma; decreased cerebral or cardiac circulation.
- *Physical:* Body weight, skin integrity, swelling or limited motion in joints, earlobes; P, BP, edema, peripheral perfusion; R, pattern, adventitious sounds; intake and output; CBC, blood glucose, serum electrolytes and uric acid, urinalysis, urine glucose and ketones, kidney and liver function tests

### Implementation

- Monitor intake and output and weigh patient daily at the same time to check for fluid retention.
- Check urine glucose and ketones daily.
- Have insulin and tolbutamide on standby in case hyperglycemic reaction occurs.
- Have dopamine, norepinephrine on standby in case of severe hypotensive reaction.

*Oral Diazoxide*

- Decrease dose in renal disease.
- Protect oral drug suspensions from light.
- Reassure patient that hirsutism will resolve when drug is discontinued.

*Parenteral Diazoxide*

- Monitor BP closely during administration until stable and then q1/2–1h.
- Protect drug from freezing and light.
- Patient should remain supine for 1 h after last injection.

### Drug-specific teaching points

*Oral Diazoxide*

- Check urine daily for glucose and ketones; report elevated levels.
- Weigh yourself daily at the same time and with the same clothes, and record the results.
- Excessive hair growth may appear on your forehead, back, or limbs; growth will end after drug is stopped.
- Report weight gain of more than 5 lb in 2–3 d, increased thirst, nausea, vomiting, confusion, fruity odor on breath, abdominal pain, swelling of extremities, difficulty breathing, bruising, bleeding.

*Parenteral Diazoxide*

- Report increased thirst, nausea, headache, dizziness, hearing or vision changes, difficulty breathing, pain at injection site.

# Diclofenac

## diclofenac sodium

*(dye **kloe'** fen ak)*

Voltaren, Voltaren-XR, Voltaren Rapide (CAN)

## diclofenac potassium

Cataflam

**Pregnancy Category B**

**Drug classes**

Analgesic (non-narcotic)
Antipyretic
Anti-inflammatory agent
Nonsteroidal anti-inflammatory drug (NSAID)

**Therapeutic actions**

Inhibits prostaglandin synthetase to cause antipyretic and anti-inflammatory effects; the exact mechanism is unknown.

### Indications

- Acute or long-term treatment of mild to moderate pain, including dysmenorrhea
- Rheumatoid arthritis
- Osteoarthritis
- Ankylating spondylitis

### Contraindications/cautions

- Contraindications: significant renal impairment, pregnancy, lactation.
- Use cautiously with impaired hearing, allergies, hepatic, cardiovascular, and GI conditions.

### Dosage

**Available Forms:** Tablets—50 mg; DR tablets—25, 50 ,75 mg; ER tablets—100 mg

ADULT

- *Pain, including dysmennorhea:* 50 mg tid PO; initial dose of 100 mg may help some patients (Cataflam)
- *Osteoarthritis:* 100–150 mg/d PO in divided doses (Voltaren); 50 mg bid–tid PO (Cataflam)
- *Rheumatoid arthritis:* 150–200 mg/d PO in divided doses (Voltaren); 50 mg bid–tid PO (Cataflam)
- *Ankylosing spondylitis:* 100–125 mg/d PO. Give as 25 mg 4×/d, with an extra 25-mg dose at HS (Voltaren); 25 mg qid PO with an additional 25 mg hs if needed (Cataflam)

PEDIATRIC: Safety and efficacy not established.

### Pharmacokinetics

| Route | Onset | Peak | Duration |
|---|---|---|---|
| Oral (sodium) | Varies | 2–3 h | 12–15 h |
| Oral (potassium) | Rapid | 20–120 min | 12–15 h |

*Metabolism:* Hepatic; $T_{1/2}$: 1.5–2 h
*Distribution:* Crosses placenta; enters breast milk
*Excretion:* Urine and feces

### Adverse effects

- CNS: *Headache, dizziness,* somnolence, insomnia, fatigue, tiredness, dizziness, tinnitus, ophthamologic effects
- GI: *Nausea, dyspepsia, GI pain, diarrhea*, vomiting, *constipation*, flatulence
- **Hematologic**: Bleeding, platelet inhibition with higher doses
- GU: Dysuria, renal impairment
- **Dermatologic**: Rash, pruritus, sweating, dry mucous membranes, stomatitis
- **Other**: Peripheral edema, anaphylactoid reactions to fatal anaphylactic shock

### Clinically important drug-drug interactions

- Increased serum levels and increased risk of lithium toxicity.

## ■ Nursing Considerations

### Assessment

- *History:* Renal impairment; impaired hearing; allergies; hepatic, CV, and GI conditions; lactation.
- *Physical:* Skin color and lesions; orientation, reflexes, ophthalmologic and audiometric evaluation, peripheral sensation; P, edema; R, adventitious sounds; liver evaluation; CBC, clotting times, renal and liver function tests; serum electrolytes, stool guaiac.

### Implementation

- Administer drug with food or after meals if GI upset occurs.
- Arrange for periodic ophthalmologic exam during long term therapy.
- Institute emergency procedures if overdose occurs (gastric lavage, induction of emesis, supportive therapy).

### Drug-specific teaching points

- Take drug with food or meals if GI upset occurs.
- Take only the prescribed dosage.
- Dizziness, drowsiness can occur (avoid driving or using dangerous machinery while on this drug).
- Report sore throat, fever, rash, itching, weight gain, swelling in ankles or fingers, changes in vision; black, tarry stools.

## dicloxacillin sodium

*(dye klox a **sill'** in)*

Dynapen, Dycill, Pathocil

**Pregnancy Category B**

### Drug classes
Antibiotic
Penicillinase-resistant pencillin

### Therapeutic actions
Bactericidal: inhibits cell wall synthesis of sensitive organisms, causing cell death.

### Indications
- Infections due to penicillanase producing staphylococci

### Contraindications/cautions
- Contraindications: allergies to penicillins, cephalosporins, or other allergens.
- Use cautiously with renal disorders, lactation (may cause diarrhea or candidiasis in the infant).

### Dosage
**Available Forms:** Capsules—125 250, 500 mg; powder for oral suspension—62.5 mg/5 ml

*ADULT:* 125 mg q6h PO. Up to 250 mg q6h PO in severe infections.

*PEDIATRIC*
- *< 40 kg:* 12.5 mg/kg per day PO in equally divided doses q6h. Up to 25 mg/kg per day PO in equally divided doses q6h in severe infections.

### Pharmacokinetics

| Route | Onset | Peak | Duration |
|---|---|---|---|
| Oral | Varies | 0.5–1 h | 4–6 h |

*Metabolism:* Hepatic; $T_{1/2}$: 30–60 min
*Distribution:* Crosses placenta; enters breast milk
*Excretion:* Urine

### Adverse effects
- CNS: Lethargy, hallucinations, seizures, decreased reflexes
- GI: *Glossitis, stomatitis, gastritis, sore mouth*, furry tongue, black
- **Hematologic**: Anemia, thrombocytopenia, leukopenia, neutropenia, prolonged bleeding time, hemorrhagic episodes at high doses
- GU: Nephritis: oliguria, proteinuria, hematuria, casts, azotemia, pyuria
- **Hypersensitivity reactions**: *Rash, fever, wheezing*, anaphylaxis
- Other: *Superinfections*: oral and rectal moniliasis, vaginitis

### Clinically important drug-drug interactions
- Decreased effectiveness if taken with tetracyclines

### Clinically important drug-food interactions
- Decreased absorption and decreased serum levels if taken with food

## ■ Nursing Considerations

### Assessment
- ***History:*** Allergies; renal disorders; lactation
- ***Physical:*** Culture infected area; skin color, lesion; R, adventitious sounds; bowel sounds; CBC, liver and renal function tests, serum electrolytes, Hct, urinalysis.

### Implementation
- Culture infection before treatment; reculture if response is not as expected.
- Administer by oral route only.
- Continue oral treatment for 10 full d.
- Administer on an empty stomach, 1 h before or 2 h after meals.
- Do not administer with fruit juices or soft drinks; a full glass of water is preferable.

### Drug-specific teaching points
- Take drug around the clock; take the full course of therapy, usually 10 d.
- Take the drug on an empty stomach, 1 h before or 2 h after meals, with a full glass of water.
- This antibiotic is only for this infection; do not use it to self-treat other infections.
- The following side effects may occur: stomach upset, nausea, diarrhea, mouth sores.
- Report unusual bleeding or bruising, fever, chills, sore throat, hives, rash, severe diarrhea, difficulty breathing.

# dicyclomine hydrochloride

*(dye sye' kloe meen)*

Antispas, Bentyl, Bentylol (CAN), Byclomine, Dibent, Formulex (CAN), Or-Tyl, Viscerol (CAN)

**Pregnancy Category C**

## Drug classes

Antispasmodic
Anticholinergic
Antimuscarinic agent
Parasympatholytic

## Therapeutic actions

Direct GI smooth muscle relaxant; competitively blocks the effects of acetylcholine at muscarinic cholinergic receptors that mediate the effects of parasympathetic postganglionic impulses, thus relaxing the GI tract.

## Indications

- Treatment of functional bowel or irritable bowel syndrome (irritable colon, spastic colon, mucous colitis)

## Contraindications/cautions

- Contraindications: glaucoma; adhesions between iris and lens, stenosing peptic ulcer, pyloroduodenal obstruction, paralytic ileus, intestinal atony, severe ulcerative colitis, toxic megacolon, symptomatic prostatic hypertrophy, bladder neck obstruction, bronchial asthma, COPD, cardiac arrhythmias, tachycardia, myocardial ischemia; impaired metabolic, liver, or kidney function, myasthenia gravis; lactation.
- Use cautiously with Down's syndrome, brain damage, spasticity, hypertension, hyperthyroidism.

## Dosage

**Available Forms:** Capsules—10, 20 mg; tablets—20 mg; syrup—10 mg/5 ml; injection 10 mg/ml

**ADULT**

- ***Oral:*** The only effective dose is 160 mg/d PO divided into four equal doses; however, begin with 80 mg/d divided into four equal doses; increase to 160 mg/d unless side effects limit dosage.
- ***Parenteral:*** 80 mg/d IM in four divided doses; **do not give IV**.

**PEDIATRIC:** Not recommended.

## Pharmacokinetics

| Route | Onset | Duration |
|---|---|---|
| Oral | 1–2 h | 4 h |

*Metabolism:* Hepatic; $T_{1/2}$: 9–10 h
*Distribution:* Crosses placenta; enters breast milk
*Excretion:* Urine

## Adverse effects

- CNS: *Blurred vision*, mydriasis, cycloplegia, photophobia, increased intraocular pressure
- GI: *Dry mouth, altered taste perception, nausea, vomiting, dysphagia*, heartburn, constipation, bloated feeling, paralytic ileus, gastroesophageal reflux
- CV: Palpitations, tachycardia
- GU: *Urinary hesitancy and retention*; impotence
- Local: *Irritation at site of IM injection*
- Other: Decreased sweating and predisposition to heat prostration, suppression of lactation

## Clinically important drug-drug interactions

• Decreased antipsychotic effectiveness of haloperidol when given with anticholinergic drugs • Decreased effectiveness of phenothiazines given with anticholinergic drugs, but increased incidence of paralytic ileus

## ■ Nursing Considerations

### Assessment

- *History:* Glaucoma; adhesions between iris and lens, stenosing peptic ulcer, pyloroduodenal obstruction, paralytic ileus, intestinal atony, severe ulcerative colitis, toxic megacolon, symptomatic prostatic hypertrophy, bladder neck obstruction, bronchial asthma, COPD, cardiac arrhythmias, myocardial ischemia; impaired metabolic, liver, or kidney function, myasthenia gravis; Down's syndrome, brain damage, spasticity, hypertension, hyperthyroidism; lactation

- *Physical:* Bowel sounds, normal output; normal urinary output, prostate palpation; R, adventitious sounds; pulse, BP; intraocular pressure, vision; bilateral grip strength, reflexes; liver palpation, liver and renal function tests; skin color, lesions, texture.

### Implementation
- Ensure adequate hydration; provide environmental control (temperature) to prevent hyperpyrexia.
- Have patient void before each drug dose if urinary retention is a problem.
- Monitor lighting to minimize discomfort of photophobia.

### Drug-specific teaching points
- Take drug exactly as prescribed.
- Avoid hot environments while taking this drug (heat intolerance may lead to dangerous reactions).
- The following side effects may occur: constipation (ensure adequate fluid intake, proper diet); dry mouth (sugarless lozenges, frequent mouth care may help; may lessen with time); blurred vision, sensitivity to light (transient effects; avoid tasks that require acute vision; wear sunglasses); impotence (reversible); difficulty in urination (empty bladder immediately before taking drug).
- Report skin rash, flushing, eye pain, difficulty breathing, tremors, loss of coordination, irregular heartbeat, palpitations, headache, abdominal distention, hallucinations, severe or persistent dry mouth, difficulty swallowing, difficulty in urination, severe constipation, sensitivity to light.

## didanosine

*(dye **dan'** oh seen)*

ddI, dideoxyinosine

Videx

**Pregnancy Category B**

### Drug classes
Antiviral

### Therapeutic actions
A synthetic nucleoside that inhibits replication of HIV, leading to viral death.

### Indications
- Treatment of adult patients with advanced HIV infection who have received prolonged prior zidovudine therapy
- Treatment of adults and children >6 mo with advanced infection who would benefit from antiretroviral therapy

### Contraindications/cautions
- Contraindications: allergy to any component of the formulation, lactation.
- Use cautiously with impaired hepatic or renal function; history of alcohol abuse.

### Dosage
**Available Forms:** Tablets—25, 50, 100, 150 mg; powder for oral solution—100, 167, 250, 375 mg; powder for pediatric solution—2, 4 g

*ADULT:* 125–200 mg PO bid; buffered powder: 167–250 mg PO bid.

*PEDIATRIC*

| *Body Surface ($m^2$)* | *Tablets (bid)* | *Pediatric Powder ($m^2$)* |
|---|---|---|
| 1.1–1.4 | 100 mg | 125 mg bid (12.5 ml) |
| 0.8–1 | 75 mg | 94 mg bid (9.5 ml) |
| 0.5–0.7 | 50 mg | 62 mg bid (6 ml) |
| <0.4 | 25 mg | 31 mg bid (3 ml) |

### Pharmacokinetics

| *Route* | *Onset* |
|---|---|
| Oral | Varies |

*Metabolism:* Hepatic; $T_{1/2}$: 1.6 h

*Distribution:* Crosses placenta; enters breast milk

*Excretion:* Urine

### Adverse effects
- CNS: Headache, pain, anxiety, confusion, nervousness, twitching, depression
- GI: *Nausea, vomiting, hepatotoxicity, abdominal pain*, **pancreatitis,** stomatitis, oral thrush, melena, dry mouth

- Hematologic: *Hemopoietic depression*, elevated bilirubin, elevated uric acid
- Dermatologic: Rash, pruritus
- Other: Chills, fever, infections, dyspnea, myopathy

**Clinically important drug-drug interactions**

- Decreased effectiveness of tetracycline, fluoroquinolone antibiotics

**Clinically important drug-food interactions**

- Decreased absorption and effectiveness of didanosine if taken with food

## ■ Nursing Considerations

### Assessment

- *History:* Allergy to any components of formulation, impaired hepatic or renal function, lactation, history of alcohol abuse.
- *Physical:* Weight; T; skin color, lesions; orientation, reflexes, muscle strength, affect; abdominal exam; CBC, pancreatic enzymes, renal and liver function tests

### Implementation

- Arrange for lab tests (CBC, SMA 12) before and frequently during therapy; monitor for bone marrow depression.
- Administer drug on an empty stomach, 1 h before or 2 h after meals.
- Instruct patient to chew tablets thoroughly or crush tablets and disperse 2 tablets in at least 1 ounce of water; stir until a uniform dispersion forms. For buffered powder, pour contents of packet into 4 oz of water. Do not mix with fruit juice or acid-containing liquid. Stir until powder completely dissolves; have patient drink entire solution immediately. Pediatric solution should be reconstituted by the pharmacy. Shake admixture thoroughly. Store tightly closed in the refrigerator.
- Avoid generating dust. When cleaning up powdered products, use a wet mop or damp sponge. Clean surface with soap and water. Contain large spills. Avoid inhaling dust.
- Monitor patient for signs of pancreatitis—abdominal pain, elevated enzymes, nausea, vomiting. Stop drug, resume only if pancreatitis has been ruled out.
- Monitor patients with hepatic or renal impairment; decreased doses may be needed if toxicity occurs.

### Drug-specific teaching points

- Take drug on an empty stomach, 1 h before or 2 h after meals.
- Chew tablets thoroughly, or crush tablets and disperse 2 tablets in at least 1 ounce of water; stir until a uniform dispersion forms. For buffered powder, pour contents of packet into 4 oz of water. Do not mix with fruit juice or acid-containing liquid. Stir until powder completely dissolves; drink entire solution immediately. Pediatric solution should be reconstituted by the pharmacy. Shake admixture thoroughly. Store tightly closed in the refrigerator.
- The following side effects may occur: loss of appetite, nausea, vomiting (frequent mouth care, small frequent meals may help); rash; chills, fever; headache.
- Have regular blood tests and physical exams to monitor drug's effects and progress of disease.
- Report abdominal pain, nausea, vomiting, cough, sore throat, change in color of urine or stools.

## dienestrol

*(dye en ess' trol)*

DV, Ortho Dienestrol

**Pregnancy Category X**

**Drug classes**

Estrogen
Hormone

**Therapeutic actions**

Intravaginal application delivers replacement estrogenic hormone to vulvovaginal area, showing symptomatic epithelial atrophy resulting from the postmenopausal withdrawal of endogenous estrogens; estrogens induce proliferation of vaginal epithelium, deposition of glycogen in vaginal epithelium, cornification of superficial vaginal cells, acidification of vaginal secretions.

### Indications

- Treatment of atrophic vaginitis and kraurosis vulvae associated with menopause

### Contraindications/cautions

- Contraindications: allergy to estrogens or any component of product; pregnancy; lactation.
- Use cautiously with endometriosis.

### Dosage

**Available Forms:** Vaginal cream—0.01%

Available as topical vaginal cream only. Administer cyclically for short-term use; attempt to discontinue or taper medication at 3- to 6-mo intervals.

*ADULT:* 1–2 applicators intravaginally daily for 1–2 wk; then reduce to half initial dosage or 1 applicator every other day for 1–2 wk. Maintenance dose of 1 applicator one to three times per week after vaginal mucosa is restored.

### Pharmacokinetics

| *Route* | *Onset* |
|---|---|
| Vaginal | Rapid |

*Metabolism:* Hepatic; $T_{1/2}$: unknown

*Distribution:* Crosses placenta; enters breast milk

### Adverse effects

- GU: *Uterine bleeding* (if absorbed through the vaginal mucosa and with sudden discontinuation), serious bleeding in sterilized women with endometriosis, vaginal discharge due to mucus hypersecretion with overdosage
- Other: Breast tenderness

## ■ Nursing Considerations

### Assessment

- *History:* Allergy to estrogens or any component of product, endometriosis, pregnancy, lactation.
- *Physical:* Breast exam; pelvic exam; abdominal palpation.

### Implementation

- Arrange for complete pelvic exam and Pap smear before beginning therapy and periodically throughout therapy.
- Administer cyclically and for short terms only; attempt to discontinue or taper medication at 3- to 6-mo intervals.
- Administer high into the vagina with the applicator provided with the product.
- Have patient lie down for 15 min after application.
- Provide patient with pad or protection for clothing after administration.

### Drug-specific teaching points

- Apply high into vagina with product applicator; lie down for 15 min after application; wear a pad or other protection for your clothing after application.
- Do not use if you are pregnant; if you think you are pregnant or wish to become pregnant, consult with your physician.
- Report breast tenderness, vaginal bleeding, vaginal discharge.

## diethylstilbestrol diphosphate

*(dye eth il stil* ***bess'trol****)*

DES, Honvol (CAN), Stilphostrol

**Pregnancy Category X**

### Drug classes

Hormone

Estrogen

### Therapeutic actions

Estrogens are endogenous female sex hormones; important in the development of the female reproductive system and secondary sex characteristics; cause capillary dilatation, fluid retention, protein anabolism, and thin cervical mucus; conserve calcium and phosphorus, and encourage bone formation; efficacy as palliation in male patients with androgen-dependent prostatic carcinoma is attributable to their competition with androgens for receptor sites.

## Indications

- Palliation in prostatic carcinoma (inoperable and progressing)
- Inoperable and progressing breast cancer

## Contraindications/cautions

- Contraindications: allergy to estrogens; breast cancer (except in specific, selected patients); estrogen-dependent neoplasm; active thrombophlebitis or thromboembolic disorders or history of such from previous estrogen use; pregnancy.
- Use cautiously with metabolic bone disease, renal insufficiency, CHF, lactation.

## Dosage

**Available Forms:** Tablets—50 mg; injection—0.25 g

ADULT

- *Prostatic cancer*
  - ***Oral:*** Initially, 50 mg tid PO; increase to > 200 mg tid, based on patient tolerance. Do not exceed 1 g/d. If relief is not obtained with high oral doses, use IV route. DES (not disphosphate) 3 mg/d PO, average dose 1 mg/d.
  - ***Parenteral:*** On the first day, give 0.5 g IV dissolved in 250 ml saline or 5% dextrose. On subsequent days, give 1 g dissolved in 250–500 ml of saline or dextrose. Administer slowly (20–30 drops/min) during the first 10–15 min and then adjust flow rate so the entire dose is infused within 1 h. Follow the procedure for > 5 d, based on response. Then administer 0.25–0.5 g in a similar manner once or twice weekly, or obtain maintenance using oral drug.
- *Inoperable breast cancer (DES, not diphosphate):* 15 mg/d PO.

PEDIATRIC: Not recommended due to effect on the growth of the long bones.

## Pharmacokinetics

| Route | Onset |
|---|---|
| Oral | Rapid |

*Metabolism:* Hepatic; $T_{1/2}$: unknown
*Distribution:* Crosses placenta; enters breast milk
*Excretion:* Urine

### IV facts

**Preparation:** Dissolve 0.5 g in 250 ml saline or 5% dextrose; on subsequent days give 1 g dissolved in 250–500 ml saline or dextrose. Store at room temperature, away from direct light. Stable for 5 d. Do not use if cloudy or precipitates have formed.

**Infusion:** Administer slowly: 20–30 drops/min during the first 10–15 min and then adjust rate so entire amount is given in 1 h.

## Adverse effects

- CNS: *Steepening of the corneal curvature with a resultant change in visual acuity and intolerance to contact lenses, headache*, migraine, dizziness, mental depression, chorea, convulsions
- GI: Hepatic adenoma, *nausea, vomiting, abdominal cramps*, bloating, cholestatic jaundice, colitis, acute pancreatitis
- CV: Increased BP, **thromboembolic and thrombotic disease**, peripheral edema
- Dermatologic: *Photosensitivity*, chloasma, erythema nodosum or multiforme, hemorrhagic eruption, loss of scalp hair, hirsutism, urticaria, dermatitis
- Endocrine: Decreased glucose tolerance, reduced carbohydrate tolerance
- Other: Weight changes, aggravation of porphyria, breast tenderness

## Clinically important drug-drug interactions

• Enhanced hepatic metabolism of diethylstilbestrol: barbiturates, phenytoin, rifampin • Increased therapeutic and toxic effects of corticosteroids if taken concurrently

## Drug-lab test interferences

• Increased sulfobromophthalein retention; increased prothrombin and factors VII, VIII,

IX, and X; decreased antithrombin III; increased thyroid-binding globulin with increased PBI, $T_4$, increased uptake of free $T_3$ resin (free $T_4$ is unaltered); impaired glucose tolerance; reduced response to metyrapone test; reduced serum folate concentration; increased serum triglycerides and phospholipid concentration

## ■ Nursing Considerations

### Assessment

- ***History:*** Allergy to estrogens; breast cancer; estrogen-dependent neoplasm; active thrombophlebitis or thromboembolic disorders; metabolic bone disease, renal insufficiency, CHF, pregnancy, lactation.
- ***Physical:*** Skin color, lesions, edema; orientation, affect, reflexes; P, auscultation, BP, peripheral perfusion; R, adventitious sounds; bowel sounds, liver evaluation, abdominal exam; serum calcium, phosphorus; liver and renal function tests; glucose tolerance test.

### Implementation

- Alert patient before therapy to the risks of estrogen use, including frequent medical followup, periodic rests from treatment.

### Drug-specific teaching points

- Arrange for periodic medical exams because many potentially serious problems have occurred with the use of this drug, including development of cancers, blood clots, liver problems.
- The following side effects may occur: nausea, vomiting, bloating; headache, dizziness, mental depression (use caution if driving or performing tasks that require alertness); sensitivity to sunlight (use a sunscreen and wear protective clothing); skin rash, loss of scalp hair, darkening of the skin on the face.
- Report pain in the groin or calves of the legs, chest pain or sudden shortness of breath, sudden severe headache, dizziness or fainting, changes in vision or speech, weakness or numbness in the arm or leg, severe abdominal pain, yellowing of the skin or eyes, severe mental depression.

# diflunisal

*(dye **floo'** ni sal)*
Dolobid
**Pregnancy Category C**

d

### Drug classes

Analgesic (non-narcotic)
Antipyretic
Anti-inflammatory agent
Nonsteroidal anti-inflammatory drug (NSAID)

### Therapeutic actions

Exact mechanism of action not known: inhibition of prostaglandin synthetase, the enzyme that breaks down prostaglandins, may account for its antipyretic and anti-inflammatory effects.

### Indications

- Acute or long-term treatment of mild to moderate pain
- Rheumatoid arthritis
- Osteoarthritis

### Contraindications/cautions

- Contraindications: allergy to diflunisal-salicylates or other NSAID, pregnancy, lactation.
- Use cautiously with CV dysfunction, peptic ulceration, GI bleeding, impaired hepatic or renal function.

### Dosage

**Available Forms:** Tablets—250, 500 mg

ADULT

- ***Mild to moderate pain:*** 1,000 mg PO initially, followed by 500 mg q12h PO.
- ***Osteoarthritis/rheumatoid arthritis:*** 500–1,000 mg/d PO in two divided doses; maintenance dosage should not exceed 1,500 mg/d.

PEDIATRIC: Safety and efficacy has not been established.

### Pharmacokinetics

| Route | Onset | Peak | Duration |
|---|---|---|---|
| Oral | 30–60 min | 2–3 h | 12 h |

*Metabolism:* Hepatic; $T_{1/2}$: 8–12 h
*Distribution:* Crosses placenta; enters breast milk
*Excretion:* Urine

**Adverse effects**

- CNS: *Headache, dizziness, somnolence, insomnia*, fatigue, tiredness, dizziness, tinnitus, ophthamologic effects
- GI: *Nausea, dyspepsia, GI pain, diarrhea*, vomiting, constipation, flatulence
- GU: Dysuria, renal impairment
- Hematologic: Bleeding, platelet inhibition with higher doses
- Dermatologic: *Rash*, pruritus, sweating, dry mucous membranes, stomatitis
- Other: Peripheral edema, **anaphylactoid reactions to fatal anaphylactic shock**

**Clinically important drug-drug interactions**

• Decreased absorption with antacids (especially aluminum salts) • Decreased serum diflunisal levels with multiple doses of aspirin

## ■ Nursing Considerations

### Assessment

- *History:* Allergy to diflunisalsalicylates or other NSAID, CV dysfunction, peptic ulceration, GI bleeding, impaired hepatic or renal function, lactation.
- *Physical:* Skin color, lesions; T; orientation, reflexes, ophthalmologic evaluation; P, BP, edema; R, adventitious sounds; liver evaluation, bowel sounds; CBC, clotting times, urinalysis, renal and liver function tests

### Implementation

- Give drug with food or after meals if GI upset occurs.
- Do not crush, and ensure that patient does not chew tablets.
- Institute emergency procedures if overdose occurs—gastric lavage, induction of emesis, supportive therapy.
- Arrange for ophthalmologic exam if patient offers any eye complaints.

### Drug-specific teaching points

- Take the drug only as recommended to avoid overdose.
- Take the drug with food or after meals if GI upset occurs. Swallow the tablet whole; do not chew or crush it.
- The following side effects may occur: nausea, GI upset, dyspepsia (take drug with food); diarrhea or constipation; dizziness, vertigo, insomnia (use caution if driving or operating dangerous machinery).
- Report eye changes, unusual bleeding or bruising, swelling of the feet or hands, difficulty breathing, severe GI pain.

## digoxin

*(di jox' in)*

Lanoxicaps, Lanoxin, Novo-Digoxin (CAN)

**Pregnancy Category A**

**Drug classes**

Cardiac glycoside
Cardiotonic agent

**Therapeutic actions**

Increases intracellular calcium and allows more calcium to enter the myocardial cell during depolarization via a sodium–potassium pump mechanism; this increases force of contraction (positive inotropic effect), increases renal perfusion (seen as diuretic effect in patients with CHF), decreases heart rate (negative chronotropic effect), and decreases AV node conduction velocity.

**Indications**

- CHF
- Atrial fibrillation
- Atrial flutter
- Paroxysmal atrial tachycardia

**Contraindications/cautions**

- Contraindications: allergy to digitalis preparations, ventricular tachycardia, ventricular fibrillation, heart block, sick sinus syndrome, IHSS, acute MI, renal insufficiency and electrolyte abnormalities (decreased $K^+$, decreased $Mg^{++}$, increased $Ca^{++}$).
- Use cautiously with pregnancy and lactation.

### Dosage

**Available Forms:** Lanoxicaps capsules—0.05, 0.1, 0.2 mg; tablets—0.25, 0.5 mg; elixir—0.05 mg/ml; injection—0.1, 0.25 mg/ml

Patient response is quite variable. Evaluate patient carefully to determine the appropriate dose.

### ADULT

- *Loading dose:* 0.75–1.25 mg PO or 0.125–0.25 mg IV. Maintenance dose: 0.125–0.25 mg/d PO.

### PEDIATRIC

- *Loading dose:*

| | Oral (mcg/kg) | IV (mcg/kg) |
|---|---|---|
| Premature | 20–30 | 15–25 |
| Neonate | 25–35 | 20–30 |
| 1–24 mo | 35–60 | 30–50 |
| 2–5 y | 30–40 | 25–35 |
| 5–10 y | 20–35 | 15–30 |
| >10 y | 10–15 | 8–12 |

- *Maintenance dose:* 25%–35% of loading dose in divided daily doses.

### GERIATRIC PATIENTS WITH IMPAIRED RENAL FUNCTION:

| Creatinine Clearance (ml/min) | Dose |
|---|---|
| 10–25 | 0.125 mg/d |
| 26–49 | 0.1875 mg/d |
| 50–79 | 0.25 mg/d |

## Pharmacokinetics

| Route | Onset | Peak | Duration |
|---|---|---|---|
| Oral | 30–120 min | 2–6 h | 6–8 d |
| IV | 5–30 min | 1–5 h | 4–5 d |

*Metabolism:* Some Hepatic; $T_{1/2}$: 30–40 h
*Distribution:* May cross placenta; enters breast milk
*Excretion:* Largely unchanged in the urine

### IV facts

**Preparation:** Give undiluted or diluted in fourfold or greater volume of Sterile Water for Injection, 0.9% Sodium Chloride Injection, 5% Dextrose Injection or Lactated Ringer's Injection. Use diluted product promptly. Do not use if solution contains precipitates.
**Infusion:** Inject slowly over 5 min or longer.

## Adverse effects

- CNS: *Headache, weakness*, drowsiness, visual disturbances
- GI: *GI upset*, anorexia
- CV: *Arrhythmias*

## Clinically important drug-drug interactions

• Increased therapeutic and toxic effects of digoxin with thioamines, verapamil, amiodarone, quinidine, quinine, erythromycin, cyclosporine (a decrease in digoxin dosage may be necessary to prevent toxicity; when the interacting drug is discontinued, an increase in the digoxin dosage may be necessary) • Increased incidence of cardiac arrhythmias with potassium-losing (loop and thiazide) diuretics • Increased absorption or increased bioavailability of oral digoxin, leading to increased effects with tetracyclines, erythromicin • Decreased therapeutic effects with thyroid hormones, metoclopramide, penicillamine • Decreased absorption of oral digoxin if taken with cholestyramine, charcoal, colestipol, antineoplastic agents (bleomycin, cyclophosphamide, methotrexate) • Increased or decreased effects of oral digoxin (adjust the dose of digoxin during concomitant therapy) with oral aminoglycosides.

## ■ Nursing Considerations

### Assessment

- *History:* Allergy to digitalis preparations, ventricular tachycardia, ventricular fibrillation, heart block, sick sinus syndrome, IHSS, acute MI, renal insufficiency, decreased $K^+$, decreased $Mg^{++}$, increased $Ca^{++}$
- *Physical:* Weight; orientation, affect, reflexes,vision; P, BP, baseline ECG, cardiac auscultation, peripheral pulses, peripheral perfusion, edema; R, adventitious sounds; abdominal percussion, bowel sounds, liver evaluation; urinary output; electrolyte levels, liver and renal function tests

### Implementation

- Monitor apical pulse for 1 min before administering; hold dose if pulse <60 in adult or <90 in infant, retake pulse in 1 h. If adult pulse remains <60 or infant <90, hold drug and notify prescriber. Note any change from baseline rhythm or rate.
- Check dosage and preparation carefully.
- Avoid IM injections, which may be very painful.

- Follow diluting instructions carefully, and use diluted solution promptly.
- Avoid giving with meals; this will delay absorption.
- Have emergency equipment ready; have $K^+$ salts, lidocaine, phenytoin, atropine, cardiac monitor on standby in case toxicity develops.
- Monitor for therapeutic drug levels: 0.5–2 ng/ml.

### Drug-specific teaching points

- Do not stop taking this drug without notifying your health care provider.
- Take pulse at the same time each day, and record it on a calendar (normal pulse for you is ___________); call your health care provider if your pulse rate falls below ___________.
- Weigh yourself every other day with the same clothing and at the same time. Record this on the calendar.
- Wear or carry a medical alert tag stating that you are on this drug.
- Have regular medical checkups, which may include blood tests, to evaluate the effects and dosage of this drug.
- Report unusually slow pulse, irregular pulse, rapid weight gain, loss of appetite, nausea, vomiting, blurred or "yellow" vision, unusual tiredness and weakness, swelling of the ankles, legs or fingers, difficulty breathing.

## digoxin immune fab (ovine)

*(di **jox'** in)*

dixogin-specific antibody fragments

Digibind

**Pregnancy Category C**

### Drug classes

Antidote

### Therapeutic actions

Antigen-binding fragments (fab) derived from specific antidigoxin antibodies; binds molecules of digoxin, making them unavailable at the site of action; fab-fragment complex accumulates in the blood and is excreted by the kidneys.

### Indications

- Treatment of life-threatening digoxin intoxication (serum digoxin levels > 10 ng/ml, serum $K^+$ > 5 mEq/L in setting of digitalis intoxication)
- Treatment of life-threatening digitoxin overdose

### Contraindications/cautions

- Contraindications: allergy to sheep products.
- Use cautiously with pregnancy or lactation.

### Dosage

**Available Forms:** Powder for injection—38 mg/vial

**ADULT/PEDIATRIC:** Dosage is determined by serum digoxin level or estimate of the amount of digoxin ingested. If no estimate is available and serum digoxin levels cannot be obtained, use 800 mg (20 vials), which should treat most life-threatening ingestions in adults and children.

- ***Estimated fab fragment dose based on amount of digoxin ingested:***

| Est. # of 0.25-mg Caps Ingested | Dose of fab Fragments |
|---|---|
| 25 | 340 mg (8.5 vials) |
| 50 | 680 mg (17 vials) |
| 75 | 1000 mg (25 vials) |
| 100 | 1360 mg (34 vials) |
| 150 | 2000 mg (50 vials) |
| 200 | 2680 mg (67 vials) |

- ***Estimated fab fragments dose based on serum digoxin concentration:***

| | Wt (Kg) | Serum digoxin concentration (ng/ml) 1 | 2 | 4 | 8 | 12 | 16 | 20 |
|---|---|---|---|---|---|---|---|---|
| Pediatric (dose in mg) | 1 | 0.4 | 1 | 1.5 | 3 | 5 | 6 | 8 |
| | 3 | 1 | 2 | 5 | 9 | 14 | 18 | 23 |
| | 5 | 2 | 4 | 8 | 15 | 23 | 30 | 38 |
| | 10 | 4 | 8 | 15 | 30 | 46 | 61 | 76 |
| | 20 | 8 | 15 | 30 | 61 | 91 | 122 | 152 |
| Adult (dose in vials) | 40 | 0.5 | 1 | 2 | 3 | 5 | 7 | 8 |
| | 60 | 0.5 | 1 | 3 | 5 | 7 | 10 | 12 |
| | 70 | 1 | 2 | 3 | 6 | 9 | 11 | 14 |
| | 80 | 1 | 2 | 3 | 7 | 10 | 13 | 16 |
| | 100 | 1 | 2 | 4 | 8 | 12 | 16 | 20 |

Equations also are available for calculating exact dosage from serum digoxin or digitoxin concentrations.

**Pharmacokinetics**

| *Route* | *Onset* | *Duration* |
|---|---|---|
| IV | 15–30 min | 4–6 h |

*Metabolism:* $T_{1/2}$: 15–20 h
*Distribution:* Crosses placenta; enters breast milk
*Excretion:* Urine

**IV facts**

**Preparation:** Dissolve the contents in each vial with 4 ml of Sterile Water for Injection. Mix gently to give an approximate isosmotic solution with a protein concentration of 10 mg/ml. Use reconstituted solution promptly. Store in refrigerator for up to 4 h. Discard after that time. Reconstituted solution may be further diluted with Sterile Isotonic Saline.
**Infusion:** Administer IV over 30 min through a 0.22-$\mu$m filter; administer as a bolus injection if cardiac arrest is imminent.

**Adverse effects**

- CV: *Low cardiac output states*, CHF, rapid ventricular response in patients with atrial fibrillation
- Hematologic: Hypokalemia due to reactivation of $Na^+$, $K^+$, ATPase
- Hypersensitivity: Allergic reactions: drug fever to **anaphylaxis**

## ■ Nursing Considerations

### Assessment

- *History:* Allergy to sheep products, digoxin drug history, lactation
- *Physical:* P, BP, auscultation, baseline ECG, serum digoxin levels, serum electrolytes

### Implementation

- Arrange for serum digoxin concentration determinations before administration.
- Monitor patient's cardiac response to digoxin overdose and therapy—cardiac rhythm, serum electrolytes, T, BP.
- Maintain life-support equipment and emergency drugs (IV inotropes) on standby for severe overdose.
- Do not redigitalize patient until digoxin immune-fab has been cleared from the body; several days to a week or longer in cases of renal insufficiency. Serum digoxin levels will be very high and will be unreliable for up to 3 days after administration.

### Drug-specific teaching points

- Report muscle cramps, dizziness, palpitations.

## dihydroergotamine mesylate

*(dye hye droe er* ***got'*** *a meen)*

DHE 45, Dihydroergotamine-Sandoz (CAN), Migranol

**Pregnancy Category X**

**Drug classes**

Ergot derivative
Antimigraine agent

**Therapeutic actions**

Mechanism of action not understood; constricts cranial blood vessels; decreases pulsation in cranial arteries and decreases hyperperfusion of basilar artery vascular bed.

**Indications**

- Rapid control of vascular headaches
- Prevention or abortion of vascular headaches when other routes of administration are not feasible (parenteral)

**Contraindications/cautions**

- Contraindications: allergy to ergot preparations, peripheral vascular disease, severe hypertension, coronary artery disease, impaired liver or renal function, sepsis, pruritus, malnutrition, pregnancy.
- Use extreme caution if lactating.

### Dosage

**Available Forms:** Injection—1 mg/ml; nasal spray—0.5 mg/spray

**ADULT:** 1 mg IM at first sign of headache; repeat at 1-h intervals to a total of 3 mg. Use the minimum effective dose based on patient's experience. For IV use, up to a maximum of 2 mg; do not exceed 6 mg/wk. Nasal spray: 2 mg dose given as one spray in each nostril; may be repeated in

15–30 min as needed at first sign of headache or aura.

*PEDIATRIC:* Safety and efficacy not established.

**Pharmacokinetics**

| *Route* | *Onset* | *Peak* | *Duration* |
|---|---|---|---|
| IM | 15–30 min | 2 h | 3–4 h |
| IV | Immediate | 1–2 h | 3–4 h |
| Nasal | Immediate | 0.9 h | 2–4 h |

*Metabolism:* Hepatic; $T_{1/2}$: 21–32 h
*Distribution:* Crosses placenta; enters breast milk
*Excretion:* Bile

**IV facts**

**Preparation:** No preparation necessary.

**Infusion:** Give by direct injection, or into running IV, each 1 mg over 1 min; administer a maximum of 2 mg.

**Adverse effects**

- CNS: *Numbness, tingling of fingers and toes*
- GI: *Nausea, vomiting*
- CV: Pulselessness, weakness in the legs; precordial distress and pain; transient tachycardia, bradycardia; localized edema and itching; increased arterial pressure, arterial insufficiency, coronary vasoconstriction, bradycardia; hypoperfusion, chest pain, BP changes, confusion
- Nasal Spray: nasal congestion, rhinorrhea, sneezing, throat discomfort
- Other: Muscle pain in the extremities; ergotism (nausea, vomiting, diarrhea, severe thirst); drug dependency and abuse with extended use

**Clinically important drug-drug interactions**

• Increased bioavailability with nitroglycerin, nitrates • Increased risk of peripheral ischemia with beta-blockers

## ■ Nursing Considerations

### Assessment

- *History:* Allergy to ergot preparations, peripheral vascular disease, severe hypertension, CAD, impaired liver or renal function, sepsis, pruritus, malnutrition, pregnancy, lactation.
- *Physical:* Skin color, edema, lesions; peripheral sensation; P, BP, peripheral pulses, peripheral perfusion; liver evaluation, bowel sounds; CBC, liver and renal function tests

### Implementation

- Avoid prolonged administration or excessive dosage.
- Use atropine or phenothiazine antiemetics if nausea and vomiting are severe.
- Examine extremities carefully for gangrene or decubitus ulcer formation.

### Drug-specific teaching points

- Take this drug as soon as possible after the first symptoms of an attack.
- The following side effects may occur: nausea, vomiting (if severe, medication may be ordered); numbness, tingling, loss of sensation in the extremities (use caution to avoid injury, and examine extremities daily for injury).
- Do not take during pregnancy; if you become or desire to become pregnant, consult with your physician.
- Report irregular heartbeat, pain or weakness of extremities, severe nausea or vomiting, numbness or tingling of fingers or toes.

# diltiazem hydrochloride

*(dil tye' a zem)*

Apo-Diltiaz (CAN), Cardizem, Cardizem CD, Cardizem SR, Dilacor XR, Novo-Diltazem (CAN), Nu-Diltiaz (CAN), Syn-Diltiazem (CAN), Tiamate, Tiazac

**Pregnancy Category C**

**Drug classes**

Calcium channel blocker
Antianginal agent
Antihypertensive

**Therapeutic actions**

Inhibits the movement of calcium ions across the membranes of cardiac and arterial muscle cells, resulting in the depression of impulse formation in specialized cardiac pacemaker cells, slowing of the velocity of conduction of the cardiac impulse, depression of myocardial contractility, and dilation of coronary arteries and arterioles and peripheral arterioles; these effects lead to decreased cardiac work, decreased cardiac energy consumption, and in patients with vasospastic (Prinzmetal's) angina, increased delivery of oxygen to myocardial cells.

**Indications**

- Angina pectoris due to coronary artery spasm (Prinzmetal's variant angina)
- Effort-associated angina; chronic stable angina in patients not controlled by beta-adrenergic blockers, nitrates
- Essential hypertension (sustained release)
- Treatment of hypertension (sustained release, Tiamate)
- Paroxysmal supraventricular tachycardia (parenteral)

**Contraindications/cautions**

- Allergy to diltiazem, impaired hepatic or renal function, sick sinus syndrome, heart block (second or third degree), lactation.

**Dosage**

**Available Forms:** Tablets—30, 60, 90, 120 mg; SR capsules—60, 90, 120, 180, 240, 300 mg; injection—25, 50 mg as 5 mg/ml

Evaluate patient carefully to determine the appropriate dose of this drug.

ADULT: Initially 30 mg PO qid before meals and hs; gradually increase dosage at 1- to 2-d intervals to 180–360 mg PO in 3–4 divided doses.

- ***Sustained release:*** Cardizem SR: Initially 60–120 mg PO bid; adjust dosage when maximum antihypertensive effect is achieved (around 14 d); optimum range is 240–360 mg/d. Cardizem CD: 180–240 mg qid PO for hypertension; 120–180 mg qd PO for angina. Dilacor XR: 180–240 mg qd PO as needed; up to 480 mg has been used. Tiazac: 120–240 mg qd PO for hypertension—once daily dose.
- ***IV:*** *Direct IV bolus*—0.25 mg/kg (20 mg for the average patient); second bolus of 0.35 mg/kg. *Continuous IV infusion:* 5–10 mg/h with increases up to 15 mg/h; may be continued for up to 24 h.

PEDIATRIC: Safety and efficacy not established.

**Pharmacokinetics**

| *Route* | *Onset* | *Peak* |
|---|---|---|
| Oral | 30–60 min | 2–3 h |
| SR | 30–60 min | 6–11 h |
| IV | Immediate | 2–3 min |

*Metabolism:* Hepatic; $T_{1/2}$: 3 1/2–6 h; 5–7 h (SR)

*Distribution:* Crosses placenta; enters breast milk

*Excretion:* Urine

**IV facts**

**Preparation:** For continuous infusion, transfer to Normal Saline, D5W, D5W/0.45% NaCl as below. Mix thoroughly. Use within 24 h. Keep refrigerated.

| *Diluent Volume (ml)* | *Quantity of Injection* | *Final conc. (mg/ml)* | *Dose (mg/h)* | *Infusion Rate (ml/h)* |
|---|---|---|---|---|
| 100 | 125 mg (25 ml) | 1 | 10 | 10 |
| | | | 15 | 15 |
| 250 | 250 mg (50 ml) | 0.83 | 10 | 12 |
| | | | 15 | 18 |
| 500 | 250 mg (50 ml) | 0.45 | 10 | 22 |
| | | | 15 | 33 |

**Infusion:** Administer bolus dose over 2 min. For continuous infusion, rate of 10 ml/h is the recommended rate. Do not use continuous infusion longer than 24 h.

**Incompatibilities:** Do not mix in the same solution with furosemide solution.

### Adverse effects

- CNS: *Dizziness, lightheadedness, headache, asthenia,* fatigue
- GI: *Nausea*, hepatic injury
- CV: *Peripheral edema*, hypotension, arrhythmias, *bradycardia*, *AV block,* asystole
- Dermatologic: *Flushing*, rash

### Clinically important drug-drug interactions

- Increased serum levels and toxicity of cyclosporine if taken concurrently with diltiazem

## ■ Nursing Considerations

### Assessment

- ***History:*** Allergy to diltiazem, impaired hepatic or renal function, sick sinus syndrome, heart block, lactation
- ***Physical:*** Skin lesions, color, edema; P, BP, baseline ECG, peripheral perfusion, auscultation; R, adventitious sounds; liver evaluation, normal output; liver and renal function tests, urinalysis

### Implementation

- Monitor patient carefully (BP, cardiac rhythm, and output) while drug is being titrated to therapeutic dose; dosage may be increased more rapidly in hospitalized patients under close supervision.
- Monitor BP carefully if patient is on concurrent doses of nitrates.
- Monitor cardiac rhythm regularly during stabilization of dosage and periodically during long-term therapy.

### Drug-specific teaching points

- The following side effects may occur: nausea, vomiting (small, frequent meals may help); headache (regulate light, noise, and temperature; medicate if severe).
- Report irregular heart beat, shortness of breath, swelling of the hands or feet, pronounced dizziness, constipation.

## dimenhydrinate

*(dye men **bye'** dri nate)*

*Oral preparations:* Calm-X, Dimetabs, Dramamine, Gravol (CAN), Nauseatol (CAN), Travel Aid (CAN), Travel Eze (CAN), Travel Tabs (CAN)

*Parenteral preparations:* Dinate, Dramanate, Dymenate, Hydrate

**Pregnancy Category B**

### Drug classes

Anti-motion sickness agent (antihistamine, anticholinergic)

### Therapeutic actions

Antihistamine with antiemetic and anticholinergic activity; depresses hyperstimulated labyrinthine function; may block synapses in the vomiting center; peripheral anticholinergic effects may contribute to antimotion sickness efficacy.

### Indications

- Prevention and treatment of nausea, vomiting, or vertigo of motion sickness

### Contraindications/cautions

- Contraindications: allergy to dimenhydrinate or its components, lactation.
- Use cautiously with narrow-angle glaucoma, stenosing peptic ulcer, symptomatic prostatic hypertrophy, bronchial asthma, bladder neck obstruction, pyloroduodenal obstruction, cardiac arrhythmias.

### Dosage

**Available Forms:** Tablets—50 mg; chewable tablets—50 mg; capsules—50 mg; injection—50 mg/ml; liquid—12.5 mg/4 ml, 15.62 mg/5 ml

*ADULT*

- ***Oral:*** 50–100 mg q4–6h PO; for prophylaxis, first dose should be taken 1/2 h before exposure to motion. Do not exceed 400 mg in 24 h.
- ***Parenteral:*** 50 mg IM as needed; 50 mg in 10 ml Sodium Chloride Injection given IV over 10 min.

*PEDIATRIC*

- *6–12 Y:* 25–50 mg PO q6–8h, not to exceed 150 mg/24 h.
- *2–6 Y:* Up to 25 mg PO q6–8h, not to exceed 75 mg/24 h.
- *<2 Y:* Only on advice of physician; 1.25 mg/kg IM qid, not to exceed 300 mg/24 h.
- *Neonates:* Not recommended.

*GERIATRIC:* Can cause dizziness, sedation, syncope, confusion and hypotension in elderly patients; use with caution.

### Pharmacokinetics

| *Route* | *Onset* | *Peak* | *Duration* |
|---|---|---|---|
| Oral | 15–30 min | 2 h | 3–6 h |
| IM | 20–30 min | 1–2 h | 3–6 h |
| IV | Immediate | 1–2 h | 3–6 h |

*Metabolism:* Hepatic; $T_{1/2}$: unknown
*Distribution:* Crosses placenta; enters breast milk
*Excretion:* Urine

### IV facts

**Preparation:** Dilute 50 mg in 10 ml Sodium Chloride Injection.
**Infusion:** Administer by direct IV injection over 2 min.

### Adverse effects

- CNS: *Drowsiness, confusion, nervousness, restlessness, headache, dizziness, vertigo, lassitude, tingling, heaviness and weakness of hands; insomnia* and excitement (especially in children), hallucinations, convulsions, **death**, blurring of vision, diplopia
- GI: Epigastric distress, anorexia, nausea, vomiting, diarrhea or constipation; dryness of mouth, nose, and throat
- CV: Hypotension, palpitations, tachycardia
- Respiratory: Nasal stuffiness, chest tightness, thickening of bronchial secretions
- Dermatologic: Urticaria, drug rash, photosensitivity

### Clinically important drug-drug interactions

- Increased depressant effects with alcohol, other CNS depressants

## ■ Nursing Considerations

### Assessment

- *History:* Allergy to dimenhydrinate or its components, lactation, narrow-angle glaucoma, stenosing peptic ulcer, symptomatic prostatic hypertrophy, bronchial asthma, bladder neck obstruction, pyloroduodenal obstruction, cardiac arrhythmias
- *Physical:* Skin color, lesions, texture; orientation, reflexes, affect; vision exam; P, BP; R, adventitious sounds; bowel sounds; prostate palpation; CBC

### Implementation

- Maintain epinephrine 1:1,000 readily available when using parenteral preparations; hypersensitivity reactions, including anaphylaxis, have occurred.

### Drug-specific teaching points

- Take drug as prescribed; avoid excessive dosage.
- Drug works best if taken before motion sickness occurs.
- The following side effects may occur: dizziness, sedation, drowsiness (use caution if driving or performing tasks that require alertness); epigastric distress, diarrhea or constipation (take drug with food); dry mouth (use frequent mouth care, suck sugarless lozenges); thickening of bronchial secretions, dryness of nasal mucosa (try another motion sickness remedy).
- Avoid alcohol; serious sedation could occur.
- Report difficulty breathing, hallucinations, tremors, loss of coordination, unusual bleeding or bruising, visual disturbances, irregular heartbeat.

## dimercaprol

*(dye mer **kap'** role)*
BAL in Oil
**Pregnancy Category D**

### Drug classes

Antidote
Chelating agent

### Therapeutic actions
Forms complexes with arsenic, gold, mercury, which increase the urinary and fecal elimination of these metals.

### Indications
- Treatment of arsenic, gold, and mercury poisoning
- Acute lead poisoning when used with calcium edetate disodium
- Acute mercury poisoning if therapy is begun within 1–2 h

### Contraindications/cautions
- Contraindications: hepatic insufficiency; iron, cadmium, or selenium poisoning.

### Dosage
**Available Forms:** Injection—100 mg/ml

ADULT
- ***Mild arsenic or gold poisoning:*** 2.5 mg/kg qid IM for 2 d, then 2× on the third day; once daily thereafter for 10 d.
- ***Severe arsenic or gold poisoning:*** 3 mg/kg q4h IM for 2 d, then 4× on the third day, then bid for 10 d.
- ***Mercury poisoning:*** 5 mg/kg IM followed by 2.5 mg/kg 1–2× per day for 10 d.
- ***Acute lead encephalopathy:*** 3–4 mg/kg IM and then at 4-h intervals in combination with calcium edetate disodium. Maintain treatment for 2–7 d.

PEDIATRIC: Same as adults, use caution–fever and decreased white cells may occur.

### Pharmacokinetics

| *Route* | *Onset* | *Peak* | *Duration* |
|---|---|---|---|
| IM | Rapid | 30–60 min | 3–4 h |

*Metabolism:* Hepatic; $T_{1/2}$: short
*Distribution:* Crosses placenta; may enter breast milk
*Excretion:* Feces and urine

### Adverse effects
- GI: *Nausea, vomiting,* burning of lips and throat, salivation, abdominal pain, anxiety, weakness, unrest
- CNS: *Headache*, conjunctivitis, lacrimation, tingling of hands
- CV: *Rise in BP, tachycardia*
- Other: Burning sensation in penis, sweating of forehead and hands, feeling of constriction in chest, throat, *pain at site of injection,* ***renal damage***

### Clinically important drug-drug interactions
- Increased risk of toxicity if taken with iron

## ■ Nursing Considerations
### Assessment
- *History:* Hepatic insufficiency; iron, cadmium or selenium poisoning
- *Physical:* Skin color, edema, lesions; peripheral sensation; P, BP, abdominal exam; CBC, liver function tests, serum levels of heavy metals

### Implementation
- Administer by deep IM injection only.
- Begin therapy as soon as possible after poisoning.
- Monitor BP and P when treatment has begun, increased BP and P can occur.
- Alkalinize urine to increase excretion of chelated complex.
- Monitor intake and output to detect any alteration in renal function.

### Drug-specific teaching points
- Treatment will need to be continued for 2–10 d.
- Drug can be given only IM.
- The following side effects may occur: nausea, vomiting (if severe, medication may be ordered); numbness, tingling, loss of sensation in the extremities (use caution to avoid injury, and examine extremities daily for injury); headache; pain at site of injection.
- Report irregular heartbeat, pain or weakness of extremities, severe nausea or vomiting, severe pain at injection site; changes in voiding patterns.

## dinoprostone

*(dye noe **prost'** one)*
prostaglandin $E_2$
Cervidil, Prepidil Gel, Prostin E2
**Pregnancy Category C**

**Drug classes**
Prostaglandin
Abortifacient

**Therapeutic actions**
Stimulates the myometrium of the pregnant uterus to contract, similar to the contractions of the uterus during labor, thus evacuating the contents of the uterus.

**Indications**
- Termination of pregnancy 12–20 wk from the first day of the last menstrual period
- Evacuation of the uterus in the management of missed abortion or intrauterine fetal death up to 28 wk gestational age
- Management of nonmetastatic gestational trophoblastic disease (benign hydatidiform mole)
- Initiation of cervical ripening before induciton of labor.

**Contraindications/cautions**
- Contraindications: allergy to prostaglandin preparations, acute PID, active cardiac, hepatic, pulmonary, renal disease.
- Use cautiously with history of asthma; hypotension; hypertension; CV, adrenal, renal, or hepatic disease; anemia; jaundice; diabetes; epilepsy; scarred uterus; cervicitis, infected endocervical lesions, acute vaginitis.

## Dosage

**Available Forms:** Vaginal suppository—20 mg; vaginal gel—0.5 mg; vaginal insert—10 mg

**ADULT**
- *Termination of pregnancy:* Insert one suppository (20 mg) high into the vagina; keep supine for 10 min after insertion. Additional suppositories may be given at 3- to 5-h intervals based on uterine response and tolerance. Do not give longer than 2 d.
- *Cervical ripening:* Give 0.5 mg gel via cervical catheter provided with patient in the dorsal position and cervix visulaized using a speculum. Repeat dose may be given if no response in 6 h. Wait 6–12 h before beginning oxytocin IV to initiate labor.

**Pharmacokinetics**

| Route | Onset | Peak | Duration |
|---|---|---|---|
| Intravaginal | 10 min | 15 min | 2–3 h |

*Metabolism:* Tissue; $T_{1/2}$: 5–10 h
*Distribution:* Crosses placenta; enters breast milk
*Excretion:* Urine

**Adverse effects**
- CNS: *Headache*, paresthesias, anxiety, weakness, syncope, dizziness
- GI: *Vomiting, diarrhea, nausea*
- CV: *Hypotension*, arrhythmias, chest pain
- **Respiratory**: Coughing, dyspnea
- GU: Endometritis, perforated uterus, uterine rupture, uterine or vaginal pain, incomplete abortion
- **Other**: Chills, diaphoresis, backache, breast tenderness, eye pain, skin rash, pyrexia

## ■ Nursing Considerations

### Assessment
- ***History:*** Allergy to prostaglandin preparations; acute PID; active cardiac, hepatic, pulmonary, renal disease; history of asthma; hypotension; hypertension; anemia; jaundice; diabetes; epilepsy; scarred uterus; cervicitis, infected endocervical lesions, acute vaginitis
- ***Physical:*** T; BP, P, auscultation; R, adventitious sounds; bowel sounds, liver evaluation; vaginal discharge, pelvic exam, uterine tone; liver and renal function tests, WBC, urinalysis, CBC

### Implementation
- Store suppositories in freezer; bring to room temperature before insertion.
- Arrange for pre- or concurrent treatment with antiemetic and antidiarrheal drugs to decrease the incidence of GI side effects.
- Ensure that abortion is complete or that other measures are used to complete the abortion if drug effects are not sufficient.

- Monitor T, using care to differentiate prostaglandin-induced pyrexia from postabortion endometritis pyrexia.
- Give gel using aseptic technique via cervical catheter to patient in dorsal position. Patient should remain in this position 15–30 min.
- Monitor uterine tone and vaginal discharge throughout procedure and several days after the procedure.
- Ensure adequate hydration throughout procedure.
- Be prepared to support patient through labor (cervical ripening). Give oxytocin infusion 6–12 h after dinoprostone.

### Drug-specific teaching points

Teaching about dinoprostone should be incorporated into the total teaching plan, including the following:

- If the patient has never had a vaginal suppository, explain the procedure and that she will need to lie down for 10 min after insertion.
- You will need to stay on your side for 15–30 min after injection of gel.
- The following side effects may occur: nausea, vomiting, diarrhea, uterine or vaginal pain, fever, headache, weakness, dizziness.
- Report severe pain, difficulty breathing, palpitations, eye pain, rash.

## diphenhydramine hydrochloride

*(dye fen* ***bye'*** *dra meen)*

*Oral:* Benadryl, Benylin Cough, Bydramine, Compoz, Diphen Cough, Dormarex 2, Nytol, Sleep-Eze 3, Sominex 2

*Oral prescription preparations:* Benadryl

*Parenteral preparations:* Benadryl

**Pregnancy Category B**

### Drug classes

Antihistamine
Anti-motion sickness agent
Sedative/hypnotic
Antiparkinsonism agent
Cough suppressant

### Therapeutic actions

Competitively blocks the effects of histamine at $H_1$ receptor sites, has atropine-like, antipruritic, and sedative effects.

### Indications

- Relief of symptoms associated with perennial and seasonal allergic rhinitis; vasomotor rhinitis; allergic conjunctivitis; mild, uncomplicated urticaria and angioedema; amelioraton of allergic reactions to blood or plasma; dermatographism; adjunctive therapy in anaphylactic reactions
- Active and prophylactic treatment of motion sickness
- Nighttime sleep aid
- Parkinsonism (including drug-induced parkinsonism and extrapyramidal reactions), in the elderly intolerant of more potent agents, for milder forms of the disorder in other age groups, and in combination with centrally acting anticholinergic antiparkinsonism drugs
- Suppression of cough due to colds or allergy (syrup formulation)

### Contraindications/cautions

- Contraindications: allergy to any antihistamines, third trimester of pregnancy, lactation.
- Use cautiously with narrow-angle glaucoma, stenosing peptic ulcer, symptomatic prostatic hypertrophy, asthmatic attack, bladder neck obstruction, pyloroduodenal obstruction, pregnancy.

### Dosage

**Available Forms:** Capsules—25, 50 mg; tablets—25, 50 mg; elixir—12.5 mg/5 ml; syrup—12.5 mg/5 ml; injection—10, 50 mg/ml

ADULT

- ***Oral:*** 25–50 mg q4–6h PO.
  - *Motion sickness:* Give full dose prophylactically 1/2 h before exposure to motion, and repeat before meals and at bedtime.
  - *Nighttime sleep aid:* 50 mg PO at bedtime.

– *Cough suppression:* 25 mg q4h PO, not to exceed 150 mg in 24 h.
- ***Parenteral:*** 10–50 mg IV or deep IM or up to 100 mg if required. Maximum daily dose is 400 mg.

*PEDIATRIC (> 10 KG, 20 LB)*
- ***Oral:*** 12.5–25 mg tid–qid PO or 5 mg/kg per day PO or 150 mg/m$^2$ per day PO. Maximum daily dose 300 mg.
  – *Motion sickness:* Give full dose prophylactically 1/2 h before exposure to motion and repeat before meals and at bedtime.
  – *Cough suppression* (6–12 y): 12.5 mg q4h PO, not to exceed 75 mg in 24 h. *2–6 y:* 6.25 mg q4h, not to exceed 25 mg in 24 h.
- ***Parenteral:*** 5 mg/kg per day or 150 mg/m$^2$ per day IV or by deep IM injection. Maximum daily is 300 mg divided into four doses.

*GERIATRIC:* More likely to cause dizziness, sedation, syncope, toxic confusional states, and hypotension in elderly patients; use with caution.

## Pharmacokinetics

| Route | Onset | Peak | Duration |
|---|---|---|---|
| Oral | 15–30 min | 1–4 h | 4–7 h |
| IM | 20–30 min | 1–4 h | 4–8 h |
| | | 30–60 min | |
| IV | Rapid | | 4–8 h |

*Metabolism:* Hepatic; $T_{1/2}$: 2.5–7 h
*Distribution:* Crosses placenta; enters breast milk
*Excretion:* Urine

### IV facts

**Preparation:** No additional preparation required.
**Infusion:** Administer slowly each 25 mg over 1 min by direct injection or into tubing of running IV.

## Adverse effects

- CNS: *Drowsiness, sedation, dizziness, disturbed coordination*, fatigue, confusion, restlessness, excitation, nervousness, tremor, headache, blurred vision, diplopia
- GI: *Epigastric distress,* anorexia, increased appetite and weight gain, nausea, vomiting, diarrhea or constipation
- CV: Hypotension, palpitations, bradycardia, tachycardia, extra systoles
- Respiratory: *Thickening of bronchial secretions,* chest tightness, wheezing, nasal stuffiness, dry mouth, dry nose, dry throat, sore throat
- Hematologic: Hemolytic anemia, hypoplastic anemia, thrombocytopenia, leukopenia, agranulocytosis, pancytopenia
- GU: Urinary frequency, dysuria, urinary retention, early menses, decreased libido, impotence
- Other: Urticaria, rash, **anaphylactic shock**, photosensitivity, excessive perspiration

## Clinically important drug-drug interactions

- Possible increased and prolonged anticholinergic effects with MAO inhibitors

## ■ Nursing Considerations

### Assessment

- *History:* Allergy to any antihistamines, narrow-angle glaucoma, stenosing peptic ulcer, symptomatic prostatic hypertrophy, asthmatic attack, bladder neck obstruction, pyloroduodenal obstruction, third trimester of pregnancy, lactation
- *Physical:* Skin color, lesions, texture; orientation, reflexes, affect; vision exam; P, BP; R, adventitious sounds; bowel sounds; prostate palpation; CBC with differential

### Implementation

- Administer with food if GI upset occurs.
- Administer syrup form if patient is unable to take tablets.
- Monitor patient response, and arrange for adjustment of dosage to lowest possible effective dose.

### Drug-specific teaching points

- Take as prescribed; avoid excessive dosage.
- Take with food if GI upset occurs.
- The following side effects may occur: dizziness, sedation, drowsiness (use caution

driving or performing tasks requiring alertness); epigastric distress, diarrhea or constipation (take drug with meals); dry mouth (use frequent mouth care, suck sugarless lozenges); thickening of bronchial secretions, dryness of nasal mucosa (use a humidifier).
- Avoid alcohol; serious sedation could occur.
- Report difficulty breathing, hallucinations, tremors, loss of coordination, unusual bleeding or bruising, visual disturbances,irregular heartbeat.

## dipyridamole

*(dye peer **id'** a mole)*

Persantine, Persantine IV

**Pregnancy Category B**

### Drug classes
Antianginal agent
Antiplatelet agent

### Therapeutic actions
Decreases coronary vascular resistance and increases coronary blood flow without increasing myocardial oxygen consumption; inhibits platelet aggregation.

### Indications
- "Possibly effective" for long-term therapy of angina pectoris; use withdrawn by the FDA; further hearings are pending
- With warfarin to prevent thromboembolism in patients with prosthetic heart valves
- Unlabeled uses: prevention of MI or reduction of mortality post-MI; with aspirin to prevent coronary bypass graft occlusion
- IV use: diagnostic aid in evaluation of CAD in patients who cannot exercise, as an alternative to exercise in thallium myocardial perfusion imaging studies

### Contraindications/cautions
- Contraindications: allergy to dipyridamole, pregnancy, lactation.
- Use cautiously with hypotension (drug can cause peripheral vasodilation that could exacerbate hypotension).

### Dosage
**Available Forms:** Tablets—25, 50, 75 mg; injection—10 mg

ADULT
- *Angina:* 50 mg tid PO at least 1 h before meals. Clinical response may not be evident before second or third month.
- ***Prophylaxis in thromboembolism following cardiac valve surgery:*** 75–100 mg qid PO as an adjunct to warfarin therapy.
- ***Diagnostic agent in thallium myocardial perfusion imaging:*** 0.142 mg/kg per minute (0.57 mg total) infused over 4 min. Inject thallium-201 within 5 min following the 4-min infusion of dipyridamole.

### Pharmacokinetics

| Route | Onset | Peak | Duration |
|---|---|---|---|
| Oral | Varies | 75 min | 3–4 h |
| IV | Rapid | 6.5 min | 30 min |

*Metabolism:* Hepatic; $T_{1/2}$: 40 min, then 10 h

*Distribution:* Crosses placenta; enters breast milk

*Excretion:* Bile

### IV facts
**Preparation:** Dilute dose based on weight in at least a 1:2 ration with 0.5N Sodium Chloride Injection, 1N Sodium Chloride Injection, or 5% Dextrose Injection for a total volume of about 20–50 ml. Protect from direct light.

**Infusion:** Infuse slowly over 4 min. Do not infuse undiluted drug; local irritation can occur.

### Adverse effects
- CNS: *Headache, dizziness*, weakness, syncope, flushing
- GI: Nausea, *GI distress,* constipation, diarrhea
- CV: **Fatal and nonfatal MI, ventricular fibrillation** (IV)
- Respiratory: **Bronchospasm** (IV)
- GU: Possible decreased fertility and loss of eggs in women

- Dermatologic: *Skin rash*, pruritus
- Local: Pain and burning at injection site

**Clinically important drug-drug interactions**

- Decreased coronary vasodilation effects if IV use with theophylline

## ■ Nursing Considerations

### Assessment

- *History:* Allergy to dipyridamole, hypotension, lactation
- *Physical:* Skin color, temperature, lesions; orientation, reflexes, affect; P, BP, orthostatic BP, baseline ECG, peripheral perfusion; R, adventitious sounds

### Implementation

- Provide continual monitoring of ECG, BP, and orientation during administration of IV dipyridamole.
- Administer oral drug at least 1 h before meals with a full glass of fluid.

### Drug-specific teaching points

- Take dipyridamole at least 1 h before meals with a full glass of fluid.
- The following side effects may occur: dizziness, lightheadedness (transient; change positions slowly; lie or sit down when you take your dose to decrease the risk of falling); headache (lie down and rest in a cool environment; OTC drugs may help); flushing of the neck or face (transient); nausea, gastric distress (small, frequent meals may help).
- Report skin rash, chest pain, fainting, severe headache; pain at injection site (IV).

## dirithromycin

*(dir **ith'** ro my sin)*
Dynabac
**Pregnancy Category C**

**Drug classes**

Macrolide antibiotic

**Therapeutic actions**

Inhibits protein synthesis in susceptible bacteria, causing cell death.

**Indications**

- Treatment of upper or lower respiratory infections caused by *Streptococcus pneumoniae, Moraxella catarrhalis, Mycoplasma pneumoniae, Legionella pneumophila*
- Treatment of pharyngitis/tonsillitis caused by *Streptococcus pyogenes*
- Treatment of skin and structure infections caused by *Staphylococcus aureus*

**Contraindications/cautions**

- Contraindications: hypersensitivity to dirithromycin, erythromycin, or any macrolide antibiotic, bacteremia
- Use cautiously with colitis, hepatic or renal impairment, pregnancy, lactation

### Dosage

**Available Forms:** Tablets—250 mg

*ADULT:* 500 mg PO qd. Bronchitis, skin, and skin structure infections—treat for 7 d; pharyngitis/tonsillitis—treat for 10 d; pneumonia—treat for 14 d.

*PEDIATRIC:* Safety and efficacy not established in children <12 years.

**Pharmacokinetics**

| *Route* | *Onset* | *Peak* |
|---|---|---|
| Oral | slow | 4 h |

*Metabolism:* Hepatic metabolism, $T_{1/2}$: 44 h
*Distribution:* Crosses placenta; passes into breast milk
*Excretion:* Feces, bile

**Adverse effects**

- GI: *diarrhea, abdominal pain, nausea*, dyspepsia, flatulence, vomiting, melena, **pseudomembranous colitis**
- CNS: dizziness, headache, vertigo, somnolence, fatigue
- Other: *superinfections*, cough, rash, **electrolyte imbalance**

**Clinically important drug-drug interactions**

- Possible risk of cardiac arrhythmias and sudden cardiac death with terfenadine, astemizole

## Nursing Considerations

### Assessment

- ***History:*** hypersensitivity to erythromycin or any macrolide antibiotic; pseudomembranous colitis, hepatic or renal impairment, bacteremia, lactation
- ***Physical:*** site of infection, skin color, lesions; orientation, GI output, bowel sounds, liver evaluation; culture and sensitivity tests of infection, urinalysis, liver and renal function tests

### Implementation

- Culture site of infection before beginning therapy.
- Give with food to increase GI effects and absorption.
- Assure that patient swallows tablet whole; continue therapy for complete course.
- Institute appropriate hygiene measures and arrange treatment if superinfections occur.
- Provide small, frequent meals and good mouth care if GI problems occur.

### Drug-specific teaching points

- Drug should be taken once a day with food. Swallow tablet whole, do not cut or crush. Take full course of therapy prescribed.
- The following side effects may occur: stomach cramping, discomfort, diarrhea; fatigue, headache (medication may help); additional infections in mouth or vagina (consult with health care provider for appropriate treatment).
- Report severe or watery diarrhea, severe nausea or vomiting, skin rash or itching, mouth or vaginal sores.

# disopyramide phosphate

*(dye soe* ***peer'*** *a mide)*

Norpace, Norpace CR, Rythmodan (CAN)

**Pregnancy Category C**

### Drug classes

Antiarrhythmic

### Therapeutic actions

Type 1a antiarrhythmic: decreases rate of diastolic depolarization, decreases automaticity, decreases the rate of rise of the action potential, prolongs the refractory period of cardiac muscle cells.

### Indications

- Treatment of ventricular arrhythmias considered to be life threatening
- Unlabeled use: treatment of paroxysmal supraventricular tachycardia

### Contraindications/cautions

- Allergy to disopyramide, CHF, hypotension, cardiac conduction abnormalities (eg, Wolff-Parkinson-White syndrome, sick sinus syndrome, heart block), cardiac myopathies, urinary retention, glaucoma, myasthenia gravis, renal or hepatic disease, potassium imbalance, pregnancy, lactation.

### Dosage

**Available Forms:** Capsules—100, 150 mg; ER capsules—100, 150 mg

Evaluate patient carefully and monitor cardiac response closely to determine the correct dosage for each patient.

*ADULT:* 400–800 mg/d PO given in divided doses q6h or q12h if using the controlled-release products.

*PEDIATRIC:* Give in equal, divided doses q6h PO, titrating the dose to the patient's need.

| *Age* | *Daily Dosage (mg/kg)* |
|---|---|
| <1 y | 10–30 |
| 1–4 y | 10–20 |
| 4–12 y | 10–15 |
| 12–18 y | 6–15 |

*GERIATRIC:* Loading dose of 150 mg PO may be given, followed by 100 mg at the intervals shown.

| *Creatinine Clearance (ml/min)* | *Interval* |
|---|---|
| 30–40 | q8h |
| 15–30 | q12h |
| <15 | q24h |

### Pharmacokinetics

| *Route* | *Onset* | *Peak* | *Duration* |
|---|---|---|---|
| Oral | 30–60 min | 2 h | 1.5–8.5 h |

*Metabolism:* Hepatic; $T_{1/2}$: 4–10 h
*Distribution:* Crosses placenta; enters breast milk
*Excretion:* Urine

**Adverse effects**
- CNS: Dizziness, fatigue, headache, *blurred vision*
- CV: CHF, hypotension, cardiac conduction disturbances
- GI: *Dry mouth, constipation*, nausea, abdominal pain, gas
- GU: *Urinary hesitancy and retention, impotence*
- Other: *Dry mose, eyes, and throat; rash*; itching; *muscle weakness; malaise; aches and pains*

**Clinically important drug-drug interactions**
- Decreased disopyramide plasma levels if used with phenytoins, rifampin

## ■ Nursing Considerations

### Assessment
- *History:* Allergy to disopyramide, CHF, hypotension, Wolff-Parkinson-White syndrome, sick sinus syndrome, heart block, cardiac myopathies, urinary retention, glaucoma, myasthenia gravis, renal or hepatic disease, potassium imbalance, labor or delivery, lactation
- *Physical:* Weight; orientation, reflexes; P, BP, auscultation, ECG, edema; R, adventitious sounds; bowel sounds, liver evaluation; urinalysis, renal and liver function tests, blood glucose, serum $K^+$

### Implementation
- Check that patients with supraventricular tachyarrhythmias have been digitalized before starting disopyramide.
- Reduce dosage in patients $<$ 110 lb.
- Reduce dosage in patients with hepatic or renal failure.
- Monitor patients with severe refractory tachycardia who may be given up to 1,600 mg/d continuously.
- Make a pediatric suspension form (1–10 mg/ml) by adding the contents of the immediate release capsule to cherry syrup, NF if desired. Store in dark bottle, and refrigerate. Shake well before using. Stable for 1 mo.
- Take care to differentiate the controlled release form from the immediate-release preparation.
- Monitor BP, orthostatic pressure.
- Evaluate for safe and effective serum levels (2–8 $\mu$g/ml).

### Drug-specific teaching points
- You will require frequent monitoring of cardiac rhythm, BP.
- The following side effects may occur: dry mouth (try frequent mouth care, suck sugarless lozenges); constipation (laxatives may be ordered); difficulty voiding (empty the bladder before taking drug); muscle weakness or aches and pains.
- Do not stop taking this drug for any reason without checking with your health care provider.
- Return for regular follow-up visits to check your heart rhythm and blood pressure.
- Report swelling of fingers or ankles, difficulty breathing, dizziness, urinary retention, severe headache or visual changes.

# disulfiram

*(dye* ***sul'*** *fi ram)*
Antabuse
**Pregnancy Category C**

**Drug classes**
Antialcoholic agent
Enzyme inhibitor

**Therapeutic actions**
Inhibits the enzyme aldehyde dehydrogenase, blocking oxidation of alcohol and allowing acetaldehyde to accumulate to concentrations in the blood 5–10 times higher than normally achieved during alcohol metabolism; accumulation of acetaldehyde produces the highly unpleasant reaction described below that deters consumption of alcohol.

## Indications

- Aids in the management of selected chronic alcoholics who want to remain in a state of enforced sobriety

## Contraindications/cautions

- Contraindications: allergy to disulfiram or other thiuram derivatives used in pesticides and rubber vulcanization, severe myocardial disease or coronary occlusion; psychoses, current or recent treatment with metrondiazole, paraldehyde, alcohol, alcohol-containing preparations (eg, cough syrups, tonics).
- Use cautiously with diabetes mellitus, hypothyroidism, epilepsy, cerebral damage, chronic and acute nephritis, hepatic cirrhosis or dysfunction.

## Dosage

**Available Forms:** Tablets—250, 500 mg

Never administer to an intoxicated patient or without patient's knowledge. Do not administer until patient has abstained from alcohol for at least 12 h.

### Adult

- *Initial dosage:* Administer maximum of 500 mg/d PO in a single dose for 1–2 wk. If a sedative effect occurs, administer at bedtime or decrease dosage.
- *Maintenance regimen:* 125–500 mg/d PO. Do not exceed 500 mg/d. Continue use until patient is fully recovered socially and a basis for permanent self-control is established.
- *Trial with alcohol (do not administer to anyone > 50 y):* After 1–2 wk of therapy with 500 mg/d PO, a drink of 15 ml of 100 proof whiskey or its equivalent is taken slowly. Dose may be repeated once, if patient is hospitalized and supportive facilities are available.

## Pharmacokinetics

| *Route* | *Onset* | *Peak* | *Duration* |
|---|---|---|---|
| Oral | Slow | 12 h | 1–2 wk |

*Metabolism:* Hepatic; $T_{1/2}$: unclear
*Distribution:* Crosses placenta; enters breast milk
*Excretion:* Feces, lungs

## Adverse effects

- **Disulfiram-alcohol reaction:** Flushing, throbbing in head and neck, throbbing headaches, respiratory difficulty, nausea, copious vomiting, sweating, thirst, chest pain, palpitations, dyspnea, hyperventilation, tachycardia, hypotension, syncope, weakness, vertigo, blurred vision, confusion; severe reactions may include arrhythmias, CV collapse, acute CHF, unconsciousness, **convulsions, MI, death**

*Adverse Effects of Disulfiram Alone*

- CNS: *Drowsiness, fatigability, headache*, restlessness, peripheral neuropathy, optic or retrobulbar neuritis
- GI: *Metallic or garliclike aftertaste*, hepatotoxicity
- Dermatologic: *Skin eruptions*, anceiform eruptions, allergic dermatitis

## Clinically important drug-drug interactions

• Increased serum levels and risk of toxicity of phenytoin and its congeners, diazepam, chlordiazepoxide • Increased therapeutic and toxic effects of theophyllines • Increased PT caused by disulfiram may lead to a need to adjust dosage of oral anticoagulants • Severe alcohol-intolerance reactions with any alcohol-containing liquid medications (eg, elixirs, tinctures) • Acute toxic psychosis with metronidazole

## ■ Nursing Considerations

### Assessment

- *History:* Allergy to disulfiram or other thiuram derivatives; severe myocardial disease or coronary occlusion; psychoses; current or recent treatment with metrondiazole, paraldehyde, alcohol, alcohol-containing preparations (eg, cough syrups, tonics); diabetes mellitus, hypothyroidism, epilepsy, cerebral damage, chronic and acute nephritis, hepatic cirrhosis or dysfunction
- *Physical:* Skin color, lesions; thyroid palpation; orientation, affect, reflexes; P, auscultation, BP ; R, adventitious sounds; liver evaluation; renal and liver function tests, CBC, SMA-12

### Implementation

- Do not administer until patient has abstained from alcohol for at least 12 h.
- Administer orally; tablets may be crushed and mixed with liquid beverages.
- Monitor liver function tests before, in 10–14 d, and every 6 mo during therapy to evaluate for hepatic dysfunction.
- Monitor CBC, SMA-12 before and every 6 mo during therapy.
- Inform patient of the seriousness of disulfiram-alcohol reaction and the potential consequences of alcohol use: disulfiram should not be taken for at least 12 h after alcohol ingestion, and a reaction may occur up to 2 wk after disulfiram therapy is stopped; all forms of alcohol must be avoided.
- Arrange for treatment with antihistamines if skin reaction occurs.

### Drug-specific teaching points

- Take drug daily; if drug makes you dizzy or tired, take it at bedtime. Tablets may be crushed and mixed with liquid.
- Abstain from forms of alcohol (beer, wine, liquor, vinegars, cough mixtures, sauces, aftershave lotions, liniments, colognes). Taking alcohol while on this drug can cause severe, unpleasant reactions—flushing, copious vomiting, throbbing headache, difficulty breathing, even death.
- Wear or carry a medical ID while you are on this drug to alert any medical emergency personnel that you are on this drug.
- Have periodic blood tests while on drug to evaluate its effects on the liver.
- The following side effects may occur: drowsiness, headache, fatigue, restlessness, blurred vision (use caution driving or performing tasks that require alertness); metallic aftertaste (transient).
- Report unusual bleeding or bruising, yellowing of skin or eyes, chest pain, difficulty breathing, ingestion of any alcohol.

## dobutamine hydrochloride

*(doe' byoo ta meen)*

Dobutrex

**Pregnancy Category C**

### Drug classes

Sympathomimetic

Beta-1 selective adrenergic agonist

### Therapeutic actions

Positive inotropic effects are mediated by beta-1 adrenergic receptors in the heart; increases the force of mycocardial contraction with relatively minor effects on heart rate, arrhythmogenesis; has minor effects on blood vessels.

### Indications

- For inotropic support in the short-term treatment of adults with cardiac decompensation due to depressed contractility, resulting from either organic heart disease or from cardiac surgical procedures
- Investigational use in children with congenital heart disease undergoing diagnostic cardiac catheterization, to augment CV function

### Contraindications/cautions

- Contraindications: IHSS; hypovolemia (dobutamine is not a substitute for blood, plasma, fluids, electrolytes, which should be restored promptly when loss has occurred and in any case before treatment with dobutamine); acute MI (may increase the size of an infarct by intensifying ischemia); general anesthesia with halogenated hydrocarbons or cyclopropane, which sensitize the myocardium to catecholamines.
- Use cautiously with diabetes, lactation.

### Dosage

**Available Forms:** Injection 12.5 mg/ml

Administer only by IV infusion. Titrate on the basis of the patient's hemodynamic/renal response. Close monitoring is necessary.

*ADULT:* 2.5–15 μg/kg/min IV is usual rate to increase cardiac output; rarely, rates up to 40 μg/kg per minute are needed.

*PEDIATRIC:* Safety and efficacy not established. When used investigationally in children undergoing cardiac catheterization (see above), doses of 2.0 and 7.75 μg/kg per minute were infused for 10 min.

### Pharmacokinetics

| Route | Onset | Peak | Duration |
|---|---|---|---|
| IV | 1–2 min | 10 min | Length of infusion |

*Metabolism:* Hepatic; $T_{1/2}$: 2 min
*Distribution:* Crosses placenta; enters breast milk
*Excretion:* Urine

### IV facts

**Preparation:** Reconstitute by adding 10 ml Sterile Water for Injection or 5% Dextrose Injection to 250-mg vial. If material is not completely dissolved, add 10 ml of diluent. Further dilute to at least 50 ml with 5% Dextrose Injection, 0.9% Sodium Chloride Injection, or Sodium Lactate Injection. Store reconstituted solution under refrigeration for 48 h or at room temperature for 6 h. Store final diluted solution in glass or Viaflex container at room temperature. Stable for 24 h. Do not freeze. (Note: drug solutions may exhibit a color that increases with time; this indicates oxidation of the drug, not a loss of potency.)
**Infusion:** May be administered through common IV tubing with dopamine, lidocaine, tobramycin, nitroprusside, potassium chloride, or protamine sulfate. Titrate rate based on patient response—P, BP, rhythm; use of an infusion pump is suggested.
**Incompatibilities:** Do *not* mix drug with alkaline solutions, such as 5% Sodium Bicarbonate Injection; do *not* mix with hydrocortisone sodium succinate, cefazolin, cefamandole, neutral cephalothin, penicillin, sodium ethacrynate; sodium heparin.

### Adverse effects

- CNS: *Headache*
- GI: *Nausea*
- CV: *Increase in heart rate, increase in systolic blood pressure, increase in ventricular ectopic beats (PVCs)*, anginal pain, palpitations, shortness of breath

### Clinically important drug-drug interactions

• Increased effects with TCAs (eg, imipramine), furazolidone, methyldopa • Risk of severe hypertension with beta-blockers (alseroxylon) • Decreased effects of guanethidine with dobutamine

## ■ Nursing Considerations

### Assessment

- *History:* IHSS, hypovolemia, acute MI, general anesthesia with halogenated hydrocarbons or cyclopropane, diabetes, lactation
- *Physical:* Weight, skin color, T; P, BP, pulse pressure, auscultation; R, adventitious sounds; urine output; serum electrolytes, Hct, ECG

### Implementation

- Arrange to digitalize patients who have atrial fibrillation with a rapid ventricular rate before giving dobutamine—dobutamine facilitates AV conduction.
- Monitor urine flow, cardiac output, pulmonary wedge pressure, ECG, and BP closely during infusion; adjust dose/rate accordingly.

### Drug-specific teaching points

- Used only in acute emergency care situations; teaching will depend on patient's awareness and will emphasize need for the drug rather than the drug itself.

## docetaxel

*(dohs eh **tax'** ell)*

Taxotere

**Pregnancy Category D**

### Drug classes

Antineoplastic

### Therapeutic actions

Inhibits the normal dynamic reorganization of the microtubule network that is essential for dividing cells; leads to cell death in rapidly dividing cells.

### Indications

- Treatment of patients with locally advanced or metastatic breast cancer who have progressed during anthracycline therapy or relapsed during anthracycline adjuvant therapy

### Contraindications/cautions

- Contraindications: hypersensitivity to docetaxel or drugs using polysorbate 80;

bone marrow depression with neutrophil counts <1500 cells/mm$^2$
- Use cautiously with hepatic dysfunction, pregnancy, lactation

### Dosage

**Available Forms:** Injection—20, 80 mg

*ADULT:* 60–100 mg/m$^2$ IV infused over 1 h every 3 wk.

*PEDIATRIC:* Safety and efficacy not established.

### Pharmacokinetics

| *Route* | *Onset* | *Duration* |
|---|---|---|
| IV | Slow | 20–24 h |

*Metabolism:* Hepatic; $T_{1/2}$: 36 min and 11.1 h

*Distribution:* Crosses placenta; enters breast milk

*Excretion:* Feces and urine

### IV facts

**Preparation:** Dilute with 0.9% Sodium Chloride Injection or 5% Dextrose Injection, stand vials at room temperature for 5 min before diluting; stable at room temperature for 8 h; refrigerate unopened vials, protect from light; avoid use of PVC infusion bags and tubing. Premedicate patient with oral corticosteroids before beginning infusion.

**Infusion:** Administer over 1 h.

### Adverse effects

- CNS: Neurosensory disturbances including paresthesias, pain, *asthenia*
- GI: *Nausea, vomiting, diarrhea, stomatitis,* constipation
- CV: Sinus tachycardia, hypotension, arrhythmias, **fluid retention**
- Hematologic: **Bone marrow depression,** *infection*
- Other: *Hypersensitivity reactions, myalgia, arthralgia, alopecia*

### Clinically important drug-drug interactions

- Possible increase in effectiveness and toxicity with cyclosporine, terfenadine, ketoconazole, erthyromycin, troleandomycin; avoid these combinations

## ■ Nursing Considerations

### Assessment

- *History:* Hypersensitivity to docetaxel, polysorbate 80; bone marrow depression; hepatic impairment, pregnancy, lactation
- *Physical:* Neurologic status, T; P, BP, peripheral perfusion; abdominal exam, mucous membranes; liver function tests, CBC

### Implementation

- Do not give drug unless blood counts are within acceptable parameters (neutrophils >1500 cells/mm$^2$).
- Handle drug with great care; use of gloves is recommended; if drug comes into contact with skin, wash immediately with soap and water.
- Premedicate patient before administration with oral corticosteroids (eg, dexamethasone 16 mg/d PO for 5 d starting 1 d before docetaxel administration) to reduce severity of fluid retention.
- Monitor BP and P during administration.
- Arrange for blood counts before and regularly during therapy.
- Monitor patient's neurologic status frequently during treatment; provide safety measures as needed.

### Drug-specific teaching points

- This drug will need to be given once every 3 wk; mark calendar with days to return for treatment.
- The following side effects may occur: nausea and vomiting (if severe, antiemetics may be helpful; eat small, frequent meals); weakness, lethargy (take frequent rest periods); increased susceptibility to infection (avoid crowds, exposure to many people or diseases); numbness and tingling in fingers or toes (avoid injury to these areas; use care if performing tasks that require precision); loss of hair (arrange for a wig or other head covering; keep the head covered at extremes of temperature).
- Report severe nausea and vomiting; fever, chills, sore throat; unusual bleeding or bruising; numbness or tingling in fingers or toes; fluid retention or swelling.

# dolasetron mesylate

*(doe **laz'** e tron)*
Anzemet, Anzemet Injection
**Pregnancy Category B**

## Drug classes
Antiemetic

## Therapeutic actions
Selectively binds to serotonin receptors in the CTZ, blocking the nausea and vomiting caused by the release of serotonin by mucosal cells during chemotherapy, radiotherapy, or surgical invasion (an action that stimulates the CTZ and causes nausea and vomiting).

## Indications
- Prevention and treatment of nausea and vomiting associated with emetogenic chemotherapy
- Prevention of postoperative nausea and vomiting
- Treatment of post-op nausea and vomiting (injection only)

## Contraindications/cautions
- Contraindications: allergy to dolasetron or any of its components.
- Use cautiously in any patient at risk of developing prolongation of cardiac conduction intervals, especially Q-T interval (congenital Q-T syndrome, hypokalemia, hypomagnesemia), pregnancy, lactation.

## Dosage
**Available Forms:** Tablets—50, 100 mg; injection—20 mg/ml

*ADULT:* 100 mg PO within 1 h before chemotherapy or within 2 h before surgery; or 1.8 mg/kg IV about 30 min before chemotherapy or 100 mg IV injection: prevention of post-op nausea and vomiting—12.5 mg IV about 15 min before stopping anesthesia; treatment of post-op nausea and vomiting—12.5 mg IV as soon as needed.

*PEDIATRIC < 2 Y:* Not recommended.

*PEDIATRIC (2–16 Y):* 1.8 mg/kg PO tablets or injection diluted in apple or apple-grape juice within 1 h before chemotherapy; or 1.2 mg/kg PO tablets or injection diluted in apple or apple-grape juice within 2 h before surgery; or 1.8 mg/kg IV for chemotherapy-induced nausea and vomiting about 30 min before chemotherapy; 1.2 mg/kg IV about 15 min before stopping anesthesia to prevent post-op nausea and vomiting; 0.35 mg/kg IV as soon as needed to treat post-op nausea and vomiting.

## Pharmacokinetics

| Route | Onset | Peak |
|---|---|---|
| Oral | Rapid | 1–2 h |
| IV | Immediate | End of infusion |

*Metabolism:* Hepatic; T $_{1/2}$: 3.5–5 h
*Distribution:* Crosses placenta; passes into breast milk
*Excretion:* Urine, feces

### IV facts
**Preparation:** Dilute in 50 ml 5% Dextrose Injection, 0.9% Sodium Chloride Injection, 5% Dextrose and 0.9% Sodium Chloride Injection, 5% Dextrose and 0.45% Sodium Chloride Injection; 3% Sodium Chloride Injection; do not mix in any alkaline solution, precipitates may form. Stable at room temperature for 48 h after dilution.
**Infusion:** Inject 100 mg undiluted over 30 sec, or infuse diluted over up to 15 min.
**Compatibilities:** Dilute only in recommended solutions.

## Adverse effects
- CNS: *Headache, dizziness,* somnolence, drowsiness, sedation, *fatigue*
- CV: *Tachycardia,* EKG changes
- GI: *Diarrhea,* constipation, abdominal pain
- Other: Fever, pruritus, injeciton site reaction

## Clinically important drug-drug interactions
- Possible cardiac arrhythmias with drugs which cause EKG interval prolongation
- Potential for severe toxic reaction with high-dose anthracycline therapy

## ■ Nursing Considerations

### Assessment

- ***History:*** Allergy to dolasetron, pregnancy, lactation, QT prolongation
- ***Physical:*** Orientation, reflexes, affect; BP; P, baseline EKG

### Implementation

- Dilute injection in apple or apple-grape juice if patient is unable to swallow tablets; dosage remains the same.
- Provide mouth care, sugarless lozenges to suck to help alleviate nausea.
- Obtain baseline EKG and periodically monitor EKG in any patient at risk for QT prolongation.
- Provide appropriate analgesics for headache.

### Drug-specific teaching points

- This drug may be given IV or orally when you are receiving your chemotherapy; it will help decrease nausea and vomiting.
- The following side effects may occur: dizziness, drowsiness (use caution if driving or performing tasks that require alertness) diarrhea; headache (appropriate medication will be arranged to alleviate this problem).
- Report severe headache, fever, numbness or tingling, palpitations, fainting episodes, change in color of stools or urine.

# donepezil hydrochloride

*(doe **nep'** ah zill)*

Aricept

**Pregnancy Category C**

### Drug classes

Cholinesterase inhibitors
Alzheimer's drug

### Therapeutic actions

Centrally acting reversible cholinesterase inhibitor leading to elevated acetylcholine levels in the cortex, which slows the neuronal degradation that occurs in Alzheimer's disease.

### Indications

- Treatment of mild to moderate dementia of the Alzheimer's type

### Contraindications/cautions

- Contraindications: allergy to donepezil, pregnancy, lactation
- Use cautiously with sick sinus syndrome, GI bleeding, seizures, asthma



### Dosage

**Available Forms:** Tablets—5, 10 mg

*ADULT:* 5 mg PO qd hs. May be increased to 10 mg qd after 4–6 wk.

*PEDIATRIC:* Safety and efficacy not established.

### Pharmacokinetics

| *Route* | *Onset* | *Peak* |
|---|---|---|
| Oral | Varies | 2–4 h |

*Metabolism:* Hepatic; $T_{1/2}$: 70 h
*Distribution:* Crosses placenta; may enter breast milk
*Excretion:* Urine

### Adverse effects

- CNS: *Insomnia, fatigue,* dizziness, confusion, ataxia, insomnia, somnolence, tremor, agitation, depression, anxiety, abnormal thinking
- GI: *Nausea, vomiting, diarrhea, dyspepsia, anorexia, abdominal pain,* flatulence, constipation, **hepatotoxicity**
- Dermatologic: *Skin rash,* flushing, purpura
- Other: *Muscle cramps*

### Clinically important drug-drug interactions

- Increased effects and risk of toxicity with theophylline, cholinesterase inhibitors
- Decreased effects of anticholinergics
- Increased risk of GI bleeding with NSAIDs

## ■ Nursing Considerations

### Assessment

- ***History:*** Allergy to donepezil, pregnancy, lactation, sick sinus syndrome, GI bleeding, seizures, asthma
- ***Physical:*** Orientation, affect, reflexes; BP, P; abdominal exam; renal and liver function tests

## Implementation

- Administer hs each day.
- Provide small, frequent meals if GI upset is severe.
- Notify surgeons that patient is on donepezil; exaggerated muscle relaxation may occur if succinylcholine-type drugs are used.

## Drug-specific teaching points

- Take this drug exactly as prescribed, at bedtime.
- This drug does not cure the disease but is thought to slow down the degeneration associated with the disease.
- Arrange for regular blood tests and follow-up visits while adjusting to this drug.
- The following side effects may occur: nausea, vomiting (eat small, frequent meals); insomnia, fatigue, confusion (use caution if driving or performing tasks that require alertness).
- Report severe nausea, vomiting, changes in stool or urine color, diarrhea, changes in neurologic functioning, yellowing of eyes or skin.

# dopamine hydrochloride

*(doe' pa meen)*

Intropin, Revimine (CAN)

**Pregnancy Category C**

## Drug classes

Sympathomimetic
Alpha adrenergic agonist
Beta-1 selective adrenergic agonist
Dopaminergic blocking agent

## Therapeutic actions

Drug acts directly and by the release of norepinephrine from sympathetic nerve terminals; dopaminergic receptors mediate dilation of vessels in the renal and splanchnic beds, which maintains renal perfusion and function; alpha receptors, which are activated by higher doses of dopamine, mediate vasoconstriction, which can override the vasodilating effects; beta-1 receptors mediate a positive inotropic effect on the heart.

## Indications

- Correction of hemodynamic imbalances present in the shock syndrome due to MI, trauma, endotoxic septicemia, open heart surgery, renal failure, and chronic cardiac decompensation in CHF

## Contraindications/cautions

- Contraindications: pheochromocytoma, tachyarrhythmias, ventricular fibrillation, hypovolemia (dopamine is not a substitute for blood, plasma, fluids, electrolytes, which should be restored promptly when loss has occurred), general anesthesia with halogenated hydrocarbons or cyclopropane, which sensitize the myocardium to catecholamines.
- Use cautiously with atherosclerosis, arterial embolism, Reynaud's disease, cold injury, frostbite, diabetic endarteritis, Buerger's disease (monitor color and temperature of extremities).

## Dosage

**Available Forms:** Injection—40, 80, 160 mg/ml; injection in 5% dextrose—80, 160, 320 mg/100 ml

Dilute before using; administer only by IV infusion, using a metering device to control the rate of flow. Titrate on the basis of patient's hemodynamic/renal response. Close monitoring is necessary. In titrating to desired systolic BP response, optimum administration rate for renal response may be exceeded, thus necessitating a reduction in rate after hemodynamic stabilization.

ADULT

- *Patients likely to respond to modest increments of cardiac contractility and renal perfusion:* Initially, 2–5 μg/kg per min IV.
- *Patients who are more seriously ill:* Initially, 5 μg/kg per min IV. Increase in increments of 5–10 μg/kg per minute up to a rate of 20–50 μg/kg per minute. Check urine output frequently if doses > 16 μg/kg per minute.

PEDIATRIC: Safety and efficacy not established.

## Pharmacokinetics

| Route | Onset | Peak | Duration |
|---|---|---|---|
| IV | 1–2 min | 10 min | Length of infusion |

*Metabolism:* Hepatic; $T_{1/2}$: 2 min
*Distribution:* Crosses placenta; enters breast milk
*Excretion:* Urine

### IV facts

**Preparation:** Prepare solution for IV infusion as follows: Add 200–400 mg dopamine to 250–500 ml of one of the following IV solutions: Sodium Chloride Injection; 5% Dextrose Injection; 5% Dextrose and 0.45% or 0.9% Sodium Chloride Solution; 5% Dextrose in Lactated Ringer's Solution; Sodium Lactate (1/5 Molar) Injection; Lactated Ringer's Injection. Commonly used concentrations are 800 $\mu$g/ml (200 mg in 250 ml) and 1,600 $\mu$g/ml (400 mg in 250 ml). The 160 mg/ml concentrate may be preferred in patients with fluid retention. Protect drug solutions from light; drug solutions should be clear and colorless.
**Infusion:** Determine infusion rate based on patient response.
**Incompatibilities:** Do *not* mix with other drugs; do *not* add to 5% Sodium Bicarbonate or other alkaline IV solutions, oxidizing agents, or iron salts because drug is inactivated in alkaline solution (solutions become pink to violet).

### Adverse effects

- GI: *Nausea, vomiting*
- CV: *Ectopic beats, tachycardia, anginal pain, palpitations, hypotension, vasoconstriction, dyspnea*, bradycardia, hypertension, widened QRS
- Other: Headache, piloerection, azotemia, gangrene with prolonged use

### Clinically important drug-drug interactions

• Increased effects with MAO inhibitors, TCAs (imipramine) • Increased risk of hypertension with alseroxylon, deserpidine, furazolidone, methyldopa • Seizures, hypotension, bradycardia when infused with phenytoin • Decreased cardiostimulating effects with guanethidine

## ■ Nursing Considerations

### Assessment

- ***History:*** Pheochromocytoma, tachyarrhythmias, ventricular fibrillation, hypovolemia, general anesthesia with halogenated hydrocarbons or cyclopropane, occlusive vascular disease, labor and delivery
- ***Physical:*** Body weight; skin color, T; P, BP, pulse pressure; R, adventitious sounds; urine output; serum electrolytes, Hct, ECG

### Implementation

- Exercise extreme caution in calculating and preparing doses; dopamine is a very potent drug; small errors in dosage can cause serious adverse effects. Drug should always be diluted before use if not prediluted.
- Arrange to reduce initial dosage by 1/10 in patients who have been on MAO inhibitors.
- Administer into large veins of the antecubital fossa in preference to veins in hand or ankle.
- Provide phentolamine on standby in case extravasation occurs (infiltration with 10–15 ml saline containing 5–10 mg phentolamine is effective).
- Monitor urine flow, cardiac output, and BP closely during infusion.

### Drug-specific teaching points

- Used only in acute emergency; teaching will depend on patient's awareness and will relate mainly to patient's status, monitors, rather than to drug. Instruct patient to report any pain at injection site.

## dornase alfa

***(door' nace)***

recombinant human deoxyribonuclease, DNase

Pulmozyme

**Pregnancy Category B**

**Drug classes**
Cystic fibrosis drug

**Therapeutic actions**
Breaks down DNA molecules in sputum, resulting in a break up of thick, sticky mucus that clogs airways.

**Indications**
- Management of respiratory symptoms associated with cystic fibrosis
- Treatment of advanced cystic fibrosis

**Contraindications/cautions**
- Contraindications: allergy to dornase, Chinese hamster ovary products
- Use cautiously with lactation.

**Dosage**
**Available Forms:** Solution for inhalation—1 mg/ml
2.5 mg qid inhaled through nebulizer for adults and children >5 y with cystic fibrosis; may increase to 2.5 mg bid.

**Pharmacokinetics**

| *Route* | *Onset* | *Peak* | *Duration* |
|---|---|---|---|
| Inhal. | Slow | 3–4 h | Up to 1 wk |

*Metabolism:* Tissue; $T_{1/2}$: unknown

**Adverse effects**
- Respiratory: Increased cough, dyspnea, hemoptysis, *pharyngitis*, rhinitis, sputum increase, wheezes, voice changes
- Other: Conjunctivitis, chest pain

## ■ Nursing Considerations

**Assessment**
- *History:* Diagnosis of cystic fibrosis, allergy to dornase, Chinese hamster ovary cell products; lactation
- *Physical:* R, auscultation

**Implementation**
- Store drug in refrigerator and protect from light.
- Monitor patient closely.
- Ensure proper use of inhalation device.

**Drug-specific teaching points**
- This drug does not cure the disease but improves the respiratory symptoms.
- Review the use of nebulizer with health care provider; store in refrigerator and protect from light.
- Report worsening of disease, difficulty breathing, increased productive cough.

## doxapram hydrochloride

*(docks' a pram)*
Dopram
**Pregnancy Category B**

**Drug classes**
Analeptic

**Therapeutic actions**
Stimulates the peripheral carotid chemoreceptors to cause an increase in tidal volume and slight increase in respiratory rate; this stimulation also has a pressor effect.

**Indications**
- To stimulate respiration in patients with drug-induced postanesthesia respiratory depression or apnea; also used to "stir up" patients in combination with oxygen postoperatively.
- To stimulate respiration, hasten arousal in patients experiencing drug-induced CNS depression.
- As a temporary measure in hospitalized patients with acute respiratory insufficiency superimposed on COPD
- Unlabeled use: treatment of apnea of prematurity when methylxanthines have failed

**Contraindications/cautions**
- Contraindications: newborns (contains benzyl alcohol), epilepsy, incompetence of the ventilatory mechanism, flail chest, hypersensitivity to doxapram, head injury, pneumothorax, acute bronchial asthma, pulmonary fibrosis, severe hypertension, CVA.
- Use cautiously with pregnancy, lactation.

**Dosage**
**Available Forms:** Injection—20 mg/ml

*ADULT*

- ***Postanesthetic use:*** Single injection of 0.5–1 mg/kg IV; do not exceed 1.5 mg/kg as a total single injection or 2 mg/kg when given as mutiple injections at 5-min intervals. *Infusion:* 250 mg in 250 ml of dextrose or saline solution; initiate at 5 mg/min until response is seen; maintain at 1–3 mg/min; recommended total dose is 300 mg.
- ***Management of drug-induced CNS depression:***
  - ***Intermittent injection:*** Priming dose of 2 mg/kg IV; repeat in 5 min. Repeat every 1–2 h until patient awakens; if relapse occurs, repeat at 1–2 h intervals.
  - ***Intermittent IV infusion:*** Priming dose of 2 mg/kg IV; if no response, infuse 250 mg in 250 ml of dextrose or saline solution at a rate of 1–3 mg/min, discontinue at end of 2 h if patient awakens; repeat in 1/2–2 h if relapse occurs; do not exceed 3 g/d.
- ***Chronic obstructive pulmonary disease associated with acute hypercapnia:*** Mix 400 mg in 180 ml of IV infusion; start infusion at 1–2 mg/min (0.5–1 ml/min); check blood gases, and adjust rate accordingly. Do not use for longer than 2 h.

*PEDIATRIC:* Do not give if $< 12$ y.

### Pharmacokinetics

| *Route* | *Onset* | *Peak* | *Duration* |
|---|---|---|---|
| IV | 20–40 sec | 1–2 min | 5–12 min |

*Metabolism:* Hepatic; $T_{1/2}$: 2.4–4.1 h
*Distribution:* May cross placenta; may enter breast milk
*Excretion:* Urine

### IV facts

**Preparation:** Add 250 mg doxapram to 250 ml of 5 or 10% DW or normal saline.

**Infusion:** Initiate infusion at 5 mg/min; once response is seen, 1–3 mg/min is satisfactory.

**Incompatibilities:** Do not mix in alkaline solutions—precipitate or gas may form.

### Adverse effects

- CNS: Headache, dizziness, apprehension, disorientation, pupillary dilation, *increased reflexes*, hyperactivity, **convulsions**, muscle spasticity, clonus, pyrexia, flushing, sweating
- GI: Nausea, vomiting, diarrhea
- CV: Arrhythmias, chest pain, tightness in the chest, *increased blood pressure*
- Respiratory: Cough, dyspnea, tachypnea, laryngospasm, **bronchospasm**, hiccups, rebound hyperventilation
- Hematologic: Decreased hemoglobin, hematocrit
- GU: Urinary retention, spontaneous voiding, proteinuria

### Clinically important drug-drug interactions

• Increased pressor effect with sympathomimetics, MAO inhibitors • Increased effects with halothane, cyclopropane, enflurane (delay treatment for at least 10 min after discontinuance of anesthesia)

## ■ Nursing Considerations

### Assessment

- *History:* Epilepsy, incompetence of the ventilatory mechanism, flail chest, hypersensitivity to doxapram, head injury, pneumothorax, acute bronchial asthma, pulmonary fibrosis, severe hypertension, CVA, lactation
- *Physical:* T; skin color; weight; R, adventitious sounds; P, BP, ECG; reflexes; urinary output; arterial blood gases, CBC

### Implementation

- Administer IV only.
- Monitor injection site for extravasation. Discontinue, and restart in another vein; apply cold compresses.
- Monitor patient carefully until fully awake—P, PB, ECG, reflexes and respiratory status. Patients with COPD should have arterial blood gases monitored during drug use.
- Do not use longer than 2 h.
- Discontinue drug and notify physician if deterioration, sudden hypotension, dyspnea occur.

### Drug-specific teaching points

- Used in emergency; patient teaching should be general and include procedure and drug.

## doxazosin mesylate

*(dox ay' zoe sin)*

Cardura

**Pregnancy Category B**

### Drug classes

Alpha adrenergic blocker
Antihypertensive

### Therapeutic actions

Reduces total peripheral resistance through $alpha_1$-blockade; does not affect cardiac output or heart rate; increases HDL and the HDL to cholesterol ratio, while lowering total cholesterol and LDL, making it desirable for patients with atherosclerosis or hyperlipidemia.

### Indications

- Treatment of mild to moderate hypertension
- Benign prostatic hyperplasia (BPH)

### Contraindications/cautions

- Contraindication: lactation.
- Use cautiously with allergy to doxazosin, CHF, renal failure, hepatic impairment.

### Dosage

**Available Forms:** Tablets—1, 2, 4, 8 mg

**ADULT**

- *Hypertension:* Initially 1 mg qd PO, given once daily. *Maintenance:* 2, 4, 8, or 16 mg qd PO, given once a day.
- *BPH:* Initially: 1 mg PO qd; maintenance: may increase to 2 mg, 4 mg, and 8 mg qd, titrate at 1–2 wk intervals

**PEDIATRIC:** Safety and efficacy not established.

### Pharmacokinetics

| *Route* | *Onset* | *Peak* |
|---|---|---|
| Oral | Varies | 2–3 h |

*Metabolism:* Hepatic; $T_{1/2}$: 22 h
*Distribution:* Crosses placenta; enters breast milk
*Excretion:* Bile/feces, urine

### Adverse effects

- CNS: *Headache, fatigue, dizziness, postural dizziness, lethargy, vertigo*, rhinitis, asthemia, anxiety, parasthesia, increased sweating, muscle cramps, insomnia, eye pain, conjunctivitis
- GI: *Nausea, dyspepsia, diarrhea,* abdominal pain, flatulence, constipation
- CV: *Tachycardia, palpitations, edema, orthostatic hypotension,* chest pain
- GU: *Sexual dysfunction*, increased urinary frequency
- Other: Dyspnea, increased sweating, rash

### Clinically important drug-drug interactions

- Increased hypotensive effects if taken with alcohol, nitrates, other antihypertensives

## ■ Nursing Considerations

### Assessment

- *History:* Allergy to doxazosin, CHF, renal failure, hepatic impairment, lactation
- *Physical:* Weight; skin color, lesions; orientation, affect, reflexes; ophthalmologic exam; P, BP, orthostatic BP, supine BP, perfusion, edema, auscultation; R, adventitious sounds, status of nasal mucous membranes; bowel sounds, normal output; voiding pattern, normal output; kidney function tests, urinalysis

### Implementation

- Monitor edema, weight in patients with incipient cardiac decompensation, and arrange to add a thiazide diuretic to the drug regimen if sodium and fluid retention, signs of impending CHF occur.
- Monitor patient carefully with first dose; chance of orthostatic hypotension, dizziness and syncope are great with the first dose. Establish safety precautions.

- Monitor signs and symptoms of BPH to titrate dosage.

### Drug-specific teaching points

- Take this drug exactly as prescribed, once a day. Dizziness, syncope may occur at beginning of therapy. Change position slowly to avoid increased dizziness.
- The following side effects may occur: dizziness, weakness (when changing position, in the early morning, after exercise, in hot weather, and after consuming alcohol; some tolerance may occur after a while; avoid driving or engaging in tasks that require alertness; change position slowly, use caution in climbing stairs, lie down if dizziness persists); GI upset (frequent, small meals may help); impotence; stuffy nose; most of these effects gradually disappear with continued therapy.
- Report frequent dizziness or fainting.

## doxepin hydrochloride

*(dox' e pin)*

Novo-Doxepin (CAN), Sinequan, Triadapin (CAN)

**Pregnancy Category C**

### Drug classes

Tricyclic antidepressant (TCA) (tertiary amine)
Antianxiety agent

### Therapeutic actions

Mechanism of action unknown; TCAs inhibit the reuptake of the neurotransmitters norepinephrine and serotonin, leading to an increase in their effects; anticholinergic at CNS and peripheral receptors; sedative.

### Indications

- Relief of symptoms of depression (endogenous depression most responsive); sedative effects may help depression associated with anxiety and sleep disturbance
- Treatment of depression in patients with manic-depressive illness
- Antianxiety agent

### Contraindications/cautions

- Contraindications: hypersensitivity to any tricyclic drug; concomitant therapy with an MAO inhibitor; recent MI; myelography within previous 24 h or scheduled within 48 h; lactation.
- Use cautiously with EST; preexisting CV disorders (severe coronary heart disease, progressive heart failure, angina pectoris, paroxysmal tachycardia); angle-closure glaucoma, increased intraocular pressure, urinary retention, ureteral or urethral spasm; seizure disorders; hyperthyroidism; impaired hepatic, renal function; psychiatric patients (schizophrenic or paranoid patients may exhibit a worsening of psychosis); manic-depressive patients; elective surgery (TCAs should be discontinued as long as possible before surgery).

### Dosage

**Available Forms:** Capsules—10, 20, 50, 75, 100, 150 mg; oral concentrate—10 mg/ml

ADULT

- *Mild to moderate anxiety or depression:* Initially 25 mg tid PO; individualize dosage. Usual optimum dosage is 75–150 mg/d; alternatively, total daily dosage, up to 150 mg, may be given at bedtime.
- *More severe anxiety or depression:* Initially 50 mg tid PO; if needed, may gradually increase to 300 mg/d.
- *Mild symptomatology or emotional symptoms accompanying organic disease:* 25–50 mg PO is often effective.

PEDIATRIC: Not recommended if < 12 y.

### Pharmacokinetics

| Route | Onset | Peak |
|---|---|---|
| Oral | Varies | 2–8 h |

*Metabolism:* Hepatic; $T_{1/2}$: 8–25 h
*Distribution:* Crosses placenta; enters breast milk
*Excretion:* Urine

### Adverse effects

- CNS: *Sedation and anticholinergic (atropine-like) effects*; *confusion* (especially in elderly), *disturbed concentration*, hallucinations, disorientation, decreased memory, feelings of unreality, delusions, anxiety, nervousness, restlessness, agitation, panic, insomnia, nightmares, hypomania, mania, exacerbation of psychosis, drowsiness, weakness, fatigue, headache, numbness, tingling, paresthesias of extremities, incoordination, motor hyperactivity, akathisia, ataxia, tremors, peripheral neuropathy, extrapyramidal symptoms, seizures, speech blockage, dysarthria, tinnitus, altered EEG
- GI: *Dry mouth, constipation*, paralytic ileus, *nausea*, vomiting, anorexia, epigastric distress, diarrhea, flatulence, dysphagia, peculiar taste, increased salivation, stomatitis, glossitis, parotid swelling, abdominal cramps, black tongue, hepatitis, jaundice (rare); elevated transaminase, altered alkaline phosphatase
- CV: *Orthostatic hypotension*, hypertension, syncope, tachycardia, palpitations, MI, arrhythmias, heart block, precipitation of CHF, stroke
- **Hematologic**: Bone marrow depression, including agranulocytosis; eosinophila, purpura, thrombocytopenia, leukopenia
- GU: Urinary retention, delayed micturition, dilation of the urinary tract, gynecomastia, testicular swelling; breast enlargement, menstrual irregularity and galactorrhea; changes in libido; impotence
- **Endocrine**: Elevated or depressed blood sugar; elevated prolactin levels; inappropriate ADH secretion
- **Hypersensitivity**: Skin rash, pruritus, vasculitis, petechiae, photosensitization, edema (generalized or of face and tongue), drug fever
- **Withdrawal**: Symptoms on abrupt discontinuation of prolonged therapy: nausea, headache, vertigo, nightmares, malaise
- **Other**: Nasal congestion, excessive appetite, weight gain or loss; sweating (paradoxical effect in a drug with prominent anticholinergic effects), alopecia, lacrimation, hyperthermia, flushing, chills

### Clinically important drug-drug interactions

• Increased TCA levels and pharmacologic (especially anticholinergic) effects with cimetidine, fluoxetine • Increased TCA levels (due to decreased metabolism) with methylphenidate, phenothiazines, oral contraceptives, disulfiram • Hyperpyretic crises, severe convulsions, hypertensive episodes and deaths with MAO inhibitors • Increased antidepressant response and cardiac arrhythmias with thyroid medication • Increased or decreased effects with estrogens • Delirium with disulfiram • Sympathetic hyperactivity, sinus tachycardia, hypertension, agitation with levodopa • Increased biotransformation of TCAs in patients who smoke cigarettes • Increased sympathomimetic (especially $\alpha$-adrenergic) effects of direct-acting sympathomimetic drugs (norepinephrine, epinephrine), due to inhibition of uptake into adrenergic nerves • Increased anticholinergic effects of anticholinergic drugs (including anticholinergic antiparkisonism drugs) • Increased response (especially CNS depression) to barbiturates • Increased effects of dicumarol (oral anticoagulant) • Decreased antihypertensive effect of guanethidine, clonidine, other antihypertensives (because the uptake of the antihypertensive drug into adrenergic neurons is inhibited) • Decreased effects of indirect-acting sympathomimetic drugs (ephedrine) because of inhibition of uptake into adrenergic nerves

## ■ Nursing Considerations

### Assessment

- ***History:*** Hypersensitivity to any tricyclic drug; concomitant therapy with an MAO inhibitor; recent MI; myelography within previous 24 h or scheduled within 48 h; lactation; EST; preexisting CV disorders; angle-closure glaucoma, increased intraocular pressure, urinary retention, ureteral or urethral spasm; seizure disorders;

hyperthyroidism; impaired hepatic, renal function; psychiatric patients; manic-depressive patients; elective surgery
- *Physical:* Weight; T; skin color, lesions; orientation, affect, reflexes, vision and hearing; P, BP, orthostatic BP, perfusion; bowel sounds, normal output, liver evaluation; urine flow, normal output; usual sexual function, frequency of menses, breast and scrotal exam; liver function tests, urinalysis, CBC, ECG

### Implementation
- Limit drug access to depressed and potentially suicidal patients.
- Give major portion of dose hs if drowsiness, severe anticholinergic effects occur.
- Dilute oral concentrate with approximately 120 ml of water, milk, or fruit juice just prior to administration; do not prepare or store bulk dilutions.
- Expect clinical antianxiety response to be rapidly evident, although antidepressant response may require 2–3 wk.
- Reduce dosage if minor side effects develop; discontinue the drug if serious side effects occur.
- Arrange for CBC if patient develops fever, sore throat, or other sign of infection during therapy.

### Drug-specific teaching points
- Take drug exactly as prescribed; do not stop abruptly or without consulting the health care provider.
- Avoid alcohol, sleep-inducing drugs, OTC drugs.
- Avoid prolonged exposure to sunlight or sunlamps; use a sunscreen or protective garments for exposure to sunlight.
- The following side effects may occur: headache, dizziness, drowsiness, weakness, blurred vision (reversible; safety measures will be needed if severe; avoid driving or performing tasks that require alertness while these persist); nausea, vomiting, loss of appetite, dry mouth (small frequent meals, frequent mouth care, and sucking sugarless candies may help); nightmares, inability to concentrate, confusion; changes in sexual function.
- Report dry mouth, difficulty in urination, excessive sedation.

## doxorubicin hydrochloride

*(dox oh **roo'** bi sin)*

ADR

Adriamycin PFS, Adriamycin RDF, Doxil, Rubex

**Pregnancy Category D**

### Drug classes
Antibiotic
Antineoplastic

### Therapeutic actions
Cytotoxic: binds to DNA and inhibits DNA synthesis in susceptible cells, causing cell death.

### Indications
- To produce regression in the following neoplasms: acute lymphoblastic leukemia, acute myeloblastic leukemia, Wilm's tumor, neuroblastoma, soft tissue and bone sarcoma, breast carcinoma, ovarian carcinoma, transitional cell bladder carcinoma, thyroid carcinoma, Hodgkin's and non-Hodgkin's lymphomas, bronchogenic carcinoma
- Liposomal form: treatment of AIDS-related Kaposi's sarcoma

### Contraindications/cautions
- Contraindications: allergy to doxorubicin hydrochloride, malignant melanoma, kidney carcinoma, large bowel carcinoma, brain tumors, CNS metastases, myelosuppression, cardiac disease (may predispose to cardiac toxicity) pregnancy, lactation.
- Use cautiously with impaired hepatic function, previous courses of doxorubicin or daunorubicin therapy (may predispose to cardiac toxicity), prior mediastinal irradiation, concurrent cyclophosphamide therapy (predispose to cardiac toxicity).

### Dosage
**Available Forms:** Powder for injection—10, 20, 50, 100 mg; injection (acqueous)—

2 mg/ml; preservative-free injection—2 mg/ml; injection (lipid)—20 mg

*ADULT:* 60–75 mg/m$^2$ as a single IV injection administered at 21-d intervals. Alternate schedule: 30 mg/m$^2$ IV on each of 3 successive days, repeated every 4 wk.

- *Liposomal form:* 20 mg/m$^2$ IV over 30 min once every 3 wk.

*PATIENTS WITH ELEVATED BILIRUBIN:* *Serum bilirubin 1.2–3.0 mg/100 ml:* 50% of normal dose. *Serum bilirubin > 3 mg/100 ml:* 25% of normal dose

- *Liposomal form: Serum bilirubin 1.2–3.0 mg/100 ml:* 50% of normal dose. *Serum bilirubin >3 mg/100 ml:* 25% of normal dose.

### Pharmacokinetics

| *Route* | *Onset* | *Peak* | *Duration* |
|---|---|---|---|
| IV | Rapid | 2 h | 24–36 h |

*Metabolism:* Hepatic; $T_{1/2}$: 12 min, then 3.3 h, then 29.6 h

*Distribution:* Crosses placenta; enters breast milk

*Excretion:* Bile/feces and urine

### IV facts

**Preparation:** Reconstitute the 10-mg vial with 5 ml, the 50-mg vial with 25 ml of 0.9% Sodium Chloride or Sterile Water for Injection to give a concentration of 2 mg/ml doxorubicin. Reconstituted solution is stable for 24 h at room temperature or 48 h if refrigerated. Protect from sunlight. Liposomal form: dilute dose to maximum of 90 mg in 250 ml of 5% Dextrose Injection; do not use in-line filters; refrigerate and use within 24 h.

**Infusion:** Administer slowly into tubing of a freely running IV infusion of Sodium Chloride Injection or 5% Dextrose Injection; attach the tubing to a butterfly needle inserted into a large vein; avoid veins over joints or in extremities with poor perfusion. Rate of administration will depend on the vein and dosage; do not give in less than 3–5 min; red streaking over the vein and facial flushing are often signs of too rapid administration. Liposomal form: single dose infused over 30 min; rapid infusion increases risk of reaction.

**Incompatibilities:** Heparin, cephalothin, dexamethasone sodium phosphatase (a precipitate forms and the IV solution must not be used), aminophylline, and 5–fluorouracil (doxorubicin decomposes) denoted by a color change from red to blue-purple.

### Adverse effects

- GI: *Nausea, vomiting, mucositis,* anorexia, diarrhea
- CV: Cardiac toxicity, CHF, phlebosclerosis
- Hematologic: *Myelosuppression*, hyperuricemia due to cell lysis
- GU: *Red urine*
- Dermatologic: *Complete but reversible alopecia*; hyperpigmentation of nailbeds and dermal creases, facial flushing
- Local: **Severe local cellulitis**, vesication and tissue necrosis if extravasation occurs
- Hypersensitivity: Fever, chills, urticaria, anaphylaxis
- Other: Carcinogenesis (documented in experimental models)

### Clinically important drug-drug interactions

- Decreased serum levels and actions of digoxin if taken concurrently with doxorubicin

## ■ Nursing Considerations

### Assessment

- *History:* Allergy to doxorubicin hydrochloride, malignant melanoma, kidney carcinoma, large bowel carcinoma, brain tumors, CNS metastases, myelosuppression, cardiac disease, impaired hepatic function, previous courses of doxorubicin or daunorubicin therapy, prior mediastinal irradiation, concurrent cyclophosphamide therapy, lactation.
- *Physical:* T; skin color, lesions; weight; hair; nailbeds; local injection site; auscultation, peripheral perfusion, pulses, ECG; R, adventitious sounds; liver eval-

uation, mucus membranes; CBC, liver function tests, uric acid levels.

### Implementation

- Do not give IM or SC because severe local reaction and tissue necrosis occur.
- Monitor injection site for extravasation: reports of burning or stinging. Discontinue, and restart in another vein. Local SC extravasation: local infiltration with corticosteroid may be ordered; flood area with normal saline; apply cold compress to area. If ulceration begins, arrange consultation with plastic surgeon.
- Monitor patient's response frequently at beginning of therapy: serum uric acid level, cardiac output (listen for $S_3$); CBC changes may require a decrease in the dose; consult with physician.
- Record doses received to monitor total dosage; toxic effects are often dose related, as total dose approaches 550 mg/m$^2$.
- Ensure adequate hydration during the course of therapy to prevent hyperuricemia.

### Drug-specific teaching points

- Prepare a calendar of days to return for drug therapy.
- The following side effects may occur: rash, skin lesions, loss of hair, changes in nails (you may want to invest in a wig before hair loss occurs; skin care may help); loss of appetite, nausea, mouth sores (frequent mouth care, small frequent meals may help; try to maintain good nutrition; a dietician may be able to help; an antiemetic may be ordered); red urine (transient).
- Arrange for regular medical followup, including blood tests.
- Report difficulty breathing, sudden weight gain, swelling, burning or pain at injection site, unusual bleeding or bruising.

## doxycycline

*(dox i sye' kleen)*

Apo-Doxy (CAN), Doryx, Doxy-Caps, Doxycin (CAN), Doxychel Hyclate, Vibra-Tabs, Vibramycin

**Pregnancy Category D**

### Drug classes

Antibiotic
Tetracycline antibiotic

### Therapeutic actions

Bacteriostatic: inhibits protein synthesis of susceptible bacteria, causing cell death.



### Indications

- Infections caused by rickettsiae; *M. pneumoniae;* agents of psittacosis, ornithosis, lymphogranuloma venereum and granuloma inguinale; *B. recurrentis; H. ducreyi; P. pestis; P. tularensis; B. bacilliformis; Bacteroides; V. comma; V. fetus; Brucella; E. coli; E. aerogenes; Shigella; A. calcoaceticus; H. influenzae; Klebsiella; D. pneumoniae; S. aureus*
- When penicillin is contraindicated, infections caused by *N. gonorrhoeae, T. pallidum, T. pertenue, L. monocytogenes, Clostridium, B. anthracis;* adjunct to amebicides in acute intestinal amebiasis
- Oral tetracyclines used for acne, uncomplicated adult urethral, endocervical or rectal infections caused by *C. trachomatis*
- Unlabeled use: prevention of "traveler's diarrhea" commonly caused by enterotoxigenic *E. coli*

### Contraindications/cautions

- Allergy to tetracyclines, renal or hepatic dysfunction, pregnancy, lactation.

### Dosage

**Available Forms:** Tablets—100 mg; powder for oral suspension—25 mg; syrup—50 mg; powder for injection—100, 200 mg

*ADULT:* 200 mg IV in one or two infusions (each over 1–4 h) on the first treatment day, followed by 100–200 mg/d IV, depending on the severity of the infection.

- *Primary or secondary syphilis:* 300 mg/d IV for 10 d; or 100 mg q12h PO on the first day, followed by 100 mg/d as one dose or 50 mg q12h PO.
- *Acute gonococcal infection:* 200 mg PO, then 100 mg at bedtime, followed by 100 mg bid for 3 d; or 300 mg PO followed by 300 mg in 1 h.
- *Primary and secondary syphilis:* 300 mg/d PO in divided doses for at least 10 d.

- *Traveler's diarrhea:* 100 mg/d PO as prophylaxis.
- *CDC recommendations for STDs:* 100 mg bid PO for 7–10 d.

PEDIATRIC

- *> 8 Y AND < 100 LB:* 4.4 mg/kg, IV in one or two infusions, followed by 2.2–4.4 mg/kg per day IV in one or two infusions; or 4.4 mg/kg, PO in two divided doses the first day of treatment, followed by 2.2–4.4 mg/kg per day on subsequent days.
- *> 100 LB:* Give adult dose.

*GERIATRIC OR RENAL FAILURE PATIENTS:* IV doses of doxycycline are not as toxic as other tetracyclines in these patients.

### Pharmacokinetics

| Route | Onset | Peak |
|---|---|---|
| Oral | Varies | 1.5–4 h |
| IV | Rapid | End of infusion |

*Metabolism:* $T_{1/2}$: 15–25 h
*Distribution:* Crosses placenta; enters breast milk
*Excretion:* Urine and feces

### IV facts

**Preparation:** Prepare solution of 10 mg/ml reconstitute with 10 ml (100-mg vial): 20 ml (200 mg vial) of Sterile Water for Injection; dilute further with 100–1,000 ml (100-mg vial) or 200–2,000 ml (200-mg vial) of Sodium Chloride Injection, 5% Dextrose Injection, Ringer's Injection, 10% Invert Sugar in Water, Lactated Ringer's Injection, 5% Dextrose in Lactated Ringer's, Normosol-M in D5-W, Normosol-R in D5-W, or Plasma-Lyte 56 or 148 in 5% Dextrose. If mixed in Lactated Ringer's or 5% Dextrose in Lactated Ringer's, infusion must be completed within 6 h after reconstitution; otherwise, may be stored up to 72 h if refrigerated and protected from light, but infusion should then be completed within 12 h; discard solution after that time.
**Infusion:** Infuse slowly over 1–4 h.

### Adverse effects

- GI: Fatty liver, liver failure, *anorexia, nausea, vomiting, diarrhea, glossitis,* dysphagia, enterocolitis, esophageal ulcer
- **Hematologic**: Hemolytic anemia, thrombocytopenia, neutropenia, eosinophilia, leukocytosis, leukopenia
- **Dermatologic**: *Phototoxic reactions, rash*, exfoliative dermatitis (more frequent and more severe with this tetracycline than with any others)
- **Dental**: *Discoloring and inadequate calcification of primary teeth of fetus if used by pregnant women, discoloring and inadequate calcification of permanent teeth if used during period of dental development*
- **Local**: Local irritation at injection site
- **Other**: Superinfections, nephrogenic diabetes insipidus syndrome

### Clinically important drug-drug interactions

• Decreased absorption with antacids, iron, alkali • Decreased therapeutic effects with barbiturates, carbamazepine, phenytoins • Increased digoxin toxicity with doxycycline • Increased nephrotoxicity with methoxyflurane • Decreased activity of penicillins.

### Clinically important drug-food interactions

• Decreased effectiveness of doxycycline if taken with food, dairy products

### Drug-lab test interferences

• Interference with culture studies for several days following therapy

## ■ Nursing Considerations

### Assessment

- *History:* Allergy to tetracyclines, renal or hepatic dysfunction, pregnancy, lactation.
- *Physical:* Skin status, R and sounds, GI function and liver evaluation, urinary output and concentration, urinalysis and BUN, liver and renal function tests; culture infected area before beginning therapy.

### Implementation

- Administer the oral medication without regard to food or meals; if GI upset occurs, give with meals.
- Protect patient from light and sun exposure.

### Drug-specific teaching points

- Take drug throughout the day for best results; if GI upset occurs, take drug with food.
- The following side effects may occur: sensitivity to sunlight (wear protective clothing, use sunscreen), diarrhea.
- Report rash, itching; difficulty breathing; dark urine or light-colored stools; pain at injection site.

## dronabinol

*(droe **nab'** i nol)*

delta-9-tetrahydrocannabinol, delta-9-THC

Marinol

**Pregnancy Category B**
**C-II controlled substance**

### Drug classes

Antiemetic

### Therapeutic actions

Principal psychoactive substance in marijuana; has complex CNS effects; mechanism of action as antiemetic is not understood.

### Indications

- Treatment of nausea and vomiting associated with cancer chemotherapy in patients who have failed to respond adequately to conventional antiemetic treatment (should be used only under close supervision by a responsible individual because of potential to alter the mental state)
- Treatment of anorexia associated with weight loss in patients with AIDS

### Contraindications/cautions

- Contraindications: allergy to dronabinol or sesame oil vehicle in capsules, nausea and vomiting arising from any cause other than cancer chemotherapy, lactation.
- Use cautiously with hypertension; heart disease; manic, depressive, schizophrenic patients (dronabinol may unmask symptoms of these disease states).

### Dosage

**Available Forms:** Capsules—2.5, 5, 10 mg

**ADULT**

- ***Antiemetic:*** Initially, 5 mg/m$^2$ PO 1–3 h prior to the administration of chemotherapy. Repeat dose q2–4h after chemotherapy is given, for a total of 4–6 doses per day. If the 5 mg/m$^2$ dose is ineffective and there are no significant side effects, increase dose by 2.5 mg/m$^2$ increments to a maximum of 15 mg/m$^2$ per dose.
- ***Appetite stimulation:*** Initially give 2.5 mg PO bid before lunch and supper. May reduce dose to 2.5 mg/d as a single hs dose; up to 10 mg PO bid.

### Pharmacokinetics

| *Route* | *Onset* | *Peak* | *Duration* |
|---|---|---|---|
| Oral | 30–60 min | 2–4 h | 4–6 h |

*Metabolism:* Hepatic; $T_{1/2}$: 25–36 h
*Distribution:* Crosses placenta; enters breast milk
*Excretion:* Bile/feces and urine

### Adverse effects

- CNS: *Drowsiness; easy laughing, elation, heightened awareness, often termed a "high;" dizziness; anxiety; muddled thinking; perceptual difficulties; impaired coordination; irritability, weird feeling, depression; weakness, sluggishness, headache; hallucinations, memory lapse; unsteadiness*, ataxia; paresthesia, visual disortions; paranoia, depersonalization; disorientation, confusion; tinnitus, nightmares, speech difficulty
- GI: *Dry mouth*
- CV: Tachycardia, postural hypotension; syncope

- GU: Decrease in pregnancy rate, spermatogenesis when doses higher than those used clinically were given in preclinical studies
- **Dermatologic**: Facial flushing, perspiring
- **Dependence**: Psychological and physical dependence; tolerance to CVS and subjective effects after 30 d of use; withdrawal syndrome (irritability, insomnia, restlessness, hot flashes, sweating, rhinorrhea, loose stools, hiccups, anorexia) beginning 12 h and ending 96 h after discontinuation of high doses of the drug

### Clinically important drug-drug interactions

• Do not give with alcohol, sedatives, hypnotics, other psychotomimetic substances
• Increased tachycardia, hypertension, drowsiness with anticholinergics, antihistamines, TCAs

## ■ Nursing Considerations

### Assessment

- *History:* Allergy to dronabinol or sesame oil vehicle in capsules, nausea and vomiting arising from any cause other than cancer chemotherapy, hypertension, heart disease, manic, depressive, schizophrenic patients, lactation.
- *Physical:* Skin—color, texture; orientation, reflexes, bilateral grip strength, affect; P, BP, orthostatic BP; status of mucous membranes.

### Implementation

- Store capsules in refrigerator.
- Limit prescriptions to the minimum necessary for a single cycle of chemotherapy because of abuse potential.
- Warn patient about drug's profound effects on mental status, abuse potential before giving drug; patient needs full information regarding the use of this drug.
- Warn patient about drug's potential effects on mood and behavior to prevent panic in case these occur.
- Patient should be supervised by a responsible adult while on drug; monitor during the first cycle of chemotherapy in which dronabinol is used to determine how long patient will need supervision.
- Discontinue drug if psychotic reaction occurs; observe patient closely until evaluated and counseled; patient should participate in decision about further use of drug, perhaps at lower dosage.

### Drug-specific teaching points

- Take drug exactly as prescribed; a responsible adult should be with you at all times while you are taking this drug.
- Avoid alcohol, sedatives, OTC drugs, including nose drops, cold remedies, while you are taking this drug.
- The following side effects may occur: mood changes (euphoria, laughing, feeling "high," anxiety, depression, weird feeling, hallucinations, memory lapse, impaired thinking); weakness, faintness (change postion slowly to avoid injury); dizziness, drowsiness (do not drive or perform tasks that require alertness if you experience these effects).
- Report bizarre thoughts, uncontrollable behavior or thought processes, fainting, dizziness, irregular heart beat.

## ☆ dyphylline

*(dye' fi lin)*

dihydroxypropyl theophyllin

Dilor, Dyflex, Lufyllin, Neothylline, Protophylline (CAN)

**Pregnancy Category C**

### Drug classes

Bronchodilator
Xanthine

### Therapeutic actions

A theophylline derivative that is not metabolized to theophylline; relaxes bronchial smooth muscle, causing bronchodilation and increasing vital capacity, which has been impaired by bronchospasm and air trapping; at high doses it also inhibits the release of slow reacting substance of anaphylaxis and histamine.

### Indications

- Symptomatic relief or prevention of bronchial asthma and reversible bronchospasm associated with chronic bronchitis and emphysema

### Contraindications/cautions

- Contraindications: hypersensitivity to any xanthine or to ethylenediamine, peptic ulcer, active gastritis.
- Use cautiously with cardiac arrhythmias, acute myocardial injury, CHF, cor pulmonale, severe hypertension, severe hypoxemia, renal or hepatic disease, hyperthyroidism, alcoholism, labor, lactation.

### Dosage

**Available Forms:** Tablets—200, 400 mg; elixir—100, 160 mg/5ml; injection—250 mg/ml

Individualize dosage based on clinical responses with monitoring of serum dyphylline levels; serum theophylline levels do *not* measure dyphylline; equivalence of dyphylline to theophylline is not known.

**ADULT:** Up to 15 mg/kg, PO qid or 250–500 mg injected slowly IM (not for IV use); do not exceed 15 mg/kg per 6 h.

**PEDIATRIC:** Use in children >6 mo; children are very sensitive to CNS stimulant action of xanthines. Use caution in younger children who cannot complain of minor side effects. 2–3 mg/lb (4.4–6.6 mg/kg) daily in divided doses.

**GERIATRIC OR IMPAIRED ADULT:** Use caution: in elderly men, cor pulmonale, CHF, kidney disease.

### Pharmacokinetics

| *Route* | *Peak* | *Duration* |
|---|---|---|
| Oral | 1 h | 6 h |
| IM | 30–45 min | 6 h |

*Metabolism:* Hepatic; $T_{1/2}$: 2 h

*Distribution:* Crosses placenta; enters breast milk

*Excretion:* Urine

### Adverse effects

- CNS: *Headache*, *insomnia*, irritability; restlessness, dizziness, muscle twitching, convulsions, severe depression, stammering speech; abnormal behavior: withdrawal, mutism, and unresponsiveness alternating with hyperactivity; brain damage, death
- GI: *Nausea, vomiting, diarrhea,* loss of appetite, hematemesis, epigastric pain, gastroesophageal reflux during sleep, increased SGOT
- CV: Palpitations, sinus tachycardia, ventricular tachycardia, life-threatening ventricular arrhythmias, circulatory failure, hypotension
- **Respiratory**: Tachypnea, respiratory arrest
- GU: Proteinuria, increased excretion of renal tubular cells and RBCs; diuresis (dehydration), urinary retention in men with prostate enlargement
- **Other**: Fever, flushing, hyperglycemia, SIADH, rash

### Clinically important drug-drug interactions

• Increased effects with probenecid, mexiletine • Increased cardiac toxicity with halothane • Decreased effects of benzodiazepines, nondepolarizing neuromuscular blockers • Mutually antagonistic effects of beta-blockers and dyphylline

## ■ Nursing Considerations

### Assessment

- *History:* Hypersensitivity to any xanthine or to ethylenediamine, peptic ulcer, active gastritis, cardiac arrhythmias, acute myocardial injury, CHF, cor pulmonale, severe hypertension, severe hypoxemia, renal or hepatic disease, hyperthyroidism, alcoholism, labor, lactation.
- *Physical:* Bowel sounds, normal output; P, auscultation, BP, perfusion, ECG; R, adventitious sounds; frequency, voiding, normal output pattern, urinalysis, renal function tests; liver palpation, liver function tests; thyroid function tests; skin color, texture, lesions; reflexes, bilateral grip strength, affect, EEG.

### Implementation

- Give oral dosage forms with food if GI effects occur.

- Monitor patient carefully for clinical signs of adverse effects.
- Maintain diazepam on standby to treat seizures.
- Monitor for therapeutic serum level: 12 mcg/ml.

### Drug-specific teaching points

- Take this drug exactly as prescribed (around the clock for adequate control of asthma attacks).
- Avoid excessive intake of coffee, tea, cocoa, cola beverages, chocolate.
- Keep all appointments for monitoring of response to this drug.
- The following side effects may occur: nausea, loss of appetite (take with food); difficulty sleeping, depression, emotional lability.
- Report nausea, vomiting, severe GI pain, restlessness, convulsions, irregular heartbeat.

# Edetate

## edetate calcium disodium

*(ed' e tate)*

calcium EDTA

Calcium Disodium Versenate

## edetate disodium

Disotate, Endrate

**Pregnancy Category C**

### Drug classes

Antidote

### Therapeutic actions

Calcium in this compound is easily displaced by heavy metals, such as lead, to form stable complexes that are excreted in the urine; edetate disodium has strong affinity to calcium, lowering calcium levels and pulling calcium out of extracirculatory stores during slow infusion.

### Indications

- Acute and chronic lead poisoning and lead encephalopathy (edetate calcium disodium)
- Emergency treatment of hypercalcemia (edetate disodium)
- Control of ventricular arrhythmias associated with digitalis toxicity (edetate disodium)

### Contraindications/cautions

- Contraindications: sensitivity to EDTA preparations, anuria, increased intracranial pressure (rapid IV infusion).
- Use cautiously with cardiac disease, CHF, lactation, renal impairment, pregnancy.

### Dosage

**Available Forms:** Injection—150 mg/ml (edetate disodium), 200 mg/ml (edetate calcium disodium)

Effective by IM, SC, IV routes. IM route is safest in children and patients with lead encephalopathy.

#### Adult

- *Lead poisoning:* Edetate calcium disodium.
  - **IV:** Asymptomatic patients: 5 ml diluted IV bid for up to 5 d. Interrupt therapy for 2 d; follow with another 5 d of treatment if indicated. Do not exceed 50 mg/kg per day. Symptomatic adults: Keep fluids to basal levels; administer above dilution over 2 h. Give second daily infusion 6 h or more after the first.
  - **IM:** Do not exceed 35 mg/kg bid, total of approximately 75 mg/kg per day.
  - **Hypercalcemia, treatment of ventricular arrhythmias due to digitalis toxicity:** Edetate disodium: Administer 50 mg/kg per day IV to a maximum dose of 3 g in 24 h. A suggested regimen includes five consecutive daily doses followed by 2 d without medication. Repeat courses as necessary to a total of 15 doses.

#### Pediatric

- *Lead poisoning:* Edetate calcium disodium.
  - **IM:** Do not exceed 35 mg/kg bid, total of approximately 75 mg/kg per day. In mild cases do not exceed 50 mg/kg per day. For younger children, give total daily dose in divided doses q8–12h for 3–5 d. Give a second course after a rest period of 4 d or more.

- *Lead encephalopathy:* Use above IM dosage. If used in combination with dimercaprol, give at separate deep IM sites.
- *Hypercalcemia, treatment of ventricular arrhythmias due to digitalis toxicity:* Edetate disodium. Administer 40 mg/kg per day IV to a maximum dose of 70 mg/kg per day, or give 15–50 mg/kg per day to a maximum of 3 g/d, allowing 5 d between courses of therapy.

### Pharmacokinetics

| *Route* | *Onset* | *Peak* |
|---|---|---|
| IM/IV | 1 h | 24–48 h |

*Metabolism:* $T_{1/2}$: 20–60 min (IV), 90 min (IM)
*Excretion:* Urine

### IV facts

**Preparation:** Lead poisoning: Dilute the 5-ml ampul with 250–500 ml of Normal Saline or 5% Dextrose Solution. Hypercalcemia: Dissolve dose in 500 ml of 5% Dextrose Injection or 0.9% Sodium Chloride Injection. Pediatric: Dissolve dose in a sufficient volume of 5% Dextrose Injection or 0.9% Sodium Chloride Injection to bring the final concentration to not more than 3%.
**Infusion:** Lead poisoning: Administer prepared solution over at least 1 h. Hypercalcemia: Infuse over 3 h or more, and do not exceed the patient's cardiac reserve. Pediatric: Infuse over 3 h or more. Do not exceed patient's cardiac reserve.

### Adverse effects

- CNS: Headache, transient circumoral paresthesia, numbness
- GI: *Nausea, vomiting, diarrhea* (edetate disodium)
- CV: CHF, blood pressure changes, thrombophlebitis
- **Hematologic**: *Electrolyte imbalance* (hypocalcemia, hypokalemia, hypomagnesemia, altered blood sugar)
- GU: Renal tubular necrosis

## ■ Nursing Considerations

### Assessment

- *History:* Sensitivity to EDTA preparations; anuria; increased intracranial pressure; cardiac disease, CHF, lactation
- *Physical:* Pupillary reflexes, orientation; P, BP; urinalysis, BUN, serum electrolytes

### Implementation

- Administer edetate calcium disodium IM.
- Avoid rapid IV infusion, which can cause fatal increases in intracranial pressure or fatal hypocalcemia with edetate disodium.
- Avoid excess fluids in patients with lead encephalopathy and increased intracranial pressure; for these patients, mix edetate calcium disodium 20% solution with procaine to give a final concentration of 0.5% procaine, and administer IM.
- Monitor patient response and electrolytes carefully during slow IV infusion of edetate disodium.
- Establish urine flow by IV infusion prior to first dose to those dehydrated from vomiting. Once urine flow is established, restrict further IV fluid. Stop EDTA when urine flow ceases.
- Arrange for periodic BUN and serum electrolyte determinations before and during each course of therapy. Stop drug if signs of increasing renal damage occur.
- Do not administer in larger than recommended doses.
- Arrange for cardiac monitoring if edetate disodium is being used to treat digitalis-induced ventricular arrhythmias. Patient should be carefully monitored for signs of CHF and other adverse effects as digitalis is withdrawn.
- Keep patient supine for a short period because of the possibility of postural hypotension.
- Do not administer edetate disodium as a chelating agent for treatment of atherosclerosis; such therapy is not approved and is suspect.

**Drug-specific teaching points**

- Prepare a schedule of rest and drug days.
- Arrange for periodic blood tests during the course of therapy.
- Constant monitoring of heart rhythm may be needed during drug administration.
- Report pain at injection site, difficulty voiding.

## edrophonium chloride

*(ed roe foe' nee um)*

Enlon, Reversol, Tensilon

**Pregnancy Category C**

### Drug classes

Cholinesterase inhibitor (anticholinesterase)
Diagnostic agent
Antidote

### Therapeutic actions

Increases the concentration of acetylcholine at the sites of cholinergic transmission; prolongs and exaggerates the effects of acetylcholine by reversibly inhibiting the enzyme acetylcholinesterase, facilitating transmission at the skeletal neuromuscular junction.

### Indications

- Differential diagnosis and adjunct in evaluating treatment of myasthenia gravis
- Antidote for nondepolarizing neuromuscular junction blockers (curare, tubocurarine, gallamine) after surgery

### Contraindications/cautions

- Contraindications: hypersensitivity to anticholinesterases, intestinal or urogenital tract obstruction, peritonitis, lactation.
- Use cautiously with asthma, peptic ulcer, bradycardia, cardiac arrhythmias, recent coronary occlusion, vagotonia, hyperthyroidism, epilepsy, pregnancy near term.

### Dosage

**Available Forms:** Injection—10 mg/ml

ADULT

- *Differential diagnosis of myasthenia gravis:*
  - **IV:** Prepare tuberculin syringe containing 10 mg edrophonium with IV needle. Inject 2 mg IV in 15–30 sec; leave needle in vein. If no reaction occurs after 45 sec, inject the remaining 8 mg. If a cholinergic reaction (parasympathomimetic effects, muscle fasciculations, or increased muscle weakness) occurs after 2 mg, discontinue the test, and administer atropine sulfate 0.4–0.5 mg IV. May repeat test after 1/2 h.
  - **IM:** If veins are inaccessible, inject 10 mg IM. Patients who demonstrate cholinergic reaction (see above) should be retested with 2 mg IM after 1/2 h to rule out false-negative results.
- *Evaluation of treatment requirements in myasthenia gravis:* 1–2 mg IV 1 h after oral intake of the treatment drug. Responses are summarized below:

| *Response to Edrophonium Test* | *Myasthenic (Under-treated)* | *Cholinergic (Over-treated)* |
|---|---|---|
| *Muscle strength*: ptosis, diplopia, respiration, limb strength | Increased | Decreased |
| *Fasciculations*: orbicularis oculi, facial and limb muscles | Absent | Present or absent |
| *Side reactions*: lacrimination, sweating, salivating, nausea, vomiting, diarrhea, abdominal cramps | Absent | Severe |

- *Edrophonium test in crisis:* Secure controlled respiration immediately if patient is apneic, then administer test. If patient is in cholinergic crisis, administration of edrophonium will increase oropharyngeal secretions and further weaken respiratory muscles. If crisis is myasthenic, administration of edrophonium will improve respiration, and patient can be treated with longer-acting IV anticholinesterase medication. To administer the test, draw up no more than 2 mg edrophonium into the syringe. Give

1 mg IV initially. Carefully observe cardiac response. If after 1 min this dose does not further impair the patient, inject the remaining 1 mg. If after a 2-mg dose no clear improvement in respiration occurs, discontinue all anticholinesterase drug therapy, and control ventilation by tracheostomy and assisted respiration.

- ***Antidote for curare:*** 10 mg given slowly IV over 30–45 sec so that onset of cholinergic reaction can be detected; repeat when necessary. Maximal dose for any patient is 40 mg.

PEDIATRIC

- ***Differential diagnosis of myasthenia gravis***
  - ***IV:*** *Children up to 75 lb (34 kg)*: 1 mg. Children over 75 lb: 2 mg. *Infants*: 0.5 mg. If children do not respond in 45 sec, dose may be titrated up to 5 mg in children under 75 lb, up to 10 mg in children over 75 lb, given in increments of 1 mg q 30–45 sec.
  - ***IM:*** Up to 75 lb (34 kg): 2 mg. Over 75 lb: 5 mg. A delay of 2–10 min occurs until reaction.

## Pharmacokinetics

| *Route* | *Onset* | *Duration* |
|---|---|---|
| IM | 2–10 min | 5–30 min |
| IV | 30–60 sec | 5–10 min |

*Metabolism:* $T_{1/2}$: 5–10 min
*Distribution:* Crosses placenta; enters breast milk
*Excretion:* Unknown

### IV facts

**Preparation:** Drug is used directly; no preparation is required.
**Infusion:** Rate of infusion varies with reason for administration; see Dosage section above.

## Adverse effects

*Parasympathomimetic Effects*

- GI: *Salivation, dysphagia, nausea, vomiting, increased peristalsis, abdominal cramps,* flatulence, diarrhea
- CV: *Bradycardia, cardiac arrhythmias,* AV block and nodal rhythm, cardiac arrest; decreased cardiac output, leading to hypotension, syncope
- **Respiratory**: *Increased pharyngeal and tracheobronchial secretions*, laryngospasm, bronchospasm, bronchiolar constriction, dyspnea
- GU: *Urinary frequency and incontinence*, urinary urgency
- EENT: *Lacrimation, miosis,* spasm of accommodation, diplopia, conjunctival hyperemia
- **Dermatologic**: Diaphoresis, flushing

*Skeletal Muscle Effects*

- CNS: Convulsions, dysarthria, dysphonia, drowsiness, dizziness, headache, loss of consciousness
- **Respiratory**: Respiratory muscle paralysis, central respiratory paralysis
- **Peripheral**: Skeletal muscle weakness, fasciculations, muscle cramps, arthralgia

*Other*

- **Dermatologic**: Skin rash, urticaria, anaphylaxis
- **Local**: Thrombophlebitis after IV use

## Clinically important drug-drug interactions

- Risk of profound muscular depression refractory to anticholinesterases if given concurrently with corticosteroids, succinylcholine.

## ■ Nursing Considerations

### Assessment

*Note:* The administration of edrophonium for diagnostic purposes would generally be supervised by a neurologist or other physician skilled and experienced in dealing with myasthenic patients; the administration of edrophonium to reverse neuromuscular blocking agents would generally be supervised by an anesthesiologist. The following are points that any nurse participating in the care of a patient receiving anticholinesterases should keep in mind.

- ***History:*** Hypersensitivity to anticholinesterases; intestinal or urogenital tract obstruction, peritonitis, lactation, asthma, peptic ulcer, cardiac arrhythmias, recent coronary occlusion, vagotonia, hyperthyroidism, epilepsy, pregnancy near term

- *Physical:* Bowel sounds, normal output; frequency, voiding pattern, normal output; R, adventitious sounds; P, auscultation, blood pressure; reflexes, bilateral grip strength, EEG; thyroid function tests; skin color, texture, lesions

### Implementation

- Administer IV slowly with constant monitoring of patient's response.
- Be aware that overdosage with anticholinesterase drugs can cause muscle weakness (cholinergic crisis) that is difficult to differentiate from myasthenic weakness; edrophonium is used to help make this diagnostic distinction. The administration of atropine may mask the parasympathetic effects of anticholinesterases and confound the diagnosis.
- Maintain atropine sulfate on standby as an antidote and antagonist to edrophonium.

### Drug-specific teaching points

- The patient should know what to expect during diagnostic test with edrophonium (patients receiving drug to reverse neuromuscular blockers will not be aware of drug effects and do not require specific teaching about the drug).

## enalapril maleate

*(e **nal'** a pril)*

Vasotec

## enalaprilat

Vasotec I.V.

**Pregnancy Category C**

### Drug classes

Antihypertensive
ACE inhibitor

### Therapeutic actions

Renin, synthesized by the kidneys, is released into the circulation where it acts on a plasma precursor to produce angiotensin I, which is converted by angiotensin-converting enzyme to angiotensin II, a potent vasoconstrictor that also causes release of aldosterone from the adrenals; both of these actions increase BP. Enalapril blocks the conversion of angiotensin I to angiotensin II, decreasing BP, decreasing aldosterone secretion, slightly increasing serum $K^+$ levels, and causing $Na^+$ and fluid loss; increased prostaglandin synthesis also may be involved in the antihypertensive action.

### Indications

- Treatment of hypertension alone or in combination with thiazide-type diuretics
- Treatment of acute and chronic CHF
- Treatment of asymptomatic left ventricular dysfunction (LVD)

### Contraindications/cautions

- Contraindication: allergy to enalapril.
- Use cautiously with impaired renal function; salt/volume depletion—hypotension may occur; lactation.

### Dosage

**Available Forms:** Tablets—2.5, 5, 10, 20 mg; injection—1.25 mg/ml

ADULT

- *Hypertension*
  - **Oral:** *Patients not taking diuretics:* Initial dose—5 mg/d PO. Adjust dosage based on patient response. Usual range is 10–40 mg/d as a single dose or in two divided doses. *Patient taking diuretics:* Discontinue diuretic for 2–3 d if possible. If it is not possible to discontinue diuretic, give initial dose of 2.5 mg, and monitor for excessive hypotension. *Converting to oral therapy from IV therapy:* 5 mg qd with subsequent doses based on patient response.
  - **Parenteral:** Give IV only. 1.25 mg q6h given IV over 5 min. A response is usually seen within 15 min, but peak effects may not occur for 4h. *Converting to IV therapy from oral therapy:* 1.25 mg q6h; monitor patient response. *Patients taking diuretics:* 0.625 mg IV over 5 min. If adequate response is not seen after 1 h, repeat the 0.625-mg dose. Give additional doses of 1.25 mg q6h.
- *Heart failure*
  - **Oral:** 2.5 mg qd or bid in conjunction with diuretics and digitalis. Maintenance dose is 5–20 mg/d given in two divided doses. Maximum daily dose is 40 mg.

- *Asymptomatic LVD*
  - ***Oral:*** 2.5 mg bid; target maintenance dose 20 mg/d in two divided doses.

PEDIATRIC: Safety and efficacy not established.

GERIATRIC AND RENAL IMPAIRED: Excretion is reduced in renal failure; use smaller initial dose, and titrate upward to a maximum of 40 mg/d PO.

| *Creatinine Clearance (ml/min)* | *Serum Creatinine* | *Initial Dose* |
|---|---|---|
| >80 | | 5 mg/d |
| ≤80 to >30 | <3 mg/dl | 5 mg/d |
| ≤30 | >3 mg/dl | 2.5 mg/d |
| Dialysis | | 2.5 mg on dialysis days |

- ***IV:*** Give 0.625 mg, which may be repeated. Additional doses of 1.25 mg q6h may be given with careful patient monitoring.

### Pharmacokinetics

| *Route* | *Onset* | *Peak* | *Duration* |
|---|---|---|---|
| Oral | 60 minutes | 4–6 h | 24 h |
| IV | 15 min | 3–4 h | 6 h |

*Metabolism:* $T_{1/2}$: 11 h

*Distribution:* Crosses placenta; enters breast milk

*Excretion:* Urine

### IV facts

**Preparation:** Enalaprilat can be given as supplied or mixed with up to 50 ml of 5% Dextrose Injection, 0.9% Sodium Chloride Injection, 0.9% Sodium Chloride Injection in 5% Dextrose, 5% Dextrose in Lactated Ringer's, Isolyte E. Stable at room temperature for 24 h.

**Infusion:** Give by slow IV infusion over at least 5 min.

### Adverse effects

- CNS: *Headache, dizziness, fatigue,* insomnia, paresthesias
- GI: Gastric irritation, *nausea*, vomiting, *diarrhea*, abdominal pain, dyspepsia, elevated liver enzymes
- CV: Syncope, chest pain, palpitations, hypotension in salt/volume depleted patients
- Hematologic: *Decreased hematocrit and hemoglobin*
- GU: Proteinuria, renal insufficiency, renal failure, polyuria, oliguria, urinary frequency, impotence
- Other: *Cough,* muscle cramps, hyperhidrosis

### Clinically important drug-drug interactions

- Decreased hypotensive effect if taken concurrently with indomethacin

## ■ Nursing Considerations

### Assessment

- *History:* Allergy to enalapril, impaired renal function, salt/volume depletion, lactation
- *Physical:* Skin color, lesions, turgor; T; orientation, reflexes, affect, peripheral sensation; P, BP, peripheral perfusion; mucous membranes, bowel sounds, liver evaluation; urinalysis, renal and liver function tests, CBC, and differential

### Implementation

- Alert surgeon, and mark patient's chart with notice that enalapril is being taken; the angiotensin II formation subsequent to compensatory renin release during surgery will be blocked; hypotension may be reversed with volume expansion.
- Monitor patients on diuretic therapy for excessive hypotension following the first few doses of enalapril.
- Monitor patient closely in any situation that may lead to a fall in BP secondary to reduced fluid volume (excessive perspiration and dehydration, vomiting, diarrhea) because excessive hypotension may occur.
- Arrange for reduced dosage in patients with impaired renal function.
- Monitor patient carefully because peak effect may not be seen for 4 h. Do not administer second dose until checking BP.



e

### Drug-specific teaching points

- Do not stop taking the medication without consulting your nurse or physician.
- The following side effects may occur: GI upset, loss of appetite, change in taste perception (will pass with time); mouth sores (frequent mouth care may help); skin rash; fast heart rate; dizziness, lightheadedness (usually passes in a few days; change position slowly, limit activities to those not requiring alertness and precision).
- Be careful in any situation that may lead to a drop in blood pressure (diarrhea, sweating, vomiting, dehydration).
- Avoid OTC medications, especially cough, cold, allergy medications that may interact with this drug.
- Report mouth sores; sore throat, fever, chills; swelling of the hands, feet; irregular heartbeat, chest pains; swelling of the face, eyes, lips, tongue, difficulty breathing.

## enoxacin

*(en **ox'** a sin)*

Penetrex

**Pregnancy Category C**

### Drug classes

Antibacterial

Flouroquinolone

### Therapeutic actions

Bactericidal: interferes with DNA replication in susceptible gram-negative bacteria, preventing cell reproduction.

### Indications

- For the treatment of infections in adults caused by susceptible organisms: caused by *Neisseria gonorrhoeae*; urinary tract infections due to *Escherichia coli, Staphylococcus epidermidis, Klebsiella pneumoniae, Proteus mirabilis, Pseudomonas aeruginosa, Enterobacter cloacae*

### Contraindications/cautions

- Contraindications: allergy to enoxacin, norfloxacin; syphilis; pregnancy; lactation.
- Use cautiously with renal dysfunction, seizures.

### Dosage

**Available Forms:** Tablet—200, 400 mg

*ADULT*

- ***Uncomplicated urinary tract infections:*** 200 mg q12h PO for 7 d.
- ***Complicated urinary tract infections:*** 400 mg q12h PO for 14 d.
- ***Sexually transmitted diseases:*** 400 mg qd PO once.

*PEDIATRIC:* Not recommended for children; produced lesions of joint cartilage in immature experimental animals.

*IMPAIRED RENAL FUNCTION:* Creatinine clearance < 30 ml/min/1.73 $m^2$; after a normal dose, use a 12-h interval and half the recommended dose.

### Pharmacokinetics

| *Route* | *Onset* | *Peak* | *Duration* |
|---|---|---|---|
| Oral | Varies | 1–1 1/2 h | 4–5 h |

*Metabolism:* Hepatic, $T_{1/2}$: 4–6 h

*Distribution:* Crosses placenta; enters breast milk

*Excretion:* Urine and bile

### Adverse effects

- CNS: *Headache, dizziness*, insomnia, fatigue, somnolence, depression, blurred vision
- GI: *Nausea, vomiting*, dry mouth, diarrhea, abdominal pain
- Hematologic: Elevated BUN, SGOT, SGPT, serum creatinine and alkaline phosphatase; decreased WBC, neutrophil count, Hct
- Other: Fever, rash, photosensitivity

### Clinically important drug-drug interactions

• Decreased therapetic effect with iron salts • Decreased absorption if taken with antacids • Increased serum levels and toxic effects of theophyllines if taken concurrently with enoxacin

## ■ Nursing Considerations

### Assessment

- *History:* Allergy to enoxacin, ciprofloxacin, norfloxacin; renal dysfunction; seizures; lactation
- *Physical:* Skin color, lesions; T; orientation, reflexes, affect; mucous membranes, bowel sounds; renal and liver function tests

### Implementation

- Arrange for culture and sensitivity tests before beginning therapy.
- Continue therapy for 2 d after the signs and symptoms of infection have disappeared.
- Administer oral drug 1 h before or 2 h after meals with a glass of water.
- Ensure that patient is well hydrated during course of drug therapy.
- Administer antacids, if needed, at least 2 h after dosing.
- Monitor clinical response; if no improvement is seen or a relapse occurs, repeat culture and sensitivity.
- Encourage patient to complete full course of therapy.

### Drug-specific teaching points

- Take oral drug on an empty stomach, 1 h before or 2 h after meals. If an antacid is needed, take it 2 h after dose.
- Drink plenty of fluids.
- The following side effects may occur: nausea, vomiting, abdominal pain (try small, frequent meals); drowsiness, blurring of vision, dizziness (use caution if driving or using dangerous equipment).
- Report rash, visual changes, severe GI problems, weakness, tremors.

# enoxaparin

*(en **ocks'** a pah in)*

Lovenox

**Pregnancy Category B**

### Drug classes

Antiplatelet agent
Low-molecular-weight heparin

### Therapeutic actions

Low molecular weight heparin that inhibits thrombus and clot formation by blocking factor Xa, factor IIa, preventing the formation of clots.

### Indications

- Prevention of deep vein thrombosis, which may lead to pulmonary embolism following hip replacement
- Unlabeled use: prevention of deep vein thrombosis following hip, knee, or abdominal surgery; reduction of mortality, MI, and recurrent angina in patients with unstable angina and non–Q-wave MI

### Contraindications/cautions

- Contraindications: hypersensitivity to enoxaparin, heparin, pork products; severe thrombocytopenia; uncontrolled bleeding.
- Use cautiously with pregnancy or lactation, history of GI bleed.

### Dosage

**Available Forms:** Injection—30 mg/0.3 ml; 40 mg/0.4 ml

*ADULT:* 30 mg SC bid initial dose soon as possible after surgery, not more than 24 h. Continue throughout the postoperative period for 7–10 d; then 40 mg qd SC for up to 3 wk may be used.

*PEDIATRIC:* Safety and efficacy not established.

### Pharmacokinetics

| *Route* | *Onset* | *Peak* | *Duration* |
|---|---|---|---|
| SC | 20–60 min | 3–5 h | 12 h |

*Metabolism:* $T_{1/2}$: 4 1/2 h
*Distribution* : May cross placenta; may enter breast milk
*Excretion:* Urine

### Adverse effects

- **Hematologic**: Hemorrhage; *bruising;* thrombocytopenia; elevated SGOT, SGPT levels; hyperkalemia
- **Hypersensitivity**: Chills, fever, urticaria, asthma
- **Other**: Fever; pain; local irritation, hematoma, erythema at site of injection

**Clinically important drug-drug interactions**
• Increased bleeding tendencies with oral anticoagulants, salicylates, penicillins, cephalosporins

**Drug-lab test interferences**
• Increased AST, ALT levels

## ■ Nursing Considerations

### Assessment
• *History:* Recent surgery or injury; sensitivity to heparin, pork products, enoxaparin; lactation; history of GI bleed
• *Physical:* Peripheral perfusion, R, stool guaiac test, PTT or other tests of blood coagulation, platelet count, kidney function tests

### Implementation
• Give drug as soon as possible after hip surgery.
• Give deep SC injections; *do not* give enoxaparin by IM injection.
• Administer by deep SC injection; patient should be lying down. Alternate between the left and right anterolateral and posterolateral abdominal wall. Introduce the whole length of the needle into a skin fold held between the thumb and forefinger; hold the skin fold throughout the injection.
• Apply pressure to all injection sites after needle is withdrawn; inspect injection sites for signs of hematoma; do not massage injection sites.
• Do not mix with other injections or infusions.
• Store at room temperature; fluid should be clear, colorless to pale yellow.
• Provide for safety measures (electric razor, soft toothbrush) to prevent injury to patient who is at risk for bleeding.
• Check patient for signs of bleeding; monitor blood tests.
• Alert all health care providers that patient is on enoxaparin.
• Discontinue and initiate appropriate therapy if thromboembolic episode occurs despite enoxaparin therapy.
• Have protamine sulfate (enoxaparin antidote) on standby in case of overdose.
• Treat overdose as follows: Protamine sulfate (1% solution). Each mg of protamine neutralizes 1 mg enoxaparin. Give very slowly IV over 10 min.

### Drug-specific teaching points
• Have periodic blood tests needed to monitor your response to this drug.
• Avoid injury while you are on this drug: Use an electric razor; avoid activities that might lead to injury.
• Report nose bleed, bleeding of the gums, unusual bruising, black or tarry stools, cloudy or dark urine, abdominal or lower back pain, severe headache.

## ephedrine sulfate

*(e fed' rin)*

*Nasal decongestant:* **Kondon's Nasal, Pretz-D**

**Pregnancy Category C**

**Drug classes**
Sympathomimetic drug
Vasopressor
Bronchodilator
Antiasthmatic drug
Nasal decongestant

**Therapeutic actions**
Peripheral effects are mediated by receptors in target organs and are due in part to the release of norepinephrine from nerve terminals. Effects mediated by these receptors include vasoconstriction (increased BP, decreased nasal congestion alpha receptors); cardiac stimulation (beta-1), and bronchodilation (beta-2). Longer acting but less potent than epinephrine; also has CNS stimulant properties.

**Indications**
• Treatment of hypotensive states, especially those associated with spinal anesthesia; Stokes-Adams syndrome with complete heart block; CNS stimulant in narcolepsy and depressive states; acute bronchospasm (parenteral)
• Pressor agent in hypotensive states following sympathectomy, overdosage with ganglionic-blocking agents, antiadrenergic agents, or other drugs used for lowering BP (parenteral)
• Relief of acute bronchospasm (parenteral; epinephrine is the preferred drug)

- Treatment of allergic disorders, such as bronchial asthma, and local treatment of nasal congestion in acute coryza, vasomotor rhinitis, acute sinusitis, hay fever (oral)
- Symptomatic relief of nasal and nasopharyngeal mucosal congestion due to the common cold, hay fever, or other respiratory allergies (topical)
- Adjunctive therapy of middle ear infections by decreasing congestion around the eustachian ostia (topical)

## Contraindications/cautions

- Contraindications: allergy to ephedrine, angle-closure glaucoma, anesthesia with cyclopropane or halothane, thyrotoxicosis, diabetes, hypertension, CV disorders, women in labor whose BP < 130/80.
- Use cautiously with angina, arrhythmias, prostatic hypertrophy, unstable vasomotor syndrome, lactation.

## Dosage

**Available Forms:** Nasal spray—0.25%; nasal jelly—1%; injection—50 mg/ml

May be given IM, SC, or slow IV; nasally.

ADULT

- ***Hypotensive episodes, allergic disorders, asthma:*** 25–50 mg IM (fast absorption), SC (slower absorption), or IV (emergency administration).
- ***Labor:*** Titrate parenteral doses to maintain BP at or below 130/80.
- ***Acute asthma:*** Administer the smallest effective dose (0.25–0.5 ml or 12.5–25 mg).
- ***Maintenance dosage—allergic disorders, asthma:*** 25–50 mg PO q3–4h as necessary.
- ***Topical nasal decongestant:*** Instill solution or apply a small amount of jelly in each nostril q4h. Do not use longer than 3–4 consecutive days.

PEDIATRIC: 25–100 mg/m$^2$ IM or SC divided into 4 to 6 doses; 3 mg/kg per day or 100 mg/m$^2$ per day divided into 4 to 6 doses, PO, SC, or IV for bronchodilation.

- ***Topical nasal decongestant (> 6 y):*** Instill solution or apply a small amount of jelly in each nostril q4h. Do not use for longer than 3–4 consecutive d. Do not use in children <6 y unless directed by physician.

GERIATRIC: More likely to experience adverse reactions; use with caution.

## Pharmacokinetics

| Route | Onset | Duration |
|---|---|---|
| Oral | 15–60 min | 3–5 h |
| SC | 30–40 min | 1 h |
| IM | 10–20 min | 1 h |
| IV | Instant | 1 h |
| Nasal | Rapid | 4–6 h |

*Metabolism:* Hepatic, $T_{1/2}$: 3–6 h

*Distribution:* Crosses placenta; enters breast milk

*Excretion:* Urine

## IV facts

**Preparation:** Administer as provided; no preparation required.

**Infusion:** Administer directly into vein or tubing of running IV; administer slowly, each 10 mg over at least 1 min.

## Adverse effects

Systemic effects are less likely with topical administration, but can take place, and should be considered.

- CNS: *Fear, anxiety, tenseness, restlessness, headache, lightheadedness, dizziness,* drowsiness, tremor, insomnia, hallucinations, psychological disturbances, convulsions, CNS depression, weakness, blurred vision, ocular irritation, tearing, photophobia, symptoms of paranoid schizophrenia
- GI: *Nausea,* vomiting, anorexia
- CV: Arrhythmias, hypertension resulting in intracranial hemorrhage, CV collapse with hypotension, palpitations, tachycardia, precordial pain in patients with ischemic heart disease
- GU: Constriction of renal blood vessels and *decreased urine formation* (initial parenteral administration), *dysuria, vesical sphincter spasm* resulting in difficult and painful urination, urinary retention in males with prostatism
- Local: *Rebound congestion* with topical nasal application
- Other: *Pallor,* respiratory difficulty, orofacial dystonia, sweating

**Clinically important drug-drug interactions**

• Severe hypertension with MAO-inhibitors, TCAs, furazolidone • Additive effects and increased risk of toxicity with urinary alkalinizers • Decreased vasopressor response with reserpine, methyldopa, urinary acidifiers • Decreased hypotensive action of guanethidine with ephedrine

## ■ Nursing Considerations

### Assessment

- ***History:*** Allergy to ephedrine; angle-closure glaucoma; anesthesia with cyclopropane or halothane; thyrotoxicosis, diabetes, hypertension, CV disorders; prostatic hypertrophy, unstable vasomotor syndrome; lactation.
- ***Physical:*** Skin color, temperature; orientation, reflexes, peripheral sensation, vision; P, BP, auscultation, peripheral perfusion; R, adventitious sounds; urinary output pattern, bladder percussion, prostate palpation

### Implementation

- Protect solution from light; give only if clear; discard any unused portion.
- Monitor urine output with parenteral administration; initially renal blood vessels may be constricted and urine formation decreased.
- Do not use nasal decongestant for longer than 3–5 d.
- Avoid prolonged use of systemic ephedrine (a syndrome resembling an anxiety effect may occur); temporary cessation of the drug usually reverses this syndrome.
- Monitor CV effects carefully; patients with hypertension may experience changes in BP because of the additional vasoconstriction. If a nasal decongestant is needed, give pseudoephedrine.

### Drug-specific teaching points

- Do not exceed recommended dose. Demonstrate proper topical nasal application. Avoid prolonged use because underlying medical problems can be disguised. Use nasal decongestant no longer than 3–5 d.
- Avoid OTC medications. Many of them contain the same or similar drugs and serious overdosage can occur.
- The following side effects may occur: dizziness, weakness, restlessness, lightheadedness, tremor (avoid driving or operating dangerous equipment); urinary retention (emptying the bladder before taking drug).
- Report nervousness, palpitations, sleeplessness, sweating.

# Epinephrine

***(ep i nef' rin)***

**adrenaline**

*Injection:* Sus-Phrine

## epinephrine bitartrate

*Aerosols:* AsthmaHaler, Bronitin, Bronkaid Mist, Primatene Mist

## epinephrine borate

*Ophthalmic solution:* Epinal

## epinephrine hydrochloride

*Injection, OTC nasal solution:* Adrenalin Chloride

*Ophthalmic solution:* Epifrin, Glaucon

*Insect sting emergencies:* EpiPen Auto-Injector (delivers 0.3 mg IM adult dose), EpiPen Jr. Auto-Injector (delivers 0.15 mg IM for children).

*OTC solutions for nebulization:* AsthmaNefrin, microNefrin, Nephron, S-2, Vaponefrin

**Pregnancy Category C**

**Drug classes**

Sympathomimetic drug
Alpha-adrenergic agonist
Beta-1 and beta-2 adrenergic agonist
Cardiac stimulant
Vasopressor
Bronchodilator
Antiasthmatic drug
Nasal decongestant
Mydriatic
Antiglaucoma drug

### Therapeutic actions

Naturally occurring neurotransmitter, the effects of which are mediated by alpha or beta receptors in target organs. Effects on alpha receptors include vasoconstriction, contraction of dilator muscles of iris. Effects on beta receptors include positive chronotropic and inotropic effects on the heart (beta-1 receptors); bronchodilation, vasodilation, and uterine relaxation (beta-2 receptors); decreased production of aqueous humor.

### Indications

- *Intravenous:* In ventricular standstill after other measures have failed to restore circulation, given by trained personnel by intracardiac puncture and intramyocardial injection; treatment and prophylaxis of cardiac arrest and attacks of transitory AV heart block with syncopal seizures (Stokes-Adams syndrome); syncope due to carotid sinus syndrome; acute hypersensitivity (anaphylactoid) reactions, serum sickness, urticaria, angioneurotic edema; in acute asthmatic attacks to relieve bronchospasm not controlled by inhalation or SC injection; relaxation of uterine musculature; additive to local anesthetic solutions for injection to prolong their duration of action and limit systemic absorption
- *Injection:* Relief from respiratory distress of bronchial asthma, chronic bronchitis, emphysema, other COPD
- *Aerosols and solutions for nebulization:* Temporary relief from acute attacks of bronchial asthma
- *Topical nasal solution:* Temporary relief from nasal and nasopharyngeal mucosal congestion due to a cold, sinusitis, hay fever, or other upper respiratory allergies; adjunctive therapy in middle ear infections by decreasing congestion around eustachian ostia
- *0.25%–2% ophthalmic solutions:* Management of open-angle (chronic simple) glaucoma, often in combination with miotics or other drugs
- *0.1% ophthalmic solution:* Conjunctivitis, during eye surgery to control bleeding, to produce mydriasis

### Contraindications/cautions

- Contraindications: allergy or hypersensitivity to epinephrine or components of preparation (many of the inhalant and ophthalmic products contain sulfites: sodium bisulfite, sodium or potassium metabisulfite; check label before using any of these products in a sulfite-sensitive patient); narrow-angle glaucoma; shock other than anaphylactic shock; hypovolemia; general anesthesia with halogenated hydrocarbons or cyclopropane; organic brain damage, cerebral arteriosclerosis; cardiac dilation and coronary insufficiency; tachyarrhythmias; ischemic heart disease; hypertension; renal dysfunction (drug may initially decrease renal blood flow); COPD patients who have developed degenerative heart disease; diabetes mellitus; hyperthyroidism; lactation.
- Use cautiously with prostatic hypertrophy (may cause bladder sphincter spasm, difficult and painful urination), history of seizure disorders, psychoneurotic individuals, labor and delivery (may delay second stage of labor; can accelerate fetal heart beat; may cause fetal and maternal hypoglycemia), children (syncope has occurred when epinephrine has been given to asthmatic children).
- Route-specific contraindications for ophthalmic preparations: wearing contact lenses (drug may discolor the contact lens), aphakic patients (maculopathy with decreased visual acuity may occur)

## Dosage

**Available Forms:** Solution for inhalation—1:100, 1.125%, 1%; aerosol—0.3 mg, 0.5%, 0.2 mg; injection—1, 5 mg/ml; solution for injection—1:1,000, 1:2,000, 1:10,000, 1:100,000; suspension for injection—1:200; ophthalmic solution—0.1%, 0.5%, 1%, 2%

ADULT

- ***Epinephrine injection***
  - *Cardiac arrest:* 0.5–1.0 mg (5–10 ml of 1:10,000 solution) IV or by intracardiac injection into left ventricular chamber; during resuscitation, 0.5 mg q5 min.

- ***Intraspinal:*** 0.2–0.4 ml of a 1:1,000 solution added to anesthetic spinal fluid mixture.
  - *Other use with local anesthetic:* Concentrations of 1:100,000–1:20,000 are usually used.
- ***1:1,000 solution***
  - *Respiratory distress:* 0.3–0.5 ml of 1:1,000 solution (0.3–0.5 mg), SC or IM, q20 min for 4 h.
- ***1:200 suspension (for SC administration only)***
  - *Respiratory distress:* 0.1–0.3 ml (0.5–1.5 mg) SC.
- ***Inhalation (aerosol):*** Begin treatment at first symptoms of bronchospasm. Individualize dosage. Wait 1–5 min between inhalations to avoid overdose.
- ***Inhalation (nebulization):*** Place 8–15 drops into the nebulizer reservoir. Place nebulizer nozzle into partially opened mouth. Patient inhales deeply while bulb is squeezed one to three times. If no relief in 5 min, give 2–3 additional inhalations. Use four to six times per day usually maintains comfort.
- ***Topical nasal solution:*** Apply locally as drops or spray or with a sterile swab, as required.
- ***Ophthalmic solution for glaucoma:*** Instill 1–2 drops into affected eye(s) qd–bid. May be given as infrequently as every 3 d; determine frequency by tonometry. When used in conjunction with miotics, instill miotic first.
- ***Ophthalmic solution for vasoconstriction, mydriasis:*** Instill 1–2 drops into the eye(s); repeat once if necessary.

PEDIATRIC

- ***Epinephrine injection:*** 1:1,000 solution, children and infants except premature infants and full-term newborns: 0.01 mg/kg or 0.3 ml/m$^2$ (0.01 mg/kg or 0.3 mg/m$^2$) SC q20 min (or more often if needed) for 4 h. Do not exceed 0.5 ml (0.5 mg) in a single dose. 1:200 suspension, infants and children (1 mo–1 y): 0.005 ml/kg (0.025 mg/kg) SC. Children 30 kg or less: Maximum single dose is 0.15 ml (0.75 mg). Administer subsequent doses only when necessary and not more often than q6h.
- ***Topical nasal solution (children > 6 y):*** Apply locally as drops or spray or with a sterile swab, as required.
- ***Ophthalmic solutions:*** Safety and efficacy for use in children not established.

GERIATRIC OR RENAL FAILURE PATIENTS: Use with caution; patients > 60 y are more likely to develop adverse effects.

## Pharmacokinetics

| *Route* | *Onset* | *Peak* | *Duration* |
|---|---|---|---|
| SC | 5–10 min | 20 min | 20–30 min |
| IM | 5–10 min | 20 min | 20–30 min |
| IV | instant | 20 min | 20–30 min |
| Inhal. | 3–5 min | 20 min | 1–3 h |
| Eye | < 1 h | 4–8 h | 24 h |

*Metabolism:* Neural

*Distribution:* Crosses placenta; passes into breast milk

### IV facts

**Preparation:** 0.5 ml dose may be diluted to 10 ml with Sodium Chloride Injection for direct injection; prepare infusion by mixing 1 mg in 250 ml D5W (4 μg/ml).

**Infusion:** Adminster by direct IV injection or into the tubing of a running IV, each 1 mg over 1 min, or run infusion at 1–4 μg/min (15–60 ml/h).

## Adverse effects

*Systemic Administration*

- CNS: *Fear, anxiety, tenseness, restlessness, headache, lightheadedness, dizziness,* drowsiness, tremor, insomnia, hallucinations, psychological disturbances, convulsions, CNS depression, weakness, blurred vision, ocular irritation, tearing, photophobia, symptoms of paranoid schizophrenia
- GI: *Nausea*, vomiting, anorexia
- CV: Arrhythmias, hypertension resulting in intracranial hemorrhage, cardiovascular collapse with hypotension, palpitations, tachycardia, precordial pain in patients with ischemic heart disease

- **GU**: Constriction of renal blood vessels and *decreased urine formation* (initial parenteral administration), *dysuria, vesical sphincter spasm* resulting in difficult and painful urination, urinary retention in males with prostatism
- **Other**: *Pallor*, respiratory difficulty, orofacial dystonia, sweating

*Local Injection*

- **Local**: Necrosis at sites of repeat injections (due to intense vasoconstriction)

*Nasal Solution*

- **Local**: Rebound congestion, local burning and stinging

*Ophthalmic Solutions*

- **CNS**: *Headache, browache, blurred vision*, photophobia, difficulty with night vision, pigmentary (adrenochrome) deposits in the cornea, conjunctiva, or lids with prolonged use
- **Local**: *Transitory stinging on initial instillation,* eye pain or ache, conjunctival hyperemia

## Clinically important drug-drug interactions

• Increased sympathomimetic effects with other TCAs (eg, imipramine) • Excessive hypertension with propranolol, beta-blocker, furazolidone • Decreased cardiostimulating and bronchodilating effects with beta-adrenergic blockers (eg, propranolol) • Decreased vasopressor effects with chlorpromazine, phenothiazines • Decreased antihypertensive effect of guanethidine, methyldopa

## ■ Nursing Considerations

### Assessment

- ***History:*** Allergy or hypersensitivity to epinephrine or components of drug preparation; narrow-angle glaucoma; shock other than anaphylactic shock; hypovolemia; general anesthesia with halogenated hydrocarbons or cyclopropane; oganic brain damage, cerebral arteriosclerosis; cardiac dilation and coronary insufficiency; tachyarrhythmias; ischemic heart disease; hypertension; renal dysfunction; COPD; diabetes mellitus; hyperthyroidism; prostatic hypertrophy; history of seizure disorders; psychoneuroses; labor and delivery; lactation; contact lens use, aphakic patients (ophthalmic prep)
- ***Physical:*** Weight; skin color, temperature, turgor; orientation, reflexes, intraocular pressure; P, BP; R, adventitious sounds; prostate palpation, normal urine output; urinalysis, kidney function tests, blood and urine glucose, serum electrolytes, thyroid function tests, ECG

e

### Implementation

- Use extreme caution when calculating and preparing doses; epinephrine is a very potent drug; small errors in dosage can cause serious adverse effects. Double-check pediatric dosage.
- Use minimal doses for minimal periods of time; "epinephrine-fastness" (a form of drug tolerance) can occur with prolonged use.
- Protect drug solutions from light, extreme heat, and freezing; do not use pink or brown solutions. Drug solutions should be clear and colorless (does not apply to suspension for injection).
- Shake the suspension for injection well before withdrawing the dose.
- Rotate SC injection sites to prevent necrosis; monitor injection sites frequently.
- Maintain a rapidly acting alpha-adrenergic blocker (phentolamine) or a vasodilator (a nitrite) on standby in case of excessive hypertensive reaction.
- Maintain an alpha-adrenergic blocker or facilities for intermittent positive pressure breathing on standby in case pulmonary edema occurs.
- Maintain a beta-adrenergic blocker (propranolol; a cardioselective beta-blocker, such as atenolol, should be used in patients with respiratory distress) on standby in case cardiac arrhythmias occur.
- Do not exceed recommended dosage of inhalation products; administer pressurized inhalation drug forms during second half of inspiration, because the airways are open wider and the aerosol distribution is more extensive. If a second in-

halation is needed, administer at peak effect of previous dose, 3–5 min.

- Use topical nasal solutions only for acute states; do not use for longer than 3–5 d, and do not exceed recommended dosage. Rebound nasal congestion can occur after vasoconstriction subsides.

### Drug-specific teaching points

- Do not exceed recommended dosage; adverse effects or loss of effectiveness may result. Read the instructions that come with respiratory inhalant products, and consult your health care provider or pharmacist if you have any questions.
- To give eye drops: Lie down or tilt head backward, and look up. Hold dropper above eye; drop medicine inside lower lid while looking up. Do not touch dropper to eye, fingers, or any surface. Release lower lid; keep eye open, and do not blink for at least 30 sec. Apply gentle pressure with fingers to inside corner of the eye for about 1 min; wait at least 5 min before using other eye drops.
- The following side effects may occur: dizziness, drowsiness, fatigue, apprehension (use caution if driving or performing tasks that require alertness); anxiety, emotional changes; nausea, vomiting, change in taste (small, frequent meals may help); fast heart rate. *Nasal solution:* burning or stinging when first used (transient). *Ophthalmic solution:* slight stinging when first used (transient); headache or browache (only during the first few days).
- Report chest pain, dizziness, insomnia, weakness, tremor or irregular heart beat (respiratory inhalant, nasal solution), difficulty breathing, productive cough, failure to respond to usual dosage (respiratory inhalant), decrease in visual acuity (ophthalmic).

## epoetin alfa

*(e poe e' tin)*

EPO, erythropoietin

Epogen, Procrit

**Pregnancy Category C**

### Drug classes

Recombinant human erythropoietin

### Therapeutic actions

A natural glycoprotein produced in the kidneys, which stimulates red blood cell production in the bone marrow.

### Indications

- Treatment of anemia associated with chronic renal failure, including patients on dialysis
- Treatment of anemia related to therapy with AZT in HIV-infected patients
- Treatment of anemia related to chemotherapy in cancer patients (Procrit only)
- Reduction of allogenic blood transfusions in surgical patients
- Unlabeled use: pruritus associated with renal failure

### Contraindications/cautions

- Uncontrolled hypertension; hypersensitivity to mammalian cell-derived products or to albumin human; lactation.

### Dosage

**Available Forms:** Injection—2,000, 3,000, 4,000, 10,000, 20,000 units/ml

*ADULT:* Starting dose: 50–100 U/kg three times weekly, IV for dialysis patients and IV or SC for nondialysis patients. Reduce dose if Hct increases > 4 points in any 2-wk period. Increase dose if Hct does not increase by 5–6 points after 8 wk of therapy. Maintenance dose: individualize based on Hct, generally 25 U/kg three times weekly. Target Hct range 30%–33%.

- *HIV-infected patients on AZT therapy:* Patients receiving < 4,200 mg/wk with serum erythopoietin levels < 500 mU/ml: 100 U/kg IV or SC 3x/w for 8 wk; when desired response is achieved, titrate dose to maintain HCT with lowest possible dose.
- *Cancer patients on chemotherapy (Procrit only):* 150 U/kg SC three times per week; after 8 wk, can be increased to 300 U/kg.
- *Surgery:* 300 U/kg/day SC for 10 days before surgery, on day of surgery and 4 days after surgery. Assure Hgb is > 10 to < 13 g/dl

*PEDIATRIC:* Safety and efficacy not established.

### Pharmacokinetics

| *Route* | *Onset* | *Peak* | *Duration* |
|---|---|---|---|
| SC | 7–14 d | 5–24 h | 24 h |

*Metabolism:* Serum, $T_{1/2}$: 4–13 h
*Distribution:* Crosses placenta; enters breast milk
*Excretion:* Urine

### IV facts

**Preparation:** As provided; no additional preparation. Enter vial only once; do not shake vial. Discard any unused solution. Refrigerate.
**Infusion:** Administer by direct IV injection or into tubing of running IV.
**Incompatibilities:** Do not mix with any other drug solution.

### Adverse effects

- CNS: *Headache, arthralgias, fatigue, asthenia, dizziness,* seizure, CVA/TIA
- GI: *Nausea, vomiting, diarrhea*
- CV: *Hypertension, edema, chest pain*
- Other: Clotting of access line

## ■ Nursing Considerations

### Assessment

- *History:* Uncontrolled hypertension, hypersensitivity to mammalian cell-derived products or to albumin human, lactation
- *Physical:* Reflexes, affect; BP, P; urinary output, renal function; tests, CBC, Hct, iron levels, electrolytes

### Implementation

- Confirm chronic, renal nature of anemia; not intended as a treatment of severe anemia or substitute for emergency transfusion.
- Gently mix; do not shake, shaking may denature the glycoprotein. Use only one dose per vial; do not reenter the vial. Discard unused portions.
- Do not give with any other drug solution.
- Administer dose 3x/w. If administered independent of dialysis, administer into venous access line. If patient is not on dialysis, administer IV or SC.
- Monitor access lines for signs of clotting.
- Arrange for Hct reading before administration of each dose to determine dosage. If patient fails to respond within 8 wk of therapy, evaluate patient for other etiologies of the problem.
- Evaluate iron stores prior to and periodically during therapy. Supplemental iron may need to be ordered.
- Maintain seizure precautions on standby.

### Drug-specific teaching points

- Drug will need to be given 3x/w and can only be given IV or SC or into a dialysis access line. Prepare a schedule of administration dates.
- Keep appointments for blood tests necessary to determine the effects of the drug on your blood count and to determine dosage.
- The following side effects may occur: dizziness, headache, seizures (avoid driving or performing hazardous tasks); fatigue, joint pain (may be medicated); nausea, vomiting, diarrhea (proper nutrition is important).
- Report difficulty breathing, numbness or tingling, chest pain, seizures, severe headache.
- Maintain all of the usual activities and restrictions that apply to your chronic renal failure. If this becomes difficult, consult with your health care provider.

## epoprostenol

*(ee poh **proz'** tin ohl)*
prostacyclin
Flolan
**Pregnancy Category C**

### Drug classes

Prostaglandin

### Therapeutic actions

Naturally occurring prostacyclin that acts as both a pulmonary and systemic vasodilator, inhibits platelet aggregation and has antiproliferative effects.

### Indications

- Treatment of primary pulmonary hypertension in patients unresponsive to standard therapy

### Contraindications/cautions

- Contraindications: nonidiopathic pulmonary hypertension, pregnancy.
- Use cautiously with bleeding tendencies (drug inhibits platelet aggregation).

### Dosage

**Available Forms:** Powder for reconstitution—0.5, 1.5 mg

Preferred administration is through continuous IV infusion through a central venous catheter using a portable infusion pump. Begin infusion with 2 ng/kg/min with subsequent increments of 2 ng/kg as tolerated. Dosage requirements increase over time; average dose after 6 mo of continuous therapy is 20–40 ng/kg/min.

### Pharmacokinetics

| *Route* | *Onset* |
|---|---|
| IV | Immediate |

*Metabolism:* Tissue; $T_{1/2}$: 6 min
*Excretion:* Renal

### IV facts

**Preparation:** Prepare solution as directed by manufacturer; dilute to volumes appropriate for pump delivery system being used; discard and prepare fresh infusion solutions q24h; refrigerate drug ampules.

**Infusion:** Infuse continuously through a central venous line using an infusion pump; check manufacturer's directions for each dilution and system.

### Adverse effects

- CNS: *Headache,* dizziness
- CV: *Bradycardia, flushing, tachycardia, hypotension,* **cardiac arrest**
- GI: *Nausea, vomiting*
- Respiratory: *dyspnea,* respiratory distress
- Other: Delivery system problems—**catheter-associated sepsis, death**

## ■ Nursing Considerations

### Assessment

- ***History:*** Respiratory disease diagnosis, bleeding tendencies
- ***Physical:*** T; reflexes; P, auscultation, peripheral perfusion; R, adventitious sounds; bleeding times

### Implementation

- Ensure diagnosis of primary pulmonary hypertension before beginning therapy.
- Continue all measures necessary for severe pulmonary disease.
- Monitor catheter insertion site for signs of infection.
- Observe patient or significant other preparing dosage and infusion pump.
- Consult with physician and limit dose if adverse effects become severe.

### Drug-specific teaching points

- This drug will be given by continuous IV infusion through a portable infusion pump. You and a significant other will need to know how to prepare the drug, how to prime and use the pump, and signs of problems to watch for.
- This drug must be given continuously. If any problem interferes with continuous administration, contact your health care provider immediately.
- The following side effects may occur: nausea, vomiting; headache, dizziness; muscle aches and pains (analgesic may help).
- Report severe headache, unusual bleeding or bruising, swelling or redness at catheter insertion site, increased difficulty in breathing.

## ergonovine maleate

*(er goe **noe'** veen)*

Ergotrate Maleate

**Pregnancy Category Unknown**

### Drug classes

Oxytocic

### Therapeutic actions

Increases the strength, duration, and frequency of uterine contractions, and decreases postpartum uterine bleeding by direct effects at neuroreceptor sites.

### Indications

- Prevention and treatment of postpartum and postabortal hemorrhage due to uterine atony
- Unlabeled use: diagnostic test for Printzmetal's angina; doses of 0.05–0.2 mg IV during coronary arteriography provoke coronary artery spasm (reversible with nitroglycerin; arrhythmias, ventricular tachycardia, MI have occurred)

### Contraindications/cautions

- Contraindications: allergy to ergonovine, induction of labor, threatened spontaneous abortion.
- Use cautiously with hypertension, heart disease, venoatrial shunts, mitral-valve stenosis, obliterative vascular disease, sepsis, hepatic or renal impairment, lactation.

### Dosage

**Available Forms:** Injection—0.2 mg/ml

*ADULT*

- ***Parenteral:*** 0.2 mg IM (IV in emergency situations). Severe bleeding may require repeat doses q2–4h.
- ***Diagnostic:*** 0.1–0.4 mg IV.

### Pharmacokinetics

| *Route* | *Onset* | *Duration* |
|---|---|---|
| IM | 2–5 min | 3 h |
| IV | Immediate | 45 min |

*Metabolism:* Hepatic, $T_{1/2}$: 0.5–2 h
*Distribution:* Crosses placenta; enters breast milk
*Excretion:* Feces, urine

### IV facts

**Preparation:** No preparation required.
**Infusion:** Administer by direct IV or into tubing of running IV; reserve IV use for emergency situation or diagnostic test, 0.2 mg over 1 min.

### Adverse effects

- CNS: *Dizziness, headache*, ringing in the ears
- GI: *Nausea, vomiting*, diarrhea
- CV: Elevation of BP—more common with ergonovine than other oxytocics
- **Hypersensitivity**: Allergic response, including shock
- **Other**: Ergotism—nausea, BP changes, weak pulse, dyspnea, chest pain, numbness and coldness of the extremities, confusion, excitement, delirium, hallucinations, convulsions, coma

## ■ Nursing Considerations

### Assessment

- *History:* Allergy to ergonovine, induction of labor, threatened spontaneous abortion, hypertension, heart disease, venoatrial shunts, obliterative vascular disease, sepsis, hepatic or renal impairment, lactation
- *Physical:* Uterine tone; orientation, reflexes, affect; P, BP, edema; R, adventitious sounds; CBC, renal and liver function tests

### Implementation

- Administer by IM injection unless emergency requires IV use; complications are more frequent with IV use.
- Monitor postpartum women for BP changes and amount and character of vaginal bleeding.
- Arrange for discontinuation of drug if signs of ergotism occur.
- Avoid prolonged use of the drug.

### Drug-specific teaching points

Usually part of an immediate medical situation. Teaching about the complication of delivery or abortion should include drug. The patient needs to know the name of the drug and what she can expect once it is administered.

- The following side effects may occur: nausea, vomiting, dizziness, headache, ringing in the ears.
- Report difficulty breathing, headache, numb or cold extremities, severe abdominal cramping.

# ergotamine tartrate

*(er got' a meen)*

*Sublingual preparations:*
Gynergen (CAN)

**Pregnancy Category X**

## Drug classes
Ergot derivative
Antimigraine drug

## Therapeutic actions
Mechanism of action not understood; constricts cranial blood vessels; decreases pulsation in cranial arteries, and decreases hyperperfusion of basilar artery vascular bed.

## Indications
- Prevention or abortion of vascular headaches, such as migraine, migraine variant, cluster headache

## Contraindications/cautions
- Allergy to ergot preparations; peripheral vascular disease, severe hypertension, CAD, impaired liver or renal function, sepsis, pruritus, malnutrition; pregnancy; lactation (can cause ergotism—vomiting, diarrhea, seizures—in infant).

## Dosage
**Available Forms:** Sublingual tablets—2 mg

ADULT: 1 tablet under the tongue soon after the first symptoms of an attack; take subsequent doses at 1/2-h intervals if necessary. Do not exceed 3 tablets/d; do not exceed 10 mg/wk.

PEDIATRIC: Safety and efficacy not established.

## Pharmacokinetics

| Route | Onset | Peak |
|---|---|---|
| Sublingual | Rapid | 1/2–3 h |

*Metabolism:* Hepatic, $T_{1/2}$: 2.7 h, then 21 h
*Distribution:* Crosses placenta; enters breast milk
*Excretion:* Feces

## Adverse effects
- CNS: *Numbness, tingling of fingers and toes, muscle pain in the extremities*
- GI: *Nausea, vomiting* (drug stimulates CTZ)
- CV: *Pulselessness, weakness in the legs; precordial distress and pain, transient tachycardia, bradycardia, localized edema and itching*; increased arterial pressure, arterial insufficiency, coronary vasoconstriction, bradycardia
- Other: Ergotism—nausea, vomiting, diarrhea, severe thirst, hypoperfusion, chest pain, BP changes, confusion (with prolonged use); drug dependency and abuse (extended use); may require increasing doses for relief of headaches and for prevention of dysphoric effects of drug withdrawal

## Clinically important drug-drug interactions
- Peripheral ischemia manifested by cold extremities; possible peripheral gangrene if taken concurrently with beta-blockers

## ■ Nursing Considerations

### Assessment
- ***History:*** Allergy to ergot preparations, peripheral vascular disease, severe hypertension, coronary artery disease, impaired liver or renal function, sepsis, pruritis, malnutrition, pregnancy, lactation
- ***Physical:*** Skin color, edema, lesions; T; peripheral sensation; P, BP, peripheral pulses, peripheral perfusion; liver evaluation, bowel sounds; CBC, liver and renal function tests

### Implementation
- Avoid prolonged administration or excessive dosage.
- Arrange for use of atropine or phenothiazine antiemetics if nausea and vomiting are severe.
- Check extremities carefully for gangrene or decubitus ulcer formation.
- Provide supportive measures if acute overdose occurs.

### Drug-specific teaching points
- Take the drug soon after the first symptoms of an attack. Do not exceed the recommended dosage; if relief is not obtained, contact your physician.

- The following side effects may occur: vomiting (if severe, may be medicated); numbness, tingling, loss of sensation in the extremities (avoid injury and examine extremities daily for injury).
- Do not take this drug during pregnancy. If you become or desire to become pregnant, consult with your physician.
- Report irregular heartbeat, pain or weakness of extremities, severe nausea or vomiting, numbness or tingling of fingers or toes.

## Erythromycin

### erythromycin base

*(er ith roe* ***mye'*** *sin)*

*Oral, ophthalmic ointment, topical dermatologic solution for acne, topical dermatologic ointment:* Akne-mycin, A/T/S, E-Mycin, Eryc, Eryderm, Erymax, Ery-Tab, Erythromid (CAN), Ilotycin, Novorythro (CAN), Robimycin, Staticin, T-Stat

### erythromycin estolate

*Oral:* Ilosone, Novorythro (CAN)

### erythromycin ethylsuccinate

*Oral:* E.E.S., E-Mycin, EryPed

### erythromycin gluceptate

*Parenteral, IV:* Ilotycin Gluceptate

### erythromycin lactobionate

*Oral:* Eramycin

### erythromycin stearate

**Pregnancy Category B**

**Drug classes**

Macrolide antibiotic

**Therapeutic actions**

Bacteriostatic or bactericidal in susceptible bacteria; binds to cell membrane, causing change in protein function, leading to cell death.

**Indications**

*Systemic Administration*

- Acute infections caused by sensitive strains of *Streptococcus pneumoniae, Mycoplasma pneumoniae, Listeria monocytogenes, Legionella pneumophila*
- URIs, LRIs, skin and soft-tissue infections caused by group A beta-hemolytic streptococci when oral treatment is preferred to injectable benzathine penicillin
- PID caused by *N. gonorrhoeae* in patients allergic to penicillin
- In conjunction with sulfonamides in URIs caused by *Haemophilus influenzae*
- As an adjunct to antitoxin in infections caused by *Corynebacterium diphtheriae* and *Corynebacterium minutissimum*
- Prophylaxis against alpha-hemolytic streptococcal endocarditis before dental or other procedures in patients allergic to penicillin who have valvular heart disease

*Oral Erythromycin*

- Treatment of intestinal amebiasis caused by *Entamoeba histolytica*; infections in the newborn and in pregnancy that are caused by *Chlamydia trachomatis* and in adult chlamydial infections when tetracycline cannot be used; primary syphilis (*Treponema pallidum*) in penicillin-allergic patients; eliminating *Bordetella pertussis* organisms from the nasopharynx of infected individuals and as prophylaxis in exposed and susceptible individuals.
- Unlabeled uses: erythromycin base is used with neomycin before colorectal surgery to reduce wound infection; treatment of severe diarrhea associated with *Campylobacter* enteritis or enterocolitis; treatment of genital, inguinal, or anorectal lymphogranuloma venereum infection; treatment of *Haemophilus ducreyi* (chancroid)

*Ophthalmic Ointment*

- Treatment of superficial ocular infections caused by susceptible strains of microorganisms; prophylaxis of ophthalmia neonatorum caused by *N. gonorrhoeae* or *C. trachomatis*

*Topical Dermatologic Solutions for Acne*

- Treatment of acne vulgaris

*Topical Dermatologic Ointment*

- Prophylaxis against infection in minor skin abrasions
- Treatment of skin infections caused by sensitive microorganisms

## Contraindications/cautions

*Systemic Administration*

- Contraindication: allergy to erythromycin.
- Use cautiously with hepatic dysfunction, lactation (secreted and may be concentrated in breast milk; may modify bowel flora of nursing infant and interfere with fever workups).

*Ophthalmic Ointment*

- Contraindications: allergy to erythromycin; viral, fungal, mycobacterial infections of the eye.

## Dosage

**Available Forms:** Base: Tablets—250, 333, 500 mg; DR capsules—250 mg; ophthalmic ointment—5 mg/g Estolate: Tablets—500 mg; capsules—250 mg; suspension—125, 250 mg/5 ml Stearate: Tablets—200, 400 mg; suspension—200, 400 mg/5 ml, 100 mg/2–5 ml; powder for suspension—200 mg/5 ml; granules for suspension—400 mg/5 ml

***Systemic administration:*** Oral preparations of the different erythromycin salts differ in pharmacokinetics: 400 mg erythromycin ethylsuccinate produces the same free erythromycin serum levels as 250 mg of erythromycin base, sterate, or estolate.

- *ADULT:* 15–20 mg/kg per day in continuous IV infusion or up to 4 g/d in divided doses q6h; 250 mg (400 mg of ethylsuccinate) q6h PO or 500 mg q12h PO or 333 mg q8h PO, up to 4 g/d, depending on the severity of the infection.
  - *Streptococcal infections:* 20–50 mg/kg per day PO in divided doses (for group A beta-hemolytic streptococcal infections, continue therapy for at least 10 d).
  - *Legionnaire's disease:* 1–4 g/d PO or IV in divided doses (ethylsuccinate 1.6 g/d; optimal doses not established).
  - *Dysenteric amebiasis:* 250 mg (400 mg of ethylsuccinate) PO qid or 333 mg q8h for 10–14 d.
  - *Acute pelvic inflammatory disease* (N. gonorrhoeae): 500 mg of lactobionate or gluceptate IV q6h for 3 d and then 250 mg stearate or base PO q6h or 333 mg q8h for 7 d.
  - *Pertussis:* 40–50 mg/kg per day PO in divided doses for 5–14 d (optimal dosage not established).
  - *Prophylaxis against bacterial endocarditis before dental or upper respiratory procedures:* 1 g (1.6 g of ethylsuccinate) 6 h later.
  - *Chlamydial infections:* Urogenital infections during pregnancy: 500 mg PO qid or 666 mg q8h for at least 7 d, 1/2 this dose q8h for at least 14 d if intolerant to first regimen. Urethritis in males: 800 mg of ethylsuccinate PO tid for 7 d.
  - *Primary syphilis:* 30–40 g (48–64 g of ethylsuccinate) in divided doses over 10–15 d.
  - *CDC recommendations for STDs:* 500 mg PO qid for 7–30 d, depending on the infection.
- *PEDIATRIC:* 30–50 mg/kg per day PO in divided doses. Specific dosage determined by severity of infection, age and weight.
  - *Dysenteric amebiasis:* 30–50 mg/kg per day in divided doses for 10–14 d.
  - *Prophylaxis against bacterial endocarditis:* 20 mg/kg before procedure and then 10 mg/kg 6 h later.
  - *Chlamydial infections:* 50 mg/kg per day PO in divided doses, for at least 2 (conjunctivitis of newborn) or 3 (pneumonia of infancy) wk.

***Ophthalmic ointment:*** 1/2-in ribbon instilled into conjunctival sac of affected eye two to six times per day, depending on severity of infection.

***Topical dermatologic solution of acne:*** Apply to affected areas morning and evening.

***Topical dermatologic ointment:*** Apply to affected area 1–5 x/d.

**Pharmacokinetics**

| *Route* | *Onset* | *Peak* |
|---|---|---|
| Oral | 1–2 h | 1–4 h |
| IV | Rapid | 1 h |

*Metabolism:* Hepatic, $T_{1/2}$: 3–5 h
*Distribution:* Crosses placenta; enters breast milk
*Excretion:* Bile and urine

### IV facts

**Preparation:** Reconstitute powder for IV infusion only with Sterile Water for Injection without preservatives—10 ml for 250- and 500-mg vials, 20 ml for 1-g vials. Prepare intermittent infusion as follows: Dilute 250–500 mg in 100–250 ml of 0.9% Sodium Chloride Injection or 5% Dextrose in Water. Prepare for continuous infusion by adding reconstituted drug to 0.9% Sodium Chloride Injection, Lactated Ringer's injection, or D5 W that will make a solution of 1 g/L.
**Infusion:** Intermittent infusion: administer over 20–60 min qid; infuse slowly to avoid vein irritation. Administer continuous infusion within 4 h, or buffer the solution to neutrality if administration is prolonged.

**Adverse effects**
*Systemic Administration*
- CNS: Reversible hearing loss, confusion, uncontrollable emotions, abnormal thinking
- GI: *Abdominal cramping, anorexia, diarrhea, vomiting*, pseudomembranous colitis, hepatotoxicity
- Hypersensitivity: Allergic reactions ranging from rash to anaphylaxis
- Other: *Superinfections*

*Ophthalmic Ointment*
- Dermatologic: Edema, utricaria, dermatitis, angioneurotic edema
- Local: *Irritation, burning, itching* at site of application

*Topical Dermatologic Preparations*
- Local: *Superinfections*, particularly with long-term use

**Clinically important drug-drug interactions**
*Systemic Administration*
Increased serum levels of digoxin• Increased effects of oral anticoagulants, theophyllines, carbamazepine • Increased therapeutic and toxic effects of corticosteroids • Increased levels of cyclosporine and risk of renal toxicity • Potentially fatal cardiac arrhythmias with astemizde, terfenadine
*Topical Dermatologic Solution for Acne*
• Increased irritant effects with peeling, desquamating, or abrasive agents

**Drug-lab test interferences**
*Systemic Administration*
• Interferes with fluorometric determination of urinary catecholamines • Decreased urinary estriol levels due to inhibition of hydrolysis of steroids in the gut

## ■ Nursing Considerations

### Assessment
- ***History:*** Allergy to erythromycin, hepatic dysfunction, lactation; viral, fungal, mycobacterial infections of the eye (ophthalmologic)
- ***Physical:*** Site of infection; skin color, lesions; orientation, affect, hearing tests; R, adventitious sounds; GI output, bowel sounds, liver evaluation; culture and sensitivity tests of infection, urinalysis, liver function tests

### Implementation
*Systemic Administration*
- Culture site of infection before therapy.
- Administer oral erythromycin base or stearate on an empty stomach, 1 h before or 2–3 h after meals, with a full glass of water (oral erythromycin estolate, ethylsuccinate, and certain enteric-coated tablets [see manufacturer's instructions] may be given without regard to meals).
- Administer around the clock to maximize effect; adjust schedule to minimize sleep disruption.

- Monitor liver function in patients on prolonged therapy.
- Give some preparations (see above) with meals, or substitute one of these preparations, if GI upset occurs with oral therapy.

*Topical Dermatologic Solution for Acne*
- Wash affected area, rinse well, and dry before application.

*Ophthalmic and Topical Dermatologic Preparation*
- Use topical products only when needed. Sensitization produced by the topical use of an antibiotic may preclude its later systemic use in serious infections. Topical antibiotic preparations not normally used systemically are best.
- Culture site before beginning therapy.
- Cover the affected area with a sterile bandage if needed (topical).

### Drug-specific teaching points

*Systemic Administration*
- Take oral drug on an empty stomach, 1 h before or 2–3 h after meals, with a full glass of water; some forms may be taken without regard to meals. The drug should be taken around the clock; schedule to minimize sleep disruption. Finish the *full course* of the drug therapy.
- The following side effects may occur: stomach cramping, discomfort (take the drug with meals, if appropriate); uncontrollable emotions, crying, laughing, abnormal thinking (reversible).
- Report severe or watery diarrhea, severe nausea or vomiting, dark urine, yellowing of the skin or eyes, loss of hearing, skin rash or itching.

*Ophthalmic Ointment*
- Pull the lower eyelid down gently and squeeze a 1/2-in ribbon of the ointment into the sac, avoid touching the eye or lid. A mirror may be helpful. Gently close the eye, and roll the eyeball in all directions.
- Drug may cause temporary blurring of vision, stinging, or itching.
- Report stinging or itching that becomes pronounced.

*Topical Dermatologic Solution for Acne*
- Wash and rinse area, and pat it dry before applying solution.
- Use fingertips or an applicator to apply; wash hands thoroughly after application.

## esmolol hydrochloride

*(ess' moe lol)*

Brevibloc

**Pregnancy Category C**

### Drug classes

Beta-adrenergic blocking agent ($\beta_1$ selective)

### Therapeutic actions

Blocks beta-adrenergic receptors in the heart and juxtaglomerular apparatus, reducing the influence of the sympathetic nervous system on these tissues; decreasing the excitability of the heart, cardiac output, and release of renin; and lowering BP. At low doses, acts relatively selectively at the $\beta_1$-adrenergic receptors of the heart; has very rapid onset and short duration.

### Indications

- Supraventricular tachycardia, when rapid but short-term control of ventricular rate is desirable (atrial fibrillation, flutter, perioperative or postoperative situations)
- Noncompensatory tachycardia when heart rate requires specific intervention

### Contraindications/cautions

- Because this drug is reserved for emergency situations, there are no contraindications to its use.

### Dosage

**Available Forms:** Injection—10 mg/ml, 250 mg/ml

**ADULT:** Individualize dosage by titration (loading dose followed by a maintenance dose): initial loading dose of 500 μg/kg/min IV for 1 min followed by a maintenance dose of 50 μg/kg/min for 4 min. If adequate response is not observed in 5 min, repeat loading dose and follow with maintenance infusion of 100 μg/kg/min. Repeat titration as necessary, increasing rate of maintenance dose in increments of 50 μg/kg/min. As desired heart rate or safe end point is approached, omit loading infusion and decrease incremental dose in maintenance infusion to 25 μg/kg/min (or less), or increase interval between titration steps from 5 to 10 min. Infusions for up to 24 h have been used; up to 48 h may be well tolerated.

*PEDIATRIC:* Safety and efficacy not established.

### Pharmacokinetics

| Route | Onset | Peak | Duration |
|---|---|---|---|
| IV | < 5 min | 10–20 min | 10–30 min |

*Metabolism:* RBC esterases, $T_{1/2}$: 9 min
*Distribution:* Crosses placenta; enters breast milk
*Excretion:* Urine

### IV facts

**Preparation:** Dilute drug before infusing as follows: Add the contents of 2 ampuls of esmolol (2.5 g) to 20 ml of a compatible diluent: 5% Dextrose Injection, 5% Dextrose in Ringer's Injection; 5% Dextrose and 0.9% or 0.45% Sodium Chloride Injection; Lactated Ringer's Injection; 0.9% or 0.45% Sodium Chloride Injection to make a drug solution with a concentration of 10 mg/ml. Diluted solution is stable for 24 h at room temperature. May be further diluted with same solution for continuous infusion.
**Infusion:** Rate of infusion is determined by patient response; see Dosage section above.
**Compatibility:** Do not mix in solution with other drugs.

### Adverse effects

- CNS: *Light-headedness, speech disorder, midscapular pain, weakness, rigors,* somnolence, confusion
- GI: *Taste perversion*
- CV: *Hypotension,* pallor
- GU: *Urinary retention*
- **Local:** *Inflammation,* induration, edema, erythema, burning at the site of infusion
- **Other:** Fever, rhonchi, flushing

### Clinically important drug-drug interactions

• Increased therapeutic and toxic effects with verapamil • Impaired antihypertensive effects with ibuprofen, indomethacin, piroxicam

## ■ Nursing Considerations

### Assessment

- *History:* Cardiac disease, cerebrovascular disease
- *Physical:* P, BP, ECG; orientation, reflexes; R, adventitious sounds; urinary output

### Implementation

- Ensure that drug is not used in chronic settings when transfer to another agent is anticipated.
- Do not give undiluted drug.
- Do not mix with sodium bicarbonate; do not mix undiluted esmolol with other drug solutions.
- Monitor BP closely.

### Drug-specific teaching points

- This drug is reserved for emergency use; incorporate information about this drug into an overall teaching plan.

## estazolam

*(es **taz'** e lam)*

ProSom

**Pregnancy Category X**
**C-IV controlled substance**

### Drug classes

Benzodiazepine
Sedative/hypnotic

### Therapeutic actions

Exact mechanisms of action not understood; acts mainly at subcortical levels of the CNS, leaving the cortex relatively unaffected; potentiates the effects of GABA, an inhibitory neurotransmitter.

## Indications

- Insomnia characterized by difficulty in falling asleep, frequent nocturnal awakenings, or early morning awakening
- Recurring insomnia or poor sleeping habits
- Acute or chronic medical situations requiring restful sleep

## Contraindications/cautions

- Contraindications: hypersensitivity to benzodiazepines, psychoses, acute narrow-angle glaucoma, shock, coma, acute alcoholic intoxication with depression of vital signs, pregnancy (increased risk of congenital malformations, neonatal withdrawal syndrome), labor and delivery ("floppy infant" syndrome reported, lactation (secreted in breast milk; chronic administration of diazepam, another benzodiazepine, to nursing mothers has caused infants to become lethargic and lose weight).
- Use cautiously with impaired liver or kidney function, debilitation, depression, suicidal tendencies.

## Dosage

**Available Forms:** Tablets—1, 2 mg

Individualize dosage.

*ADULT:* 1 mg PO before bedtime; up to 2 mg may be needed.

*PEDIATRIC:* Not for use in children $<$ 15 y.

*GERIATRIC PATIENTS OR THOSE WITH DEBILITATING DISEASE:* 1 mg PO if healthy; start with 0.5 mg in debilitated patients.

## Pharmacokinetics

| *Route* | *Onset* | *Peak* |
|---|---|---|
| Oral | 45–60 min | 2 h |

*Metabolism:* Hepatic, $T_{1/2}$: 10–24 h

*Distribution:* Crosses placenta; enters breast milk

*Excretion:* Urine

## Adverse effects

- CNS: *Transient, mild drowsiness initially; sedation, depression, lethargy, apathy, fatigue, lightheadedness, disorientation, restlessness, asthenia*, crying, delirium, headache, slurred speech, dysarthria, stupor, rigidity, tremor, dystonia, vertigo, euphoria, nervousness, difficulty in concentration, vivid dreams, psychomotor retardation, extrapyramidal symptoms, *mild paradoxical excitatory reactions, during first 2 wk of treatment* (especially in psychiatric patients, aggressive children, and with high dosage), visual and auditory disturbances, diplopia, nystagmus, depressed hearing, nasal congestion
- GI: *Constipation, diarrhea, dyspepsia*, dry mouth, salivation, nausea, anorexia, vomiting, difficulty in swallowing, gastric disorders, elevations of blood enzymes: LDH, alkaline phosphatase, SGOT, SGPT, hepatic dysfunction, jaundice
- CV: *Bradycardia, tachycardia*, cardiovascular collapse, hypertension and hypotension, palpitations, edema
- **Hematologic**: Decreased hematocrit, blood dyscrasias
- GU: *Incontinence, urinary retention, changes in libido*, menstrual irregularities
- **Dermatologic**: Urticaria, pruritus, skin rash, dermatitis
- **Dependence**: *Drug dependence with withdrawal syndrome* when drug is discontinued (more common with abrupt discontinuation of higher dosage used for longer than 4 mo)
- **Other**: Hiccups, fever, diaphoresis, paresthesias, muscular disturbances, gynecomastia

## Clinically important drug-drug interactions

• Increased CNS depression when taken with alcohol, omeprazole • Increased pharmacologic effects of estazolam when given with cimetidine • Decreased sedative effects of estazolam if taken concurrently with theophylline, aminophylline, dyphylline, oxitriphylline

# ■ Nursing Considerations

## Assessment

- *History:* Hypersensitivity to benzodiazepines; psychoses; acute narrow-angle

glaucoma; shock; coma; acute alcoholic intoxication; pregnancy; labor; lactation; impaired liver or kidney function, debilitation, depression, suicidal tendencies.
- *Physical:* Skin color, lesions; T, orientation, reflexes, affect, ophthalmologic exam; P, BP; R, adventitious sounds; liver evaluation, abdominal exam, bowel sounds, normal output; CBC, liver and renal function tests.

### Implementation
- Arrange to monitor liver and kidney function, CBC during long-term therapy.
- Taper dosage gradually after long-term therapy, especially in epileptic patients.

### Drug-specific teaching points
- Take drug exactly as prescribed; do not stop taking this drug without consulting the health care provider.
- Avoid alcohol, sleep-inducing, or OTC drugs while on this drug.
- The following side effects may occur: transient drowsiness, dizziness (avoid driving or engaging in dangerous activities); GI upset (take the drug with water); depression, dreams, emotional upset, crying; sleep may be disturbed for several nights after discontinuing the drug.
- Report severe dizziness, weakness, drowsiness that persists, rash or skin lesions, palpitations, swelling of the extremities, visual changes, difficulty voiding.

# Estradiols

## estradiol oral
*(ess tra **dye'** ole)*

Estrace

## estradiol transdermal system

Alora, Climara, Estraderm, FemPatch, Vivelle

## estradiol topical vaginal cream

Estrace

## estradiol vaginal ring

Estring

## estradiol cypionate in oil

Depo-Estradiol Cypionate, dep Gynogen, Depogen, Estro-Cyp

## estradiol valerate in oil

Delestrogen, Dioval, Estra-L 40, Gynogen L.A., Valergen

**Pregnancy Category X**

### Drug classes
Hormone
Estrogen

### Therapeutic actions
Estradiol is the most potent endogenous female sex hormone. Estrogens are important in the development of the female reproductive system and secondary sex characteristics; affect the release of pituitary gonadotropins; cause capillary dilatation, fluid retention, protein anabolism and thin cervical mucus; conserve calcium and phosphorus and encourage bone formation; inhibit ovulation and prevent postpartum breast discomfort. They are responsible for the proliferation of the endometrium; absence or decline of estrogen produces signs and symptoms of menopause on the uterus, vagina, breasts, cervix; relief in androgen-dependent prostatic carcinoma is attributable to competition with androgens for receptor sites, decreasing the influence of androgens.

### Indications
- Palliation of moderate to severe vasomotor symptoms, atrophic vaginitis or kraurosis vulvae associated with menopause (estradiol oral, transdermal, cream, estradiol valerate)
- Treatment of female hypogonadism, female castration, primary ovarian failure (estradiol oral, transdermal, estradiol cypionate, valerate)

- Palliation of inoperable prostatic cancer (estradiol oral, estradiol valerate)
- Palliation of inoperable, progressing breast cancer (estradiol oral)
- Prevention of postpartum breast engorgement (estradiol valerate)

## Contraindications/cautions

- Contraindications: allergy to estrogens, allergy to tartrazine (in 2-mg oral tablets), breast cancer (with exceptions), estrogen-dependent neoplasm, undiagnosed abnormal genital bleeding, active or past history of thrombophlebitis or thromboembolic disorders (potential serious fetal defects; women of childbearing age should be advised of risks and birth control measures suggested).
- Use cautiously with metabolic bone disease, renal insufficiency, CHF, lactation.

## Dosage

**Available Forms:** Transdermal—release rates of 0.025, 0.0375, 0.05, 0.075, 0.1 mg/24 h; tablets—0.5, 1, 2 mg; injection—10, 20, 40 mg/ml; vaginal cream—0.1 mg

**ADULT**

- ***Moderate to severe vasomotor symptoms, atrophic vaginitis, kraurosis vulvae associated with menopause:*** 1–2 mg/d PO. Adjust dose to control symptoms. Cyclic therapy (3 wk on/1 wk off) is recommended, especially in women who have not had a hysterectomy. 1–5 mg estradiol cypionate in oil IM every 3–4 wk. 10–20 mg estradiol valerate in oil IM, every 4 wk. 0.05-mg system applied to the skin twice weekly. If women oral estrogens have been used, start transdermal system 1 wk after withdrawal of oral form. Given on a cyclic schedule (3 wk on/1wk off). Attempt to taper or discontinue medication every 3–6 mo.
  - ***Vaginal cream:*** 2–4 g intravaginally daily for 1–2 wk, then reduce to 1/2 dosage for similar period followed by maintenance doses of 1 g 1–3×/wk thereafter. Discontinue or taper at 3– 6-mo intervals.
  - ***Vaginal ring:*** Insert one ring high into vagina. Replace every 90 days.
- *Female hypogonadism, female castration, primary ovarian failure:* 1–2 mg/d PO. Adjust dose to control symptoms. Cyclic therapy (3 wk on/1 wk off) is recommended. 1.5–2 mg estradiol cypionate in oil IM at monthly intervals. 10–20 mg estradiol valerate in oil IM every 4 wk. 0.05 mg system applied to skin twice weekly as above.
- *Prostatic cancer (inoperable):* 1–2 mg PO tid. Administer chronically. 30 mg or more estradiol valerate in oil IM every 1–2 wk.
- *Breast cancer (inoperable, progressing):* 10 mg tid PO for at least 3 mo.
- *Prevention of postpartum breast engorgement:* 10–25 mg estradiol valerate in oil IM as a single injection at the end of the first stage of labor.

**PEDIATRIC:** Not recommended due to effect on the growth of the long bones.

## Pharmacokinetics

| *Route* | *Onset* | *Peak* |
|---|---|---|
| Oral | Slow | Days |

*Metabolism:* Hepatic, $T_{1/2}$: not known
*Distribution:* Crosses placenta; enters breast milk
*Excretion:* Urine

## Adverse effects

- CNS: Steepening of the corneal curvature with a resultant change in visual acuity and intolerance to contact lenses, *headache*, migraine, dizziness, mental depression, chorea, convulsions
- GI: Gallbladder disease (in postmenopausal women), **hepatic adenoma, *nausea, vomiting, abdominal cramps, bloating*, cholestatic jaundice, colitis, acute pancreatitis**
- CV: Increased blood pressure, thromboembolic and thrombotic disease
- Hematologic: Hypercalcemia, decreased glucose tolerance

- **GU**: Increased risk of postmenopausal endometrial cancer, *breakthrough bleeding, change in menstrual flow, dysmenorrhea, premenstrual-like syndrome*, amenorrhea, vaginal candidiasis, cystitis-like syndrome, endometrial cystic hyperplasia
- **Dermatologic**: *Photosensitivity, peripheral edema, chloasma*, erythema nodosum or multiforme, hemorrhagic eruption, loss of scalp hair, hirsutism, urticaria, dermatitis
- **Local**: *Pain at injection site*, sterile abscess, postinjection flare
- **Other**: Weight changes, reduced carbohydrate tolerance, aggravation of porphyria, edema, changes in libido, breast tenderness

*Topical Vaginal Cream*

Systemic absorption may cause uterine bleeding in menopausal women and may cause serious bleeding of remaining endometrial foci in sterilized women with endometriosis.

### Clinically important drug-drug interactions

• Increased therapeutic and toxic effects of corticosteroids • Decreased serum levels of estradiol with drugs that enhance hepatic metabolism of the drug: barbiturates, phenytoin, rifampin

### Drug-lab test interferences

• Increased sulfobromophthalein retention; prothrombin and factors VII, VIII, IX, and X; thyroid-binding globulin with increased PBI, $T_4$, increased uptake of free $T_3$ resin (free $T_4$ is unaltered), serum triglycerides and phospholipid concentration • Decreased antithrombin III, pregnanediol excretion, response to metyrapone test, serum folate concentration • Impaired glucose tolerance

## ■ Nursing Considerations

### Assessment

- *History:* Allergy to estrogens, tartrazine; breast cancer, estrogen-dependent neoplasm; undiagnosed abnormal genital bleeding; active or previous thrombophlebitis or thromboembolic disorders; pregnancy; lactation; metabolic bone disease; renal insufficiency; CHF
- *Physical:* Skin color, lesions, edema; breast exam; injection site; orientation, affect, reflexes; P, auscultation, BP, peripheral perfusion; R, adventitious sounds; bowel sounds, liver evaluation, abdominal exam; pelvic exam; serum calcium, phosphorus; liver and renal function tests; Pap smear; glucose tolerance test

### Implementation

- Arrange for pretreatment and periodic (at least annual) history and physical, which should include BP, breasts, abdomen, pelvic organs, and a Pap smear.
- Caution patient of the risks of estrogen use, the need to prevent pregnancy during treatment, for frequent medical follow-up, and for periodic rests from drug treatment.
- Administer cyclically for short-term only when treating postmenopausal conditions because of the risk of endometrial neoplasm; taper to the lowest effective dose, and provide a drug-free week each month.
- Apply transdermal system to a clean, dry area of skin on the trunk of the body, preferably the abdomen; do not apply to breasts; rotate the site at least 1 wk between applications; avoid the waistline because clothing may rub the system off; apply immediately after opening and compress for about 10 sec to attach.
- Arrange for the concomitant use of progestin therapy during chronic estrogen therapy; this will mimic normal physiologic cycling and allow for a cyclic uterine bleeding that may decrease the risk of endometrial cancer.
- Administer parenteral preparations by deep IM injection only. Monitor injection sites and rotate with each injection to decrease development of abscesses.

### Drug-specific teaching points

- Use this drug in cycles or short term; prepare a calendar of drug days, rest days, and drug-free periods.

- Apply transdermal system and vaginal cream properly.
- Potentially serious side effects: cancers, blood clots, liver problems; it is very important to have periodic medical exams throughout therapy.
- This drug cannot be given to pregnant women because of serious toxic effects to the baby.
- The following side effects may occur: nausea, vomiting, bloating; headache, dizziness, mental depression (use caution if driving or performing tasks that require alertness); sensitivity to sunlight (use a sunscreen and wear protective clothing); skin rash, loss of scalp hair, darkening of the skin on the face; changes in menstrual patterns.
- Report pain in the groin or calves of the legs, chest pain or sudden shortness of breath, abnormal vaginal bleeding, lumps in the breast, sudden severe headache, dizziness or fainting, changes in vision or speech, weakness or numbness in the arm or leg, severe abdominal pain, yellowing of the skin or eyes, severe mental depression, pain at injection site.

## estramustine phosphate sodium

*(ess tra* ***muss'*** *teen)*

Emcyt

**Pregnancy Category X**

### Drug classes

Hormonal agent
Estrogen
Antineoplastic agent

### Therapeutic actions

Estradiol and an alkylating agent are linked in each molecule of drug; the drug binds preferentially to cells with estrogen (steroid) receptors, where alkylating effect is enhanced and cell death occurs.

### Indications

- Palliative treatment of metastatic or progressive carcinoma of the prostate

### Contraindications/cautions

- Contraindications: allergy to estradiol or nitrogen mustard; active thrombophlebitis or thromboembolic disorders (except when the tumor mass is the cause of the thromboembolic phenomenon, and the benefits outweigh the risks).
- Use cautiously with cerebral vascular and coronary artery disorders; epilepsy, migraine, renal dysfunction, CHF; impaired hepatic function; metabolic bone diseases with hypercalcemia; diabetes mellitus.

### Dosage

**Available Forms:** Capsules—140 mg

*ADULT:* 10–16 mg/kg per day PO in 3–4 divided doses. Treat for 30–90 d before assessing benefits. Continue therapy as long as response is favorable.

### Pharmacokinetics

| *Route* | *Onset* | *Peak* |
|---|---|---|
| Oral | Varies | 2–3 h |

*Metabolism:* Hepatic, $T_{1/2}$: 20 h
*Excretion:* Feces

### Adverse effects

- CNS: *Lethargy, emotional lability, insomnia, headache, anxiety*, chest pain, tearing of the eyes
- GI: *Nausea, vomiting, diarrhea, anorexia,* flatulence, GI bleeding, burning throat, thirst
- CV: CVA, MI, thrombophlebitis, pulmonary emboli, *CHF, edema, dyspnea, leg cramps, elevated blood pressure*
- **Respiratory**: Upper respiratory discharge, hoarseness
- **Hematologic**: Leukopenia, thrombopenia, abnormalities in bilirubin, LDH, SGOT; decreased glucose tolerance
- **Dermatologic**: *Rash, pruritus, dry skin, peeling skin or fingertips*, easy bruising, flushing, thinning hair
- **Other**: *Breast tenderness, mild to moderate breast enlargement*, carcinoma of the liver, breast

## Nursing Considerations

### Assessment

- *History:* Allergy to estradiol or nitrogen mustard; active thrombophlebitis or thromboembolic disorder; cerebrovascular and coronary artery disorders; epilepsy, migraine, renal dysfunction, CHF; impaired hepatic function; metabolic bone diseases with hypercalcemia; diabetes mellitus
- *Physical:* Skin lesions, color, turgor; hair; breast exam; body weight; orientation, affect, reflexes; P, BP, auscultation, peripheral pulses, edema; R, adventitious sounds; liver evaluation, bowel sounds; stool guaiac, renal and liver function tests, blood glucose

### Implementation

- Administer the drug for 30–90 d before assessing the possible benefits of continued therapy; therapy can be continued as long as response is favorable.
- Refrigerate capsules; capsules may be left out of the refrigerator for up to 48 h without loss of potency.
- Monitor diabetic patients carefully, glucose tolerance may change, affecting need for insulin.
- Arrange to monitor hepatic function periodically during therapy.
- Monitor BP regularly throughout therapy.
- Caution patient to use some contraceptive method while on this drug, because mutagenesis has been reported.

### Drug-specific teaching points

- The effects may not be seen for several weeks. Capsules should be stored in the refrigerator; they will be stable for up to 48 h out of the refrigerator.
- The following side effects may occur: nausea, vomiting, diarrhea, flatulence; dry, peeling skin and rash; headache, emotional lability, lethargy (reversible).
- Use contraceptive measures; there is a risk of fetal deformity with this drug.
- Report pain or swelling in the legs, chest pain, difficulty breathing, edema, leg cramps.

# estrogens, conjugated

*(ess' troe jenz)*

*Oral, topical vaginal cream:* C.E.S. (CAN), C.S.D. (CAN), Premarin

*Parenteral:* Premarin Intravenous

**Pregnancy Category X**

### Drug classes

Hormone
Estrogen

### Therapeutic actions

Estrogens are endogenous female sex hormones important in the development of the female reproductive system and secondary sex characteristics. They affect the release of pituitary gonadotropins; cause capillary dilatation, fluid retention, protein anabolism, and thin cervical mucus; conserve calcium and phosphorus; encourage bone formation; inhibit ovulation and prevent postpartum breast discomfort. They are responsible for the proliferation of the endometrium; absence or decline of estrogen produces signs and symptoms of menopause on the uterus, vagina, breasts, cervix. Their efficacy as palliation in male patients with androgen-dependent prostatic carcinoma is attributable to their competition with androgens for receptor sites, thus decreasing the influence of androgens.

### Indications

- *Oral:* palliation of moderate to severe vasomotor symptoms, atrophic vaginitis, or kraurosis vulvae associated with menopause
- Treatment of female hypogonadism; female castration; primary ovarian failure
- Osteoporosis: to retard progression
- Palliation of inoperable prostatic cancer
- Palliation of mammary cancer
- Prevention of postpartum breast engorgement
- Unlabeled use: postcoital contraceptive
- *Parenteral:* treatment of uterine bleeding due to hormonal imbalance in the absence of organic pathology

- *Vaginal cream:* treatment of atrophic vaginitis and kraurosis vulvae associated with menopause

## Contraindications/cautions

- Contraindications: allergy to estrogens, breast cancer ( with exceptions), estrogen-dependent neoplasm, undiagnosed abnormal genital bleeding, active or past thrombophlebitis or thromboembolic disorders from previous estrogen use, pregnancy (serious fetal defects; women of childbearing age should be advised of risks and birth control measures suggested).
- Use cautiously with metabolic bone disease, renal insufficiency, CHF, lactation.

## Dosage

**Available Forms:** Tablets—0.3, 0.625, 0.9, 1.25, 2.5 mg; injection—25 mg; vaginal cream—0.625 mg

Oral drug should be given cyclically (3 wk on/1 wk off) except in selected cases of carcinoma and prevention of postpartum breast engorgement.

**ADULT**

- ***Moderate to severe vasomotor symptoms associated with menopause and to retard progression of:*** 1.25 mg/d PO. If patient has not menstruated in 2 mo, start at any time. If patient is menstruating, start therapy on day 5 of bleeding.
- ***Atrophic vaginitis, kraurosis vulvae associated with menopause:*** 0.3–1.25 mg/day PO or more if needed. 2–4 g vaginal cream daily intravaginally or topically, depending on severity of condition. Taper or discontinue at 3- to 6-mo intervals.
- ***Female hypogonadism:*** .5 mg/d PO in divided doses for 20 d followed by 10 d of rest. If bleeding does not appear at the end of this time, repeat course. If bleeding does occur before the end of the 10-d rest, begin a 20-d 2.5–7.5 mg estrogen with oral progestin given during the last 5 d of therapy. If bleeding occurs before this cycle is finished, restart course of day 5 of bleeding.
- ***Female castration, primary ovarian failure:*** 1.25 mg/d PO. Adjust dosage by patient response to lowest effective dose.
- ***Prostatic cancer (inoperable):*** 1.25–2.5 mg tid PO. Judge effectiveness by phosphatase determinations and by symptomatic improvement.
- ***Breast cancer (inoperable, progressing):*** 10 mg tid PO for at least 3 mo.
- ***Prevention of postpartum breast engorgement:*** 3.75 mg q4h PO for 5 doses, or 1.25 mg q4h for 5 d.
- ***Abnormal uterine bleeding due to hormonal imbalance:*** 25 mg IV or IM. Repeat in 6–12 h as needed. IV route provides a more rapid response.
- ***Postcoital contraceptive:*** 30 mg/d PO in divided doses for 5 consecutive days within 72 h after intercourse.

**PEDIATRIC:** Not recommended due to effect on the growth of the long bones.

## Pharmacokinetics

| *Route* | *Onset* | *Peak* |
|---|---|---|
| Oral | Slow | Days |
| IV | Gradual | Hours |

*Metabolism:* Hepatic, $T_{1/2}$: not known

*Distribution:* Crosses placenta; enters breast milk

*Excretion:* Urine

### IV facts

**Preparation:** Reconstitute with provided diluent; add to Normal Saline, dextrose, and invert sugar solutions. Refrigerate unreconstituted parenteral solution; use reconstituted solution within a few hours. Refrigerated reconstituted solution is stable for 60 d; do not use solution if darkened or precipitates have formed.

**Infusion:** Inject slowly over 2–5 min.

**Incompatibilities:** Do *not* mix with protein hydrolysate, ascorbic acid or any solution with an acid pH.

## Adverse effects

- CNS: Steepening of the corneal curvature with a resultant change in visual acuity and intolerance to contact lenses, *headache*, migraine, dizziness, mental depression, chorea, convulsions
- GI: Gallbladder disease (in postmenopausal women), **hepatic adenoma,**

***nausea, vomiting, abdominal cramps, bloating*, cholestatic jaundice, colitis, acute pancreatitis**

- CV: Increased blood pressure, thromboembolic and thrombotic disease
- Hematologic: Hypercalcemia, decreased glucose tolerance
- GU: Increased risk of endometrial cancer in postmenopausal women, *breakthrough bleeding, change in menstrual flow, dysmenorrhea, premenstrual-like syndrome*, amenorrhea, vaginal candidiasis, cystitis-like syndrome, endometrial cystic hyperplasia
- Dermatologic: *Photosensitivity, peripheral edema, chloasma*, erythema nodosum or multiforme, hemorrhagic eruption, loss of scalp hair, hirsutism, urticaria, dermatitis
- Local: *Pain at injection site*, sterile abscess, postinjection flare
- Other: Weight changes, reduced carbohydrate tolerance, aggravation of porphyria, edema, changes in libido, breast tenderness

*Topical Vaginal Cream*

Systemic absorption may cause uterine bleeding in menopausal women and serious bleeding of remaining endometrial foci in sterilized women with endometriosis.

### Clinically important drug-drug interactions

• Increased therapeutic and toxic effects of corticosteroids • Decreased serum levels of estrogen with drugs that enhance hepatic metabolism of the drug: barbiturates, phenytoin, rifampin

### Drug-lab test interferences

• Increased sulfobromophthalein retention; prothrombin and factors VII, VIII, IX, and X; thyroid-binding globulin with increased PBI, $T_4$, increased uptake of free $T_3$ resin (free $T_4$ is unaltered), serum triglycerides and phospholipid concentration • Decreased antithrombin III, pregnanediol excretion, response to metyrapone test, serum folate concentration • Impaired glucose tolerance

## ■ Nursing Considerations

### Assessment

- *History:* Allergy to estrogens; breast cancer, estrogen-dependent neoplasm; undiagnosed abnormal genital bleeding; active or previous thrombophlebitis or thromboembolic disorders; pregnancy; lactation; metabolic bone disease; renal insufficiency; CHF
- *Physical:* Skin color, lesions, edema; breast exam; injection site; orientation, affect, reflexes; P, auscultation, BP, peripheral perfusion; R, adventitious sounds; bowel sounds, liver evaluation, abdominal exam; pelvic exam; serum calcium, phosphorus; liver and renal function tests; Pap smear; glucose tolerance test

### Implementation

- Arrange for pretreatment and periodic (at least annual) history and physical, which should include BP, breasts, abdomen, pelvic organs, and a Pap smear.
- Caution patient of the risks involved with estrogen use, the need to prevent pregnancy during treatment, for frequent medical follow-up, and periodic rests from drug treatment.
- Give cyclically for short term only when treating postmenopausal conditions because of the risk of endometrial neoplasm; taper to the lowest effective dose, and provide a drug-free week each month.
- Refrigerate unreconstituted parenteral solution; use reconstituted solution within a few hours.
- Refrigerated reconstituted solution is stable for 60 d; do not use solution if darkened or precipitates have formed.
- Arrange for the concomitant use of progestin therapy during chronic estrogen therapy in women; this will mimic normal physiologic cycling and allow for cyclic uterine bleeding, which may decrease the risk of endometrial cancer.

### Drug-specific teaching points

- Use this drug cyclically or short term; prepare a calendar of drug days, rest days, and drug-free periods.



e

- Apply transdermal system, use vaginal cream properly.
- Potentially serious side effectscan occur: cancers, blood clots, liver problems; it is very important that you have periodic medical exams throughout therapy.
- This drug cannot be given to pregnant women because of serious toxic effects to the baby.
- The following side effects may occur: nausea, vomiting, bloating; headache, dizziness, mental depression (use caution if driving or performing tasks that require alertness); sensitivity to sunlight (use a sunscreen and wear protective clothing); skin rash, loss of scalp hair, darkening of the skin on the face; changes in menstrual patterns.
- Report pain in the groin or calves of the legs, chest pain or sudden shortness of breath, abnormal vaginal bleeding, lumps in the breast, sudden severe headache, dizziness or fainting, changes in vision or speech, weakness or numbness in the arm or leg, severe abdominal pain, yellowing of the skin or eyes, severe mental depression, pain at injection site.

## estrogens, esterified

*(ess' troe jenz)*

Climestrone (CAN), Estratab, Estromed (CAN), Menest

**Pregnancy Category X**

### Drug classes

Hormone
Estrogen

### Therapeutic actions

Estrogens are endogenous hormones important in the development of the female reproductive system and secondary sex characteristics. They cause capillary dilatation, fluid retention, protein anabolism, and thin cervical mucus; conserve calcium and phosphorus and encourage bone formation; inhibit ovulation and prevent postpartum breast discomfort. They are responsible for the proliferation of the endometrium; absence or decline of estrogen produces signs and symptoms of menopause on the uterus, vagina, breasts, cervix. Palliation with androgen-dependent prostatic carcinoma is attributable to competition for androgen receptor sites, decreasing the influence of androgens.

### Indications

- Palliation of moderate to severe vasomotor symptoms, atrophic vaginitis, or kraurosis vulvae associated with menopause
- Treatment of female hypogonadism; female castration; primary ovarian failure
- Palliation of inoperable prostatic cancer
- Palliation of inoperable, progressing breast cancer in men, postmenopausal women

### Contraindications/cautions

- Contraindications: allergy to estrogens, breast cancer (with exceptions), estrogen-dependent neoplasm, undiagnosed abnormal genital bleeding, active or past thrombophlebitis or thromboembolic disorders from previous estrogen use, pregnancy (serious fetal defects; women of childbearing age should be advised of the risks and birth control measures suggested).
- Use cautiously with metabolic bone disease, renal insufficiency, CHF, lactation.

### Dosage

**Available Forms:** Tablets—0.3, 0.625, 1.25, 2.5 mg

Administer PO only.

**ADULT**

- ***Moderate to severe vasomotor symptoms, atrophic vaginitis, kraurosis vulvae associated with menopause:*** 0.3–1.25 mg/d PO. Adjust to lowest effective dose. Cyclic therapy (3 wk of daily estrogen followed by 1 wk of rest from drug therapy) is recommended.
- ***Female hypogonadism:*** 2.5–7.5 mg/d PO in divided doses for 20 d on/10 d off. If bleeding does not occur by the end of that period, repeat the same dosage schedule. If bleeding does occur before the end of the 10-d rest, begin a 20-d estrogen-progestin cyclic regimen with progestin given orally during the last

5 d of estrogen therapy. If bleeding occurs before end of 10-d rest period, begin a 20-d estrogen-progestin cyclic regimen.
- *Female castration, primary ovarian failure:* Begin a 20-d estrogen-progestin regimen of 2.5–7.5 mg/d PO estrogen in divided doses for 20 d with oral progestin given during the last 5 d of estrogen therapy. If bleeding occurs before the regimen is completed, discontinue therapy and resume on the fifth day of bleeding.
- *Prostatic cancer (inoperable):* 1.25–2.5 mg tid PO. Chronic therapy: judge effectiveness by symptomatic response and serum phosphatase determinations.
- *Breast cancer (inoperable, progressing):* 10 mg tid PO for at least 3 mo in selected men and postmenopausal women.

*PEDIATRIC:* Not recommended due to effect on the growth of the long bones.

### Pharmacokinetics

| *Route* | *Onset* | *Peak* |
|---|---|---|
| Oral | Slow | Days |

*Metabolism:* Hepatic, $T_{1/2}$: not known
*Distribution:* Crosses placenta; enters breast milk
*Excretion:* Urine

### Adverse effects

- CNS: Steepening of the corneal curvature with a resultant change in visual acuity and intolerance to contact lenses, *headache*, migraine, dizziness, mental depression, chorea, convulsions
- GI: Gallbladder disease (in postmenopausal women), hepatic adenoma (rarely occurs, but may rupture and cause death), *nausea, vomiting, abdominal cramps, bloating*, cholestatic jaundice, colitis, acute pancreatitis
- CV: Increased BP, thromboembolic and thrombotic disease (with high doses in certain groups of susceptible women and in men receiving estrogens for prostatic cancer)
- **Hematologic:** Hypercalcemia (in breast cancer patients with bone metastases), decreased glucose tolerance
- GU: Increased risk of endometrial cancer in postmenopausal women, *breakthrough bleeding, change in menstrual flow, dysmenorrhea, premenstrual-like syndrome*, amenorrhea, vaginal candidiasis, cystitis-like syndrome, endometrial cystic hyperplasia
- **Dermatologic:** *Photosensitivity, peripheral edema, chloasma*, erythema nodosum or multiforme, hemorrhagic eruption, loss of scalp hair, hirsutism, urticaria, dermatitis
- **Other:** Weight changes, reduced carbohydrate tolerance, aggravation of porphyria, edema, changes in libido, breast tenderness

### Clinically important drug-drug interactions

• Increased therapeutic and toxic effects of corticosteroids • Decreased serum levels of estrogen if taken with drugs that enhance hepatic metabolism of the drug: barbiturates, phenytoin, rifampin

### Drug-lab test interferences

• Increased sulfobromophthalein retention; prothrombin and factors VII, VIII, IX, and X; thyroid-binding globulin with increased PBI, $T_4$, increased uptake of free $T_3$ resin (free $T_4$ is unaltered), serum triglycerides and phospholipid concentration • Decreased antithrombin III, pregnanediol excretion, response to metyrapone test, serum folate concentration • Impaired glucose tolerance

## ■ Nursing Considerations

### Assessment

- *History:* Allergy to estrogens; breast cancer, estrogen-dependent neoplasm; undiagnosed abnormal genital bleeding; thrombophlebitis or thromboembolic disorders; pregnancy; lactation; metabolic bone disease; renal insufficiency; CHF
- *Physical:* Skin—color, lesions, edema; breast exam; injection site; orientation, affect, reflexes; P, auscultation, BP, peripheral perfusion; R, adventitious sounds; bowel sounds, liver evaluation, abdominal exam; pelvic exam; serum

calcium, phosphorus; liver and renal function tests; Pap smear; glucose tolerance test

### Implementation

- Arrange for pretreatment and periodic (at least annual) history and physical, which should include BP, breasts, abdomen, pelvic organs, and a Pap smear.
- Caution patient of the risks involved with estrogen use; the need to prevent pregnancy during treatment, for frequent medical follow-up, and for periodic rests from drug treatment.
- Give cyclically for short term only when treating postmenopausal conditions because of the risk of endometrial neoplasm; taper to the lowest effective dose, and provide a drug-free week each month.
- Arrange for the concomitant use of progestin therapy during chronic estrogen therapy in women; this will mimic normal physiologic cycling and allow for cyclic uterine bleeding, which may decrease the risk of endometrial cancer.

### Drug-specific teaching points

- Use this drug in cycles or short term; prepare a calendar of drug days, rest days, and drug-free periods.
- Potentially serious side effects can occur: cancers, blood clots, liver problems; it is very important that you have periodic medical exams throughout therapy.
- This drug cannot be given to pregnant women because of serious toxic effects to the baby.
- The following side effects may occur: nausea, vomiting, bloating; headache, dizziness, mental depression (use caution if driving or performing tasks that require alertness); sensitivity to sunlight (use a sunscreen and wear protective clothing); skin rash, loss of scalp hair, darkening of the skin on the face; changes in menstrual patterns.
- Report pain in the groin or calves of the legs, chest pain or sudden shortness of breath, abnormal vaginal bleeding, lumps in the breast, sudden severe headache, dizziness or fainting, changes in vision or speech, weakness or numbness in the arm or leg, severe abdominal pain, yellowing of the skin or eyes, severe mental depression.

## estrone

*(ess' trone)*

Aquest, Estrone 5, Femogen (CAN), Kestrone 5

estrogenic substance (mainly estrone)

**Pregnancy Category X**

### Drug classes

Hormone
Estrogen

### Therapeutic actions

Estrogens are endogenous hormones important in the development of the female reproductive system and secondary sex characteristics. They cause capillary dilatation, fluid retention, protein anabolism, and thin cervical mucus; conserve calcium and phosphorus and encourage bone formation; inhibit ovulation and prevent postpartum breast discomfort. They are responsible for the proliferation of the endometrium; absence or decline of estrogen produces signs and symptoms of menopause on the uterus, vagina, breasts, cervix. Palliation with androgen-dependent prostatic carcinoma is attributable to competition with androgens for receptor sites, decreasing the influence of androgens.

### Indications

- Palliation of moderate to severe vasomotor symptoms, atrophic vaginitis or kraurosis vulvae associated with menopause
- Treatment of female hypogonadism, female castration, primary ovarian failure
- Palliation of inoperable prostatic cancer and breast cancer
- Treatment of abnormal uterine bleeding due to hormone imbalance

### Contraindications/cautions

- Contraindications: allergy to estrogens, breast cancer (with exceptions), estrogen-dependent neoplasm, undiagnosed ab-

normal genital bleeding, active or previous thrombophlebitis or thromboembolic disorders from estrogen use, pregnancy (serious fetal defects; women of childbearing age should be advised of risks and birth control measures suggested).
- Use cautiously with metabolic bone disease, renal insufficiency, CHF, lactation.

## Dosage

**Available Forms:** Injection—2, 5 mg/ml

Administer IM only.

ADULT

- *Moderate to severe vasomotor symptoms, atrophic vaginitis, kraurosis vulvae associated with menopause:* 0.1–0.5 mg 2–3X/wk IM.
- *Female hypogonadism, female castration, primary ovarian failure:* Initially, 0.1–1 mg/wk in single or divided doses IM. 0.5–2 mg/wk has been used in some cases.
- *Prostatic cancer (inoperable):* 2–4 mg, 2–3X/wk IM. Response should occur within 3 mo. If a response does occur, continue drug until disease is again progressive.
- *Breast cancer (inoperable):* 5 mg IM 3 or more X/wk based on pain.
- *Abnormal uterine bleeding due to hormone imbalance:* 2–5 mg IM for several days.

PEDIATRIC: Not recommended due to effect on the growth of the long bones.

## Pharmacokinetics

| Route | Onset | Peak |
|---|---|---|
| IM | Slow | Days |

*Metabolism:* Hepatic, $T_{1/2}$: not known

*Distribution:* Crosses placenta; enters breast milk

*Excretion:* Urine

## Adverse effects

- CNS: Steepening of the corneal curvature with a resultant change in visual acuity and intolerance to contact lenses, *headache*, migraine, dizziness, mental depression, chorea, convulsions
- GI: Gallbladder disease (in postmenopausal women), **hepatic adenoma,** ***nausea, vomiting, abdominal cramps, bloating,*** **cholestatic jaundice, colitis, acute pancreatitis**
- CV: Increased BP, thromboembolic and thrombotic disease
- **Hematologic**: Hypercalcemia, decreased glucose tolerance
- GU: Increased risk of endometrial cancer in postmenopausal women, *breakthrough bleeding, change in menstrual flow, dysmenorrhea, premenstrual-like syndrome,* amenorrhea, vaginal candidiasis, cystitis-like syndrome, endometrial cystic hyperplasia
- **Dermatologic**: *Photosensitivity, peripheral edema, chloasma,* erythema nodosum or multiforme, hemorrhagic eruption, loss of scalp hair, hirsutism, urticaria, dermatitis
- **Local**: *Pain at injection site,* sterile abscess, postinjection flare
- **Other**: weight changes, reduced carbohydrate tolerance, aggravation of porphyria, edema, changes in libido, breast tenderness

## Clinically important drug-drug interactions

• Increased therapeutic and toxic effects of corticosteroids • Decreased serum levels of estrogens if taken with drugs that enhance hepatic metabolism of the drug: barbiturates, phenytoin, rifampin

## Drug-lab test interferences

• Increased sulfobromophthalein retention; prothrombin and factors VII, VIII, IX, and X; thyroid-binding globulin with increased PBI, $T_4$, increased uptake of free $T_3$ resin (free $T_4$ is unaltered), serum triglycerides and phospholipid concentration • Decreased antithrombin III, pregnanediol excretion, response to metyrapone test, serum folate concentration • Impaired glucose tolerance

## ■ Nursing Considerations

### Assessment

- *History:* Allergy to estrogens; breast cancer, estrogen-dependent neoplasm; undiagnosed abnormal genital bleeding; thrombophlebitis or thromboembolic disorders; pregnancy; lactation; metabolic bone disease; renal insufficiency; CHF

- *Physical:* Skin—color, lesions, edema; breast exam; injection site; orientation, affect, reflexes; P, auscultation, BP, peripheral perfusion; R, adventitious sounds; bowel sounds, liver evaluation, abdominal exam; pelvic exam; serum calcium, phosphorus; liver and renal function tests; Pap smear; glucose tolerance test

### Implementation

- Arrange for pretreatment and periodic (at least annual) history and physical, which should include BP, breasts, abdomen, pelvic organs, and a Pap smear.
- Caution patient of the risks involved with estrogen use, the need to prevent pregnancy during treatment, for frequent medical follow-up, and for periodic rests from drug treatment.
- Give cyclically for short term only when treating postmenopausal conditions because of the risk of endometrial neoplasm. Taper to the lowest effective dose, and provide a drug-free week each month.
- Arrange for the concomitant use of progestin therapy during chronic estrogen therapy in women; this will mimic normal physiologic cycling and allow for a cyclic uterine bleeding, which may decrease the risk of endometrial cancer.
- Administer by deep IM injection only; monitor and rotate injection sites to decrease development of abscesses.

### Drug-specific teaching points

- This drug can only be given IM. Keep a calendar of drug days, rest days, and drug-free periods.
- Potentially serious side effects: cancers, blood clots, liver problems; it is very important that you have periodic medical exams throughout therapy.
- This drug cannot be given to pregnant women because of serious toxic effects to the baby.
- The following side effects may occur: nausea, vomiting, bloating; headache, dizziness, mental depression (use caution driving or performing tasks that require alertness); sensitivity to sunlight (use a sunscreen and wear protective clothing); skin rash, loss of scalp hair, darkening of the skin on the face; changes in menstrual patterns.
- Report pain in the groin or calves of the legs, chest pain or sudden shortness of breath, abnormal vaginal bleeding, lumps in the breast, sudden severe headache, dizziness or fainting, changes in vision or speech, weakness or numbness in the arm or leg, severe abdominal pain, yellowing of the skin or eyes, severe mental depression, pain at injection site.

## estropipate

*(ess' troe **pi'** pate)*

piperazine estrone sulfate

Ogen, Ortho-Est

**Pregnancy Category X**

### Drug classes

Hormone

Estrogen

### Therapeutic actions

Estrogens are endogenous female sex hormones important in the development of the female reproductive system and secondary sex characteristics. They cause capillary dilatation, fluid retention, protein anabolism, and thin cervical mucus; conserve calcium and phosphorus and encourage bone formation; inhibit ovulation and prevent postpartum breast discomfort. They are responsible for the proliferation of the endometrium; absence or decline of estrogen produces signs and symptoms of menopause on the uterus, vagina, breasts, cervix. Palliation with androgen-dependent prostatic carcinoma is attributable to competition with androgens for receptor sites, decreasing the influence of androgens.

### Indications

- Palliation of moderate to severe vasomotor symptoms, atrophic vaginitis, or kraurosis vulvae associated with menopause

- Treatment of female hypogonadism, female castration, primary ovarian failure
- Prevention of osteoporosis

### Contraindications/cautions

- Contraindications: allergy to estrogens, breast cancer (with exceptions), estrogen-dependent neoplasm, undiagnosed abnormal genital bleeding, active or past thrombophlebitis or thromboembolic disorders from previous estrogen use, pregnancy (serious fetal defects; women of childbearing age should be advised of the potential risks and birth control measures suggested).
- Use cautiously with metabolic bone disease, renal insufficiency, CHF, lactation.

### Dosage

**Available Forms:** Tablets—0.625, 1.25, 2.5 mg; vaginal cream—1.5 mg

**ADULT**

- *Moderate to severe vasomotor symptoms, atrophic vaginitis, kraurosis vulvae associated with menopause:* 0.625–5 mg/d PO given cyclically; 2–4 g/d intravaginally given cyclically, 3 wk on, 1 wk off
- *Female hypogonadism, female castration, primary ovarian failure:* 1.25–7.5 mg/d PO for the first 3 wk, followed by a rest period of 8–10 d. Repeat if bleeding does not occur at end of rest period.
- *Prevention of osteoporosis:* 0.625 mg qd PO for 25 d of a 31-d cycle per month

**PEDIATRIC:** Not recommended due to effect on the growth of the long bones.

### Pharmacokinetics

| Route | Onset | Peak |
|---|---|---|
| PO | Slow | Days |

*Metabolism:* Hepatic, $T_{1/2}$: not known
*Distribution:* Crosses placenta; enters breast milk
*Excretion:* Urine

### Adverse effects

- CNS: Steepening of the corneal curvature with a resultant change in visual acuity and intolerance to contact lenses, *headache*, migraine, dizziness, mental depression, chorea, convulsions
- GI: Gallbladder disease (in postmenopausal women), **hepatic adenoma, *nausea, vomiting, abdominal cramps, bloating*, cholestatic jaundice, colitis, acute pancreatitis**
- CV: Increased BP, thromboembolic and thrombotic disease
- Hematologic: Hypercalcemia, decreased glucose tolerance
- GU: Increased risk of endometrial cancer in postmenopausal women, *breakthrough bleeding, change in menstrual flow, dysmenorrhea, premenstrual-like syndrome*, amenorrhea, vaginal candidiasis, cystitis-like syndrome, endometrial cystic hyperplasia
- Dermatologic: *Photosensitivity, peripheral edema, chloasma*, erythema nodosum or multiforme, hemorrhagic eruption, loss of scalp hair, hirsutism, urticaria, dermatitis
- Other: Weight changes, reduced carbohydrate tolerance, aggravation of porphyria, edema, changes in libido, breast tenderness

### Clinically important drug-drug interactions

• Increased therapeutic and toxic effects of corticosteroids • Decreased serum levels of estrogens if taken with drugs that enhance hepatic metabolism of the drug: barbiturates, phenytoin, rifampin

### Drug-lab test interferences

• sed sulfobromophthalein retention; prothrombin and factors VII, VIII, IX, and X; thyroid-binding globulin with increased PBI, $T_4$, increased uptake of free $T_3$ resin (free $T_4$ is unaltered), serum triglycerides and phospholipid concentration • Decreased antithrombin III, pregnanediol excretion, response to metyrapone test, serum folate concentration • Impaired glucose tolerance

## ■ Nursing Considerations

### Assessment

- *History:* Allergy to estrogens; breast cancer, estrogen-dependent neoplasm; undi-

agnosed abnormal genital bleeding; thrombophlebitis or thromboembolic disorders; pregnancy; lactation; metabolic bone disease; renal insufficiency; CHF
- *Physical:* Skin—color, lesions, edema; breast exam; injection site; orientation, affect, reflexes; P, auscultation, BP, peripheral perfusion; R, adventitious sounds; bowel sounds, liver evaluation, abdominal exam; pelvic exam; serum calcium, phosphorus; liver and renal function tests; Pap smear; glucose tolerance test

### Implementation
- Arrange for pretreatment and periodic (at least annual) history and physical, which should include BP, breasts, abdomen, pelvic organs, and a Pap smear.
- Caution patient of the risks involved with estrogen use, the need to prevent pregnancy during treatment, for frequent medical follow-up, and for periodic rests from drug treatment.
- Give cyclically for short term only when treating postmenopausal conditions because of the risk of endometrial neoplasm. Taper to the lowest effective dose and provide a drug-free week each month.
- Arrange for the concomitant use of progestin therapy during chronic estrogen therapy in women; this will mimic normal physiologic cycling and allow for a cyclic uterine bleeding, which may decrease the risk of endometrial cancer.

### Drug-specific teaching points
- Prepare a calendar of drug days, rest days, and drug-free periods.
- Potentially serious side effects can occur: cancers, blood clots, liver problems; it is very important that you have periodic medical exams throughout therapy.
- This drug cannot be given to pregnant women because of serious toxic effects to the baby.
- The following side effects may occur: nausea, vomiting, bloating; headache, dizziness, mental depression (use caution driving or performing tasks that require alertness); sensitivity to sunlight (use a sunscreen and wear protective clothing); skin rash, loss of scalp hair, darkening of the skin on the face; changes in menstrual patterns.
- Report pain in the groin or calves of the legs, chest pain or sudden shortness of breath, abnormal vaginal bleeding, lumps in the breast, sudden severe headache, dizziness or fainting, changes in vision or speech, weakness or numbness in the arm or leg, severe abdominal pain, yellowing of the skin or eyes, severe mental depression.

## Ethacrynic acid

## ethacrynic acid
*(eth a **krin'** ik)*

Edecrin

## ethacrynate sodium

Sodium Edecrin

**Pregnancy Category B**

### Drug classes
Loop (high ceiling) diuretic

### Therapeutic actions
Inhibits the reabsorption of sodium and chloride from the proximal and distal renal tubules and the loop of Henle, leading to a sodium-rich diuresis.

### Indications
- Edema associated with CHF, cirrhosis, renal disease
- Acute pulmonary edema (IV)
- Ascites due to malignancy, idiopathic edema, lymphedema
- Short-term management of pediatric patients with congenital heart disease

### Contraindications/cautions
- Contraindications: allergy to ethacrynic acid, electrolyte depletion, anuria, severe renal failure, hepatic coma, SLE, gout, diabetes mellitus, lactation.
- Use cautiously with hypoproteinemia (reduces response to drug).

### Dosage
**Available Forms:** Tablet—25, 50 mg; powder for injection—50 mg/vial

**ADULT**

- *Edema:* Initial dose: 50–100 mg/d PO. Adjust dose in 25- to 50-mg intervals. Higher doses, up to 200 mg/d, may be required in refractory patients. Intermittent maintenance dosage is best. When used with other diuretics, give initial dose of 25 mg/d and adjust dosage in 25-mg increments.
- *Parenteral therapy:* Do not give IM or SC–causes pain and irritation. Usual adult dose is 50 mg or 0.5–1 mg/kg run slowly through IV tubing or by direct injection over several minutes. *Not recommended for pediatric patients.*

**PEDIATRIC:** Initial dose of 25 mg PO with careful adjustment of dose by 25-mg increment. Maintain at lowest effective dose. Avoid use in infants.

### Pharmacokinetics

| Route | Onset | Peak | Duration |
|---|---|---|---|
| Oral | 30 min | 2 h | 6–8 h |
| IV | 5 min | 15–30 min | 2 h |

*Metabolism:* Hepatic, $T_{1/2}$: 30–70 min
*Distribution:* Crosses placenta; enters breast milk
*Excretion:* Urine and bile

### IV facts

**Preparation:** Add 50 ml of 5% Dextrose Injection or Sodium Chloride Injection to the vial of parenteral solution; do not use solution diluted with dextrose if it appears hazy or opalescent. Dextrose solutions may have a low pH. Discard unused solution after 24 h.

**Infusion:** Give slowly over several minutes by direct IV injection or into the tubing of actively running IV over 30 min.

**Incompatibilities:** Do not mix IV solution with whole blood or its derivatives.

### Adverse effects

- CNS: *Dizziness, vertigo, paresthesias, confusion*, apprehension, fatigue, nystagmus, weakness, headache, drowsiness, blurred vision, tinnitus, irreversible hearing loss
- GI: *Nausea, anorexia, vomiting, GI bleeding, dysphagia; sudden, profuse watery diarrhea,* acute pancreatitis, jaundice
- CV: *Orthostatic hypotension,* volume depletion, cardiac arrhythmias, thrombophlebitis
- **Hematologic:** Leukopenia, anemia, thrombocytopenia, fluid and electrolyte imbalances (hyperuricemia, metabolic alkalosis, hypokalemia, hyponatremia, hypochloremia, hypocalcemia, hyperuricemia, hyperglycemia, increased serum creatinine)
- GU: *Polyuria, nocturia, glycosuria,* hematuria
- Dermatologic: *Photosensitivity, rash,* pruritus, urticaria, purpura
- Other: Muscle cramps and muscle spasms

### Clinically important drug-drug interactions

• Increased risk of cardiac glycoside (digitalis) toxicity (secondary to hypokalemia) • Increased risk of ototoxicity with aminoglycoside antibiotics, cisplatin • Decreased diuretic effect with NSAIDs

## ■ Nursing Considerations

### Assessment

- *History:* Allergy to ethacrynic acid; electrolyte depletion; anuria, severe renal failure; hepatic coma; SLE; gout; diabetes mellitus; hypoproteinemia; lactation
- *Physical:* Skin color, lesions, edema; orientation, reflexes, hearing; P, baseline ECG, BP, orthostatic BP, perfusion; R, pattern, adventitious sounds; liver evaluation, bowel sounds; output patterns; CBC, serum electrolytes (including calcium), blood sugar, liver and renal function tests, uric acid, urinalysis

### Implementation

- Administer oral doses with food or milk to prevent GI upset.
- Mark calendars for outpatients if every other day or 3–5 d/wk therapy is the most effective for treating edema.
- Administer early in the day so that increased urination does not disturb sleep.
- Avoid IV use if oral use is at all possible.



e

- Change injection sites to prevent thrombophlebitis if more than one IV injection is needed.
- Measure and record regular body weights to monitor fluid changes.
- Arrange to monitor serum electrolytes, hydration, liver function during long-term therapy.
- Provide potassium-rich diet or supplemental potassium.

### Drug-specific teaching points

- Record alternate day therapy on calendar or dated envelopes. Take the drug early in the day, as increased urination will occur. The drug should be taken with food or meals to prevent GI upset.
- Weigh yourself regularly at the same time and in the same clothing; record weight on calendar.
- The following side effects may occur: increased volume and frequency of urination; dizziness, feeling faint on arising, drowsiness (avoid rapid position changes; hazardous activities, driving a car; and consumption of alcohol, which can intensify these problems); sensitivity to sunlight (use sunglasses, sunscreen, and wear protective clothing); increased thirst (suck on sugarless lozenges; frequent mouth care may help); loss of body potassium (a potassium-rich diet or potassium supplement will be necessary).
- Report loss or gain of more than 3 lb in one day, swelling in your ankles or fingers, unusual bleeding or bruising, dizziness, trembling, numbness, fatigue, muscle weakness or cramps.

## ethambutol hydrochloride

*(e **tham'** byoo tole)*

Etibi (CAN), Myambutol

**Pregnancy Category B**

### Drug classes

Antituberculous drug ("second line")

### Therapeutic actions

Inhibits the synthesis of metabolites in growing mycobacterium cells, impairing cell metabolism, arresting cell multiplication, and causing cell death.

### Indications

- Treatment of pulmonary tuberculosis in conjunction with at least one other antituberculous drug

### Contraindications/cautions

- Contraindications: allergy to ethambutol; optic neuritis; pregnancy (the safest antituberculous regimen for use in pregnancy is considered to be ethambutol, isoniazid, and rifampin).
- Use cautiously with impaired renal function.

### Dosage

Available Forms: Tablets—100, 400 mg

Ethambutol is not administered alone; use in conjunction with four other antituberculosis agents.

ADULT: *Initial treatment:* 15 mg/kg per day PO as a single daily oral dose. Continue therapy until bacteriologic conversion has become permanent and maximal clinical improvement has occurred. *Retreatment:* 25 mg/kg per day as a single daily oral dose. After 60 d, reduce dose to 15 mg/kg per day as a single daily dose.

PEDIATRIC: Not recommended for children <13 y.

### Pharmacokinetics

| Route | Onset | Peak | Duration |
|---|---|---|---|
| Oral | Rapid | 2–4 h | 20–24 h |

*Metabolism:* Hepatic, $T_{1/2}$: 3.3 h

*Distribution:* Crosses placenta; enters breast milk

*Excretion:* Urine, feces

### Adverse effects

- CNS: *Optic neuritis* (loss of visual acuity, changes in color perception), *fever, malaise, headache*, dizziness, mental confusion, disorientation, hallucinations, peripheral neuritis

- GI: *Anorexia, nausea, vomiting,* GI upset, abdominal pain, transient liver impairment
- Hypersensitivity: Allergic reactions—dermatitis, pruritus, anaphylactoid reaction
- Other: Toxic epidermal necrolysis, thrombocytopenia, joint pain, acute gout

**Clinically important drug-drug interactions**

- Decreased absorption with aluminum salts

## ■ Nursing Considerations

### Assessment

- *History:* Allergy to ethambutol, optic neuritis, impaired renal function
- *Physical:* Skin color, lesions; T, orientation, reflexes, ophthalmologic examination; liver evaluation, bowel sounds; CBC, liver and renal function tests

### Implementation

- Administer with food if GI upset occurs.
- Administer in a single daily dose; must be used in combination with other antituberculous agents.
- Arrange for follow-up of liver and renal function tests, CBC, ophthalmologic examinations.

### Drug-specific teaching points

- Take drug in a single daily dose; it may be taken with meals if GI upset occurs.
- Take this drug regularly; avoid missing doses. *Do not* discontinue this drug without first consulting your physician.
- The following side effects may occur: nausea, vomiting, epigastric distress; skin rashes or lesions; disorientation, confusion, drowsiness, dizziness (use caution if driving or operating dangerous machinery; use precautions to avoid injury).
- Arrange to have periodic medical checkups, which will include an eye examination and blood tests.
- Report changes in vision (blurring, altered color perception), skin rash.

# ethchlorvynol

*(eth klor **vi'** nole)*

Placidyl

**Pregnancy Category C**

**C-IV controlled substance**

**Drug classes**

Sedative-hypnotic (nonbarbiturate)

**Therapeutic actions**

Has sedative-hypnotic, anticonvulsant and muscle relaxant properties; produces EEG patterns similar to those produced by the barbiturates.

**Indications**

- Short-term hypnotic therapy for periods up to 1 wk in the management of insomnia; repeat only after drug free interval of 1 wk or more and further evaluation of the patient
- Unlabeled use: sedative: dosage of 100–200 mg bid–tid PO

**Contraindications/cautions**

- Contraindications: hypersensitivity to ethchlorvynol, allergy to tartrazine, acute intermittent porphyria, insomnia in the presence of pain, lactation.
- Use cautiously with those known to exhibit unpredictable behavior or paradoxical restlessness or excitement to barbiturates or alcohol; impaired hepatic or renal function; addiction-prone and emotionally depressed patients with or without suicidal tendencies.

### Dosage

**Available Forms:** Capsules—200, 500, 750 mg

**ADULT:** Individualize dosage. Usual hypnotic dosage is 500 mg PO at bedtime. 750–1,000 mg may be needed for severe insomnia. May supplement with 200 mg PO to reinstitute sleep in patients who awaken during early morning hours after the original bedtime dose of 500 or 750 mg. Do not prescribe for longer than 1 wk.

**PEDIATRIC:** Safety and efficacy not established; not recommended.

*Geriatric or Debilitated:* Give the smallest effective dose.

### Pharmacokinetics

| *Route* | *Onset* | *Peak* | *Duration* |
|---|---|---|---|
| Oral | 15–60 min | 2 h | 5 h |

*Metabolism:* Hepatic, $T_{1/2}$: 10–20 h
*Distribution:* Crosses placenta; enters breast milk
*Excretion:* Urine

### Adverse effects

- CNS: *Dizziness, facial numbness, transient giddiness and ataxia*, mild hangover, blurred vision
- GI: *Vomiting, gastric upset, nausea*, aftertaste, cholestatic jaundice
- **Hematologic**: Thrombocytopenia
- **Dermatologic**: Urticaria, rash
- **Other**: Idiosyncratic reactions: syncope without marked hypotension; mild stimulation; marked excitement, hysteria; prolonged hypnosis; profound muscular weakness; physical, psychological dependence; tolerance; withdrawal reaction

### Clinically important drug-drug interactions

• Decreased PT response to coumarin anticoagulants, dosage adjustment may be necessary when ethchlorvynol therapy is inititated or discontinued • Exaggerated depressant effects with alcohol, barbiturates, narcotics

## ■ Nursing Considerations

### Assessment

- *History:* Hypersensitivity to ethchlorvynol, tartrazine, acute intermittent porphyria, insomnia in the presence of pain, unpredictable behavior or paradoxical restlessness or excitement in response to barbiturates or alcohol, impaired hepatic or renal function, addiction-prone patients, emotionally depressed patients with or without suicidal tendencies, lactation
- *Physical:* Skin color, lesions; orientation, affect, reflexes, vision exam; P, BP; bowel sounds, normal output, liver evaluation; CBC with differential, hepatic and renal function tests

### Implementation

- Supervise prescription for patients who are addiction prone or likely to increase dosage on their own initiative.
- Dispense least effective amount of drug to patients who are depressed or suicidal.
- Withdraw drug gradually if patient has used drug long term or developed tolerance; supportive therapy similar to that for withdrawal from barbiturates may be necessary.

### Drug-specific teaching points

- Take this drug exactly as prescribed. Take drug with food to reduce GI upset, giddiness, ataxia. Do not exceed prescribed dosage.
- Avoid alcohol, sleep-inducing, or OTC drugs while you are on this drug.
- The following side effects may occur: drowsiness, dizziness, blurred vision (avoid driving or performing tasks requiring alertness or visual acuity), GI upset (frequent small meals may help).
- Report skin rash, yellowing of the skin or eyes, bruising.

## ethionamide

*(e thye on **am'** ide)*

Trecator S.C.

**Pregnancy Category D**

### Drug classes

Antituberculous drug ("third line")

### Therapeutic actions

Bacteriostatic against *Mycobacterium tuberculosis*; mechanism of action is not known.

### Indications

- Tuberculosis—any form that is not responsive to first-line antituberculous agents—in conjunction with other antituberculous agents

### Contraindications/cautions

- Contraindications: allergy to ethionamide, pregnancy.
- Use cautiously with hepatic impairment, diabetes mellitus.

### Dosage

**Available Forms:** Tablets—250 mg

*ADULT:* Always use with at least one other antituberculous agent: 0.5–1.0 g/d in divided doses PO. Concomitant use of pyridoxine is recommended

*PEDIATRIC:* 15–20 mg/kg per day PO; maximum dose of 1 g/d.

### Pharmacokinetics

| *Route* | *Peak* | *Duration* |
|---|---|---|
| Oral | 3 h | 9 h |

*Metabolism:* Hepatic, $T_{1/2}$: h
*Distribution:* Crosses placenta; enters breast milk
*Excretion:* Urine

### Adverse effects

- CNS: *Depression, drowsiness, asthenia,* convulsions, peripheral neuritis, neuropathy, olfactory disturbances, blurred vision, diplopia, optic neuritis, dizziness, headache, restlessness, tremors, psychosis
- GI: *Anorexia, nausea, vomiting, diarrhea, metallic taste,* stomatitis, hepatitis
- CV: Postural hypotension
- Dermatologic: Skin rash, acne, alopecia, thrombocytopenia, pellagra-like syndrome
- Other: Gynecomastia, impotence, menorrhagia, difficulty managing diabetes mellitus

## ■ Nursing Considerations

### Assessment

- *History:* Allergy to ethionamide; hepatic impairment, diabetes mellitus; pregnancy
- *Physical:* Skin color, lesions; orientation, reflexes, ophthalmologic exam, affect; BP, orthostatic BP; liver evaluation; liver function tests, blood and urine glucose

### Implementation

- Arrange for culture and sensitivity tests before use.
- Give only with other antituberculous agent.
- Arrange for follow-up of liver function tests prior to and every 2–4 wk during therapy.

### Drug-specific teaching points

- Take drug three to four times each day; take with food if GI upset occurs.
- Take this drug regularly; avoid missing doses. *Do not* discontinue this drug without first consulting health care provider.
- The following side effects may occur: loss of appetite, nausea, vomiting, metallic taste in mouth, increased salivation (take the drug with food, frequent mouth care, small frequent meals may help) diarrhea; drowsiness, depression, dizziness, blurred vision (use caution operating a car or dangerous machinery; change position slowly; avoid injury); impotence, menstrual difficulties.
- Arrange to have regular, periodic medical checkups, including blood tests.
- Report unusual bleeding or bruising, severe GI upset, severe changes in vision.

e

## ethosuximide

*(eth oh* ***sux'*** *i mide)*

Zarontin

**Pregnancy Category C**

### Drug classes

Antiepileptic
Succinimide

### Therapeutic actions

Suppresses the EEG pattern associated with lapses of consciousness in absence (petit mal) seizures; reduces frequency of attacks; mechanism of action not understood, but may act in inhibitory neuronal systems.

### Indications

- Control of absence (petit mal) seizures

### Contraindications/cautions

- Contraindications: hypersensitivity to succinimides, lactation.

- Use cautiously with hepatic, renal abnormalities; pregnancy.

### Dosage

**Available Forms:** Capsules—250 mg; syrup—250 mg/5 ml

*ADULT:* Initial dosage is 500 mg/d PO. Increase by small increments to maintenance level. One method is to increase the daily dose by 250 mg every 4–7 d until control is achieved with minimal side effects. Administer dosages > 1.5 g/d in divided doses only under strict supervision (compatible with other antiepileptics when other forms of epilepsy coexist with absence seizures).

*PEDIATRIC:* 3–6 y: Initial dose is 250 mg/d PO. Increase as described for adults above. > 6 y: Adult dosage.

### Pharmacokinetics

| Route | Peak |
|---|---|
| Oral | 3–7 h |

*Metabolism:* Hepatic, $T_{1/2}$: 30 h in children, 60 h in adults

*Distribution:* Crosses placenta; enters breast milk

*Excretion:* Urine, bile

### Adverse effects

*Succinimides*

- CNS: *Drowsiness, ataxia, dizziness, irritability, nervousness, headache, blurred vision*, myopia, photophobia, hiccups, euphoria, dreamlike state, lethargy, hyperactivity, fatigue, insomnia, increased frequency of grand mal seizures may occur when used alone in some patients with mixed types of epilepsy, confusion, instability, mental slowness, depression, hypochondriacal behavior, sleep disturbances, night terrors, aggressiveness, inability to concentrate
- GI: *Nausea, vomiting, vague gastric upset, epigastric and abdominal pain, cramps, anorexia, diarrhea, constipation, weight loss*, swelling of tongue, gum hypertrophy
- Hematologic: Eosinophilia, granulocytopenia, leukopenia, agranulocytosis, aplastic anemia, monocytosis, **pancytopenia**
- Dermatologic: *Pruritus, urticaria*, Stevens-Johnson syndrome, pruritic erythematous rashes, skin eruptions, erythema multiforme, systemic lupus erythmatosus, alopecia, hirsutism
- Other: Vaginal bleeding, periorbital edema, hyperemia, muscle weakness, abnormal liver and kidney function tests

### Clinically important drug-drug interactions

- Decreased serum levels of primidone

## ■ Nursing Considerations

### Assessment

- *History:* Hypersensitivity to succinimides; hepatic, renal abnormalities; lactation
- *Physical:* Skin color, lesions; orientation, affect, reflexes, bilateral grip strength, vision exam; bowel sounds, normal output, liver evaluation; liver and kidney function tests, urinalysis, CBC with differential, EEG

### Implementation

- Reduce dosage, discontinue, or substitute other antiepileptic medication gradually; abrupt discontinuation may precipitate absence (petit mal) status.
- Monitor CBC and differential before and frequently during therapy.
- Discontinue drug if skin rash, depression of blood count, or unusual depression, aggressiveness, or behavioral alterations occur.
- Arrange counseling for women of childbearing age who need chronic maintenance therapy with antiepileptic drugs and who wish to become pregnant.
- Evaluate for therapeutic serum levels (40–100 $\mu$g/ml).

### Drug-specific teaching points

- Take this drug exactly as prescribed. Do not discontinue this drug abruptly or change dosage.
- Avoid alcohol, sleep-inducing, or OTC drugs while you are on this drug.

- Arrange for frequent checkups to monitor this drug; keep all appointments for checkups.
- The following side effects may occur: drowsiness, dizziness, confusion, blurred vision (avoid driving or performing tasks requiring alertness or visual acuity); GI upset (take the drug with food or milk and eat frequent small meals).
- Wear a medical ID at all times so that any emergency medical personnel will know that you are an epileptic taking antiepileptic medication.
- Report skin rash, joint pain, unexplained fever, sore throat, unusual bleeding or bruising, drowsiness, dizziness, blurred vision, pregnancy.

## ethotoin

***(eth' i toe in)***

Peganone

**Pregnancy Category D**

### Drug classes

Antiepileptic
Hydantoin

### Therapeutic actions

Has antiepileptic activity without causing general CNS depression; stabilizes neuronal membranes and prevents hyperexcitability caused by excessive stimulation; limits the spread of seizure activity from an active focus.

### Indications

- Control of grand mal (tonic-clonic) and psychomotor seizures

### Contraindications/cautions

- Contraindications: hypersensitivity to hydantoins, pregnancy, lactation, hepatic abnormalities, hematologic disorders.
- Use cautiously with acute intermittent porphyria; hypotension, severe myocardial insufficiency; diabetes mellitus, hyperglycemia.

### Dosage

Available Forms: Tablets—250, 500 mg

Administer in 4–6 divided doses daily. Take after eating; space as evenly as possible.

*ADULT:* Initial dose should be $<$ 1 g/d PO. Increase gradually over several days; maintenance from 2–3 g/d PO; $<$ 2 g/d is ineffective in most adults. If replacing another drug, reduce the dose of the other drug gradually as ethotoin dose is increased.

*PEDIATRIC:* Initial dose should not exceed 750 mg/d PO; maintenance doses range from 500 mg/d to 1 g/d PO.

### Pharmacokinetics

| *Route* | *Onset* | *Peak* |
|---|---|---|
| Oral | Rapid | 1–3 h |

*Metabolism:* Hepatic, $T_{1/2}$: 3–9 h
*Distribution:* Crosses placenta; enters breast milk
*Excretion:* Urine

### Adverse effects

- CNS: *Nystagmus, ataxia, dysarthria, slurred speech, mental confusion, dizziness, drowsiness, insomnia, transient nervousness, motor twitchings, fatigue, irritability, depression, numbness, tremor, headache*, photophobia, diplopia, conjunctivitis
- GI: *Nausea*, vomiting, diarrhea, constipation, *gingival hyperplasia*, toxic hepatitis, liver damage, sometimes fatal; hypersensitivity reactions with hepatic involvement, including hepatocellular degeneration and fatal hepatocellular necrosis
- Respiratory: **Pulmonary fibrosis**, acute pneumonitis
- Hematologic: Hematopoietic complications, sometimes fatal: thrombocytopenia, leukopenia, granulocytopenia, agranulocytosis, pancytopenia; macrocytosis and megaloblastic anemia that usually respond to folic acid therapy; eosinophilia, monocytosis, leukocytosis, simple anemia, hemolytic anemia, aplastic anemia, hyperglycemia
- GU: Nephrosis

- **Dermatologic**: Scarlatiniform, morbilliform, maculopapular, urticarial and nonspecific rashes; also serious and sometimes fatal dermatologic reactions: bullous, exfoliative, or purpuric dermatitis, lupus erythematosus, and Stevens-Johnson syndrome; toxic epidermal necrolysis, hirsutism, alopecia, coarsening of the facial features, enlargement of the lips, Peyronie's disease
- **Other**: Lymph node hyperplasia, sometimes progressing to frank malignant lymphoma, monoclonal gammopathy and multiple myeloma (prolonged therapy), polyarthropathy, osteomalacia, weight gain, chest pain, periarteritis nodosa

### Clinically important drug-drug interactions

• Increased pharmacologic effects with chloramphenicol, cimetidine, disulfiram, isoniazid, phenacemide, phenylbutazone, sulfonamides, trimethoprim • Complex interactions and effects when hydantoins and valproic acid are given together: toxicity with apparently normal serum ethotoin levels; decreased plasma levels of valproic acid given with hydantoins; breakthrough seizures when the two drugs are given together • Decreased pharmacologic effects with antineoplastics, diazoxide, folic acid, rifampin, theophyllines • Increased pharmacologic effects and toxicity with primidone, oxyphenbutazone, fluconazole, amiodarone • Increased hepatotoxicity with acetaminophen • Decreased pharmacologic effects of the following drugs: corticosteroids, cyclosporine, dicumarol, disopyramide, doxycycline, estrogens, levodopa, methadone, metyrapone, mexiletine, oral contraceptives, quinestrol, carbamazepine

### Drug-lab test interferences

• Interference with the metyrapone and the 1-mg dexamethasone tests; avoid the use of hydantoins for at least 7 d prior to metyrapone testing

## ■ Nursing Considerations

### Assessment

- *History:* Hypersensitivity to hydantoins; hepatic abnormalities; hematologic disorders; acute intermittent porphyria; hypotension, severe myocardial insufficiency; diabetes mellitus, hyperglycemia; pregnancy; lactation
- *Physical:* T; skin color, lesions; lymph node palpation; orientation, affect, reflexes, vision exam; P, BP; R, adventitious sounds; bowel sounds, normal output, liver evaluation; periodontal exam; liver function tests, urinalysis, CBC and differential, blood proteins, blood and urine glucose, EEG and ECG

### Implementation

- Give after food to enhance absorption and reduce GI upset.
- Administer with other anticonvulsants to regulate seizures; not compatible with phenacemide.
- Reduce dosage, discontinue, or substitute other antiepileptic medication gradually; abrupt discontinuation may precipitate status epilepticus.
- Discontinue drug if skin rash, depression of blood count, enlarged lymph nodes, hypersensitivity reaction, signs of liver damage, or Peyronie's disease (induration of the corpora cavernosa of the penis) occurs. Institute another antiepileptic drug promptly.
- Monitor hepatic function periodically during chronic therapy; monitor blood counts, urinalysis monthly.
- Monitor urine sugar of patients with diabetes mellitus regularly. Adjustment of dosage of hypoglycemic drug may be necessary because antiepileptic drug may inhibit insulin release and induce hyperglycemia.
- Arrange to have lymph node enlargement occurring during therapy evaluated carefully. Lymphadenopathy, which simulates Hodgkin's disease, has occurred. Lymph node hyperplasia may progress to lymphoma.
- Monitor blood proteins to detect early malfunction of the immune system (multiple myeloma).
- Arrange dental consultation for patients on long-term therapy; proper oral hy-

giene can prevent development of gum hyperplasia.

- Arrange counseling for women of child-bearing age who need chronic maintenance therapy with antiepileptic drugs and who wish to become pregnant.

### Drug-specific teaching points

- Take this drug exactly as prescribed, after food to enhance absorption and reduce GI upset. Be especially careful not to miss a dose if you are on once-a-day therapy.
- Do not discontinue this drug abruptly or change dosage.
- Maintain good oral hygiene—regular brushing and flossing—to prevent gum disease while you are taking this drug.
- Arrange frequent dental checkups to prevent serious gum disease.
- Arrange for frequent checkups to monitor your response to this drug; keep all appointments for checkups.
- Monitor your urine sugar regularly, and report any abnormality if you are a diabetic.
- Use some form of contraception, other than birth control pills, while you are on this drug. This drug is not recommended for use during pregnancy. If you wish to become pregnant, discuss with health care provider.
- The following side effects may occur: drowsiness, dizziness, confusion, blurred vision (avoid driving or performing tasks requiring alertness or visual acuity); GI upset (take the drug with food and eat frequent small meals).
- Wear a medical alert tag at all times so that any emergency medical personnel will know that you are an epileptic taking antiepileptic medication.
- Report skin rash, severe nausea or vomiting, drowsiness, slurred speech, impaired coordination, swollen glands, bleeding, swollen or tender gums, yellowish discoloration of the skin or eyes, joint pain, unexplained fever, sore throat, unusual bleeding or bruising, persistent headache, malaise, any indication of an infection or bleeding tendency, abnormal erection, pregnancy.

## etidronate disodium

*(e **tid'** ro nate)*

Didronel, Didronel IV

**Pregnancy Category C (parenteral)**

**Pregnancy Category B (oral)**



### Drug classes

Bisphosphonate
Calcium regulator

### Therapeutic actions

Slows normal and abnormal bone resorption; reduces bone formation.

### Indications

- Treatment of Paget's disease of bone (oral)
- Treatment of heterotopic ossification (oral)
- Treatment of hypercalcemia of malignancy in patients inadequately managed by diet or oral hydration (parenteral)
- Treatment of hypercalcemic of malignancy which persists after adequate hydration has been restored (parenteral)

### Contraindications/cautions

- Contraindications:allergy to bisphosphonates; hypocalcemia, pregnancy, lactation, severe renal impairment.
- Use cautiously with renal dysfunction, upper GI disease.

### Dosage

**Available Forms:** Tablets—200, 400 mg; injection—300 mg/amp

**ADULT**

- *Paget's Disease:* 5–10 mg/kg/d PO for up to 6 mo; or 11 mg/kg/d PO for up to 3 mo. If retreatment is needed, wait at least 90 d between treatment regimens.
- *Heterotopic ossification:* 20 mg/kg/d PO for 2 wk followed by 10 mg/kg/d PO for 10 wk (following spinal cord injury); 20 mg/kg/d PO for 1 mo preoperatively if due to total hip replacement, then 20 mg/kg/d PO for 3 mo post-op.
- *Hypercalcemia of malignancy:* 7.5 mg/kg/d IV for 3 successive d.

*Pediatric:* Safety and efficacy not established.

*Renal Impaired:* Use caution and monitor patient frequently.

### Pharmacokinetics

| *Route* | *Onset* | *Duration* |
|---|---|---|
| PO | Slow | 90 d |
| IV | Rapid | Days |

*Metabolism:* Not metabolized; $T_{1/2}$: 6 h

*Distribution:* Crosses placenta; may pass into breast milk

*Excretion:* Urine

### IV Facts

**Preparation:** Dilute daily dose in 250 ml normal saline for infusion; store at room temperature.

**Infusion:** Infuse over at least 2 h.

### Adverse effects

- CNS: *Headache*
- GI: *Nausea, diarrhea*, altered taste, metallic taste
- Hematological: Elevated BUN, serum creatinine
- Skeletal: *Increased or recurrent bone pain*, focal osteomalacia

### Clinically important drug-drug interactions

- Increased risk of GI distress with aspirin
- Decreased absorption with antacids, calcium, iron, multivalent cations; separate dosing by at least 30 min

### Clinically important drug-food interactions

- Significantly decreased absorption and serum levels if taken with any food; administer on an empty stomach 2 h before meals

## ■ Nursing Considerations

### Assessment

- *History:* Allergy to bisphosphonates, renal failure, upper GI disease, lactation, pregnancy
- *Physical:* Muscle tone, bone pain; bowel sounds; urinalysis, serum calcium, renal funciton tests

### Implementation

- Administer with a full glass of water, 2 h before meals.
- Monitor serum calcium levels before, during, and after therapy.
- Ensure 3-mo rest period after treatment for Paget's disease if retreatment is required, 7 d between treatments for hypercalcemia of malignancy.
- Ensure adequate vitamin D and calcium intake.
- Provide comfort measures if bone pain returns.

### Drug-specific teaching points

- Take this drug with a full glass of water 2 h before meals.
- Periodic blood tests may be required to monitor your calcium levels.
- The following side effects may occur: nausea, diarrhea, bone pain, headache (analgesics may be available to help).
- Report twitching, muscle spasms, dark-colored urine, severe diarrhea.

## etodolac

*(ee toe **doe'** lak)*

Lodine, Lodine XL

**Pregnancy Category C**

### Drug classes

Analgesic (non-narcotic)
Antipyretic
NSAID

### Therapeutic actions

Inhibits prostaglandin synthetase to cause antipyretic and anti-inflammatory effects; the exact mechnanism of action is not known.

### Indications

- Acute or long-term use in the management of signs and symptoms of osteoarthritis
- Management of pain
- Treatment of rheumatoid arthritis
- Unlabeled uses: ankylosing spondylitis, tendinitis, bursitis, gout

### Contraindications/cautions

- Contraindications: significant renal impairment, pregnancy, lactation.
- Use cautiously with impaired hearing, allergies, hepatic, cardiovascular, and GI conditions.

### Dosage

**Available Forms:** Capsules—200, 300 mg; tablets—400 mg; ER capsules—400, 600 mg

ADULT

- *Osteoarthritis:* Initially 800–1,200 mg/d PO in divided doses; maintenance ranges 600–1,200 mg/d in divided doses. Do not exceed 1,200 mg/d. Patients <60 kg: Do not exceed 20 mg/kg. Sustained release: 400–1000 mg/d PO; titrate based on patient response.
- *Analgesia, acute pain:* 200–400 mg q6–8h PO. Do not exceed 1,200 mg/d. Patients < 60 kg: Do not exceed 20 mg/kg.
- *Rheumatoid arthritis:* 500 mg PO q6–8h.

PEDIATRIC: Safety and efficacy not established.

### Pharmacokinetics

| Route | Onset | Peak |
|---|---|---|
| Oral | Varies | 1–2 h |
| Oral (SR) | Slow | 7.3 h |

*Metabolism:* Hepatic, $T_{1/2}$: 7.3 h, 8.3 h (SR)
*Distribution:* Crosses placenta; enters breast milk
*Excretion:* Urine and feces

### Adverse effects

- CNS: *Dizziness,* somnolence, insomnia, fatigue, tiredness, dizziness, tinnitus, ophthalmologic effects
- GI: *Nausea, dyspepsia, GI pain, diarrhea*, vomiting, *constipation*, flatulence
- Hematologic: Bleeding, platelet inhibition with higher doses
- GU: Dysuria, renal impairment
- Dermatologic: Rash, pruritus, sweating, dry mucous membranes, stomatitis
- Other: Peripheral edema, **anaphylactoid reactions** to fatal anaphylactic shock

## ■ Nursing Considerations

### Assessment

- *History:* Renal impairment, impaired hearing, allergies, hepatic, CV, and GI conditions, lactation
- *Physical:* Skin color and lesions; orientation, reflexes, ophthalmologic and audiometric evaluation, peripheral sensation; P, edema; R, adventitious sounds; liver evaluation; CBC, clotting times, renal and liver function tests; serum electrolytes, stool guaiac

### Implementation

- Give with food or after meals if GI upset occurs.
- Arrange for periodic ophthalmologic examination during long-term therapy.
- Institute emergency procedures if overdose occurs (gastric lavage, induction of emesis, supportive therapy).

### Drug-specific teaching points

- Take with food or meals if GI upset occurs.
- Take only the prescribed dosage.
- Dizziness, drowsiness can occur (avoid driving or the use of dangerous machinery while on this drug).
- Report sore throat, fever, rash, itching, weight gain, swelling in ankles or fingers; changes in vision; black, tarry stools.

## etoposide

*(e toe **poe'** side)*
VP-16-213
Toposar, VePesid
**Pregnancy Category D**

### Drug classes

Mitotic inhibitor
Antineoplastic agent

### Therapeutic actions

$G_2$ specific cell toxic: lyses cells entering mitosis; inhibits cells from entering prophase; inhibits DNA synthesis, leading to cell death.

## Indications
- Refractory testicular tumors as part of combination therapy
- Treatment of small cell lung carcinoma as part of combination therapy

## Contraindications/cautions
- Allergy to etoposide, bone marrow suppression, pregnancy, lactation.

## Dosage
**Available Forms:** Capsules—50 mg; injection—20 mg/ml

Modify dosage based on myelosuppression.

ADULT
- ***Testicular cancer:*** 50–100 mg/m$^2$ per day IV on days 1 to 5 or 100 mg/m$^2$ per day IV on days 1, 3, and 5, every 3–4 wk in combination with other agents.
- ***Small-cell lung cancer:*** 35 mg/m$^2$ per day IV for 4 d to 50 mg/m$^2$ for day for 5 d; repeat every 3–4 wk after recovery from toxicity.
- ***Oral:*** Two times the IV dose rounded to the nearest 50 mg.

PEDIATRIC: Safety and efficacy not established.

## Pharmacokinetics

| *Route* | *Onset* | *Peak* | *Duration* |
|---|---|---|---|
| Oral | 30–60 min | 1–1 1/2 h | 20–30 h |
| IV | 30 min | 60 min | 20–30 h |

*Metabolism:* Hepatic, $T_{1/2}$: 4–11 h

*Distribution:* Crosses placenta; enters breast milk

*Excretion:* Urine and bile

### IV facts
**Preparation:** Dilute with 5% Dextrose Injection or 0.9% Sodium Chloride Injection to give a concentration of 0.2 or 0.4 mg/ml. Unopened vials are stable at room temperature for 2 y; diluted solutions are stable at room temperature for 2 (0.4 mg/ml) or 4 (0.2 mg/ml) d.

**Infusion:** Administer slowly over 30–60 min. *Do not give by rapid IV push.*

## Adverse effects
- CNS: *Somnolence, fatigue,* peripheral neuropathy
- GI: *Nausea, vomiting, anorexia, diarrhea,* stomatitis, aftertaste, liver toxicity
- CV: Hypotension (after rapid IV administration)
- **Hematologic:** *Myelotoxicity*
- Dermatologic: *Alopecia*
- **Hypersensitivity:** Chills, fever, tachycardia, bronchospasm, dyspnea, anaphylactic-like reaction
- **Other:** Potentially, carcinogenesis

## ■ Nursing Considerations

### Assessment
- ***History:*** Allergy to etoposide; bone marrow suppression; pregnancy; lactation
- ***Physical:*** T; weight; hair; orientation, reflexes; BP, P; mucous membranes, abdominal exam; CBC

### Implementation
- Do not administer IM or SC; severe local reaction and tissue necrosis occur.
- Avoid skin contact with this drug; use rubber gloves; if contact occurs, immediately wash with soap and water.
- Monitor BP during administration; if hypotension occurs, discontinue dose and consult with physician. Fluids and other supportive therapy may be needed.
- Obtain platelet count, Hgb, WBC count, differential before starting therapy and prior to each dose. If severe response occurs, discontinue therapy and consult with physician.
- Arrange for an antiemetic for severe nausea and vomiting.
- Arrange for wig or other suitable head covering before alopecia occurs. Teach patient the importance of covering the head at extremes of temperature.

### Drug-specific teaching points
- Keep a calendar for specific treatment days and additional courses of therapy.
- The following side effects may occur: loss of appetite, nausea, vomiting, mouth sores (frequent mouth care, small frequent meals may help; try to maintain good nutrition; a dietician may be able to help, and an antiemetic may be ordered); loss of hair (arrange for a wig or

other suitable head covering before the hair loss occurs; it is important to keep the head covered at extremes of temperature).
- Have regular blood tests to monitor the drug's effects.
- Report severe GI upset, diarrhea, vomiting, unusual bleeding or bruising, fever, chills, sore throat, difficulty breathing.

## etretinate

*(e **tret'** i nate)*
Tegison
**Pregnancy Category X**

### Drug classes
Antipsoriatic (systemic)

### Therapeutic actions
Related to retinoic acid vitamin A; mechanism of action is not known, but improvement seems to be related to a decrease in scale, erythema, and thickness of lesions; normalization of epidermal differentiation and decreased inflammation in the epidermis and dermis.

### Indications
- Treatment of severe recalcitrant psoriasis in patients who are unresponsive to standard treatment

### Contraindications/cautions
- Contraindications: allergy to etretinate, retinoids, pregnancy, lactation.
- Use cautiously with CV disease (drug increases triglycerides); diabetes mellitus, obesity, large alcohol intake, familial history of same (may have a tendency to develop hypertriglyceridemia and be at greater risk of developing this condition with etretinate therapy); pregnancy (severe fetal malformations and spontaneous abortions); lactation.

### Dosage
**Available Forms:** Capsules—10.25 mg

*ADULT:* Individualize dosage based on side effects and disease response. Initial dose: 0.75–1 mg/kg per day PO in divided doses. Maximum daily dose: 1.5 mg/kg. Erythrodermic psoriasis may respond to lower initial doses of 0.25 mg/kg per day, PO increased by 0.25 mg/kg per day each wk until optimal initial response is attained. Maintenance doses of 0.5–0.75 mg/kg per day PO may be initiated after initial response, generally after 8–16 wk of therapy. Therapy is usually terminated in patients whose lesions have sufficiently resolved; relapses may be treated as for initial therapy.

*PEDIATRIC:* Use only if all other treatments have proven unsuccessful; may cause premature closure of the epiphyses.

### Pharmacokinetics

| Route | Onset | Peak | Duration |
|---|---|---|---|
| Oral | Slow | 2–6 h | Weeks–months |

*Metabolism:* Hepatic, $T_{1/2}$: 120 d

*Distribution:* Crosses placenta; may enter breast milk

*Excretion:* Bile and urine

### Adverse effects
- CNS: *Lethargy, insomnia, fatigue, headache, fever, dizziness, amnesia*, abnormal thinking, pseudotumor cerebri
- GI: *Cheilitis, chapped lips; dry mouth, thirst; sore mouth and tongue, gingival bleeding and inflammation, nausea,* vomiting, abdominal pain, anorexia, inflammatory bowel disease, **hepatitis** (including fatalities)
- CV: *Cardiovascular, thrombotic or obstructive events,* edema, *dyspnea*
- Hematologic: *Elevated mean corpuscular hemoglobin concentration*, mean corpuscular hemoglobin, reticulocytes, partial thromboplastin time, erythrocyte sedimentation rate; decreased Hgb/Hct, RBC and mean corpuscular volume, increased platelets, *increased or decreased WBC or prothrombin time,* elevated triglycerides, AST, ALT, alkaline phosphatase, GGTP, globulin, cholesterol, bilirubin abnormal liver function tests, increased fasting serum glucose, increased BUN and creatinine, increased or decreased potassium

- GU: *White cells in the urine, proteinuria, red blood cells in the urine, hematuria,* glycosuria, aceetonuria
- MS: *Skeletal hyperostosis, arthralgia, muscle cramps,* bone and joint pain and stiffness
- EENT: Epistaxis, *dry nose, eye irritation, conjunctivitis, corneal opacities, eyeball pain; abnormalities of eyelid, cornea, lens, and retina; decreased visual acuity, double vision;* abnormalities of lacrimation, vision, extraocular musculature, ocular tension, pupil and vitreous, earache, otitis externa
- Dermatologic: *Skin fragility, dry skin, pruritus, rash, thinning of hair, peeling of palms and soles,* skin infections, nail brittleness, petechiae, sunburn, changes in perspiration

### Clinically important drug-food interactions

- Increased absorption with milk

## ■ Nursing Considerations

### Assessment

- ***History:*** Allergy to etretinate, retinoids; cardiovascular disease; diabetes mellitus, obesity, increased alcohol intake; pregnancy, lactation
- ***Physical:*** Weight; skin color, lesions, turgor, texture; joints—range of motion; orientation, reflexes, affect, ophthalmologic exam; mucous membranes, bowel sounds; hepatic function tests (AST, ALT, LDH), serum triglycerides, cholesterol, HDL, sedimentation rate, CBC and differential, urinalysis, serum electrolytes, pregnancy test

### Implementation

- Ensure that patient is not pregnant before administering; arrange for a pregnancy test 2 wk before beginning therapy. Advise patient to use contraceptive measures during treatment and for an indefinite period after treatment is discontinued (the exact length of time after treatment when pregnancy should be avoided is not known; etretinate has been detected in the blood of some patients 2–3 y after therapy was discontinued).
- Arrange for patient to have hepatic function tests prior to therapy and at 1- to 2-wk intervals for the first 1–2 mo of therapy and at intervals of 1–3 mo thereafter.
- Arrange for patient to have blood lipid determinations before therapy and at intervals of 1 or 2 wk until the lipid response is established (usually within 4–8 wk). If elevations occur, institute other measures to lower serum triglycerides: weight reduction, reduction in dietary fat, exercise, increased intake of insoluble fiber, decreased alcohol consumption.
- Administer drug with meals; do not crush capsules.
- Discontinue drug if signs of papilledema occur, and arrange for patient to consult a neurologist for further care.
- Discontinue drug if visual disturbances occur, and arrange for an ophthalmologic exam.
- Discontinue drug if abdominal pain, rectal bleeding, or severe diarrhea occurs, and consult with physician.
- Do not allow blood donation from patients taking etretinate due to the teratogenic effects of the drug.

### Drug-specific teaching points

- Take drug with meals. Do not crush capsules.
- This drug has been associated with severe birth defects and miscarriages, it is contraindicated in pregnant women. It is important to use contraceptive measures during treatment and for 1 mo after treatment is discontinued. If you think that you have become pregnant, consult with your physician immediately.
- Do not take vitamin A supplements while you are taking this drug.
- Do not donate blood while on this drug because of its possible effects on the fetus of a blood recipient.
- The following side effects may occur: exacerbation of psoriasis during initial therapy; dizziness, lethargy, headache, visual changes (avoid driving or performing tasks that require alertness); sensitivity to the sun (avoid sunlamps, use sunscreens,

protective clothing); diarrhea, abdominal pain, loss of appetite (take with meals); dry mouth (suck sugarless lozenges); eye irritation and redness, inability to wear contact lenses; dry skin, itching, redness.
- Report headache with nausea and vomiting, yellowing of the skin, eyes; pale stools, visual difficulties.

## factor IX concentrates

*(fac' tor nin)*

AlphaNine SD, Benefix, Hemonyne, Konyne-80, Mononine, Profilnine SD, Proplex T

**Pregnancy Category C**

### Drug classes
Antihemophilic agent

### Therapeutic actions
Human factor IX complex consists of plasma fractions involved in the intrinsic pathway of blood coagulation; causes an increase in blood levels of clotting factors II, VII, IX, and X.

### Indications
- Factor IX deficiency (hemophilia B, Christmas disease) to prevent or control bleeding
- Bleeding episodes in patients with inhibitors to factor VIII
- Bleeding episodes in patients with hemophilia A (Proplex T, Konyne-80 only)
- Prevention or control of bleeding episodes in patients with factor VII deficiency (Proplex T only)

### Contraindications/cautions
- Factor VII deficiencies (except as listed above for Proplex T, Konye-80); liver disease with signs of intravascular coagulation or fibrinolysis

### Dosage
**Available Forms:** Injection—varies with brand, see label

Dosage depends on severity of deficiency and severity of bleeding; follow treatment carefully with factor IX level assays. To calculate dosage, use the following formula: Dose 1 U/kg × body weight (kg) × desired increase (% of normal). Administer qd–bid (once every 2–3 d may suffice to maintain lower effective levels) IV.

**ADULT/PEDIATRIC**
- *Surgery:* Maintain levels > 25% for at least 1 wk. Calculate dose to raise level to 40%–60% of normal.
- *Hemarthroses:* In hemophiliacs with inhibitors to factor VIII, dosage levels approximate 75 U/kg IV. Give a second dose after 12 h if needed.
- *Maintenance dose:* Dose is usually 10–20 U/kg per day IV. Individualize dose based on patient response.
- *Inhibitor patients (hemophilia A patients with inhibitors to factor VIII):* 75 U/kg IV; give a second dose after 12 h if needed.
- *Reversal of coumadin effect:* 15 U/kg IV is suggested.
- *Prophylaxis:* 10–20 U/kg IV once or twice a week may prevent spontaneous bleeding in hemophilia B patients. Individualize dose. Increase dose if patient is exposed to trauma or surgery.

### Pharmacokinetics

| *Route* | *Onset* | *Duration* |
|---|---|---|
| IV | Immediate | 1–2 d |

*Metabolism:* Plasma, $T_{1/2}$: 24–32 h

*Distribution:* Crosses placenta; enters breast milk

### IV facts
**Preparation:** Prepare using diluents and needles supplied with product. Refrigerate.

**Infusion:** Infuse slowly. 100 U/min and 2–3 ml/min have been suggested. Do not exceed 3 ml/min, and stop or slow the infusion at any sign of headache, pulse, or BP changes.

### Adverse effects
- CNS: *Headache,* flushing, chills, tingling, somnolence, lethargy
- GI: *Nausea,* vomiting, hepatitis—risk associated with use of blood products

- Hematologic: *Thrombosis*, DIC, AIDS—risk associated with use of blood products (not as common with SD [solvent deter-gent)]–treated preparations)
- Other: Chills, fever; blood pressure changes, urticaria

## ■ Nursing Considerations

### Assessment

- *History:* Factor VII deficiencies; liver disease with signs of intravascular coagulation or fibrinolysis
- *Physical:* Skin color, lesions; T; orientation, reflexes, affect; P, BP, peripheral perfusion; clotting factors levels, liver function tests

### Implementation

- Administer by IV route only.
- Decrease rate of infusion if headache, flushing, fever, chills, tingling, urticaria occur; in some individuals, the drug will need to be discontinued.
- Monitor patient's clinical response and factors IX, II, VII, X levels regularly, and regulate dosage based on response.
- Monitor patient for any sign of thrombosis; use comfort and preventive measures when possible (exercise, support stockings, ambulation, positioning).

### Drug-specific teaching points

- Dosage varies widely. Safety precautions are taken to ensure that this blood product is pure and the risk of AIDS and hepatitis is minimal.
- Wear or carry a medical ID to alert emergency medical personnel that you require this treatment.
- Report headache, rash, chills, calf pain, swelling, unusual bleeding, or bruising.

## famciclovir sodium

*(fam sye' kloe vir)*

Famvir

**Pregnancy Category C**

### Drug classes

Antiviral

### Therapeutic actions

Antiviral activity; inhibits viral DNA replication in acute herpes zoster.

### Indications

- Management of acute herpes zoster (shingles)
- Suppression of recurrent episodes of genital herpes

### Contraindications/cautions

- Contraindications: hypersensitivity to famciclovir or acyclovir, lactation.
- Use cautiously with cytopenia, history of cytopenic reactions, impaired renal function.

### Dosage

**Available Forms:** Tablets—125, 250, 500 mg

ADULT

- *Herpes zoster:* 500 mg q8h PO for 7 d.
- *Genital herpes:* 125 mg PO bid for 5 d. Suppression of recurrent episodes of genital herpes: 250 mg PO bid.

PEDIATRIC: Safety and efficacy not established.

RENAL IMPAIRMENT

- *Herpes zoster*

| CCr (ml/min) | Dose |
|---|---|
| >60 | 500 mg q8h |
| 40–59 | 500 mg q12h |
| 20–39 | 500 mg qd |
| <20 | 250 mg q48h |

- *Genital herpes*

| CCr (ml/min) | Dose |
|---|---|
| >40 | 125 mg q12h |
| 20–39 | 125 mg q24h |
| <20 | 125 mg q48h |

### Pharmacokinetics

| Route | Onset | Peak |
|---|---|---|
| Oral | Varies | 0.5–1 h |

*Metabolism:* $T_{1/2}$: 2 h
*Distribution* : Crosses placenta; may enter breast milk
*Excretion* : Urine

### Adverse effects

- CNS: Dreams, ataxia, coma, confusion, dizziness, *headache*
- GI: Abnormal liver function tests, nausea, vomiting, anorexia, *diarrhea*, abdominal pain
- CV: Arrhythmia, hypertension, hypotension
- Hematologic: Granulocytopenia, thrombocytopenia, anemia
- Dermatologic: *Rash,* alopecia, pruritus, urticaria
- Other: *Fever*, chills, **cancer, sterility**

### Clinically important drug-drug interactions

• Increased serum concentration of famciclovir if taken with cimetidine • Increased digoxin levels if taken together

## ■ Nursing Considerations

### Assessment

- *History:* Hypersensitivity to famciclovir or acyclovir; cytopenia; impaired renal function; lactation
- *Physical:* Skin color, lesions; orientation; BP, P, auscultation, perfusion, edema; R, adventitious sounds; urinary output; CBC, Hct, BUN, creatinine clearance, liver function tests

### Implementation

- Decrease dosage in patients with impaired renal function.
- Arrange for CBC before and every 2 d during therapy and at least weekly thereafter. Consult with physician to reduce dosage if WBCs or platelets fall.

### Drug-specific teaching points

- Take this drug for 5 or 7 full days as prescribed.
- The following side effects may occur: decreased blood count leading to susceptibility to infection (blood tests may be needed; avoid crowds and exposure to disease), headache (analgesics may be ordered), diarrhea.
- Famciclovir is not a cure for genital herpes; use appropriate precautions to prevent transmission
- Report bruising, bleeding, worsening of condition, fever, infection.

## famotidine

*(fa moe' ti deen)*
Pepcid, Pepcid AC
**Pregnancy Category B**

### Drug classes

Histamine 2 ($H_2$) antagonist

### Therapeutic actions

Competitively blocks the action of histamine at the histamine ($H_2$) receptors of the parietal cells of the stomach; inhibits basal gastric acid secretion and chemically induced gastric acid secretion.

### Indications

- Short-term treatment and maintenance of duodenal ulcer
- Short-term treatment of benign gastric ulcer
- Treatment of pathologic hypersecretory conditions
- Short-term treatment of gastroesophageal reflux disease (GERD), esophagitis due to GERD
- Heartburn, acid indigestion, sour stomach (OTC)

### Contraindications/cautions

- Allergy to famotidine; renal failure; pregnancy; lactation.

### Dosage

**Available Forms:** Tablets—10, 20, 40 mg; powder for oral suspension—40 mg/5 ml; injection—10 mg/ml; injection, premixed—20 mg/50 ml in 0.9% sodium chloride

**ADULT**

- *Active duodenal ulcer:* 40 mg PO or IV at bedtime *or* 20 mg bid PO or IV. Therapy at full dosage should generally be discontinued after 6–8 wk.
- *Maintenance therapy, duodenal ulcer:* 20 mg PO at bedtime.
- *Benign gastric ulcer:* 40 mg PO qd at bedtime.

- *Hypersecretory syndrome:* 20 mg q6h PO initially. Doses up to 160 mg q6h have been administered.
- *GERD:* 20 mg bid PO for up to 6 wk.
- *Esophagitis:* 20–40 mg bid PO for up to 12 wk.
- *Heatburn, acid indigestion:* 10 mg PO for relief; 10 mg PO 1h before eating for prevention. Do not exceed 20 mg/24h.

PEDIATRIC: Safety and efficacy not established.

GERIATRIC OR RENAL INSUFFICIENCY: Reduce dosage to 20 mg PO at bedtime *or* 40 mg PO q36–48h.

### Pharmacokinetics

| *Route* | *Onset* | *Peak* | *Duration* |
|---|---|---|---|
| Oral | Slow | 1–3 h | 6–12 h |
| IV | < 1 h | 1/2–3 h | 8–15 h |

*Metabolism:* Hepatic, $T_{1/2}$: 2 1/2–3 1/2 h
*Distribution:* Crosses placenta; enters breast milk
*Excretion:* Urine

#### IV facts

**Preparation:** For direct injection, dilute 2 ml (solution contains 10 mg/ml) with 0.9% Sodium Chloride Injection, Water for Injection, 5% or 10% Dextrose Injection, Lactated Ringer's Injection, or 5% Sodium Bicarbonate Injection to a total volume of 5–10 ml. For infusion, 2 ml diluted with 100 ml 5% Dextrose Solution or other IVs. Stable for 48 h at room temperature, 14 d if refrigerated.
**Infusion:** Inject directly slowly, over not less than 2 min. Infuse over 15–30 min; continuous infusion: 40 mg/24 hr.

### Adverse effects

- CNS: *Headache,* malaise, *dizziness*, somnolence, insomnia
- GI: *Diarrhea, constipation*, anorexia, abdominal pain
- **Dermatologic**: Skin rash
- **Other**: Muscle cramp, increase in total bilirubin, sexual impotence

## ■ Nursing Considerations

### Assessment

- *History:* Allergy to famotidine; renal failure; lactation
- *Physical:* Skin lesions; liver evaluation, abdominal exam, normal output; renal function tests, serum bilirubin

### Implementation

- Administer drug at bedtime.
- Decrease doses with renal failure.
- Arrange for administration of concurrent antacid therapy to relieve pain.

### Drug-specific teaching points

- Take this drug at bedtime (or in the morning and at bedtime). Therapy may continue for 4–6 wk or longer.
- Take antacid exactly as prescribed, being careful of the times of administration.
- Have regular medical follow-up while on this drug to evaluate your response.
- Take OTC drug 1h before eating to prevent indigestion. Do not take more than 2/day.
- The following side effects may occur: constipation or diarrhea; loss of libido or impotence (reversible); headache (adjust lights, temperature, noise levels).
- Report sore throat, fever, unusual bruising or bleeding, severe headache, muscle or joint pain.

## fat emulsion, intravenous

*(fat ee **mul'** shun)*

Intralipid 10%, 20%; Liposyn II 10%, 20%; Liposyn III 10%, 20%

**Pregnancy Category C**

### Drug classes

Caloric agent

### Therapeutic actions

A preparation from soybean or safflower oil that provides neutral triglycerides, mostly unsaturated fatty acids; these are used as a source of energy, causing an increase in heat production, decrease in respiratory quotient, and increase in oxygen consumption.

## Indications

- Source of calories and essential fatty acids for patients requiring parental nutrition for extended periods
- Essential fatty acid deficiency

## Contraindications/cautions

- Contraindications: disturbance of normal fat metabolism (hyperlipemia, lipoid nephrosis, acute pancreatitis), allergy to eggs.
- Use cautiously with severe liver damage, pulmonary disease, anemia, blood coagulation disorders, pregnancy, jaundiced or premature infants.

## Dosage

**Available Forms:** Injection—10% (50, 100, 200, 250, 300 ml), 20% (50, 100, 200, 250, 500 ml)

***Adult parenteral nutrition:*** Should not comprise more than 60% of total calorie intake. *10%*: infuse IV at 1 ml/min for the first 15–30 min; may be increased to 2 ml/min. Infuse only 500 ml the first day, and increase the following day. Do not exceed 2.5 g/kg per day. *20%*: infuse at 0.5 ml/min for the first 15–30 min; infuse only 250 ml Liposyn II or 500 ml Intralipid the first day, and increase the following day. Do not exceed 3 g/kg per day.

***Fatty acid deficiency:*** Supply 8%–10% of the caloric intake by IV fat emulsion.

***Pediatric parenteral nutrition:*** Should not comprise more than 60% of total calorie intake. *10%*: initial IV infusion rate is 0.1 ml/min for the first 10–15 min. *20%*: initial infusion rate is 0.05 ml/min for the first 10–15 min. If no untoward reactions occur, increase rate to 1 g/kg in 4 h. Do not exceed 3 g/kg per day.

## Pharmacokinetics

| *Route* | *Onset* |
|---|---|
| IV | Rapid |

*Metabolism:* Hepatic and tissue, $T_{1/2}$: varies

*Distribution:* Crosses placenta; may enter breast milk

## IV facts

**Preparation:** Supplied in single-dose containers; do not store partially used bottles; do not resterilize for later use; do not use with filters; do not use any bottle in which there appears to be separation from the emulsion.

**Infusion:** Infusion rate is 1 ml/min for 10% solution, monitor for 15–30 min; if no adverse reaction occurs, may be increased to 2 ml/min; 0.5 ml/min for 20% solution, may be increased if no adverse reactions. May be infused simultaneously with Amino Acid-Dextrose mixtures by means of Y-connector located near the infusion site using separate flow rate; keep the Lipid Solution higher than the Amino Acid-Dextrose line.

**Incompatibilities:** Do not mix with amikacin, tetracycline. Monitor electrolyte and acid content; fat emulsion seperates in acid solution.

## Adverse effects

- CNS: *Headache,* flushing, fever, sweating, sleepiness, pressure over the eyes, dizziness
- GI: *Nausea,* vomiting
- Hematologic: *Thrombophlebitis,* ***sepsis****, hyperlipemia, hypercoagulability, thrombocytopenia, leukopenia, elevated liver enzymes*
- Other: Irritation at infusion site, brown pigmentation in RES (IV fat pigment), cyanosis

## ■ Nursing Considerations

### Assessment

- *History:* Disturbance of normal fat metabolism, allergy to eggs, severe liver damage, pulmonary disease, anemia, blood coagulation disorders, pregnancy, jaundiced or premature infants
- *Physical:* Skin color, lesions; T; orientation; P, BP, peripheral perfusion; CBC, plasma lipid profile, clotting factors levels, liver function tests

### Implementation

- Administer by IV route only.
- Inspect admixture for "breaking or oiling out" of the emulsion—seen as yellow streaking or accumulation of yellow droplets—or for the formation of any particulates; discard any admixture if these occur.
- Monitor patient carefully for fluid or fat overloading during infusion: diluted serum electrolytes, overhydration, pulmonary edema, elevated JVP, metabolic acidosis, impaired pulmonary diffusion capacity. Discontinue the infusion; reevaluate patient before restarting infusion at a lower rate.
- Monitor patient's clinical response, serum lipid profile, weight gain, improved nitrogen balance.
- Monitor patient for thrombosis or sepsis; use comfort and preventive measures (exercise, support stockings, ambulation, positioning).

### Drug-specific teaching points

- Report pain at infusion site, difficulty breathing, chest pain, calf pain, excessive sweating.

## felodipine

*(fell oh' di peen)*

Plendil

**Pregnancy Category C**

### Drug classes

Calcium channel blocker
Antihypertensive

### Therapeutic actions

Inhibits the movement of calcium ions across the membranes of cardiac and arterial muscle cells; inhibition of transmembrane calcium flow results in the depression of impulse formation in pacemaker cells, slowing of velocity of conduction of cardiac impulse, depression of myocardial contractility, dilation of coronary arteries, arterioles and peripheral arterioles; these effects lead to decreased cardiac work, energy consumption, and decreased BP.

### Indications

- Essential hypertension, alone or in combination with other antihypertensives

### Contraindications/cautions

- Allergy to felodipine or other calcium channel-blockers, impaired hepatic or renal function, sick sinus syndrome, heart block (second or third degree), lactation.

### Dosage

**Available Forms:** ER tablets—2.5, 5, 10 mg

*ADULT:* Initially 5 mg PO qd; dosage may be gradually increased over 10–14 d to an average 10–15 mg PO qd. Maximum effective dose is 20 mg qd.

*PEDIATRIC:* Safety and efficacy not established.

*GERIATRIC OR HEPATIC IMPAIRMENT:* Carefully monitor; do not exceed 10 mg qd PO.

### Pharmacokinetics

| *Route* | *Onset* | *Peak* |
|---|---|---|
| Oral | 120–130 min | 2 1/2–5 h |

*Metabolism:* Hepatic metabolism, $T_{1/2}$: 11–16 h

*Distribution:* Crosses placenta; may pass into breast milk

*Excretion:* Urine

### Adverse effects

- CNS: *Dizziness, lightheadedness, headache*, asthenia, *fatigue, lethargy*
- GI: *Nausea*, abdominal discomfort
- CV: *Peripheral edema*, arrhythmias
- Dermatologic: *Flushing*, rash

### Clinically important drug-drug interactions

• Decreased serum levels with barbiturates, hydantoins • Increased serum levels and toxicity with erythromycin, cimetidine, ranitidine

## ■ Nursing Considerations

### Assessment

- *History:* Allergy to felodipine, impaired hepatic or renal function, sick sinus syndrome, heart block, lactation

- *Physical:* Skin lesions, color, edema; P, BP, baseline ECG, peripheral perfusion, auscultation, R, adventitious sounds; liver evaluation, GI normal output; liver and renal function tests, urinalysis

### Implementation
- Have patient swallow tablet whole; do not chew or crush.
- Monitor patient carefully (BP, cardiac rhythm and output) while drug is being titrated to therapeutic dose.
- Monitor cardiac rhythm regularly during stabilization of dosage and periodically during long-term therapy.
- Administer drug without regard to meals.

### Drug-specific teaching points
- Take this drug with meals if upset stomach occurs.
- The following side effects may occur: nausea, vomiting (small, frequent meals may help); headache (adjust lighting, noise, and temperature; medication may be ordered if severe).
- Report irregular heart beat, shortness of breath, swelling of the hands or feet, pronounced dizziness, constipation.

## fenoprofen

*(fen oh **proe'** fen)*
Nalfon
**Pregnancy Category B**

### Drug classes
Nonsteroidal anti-inflammatory drug (NSAID)
Analgesic (non-narcotic)
Propionic acid derivative

### Therapeutic actions
Analgesic, anti-inflammatory, and antipyretic activities largely related to inhibition of prostaglandin synthesis; exact mechanisms of action are not known.

### Indications
- Acute and long-term treatment of rheumatoid arthritis and osteoarthritis
- Mild to moderate pain

### Contraindications/cautions
- Contraindications: significant renal impairment, pregnancy, lactation.
- Use cautiously with impaired hearing, allergies, hepatic, CV, and GI conditions.

### Dosage
**Available Forms:** Capsules—200, 300 mg; tablets—600 mg
Do not exceed 3,200 mg/d.

ADULT
- *Rheumatoid arthritis/osteoarthritis:* 300–600 mg PO tid or qid. 2–3 wk may be required to see improvement.
- *Mild to moderate pain:* 200 mg q4–6h PO, as needed.

PEDIATRIC: Safety and efficacy have not been established.

### Pharmacokinetics

| Route | Onset | Peak |
|---|---|---|
| Oral | 30–60 min | 1–2 h |

*Metabolism:* Hepatic, $T_{1/2}$: 2–3 h
*Distribution:* Crosses placenta; enters breast milk
*Excretion:* Urine

### Adverse effects
*NSAIDs*
- CNS: *Headache, dizziness, somnolence, insomnia*, fatigue, tiredness, dizziness, tinnitus, ophthalmologic effects
- GI: *Nausea, dyspepsia, GI pain,* diarrhea, vomiting, *constipation*, flatulence
- Respiratory: Dyspnea, hemoptysis, pharyngitis, bronchospasm, rhinitis
- Hematologic: Bleeding, platelet inhibition with higher doses, neutropenia, eosinophilia, leukopenia, pancytopenia, thrombocytopenia, agranulocytosis, granulocytopenia, aplastic anemia, decreased hemoglobin or hematocrit, bone marrow depression, menorrhagia
- GU: Dysuria, **renal impairment** (fenoprofen is one of the most nephrotoxic NSAIDs)
- Dermatologic: *Rash*, pruritus, sweating, dry mucous membranes, stomatitis
- Other: Peripheral edema, **anaphylactoid reactions to fatal anaphylactic shock**

## Nursing Considerations

### Assessment

- *History:* Renal impairment, impaired hearing, allergies, hepatic, cardiovascular, and GI conditions, lactation
- *Physical:* Skin color and lesions; orientation, reflexes, ophthalmologic and audiometric evaluation, peripheral sensation; P, edema; R, adventitious sounds; liver evaluation; CBC, clotting times, renal and liver function tests; serum electrolytes, stool guaiac

### Implementation

- Administer drug with food or after meals if GI upset occurs.
- Arrange for periodic ophthalmologic examination during long-term therapy.
- Institute emergency procedures if overdose occurs—gastric lavage, induction of emesis, supportive therapy.

### Drug-specific teaching points

- Take drug with food or meals if GI upset occurs.
- Take only the prescribed dosage.
- Dizziness, drowsiness can occur (avoid driving or using dangerous machinery).
- Report sore throat, fever, rash, itching, weight gain, swelling in ankles or fingers; changes in vision, black, tarry stools.

## fentanyl

*(fen' ta nil)*

Duragesic, Fentanyl Oralet, Fentanyl Transdermal, Fentanyl Transmucosal, Sublimaze

**Pregnancy Category B**
**C-II controlled substance**

### Drug classes

Narcotic agonist analgesic

### Therapeutic actions

Acts at specific opioid receptors, causing analgesia, respiratory depression, physical depression, euphoria.

### Indications

- Analgesic action of short duration during anesthesia and in the immediate postoperative period
- Analgesic supplement in general or regional anesthesia
- Administration with a neuroleptic as an anesthetic premedication, for induction of anesthesia, and as an adjunct in maintenance of general and regional anesthesia
- For use as an anesthetic agent with oxygen in selected high-risk patients
- Transdermal system: management of chronic pain in patients requiring opioid analgesia

### Contraindications/cautions

- Contraindications: hypersensitivity to narcotics, diarrhea caused by poisoning, acute bronchial asthma, upper airway obstruction, pregnancy.
- Use cautiously with bradycardia, history of seizures, lactation.

### Dosage

**Available Forms:** Lozenges—100, 200, 300, 400 μg; transdermal—25, 50, 75, 100 μg/h; injection—0.05 mg/ml

Individualize dosage; monitor vital signs.

**ADULT**

- *Premedication:* 0.05–0.1 mg IM 30–60 min prior to surgery.
- *Adjunct to general anesthesia:* Total dosage is 0.002 mg/kg. Maintenance dose: 0.025–0.1 mg IV or IM when changes in vital signs indicate surgical stress or lightening of analgesia.
- *With oxygen for anesthesia:* Total high dose is 0.05–0.1 mg/kg IV; up to 0.12 mg/kg may be necessary.
- *Adjunct to regional anesthesia:* 0.05–0.1 mg IM or slowly IV over 1–2 min.
- *Postoperatively:* 0.05–0.1 mg IM for the control of pain, tachypnea or emergence delirium; repeat in 1–2 h if needed.
- *Transdermal:* Apply to nonirritated and nonirradiated skin on a flat surface of the upper torso; may require replacement in 72 h if pain has not subsided.
- *Lozenges:* Place in mouth and suck, 20–40 min before desired effect.

**PEDIATRIC (2–12 Y):** 2–3 μg/kg IV as vital signs indicate. Transdermal: do not exceed 15 μg/kg.

**Pharmacokinetics**

| *Route* | *Onset* | *Duration* |
|---|---|---|
| IM | 7–8 min | 1–2 h |
| Transdermal | Gradual | 72 h |

*Metabolism:* Plasma, $T_{1/2}$: 1 1/2–6 h
*Distribution:* Crosses placenta; enters breast milk

### IV facts

**Preparation:** May be used undiluted or diluted with 250 ml of $D_5W$. Protect vials from light.

**Infusion:** Administer slowly by direct injection, each ml over at least 1 min, or into running IV tubing.

### Adverse effects

- CNS: *Sedation, clamminess, sweating, headache, vertigo, floating feeling, dizziness, lethargy, confusion, lightheadedness,* nervousness, unusual dreams, agitation, euphoria, hallucinations, delirium, insomnia, anxiety, fear, disorientation, impaired mental and physical performance, coma, mood changes, weakness, headache, tremor, convulsions
- GI: *Nausea, vomiting,* dry mouth, anorexia, constipation, biliary tract spasm
- CV: Palpitation, increase or decrease in BP, circulatory depression, **cardiac arrest, shock**, tachycardia, bradycardia, arrhythmia, palpitations
- Respiratory: Slow, shallow respiration, apnea, suppression of cough reflex, laryngospasm, bronchospasm
- GU: Ureteral spasm, spasm of vesical sphincters, urinary retention or hesitancy, oliguria, antidiuretic effect, reduced libido or potency
- EENT: Diplopia, blurred vision
- Dermatologic: Rash, hives, pruritus, flushing, warmth, sensitivity to cold
- Local: Phlebitis following IV injection, pain at injection site; tissue irritation and induration (SC injection)
- Other: Physical tolerance and dependence, psychological dependence; local skin irritation with transdermal system

### Clinically important drug-drug interactions

- Potentiation of effects when given with barbiturate anesthetics; decrease dose of fentanyl when coadministering

### Drug-lab test interferences

- Elevated biliary tract pressure may cause increases in plasma amylase, lipase; determinations of these levels may be unreliable for 24 h after administration of narcotics

## ■ Nursing Considerations

### Assessment

- *History:* Hypersensitivity to fentanyl or narcotics, physical dependence on a narcotic analgesic, pregnancy, labor, lactation, COPD, respiratory depression, anoxia, increased intracranial pressure, acute MI, ventricular failure, coronary insufficiency, hypertension, biliary tract surgery, renal or hepatic dysfunction
- *Physical:* Orientation, reflexes, bilateral grip strength, affect; pupil size, vision; P, auscultation, BP; R, adventitious sounds; bowel sounds, normal output; liver and kidney function tests

### Implementation

- Administer to women who are nursing a baby 4–6 h before the next scheduled feeding to minimize the amount in milk.
- Provide narcotic antagonist, facilities for assisted or controlled respiration on standby during parenteral administration.
- Prepare site by clipping (not shaving) hair at site; do not use soap, oils, lotions, alcohol; allow skin to dry completely before application. Apply immediately after removal from the sealed package; firmly press the transdermal system in place with the palm of the hand for 10–20 sec, making sure the contact is complete. Must be worn continually for 72 h.

### Drug-specific teaching points

- The following side effects may occur: dizziness, sedation, drowsiness, impaired visual acuity (ask for assistance if you need to move); nausea, loss of appetite (lie

quietly, eat frequent small meals); constipation (a laxative may help).
- Report severe nausea, vomiting, palpitations, shortness of breath or difficulty breathing.

## Ferrous salts

### ferrous fumarate

*(fair' us)*

Feostat, Ferrous fumarate, Fersamal (CAN), Fumerin, Fumasorb, Hemocyte, Ircon, Novofumar (CAN), Palafer (CAN)

### ferrous gluconate

Fergon, Ferralet, Fertinic (CAN), Novoferrogluc (CAN), Simron

### ferrous sulfate

Feosol, Fer-In-Sol, Fer-Iron, Fero-Gradumet Filmtabs, Ferospace, Fesofor (CAN), Mol-Iron, Novoferrosulfa (CAN)

### ferrous sulfate exsiccated

Feosol, Fer-In-Sol, Ferralyn Lanacaps, Slow FE

**Pregnancy Category A**

### Drug classes

Iron preparation

### Therapeutic actions

Elevates the serum iron concentration and is then converted to hemoglobin or trapped in the reticuloendothelial cells for storage and eventual conversion to a usable form of iron.

### Indications

- Prevention and treatment of iron deficiency anemias
- Unlabeled use: supplemental use during epoetin therapy to ensure proper hematologic response to epoetin

### Contraindications/cautions

- Allergy to any ingredient; tartrazine allergy (tartrazine is contained in timed-release capsules marketed as Mol-Iron); sulfite allergy; hemochromatosis, hemosiderosis, hemolytic anemias; normal iron balance; peptic ulcer, regional enteritis, ulcerative colitis

### Dosage

**Available Forms:** Tablets—sulfate, 195, 300, 324 mg; sulfate exsiccated, 200 mg; gluconate, 300, 320, 325 mg; fumarate, 63, 195, 200, 324, 325, 350 mg; capsules—sulfate, 250 mg; gluconate, 86 mg; TR capsules—sulfate exsiccated, 150, 250 mg; fumarate, 325 mg; TR tablets—sulfate, 525 mg; sulfate exsiccated, 160 mg; gluconate, 320 mg; syrup—sulfate, 90 mg; elixir—sulfate, 220 mg; gluconate, 300 mg; drops—sulfate, 75 mg/0.5 ml, 125 mg/ml; fumarate, 45 mg/0.5 ml

**ADULT**

- *Daily requirements:* Males, 10 mg/d PO; females, 18 mg/d PO; pregnancy and lactation, 30–60 mg/d PO.
- *Replacement in deficiency states:* 90–300 mg/d (6 mg/kg per day) PO for approximately 6–10 mo may be required.

**PEDIATRIC:** Daily requirement: 10–15 mg/d PO.

### Pharmacokinetics

| *Route* | *Onset* | *Peak* | *Duration* |
|---|---|---|---|
| Oral | 4 d | 7–10 d | 2–4 mo |

*Metabolism:* Recycled for use, $T_{1/2}$: not known

*Distribution:* Crosses placenta; enters breast milk

### Adverse effects

- CNS: CNS toxicity, acidosis, **coma and death**—overdose
- GI: *GI upset, anorexia, nausea, vomiting, constipation*, diarrhea, dark stools, temporary staining of the teeth (liquid preparations)

### Clinically important drug-drug interactions

• Decreased anti-infective response to ciprofloxacin, enoxacin, norfloxacin, ofloxacin • Decreased absorption with antacids, cimetidine • Decreased effects of levodopa if taken with iron • Increased serum iron levels with chloramphenicol

### Clinically important drug-food interactions

• Decreased absorption with antacids, eggs or milk, coffee and tea; to avoid concurrent administration of any of these

## ■ Nursing Considerations

### Assessment

- *History:* Allergy to any ingredient, sulfite; hemochromatosis, hemosiderosis, hemolytic anemias; normal iron balance; peptic ulcer, regional enteritis, ulcerative colitis
- *Physical:* Skin lesions, color; gums, teeth (color); bowel sounds; CBC, Hgb, Hct, serum ferritin assays

### Implementation

- Confirm that patient does have iron deficiency anemia before treatment.
- Give drug with meals (avoiding milk, eggs, coffee, and tea) if GI discomfort is severe, and slowly increase to build up tolerance.
- Administer liquid preparations in water or juice to mask the taste and prevent staining of teeth; have the patient drink solution with a straw.
- Warn patient that stool may be dark or green.
- Arrange for periodic monitoring of hematocrit and hemoglobin levels.

### Drug-specific teaching points

- Take drug on an empty stomach with water. Take after meals if GI upset is severe (avoid milk, eggs, coffee, and tea).
- Take liquid preparations diluted in water or juice and sipped through a straw to prevent staining of the teeth.
- Treatment may not be necessary if cause of anemia can be corrected. Treatment may be needed for several months to reverse the anemia.
- Have periodic blood tests during therapy to determine the appropriate dosage.
- Do not take this preparation with antacids or tetracyclines. If these drugs are needed, they will be prescribed.
- The following side effects may occur: GI upset, nausea, vomiting (take drug with meals); diarrhea or constipation; dark or green stools.
- Report severe GI upset, lethargy, rapid respirations, constipation.



# fexofenadine hydrochloride

*(fecks oh **fen'** a deen)*

Allegra

**Pregnancy Category C**

### Drug classes

Antihistamine (non-sedating type)

### Therapeutic actions

Competitively blocks the effects of histamine at peripheral $H_1$ receptor sites; has no anticholinergic (atropine-like) or sedating effects.

### Indications

- Symptomatic relief of symptoms associated with seasonal allergic rhinitis in adults and children >12 y

### Contraindications/cautions

- Contraindications: allergy to any antihistamines, pregnancy, lactation
- Use cautiously with hepatic or renal impairment, geriatric patients

### Dosage

**Available Forms:** Capsules—60 mg

***Adult and Children > 12 y:*** 60 mg PO bid.

***Pediatric:*** Not recommended in children <12 y.

***Geriatric or Renal Impaired:*** 60 mg PO qd.

### Pharmacokinetics

| *Route* | *Onset* | *Peak* |
|---|---|---|
| Oral | Rapid | 2.6 h |

*Metabolism:* Hepatic; $T_{1/2}$: 14.4 h
*Distribution:* Crosses placenta; may enter breast milk
*Excretion:* Feces and urine

### Adverse effects
- CNS: Fatigue, drowsiness
- GI: Nausea, dyspepsia
- Other: Dysmenorrhea, flulike illness

### Clinically important drug-drug interactions
- Increased levels and possible toxicity with ketoconazole, erythromycin; fexofenadine dose may need to be decreased

## ■ Nursing Considerations

### Assessment
- ***History:*** Allergy to any antihistamines, renal or hepatic impairment, pregnancy, lactation
- ***Physical:*** Mucous membranes, oropharynx, R, adventitious sounds; orientation, affect; renal and liver function tests

### Implementation
- Arrange for use of humidifier if thickening of secretions, nasal dryness become bothersome; encourage adequate intake of fluids.
- Provide supportive care if flulike symptoms occur.

### Drug-specific teaching points
- Avoid excessive dosage; take only the dosage prescribed.
- The following side effects may occur: dizziness, sedation, drowsiness (use caution if driving or performing tasks that require alertness); thickening of bronchial secretions, dryness of nasal mucosa (use of a humidifier may help); menstrual irregularities; flulike symptoms (medication may be helpful).
- Report difficulty breathing, severe nausea, fever.

## fibrinolysin and desoxyribonuclease

*(fye brin oh **lye'** sin and dez ox ee rye boe **nuke'** lee ase)*
Elase

### Drug classes
Enzyme

### Therapeutic actions
Fibrinolysin attacks fibrin of blood clots and exudates; desoxyribonuclease attacks DNA found in purulent exudates.

### Indications
- Debriding agent in general surgical wounds; ulcerative lesions; second- and third-degree burns; circumcision; episiotomy
- Cervicitis and vaginitis
- Irrigation agent for infected wounds, superficial hematomas, otorhinolaryngologic wounds

### Contraindications/cautions
- Allergy to any component of the preparation, bovine products.

### Dosage
**Available Forms:** Powder—254 fibrinolysin with 15,000 U desoxyribonuclease/vial; ointment—1 U fibrinolysin and 666.6 U desoxyribonuclease/g
***Topical:*** Apply a thin layer of ointment, and cover with petrolatum gauze or other nonadhering agent 2–3 ×/d or mix solution and saturate strips of gauze. Pack ulcerated area with gauze; allow to dry, 6–8 h. Remove dry gauze; repeat 3–4 ×/d.
***Intravaginal:*** Apply 5 g of ointment deep into vagina hs for five applications. In severe cases, insert 10 ml of solution intravaginally, wait 1–2 min, then insert cotton tampon; remove the next day.
*Abscesses:* Irrigate with solution; drain and replace solution every 6–10 h.

### Pharmacokinetics

| *Route* | *Onset* | *Duration* |
|---|---|---|
| Topical | Slow | 24 h |

Negligible systemic absorption.

### Adverse effects
- **Local:** Hyperemia with high concentrations

## ■ Nursing Considerations

### Assessment

- *History:* Allergy to bovine products, drug or components of preparation
- *Physical:* Affected site—lesions, color, edema

### Implementation

- Clean wound with water, peroxide, or normal saline, and dry area gently. Surgically remove dense, dry eschar before applying ointment. Apply a thin layer of ointment, and cover with petrolatum gauze or other nonadhering dressing. Change dressing at least once a day, preferably 2–3 ×. Flush away the necrotic debris and fibrinous exudates with saline, peroxide, or warm water.
- Prepare solution by reconstituting contents of each vial with 10 ml isotonic sodium chloride solution. Higher or lower concentrations can be made by varying diluent. Solutions should be prepared fresh before each use; refrigerate for up to 24 h; discard after that time.
- Prepare wet to dry dressing by mixing 1 vial of powder with 10–50 ml saline, and saturate strips of fine-mesh gauze or unfolded sterile gauze sponge with solution. Pack area with gauze, and allow to dry. Remove dried gauze; this débrides the area. Repeat 3–4 ×/d. After 2–4 d, the area will be clean and will begin to fill in with granulation tissue.
- Apply vaginally very high in the vagina, preferably hs when patient will remain supine.
- Irrigate abscesses as above. Traces of blood in discharge with irrigation usually indicates active filling of the cavity.
- Maintain epinephrine 1:1,000 on standby in case of severe allergic reaction.

### Drug-specific teaching points

Incorporate teaching about this drug into the explanation of wound care while changing dressing, irrigating.

- Insert high into vagina just before bedtime. You may wish to wear a sanitary pad to protect clothing while using this drug.
- Be aware that some discomfort may occur at site of infection.
- Report difficulty breathing, fast heart rate, pain at site of infection.

## filgrastim

*(fill **grass'** stim)*

granulocyte colony-stimulating factor, G-CSF

Neupogen

**Pregnancy Category C**

### Drug classes

Colony stimulating factor

### Therapeutic actions

Human granulocyte colony-stimulating factor produced by recombinant DNA technology; increases the production of neutrophils within the bone marrow with little effect on the production of other hematopoietic cells.

### Indications

- To decrease the incidence of infection in patients with nonmyeloid malignancies receiving myelosuppressive anticancer drugs associated with a significant incidence of severe neutropenia with fever
- To reduce the duration of neutropenia following bone marrow transplant
- Treatment of severe chronic neutropenia
- Mobilization of hematopoietic progenitor cells into the blood for leukapheresis collection
- Orphan drug uses: treatment of myelodysplastic syndrome, aplastic anemia

### Contraindications/cautions

- Contraindications: hypersensitivity to *Escherichia coli* products, pregnancy.
- Use cautiously with lactation.

### Dosage

**Available Forms:** Injection—300 μg/ml

**ADULT:** Starting dose is 5 μg/kg per day SC or IV as a single daily injection. May be increased in increments of 5 μg/kg for each chemotherapy cycle. 4–8 μg/kg per day is usually effective.

- *Bone marrow transplant:* 10 $\mu$g/kg/day IV or continuous SC infusion
- *Severe chronic neutropenia:* 6 $\mu$g/kg SC bid.
- *Mobilization for harvesting:* 10 mcg/kg/d SC at least 4 d before first leukapheresis; continue to last leukapheresis.

*PEDIATRIC:* Safety and efficacy not established.

### Pharmacokinetics

| *Route* | *Peak* | *Duration* |
|---|---|---|
| SC | 8 h | 4 d |
| IV | 2 h | 4 d |

*Metabolism:* Unknown; $T_{1/2}$: 210–231 min
*Distribution:* Crosses placenta; may enter breast milk

### IV facts

**Preparation:** No special preparation required. Refrigerate; avoid shaking. Prior to injection, allow to warm to room temperature. Discard vial after one use, and do not reenter vial; discard any vial that has been at room temperature > 6 h.

**Infusion:** Inject directly IV slowly over 15–30 min, or inject slowly into tubing of running IV over 4–24 h.

**Incompatibilities:** Do not mix in solutions other than $D_5W$. Incompatible with numerous drugs in solution; check manufacturer's details before any combination.

### Adverse effects

- CNS: Headache, fever, generalized weakness, fatigue
- GI: *Nausea, vomiting*, stomatitis, anorexia, *diarrhea*, constipation
- Dermatologic: *Alopecia*, rash, mucositis
- Other: *Bone pain*, generalized pain, sore throat, cough

## ■ Nursing Considerations

### Assessment

- *History:* Hypersensitivity to *E. coli* products, pregnancy, lactation.
- *Physical:* Skin color, lesions, hair; T; abdominal exam, status of mucous membranes; CBC, platelets

### Implementation

- Obtain CBC and platelet count prior to and twice weekly during therapy; doses may be increased after chemotherapy cycles according to the duration and severity of bone marrow suppression.
- Do not give within 24 h before and after chemotherapy.
- Give daily for up to 2 wk until the neutrophil count is 10,000/mm$^3$; discontinue therapy if this number is exceeded.
- Store in refrigerator; allow to warm to room temperature before use; if vial is at room temperature for > 6 h, discard. Use each vial for one dose; do not reenter the vial. Discard any unused drug.
- Do not shake vial before use. If SC dose exceeds 1 ml, consider using two sites.

### Drug-specific teaching points

- Store drug in refrigerator; do not shake vial. Each vial can be used only once; do not reuse syringes or needles (proper container for disposal will be provided). Another person should be instructed in the proper administration technique. Use sterile technique.
- Avoid exposure to infection while you are receiving this drug (eg, crowds).
- The following side effects may occur: bone pain (analgesia may be ordered), nausea and vomiting (eat small, frequent meals), loss of hair (it is very important to cover head in extreme temperatures).
- Keep appointments for frequent blood tests to evaluate effects of drug on your blood count.
- Report fever, chills, severe bone pain, sore throat, weakness, pain or swelling at injection site.

## finasteride

*(fin **as'** teh ride)*

Proscar, Propecia

**Pregnancy Category X**

### Drug classes

Androgen hormone inhibitor

### Therapeutic actions
Inhibits the intracellular enzyme that coverts testosterone into a potent androgen (DHT); does not affect androgen receptors in the body; the prostate gland depends on DHT for its development and maintenance.

### Indications
- Treatment of symptomatic benign prostatic hyperplasia (BPH); most effective with long-term use
- Prevention of male pattern baldness in patients with family history or early signs of loss
- Unlabeled uses: adjuvant monotherapy following radical prostatectomy; prevention of the progression of first-stage prostate cancer; treatment of acne, hirsutism

### Contraindications/cautions
- Contraindications: allergy to finasteride or any component of the product, pregnancy, lactation.
- Use cautiously with hepatic impairment.

### Dosage
**Available Forms:** Tablets—1, 5 mg

ADULT
- *BPH:* 5 mg qd PO with or without meals; may take 6–12 mo for response.
- *Male pattern baldness:* 1 mg/d PO

PEDIATRIC: Safety and efficacy not established.

GERIATRIC OR RENAL INSUFFICIENCY: No dosage adjustment is needed.

### Pharmacokinetics

| Route | Onset | Peak | Duration |
|---|---|---|---|
| Oral | Rapid | 8 h | 24 h |

*Metabolism:* Hepatic, $T_{1/2}$: 6 h
*Distribution:* Crosses placenta; may enter breast milk (not used in women)
*Excretion:* Feces and urine

### Adverse effects
- GI: Abdominal upset
- GU: Impotence, decreased libido, decreased volume of ejaculation

### Clinically important drug-drug interactions
- Possible decreased levels of theophylline

### Drug-lab test interferences
- Decreased PSA levels when measured; false decrease does not mean patient is free of risk of prostate cancer

## ■ Nursing Considerations

### Assessment
- ***History:*** Allergy to finasteride or any component, hepatic impairment
- ***Physical:*** Liver evaluation, abdominal exam; renal function tests, normal urine output, prostate exam

### Implementation
- Confirm that problem is BPH, and other disorders (prostate cancer, infection, strictures, hypotonic bladder) have been ruled out.
- Administer without regard to meals; protect container from light.
- Arrange for regular follow-up, including prostate exam, PSA levels, and evaluation of urine flow.
- Monitor urine flow and output; increase in urine flow may not occur in all situations.
- Do not allow pregnant women to handle finasteride tablets or crushed tablets, because of risk of inadvertent absorption, adversely affecting the fetus.
- Caution patients that if their sexual partner is or may become pregnant, she should be protected from exposure to his semen, which contains drug and adversely affects the fetus. The patient should use a condom or discontinue therapy.
- Alert patient that libido may be decreased as well as the volume of ejaculate; usually reversible when the drug is stopped.

### Drug-specific teaching points
- Take this drug once a day without regard to meals; protect from light.
- Have regular medical follow-up to evaluate your response.
- The following side effects may occur: loss of libido, impotence, decreased amount of ejaculate (usually reversible when the drug is stopped).

f

- This drug has serious adverse effects on unborn babies. Do not allow a pregnant woman to handle the drug; if your sexual partner is or may become pregnant, protect her from exposure to semen by using a condom or discontinuing drug if this is not acceptable.
- Report inability to void, groin pain, sore throat, fever, weakness

## flavoxate hydrochloride

*(fla vox' ate)*
Urispas
**Pregnancy Category C**

### Drug classes
Urinary antispasmodic
Parasympathetic blocking agent

### Therapeutic actions
Counteracts smooth muscle spasm of the urinary tract by relaxing the detrusor and other muscles through action at the parasympathetic receptors; has local anesthetic and analgesic properties.

### Indications
- Symptomatic relief of dysuria, urgency, nocturia, suprapubic pain, frequency and incontinence due to cystitis, prostatitis, urethritis, urethrocystitis/urethrotrigonitis

### Contraindications/cautions
- Contraindications: allergy to flavoxate, pyloric or duodenal obstruction, obstructive intestinal lesions or ileus, achalasia, GI hemorrhage, obstructive uropathies of the lower urinary tract.
- Use cautiously with glaucoma.

### Dosage
**Available Forms:** Tablets—100 mg

*ADULT AND PEDIATRIC > 12 Y:* 100–200 mg PO tid or qid. Reduce dose when symptoms improve. Use of up to 1,200 mg/d in severe urinary urgency following pelvic radiotherapy.

*PEDIATRIC (< 12 Y):* Safety and efficacy not established.

### Pharmacokinetics

| Route | Onset | Duration |
|---|---|---|
| Oral | Slow | 6 h |

*Metabolism:* $T_{1/2}$: 2–3 h
*Distribution:* May cross placenta
*Excretion:* Urine

### Adverse effects
- GI: *Nausea, vomiting, dry mouth*
- CNS: *Nervousness, vertigo, headache, drowsiness*, mental confusion, hyperpyrexia, *blurred vision*, increased ocular tension, disturbance in accommodation
- **Dermatologic**: Urticaria, dermatoses
- GU: Dysuria
- CV: Tachycardia, palpitations
- **Hematologic**: Eosinophilia, leukopenia

## ■ Nursing Considerations

### Assessment
- *History:* Allergy to flavoxate, pyloric or duodenal obstruction, obstructive intestinal lesions or ileus, achalasia, GI hemorrhage, obstructive uropathies of the lower urinary tract, glaucoma
- *Physical:* Skin color, lesions; T; orientation, affect, reflexes, ophthalmic exam, ocular pressure measurement; P; bowel sounds, oral mucous membranes; CBC, stool guaiac

### Implementation
- Arrange for definitive treatment of urinary tract infections causing the symptoms being managed by flavoxate.
- Arrange for ophthalmic exam before and during therapy.

### Drug-specific teaching points
- Take drug three to four times a day.
- This drug is meant to relieve the symptoms you are experiencing; other medications will be used to treat the cause.
- The following side effects may occur: dry mouth, GI upset (suck on sugarless lozenges and use frequent mouth care); drowsiness, blurred vision (avoid driving or performing tasks requiring alertness).
- Report blurred vision, fever, skin rash, nausea, vomiting.

## flecainide acetate

*(fle kay' nide)*

Tambocor

**Pregnancy Category C**

### Drug classes
Antiarrhythmic

### Therapeutic actions
Type 1c antiarrhythmic: acts selectively to depress fast sodium channels, decreasing the height and rate of rise of cardiac action potentials and slowing conduction in all parts of the heart.

### Indications
- Treatment of life-threatening ventricular arrhythmias, such as sustained ventricular tachycardia (not recommended for less severe ventricular arrhythmias)
- Prevention of paroxysmal atrial fibrillation/flutter (PAF) associated with symptoms and paroxysmal supraventricular tachycardias (PSVT), including atrioventricular nodal and atrioventricular reentrant tachycardia; other supraventricular tachycardias of unspecified mechanism with disabling symptoms in patients without structural heart disease

### Contraindications/cautions
- Contraindications: allergy to flecainide; CHF; cardiogenic shock; cardiac conduction abnormalities (heart blocks of any kind, unless an artificial pacemaker is present to maintain heart beat); sick sinus syndrome; lactation.
- Use cautiously with endocardial pacemaker (permanent or temporary—stimulus parameters may need to be increased); hepatic or renal disease; potassium imbalance.

### Dosage
**Available Forms:** Tablets—50, 100, 150 mg

Evaluation with close monitoring of cardiac response necessary for determining the correct dosage.

ADULT
- *PSVT and PAF:* Starting dose of 50 mg q12h PO; may be increased in increments of 50 mg bid q4d until efficacy is achieved; max dose is 300 mg/d.
- *Sustained ventricular tachycardia:* 100 mg q12h PO. Increase in 50-mg increments twice a day every fourth day until efficacy is achieved. Maximum dose is 400 mg/d.
- *Recent MI or CHF:* Initial dose of no more than 100 mg q12h PO. May increase in 50-mg increments bid every fourth day to a max of 200 mg/d; higher doses associated with increased CHF.

PEDIATRIC: Safety and efficacy in children < 18 y has not been established.

GERIATRIC AND RENAL IMPAIRED: *Initial dose:* 100 mg qd PO or 50 mg q12h. Wait about 4 d to reach a steady state and then increase dose cautiously. Creatinine clearance < 20 ml/min: decrease dose by 25%–50%.

*Transfer to flecainide:* Allow at least 2–4 plasma half-lives to elapse of drug being discontinued before starting flecainide. Consider hospitalization for withdrawal of a previous antiarrhythmic is likely to produce life-threatening arrhythmias.

### Pharmacokinetics

| *Route* | *Onset* | *Peak* | *Duration* |
|---|---|---|---|
| Oral | 30–60 min | 3 h | 24 h |

*Metabolism:* Hepatic, $T_{1/2}$: 20 h
*Distribution:* Crosses placenta; may enter breast milk
*Excretion:* Urine and feces

### Adverse effects
- CNS: *Dizziness, fatigue, drowsiness, visual changes, headache*, tinnitus, paresthesias
- GI: *Nausea, vomiting, abdominal pain, constipation*, diarrhea
- CV: *Cardiac arrhythmias*, congestive heart failure, slowed cardiac conduction, *palpitations, chest pain*
- GU: Polyuria, urinary retention, decreased libido

- **Other:** *Dyspnea,* sweating, hot flashes, night sweats, leukopenia

## ■ Nursing Considerations

### Assessment

- *History:* Allergy to flecainide, CHF, cardiogenic shock, cardiac conduction abnormalities, sick sinus syndrome, endocardial pacemaker, hepatic or renal disease, potassium imbalance, lactation
- *Physical:* Weight; orientation, reflexes, vision; P, BP, auscultation, ECG, edema, R, adventitious sounds; bowel sounds, liver evaluation; urinalysis, CBC, serum electrolytes, liver and renal function tests

### Implementation

- Monitor patient response carefully, especially when beginning therapy.
- Reduce dosage in patients with renal disease, hepatic failure, CHF, or recent MI.
- Check serum $K^+$ levels before giving.
- Monitor cardiac rhythm carefully.
- Evaluate for therapeutic serum levels of 0.2–1 $\mu$g/ml.
- Provide life support equipment, including pacemaker, on standby in case serious CVS, CNS effects occur—also dopamine, dobutamine, isoproterenol, or other positive inotropic agents.

### Drug-specific teaching points

- You will need frequent monitoring of cardiac rhythm.
- The following side effects may occur: drowsiness, dizziness, numbness, visual disturbances (avoid driving or using dangerous machinery); nausea, vomiting (small, frequent meals may help); diarrhea, polyuria; sweating, night sweats, hot flashes, loss of libido (reversible after stopping the drug).
- Do not stop taking this drug for any reason without checking with your health care provider. Drug is taken at 12-h intervals; work out a schedule so you take the drug as prescribed without waking up at night.
- Return for regular follow-up visits to check your heart rhythm and have a blood test to check your blood levels of this drug.
- Report swelling of ankles or fingers, palpitations, fainting, chest pain.

## floxuridine

*(flox* ***yoor'*** *i deen)*

FUDR

**Pregnancy Category D**

### Drug classes

Antimetabolite

Antineoplastic

### Therapeutic actions

Converted in the body to fluorouracil, another antineoplastic drug; inhibits the enzyme thymidylate synthetase, leading to inhibition of DNA synthesis.

### Indications

- Palliative management of GI adenocarcinoma metastatic to the liver in patients considered to be incurable by surgery or other means (given only by regional intra-arterial perfusion)

### Contraindications/cautions

- Allergy to floxuridine; poor nutritional status; serious infections; hematopoietic depression secondary to radiation or chemotherapy; impaired liver function; pregnancy; lactation.

### Dosage

**Available Forms:** Powder for injection—500 mg/10 ml, 500 mg/5 ml; preservative-free injection—100 mg/ml

**ADULT:** Given by intra-arterial infusion only: continuous arterial infusion of 0.1–0.6 mg/kg per day (larger doses of 0.4–0.6 mg/kg per day are used for infusion into the hepatic artery as the liver metabolizes the drug). Continue until adverse reactions occur; resume therapy when side effects subside. Maintain use as long as patient is responding to therapy.

**Pharmacokinetics**

| *Route* | *Onset* | *Peak* | *Duration* |
|---|---|---|---|
| Intra-arterial | Immediate | 1–2 h | 3 h |

*Metabolism:* Hepatic, $T_{1/2}$: 20 h
*Distribution:* Crosses placenta; enter breast milk
*Excretion:* Urine

**Adverse effects**

- CNS: *Lethargy, malaise, weakness*, euphoria, acute cerebellar syndrome, photophobia, lacrimation, decreased vision, nystagmus, diplopia, fever, epistaxis
- GI: *Diarrhea, anorexia, nausea, vomiting*, cramps, enteritis, duodenal ulcer, duodenitis, gastritis, glossitis, stomatitis, pharyngitis, esophagopharyngitis
- CV: Myocardial ischemia, angina
- Hematologic: *Leukopenia, thrombocytopenia*, elevations of alkaline phosphatase, serum transaminase, serum bilirubin, lactic dehydrogenase
- Dermatologic: *Alopecia, dermatitis*, maculopapular rash, photosensitivity, nail changes, including nail loss, dry skin, fissures
- Regional arterial infusion: Arterial aneurysm, arterial ischemia, arterial thrombosis, bleeding at catheter site, embolism, fibromyositis, abscesses, infection at catheter site, thrombophlebitis

**Drug-lab test interferences**

• 5-hydroxyindoleacetic acid (5-HIAA) urinary excretion may increase • Plasma albumin may decrease due to protein malabsorption

## ■ Nursing Considerations

### Assessment

- ***History:*** Allergy to floxuridine, poor nutritional status, serious infections, hematopoietic depression secondary to radiation or chemotherapy, impaired liver function, pregnancy, lactation
- ***Physical:*** Weight; T; skin lesions, color; hair; vision, speech, orientation, reflexes, sensation; R, adventitious sounds; mucous membranes, liver evaluation, abdominal exam; CBC, differential; renal and liver function tests; urinalysis, chest x-ray

### Implementation

- Evaluate hematologic status prior to therapy and before each dose.
- Arrange for discontinuation of drug therapy if any sign of toxicity occurs (stomatitis, esophagopharyngitis, rapidly falling WBC count, intractable vomiting, diarrhea, GI ulceration and bleeding, thrombocytopenia, hemorrhage); consult with physician.
- Reconstitute with 5 ml sterile water; refrigerate no more than 2 wk.
- Administer by intra-arterial line only; use an infusion pump to ensure continual delivery and overcome pressure of arteries.

### Drug-specific teaching points

- Prepare a calendar of treatment days.
- The following side effects may occur: nausea, vomiting, loss of appetite (medication may be ordered; small, frequent meals may help; try to maintain your nutrition while you are on this drug); decreased vision, tearing, double vision, malaise, weakness, lethargy (it is advisable to avoid driving or operating dangerous machinery); mouth sores (use frequent mouth care); diarrhea; loss of hair (obtain a wig or other suitable head covering; keep head covered in extremes of temperature); skin rash, sensitivity of skin and eyes to sunlight and UV light (avoid exposure or use a sunscreen and protective clothing).
- Use birth control while on this drug; may cause birth defects or miscarriages.
- Arrange to have frequent, regular medical follow-up, including frequent blood tests.
- Report black, tarry stools; fever; chills; sore throat; unusual bleeding or bruising; chest pain; mouth sores.

# fluconazole

*(floo **kon'** a zole)*

Diflucan

**Pregnancy Category C**

**Drug classes**
Antifungal

**Therapeutic actions**
Binds to sterols in the fungal cell membrane, changing membrane permeability; fungicidal or fungistatic depending on concentration and organism.

**Indications**
- Treatment of oropharyngeal and esophageal candidiasis
- Treatment of cryptococcal meningitis
- Treatment of systemic fungal infections
- Prophylaxis to decrease incidence of candidiasis in bone marrow transplants

**Contraindications/cautions**
- Contraindications: hypersensitivity to fluconazole, lactation.
- Use cautiously with renal impairment.

**Dosage**
**Available Forms:** Tablets—50, 100, 150, 200 mg; powder for oral suspension—10, 40 mg/ml; injection—2 mg/ml
Individualize dosage; same for oral or IV routes because of rapid and almost complete absorption.
ADULT
- *Oropharyngeal candidiasis:* 200 mg PO or IV on the first day, followed by 100 mg qd. Continue treatment for at least 2 wk to decrease likelihood of relapse.
- *Esophageal candidiasis:* 200 mg PO or IV on the first day, followed by 100 mg qd. Dosage up to 400 mg/d may be used in severe cases. Treat for a minimum of 3 wk; at least 2 wk after resolution.
- *Systemic candidiasis:* 400 mg PO or IV on the first day, followed by 200 mg qd. Treat for a minimum of 4 wk; at least 2 wk after resolution.
- *Vaginal candidiasis:* 150 mg PO as a single dose.
- *Cryptococcal meningitis:* 400 mg PO or IV on the first day, followed by 200 mg qd. 400 mg qd may be needed. Continue treatment for 10–12 wk.
- *Suppression of cryptococcal meningitis in AIDS patients:* 200 mg qd PO or IV.
- *Prevention of candidiasis in bone marrow transplants:* 400 mg PO qd for several d before and 7 d after neutropenia.

PEDIATRIC
- *Oropharyngeal candidiasis:* 6 mg/kg PO or IV on the first day, followed by 3 mg/kg once daily for at least 2 wk.
- *Esophageal candidiasis:* 6 mg/kg PO or IV on the first day, followed by 3 mg/kg once daily. Treat for a minimum of 3 wk; at least 2 wk after resolution.
- *Systemic Candida infections:* Daily doses of 6–12 mg/kg/d PO or IV.
- *Cryptococcal meningitis:* 12 mg/kg PO or IV on the first day, followed by 6 mg/kg once daily. Continue treatment for 10–12 wk.

GERIATRIC OR RENAL IMPAIRED: Initial dose of 50–400 mg PO or IV. If creatinine clearance > 50 ml/min, use 100% recommended dose; creatinine clearance 21–50 ml/min, use 50% of the recommended dose; creatinine clearance 11–20, use 25% of recommended dose; patients on hemodialysis, use one dose after each dialysis.

**Pharmacokinetics**

| *Route* | *Onset* | *Peak* | *Duration* |
|---|---|---|---|
| Oral | Slow | 1–2 h | 2–4 d |
| IV | Rapid | 1 h | 2–4 d |

*Metabolism:* Hepatic, $T_{1/2}$: 30 h
*Distribution:* Crosses placenta; may enter breast milk
*Excretion:* Urine

**IV facts**
**Preparation:** Do not remove overwrap until ready for use. Inner bag maintains sterility of product. Do not use plastic containers in series connections. Tear overwrap down side at slit, and remove solution container. Some opacity of plastic may occur; check for minute leaks, squeezing bag firmly. Discard solution if any leaks are found.
**Infusion:** Infuse at a maximum rate of 200 mg/h given as a continuous infusion.
**Incompatibilities:** Do not add any supplementary medications.

**Adverse effects**

- CNS: *Headache*
- GI: *Nausea, vomiting, diarrhea, abdominal pain*
- Other: Skin rash

**Clinically important drug-drug interactions**

• Increased serum levels and therefore therapeutic and toxic effects of cyclosporine, phenytoin, oral hypoglycemics, warfarin anticoagulants • Decreased serum levels with rifampin

## ■ Nursing Considerations

### Assessment

- *History:* Hypersensitivity to fluconazole, renal impairment, lactation
- *Physical:* Skin color, lesions; T; injection site; orientation, reflexes, affect; bowel sounds; renal function tests; CBC and differential; culture of area involved

### Implementation

- Culture infection prior to therapy; begin treatment before lab results are returned.
- Decrease dosage in cases of renal failure.
- Infuse IV only; not intended for IM or SC use.
- Do not add supplement medication to fluconazole.
- Administer through sterile equipment at a maximum rate of 200 mg/h given as a continuous infusion.
- Monitor renal function tests weekly, discontinue or decrease dosage of drug at any sign of increased renal toxicity.

### Drug-specific teaching points

- Drug may be given orally or IV as needed. The drug will need to be taken for the full course and may need to be long term.
- Use hygiene measures to prevent reinfection or spread of infection.
- Arrange for frequent follow-up while you are on this drug. Be sure to keep all appointments, including blood tests.
- The following side effects may occur: nausea, vomiting, diarrhea (small frequent meals may help); headache (analgesics may be ordered).
- Report rash, changes in stool or urine color, difficulty breathing, increased tears or salivation.

## flucytosine

*(floo sye' toe seen)*

5-FC, 5-fluorocytosine

Ancobon, Ancotil (CAN)

**Pregnancy Category C**

**Drug classes**

Antifungal

**Therapeutic actions**

Affects cell membranes of susceptible fungi to cause fungus death; exact mechanism of action is not understood.

**Indications**

- Treatment of serious infections caused by susceptible strains of *Candida, Cryptococcus*
- Unlabeled use: treatment of chromomycosis

**Contraindications/cautions**

- Contraindications: allergy to flucytosine, pregnancy, lactation.
- Use cautiously with renal impairment (drug accumulation and toxicity may occur), bone marrow depression.

### Dosage

**Available Forms:** Capsules—250, 500 mg

ADULT: 50–150 mg/kg per day PO at 6-h intervals.

GERIATRIC OR RENAL IMPAIRED: Initial dose should be at the lower level.

**Pharmacokinetics**

| Route | Onset | Peak | Duration |
|---|---|---|---|
| Oral | Varies | 2 h | 10–12 h |

*Metabolism:* $T_{1/2}$: 2–5 h

*Distribution:* Crosses placenta; may enter breast milk

*Excretion:* Urine and feces

**Adverse effects**

- CNS: Confusion, hallucinations, headache, sedation, vertigo

- GI: *Nausea, vomiting, diarrhea*
- Hematologic: *Anemia, leukopenia, thrombopenia*, elevation of liver enzymes, BUN and creatinine
- Dermatologic: *Rash*

## ■ Nursing Considerations

### Assessment
- *History:* Allergy to flucytosine, renal impairment, bone marrow depression, lactation
- *Physical:* Skin color, lesions; orientation, reflexes, affect; bowel sounds, liver evaluation; renal and liver function tests; CBC and differential

### Implementation
- Administer capsules a few at a time over a 15-min period to decrease the GI upset and diarrhea.
- Monitor hepatic and renal function tests and hematologic function periodically throughout treatment.

### Drug-specific teaching points
- Take the capsules a few at a time over a 15-min period to decrease GI upset.
- The following side effects may occur: nausea, vomiting, diarrhea (take capsules a few at a time over 15 min); sedation, dizziness, confusion (avoid driving or performing tasks that require alertness).
- Report skin rash, severe nausea, vomiting, diarrhea, fever, sore throat, unusual bleeding or bruising.

## fludarabine

*(floo dar' a been)*
Fludara
**Pregnancy Category D**

### Drug classes
Antimetabolite
Antineoplastic

### Therapeutic actions
Inhibits DNA polymerase alpha, ribonucleotid reductase and DNA primase, which inhibits DNA synthesis and prevents cell replication.

### Indications
- Chronic lymphocytic leukemia (CLL); unresponsive B-cell CLL or no progress during treatment with at least one standard regimen that contains an alkylating agent
- Unlabeled uses: non-Hodgkin's lymphoma, macroglobulinemic lymphoma, prolymphocytic leukemia or prolymphocytoid variant of CLL, mycosis fungoides, hairy-cell leukemia, Hodgkin's disease.

### Contraindications/cautions
- Contraindications: allergy to fludarabine or any component, lactation, pregnancy, severe bone marrow depression.
- Use cautiously with renal impairment.

### Dosage
**Available Forms:** Powder for reconstitution—50 mg

ADULT: 25 $mg/m^2$ IV over 30 min for 5 consecutive d. Begin each 5-d course every 28 d. It is recommended that three additional cycles follow the achievement of a maximal response, then discontinue drug.

### Pharmacokinetics

| Route | Onset | Peak |
|---|---|---|
| IV | Rapid | 1–2 h |

*Metabolism:* Hepatic, $T_{1/2}$: 10 h
*Distribution:* Crosses placenta; enters breast milk
*Excretion:* Urine

### IV facts
**Preparation:** Reconstitute with 2 ml of Sterile Water for Injection; the solid cake should dissolve in < 15 sec; each ml of resulting solution will contain 25 mg fludarabine, 25 mg mannitol and sodium hydroxide; may be further diluted in 100 or 125 ml of 5% Dextrose Injection or 0.9% Sodium Chloride; use within 8 h of reconstitution; discard after that time. Store unreconstituted drug in refrigerator.
**Infusion:** Infuse slowly over no less than 30 min.

**Adverse effects**

- CNS: *Weakness, paresthesia, headache, visual disturbance,* hearing loss, sleep disorder, depression, **CNS toxicity**
- GI: *Diarrhea, anorexia, nausea, vomiting, stomatitis,* esophagopharyngitis, GI bleeding, mucositis
- CV: *Edema,* angina
- Respiratory: *Cough, pneumonia, dyspnea, sinusitis,* upper respiratory infection, epistaxis, bronchitis, hypoxia
- Hematologic: *Bone marrow toxicity*
- GU: Dysuria, urinary infection, hematuria, **renal failure**
- Dermatologic: *Rash, pruritus,* seborrhea
- General: *Fever, chills, fatigue, infection, pain, malaise,* diaphoresis, hemorrhage, myalgia, arthralgia, osteoporosis, **tumor lysis syndrome**

## ■ Nursing Considerations

### Assessment

- *History:* Allergy to fludarabine or any component, lactation, pregnancy, severe bone marrow depression, renal impairment
- *Physical:* Weight; T; skin lesions, color, edema; hair; vision, speech, orientation, reflexes, sensation; R, adventitious sounds; mucous membranes, liver evaluation, abdominal exam; CBC, differential; renal and liver function tests; urinalysis, chest x-ray

### Implementation

- Evaluate hematologic status prior to therapy and before each dose.
- Discontinue therapy if any sign of toxicity occurs (CNS complaints, stomatitis, esophagopharyngitis, rapidly falling WBC count, intractable vomiting, diarrhea, GI ulceration and bleeding, thrombocytopenia, hemorrhage); consult with physician.
- Caution patient to avoid pregnancy while on this drug.

### Drug-specific teaching points

- Prepare a calendar of treatment days.
- The following side effects may occur: nausea, vomiting, loss of appetite (medication; small, frequent meals may help; maintain your nutrition while you are on this drug); headache, fatigue, malaise, weakness, lethargy (avoid driving or operating dangerous machinery); mouth sores (use frequent mouth care); diarrhea; increased susceptibility to infection (avoid crowds, exposure to infection; report any sign of infection, eg, fever, fatigue)
- Use birth control while on this drug; may cause birth defects or miscarriages.
- Have frequent, regular medical follow-up, including blood tests.
- Report black, tarry stools; fever; chills; sore throat; unusual bleeding or bruising; chest pain; mouth sores; changes in vision; dizziness.

f

## fludrocortisone acetate

*(floo droe **kor'** ti sone)*

Florinef Acetate

**Pregnancy Category C**

**Drug classes**

Corticosteroid
Mineralocorticoid
Hormone

**Therapeutic actions**

Increases sodium reabsorption in renal tubules and increases potassium and hydrogen excretion, leading to sodium and water retention.

**Indications**

- Partial replacement therapy in primary and secondary cortical insufficiency and for the treatment of salt-losing adrenogenital syndrome (therapy must be accompanied by adequate doses of glucocorticoids).
- Unlabeled use: management of servere orthostatic hypotension

**Contraindications/cautions**

- Contraindications: CHF, hypertension, cardiac disease.

- Use cautiously with infections, high sodium intake, lactation.

## Dosage

**Available Forms:** Tablets—0.1 mg

*ADULT*

- ***Addison's disease:*** 0.1 mg/d (range 0.1 mg 3 ×/wk to 0.2 mg/d) PO. Reduce dose to 0.05 mg/d if transient hypertension develops. Administration with hydrocortisone (10–30 mg/d) or cortisone (10.0–37.5 mg/d) is preferable.
- ***Salt-losing adrenogenital syndrome:*** 0.1–0.2 mg/d PO.

*PEDIATRIC:* Safety and efficacy not established. If infants or children are maintained on prolonged therapy, their growth and development must be carefully observed.

## Pharmacokinetics

| *Route* | *Onset* | *Peak* | *Duration* |
|---|---|---|---|
| Oral | Gradual | 1.7 h | 18–36 h |

*Metabolism:* Hepatic, $T_{1/2}$: 3 1/2 h
*Distribution:* Crosses placenta; enters breast milk

## Adverse effects

- CNS: *Frontal and occipital headaches, arthralgia*, tendon contractures, weakness of extremities with ascending paralysis
- CV: *Increased blood volume, edema, hypertension*, CHF, cardiac arrhythmias, enlargement of the heart
- Hypersensitivity: Rash to **anaphylaxis**

## Clinically important drug-drug interactions

• Decreased effects with barbiturates, hydantoins, rifampin • Decreased effects of anticholinesterases with resultant muscular depression in myasthenia gravis • Decreased serum levels and effectiveness of salicylates

## ■ Nursing Considerations

### Assessment

- *History:* CHF, hypertension, cardiac disease, infections, high sodium intake, lactation
- *Physical:* P, BP, chest sounds, weight, T, tissue turgor, reflexes and bilateral grip strength, serum electrolytes

### Implementation

- Use only in conjunction with glucocorticoid therapy and control of electrolytes and infection.
- Increase dosage during times of stress to prevent drug-induced adrenal insufficiency.
- Monitor BP and serum electrolytes regularly to prevent overdosage.
- Discontinue if signs of overdosage (hypertension, edema, excessive weight gain, increased heart size) appear.
- Treat muscle weakness due to excessive $K^+$ loss with supplements.
- Restrict sodium intake if edema develops.

### Drug-specific teaching points

- Use range-of-motion exercises, positioning to deal with musculoskeletal effects.
- Take drug exactly as prescribed; do not stop without notifying health care provider; if a dose is missed, take it as soon as possible unless it is almost time for the next dose—do not double the next dose.
- Keep appointments for frequent follow-up visits so response may be determined and dosage adjusted.
- Wear a medical alert ID so that any emergency medical personnel will know about this drug therapy.
- Report unusual weight gain, swelling of the lower extremities, muscle weakness, dizziness, and severe or continuing headache.

# flumazenil

*(floo **maz'** eh nill)*

Romazicon

**Pregnancy Category C**

## Drug classes

Antidote
Benzodiazepine receptor antagonist

**Therapeutic actions**

Antagonizes the actions of benzodiazepines on the CNS and inhibits activity at GABA/benzodiazepine receptor sites.

**Indications**

- Complete or partial reversal of the sedative effects of benzodiazepines when general anesthesia has been induced or maintained with them, and when sedation has been produced for diagnostic and therapeutic procedures; management of benzodiazepine overdose.

**Contraindications/cautions**

- Contraindications: hypersensitivity to flumazenil or benzodiazepines; patients who have been given benzodiazepines to control potentially life threatening conditions; patients showing signs of serious cyclic antidepressant overdose.
- Use cautiously with history of seizures, hepatic impairment, panic disorders, head injury, history of drug or alcohol dependence.

**Dosage**

**Available Forms:** Injection—0.1 mg/ml

Use smallest effective dose possible.

ADULTS

- ***Reversal of conscious sedation or in general anesthesia:*** Initial dose of 0.2 mg (2 ml) IV; wait 45 sec; if ineffectual, repeat dose at 60-sec intervals. Maximum dose of 1 mg (10 ml).
- ***Management of suspected benzodiazepine overdose:*** Initial dose of 0.2 mg IV; repeat with 0.3 mg IV q30 sec, up to a maximum dose of 3 mg.

PEDIATRIC: Safety and efficacy not established.

GERIATRIC: No reduction of dosage.

**Pharmacokinetics**

| *Route* | *Onset* | *Peak* | *Duration* |
|---|---|---|---|
| IV | 20–30 sec | 6–10 min | 72 h |

*Metabolism:* Hepatic, $T_{1/2}$: 7–15 min, then 41–79 min

*Distribution:* Crosses placenta; may enter breast milk

**IV facts**

**Preparation:** Can be drawn into syringe with 5% Dextrose in Water, Lactated Ringer's, and normal saline solutions. Discard within 24 h if mixed in solution. Do not remove from vial until ready for use.

**Infusion:** Infuse slowly over 15 sec for general anesthesia, over 30 sec for overdose. To reduce pain of injection, administer through a freely running IV infusion in a large vein.

**Adverse effects**

- CNS: *Dizziness, vertigo*, agitation, nervousness, dry mouth, tremor, palpitations, emotional lability, confusion, crying, vision changes
- GI: *Nausea, vomiting,* hiccups
- CV: Vasodilation, flushing, arrhythmias, chest pain
- Other: *Headache, pain at injection site, increased sweating,* fatigue

**Clinically important drug-food interactions**

- Ingestion of food during IV infusion decreases serum levels and effectiveness

## ■ Nursing Considerations

**Assessment**

- ***History:*** Hypersensitivity to flumazenil or benzodiazepines; use of benzodiazepines for control of potentially life threatening conditions; signs of serious cyclic antidepressant overdose, history of seizures, hepatic impairment, panic disorders, head injury, history of drug or alcohol dependence
- ***Physical:*** Skin color, lesions; T; orientation, reflexes, affect; P, BP, peripheral perfusion; serum drug levels

**Implementation**

- Administer by IV route only.
- Have emergency equipment, secure airway ready during administration.
- Monitor clinical response carefully to determine effects of drug and need for repeated doses.

- Inject into running IV in a large vein to decrease pain of injection.
- Provide patient with written information after use; amnesia may be long-term, and teaching may not be remembered, including safety measures.

**Drug-specific teaching points**

- Drug may cause changes in vision, dizziness, changes in alertness (avoid driving or operating hazardous machinery for at least 18–24 h after drug use).
- Do not use any alcohol or OTC drugs for 18–24 h after use of this drug.
- Report difficulty breathing, pain at IV site, changes in vision, severe headache.

## flunisolide

*(floo **niss'** oh lide)*

AeroBid, Nasalide, Nasarel

**Pregnancy Category C**

### Drug classes

Corticosteroid
Glucocorticoid
Hormone

### Therapeutic actions

Anti-inflammatory effect; local administration into lower respiratory tract or nasal passages maximizes beneficial effects while decreasing possible adverse effects from systemic absorption.

### Indications

- Respiratory inhalant: control of bronchial asthma that requires corticosteroids
- Intranasal: relief of symptoms of seasonal or perennial rhinitis that respond poorly to other treatments

### Contraindications/cautions

- Presence of systemic fungal infections, untreated local nasal infections, epistaxis, nasal trauma, septal ulcers, recent nasal surgery, lactation.

### Dosage

**Available Forms:** Aerosal—250 μg/actuation; spray—25 μg/actuation

***Respiratory inhalant:*** Each actuation delivers 250 μg.

- *ADULT:* Two inhalations (500 μg) bid morning and evening (total dose 1 mg), not to exceed 4 bid (2 mg).
- *PEDIATRIC (6–12 Y):* Two inhalations bid morning and evening. Do not use in children < 6 y.

***Intranasal:*** Each actuation of the inhaler delivers 25 μg.

- *ADULT:* Initial dosage 2 sprays (50 μg) in each nostril bid (total dose 200 μg/d); may be increased to 2 sprays in each nostril tid (total dose 300 μg/d). Maximum daily dose, 8 sprays in each nostril (400 μg/d).
- *PEDIATRIC (6–14 Y):* Initial dosage 1 spray in each nostril tid or 2 sprays in each nostril bid (total dose 150–200 μg/d). Maximum daily dose 4 sprays in each nostril (200 μg/d). Not recommended for children younger than 6 y.
  - *Maintenance dosage:* Reduce to smallest effective dose. Discontinue therapy after 3 wk if no significant symptomatic improvement.

### Pharmacokinetics

| *Route* | *Onset* | *Peak* | *Duration* |
|---|---|---|---|
| Intranasal | Slow | 10–30 min | 4–6 h |

*Metabolism:* Hepatic, $T_{1/2}$: 1–2 h
*Distribution:* Crosses placenta; enters breast milk
*Excretion:* Urine and feces

### Adverse effects

*Respiratory Inhalant*

- Endocrine: **Suppression of hypothalamic-pituitary-adrenal (HPA) function due to systemic absorption**
- Local: *Oral, laryngeal, pharyngeal irritation*; fungal infections

*Intranasal*

- CNS: *Headache*
- GI: Nausea
- Respiratory: *Epistaxis, rebound congestion*, perforation of the nasal septum, anosmia
- Dermatologic: Urticaria

- Endocrine: HPA suppression, Cushing's syndrome with overdosage
- Local: *Nasal irritation, fungal infection*

## ■ Nursing Considerations

### Assessment

- *History:* Systemic fungal infections, untreated local nasal infections, epistaxis, nasal trauma, septal ulcers, recent nasal surgery, lactation
- *Physical:* Weight, T; BP, P, auscultation, R, adventitious sounds, examination of nares

### Implementation

- Do not use during an acute asthmatic attack or to manage status asthmaticus.
- Taper systemic steroids carefully during transfer to inhalational steroids; deaths from adrenal insufficiency have occurred.
- Use decongestant nose drops to facilitate penetration if edema, excessive secretions are present.

### Drug-specific teaching points

- Do not use this drug more often than prescribed.
- Do not stop using this drug without consulting your health care provider.
- Use inhalational bronchodilator drug before oral inhalant if receiving concomitant bronchodilator therapy. Allow at least 1 min between puffs.
- Rinse your mouth after using.
- Use decongestant nose drops first if nasal passages are blocked when using intranasal form.
- Know that the following side effects may occur: local irritation (make sure you are using your device correctly), headache.
- Report sore mouth, sore throat.

## fluorouracil

*(flure oh **yoor'** a sill)*

5-fluorouracil, 5-FU

Adrucil, Efudex, Fluoroplex

**Pregnancy Category D**

### Drug classes

Antimetabolite
Antineoplastic

### Therapeutic actions

Inhibits thymidylate synthetase, leading to inhibition of DNA synthesis and cell death.

### Indications

- Palliative management of carcinoma of the colon, rectum, breast, stomach, pancreas in selected patients considered incurable by surgery or other means (parenteral)
- Topical treatment of multiple actinic or solar keratoses
- Topical treatment of superficial basal cell carcinoma
- Unlabeled use: topical treatment of condylomata acuminata
- Orphan drug uses: in combination with interferon alpha 2-a recombinant for esophageal and advanced colorectal carcinoma; with leucovorin for colon/rectum metastatic adenocarcinoma

### Contraindications/cautions

- Allergy to fluorouracil; poor nutritional status; serious infections; hematopoietic depression secondary to radiation or chemotherapy; impaired liver function; pregnancy; lactation.

### Dosage

**Available Forms:** Injection—50 mg/ml; cream—1%, 5%; solution—1%, 2%, 5%

**ADULT:** Initial dosage: 12 mg/kg IV daily for 4 successive d; do not exceed 800 mg/d. If no toxicity occurs, give 6 mg/kg on the sixth, eighth, 10th, and 12th day with no drug therapy on days 5, 7, 9, and 11. Discontinue therapy at end of 12th day, even if no toxicity is apparent.

***Poor-risk Patients, Undernourished***

6 mg/kg per day IV for 3 d. If no toxicity develops, give 3 mg/kg on the fifth, seventh, and ninth days. No drug is given on days 4, 6, and 8. Do not exceed 400 mg/d.

***Maintenance Therapy***

Continue therapy on appropriate schedules:
1. Without toxicity, repeat dosage every

30 d after the last day of the previous treatment. 2. With toxicity, give 10–15 mg/kg per week as a single dose after signs of toxicity subside. Do not exceed 1 g/wk. Adjust dosage based on patient response; therapy may be prolonged (12–60 mo).

***Hepatic Failure***

If serum bilirubin > 5, do not administer fluorouracil.

***Topical Use***

- *Actinic or solar keratoses:* Apply bid to cover lesions. Continue until inflammatory response reaches erosion, necrosis, and ulceration stage, then discontinue. Usual course of therapy is 2–6 wk. Complete healing may not be evident for 1–2 mo after cessation of therapy.
- *Superficial basal cell carcinoma:* Apply 5% strength bid in an amount sufficient to cover the lesions. Continue treatment for at least 3–6 wk. Treatment may be required for 10–12 wk.

## Pharmacokinetics

| *Route* | *Onset* | *Peak* | *Duration* |
|---|---|---|---|
| IV | Immediate | 1–2 h | 6 h |
| Topical | Minimal absorption | | |

*Metabolism:* Hepatic, $T_{1/2}$: 18–20 min
*Distribution:* Crosses placenta; enters breast milk
*Excretion:* Urine and lungs

### IV facts

**Preparation:** Store vials at room temperature; solution may discolor during storage with no adverse effects. Protect ampule from light. Precipitate may form during storage, heat to 60°C, and shake vigorously to dissolve. Cool to body temperature before administration. No dilution is required.
**Infusion:** Infuse slowly over 24 h; inject into tubing of running IV to avoid pain on injection; direct injection over 1–3 min.
**Incompatibilities:** Do not mix with IV additives or other chemotherapeutic agents.

## Adverse effects

*Parenteral*

- CNS: *Lethargy, malaise, weakness,* euphoria, acute cerebellar syndrome, photophobia, lacrimation, decreased vision, nystagmus, diplopia
- GI: *Diarrhea, anorexia, nausea, vomiting, cramps, enteritis, duodenal ulcer, duodenitis, gastritis, glossitis, stomatitis,* pharyngitis, esophagopharyngitis
- CV: Myocardial ischemia, angina
- **Hematologic**: *Leukopenia, thrombocytopenia,* elevations in alkaline phosphatase, serum transaminase, serum bilirubin, lactic dehydrogenase
- **Dermatologic**: *Alopecia, dermatitis, maculopapular rash, photosensitivity,* nail changes including nail loss, dry skin, fissures
- **Other**: Fever, epistaxis

*Topical*

- **Hematologic**: Leukocytosis, thrombocytopenia, toxic granulation, eosinophilia
- **Local**: *Local pain, pruritus, hyperpigmentation, irritation, inflammation and burning at the site of application,* allergic contact dermatitis, scarring, soreness, tenderness, suppuration, scaling and swelling

## Drug-lab test interferences

• 5-hydroxyindoleacetic acid (5-HIAA) urinary excretion may increase • Plasma albumin may decrease due to protein malabsorption

## ■ Nursing Considerations

### Assessment

- *History:* Allergy to fluorouracil, poor nutritional status, serious infections, hematopoietic depression, impaired liver function, pregnancy, lactation
- *Physical:* Weight; T; skin lesions, color; hair; vision, speech, orientation, reflexes, sensation; R, adventitious sounds; mucous membranes, liver evaluation, abdominal exam; CBC, differential; renal and liver function tests; urinalysis, chest x-ray

### Implementation

- Evaluate hematologic status before beginning therapy and before each dose.
- Discontinue drug therapy at any sign of toxicity (stomatitis, esophagopharyngitis, rapidly falling WBC count, intractable vomiting, diarrhea, GI ulceration and bleeding, thrombocytopenia, hemorrhage); consult with physician.
- Arrange for biopsies of skin lesions to rule out frank neoplasm before beginning topical therapy and in all patients who do not respond to topical therapy.
- Wash hands thoroughly immediately after application of topical preparations. Use caution in applying near the nose, eyes, and mouth.
- Avoid occlusive dressings with topical application; the incidence of inflammatory reactions in adjacent skin areas is increased with these dressings. Use porous gauze dressings for cosmetic reasons.

### Drug-specific teaching points

- Prepare a calendar of treatment days. If using the topical application, wash hands thoroughly after application. Do not use occlusive dressings, a porous gauze dressing may be used for cosmetic reasons.
- The following side effects may occur: nausea, vomiting, loss of appetite (request medication; small, frequent meals may help; maintain nutrition); decreased vision, tearing, double vision, malaise, weakness, lethargy (reversible; avoid driving or operating dangerous machinery); mouth sores (frequent mouth care is needed); diarrhea; loss of hair (obtain a wig or other head covering; keep the head covered in extremes of temperature); skin rash, sensitivity of skin and eyes to sun and ultraviolet light (avoid exposure to the sun; use a sunscreen and protective clothing; topical application: ultraviolet will increase the severity of the local reaction); birth defects or miscarriages (use birth control); unsightly local reaction to topical application (transient; use a porous gauze dressing to cover areas); pain, burning, stinging, swelling at local application.
- Have frequent, regular medical follow-up, including frequent blood tests to evaluate drug effects.
- Report black, tarry stools; fever; chills; sore throat; unusual bleeding or bruising; chest pain; mouth sores; severe pain; tenderness; scaling at sight of local application.

## fluoxetine hydrochloride

*(floo **ox'** e teen)*

Prozac

**Pregnancy Category B**

### Drug classes

Antidepressant

Selective serotinin reuptake inhibitor (SSRI)

### Therapeutic actions

Acts as an antidepressant by inhibiting CNS neuronal uptake of serotonin; blocks uptake of serotonin with little effect on norepinephrine; little affinity for muscarinic, histaminergic and $\alpha_1$-adrenergic receptors.

### Indications

- Treatment of depression; most effective in patients with major depressive disorder
- Treatment of obsessive-compulsive disorder
- Treatment of bulimia
- Unlabeled use: treatment of obesity, alcoholism, numerous psychiatric disorders

### Contraindications/cautions

- Contraindications: hypersensitivity to fluoxetine; pregnancy.
- Use cautiously with impaired hepatic or renal function, diabetes mellitus, lactation.

### Dosage

**Available Forms:** Pulvules—10, 20 mg; liquid—20 mg/5 ml

ADULT

- *Antidepressant:* The full antidepressant effect may not be seen for up to 4 wk. Initial: 20 mg/d PO in the morning. If no clinical improvement is seen, increase dose after several weeks. Administer doses > 20 mg/d on a bid schedule. Do not exceed 80 mg/d.

- ***Obesessive-compulsive disorder and bulimia:*** 20–60 mg/day PO; may require up to 5 wk for effectiveness

PEDIATRIC: Safety and efficacy not established.

GERIATRIC OR RENAL IMPAIRED: Give a lower or less frequent dose. Monitor response to guide dosage.

### Pharmacokinetics

| *Route* | *Onset* | *Peak* |
|---|---|---|
| Oral | Slow | 6–8 h |

*Metabolism:* Hepatic, $T_{1/2}$: 2–9 d
*Distribution:* Crosses placenta; enters breast milk
*Excretion:* Urine and feces

### Adverse effects

- CNS: *Headache, nervousness, insomnia, drowsiness, anxiety, tremor, dizziness, lightheadedness,* agitation, sedation, abnormal gait, convulsions
- GI: *Nausea, vomiting, diarrhea, dry mouth, anorexia, dyspepsia, constipation, taste changes,* flatulence, gastroenteritis, dysphagia, gingivitis
- CV: Hot flashes, palpitations
- Respiratory: *Upper respiratory infections, pharyngitis,* cough, dyspnea, bronchitis, rhinitis
- GU: *Painful menstruation, sexual dysfunction, frequency,* cystitis, impotence, urgency, vaginitis
- Dermatologic: *Sweating, rash, pruritus,* acne, alopecia, contact dermatitis
- Other: *Weight loss, asthenia, fever*

### Clinically important drug-drug interactions

• Increased therapeutic and toxic effects of TCAs • Decreased therapeutic effects if taken with cyproheptadine

## ■ Nursing Considerations

### Assessment

- *History:* Hypersensitivity to fluoxetine, impaired hepatic or renal function, diabetes mellitus, lactation, pregnancy
- *Physical:* Weight, T; skin rash, lesions; reflexes, affect; bowel sounds, liver evaluation; P, peripheral perfusion; urinary output, renal function; renal and liver function tests, CBC

### Implementation

- Arrange for lower or less frequent doses in elderly patients and patients with hepatic or renal impairment.
- Establish suicide precautions for severely depressed patients. Limit quantity of capsules dispensed.
- Administer drug in the morning. If dose of > 20 mg/d is needed, administer in divided doses.
- Monitor patient for response to therapy for up to 4 wk before increasing dose.

### Drug-specific teaching points

- It may take up to 4 wk before the full effect occurs. Take in the morning (or in divided doses if necessary).
- The following side effects may occur: dizziness, drowsiness, nervousness, insomnia (avoid driving or performing hazardous tasks); nausea, vomiting, weight loss (small, frequent meals may help; monitor your weight loss); sexual dysfunction; flulike symptoms.
- Do not take this drug during pregnancy. If you think that you are pregnant or wish to become pregnant, consult with your physician.
- Report rash, mania, seizures, severe weight loss.
- Keep this drug, and all medications, out of the reach of children.

# fluoxymesterone

*(floo ox i **mes'** te rone)*
Halotestin
**Pregnancy Category X**
**C-III controlled substance**

### Drug classes

Androgen
Hormone

**Therapeutic actions**

Analog of testosterone, the primary natural androgen; endogenous androgens are responsible for growth and development of male sex organs and the maintenance of secondary sex characteristics; administration of androgen analogs increases the retention of nitrogen, sodium, potassium, phosphorus, and decreases urinary excretion of calcium; increases protein anabolism and decreases protein catabolism; stimulates the production of red blood cells.

**Indications**

- Male: replacement therapy in hypogonadism—primary hypogonadism, hypogonadotropic hypogonadism, delayed puberty
- Female: metastatic cancer—breast cancer in women who are 1–5 years postmenopausal; postpartum breast pain/engorgement

**Contraindications/cautions**

- Contraindications: known sensitivity to androgens, allergy to tartrazine or aspirin (in products marketed under the brand name *Halotestin*), prostate or breast cancer in males, pregnancy, lactation.
- Use cautiously with MI, liver disease.

**Dosage**

**Available Forms:** Tablets—2, 5, 10 mg

ADULT

- *Hypogonadism:* 5–20 mg/d PO.
- *Delayed puberty:* 2.5–20 mg/d PO, although generally 2.5–10 mg/d PO for 4–6 mo is sufficient.
- *Postpartum breast pain/engorgement:* 2.5 mg PO shortly after delivery, then 5–10 mg/d PO in divided doses for 4–5 d.
- *Carcinoma of the breast:* 10–40 mg/d PO in divided doses. Continue for 1 mo for a subjective response and 2–3 mo for an objective response.

**Pharmacokinetics**

| Route | Onset | Peak |
|---|---|---|
| Oral | Rapid | 2 h |

*Metabolism:* Hepatic, $T_{1/2}$: 9.5 h

*Distribution:* Crosses placenta; enters breast milk

*Excretion:* Urine and feces

**Adverse effects**

- CNS: *Dizziness, headache, sleep disorders, fatigue,* tremor, sleeplessness, generalized paresthesia, sleep apnea syndrome, CNS hemorrhage
- GI: *Nausea,* hepatic dysfunction; hepatocellular carcinoma, **potentially life threatening peliosis hepatitis**
- Hematologic: *Polycythemia, leukopenia,* hypercalcemia, altered serum cholesterol levels; retention of sodium, chloride, water, potassium, phosphates, and calcium
- GU: Fluid retention, decreased urinary output
- Dermatologic: *Rash,* dermatitis, anaplylactoid reactions
- Endocrine: *Androgenic effects* (acne, edema, mild hirsutism, decrease in breast size, deepening of the voice, oily skin or hair, weight gain, clitoral hypertrophy or testicular atrophy), *hypoestrogenic effects* (flushing, sweating, vaginitis, nervousness, emotional lability)
- Other: Chills, premature closure of the epiphyses

**Clinically important drug-drug interactions**

• Potentiation of oral anticoagulants with androgens; anticoagulant dosage may need to be decreased

**Drug-lab test interferences**

• Altered glucose tolerance tests • Decrease in thyroid function tests, may persist for 2–3 wk after stopping therapy • Suppression of clotting factors II, V, VII, and X • Increased creatinine, creatinine clearance, may last for 2 wk after therapy

## ■ Nursing Considerations

**Assessment**

- *History:* Sensitivity to androgens, allergy to tartrazine or aspirin, prostate or breast cancer in males, MI, liver disease, pregnancy, lactation

- *Physical:* Skin color, lesions, texture; hair distribution pattern; affect, orientation, peripheral sensation; abdominal exam, liver evaluation; serum electrolytes, serum cholesterol levels, liver function tests, glucose tolerance tests, thyroid function tests, long bone x-ray (in children)

### Implementation
- Administer drug with meals or snacks to decrease GI upset.
- Monitor effect on children with long bone x-rays every 3–6 mo. Stop drug well before the bone age reaches the norm for the patient's chronologic age.
- Monitor patient for occurrence of edema; arrange for diuretic therapy.
- Monitor liver function, serum electrolytes periodically, and consult with physician for corrective measures.
- Measure cholesterol levels in those at high risk for CAD.
- Monitor diabetic patients closely as glucose tolerance may change. Adjust insulin, oral hypoglycemic dosage and diet.
- Arrange for periodic monitoring of urine and serum calcium of disseminated breast carcinoma, and arrange for treatment or stop drug.
- Monitor geriatric males for prostatic hypertrophy and carcinoma.
- Stop drug and arrange for consultation if abnormal vaginal bleeding occurs.

### Drug-specific teaching points
- Take drug with meals or snacks to decrease the GI upset.
- The following side effects may occur: body hair growth, baldness, deepening of the voice, loss of libido, impotence (reversible); excitation, confusion, insomnia (avoid driving, performing tasks that require alertness); swelling of the ankles, fingers (request medication).
- Diabetic patients need to monitor urine or blood sugar closely as glucose tolerance may change. Report any abnormalities to physician, for corrective action.
- Report ankle swelling, nausea, vomiting, yellowing of skin or eyes, unusual bleeding or bruising, penile swelling or pain, hoarseness, body hair growth, deepening of the voice, acne, menstrual irregularities.

# Fluphenazine

## fluphenazine decanoate

*(floo* ***fen'*** *a zeen)*

*Injection:* Modecate Deconoate (CAN), Prolixin Decanoate

## fluphenazine enanthate

*Injection:* Moditen Enanthate (CAN), Prolixin Enanthate

## fluphenazine hydrochloride

*Oral tablets, concentrate, elixir, injection:* Apo-Fluphenazine (CAN), Moditen Hydrochloride (CAN), Permitil, Prolixin

**Pregnancy Category C**

### Drug classes
Phenothiazine
Dopaminergic blocking agent
Antipsychotic

### Therapeutic actions
Mechanism not fully understood: antipsychotic drugs block postsynaptic dopamine receptors in the brain, depress the RAS, including the parts of the brain involved with wakefulness and emesis; anticholinergic, antihistaminic ($H_1$), and alpha-adrenergic blocking activity also may contribute to some of its therapeutic (and adverse) actions.

### Indications
- Management of manifestations of psychotic disorders; the longer acting parenteral dosage forms, fluphenazine enanthate and fluphenazine decanoate, indicated for management of patients (chronic schizophrenics) who require prolonged parenteral therapy

### Contraindications/cautions
- Contraindications: coma or severe CNS depression, bone marrow depression, blood dyscrasia, circulatory collapse, subcortical brain damage, Parkinson's

disease, liver damage, cerebral arteriosclerosis, coronary disease, severe hypotension or hypertension.

- Use cautiously with respiratory disorders ("silent pneumonia"); glaucoma, prostatic hypertrophy (anticholinergic effects may exacerbate glaucoma and urinary retention); epilepsy or history of epilepsy (drug lowers seizure threshold); breast cancer (elevations in prolactin may stimulate a prolactin-dependent tumor); thyrotoxicosis; peptic ulcer, decreased renal function; myelography within previous 24 h or myelography scheduled within 48 h; exposure to heat or phosphorous insecticides; pregnancy; lactation; children younger than 12 y, especially those with chickenpox, CNS infections (children are especially susceptible to dystonias that may confound the diagnosis of Reye's syndrome).

### Dosage

**Available Forms:** Tablets—1, 2.5, 5, 10 mg; elixir—2.5 mg/5 ml; concentrate—5 mg/ml; injection—2.5 mg/ml

Full clinical effects may require 6 wk–6 mo of therapy. Patients who have never taken phenothiazines, "poor-risk" patients (those disorders that predispose to undue reactions) should be treated initially with this shorter acting dosage form and then switched to the longer acting parenteral forms, fluphenazine enanthate or decanoate.

The duration of action of the esterified forms of fluphenazine is *markedly* longer than those of fluphenazine hydrochloride; the duration of action of fluphenazine enanthate is estimated to be 1–3 wk; the duration of action of fluphenazine decaonate is estimated to be 4 wk. No precise formula is available for the conversion of fluphenazine hydrochloride dosage to fluphenazine dicanoate dosage, but one study suggests that 20 mg of fluphenazine hydrochloride daily was equivalent to 25 mg decanoate every 3 wk.

***Fluphenazine hydrochloride***

- Adult: Individualize dosage, begin with low dosage, gradually increase.
  - ***Oral:*** 0.5–10.0 mg/d in divided doses q6–8h; usual daily dose is less than 3 mg. Give daily doses greater than 20 mg with caution. When symptoms are controlled, gradually reduce dosage.
  - ***IM:*** Average starting dose is 1.25 mg (range 2.5–10.0 mg), divided and given q6–8h; parenteral dose is one-third to one-half the oral dose. Give daily doses greater than 10 mg with caution.
- Pediatric: Generally not recommended for children < 12 y.
- Geriatric: Initial oral dose is 1.0–2.5 mg/d.

***Fluphenazine enanthate, fluphenazine decanoate***

- Adult: Initial dose 12.5–25.0 mg IM or SC; determine subsequent doses and dosage interval based on patient response. Dose should not exceed 100 mg.

### Pharmacokinetics

| Route | Onset | Peak | Duration |
|---|---|---|---|
| Oral | 60 min | 2 h | 6–8 h |
| IM (HCl) | 60 min | 1–2 h | 6–8 h |
| IM (enanthate) | 24–72 h | | 2 wk |
| IM (decanoate) | 24–72 h | | 1–6 wk |

*Metabolism:* Hepatic, $T_{1/2}$: 4.5-15.3 h (fluphenazine), 3.7 d (fluphenazine enanthate), 6.8–9.6 d (fluphenazine decanoate)

*Distribution:* Crosses placenta; enters breast milk

*Excretion:* Unchanged in the urine

### Adverse effects

- CNS: *Drowsiness*, insomnia, vertigo, headache, weakness, tremor, ataxia, slurring, cerebral edema, seizures, exacerbation of psychotic symptoms, extrapyramidal syndromes *(pseudoparkinsonism); dystonias; akathisia*, tardive dyskinesias, potentially irreversible, neuroleptic malignant syndrome (extrapyramidal symptoms), hyperthermias, **autonomic disturbances** (rare, but 20% fatal)
- CV: Hypotension, orthostatic hypotension, hypertension, tachycardia, bradycardia, cardiac arrest, CHF, cardiomegaly, **refractory arrhythmias** (some fatal), pulmonary edema

- **Respiratory**: Bronchospasm, laryngospasm, dyspnea; suppression of cough reflex and potential for aspiration **(sudden death related to asphyxia or cardiac arrest has been reported)**
- **Hematologic**: Eosinophilia, leukopenia, leukocytosis, anemia; aplastic anemia; hemolytic anemia; thrombocytopenic or nonthrombocytopenic purpura; pancytopenia
- **Hypersensitivity**: Jaundice, urticaria, angioneurotic edema, laryngeal edema, photosensitivity, eczema, asthma, anaphylactoid reactions, exfoliative dermatitis
- **Endocrine**: Lactation, breast engorgement in females, galactorrhea; syndrome of inappropriate ADH secretion; amenorrhea, menstrual irregularities; gynecomastia in males; changes in libido; hyperglycemia or hypoglycemia; glycosuria; hyponatremia; pituitary tumor with hyperprolactinemia; inhibition of ovulation, infertility, pseudopregnancy; reduced urinary levels of gonadotropins, estrogens, progestins
- **Autonomic**: Dry mouth, salivation, nasal congestion, nausea, vomiting, anorexia, fever, pallor, flushed facies, sweating, constipation, paralytic ileus, urinary retention, incontinence, polyuria, enuresis, priapism, ejaculation inhibition, male impotence

### Clinically important drug-drug interactions

• Additive CNS depression with alcohol • Additive anticholinergic effects and possibly decreased antipsychotic efficacy with anticholinergic drugs • Increased likelihood of seizures with metrizamide (contrast agent used in myelography) • Decreased antihypertensive effect of guanethidine with antipsychotic drugs

### Drug-lab test interferences

• False-positive pregnancy tests (less likely if serum test is used) • Increase in PBI, not attributable to an increase in thyroxine

## ■ Nursing Considerations

### Assessment

- ***History:*** Coma or severe CNS depression; bone marrow depression; blood dyscrasia; circulatory collapse; subcortical brain damage; Parkinson's disease; liver damage; cerebral arteriosclerosis; coronary disease; severe hypotension or hypertension; respiratory disorders; glaucoma, prostatic hypertrophy; epilepsy; breast cancer; thyrotoxicosis; peptic ulcer, decreased renal function; myelography within previous 24 h or myelography scheduled within 48 h; exposure to heat or phosphorous insecticides; children $<$ 12 y, chickenpox, CNS infections
- ***Physical:*** Weight, T; reflexes, orientation, intraocular pressure; P, BP, orthostatic BP; R, adventitious sounds; bowel sounds and normal output, liver evaluation; urinary output, prostate size; CBC, urinalysis, thyroid, liver and kidney function tests

### Implementation

- Use the oral elixir or the oral concentrate for those unable or unwilling to swallow tablets.
- Dilute the oral concentrate *only* in the following: water, saline, Seven-Up, homogenized milk, carbonated orange beverage, and pineapple, apricot, prune, orange, V-8, tomato, and grapefruit juices.
- Do *not* mix the oral concentrate with beverages containing caffeine (coffee, cola), tannics (tea), or pectinates (apple juice), because drug may be physically incompatible with these liquids.
- Avoid skin contact with oral solution; contact dermatitis has occurred.
- Arrange for discontinuation of drug if serum creatinine, BUN become abnormal or if WBC count is depressed.
- Monitor elderly patients for dehydration, institute remedial measures promptly. Sedation and decreased sensation of thirst related to CNS effects can lead to severe dehydration.
- Consult physician regarding appropriate warning of patient or patient's guardian about tardive dyskinesias.
- Consult physician about dosage reduction, use of anticholinergic antiparkinsonian drugs (controversial) if extrapyramidal effects occur.

### Drug-specific teaching points

- Take drug exactly as prescribed.
- Avoid driving or engaging in other dangerous activities if CNS, vision changes occur.
- Avoid prolonged exposure to sun; use a sunscreen or covering garments if exposure is unavoidable.
- Maintain fluid intake, and use precautions against heatstroke in hot weather.
- Report sore throat, fever, unusual bleeding or bruising, rash, weakness, tremors, impaired vision, dark urine (pink or reddish brown urine is expected), pale stools, yellowing of skin or eyes.

## flurazepam hydrochloride

*(flur az' e pam)*

Dalmane, Somnal (CAN)

**Pregnancy Category X**
**C-IV controlled substance**

### Drug classes

Benzodiazepine
Sedative/hypnotic

### Therapeutic actions

Exact mechanisms not understood; acts mainly at subcortical levels of the CNS, leaving the cortex relatively unaffected; potentiates the effects of gamma-aminobutyate, an inhibitory neurotransmitter.

### Indications

- Insomnia characterized by difficulty in falling asleep, frequent nocturnal awakenings, or early morning awakening
- Recurring insomnia or poor sleeping habits
- Acute or chronic medical situations requiring restful sleep

### Contraindications/cautions

- Contraindications: hypersensitivity to benzodiazepines, psychoses, acute narrow-angle glaucoma, shock, coma, acute alcoholic intoxication with depression of vital signs, pregnancy (risk of congenital malformations, neonatal withdrawal syndrome), labor and delivery ("floppy infant" syndrome), lactation (infants become lethargic and lose weight).
- Use cautiously with impaired liver or kidney function, debilitation, depression, suicidal tendencies.

### Dosage

**Available Forms:** Capsules—15, 30 mg

Individualize dosage.

**ADULT:** 30 mg PO before HS; 15 mg may suffice.

**PEDIATRIC:** Not for use in children < 15 y.

**GERIATRIC PATIENTS OR THOSE WITH DEBILITATING DISEASE:** Initially, 15 mg; adjust as needed and tolerated.

### Pharmacokinetics

| Route | Onset | Peak |
|---|---|---|
| Oral | Varies | 30–60 min |

*Metabolism:* Hepatic, $T_{1/2}$: 47–100 h

*Distribution:* Crosses placenta; enters breast milk

*Excretion:* Urine

### Adverse effects

- CNS: *Transient, mild drowsiness initially; sedation, depression, lethargy, apathy, fatigue, lightheadedness, disorientation, restlessness, asthenia*, crying, delirium, headache, slurred speech, dysarthria, stupor, rigidity, tremor, dystonia, vertigo, euphoria, nervousness, difficulty in concentration, vivid dreams, psychomotor retardation, extrapyramidal symptoms; *mild paradoxical excitatory reactions during first 2 wk of treatment* (psychiatric patients, aggressive children, with high dosage), visual and auditory disturbances, diplopia, nystagmus, depressed hearing, nasal congestion
- GI: *Constipation, diarrhea, dyspepsia*, dry mouth, salivation, nausea, anorexia, vomiting, difficulty in swallowing, gastric disorders, elevations of blood enzymes: LDH, alkaline phosphatase, SGOT, SGPT, hepatic dysfunction, jaundice

- CV: *Bradycardia, tachycardia*, CV collapse, hypertension and hypotension, palpitations, edema
- **Hematologic**: Decreased hematocrit, blood dyscrasias
- GU: *Incontinence, urinary retention, changes in libido,* menstrual irregularities
- **Dermatologic**: Urticaria, pruritus, skin rash, dermatitis
- **Dependence**: *Drug dependence with withdrawal syndrome* when drug is discontinued (common with abrupt cessation of high dosage used more than 4 mo)
- **Other**: Hiccups, fever, diaphoresis, paresthesias, muscular disturbances, gynecomastia

### Clinically important drug-drug interactions

• Increased CNS depression with alcohol, omeprazole • Increased pharmacologic effects of chlordiazepoxide with cimetidine, disulfiram, oral contraceptives • Decreased sedative effects of chlordiazepoxide with theophylline, aminophylline, dyphylline, oxitriphylline

## ■ Nursing Considerations

### Assessment

- *History:* Hypersensitivity to benzodiazepines; psychoses; acute narrow-angle glaucoma; shock; coma; acute alcoholic intoxication; pregnancy; labor; lactation; impaired liver or kidney function, debilitation, depression, suicidal tendencies
- *Physical:* Skin color, lesions; T; orientation, reflexes, affect, ophthalmologic exam; P, BP; R, adventitious sounds; liver evaluation, abdominal exam, bowel sounds, normal output; CBC, liver and renal function tests

### Implementation

- Monitor liver and kidney function, CBC during long-term therapy.
- Taper dosage gradually after long-term therapy, especially in epileptics.

### Drug-specific teaching points

- Take drug exactly as prescribed.
- Do not stop taking (long-term therapy) without consulting the health care provider.
- The following side effects may occur: drowsiness, dizziness (may lessen; avoid driving or engaging in other dangerous activities); GI upset (take with water); depression, dreams, emotional upset, crying; nocturnal sleep disturbance (may be prolonged after drug cessation).
- Report severe dizziness, weakness, drowsiness that persists, rash or skin lesions, palpitations, swelling of the extremities, visual changes, difficulty voiding.

## flurbiprofen

*(flure* ***bi'*** *proe fen)*

Ophthalmic solution: Ocufen

Oral: Ansaid

**Pregnancy Category B**

### Drug classes

Nonsteroidal anti-inflammatory drug (NSAID)
Analgesic (non-narcotic)
Anti-inflammatory agent

### Therapeutic actions

Analgesic, anti-inflammatory, and antipyretic activities largely related to inhibition of prostaglandin synthesis; exact mechanisms of action are not known.

### Indications

- Acute or long-term treatment of the signs and symptoms of rheumatoid arthritis and osteoarthritis (oral)
- Inhibition of intraoperative miosis (ophthalmic solution)
- Unlabeled uses of ophthalmic solution: topical treatment of cystoid macular edema, inflammation after cataract surgery and uveitis syndromes

### Contraindications/cautions

- Contraindications: significant renal impairment, pregnancy, lactation.
- Use cautiously with impaired hearing, allergies, hepatic, CV, and GI conditions.

### Dosage

**Available Forms:** Tablets—50, 100 mg

**ADULT**

- ***Oral:*** Initial recommended daily dose of 200—300 mg PO, give in divided doses 2, 3, 4 ×/d. Largest recommended single dose is 100 mg. Doses above 300 mg/d PO are not recommended. Taper to lowest possible dose.
- ***Ophthalmic solutions:*** Instill 1 drop approximately every 1/2 h, beginning 2 h before surgery (total of 4 drops).

**PEDIATRIC:** Safety and efficacy not established.

### Pharmacokinetics

| *Route* | *Onset* | *Peak* |
|---|---|---|
| Oral | 30–60 min | 1 1/2 h |
| Ophthalmologic | Minimal systemic absorption | |

*Metabolism:* Hepatic, $T_{1/2}$: 5.7 h
*Distribution:* Crosses placenta; enters breast milk
*Excretion:* Urine

### Adverse effects

*NSAIDs*

- CNS: *Headache, dizziness, somnolence, insomnia*, fatigue, tiredness, dizziness, tinnitus, ophthamological effects
- GI: *Nausea, dyspepsia, GI pain,* diarrhea, vomiting, *constipation,* flatulence
- Respiratory: Dyspnea, hemoptysis, pharyngitis, bronchospasm, rhinitis
- Hematologic: Bleeding, platelet inhibition with higher doses, neutropenia, eosinophilia, leukopenia, pancytopenia, thrombocytopenia, agranulocytosis, granulocytopenia, aplastic anemia, decreased hemoglobin or hematocrit, bone marrow depression, menorrhagia
- GU: Dysuria, **renal impairment**
- Dermatologic: *Rash,* pruritus, sweating, dry mucous membranes, stomatitis
- Other: Peripheral edema, **fatal anaphylactic shock**

*Ophthalmic Solution*

- Local: *Transient stinging and burning on instillation, ocular irritation*

## ■ Nursing Considerations

### Assessment

- *History:* Renal impairment; impaired hearing; allergies; hepatic, CV, and GI conditions; lactation
- *Physical:* Skin color and lesions; orientation, reflexes, ophthalmologic and audiometric evaluation, peripheral sensation; P, edema; R, adventitious sounds; liver evaluation; CBC, clotting times, renal and liver function tests; serum electrolytes, stool guaiac

### Implementation

- Administer drug with food or after meals if GI upset occurs.
- Assess patient receiving ophthalmic solutions for systemic effects, because absorption does occur.
- Arrange for periodic ophthalmologic examination during long-term therapy.
- Institute emergency procedures if overdose occurs: gastric lavage, induction of emesis, supportive therapy.

### Drug-specific teaching points

- Take drug with food or meals if GI upset occurs; take only the prescribed dosage.
- Dizziness, drowsiness can occur (avoid driving or using dangerous machinery).
- Report sore throat, fever, rash, itching, weight gain, swelling in ankles or fingers, changes in vision, black, tarry stools.

## flutamide

***(floo' ta mide)***

Eulexin

**Pregnancy Category D**

### Drug classes

Antiandrogen

### Therapeutic actions

A nonsteroidal agent, it exerts potent antiandrogenic activity by inhibiting androgen uptake or by inhibiting nuclear binding of androgen in target tissues.

## Indications

- Treatment of early-stage and metastatic prostatic carcinoma in combination with LHRH agonistic analogs (leuprolide acetate)

## Contraindications/cautions

- Hypersensitivity to flutamide or any component of the preparation, pregnancy, lactation.

## Dosage

**Available Forms:** Capsules—125 mg

*ADULT*

- ***Early-stage prostatic cancer:*** 125 mg PO tid.
- ***Metastatic prostatic cancer:*** Two capsules 3 ×/d PO at 8-h intervals; total daily dosage of 750 mg.

*PEDIATRIC:* Safety and efficacy not established.

## Pharmacokinetics

| *Route* | *Onset* | *Peak* | *Duration* |
|---|---|---|---|
| Oral | Varies | 2 h | 72 h |

*Metabolism:* Hepatic, $T_{1/2}$: 6 h
*Distribution:* Crosses placenta; enters breast milk
*Excretion:* Urine

## Adverse effects

- CNS: Drowsiness, confusion, depression, anxiety, nervousness
- GI: *Nausea, vomiting, diarrhea, GI disturbances*, jaundice, hepatitis, hepatic necrosis
- Hematologic: *Anemia, leukopenia,* thrombocytopenia, elevated AST, ALT
- GU: *Impotence, loss of libido*
- Dermatologic: *Rash*, photosensitivity
- Endocrine: *Gynecomastia, hot flashes*
- Other: Carcinogenesis, mutagenesis

## ■ Nursing Considerations

### Assessment

- ***History:*** Hypersensitivity to flutamide or any component of the preparation, pregnancy, lactation
- ***Physical:*** Skin color, lesions; reflexes, affect; urinary output; bowel sounds, liver evaluation; CBC, Hct, electrolytes, liver function tests

### Implementation

- Give flutamide with other drugs used for medical castration.
- Arrange for periodic monitoring of liver function tests during long-term therapy.

### Drug-specific teaching points

- Take this drug with other drugs to treat your problem. Do not interrupt dosing or stop taking these medications without consulting your health care provider.
- Periodic blood tests will be necessary to monitor the drug effects. Keep appointments for these tests.
- The following side effects may occur: dizziness, drowsiness (avoid driving or performing hazardous tasks); nausea, vomiting, diarrhea (maintain nutrition, consult dietician); impotence, loss of libido (reversible).
- Report change in stool or urine color, yellow skin, difficulty breathing, malaise.

# fluticasone propionate

*(flew **tick'** ah zone)*

Flonase, Flovent, Flovent Rotadisk

**Pregnancy Category C**

## Drug classes

Corticosteroid

## Therapeutic actions

Anti-inflammatory effect; local administration into nasal passages maximizes beneficial effects on these tissues while decreasing the likelihood of adverse effects from systemic absorption.

## Indications

- Maintenance treatment of asthma as prophylactic therapy
- Maintenance treatment of asthma patients requiring oral corticosteroid therapy
- Preventative treatment of asthma in children 4–11 y

**Contraindications/cautions**

- Contraindications: varicella, vaccinia, tuberculosis, untreated systemic fungal, bacterial, viral, or parasitic infections or ocular herpes simplex; pregnancy
- Use cautiously with adrenocortical impairment, lactation

### Dosage

**Available Forms:** Nasal spray—50 μg/actuation; aerosal spray—44, 10, 220 μg/actuation; dischaler—50, 100 μg

ADULT

*Previously on bronchodilators alone:* 88–440 mcg intranasal bid. *Previously on inhaled corticosteroids:* 88–220 mcg intranasal bid. *Previously on oral corticosteroids:* 880 mcg nasal bid.

PEDIATRIC: 50–600 μg bid via dischaler (Flovent Rotadisk)

**Pharmacokinetics**

| *Route* | *Onset* | *Peak* | *Duration* |
|---|---|---|---|
| Intranasal | Immediate | Rapid | 8–12 h |

*Metabolism:* Hepatic; $T_{1/2}$: unknown

*Distribution:* Crosses placenta; may enter breast milk

*Excretion:* Unchanged in urine

**Adverse effects**

- CNS: *Headache*
- Respiratory: *Upper respiratory infections,* epistaxis, rebound congestion, pharyngitis, cough, **bronchospasm**
- Endocrine: HPA suppression, Cushing's syndrome with overdosage and systemic absorption
- Local: *Nasal irritation, rhinitis, nasal congestion/discharge, sinusitis, oral candidiasis,* fungal infection
- Other: *Flulike illness*

## ■ Nursing Considerations

### Assessment

- *History:* Untreated local or systemic infections, nasal trauma, septal ulcers, recent nasal surgery, pregnancy, lactation, adrenocortical impairment
- *Physical:* BP, P, auscultation, R, adventitious sounds, examination of nares

### Implementation

- Do not administer as primary treatment for acute asthma attack.
- Avoid contact with eyes.
- Monitor adrenocortical function before and periodically during thrapy.
- Arrange to taper systemic steroids carefully during transfer to inhalational steroids; deaths owing to adrenal insufficiency have occurred.
- Arrange for use of decongestant nose drops to facilitate penetration if edema occurs or excessive secretions are present.
- Provide positioning to facilitate breathing.

### Drug-specific teaching points

- Do not take this drug as primary treatment during an acute asthma attack.
- Take this drug as prescribed. Do not stop using this drug without consulting your health care provider.
- Avoid contact with eyes.
- It may take several weeks to achieve maximum effects; do not stop taking the drug if effects are not immediate.
- You should administer decongestant nose drops first if nasal passages are blocked.
- The following side effects may occur: local irritation (make sure that you are using your device correctly); upper respiratory infections, flush (notify health care provider).
- Report sore mouth, sore throat, thrush, severe headache, fatigue, flulike illness.

# fluvastatin

*(flue va **sta'** tin)*

Lescol

**Pregnancy Category X**

**Drug classes**

Antihyperlipidemic

**Therapeutic actions**

A fungal metabolite that inhibits the enzyme HMG-CoA that catalyzes the first step in the cholesterol synthesis pathway, resulting in a decrease in serum cholesterol, serum LDLs (associated with increased risk of CAD), and either an increase or no change in serum HDLs (associated with decreased risk of CAD).

### Indications

- Adjunct to diet in the treatment of elevated total cholestrol and LDL cholesterol with primary hypercholesterolemia (types IIa and IIb) where response to dietary restriction of satruated fat and cholesterol and other nonpharmacologic measures has not been adequate.

### Contraindications/cautions

- Contraindications: allergy to fluvastatin, fungal byproducts, pregnancy, lactation.
- Use cautiously with impaired hepatic function, cataracts.

### Dosage

**Available Forms:** Capsules—20, 40 mg

*ADULT:* Initial dosage: 20 mg/d PO administered in the evening. Maintenance doses: 20–40 mg/d PO as a single evening dose.

*PEDIATRIC:* Safety and efficacy not established.

### Pharmacokinetics

| *Route* | *Onset* | *Peak* |
|---|---|---|
| Oral | Slow | 4–6 wk |

*Metabolism:* Hepatic, $T_{1/2}$: unknown
*Distribution:* Crosses placenta; enters breast milk
*Excretion:* Bile and feces

### Adverse effects

- CNS: *Headache, blurred vision*, dizziness, insomnia, fatigue, muscle cramps, cataracts
- GI: *Flatulence, abdominal pain, cramps, constipation, nausea,* dyspepsia, heartburn
- **Hematologic**: Elevations of CPK, alkaline phosphatase and transaminiases

### Clinically important drug-drug interactions

- Possible severe myopathy or rhabdomyolysis if taken with cyclosporine, erythromycin, gemfibrozil, niacin

## ■ Nursing Considerations

### Assessment

- ***History:*** Allergy to fluvastatin, fungal byproducts; impaired hepatic function; cataracts (use caution); pregnancy; lactation
- ***Physical:*** Orientation, affect, ophthalmologic exam; liver evaluation; lipid studies, liver function tests

### Implementation

- Give in the evening; highest rates of cholesterol synthesis are between midnight and 5 AM.
- Arrange for regular follow-up during long-term therapy.
- Arrange for periodic ophthalmologic exam to check for cataract development.

### Drug-specific teaching points

- Take drug in the evening.
- Institute dietary changes.
- The following side effects may occur: nausea (small, frequent meals may help); headache, muscle and joint aches and pains (may lessen).
- Arrange to have periodic ophthalmic exams while you are on this drug.
- Report severe GI upset, changes in vision, unusual bleeding or bruising, dark urine or light-colored stools.

## fluvoxamine maleate

*(floo **vox'** a meen)*

Luvox

**Pregnancy Category C**

### Drug classes

Selective serotinin reuptake inhibitor (SSRI)

### Therapeutic actions

Selectively inhibits CNS neuronal uptake of serotonin; blocks uptake of serotonin with weak effect on norepinephrine; little affinity for muscarinic, histaminergic and $a_1$-adrenergic receptors.

### Indications
- Treatment of obsessive-compulsive disorder
- Unlabeled use—treatment of depression

### Contraindications/cautions
- Contraindications: hypersensitivity to fluvoxamine, lactation.
- Use cautiously with impaired hepatic or renal function, suicidal tendencies, seizures, mania, ECT therapy, CV disease, labor and delivery, pregnancy.

### Dosage
**Available Forms:** Tablets—50, 100 mg

ADULT: Initially 50 mg PO hs. Increase in 50 mg increments at 4–7 d intervals. Usual range 100–300 mg/d. Divide doses over 100 mg and give larger dose hs.

PEDIATRIC: Safety and efficacy not established for < 18 y.

GERIATRIC OR HEPATIC IMPAIRED: Give a reduced dose, titrate more slowly.

### Pharmacokinetics

| *Route* | *Onset* | *Peak* |
|---|---|---|
| Oral | Rapid | 2–8 h |

*Metabolism:* Hepatic metabolism; $T_{1/2}$: 15 h

*Distribution* : Crosses placenta; passes into breast milk

*Excretion* : Urine

### Adverse effects
- CNS: *Headache, nervousness, insomnia, drowsiness, anxiety, tremor, dizziness, lightheadedness,* agitation, sedation, abnormal gait, convulsions
- GI: *Nausea, vomiting, diarrhea, dry mouth, anorexia, dyspepsia, constipation, taste changes,* flatulence, gastroenteritis, dysphagia, gingivitis
- **Dermatologic**: *Sweating, rash, pruritus,* acne, alopecia, contact dermatitis
- **Respiratory**: *Upper respiratory infections, pharyngitis,* cough, dyspnea, bronchitis, rhinitis
- GU: *sexual dysfunction, frequency,* cystitis, impotence, urgency, vaginitis

### Clinically important drug-drug interactions
• Do not administer with terfenadine, astemizole, MAO inhibitors (during or within 14 d). • Increased effects of triazolam, alprazolam, warfarin, carbamazepine, methadone, beta blockers, diltiazem. Reduced dosages of these drugs will be needed. • Decreased effects due to increased metabolism in cigarette smokers.

f

## ■ Nursing Considerations

### Assessment
- ***History:*** Hypersensitivity to fluvoxamine; lactation; impaired hepatic or renal function; suicidal tendencies; seizures; mania; ECT therapy; CV disease; labor and delivery; pregnancy
- ***Physical:*** Weight; T; skin rash, lesions; reflexes; affect; bowel sounds; liver evaluation; P, peripheral perfusion; urinary output; renal function; renal and liver function tests; CBC

### Implementation
- Give lower or less frequent doses in elderly patients, and with hepatic or renal impairment.
- Establish suicide precautions for severly depressed patients. Limit quantity of capsules dispensed.
- Administer drug at bedtime, if dose exceeds 100 mg, divide dose and administer the largest dose at bedtime.
- Monitor patient for therapeutic response for up to 4–7 d before increasing dose.

### Drug-specific teaching points
- Take this drug at bedtime; if a large dose is needed, the dose may be divided, but take the largest dose at bedtime.
- The following side effects may occur: dizziness, drowsiness, nervousness, insomnia (avoid driving or performing hazardous tasks), nausea, vomiting, weight loss (small frequent meals may help), sexual dysfunction (reversible).
- Report rash, mania, seizures, severe weight loss.

# folic acid

*(foe' lik)*

folacin, pteroylglutamic acid, folate

Rolvite

**Pregnancy Category A**

## Drug classes
Folic acid

## Therapeutic actions
Active reduced form of folic acid; required for nucleoprotein synthesis and maintenence of normal erythropoiesis.

## Indications
- Treatment of megoblastic anemias due to sprue, nutritional deficiency, pregnancy, infancy, and childhood

## Contraindications/cautions
- Contraindications: allergy to folic acid preparations; pernicious, aplastic, normocytic anemias.
- Use cautiously during lactation.

## Dosage
**Available Forms:** Tablets—0.4, 0.8, 1 mg; injection—5 mg/ml

Administer orally unless severe intestinal malabsorption is present.

ADULT
- *Therapeutic dose:* Up to 1 mg/d PO, IM, IV, or SC. Larger doses may be needed in severe cases.
- *Maintainence dose:* 0.4 mg/d.
- *Pregnancy and lactation:* 0.8 mg/d.

PEDIATRIC
- *Maintenance*
  - *INFANTS:* 0.1 mg/d.
  - *<4 Y:* Up to 0.3 mg/d.
  - *>4 Y:* 0.4 mg/d.

## Pharmacokinetics

| Route | Onset | Peak |
|---|---|---|
| Oral, IM, SC, IV | Varies | 30–60 min |

*Metabolism:* Hepatic, $T_{1/2}$: unknown
*Distribution:* Crosses placenta; enters breast milk
*Excretion:* Urine

## IV facts
**Preparation:** Solution is yellow to yellow-orange; may be added to hyperalimentation solution or dextrose solutions.
**Infusion:** Infuse at rate of 5 mg/min by direct IV injection; may be diluted in hyperalimentation for continuous infusion.

## Adverse effects
- Hypersensitivity: Allergic reactions
- Local: *Pain and discomfort at injection site*

## Clinically important drug-drug interactions
• Decrease in serum phenytoin and increase in seizure activity with folic acid preparations • Decreased absorption with sulfasalazine, aminosalicyclic acid

## ■ Nursing Considerations

### Assessment
- *History:* Allergy to folic acid preparations; pernicious, aplastic, normocytic anemias; lactation
- *Physical:* Skin lesions, color; R, adventitious sounds; CBC, Hgb, Hct, serum folate levels, serum vitamin $B_{12}$ levels, Schilling test

### Implementation
- Administer orally if at all possible. With severe GI malabsorption or very severe disease, give IM, SC, or IV.
- Test using Schilling test and serum vitamin $B_{12}$ levels to rule out pernicious anemia. Therapy may mask signs of pernicious anemia while the neurologic deterioration continues.
- Use caution when giving the parenteral preparations to premature infants. These preparations contain benzyl alcohol, may produce a fatal gasping syndrome in premature infants.
- Monitor patient for hypersensitivity reactions, especially if drug previously taken. Maintain supportive equipment and emergency drugs on standby in case of serious allergic response.

### Drug-specific teaching points

- When the cause of megaloblastic anemia is treated or passes (infancy, pregnancy), there may be no need for foic acid because it normally exists in sufficient quantities in the diet.
- Report rash, difficulty breathing, pain or discomfort at injection site.

## follitropin alfa

*(fol i **tro'** pin)*
Gonal-F
**Pregnancy Category X**

### Drug classes
Fertility drug
GnRH (gonadotropic releasing hormone)

### Therapeutic actions
Human follicle stimulating hormone (FSH) made from recombinant DNA technology; stimulates ovarian follicular growth and maturation in women who do not have primary ovarian failure; to effect ovulation, human chorionic gonadotropin (HCG) must be given when the follicles are sufficiently mature.

### Indications
- Induction of ovulation and pregnancy in anovulatory infertile patients in whom the cause of the infertility is functional and not caused by primary ovarian failure
- Stimulation and development of multiple follicles in ovulatory patients undergoing in vitro fertilization

### Contraindications/cautions
- Contraindications: primary ovarian failure; overt thyroid or adrenal dysfunction; organic cranial lesion; abnormal uterine bleeding of undertermined origin; ovarian cysts or enlargement not due to polycystic ovary syndrome, pregnancy (fetal defects have occurred), hypersensitivity to follitropins.
- Use cautiously with lactation, respiratory disease, history of thrombi.

### Dosage
**Available Forms:** Powder for injection—75, 150 IU

***Ovulation induction:*** Initial dose of the first cycle—75 IU/d SC; increase by 37.5 IU/d after 14 d; further dosage increases may be made after 7 d if needed. Do not exceed 35 d of treatment. If serum estradiol levels indicate follicular development (>2,000 pg/ml), 5,000 U HCG should be give 1 d after the last dose of follitropin alfa to complete follicular development and effect ovulation. Doses of subsequent cycles of follitropin alfa should be based on response to preceding cycle. > 300 IU/d is not recommended.

***Follicle stimulation:*** Initial dose of 150 IU/d SC should be given on cycle day 2 or 3; continue for up to 10 d. Administer 5,000–10,000 U HCG once adequate follicular development has occurred. Up to 225 IU/d may be necessary in some cases.

### Pharmacokinetics

| *Route* | *Onset* | *Peak* |
|---|---|---|
| SC | Slow | 16 h |

*Metabolim:* Hepatic; $T_{1/2}$: 24–32 h
*Distribution:* Crosses placenta; passes into breast milk
*Excretion:* Urine

### Adverse effects
- CNS: Headache
- GI: *Abdominal discomfort,* distention, bloating, nausea, vomiting, diarrhea
- CV: **Arterial thromboembolism**
- GU: Uterine bleeding, *ovarian enlargement,* breast tenderness, ectopic pregnancy, *ovarian overstimulation* (abdominal distention, pain, accompaied in more serious cases by ascites, pleural effusion), multiple births, birth defects in resulting pregnancies
- **Local:** *Pain, rash, swelling or irritation at injection site*
- **Other:** Febrile reaction—fever, chills, musculoskeletal aches or pain, malaise, fatigue

## ■ Nursing Considerations

### Assessment

- *History:* Known sensitivity to follitropin, high levels of FSH, LH indicating primary ovarian failure; overt thyroid or adrenal dysfunction; organic cranial lesion; abnormal uterine bleeding of undetermined origin; ovarian cysts or enlargement not due to polycystic ovary syndrome, pregnancy, lactation, history of pulmonary disorders, thrombi
- *Physical:* Skin color, temperature; injection site; R, adventitious sounds; abdominal exam, pelvic exam; urinary pregnanandiol and gonadotropin, abdominal ultrasound

### Implementation

- Arrange for a complete pelvic exam before each course of treatment to rule out ovarian enlargement, pregnancy, other uterine difficulties.
- Caution patient about the risks of multiple births, drug effects, and need for medical evaluation and follow-up.
- Dissolve contents of 1 or more ampules in 0.5–1 ml of Sterile Water for Injection; do not exceed concentration of 225 IU/0.5 ml. Store in refrigerator and protect from light. Use immediately after reconstitution; discard any unused portions.
- Administer SC only; monitor injection sites for signs of swelling, irritation.
- Discontinue drug at any sign of ovarian overstimulation and arrange to have patient admitted to the hospital for observation and supportive measures.
- Examine patient at least every other day for signs of excessive ovarian stimulation during treatment and during a 2 wk posttreatment period.
- Provide women with calendar of treatment days and explanations about what to watch for for signs of ovulation. Caution patient that 24 h urine collections, serum blood tests or abdominal ultrasound will be needed periodically to determine drug effects on the ovaries and that timing of intercourse is important for achieving pregnancy. Patient should engage in intercourse daily beginning on the day prior to HCG administration until ovulation is apparent from determination of progestational activity.

### Drug-specific teaching points

- Prepare a calendar showing the treatment schedule and plotting out ovulation, etc.
- The following side effects may occur: abdominal distention, flushing, breast tenderness, pain, rash, swelling at injection site.
- There is an increased incidence of multiple births in women using this drug.
- Report bloating, stomach pain, fever, chills, muscle aches or pains, abdominal swelling, back pain, swelling or pain in the legs, pain at injection sites, difficulty breathing.

## follitropin beta

*(fol i **tro'** pin)*

Follistin

**Pregnancy Category X**

### Drug classes

Fertility drug
Gonadotropin

### Therapeutic actions

Human follicle stimulating hormone (FSH) made from recombinant DNA technology; stimulates ovarian follicular growth and maturation in women who do not have primary ovarian failure; to effect ovulation, human chorionic gonadotropin (HCG) must be given when the follicles are sufficiently mature.

### Indications

- Induction of ovulation and pregnancy in anovulatory infertile patient in whom the cause of the infertility is functional and not caused by primary ovarian failure
- Stimulation and development of multiple follicles in ovulatory patients undergoing in vitro fertilization

### Contraindications/cautions

- Contraindications: primary ovarian failure; overt thyroid or adrenal dysfunction; organic cranial lesion; abnormal uterine bleeding of undertermined origin; ovarian cysts or enlargement not due to poly-

cystic ovary syndrome, pregnancy (fetal defects have occurred), hypersensitivity to follitropins.
- Use cautiously with lactation, respiratory disease, history of thrombi.

### Dosage

**Available Forms:** Powder for injection—75 IU

***Ovulation induction:*** Initial dose of the first cycle—75 IU/d SC or IM; increase by 37.5 IU/d after 14 d; further dosage increases may be made after 7 d if needed. Do not exceed 35 d of treatment. If serum estradiol levels indicate follicular development (> 2,000 pg/ml), 5,000–10,000 U HCG should be given 1 d after the last dose of follitropin alfa to complete follicular development and effect ovulation. Doses of subsequent cycles of follitropin alfa should be based on response to preceding cycle. > 300 IU/d is not recommended.

***Follicle stimulation:*** Initial dose of 150–225 IU/d SC or IM should be given on cycle day 2 or 3; continue for up to 10 d. Adminster 5,000–10,000 U HCG once adequate follicular development has occurred. Maintenance doses of 375–600 IU/d SC or IM may be necessary.

### Pharmacokinetics

| *Route* | *Onset* | *Peak* |
|---|---|---|
| SC, IM | Slow | 27 h |

*Metabolism:* $T_{1/2}$: 30 h
*Distribution:* Crosses placenta; passes into breast milk
*Excretion:* Urine

### Adverse effects

- CNS: Headache
- GI: *Abdominal discomfort,* distention, bloating, nausea, vomiting, diarrhea
- CV: **Arterial thromboembolism**
- GU: Uterine bleeding, *ovarian enlargement,* breast tenderness, ectopic pregnancy, *ovarian overstimulation* (abdominal distention, pain, accompanied in more serious cases by ascites, pleural effusion), multiple births, birth defects in resulting pregnancies
- **Local:** *Pain, rash, swelling or irritation at injection site*
- **Other:** Febrile reaction—fever, chills, musculoskeletal aches or pain, malaise, fatigue

## ■ Nursing Considerations

### Assessment

- ***History:*** Known sensitivity to follitropin, high levels of FSH, LH indicating primary ovarian failure; overt thyroid or adrenal dysfunction; organic cranial lesion; abnormal uterine bleeding of undetermined origin; ovarian cysts or enlargement not due to polysystic ovary syndrome, pregnancy, lactation, history of pulmonary disorders, thrombi
- ***Physical:*** Skin color, temperature; T; injection site; R, adventitious sounds; abdominal exam, pelvic exam; urinary pregnanadiol and gonadotropin, abdominal ultrasound

### Implementation

- Arrange for a complete pelvic exam before each course of treatment to rule out ovarian enlargement, pregnancy, other uterine difficulties.
- Caution patient of the risks of multiple births, drug effects, and need for medical evaluation and follow-up.
- Inject 1 ml of 0.45% Sodium Chloride Injection into the vial, *do not shake,* gently swirl until solution is clear. Store powder in refrigerator, protect from light. Use immediately after reconstitution and discard any unused portion.
- Administer SC in the abdomen or naval or inject IM, preferably in the upper outer buttocks muscle; stretch skin and inject swiftly to decrease pain; monitor injection sites for signs of swelling, irritation.
- Teach patient and significant other proper technique for storage, reconstitution and administration if home administration will be used.
- Discontinue drug at any sign of ovarian overstimulation and arrange to have pa-

tient admitted to the hospital for observation and supportive measures.

- Examine patient at least every other day for signs of excessive ovarian stimulation during treatment and during a 2 wk post-treatment period.
- Provide women with calendar of treatment days and explanations about what to watch for for signs of ovulation.
- Caution patient that 24 h urine collections, serum blood tests or abdominal ultrasound will be needed periodically to determine drug effects on the ovaries and that timing of intercourse is important for achieving pregnancy. Patient should engage in intercourse daily beginning on the day prior to HCG administration until ovulation is apparent from determination of progestational activity.

### Drug-specific teaching points

- Prepare a calendar showing the treatment schedule and plotting out ovulation, etc.
- The following side effects may occur: abdominal distention, flushing, breast tenderness, pain, rash swelling at injection site.
- There is an increased incidence of multiple births in women using this drug.
- Report bloating, stomach pain, fever, chills, muscle aches or pain, abdominal swelling, back pain, swelling or pain in the legs, pain at injection sites, difficulty breathing.

## foscarnet sodium

*(foss **kar'** net)*

Foscavir

**Pregnancy Category C**

### Drug classes

Antiviral

### Therapeutic actions

Inhibits replication of all known herpes viruses by selectively inhibiting specific DNA and RNA enzymes.

### Indications

- Treatment of CMV retinitis in patients with AIDS; combination therapy with ganciclovir for patients who have relapsed after monotherapy with either drug
- Treatment of cyclovir-resistant HSV infections in immunocompromised patients

### Contraindications/cautions

- Allergy to foscarnet.
- Use cautiously during lactation.

### Dosage

**Available Forms:** Injection—24 mg/ml

ADULT

- ***CMV retinitis***
  - *Induction:* 60 mg/kg q8h IV for 2–3 wk.
  - *Maintenance:* 90–120 mg/kg IV.
- ***HSV infection***
  - *Induction:* 40 mg/kg IV q8–12 h for 2–3 wk or until healed.

GERIATRIC OR RENAL IMPAIRED: Monitor patient carefully; if Ccr falls below 0.4 ml/min/kg, discontinue therapy.

### Pharmacokinetics

| Route | Onset |
|---|---|
| IV | Immediate |

*Metabolism:* $T_{1/2}$: 1.4–3 h

*Distribution:* Crosses placenta; enters breast milk

*Excretion:* Urine

### IV facts

**Preparation:** Give with Normal Saline, 5% Dextrose Solution.

**Infusion:** Infuse slowly. Induction dose infuse over a minimum of 1 h using an infusion pump. Maintenance dose: infuse over 2 h using an infusion pump to control rate.

**Incompatibilities:** Do not mix in the same catheter with anything but Normal Saline or 5% Dextrose Solution. Incompatible with 30% Dextrose, amphotericin B, solutions containing calcium; acyclovir sodium, ganciclovir, trimetrexate, pentamidine, vancomycin, trimethoprim/sulfamethoxazole, diazepam, disazolam, digoxin, phenytoin, leucovorin, prochlorperazine.

**Adverse effects**

- CNS: *Headache, seizures,* paresthesia, tremor, ataxia, abnormal coordination, **coma, death**, depression, confusion, anxiety, insomnia, nervousness, emotional lability, vision changes, taste abnormalities
- GI: *Nausea, vomiting, diarrhea,* abdominal pain, dry mouth, melena, pancreatitis
- Respiratory: Cough, dyspnea, pneumonia, sinusitis, pharyngitis
- Hematologic: **Bone marrow suppression**, *anemia*, mineral and electrolyte imbalance
- Renal: **Acute renal failure, *abnormal renal functions,* dysuria, polyuria, urinary retention, urinary tract infections**
- Other: *Fever;* fatigue, rash, pain, edema, pain at site of injection

**Clinically important drug-drug interactions**

• Increased risk of renal problems with other renal toxic drugs • Risk of hypocalcemia with pentamidine

## ■ Nursing Considerations

### Assessment

- *History:* Presence of allergy to foscarnet, lactation
- *Physical:* Skin color, lesions; T; orientation, reflexes, affect; urinary output; R, adventitious sounds; CBC, serum electrolytes, renal function tests

### Implementation

- Give by IV route only; do give by bolus or rapid injection.
- Monitor serum creatinine and renal function carefully during treatment; dosage adjustment may be necessary.
- Stop infusion immediately at any report of tingling, paresthesias, numbness. Monitor electrolytes.
- Ensure adequate hydration during treatment; push fluids to ensure diuresis and decrease the risk of renal impairment.
- Arrange for periodic ophthalmic exams for retinitis; foscarnet is not a cure.

### Drug-specific teaching points

- This drug must be given IV using a special pump.
- Foscarnet is not a cure for retinitis; symptoms may continue. Arrange for periodic ophthalmic exams.
- Drink a lot of fluids, and you may also receive a lot of IV fluids.
- Arrange for periodic medical exams, including blood tests.
- The following side effects may occur: fever, headache (medication may be ordered); dizziness, fatigue, vision changes (do not drive or operate dangerous machinery); nausea, vomiting, diarrhea.
- Report tingling around the mouth, numbness, "heavy" extremities, difficulty breathing, leg cramps, tremors, pain at injection site.



## fosfomycin tromethamine

*(foss foe my' sin)*

Monurol

**Pregnancy Category B**

**Drug classes**

Antibacterial
Urinary tract anti-infective

**Therapeutic actions**

Bactericidal; interferes with bacterial cell wall synthesis, blocks adherence of bacteria to uroepithelial cells.

**Indications**

- Uncomplicated urinary tract infections in women caused by susceptible strains of *E. coli* and *E. Faecalis*; not indicated for the treatment of pyelonephritis or perinephric abscess

**Contraindications/cautions**

- Contraindications: allergy to fosfomycin.
- Use cautiously with pregnancy, lactation.

### Dosage

**Available Forms:** Granule packet—3 g

*ADULT:* 1 packet dissolved in water PO.

*PEDIATRIC < 18 Y:* Not recommended.

## Pharmacokinetics

| Route | Onset | Peak |
| --- | --- | --- |
| Oral | Rapid | 2–4 h |

*Metabolism:* Hepatic; $T_{1/2}$: 5.7 h
*Distribution:* Crosses placenta; passes into breast milk
*Excretion:* Urine and feces

## Adverse effects

- CNS: *Headache, dizziness,* back pain, asthenisa
- GI: *Nausea,* abdominal cramps, dyspepsia
- GU: Vaginitis, dysmenorrhea
- Other: Rhinitis, rash

## Clinically important drug-drug interactions

- Lowered serum concentration and urinary tract excretion with metoclopramide

## ■ Nursing Considerations

### Assessment

- ***History:*** Allergy to fosfomycin, pregnancy, lactation
- ***Physical:*** Skin color, lesions; orientation, reflexes; urine for analysis

### Implementation

- Arrange for culture and sensitivity tests.
- Administer drug with food if GI upset occurs.
- Do not administer dry; mix a single dose packet in 90–120 ml of water and stir to dissolve; do not use hot water. Administer immediately.
- Monitor clinical response; if no improvement is seen or a relapse occurs, send urine for repeat culture and sensitivity.
- Encourage patient to observe other measures (avoid bubble baths, alkaline ash foods, sexual intercourse; drink lots of fluids) to decrease risk of urinary tract infection.

### Drug-specific teaching points

- This drug is meant to be a one dose treatment for urinary tract infection; improvement should be seen in 2–3 days. If no improvement occurs, consult your health care provider.
- Take drug with food if GI upset occurs. Do not take in the dry form; mix a single dose packet in 90–120 ml of water and stir to dissolve; do not use hot water. Drink immediately after mixing.
- The following side effects may occur: nausea, abdominal pain (eat small, frequent meals; take the drug with meals); dizziness (observe caution if driving or using dangerous equipment).
- Report rash, visual changes, severe GI problems, weakness, tremors, worsening of urinary tract symptoms.

# fosinopril sodium

*(foh **sin'** oh pril)*

Monopril

**Pregnancy Category D**

## Drug classes

Antihypertensive
Angiotensin converting enzyme inhibitor (ace inhibitor)

## Therapeutic actions

Renin, synthesized by the kidneys, is released into the circulation where it acts on a plasma precursor to produce angiotensin I, which is converted by angiotensin-converting enzyme to angiotensin II, a potent vasoconstrictor that also causes release of aldosterone from the adrenals; fosinopril blocks the conversion of angiotensin I to angiotensin II, leading to decreased BP, decreased aldosterone secretion, a small increase in serum potassium levels, and sodium and fluid loss; increased prostaglandin synthesis may be involved in the antihypertensive action.

## Indications

- Treatment of hypertension, alone or in combination with thiazide-type diuretics
- Management of CHF as adjunctive therapy

## Contraindications/cautions

- Contraindications in the presence of allergy to fosinopril or other ACE inhibitors.

- Use cautiously with impaired renal function, CHF, salt/volume depletion, lactation.

Dosage

Available Forms: Tablets—10, 20, 40 mg

ADULT: Initial dose: 10 mg PO qd. Maintenance dose: 20–40 mg/d PO as a single dose or two divided doses. Discontinue diuretics 2–3 d before beginning fosinopril. If BP is not controlled, add diuretic slowly. If diuretic cannot be discontinued, begin fosinopril therapy with 10 mg.

PEDIATRIC: Safety and efficacy not established.

### Pharmacokinetics

| *Route* | *Onset* | *Peak* | *Duration* |
|---|---|---|---|
| Oral | 1 h | 3 h | 24 h |

*Metabolism:* Hepatic, $T_{1/2}$: 12 h

*Distribution:* Crosses placenta; enters breast milk

*Excretion:* Urine and feces

### Adverse effects

- GI: *Nausea*, abdominal pain, vomiting, diarrhea
- CV: Angina pectoris, orthostatic hypotension in salt/volume depleted patients, palpitations
- **Respiratory**: *Cough,* asthma, bronchitis, dyspnea, sinusitis
- **Dermatologic**: Rash, pruritus, diaphoresis, flushing
- **Other**: Angioedema, asthenia, myalgia, arthralgia

## ■ Nursing Considerations

### Assessment

- *History:* Allergy to fosinopril and other ACE inhibitors, impaired renal function, CHF, salt/volume depletion, lactation
- *Physical:* Skin color, lesions, turgor; T; P, BP, peripheral perfusion; mucous membranes, bowel sounds, liver evaluation; urinalysis, renal and liver function tests, CBC, and differential

### Implementation

- Alert surgeon and mark patient's chart with notice that fosinopril is being taken; the angiotensin II formation subsequent to compensatory renin release during surgery will be blocked; hypotension may be reversed with volume expansion.
- Monitor patient closely for a fall in BP secondary to reduction in fluid volume (excessive perspiration and dehydration, vomiting, diarrhea) because excessive hypotension may occur.

### Drug-specific teaching points

- Do not stop taking the medication without consulting your prescriber.
- The following side effects may occur: GI upset, loss of appetite (these may be transient); lightheadedness (transient; change position slowly and limit activities to those that do not require alertness and precision); dry cough (not harmful).
- Be careful in any situation that may lead to a drop in BP (diarrhea, sweating, vomiting, dehydration); if lightheadedness or dizziness occurs, consult your care provider.
- Report mouth sores; sore throat, fever, chills; swelling of the hands, feet; irregular heartbeat, chest pains; swelling of the face, eyes, lips, tongue, difficulty in breathing, persistent cough.

## fosphenytoin sodium

*(faws **fen'** i toe in)*

Cerebyx

**Pregnancy Category D**

### Drug classes

Antiepileptic agent

Hydantoin

### Therapeutic actions

A metabolite of phenytoin that has antiepileptic activity without causing general CNS depression; stabilizes neuronal membranes and prevents hyperexcitability caused by excessive stimulation; limits the spread of seizure activity from an active focus.

## Indications

- Short-term control of general convulsive status epilepticus
- Prevention and treatment of seizures occurring during or following neurosurgery

## Contraindications/cautions

- Contraindications: hypersensitivity to hydantoins, sinus bradycardia, sinoatrial block, second- or third-degree AV heart block, Stokes-Adams syndrome, pregnancy (data suggest an association between use of antiepileptic drugs by women with epilepsy and an elevated incidence of birth defects in children born to these women; however, do not discontinue antiepileptic therapy in pregnant women who are receiving therapy to prevent major seizures—this is likely to precipitate status epilepticus, with attendant hypoxia and risk to both mother and unborn child); lactation
- Use cautiously with hypotension, hepatic dysfunction

### Dosage

**Available Forms:** Injection—150, 750 mg/vial

Dosage is given as phenytoin equivalents (PE) to facilitate transfer from phenytoin.

ADULT

- ***Status epilepticus:*** Loading dose of 15–20 mg PE/kg administered at 100–150 mg PE/min.
- ***Neurosurgery (prophylaxis):*** Loading dose of 10–20 mg PE/kg IM or IV; maintenance dose of 4–6 mg PE/kg/d.

PEDIATRIC: Not recommended.

RENAL AND HEPATIC IMPAIRMENT: Use caution and monitor for early signs of toxicity—handling of the metabolism of the drug may result in increased risk of adverse effects.

## Pharmacokinetics

| Route | Onset | Peak |
|---|---|---|
| IV | Rapid | End of infusion |

*Metabolism:* Hepatic; $T_{1/2}$: 15 min

*Distribution:* Crosses placenta; enters breast milk

*Excretion:* Urine

### IV facts

**Preparation:** Dilute in 5% Dextrose or 0.9% Saline Solution to a concentration of 1.5–25 mg PE/mL. Refrigerate; stable at room temperature for $<$48 h.

**Infusion:** Infuse for status epilepticus at rate of 100–150 mg PE/min; never administer at a rate $>$150 mg PE/min.

## Adverse effects

- CNS: *Nystagmus, ataxia, dizziness, somnolence,* drowsiness, insomnia, transient nervousness, motor twitchings, fatigue, irritability, depression, numbness, tremor, headache, photophobia, diplopia, asthenia, back pain
- GI: *Nausea,* vomiting, dry mouth, taste perversion
- CV: *Hypotension,* vasodilation, tachycardia
- **Dermatologic:** *Pruritus*
- **Other:** Lymph node hyperplasia, sometimes progressing to frank malignant lymphoma, monoclonal gammopathy and multiple myeloma (prolonged therapy), polyarthropathy, osteomalacia, weight gain, chest pain, periarteritis nodosa

## Clinically important drug-drug interactions

No specific drug interactions have been reported, but since fosphenytoin is a metabolite of phenytoin, documented interactions with that drug should be considered.

• Increased pharmacologic effects or hydantoins with chloramphenicol, cimetidine, disulfiram, phenacemide, phenylbutazone, sulfonamides, trimethoprim; reduced fosphenytoin dose may be needed • Complex interactions and effects when phenytoin and valproic acid are given together; phenytoin toxicity with apparently normal serum phenytoin levels; decreased plasma levels of valproic acid given with phenytoin; breakthrough seizures when the two drugs are given together • Increased pharmacologic effects and toxicity when primidone, oxyphenbutazone, amiodarone, chloramphenicol, fluconazole, isoniazid are given with hydantoins • Decreased pharmacologic effects of the following with hydantoins: corticosteroids, cyclosporine, dicumarol, disopyramide, doxycycline, estrogens, furosemide, levodopa, methadone, metyrapone, mexiletine, oral contraceptives, quinidine, atracurium, gallamine triethiodide, metocurine, pancuronium, tubocurarine, vecuronium, carbamazepine, diazoxide

**Drug-lab test interferences**

• Interference with metyrapone and 1-mg dexamethasone tests for at least 7 d

## ■ Nursing Considerations

### Assessment

- *History:* Hypersensitivity to hydantoins; sinus bradycardia, sinoatrial block, second- or third-degree AV heart block, Stokes-Adams syndrome, pregnancy, lactation, hepatic failure
- *Physical:* T; skin color, lesions; orientation, affect, reflexes, vision exam; P, BP; bowel sounds, normal output, liver evaluation; liver function tests, urinalysis, CBC and differential, EEG and ECG

### Implementation

- Continue supportive measures, including use of an IV benzodiazepine, until drug becomes effective against seizures.
- Administer IV slowly to prevent severe hypotension; margin of safety between full therapeutic and toxic doses is small. Continually monitor cardiac rhythm and check BP frequently and regularly during IV infusion and for 10–20 min after infusion.
- Monitor infusion site carefully—drug solutions are very alkaline and irritating.
- This drug is recommended for short-term use only (up to 5 d); switch to oral phenytoin as soon as possible.

### Drug-specific teaching points

- This drug can only be given IV and will be stopped as soon as you are able to take an oral drug.
- The following side effects may occur: drowsiness, dizziness, GI upset.
- Report skin rash, severe nausea or vomiting, drowsiness, slurred speech, impaired coordination (ataxia), sore throat, unusual bleeding or bruising, persistent headache, malaise, pain at injection site.

# furosemide

*(fur oh' se mide)*

Lasix, Novosemide (CAN), Uritol (CAN)

**Pregnancy Category C**

**Drug classes**

Loop diuretic

**Therapeutic actions**

Inhibits the reabsorption of sodium and chloride from the proximal and distal renal tubules and the loop of Henle, leading to a sodium-rich diuresis.

**Indications**

- Edema associated with CHF, cirrhosis, renal disease (oral, IV)
- Acute pulmonary edema (IV)
- Hypertension (oral)

**Contraindications/cautions**

- Contraindications: allergy to furosemide, sulfonamides; allergy to tartrazine (in oral solution); electrolyte depletion; anuria, severe renal failure; hepatic coma; pregnancy; lactation.
- Use cautiously with SLE, gout, diabetes mellitus.

### Dosage

**Available Forms:** Tablets—20, 40, 80 mg; oral solution—10 mg/ml, 40 mg/5 ml; injection—10 mg/ml

ADULT

- *Edema:* Initially, 20–80 mg/d PO as a single dose. If needed, a second dose may be given in 6–8 h. If response is unsatisfactory, dose may be increased in 20- to 40-mg increments at 6- to 8-h intervals. Up to 600 mg/d may be given. Intermittent dosage schedule (2–4 consecutive d/wk) is preferred for maintenance, *or* 20–40 mg IM or IV (slow IV injection over 1–2 min). May increase dose in increments of 20 mg in 2 h. High-dose therapy should be given as infusion at rate not exceeding 4 mg/min.

- *Acute pulmonary edema:* 40 mg IV over 1–2 min. May be increased to 80 mg IV given over 1–2 min if response is unsatisfactory after 1 h.
- *Hypertension:* 40 mg bid PO. If needed, additional antihypertensive agents may be added at 50% usual dosage.

PEDIATRIC: Avoid use in premature infants: stimulates $PGE_2$ synthesis and may increase incidence of patent ductus arteriosus and complicate respiratory distress syndrome.

- *Hypertension:* Initially, 2 mg/kg per day PO. If needed, increase by 1–2 mg/kg in 6–8 h. *Do not exceed* 6 mg/kg. Adjust maintenance dose to lowest effective level.
- *Edema:* 1 mg/kg IV or IM. May increase by 1 mg/kg in 2 h until the desired effect is seen. *Do not exceed* 6 mg/kg.

GERIATRIC OR RENAL IMPAIRED: Up to 2–2.5 g/d has been tolerated. IV bolus injection should not exceed 1 g/d given over 30 min.

## Pharmacokinetics

| *Route* | *Onset* | *Peak* | *Duration* |
|---|---|---|---|
| Oral | 60 min | 60–120 min | 6–8 h |
| IV/IM | 5 min | 30 min | 2 h |

*Metabolism:* Hepatic, $T_{1/2}$: 120 min
*Distribution:* Crosses placenta; enters breast milk
*Excretion:* Urine

### IV facts

**Preparation:** Store at room temperature; exposure to light may slightly discolor solution.
**Infusion:** Inject directly or into tubing of actively running IV; inject slowly over 1–2 min.
**Incompatibilites:** Do not mix with acidic solutions. Isotonic saline, Lactated Ringer's Injection, and 5% Dextrose Injection may be used after pH has been adjusted (if necessary); precipitates form with gentamicin, netilimicin, milrinone in 5% Dextrose, 0.9% Sodium Chloride.

## Adverse effects

- CNS: *Dizziness, vertigo, paresthesias, xanthopsia, weakness,* headache, drowsiness, fatigue, blurred vision, tinnitus, irreversible hearing loss
- GI: *Nausea, anorexia, vomiting, oral and gastric irritation, constipation;* diarrhea, acute pancreatitis, jaundice
- CV: *Orthostatic hypotension,* volume depletion, cardiac arrhythmias, *thrombophlebitis*
- **Hematologic:** *Leukopenia, anemia, thrombocytopenia,* fluid and electrolyte imbalances
- GU: Polyuria, nocturia, *glycosuria, urinary bladder spasm*
- **Dermatologic:** *Photosensitivity, rash, pruritus, urticaria,* purpura, exfoliative dermatitis, erythema multiforme
- **Other:** *Muscle cramps and muscle spasms*

## Clinically important drug-drug interactions

• Increased risk of cardiac arrhythmias with digitalis glycosides (due to electrolyte imbalance) • Increased risk of ototoxicity with aminoglycoside antibiotics, cisplatin • Decreased absorption of furosemide with phenytoin • Decreased natriuretic and antihypertensive effects with indomethacin, ibuprofen, other NSAIDs • Decreased GI absorption with charcoal

## ■ Nursing Considerations

### Assessment

- *History:* Allergy to furosemide, sulfonamides, tartrazine; electrolyte depletion anuria, severe renal failure; hepatic coma; SLE; gout; diabetes mellitus; lactation
- *Physical:* Skin color, lesions, edema; orientation, reflexes, hearing; pulses, baseline ECG, BP, orthostatic BP, perfusion; R, pattern, adventitious sounds; liver evaluation, bowel sounds; urinary output patterns; CBC, serum electrolytes (including calcium), blood sugar, liver and renal function tests, uric acid, urinalysis

### Implementation

- Administer with food or milk to prevent GI upset.
- Reduce dosage if given with other antihypertensives; readjust dosages gradually as BP responds.
- Give early in the day so that increased urination will not disturb sleep.
- Avoid IV use if oral use is at all possible.
- Do not mix parenteral solution with highly acidic solutions with pH below 3.5.
- Do not expose to light, may discolor tablets or solution; do not use discolored drug or solutions.
- Discard diluted solution after 24 h.
- Refrigerate oral solution.
- Measure and record weight to monitor fluid changes.
- Arrange to monitor serum electrolytes, hydration, liver function.
- Arrange for potassium-rich diet or supplemental potassium as needed.

### Drug-specific teaching points

- Record intermittent therapy on a calendar or dated envelopes. When possible, take the drug early so increased urination will not disturb sleep. Take with food or meals to prevent GI upset.
- Weigh yourself on a regular basis, at the same time and in the same clothing, and record the weight on your calendar.
- The following side effects may occur: increased volume and frequency of urination; dizziness, feeling faint on arising, drowsiness (avoid rapid position changes; hazardous activities, like driving; and consumption of alcohol); sensitivity to sunlight (use sunglasses, wear protective clothing, or use a sunscreen); increased thirst (suck on sugarless lozenges; use frequent mouth care); loss of body potassium (a potassium-rich diet or potassium supplement, will be necessary).
- Report loss or gain of more than 3 lb in one day, swelling in your ankles or fingers, unusual bleeding or bruising, dizziness, trembling, numbness, fatigue, muscle weakness or cramps.

## gabapentin

*(gab ah **pen'** tin)*

Neurontin

**Pregnancy Category C**

### Drug classes

Antiepileptic agent

### Therapeutic actions

Mechanism of action not understood; antiepileptic activity may be related to its ability to inhibit polysynaptic responses and block post-tetanic potentiation.

### Indications

- Adjunctive therapy in the treatment of partial seizures with and without secondary generalization in adults with epilepsy

### Contraindications/cautions

- Hypersensitivity to gabapentin, lactation.

### Dosage

**Available Forms:** Capsules—100, 300, 400 mg

**ADULT:** 900–1,800 mg/d PO in divided doses 3×/d PO; maximum time between doses should not exceed 12 h. Up to 2,400–3,600 mg/d has been used. Initial dose of 300 mg/d PO; 300 mg bid PO on day 2; 300 tid PO on day 3.

**PEDIATRIC:** Safety and efficacy not established.

**GERIATRIC OR RENAL IMPAIRED:** Creatinine clearance > 60 ml/min: 400 mg tid PO; 30–60 ml/min: 300 mg bid PO; 15–30 ml/min: 300 mg qd PO; < 15 ml/min: 300 mg qod PO; dialysis: 200–300 mg PO following each 4 h of dialysis.

### Pharmacokinetics

| *Route* | *Onset* | *Duration* |
|---|---|---|
| Oral | Varies | 6–8 h |

*Metabolism:* $T_{1/2}$: 5–7 h

*Distribution:* Crosses placenta; enters breast milk

*Excretion:* Urine

### Adverse effects

- CNS: *Dizziness, insomnia,* nervousness, fatigue, *somnolence, ataxia,* diplopia
- GI: Dyspepsia, vomiting, nausea, constipation
- Respiratory: Rhinitis, pharyngitis
- Dermatologic: Pruritus, abrasion
- Other: Weight gain, facial edema, cancer, impotence

### Clinically important drug-drug interactions

- Decreased serum levels with antacids

## ■ Nursing Considerations

### Assessment

- *History:* Hypersensitivity to gabapentin; lactation
- *Physical:* Weight; T; skin color, lesions; orientation, affect, reflexes; P; R, adventitious sounds; bowel sounds, normal output

### Implementation

- Give drug with food to prevent GI upset.
- Arrange for consultation with support groups for epileptics.

### Drug-specific teaching points

- Take this drug exactly as prescribed; do not discontinue abruptly or change dosage, except on the advice of your physician.
- The following side effects may occur: dizziness, blurred vision (avoid driving or performing other tasks requiring alertness or visual acuity); GI upset (take drug with food or milk, eat frequent small meals); headache, nervousness, insomnia; fatigue (periodic rest periods may help).
- Wear a medical alert tag at all times so that any emergency medical personnel will know that you are an epileptic taking antiepileptic medication.
- Report severe headache, sleepwalking, skin rash, severe vomiting, chills, fever, difficulty breathing.

## gallium nitrate

*(gal' ee um)*

Ganite

**Pregnancy Category C**

### Drug classes

Antihypercalcemic

### Therapeutic actions

Inhibits calcium resorption from bone, reduces bone turnover, resulting in lower serum calcium levels.

### Indications

- Treatment of cancer-related hypercalcemia (clearly symptomatic) unresponsive to adequate hydration

### Contraindications/cautions

- Contraindications: severe renal impairment, lactation.
- Use cautiously with asymptomatic or mild to moderate hypocalcemia, visual and auditory disturbances, pregnancy.

### Dosage

**Available Forms:** Injection—25 mg/ml

ADULT: 200 mg/$m^2$ IV per day for 5 consecutive d; 100 mg/$m^2$ IV per day may be effective in mild hypercalcemia.

PEDIATRIC: Safety and efficacy not established.

### Pharmacokinetics

| Route | Onset | Peak | Duration |
|---|---|---|---|
| IV | Slow | 2 d | 3–4 d |

*Metabolism:* $T_{1/2}$: unknown

*Distribution:* May cross placenta; may enter breast milk

*Excretion:* Urine

### IV facts

**Preparation:** Dilute daily dose in 1 L 0.9% Sodium Chloride Injection or 5% Dextrose Injection. Stable for 48 h at room temperature and 7 d refrigerated; discard any unused portion after that time.

**Infusion:** Infuse slowly over 24 h.

**Incompatibilities:** Do not mix with IV anesthetics; precipitates may form.

### Adverse effects

- CNS: Acute optic neuritis, visual impairment, decreased hearing
- GI: Nausea, vomiting, diarrhea, constipation

- GU: *Rising BUN, creatinine*; **acute renal failure**
- CV: Tachycardia, edema, decreased BP
- Respiratory: Dyspnea, rales and rhonchi, pleural effusion, pulmonary infiltrates
- Metabolic: *Hypocalcemia; decreased serum bicarbonate*

### Clinically important drug-drug interactions

- Increased risk of nephrotoxicity with other nephrotoxic drugs: aminoglycosides, amphotericin B

## ■ Nursing Considerations

### Assessment

- ***History:*** Severe renal impairment, lactation, hypocalcemia, visual and auditory disturbances, pregnancy
- ***Physical:*** Weight, skin condition, hydration, reflexes, P, BP, R and adventitious sounds, kidney function tests, serum electrolytes, especially calcium, phosphorus

### Implementation

- Monitor serum calcium, phosphorus, renal function daily during therapy and twice weekly thereafter.
- Discontinue gallium if serum creatinine exceeds 2.5 mg/dl.
- Discontinue gallium therapy if serum calcium levels return to normal before the 5-d course is finished.
- Maintain adequate hydration; use caution to avoid overhydraton if patient is cardiac compromised.

### Drug-specific teaching points

- This drug can be given only IV and must be given for 5 consecutive d; frequent blood tests will be needed to evaluate the drug effects.
- Report difficulty breathing, very slow breathing, changes in vision or hearing, numbness or tingling.

## ganciclovir sodium

*(gan sye' kloe vir)*

DHPG

Cytovene

**Pregnancy Category C**

### Drug classes

Antiviral

### Therapeutic actions

Antiviral activity; inhibits viral DNA replication in CMV.

### Indications

- Treatment of CMV retinitis in immunocompromised patients, including patients with AIDS (IV)
- Prevention of CMV disease in transplant recipients at risk for CMV disease (IV)
- Alternative to IV for maintenance treatment of CMV retinitis (PO)
- Prevention of CMV disease in individuals with advanced HIV infection at risk of developing CMV disease (oral)
- Unlabeled use: Treatment of other CMV infections in immunocompromised patients

### Contraindications/cautions

- Contraindications: hypersensitivity to ganciclovir or acyclovir, lactation.
- Use cautiously with cytopenia, history of cytopenic reactions, impaired renal function.

### Dosage

**Available Forms:** Capsules—250 mg; powder for injection—500 mg/vial

**ADULT**

- ***CMV retinitis:*** Initial dose: 5 mg/kg given IV at a constant rate over 1 h, q12h for 14–21 d. Maintenance: 5 mg/kg given by IV infusion over 1 h once/d, 7 d/wk *or* 6 mg/kg once/d, 5 d/wk; or 1000 mg PO tid with food or 500 mg PO 6×/d every 3 h with food while awake.
- ***Prevention of CMV disease in transplant recipients:*** 5 mg/kg IV over 1 h q12h for 7–14 d; then 5 mg/kg/d once daily for 7 d/wk, or 6 mg/kg/d once daily for 5 d/wk.
- ***Prevention of CMV disease with advanced AIDS:*** 1000 mg PO tid with food.

**PEDIATRIC:** Safety and efficacy not established. Use only if benefit outweighs potential carcinogenesis and reproductive toxicity.

*GERIATRIC OR RENAL IMPAIRED:* Reduce initial dose by up to 50%, monitoring patient response. Maintenance dose:

| *Creatinine Clearance* | *Dose IV (mg/kg)* | *Dosing Intervals (h)* |
|---|---|---|
| ≥80 | 5 | 12 |
| 50–79 | 2.5 | 12 |
| 25–49 | 2.5 | 24 |
| <25 | 1.25 | 24 |

| *Creatinine Clearance* | *Dose PO (mg)* |
|---|---|
| ≥70 | 1000 tid or 500 q3h 6×/d |
| 50–69 | 1500 qd or 500 tid |
| 25–49 | 1000 qd or 500 bid |
| 10–24 | 500 qd |
| <10 | 500 3×/wk followed by dialysis |

### Pharmacokinetics

| *Route* | *Onset* | *Peak* |
|---|---|---|
| IV | Slow | 1 h |
| Oral | Slow | 2–4 h |

*Metabolism:* $T_{1/2}$: 2–4 h (IV), 4.8 h (PO)
*Distribution:* Crosses placenta; may enter breast milk
*Excretion:* Urine and feces

### IV facts

**Preparation:** Reconstitute vial by injecting 10 ml of Sterile Water for Injection into vial; *do not* use Bacteriostatic Water for Injection; shake vial to dissolve the drug. Discard vial if any particulate matter or discoloration is seen. Reconstituted solution in the vial is stable at room temperature for 12 h. *Do not refrigerate* reconstituted solution.
**Infusion:** Infuse slowly over 1 h.
**Compatibilities:** Compatible with 0.9% Sodium Chloride, 5% Dextrose, Ringer's Injection, and Lactated Ringer's Injection.

### Adverse effects

- CNS: Dreams, ataxia, coma, confusion, dizziness, headache
- GI: *Abnormal liver function tests*, nausea, vomiting, anorexia, diarrhea, abdominal pain
- CV: Arrhythmia, hypertension, hypotension
- Hematologic: *Granulocytopenia, thrombocytopenia, anemia*
- Dermatologic: *Rash,* alopecia, pruritus, urticaria
- Local: *Pain, inflammation at injection site*, phlebitis
- Other: *Fever*, chills, **cancer, sterility**

### Clinically important drug-drug interactions

• Increased effects if taken with probenecid • Use with extreme caution with cytotoxic drugs because the accumulation effect could cause severe bone marrow depression and other GI and dermatologic problems • Increased risk of seizures with imipenem-cilastatin • Extreme drowsiness and risk of bone marrow depression with zidovudine

## ■ Nursing Considerations

### Assessment

- *History:* Hypersensitivity to ganciclovir or acyclovir; cytopenia; impaired renal function; lactation
- *Physical:* Skin color, lesions; orientation; BP, P, auscultation, perfusion, edema; R, adventitious sounds; urinary output; CBC, Hct, BUN, creatinine clearance, liver function tests

### Implementation

- Give by IV infusion only. Do not give IM or SC; drug is very irritating to tissues.
- Do not exceed the recommended dosage, frequency, or infusion rates.
- Monitor infusion carefully; infuse at concentrations no greater than 10 mg/ml.
- Decrease dosage in patients with impaired renal function.
- Give oral doses with food.
- Obtain CBC before therapy, every 2 d during daily dosing, and at least weekly thereafter. Consult with physician and arrange for reduced dosage if WBCs or platelets fall.
- Consult with pharmacy for proper disposal of unused solution. Precautions are required for disposal of nucleoside analogues.

- Provide patient with a calendar of drug days, and arrange convenient times for the IV infusion in outpatients.
- Arrange for periodic ophthalmic examinations. Drug is not a cure for the disease, and deterioration may occur.
- Advise patients that ganciclovir can decrease sperm production and cause birth defects in fetuses. Advise the patient to use contraception during ganciclovir therapy. Men receiving ganciclovir therapy should use barrier contraception during and for at least 90 d after ganciclovir therapy.
- Advise patient that ganciclovir has caused cancer in animals and that risk is possible in humans.

### Drug-specific teaching points

- This drug will need to be given daily and can be given only via IV line. Appointments will be made for outpatients on IV therapy. Long-term therapy is frequently needed. Take the oral drug with food.
- Frequent blood tests will be necessary to determine drug effects on your blood count and to adjust drug dosage. Keep appointments for these tests.
- Arrange for periodic ophthalmic examinations during therapy to evaluate progress of the disease. This drug is not a cure for your retinitis.
- If you also are receiving zidovudine, the two drugs cannot be given concomitantly; severe adverse effects may occur.
- The following side effects may occur: rash, fever, pain at injection site; decreased blood count leading to susceptibility to infection (frequent blood tests will be needed; avoid crowds and exposure to disease); birth defects and decreased sperm production (drug must not be taken during pregnancy; if pregnant or intending to become pregnant, consult with your physician; use some form of contraception during therapy; male patients should use barrier contraception during therapy and for at least 90 d after therapy).
- Report bruising, bleeding, pain at injection site, fever, infection.

## gemcitabine hydrochloride

*(jem site' ah ben)*

Gemzar

**Pregnancy Category D**

### Drug classes

Antineoplastic

### Therapeutic actions

Cytotoxic: a nucleoside analog that is cell cycle S specific; causes cell death by disrupting and inhibiting DNA synthesis

### Indications

- First-line treatment of locally advanced or metastatic adenocarcinoma of pancreas; indicated for patients who have previously received 5-FU

### Contraindications/cautions

- Contraindication: hypersensitivity to gemcitabine
- Use cautiously with bone marrow suppression, renal or hepatic impairment, pregnancy, lactation

### Dosage

**Available Forms:** Powder—20 mg/ml

**ADULT:** 1000 mg/m$^2$ IV over 30 min given once weekly for up to 7 wk or until bone marrow suppression requires withholding treatment; subsequent cycles of once weekly for 3 consecutive wk out of 4 can be given after 1-wk rest from treatment. Patients who require further therapy and have not experienced severe toxicity may be given 25% larger dose with careful monitoring.

**PEDIATRIC:** Safety and efficacy not established.

### Pharmacokinetics

| Route | Onset | Peak |
|---|---|---|
| IV | Rapid | 30 min |

*Metabolism:* Hepatic; $T_{1/2}$: 42–70 min

*Distribution:* Crosses placenta; may enter breast milk

*Excretion:* Bile and urine

g

### IV facts

**Preparation:** Use 0.9% Sodium Chloride Injection as diluent for reconstitution of powder, 5 ml of 0.9% Sodium Chloride Injection added to the 200-mg vial or 25 ml added to the 1-g vial. This will yield a concentration of 40 mg/ml; higher concentrations may lead to inadequate dissolution of powder. Resultant drug can be injected as reconstituted or further diluted in 0.9% Sodium Chloride Injection. Stable for 24 h at room temperature after reconstitution.

**Infusion:** Infuse slowly over 30 min.

### Adverse effects

- CNS: Somnolence, paresthesias
- GI: *Nausea, vomiting,* diarrhea, constipation, mucositis, GI bleeding, stomatitis, hepatic dysfunction
- Hematologic: **Bone marrow depression,** *infections*
- Pulmonary: Dyspnea
- Renal: Hematuria, proteinuria, elevated BUN and creatinine
- Other: *Fever, alopecia, pain, rash*

## ■ Nursing Considerations

### Assessment

- ***History:*** Hypersensitivity to gemcitabine; bone marrow depression; renal or hepatic dysfunction; pregnancy, lactation
- ***Physical:*** T; skin color, lesions; R, adventitious sounds; abdominal exam, mucous membranes; liver and renal function tests, CBC with differential, UA

### Implementation

- Follow CBC, renal and liver function tests carefully before and frequently during therapy; dosage adjustment may be needed if myelosuppression becomes severe or hepatic or renal dysfunction occurs.
- Protect patient from exposure to infection; monitor occurrence of infection at any site and arrange for appropriate treatment.
- Provide medication, frequent small meals for severe nausea and vomiting; monitor nutritional status.

### Drug-specific teaching points

- This drug will need to be given IV over 30 min once a wk. Mark calendar with days to return for treatment. Regular blood tests will be needed to evaluate the effects of treatment.
- The following side effects may occur: nausea and vomiting (may be severe; antiemetics may be helpful; eat small, frequent meals); increased susceptibility to infection (avoid crowds and situations that may expose you to diseases); loss of hair (arrange for a wig or other head covering; keep the head covered at extremes of temperature).
- Report severe nausea and vomiting, fever, chills, sore throat, unusual bleeding or bruising, changes in color of urine or stool.

## gemfibrozil

*(jem fi' broe zil)*

Apo-Gemfibrozil (CAN), Lopid, NOVO-Gemfibrozil (CAN)

**Pregnancy Category B**

### Drug classes

Antihyperlipidemic

### Therapeutic actions

Inhibits peripheral lipolysis and decreases the hepatic excretion of free fatty acids; this reduces hepatic triglyceride production; inhibits synthesis of VLDL carrier apolipoprotein; decreases VLDL production; increases HDL concentration.

### Indications

- Hypertriglyceridemia in adult patients with triglyceride levels > 750 mg/dl (type IV and V hyperlipidemia) at risk of abdominal pain and pancreatitis unresponsive to diet therapy
- Reduction of coronary heart disease risk, possibly effective

### Contraindications/cautions

- Allergy to gemfibrozil, hepatic or renal dysfunction, primary biliary cirrhosis, gallbladder disease, pregnancy, lactation.

### Dosage

**Available Forms:** Tablets—60 mg

*ADULT:* 1,200 mg/d PO in two divided doses, 30 min before morning and evening meals. Adjust dosage to patient response; dosages may range from 900–1,500 mg/d. *Caution:* Use only if strongly indicated and lipid studies show a definite response; hepatic tumorigenicity occurs in laboratory animals.

*PEDIATRIC:* Safety and efficacy not established.

### Pharmacokinetics

| Route | Onset | Peak |
|---|---|---|
| Oral | Varies | 1–2 h |

*Metabolism:* Hepatic, $T_{1/2}$: 1 1/2 h

*Distribution:* Crosses placenta; enters breast milk

*Excretion:* Urine and feces

### Adverse effects

- CNS: *Headache, dizziness, blurred vision*, vertigo, insomnia, paresthesia, tinnitus, *fatigue*, malaise, syncope
- GI: *Abdominal pain, epigastric pain, diarrhea, nausea, vomiting*, flatulence, dry mouth, constipation, anorexia, *dyspepsia*, cholelithiasis
- **Hematologic**: Anemia, eosinophilia, leukopenia, hypokalemia, liver function changes, hyperglycemia
- GU: Impairment of fertility
- **Dermatologic**: *Eczema, rash*, dermatitis, pruritus, urticaria
- **Other**: Painful extremities, back pain, arthralgia, muscle cramps, myalgia, swollen joints

### Clinically important drug-drug interactions

- Risk of rhabdomyolysis from 3wk to several mo after therapy when combined with Hmg-CoA inhibitors (lovastatin, simvastatin)

## ■ Nursing Considerations

### Assessment

- *History:* Allergy to gemfibrozil, hepatic or renal dysfunction, primary biliary cirrhosis, gallbladder disease, pregnancy, lactation
- *Physical:* Skin lesions, color, temperature; gait, range of motion; orientation, affect, reflexes; bowel sounds, normal output, liver evaluation; lipid studies, CBC, liver and renal function tests, blood glucose

### Implementation

- Administer drug with meals or milk if GI upset occurs.
- Arrange for regular follow-up, including blood tests for lipids, liver function, CBC, blood glucose during long-term therapy.

### Drug-specific teaching points

- Take the drug with meals or with milk if GI upset occurs; diet changes will need to be made.
- The following side effects may occur: diarrhea, loss of appetite, flatulence (small, frequent meals may help); muscular aches and pains, bone and joint discomfort; dizziness, faintness, blurred vision (use caution if driving or operating dangerous equipment).
- Have regular follow-up visits to your doctor for blood tests to evaluate drug effectiveness.
- Report severe stomach pain with nausea and vomiting, fever and chills or sore throat, severe headache, vision changes.

g

# gentamicin sulfate

*(jen ta **mye'** sin)*

*Parenteral, intrathecal:* Alcomicin (CAN), Cidomycin (CAN), Garamycin, Jenamicin

*Topical dermatologic cream, ointment:* Garamycin, G-myticin

*Ophthalmic:* Garamycin, Gentak, Gentacidin, Genoptic

*Gentamicin impregnated PMMA beads:* Septopal, Gentamicin Liposome injection

**Pregnancy Category C**

## Drug classes
Aminoglycoside

## Therapeutic actions
Bactericidal: inhibits protein synthesis in susceptible strains of gram-negative bacteria; appears to disrupt functional integrity of bacterial cell membrane, causing cell death.

## Indications
*Parenteral*
- Serious infections caused by susceptible strains of *Pseudomonas aeruginosa, Proteus, Escherichia coli, Klebsiella-Enterobacter-Serratia* species, *Citrobacter,* staphylococci
- In serious infections when causative organisms are not known (often in conjunction with a penicillin or cephalosporin)
- Unlabeled use: with clindamycin as alternative regimen in PID

*Intrathecal*
- For serious CNS infections caused by susceptible *Pseudomonas* species

*Ophthalmic Preparations*
- Treatment of superficial ocular infections due to strain of microorganisms susceptible to gentamicin

*Topical Dermatologic Preparation*
- Infection prophylaxis in minor skin abrasions and treatment of superficial infections of the skin due to susceptible organisms amenable to local treatment

*Gentamicin-Impregnated PMAA Beads on Surgical Wire*
- Orphan drug use: treatment of chronic osteomyelitis of post-traumatic, postoperative, or hematogenous origin

*Gentamicin Liposome Injection*
- Orphan drug use: treatment of disseminated *Myobacterium avium-intracellulare* infection

## Contraindications/cautions
- Contraindications: allergy to any aminoglycosides; renal or hepatic disease; preexisting hearing loss; active infection with herpes, vaccinia, varicella, fungal infections, myobacterial infections (ophthalmic preparations); myasthenia gravis; parkinsonism; infant botulism; lactation.
- Use caution during pregnancy.

## Dosage
**Available Forms:** Injection—2, 10, 40 mg/ml; ophthamic solution—3 mg/ml; ophthamic ointment—3 mg/g; topical ointment—0.1%; topical cream—0.1%; ointment—1 mg; cream—1 mg

ADULT: 3 mg/kg per day in 3 equal doses q8h IM or IV. Up to 5 mg/kg per day in 3–4 equal doses in severe infections. For IV use, a loading dose of 1–2 mg/kg may be infused over 30–60 min, followed by a maintenance dose.
- *PID:* 2 mg/kg IV followed by 1.5 mg/kg tid plus clindamycin 600 mg IV qid. Continue for at least 4 d and at least 48 h after patient improves, then continue clindamycin 450 mg orally qid for 10–14 d total therapy.
- ***Surgical prophylaxis regimens:*** Several complex, multidrug prophylaxis regimens are available for preoperative use; consult manufacturer's instructions.

PEDIATRIC: 2–2.5 mg/kg q8h IM or IV. Infants and neonates: 2.5 mg/kg q8h. Premature or full-term neonates: 2.5 mg/kg q12h.

GERIATRIC OR RENAL FAILURE PATIENTS: Reduce dosage or extend time dosage intervals, and carefully monitor serum drug levels and renal function tests.

***Ophthalmic solution:*** 1–2 drops into affected eye(s) q4h; up to 2 drops hourly in severe infections.

***Ophthalmic ointment:*** Apply small amount to affected eye bid–tid.

***Dermatologic preparations:*** Apply 1–5×/d. Cover with sterile bandage if needed.

## Pharmacokinetics

| *Route* | *Onset* | *Peak* |
|---|---|---|
| IM/IV | Rapid | 30–90 min |

*Metabolism:* $T_{1/2}$: 2–3 h

*Distribution:* Crosses placenta; enters breast milk

*Excretion:* Urine

### IV facts
**Preparation:** Dilute single dose in 50–200 ml of sterile isotonic saline or 5% Dextrose in Water. Do not mix in solution with any other drugs.

**Infusion:** Infuse over 1/2–2 h.
**Incompatibilities:** Do not mix in solution with any other drugs.

### Adverse effects

- CNS: Ototoxicity—*tinnitus, dizziness,* vertigo, **deafness** (partially reversible to irreversible), vestibular paralysis, confusion, disorientation, depression, lethargy, nystagmus, visual disturbances, headache, *numbness, tingling*, tremor, paresthesias, muscle twitching, convulsions, muscular weakness, neuromuscular blockade
- GI: Hepatic toxicity, *nausea, vomiting, anorexia,* weight loss, stomatitis, increased salivation
- CV: Palpitations, hypotension, hypertension
- Hematologic: *Leukemoid reaction,* agranulocytosis, granulocytosis, leukopenia, leukocytosis, thrombocytopenia, eosinophilia, pancytopenia, anemia, hemolytic anemia, increased or decreased reticulocyte count, electrolyte disturbances
- GU: *Nephrotoxicity*
- Hypersensitivity: *Purpura, rash*, urticaria, exfoliative dermatitis, itching
- Local: *Pain, irritation, arachnoiditis at IM injection sites*
- Other: Fever, apnea, splenomegaly, joint pain, *superinfections*

*Ophthalmic Preparations*

- Local: *Transient irritation, burning, stinging, itching,* angioneurotic edema, urticaria, vesicular and maculopapular dermatitis

*Topical Dermatologic Preparations*

- Local: *photosensitization,* superinfections

### Clinically important drug-drug interactions

• Increased ototoxic, nephrotoxic, neurotoxic effects with other aminoglycosides, cephalothin, potent diuretics • Increased neuromuscular blockade and muscular paralysis with anesthetics, nondepolarizing neuromuscular blocking drugs, succinylcholine, citrate-anticoagulated blood • Potential inactivation of both drugs if mixed with beta-lactam-type antibiotics (space doses with concomitant therapy) • Increased bactericidal effect with penicillins, cephalopsorins (to treat some gram-negative organisms and enterococci) carbenicillin, ticarcillin (to treat *Pseudomonas* infections)

## ■ Nursing Considerations

### Assessment

- ***History:*** Allergy to any aminoglycosides; renal or hepatic disease; preexisting hearing loss; active infection with herpes, vaccinia, varicella, fungal infections, myobacterial infections (ophthalmic preparations); myasthenia gravis; parkinsonism; infant botulism; lactation
- ***Physical:*** Site of infection; skin color, lesions; orientation, reflexes, eighth cranial nerve function; P, BP ; R, adventitious sounds; bowel sounds, liver evaluation; urinalysis, BUN, serum creatinine, serum electrolytes, liver function tests, CBC

### Implementation

- Give by IM route if at all possible; give by deep IM injection.
- Culture infected area before therapy.
- Use 2 mg/ml intrathecal preparation without preservatives, for intrathectal use.
- Cleanse area before application of dermatologic preparations.
- Ensure adequate hydration of patient before and during therapy.
- Monitor renal function tests, complete blood counts, serum drug levels during long-term therapy. Consult with prescriber to adjust dosage.

### Drug-specific teaching points

- Apply ophthalmic preparations by tilting head back; place medications into conjunctival sac and close eye; apply light pressure on lacrimal sac for 1 min. Cleanse area before applying dermatologic preparations; area may be covered if necessary.
- The following side effects may occur: ringing in the ears, headache, dizziness (reversible; use safety measures if severe); nausea, vomiting, loss of appetite (small frequent meals, frequent mouth care may

help); burning, blurring of vision with ophthalmic preparations (avoid driving or performing dangerous activities if visual effects occur); photosensitization with dermatologic preparations (wear sunscreen and protective clothing).
- Report pain at injection site, severe headache, dizziness, loss of hearing, changes in urine pattern, difficulty breathing, rash or skin lesions; itching or irritation (ophthalmic preparations); worsening of the condition, rash, irritation (dermatologic preparation).

## glatiramer acetate

*(gla **tear'** ah mer)*

Copaxone

**Pregnancy Category B**

### Drug classes
Multiple sclerosis agent

### Therapeutic actions
Mechanism of action is unknown; it is thought to modify the immune process that is thought to be responsible for the pathogenesis of multiple sclerosis.

### Indications
- Reduction of the frequency of relapses in patients with relapsing/remitting multiple sclerosis

### Contraindications/cautions
- Contraindications: allergy to glatiramer or mannitol.
- Use cautiously with pregnancy and lactation.

### Dosage
**Available Forms:** Injection—20 mg

**ADULT:** 20 mg/d SC.

**PEDIATRIC:** Safety and efficacy not established.

### Pharmacokinetics

| Route | Onset | Duration |
|---|---|---|
| SC | Slow | Unknown |

*Metabolism:* Local; $T_{1/2}$: unknown

*Distribution:* May cross placenta; may pass into breast milk

*Excretion:* Unknown

### Adverse effects
- CNS: *Anxiety, hypertonia,* tremor, vertigo, agitation
- GI: *Nausea,* GI distress, *diarrhea,* vomiting, anorexia
- CV: *Vasodilation, palpitations,* tachycardia
- Dermatologic: *Rash, pruritus, sweating,* erythema, uticaria
- Local: *Pain at injection site, erythema, inflammation, induration, mass*
- Other: *Infection, asthenia, pain, chest pain, flulike syndrome, back pain,* fever, chills, *arthralgias*

### ■ Nursing Considerations

#### Assessment
- ***History:*** Allergy to glatiramer, mannitol; pregnancy, lactation
- ***Physical:*** T; orientation, affect, reflexes; skin color, lesions; P, BP, peripheral perfusion; evaluate sites for injection

#### Implementation
- Reconstitute with diluent supplied, Sterile Water for Injection; gently swirl bottle and let stand at room temperature until all solid material is dissolved; use immediately. Refrigerate unreconstituted vial.
- Administer by SC injection in the arms, abdomen, hips and thighs. Rotate sites and keep chart of areas used.
- Encourage patient to avoid pregnancy while on this drug; use of barrier contraceptives is recommended.
- Offer supportive care to deal with the unpleasant side effects of this drug.

#### Drug-specific teaching points
- This drug must be give by SC injection; you and a significant other should learn to administer the drug. Refrigerate drug until ready to use; dilute with diluent provided, gently swirl bottle and let stand at room temperature until all solid material is dissolved. Use immediately.

- Keep chart of sites used for injection, rotate sites; abdomen, arms, thigh and hips can be used.
- Do not become pregnant while on this drug; use of barrier contraceptives is advised. If you think that you are pregnant, consult your health care provider immediately.
- The following side effects may occur: nausea, diarrhea, GI distress (take the drug with meals); sweating, flushing, rash (temperature control and frequent skin care may help); pain and swellling at the injection site (rotate sites daily, observe sterile technique).
- Report chest pain, difficulty breathing, sever GI upset, rash, sever pain at injection site, continued swelling or hardening of injection sites.

## glimepiride

*(glye **meh'** per ide)*
Amaryl
**Pregnancy Category B**

### Drug classes
Antidiabetic agent
Sulfonylurea (second generation)

### Therapeutic actions
Stimulates insulin release from functioning beta cells in the pancreas; may improve binding between insulin and insulin receptors or increase the number of insulin receptors; thought to be more potent in effect than first-generation sulfonylureas.

### Indications

### Contraindications/cautions
- Contraindications: allergy to sulfonylureas; diabetes complicated by fever, severe infections, severe trauma, major surgery, ketosis, acidosis, coma (insulin is indicated in these conditions); Type I or juvenile diabetes, serious hepatic or renal impairment, uremia, thyroid or endocrine impairment, glycosuria, hyperglycemia associated with primary renal disease; labor and delivery—if glimepride is used during pregnancy, discontinue drug at least 1 mo before delivery; lactation, safety not established.

### Dosage
**Available Forms:** Tablets—1, 2, 4 mg

**ADULT:** Usual starting dose is 1–2 mg PO once daily with breakfast or first meal of the day; usual maintenance dose is 1–4 mg PO once daily, depending on patient response and glucose levels. Do not exceed 8 mg/d.
- ***Combination with insulin therapy:*** 8 mg PO qd with first meal of the day with low-dose insulin.
- ***Transfer from other hypoglycemic agents:*** No transition period is necessary.

**PEDIATRIC:** Safety and efficacy not established.

**RENAL IMPAIRED:** Usual starting dose is 1 mg PO once daily; titrate dose carefully, lower maintenance doses may be sufficient to control blood sugar.

### Pharmacokinetics

| Route | Onset | Peak |
|---|---|---|
| Oral | 1 h | 2–3 h |

*Metabolism:* Hepatic; $T_{1/2}$: 5.5–7 h
*Distribution:* Crosses placenta; enters breast milk
*Excretion:* Bile and urine

### Adverse effects
- CV: **Increased risk of cardiovascular mortality**
- GI: *Anorexia, nausea,* vomiting, *epigastric discomfort, heartburn, diarrhea*
- Hematologic: Leukopenia, thrombocytopenia, anemia
- Endocrine: *Hypoglycemia*
- Hypersensitivity: *Allergic skin reactions,* eczema, pruritus, erythema, urticaria, photosensitivity, fever, eosinophilia, jaundice

### Clinically important drug-drug interactions
- Increased risk of hypoglycemia with sulfonamides, chloramphenicol, fenfluramine, oxyphenbutazone, phenylbutazone, salicy-

lates, clofibrate • Decreased effectiveness of both glimepride and diazoxide if taken concurrently • Increased risk of hyperglycemia with rifampin, thiazides • Risk of hypoglycemia and hyperglycemia with ethanol; "disulfiram reaction" has also been reported

## ■ Nursing Considerations

### Assessment

- *History:* Allergy to sulfonylureas; diabetes complicated by fever, severe infections, severe trauma, major surgery, ketosis, acidosis, coma (insulin is indicated in these conditions): Type I or juvenile diabetes, serious hepatic or renal impairment, uremia, thyroid or endocrine impairment, glycosuria, hyperglycemia associated with primary renal disease
- *Physical:* Skin color, lesions; T; orientation, reflexes, peripheral sensation; R, adventitious sounds; liver evaluation, bowel sounds; urinalysis, BUN, serum creatinine, liver function tests, blood glucose, CBC

### Implementation

- Monitor urine and serum glucose levels frequently to determine effectiveness of drug and dosage being used.
- Transfer to insulin therapy during periods of high stress (infections, surgery, trauma, etc.).
- Use IV glucose if severe hypoglycemia occurs as a result of overdose.
- Arrange for consultation with dietician to establish weight-loss program and dietary control.
- Arrange for thorough diabetic teaching program, including disease, dietary control, exercise, signs and symptoms of hypoglycemia and hyperglycemia, avoidance of infection, hygiene.

### Drug-specific teaching points

- Take this drug once a day with breakfast or the first main meal of the day.
- Do not discontinue this drug without consulting your health care provider; continue with diet and exercise program for diabetes control.
- Monitor urine or blood for glucose and ketones as prescribed.
- Do not use this drug if you are pregnant.
- Avoid alcohol while on this drug.
- Report fever, sore throat, unusual bleeding or bruising, skin rash, dark urine, light-colored stools, hypoglycemic or hyperglycemic reactions.

# glipizide

***(glip' i zide)***
Glucotrol, Glucotrol XL
**Pregnancy Category C**

### Drug classes

Antidiabetic agent
Sulfonylurea (second generation)

### Therapeutic actions

Stimulates insulin release from functioning beta cells in the pancreas; may improve binding between insulin and insulin receptors or increase the number of insulin receptors; more potent in effect than first-generation sulfonylureas.

### Indications

- Adjunct to diet to lower blood glucose with non–insulin-dependent diabetes mellitus (Type II)
- Adjunct to insulin therapy in the stabilization of certain cases of insulin-dependent maturity-onset diabetes, reducing the insulin requirement and decreasing the chance of hypoglycemic reactions

### Contraindications/cautions

- Allergy to sulfonylureas; diabetes complicated by fever, severe infections, severe trauma, major surgery, ketosis, acidosis, coma (insulin is indicated); Type I or juvenile diabetes, serious hepatic impairment, serious renal impairment, uremia, thyroid or endocrine impairment, glycosuria, hyperglycemia associated with primary renal disease; labor and delivery (if glipizide is used during pregnancy, discontinue drug at least 1 mo before delivery); lactation.

### Dosage

**Available Forms:** Tablets—5, 10 mg; ER tablets—5, 10 mg

Give approximately 30 min before meal to achieve greatest reduction in postprandial hyperglycemia.

ADULT

- *Initial therapy:* 5 mg PO before breakfast. Adjust dosage in increments of 2.5–5 mg as determined by blood glucose response. At least several days should elapse between titration steps. Maximum once-daily dose should not exceed 15 mg; above 15 mg, divide dose, and administer before meals. Do not exceed 40 mg/d.
- *Maintenance therapy:* Total daily doses above 15 mg PO should be divided; total daily doses above 30 mg are given in divided doses bid.

PEDIATRIC: Safety and efficacy not established.

GERIATRIC AND HEPATIC IMPAIRED: Geriatric patients tend to be more sensitive to the drug. Start with initial dose of 2.5 mg/d PO. Monitor for 24 h and gradually increase dose after several days as needed.

### Pharmacokinetics

| Route | Onset | Peak | Duration |
|---|---|---|---|
| Oral | 1–1.5 h | 1–3 h | 10–16 h |

*Metabolism:* Hepatic, $T_{1/2}$: 2–4 h
*Distribution:* Crosses placenta; enters breast milk
*Excretion:* Bile and urine

### Adverse effects

- GI: *Anorexia, nausea,* vomiting, *epigastric discomfort, heartburn, diarrhea*
- CV: Increased risk of CV mortality
- **Hematologic**: Leukopenia, thrombocytopenia, anemia
- **Hypersensitivity**: *Allergic skin reactions,* eczema, pruritus, erythema, urticaria, photosensitivity, fever, eosinophilia, jaundice
- Endocrine: *Hypoglycemia*

### Clinically important drug-drug interactions

• Increased risk of hypoglycemia with sulfonamides, chloramphenicol, fenfluramine, oxyphenbutazone, phenylbutazone, salicylates, clofibrate • Decreased effectiveness of glipizide and diazoxide if taken concurrently • Increased risk of hyperglycemia with rifampin, thiazides • Risk of hypoglycemia and hyperglycemia with ethanol; "disulfiram reaction" also has been reported

## ■ Nursing Considerations

### Assessment

- *History:* Allergy to sulfonylureas; diabetes with complications; Type I or juvenile diabetes, serious hepatic or renal impairment, uremia, thyroid or endocrine impairment, glycosuria, hyperglycemia associated with primary renal disease
- *Physical:* Skin color, lesions; T; orientation, reflexes, peripheral sensation; R, adventitious sounds; liver evaluation, bowel sounds; urinalysis, BUN, serum creatinine, liver function tests, blood glucose, CBC

### Implementation

- Give drug 30 min before breakfast; if severe GI upset occurs or more than 15 mg/d is required, dose may be divided and given before meals.
- Monitor urine and serum glucose levels frequently to determine drug effectiveness and dosage.
- Transfer to insulin therapy during periods of high stress (eg, infections, surgery, trauma).
- Use IV glucose if severe hypoglycemia occurs as a result of overdose.

### Drug-specific teaching points

Take this drug 30 min before breakfast for best results.

- Do not discontinue this medication without consulting physician.
- Monitor urine or blood for glucose and ketones.
- Do not use this drug during pregnancy.
- Avoid alcohol while on this drug.
- Report fever, sore throat, unusual bleeding or bruising, skin rash, dark urine,

g

light-colored stools, hypoglycemic or hyperglycemic reactions.

## glucagon

*(gloo' ka gon)*

**Pregnancy Category B**

### Drug classes

Glucose elevating agent
Hormone
Diagnostic agent

### Therapeutic actions

Accelerates the breakdown of glycogen to glucose (glycogenolysis) in the liver, causing an increase in blood glucose level; relaxes smooth muscle of the GI tract.

### Indications

- Hypoglycemia: counteracts severe hypoglycemic reactions in diabetic patients or during insulin shock therapy in psychiatric patients
- Diagnostic aid in the radiologic examination of the stomach, duodenum, small bowel, or colon when a hypotonic state is advantageous
- Unlabeled use: treatment of propranolol overdose

### Contraindications/cautions

- Insulinoma (drug releases insulin), pheochromocytoma (drug releases catecholamines), pregnancy, lactation.

### Dosage

**Available Forms:** Powder for injection—1, 10 mg

**ADULT**

- ***Hypoglycemia:*** 0.5–1.0 mg SC, IV, or IM. Response is usually seen in 5–20 min. If response is delayed, dose may be repeated one to two times.
- ***Insulin shock therapy:*** 0.5–1.0 mg SC, IV, or IM after 1 h of coma. Dose may be repeated if no response.
- ***Diagnostic aid:*** Suggested dose, route, and timing of dose vary with the segment of GI tract to be examined and duration of effect needed. Carefully check manufacturer's literature before use.

### Pharmacokinetics

| *Route* | *Onset* | *Peak* | *Duration* |
|---|---|---|---|
| IV | 1 min | 15 min | 9–20 min |
| IM | 8–10 min | 20–30 min | 19–32 min |

*Metabolism:* Hepatic, $T_{1/2}$: 3–10 min
*Distribution:* Crosses placenta; enters breast milk
*Excretion:* Bile and urine

### IV facts

**Preparation:** Reconstitute with vial provided. Use immediately; refrigerated solution stable for 48 h. If doses higher than 2 mg, reconstitute with Sterile Water for Injection and use immediately.
**Infusion:** Inject directly into the IV tubing of an IV drip infusion, each 1 mg over 1 min.
**Incompatibilities:** Compatible with dextrose solutions, but precipitates may form in solutions of sodium chloride, potassium chloride, or calcium chloride.

### Adverse effects

- **GI**: *Nausea, vomiting*
- **Hematologic**: Hypokalemia in overdose
- **Hypersensitivity**: Urticaria, respiratory distress, hypotension

### Clinically important drug-drug interactions

- Increased anticoagulant effect and risk of bleeding with oral anticoagulants

## ■ Nursing Considerations

### Assessment

- ***History:*** Insulinoma, pheochromocytoma, lactation
- ***Physical:*** Skin color, lesions, temperature; orientation, reflexes; P, BP, peripheral perfusion; R; liver evaluation, bowel sounds; blood and urine glucose, serum potassium

### Implementation

- Arouse hypoglycemic patient as soon as possible after drug injection, and provide supplemental carbohydrates to restore

liver glycogen and prevent secondary hypoglycemia.
- Arouse patient from insulin shock therapy as soon as possible, and provide oral carbohydrates and reinstitute regular dietary regimen.
- Arrange for evaluation of insulin dosage in cases of hypoglycemia as a result of insulin overdosage; insulin dosage may need to be adjusted.

### Drug-specific teaching points

- Diabetic and significant others should learn to administer the drug SC in case of hypoglycemia. They also should learn how to give drug, its use, and notification of physician.

## glutethimide

*(gloo **teth'** i mide)*

**Pregnancy Category C**
**C-II controlled substance**

### Drug classes

Sedative/hypnotic (nonbarbiturate)

### Therapeutic actions

Mechanism by which CNS is affected is not known; causes CNS depression similar to barbiturates; anticholinergic.

### Indications

- Short-term relief of insomnia (3–7 d); not indicated for chronic administration; allow a drug-free interval of 1 wk or more before retreatment

### Contraindications/cautions

- Hypersensitivity to glutethimide, porphyria, lactation.

### Dosage

**Available Forms:** Tablets—250 mg

**ADULT:** Usual dosage: 250–500 mg PO hs.

**PEDIATRIC:** Not recommended.

**GERIATRIC OR DEBILITATED:** Initial daily dosage should not exceed 500 mg PO hs to avoid oversedation.

### Pharmacokinetics

| *Route* | *Onset* | *Peak* |
|---|---|---|
| Oral | Erratic | 1–6 h |

*Metabolism:* Hepatic, $T_{1/2}$: 10–12 h

*Distribution:* Crosses placenta; enters breast milk

*Excretion:* Urine

### Adverse effects

- CNS: *Drowsiness, hangover*, suppression of REM sleep; REM rebound when drug is discontinued, mydriasis
- GI: *Nausea*, dry mouth, decreased intestinal motility
- **Hematologic:** Porphyria, blood dyscrasias
- Dermatologic: *Skin rash*
- Other: Physical, psychological dependence; tolerance; withdrawal reaction

### Clinically important drug-drug interactions

• Additive CNS depression when given with alcohol • Increased metabolism and decreased effectiveness of oral (coumarin) anticoagulants • Reduced absorption and decreased circulating levels with charcoal interactants

## ■ Nursing Considerations

### Assessment

- ***History:*** Hypersensitivity to glutethimide, porphyria, lactation
- ***Physical:*** Skin color, lesions; orientation, affect, reflexes; bowel sounds

### Implementation

- Supervise dose and amount prescribed carefully in patients who are addiction prone or alcoholic; normally a week's supply is sufficient; patient should then be reevaluated.
- Dispense least amount of drug feasible to patients who are depressed or suicidal.
- Withdraw drug gradually in long-term use or if tolerance has developed; supportive therapy similar to that for barbiturate withdrawal may be necessary to prevent dangerous withdrawal symptoms (nausea, abdominal discomfort, tremors, convulsions, delirium).
- Arrange for reevaluation of patients with prolonged insomnia. Therapy of the underlying cause (eg, pain, depression) is

preferable to prolonged therapy with sedative/hypnotic drugs.

### Drug-specific teaching points

- Take this drug exactly as prescribed. Do not exceed prescribed dosage; do not use for longer than 1 wk.
- Do not discontinue the drug abruptly; consult your health care provider if you wish to stop before instructed to do so.
- Avoid alcohol, sleep-inducing, or OTC drugs; these could cause dangerous effects.
- The following side effects may occur: drowsiness, dizziness, blurred vision (avoid driving or performing other tasks requiring alertness or visual acuity), GI upset (frequent small meals may help).
- Report skin rash.

## glyburide

*(glye' byoor ide)*

DiaBeta, Micronase, Glynase PresTab

**Pregnancy Category B**

### Drug classes

Antidiabetic agent

### Therapeutic actions

Stimulates insulin release from functioning beta cells in the pancreas; may improve binding between insulin and insulin receptors or increase the number of insulin receptors; more potent in effect than first-generation sulfonylureas.

### Indications

- Adjunct to diet to lower blood glucose with non–insulin-dependent diabetes mellitus (type II)
- Adjunct to insulin therapy in the stabilization of certain cases of insulin-dependent, maturity-onset diabetes, reducing the insulin requirement, and decreasing the chance of hypoglycemic reactions

### Contraindications/cautions

- Allergy to sulfonylureas; diabetes complicated by fever, severe infections, severe trauma, major surgery, ketosis, acidosis, coma (insulin is indicated); type I or juvenile diabetes, serious hepatic or renal impairment, uremia, thyroid or endocrine impairment, glycosuria, hyperglycemia associated with primary renal disease; labor and delivery (if glyburide is used during pregnancy, discontinue drug at least 1 mo before delivery); lactation.

### Dosage

**Available Forms:** Tablets—1.25, 1.5, 2.5, 3, 5, 6 mg

ADULT

- ***Initial therapy:*** 2.5–5 mg PO with breakfast (DiaBeta, Micronase); 1.5–3 mg/d PO (Glynase).
- ***Maintenance therapy:*** 1.25–20 mg/d PO given as a single dose or in divided doses. Increase in increments of no more than 2.5 mg at weekly intervals based on patient's blood glucose response (DiaBeta, Micronase); 0.75–12 mg/d PO (Glynase).

PEDIATRIC: Safety and efficacy not established.

GERIATRIC: Geriatric patients tend to be more sensitive to the drug; start with initial dose of 1.25 mg/d PO. Monitor for 24 h, and gradually increase dose after at least 1 wk as needed.

### Pharmacokinetics

| *Route* | *Onset* | *Duration* |
|---|---|---|
| Oral | 1 h | 24 h |

*Metabolism:* Hepatic, $T_{1/2}$: 4 h
*Distribution:* Crosses placenta; enters breast milk
*Excretion:* Bile and urine

### Adverse effects

- GI: *Anorexia, nausea*, vomiting, *epigastric discomfort, heartburn, diarrhea*
- CV: Increased risk of CV mortality
- **Hematologic**: Leukopenia, thrombocytopenia, anemia
- Hypersensitivity: *Allergic skin reactions*, eczema, pruritus, erythema, urticaria, photosensitivity, fever, eosinophilia, jaundice
- Endocrine: *Hypoglycemia*

### Clinically important drug-drug interactions

• Increased risk of hypoglycemia with sulfonamides, chloramphenicol, fenfluramine, oxyphenbutazone, phenylbutazone, salicylates, clofibrate • Decreased effectiveness of glyburide and diazoxide if taken concurrently • Increased risk of hyperglycemia with rifampin, thiazides • Risk of hypoglycemia and hyperglycemia with ethanol; "disulfiram reaction" has been reported

## ■ Nursing Considerations

### Assessment

- *History:* Allergy to sulfonylureas; diabetes with complications; Type I or juvenile diabetes, serious hepatic or renal impairment, uremia, thyroid or endocrine impairment, glycosuria, hyperglycemia associated with primary renal disease
- *Physical:* Skin color, lesions; T; orientation, reflexes, peripheral sensation; R, adventitious sounds; liver evaluation, bowel sounds; urinalysis, BUN, serum creatinine, liver function tests, blood glucose, CBC

### Implementation

- Give drug before breakfast. If severe GI upset occurs, dose may be divided and given before meals.
- Monitor urine and serum glucose levels frequently to determine drug effectiveness and dosage.
- Monitor dosage carefully if switching to or from Glynase.
- Transfer to insulin therapy during periods of high stress (eg, infections, surgery, trauma).
- Use IV glucose if severe hypoglycemia occurs as a result of overdose.

### Drug-specific teaching points

- Do not discontinue this medication without consulting physician.
- Monitor urine or blood for glucose and ketones.
- Do not use this drug during pregnancy.
- Avoid alcohol while on this drug.
- Report fever, sore throat, unusual bleeding or bruising, skin rash, dark urine, light-colored stools, hypoglycemic or hyperglycemic reactions.

## glycerin

*(gli' ser in)*

glycerol

Fleet Babylax, Osmoglyn, Sani-Supp

**Pregnancy Category C**

### Drug classes

Osmotic diuretic
Hyperosmolar laxative

### Therapeutic actions

Elevates the osmolarity of the glomerular filtrate, thereby hindering the reabsorption of water and leading to a loss of water, sodium, and chloride; creates an osmotic gradient in the eye between plasma and ocular fluids, thereby reducing intraocular pressure; causes the local absorption of sodium and water in the stool, leading to a more liquid stool and local intestinal movement.

### Indications

- Glaucoma: to interrupt acute attacks, or when a temporary drop in intraocular pressure is required (Osmoglyn)
- Prior to ocular surgery performed under local anesthetic when a reduction in intraocular pressure is indicated (Osmoglyn)
- Temporary relief of constipation
- Unlabeled use: IV (with proper preparation) to lower intracranial or intraocular pressure

### Contraindications/cautions

- Contraindications: hypersensitivity to glycerin.
- Use cautiously with hypervolemia, CHF, confused mental states, severe dehydration, elderly, senility, diabetes, lactation.

### Dosage

**Available Forms:** Oral solution—50% 0.6 mg/ml; liquid suppositories—4 ml/applicator

ADULT

- ***Reduction of intraocular pressure:*** Osmoglyn: Given PO only: 1–1.5 g/kg, 1–1 1/2 h prior to surgery.

- *Laxative:* Insert one suppository high in rectum and retain 15 min; rectal liquid: insert stem with tip pointing toward navel; squeeze unit until nearly all liquid is expelled, then remove.

*PEDIATRIC:* Safety and efficacy not established.

### Pharmacokinetics

| *Route* | *Onset* | *Peak* | *Duration* |
|---|---|---|---|
| Oral (Osmoglyn) | Varies | 1 h | 5 h |

*Metabolism:* $T_{1/2}$: 2–3 h
*Distribution:* Crosses placenta; may enter breast milk
*Excretion:* Urine

### Adverse effects

- CNS: *Confusion, headache, syncope,* disorientation
- GI: *Nausea, vomiting*
- CV: Cardiac arrhythmias
- **Endocrine**: Hyperosmolar nonketotic coma
- **Other**: Severe dehydration, weight gain with continued use

## ■ Nursing Considerations

### Assessment

- *History:* Hypersensitivity to glycerin, hypervolemia, CHF, confused mental states, severe dehydration, elderly, senility, diabetes, lactation
- *Physical:* Skin color, edema; orientation, reflexes, muscle strength, pupillary reflexes; P, BP, perfusion; R, pattern, adventitious sounds; urinary output patterns; serum electrolytes, urinalysis

### Implementation

- Give Osmoglyn orally only; not for injection.
- Give laxative as follows: Insert one suppository high in rectum, and have patient retain 15 min; rectal liquid—insert stem with tip pointint toward navel; squeeze unit until nearly all liquid is expelled, then remove.
- Monitor urinary output carefully.
- Monitor BP regularly.

### Drug-specific teaching points

- Take laxative as follows: Insert one suppository high in rectum and retain 15 min; rectal liquid—insert stem with tip pointing toward navel; squeeze unit until nearly all liquid is expelled, then remove.
- The following side effects may occur: increased urination, GI upset (small frequent meals may help), dry mouth (sugarless lozenges to suck may help), headache, blurred vision (use caution when moving around; ask for assistance).
- Report severe headache, chest pain, confusion, rapid respirations, violent diarrhea.

## glycopyrrolate

*(glye koe **pye'** roe late)*

Robinul, Robinul Forte

**Pregnancy Category C (parenteral)**

**Pregnancy Category B**

### Drug classes

Anticholinergic (quaternary)
Antimuscarinic agent
Parasympatholytic
Antispasmodic

### Therapeutic actions

Competitively blocks the effects of acetylcholine at receptors that mediate the effects of parasympathetic postganglionic impulses; depresses salivary and bronchial secretions; dilates the bronchi; inhibits vagal influences on the heart; relaxes the GI and GU tracts; inhibits gastric acid secretion.

### Indications

- Adjunctive therapy in the treatment of peptic ulcer (oral)
- Reduction of salivary, tracheobronchial, and pharyngeal secretions preoperatively; reduction of the volume and free acidity of gastric secretions; and blocking of cardiac vagal inhibitory reflexes during induction of anesthesia and intubation; may be used intraoperatively to counter-

act drug-induced or vagal traction reflexes with the associated arrhythmias (parenteral)
- Protection against the peripheral muscarinic effects (eg, bradycardia, excessive secretions) of cholinergic agents (neostigmine, pyridostigmine) that are used to reverse the neuromuscular blockade produced by nondepolarizing neuromuscular junction blockers (parenteral)

## Contraindications/cautions

- Contraindications: glaucoma; adhesions between iris and lens; stenosing peptic ulcer; pyloroduodenal obstruction; paralytic ileus; intestinal atony; severe ulcerative colitis; toxic megacolon; symptomatic prostatic hypertrophy; bladder neck obstruction; bronchial asthma; COPD; cardiac arrhythmias; tachycardia; myocardial ischemia; lactation; impaired metabolic, liver, or kidney function; myasthenia gravis.
- Use cautiously with Down's syndrome, brain damage, spasticity, hypertension, hyperthyroidism.

## Dosage

**Available Forms:** Tablets—1, 2, mg; injection 0.2 mg/ml

### ADULT

- ***Oral:*** 1 mg tid or 2 mg bid–tid; maintenance: 1 mg bid.
- ***Parenteral***
  - *Peptic ulcer:* 0.1–0.2 mg IM or IV tid–qid.
  - *Preanesthetic medication:* 0.004 mg/kg (0.002 mg/lb) IM 30–60 min prior to anesthesia.
  - *Intraoperative:* 0.1 mg IV; repeat as needed at 2- to 3-min intervals. With neostigmine, pyridostigmine: 0.2 mg for each 1 mg neostigmine or 5 mg pyridostigmine; administer IV simultaneously.

**PEDIATRIC:** Not recommended for children <12 y for peptic ulcer.

- ***Parenteral***
  - *Preanesthetic medication (<2 y):* 0.004 mg/lb IM 30 min to 1 h prior to anesthesia. <12 y: 0.002–0.004 mg/lb IM.
  - *Intraoperative:* 0.004 mg/kg (0.002 mg/lb) IV, not to exceed 0.1 mg in a single dose. May be repeated at 2- to 3-min intervals.
  - *With neostigmine, pyridostigmine:* 0.2 mg for each 1 mg neostigmine or 5 mg pyridostigmine. Give IV simultaneously.

## Pharmacokinetics

| *Route* | *Onset* | *Peak* | *Duration* |
|---|---|---|---|
| Oral | 60 min | 60 min | 8–12 h |
| IM/SC | 15–30 min | 30–45 min | 2–7 h |
| IV | 1 min | | |

*Metabolism:* Hepatic, $T_{1/2}$: 2.5 h
*Distribution:* Crosses placenta; enters breast milk
*Excretion:* Urine

### IV facts

**Preparation:** No additional preparation required.
**Infusion:** Administer slowly into tubing of a running IV, each 0.2 mg over 1–2 min.

## Adverse effects

- CNS: *Blurred vision*, mydriasis, cycloplegia, photophobia, increased intraocular pressure
- GI: *Dry mouth, altered taste perception, nausea, vomiting, dysphagia*, heartburn, constipation, bloated feeling, paralytic ileus, gastroesophageal reflux
- CV: Palpitations, tachycardia
- GU: *Urinary hesitancy and retention*, impotence
- Local: *Irritation at site of IM injection*
- Other: Decreased sweating and predisposition to heat prostration, suppression of lactation, nasal congestion

## Clinically important drug-drug interactions

- Decreased antipsychotic effectiveness of haloperidol with anticholinergic drugs

## ■ Nursing Considerations

### Assessment

- *History:* Glaucoma; adhesions between iris and lens, stenosing peptic ulcer, pyloroduodenal obstruction, paralytic ileus, intestinal atony, severe ulcerative colitis, toxic megacolon, symptomatic prostatic hypertrophy, bladder neck obstruction, COPD, cardiac arrhythmias, myocardial ischemia, impaired metabolic, liver or kidney function, myasthenia gravis; lactation; Down's syndrome, brain damage, spasticity, hypertension, hyperthyroidism

- *Physical:* Bowel sounds, normal output; normal urinary output, prostate palpation; R, adventitious sounds; P, BP; intraocular pressure, vision; bilateral grip strength, reflexes; hepatic palpation, liver and renal function tests; skin color, lesions, texture

### Implementation

- Ensure adequate hydration; provide environmental control (temperature) to prevent hyperpyrexia.
- Have patient void before each dose if urinary retention is a problem.

### Drug-specific teaching points

- Take this drug exactly as prescribed.
- Avoid hot environments (you will be heat-intolerant, and dangerous reactions may occur).
- The following side effects may occur: constipation (ensure adequate fluid intake, proper diet); dry mouth (sugarless lozenges, frequent mouth care may help; effect may lessen); blurred vision, sensitivity to light (reversible; avoid tasks that require acute vision; wear sunglasses in bright light); impotence (reversible); difficulty in urination (empty bladder immediately before taking each dose).
- Report skin rash, flushing, eye pain, difficulty breathing, tremors, loss of coordination, irregular heartbeat, palpitations, headache, abdominal distention, hallucinations, severe or persistent dry mouth, difficulty swallowing, difficulty urinating, severe constipation, sensitivity to light.

## gold sodium thiomalate (gold)

Aurolate

**Pregnancy Category C**

### Drug classes

Antirheumatic
Gold compound

### Therapeutic actions

Suppresses and prevents arthritis and synovitis: taken up by macrophages, this results in inhibition of phagocytosis and inhibition of activities of lysosomal enzymes; decreases concentrations of rheumatoid factor and immunoglobulins.

### Indications

- Treatment of selected cases of adult and juvenile rheumatoid arthritis; most effective early in disease; late in the disease when damage has occurred, gold can only prevent further damage.

### Contraindications/cautions

- Allergy to gold preparations, uncontrolled diabetes mellitus, severe debilitation, renal disease, hepatic dysfunction, history of infectious hepatitis, marked hypertension, uncontrolled CHF, SLE, agranulocytosis, hemorrhagic diathesis, blood dyscrasias, recent radiation treatment, previous toxic response to gold or heavy metals (urticaria, eczema, colitis), pregnancy, lactation.

### Dosage

**Available Forms:** Injection—50 mg/ml

Contains approximately 50% gold. Administer by IM injection only, preferably intragluteally.

#### Adult

- ***Weekly injections:*** First injection, 10 mg, IM; Second injection, 25 mg, IM; Third and subsequent injections, 25–50 mg IM until major clinical improvement is seen, toxicity occurs, or cumulative dose reaches 1 g.
- ***Maintenance:*** 25–50 mg IM every other week for 2–20 wk. If clinical course remains stable, give 25–50 mg every third and then every fourth week indefinitely. Some patients require maintenance intervals of 1–3 wk. If arthritis is exacerbated, resume weekly injections. In severe cases, dosage can be increased by 10-mg increments; do not exceed 100 mg in a single injection.

*PEDIATRIC:* Initial test dose of 10 mg IM, then give 1 mg/kg, not to exceed 50 mg as a single injection. Adult guidelines for dosage apply.

*GERIATRIC:* Monitor patients carefully; tolerance to gold decreases with age.

### Pharmacokinetics

| *Route* | *Onset* | *Peak* |
|---|---|---|
| IM | Slow | 3–6 h |

*Metabolism:* $T_{1/2}$: 14–40 d, then 168 d
*Distribution:* Crosses placenta; enters breast milk
*Excretion:* Urine and feces

### Adverse effects

- **GI**: *Stomatitis, glossitis, gingivitis,* metallic taste, pharyngitis, gastritis, colitis, tracheitis, nausea, vomiting, anorexia, abdominal cramps, *diarrhea,* hepatitis with jaundice
- **Respiratory**: Gold bronchitis, interstitial pneumonitis and fibrosis, cough, shortness of breath
- **Hematologic**: Granulocytopenia, thrombocytopenia, leukopenia, eosinophilia, anemias
- **GU**: Vaginitis, nephrotic syndrome or glomerulitis with proteinuria and hematuria, acute tubular necrosis and renal failure
- **Dermatologic**: *Dermatitis; pruritus, erythema, exfoliative dermatitis,* chrysiasis (gray-blue color to the skin due to gold deposition), rash
- **Hypersensitivity**: Nitritoid or allergic reactions: flushing, fainting, dizziness, sweating, nausea, vomiting, malaise, weakness
- **Immediate postinjection effects**: **Anaphylactic shock**, syncope, bradycardia, thickening of the tongue, dysphagia, dyspnea, angioneurotic edema
- **Other**: Fever, nonvasomotor postinjection reaction: arthralgia for 1–2 d after the injection, usually subsides after the first few injections; carcinogenesis, mutagenesis, impairment of fertility (reported in preclinical studies)

## ■ Nursing Considerations

### Assessment

- ***History:*** Allergy to gold preparations, uncontrolled diabetes mellitus, severe debilitation, renal or hepatic dysfunction, history of infectious hepatitis, marked hypertension, uncontrolled CHF, SLE, hemorrhagic diathesis, blood dyscrasias, recent radiation treatment, previous toxic response to gold or heavy metals, lactation
- ***Physical:*** Skin color, lesions; T; edema; P, BP; R, adventitious sounds; mucous membranes, bowel sounds, liver evaluation; CBC, renal and liver function tests, chest x-ray

### Implementation

- Do not give to patients with history of idiosyncratic or severe reactions to gold therapy.
- Monitor hematologic status, liver and kidney function, respiratory status regularly.
- Do not use if material has darkened; color should be a pale yellow.
- Give by intragluteal IM injection; have patient remain recumbent for 10 min after injection.
- Discontinue at first sign of toxic reaction.
- Use systemic corticosteroids for treatment of severe stomatitis, dermatitis, renal, hematologic, pulmonary, enterocolitic complications.
- Protect from sunlight or ultraviolet light to decrease risk of chrysiasis.

### Drug-specific teaching points

- Prepare a calendar of projected injection dates. This drug's effects are not seen immediately; several months of therapy are needed to see results. You will be asked to stay in the recumbent position for about 10 min after each injection.
- This drug does not cure the disease, but only stops its effects.
- The following side effects may occur: increased joint pain for 1–2 d after injection (usually subsides after first few injections); diarrhea; mouth sores, metallic

taste (frequent mouth care will help); rash, gray-blue color to the skin (avoid exposure to sun or ultraviolet light); nausea, loss of appetite (small, frequent meals may help).

- Do not become pregnant while on this drug; if you decide to become pregnant, consult with physician about discontinuing drug.
- Report unusual bleeding or bruising, sore throat, fever, severe diarrhea, skin rash, mouth sores.

# Gonadorelin

## gonadorelin acetate

*(goe nad oh **rell' in**)*

GnRH

Lutrepulse

## gonadorelin hydrochloride

Factrel

**Pregnancy Category B**

### Drug classes

GnRH (gonadotropic releasing hormone)
Hormone
Diagnostic agent

### Therapeutic actions

A synthetic polypeptide that is identical to gonadotropic releasing hormone (GnRH) which is released from the hypothalamus in a pulsatile fashion to stimulate LH (leutinizing hormone) and FSH (follicle stimulating hormone) release from the pituitary; these hormones in turn are responsible for regulating reproductive status.

### Indications

- Treatment of primary hypothalamic amenorrhea (gonadorelin acetate)
- Evaluation of functional capacity and response of the gonadotropes of the anterior pituitary; testing suspected gonadotropin deficiency; evaluating residual gonadotropic function of the pituitary following removal of a pituitary tumor by surgery or irradiation (gonadorelin hydrochloride)
- Unlabeled uses of gonadorelin hydrochloride: induction of ovulation (by IV, SC, and intranasal routes); ovulation inhibition; treatment of precocious puberty

### Contraindications/cautions

- Hypersensitivity to gonadorelin or any of the components; ovarian cyst, causes of anovulation other than those of hypothalamic origin; hormone-dependent tumors; lactation.

### Dosage

**Available Forms:** Powder for injection—0.8, 3.2 mg (Lutrepulse), 100 $\mu$g/vial (Factrel)

ADULT

**Gonadorelin acetate**

- *Primary hypothalamic amenorrhea:* 5 $\mu$g q90 min (range 1–20 $\mu$g). This is delivered by the *Lutrepulse* pump using the 0.8-mg solution at 50 $\mu$l per pulse; 68% of the 5 $\mu$g q90 min regimens induced ovulation. For individualization of dose, see manufacturer's instructions.

**Gonadorelin hydrochloride:** 100 $\mu$g SC or IV. In females, perform the test in the early follicular phase (days 1–7) of the menstrual cycle.

PEDIATRIC

**Gonadorelin acetate:** Safety and efficacy not established.

### Pharmacokinetics

| Route | Onset | Duration |
|---|---|---|
| IV, SC | Slow | 3–5 h |

*Metabolism:* Plasma, $T_{1/2}$: 10–40 min
*Distribution:* Crosses placenta; enters breast milk
*Excretion:* Urine

### IV facts

**Preparation:** Reconstitute gonadorelin acetate using aseptic technique with 8 ml of diluent immediately prior to use, and transfer to plastic reservoir. Shake for a few seconds to produce a clear, colorless solution with no particulate matter. Prepare gonadorelin hydrochloride by reconstituting 100-$\mu$g vial with 1 ml and the 500-$\mu$g vial with 2 ml of the accompanying diluent. Prepare immediately before use. Store at room temperature; use within 1 d. Discard any unused solution and diluent.

**Infusion:** Administer gonadorelin acetate IV using the Lutrepulse pump set at pulse period of 1 min at a frequency of 90 min. The 8-ml solution will supply 90-min pulsatile doses for approximately 7 consecutive d. Inject gonadorelin HCl directly into vein or into tubing of running IV over 15–30 sec.

### Adverse effects

- CNS: Headache, lightheadedness
- GI: Nausea, abdominal discomfort
- GU: *Ovarian hyperstimulation, multiple pregnancies* (gonadorelin acetate)
- Local: *Inflammation, infection, mild phlebitis, hematoma at injection site*

## ■ Nursing Considerations

### Assessment

- *History:* Hypersensitivity to gonadorelin or any of the components, ovarian cyst, hormone-dependent tumors, lactation
- *Physical:* Reflexes, affect; Pap smear, pelvic exam; pregnancy test

### Implementation

- Determine cause of amenorrhea before treatment.
- Monitor for response to gonadorelin acetate within 2–3 wk after therapy started. Continue infusion pump for another 2 wk to maintain the corpus luteum.
- Monitor injection sites; pump access line for signs of local irritation and inflammation.
- Monitor patients on infusion pumps for signs of infection; change the cannula and IV sites q48h.

### Drug-specific teaching points

*Gonadorelin acetate*

- Gonadorelin acetate needs to be delivered in a pulsating fashion using the Lutrepulse pump. Care of the pump and injection site will be covered in the information kit provided by the manufacturer.
- Ovulation may occur within 2–3 wk of the beginning of therapy. You will need to be followed closely. If pregnancy does occur, the therapy will be continued for 2 wk to help maintain the pregnancy.
- The following side effects may occur: headache, abdominal discomfort; multiple pregnancies (you need to be aware of this possibility and its implications); pain or discomfort at injection site.
- Report difficulty breathing, rash, fever, redness or swelling at injection site, pain at injection site, severe abdominal pain.

*Gonadorelin HCl*

- Patients receiving gonadorelin hydrochloride for diagnostic testing should be informed about the drug as part of their teaching about their condition and testing.
- Report difficulty breathing, rash, pain or inflammation at injection site.

g

## goserelin acetate

*(goe' se rel in)*

Zoladex

**Pregnancy Category X**

### Drug classes

Antineoplastic

Hormone

### Therapeutic actions

An analog of LHRH or GnRH; potent inhibitor of pituitary gonadotropin secretion; initial administration causes an increase in FSH and LH and resultant increase in testosterone levels; with chronic administration, these hormone levels fall to levels normally seen with surgical castration within 2–4 wk, as pituitary is inhibited.

### Indications

- Palliative treatment of advanced prostatic cancer when orchiectomy or estrogen administration is not indicated or is unacceptable
- Management of endometriosis, including pain relief and reduction of endometriotic lesions
- Palliative treatment of advanced breast cancer

### Contraindications/cautions

- Pregnancy, lactation, hypersensitivity to LHRH or any component.

### Dosage

Available Forms: Implant—3.6 mg

ADULT: 3.6 mg SC every 28 d into the upper abdominal wall.

- *Prostatic/breast carcinoma:* Long-term use.
- *Endometriosis:* Continue therapy for 6 mo.

PEDIATRIC: Safety and efficacy not established.

### Pharmacokinetics

| Route | Onset | Peak |
|---|---|---|
| SC | Slow | 12–15 d |

*Metabolism:* Hepatic, $T_{1/2}$: 4.2 h

*Distribution:* Crosses placenta; may enter breast milk

*Excretion:* Urine

### Adverse effects

- CNS: Insomnia, dizziness, lethargy, anxiety, depression
- GI: Nausea, anorexia
- CV: CHF, edema, hypertension, arrhythmia, chest pain
- GU: *Hot flashes, sexual dysfunction, decreased erections, lower urinary tract symptoms*
- Other: Rash, sweating, cancer

## ■ Nursing Considerations

### Assessment

- *History:* Pregnancy, lactation
- *Physical:* Skin temperature, lesions; reflexes, affect; BP, P; urinary output; pregnancy test if appropriate

### Implementation

- Use syringe provided. Discard if package is damaged. Remove sterile syringe immediately before use. Use a local anesthetic prior to injection to decrease pain and discomfort.
- Administer using aseptic technique under the supervision of a physician familiar with the implant technique.
- Bandage area after implant has been injected.
- Repeat injection in 28 d; keep as close to this schedule as possible.

### Drug-specific teaching points

- This drug will be implanted into your upper abdomen every 28 d. It is important to keep to this schedule. Mark a calendar of injection dates.
- The following side effects may occur: hot flashes (a cool temperature may help); sexual dysfunction—regression of sex organs, impaired fertility, decreased erections; pain at injection site (a local anesthetic will be used; if discomfort is severe, analgesics may be ordered).
- Do not take this drug if pregnant; if you are pregnant or wish to become pregnant, consult with your physician.
- Report chest pain, increased signs and symptoms of your cancer, difficulty breathing, dizziness, severe pain at injection site.

## granisetron hydrochloride

*(gran iz' e tron)*

Kytril

**Pregnancy Category B**

### Drug classes

Antiemetic

### Therapeutic actions

Selectively binds to serotonin receptors in the CTZ, blocking the nausea and vomiting caused by the release of serotonin by mucosal cells during chemotherapy, which stimulates the CTZ and causes nausea and vomiting.

### Indications

- Prevention and treatment of nausea and vomiting associated with emetogenic chemotherapy

### Contraindications/cautions

- Contraindicated in pregnancy, lactation.

### Dosage

**Available Forms:** Tablets—1 mg; injection—1 mg/ml, 1.12 mg/4 ml

*ADULT AND PEDIATRIC >2 Y:* IV: 10 μg/kg IV over 5 min starting within 30 min of chemotherapy; only on days of chemotherapy. Oral: 1 mg PO bid beginning up to 1 h before chemotherapy and second dose 12 h after chemotherapy; only on days of chemotherapy.

*PEDIATRIC <2 Y:* Not recommended.

### Pharmacokinetics

| *Route* | *Onset* | *Peak* |
|---|---|---|
| IV | Rapid | 30–45 min |
| Oral | Moderate | 60–90 min |

*Metabolism:* Hepatic, $T_{1/2}$: 5 h (IV), 6.2 h (oral)

*Distribution:* Crosses placenta; enters breast milk

*Excretion:* Urine

#### IV facts

**Preparation:** Dilute in 0.9% sodium chloride or 5% Dextrose to a total volume of 20–50 ml; stable up to 24h refrigerated; protect from light

**Infusion:** Inject slowly over 5 min.

**Compatibility:** Do not mix in solution with other drugs.

### Adverse effects

- CNS: *Headache,* asthenia, somnolence
- GI: Diarrhea or constipation
- CV: Hypertension
- Other: Fever

## ■ Nursing Considerations

### Assessment

- ***History:*** Allergy to granisetron, pregnancy, lactation, liver or renal impairment
- ***Physical:*** Orientation, reflexes, affect; BP; bowel sounds; T

### Implementation

- Provide mouth care, sugarless lozenges to suck to help alleviate nausea.
- Give drug only on days of chemotherapy.

### Drug-specific teaching points

- This drug may be given IV or orally when you are receiving your chemotherapy; it will help decrease nausea and vomiting.
- The following side effects may occur: lack of sleep, drowsiness (use caution if driving or performing tasks that require alertness); diarrhea or constipation; headache (request medication).
- Report severe headache, fever, numbness or tingling, severe diarrhea or constipation.

g

## grepafloxacin hydrochloride

*(grep ah **flox'** a sin)*

Raxar

**Pregnancy Category C**

### Drug classes

Antibiotic

Flouroquinolone

### Therapeutic actions

Bactericidal, broad spectrum; interferes with DNA replication in susceptible gram-negative and gram-positive bacteria, preventing cell reproduction.

### Indications

- Treatment of adults with community-acquired pneumonia caused by *H. influenzae, S. pneumoniae, M. catarrhalis*
- Treatment of acute exacerbation of chronic bronchitis caused by *H. influenzae, S. pneumoniae, M. catarrhalis*
- Treatment of uncomplicated gonorrhea, nongonoccoccal urethritis, and cervicitis caused by *C. trachomatis*

### Contraindications/cautions

- Contraindications: allergy to fluoroquinolones, hepatic failure, QT prolongation, pregnancy, lactation, hepatic failure.
- Use cautiously with hypokalemia, bradycardia, CHF, myocardial ischemia, atrial fibrillation, predisposition to seizures.

### Dosage

**Available Forms:** Tablets—200 mg

ADULT

- *Community-acquired pneumonia:* 600 mg PO once daily for 10 d.
- *Chronic bronchitis:* 400–600 mg PO once daily for 10 d.
- *Urethritis, cervicitis:* 400 mg PO once daily for 7 d.
- *Gonorrhea:* 400 mg PO as a single dose.

PEDIATRIC: Not recommended for children < 18 y.

### Pharmacokinetics

| *Route* | *Onset* | *Duration* |
|---|---|---|
| Oral | Slow | 14–20 h |

*Metabolism:* Hepatic: $T_{1/2}$: 15 h

*Distribution:* Crosses placenta; passes into breast milk

*Excretion:* Urine and bile

### Adverse effects

- CNS: *Headache, dizziness, insomnia,* fatigue, somnolence, depression, blurred vision
- GI: *Nausea, taste perversion,* vomiting, dry mouth, *diarrhea,* abdominal pain
- Dermatologic: **Severe photosensitivity reactions,** rash, pruritus
- Other: Fever, superinfections, vaginitis

### Clinically important drug-drug interactions

• Decreased therapeutic effect with iron salts, sulcrafate, mineral supplements • Decreased absorption with antacids; separate by at least 4 h • Possibility of severe to fatal cardiac reactions with drugs that increase QT intervals or cause torsades de pointes (quinidine, procainamide, amiodarone, sotalol, bepridil, erythromycin, terfenadine, astemizole, cisapride, pentamidine, tricyclics, phenothiazines); avoid these combinations, hospitalize patient and provide continual cardiac monitoring if unavoidable • Increased theophylline levels if combined; decrease theophylline dose by half and monitor serum levels carefully • Possible increased risk of CNS stimulation with NSAIDs

## ■ Nursing Considerations

### Assessment

- *History:* Allergy to fluoroquinolones; hepatic failure, QT prolongation, pregnancy, lactation, hypokalemia, bradycardia, CHF, myocardial ischemia, atrial fibrillation, predisposition to seizures.
- *Physical:* Skin color, lesions; T; orientation, reflexes, affect; mucous membranes, bowel sounds; P, BP, baseline EKG; renal and liver function tests, serum electrolytes.

### Implementation

- Arrange for culture and sensitivity tests before beginning therapy.
- Continue therapy for full 10 d even if signs and symptoms of infection have disappeared.
- Ensure that patient is well hydrated during course of drug therapy.
- Administer antacids (if needed) at least 4 h after dosing.
- Discontinue drug if tendon pain, inflammation, rupture, skin rash, photosensitivity, or other severe reactions occur.
- Protect patient from exposure to ultraviolet light (use protective clothing, sunblock, etc.); photosensitivity reaction can be severe.
- Monitor clinical response; if no improvement is seen or a relapse occurs, repeat culture and sensitivity.

### Drug-specific teaching points

- Drink plenty of fluids while you are on this drug.
- The following side effects may occur: nausea, vomiting, abdominal pain (eat small, frequent meals); diarrhea or constipation (consult nurse or physician); drowsiness, blurring of vision, dizziness (use caution if driving or using dangerous equipment); sensitivity to ultraviolet light (sunlight and indoor light) (wear protective clothing, use a sunblock at all times; report any severe skin rash immediately).

- Report rash, visual changes, severe GI problems, weakness, tremors, palpitations, fainting spells.

## guaifenesin

*(gwye fen' e sin)*

Anti-Tuss, Breonesin, Genatuss, GG-Cen, Glyate, Halotussin, Hytuss 2X, Humibid Sprinkle, Mytussin, Naldecon-EX, Robitussin, Scot-tussin Expectorant, Uni-tussin

**Pregnancy Category C**

### Drug classes

Expectorant

### Therapeutic actions

Enhances the output of respiratory tract fluid by reducing adhesiveness and surface tension, facilitating the removal of viscous mucus.

### Indications

- Symptomatic relief of respiratory conditions characterized by dry, nonproductive cough and in the presence of mucus in the respiratory tract.

### Contraindications/cautions

- Allergy to guaifenesin.

### Dosage

**Available Forms:** Syrup—100 mg/5 ml; liquid—200 mg/5 ml; capsules—200 mg; SR capsules—300 mg; tablets—100, 200 mg; SR tablets—600 mg

*ADULT AND PEDIATRIC > 12 Y:* 100–400 mg PO q4h. Do not exceed 2.4 g/d.

*PEDIATRIC:*

- *6–12 y:* 100–200 mg PO q4h. Do not exceed 1.2 g/d.
- *2–6 y:* 50–100 mg PO q4h. Do not exceed 600 mg/d.

### Pharmacokinetics

| Route | Onset | Duration |
|---|---|---|
| Oral | 30 min | 4–6 h |

*Metabolism:* Not known, $T_{1/2}$: not known
*Distribution and Excretion:* Unknown

### Adverse effects

- CNS: Headache, dizziness
- GI: *Nausea, vomiting*
- Dermatologic: Rash

### Drug-lab test interferences

- Color interference and false results of 5-HIAA and VMA urinary determinations

### ■ Nursing Considerations

#### Assessment

- *History:* Allergy to guaifenesin; persistent cough due to smoking, asthma, or emphysema; very productive cough
- *Physical:* Skin lesions, color; T; orientation, affects; R, adventitious sounds

#### Implementation

- Monitor reaction to drug; persistent cough for more than 1 wk, fever, rash, or persistent headache may indicate a more serious condition.

#### Drug-specific teaching points

- Do not take for longer than 1 wk; if fever, rash, headache occur, consult physician.
- The following side effects may occur: nausea, vomiting (small, frequent meals may help); dizziness, headache (avoid driving or operating dangerous machinery).
- Report fever, rash, severe vomiting, persistent cough.

## guanabenz acetate

*(gwahn' a benz)*

Wytensin

**Pregnancy Category C**

### Drug classes

Antihypertensive
Sympatholytic, centrally acting

### Therapeutic actions

Stimulates central (CNS) $alpha_2$-adrenergic receptors, reduces sympathetic nerve impulses from the vasomotor center to the heart and blood vessels, decreases peripheral vascular resistance, and lowers systemic blood pressure.

### Indications

- Management of hypertension, alone or in combination with a thiazide diuretic

### Contraindications/cautions

- Contraindications: hypersensitivity to guanabenz, lactation.
- Use cautiously with severe coronary insufficiency, recent MI, CV disease, severe renal or hepatic failure, pregnancy.

### Dosage

**Available Forms:** Tablets—4, 8 mg

*ADULT:* Individualize dosage. Initial dose of 4 mg PO bid, alone or with a thiazide diuretic; increase in increments of 4–8 mg/d every 1–2 wk. Maximum dose 32 mg bid, but doses this high are rarely needed.

*PEDIATRIC:* Safety and efficacy not established for children <12 y; therefore, not recommended for use in this age group.

### Pharmacokinetics

| *Route* | *Onset* | *Peak* | *Duration* |
|---|---|---|---|
| Oral | 45–60 min | 2–5 h | 6–12 h |

*Metabolism:* Unknown, $T_{1/2}$: 6 h

*Distribution:* Crosses placenta; enters breast milk

*Excretion:* Urine and feces

### Adverse effects

- CNS: *Sedation, weakness, dizziness, headache*
- GI: *Dry mouth*
- CV: Chest pain, edema, **arrhythmias**

## ■ Nursing Considerations

### Assessment

- *History:* Hypersensitivity to guanabenz; severe coronary insufficiency, cerebrovascular disease, severe renal or hepatic failure; lactation
- *Physical:* Orientation, affect, reflexes; P, BP, orthostatic BP, perfusion, auscultation; liver and kidney function tests, ECG

### Implementation

- Store tightly sealed, protected from light.
- Do not discontinue drug abruptly; discontinue therapy by reducing the dosage gradually over 2–4 d to avoid rebound hypertension, increased blood and urinary catecholamines, anxiety, nervousness, and other subjective effects.
- Assess compliance with drug regimen in a nonthreatening, supportive manner.

### Drug-specific teaching points

- Take this drug exactly as prescribed; do not miss doses. Do not discontinue unless instructed to do so. Do not discontinue abruptly. Store tightly sealed, protected from light.
- The following side effects may occur: drowsiness, dizziness, lightheadedness, headache, weakness (transient; observe caution while driving or performing other tasks that require alertness or physical dexterity).
- Report persistent or severe drowsiness, dry mouth.

## guanadrel sulfate

*(gwahn' a drel)*

Hylorel

**Pregnancy Category B**

### Drug classes

Antihypertensive

Adrenergic neuron blocker

### Therapeutic actions

Antihypertensive effects depend on inhibition of norepinephrine release and depletion of norepinephrine from postganglionic sympathetic adrenergic nerve terminals.

### Indications

- Treatment of hypertension in patients not responding adequately to a thiazide-type diuretic

### Contraindications/cautions

- Contraindications: hypersensitivity to guanadrel; known or suspected pheochromocytoma, frank CHF not due to hypertension; lactation.
- Use cautiously with CAD with insufficiency or recent MI, CV disease (special risk if orthostatic hypotension occurs); history of bronchial asthma; active peptic

ulcer, ulcerative colitis (may be aggravated by a relative increase in parasympathetic tone); renal dysfunction (drug-induced hypotension may further compromise renal function).

### Dosage

**Available Forms:** Tablets—10, 25 mg

Individualize dosage.

*ADULT:* Usual starting dose is 10 mg/d PO. Most patients require a daily dosage of 20–75 mg, usually in twice daily doses. For larger doses, 3–4× daily dosing may be needed. Administer in divided doses; adjust dosage weekly or monthly until BP is controlled. In long-term therapy, some tolerance may occur, and dosage may need to be increased.

*PEDIATRIC:* Safety and efficacy not established.

*GERIATRIC OR RENAL IMPAIRED:* Reduce initial dosage to 5 mg q24h PO for Ccr of 30–60 ml/min; Ccr < 30 ml/min: give 5 mg q48h PO. Cautiously adjust dosage at intervals of 7–14 d.

## Pharmacokinetics

| *Route* | *Onset* | *Peak* | *Duration* |
|---|---|---|---|
| Oral | 1 1/2–2 h | 4–6 h | 4–14 h |

*Metabolism:* $T_{1/2}$: 10 h

*Distribution:* May cross placenta; may enter breast milk

*Excretion:* Urine

## Adverse effects

Incidence is higher during the first 8 wk of therapy.

- CNS: *Fatigue, headache, faintness, drowsiness, visual disturbances, paresthesias, confusion,* psychological problems
- GI: *Increased bowel movements, gas pain/indigestion, constipation, anorexia,* glossitis
- CV/Respiratory: *Shortness of breath on exertion,* ***palpitations,*** *chest pain, coughing,* shortness of breath at rest
- GU: *Nocturia, urinary urgency or frequency, peripheral edema, ejaculation disturbances,* impotence
- Other: *Excessive weight loss, excessive weight gain, aching limbs,* leg cramps

## ■ Nursing Considerations

### Assessment

- ***History:*** Hypersensitivity to guanadrel; known or suspected pheochromocytoma; frank CHF; CAD, cerebrovascular disease; history of bronchial asthma; active peptic ulcer, ulcerative colitis; renal dysfunction; lactation
- ***Physical:*** Weight; skin color, lesions; orientation, affect, reflexes; P, BP, orthostatic BP, supine BP, perfusion, edema, auscultation; R, adventitious sounds, status of nasal mucous membranes; bowel sounds, normal output, palpation of salivary glands; voiding pattern, normal output; kidney function tests, urinalysis

### Implementation

- Discontinue drug if diarrhea is severe.
- Discontinue guanadrel therapy 48–72 h prior to surgery to reduce the possibility of vascular collapse and cardiac arrest during anesthesia.
- Note prominently on patient's chart that patient is receiving guanadrel if emergency surgery is needed; a reduced dosage of preanesthetic medication and anesthetics will be needed.
- Monitor patient for orthostatic hypotension, which is most marked in the morning, and is accentuated by hot weather, alcohol, exercise.
- Monitor edema, weight with incipient cardiac decompensation; arrange to add a thiazide diuretic if sodium and fluid retention, signs of impending CHF, occur.

### Drug-specific teaching points

- Take this drug exactly as prescribed.
- Do not get out of bed without help while dosage is being adjusted.
- The following side effects may occur: dizziness, weakness (most likely to occur when you change position, in the early morning, after exercise, in hot weather, and when you have consumed alcohol; some tolerance may occur over time; avoid driving or engaging in tasks that require alertness; remember to change position slowly; use caution when climbing stairs); diarrhea; GI upset (frequent small meals may help); im-

potence, failure of ejaculation; emotional depression; stuffy nose.
- Report severe diarrhea, frequent dizziness or fainting.

## guanethidine monosulfate

*(gwahn eth' i deen)*

Ismelin

**Pregnancy Category C**

### Drug classes
Antihypertensive
Adrenergic neuron blocker

### Therapeutic actions
Antihypertensive effects depend on inhibition of norepinephrine release and depletion of norepinephrine from postganglionic sympathetic adrenergic nerve terminals.

### Indications
- Moderate to severe hypertension either alone or as an adjunct
- Renal hypertension, including that secondary to pyelonephritis, renal amyloidosis, and renal artery stenosis
- Orphan drug use: treatment of moderate to severe reflex sympathetic dystrophy and causalgia

### Contraindications/cautions
- Contraindications: hypersensitivity to guanethidine; known or suspected pheochromocytoma; frank CHF; lactation.
- Use cautiously with CAD with insufficiency or recent MI; CV disease, especially with encephalopathy; history of bronchial asthma (increased likelihood to be hypersensitive to catecholamine depletion); active peptic ulcer, ulcerative colitis (may be aggravated by a relative increase in parasympathetic tone); renal dysfunction (drug-induced hypotension may further compromise renal function).

### Dosage
**Available Forms:** Tablets—10, 25 mg

Initial doses should be small, and dosage should be increased slowly. It may take 2 wk to adequately evaluate the response to daily administration.

**ADULT**
- *Ambulatory patients:* 10 mg/d PO initially. Do not increase dosage more often than every 5–7 d. Take BP in supine position, after standing for 10 min, and immediately after exercise if feasible. Increase dosage only if there has been no decrease in standing BP from the previous levels. Average dose is 25–50 mg qd. Reduce dosage with the following: normal supine pressure, excessive orthostatic fall in pressure, severe diarrhea.
- *Hospitalized patients:* Initial dose of 25–50 mg PO. Increase by 25 or 50 mg daily or every other day as indicated.
- *Combination therapy:* Diuretics enhance guanethidine effectiveness, may reduce incidence of edema, and may allow reduction of guanethidine dosage. Withdraw MAO inhibitors at least 1 wk before starting guanethidine. It may be advisable to withdraw ganglionic blockers gradually to prevent spiking BP response during the transfer.

**PEDIATRIC:** Initial dose of 0.2 mg/kg per hour (6 mg/$m^2$ per 24 h) as a single oral dose. Increase by 0.2 mg/kg per 24 h PO every 7–10 d. Maximum dosage: 3 mg/kg per 24 h PO.

**GERIATRIC OR IMPAIRED RENAL FUNCTION:** Use reduced dosage.

### Pharmacokinetics

| Route | Onset | Peak | Duration |
|---|---|---|---|
| Oral | Slow | 1–3 wk | up to 2 wk |

*Metabolism:* Hepatic, $T_{1/2}$: 4–8 d
*Distribution:* Crosses placenta; enters breast milk
*Excretion:* Urine

### Adverse effects
- CNS: *Dizziness, weakness, lassitude, syncope resulting from either postural or exertional hypotension,* fatigue, myalgia, muscle tremor, emotional depression, ptosis of the lids and blurring of vision
- GI: *Increase in bowel movements and diarrhea,* nausea, vomiting, dry mouth, parotid tenderness

- CV: *Bradycardia*, angina, chest paresthesias, *fluid retention and edema with occasional development of CHF*
- **Respiratory**: Dyspnea, nasal congestion, asthma,
- GU: *Inhibition of ejaculation*, nocturia, urinary incontinence
- **Dermatologic**: Dermatitis, alopecia

**Clinically important drug-drug interactions**

• Decreased antihypertensive effect with anorexiants (eg, amphetamines), TCAs (imipramine, etc), phenothiazines (chlorpromazine), indirect-acting sympathomimetics (ephedrine, phenylpropanolamine, pseudoephedrine) • Increased pressor response and arrhythmogenic potential of direct-acting sympathomimetics (epinephrine, norepinephrine, phenylephrine), metaraminol, methoxamine

## ■ Nursing Considerations

### Assessment

- ***History:*** Hypersensitivity to guanethidine; known or suspected pheochromocytoma; frank CHF; CAD; cerebrovascular disease; history of bronchial asthma; active peptic ulcer, ulcerative colitis; renal dysfunction; lactation
- ***Physical:*** Weight; skin color, lesions; orientation, affect, reflexes; P, BP, orthostatic BP, supine BP, perfusion, edema, auscultation; R, adventitious sounds, status of nasal mucous membranes; bowel sounds, normal output, palpation of salivary glands; voiding pattern, normal output; kidney function tests, urinalysis

### Implementation

- Discontinue drug if diarrhea is severe.
- Discontinue guanethidine therapy at least 2 wk prior to surgery to reduce the possibility of vascular collapse and cardiac arrest during anesthesia.
- Note prominently on patient's chart that patient is receiving guanethidine if emergency surgery is needed; a reduced dosage of preanesthetic medication and anesthetics will be needed.
- Decrease dosage during fever, which decreases drug requirements.
- Monitor patient for orthostatic hypotension, which is most marked in the morning and is accentuated by hot weather, alcohol, exercise.
- Monitor edema, weight with incipient cardiac decompensation, and arrange to add a thiazide diuretic if sodium and fluid retention, signs of impending CHF, occur.

### Drug-specific teaching points

- Take this drug exactly as prescribed.
- Do not get out of bed without help while dosage is being adjusted.
- The following side effects may occur: dizziness, weakness (most likely to occur when you change position, in the early morning, after exercise, in hot weather, and when you have consumed alcohol; some tolerance may occur over time, but avoid driving or engaging in tasks that require alertness; remember to change positions slowly; use caution in climbing stairs); diarrhea; GI upset (frequent small meals may help); impotence, failure of ejaculation; emotional depression; stuffy nose.
- Report severe diarrhea, frequent dizziness or fainting.



# guanfacine hydrochloride

*(gwahn' fa seen)*

Tenex

**Pregnancy Category B**

**Drug classes**

Antihypertensive
Sympatholytic, centrally acting

**Therapeutic actions**

Stimulates central (CNS) alpha$_2$-adrenergic receptors, reduces sympathetic nerve impulses from the vasomotor center to the heart and blood vessels, decreases peripheral vascular resistance, and lowers systemic blood pressure.

### Indications

- Management of hypertension, alone or with a thiazide diuretic
- Unlabeled use: amelioration of withdrawal symptoms in heroin withdrawal

### Contraindications/cautions

- Contraindications: hypersensitivity to guanfacine, labor and delivery, lactation.
- Use cautiously with severe coronary insufficiency, recent MI, CV disease, chronic renal or hepatic failure, pregnancy.

### Dosage

**Available Forms:** Tablets—1, 2 mg

*ADULT:* Recommended dose is 1 mg/d PO given hs to minimize somnolence. If 1 mg/d does not give a satisfactory result after 3–4 wk of therapy, doses of 2 mg and then 3 mg may be given, although most of the drug's effect is seen at 1 mg. If BP rises toward the end of the dosing interval, divided dosage should be used. Higher daily doses (rarely up to 40 mg/d in divided doses) have been used, but adverse reactions increase with doses > 3 mg/d, and there is no evidence of increased efficacy.

*PEDIATRIC:* Safety and efficacy not established for children <12 y; therefore, not recommended for use in this age group.

### Pharmacokinetics

| *Route* | *Onset* | *Peak* | *Duration* |
|---|---|---|---|
| Oral | 2 h | 1–4 h | 24 h |

*Metabolism:* Hepatic, $T_{1/2}$: 10–30 h
*Distribution:* Crosses placenta; enters breast milk
*Excretion:* Urine

### Adverse effects

- CNS: *Sedation, weakness, dizziness,* headache, insomnia, amnesia, confusion, depression, conjunctivitis, iritis, vision disturbance, malaise, paresthesia, paresis, taste perversion, tinnitus, hypokinesia
- GI: *Dry mouth, constipation,* abdominal pain, diarrhea, dyspepsia, dysphagia, nausea
- CV: Bradycardia, palpitations, substernal pain
- GU: *Impotence*, libido decrease, testicular disorder, urinary incontinence
- **Dermatologic**: Dermatitis, pruritus, purpura, sweating
- **Other**: Rhinitis, leg cramps

## ■ Nursing Considerations

### Assessment

- ***History:*** Hypersensitivity to guanfacine; severe coronary insufficiency, cerebrovascular disease; chronic renal or hepatic failure; pregnancy; lactation
- ***Physical:*** Skin color, lesions; orientation, affect, reflexes; ophthalmologic exam; P, BP, orthostatic BP, perfusion, auscultation; R, adventitious sounds; bowel sounds, normal output; normal urinary output, voiding pattern; liver and kidney function tests, ECG

### Implementation

- Do not discontinue drug abruptly; discontinue therapy by reducing the dosage gradually over 2–4 d to avoid rebound hypertension (much less likely than with clonidine; BP usually returns to pretreatment levels in 2–4 d without ill effects).
- Assess compliance with drug regimen in a nonthreatening, supportive manner.

### Drug-specific teaching points

- Take this drug exactly as prescribed; it is important that you do not miss doses. Do not discontinue the drug unless instructed to do so. Do not discontinue abruptly.
- The following side effects may occur: drowsiness, dizziness, lightheadedness, headache, weakness (transient; observe caution while driving or performing other tasks that require alertness or physical dexterity); dry mouth (sucking on sugarless lozenges or ice chips may help); GI upset (frequent small meals may help); dizziness, lightheadedness when you change position (get up slowly; use caution when climbing stairs); impotence, other sexual dysfunction, decreased libido; palpitations.
- Report urinary incontinence, changes in vision, skin rash.

# Haloperidol

## haloperidol decanoate

*(ha loe **per'** i dole)*

Apo-Haloperidol (CAN), Haldol, Haldol Decanoate, Haldol LA (CAN), Novoperidol (CAN), Peridol (CAN)

## haloperidol lactate

**Pregnancy Category C**

### Drug classes

Dopaminergic blocking drug
Antipsychotic drug
Butyrophenone (not a phenothiazine)

### Therapeutic actions

Mechanism not fully understood: antipsychotic drugs block postsynaptic dopamine receptors in the brain, depress the RAS, including those parts of the brain involved with wakefulness and emesis; chemically resembles the phenothiazines.

### Indications

- Management of manifestations of psychotic disorders
- Control of tics and vocalizations in Gilles de la Tourette's syndrome in adults and children
- Short-term treatment of hyperactive children who also show impulsivity, difficulty sustaining attention, aggressivity, mood lability, or poor frustration tolerance
- Prolonged parenteral therapy of chronic schizophrenia (haloperidol decanoate)
- Unlabeled uses: control of nausea and vomiting, control of acute psychiatric situations (IV use)

### Contraindications/cautions

- Contraindications: coma or severe CNS depression, bone marrow depression, blood dyscrasia, circulatory collapse, subcortical brain damage, Parkinson's disease, liver damage, cerebral arteriosclerosis, coronary disease, severe hypotension or hypertension.
- Use cautiously with respiratory disorders ("silent pneumonia"); glaucoma, prostatic hypertrophy (anticholinergic effects may exacerbate glaucoma and urinary retention); epilepsy or history of epilepsy (drug lowers seizure threshold); breast cancer (elevations in prolactin may stimulate a prolactin-dependent tumor); thyrotoxicosis; peptic ulcer, decreased renal function; myelography within previous 24 h or scheduled within 48 h; exposure to heat or phosphorous insecticides; lactation; children younger than 12 y, especially those with chickenpox, CNS infections (children are especially susceptible to dystonias that may confound the diagnosis of Reye's syndrome); allergy to aspirin if giving the 1-, 2-, 5-, and 10-mg tablets (these tablets contain tartrazine).

### Dosage

**Available Forms:** Tablets—0.5, 1, 2, 5, 10, 20 mg; concentrate—2 mg/ml; injection—50, 100 mg/ml

Full clinical effects may require 6 wk–6 mo of therapy. Children, debilitated and geriatric patients, and patients with a history of adverse reactions to neuroleptic drugs may require lower dosage.

**ADULT**

- ***Initial oral dosage range:*** 0.5–2.0 mg bid–tid PO with moderate symptoms; 3–5 mg bid–tid PO for more resistant patients. Daily dosages up to 100 mg/d (or more) have been used, but safety of prolonged use has not been demonstrated. For maintenance, reduce dosage to lowest effective level.
- ***IM, haloperidol lactate injection:*** 2–5 mg (up to 10–30 mg) q30–60 min or q4–8h IM as necessary for prompt control of acutely agitated patients with severe symptoms. Switch to oral dosage as soon as feasible, using total IM dosage in previous 24 h as a guide to total daily oral dosage.
- ***IV, haloperidol lactate injection, unlabeled use for acute situations:*** 2–25 mg q30 IV or more min at a rate of 5 mg/min.
- ***Haloperidol decanoate injection (IM):*** Initial dose: 10–15 times the daily oral dose; repeat at 4-wk intervals.

*Pediatric*

- *3–12 y or 15–40 kg weight:* Initial dose of 0.5 mg/d PO; may increase in increments of 0.5 mg q5–7 d as needed. Total daily dose may be divided and given bid–tid.
- *Psychiatric disorders:* 0.05–0.15 mg/kg PO per day. Severely disturbed psychotic children may require higher dosage. There is little evidence that behavior is improved by doses greater than 6 mg/d.
- *Nonpsychotic and Gilles de la Tourette's syndromes:* 0.05–0.075 mg/kg PO per day.

*Geriatric:* Use lower doses (0.5–2.0 mg bid–tid), and increase dosage more gradually than in younger patients.

## Pharmacokinetics

| Route | Onset | Peak |
|---|---|---|
| Oral | Varies | 3–5 h |
| IM | Rapid | 20 min |
| IM, decanoate | Slow | 4–11d |

*Metabolism:* Hepatic, $T_{1/2}$: 21–24 h, 3 wk for decanoate

*Distribution:* Crosses placenta; enters breast milk

*Excretion:* Urine and bile

## Adverse effects

Not all effects have been reported with haloperidol; however, because haloperidol has certain pharmacologic similarities to the phenothiazine class of antipsychotic drugs, all adverse effects associated with phenothiazine therapy should be kept in mind when haloperidol is used.

- CNS: *Drowsiness*, insomnia, vertigo, headache, weakness, tremor, ataxia, slurring, cerebral edema, seizures, exacerbation of psychotic symptoms, extrapyramidal syndromes—*pseudoparkinsonism; dystonias; akathisia,* tardive dyskinesias, potentially irreversible (no known treatment), **neuroleptic malignant syndrome**—extrapyramidal symptoms, hyperthermia, autonomic disturbances
- CV: Hypotension, orthostatic hypotension, hypertension, tachycardia, bradycardia, cardiac arrest, CHF, cardiomegaly, **refractory arrhythmias** (some fatal), pulmonary edema
- Respiratory: Bronchospasm, laryngospasm, dyspnea; **suppression of cough reflex and potential for aspiration**
- Hematologic: Eosinophilia, leukopenia, leukocytosis, anemia; aplastic anemia; hemolytic anemia; thrombocytopenic or nonthrombocytopenic purpura; pancytopenia
- Hypersensitivity: Jaundice, urticaria, angioneurotic edema, laryngeal edema, photosensitivity, eczema, asthma, **anaphylactoid reactions**, exfoliative dermatitis
- Endocrine: Lactation, breast engorgement in females, galactorrhea; SIADH; amenorrhea, menstrual irregularities; gynecomastia in males; changes in libido; hyperglycemia or hypoglycemia; glycosuria; hyponatremia; pituitary tumor with hyperprolactinemia; inhibition of ovulation, infertility, pseudopregnancy
- Autonomic: Dry mouth, salivation, nasal congestion, nausea, vomiting, anorexia, fever, pallor, flushed facies, sweating, constipation, paralytic ileus, urinary retention, incontinence, polyuria, enuresis, priapism, ejaculation inhibition

## Clinically important drug-drug interactions

• Additive anticholinergic effects and possibly decreased antipsychotic efficacy with anticholinergic drugs • Increased risk of toxic side effects with lithium • Decreased effectiveness with carbamazepine

## Drug-lab test interferences

• False-positive pregnancy tests (less likely if serum test is used) • Increase in PBI, not attributable to an increase in thyroxine

## ■ Nursing Considerations

### Assessment

- *History:* Severe CNS depression; bone marrow depression; blood dyscrasia; circulatory collapse; subcortical brain dam-

age; Parkinson's disease; liver damage; cerebral arteriosclerosis; coronary disease; severe hypotension or hypertension; respiratory disorders; glaucoma, prostatic hypertrophy; epilepsy or history of epilepsy; breast cancer; thyrotoxicosis; peptic ulcer, decreased renal function; myelography within previous 24 h or scheduled within 48 h; exposure to heat or phosphorus insecticides; children younger than 12 y, especially those with chickenpox, CNS infections; allergy to aspirin
- *Physical:* Weight, T; reflexes, orientation, intraocular pressure; P, BP, orthostatic BP; R, adventitious sounds; bowel sounds and normal output, liver evaluation; urinary output, prostate size, CBC, urinalysis, thyroid, liver and kidney function tests

### Implementation
- Do not give children IM injections.
- Do not use haloperidol decanoate for IV injections.
- Gradually withdraw drug when patient has been on maintenance therapy to avoid withdrawal-emergent dyskinesias.
- Discontinue drug if serum creatinine, BUN become abnormal or if WBC count is depressed.
- Monitor elderly patients for dehydration; institute remedial measures promptly; sedation and decreased thirst related to CNS effects can lead to severe dehydration.
- Consult physician regarding appropriate warning of patient or patient's guardian about tardive dyskinesias.
- Consult physician about dosage reduction, use of anticholinergic antiparkinsonian drugs (controversial) if extrapyramidal effects occur.

### Drug-specific teaching points
- Take this drug exactly as prescribed.
- Avoid driving or engaging in other dangerous activities if CNS, vision changes occur.
- Avoid prolonged exposure to sun, or use a sunscreen or covering garments.
- Maintain fluid intake, and use precautions against heatstroke in hot weather.
- Report sore throat, fever, unusual bleeding or bruising, rash, weakness, tremors, impaired vision, dark-colored urine (pink or reddish brown urine is to be expected), pale stools, yellowing of the skin or eyes.

## Heparin

### heparin calcium injection
***(hep' ah rin)***

Calcilean (CAN)

### heparin sodium injection
Hepalean (CAN)

### heparin sodium and 0.9% sodium chloride
Heparin Lock Flush, Hep-Lock

### heparin sodium lock flush solution

**Pregnancy Category C**

### Drug classes
Anticoagulant

### Therapeutic actions
Inhibits thrombus and clot formation by blocking the conversion of prothrombin to thrombin and fibrinogen to fibrin, the final steps in the clotting process.

### Indications
- Prevention and treatment of venous thrombosis and pulmonary embolism
- Treatment of atrial fibrillation with embolization
- Diagnosis and treatment of DIC
- Prevention of clotting in blood samples and heparin lock sets and during dialysis procedures
- Unlabeled uses: adjunct in therapy of coronary occlusion with acute MI, prevention of left ventricular thrombi and CVA post-MI, prevention of cerebral thrombosis in the evolving stroke

### Contraindications/cautions
- Hypersensitivity to heparin; severe thrombocytopenia; uncontrolled bleeding; any patient who cannot be monitored regularly with blood coagulation tests; labor

and immediate postpartum period; women older than 60 y are at high risk for hemorrhaging; dysbetalipoproteinemia; recent surgery or injury.

## Dosage

**Available Forms:** Injection—1,000, 2,000, 2,500, 5,000, 10,000, 20,000, 40,000 U/ml; also single dose and unit-dose forms

Adjust dosage according to coagulation tests. Dosage is adequate when WBCT 2.5—3× control—or APTT 1.5—3× control value. The following are guidelines to dosage:

**ADULT**

- *For general anticoagulation:*
  - ***SC (deep SC injection):*** IV loading dose of 5,000 U and then 10,000–20,000 U SC followed by 8,000–10,000 U q8h or 15,000–20,000 U q12h.
  - ***Intermittent IV:*** Initial dose of 10,000 U and then 5,000–10,000 U q4–6h.
  - ***Continuous IV infusion:*** Loading dose of 5,000 U and then 20,000–40,000 U/d.
- *Prophylaxis of postoperative thromboembolism:* 5,000 U by deep SC injection 2 h before surgery and q8–12h thereafter for 7 d or until patient is fully ambulatory.
- *Surgery of heart and blood vessels for patients undergoing total body perfusion:* Not less than 150 U/kg; guideline often used is 300 U/kg for procedures less than 60 min, 400 U/kg for longer procedures.
- *Clot prevention in blood samples:* 70–150 U/10–20 ml of whole blood.
- *Heparin lock and extracorporal dialysis:* See manufacturer's instructions.

**PEDIATRIC:** Initial IV bolus of 50 U/kg and then 100 U/kg IV q4h, or 20,000 U/m$^2$ per 24 h by continuous IV infusion.

## Pharmacokinetics

| *Route* | *Onset* | *Peak* | *Duration* |
|---|---|---|---|
| IV | Immediate | Minutes | 2–6 h |
| SC | 20–60 min | 2–4 h | 8–12 h |

*Metabolism:* $T_{1/2}$: 30–180 min

*Distribution:* Does not cross placenta, does not enter breast milk; broken down in liver

*Excretion:* Urine

## IV facts

**Continuous infusion:** can be mixed in Normal Saline, D5W, Ringer's; mix well; invert bottle numerous times to ensure adequate mixing. Monitor patient closely; infusion pump is recommended. Single dose: direct, undiluted IV injection of up to 5,000 U (adult) or 50 U/kg (pediatric), given over 60 seconds.

**Monitoring:** blood should be drawn for coagulation testing 30 min before each intermittent IV dose or q4h if patient is on continuous infusion pump.

**Incompatibilities:** Heparin should *not* be mixed in solution with any other drug unless specifically ordered; direct incompatibilities in solution seen with amikacin, codeine, chlorpromazine, cytarabine, diazepam, dobutamine, doxorubicin, droperidol, ergotamine, erythromycin, gentamicin, haloperidol, nyaluronidase, hydrocortisone, kanamycin, levorphanol, meperidine, methadone, methicillin, methotrimeprazine, morphine, netilimicin, pentazocine, phenytoin, polymyxin B, promethazine, streptomycin, tetracycline, tobramycin, triflupromazine, vancomycin

## Adverse effects

- Hematologic: *Hemorrhage; bruising;* thrombocytopenia; elevated SGOT, SGPT levels, hyperkalemia
- Dermatologic: Loss of hair
- Hypersensitivity: Chills, fever, urticaria, asthma
- Other: Osteoporosis, suppression of renal function (long-term, high-dose therapy)
- Treatment of overdose: Protamine sulfate (1% solution). Each mg of protamine neutralizes 100 USP heparin U. Give very slowly IV over 10 min, not to exceed 50 mg. Establish dose based on blood coagulation studies.

**Clinically important drug-drug interactions**
• Increased bleeding tendencies with oral anticoagulants, salicylates, penicillins, cephalosporins • Decreased anticoagulation effects if taken concurrently with nitroglycerin

**Drug-lab test interferences**
• Increased AST, ALT levels • Increased thyroid function tests • Altered blood gas analyses, especially levels of carbon dioxide, bicarbonate concentration, and base excess

## Nursing Considerations

### Assessment
- *History:* Recent surgery or injury; sensitivity to heparin; hyerlipidemia
- *Physical:* Peripheral perfusion, R, stool guaiac test, PTT or other tests of blood coagulation, platelet count, kidney function tests

### Implementation
- Adjust dose according to coagulation test results performed just before injection (30 min before each intermittent dose or q4h if continuous IV dose). Therapeutic range: 1.5–2.5 × control.
- Use heparin lock needle to avoid repeated injections.
- Give deep subcutaneous injections; *do not* give heparin by IM injection.
- Do not give IM injections to patients on heparin therapy (heparin predisposes to hematoma formation).
- Apply pressure to all injection sites after needle is withdrawn; inspect injection sites for signs of hematoma; do not massage injection sites.
- Mix well when adding heparin to IV infusion.
- Do not add heparin to infusion lines of other drugs, and do not piggyback other drugs into heparin line. If this must be done, ensure drug compatibility.
- Provide for safety measures (electric razor, soft toothbrush) to prevent injury from bleeding.
- Check for signs of bleeding; monitor blood tests.
- Alert all health care providers of heparin use.
- Have protamine sulfate (heparin antidote) on standby in case of overdose; each mg neutralizes 100 U of heparin.

### Drug-specific teaching points
- This drug must be given by a parenteral route (cannot be taken orally).
- Frequent blood tests are necessary to determine blood clotting time is within the correct range.
- Be careful to avoid injury; use an electric razor, avoid contact sports, avoid activities that might lead to injury.
- Side effects may include the loss of hair.
- Report nose bleed, bleeding of the gums, unusual bruising, black or tarry stools, cloudy or dark urine, abdominal or lower back pain, severe headache.

h

# hetastarch

*(het' a starch)*
hydroxyethyl starch
HES
Hespan
**Pregnancy Category C**

**Drug classes**
Plasma expander

**Therapeutic actions**
Complex mixture of various molecules with colloidal properties that raise human plasma volume when administered IV; increases the erythrocyte sedimentation rate and improves the efficiency of granulocyte collection by centrifugal means.

**Indications**
- Adjunctive therapy for plasma volume expansion in shock due to hemorrhage, burns, surgery, sepsis, trauma
- Adjunctive therapy in leukapheresis to improve harvesting and increase the yield of granulocytes

**Contraindications/cautions**
- Contraindications: allergy to hetastarch, severe bleeding disorders, severe cardiac congestion, renal failure or anuria.
- Use cautiously with liver dysfunction, pregnancy.

### Dosage

**Available Forms:** Injection—6 g/100ml

*ADULT*

- *Plasma volume expansion:* 500–1,000 ml IV. Do not usually exceed 1,500 ml/d. In acute hemorrhagic shock, rates approaching 20 ml/kg per hour are often needed.
- *Leukapheresis:* 250–700 ml hetastarch infused at a constant fixed ratio of 1:8 to venous whole blood. Safety of up to 2 procedures per week and a total of 7–10 procedures using hetastarch have been established.

*PEDIATRIC:* Safety and efficacy have not been established.

### Pharmacokinetics

| *Route* | *Onset* | *Peak* | *Duration* |
|---|---|---|---|
| IV | Immediate | 24 h | 24–36 h |

*Metabolism:* Hepatic, $T_{1/2}$: 17 d, then 48 d
*Distribution:* Crosses placenta; enters breast milk
*Excretion:* Urine

#### IV facts

**Preparation:** Use as prepared by manufacturer; store at room temperature; do not use if turbid deep brown or if crystalline precipitate forms.

**Infusion:** Rate of infusion should be determined by patient response; start at approximately 20 ml/kg, reduce rate to lowest possible needed to maintain hemodynamics.

### Adverse effects

- CNS: *Headache*, muscle pain
- GI: *Vomiting, submaxillary and parotid glandular enlargement*
- Hematologic: Prolongation of PT, PTT; **bleeding and increased clotting times**
- Hypersensitivity: Periorbital edema, urticaria, wheezing
- Other: *Mild temperature elevations, chills, itching, mild influenza-like symptoms*, peripheral edema of the lower extremities

## ■ Nursing Considerations

### Assessment

- *History:* Allergy to hetastarch, severe bleeding disorders, severe cardiac congestion, renal failure or anuria; liver dysfunction
- *Physical:* T; submaxillary and parotid gland evaluation; P, BP, adventitious sounds, peripheral and periorbital edema; R, adventitious sounds; liver evaluation; urinalysis, renal and liver function tests, clotting times, PT, PTT, Hgb, Hct

### Implementation

- Administer by IV infusion only; monitor rates based on patient response.
- Maintain life support equipment on standby in cases of shock.

### Drug-specific teaching points

- This drug can only be given IV.
- Report difficulty breathing, headache, muscle pain, skin rash, unusual bleeding or bruising.

## histrelin acetate

***(his trell' in)***

Supprelin

**Pregnancy Category X**

### Drug classes

Gonadotropin-releasing hormone (GnRH) agonist

### Therapeutic actions

GnRH or LHRH agonist; inhibits gonadotropin secretion in chronic administration, resulting in decreased sex steroid levels and regression of secondary sexual characteristics.

### Indications

- Control of the biochemical and clinical manifestations of central precocious puberty

### Contraindications/cautions

- Hypersensitivity to histrelin or any of the components; pregnancy; congenital adrenal hyperplasia; steroid-secreting tumors.

### Dosage

**Available Forms:** Injection—120, 300, 600 μg/0.6 ml

*PEDIATRIC:* 10 μg/kg SC as a single daily injection. If response is not as anticipated within 3 mo, reevaluate therapy.

### Pharmacokinetics

| *Route* | *Onset* | *Duration* |
|---|---|---|
| SC | Slow | 3 mo |

*Metabolism:* Plasma, $T_{1/2}$: unknown
*Distribution:* Crosses placenta; may enter breast milk
*Excretion:* Unknown

### Adverse effects

- CNS: *Headache*, lightheadedness, mood changes, libido changes, depression, ear pain
- GI: Nausea, vomiting, abdominal pain, flatulence, dyspepsia, anorexia
- CV: *Vasodilitation*, edema, palpitations
- GU: *Vaginal dryness, irritation, odor*; leukorrhea; metrorrhagia; *vaginal bleeding* (within first 1–3 wk)
- Endocrine: Breast pain/discharge, goiter, tenderness of female genitalia
- Respiratory: URI, cough, asthma
- Other: *Chills, pyrexia, malaise*, weight gain, viral infections, joint stiffness, muscle pain
- Local: *Inflammation, infection at injection site*

## ■ Nursing Considerations

### Assessment

- *History:* Hypersensitivity to histrelin or any of the components, pregnancy, congenital adrenal hyperplasia, steroid-secreting tumors, lactation
- *Physical:* Height and weight; T; skin color, lesions; P; R, adventitious sounds; reflexes, affect; abdominal exam; injection site; wrist and hand x-rays; steroid levels; GnRH stimulation test; tomography of the head; pelvic/adrenal/testicular ultrasounds; beta-human chorionic gonadotropin levels; GnRH levels

### Implementation

- Ensure patient has only central precocious puberty before treatment: wrist and hand x-rays; steroid levels; GnRH stimulation test; tomography of the head; pelvic/adrenal/testicular ultrasounds; beta-human chorionic gonadotropin levels to rule out other problems.
- Monitor response to drug, including GnRH levels. If desired response is not seen within 3 mo, consider alternate therapy.
- Rotate injection sites daily. Monitor sites for inflammation, pain, infection. Arrange for treatment: hot soaks, steroids.
- Instruct patient and significant others in the proper techniques for SC injection.
- Refrigerate vials; use each vial only once and discard. Allow vial to warm to room temperature before injection.
- Discontinue therapy at any sign of hypersensitivity: difficulty breathing, swallowing; rash, fever, chills; tachycardia.

### Drug-specific teaching points

- Histrelin must be given by single, daily SC injections. Learn the proper technique for administering this drug. Refrigerate vials. Warm vial to room temperature before injection. Use each vial only once and then discard.
- Administer drug each day. Failure to inject daily may result in failure of therapy and return to pubertal state.
- Rotate injection sites daily. Monitor sites for any sign of infection—swelling, pain, redness.
- Arrange for regular medical follow-ups: blood tests, x-rays of bones, and monitoring of sexual development.
- Possible side effects may occur: headache, abdominal discomfort (medications may be available to help); vaginal bleeding (during the first 1–3 wk of therapy); vaginal pain, irrititation, odor; nausea, loss of appetite, vomiting (small, frequent meals may help); flushing, red face (cool environment, avoiding exposure to heat will help).
- Report difficulty breathing, rash, swelling, rapid heartbeat, difficulty swallowing, ir-

h

ritation or redness of injection sites that does not go away.

## hyaluronidase

*(hye al yoor **on'** i dase)*

Wydase

**Pregnancy Category C**

### Drug classes

Enzyme

### Therapeutic actions

Spreading factor that promotes diffusion and absorption of fluid injected in the subcutaneous tissues by breaking down the viscous substance, hyaluronic acid, that is in the interstices of tissues.

### Indications

- Adjuvant to increase absorption and dispersion of injected drugs
- Hypodermoclysis
- Adjunct in SC urography to improve resorption of radiopaques

### Contraindications/cautions

- Contraindications: allergy to bovine products; acutely inflamed or cancerous areas (avoid injection into these areas).
- Use caution if lactating.

### Dosage

**Available Forms:** Powder for injection—150, 1,500 U/vial; solution for injection—150 U/ml

ADULT

- *Absorption and dispersion of injected drugs:* Add 150 U hyaluronidase to the vehicle containing the other medication.
- *Hypodermoclysis:* Inject hyaluronidase solution into rubber tubing close to needle inserted between skin and muscle, *or* inject hyaluronidase SC before clysis; 150 U will facilitate absorption of 1,000 ml or more of solution. Individualize dose, rate of injection, and type of solution (saline, glucose, Ringer's).

PEDIATRIC

- *Hypodermoclysis: For children <3 y:* limit the volume of a single clysis to 200 ml; in premature infants or neonates, the daily dosage should not exceed 25 ml/kg; rate should not be greater than 2 ml/min.
- *Subcutaneous urography:* With the patient prone, inject 75 U hyaluronidase SC over each scapula. Inject the contrast medium at the same sites.

GERIATRIC: Do not exceed the rate and volume used for IV infusion.

### Pharmacokinetics

| *Route* | *Onset* | *Duration* |
|---|---|---|
| SC | Rapid | 36–40 h |

*Metabolism:* Tissue, $T_{1/2}$: unknown

*Distribution:* May cross placenta or enter breast milk

### Adverse effects

- Hematologic: *Hypovolemia* (if solutions devoid of inorganic electrolytes are given by hypodermoclysis)
- Hypersensitivity: Occurs infrequently (drug is a protein and potential antigen)

## ■ Nursing Considerations

### Assessment

- *History:* Allergy to bovine products, acutely inflamed or cancerous areas
- *Physical:* Skin—injection sites; turgor; P, BP, JVP to monitor hypovolemia

### Implementation

- Perform a preliminary skin test in patients prone to sensitivity reactions: intradermal injection of 0.02 ml solution. Positive reaction consists of a wheal with pseudopods appearing within 5 min and persisting for 20–30 min with itching.
- Prepare lyphilized powder for injection by adding 1 ml of 0.9% sodium chloride to a vial containing 150 U hyaluronidase and 10 ml 0.9% sodium chloride to 1,500 U hyaluronidase; resulting solution contains 150 U/ml. Refrigerate prepared solution.
- Monitor patients given hyaluronidase with epinephrine for the systemic effects of epinephrine.

- Monitor for hypovolemia; can be corrected through solution change.

**Drug-specific teaching points**

- There may be some discomfort at the injection site.
- Report itching, pain at injection site, shortness of breath, dizziness.

## hydralazine hydrochloride

*(hye **dral'** a zeen)*

Apresoline

**Pregnancy Category C**

### Drug classes

Antihypertensive drug
Vasodilator

### Therapeutic actions

Acts directly on vascular smooth muscle to cause vasodilation, primarily arteriolar; maintains or increases renal and cerebral blood flow.

### Indications

- Oral: essential hypertension alone or in combination with other agents
- Parenteral: severe essential hypertension when drug cannot be given orally or when need to lower blood pressure is urgent
- Unlabeled uses: reducing afterload in the treatment of CHF, severe aortic insufficiency, and after valve replacement (doses up to 800 mg tid)

### Contraindications/cautions

- Contraindications: hypersensitivity to hydralazine, tartrazine (in 100-mg tablets marketed as Apresoline); CAD, mitral valvular rheumatic heart disease (implicated in MI).
- Use cautiously with CVAs; increased intracranial pressure (drug-induced BP fall risks cerebral ischemia); severe hypertension with uremia; advanced renal damage; slow acetylators (higher plasma levels may be achieved; lower dosage may be adequate); lactation.

### Dosage

**Available Forms:** Tablets—10, 25, 50, 100 mg; injection 20 mg/ml

ADULT

- ***Oral:*** Inititate therapy with gradually increasing dosages. Start with 10 mg qid PO for the first 2–4 d; increase to 25 mg qid PO for the first week. Second and subsequent weeks: 50 mg qid. Maintenance: Adjust to lowest effective dosage; twice daily dosage may be adequate. Some patients may require up to 300 mg/d. Incidence of toxic reactions, particularly the LE syndrome, is high in patients receiving large doses.
- ***Parenteral:*** Patient should be hospitalized. Give IV or IM. Use parenteral therapy only when drug cannot be given orally. Usual dose is 20–40 mg, repeated as necessary. Monitor BP frequently; average maximal decrease occurs in 10–80 min.

PEDIATRIC: Although safety and efficacy have not been established by controlled clinical trials, there is experience with the use of hydralazine in children.

- ***Oral:*** 0.75–3 mg/kg per 24 h PO, given in divided doses q6–12h. Dosage may be gradually increased over the next 3–4 wk to a maximum of 7.5 mg/kg per 24 h PO or 200 mg/24 h PO.
- ***Parenteral:*** 1.7–3.5 mg/kg per 24 h IV or IM, divided into four to six doses.

### Pharmacokinetics

| *Route* | *Onset* | *Peak* | *Duration* |
|---|---|---|---|
| Oral | Varies | 1–2 h | 6–12 h |
| IM/IV | Rapid | 10–20 min | 2–4 h |

*Metabolism:* Hepatic, $T_{1/2}$: 3–7 h
*Distribution:* Crosses placenta; may enter breast milk
*Excretion:* Urine

### IV facts

**Preparation:** No further preparation required, use as provided.
**Infusion:** Inject slowly over 1 min, directly into vein or into tubing of running IV; monitor BP response continually.

**Adverse effects**

- CNS: *Headache,* lacrimation, conjunctivitis, peripheral neuritis, dizziness, tremors; psychotic reactions characterized by depression, disorientation, or anxiety
- GI: *Anorexia, nausea, vomting, diarrhea,* constipation, paralytic ileus
- CV: *Palpitations, tachycardia, angina pectoris,* hypotension, paradoxical pressor response
- GU: Difficult micturition, impotence
- **Hypersensitivity**: Rash, urticaria, pruritus; fever, chills, arthralgia, eosinophilia; rarely, hepatitis and obstructive jaundice
- **Hematologic**: Blood dyscrasias
- **Other**: Nasal congestion, flushing, edema, muscle cramps, lymphadenopathy, splenomegaly, dyspnea, lupus-like (LE) syndrome, possible carcinogenesis

**Clinically important drug-drug interactions**

• Increased bioavailability of oral hydralazine given with food • Increased pharmacologic effects of beta-adrenergic blockers and hydralazine when given concomitantly; dosage of beta-blocker may need adjusting

## ■ Nursing Considerations

### Assessment

- *History:* Hypersensitivity to hydralazine, tartrazine; heart disease; CVA; increased intracranial pressure; severe hypertension; advanced renal damage; slow acetylators; lactation
- *Physical:* Weight; T; skin color, lesions; lymph node palpation; orientation, affect, reflexes; exam of conjunctiva; P, BP, orthostatic BP, supine BP, perfusion, edema, auscultation; R, adventitious sounds, status of nasal mucous membranes; bowel sounds, normal output; voiding pattern, normal output; CBC with differential, LE cell preparations, antinuclear antibody (ANA) determinations, kidney function tests, urinalysis

### Implementation

- Give oral drug with food to increase bioavailability (drug should be given in a consistent relationship to ingestion of food for consistent response to therapy).
- Use parenteral drug immediately after opening ampul. Use as quickly as possible after drawing through a needle into a syringe. Hydralazine changes color after contact with metal, and discolored solutions should be discarded.
- Withdraw drug gradually, especially from patients who have experienced marked blood pressure reduction. Rapid withdrawal may cause a possible sudden increase in BP.
- Arrange for CBC, LE cell preparations, ANA titers before and periodically during prolonged therapy, even in the asymptomatic patient. Discontinue if blood dyscrasias occur. Reevaluate therapy if ANA or LE tests are positive.
- Discontinue or reevaluate therapy if patient develops arthralgia, fever, chest pain, continued malaise.
- Arrange for pyridoxine therapy if patient develops symptoms of peripheral neuritis.
- Monitor patient for orthostatic hypotension; most marked in the morning and in hot weather, with alcohol or exercise.

### Drug-specific teaching points

- Take this drug exactly as prescribed. Take with food. Do not discontinue or reduce dosage without consulting your health care provider.
- The following side effects may occur: dizziness, weakness (these are most likely when changing position, in the early morning, after exercise, in hot weather, and when you have consumed alcohol; some tolerance may occur; avoid driving or engaging in tasks that require alertness; change position slowly; use caution in climbing stairs; lie down for a while if dizziness persists); GI upset (frequent, small meals may help); constipation; impotence; numbness, tingling (vitamin supplements may ameliorate symptoms); stuffy nose.
- Report persistent or severe constipation; unexplained fever or malaise, muscle or joint aching; chest pain; skin rash; numbness, tingling.

# 1999 Quick Access Photo Guide to Pills and Capsules

Adapted from **Facts and Comparisons**, St. Louis, Missouri

This photo guide presents nearly 400 pills and capsules, representing the most commonly prescribed generic and trade drugs in the community. These leading products, organized alphabetically by generic name, are shown in actual size and color. Each product is labeled with its trade name, as well as its strength and manufacturer.

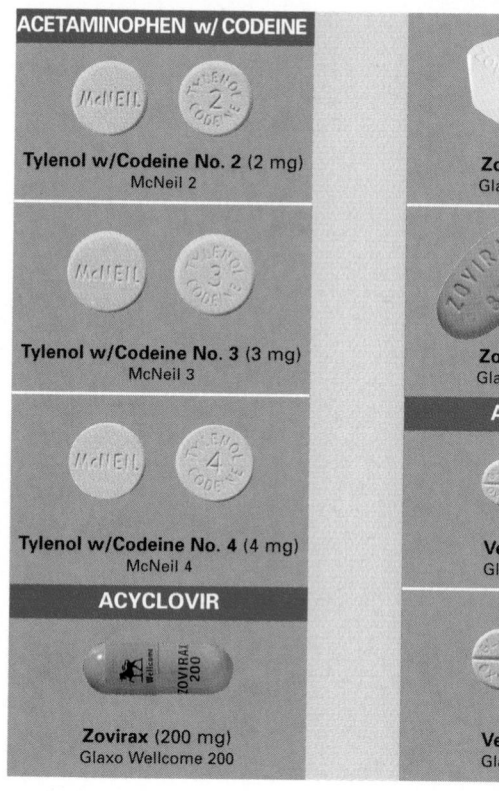

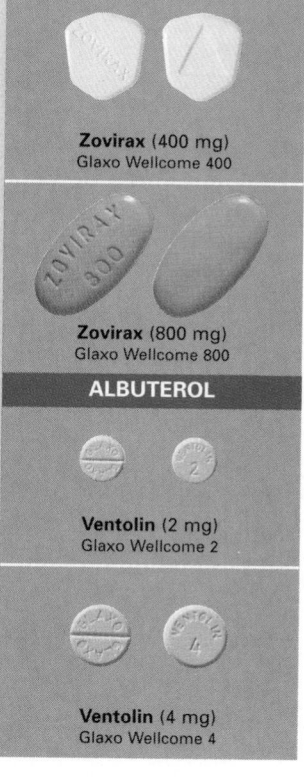

## ACETAMINOPHEN w/ CODEINE

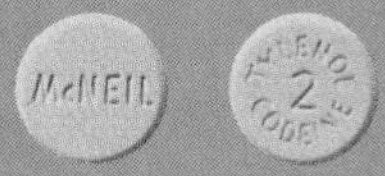


**Tylenol w/Codeine No. 2** (2 mg)
McNeil 2

**Tylenol w/Codeine No. 3** (3 mg)
McNeil 3

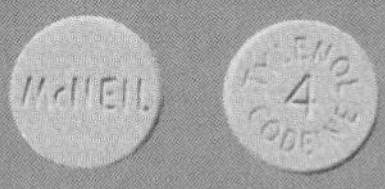


**Tylenol w/Codeine No. 4** (4 mg)
McNeil 4

## ACYCLOVIR

**Zovirax** (200 mg)
Glaxo Wellcome 200

**Zovirax** (400 mg)
Glaxo Wellcome 400

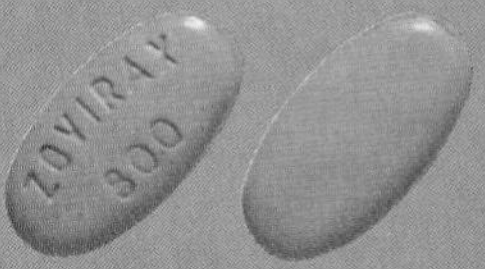


**Zovirax** (800 mg)
Glaxo Wellcome 800

## ALBUTEROL

**Ventolin** (2 mg)
Glaxo Wellcome 2

**Ventolin** (4 mg)
Glaxo Wellcome 4

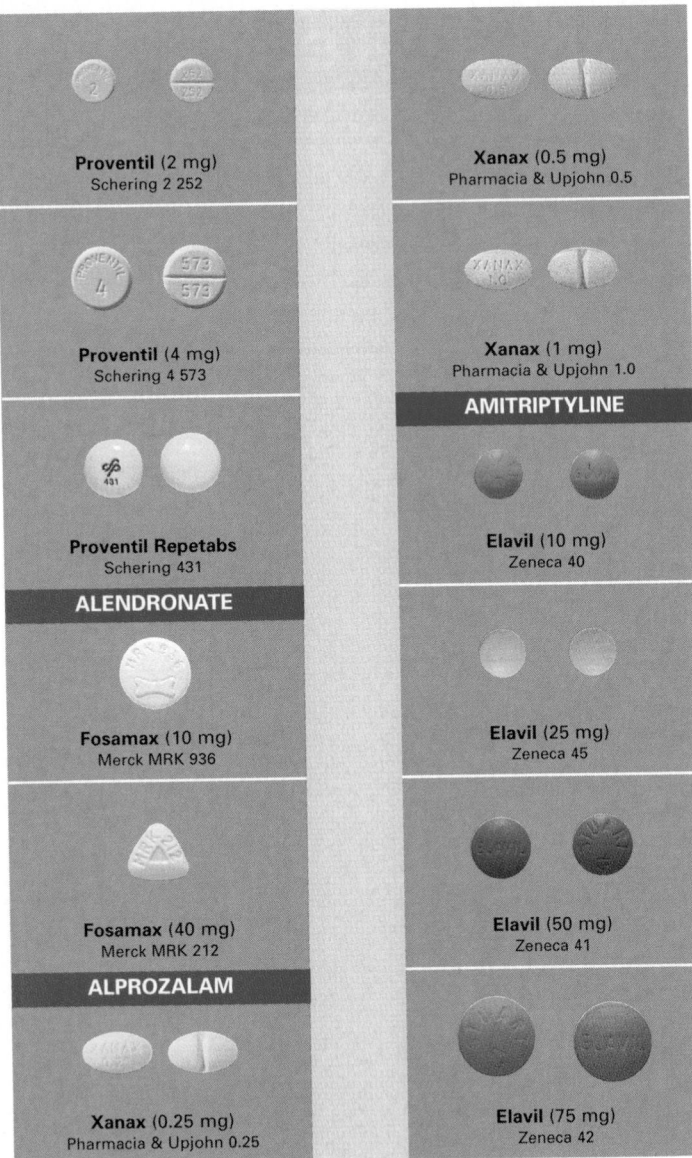

**Proventil** (2 mg)
Schering 2 252

**Proventil** (4 mg)
Schering 4 573

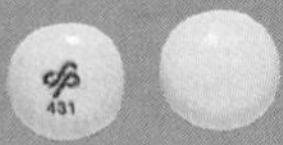

**Proventil Repetabs**
Schering 431

## ALENDRONATE

**Fosamax** (10 mg)
Merck MRK 936

**Fosamax** (40 mg)
Merck MRK 212

## ALPROZALAM

**Xanax** (0.25 mg)
Pharmacia & Upjohn 0.25

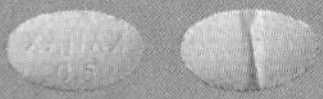

**Xanax** (0.5 mg)
Pharmacia & Upjohn 0.5

**Xanax** (1 mg)
Pharmacia & Upjohn 1.0

## AMITRIPTYLINE

**Elavil** (10 mg)
Zeneca 40

**Elavil** (25 mg)
Zeneca 45

**Elavil** (50 mg)
Zeneca 41

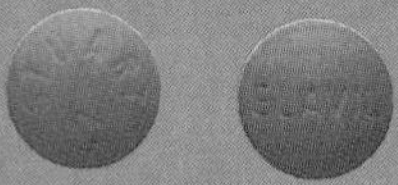

**Elavil** (75 mg)
Zeneca 42

Adapted from Facts and Comparisons, St. Louis, Missouri

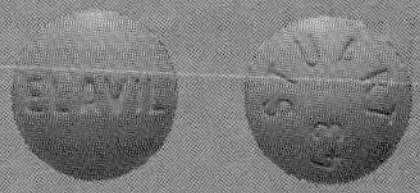

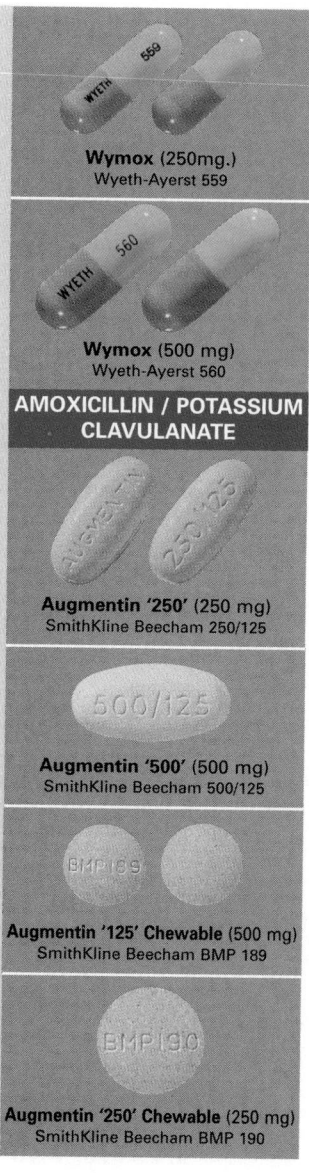


**Elavil** (100mg.)
Zeneca 43

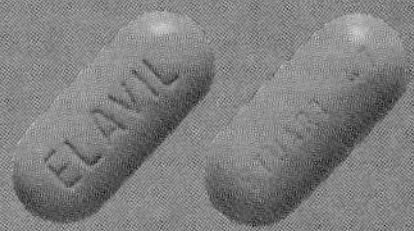


**Elavil** (150 mg)
Zeneca 47

## AMOXICILLIN

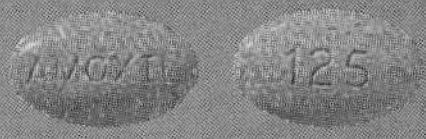


**Amoxil Chewable** (125 mg)
SmithKline Beecham 125

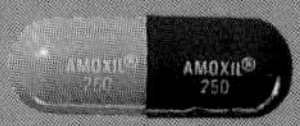


**Amoxil** (250 mg)
SmithKline Beecham 250

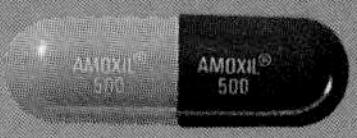


**Amoxil** (500 mg)
SmithKline Beecham 500

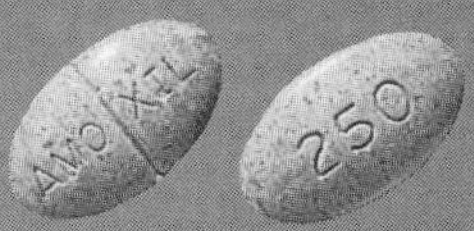


**Amoxil Chewable** (250 mg)
SmithKline Beecham 250

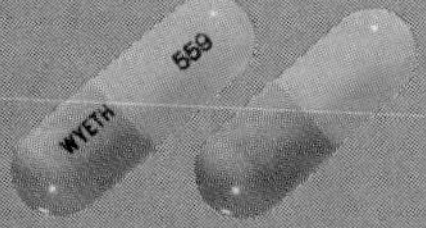


**Wymox** (250mg.)
Wyeth-Ayerst 559

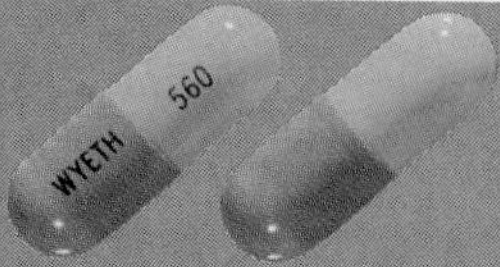


**Wymox** (500 mg)
Wyeth-Ayerst 560

## AMOXICILLIN / POTASSIUM CLAVULANATE

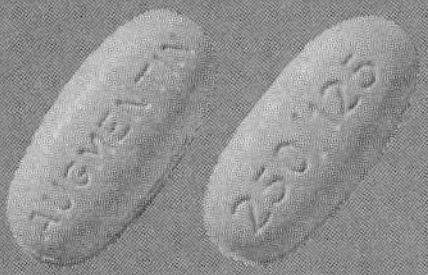


**Augmentin '250'** (250 mg)
SmithKline Beecham 250/125

**Augmentin '500'** (500 mg)
SmithKline Beecham 500/125

**Augmentin '125' Chewable** (500 mg)
SmithKline Beecham BMP 189

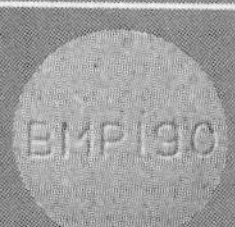


**Augmentin '250' Chewable** (250 mg)
SmithKline Beecham BMP 190

Adapted from Facts and Comparisons, St. Louis, Missouri

## AMPICILLIN

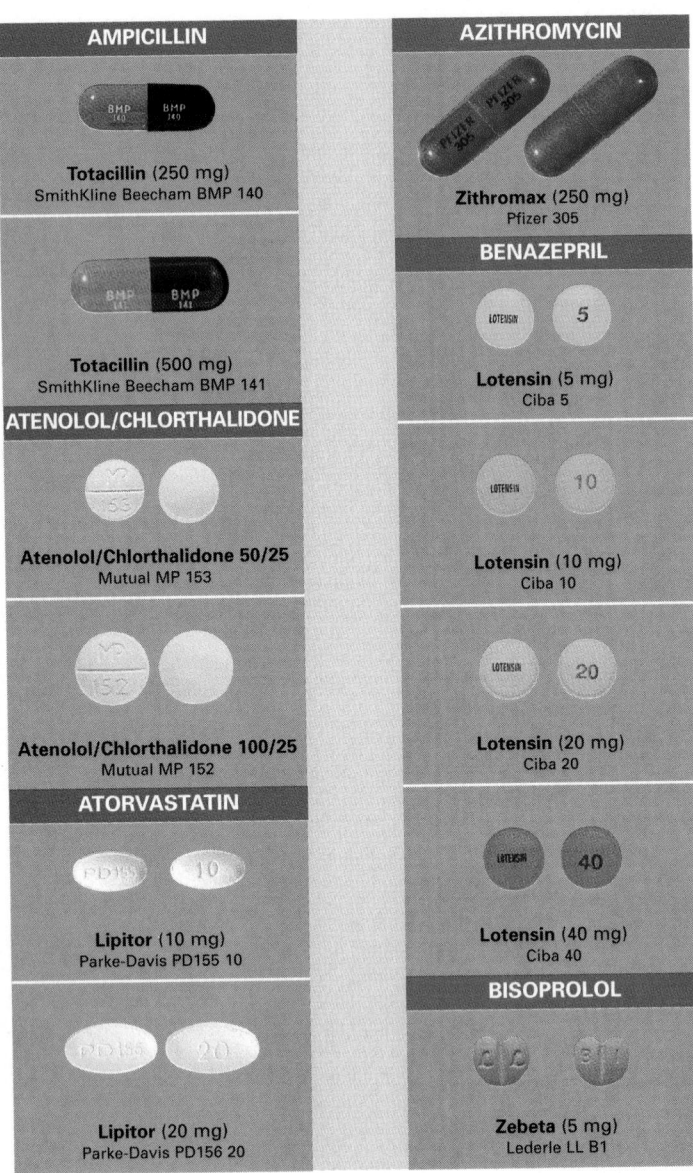


**Totacillin** (250 mg)
SmithKline Beecham BMP 140

**Totacillin** (500 mg)
SmithKline Beecham BMP 141

## ATENOLOL/CHLORTHALIDONE

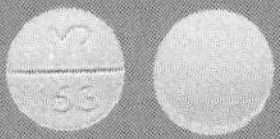


**Atenolol/Chlorthalidone 50/25**
Mutual MP 153

**Atenolol/Chlorthalidone 100/25**
Mutual MP 152

## ATORVASTATIN

**Lipitor** (10 mg)
Parke-Davis PD155 10

**Lipitor** (20 mg)
Parke-Davis PD156 20

## AZITHROMYCIN

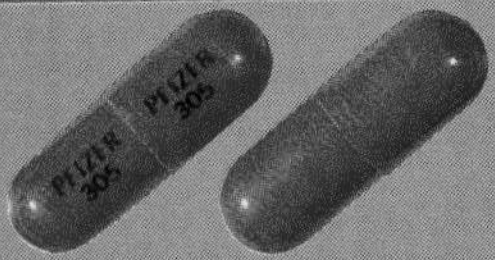


**Zithromax** (250 mg)
Pfizer 305

## BENAZEPRIL

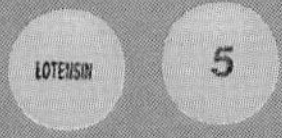


**Lotensin** (5 mg)
Ciba 5

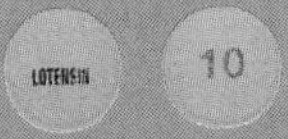


**Lotensin** (10 mg)
Ciba 10

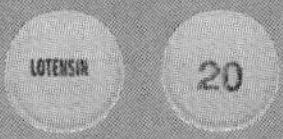


**Lotensin** (20 mg)
Ciba 20

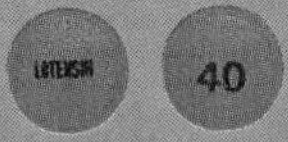


**Lotensin** (40 mg)
Ciba 40

## BISOPROLOL

**Zebeta** (5 mg)
Lederle LL B1

Adapted from Facts and Comparisons, St. Louis, Missouri

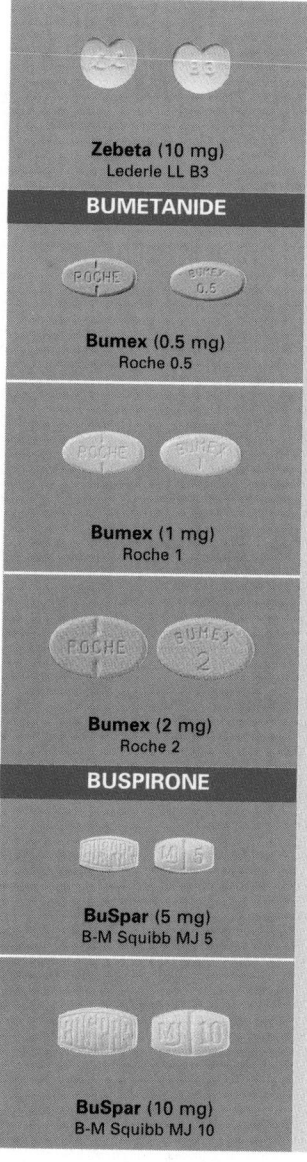


**Zebeta** (10 mg)
Lederle LL B3

## BUMETANIDE

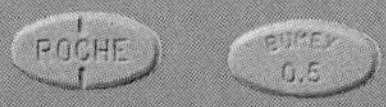


**Bumex** (0.5 mg)
Roche 0.5

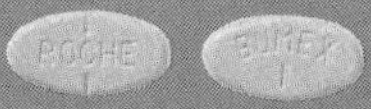


**Bumex** (1 mg)
Roche 1

**Bumex** (2 mg)
Roche 2

## BUSPIRONE

**BuSpar** (5 mg)
B-M Squibb MJ 5

**BuSpar** (10 mg)
B-M Squibb MJ 10

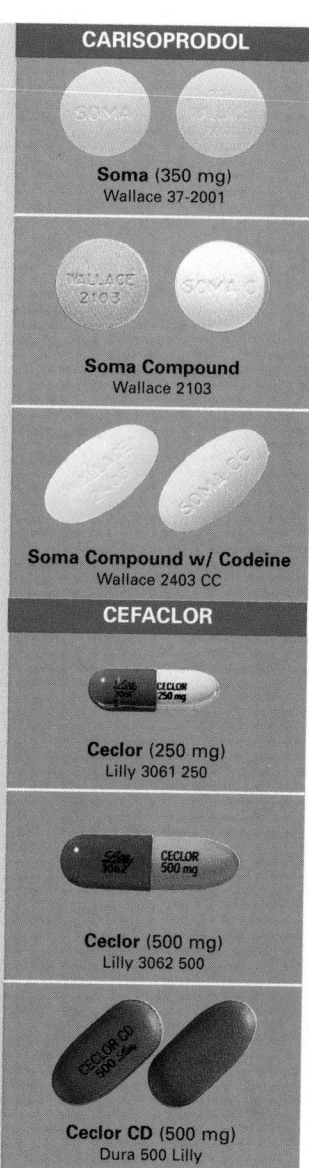

## CARISOPRODOL

**Soma** (350 mg)
Wallace 37-2001

**Soma Compound**
Wallace 2103

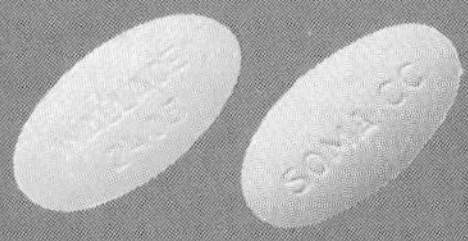


**Soma Compound w/ Codeine**
Wallace 2403 CC

## CEFACLOR

**Ceclor** (250 mg)
Lilly 3061 250

**Ceclor** (500 mg)
Lilly 3062 500

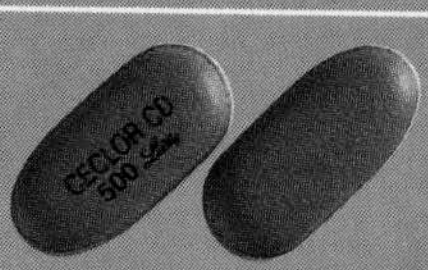


**Ceclor CD** (500 mg)
Dura 500 Lilly

Adapted from Facts and Comparisons, St. Louis, Missouri

## CEFIXIME

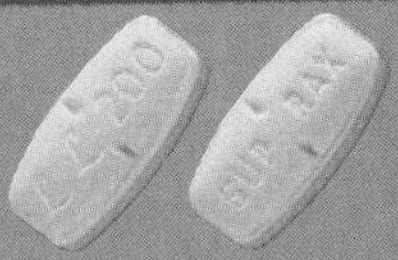

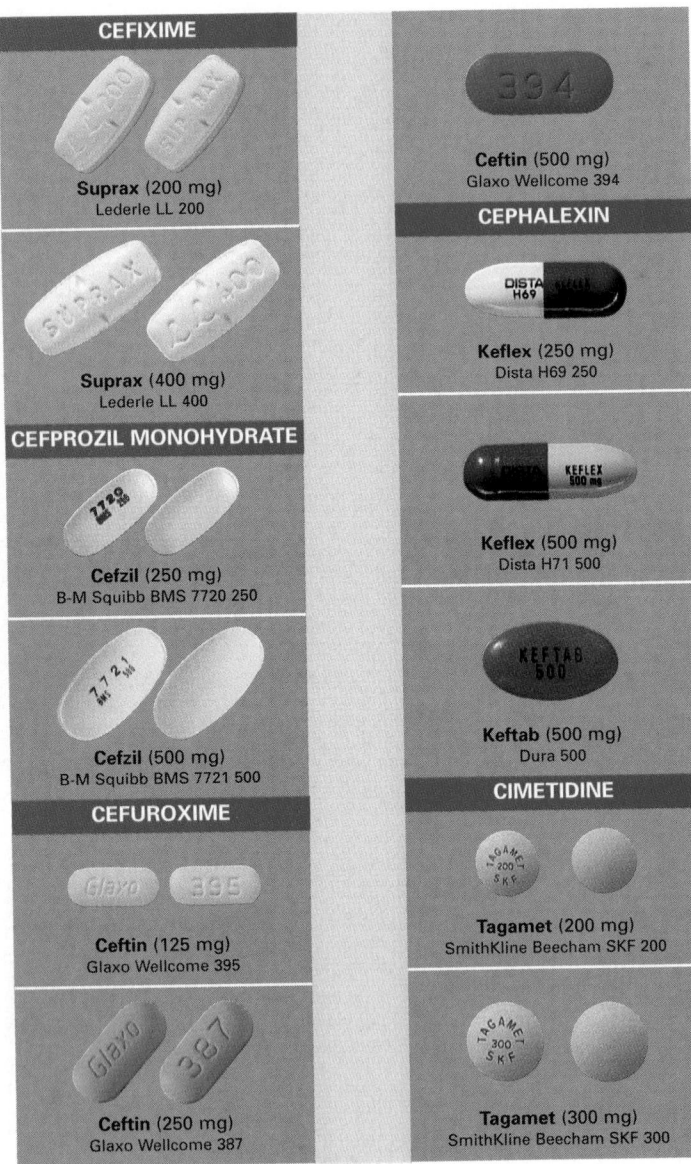


**Suprax** (200 mg)
Lederle LL 200

**Suprax** (400 mg)
Lederle LL 400

## CEFPROZIL MONOHYDRATE

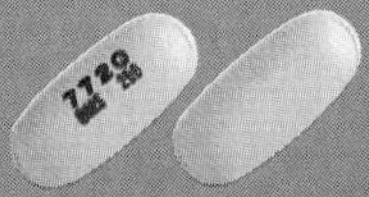

**Cefzil** (250 mg)
B-M Squibb BMS 7720 250

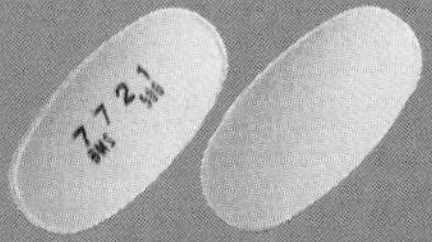

**Cefzil** (500 mg)
B-M Squibb BMS 7721 500

## CEFUROXIME

**Ceftin** (125 mg)
Glaxo Wellcome 395

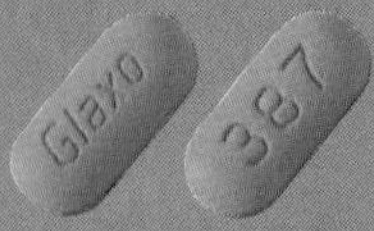


**Ceftin** (250 mg)
Glaxo Wellcome 387

**Ceftin** (500 mg)
Glaxo Wellcome 394

## CEPHALEXIN

**Keflex** (250 mg)
Dista H69 250

**Keflex** (500 mg)
Dista H71 500

**Keftab** (500 mg)
Dura 500

## CIMETIDINE

**Tagamet** (200 mg)
SmithKline Beecham SKF 200

**Tagamet** (300 mg)
SmithKline Beecham SKF 300

Adapted from Facts and Comparisons, St. Louis, Missouri

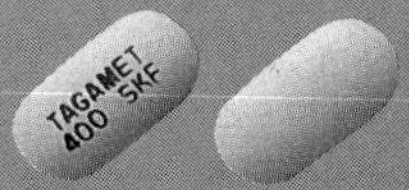

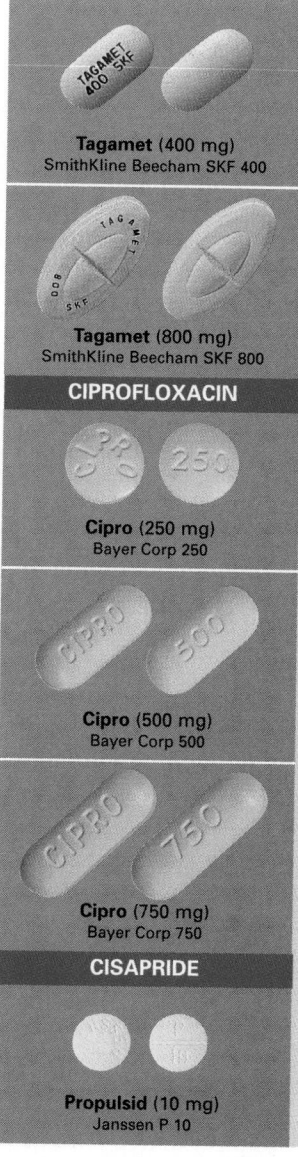


**Tagamet** (400 mg)
SmithKline Beecham SKF 400

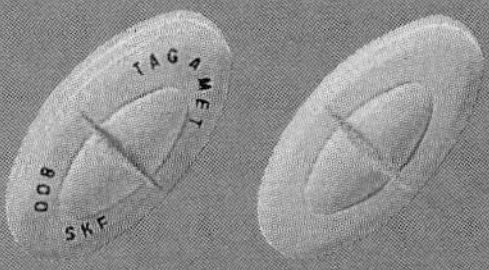

**Tagamet** (800 mg)
SmithKline Beecham SKF 800

## CIPROFLOXACIN

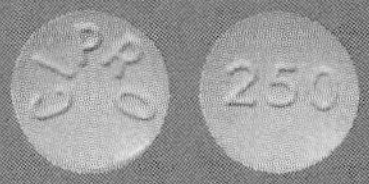


**Cipro** (250 mg)
Bayer Corp 250

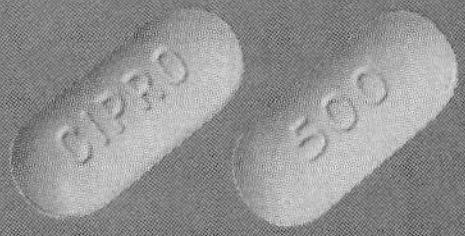


**Cipro** (500 mg)
Bayer Corp 500

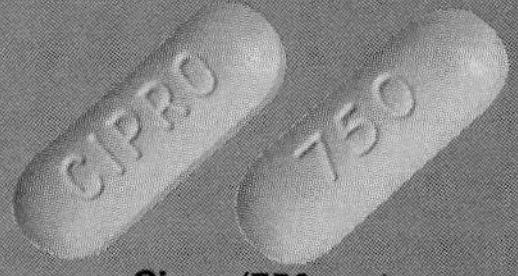


**Cipro** (750 mg)
Bayer Corp 750

## CISAPRIDE

**Propulsid** (10 mg)
Janssen P 10

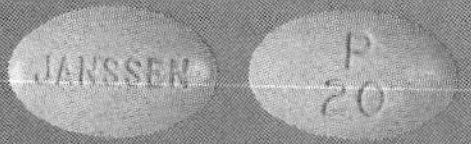

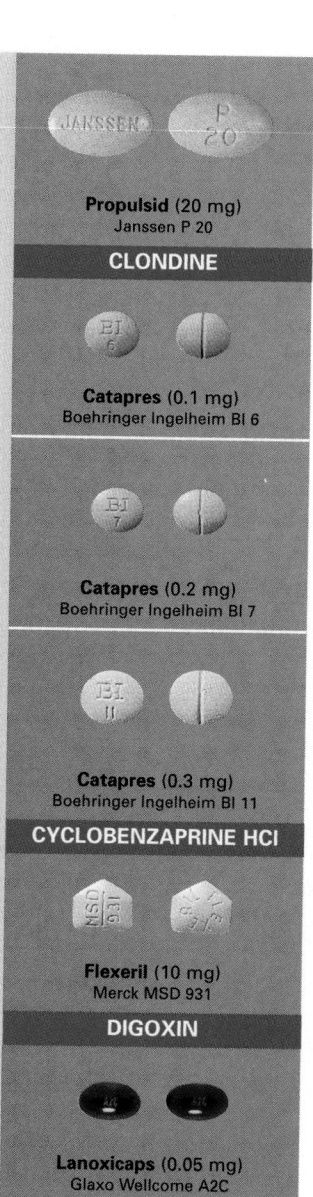


**Propulsid** (20 mg)
Janssen P 20

## CLONDINE

**Catapres** (0.1 mg)
Boehringer Ingelheim BI 6

**Catapres** (0.2 mg)
Boehringer Ingelheim BI 7

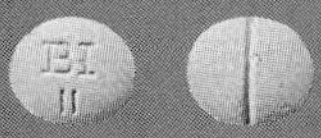

**Catapres** (0.3 mg)
Boehringer Ingelheim BI 11

## CYCLOBENZAPRINE HCl

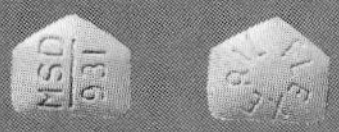


**Flexeril** (10 mg)
Merck MSD 931

## DIGOXIN

**Lanoxicaps** (0.05 mg)
Glaxo Wellcome A2C

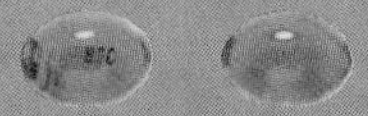

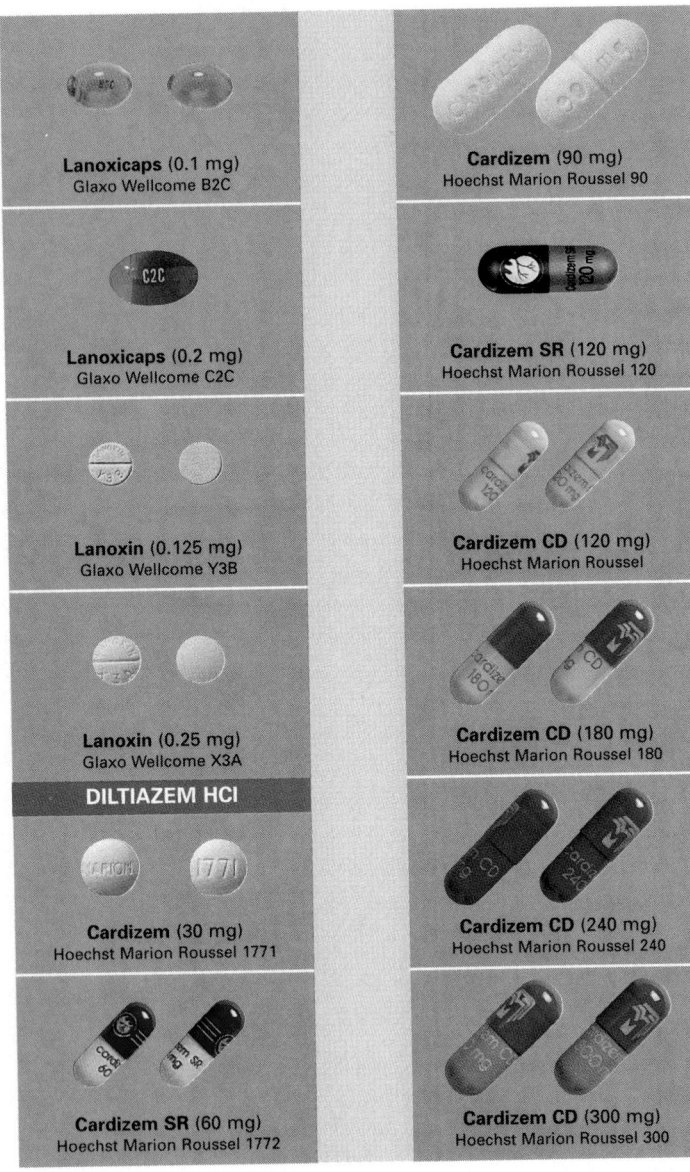

**Lanoxicaps** (0.1 mg)
Glaxo Wellcome B2C

**Lanoxicaps** (0.2 mg)
Glaxo Wellcome C2C

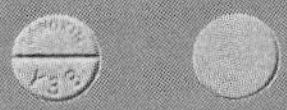

**Lanoxin** (0.125 mg)
Glaxo Wellcome Y3B

**Lanoxin** (0.25 mg)
Glaxo Wellcome X3A

## DILTIAZEM HCl

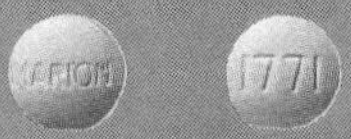


**Cardizem** (30 mg)
Hoechst Marion Roussel 1771

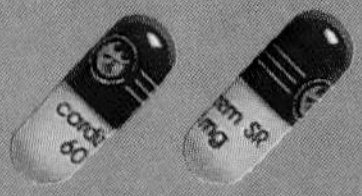

**Cardizem SR** (60 mg)
Hoechst Marion Roussel 1772

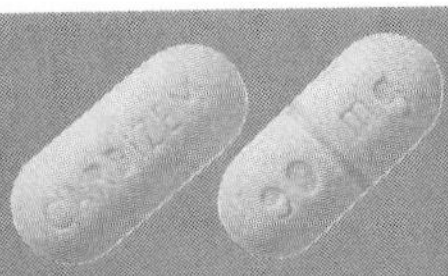

**Cardizem** (90 mg)
Hoechst Marion Roussel 90

**Cardizem SR** (120 mg)
Hoechst Marion Roussel 120

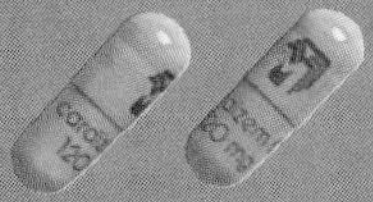

**Cardizem CD** (120 mg)
Hoechst Marion Roussel

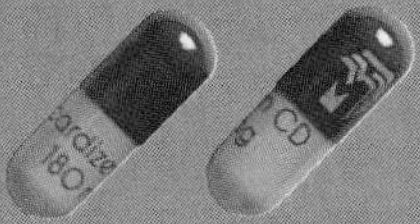

**Cardizem CD** (180 mg)
Hoechst Marion Roussel 180

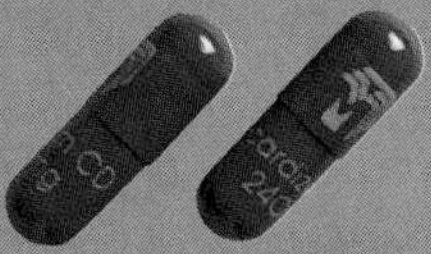

**Cardizem CD** (240 mg)
Hoechst Marion Roussel 240

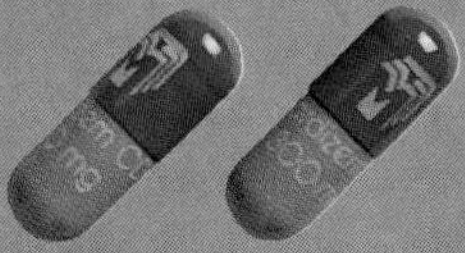

**Cardizem CD** (300 mg)
Hoechst Marion Roussel 300

Adapted from Facts and Comparisons, St. Louis, Missouri

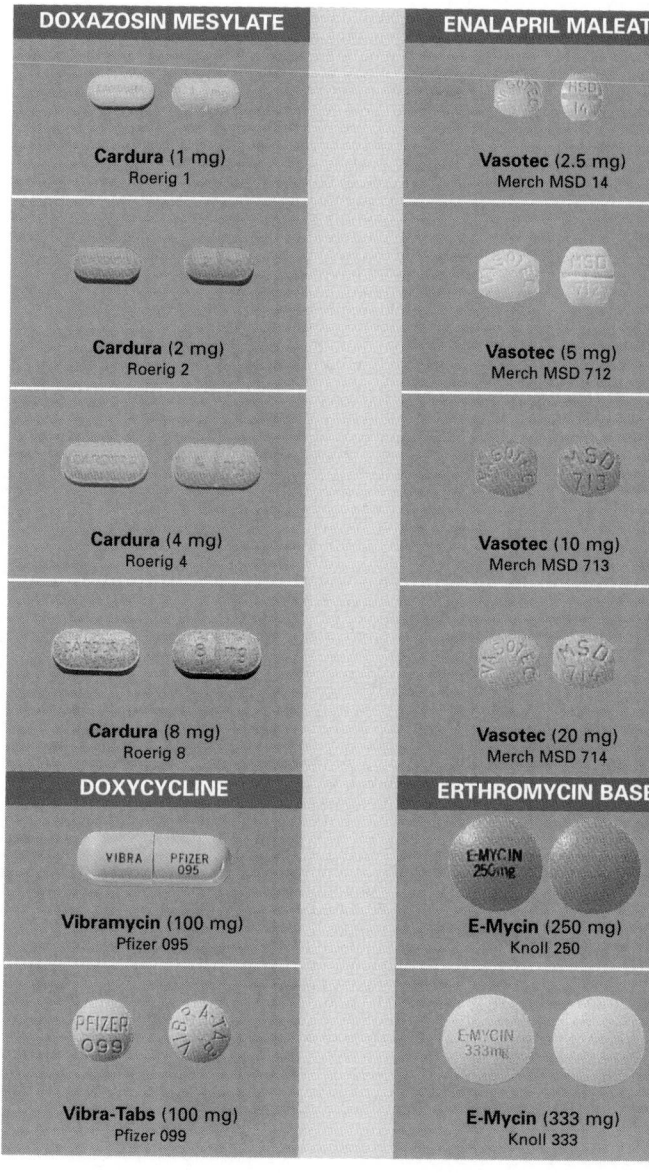

## DOXAZOSIN MESYLATE

**Cardura** (1 mg)
Roerig 1

**Cardura** (2 mg)
Roerig 2

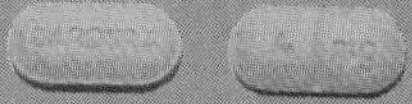

**Cardura** (4 mg)
Roerig 4

**Cardura** (8 mg)
Roerig 8

## DOXYCYCLINE

**Vibramycin** (100 mg)
Pfizer 095

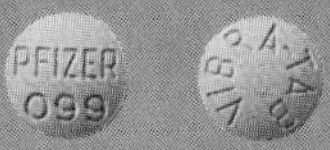


**Vibra-Tabs** (100 mg)
Pfizer 099

## ENALAPRIL MALEATE

**Vasotec** (2.5 mg)
Merch MSD 14

**Vasotec** (5 mg)
Merch MSD 712

**Vasotec** (10 mg)
Merch MSD 713

**Vasotec** (20 mg)
Merch MSD 714

## ERTHROMYCIN BASE

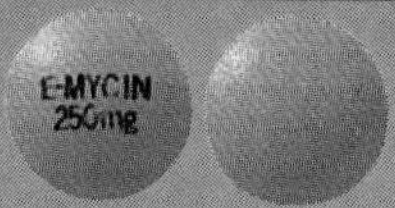


**E-Mycin** (250 mg)
Knoll 250

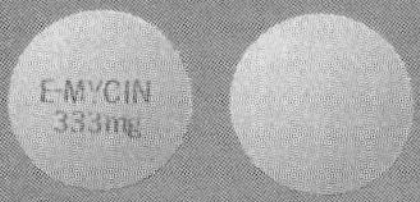


**E-Mycin** (333 mg)
Knoll 333

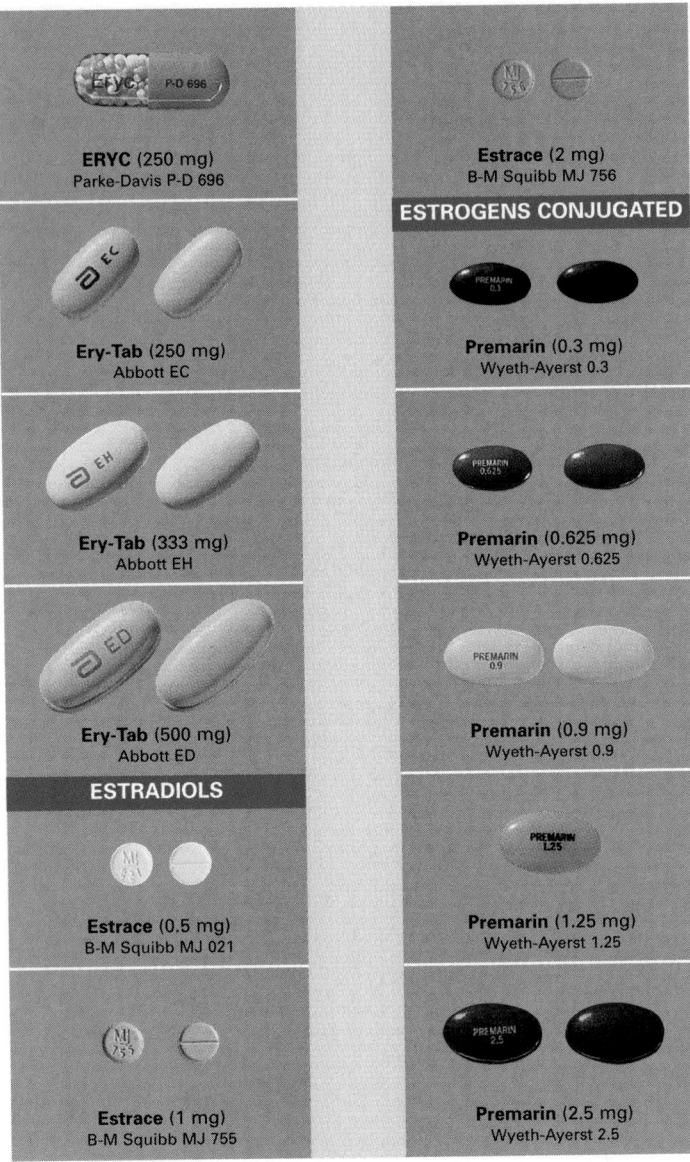


**ERYC** (250 mg)
Parke-Davis P-D 696

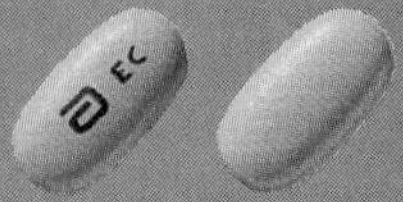


**Ery-Tab** (250 mg)
Abbott EC

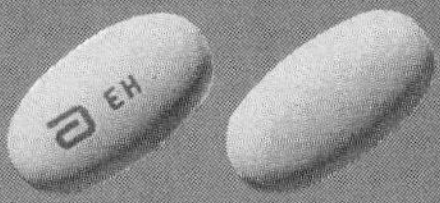


**Ery-Tab** (333 mg)
Abbott EH

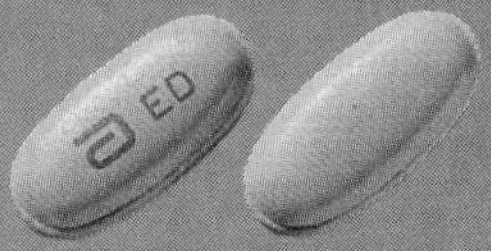


**Ery-Tab** (500 mg)
Abbott ED

## ESTRADIOLS

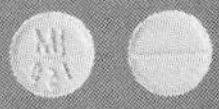

**Estrace** (0.5 mg)
B-M Squibb MJ 021

**Estrace** (1 mg)
B-M Squibb MJ 755

**Estrace** (2 mg)
B-M Squibb MJ 756

## ESTROGENS CONJUGATED

**Premarin** (0.3 mg)
Wyeth-Ayerst 0.3

**Premarin** (0.625 mg)
Wyeth-Ayerst 0.625

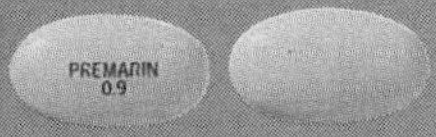


**Premarin** (0.9 mg)
Wyeth-Ayerst 0.9

**Premarin** (1.25 mg)
Wyeth-Ayerst 1.25

**Premarin** (2.5 mg)
Wyeth-Ayerst 2.5

Adapted from Facts and Comparisons, St. Louis, Missouri

## ETODOLAC

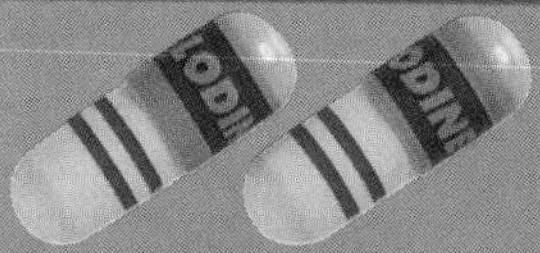

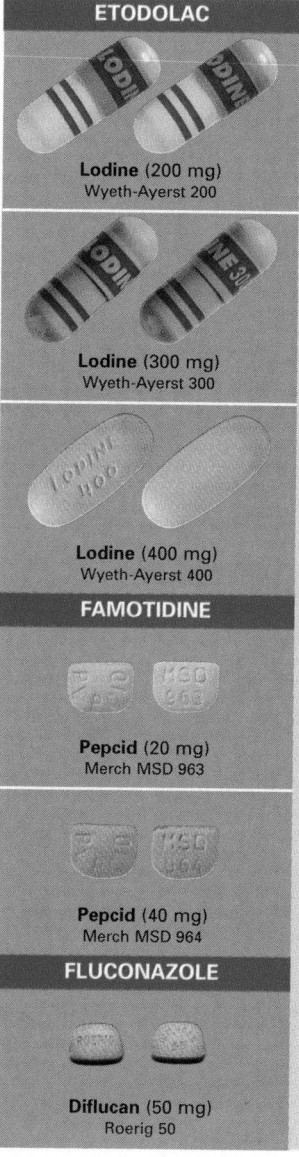

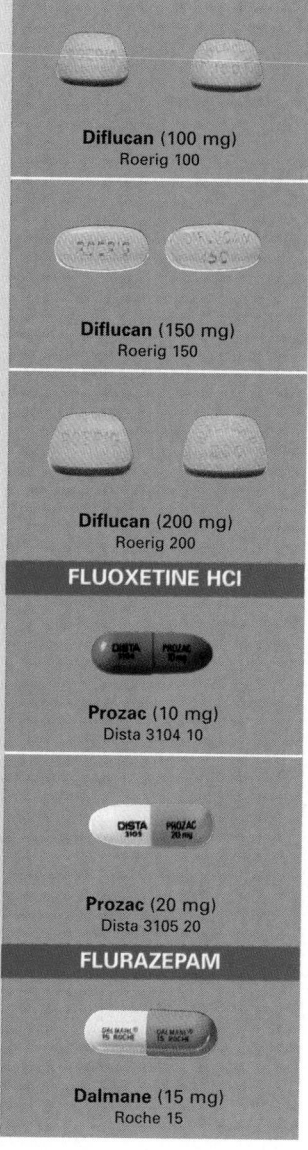

**Lodine** (200 mg)
Wyeth-Ayerst 200

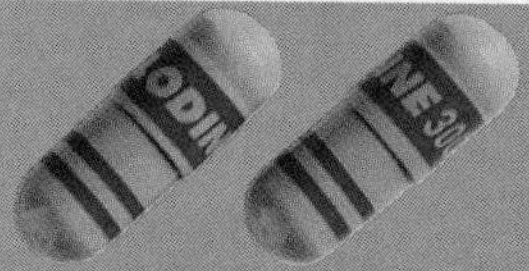

**Lodine** (300 mg)
Wyeth-Ayerst 300

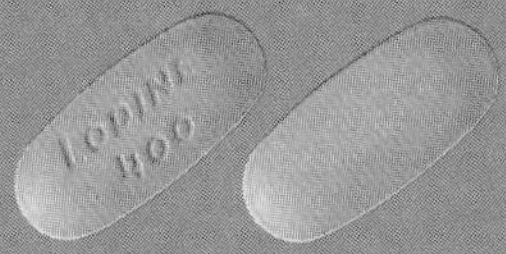


**Lodine** (400 mg)
Wyeth-Ayerst 400

## FAMOTIDINE

**Pepcid** (20 mg)
Merch MSD 963

**Pepcid** (40 mg)
Merch MSD 964

## FLUCONAZOLE

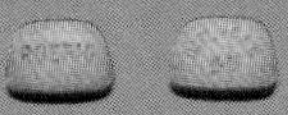

**Diflucan** (50 mg)
Roerig 50

**Diflucan** (100 mg)
Roerig 100

**Diflucan** (150 mg)
Roerig 150

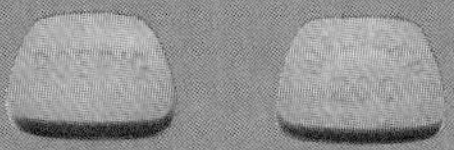

**Diflucan** (200 mg)
Roerig 200

## FLUOXETINE HCl

**Prozac** (10 mg)
Dista 3104 10

**Prozac** (20 mg)
Dista 3105 20

## FLURAZEPAM

**Dalmane** (15 mg)
Roche 15

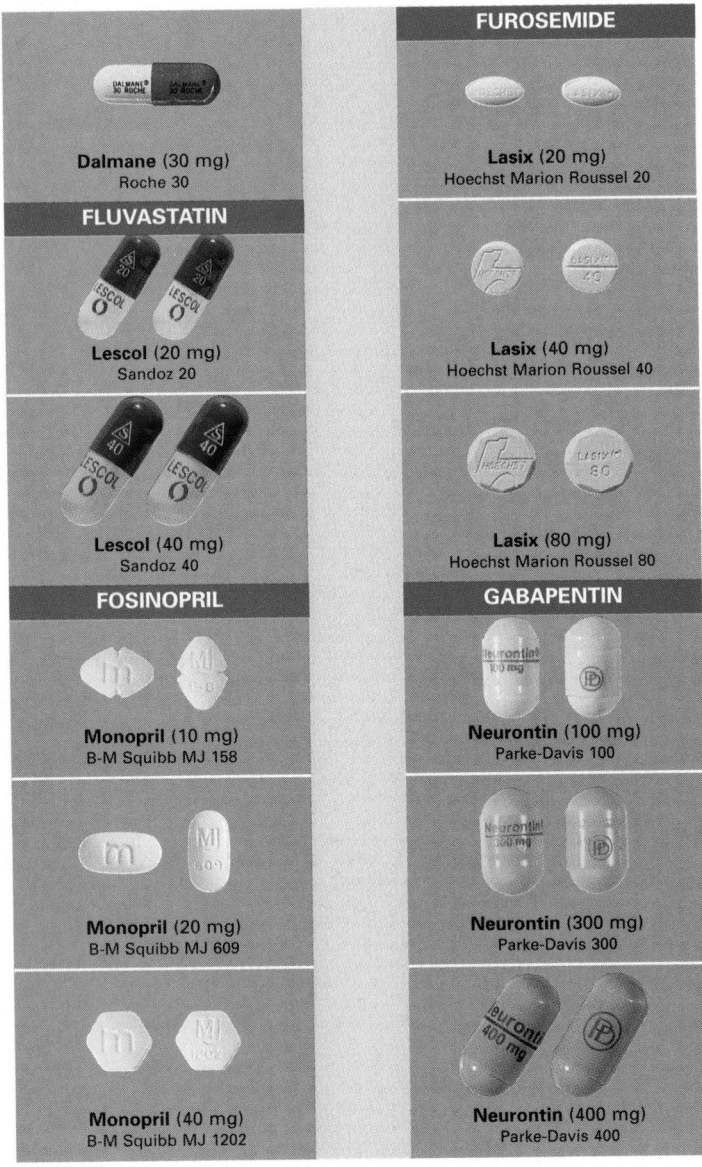

**Dalmane** (30 mg)
Roche 30

## FLUVASTATIN

**Lescol** (20 mg)
Sandoz 20

**Lescol** (40 mg)
Sandoz 40

## FOSINOPRIL

**Monopril** (10 mg)
B-M Squibb MJ 158

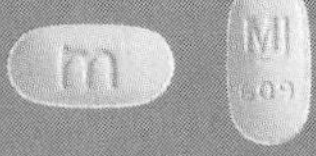

**Monopril** (20 mg)
B-M Squibb MJ 609

**Monopril** (40 mg)
B-M Squibb MJ 1202

## FUROSEMIDE

**Lasix** (20 mg)
Hoechst Marion Roussel 20

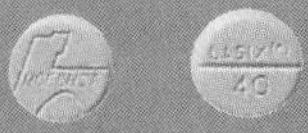


**Lasix** (40 mg)
Hoechst Marion Roussel 40

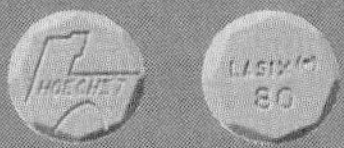


**Lasix** (80 mg)
Hoechst Marion Roussel 80

## GABAPENTIN

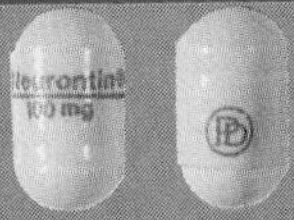

**Neurontin** (100 mg)
Parke-Davis 100

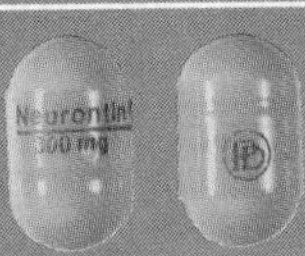

**Neurontin** (300 mg)
Parke-Davis 300

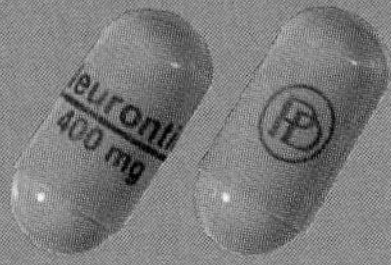


**Neurontin** (400 mg)
Parke-Davis 400

Adapted from Facts and Comparisons, St. Louis, Missouri

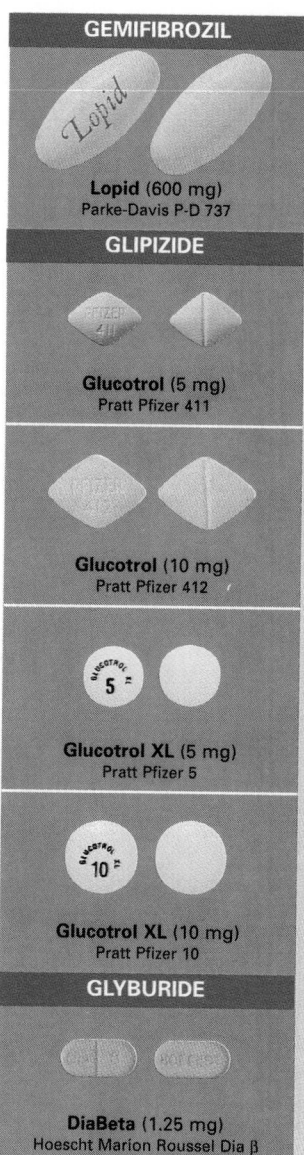

## GEMIFIBROZIL

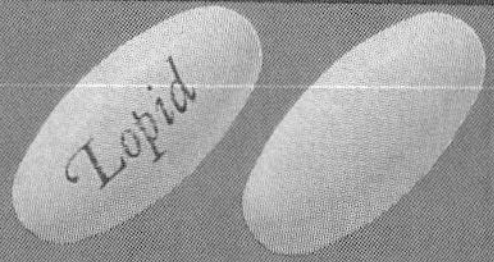


**Lopid** (600 mg)
Parke-Davis P-D 737

## GLIPIZIDE

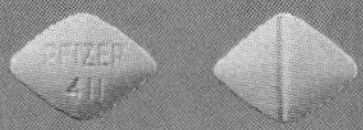

**Glucotrol** (5 mg)
Pratt Pfizer 411

**Glucotrol** (10 mg)
Pratt Pfizer 412

**Glucotrol XL** (5 mg)
Pratt Pfizer 5

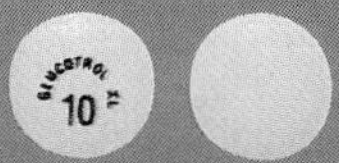


**Glucotrol XL** (10 mg)
Pratt Pfizer 10

## GLYBURIDE

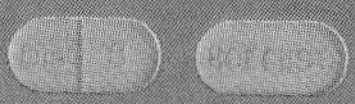

**DiaBeta** (1.25 mg)
Hoescht Marion Roussel Dia β

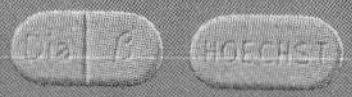

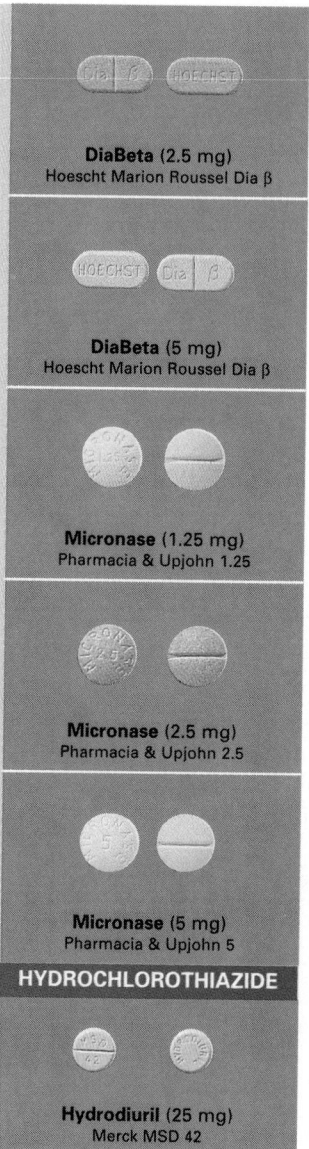


**DiaBeta** (2.5 mg)
Hoescht Marion Roussel Dia β

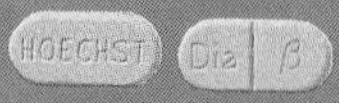


**DiaBeta** (5 mg)
Hoescht Marion Roussel Dia β

**Micronase** (1.25 mg)
Pharmacia & Upjohn 1.25

**Micronase** (2.5 mg)
Pharmacia & Upjohn 2.5

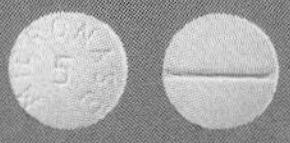

**Micronase** (5 mg)
Pharmacia & Upjohn 5

## HYDROCHLOROTHIAZIDE

**Hydrodiuril** (25 mg)
Merck MSD 42

Adapted from Facts and Comparisons, St. Louis, Missouri

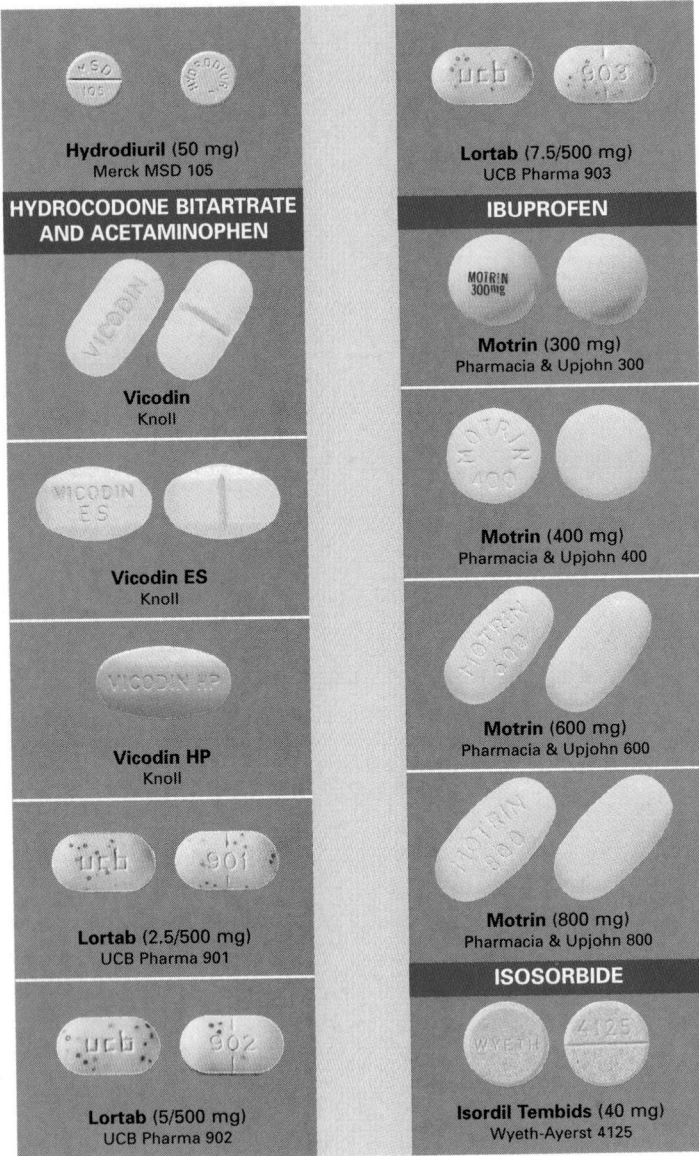


**Hydrodiuril** (50 mg)
Merck MSD 105

## HYDROCODONE BITARTRATE AND ACETAMINOPHEN

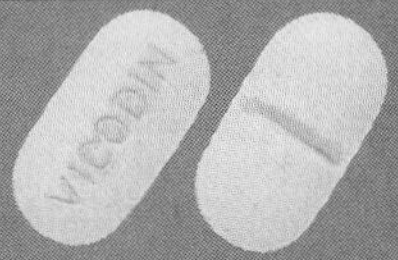


**Vicodin**
Knoll

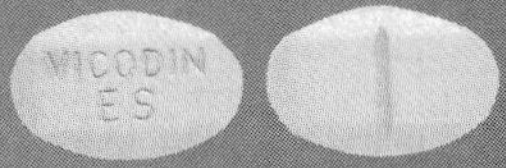


**Vicodin ES**
Knoll

**Vicodin HP**
Knoll

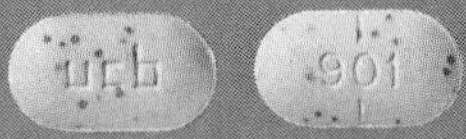


**Lortab** (2.5/500 mg)
UCB Pharma 901

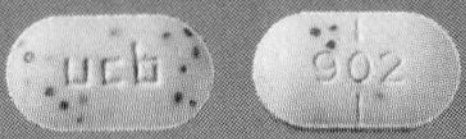


**Lortab** (5/500 mg)
UCB Pharma 902

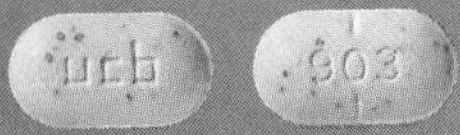


**Lortab** (7.5/500 mg)
UCB Pharma 903

## IBUPROFEN

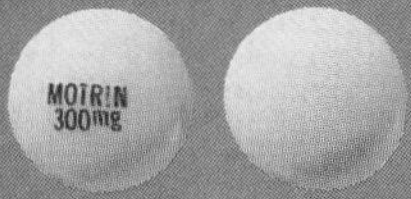


**Motrin** (300 mg)
Pharmacia & Upjohn 300

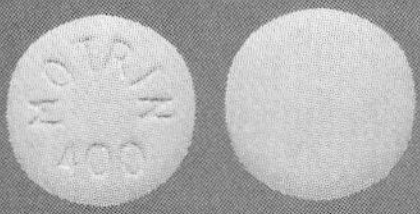


**Motrin** (400 mg)
Pharmacia & Upjohn 400

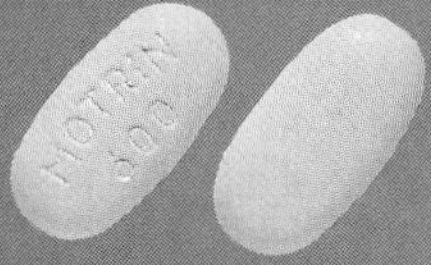


**Motrin** (600 mg)
Pharmacia & Upjohn 600

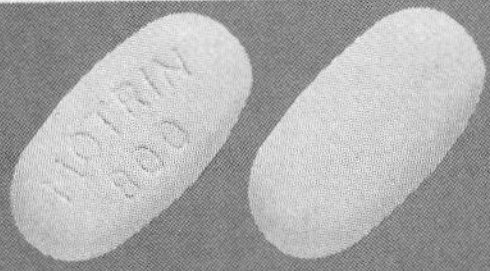


**Motrin** (800 mg)
Pharmacia & Upjohn 800

## ISOSORBIDE

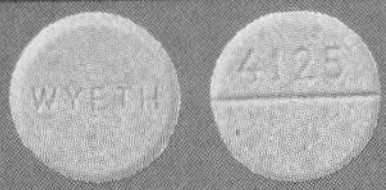


**Isordil Tembids** (40 mg)
Wyeth-Ayerst 4125

Adapted from Facts and Comparisons, St. Louis, Missouri

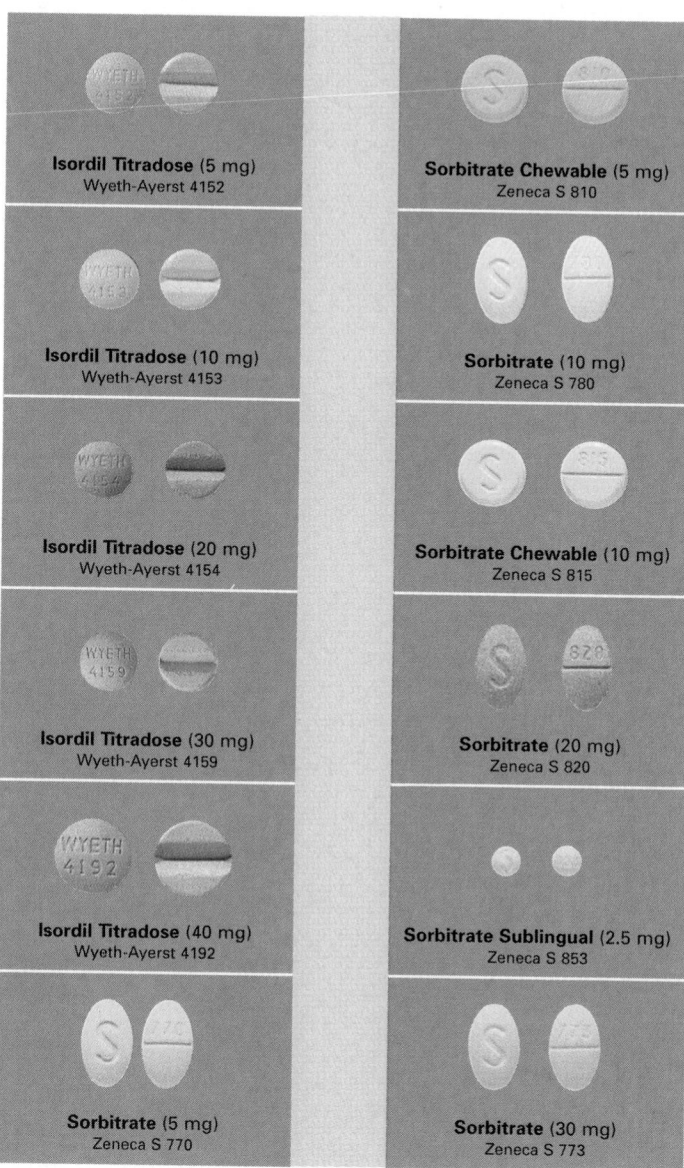


**Isordil Titradose** (5 mg)
Wyeth-Ayerst 4152

**Isordil Titradose** (10 mg)
Wyeth-Ayerst 4153

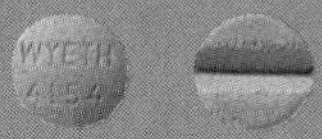


**Isordil Titradose** (20 mg)
Wyeth-Ayerst 4154

**Isordil Titradose** (30 mg)
Wyeth-Ayerst 4159

**Isordil Titradose** (40 mg)
Wyeth-Ayerst 4192

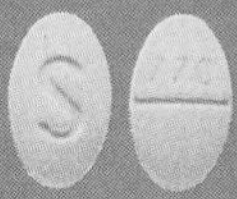


**Sorbitrate** (5 mg)
Zeneca S 770

**Sorbitrate Chewable** (5 mg)
Zeneca S 810

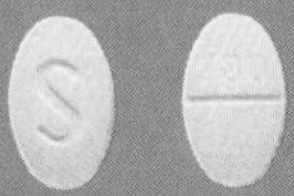


**Sorbitrate** (10 mg)
Zeneca S 780

**Sorbitrate Chewable** (10 mg)
Zeneca S 815

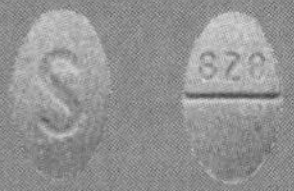


**Sorbitrate** (20 mg)
Zeneca S 820

**Sorbitrate Sublingual** (2.5 mg)
Zeneca S 853

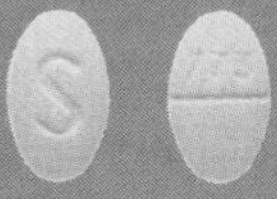


**Sorbitrate** (30 mg)
Zeneca S 773

Adapted from Facts and Comparisons, St. Louis, Missouri

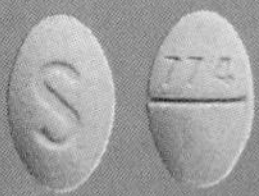

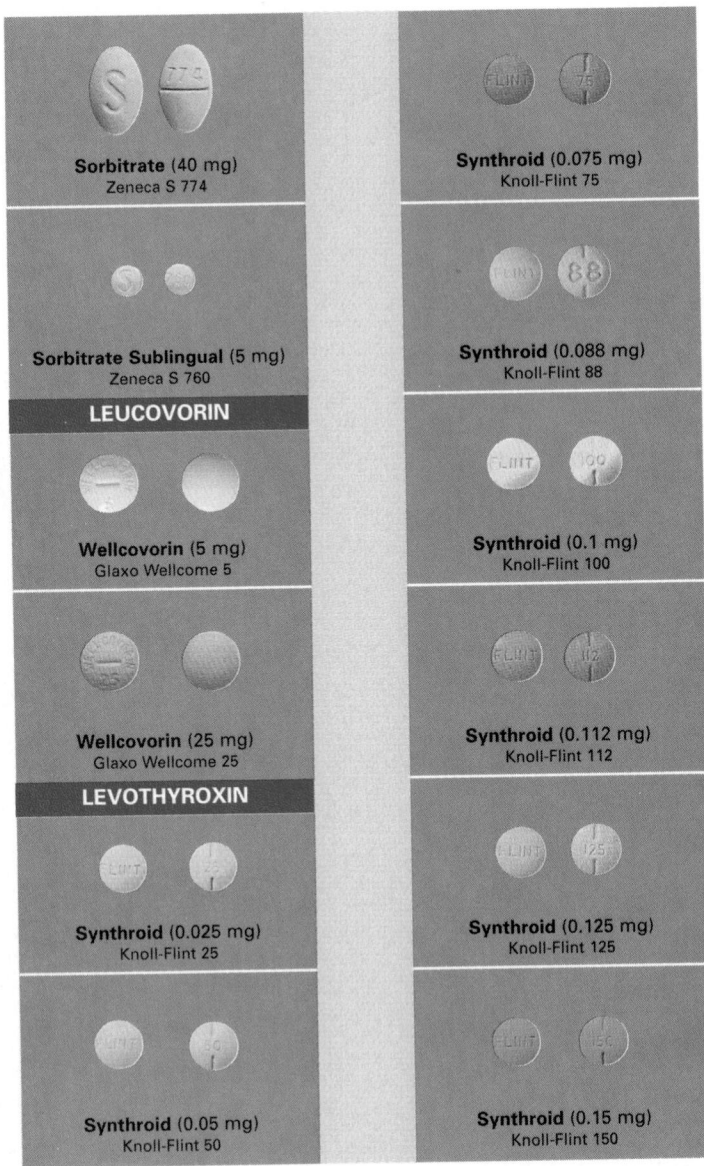


**Sorbitrate** (40 mg)
Zeneca S 774

**Sorbitrate Sublingual** (5 mg)
Zeneca S 760

## LEUCOVORIN

**Wellcovorin** (5 mg)
Glaxo Wellcome 5

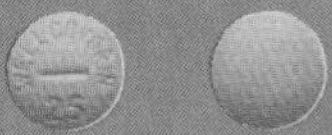

**Wellcovorin** (25 mg)
Glaxo Wellcome 25

## LEVOTHYROXIN

**Synthroid** (0.025 mg)
Knoll-Flint 25

**Synthroid** (0.05 mg)
Knoll-Flint 50

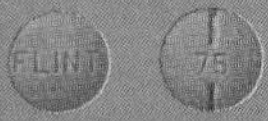


**Synthroid** (0.075 mg)
Knoll-Flint 75

**Synthroid** (0.088 mg)
Knoll-Flint 88

**Synthroid** (0.1 mg)
Knoll-Flint 100

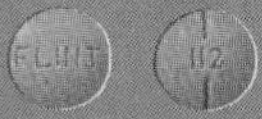

**Synthroid** (0.112 mg)
Knoll-Flint 112

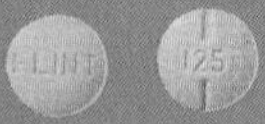


**Synthroid** (0.125 mg)
Knoll-Flint 125

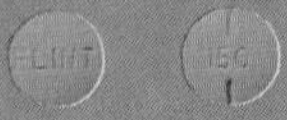

**Synthroid** (0.15 mg)
Knoll-Flint 150

Adapted from Facts and Comparisons, St. Louis, Missouri

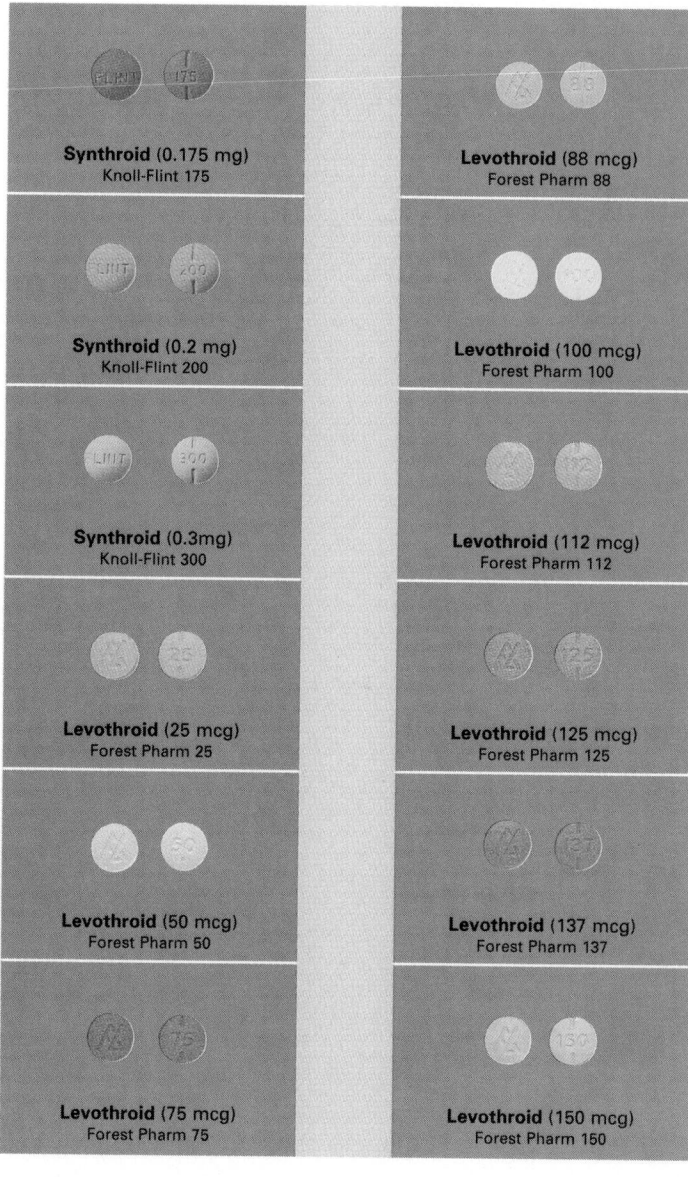

**Synthroid** (0.175 mg)
Knoll-Flint 175

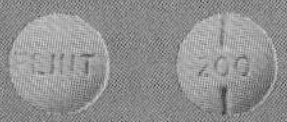

**Synthroid** (0.2 mg)
Knoll-Flint 200

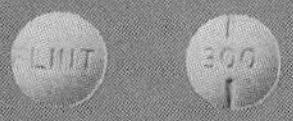

**Synthroid** (0.3mg)
Knoll-Flint 300

**Levothroid** (25 mcg)
Forest Pharm 25

**Levothroid** (50 mcg)
Forest Pharm 50

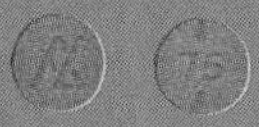

**Levothroid** (75 mcg)
Forest Pharm 75

**Levothroid** (88 mcg)
Forest Pharm 88

**Levothroid** (100 mcg)
Forest Pharm 100

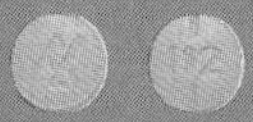

**Levothroid** (112 mcg)
Forest Pharm 112

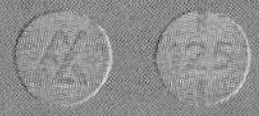

**Levothroid** (125 mcg)
Forest Pharm 125

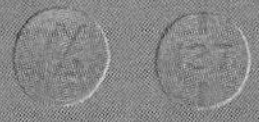

**Levothroid** (137 mcg)
Forest Pharm 137

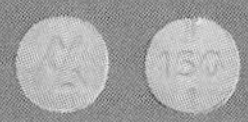

**Levothroid** (150 mcg)
Forest Pharm 150

Adapted from Facts and Comparisons, St. Louis, Missouri

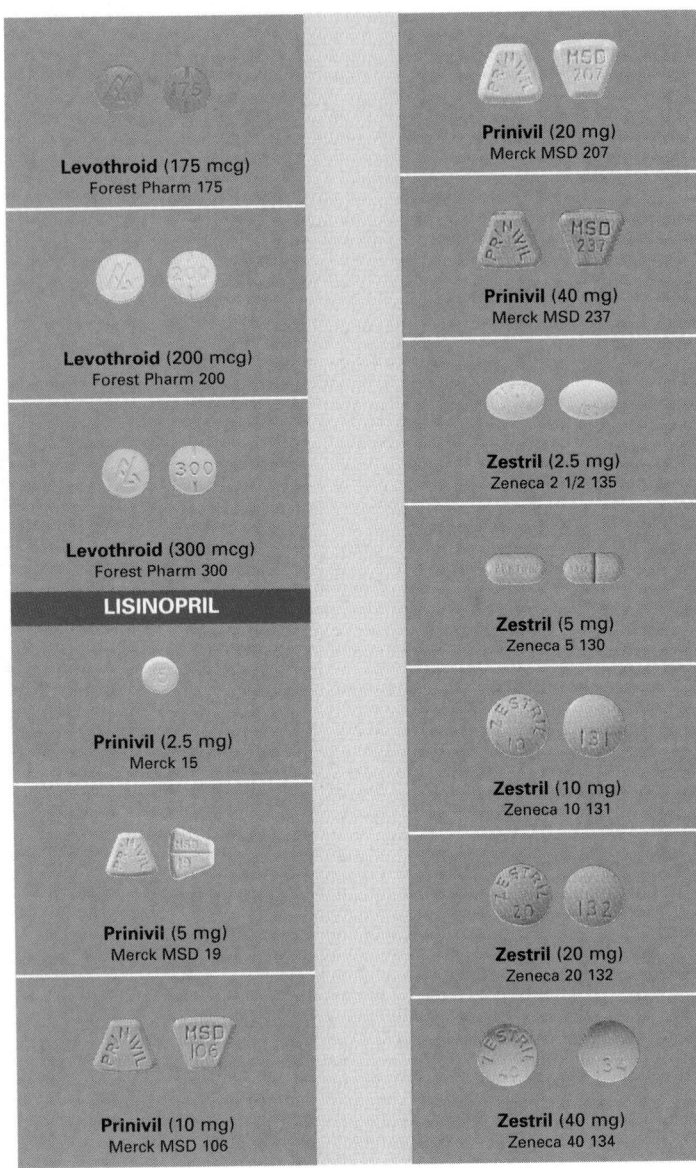

**Levothroid** (175 mcg)
Forest Pharm 175

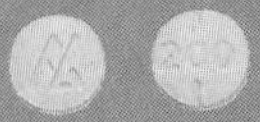

**Levothroid** (200 mcg)
Forest Pharm 200

**Levothroid** (300 mcg)
Forest Pharm 300

## LISINOPRIL

**Prinivil** (2.5 mg)
Merck 15

**Prinivil** (5 mg)
Merck MSD 19

**Prinivil** (10 mg)
Merck MSD 106

**Prinivil** (20 mg)
Merck MSD 207

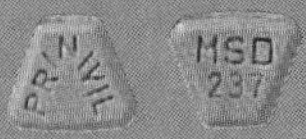

**Prinivil** (40 mg)
Merck MSD 237

**Zestril** (2.5 mg)
Zeneca 2 1/2 135

**Zestril** (5 mg)
Zeneca 5 130

**Zestril** (10 mg)
Zeneca 10 131

**Zestril** (20 mg)
Zeneca 20 132

**Zestril** (40 mg)
Zeneca 40 134

Adapted from Facts and Comparisons, St. Louis, Missouri

## LORAZEPAM

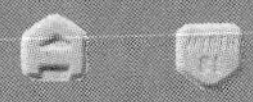

**Ativan** (0.5 mg)
Wyeth-Ayerst A 81

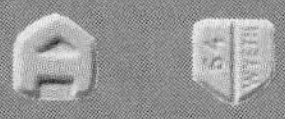

**Ativan** (1 mg)
Wyeth-Ayerst A 64

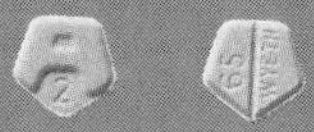

**Ativan** (2 mg)
Wyeth-Ayerst A2 65

## LOVASTATIN

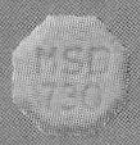

**Mevacor** (10 mg)
Merck MSD 730

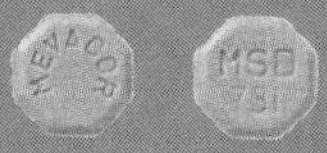

**Mevacor** (20 mg)
Merck MSD 731

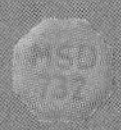

**Mevacor** (40 mg)
Merck MSD 732

## MEDROXYPROGESTERONE

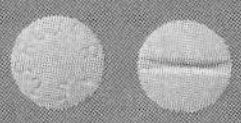

**Provera** (2.5 mg)
Pharmacia & Upjohn 2.5

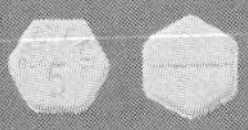

**Provera** (5 mg)
Pharmacia & Upjohn 5

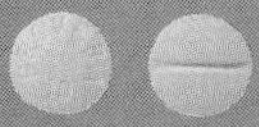

**Provera** (10 mg)
Pharmacia & Upjohn 10

## MEPERIDINE

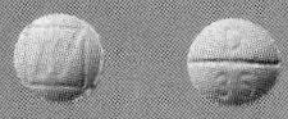

**Demerol** (50 mg)
Sanofi Winthrop WD 35

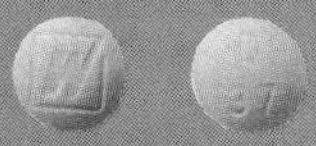

**Demerol** (100 mg)
Sanofi Winthrop WD 37

## METFORMIN

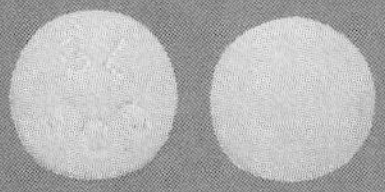

**Glucophage** (500 mg)
B-M Squibb BMS 6060 500

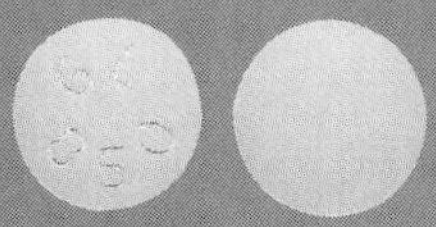

**Glucophage** (850 mg)
B-M Squibb BMS 6070 850

Adapted from Facts and Comparisons, St. Louis, Missouri

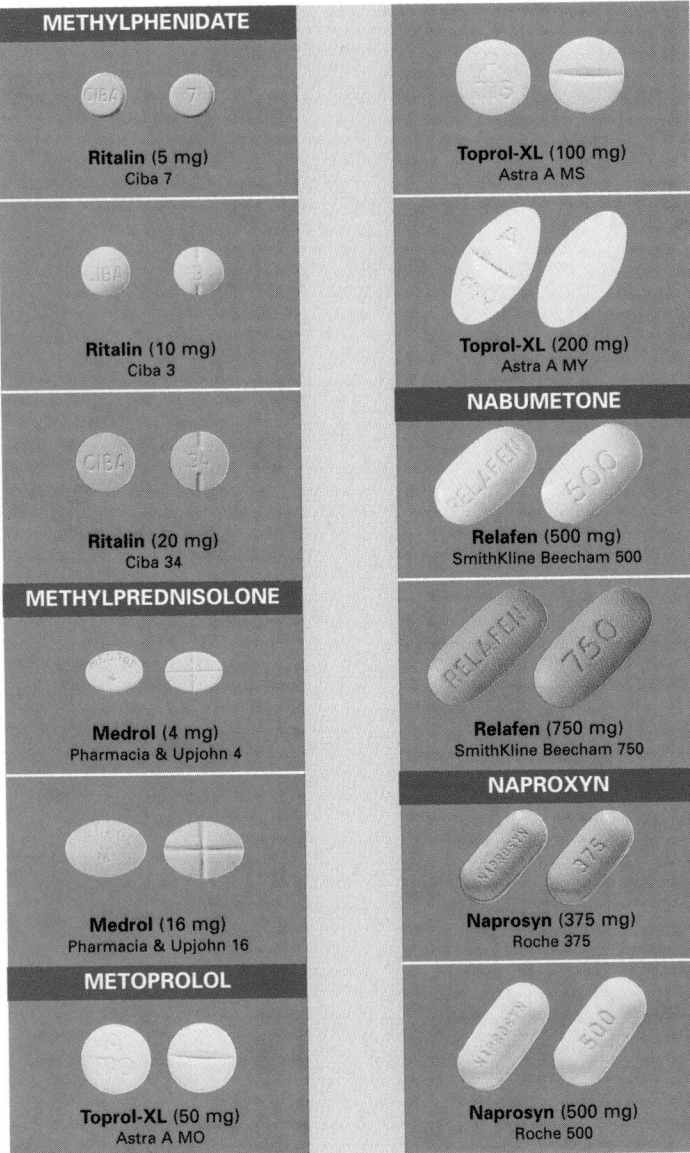

## METHYLPHENIDATE

**Ritalin** (5 mg)
Ciba 7

**Ritalin** (10 mg)
Ciba 3

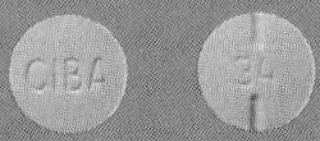

**Ritalin** (20 mg)
Ciba 34

## METHYLPREDNISOLONE

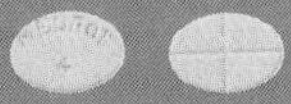

**Medrol** (4 mg)
Pharmacia & Upjohn 4

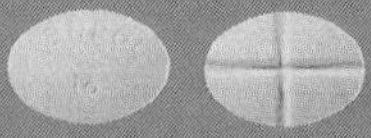

**Medrol** (16 mg)
Pharmacia & Upjohn 16

## METOPROLOL

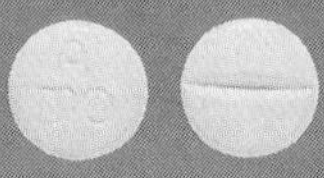

**Toprol-XL** (50 mg)
Astra A MO

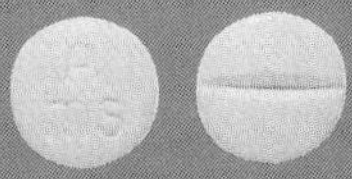

**Toprol-XL** (100 mg)
Astra A MS

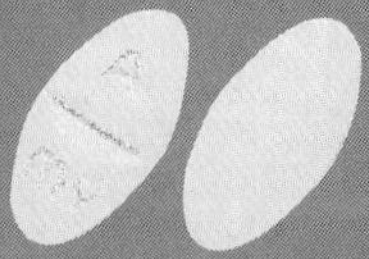

**Toprol-XL** (200 mg)
Astra A MY

## NABUMETONE

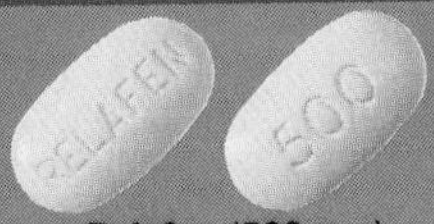


**Relafen** (500 mg)
SmithKline Beecham 500

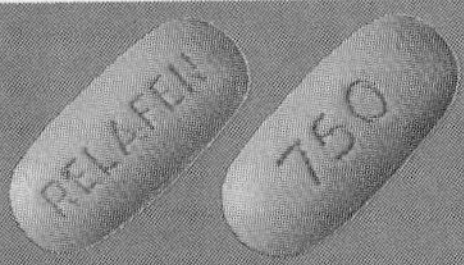


**Relafen** (750 mg)
SmithKline Beecham 750

## NAPROXYN

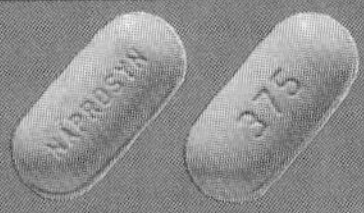

**Naprosyn** (375 mg)
Roche 375

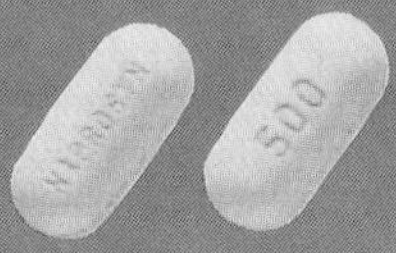

**Naprosyn** (500 mg)
Roche 500

Adapted from Facts and Comparisons, St. Louis, Missouri

## NEFAZODONE

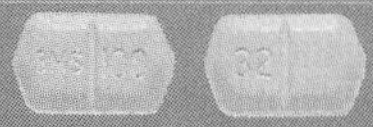

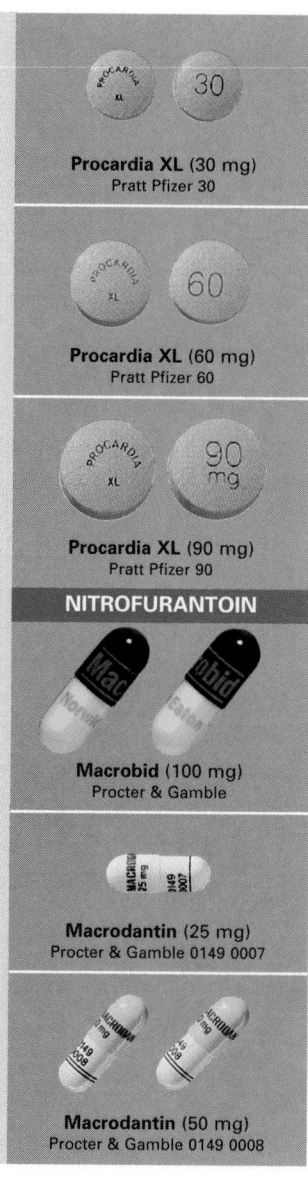

**Serzone** (100 mg)
B-M Squibb BMS 100 32

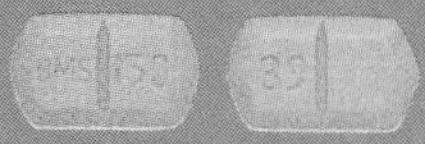

**Serzone** (150 mg)
B-M Squibb BMS 150 39

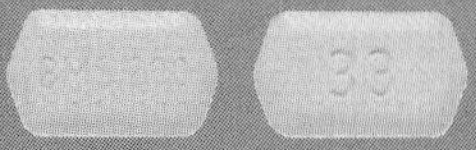

**Serzone** (200 mg)
B-M Squibb BMS 200 33

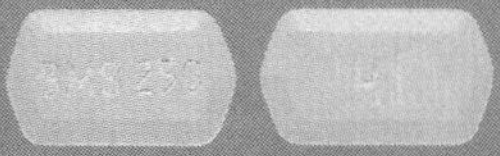

**Serzone** (250 mg)
B-M Squibb BMS 250 41

## NIFEDIPINE

**Procardia** (10 mg)
Pratt Pfizer 260

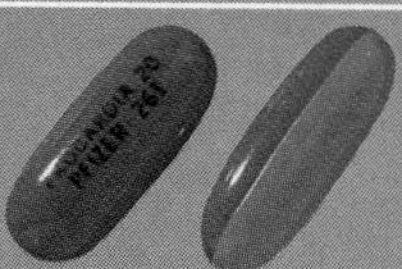

**Procardia** (20 mg)
Pratt Pfizer 20 261

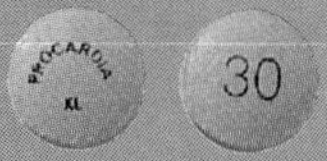


**Procardia XL** (30 mg)
Pratt Pfizer 30

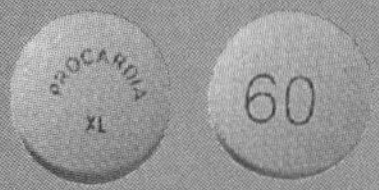


**Procardia XL** (60 mg)
Pratt Pfizer 60

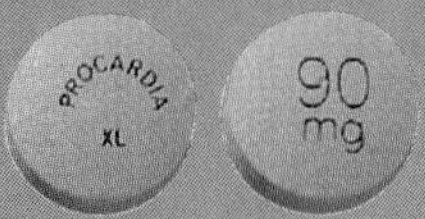


**Procardia XL** (90 mg)
Pratt Pfizer 90

## NITROFURANTOIN

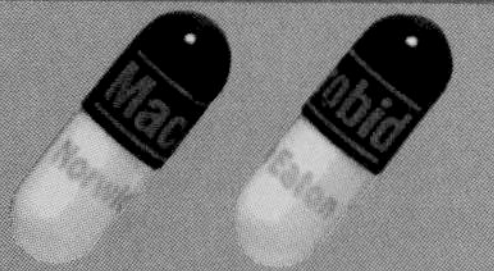

**Macrobid** (100 mg)
Procter & Gamble

**Macrodantin** (25 mg)
Procter & Gamble 0149 0007

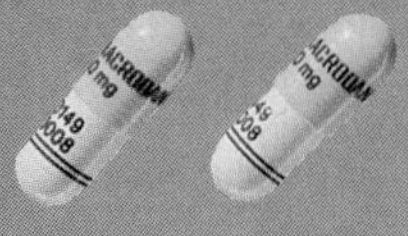

**Macrodantin** (50 mg)
Procter & Gamble 0149 0008

Adapted from Facts and Comparisons, St. Louis, Missouri

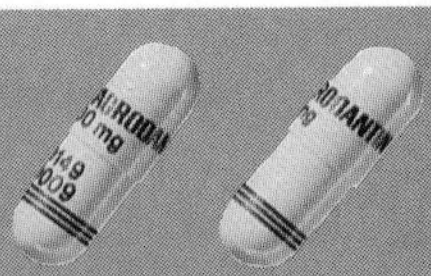

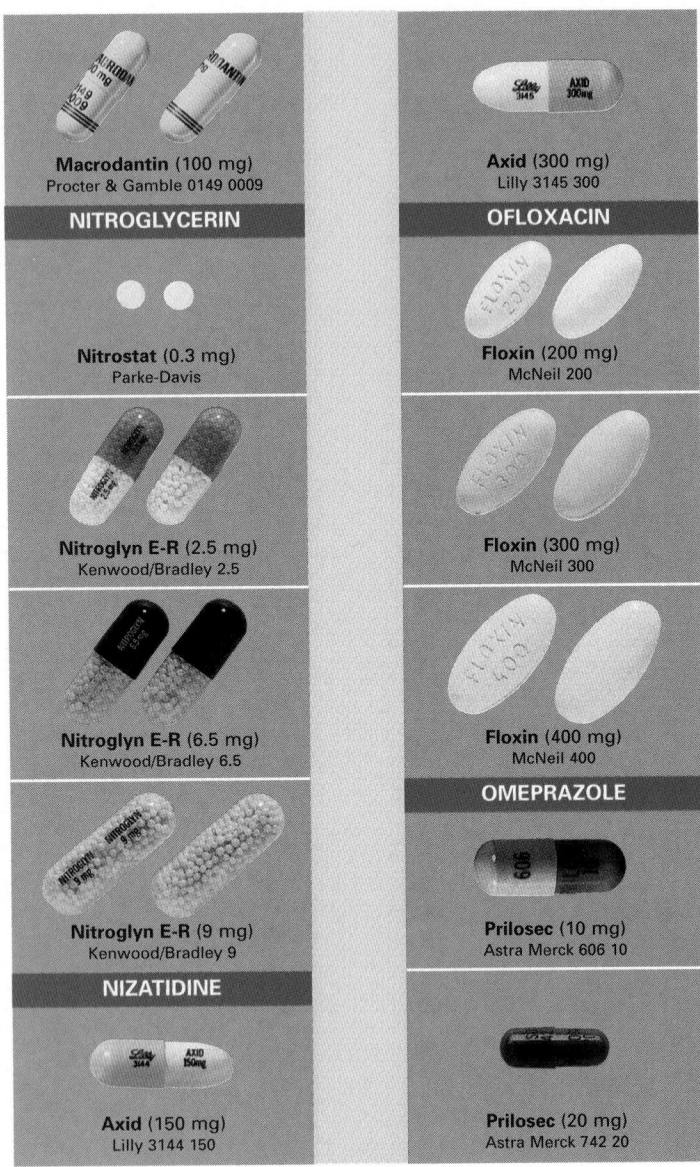

**Macrodantin** (100 mg)
Procter & Gamble 0149 0009

## NITROGLYCERIN

**Nitrostat** (0.3 mg)
Parke-Davis

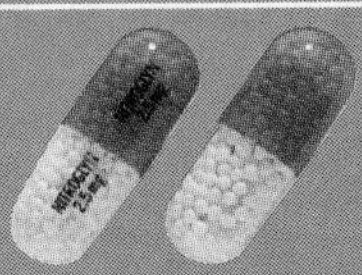

**Nitroglyn E-R** (2.5 mg)
Kenwood/Bradley 2.5

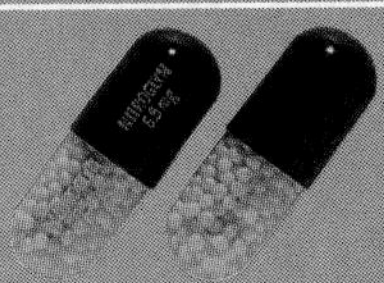

**Nitroglyn E-R** (6.5 mg)
Kenwood/Bradley 6.5

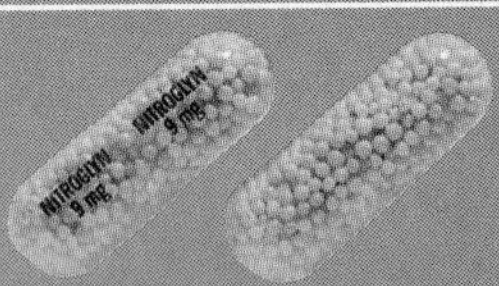


**Nitroglyn E-R** (9 mg)
Kenwood/Bradley 9

## NIZATIDINE

**Axid** (150 mg)
Lilly 3144 150

**Axid** (300 mg)
Lilly 3145 300

## OFLOXACIN

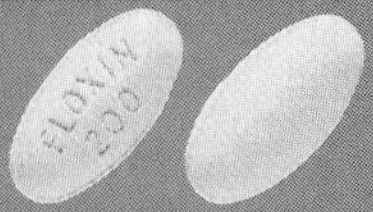


**Floxin** (200 mg)
McNeil 200

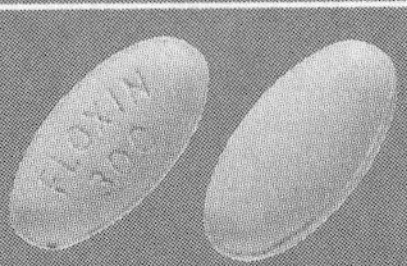


**Floxin** (300 mg)
McNeil 300

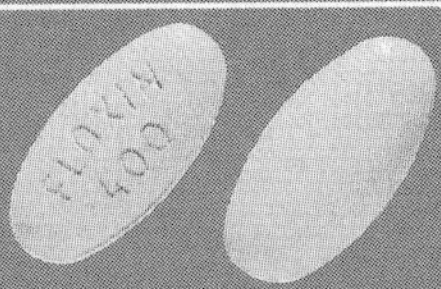


**Floxin** (400 mg)
McNeil 400

## OMEPRAZOLE

**Prilosec** (10 mg)
Astra Merck 606 10

**Prilosec** (20 mg)
Astra Merck 742 20

Adapted from Facts and Comparisons, St. Louis, Missouri

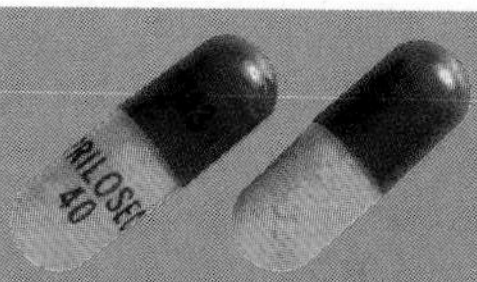

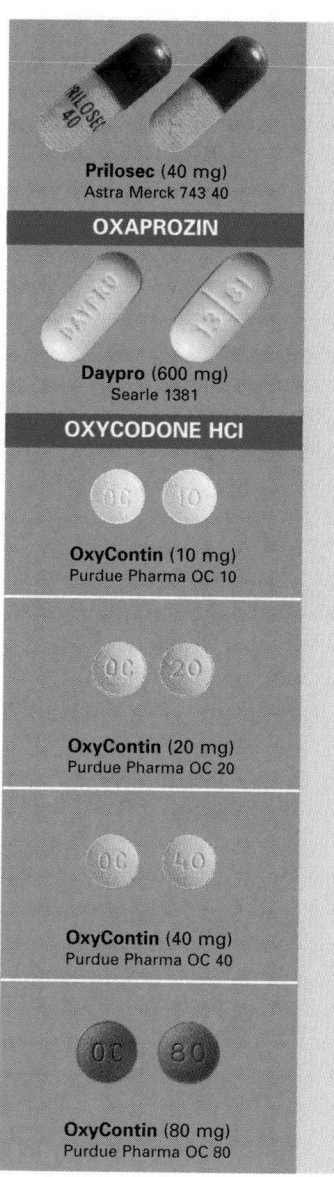

**Prilosec** (40 mg)
Astra Merck 743 40

## OXAPROZIN

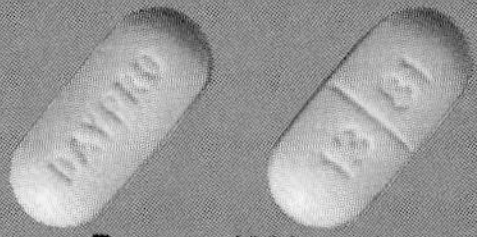


**Daypro** (600 mg)
Searle 1381

## OXYCODONE HCl

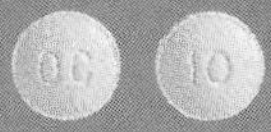


**OxyContin** (10 mg)
Purdue Pharma OC 10

**OxyContin** (20 mg)
Purdue Pharma OC 20

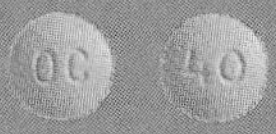


**OxyContin** (40 mg)
Purdue Pharma OC 40

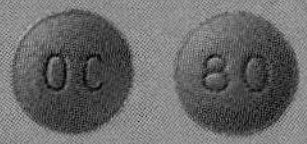


**OxyContin** (80 mg)
Purdue Pharma OC 80

## PAROXETINE

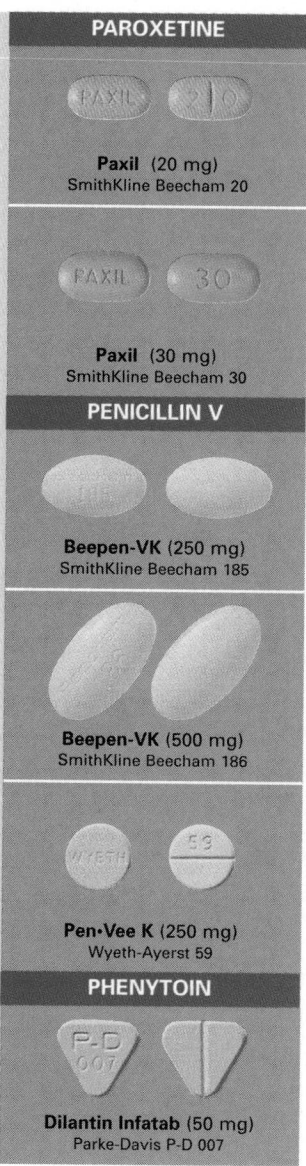


**Paxil** (20 mg)
SmithKline Beecham 20

**Paxil** (30 mg)
SmithKline Beecham 30

## PENICILLIN V

**Beepen-VK** (250 mg)
SmithKline Beecham 185

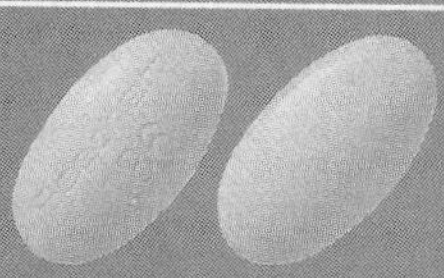

**Beepen-VK** (500 mg)
SmithKline Beecham 186

**Pen•Vee K** (250 mg)
Wyeth-Ayerst 59

## PHENYTOIN

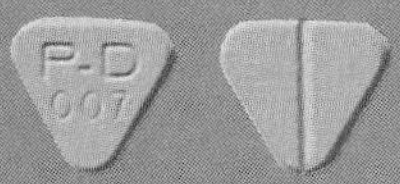


**Dilantin Infatab** (50 mg)
Parke-Davis P-D 007

Adapted from Facts and Comparisons, St. Louis, Missouri

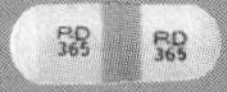

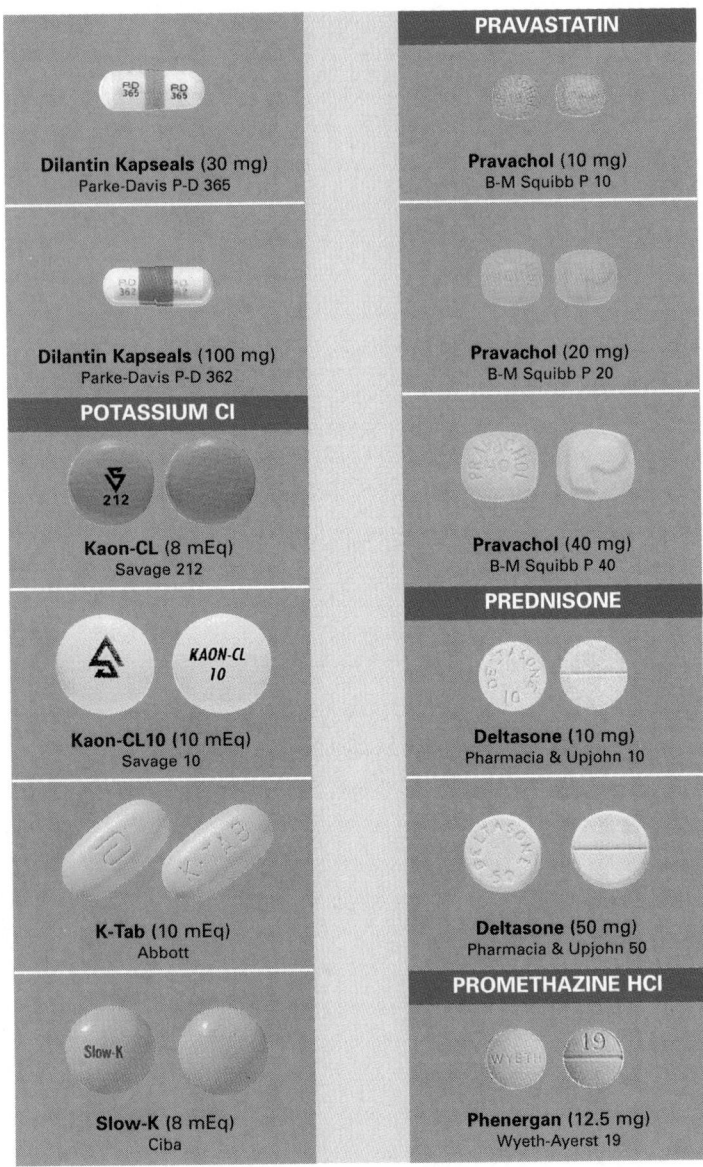


**Dilantin Kapseals** (30 mg)
Parke-Davis P-D 365

**Dilantin Kapseals** (100 mg)
Parke-Davis P-D 362

## POTASSIUM CI

**Kaon-CL** (8 mEq)
Savage 212

**Kaon-CL10** (10 mEq)
Savage 10

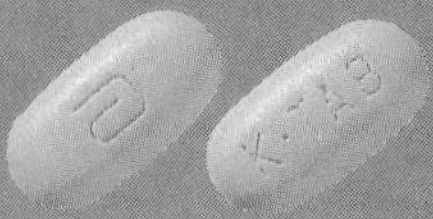

**K-Tab** (10 mEq)
Abbott

**Slow-K** (8 mEq)
Ciba

## PRAVASTATIN

**Pravachol** (10 mg)
B-M Squibb P 10

**Pravachol** (20 mg)
B-M Squibb P 20

**Pravachol** (40 mg)
B-M Squibb P 40

## PREDNISONE

**Deltasone** (10 mg)
Pharmacia & Upjohn 10

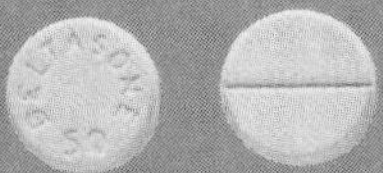

**Deltasone** (50 mg)
Pharmacia & Upjohn 50

## PROMETHAZINE HCI

**Phenergan** (12.5 mg)
Wyeth-Ayerst 19

Adapted from Facts and Comparisons, St. Louis, Missouri

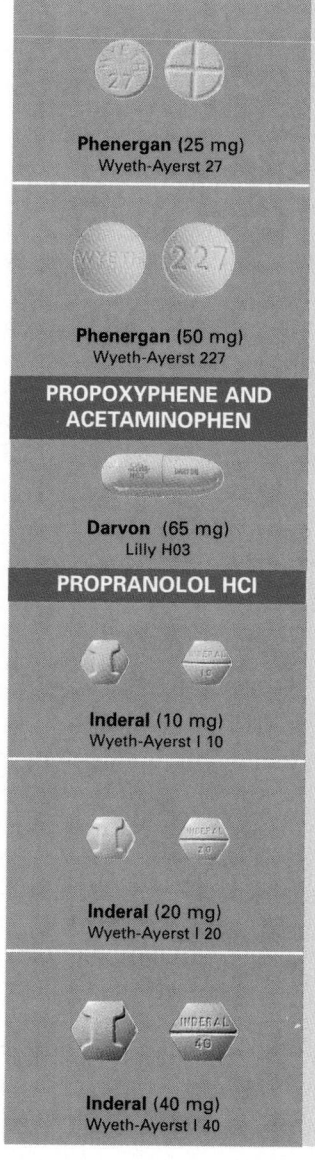

**Phenergan** (25 mg)
Wyeth-Ayerst 27

**Phenergan** (50 mg)
Wyeth-Ayerst 227

## PROPOXYPHENE AND ACETAMINOPHEN

**Darvon** (65 mg)
Lilly H03

## PROPRANOLOL HCl

**Inderal** (10 mg)
Wyeth-Ayerst I 10

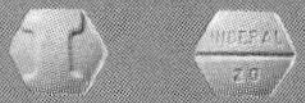

**Inderal** (20 mg)
Wyeth-Ayerst I 20

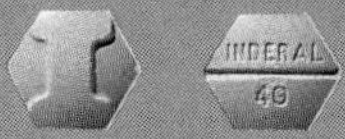

**Inderal** (40 mg)
Wyeth-Ayerst I 40

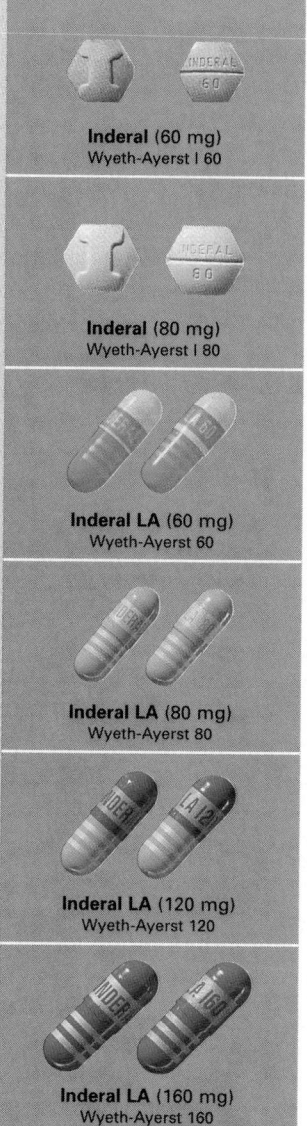

**Inderal** (60 mg)
Wyeth-Ayerst I 60

**Inderal** (80 mg)
Wyeth-Ayerst I 80

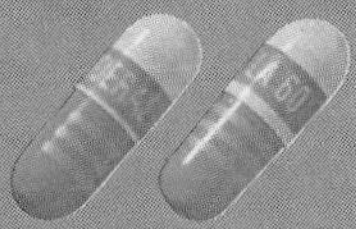

**Inderal LA** (60 mg)
Wyeth-Ayerst 60

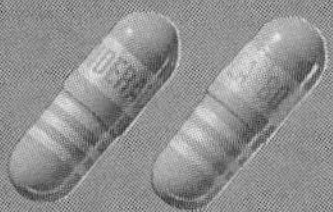

**Inderal LA** (80 mg)
Wyeth-Ayerst 80

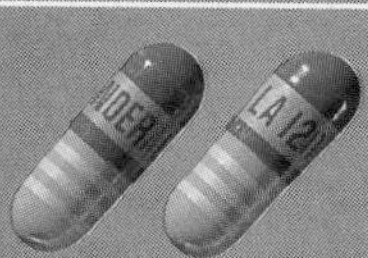

**Inderal LA** (120 mg)
Wyeth-Ayerst 120

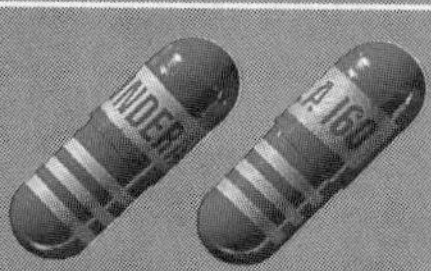

**Inderal LA** (160 mg)
Wyeth-Ayerst 160

Adapted from Facts and Comparisons, St. Louis, Missouri

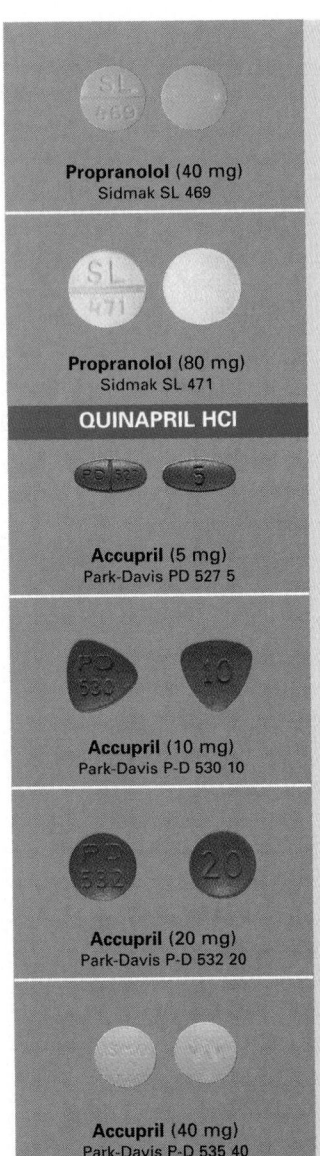


**Propranolol** (40 mg)
Sidmak SL 469

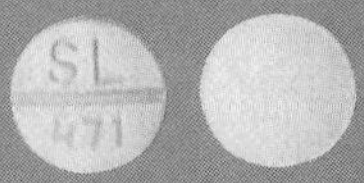


**Propranolol** (80 mg)
Sidmak SL 471

## QUINAPRIL HCl

**Accupril** (5 mg)
Park-Davis PD 527 5

**Accupril** (10 mg)
Park-Davis P-D 530 10

**Accupril** (20 mg)
Park-Davis P-D 532 20

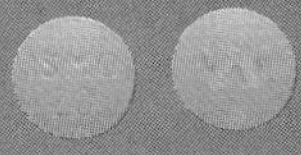

**Accupril** (40 mg)
Park-Davis P-D 535 40

## RAMIPRIL

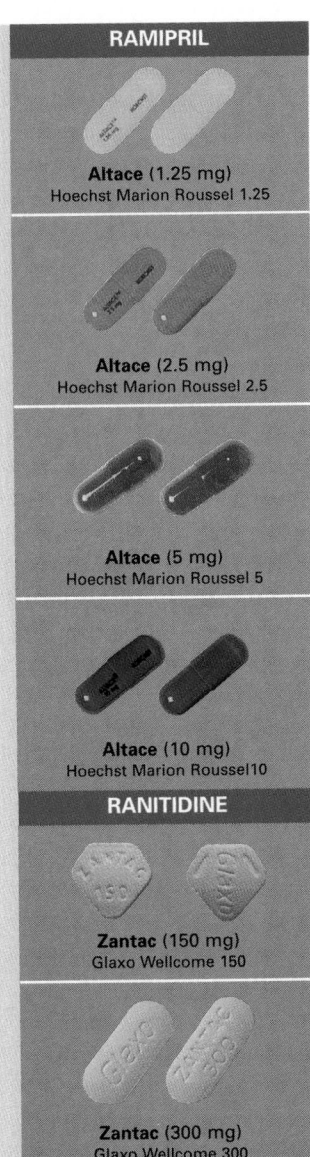

**Altace** (1.25 mg)
Hoechst Marion Roussel 1.25

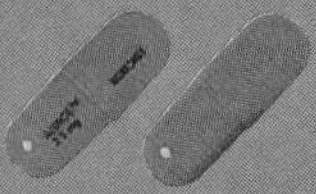

**Altace** (2.5 mg)
Hoechst Marion Roussel 2.5

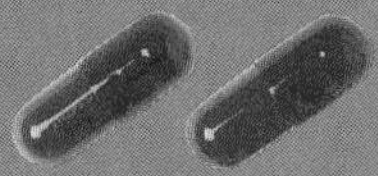

**Altace** (5 mg)
Hoechst Marion Roussel 5

**Altace** (10 mg)
Hoechst Marion Roussel10

## RANITIDINE

**Zantac** (150 mg)
Glaxo Wellcome 150

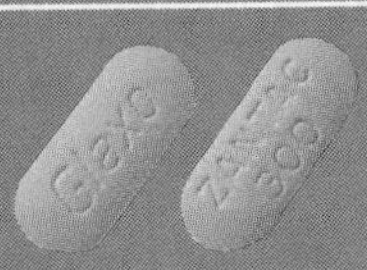


**Zantac** (300 mg)
Glaxo Wellcome 300

Adapted from Facts and Comparisons, St. Louis, Missouri

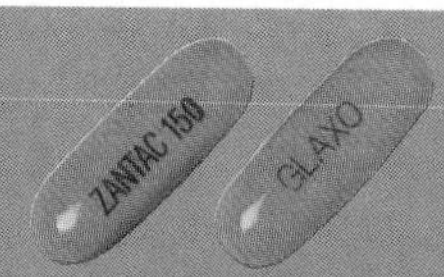

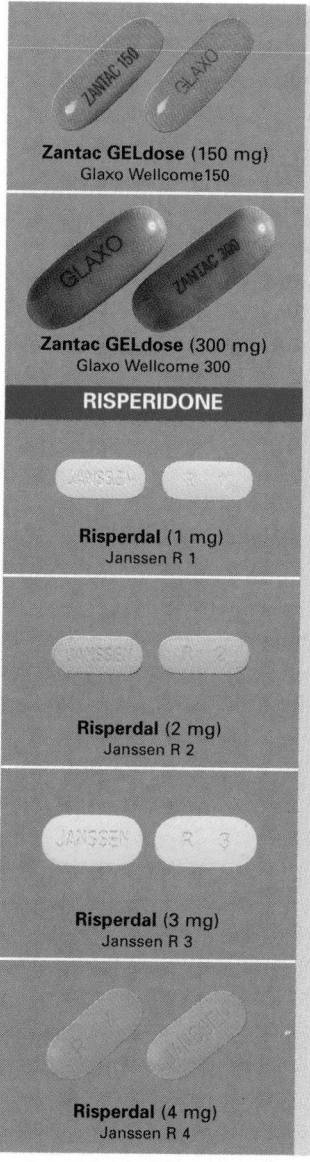


**Zantac GELdose** (150 mg)
Glaxo Wellcome150

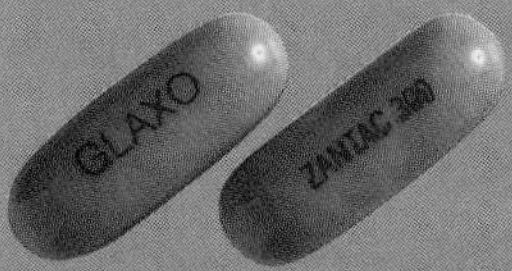


**Zantac GELdose** (300 mg)
Glaxo Wellcome 300

## RISPERIDONE

**Risperdal** (1 mg)
Janssen R 1

**Risperdal** (2 mg)
Janssen R 2

**Risperdal** (3 mg)
Janssen R 3

**Risperdal** (4 mg)
Janssen R 4

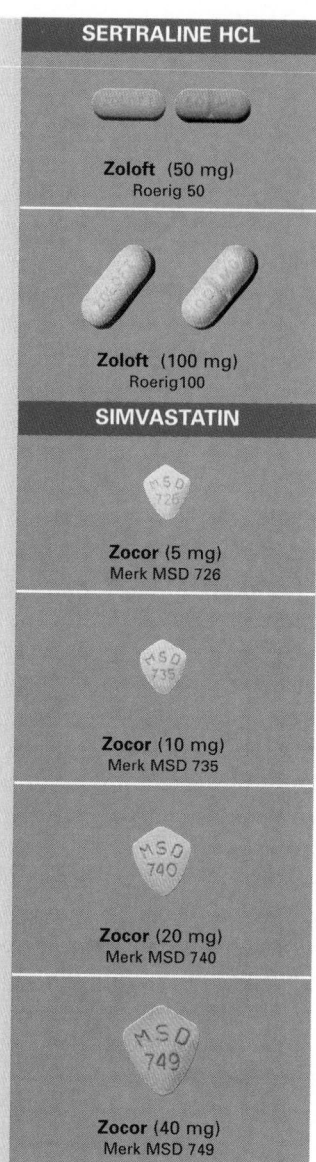

## SERTRALINE HCL

**Zoloft** (50 mg)
Roerig 50

**Zoloft** (100 mg)
Roerig100

## SIMVASTATIN

**Zocor** (5 mg)
Merk MSD 726

**Zocor** (10 mg)
Merk MSD 735

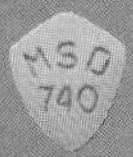


**Zocor** (20 mg)
Merk MSD 740

**Zocor** (40 mg)
Merk MSD 749

Adapted from Facts and Comparisons, St. Louis, Missouri

## SUCRALFATE

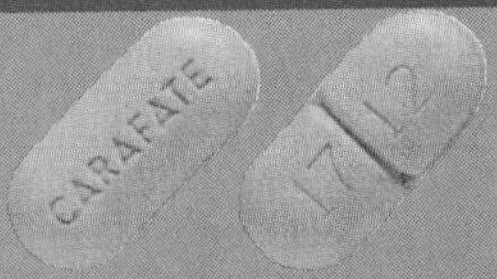

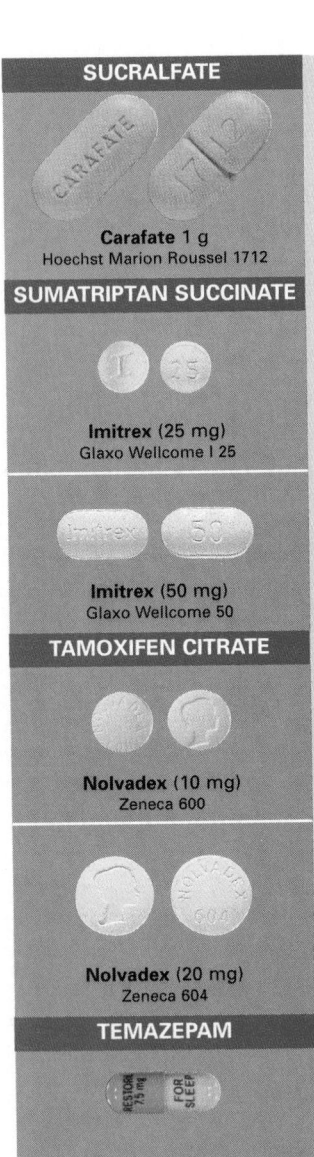


**Carafate** 1 g
Hoechst Marion Roussel 1712

## SUMATRIPTAN SUCCINATE

**Imitrex** (25 mg)
Glaxo Wellcome I 25

**Imitrex** (50 mg)
Glaxo Wellcome 50

## TAMOXIFEN CITRATE

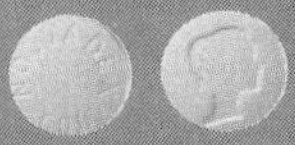

**Nolvadex** (10 mg)
Zeneca 600

**Nolvadex** (20 mg)
Zeneca 604

## TEMAZEPAM

**Restoril** (7.5 mg)
Sandoz 7.5

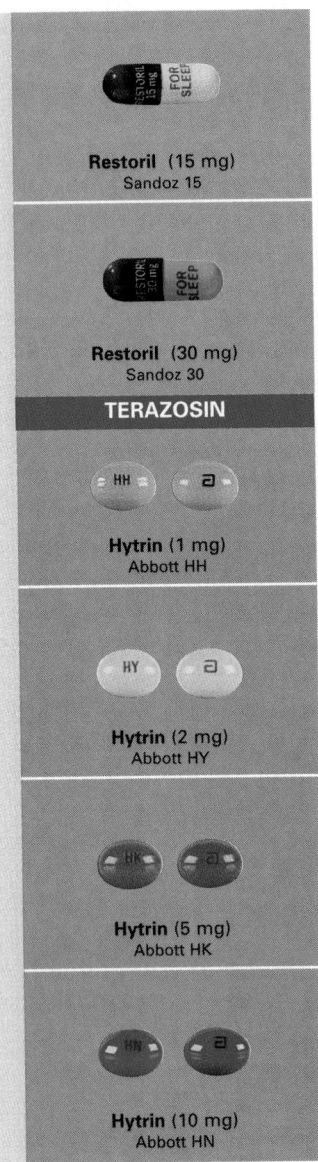


**Restoril** (15 mg)
Sandoz 15

**Restoril** (30 mg)
Sandoz 30

## TERAZOSIN

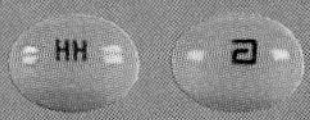


**Hytrin** (1 mg)
Abbott HH

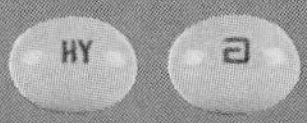


**Hytrin** (2 mg)
Abbott HY

**Hytrin** (5 mg)
Abbott HK

**Hytrin** (10 mg)
Abbott HN

Adapted from Facts and Comparisons, St. Louis, Missouri

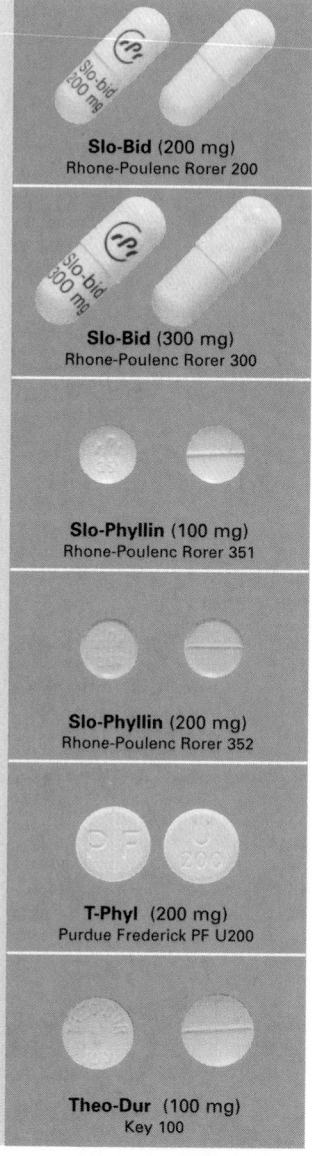

## THEOPHYLLINE

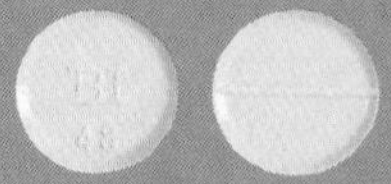

**Respbid** (250 mg)
Boehringer Ingelheim BI 48

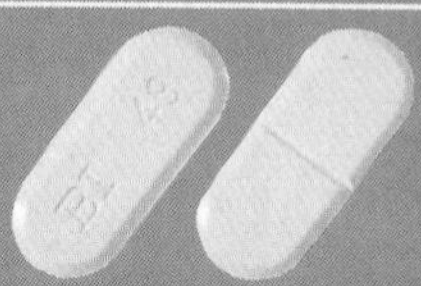

**Respbid** (500 mg)
Boehringer Ingelheim BI 49

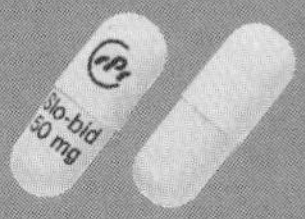


**Slo-Bid** (50 mg)
Rhone-Poulenc Rorer 50

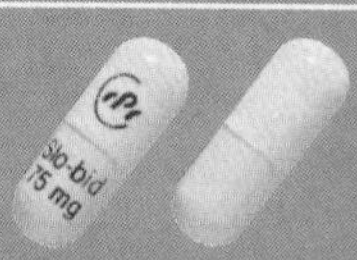


**Slo-Bid** (75 mg)
Rhone-Poulenc Rorer 75

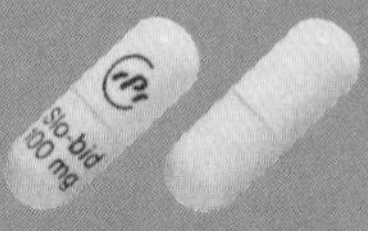

**Slo-Bid** (100 mg)
Rhone-Poulenc Rorer 100

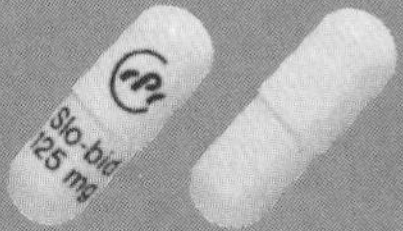

**Slo-Bid** (125 mg)
Rhone-Poulenc Rorer 125

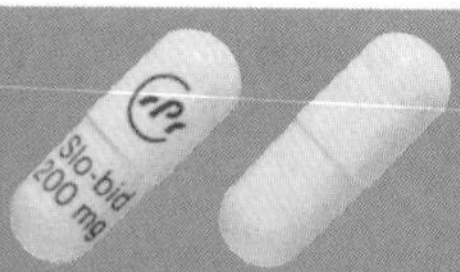


**Slo-Bid** (200 mg)
Rhone-Poulenc Rorer 200

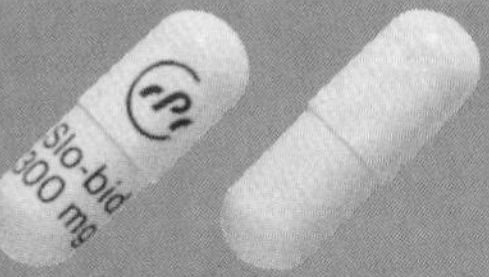


**Slo-Bid** (300 mg)
Rhone-Poulenc Rorer 300

**Slo-Phyllin** (100 mg)
Rhone-Poulenc Rorer 351

**Slo-Phyllin** (200 mg)
Rhone-Poulenc Rorer 352

**T-Phyl** (200 mg)
Purdue Frederick PF U200

**Theo-Dur** (100 mg)
Key 100

Adapted from Facts and Comparisons, St. Louis, Missouri

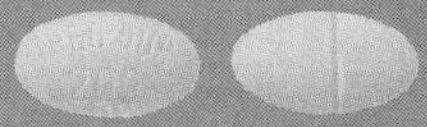

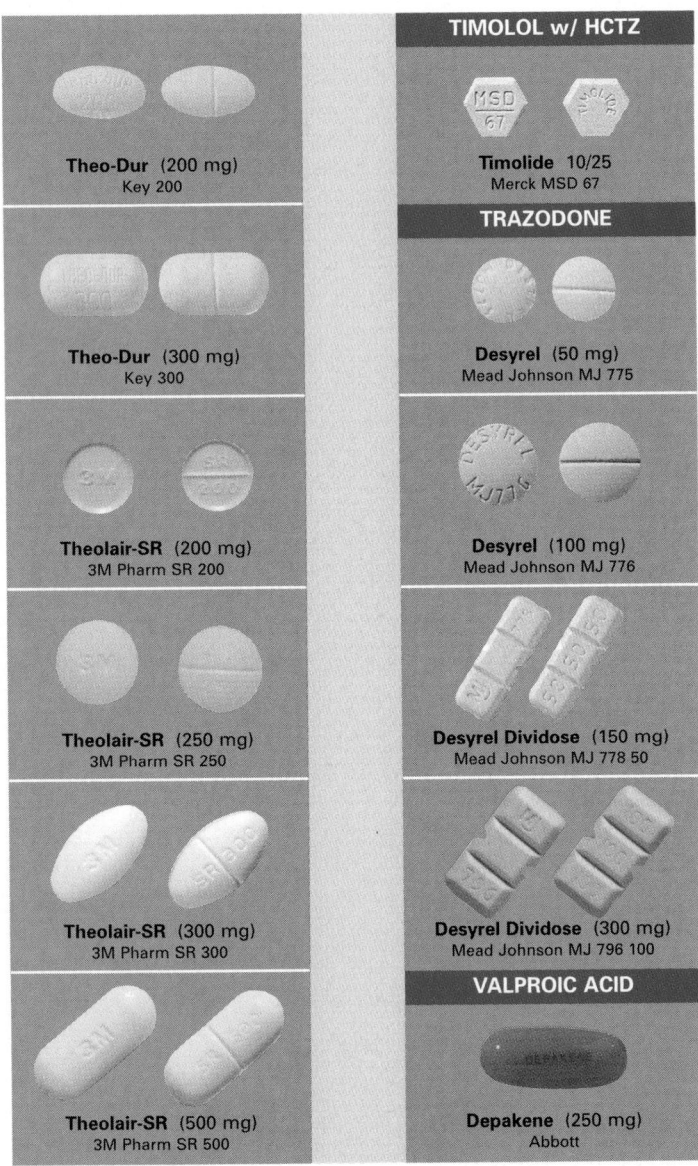

**Theo-Dur** (200 mg)
Key 200

**Theo-Dur** (300 mg)
Key 300

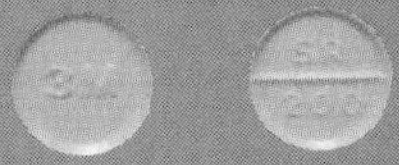

**Theolair-SR** (200 mg)
3M Pharm SR 200

**Theolair-SR** (250 mg)
3M Pharm SR 250

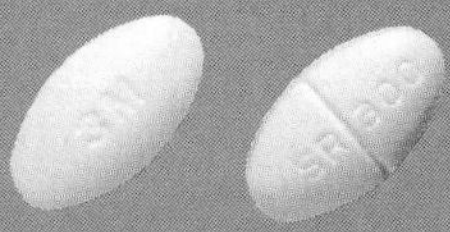

**Theolair-SR** (300 mg)
3M Pharm SR 300

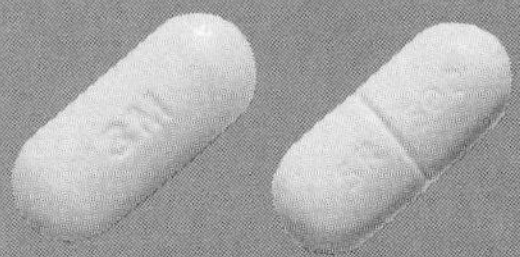

**Theolair-SR** (500 mg)
3M Pharm SR 500

## TIMOLOL w/ HCTZ

**Timolide** 10/25
Merck MSD 67

## TRAZODONE

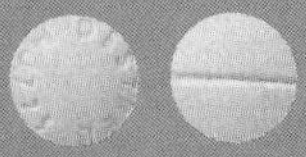

**Desyrel** (50 mg)
Mead Johnson MJ 775

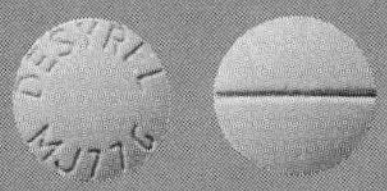


**Desyrel** (100 mg)
Mead Johnson MJ 776

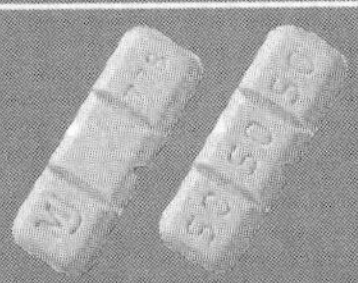

**Desyrel Dividose** (150 mg)
Mead Johnson MJ 778 50

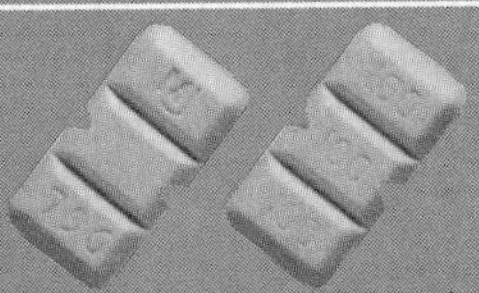

**Desyrel Dividose** (300 mg)
Mead Johnson MJ 796 100

## VALPROIC ACID

**Depakene** (250 mg)
Abbott

Adapted from Facts and Comparisons, St. Louis, Missouri

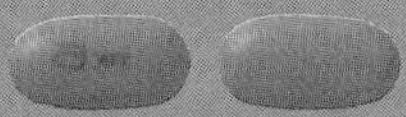

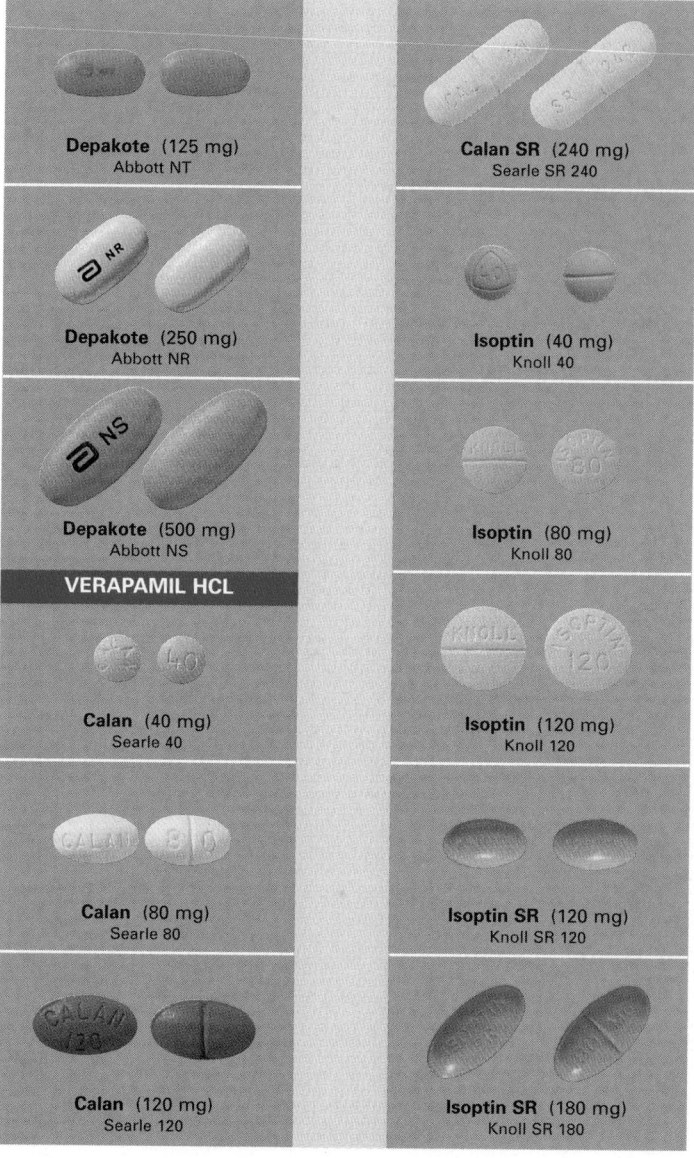

**Depakote** (125 mg)
Abbott NT

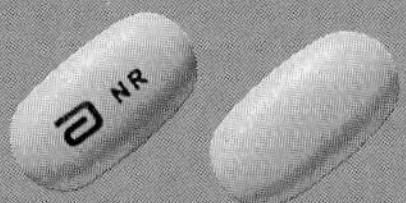


**Depakote** (250 mg)
Abbott NR

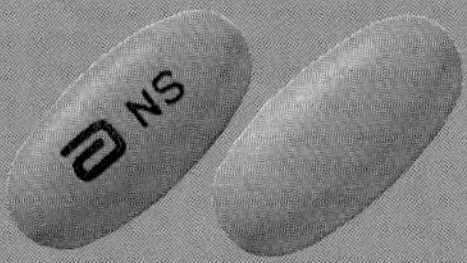


**Depakote** (500 mg)
Abbott NS

## VERAPAMIL HCL

**Calan** (40 mg)
Searle 40

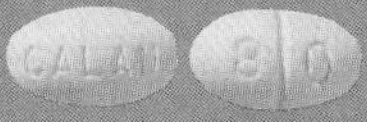

**Calan** (80 mg)
Searle 80

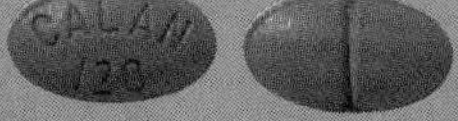

**Calan** (120 mg)
Searle 120

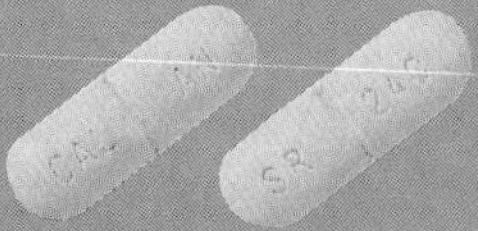

**Calan SR** (240 mg)
Searle SR 240

**Isoptin** (40 mg)
Knoll 40

**Isoptin** (80 mg)
Knoll 80

**Isoptin** (120 mg)
Knoll 120

**Isoptin SR** (120 mg)
Knoll SR 120

**Isoptin SR** (180 mg)
Knoll SR 180

Adapted from Facts and Comparisons, St. Louis, Missouri

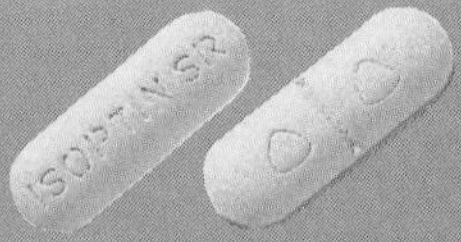

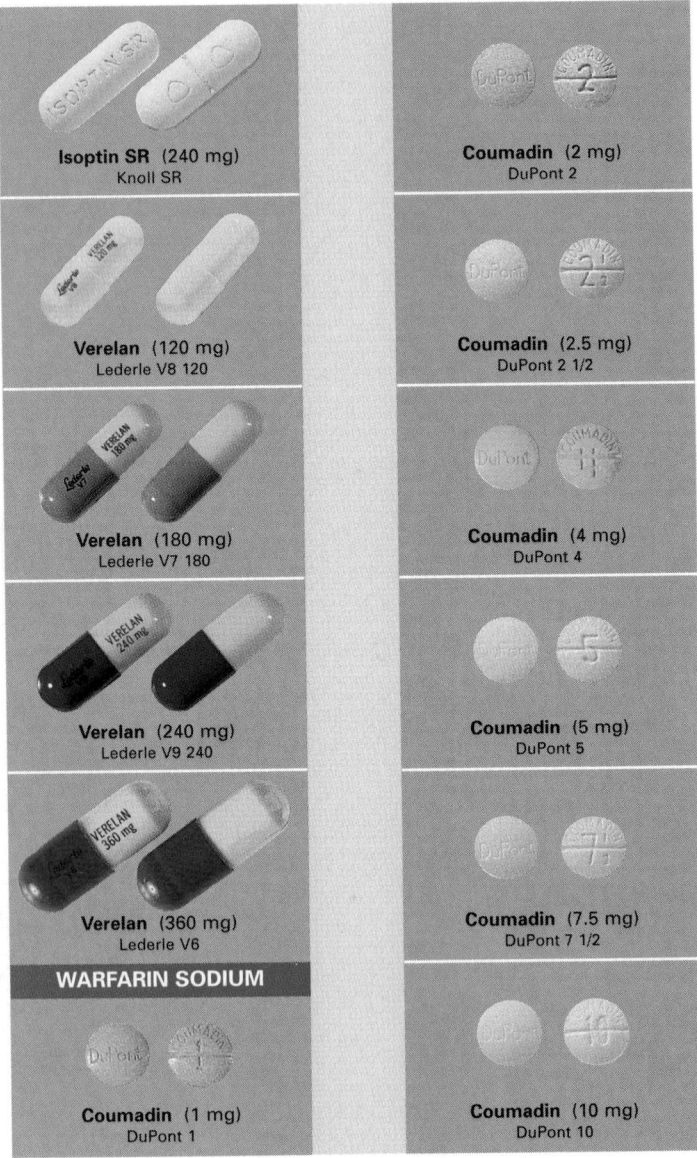


**Isoptin SR** (240 mg)
Knoll SR

**Verelan** (120 mg)
Lederle V8 120

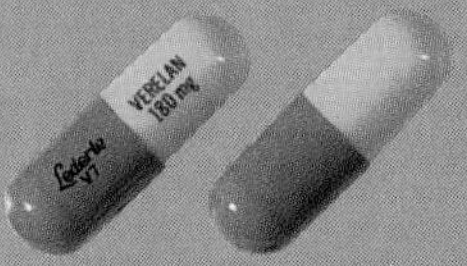


**Verelan** (180 mg)
Lederle V7 180

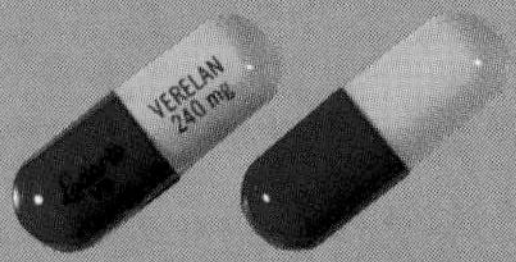


**Verelan** (240 mg)
Lederle V9 240

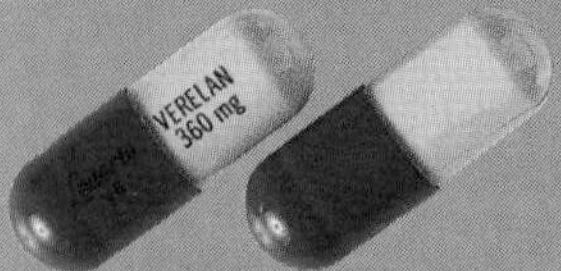


**Verelan** (360 mg)
Lederle V6

## WARFARIN SODIUM

**Coumadin** (1 mg)
DuPont 1

**Coumadin** (2 mg)
DuPont 2

**Coumadin** (2.5 mg)
DuPont 2 1/2

**Coumadin** (4 mg)
DuPont 4

**Coumadin** (5 mg)
DuPont 5

**Coumadin** (7.5 mg)
DuPont 7 1/2

**Coumadin** (10 mg)
DuPont 10

Adapted from Facts and Comparisons, St. Louis, Missouri

# hydrochlorothiazide

*(hye droe klor oh **thye'** a zide)*

Diuchlor H (CAN), Esidrix, HydroDIURIL, Hydro-Par, Hydrozide (CAN), Microzide Capsules, Neo-Codema (CAN), Novohydrazide (CAN), Oretic, Urozide (CAN)

**Pregnancy Category B**

## Drug classes

Thiazide diuretic

## Therapeutic actions

Inhibits reabsorption of sodium and chloride in distal renal tubule, increasing the excretion of sodium, chloride, and water by the kidney.

## Indications

- Adjunctive therapy in edema associated with CHF, cirrhosis, corticosteroid, and estrogen therapy; renal dysfunction
- Hypertension as sole therapy or in combination with other antihypertensives
- Unlabeled uses: calcium nephrolithiasis alone or with amiloride or allopurinal to prevent recurrences in hypercalciuric or normal calciuric patients; diabetes insipidus, especially nephrogenic diabetes insipidus; osteoporosis

## Contraindications/cautions

- Contraindications: allergy to thiazides, sulfonamides; fluid or electrolyte imbalance; renal disease (can lead to azotemia); liver disease (risk of hepatic coma); gout (risk of attack); SLE; glucose tolerance abnormalities, diabetes mellitus; hyperparathyroidism; manic-depressive disorder (aggravated by hypercalcemia); pregnancy; lactation.

## Dosage

**Available Forms:** Tablets—25, 50, 100 mg; solution—50 mg/5 ml; intensol solution 100 mg/ml; capsules—12.5 mg

**ADULT**

- *Edema:* 25–200 mg qd PO until dry weight is attained. Then, 25–100 mg qd PO or intermittently, up to 200 mg/d.
- *Hypertension:* 50–100 mg PO as a starting dose. 25–100 mg qd, maintenance.
- *Calcium nephrolithiasis:* 50 mg qd or bid PO.

**PEDIATRIC:** 2.2 mg/kg per day PO in 2 doses. *<6 mo:* Up to 3.3 mg/kg per day in 2 doses. *6 mo–2 y:* 12.5–37.5 mg/d in 2 doses. *2–12 y:* 37.5–100.0 mg/d in 2 doses.

## Pharmacokinetics

| *Route* | *Onset* | *Peak* | *Duration* |
|---|---|---|---|
| Oral | 2 h | 4–6 h | 6–12 h |

*Metabolism:* Hepatic, $T_{1/2}$: 5.6–14.8 h
*Distribution:* Crosses placenta; enters breast milk
*Excretion:* Urine

## Adverse effects

- CNS: *Dizziness, vertigo,* paresthesias, weakness, headache, drowsiness, fatigue, leukopenia, thrombocytopenia, agranulocytosis, aplastic anemia, neutropenia
- GI: *Nausea, anorexia, vomiting, dry mouth,* diarrhea, constipation, jaundice, hepatitis, pancreatitis
- CV: Orthostatic hypotension, venous thrombosis, volume depletion, cardiac arrhythmias, chest pain
- GU: *Polyuria, nocturia,* impotence, loss of libido
- Dermatologic: Photosensitivity, rash, purpura, exfoliative dermatitis, hives
- Other: Muscle cramps and muscle spasms, fever, gouty attacks, flushing, weight loss, rhinorrhea

## Clinically important drug-drug interactions

• Increased thiazide effects with diazoxide • Decreased absorption with cholestyramine, colestipol • Increased risk of cardiac glycoside toxicity if hypokalemia occurs • Increased risk of lithium toxicity • Decreased effectiveness of antidiabetic agents

## Drug-lab test interferences

• Decreased PBI levels without clinical signs of thyroid disturbance

h

## ■ Nursing Considerations

### Assessment

- *History:* Allergy to thiazides, sulfonamides; fluid or electrolyte imbalance; renal or liver disease; gout; SLE; glucose tolerance abnormalities, diabetes mellitus; hyperparathyroidism; manic-depressive disorders; lactation
- *Physical:* Skin color, lesions, edema; orientation, reflexes, muscle strength; pulses, baseline ECG, BP, orthostatic BP, perfusion; R, pattern, adventitious sounds; liver evaluation, bowel sounds urinary output patterns; CBC, serum electrolytes, blood glucose, liver and renal function tests, serum uric acid, urinalysis

### Implementation

- Give with food or milk if GI upset occurs.
- Mark calendars or provide other reminders of drug for alternate day or 3–5 d/wk therapy.
- Reduce dosage of other antihypertensives by at least 50% if given with thiazides; readjust dosages gradually as BP responds.
- Administer early in the day so increased urination will not disturb sleep.
- Measure and record weights to monitor fluid changes.

### Drug-specific teaching points

- Record intermittent therapy on a calendar, or use prepared, dated envelopes. Take drug early so increased urination will not disturb sleep. Drug may be taken with food or meals if GI upset occurs.
- Weigh yourself on a regular basis, at the same time and in the same clothing: record weight on your calendar.
- The following side effects may occur: increased volume and frequency of urination; dizziness, feeling faint on arising, drowsiness (avoid rapid position changes; hazardous activities, like driving; and alcohol); sensitivity to sunlight (use sunglasses, wear protective clothing, or use a sunscreen); decrease in sexual function; increased thirst (sucking on sugarless lozenges and frequent mouth care may help).
- Report weight change of more than 3 lb in one day, swelling in your ankles or fingers, unusual bleeding or bruising, dizziness, trembling, numbness, fatigue, muscle weakness or cramps.

## hydrocodone bitartrate

*(hye droe **koe'** done)*

Hycodan

**Pregnancy Category C**
**C-III controlled substance**

### Drug classes

Narcotic agonist analgesic
Antitussive

### Therapeutic actions

Acts at opioid receptors in the CNS to produce analgesia, euphoria, sedation; acts in medullary cough center to depress cough reflex.

### Indications

- Suppresses cough reflex by direct action on cough center in the medulla. Available only in combination products.

### Contraindications/cautions

- Use cautiously with pregnancy, labor, lactation, bronchial asthma, COPD, respiratory depression, anoxia, increased intracranial pressure, debilitation, postoperative state.

### Dosage

**Available Forms:** Capsules—5 mg; suspension—5 mg/ml; tablets—5 mg; XR tablets—10 mg

**ADULT:** 5–10 mg PO q4–6h prn; do not exceed 15 mg/dose.

**PEDIATRIC:** 2–12 y: 1.25–5 mg PO q4–6h; do not exceed 10 mg/dose.

### Pharmacokinetics

| *Route* | *Onset* | *Peak* |
|---|---|---|
| Oral | 10–20 min | 30–60 min |

*Metabolism:* Hepatic, $T_{1/2}$: 3.8 h
*Distribution:* Crosses placenta; enters breast milk
*Excretion:* Urine

### Adverse effects

- CNS: *Sedation, clamminess, sweating, headache, vertigo, floating feeling, dizziness, lethargy, confusion, lightheadedness*
- GI: Dry mouth, anorexia, *constipation, nausea*, biliary tract spasm
- **Dermatologic**: Rash, hives, pruritus, flushing, warmth, sensitivity to cold

### Clinically important drug-drug interactions

- Potentiation of effects of codeine when given with barbiturate anesthetics; decrease dose of hydrocodone when coadministering.

### Drug-lab test interferences

- Elevated biliary tract pressure may cause increases in plasma amylase, lipase; determinations of these levels may be unreliable for 24 h after administration of narcotics.

## ■ Nursing Considerations

### Assessment

- *History:* Hypersensitivity to codeine, hydrocodone, physical dependence on a narcotic analgesic, pregnancy, labor, lactation, COPD, respiratory depression, anoxia, increased intracranial pressure, recent surgery
- *Physical:* Orientation, reflexes, bilateral grip strength, affect; pupil size, vision; P, auscultation, BP; R, adventitious sounds; bowel sounds, normal output; liver and kidney function tests

### Implementation

- Give to nursing women 4–6 h before the next scheduled feeding to minimize drug in milk.
- Provide narcotic antagonist, facilities for assisted or controlled respiration on standby during parenteral administration.
- Instruct postoperative patients in pulmonary toilet; drug suppresses cough reflex.

### Drug-specific teaching points

- Take drug exactly as prescribed.
- The following side effects may occur: dizziness, sedation, drowsiness, impaired visual acuity (avoid driving, performing other tasks that require alertness); nausea, loss of appetite (lying quietly, frequent small meals may help); constipation (laxative may be used).
- Report severe nausea, vomiting, palpitations, shortness of breath or difficulty breathing.

# Hydrocortisone

## hydrocortisone butyrate

*(hye droe **kor'** ti zone)*

*Dermatologic ointment and cream:* Locoid

## hydrocortisone cypionate

*Oral suspension:* Cortef, Hycort (CAN)

## hydrocortisone sodium phosphate

*IV, IM, or SC injection:* Hydrocortisone phosphate

## hydrocortisone sodium succinate

*IV, IM injection:* A-hydroCort, Solu-Cortef

## hydrocortisone valerate

*Dermatologic cream, ointment, lotion:* Westcort

**Pregnancy Category C**

### Drug classes

Corticosteroid, short acting
Glucocorticoid
Mineralocorticoid
Adrenal cortical hormone (hydrocortisone)
Hormonal agent

### Therapeutic actions

Enters target cells and binds to cytoplasmic receptors; initiates many complex reactions

h

that are responsible for its anti-inflammatory, immunosuppressive (glucocorticoid), and salt-retaining (mineralocorticoid) actions. Some actions may be undesirable, depending on drug use.

### Indications

- Replacement therapy in adrenal cortical insufficiency
- Hypercalcemia associated with cancer
- Short-term inflammatory and allergic disorders, such as rheumatoid arthritis, collagen diseases (SLE), dermatologic diseases (pemphigus), status asthmaticus, and autoimmune disorders
- Hematologic disorders—thrombocytopenic purpura, erythroblastopenia
- Trichinosis with neurologic or myocardial involvement
- Ulcerative colitis, acute exacerbations of multiple sclerosis, and palliation in some leukemias and lymphomas
- Intra-articular or soft-tissue administration: Arthritis, psoriatic plaques.
- Retention enema: For ulcerative colitis/proctitis
- Dermatologic preparations: To relieve inflammatory and pruritic manifestations of dermatoses that are steroid responsive
- Anorectal cream, suppositories: To relieve discomfort of hemorrhoids and perianal itching or irritation

### Contraindications/cautions

- Systemic administration: infections, especially tuberculosis, fungal infections, amebiasis, hepatitis B, vaccinia, or varicella, and antibiotic-resistant infections; kidney disease (risk to edema); liver disease, cirrhosis, hypothyroidism; ulcerative colitis with impending perforation; diverticulitis; recent GI surgery; active or latent peptic ulcer; inflammatory bowel disease (risks exacerbations or bowel perforation); hypertension, CHF; thromboembolitic tendencies, thrombophlebitis, osteoporosis, convulsive disorders, metastatic carcinoma, diabetes mellitus; lactation.
- Retention enemas, intrarectal foam: systemic fungal infections, recent intestinal surgery, extensive fistulas.
- Topical dermatologic administration: fungal, tubercular, herpes simplex skin infections; vaccinia, varicella; ear application when eardrum is perforated; lactation.

### Dosage

**Available Forms:** Tablets—5, 10, 20 mg; oral suspension—10 mg/5 ml; injection—50 mg/ml, 100, 250, 500, 1,000 mg/vial; topical lotion—1%, 2%, 2.5%; topical liquid—1%; topical oil—1%; topical solution—1%; topical spray—1%; cream—0.5%

*ADULT:* Individualize dosage, based on severity and response. Give daily dose before 9 AM to minimize adrenal suppression. If long-term therapy is needed, alternate-day therapy should be considered. After long-term therapy, withdraw drug slowly to avoid adrenal insufficiency. For maintenance therapy, reduce initial dose in small increments at intervals until lowest clinically satisfactory dose is reached.

- ***IM, IV (hydrocortisone sodium succinate):*** 100–500 mg initially and q2–6h, based on condition and response.
  - *Acute adrenal insufficiency (hydrocortisone sodium phosphate):* 100 mg IV followed by 100 mg q8h in IV fluids.

*PEDIATRIC:* Individualize dosage based on severity and response rather than by to formulae that corrects adult doses for age or weight. Carefully observe growth and development in infants and children on prolonged therapy.

- ***Oral (hydrocortisone and cypionate):*** 20–240 mg/d in single or divided doses.
- ***IM or SC (hydrocortisone and sodium phosphate):*** 20–240 mg/d usually in divided doses q12h.
- ***IM, IV (hydrocortisone sodium succinate):*** Reduce dose, based on condition and response, but give no less than 25 mg/d.
  - *Acute adrenal insufficiency (hydrocortisone sodium phosphate):* Older children: 1–2 mg/kg IV bolus; then 150–250 mg/kg per day in divided doses. Infants: 1–2 mg/kg IV bolus; then 25–150 mg/kg per day in divided doses.

ADULT, PEDIATRIC

- ***IM, IV (hydrocortisone sodium succinate)***
- *Retention enema (hydrocortisone):* 100 mg nightly for 21 d.
- *Intrarectal foam (hydrocortisone acetate):* 1 applicator qd or bid for 2 wk and every second day thereafter.
- *Intra-articular, intralesional (hydrocortisone acetate):* 5–25 mg, depending on joint or soft-tissue injection site.
- *Topical dermatologic preparations:* Apply sparingly to affected area bid–qid.

**Pharmacokinetics**

| *Route* | *Onset* | *Peak* | *Duration* |
|---|---|---|---|
| Oral | 1–2 h | 1–2 h | 1–1 1/2 d |
| IM | Rapid | 4–8 h | 1–1 1/2 d |
| IV | Immediate | | 1–1 1/2 d |
| PR | Slow | 3–5 d | 4–6 d |

*Metabolism:* Hepatic, $T_{1/2}$: 80–120 min
*Distribution:* Crosses placenta; enters breast milk
*Excretion:* Urine

**IV facts**

**Preparation:** Give directly or dilute in Normal Saline or D5W. Administer within 24 h of diluting.

**Infusion:** Inject slowly, directly or dilute, and infuse hydrocortisone phosphate at a rate of 25 mg/min; hydrocortisone sodium succinate at rate of each 500 mg over 30–60 sec.

**Incompatibilities:** Do not mix with amobarbital, ampicillin, bleomycin, colistimethate, dimenhydrinate, doxapram, doxorubicin, ephedrine, ergotamine, heparin, hydralazine, metaraminol, methicillin, nafcillin, pentobarbital, phenobarbital, phenytoin, prochloperazine, promethazine, secobarbital, tetracyclines.

**Adverse effects**

*Systemic*

- CNS: *Vertigo, headache*, paresthesias, insomnia, convulsions, psychosis
- GI: *Peptic or esophageal ulcer, pancreatitis,* abdominal distention, nausea, vomiting, increased appetite and weight gain (long-term therapy)
- CV: *Hypotension, shock,* hypertension and CHF secondary to fluid retention, thromboembolism, thrombophlebitis, fat embolism, cardiac arrhythmias secondary to electrolyte disturbances
- Hematologic: *$Na^+$ and fluid retention, hypokalemia,* hypocalcemia, increased blood sugar, increased serum cholesterol, decreased serum $T_3$ and $T_4$ levels
- MS: *Muscle weakness,* steroid myopathy and loss of muscle mass, osteoporosis, spontaneous fractures (long-term therapy)
- EENT: Cataracts, glaucoma (long-term therapy), increased intraocular pressure
- Dermatologic: *Thin, fragile skin; petechiae; ecchymoses;* purpura; striae; subcutaneous fat atrophy
- Hypersensitivity: Anaphylactoid or hypersensitivity reactions
- Endocrine: *Amenorrhea, irregular menses,* growth retardation, decreased carbohydrate tolerance and diabetes mellitus, cushingoid state (long-term therapy), hypothalamic-pituitary-adrenal (HPA) suppression systemic with therapy longer than 5 d
- Other: *Immunosuppression, aggravation or masking of infections, impaired wound healing*

*Adverse Effects Related to Specific Routes of Administration*

- IM repository injections: Atrophy at injection site
- Retention enema: Local pain, burning; rectal bleeding; systemic absorption and adverse effects (above)
- Intra-articular: Osteonecrosis, tendon rupture, infection
- Intraspinal: Meningitis, adhesive arachnoiditis, conus medullaris syndrome
- Intralesional therapy, head and neck: Blindness (rare)
- Intrathecal administration: Arachnoiditis
- Topical dermatologic ointments, creams, sprays: Local burning, irritation, acneiform lesions, striae, skin atrophy

**Clinically important drug-drug interactions**

• Increased steroid blood levels with oral contraceptives, troleandomycin • Decreased steroid blood levels with phenytoin, phenobarbital, rifampin, cholestyramine • Decreased serum level of salicylates • Decreased effectiveness of anticholinesterases (ambenonium, edrophonium, neostigmine, pyridostigmine)

**Drug-lab test interferences**

• False-negative nitroblue-tetrazolium test for bacterial infection (with systemic absorption) • Suppression of skin test reactions

## ■ Nursing Considerations

### Assessment

- ***History:*** Infections; kidney disease; liver disease, hypothyroidism; ulcerative colitis with impending perforation; diverticulitis; recent GI surgery; active or latent peptic ulcer; inflammatory bowel disease; hypertension, CHF; thromboembolitic tendencies, thrombophlebitis, osteoporosis, convulsive disorders, metastatic carcinoma, diabetes mellitus; lactation. *Retention enemas, intrarectal foam:* Systemic fungal infections; recent intestinal surgery, extensive fistulas. *Topical dermatologic administration:* Fungal, tubercular, herpes simplex skin infections; vaccinia, varicella; ear application when eardrum is perforated
- ***Physical:*** *Systemic administration:* weight, T; reflexes, affect, bilateral grip strength, ophthalmologic exam; BP, P, auscultation, peripheral perfusion, discoloration, pain or prominence of superficial vessels; R, adventitious sounds, chest x-ray; upper GI x-ray (history or symptoms of peptic ulcer), liver palpation; CBC, serum electrolytes, 2-h postprandial blood glucose, urinalysis, thyroid function tests, serum cholesterol. *Topical, dermatologic preparations:* Affected area, integrity of skin

### Implementation

*Systemic Administration*

- Give daily before 9 AM to mimic normal peak diurnal corticosteroid levels and minimize HPA suppression.
- Space multiple doses evenly throughout the day.
- Do not give IM injections if patient has thrombocytopenic purpura.
- Rotate sites of IM repository injections to avoid local atrophy.
- Use minimal doses for minimal duration to minimize adverse effects.
- Taper doses when discontinuing high-dose or long-term therapy.
- Arrange for increased dosage when patient is subject to unusual stress.
- Use alternate-day maintenance therapy with short-acting corticosteroids whenever possible.
- Do not give live virus vaccines with immunosuppressive doses of hydrocortisone.
- Provide antacids between meals to help avoid peptic ulcer.

*Topical Dermatologic Administration*

- Use caution with occlusive dressings, tight or plastic diapers over affected area can increase systemic absorption.
- Avoid prolonged use, especially near eyes, in genital and rectal areas, on face, and in skin creases.

### Drug-specific teaching points

*Systemic Administration*

- Take this drug exactly as prescribed. Do not stop taking this drug without notifying your health care provider; slowly taper dosage to avoid problems.
- Take with meals or snacks if GI upset occurs.
- Take single daily or alternate-day doses before 9 AM; mark calendar or use other measures as reminder of treatment days.
- Do not overuse joint after intra-articular injections, even if pain is gone.
- Frequent follow-ups to your health care provider are needed to monitor drug response and adjust dosage.
- The following side effects may occur: increase in appetite, weight gain (some of gain may be fluid retention; monitor intake); heartburn, indigestion (small, frequent meals, use of antacids may help); increased susceptibility to infection (avoid crowds during peak cold or flu seasons, and avoid anyone with a known infection); poor wound healing (if injured or

wounded, consult health care provider); muscle weakness, fatigue (frequent rest periods may help).

- Wear a medical alert ID (chronic therapy) so that any emergency medical personnel will know that you are taking this drug.
- Report unusual weight gain, swelling of lower extremities, muscle weakness, black or tarry stools, vomiting of blood, epigastric burning, puffing of face, menstrual irregularities, fever, prolonged sore throat, cold or other infection, worsening of symptoms.
- Dosage reductions may create adrenal insufficiency. Report any of the following: fatigue, muscle and joint pains, anorexia, nausea, vomiting, diarrhea, weight loss, weakness, dizziness, low blood sugar (if you monitor blood sugar).

*Intra-articular, Intra-lesional Administration*

- Do not overuse the injected joint even if the pain is gone. Adhere to rules of proper rest and exercise.

*Topical Dermatologic Administration*

- Apply sparingly, and rub in lightly
- Avoid eye contact.
- Report burning, irritation, or infection of the site, worsening of the condition.
- Avoid prolonged use.

*Anorectal Preparations*

- Maintain normal bowel function with proper diet, adequate fluid intake, and regular exercise.
- Use stool softeners or bulk laxatives if needed.
- Notify your health care provider if symptoms do not improve in 7 d or if bleeding, protrusion, or seepage occurs.

## hydroflumethiazide

*(hye droe floo me **thye'** a zide)*

Diucardin, Saluron

**Pregnancy Category C**

### Drug classes

Thiazide diuretic

### Therapeutic actions

Inhibits reabsorption of sodium and chloride in distal renal tubule, increasing the excretion of sodium, chloride, and water by the kidney.

### Indications

- Adjunctive therapy in edema associated with CHF, cirrhosis, corticosteroid, and estrogen therapy; renal dysfunction
- Hypertension, alone or with other antihypertensives
- Unlabeled uses: calcium nephrolithiasis alone or with amiloride or allopurinal to prevent recurrences in hypercalciuric or normal calciuric patients, diabetes insipidus, especially nephrogenic diabetes insipidus, osteoporosis

### Contraindications/cautions

- Contraindications: allergy to thiazides, sulfonamides; fluid or electrolyte imbalance; renal disease (azotemia); liver disease (hepatic coma); gout (risk of attack); SLE; glucose tolerance abnormalities, diabetes mellitus; hyperparathyroidism; manic-depressive disorder (aggravated by hypercalcemia); pregnancy; lactation.

### Dosage

**Available Forms:** Tablets—50 mg

**ADULT**

- ***Edema:*** 50 mg qd–bid PO. Maintenance: 25–200 mg qd PO; divide doses if dose exceeds 100 mg/d
- ***Hypertension:*** 50 mg PO bid. Maintenance: 50–100 mg/d PO. Do not exceed 200 mg/d.

### Pharmacokinetics

| Route | Onset | Peak | Duration |
|---|---|---|---|
| Oral | 2 h | 4 h | 6–12 h |

*Metabolism:* Hepatic, $T_{1/2}$: 17 h

*Distribution:* Crosses placenta; enters breast milk

*Excretion:* Urine

### Adverse effects

- CNS: *Dizziness, vertigo,* paresthesias, weakness, headache, drowsiness, fatigue, leukopenia, thrombocytopenia, agranulocytosis, aplastic anemia, neutropenia
- GI: *Nausea, anorexia, vomiting, dry mouth,* diarrhea, constipation, jaundice, hepatitis, pancreatitis

- CV: Orthostatic hypotension, venous thrombosis, volume depletion, cardiac arrhythmias, chest pain
- GU: *Polyuria, nocturia,* impotence, loss of libido
- **Dermatologic**: Photosensitivity, rash, purpura, exfoliative dermatitis, hives
- **Other**: Muscle cramps and muscle spasms, fever, gouty attacks, flushing, weight loss, rhinorrhea

### Clinically important drug-drug interactions

• Increased thiazide effects if taken with diazoxide • Decreased absorption with cholestyramine, colestipol • Increased risk of cardiac glycoside toxicity if hypokalemia occurs • Increased risk of lithium toxicity • Decreased effectiveness of antidiabetic agents when taken concurrently with hydrochlorothiazide

### Drug-lab test interferences

• Decreased PBI levels without clinical signs of thyroid disturbance

## ■ Nursing Considerations

### Assessment

- *History:* Allergy to thiazides, sulfonamides; fluid or electrolyte imbalance; renal or liver disease; gout; SLE; glucose tolerance abnormalities; hyperparathyroidism; manic-depressive disorders; lactation
- *Physical:* Skin color, lesions, edema; orientation, reflexes, muscle strength; pulses, baseline ECG, BP, orthostatic BP, perfusion; R, pattern, adventitious sounds; liver evaluation, bowel sounds, urinary output patterns; CBC, serum electrolytes, blood glucose, liver and renal function tests, serum uric acid, urinalysis

### Implementation

- Give with food or milk if GI upset occurs.
- Mark calendars or other reminders for alternate day or 3–5 d/wk therapy for edema
- Reduce dosage of other antihypertensive drugs by at least 50% if given with thiazides; readjust dosages gradually as BP responds.
- Give early so increased urination will not disturb sleep.
- Measure and record regular body weights to monitor fluid changes.

### Drug-specific teaching points

- Record intermittent therapy on a calendar, or use prepared, dated envelopes. Take the drug early in the day so increased urination will not disturb sleep. Take drug with food or meals if GI upset occurs.
- Weigh yourself on a regular basis, at the same time and in the same clothing, record the weight on your calendar.
- The following side effects may occur: increased volume and frequency of urination; dizziness, feeling faint on arising, drowsiness (avoid rapid position changes; hazardous activities, like driving; and alcohol); sensitivity to sunlight (use sunglasses, wear protective clothing, or use a sunscreen); decrease in sexual function; increased thirst (sucking on sugarless lozenges and frequent mouth care may help).
- Report weight change of more than 3 lb in one day, swelling in your ankles or fingers, unusual bleeding or bruising, dizziness, trembling, numbness, fatigue, muscle weakness or cramps.

# hydromorphone hydrochloride

*(hye droe **mor'** fone)*

Dilaudid

**Pregnancy Category C**

**Pregnancy Category D (labor & delivery)**

**C-II controlled substance**

### Drug classes

Narcotic agonist analgesic

### Therapeutic actions

Acts as agonist at specific opioid receptors in the CNS to produce analgesia, euphoria, sedation; the receptors mediating these effects are thought to be the same as those mediating the effects of endogenous opioids (enkephalins, endorphins).

**Indications**

- Relief of moderate to severe pain

**Contraindications/cautions**

- Contraindications: hypersensitivity to narcotics, tartrazine (1-, 2-, and 4-mg tablets, Dilaudid); physical dependence on a narcotic analgesic (drug may precipitate withdrawal); lactation.
- Use cautiously with pregnancy (readily crosses placenta; neonatal withdrawal if mothers used drug during pregnancy); labor or delivery (safety to mother and fetus has not been established); bronchial asthma, COPD, respiratory depression, anoxia, increased intracranial pressure, acute MI, ventricular failure, coronary insufficiency, hypertension, biliary tract surgery, renal or hepatic dysfunction.

**Dosage**

**Available Forms:** Injection—1, 2, 3, 4, 10 mg/ml; tablets—1, 2, 3, 4 mg; suppositories—3 mg

ADULT

- ***Oral:*** 2–4 mg q4–6h.
- ***Parenteral:*** 2–4 mg IM, SC q4–6h as needed. May be given by slow IV injection if no other route is tolerated.
- ***Rectal:*** 3 mg q6–8h.

PEDIATRIC: Safety and efficacy not established. Contraindicated in premature infants.

GERIATRIC OR IMPAIRED ADULT: Use caution; respiratory depression may occur in elderly, the very ill, those with respiratory problems. Reduced dosage may be necessary.

**Pharmacokinetics**

| Route | Onset | Peak | Duration |
|---|---|---|---|
| Oral | Varies | 30–60 min | 4–5 h |
| IM | 15–30 min | 30–60 min | 4–5 h |

*Metabolism:* Hepatic, $T_{1/2}$: 2–3 h

*Distribution:* Crosses placenta; enters breast milk

*Excretion:* Urine

**IV facts**

**Preparations:** Administer undiluted or diluted in Normal Saline or D5W.

**Infusion:** Inject slowly, each 2 mg over 2–5 min, directly into vein or into tubing of running IV.

**Adverse effects**

- CNS: *Lightheadedness, dizziness, sedation,* euphoria, dysphoria, delirium, insomnia, agitation, anxiety, fear, hallucinations, disorientation, drowsiness, lethargy, impaired mental and physical performance, coma, mood changes, weakness, headache, tremor, convulsions, miosis, visual disturbances, suppression of cough reflex
- GI: *Nausea, vomiting,* dry mouth, anorexia, constipation, biliary tract spasm; increased colonic motility in patients with chronic ulcerative colitis
- CV: Facial flushing, peripheral circulatory collapse, tachycardia, bradycardia, arrhythmia, palpitations, chest wall rigidity, hypertension, hypotension, orthostatic hypotension, syncope
- GU: Ureteral spasm, spasm of vesical sphincters, urinary retention or hesitancy, oliguria, antidiuretic effect, reduced libido or potency
- Dermatologic: Pruritus, urticaria, laryngospasm, bronchospasm, edema
- Hypersensitivity: Anaphylactoid reactions (IV administration)
- Local: Phlebitis following IV injection pain at injection site; tissue irritation and induration (SC injection)
- Major hazards: **Respiratory depression, apnea, circulatory depression, respiratory arrest, shock, cardiac arrest**
- Other: *Sweating,* physical tolerance and dependence, psychological dependence

**Clinically important drug-drug interactions**

- Potentiation of effects of hydromorphone with barbiturate anesthetics; decrease dose of hydromorphone when coadministering.

h

**Drug-lab test interferences**

- Elevated biliary tract pressure (an effect of narcotics) may cause increases in plasma amylase, lipase; determinations of these levels may be unreliable for 24 h after administration of narcotics.

## ■ Nursing Considerations

### Assessment

- *History:* Hypersensitivity to narcotics, tartrazine, physical dependence on a narcotic analgesic; pregnancy; lactation; COPD, respiratory depression, anoxia, increased intracranial pressure, acute MI, ventricular failure, coronary insufficiency, hypertension, biliary tract surgery, renal or hepatic dysfunction
- *Physical:* Orientation, reflexes, bilateral grip strength, affect; pupil size, vision; P, auscultation, BP; R, adventitious sounds; bowel sounds, normal output; thyroid, liver, kidney function tests

### Implementation

- Give to nursing women 4–6 h before the next scheduled feeding to minimize drug in milk.
- Provide narcotic antagonist, facilities for assisted or controlled respiration on standby during parenteral administration.
- Use caution when injecting SC into chilled body areas or in patients with hypotension or in shock; impaired perfusion may delay absorption. With repeated doses, an excessive amount may be absorbed when circulation is restored.
- Refrigerate rectal suppositories.

### Drug-specific teaching points

- Learn how to administer rectal suppositories; refrigerate suppositories.
- Take drug exactly as prescribed.
- Avoid alcohol, antihistamines, sedatives, tranquilizers, OTC drugs.
- The following side effects may occur: nausea, loss of appetite (take drug with food and lie quietly, eat frequent small meals); constipation (laxative may help); dizziness, sedation, drowsiness, impaired visual acuity (avoid driving, performing tasks that require alertness, visual acuity).
- Do not take leftover medication for other disorders, and do not let anyone else take the prescription.
- Report severe nausea, vomiting, constipation, shortness of breath or difficulty breathing.

# hydroxocobalamin crystalline

*(hye drox oh koe **bal'** a min)*

vitamin $B_{12a}$

Hydro-Crysti 12, Hydro-Cobex, LA-12

**Pregnancy Category C**

**Drug classes**

Vitamin

**Therapeutic actions**

Essential to growth, cell reproduction, hematopoiesis, and nucleoprotein and myelin synthesis; physiologic function is associated with nucleic acid and protein synthesis; acts the same way as cyanocobalamin.

**Indications**

- Vitamin $B_{12}$ deficiency due to malabsorption; GI pathology, dysfunction, or surgery; fish tapeworm; gluten enteropathy, sprue; small bowel bacterial overgrowth; folic acid deficiency
- Increased vitamin $B_{12}$ requirements—pregnancy, thyrotoxicosis, hemolytic anemia, hemorrhage, malignancy, hepatic and renal disease
- Unlabeled use: prevention and treatment of cyanide toxicity associated with sodium nitroprusside (forms cyanocobalamin with the cyanide, thus lowering plasma and RBC cyanide concentrations)

**Contraindications/cautions**

- Contraindications: allergy to cobalt, vitamin $B_{12}$, or their components; Leber's disease.
- Use cautiously with pregnancy (safety not established, but is an essential vitamin required during pregnancy—4 $\mu$g/d); lactation—secreted in breast milk (required nutrient during lactation—4 $\mu$g/d).

### Dosage

**Available Forms:** Injection—1000 μg/ml

For IM use only; folic acid therapy should be given concurrently if needed.

*ADULT:* 30 μg/d for 5–10 d IM, followed by 100–200 μg/mo.

*PEDIATRIC:* 1–5 mg over 2 or more wk in doses of 100 μg IM, then 30–50 μg every 4 wk for maintainence.

### Pharmacokinetics

| Route | Onset | Peak |
|---|---|---|
| IM | Intermediate | 60 min |

*Metabolism:* Hepatic, $T_{1/2}$: 24–36 h
*Distribution:* Crosses placenta; enters breast milk
*Excretion:* Urine

### Adverse effects

- CNS: Severe and swift optic nerve atrophy (patients with early Leber's disease)
- GI: *Mild, transient diarrhea*
- CV: Pulmonary edema, CHF, peripheral vascular thrombosis
- Hematologic: Polycythemia vera
- Dermatologic: *Itching, transitory exanthema*, urticaria
- Hypersensitivity: **Anaphylactic shock and death**
- Local: *Pain at injection site*
- Other: Feeling of total body swelling; hypokalemia

### Drug-lab test interferences

- Invalid folic acid and vitamin $B_{12}$ diagnostic blood assays if patient is taking methotrexate, pyrimethamine, most antibiotics

## ■ Nursing Considerations

### Assessment

- *History:* Allergy to cobalt, vitamin $B_{12}$, or any component of these medications; Leber's disease
- *Physical:* Skin color, lesions; ophthalmic exam; P, BP, peripheral perfusion; R, adventitious sounds; CBC, Hct, Hgb, vitamin $B_{12}$, and folic acid levels

### Implementation

- Give in parenteral form for pernicious anemia.
- Give with folic acid if needed; check serum levels.
- Monitor serum potassium levels, especially during the first few days of treatment; arrange for appropriate treatment of hypokalemia.
- Maintain emergency drugs and life support equipment on standby in case of severe anaphylactic reaction.
- Arrange for periodic checks for stomach cancer with pernicious anemia; risk is three times greater in these patients.

### Drug-specific teaching points

- The IM route is the only one available. Monthly injections needed for life with pernicious anemia. Without it, anemia will return and irreversible neurologic damage will develop.
- The following side effects may occur: mild diarrhea (transient); rash, itching; pain at injection site.
- Report swelling of the ankles, leg cramps, fatigue, difficulty breathing, pain at injection site.

## hydroxychloroquine sulfate

*(hye drox ee **klor'** oh kwin)*
Plaquenil Sulfate
**Pregnancy Category C**

### Drug classes

Antimalarial
Antirheumatic agent
4-aminoquinoline

### Therapeutic actions

Inhibits protozoal reproduction and protein synthesis, preventing the replication of DNA, the transcription of RNA, and the synthesis of protein. Anti-inflammatory action in rheumatoid arthritis, lupus: mechanism of action is not known but is thought to involve the suppression of the formation of antigens, which cause hypersensitivity reactions and symptoms.

## Indications

- Suppression and treatment of acute attacks of malaria caused by susceptible strains of plasmodia
- Treatment of acute or chronic rheumatoid arthritis
- Treatment of chronic discoid and systemic lupus erythematosus
- *Note:* Radical cure of vivax malaria requires concomitant primaquine therapy; some strains of *Plasmodium falciparum* are resistant to chloroquine and related drugs.

## Contraindications/cautions

- Contraindications: allergy to 4-aminoquinolines, porphyria, psoriasis, retinal disease (irreversible retinal damage may occur); pregnancy.
- Use cautiously with hepatic disease, alcoholism, G-6-PD deficiency.

## Dosage

**Available Forms:** Tablets—200 mg

200 mg hydroxychloroquine sulfate is equivalent to 155 mg hydroxychloroquine base.

### ADULT

- ***Suppression of malaria:*** 310 mg base/wk PO on the same day each week, beginning 1–2 wk prior to exposure and continuing for 4 wk after leaving the endemic area. If suppressive therapy is not begun prior to exposure, double the initial loading dose (620 mg base), and give in two doses, 6 h apart.
- ***Acute attack of malaria:***

| Dose | Time | Dosage (mg Base) |
|---|---|---|
| Initial | Day 1 | 620 mg |
| 2nd dose | 6 h later | 310 mg |
| 3rd dose | Day 2 | 310 mg |
| 4th dose | Day 3 | 310 mg |

- ***Rheumatoid arthritis:*** Initial dosage 400–600 mg/d PO taken with meals or a glass of milk. From 5–10 d later, gradually increase dosage to optimum effectiveness. *Maintenance dosage:* When good response is obtained (usually 4–12 wk), reduce dosage to 200–400 mg/d PO.
- ***Lupus erythematosus:*** 400 mg qd–bid PO continued for several weeks or months; for prolonged use, 200–400 mg/d may be sufficient.

### PEDIATRIC

- ***Suppression of malaria:*** 5 mg base/kg weekly PO for adults (above).
- ***Acute attack of malaria:***

| Dose | Time | Dosage (mg Base) |
|---|---|---|
| Initial | Day 1 | 10 mg/kg |
| 2nd dose | 6 h later | 5 mg/kg |
| 3rd dose | Day 2 | 5 mg/kg |
| 4th dose | Day 3 | 5 mg/kg |

## Pharmacokinetics

| Route | Onset | Peak |
|---|---|---|
| Oral | Varies | 1–6 h |

*Metabolism:* Hepatic, $T_{1/2}$: 70–120 h

*Distribution:* Crosses placenta; enters breast milk

*Excretion:* Urine

## Adverse effects

- CNS: Tinnitus, loss of hearing (ototoxicity), exacerbation of porphyria, muscle weakness, absent or hypoactive deep tendon reflexes, irritability, nervousness, emotional changes, nightmares, psychosis, headache, dizziness, vertigo, nystagmus, convulsions, ataxia
- GI: *Nausea, vomiting, diarrhea*, abdominal cramps, loss of appetite
- **Hematologic**: *Blood dyscrasias*, immunoblastic lymphadenopathy, hemolysis in patients with G-6-PD deficiency
- EENT: *Retinal changes, corneal changes*—edema, opacities, decreased sensitivity; ciliary body changes—disturbance of accommodation, blurred vision
- **Dermatologic**: *Pruritus, bleaching of hair,* alopecia, skin and mucosal pigmentation, skin eruptions, psoriasis, exfoliative dermatitis

## ■ Nursing Considerations

### Assessment

- ***History:*** Allergy to 4-aminoquinolines, porphyria, psoriasis, retinal disease, hepatic disease, alcoholism, G-6-PD deficiency

- *Physical:* Skin color, lesions; hair; reflexes, muscle strength, auditory and ophthalmological screening, affect, reflexes; liver palpation, abdominal exam, mucous membranes; CBC, G-6-PD in deficient patients, liver function tests

### Implementation

- Administer with meals or milk.
- Titrate long-term therapy to smallest effective dose; incidence of retinopathy increases with larger doses.
- Schedule malaria suppressive doses for weekly same-day therapy on a calendar.
- Double check pediatric doses; children are very susceptible to overdosage.
- Arrange for administration of ammonium chloride (8 g/d in divided doses for adults) 3–4 d/wk for several months after therapy has been stopped if serious toxic symptoms occur.
- Arrange for ophthalmologic examinations during long-term therapy.

### Drug-specific teaching points

- Take full course of drug as prescribed.
- Take drug with meals or milk.
- Mark your calendar with the drug days for malarial prophylaxis.
- The following side effects may occur: stomach pain, loss of appetite, nausea, vomiting or diarrhea; irritability, emotional changes, nightmares, headache (reversible).
- Arrange for regular ophthalmologic exams if long-term use is indicated.
- Report blurring of vision, loss of hearing, ringing in the ears, muscle weakness, skin rash or itching, unusual bleeding or bruising, yellow color of eyes or skin, mood swings or mental changes.

## hydroxyprogesterone caproate in oil

*(hye **drox'** ee proe **jess'** te rone)*

Hylutin, Hyprogest 250

**Pregnancy Category X**

### Drug classes

Hormonal agent
Progestin

### Therapeutic actions

Progesterone derivative. Endogenous progesterone transforms proliferative endometrium into secretory endometrium; inhibits the secretion of pituitary gonadotropins, which prevents follicular maturation and ovulation; and inhibits spontaneous uterine contraction. Progestins have varying profiles of estrogenic, antiestrogenic, anabolic, and androgenic activity.

### Indications

- Treatment of amenorrhea (primary or secondary); abnormal uterine bleeding due to hormonal imbalance
- Production of secretory endometrium and desquamation

### Contraindications/cautions

- Contraindications: allergy to progestins; thrombophlebitis, thromboembolic disorders, cerebral hemorrhage, or history of these; hepatic disease, carcinoma of the breast or genital organs, undiagnosed vaginal bleeding, missed abortion; pregnancy (fetal abnormalities, including masculinization of the female fetus); lactation.
- Use cautiously with epilepsy, migraine, asthma, cardiac or renal dysfunction.

### Dosage

**Available Forms:** Injection—125, 250 mg/ml

Administer IM only.

ADULT

- ***Amenorrhea; abnormal uterine bleeding:*** 375 mg IM at any time. After 4 d of desquamation or if no bleeding occurs in 21 d after hydroxyprogesterone alone, start cyclic therapy (administer 20 mg estradiol valerate on day 1 of each cycle; 2 wk after day 1, administer 250 mg hydroxyprogesterone caproate and 5 mg estradiol valerate; 4 wk after day 1 is day 1 of the next cycle). Repeat every 4 wk, and stop after four cycles. Observe patient for onset of normal cycling for 2 to 3 cycles after cessation of therapy.
- ***Production of secretory endometrium and desquamation:*** Start cyclic therapy any time (see above); repeat every 4 wk until no longer required. Give

125–250 mg IM given on 10th day of cycle; repeat q7 d until suppression is no longer necessary.

### Pharmacokinetics

| Route | Onset | Duration |
|---|---|---|
| IM | Slow | 9–17 d |

*Metabolism:* Hepatic, $T_{1/2}$: unkown
*Distribution:* Crosses placenta; enters breast milk
*Excretion:* Urine

### Adverse effects

- CNS: Sudden, partial or complete loss of vision, proptosis, diplopia, migraine, precipitation of acute intermittent porphyria, mental depression, pyrexia, insomnia, somnolence
- GI: Cholestatic jaundice, nausea
- CV: Thrombophlebitis, cerebrovascular disorders, retinal thrombosis, pulmonary embolism, thromboembolic and thrombotic disease, increased BP
- GU: *Breakthrough bleeding, spotting, change in menstrual flow, amenorrhea,* changes in cervical erosion and cervical secretions, breast tenderness and secretion
- **Dermatologic**: *Rash with or without pruritis, acne,* melasma or chloasma, alopecia, hirsutism, photosensitivity
- General: *Fluid retention, edema, increase or decrease in weight*
- Other: Decreased glucose tolerance

### Drug-lab test interferences

- Inaccurate tests of hepatic and endocrine function

## ■ Nursing Considerations

### Assessment

- *History:* Allergy to progestins; thromboembolic disorders, cerebral hemorrhage; hepatic disease, carcinoma of the breast or genital organs, undiagnosed vaginal bleeding, missed abortion; epilepsy, migraine, asthma, cardiac or renal dysfunction
- *Physical:* Skin—color, lesions, turgor; hair; breasts; pelvic exam; orientation, affect; ophthalmologic exam; P, auscultation, peripheral perfusion, edema; R, adventitious sounds; liver evaluation; liver and renal function tests, glucose tolerance, Pap smear

### Implementation

- Arrange for pretreatment and periodic (at least annual) history and physical, which should include BP, breasts, abdomen, pelvic organs, and a Pap smear.
- Alert patient before therapy to avoid pregnancy during treatment and to have frequent medical follow-ups.
- Administer IM only.
- Discontinue medication and consult physician if sudden partial or complete loss of vision occurs; if papilledema or retinal vascular lesions are present on exam, discontinue drug.
- Arrange to discontinue medication and consult physician at the first sign of thromboembolic disease (leg pain, swelling, peripheral perfusion changes, shortness of breath).

### Drug-specific teaching points

- Prepare a calendar of drug days to remind you about doses.
- This drug can be given only by IM injection.
- The following side effects may occur: sensitivity to light (avoid exposure to the sun; use sunscreen and protective clothing); dizziness, sleeplessness, depression (use caution if driving or performing tasks that require alertness); skin rash, color changes, loss of hair; fever; nausea.
- Do not take drug during pregnancy; serious fetal abnormalities have occurred.
- Report pain or swelling and warmth in the calves, acute chest pain or shortness of breath, sudden severe headache or vomiting, dizziness or fainting, visual disturbances, numbness or tingling in the arm or leg.

## hydroxyurea

*(hye drox ee yoor **ee'** a)*
Hydrea
**Pregnancy Category D**

### Drug classes
Antineoplastic agent

### Therapeutic actions
Cytotoxic: inhibits an enzyme that is crucial for DNA synthesis, but exact mechanism of action is not fully understood.

### Indications
- Melanoma
- Resistant chronic myelocytic leukemia
- Recurrent, metastatic, or inoperable ovarian cancer
- Concomitant therapy with irradiation for primary squamous cell carcinoma of the head and neck, excluding the lip
- Treatment of sickle cell anemia

### Contraindications/cautions
- Allergy to hydroxyurea, irradiation, leukopenia, impaired hepatic and renal function, pregnancy, lactation.

### Dosage
**Available Forms:** Capsules—500 mg

*ADULT:* Base dosage on ideal or actual body weight, whichever is less. Interrupt therapy if WBC falls below 2,500/mm$^3$ or platelet count below 100,000/mm$^3$. Recheck in 3 d and resume therapy when counts approach normal.
- ***Solid tumors:*** Intermittent therapy: 80 mg/kg PO as a single dose every third day. Continuous therapy: 20–30 mg/kg PO as a single daily dose.
- ***Concomitant therapy with irradiation:*** 80 mg/kg as a single daily dose every third day. Begin hydroxyurea 7 d before irradiation, and continue during and for a prolonged period after radiotherapy.
- ***Resistant chronic myelocytic leukemia:*** 20–30 mg/kg as a single daily dose.

*PEDIATRIC:* Dosage regimen not established.

### Pharmacokinetics
| *Route* | *Onset* | *Peak* | *Duration* |
|---|---|---|---|
| Oral | Varies | 2 h | 18–20 h |

*Metabolism:* Hepatic, $T_{1/2}$: 3–4 h
*Distribution:* Crosses placenta; enters breast milk
*Excretion:* Urine

### Adverse effects
- CNS: *Headache, dizziness*, disorientation, hallucinations
- GI: *Stomatitis, anorexia, nausea, vomiting*, diarrhea, constipation, elevated hepatic enzymes
- **Hematologic**: *Bone marrow depression*
- GU: Impaired renal tubular function
- **Dermatologic**: Maculopapular rash, facial erythema
- **Local**: Mucositis at the site, especially in combination with irradiation
- **Other**: Fever, chills, malaise

### Drug-lab test interferences
- Serum uric acid, BUN and creatinine levels may increase with hydroxyurea therapy
- Drug causes self-limiting abnormalities in erythrocytes that resemble those of pernicious anemia but are not related to vitamin $B_{12}$ or folate deficiency

## ■ Nursing Considerations

### Assessment
- ***History:*** Allergy to hydroxyurea, irradiation, leukopenia, impaired hepatic and renal function, lactation
- ***Physical:*** Weight; T; skin color, lesions; reflexes, orientation, affect; mucous membranes, abdominal exam; CBC, renal and liver function tests

### Implementation
- Give in oral form only. If patient is unable to swallow capsules, empty capsules into a glass of water, and give immediately (inert products may not dissolve).
- Encourage patient to drink 10–12 glasses of fluid each day.
- Check CBC before administration of each dose of drug.

### Drug-specific teaching points
- Prepare a calendar for dates to return for diagnostic testing and treatment days. If you are unable to swallow the capsule,

h

empty the capsule into a glass of water, and take immediately (some of the material may not dissolve).

- The following side effects may occur: loss of appetite, nausea, vomiting, mouth sores (frequent mouth care, small frequent meals may help; maintain good nutrition; an antiemetic may be ordered); constipation or diarrhea (a bowel program may be established); disorientation, dizziness, headache (take precautions to avoid injury); red face, rash (reversible).
- Arrange for regular blood tests to monitor the drug's effects.
- Drink at least 10–12 glasses of fluid each day while on this drug.
- Report fever, chills, sore throat, unusual bleeding or bruising, severe nausea, vomiting, loss of appetite, sores in the mouth or on the lips, pregnancy (it is advisable to use birth control while on this drug).

## Hydroxyzine

### hydroxyzine hydrochloride

*(hye **drox'** i zeen)*

*Oral preparations:* Anxanil, Atarax, Vistaril

*Parenteral preparations:* Hyzine, Multipax (CAN), Quiess, QYS, Vistacon, Vistaquel, Vistaril

### hydroxyzine pamoate

*Oral preparations:* Vistaril

**Pregnancy Category C**

### Drug classes

Antianxiety drug
Antihistamine
Antiemetic

### Therapeutic actions

Mechanisms of action not understood; actions may be due to suppression of subcortical areas of the CNS; has clinically demonstrated antihistaminic, analgesic, antispasmodic, antiemetic, mild antisecretory, and bronchodilator activity.

### Indications

- Symptomatic relief of anxiety and tension associated with psychoneurosis; adjunct in organic disease states in which anxiety is manifested; alcoholism and asthma
- Management of pruritus due to allergic conditions, such as chronic urticaria, atopic and contact dermatosis, and in histamine-mediated pruritus
- Sedation when used as premedication and following general anesthesia
- Management of the acutely disturbed or hysterical patient; the acute or chronic alcoholic with anxiety withdrawal symptoms or delirium tremens; as preoperative and postoperative and prepartum and postpartum adjunctive medication to permit reduction in narcotic dosage, allay anxiety, and control emesis (IM administration)

### Contraindications/cautions

- Allergy to hydroxyzine; uncomplicated vomiting in children (may contribute to of Reye's syndrome or unfavorably influence its outcome; extrapyramidal effects may obscure diagnosis of Reye's syndrome); pregnancy; lactation.

### Dosage

**Available Forms:** Tablets—10, 25, 50, 100 mg; syrup—10 mg/5 ml; capsules—25, 50, 100 mg; oral suspension—25 mg/5 ml; injection 25 mg/ml

Start patients on IM therapy; use oral therapy for maintenance. Adjust dosage to patient's response.

**ADULT**

- ***Oral***
  - *Symptomatic relief of anxiety:* 50–100 mg qid.
  - *Management of pruritus:* 25 mg tid–qid.
  - *Sedative (preoperative and postoperative):* 50–100 mg.
- ***IM***
  - *Psychiatric and emotional emergencies, including alcoholism:* 50–100 mg immediately and q4–6h as needed.
  - *Nausea and vomiting:* 25–100 mg.
  - *Preoperative and postoperative, prepartum and postpartum:* 25–100 mg.

**PEDIATRIC**

- *Oral*
- *Anxiety, pruritus:* >*6 y:* 50–100 mg/d in divided doses. <*6 y:* 50 mg/d in divided doses.
- *Sedative:* 0.6 mg/kg.
- *IM*
- *Nausea, preoperative and postoperative:* 1.1 mg/kg (0.5 mg/lb).

### Pharmacokinetics

| Route | Onset | Peak | Duration |
|---|---|---|---|
| Oral/IM | 15–30 min | 3 h | 4–6 h |

*Metabolism:* Hepatic, $T_{1/2}$: 3 h
*Distribution:* Crosses placenta; may enter breast milk
*Excretion:* Urine

### Adverse effects

- CNS: *Drowsiness*, involuntary motor activity, including tremor and convulsions
- GI: *Dry mouth*
- **Hypersensitivity**: Wheezing, dyspnea, chest tightness

## ■ Nursing Considerations

### Assessment

- ***History:*** Allergy to hydroxyzine, uncomplicated vomiting in children, lactation
- ***Physical:*** Skin color, lesions, texture; orientation, reflexes, affect; R, adventitious sounds

### Implementation

- Determine and treat underlying cause of vomiting. Drug may mask signs and symptoms of serious conditions, such as brain tumor, intestinal obstruction, appendicitis.
- Do not administer parenteral solution SC, IV or intra-arterially; tissue necrosis has occurred with SC and intra-arterial injection, hemolysis with IV injection.
- Give IM injections deep into a large muscle: adults: upper outer quadrant of buttocks or midlateral thigh; children: midlateral thigh muscles; use deltoid area only if well developed.

### Drug-specific teaching points

- Take this drug as prescribed. Avoid excessive dosage.
- The following side effects may occur: dizziness, sedation, drowsiness (use caution if driving or performing tasks that require alertness); avoid alcohol, sedatives, sleep aids (serious overdosage could result); dry mouth (frequent mouth care, sucking sugarless lozenges may help).
- Report difficulty breathing, tremors, loss of coordination, sore muscles, or muscle spasms.

## hylan G-F 20

***(hye' lan)***
Synvisc
**Unknown**

### Drug classes

Hyaluronic acid derivative

### Therapeutic actions

Made of hylans, a natural complex sugar acting as a polymer for joint fluids, having elastic and viscous properties; derived from chicken combs.

### Indications

- Treatment of pain in osteoarthritis of the knee in patients who have failed to respond adequately to conservative therapy and simple analgesics

### Contraindications/cautions

- Contraindications: hypersensitivity to any component of the drug or chicken products; infection of the knee, skin or surrounding area.
- Use cautiously with pregnancy, lactation (no data are available), edema or lymphostasis of the leg.

### Dosage

**Available Forms:** Injection—16 mg/2 ml glass syringe
**ADULT:** 2 ml by intra-articular injection 1 X/wk for 3 wk; no data are available on repeat treatment cycles.

### Pharmacokinetics

Hylan G-F 20 is not thought to be absorbed systemically.

### Adverse effects

- Local: Inflammation and edema at site of infection; knee pain

### Clinically important drug-drug interactions

- Do not inject local anesthetic at same site and time as hylan G-F 20

## ■ Nursing Considerations

### Assessment

- *History:* Hypersensitivity to any component of the drug or chicken products; infection of the knee or surrounding area, pregnancy, lactation, edema or lymphostasis
- *Physical:* T; knee exam and evaluation including range of motion

### Implementation

- Use strict aseptic technique; do not use if seal is broken; each vial is for one use only, discard after use.
- Do not administer to any other joint; do not administer into severely inflamed knee.
- Do not inject any other medication or anesthetic into a knee injected with hylan G-F 20.
- Remove any synovial fluid of effusion before injection into knee.

### Drug-specific teaching points

- Little is known about the long-term effects of this drug; it will need to be injected into your knee once a week for three weeks.
- Avoid strenuous activities and prolonged weight bearing following this injection.
- Some swelling and discomfort may occur following injection; this should resolve quickly.
- Report increased swelling, redness, heat in knee, fever, worsening of knee pain.

# ibuprofen

*(eye **byoo'** proe fen)*

Advil, Amersol (CAN), Arthritis Foundation, Bayer Select Pain Relief, Children's Advil, Children's Motrin, Genpril, Haltran, IBU, Ibuprin, Ibuprohm, Menadol, Midol, Motrin, Nuprin, PediaProfen, Saleto-200, 400, 600, 800

**Pregnancy Category B**

### Drug classes

Nonsteroidal anti-inflammatory drug (NSAID)
Analgesic (non-narcotic)
Propionic acid derivative

### Therapeutic actions

Anti-inflammatory, analgesic, and antipyretic activities largely related to inhibition of prostaglandin synthesis; exact mechanisms of action are not known.

### Indications

- Relief of signs and symptoms of rheumatoid arthritis and osteoarthritis
- Relief of mild to moderate pain
- Treatment of primary dysmenorrhea
- Fever reduction

### Contraindications/cautions

- Contraindications: allergy to ibuprofen, salicylates, or other NSAIDs (more common in patients with rhinitis, asthma, chronic urticaria, nasal polyps); CV dysfunction, hypertension; peptic ulceration, GI bleeding; pregnancy; lactation.
- Use cautiously with impaired hepatic or renal function.

### Dosage

**Available Forms:** Tablets—100, 200, 300, 400, 600, 800 mg; chewable tablets—50, 100 mg; suspension—100 mg/5ml; oral drops—40 mg/ml; caplets—100 mg

Do not exceed 3200 mg/d.

**ADULT**

- *Mild to moderate pain:* 400 mg q4–6h PO.
- *Osteoarthritis/rheumatoid arthritis:* 1,200–3,200 mg/d PO (300 mg qid or 400, 600, 800 mg tid or qid; individualize dosage. Therapeutic response may occur in a few days, but often takes 2 wk).
- *Primary dysmenorrhea:* 400 mg q4h PO.
- *OTC use:* 200–400 mg q4–6h PO while symptoms persist; do not exceed 1,200 mg/d. Do not take for more than 10 d for pain or 3 d for fever, unless so directed by health care provider.

PEDIATRIC

- *Juvenile arthritis:* 30–70 mg/kg per day PO in three to four divided doses; 20 mg/kg per day for milder disease.
- *Fever:* 5–10 mg/kg PO q6–8h; do not exceed 40 mg/kg per day.

### Pharmacokinetics

| *Route* | *Onset* | *Peak* | *Duration* |
|---|---|---|---|
| Oral | 30 min | 1–2 h | 4–6 h |

*Metabolism:* Hepatic; $T_{1/2}$: 1.8–2 1/2 h
*Distribution:* Crosses placenta; may enter breast milk
*Excretion:* Urine

### Adverse effects

*NSAIDs*

- CNS: *Headache, dizziness, somnolence, insomnia,* fatigue, tiredness, dizziness, tinnitus, ophthalmologic effects
- GI: *Nausea, dyspepsia, GI pain,* diarrhea, vomiting, *constipation,* flatulence
- Respiratory: Dyspnea, hemoptysis, pharyngitis, bronchospasm, rhinitis
- Hematologic: Bleeding, platelet inhibition with higher doses, neutropenia, eosinophilia, leukopenia, pancytopenia, thrombocytopenia, agranulocytosis, granulocytopenia, aplastic anemia, decreased Hgb or Hct, bone marrow depression
- GU: Dysuria, renal impairment, menorrhagia
- Dermatologic: *Rash,* pruritus, sweating, dry mucous membranes, stomatitis
- Other: Peripheral edema, **anaphylactoid reactions to fatal anaphylactic shock**

### Clinically important drug-drug interactions

• Increased toxic effects of lithium with ibuprofen • Decreased diuretic effect with loop diuretics: bumetanide, furosemide, ethacrynic acid • Potential decrease in antihypertensive effect of beta-adrenergic blocking agents

## ■ Nursing Considerations

### Assessment

- *History:* Allergy to ibuprofen, salicylates or other NSAIDs; CV dysfunction, hypertension; peptic ulceration, GI bleeding; impaired hepatic or renal function; pregnancy; lactation
- *Physical:* Skin color, lesions; T; orientation, reflexes, ophthalmologic evaluation, audiometric evaluation, peripheral sensation; P, BP, edema; R, adventitious sounds; liver evaluation, bowel sounds; CBC, clotting times, urinalysis, renal and liver function tests, serum electrolytes, stool guaiac

### Implementation

- Administer drug with food or after meals if GI upset occurs.
- Arrange for periodic ophthalmologic examination during long-term therapy.
- Discontinue drug if eye changes, symptoms of liver dysfunction, renal impairment occur.
- Institute emergency procedures if overdose occurs: gastric lavage, induction of emesis, supportive therapy.

### Drug-specific teaching points

- Use drug only as suggested; avoid overdose. Take the drug with food or after meals if GI upset occurs. Do not exceed the prescribed dosage.
- The following side effects may occur: nausea, GI upset, dyspepsia (take drug with food); diarrhea or constipation; drowsiness, dizziness, vertigo, insomnia (use caution when driving or operating dangerous machinery).
- Avoid OTC drugs. Many of these drugs contain similar medications, and serious overdosage can occur.
- Report sore throat, fever, rash, itching, weight gain, swelling in ankles or fingers, changes in vision, black or tarry stools.

# ibutilide fumarate

*(eye **byu'** ti lyed)*

Corvert

**Pregnancy Category C**

### Drug classes

Antiarrhythmic

## Therapeutic actions

Prolongs cardiac action potential, increases atrial and ventricular refractoriness; produces mild slowing of sinus rate and AV conduction.

## Indications

- Rapid conversion of atrial fibrillation/flutter of recent onset to sinus rhythm; most effective in arrhythmias of <90 d duration

## Contraindications/cautions

- Contraindications: hypersensitivity to ibutilide; second- or third-degree AV heart block, prolonged QT intervals; pregnancy, lactation.
- Use cautiously with ventricular arrhythmias.

## Dosage

**Available Forms:** Solution—0.1 mg/ml

*ADULT:* ≤60 kg (132 lb): 1 vial (1 mg) infused over 10 min; may be repeated after 10 min if arrhythmia is not terminated. <60 kg: 0.1 ml/kg (0.01 mg/kg) infused over 10 min; may be repeated after 10 min if arrhythmia is not terminated.

*PEDIATRIC:* Not recommended.

## Pharmacokinetics

| Route | Onset | Peak |
|---|---|---|
| IV | Immediate | 10 min |

*Metabolism:* Hepatic; $T_{1/2}$: 6 h

*Distribution:* Crosses placenta, may be excreted in breast milk

*Excretion:* Urine and feces

### IV facts

**Preparation:** May be diluted in 50 ml of diluent, 0.9% Sodium Chloride or 5% Dextrose Injection; 1 10-ml vial added to 50 ml of diluent yields a concentration of 0.017 mg/ml; may also be infused undiluted; diluted solution is stable for 24 h at room temperature or for 48 h refrigerated.

**Infusion:** Infuse slowly over 10 min.

**Compatibilities:** Compatible with 5% Dextrose Injection, 0.9% Sodium Chloride Injection; do not mix in solution with other drugs.

## Adverse effects

- CNS: Headache, lightheadedness, dizziness, tingling in arms, numbness
- CV: **Ventricular arrhythmias,** hypotension, hypertension
- GI: *Nausea*

## Clinically important drug-drug interactions

• Increased risk of serious to life-threatening arrhythmias with disopyramide, quinidine, procainamide, amiodarone, sotalol; do not give together • Increased risk of proarrhythmias with phenothiazines, TCAs, antihistamines

## ■ Nursing Considerations

### Assessment

- *History:* Hypersensitivity to ibutilide; second- or third-degree AV heart block, time of onset of atrial arrhythmia; prolonged QT intervals; pregnancy, lactation; ventricular arrhythmias
- *Physical:* Orientation; BP, P, auscultation, ECG; R, adventitious sounds

### Implementation

- Determine time of onset of arrhythmia and potential benefit before beginning therapy. Conversion is more likely in patients with arrhythmias of short (<90 d) duration.
- Ensure that patient is adequately anticoagulated, generally for at least 2 wk, if atrial fibrillation is of >2–3 d duration.
- Monitor ECG continually during and for at least 4 h after administration. Be alert for possible arrhythmias, including PVCs, sinus tachycardia, sinus bradycardia, varying degrees of block at time of conversion.
- Maintain emergency equipment on standby during and for at least 4 h after administration.
- Provide appointments for continued follow-up, including ECG monitoring; tendency to revert to atrial arrhythmia after conversion increases with length of time patient was in abnormal rhythm.

### Drug-specific teaching points
- This drug can only be given by IV infusion. You will need ECG monitoring during and for 4 hours after administration.
- Arrange for follow-up medical evaluation, including ECG, which is important to monitor the effect of the drug on your heart.
- The following side effects may occur: rapid or irregular heartbeat (usually passes shortly), headache.
- Report chest pain, difficulty breathing, numbness or tingling.

## idarubicin hydrochloride

*(eye da **roo'** bi sin)*
Idamycin
**Pregnancy Category D**

### Drug classes
Antibiotic (anthracycline)
Antineoplastic

### Therapeutic actions
Cytotoxic: binds to DNA and inhibits DNA synthesis in susceptible cells.

### Indications
- In combination with other approved antileukemic drugs for the treatment of acute myeloid leukemia (AML) in adults
- Orphan drug uses: acute nonlymphocytic leukemia, acute lymphoblastic leukemia in pediatric patients

### Contraindications/cautions
- Contraindications: allergy to idarubicin, other anthracycline antibiotics; myelosuppression; cardiac disease; pregnancy; lactation.
- Use cautiously with impaired hepatic or renal function.

### Dosage
**Available Forms:** Powder for injection—5, 10 , 20 mg

ADULT
- ***Induction therapy in adults with AML:*** 12 mg/m$^2$ daily for 3 d by slow IV injections in combination with Ara-C; 100 mg/m$^2$ daily given by continuous infusion for 7 d or as a 25-mg/m$^2$ IV bolus followed by 200 mg/m$^2$ daily for 5 d by continuous infusion. A second course may be administered when toxicity has subsided, if needed.

PEDIATRIC: Safety and efficacy not established.

GERIATRIC, RENAL OR HEPATIC IMPAIRMENT: Reduce dosage by 25%. Do not administer if bilirubin level is > 5 mg/dl.

### Pharmacokinetics

| *Route* | *Onset* | *Peak* |
|---|---|---|
| IV | Rapid | Minutes |

*Metabolism:* Hepatic; $T_{1/2}$: 22 h
*Distribution:* Crosses placenta; enters breast milk
*Excretion:* Bile and urine

### IV facts
**Preparation:** Reconstitute the 5- and 10-mg vials with 5 and 10 ml, respectively of 0.9% Sodium Chloride Injection to give a final concentration of 1 mg/ml. Do not use bacteriostatic diluents. Use extreme caution when preparing drug. Use of goggles and gloves is recommended as drug can cause severe skin reactions. If skin is accidently exposed to idarubicin, wash with soap and water; use standard irrigation techniques if eyes are contaminated. Vials are under pressure; use care when inserting needle to minimize inhalation of any aerosol that is released. Reconstituted solution is stable for 7 d if refrigerated and 72 h at room temperature.
**Infusion:** Administer slowly (over 10–15 min) into tubing of a freely running IV infusion of Sodium Chloride Injection or 5% Dextrose Injection. Attach the tubing to a butterfly needle inserted into a large vein; avoid veins over joints or in extremities with poor perfusion.
**Incompatibilities:** Do not mix idarubicin with other drugs, especially heparin (a precipitate forms, and the IV solution must not be used) and any alkaline solution.

**Adverse effects**

- GI: *Nausea, vomiting, mucositis,* anorexia, diarrhea
- CV: **Cardiac toxicity,** CHF, phlebosclerosis
- Hematologic: **Myelosuppression,** hyperuricemia due to cell lysis
- Dermatologic: *Complete but reversible alopecia,* hyperpigmentation of nailbeds and dermal creases, facial flushing
- Hypersensitivity: Fever, chills, urticaria, anaphylaxis
- Local: Severe local cellulitis, vesication and tissue necrosis if extravasation occurs
- Other: Carcinogenesis, infertility

## ■ Nursing Considerations

### Assessment

- *History:* Allergy to idarubicin, other anthracycline antibiotics; myelosuppression; cardiac disease; impaired hepatic or renal function; pregnancy; lactation
- *Physical:* T; skin color, lesions; weight; hair; nailbeds; local injection site; cardiac auscultation, peripheral perfusion, pulses, ECG; R, adventitious sounds; liver evaluation, mucous membranes; CBC, liver and renal function tests, uric acid levels

### Implementation

- Do not give IM or SC because severe local reaction and tissue necrosis occur. Give IV only.
- Monitor injection site for extravasation: reports of burning or stinging. If extravasation occurs discontinue infusion immediately, and restart in another vein. For local SC extravasation, local infiltration with corticosteroid may be ordered; flood area with normal saline, and apply cold compress to area. If ulceration begins, arrange consultation with plastic surgeon.
- Monitor patient's response to therapy frequently at beginning of therapy: serum uric acid level, CBC, cardiac output (listen for $S_3$). CBC changes may require a decrease in the dose; consult with physician.
- Ensure adequate hydration to prevent hyperuricemia.

### Drug-specific teaching points

- Prepare a calendar for days to return for drug therapy. Drug can only be given IV.
- The following side effects may occur: rash, skin lesions, loss of hair, changes in nails (obtain a wig before hair loss occurs; skin care may help); loss of appetite, nausea, mouth sores (frequent mouth care, small frequent meals may help; maintain good nutrition; consult a dietician; an antiemetic may be ordered); red urine (transient).
- Have regular medical follow-up, including blood tests to monitor the drug's effects.
- Report difficulty breathing, sudden weight gain, swelling, burning or pain at injection site, unusual bleeding or bruising.

# ifosfamide

*(eye foss' fa mide)*

Ifex

**Pregnancy Category D**

**Drug classes**

Alkylating agent
Nitrogen mustard
Antineoplastic

**Therapeutic actions**

Cytotoxic: Exact mechanism of action is not known, though metabolite of ifosfamide alkylates DNA, interferes with the replication of susceptible cells; immunosuppressive: lymphocytes are especially sensitive to drug effects.

**Indications**

- In combination with other approved neoplastic agents for third-line chemotherapy of germ cell testicular cancer; should be used with an agent for hemorrhagic cystitis
- Unlabeled uses: possible effectiveness in the treatment of lung, breast, ovarian, pancreatic and gastric cancer, sarcomas, acute leukemias, malignant lymphomas

- Orphan drug uses: third-line chemotherapy in the treatment of germ cell testicular cancer, bone sarcomas, soft-tissue sarcomas

**Contraindications/cautions**

- Allergy to ifosfamide, hematopoietic depression, impaired hepatic or renal function, pregnancy, lactation.

## Dosage

**Available Forms:** Powder for injection—1, 3 g

*ADULT:* Administer IV at a dose of 1.2 mg/$m^2$ per day for 5 consecutive d. Treatment is repeated every 3 wk or after recovery from hematologic toxicity.

*PEDIATRIC:* Safety and efficacy not established.

*GERIATRIC OR RENAL OR HEPATIC IMPAIRED:* Data not available on appropriate dosage. Reduced dosage is advisable.

**Pharmacokinetics**

| Route | Onset |
|---|---|
| IV | Rapid |

*Metabolism:* Hepatic; $T_{1/2}$: 15 h

*Distribution:* Crosses placenta; enters breast milk

*Excretion:* Urine

### IV facts

**Preparation:** Add Sterile Water for Injection or Bacteriostatic Water for Injection to the vial, and shake gently. Use 20 ml diluent with 1-g vial, giving a final concentration of 50 mg/ml, or use 60-ml diluent with 3-g vial, giving a final concentration of 50 mg/ml. Solutions may be further diluted to achieve concentrations of 0.6–20 mg/ml in 5% Dextrose Injection, 0.9% Sodium Chloride Injection, Lactated Ringer's Injection, and Sterile Water for Injection. Solution is stable for at least 1 wk at room temperature or 6 wk if refrigerated. Dilutions not prepared with Bacteriostatic Water for Injection should be refrigerated and used within 6 h.

**Infusion:** Administer as a slow IV infusion lasting a minimum of 30 min.

**Adverse effects**

- CNS: *Somnolence, confusion, hallucinations,* coma, depressive psychosis, dizziness, seizures
- GI: *Anorexia, nausea, vomiting,* diarrhea, stomatitis
- **Hematologic**: *Leukopenia,* thrombocytopenia, anemia (rare), increased serum uric acid levels
- GU: *Hemorrhagic cystitis,* bladder fibrosis, *hematuria* to potentially fatal hemorrhagic cystitis, increased urine uric acid levels, gonadal suppression
- **Dermatologic**: *Alopecia,* darkening of skin and fingernails
- **Other**: Immunosuppression, secondary neoplasia

## ■ Nursing Considerations

### Assessment

- ***History:*** Allergy to ifosfamide, hematopoietic depression, impaired hepatic or renal function, pregnancy, lactation
- ***Physical:*** Reflexes, affect; skin lesions, hair; urinary output, renal function; renal and hepatic function tests, CBC, Hct

### Implementation

- Arrange for blood tests to evaluate hematopoietic function before beginning therapy and weekly during therapy.
- Arrange for extensive hydration consisting of at least 2 L of oral or IV fluid per day to prevent bladder toxicity.
- Arrange to administer a protector, such as mesna, to prevent hemorrhagic cystitis.
- Counsel male patients not to father a child during or immediately after therapy; infant cardiac and limb abnormalities have occurred. Counsel female patients not to become pregnant while on this drug; severe birth defects have occurred.

### Drug-specific teaching points

- This drug can only be given IV.
- Have frequent blood tests to monitor your response to this drug. All appointments for follow-up should be kept.
- The following side effects may occur: nausea, vomiting, loss of appetite (take



i

drug with food, have small frequent meals); maintain your fluid intake and nutrition (drink at least 10–12 glassses of fluid each day); darkening of the skin and fingernails, loss of hair (obtain a wig or arrange for some other head covering before hair loss occurs; keep head covered in extremes of temperature).

- Use birth control while on drug and for a time afterwards (male and female patients); this drug can cause severe birth defects.
- Report unusual bleeding or bruising, fever, chills, sore throat, cough, shortness of breath, blood in the urine, painful urination, unusual lumps or masses, flank, stomach or joint pain, sores in mouth or on lips, yellow discoloration of skin or eyes.

# Imipramine

## imipramine hydrochloride

*(im **ip'** ra meen)*

Apo-Imipramine (CAN), Impril (CAN), Novopramine (CAN), Tofranil

## imipramine pamoate

Tofranil-PM

**Pregnancy Category B**

### Drug classes

Tricyclic antidepressant (TCA) (tertiary amine)

### Therapeutic actions

Mechanism of action unknown; the TCAs are structurally related to the phenothiazine antipsychotic drugs (eg, chlorpromazine), but unlike the phenothiazines, TCAs inhibit the presynaptic reuptake of the neurotransmitters norepinephrine and serotonin; anticholinergic at CNS and peripheral receptors; sedative; the relation of these effects to clinical efficacy is unknown.

### Indications

- Relief of symptoms of depression (endogenous depression most responsive); sedative effects of tertiary amine TCAs may be helpful in patients whose depression is associated with anxiety and sleep disturbance
- Enuresis in children 6 y or older
- Unlabeled use: control of chronic pain (eg, intractable pain of cancer, peripheral neuropathies, postherpetic neuralgia, tic douloureux, central pain syndromes)

### Contraindications/cautions

- Contraindications: hypersensitivity to any tricyclic drug or to tartrazine (in preparations marketed as Tofranil, Tofranil PM; patients with aspirin allergy are often allergic to tartrazine); concomitant therapy with an MAO inhibitor; EST with coadministration of TCAs; recent MI; myelography within previous 24 h or scheduled within 48 h; pregnancy; lactation.
- Use cautiously with preexisting CV disorders; seizure disorders (TCAs lower the seizure threshold); hyperthyroidism; angle-closure glaucoma, increased intraocular pressure, urinary retention, ureteral or urethral spasm; impaired hepatic, renal function; psychiatric patients (schizophrenic or paranoid patients may exhibit a worsening of psychosis with TCA therapy; manic-depressive patients may shift to hypomanic or manic phase); elective surgery.

### Dosage

**Available Forms:** Capsules—75, 100, 125, 150 mg

**ADULT**

- ***Depression:*** Hospitalized patients: Initially, 100–150 mg/d PO in divided doses. Gradually increase to 200 mg/d as required. If no response after 2 wk, increase to 250–300 mg/d. Total daily dosage may be given hs. May be given IM initially only in patients unable or unwilling to take drug PO: up to 100 mg/d in divided doses. Replace with oral medication as soon as possible. Outpatients: Initially, 75 mg/d PO, increasing to 150 mg/d. Dosages > 200 mg/d not recommended. Total daily dosage may be given hs. Maintenance dose is 50–150 mg/d.
- ***Chronic pain:*** 50–200 mg/d PO.

***Pediatric Adolescent Patients:*** 30–40 mg/d PO; doses > 100mg/d generally are not needed.

- *Childhood enuresis (6 y or older):* Initially, 25 mg/d 1 h before bedtime. If response is not satisfactory after 1 wk, increase to 50 mg nightly in children <12 y, 75 mg nightly in children >12 y. Doses > 75 mg/d do not have greater efficacy but are more likely to increase side effects. Do not exceed 2.5 mg/kg per day. Early night bedwetters may be more effectively treated with earlier and divided dosage (25 mg midafternoon, repeated hs). Institute drug-free period after successful therapy, gradually tapering dosage.

***Geriatric:*** 30–40 mg/day PO; doses > 100 mg/d generally are not needed.

## Pharmacokinetics

| *Route* | *Onset* | *Peak* |
|---|---|---|
| Oral | Varies | 2–4 h |

*Metabolism:* Hepatic; $T_{1/2}$: 8–16 h
*Distribution:* Crosses placenta; enters breast milk
*Excretion:* Urine

## Adverse effects

### *Adult Use*

- CNS: *Sedation and anticholinergic effects*—dry mouth, blurred vision, disturbance of accommodation for near vision, mydriasis, increased intraocular pressure; *confusion, disturbed concentration,* hallucinations, disorientation, decreased memory, feelings of unreality, delusions, anxiety, nervousness, restlessness, agitation, panic, insomnia, nightmares, hypomania, mania, exacerbation of psychosis, drowsiness, weakness, fatigue, headache, numbness, tingling, paresthesias of extremities, incoordination, motor hyperactivity, akathisia, ataxia, tremors, peripheral neuropathy, extrapyramidal symptoms, *seizures,* speech blockage, dysarthria, tinnitus, altered EEG
- GI: *Dry mouth, constipation,* paralytic ileus, *nausea,* vomiting, anorexia, epigastric distress, diarrhea, flatulence, dysphagia, peculiar taste, increased salivation, stomatitis, glossitis, parotid swelling, abdominal cramps, black tongue, hepatitis
- CV: *Orthostatic hypotension,* hypertension, syncope, tachycardia, palpitations, MI, arrhythmias, heart block, precipitation of CHF, stroke
- **Hematologic**: Bone marrow depression, including agranulocytosis; eosinophila, purpura, thrombocytopenia, leukopenia
- GU: Urinary retention, delayed micturition, dilation of the urinary tract, gynecomastia, testicular swelling in men; breast enlargement, menstrual irregularity and galactorrhea in women; increased or decreased libido; impotence
- **Hypersensitivity**: Skin rash, pruritus, vasculitis, petechiae, photosensitization, edema (generalized, facial, tongue), drug fever
- **Endocrine**: Elevated or depressed blood sugar, elevated prolactin levels, inappropriate ADH secretion
- **Withdrawal**: Abrupt discontinuation of prolonged therapy: nausea, headache, vertigo, nightmares, malaise
- **Other**: Nasal congestion, excessive appetite, weight gain or loss; sweating (paradoxical effect in a drug with prominent anticholinergic effects), alopecia, lacrimation, hyperthermia, flushing, chills

### *Pediatric Use for Enuresis*

- CNS: *Nervousness, sleep disorders, tiredness,* convulsions, anxiety, emotional instability, syncope, collapse
- GI: Constipation, *mild GI disturbances*
- CV: ECG changes of unknown significance when given in doses of 5 mg/kg per day
- **Other**: Adverse reactions reported with adult use

## Clinically important drug-drug interactions

• Increased TCA levels and pharmacologic (especially anticholinergic) effects with cimetidine, fluoxetine, ranitidine • Increased serum levels and risk of bleeding with oral anticoagulants • Altered response, including dysrhythmias and hypertension with sympathomimetics • Risk of severe hypertension with clonidine • Hyperpyretic crises, severe convulsions, hypertensive episodes, and deaths when MAO inhibitors are given with TCAs • Decreased hypotensive activity of guanethidine with imipramine *Note:* MAOIs and TCAs have been used successfully in some patients resistant to therapy with single agents; however, the combination can cause serious and potentially fatal adverse effects.

## ■ Nursing Considerations

### Assessment

- ***History:*** Hypersensitivity to any tricyclic drug or to tartrazine; concomitant therapy with an MAO inhibitor; EST with coadministration of TCAs; recent MI; myelography within previous 24 h or scheduled within 48 h; preexisting CV disorders; seizure disorders; hyperthyroidism; angle-closure glaucoma, increased intraocular pressure, urinary retention, ureteral or urethral spasm; impaired hepatic, renal function; psychiatric patients; elective surgery; pregnancy; lactation
- ***Physical:*** Weight; T; skin color, lesions; orientation, affect, reflexes, vision and hearing; P, BP, auscultation, orthostatic BP, perfusion; bowel sounds, normal output, liver evaluation; urine flow, normal output; usual sexual function, frequency of menses, breast and scrotal examination; liver function tests, urinalysis, CBC, ECG

### Implementation

- Limit drug access for depressed and potentially suicidal patients.
- Give IM only when oral therapy is impossible. Do not give IV.
- Give major portion of dose hs if drowsiness, severe anticholinergic effects occur (note that elderly may not tolerate single daily dose therapy).
- Reduce dosage if minor side effects develop; discontinue if serious side effects occur.
- Arrange for CBC if patient develops fever, sore throat, or other sign of infection during therapy.

### Drug-specific teaching points

- Take drug exactly as prescribed. Do not stop taking drug abruptly or without consulting your health care provider.
- Avoid prolonged exposure to sunlight or sunlamps; use a sunscreen or protective garments.
- The following side effects may occur: headache, dizziness, drowsiness, weakness, blurred vision (reversible; safety measures may need to be taken if severe; avoid driving or performing tasks that require alertness); nausea, vomiting, loss of appetite (small frequent meals, frequent mouth care may help); dry mouth (sucking sugarless candies may help); disorientation, difficulty concentrating, emotional changes; changes in sexual function, impotence, changes in libido.
- Report dry mouth, difficulty in urination, excessive sedation, fever, chills, sore throat, palpitations.

# indapamide

*(in **dap'** a mide)*

Lozol

**Pregnancy Category B**

### Drug classes

Thiazide-like diuretic (actually an indoline)

### Therapeutic actions

Inhibits reabsorption of sodium and chloride in distal renal tubule, increasing excretion of sodium, chloride, and water by the kidney.

### Indications

- Edema associated with CHF
- Hypertension, as sole therapy or in combination with other antihypertensives
- Unlabeled use: diabetes insipidus, especially nephrogenic diabetes insipidus

### Contraindications/cautions

- Contraindications: allergy to thiazides, sulfonamides; fluid or electrolyte imbalance; renal disease (risk of azotemia); liver disease (may precipitate hepatic coma); gout (risk of precipitation of attack); SLE; glucose tolerance abnormalities, diabetes mellitus; hyperparathyroidism; manic-depressive disorder (aggravated by hypercalcemia); pregnancy; lactation.

### Dosage

**Available Forms:** Tablets—1.25, 2.5 mg

*ADULT*

- ***Edema:*** 2.5 mg/d PO as single dose in the morning. May be increased to 5 mg/d if response is not satisfactory after 1 wk.
- ***Hypertension:*** 2.5 mg/d PO. May be increased up to 5 mg/d if response is not satisfactory after 4 wk. If combination antihypertensive therapy is needed, reduce the dosage of other agents by 50%, then adjust according to patient's response.

### Pharmacokinetics

| *Route* | *Onset* | *Peak* | *Duration* |
|---|---|---|---|
| Oral | 1–2 h | 2 h | 36 h |

*Metabolism:* Hepatic; $T_{1/2}$: 14 h
*Distribution:* Crosses placenta; enters breast milk
*Excretion:* Urine

### Adverse effects

- CNS: *Dizziness, vertigo,* paresthesias, weakness, headache, drowsiness, fatigue, leukopenia, thrombocytopenia, agranulocytosis, aplastic anemia, neutropenia
- GI: *Nausea, anorexia, vomiting, dry mouth,* diarrhea, constipation, jaundice, hepatitis, pancreatitis
- CV: Orthostatic hypotension, venous thrombosis, volume depletion, cardiac arrhythmias, chest pain
- GU: *Polyuria, nocturia,* impotence, loss of libido
- Dermatologic: Photosensitivity, rash, purpura, exfoliative dermatitis, hives
- Other: Muscle cramps and muscle spasms, fever, gouty attacks, flushing, weight loss, rhinorrhea

### Clinically important drug-drug interactions

• Increased thiazide effects if taken with diazoxide • Decreased absorption with cholestyramine, colestipol • Increased risk of cardiac glycoside toxicity if hypokalemia occurs • Increased risk of lithium toxicity • Decreased effectiveness of antidiabetic agents

### Drug-lab test interferences

• Decreased PBI levels without clinical signs of thyroid disturbance

## ■ Nursing Considerations

### Assessment

- ***History:*** Allergy to thiazides, sulfonamides; fluid or electrolyte imbalance; renal or liver disease; gout; SLE; glucose tolerance abnormalities, diabetes mellitus; hyperparathyroidism; manic-depressive disorders; lactation
- ***Physical:*** Skin color, lesions, edema; orientation, reflexes, muscle strength; pulses, baseline ECG, BP, orthostatic BP, perfusion; R, pattern, adventitious sounds; liver evaluation, bowel sounds, urinary output patterns; CBC, serum electrolytes, blood glucose, liver and renal function tests, serum uric acid, urinalysis

### Implementation

- Give with food or milk if GI upset occurs.
- Mark calendars or provide other reminders for outpatients on alternate-day or 3–5 d/wk therapy.
- Give early in the day so increased urination will not disturb sleep.
- Measure and record regular weight to monitor fluid changes.

### Drug-specific teaching points

- Record intermittent therapy on a calendar, or use prepared, dated envelopes. Take the drug early so increased urination will not disturb sleep. The drug may be taken with food or meals if GI upset occurs.
- Weigh yourself on a regular basis, at the same time of the day and in the same clothing; record the weight on your calendar.
- The following side effects may occur: increased volume and frequency of urination; dizziness, feeling faint on arising,

drowsiness (avoid rapid position changes; hazardous activities, like driving a car, and alcohol, which can intensify these problems); sensitivity to sunlight (use sunglasses, wear protective clothing, or use a sunscreen); decrease in sexual function; increased thirst (sucking on sugarless lozenges, frequent mouth care may help).
- Report weight change of more than 3 lb in one day, swelling in ankles or fingers, unusual bleeding or bruising, dizziness, trembling, numbness, fatigue, muscle weakness or cramps.

## indinavir sulfate

*(in **din'** ah ver)*
Crixivan
**Pregnancy Category C**

### Drug classes
Antiviral

### Therapeutic actions
Antiviral activity; inhibits HIV protease activity, leading to production of immature, noninfective HIV particles

### Indications
- Treatment of HIV infection in adults when antiretroviral therapy is indicated

### Contraindications/cautions
- Contraindication: allergy to component of indinavir
- Use cautiously with pregnancy, hepatic or renal impairment, lactation

### Dosage
AVAILABLE FORMS: Capsules—200, 400 mg

ADULT: 800 mg PO q8h.

PEDIATRIC: Safety and efficacy not established in children <12 y.

HEPATIC IMPAIRMENT: 600 mg PO q8h with mild to moderate hepatic impairment.

### Pharmacokinetics

| Route | Onset | Peak |
|---|---|---|
| Oral | Rapid | 0.8 h |

*Metabolism:* Hepatic; $T_{1/2}$: 3–4 h
*Distribution:* Crosses placenta; passes into breast milk
*Excretion:* Feces and urine

### Adverse effects
- CNS: *Headache,* dizziness, insomnia, somnolence
- GI: *Nausea, vomiting, diarrhea,* anorexia, dry mouth, acid regurgitation, *hyperbilirubinemia*
- CV: Palpitations
- Respiratory: Cough, dyspnea, sinusitis
- GU: Dysuria, hematuria, nocturia, pyelonephritis, nephrolithiasis
- Dermatologic: Acne, dry skin, contact dermatitis, rash, body odor
- Other: Hypothermia, chills, back pain, flank pain, flulike illness

### Clinically important drug-drug interactions
• Potentially large increase in serum concentration of astemizole, cisapride, terfenadine, triazolam, midazolam with indinavir; potential for serious arrhythmias, seizure, and fatal reactions; do not administer indinavir with any of these drugs • Decreased effectiveness with didanosine; give these two drugs 1 h apart on empty stomach to decrease effects of interaction • Significant decrease in serum levels with nevirapine—avoid this combination; if combination is necessary, increase indinavir to 1000 mg q8h with nevirapine 200 mg bid; carefully monitor effectiveness of indinavir if starting or stopping nevirapine

### Clinically important drug-food interactions
• Absorption is decreased by presence of food and grapefruit juice; give on empty stomach with full glass of water

## ■ Nursing Considerations

### Assessment
- *History:* Allergy to indinavir, hepatic or renal dysfunction, pregnancy, lactation
- *Physical:* T; orientation, reflexes; BP, P, peripheral perfusion; R, adventitious

sounds; bowel sounds; urinary output; skin color, perfusion; liver and renal function tests

### Implementation

- Capsules should be protected from moisture; store in container provided and keep desiccant in bottle.
- Give on an empty stomach, 1 h before or 2 h after meal with a full glass of water. If GI upset is severe, give with a light meal; avoid grapefruit juice, foods high in calories, fat, or protein.
- Carefully screen drug history to avoid potentially dangerous drug–drug interactions.
- Monitor patient to maintain hydration; if nephrolithiasis occurs, therapy will need to be interrupted or stopped.

### Drug-specific teaching points

- Take this drug on an empty stomach, 1 h before or 2 h after a meal, with a full glass of water. If GI upset is severe, take with a light meal; avoid grapefruit juice, foods high in calories, fat, or protein.
- Store the capsules in the original container and leave the desiccant in the bottle. These capsules are very sensitive to moisture.
- Take the full course of therapy as prescribed; do not double up doses if one is missed; do not change dosage without consulting your physician.
- This drug does not cure HIV infection; long-term effects are not yet known; continue to take precautions as the risk of transmission is not reduced by this drug.
- Do not take any other drug, prescription or OTC, without consulting your health care provider; this drug interacts with many other drugs and serious problems can occur.
- The following side effects may occur: nausea, vomiting, loss of appetite, diarrhea, abdominal pain, headache, dizziness, insomnia.
- Report severe diarrhea, severe nausea, personality changes, changes in color of urine or stool, flank pain, fever or chills.

# Indomethacin

## indomethacin

*(in doe **meth'** a sin)*

Apo-Indomethacin (CAN), Indocin I.V., Novomethacin (CAN)

## indomethacin sodium trihydrate

Apo-Indomethacin (CAN), Indocin, Indocin-SR, Inocid (CAN), Novomethacin (CAN)

**Pregnancy Category B**

**Pregnancy Category D (third trimester)**

i

### Drug classes

Nonsteroidal anti-inflammatory drug (NSAID)

### Therapeutic actions

Anti-inflammatory, analgesic, and antipyretic activities largely related to inhibition of prostaglandin synthesis; exact mechanisms of action are not known.

### Indications

*Oral, Topical, Suppositories*

- Relief of signs and symptoms of moderate to severe rheumatoid arthritis and moderate to severe osteoarthritis, moderate to severe ankylosing spondylitis, acute painful shoulder (bursitis, tendinitis), acute gouty arthritis (*not* sustained-release form)
- Unlabeled uses for oral form: pharmacologic closure of persistent patent ductus arteriosus in premature infants; suppression of uterine activity to prevent premature labor; juvenile rheumatoid arthritis
- Unlabeled use of topical eye drops: cystoid macular edema

*IV Preparation*

- Closure of hemodynamically significant patent ductus arteriosus in premature infants weighing between 500–1,750 g, if 48 h of usual medical management is not effective

## Contraindications/cautions

- Oral and rectal preparations: allergy to indomethacin, salicylates or other NSAIDs; CV dysfunction, hypertension; peptic ulceration, GI bleeding; history of proctitis or rectal bleeding; impaired hepatic or renal function; pregnancy; labor and delivery; lactation. IV preparations: proven or suspected infection; bleeding, thrombocytopenia, coagulation defects; necrotizing enterocolitis; renal impairment; local irritation if extravasation occurs.

## Dosage

**Available Forms:** Capsules—25, 50 mg; SR capsules—75 mg; oral suspension—25 mg/5 ml; suppositories—50 mg; powder for injection—1 mg

ADULT

- ***Osteoarthritis/rheumatoid arthritis, ankylosing spondylitis:*** 25 mg PO bid or tid. If tolerated, increase dose by 25- or 50-mg increments if needed up to total daily dose of 150–200 mg/d PO.
- ***Acute painful shoulder:*** 75–150 mg/d PO, in 3–4 divided doses. Discontinue drug after inflammation is controlled, usually 7–14 d.
- ***Acute gouty arthritis:*** 50 mg PO, tid until pain is tolerable, then rapidly decrease dose until no longer needed, usually within 3–5 d.

PEDIATRIC: Safety and efficacy have not been established. When special circumstances warrant use in children older than 2 y, initial dose is 2 mg/kg per day in divided doses PO. Do not exceed 4 mg/kg per day or 150–200 mg/d, whichever is less.

- ***IV:*** Three IV doses given at 12- to 24-h intervals.

| *Age* | *1st Dose* | *2nd Dose* | *3rd Dose* |
|---|---|---|---|
| <48 h | 0.2 mg/kg | 0.1 mg/kg | 0.1 mg/kg |
| 2–7 d | 0.2 mg/kg | 0.2 mg/kg | 0.2 mg/kg |
| >7 d | 0.2 mg/kg | 0.25 mg/kg | 0.25 mg/kg |

If marked anuria or oliguria occurs, do not give additional doses. If ductus reopens, course of therapy may be repeated at 12- to 24-h intervals.

## Pharmacokinetics

| *Route* | *Onset* | *Peak* | *Duration* |
|---|---|---|---|
| Oral | 30 min | 1–2 h | 4–6 h |
| IV | Immediate | | 15–30 min |

*Metabolism:* Hepatic; $T_{1/2}$: 4 1/2–6 h
*Distribution:* Crosses placenta; enters breast milk
*Excretion:* Urine

### IV facts

**Preparation:** Reconstitute solution with 1–2 ml of 0.9% Sodium Chloride Injection or Water for Injection; diluents should be preservative free. If 1 ml of diluent is used, concentration is 0.1 mg/0.1 ml. If 2 ml of diluent is used, concentration is 0.05 mg/0.1 ml. Discard any unused portion of the solution; prepare fresh solution before each dose.

**Infusion:** Inject reconstituted solution IV over 5–10 sec; further dilution is not recommended.

## Adverse effects

NSAIDs: *Oral, Suppositories*

- CNS: *Headache, dizziness, somnolence, insomnia,* fatigue, tiredness, dizziness, tinnitus, ophthalmologic effects
- GI: *Nausea, dyspepsia, GI pain,* diarrhea, vomiting, *constipation*, flatulence
- Respiratory: Dyspnea, hemoptysis, pharyngitis, bronchospasm, rhinitis
- Hematologic: Bleeding, platelet inhibition with higher doses, neutropenia, eosinophilia, leukopenia, pancytopenia, thrombocytopenia, agranulocytosis, granulocytopenia, aplastic anemia, decreased Hgb or Hct, bone marrow depression, mennorhagia
- GU: Dysuria, renal impairment
- Dermatologic: *Rash*, pruritus, sweating, dry mucous membranes, stomatitis
- Other: Peripheral edema, **anaphylactoid reactions to fatal anaphylactic shock**

*Intravenous Preparation*

- GI: *GI bleeding, vomiting*, abdominal distention, transient ileus

- **Respiratory**: *Apnea, exacerbation of pulmonary infection,* pulmonary hemorrhage
- **Hematologic**: *Increased bleeding problems,* including intracranial bleed, disseminated intravascular coagulopathy, hyponatremia, hyperkalemia, hypoglycemia, fluid retention
- **GU**: Renal dysfunction
- **Other**: Retrolental fibroplasia

## Clinically important drug-drug interactions

• Increased toxic effects of lithium • Decreased diuretic effect with loop diuretics: bumetanide, furosemide, ethacrynic acid • Potential decrease in antihypertensive effect of beta-adrenergic blocking agents, captopril, lisinopril, enalapril

## ■ Nursing Considerations

### Assessment

- *History:* Oral and rectal preparations: allergy to indomethacin, salicylates or other NSAIDs; CV dysfunction, hypertension; peptic ulceration, GI bleeding; history of proctitis or rectal bleeding; impaired hepatic or renal function; pregnancy; labor and delivery. IV preparations: proven or suspected infection; bleeding, thrombocytopenia, coagulation defects; necrotizing enterocolitis; renal impairment; local irritation if extravasation occurs
- *Physical:* Skin color, lesions; T; orientation, reflexes, ophthalmological evaluation, audiometric evaluation, peripheral sensation; P, BP, edema; R, adventitious sounds; liver evaluation, bowel sounds; CBC, clotting times, urinalysis, renal and liver function tests, serum electrolytes, stool guaiac

### Implementation

*Oral and Rectal Preparations*

- Give drug with food or after meals if GI upset occurs.
- Do not give sustained-release tablets for gouty arthritis.
- Arrange for periodic ophthalmologic examination during long-term therapy.
- Discontinue drug if eye changes, symptoms of liver or renal dysfunction occur.
- Institute emergency procedures if overdose occurs: gastric lavage, induction of emesis, support.
- Test renal function between doses. If severe renal impairment is noted, do not give the next dose.

### Drug-specific teaching points

- Use the drug only as suggested; avoid overdose. Take the drug with food or after meals if GI upset occurs. Do not exceed the prescribed dosage
- The following side effects may occur: nausea, GI upset, dyspepsia (take drug with food); diarrhea or constipation; drowsiness, dizziness, vertigo, insomnia (use caution if driving or operating dangerous machinery).
- Report sore throat, fever, rash, itching, weight gain, swelling in ankles or fingers, changes in vision, black, tarry stools.
- Parents of infants receiving IV therapy for PDA will need support and encouragement and an explanation of the drug's action; this is best incorporated into the teaching about the disease.

# insulin

***(in' su lin)***

*Insulin injection:* Humulin R, Novolin R, Regular Iletin I, Regular Iletin II, Regular Purified Pork Insulin, Velosulin Human BR

*Insulin lispro:* Humalog

*Insulin zinc suspension, prompt (Semilente):*

*Isophane insulin suspension (NPH):* Humulin N, Novolin N, NPH Ilentin I, NPH Ilentin II, NPH-N

*Insulin zinc suspension (Lente):* Lente Humulin-L, Lente Ilentin I, Lente Ilentin II, Novolin L

*(continues)*

*Protamine zinc suspension (PZI):* Iletin PZI (CAN)

*Insulin zinc suspension, extended (Ultralente):* Humulin U (CAN), Humulin U Ultralente

*Insulin injection concentrated:* Regular (concentrated) Iletin II

**Pregnancy Category B**

## Drug classes

Antidiabetic agent
Hormone

## Therapeutic actions

Insulin is a hormone that, by receptor-mediated effects, promotes the storage of the body's fuels, facilitating the transport of metabolites and ions (potassium) through cell membranes and stimulating the synthesis of glycogen from glucose, of fats from lipids, and proteins from amino acids.

## Indications

- Treatment of diabetes mellitus type I
- Treatment of diabetes mellitus type II that cannot be controlled by diet
- Treatment of severe ketoacidosis or diabetic coma (regular insulin injection)
- Treatment of hyperkalemia with infusion of glucose to produce a shift of potassium into the cells
- Highly purified and human insulins promoted for short courses of therapy (surgery, intercurrent disease), newly diagnosed patients, patients with poor metabolic control, and patients with gestational diabetes
- Insulin injection concentrated indicated for treatment of diabetic patients with marked insulin resistance (requirements of >200 U/d)

## Contraindications/cautions

- Allergy to beef, pork products (varies with preparations; use of human insulin removes this caution); pregnancy (keep patients under close supervision; rigid control is desired; following delivery, requirements may drop for 24–72 h, rising to normal levels during next 6 wk); lactation (monitor mother carefully; insulin requirements may decrease during lactation).

## Dosage

**Available Forms:** Injection—100 units/ml

*ADULT AND PEDIATRIC:* The number and size of daily doses, times of administration, and type of insulin preparation are determined after close medical scrutiny of the patient's blood and urine glucose, diet, exercise, and intercurrent infections and other stresses. Usually given SC. Regular insulin may be given IV or IM in diabetic coma or ketoacidosis. Insulin injection concentrated may be given SC or IM, but do not administer IV.

## Pharmacokinetics

| *Type* | *Onset* | *Peak* | *Duration* |
|---|---|---|---|
| Regular | 30–60 min | 2–3 h | 6–8 h |
| Semilente | 1–1.5 h | 5–10 h | 12–16 h |
| NPH | 1–1.5 h | 4–12 h | 24 h |
| Lente | 1–2.5 h | 7–15 h | 24 h |
| PZI | 4–8 h | 14–24 h | 36 h |
| Ultralente | 4–8 h | 10–30 h | >36 h |
| Lispro | 15 min | 1 h | 3.5–4.5 h |

*Metabolism:* Cellular; $T_{1/2}$: varies with preparation

*Distribution:* Crosses placenta; does not enter breast milk

## IV facts

**Preparation:** May be mixed with standard IV solutions; use of plastic tubing or bag will change the amount of insulin delivered.

**Infusion:** Use of a monitored delivery system is suggested. Rate should be determined by patient response and glucose levels.

## Adverse effects

- Hypersensitivity: Rash, **anaphylaxis or angioedema, may be life threatening**
- Metabolic: Hypoglycemia; ketoacidosis
- Local: Allergy—local reactions at injection site—redness, swelling, itching; usually resolves in a few days to a few weeks; a change in type or species source of insulin may be tried

**Clinically important drug-drug interactions**

• Increased hypoglycemic effects of insulin with monoamine oxidase inhibitors, beta blockers, salicylates, alcohol • Altered insulin requirements in diabetics secondary to use of fenfluramine, requiring cautious administration of insulin and regular monitoring of glucose levels • Delayed recovery from hypoglycemic episodes and masked signs and symptoms of hypoglycemia if taken with beta-adrenergic blocking agents

## ■ Nursing Considerations

### Assessment

- *History:* Allergy to beef, pork products; pregnancy; lactation
- *Physical:* Skin color, lesions; eyeball turgor; orientation, reflexes, peripheral sensation; P, BP, adventitious sounds; R, adventitious sounds; urinalysis, blood glucose

### Implementation

- Ensure uniform dispersion of insulin suspensions by rolling the vial gently between hands; avoid vigorous shaking.
- Give maintenance doses SC, rotating injection sites regularly to decrease incidence of lipodystrophy; give regular insulin IV or IM in severe ketoacidosis or diabetic coma.
- Monitor patients receiving insulin IV carefully; plastic IV infusion sets have been reported to remove 20%–80% of the insulin; dosage delivered to the patient will vary.
- Do not give insulin injection concentrated IV; severe anaphylactic reactions can occur.
- Use caution when mixing two types of insulin; always draw the regular insulin into the syringe first; if mixing with insulin lispro, draw the lispro first; use mixtures of regular and NPH or regular and lente insulins within 5–15 min of combining them.
- Double-check, or have a colleague check, the dosage drawn up for pediatric patients, for patients receiving concentrated insulin injection, or patients receiving very small doses; even small errors in dosage can cause serious problems.
- Monitor patients being switched from one type of insulin to another carefully; dosage adjustments are often needed. Human insulins often require smaller doses than beef or pork insulin; monitor cautiously if patients are switched; lispro insulin is given 15 min before a meal.
- Store insulin in a cool place away from direct sunlight. Refrigeration is preferred. Do not freeze insulin. Insulin prefilled in glass or plastic syringes is stable for 1 wk refrigerated; this is a safe way of ensuring proper dosage for patients with limited vision or who have problems with drawing up insulin.
- Monitor urine and serum glucose levels frequently to determine effectiveness of drug and dosage. Patients can learn to adjust insulin dosage on a "sliding scale" based on test results.
- Monitor insulin needs during times of trauma or severe stress; dosage adjustments may be needed.
- Maintain life support equipment, glucose on standby to deal with ketoacidosis or hypoglycemic reactions.

### Drug-specific teaching points

- Use the same type and brand of syringe; use the same type and brand of insulin to avoid dosage errors.
- Do not change the order of mixing insulins. Rotate injection sites regularly (keep a chart) to prevent breakdown at injection sites.
- Dosage may vary with activities, stress, diet. Monitor blood or urine glucose levels, and consult physician if problems arise.
- Store drug in the refrigerator or in a cool place out of direct sunlight; do not freeze insulin.
- Monitor your urine or blood for glucose and ketones as prescribed.
- Wear a medical alert tag stating that you are a diabetic taking insulin so that emergency medical personnel will take proper care of you.
- Avoid alcohol; serious reactions can occur.

- Report fever, sore throat, vomiting, hypoglycemic or hyperglycemic reactions, skin rash.

## interferon alfa-2a

*(in ter feer' on)*
IFLrA, rIFN-A
Roferon-A
**Pregnancy Category C**

### Drug classes

Antineoplastic
Interferon

### Therapeutic actions

Inhibits growth of tumor cells: mechanism of action is not clearly understood; prevents tumor cells from multiplying and modulates host immune response. Interferons are produced by human leukocytes in response to viral infections and other stimuli. Interferon alfa-2a is produced by recombinant DNA technology using *Escherichia coli.*

### Indications

- Hairy cell leukemia in selected patients 18 y and older
- AIDS-related Kaposi's sarcoma in selected patients 18 y and older
- Treatment of chronic myelogenous leukemia in chronic phrase in Philadelphia chromosome–positive patient
- Unlabeled uses: treatment of several malignant and viral conditions, phase I AIDS, ARC
- Orphan drug uses: treatment of advanced colorectal cancer, esophageal carcinoma, metastatic malignant melanoma, renal cell carcinoma

### Contraindications/cautions

- Contraindications: allergy to interferon-$\alpha$ or any components of the product, pregnancy, lactation.
- Use cautiously with pancreatitis, hepatic or renal disease, seizure disorders, compromised CNS function, cardiac disease or history of cardiac disease, bone marrow depression.

### Dosage

**Available Forms:** Injection solution—3 million IU/ml, 6 million IU/ml$^2$, 9 million IU/0.9 ml, 36 million IU/ml$^2$; powder for injection—6 million IU/ml

ADULT

- ***Hairy cell leukemia:*** Induction dose: 3 million IU/d SC or IM for 16–24 wk. Maintenance dose: 3 million IU/d 3×/wk. Treat patient for approximately 6 mo, then evaluate response before continuing therapy. Treatment for up to 20 mo has been reported. Dosage may need to be adjusted downward based on adverse reactions.
- ***AIDS-related Kaposi's sarcoma:*** 36 million IU daily for 10–12 wk IM or SC. Maintenance: 36 million IU 3×/wk. Reduce dose by one-half or withhold individual doses when severe adverse reactions occur. Continue treatment until tumor disappears or until discontinuation is required.

*CML:* Induction dose: 9 million IU daily IM or SC. Continue therapy until disease progresses or adverse effects are severe.

*PEDIATRIC (< 18 Y):* Safety and efficacy not established.

### Pharmacokinetics

| *Route* | *Onset* | *Peak* |
|---|---|---|
| IM | Rapid | 3.8 h |
| SC | Slow | 7.3 h |

*Metabolism:* Hepatic and renal; $T_{1/2}$: 3.7–8.5 h
*Distribution:* Crosses placenta; may enter breast milk
*Excretion:* Urine

### Adverse effects

- CNS: *Dizziness, confusion,* paresthesias, numbness, lethargy, decreased mental status, depression, visual disturbances, sleep disturbances, nervousness
- CV: Hypotension, edema, hypertension, chest pain, arrhythmias, palpitations
- GI: *Anorexia, nausea*, diarrhea, vomiting, change in taste
- **Hematologic**: Leukopenia, neutropenia, thrombocytopenia, anemia, decreased

Hgb; increased levels of SGOT, LDH, alkaline phosphatase, bilirubin, uric acid, serum creatinine, BUN, blood sugar, serum phosphorus, neutralizing antibodies; hypocalcemia

- GU: Impairment of fertility in women, transient impotence in men
- **Dermatologic**: Rash, dryness or inflammation of the oropharnyx, dry skin, pruritus, partial alopecia
- **General**: *Flulike syndrome,* weight loss, diaphoresis, arthralgia

## ■ Nursing Considerations

### Assessment

- ***History:*** Allergy to interferon-$\alpha$ or any product components, pancreatitis, hepatic or renal disease, seizure disorders, compromised CNS function, cardiac disease or history of cardiac disease, bone marrow depression, pregnancy, lactation
- ***Physical:*** Weight; T; skin color, lesions; orientation, reflexes; P, BP, edema, ECG; liver evaluation; CBC, blood glucose, liver and renal function tests, urinalysis

### Implementation

- Obtain laboratory tests (CBC, differential, granulocytes and hairy cells, bone marrow hairy cells, and liver function tests) before therapy and monthly during therapy.
- Monitor for severe reactions; notify physician immediately; dosage reduction or discontinuation may be necessary.
- Refrigerate solution; do not shake. Use reconstituted powder within 30 d.
- Ensure that patient is well hydrated, especially during initiation of treatment.
- Provide small, frequent meals if GI problems occur.
- Counsel female patients to use some form of birth control. Drug is contraindicated in pregnancy.
- Assure patient that all steps possible are taken to ensure that there is little risk of hepatitis and AIDS from use of human blood products.

### Drug-specific teaching points

- Prepare a calendar to check off as drug is given. You and a significant other should learn the proper technique for SC or IM injection for outpatient use. Do not change brands of interferon without consulting with physician.
- Refrigerate solution; do not shake. Use reconstituted powder within 30 d.
- The following side effects may occur: loss of appetite, nausea, vomiting (frequent mouth care, small frequent meals may help; maintain good nutrition; a dietician may be able to help; an antiemetic also may be ordered); fatigue, confusion, dizziness, numbness, visual disturbances, depression (transient; avoid injury; avoid driving or using dangerous machinery); impotence (transient); fetal deformities or death (use birth control).
- Arrange for regular blood tests to monitor the drug's effects.
- Report fever, chills, sore throat, unusual bleeding or bruising, chest pain, palpitations, dizziness, changes in mental status.

## interferon alfa-2b

*(in ter **feer'** on)*

IFN-alpha 2, rIFN-a2, a-2-interferon

Intron-A

**Pregnancy Category C**

### Drug classes

Antineoplastic
Interferon

### Therapeutic actions

Inhibits growth of tumor cells; mechanism of action is not clearly understood; prevents the replication of tumor cells and enhances host immune response. Interferons are produced by human leukocytes in response to viral infections and other stimuli. Interferon alfa-2b is produced by recombinant DNA technology using *E. coli.*

### Indications

- Hairy cell leukemia
- Intralesional treatment of condylomata acuminata

- AIDS-related Kaposi's sarcoma
- Treatment of malignant melanoma in patients >18 y
- Treatment of chronic hepatitis, non-A, non B/C
- Treatment of chronic hepatitis B
- Unlabeled uses: treatment of several malignant and viral conditions
- Orphan drug uses: chronic myelogenous leukemia, metastatic renal cell carcinoma, ovarian carcinoma, invasive carcinoma of cervix, primary malignant brain tumors, laryngeal papillomatosis, carcinoma in situ of urinary bladder, chronic delta hepatitis, acute hepatitis B

## Contraindications/cautions

- Contraindications: allergy to interferon-$\alpha$ or any components of the product, lactation.
- Use cautiously with cardiac disease, pulmonary disease, diabetes mellitus prone to ketoacidosis, coagulation disorders, bone marrow depression, pregnancy.

## Dosage

**Available Forms:** Injection solution—3, 6, 9, 36 million IU/ml; powder for injection—6 million IU/ml

ADULT

- ***Hairy cell leukemia:*** 2 million IU/m$^2$ SC or IM 3×/wk. Continue for several months, depending on clinical and hematologic response.
- ***Condylomata acuminata:*** 1 million IU/lesion 3×/wk for 3 wk intralesionally. Maximum response occurs 4–8 wk after initiation of therapy.
- ***Chronic hepatitis, non-A, non B/C:*** 3 million IU SC or IM, 3×/wk.
- ***AIDS-related Kaposi's sarcoma:*** 30 million IU/m$^2$ 3×/wk SC or IM. Maintain dosage until disease progresses rapidly or severe intolerance occurs.
- ***Chronic hepatitis B:*** 30–35 million IU/wk SC or IM either as 5 million IU daily or 10 million IU 3×/wk for 16 wk.
- ***Malignant melanoma:*** 20 million IU/m$^2$ IV on 5 consecutive d/wk for 4 wk; maintenance: 10 million IU/m$^2$ IV 3×/wk for 48 wk.

PEDIATRIC: Safety and efficacy not established in children younger than 18 y.

## Pharmacokinetics

| Route | Onset | Peak |
|---|---|---|
| IM/SC | Rapid | 3–12 h |
| IV | Rapid | End of infusion |

*Metabolism:* Renal; $T_{1/2}$: 2–3 h
*Distribution:* Crosses placenta; may enter breast milk
*Excretion:* Unknown

## IV facts

**Preparation:** Inject diluent (Bacteriostatic Water for Injection) into vial using chart provided by manufacturer; agitate gently, withdraw with sterile syringe, inject into 100 ml of Normal Saline.
**Infusion:** Administer each dose slowly over 20 min.

## Adverse effects

- CNS: *Dizziness, confusion,* paresthesias, numbness, lethargy, decreased mental status, depression, visual disturbances, sleep disturbances, nervousness
- GI: *Anorexia, nausea*, diarrhea, vomiting, change in taste
- CV: Hypotension, edema, hypertension, chest pain, arrhythmias, palpitations
- **Hematologic**: Leukopenia, neutropenia, thrombocytopenia, anemia, decreased Hgb; increased levels of SGOT, LDH, alkaline phosphatase, bilirubin, uric acid, serum creatinine, BUN, blood sugar, serum phosphorus, neutralizing antibodies; hypocalcemia
- GU: Impaired fertility in women, transient impotence
- **Dermatologic**: *Rash*, dryness or inflammation of the oropharnyx, *dry skin, pruritus,* partial alopecia
- **General**: *Flulike syndrome,* weight loss, diaphoresis, arthralgia

## ■ Nursing Considerations

### Assessment

- ***History:*** Allergy to interferon-$\alpha$ or product components, cardiac or pulmonary disease, diabetes mellitus prone to ketoacidosis, coagulation disorders, bone marrow depression, pregnancy, lactation

- *Physical:* Weight; T; skin color, lesions; orientation, reflexes; P, BP, edema, ECG; liver evaluation; CBC, blood glucose, liver and renal function tests, urinalysis

### Implementation

- Obtain laboratory tests (CBC, differential, granulocytes and hairy cells, bone marrow and hairy cells) before therapy and monthly during therapy.
- Prepare solution as follows:

| *Vial Strength in Million IU* | *Amount of diluent in ml* | *Final Conc. in Million IU/ml* |
|---|---|---|
| 3 | 1 | 3 |
| 5 | 1 | 5 |
| 10 | 2 | 5 |
| 25 | 5 | 5 |
| 10 | 1 | 10 |
| 50 | 1 | 50 |

- Use Bacteriostatic Water for Injection as diluent. Agitate gently. After reconstitution, stable for 1 mo if refrigerated.
- Administer IM or SC.
- Monitor for severe reactions, including hypersensitivity reactions; notify physician immediately; dosage reduction or discontinuation may be necessary.
- Ensure that patient is well hydrated, especially during initiation of treatment.

### Drug-specific teaching points

- Prepare a calendar to check off as drug is given. You and a significant other should learn the proper technique for SC or IM injection for outpatient use. Do not change brands of interferon without consulting with physician.
- The following side effects may occur: loss of appetite, nausea, vomiting (frequent mouth care, small frequent meals may help; maintain good nutrition; a dietician may be able to help; an antiemetic also may be ordered); fatigue, confusion, dizziness, numbness, visual disturbances, depression (use special precautions to avoid injury; avoid driving or using dangerous machinery); flulike syndrome (take drug at bedtime; ensure rest periods for yourself; a medication may be ordered for fever).
- Arrange for regular blood tests to monitor the drug's effects.
- Report fever, chills, sore throat, unusual bleeding or bruising, chest pain, palpitations, dizziness, changes in mental status.

## interferon alfa-n3

*(in ter feer' on)*

Alferon N

**Pregnancy Category C**

### Drug classes

Antineoplastic
Interferon

### Therapeutic actions

Inhibits viral replication and suppresses cell proliferation; mechanism of action not completely understood. Interferons are produced by human leukocytes in response to viral infections and other stimuli. Interferon alfa-n3 is produced by harvesting human leukocytes.

### Indications

- Intralesional treatment of refractory and recurring condylomata acuminata
- Unlabeled uses: treatment of a variety of cancers and viral infections, including AIDS-related diseases

### Contraindications/cautions

- Contraindications: allergy to interferon-α or product components, egg protein or neomycin, pregnancy, lactation.
- Use cautiously with debilitating medical conditions.

### Dosage

**Available Forms:** Injection—5 mIU/vial

**ADULT**

- *Condylomata acuminata:* 0.05 ml (250,000 U) per wart. Give twice weekly for up to 8 wk. Maximum recommended dose per treatment is 0.5 ml (2.5 million U). Inject into the base of each wart, using a 30-gauge needle. Large warts may be injected at several points around their periphery, using a total dose of 0.05 ml per wart.

*PEDIATRIC (< 18 Y):* Safety and efficacy not established.

### Pharmacokinetics

Not generally absorbed systemically.

### Adverse effects

- CNS: *Dizziness, confusion,* paresthesias, numbness, lethargy, decreased mental status, depression, visual disturbances, sleep disturbances, nervousness
- GI: *Anorexia, nausea*, diarrhea, vomiting, change in taste
- CV: Hypotension, edema, hypertension, chest pain, arrhythmias, palpitations
- **Hematologic**: Leukopenia, neutropenia, thrombocytopenia, anemia, decreased Hgb; increased levels of SGOT, LDH, alkaline phosphatase
- GU: Impaired fertility in women, transient impotence
- **Dermatologic**: Rash, dryness or inflammation of the oropharnyx, dry skin, pruritus
- **General**: *Flulike syndrome*, weight loss, diaphoresis, arthralgia

## ■ Nursing Considerations

### Assessment

- *History:* Allergy to interferon-α or product components, egg protein or neomycin, debilitating medical conditions, pregnancy, lactation
- *Physical:* Weight; T; skin color, lesions; orientation, reflexes; P, BP, edema; liver evaluation; CBC, blood glucose, liver and renal function tests, urinalysis

### Implementation

- Obtain laboratory tests (CBC, differential) before therapy and monthly during therapy.
- Monitor for severe reactions; notify physician immediately; dosage reduction or discontinuation may be necessary.
- Finish the full 8-wk course of therapy; most warts will resolve by this time. If a second course of therapy is needed, wait 3 mo before beginning.
- Assure patient that all steps possible are taken to ensure that there is little risk of hepatitis or AIDS from use of human blood products.

### Drug-specific teaching points

- Prepare a calendar to check off as drug is given. You and a significant other should learn the proper technique for injection for outpatient use. Do not change brands of interferon without consulting with physician.
- The following side effects may occur: loss of appetite, nausea, vomiting (frequent mouth care, small frequent meals may help; maintain good nutrition; a dietician may be able to help; an antiemetic also may be ordered); fatigue, confusion, dizziness, numbness, visual disturbances, depression (use special precautions to avoid injury; avoid driving or using dangerous machinery); impotence (transient).
- Report hives, generalized urticaria, tightness of the chest, wheezing, fainting, dizziness, failure of warts to respond to treatment.

## interferon alfacon-1

***(in ter feer' on)***

Infergen

**Pregnancy Category C**

### Drug classes

Interferon

### Therapeutic actions

Interferons are produced by human leukocytes in response to viral infections and other stimuli; interferon alfacon-1 blocks replication of viruses and stimulates the host immunoregulatory activities; type 1 interferons exhibit antiviral, natural killer cell activation, cytokine induction activity; produced by recombinant DNA technology with *E. coli* bacteria.

### Indications

- Treatment of chronic hepatitis C infection in patients > 18 y of age with compen-

sated liver disease who have HCV antibodies
- Unlabeled uses: treatment of hairy cell leukemia in combination with G-CSF therapy

**Contraindications/cautions**
- Contraindications: allergy to alfa interferons or product dervied from *E. coli,* pregnancy, lactation.
- Use cautiously with a history of psychotic events, cardiac disease, hepatic dysfunction.

**Dosage**

**Available Forms:** Injection—9, 15 μg

*ADULT:* 9 μg SC as a single injection, 3 X/wk for 24 wk; at least 48 h must elapse between doses.

*PEDIATRIC (<18 Y):* Safety and efficacy not established.

**Pharmacokinetics**

| *Route* | *Onset* | *Peak* |
|---|---|---|
| SC | Slow | 24–36 h |

*Metabolism:* Hepatic and renal; $T_{1/2}$: unknown

*Distribution:* Crosses placenta; may pass into breast milk

*Excretion:* Urine

**Adverse effects**
- CNS: *Dizziness, insomnia,* paresthesias, anmesia, hypoesthesia, **psychotic episodes,** depression, anxiety, *nervousness*
- GI: *Anorexia, nausea, diarrhea,* vomiting, change in taste, *abdominal pain*
- CV: Hypertension, chest pain, palpitations
- GU: Impairment of fertility in women, transient impotence
- Respiratory: *Pharyngitis, upper respiratory infection, cough, sinusitis,* rhinitis, congestion, dyspnea
- Hematologic: *Granulocytosis, thrombocytopenia,* leukopenia
- Dermatologic: *Alopecia, pruritus,* rash, erythema, dry skin
- General: *Flulike syndrome,* weight loss, diaphoresis, arthralgia, *injection site reaction*

## ■ Nursing Considerations

**Assessment**
- ***History:*** Allergy to alfa interferon or *E. coli*–produced products, mental disorders, cardiac or hepatic disease, pregnancy, lactation.
- ***Physical:*** Weight; T; skin color, lesions; orientation, reflexes; P, BP edema; R, adventitious sounds; liver evaluation; CBC

**Implementation**
- Arrange for laboratory tests (CBC, differential, HCV antibodies) before beginning therapy.
- Monitor for severe reactions of any kind; notify prescriber immediately. Dosage reduction or discontinuation of drug may be necessary.
- Refrigerate vials; avoid vigorous shaking; discard any unused portions.
- Ensure that patient is well hydrated, especially during initiation of treatment.
- Arrange for supportive treatment if flulike syndrome occurs: rest, acetaminophen for fever and headache, environmental control.
- Monitor patients with any history of mental disorders or suicidal tendencies carefully for any evidence of psychotic reaction, which can be severe.
- Consult with physician for antiemetic for severe nausea and vomiting.
- Counsel female patients to use some form of birth control while on this drug. Drug is contraindicated in pregnancy.

**Drug-specific teaching points**
- Store vial in refrigerator; do not shake. Inject SC into arms, abdomen, hips, thighs. Vial is for single use only. Discard any unused portions.
- Keep a chart of injection sites to prevent overuse of one area.
- The following side effects may occur: loss of appetite, nausea, vomiting (use frequent mouth care; eat small, frequent meals; an antiemetic may also be ordered); fatigue, confusion, dizziness, numbness, visual disturbances, depression (use special precautions to avoid in-

jury; avoid driving or using dangerous machinery).
- Arrange for regular follow-up; this drug will be given for 24 weeks.
- Avoid pregnancy while on this drug; use of barrier contraceptives is advised.
- Report fever, chills, sore throat, unusual bleeding or bruising, chest pain, palpitations, dizziness, changes in mental status.

## interferon beta-1a

*(in ter feer' on)*
Avonex
**Pregnancy Category C**

### Drug classes
Interferon

### Therapeutic actions
Interferons are produced by human leukocytes in response to viral infections and other stimuli; interferon beta-1a blocks replication of viruses and stimulates the host immunoregulatory activities. It is produced by Chinese hamster ovary cells.

### Indications
- Multiple sclerosis—treatment of relapsing forms of MS to slow accumulation of physical disability and decrease frequency of clinical exacerbations
- Unlabeled uses: treatment of AIDS, AIDS-related Kaposi's sarcoma, metastatic renal-cell carcinoma, malignant melanoma, cutaneous T-cell lymphoma, acute non-A non-B hepatitis

### Contraindications/cautions
- Contraindications: allergy to beta interferon or any components of product, pregnancy, lactation
- Use cautiously with chronic progressive MS, suicidal tendencies or mental disorders, cardiac disease, seizures

### Dosage
**Available Forms:** Powder for injection—33 μg
*ADULT:* 30 μg IM once/wk.
*PEDIATRIC (< 18 Y):* Safety and efficacy not established.

### Pharmacokinetics

| *Route* | *Onset* | *Peak* | *Duration* |
|---|---|---|---|
| IM | 12 h | 48 h | 4 d |

*Metabolism:* Hepatic and renal; $T_{1/2}$: 10 h
*Distribution:* Crosses placenta; may pass into breast milk
*Excretion:* Urine

### Adverse effects
- CNS: *Dizziness, confusion,* paresthesias, numbness, lethargy, decreased mental status, depression, visual disturbances, sleep disturbances, nervousness
- GI: *Anorexia, nausea,* diarrhea, vomiting, change in taste
- CV: Hypotension, edema, hypertension, chest pain, arrhythmias, palpitations
- **Hematologic**: Leukopenia, neutropenia, thrombocytopenia, anemia, decreased Hgb; increased levels of SGOT, LDH, alkaline phosphatase, bilirubin, uric acid, serum creatinine, BUN, blood sugar, serum phosphorus, neutralizing antibodies; hypocalcemia
- GU: Impairment of fertility in women, transient impotence
- **Dermatologic**: *Photosensitivity,* rash, alopecia, sweating
- **Other**: *Flulike syndrome,* weight loss, diaphoresis, arthralgia, injection site reaction

## ■ Nursing Considerations

### Assessment
- ***History:*** Allergy to beta interferon or any component of produce, mental disorders, suicidal tendencies, cardiac disease, seizures, depression, pregnancy, lactation
- ***Physical:*** Weight; T; skin color, lesions; orientation, reflexes; P. BP, edema, ECG; liver evaluation; CBC, blood glucose, liver and renal function tests, urinalysis

### Implementation

- Arrange for laboratory tests—CBC, differential, granulocytes and hairy cells and bone marrow hairy cells and liver function tests—before and monthly during therapy.
- Reconstitute with 1.1 ml of diluent and swirl gently to dissolve; use within 6 h.
- Ensure that patient is well hydrated, especially during initiation of treatment.
- Ensure regular follow-up and treatment of MS; this drug is not a cure.
- Arrange for supportive treatment if flulike syndrome occurs: rest, acetaminophen for fever and headache, environmental control.
- Carefully monitor patients with any history of mental disorders or suicidal tendencies.
- Counsel female patients to use birth control while on this drug. Drug is contraindicated in pregnancy.

### Drug-specific teaching points

- This drug needs to be given weekly. If you or significant other can give an IM injection: store vial in refrigerator, reconstitute with 1.1 ml of diluent and swirl gently, use within 6 h. Do not give in the same site each week.
- Keep a chart of injection sites to prevent overuse of one area.
- The following side effects may occur: loss of appetite, nausea, vomiting (use frequent mouth care; eat small, frequent meals; maintain good nutrition if possible—dietician may be able to help; antiemetics may be ordered); fatigue, confusion, dizziness, numbness, visual disturbances, depression (use cautions to avoid injury; avoid driving or using dangerous machinery); impotence (usually transient); sensitivity to sunlight (use a sunscreen, wear protective clothing if exposure to sun cannot be prevented).
- Arrange for regular treatment and follow-up of MS; this drug is not a cure.
- Report fever, chills, sore throat, unusual bleeding or bruising, chest pain, palpitations, dizziness, changes in mental status.

## interferon beta-1b

*(in ter feer' on)*
rIFN-B
Betaseron
**Pregnancy Category C**

### Drug classes

Interferon

### Therapeutic actions

Interferons are produced by human leukocytes in response to viral infections and other stimuli; interferon beta-1b block replication of viruses and stimulate the host immunoregulatory activities. Interferon beta 1-b is produced by recombinant DNA technology using *E. coli.*

### Indications

- Reduce the frequency of clinical exacerbations in relapsing, remitting multiple sclerosis (MS)
- Unlabeled uses: treatment of AIDS, AIDS-related Kaposi's sarcoma, metastatic renal cell carcinoma, malignant melanoma, cutaneous T-cell lymphoma, acute non-A, non-B hepatitis

### Contraindications/cautions

- Contraindications: allergy to beta interferon, human albumin, or product components, pregnancy, lactation.
- Use cautiously with chronic progressive MS, suicidal tendencies, or mental disorders.

### Dosage

**Available Forms:** Powder for injection—0.3 mg

**ADULT:** 0.25 mg (8 ml IU) SC qod; discontinue use if disease is unremitting > 6 mo.

**PEDIATRIC (< 18 Y):** Safety and efficacy not established.

### Pharmacokinetics

| *Route* | *Onset* | *Peak* |
|---|---|---|
| SC | Slow | 1–8 h |

*Metabolism:* Hepatic and renal; $T_{1/2}$: 8 min–4.3 h
*Distribution:* Crosses placenta; may enter breast milk
*Excretion:* Urine

### Adverse effects

- CNS: *Dizziness, confusion,* paresthesias, numbness, lethargy, decreased mental status, depression, visual disturbances, sleep disturbances, nervousness
- GI: *Anorexia, nausea,* diarrhea, vomiting, change in taste
- CV: Hypotension, edema, hypertension, chest pain, arrhythmias, palpitations
- **Hematologic**: Leukopenia, neutropenia, thrombocytopenia, anemia, decreased Hgb; increased levels of SGOT, LDH, alkaline phosphatase, bilirubin, uric acid, serum creatinine, BUN, blood sugar, serum phosphorus, neutralizing antibodies; hypocalcemia
- GU: Impairment of fertility in women, transient impotence
- **Dermatologic**: *Photosensitivity,* rash, alopecia, sweating
- **General**: *Flulike syndrome*, weight loss, diaphoresis, arthralgia, injection site reaction

## ■ Nursing Considerations

### Assessment

- ***History:*** Allergy to interferon beta or any components of the product, mental disorders, suicidal tendencies, pregnancy, lactation
- ***Physical:*** Weight; T; skin color, lesions; orientation, reflexes; P, BP, edema, ECG; liver evaluation; CBC, blood glucose, liver and renal function tests, urinalysis

### Implementation

- Obtain laboratory tests (CBC, differential, granulocytes and hairy cells, bone marrow hairy cells, and liver function tests) before therapy and monthly during therapy.
- Monitor for severe reactions; notify physician immediately; dosage reduction or discontinuation may be necessary.
- Reconstitute by using a sterile syringe and needle to inject 1.2 ml supplied diluent into vial; gently swirl vial to dissolve drug completely; do not shake. Discard if any particulate matter or discoloration has occurred. After reconstitution, vial contains 0.25 mg/ml solution. Withdraw 1 ml of reconstituted solution with a sterile syringe fitted with a 27-gauge needle. Inject SC into arms, abdomen, hips, thighs. Vial is for single use only. Discard any unused portions. Refrigerate. Use reconstituted solution within 3 h.
- Ensure that patient is well hydrated, especially during initiation of treatment.
- Assure regular follow-up and treatment of MS; this drug is not a cure.
- Monitor patients with any mental disorders or suicidal tendencies carefully.
- Counsel female patients to use birth control. Drug is contraindicated in pregnancy.

### Drug-specific teaching points

- Reconstitute by using a sterile syringe and needle to inject 1.2 ml supplied diluent into vial; gently swirl the vial to dissolve the drug completely; do not shake. Discard if any particulate matter or discoloration has occurred. After reconstitution, vial contains 0.25 mg/ml solution. Withdraw 1 ml of reconstituted solution with a sterile syringe fitted with a 27-gauge needle. Inject SC into arms, abdomen, hips, thighs. Vial is for single use only. Discard any unused portions. Refrigerate. Use reconstituted solution within 3 h.
- Keep a chart of injection sites to prevent overuse of one area.
- The following side effects may occur: loss of appetite, nausea, vomiting (frequent mouth care, small frequent meals may help; maintain good nutrition; a dietician may be able to help; an antiemetic also may be ordered); fatigue, confusion, dizziness, numbness, visual disturbances, depression (use special precautions to avoid injury; avoid driving or using dangerous machinery); impotence (transient and reversible); sensitivity to the sun (use

sunscreen and wear protective clothing if exposed to sun).

- Arrange for regular treatment and follow-up of MS; this drug is not a cure.
- Report fever, chills, sore throat, unusual bleeding or bruising, chest pain, palpitations, dizziness, changes in mental status.

## interferon gamma-1b

*(in ter feer' on)*

Actimmune

**Pregnancy Category C**

### Drug classes

Interferon

### Therapeutic actions

Interferons are produced by human leukocytes in response to viral infections and other stimuli; interferon gamma-1b block has potent phagocyte-activating effects; acts as an interleukin; produced by *E. coli* bacteria.

### Indications

- For reducing the frequency and severity of serious infections associated with chronic granulomatous disease

### Contraindications/cautions

- Contraindications: allergy to interferon gamma, *E. coli*, or product components, pregnancy, lactation.
- Use cautiously with seizure disorders, compromised CNS function, cardiac disease, myelosuppression.

### Dosage

**Available Forms:** Injection—100 μg

*ADULT:* 50 μg/m² (1.5 million U/m²) SC 3×/wk in patients with body surface area > 0.5 m²; 1.5 μg/kg per dose in patients with body surface area < 0.5 m².

*PEDIATRIC (<18 Y):* Safety and efficacy not established.

### Pharmacokinetics

| *Route* | *Onset* | *Peak* |
|---|---|---|
| SC | Slow | 7 h |

*Metabolism:* Hepatic and renal; $T_{1/2}$: 2.9–5.9 h

*Distribution:* Crosses placenta; may enter breast milk

*Excretion:* Urine

### Adverse effects

- CNS: *Dizziness, confusion,* paresthesias, numbness, lethargy, decreased mental status, depression, visual disturbances, sleep disturbances, nervousness
- GI: *Anorexia, nausea*, diarrhea, vomiting, change in taste, pancreatitis
- CV: Hypotension, edema, hypertension, chest pain, arrhythmias, palpitations
- General: *Flulike syndrome,* weight loss, diaphoresis, arthralgia, injection site reaction

## Nursing Considerations

### Assessment

- *History:* Allergy to interferon gamma, *E. coli*, or product components, pregnancy, lactation, seizure disorders, compromised CNS function, cardiac disease, myelosuppression
- *Physical:* Weight; T; skin color, lesions; orientation, reflexes; P, BP, edema, ECG; liver evaluation; CBC, blood glucose, liver and renal function tests, urinalysis

### Implementation

- Obtain laboratory tests (CBC, differential, granulocytes and hairy cells, bone marrow and hairy cells, and liver function tests) before therapy and monthly during therapy.
- Monitor for severe reactions; notify physician immediately; dosage reduction or discontinuation may be necessary.
- Store in refrigerator; each vial is for one use only, discard after that time. Discard any vial that has been unrefrigerated for 12 h.
- Give drug hs if flulike symptoms become a problem.

### Drug-specific teaching points

- Store in refrigerator; each vial is for one use only; discard after that time. Discard vial that has been unrefrigerated for 12 h. You and a significant other should learn the proper technique for SC injections.

- Keep a chart of injection sites to prevent overuse of one area.
- The following side effects may occur: loss of appetite, nausea, vomiting (frequent mouth care, small frequent meals may help; maintain good nutrition; a dietician may be able to help; an antiemetic also may be ordered); fatigue, confusion, dizziness, numbness, visual disturbances, depression (use special precautions to avoid injury; avoid driving or using dangerous machinery); flulike symptoms (eg, fever, chills, aches, pains; rest, acetaminophen for fever and headache; take drug at bedtime).
- Report fever, chills, sore throat, unusual bleeding or bruising, chest pain, palpitations, dizziness, changes in mental status.

# iodine thyroid products

*(eye' oh dine)*

Lugol's Solution

potassium iodide, sodium iodide, strong iodine solution

Thyro-Block

**Pregnancy Category C**

## Drug classes
Thyroid suppressant

## Therapeutic actions
Inhibits synthesis of the active thyroid hormones $T_3$ and $T_4$ and inhibits the release of these hormones into circulation.

## Indications
- Hyperthyroidism: adjunctive therapy with antithyroid drugs in preparation for thyroidectomy, treatment of thyrotoxic crisis or neonatal thyrotoxicosis
- Thyroid blocking in a radiation emergency
- Unlabeled uses: potassium iodide has been effective with Sweet's syndrome, treatment of lymphocutaneous sporotrichosis

## Contraindications/cautions
- Allergy to iodides; pulmonary edema, pulmonary tuberculosis (sodium iodide); pregnancy; lactation.

## Dosage
**Available Forms:** Solution—5% iodine, 10% potassium iodide; tablets—130 mg

### Adult
- *RDA:* 150 $\mu$g PO.
- ***Preparation for thyroidectomy:*** 2–6 drops strong iodine solution tid PO for 10 d prior to surgery.
- ***Thyroid blocking in a radiation emergency:*** One tablet (130 mg potassium iodide) PO or 6 drops (21 mg potassium iodide/drop) added to half glass of liquid per day for 10 d.

### Pediatric
- ***Thyroid blocking in a radiation emergency***
  - *>1 y:* Adult dose.
  - *<1 y:* 1/2 crushed tablet or 3 drops in a small amount of liquid per d for 10 d. *Note;* Potassium iodide tablets and drops are available only to state and federal agencies.

## Pharmacokinetics

| *Route* | *Onset* | *Peak* | *Duration* |
|---|---|---|---|
| Oral | 24 h | 10–15 d | 6 wk |

*Metabolism:* Hepatic; $T_{1/2}$: unknown
*Distribution:* Crosses placenta; may enter breast milk
*Excretion:* Urine

## Adverse effects
- GI: *Swelling of the salivary glands, iodism* (metallic taste, burning mouth and throat, sore teeth and gums, head cold symptoms, stomach upset, diarrhea)
- Dermatologic: *Skin rash*
- Hypersensitivity: Allergic reactions-fever, joint pains, swelling of the face or body, shortness of breath
- Endocrine: Hypothyroidism, hyperthyroidism, goiter

## Clinically important drug-drug interactions
- Increased risk of hypothyroidism if taken concurrently with lithium

## ■ Nursing Considerations

### Assessment
- *History:* Allergy to iodides, pulmonary edema, pulmonary tuberculosis, lactation

- *Physical:* Skin color, lesions, edema; R, adventitious sounds; gums, mucous membranes; $T_3$, $T_4$

**Implementation**
- Test skin for idiosyncrasy to iodine before giving parenteral doses.
- Dilute strong iodine solution with fruit juice or water to improve taste.
- Crush tablets for small children.
- Discontinue drug if symptoms of acute iodine toxicity occur: vomiting, abdominal pain, diarrhea, circulatory collapse.

**Drug-specific teaching points**
- Drops may be diluted in fruit juice or water. Tablets may be crushed.
- Discontinue use and report fever, skin rash, swelling of the throat, metallic taste, sore teeth and gums, head cold symptoms, severe GI distress, enlargement of the thyroid gland.

## iodoquinol

*(eye oh doe **kwin'** ole)*
diiodohydroxyquinoline
Diodoquin (CAN), Yodoxin
**Pregnancy Category C**

### Drug classes
Amebicide

### Therapeutic actions
Direct amebicidal by an unknown mechanism; is poorly absorbed in the GI tract and is able to exert its amebicidal action directly in the large intestine.

### Indications
- Acute or chronic intestinal amebiasis

### Contraindications/cautions
- Contraindications: hepatic failure, allergy to iodine preparations or 8-hydroxyquinolines.
- Use cautiously with thyroid disease, pregnancy, lactation.

### Dosage
**Available Forms:** Tablets— 210, 650 mg
*ADULT:* 650 mg tid PO after meals for 20 d.
*PEDIATRIC:* 40 mg/kg per day PO, in 3 divided doses for 20 d. Maximum dose: 650 mg/dose. Do not exceed 1.95 g in 24 h for 20 d.

### Pharmacokinetics

| Route | Onset |
|---|---|
| Oral | Slow |

Very poorly absorbed; exerts effects locally in the intestine.

### Adverse effects
- CNS: Blurring of vision, weakness, fatigue, numbness, headache
- GI: *Nausea, vomiting, diarrhea,* anorexia
- Dermatologic: *Skin rash, pruritus*
- General: Fever, chills
- Other: Thyroid enlargement

### Drug-lab test interferences
- Interferes with many tests of thyroid function; interference may last up to 6 mo after drug is discontinued.

### ■ Nursing Considerations

**Assessment**
- *History:* Hepatic failure, allergy to iodine preparations or 8-hydroxyquinolines, thyroid disease, lactation
- *Physical:* Skin rashes, lesions; check reflexes, ophthalmologic exam; BP, P, R; liver and thyroid function tests (PBI, $T_3$, $T_4$)

**Implementation**
- Administer drug after meals.
- Administer for full course of therapy.
- Maintain patient's nutrition.

**Drug-specific teaching points**
- Take drug after meals.
- The following side effects often occur: GI upset, nausea, vomiting, diarrhea (small frequent meals, frequent mouth care often help).
- Report severe GI upset, skin rash, blurring of vision, unusual fatigue, fever.

## ipecac syrup

*(**ip'** e kak)*
**Pregnancy Category C**

**Drug classes**
Emetic agent

**Therapeutic actions**
Produces vomiting by a local GI mucosa irritant effect and a central medullary effect (CTZ stimulation).

**Indications**
- Treatment of drug overdose and certain poisonings

**Contraindications/cautions**
- Unconscious, semiconscious, convulsing states; poisoning with corrosives, such as alkalies, strong acids, petroleum distillates.

### Dosage
**Available Forms:** Syrup—1.5%–1.75% alcohol in 15 and 30 ml, 2% alcohol in 15 and 30 ml

*ADULT:* 15–30 ml PO followed by 3–4 glasses of water.

*CHILDREN < 1 Y:* 5–10 ml PO followed by 1/2–1 glass of water.

*CHILDREN > 1 Y:* 15 ml PO followed by 2–3 glasses of water. Repeat dosage if vomiting does not occur within 20 min. If vomiting does not occur within 30 min of second dose, perform gastric lavage.

**Pharmacokinetics**

| Route | Onset | Peak |
|---|---|---|
| Oral | Varies | 20–30 min |

Minimal systemic absorption occurs if taken correctly.

**Adverse effects**
- CNS: *Mild CNS depression*
- GI: *Diarrhea, mild GI upset*
- CV: Heart conduction disturbances, atrial fibrillation, fatal myocarditis if drug is not vomited

## ■ Nursing Considerations

### Assessment
- ***History:*** Unconscious, semiconscious, convulsing states; poisoning with corrosives; lactation
- ***Physical:*** Orientation, affect; P, baseline ECG, auscultation; stools, bowel sounds

### Implementation
- Give to conscious patients only.
- Give as soon after poisoning as possible.
- Ipecac syrup differs from ipecac fluid extract, which is 14 times stronger and has caused some deaths.
- Consult with a Poison Control Center if in doubt and if vomiting does not occur within 20 min of second dose.
- Give with adequate amounts of water.
- Maintain life support equipment on standby for poisoning and overdose; cardiac support will be needed if vomiting of ipecac does not occur.
- Use activated charcoal if vomiting of ipecac does not occur or if overdose of ipecac occurs.

### Drug-specific teaching points
- Drug is available in premeasured doses for emergency home use.
- Call physician, poison control center, or emergency room in cases of accidental ingestion.
- Give drug with adequate amounts of water. Do not exceed recommended dose.
- The following side effects may occur: diarrhea, GI upset, drowsiness and lethargy.

## ipratropium bromide

*(i pra **troe'** pee um)*

Atrovent

**Pregnancy Category B**

**Drug classes**
Anticholinergic
Antimuscarinic agent
Parasympatholytic

**Therapeutic actions**
Anticholinergic, chemically related to atropine, which blocks vagally mediated reflexes by antagonizing the action of acetylcholine.

**Indications**
- Bronchodilator for maintenance treatment of bronchospasm associated with COPD (solution, aerosol)

- Symptomatic relief of rhinorrhea associated with perennial rhinitis, common cold (nasal spray)

### Contraindications/cautions

- Contraindications: hypersensitivity to atropine or its derivatives, acute episodes of bronchospasm.
- Use cautiously with narrow-angle glaucoma, prostatic hypertrophy, bladder neck obstruction, pregnancy, lactation.

### Dosage

**Available Forms:** Aerosol—18 μg/actuation; solution for inhalation—0.02%; nasal spray—0.03% (21 μg/spray), 0.06% (42 μg/spray)

ADULT

- ***Inhalation:*** The usual dosage is 2 inhalations (36 μg) 4×/d. Patients may take additional inhalations as required. Do not exceed 12 inhalations/24 h. Solution for inhalation: 500 μg, 3–4×/d with doses 6–8 h apart.
- ***Nasal spray:*** 2 sprays 0.03% per nostril 2–3×/d or 2 sprays 0.06% per nostril 3–4×/d.

PEDIATRIC: Safety and efficacy in children <12 y not established.

### Pharmacokinetics

| *Route* | *Onset* | *Peak* | *Duration* |
|---|---|---|---|
| Inhalation | 15 min | 1–2 h | 3–4 h |

### Adverse effects

- CNS: *Nervousness, dizziness, headache,* fatigue, insomnia, *blurred vision*
- GI: *Nausea,* GI distress, dry mouth
- Respiratory: *Cough,* exacerbation of symptoms, hoarseness
- Other: Palpitations, rash

## ■ Nursing Considerations

### Assessment

- ***History:*** Hypersensitivity to atropine; acute bronchospasm, narrow-angle glaucoma, prostatic hypertrophy, bladder neck obstruction, pregnancy, lactation
- ***Physical:*** Skin color, lesions, texture; T; orientation, reflexes, bilateral grip strength; affect; ophthalmic exam; P, BP; R, adventitious sounds; bowel sounds, normal output; normal urinary output, prostate palpation

### Implementation

- Protect solution for inhalation from light.
- Ensure adequate hydration, provide environmental control (temperature) to prevent hyperpyrexia.
- Have patient void before taking medication to avoid urinary retention.
- Teach patient proper use of inhalator.

### Drug-specific teaching points

- Use this drug as an inhalation product. Review the proper use of inhalator; for nasal spray, initiation of pump requires 7 actuations; if not used for 24 h, 2 actuations will be needed before use.
- The following side effects may occur: dizziness, headache, blurred vision (avoid driving or performing hazardous tasks); nausea, vomiting, GI upset (proper nutrition is important; consult with your dietician to maintain nutrition); cough.
- Report rash, eye pain, difficulty voiding, palpitations, vision changes.

## irbesartan

*(er bah sar' tan)*

Avapro

**Pregnancy Category D (second & third trimesters)**

**Pregnancy Category C (first trimester)**

### Drug classes

Angiotensin II receptor antagonist
Antihypertensive

### Therapeutic actions

Selectively blocks the binding of angiotensin II to specific tissue receptors found in the vascular smooth muscle and adrenal gland; this action blocks the vasoconstriction effect of the renin-angiotensin system as well as the release of aldosterone, leading to decreased blood pressure.

### Indications

- Treatment of hypertension as monotherapy

### Contraindications/cautions

- Contraindications: hypersensitivity to irbesartan, pregnancy (use during the second or third trimester can cause inujry or even death to the fetus), lactation.
- Use cautiously with hepatic or renal dysfunction, hypovolemia.

### Dosage

**Available Forms:** Tablets—75, 150, 300 mg

*ADULT:* 75–300 mg PO qd as one dose; titrate slowly to determine effective dose.

*PEDIATRIC:* Safety and efficacy not established.

### Pharmacokinetics

| *Route* | *Onset* | *Peak* |
|---|---|---|
| Oral | Varies | 1–3 h |

*Metabolism:* Hepatic; $T_{1/2}$: 11–15 h
*Distribution:* Crosses placenta; passes into breast milk
*Excretion:* Feces and urine

### Adverse effects

- CNS: *Headache, dizziness,* syncope, muscle weakness
- GI: *Diarrhea, abdominal pain, nausea,* constipation, dry mouth, dental pain
- CV: Hypotension, orthostatic hypotension
- **Respiratory:** *URI symptoms, cough,* sinus disorders
- **Dermatologic:** Rash, inflammation, urticaria, pruritus, alopecia, dry skin
- **Other:** Cancer in preclinical studies, back pain, fever, gout, *fatigue*

## ■ Nursing Considerations

### Assessment

- *History:* Hypersensitivity to irbesartan, pregnancy, lactation, hepatic or renal dysfunction, hypovolemia.
- *Physical:* Skin lesions, turgor; T; reflexes, affect; BP; R, respiratory auscultation; liver and kidney function tests.

### Implementation

- Administer without regard to meals.
- Ensure that patient is not pregnant before beginning therapy; suggest the use of barrier birth control while using irbesartan; fetal injury and deaths have been reported.
- Find an alternative method of feeding the baby if giving drug to a nursing mother. Depression of the renin-angiotensin system in infants is potentially very dangerous.
- Alert surgeon and mark patient's chart with notice that irbesartan is being taken. The blockage of the renin-angiotensin system following surgery can produce problems. Hypotension may be reversed with volume expansion.
- Monitor patient closely in any situation that may lead to a decrease in blood pressure secondary to reduction in fluid volume (excessive perspiration, dehydration, vomiting, diarrhea); excessive hypotension can occur.

### Drug-specific teaching points

- Take this drug without regard to meals. Do not stop taking this drug without consulting your nurse or physician.
- Use a barrier method of birth control while on this drug; if you become pregnant or desire to become pregnant, consult with your physician.
- The following side effects may occur: dizziness (more likely to occur in any situation where you may be fluid depleted [extreme heat, exertion, etc.]; avoid driving or performing hazardous tasks); headache (medications may be available to help); nausea, vomiting, diarrhea (proper nutrition is important; consult with your dietician); symptoms of upper respiratory tract infection, cough (do not self-medicate; consult with your nurse or physician if this becomes uncomfortable).
- Report fever, chills, dizziness, pregnancy.

## irinotecan hydrochloride

*(eh rin oh' te kan)*

Camptosar

**Pregnancy Category D**

### Drug classes
Antineoplastic

### Therapeutic actions
Cytotoxic: causes death of cells during cell division by causing damage to the DNA strand during DNA synthesis; specific to cells using topoisomerease I, DNA and irinotecan complexes

### Indications
- Treatment of patients with metastatic colon or rectal cancer whose disease has recurred or progressed following 5-FU therapy

### Contraindications/cautions
- Contraindications: allergy to irinotecan
- Use cautiously with bone marrow depression, severe diarrhea, pregnancy, lactation

### Dosage
**Available Forms:** Injection—20 mg/ml

*ADULT:* 125 $mg/m^2$ IV over 90 min once weekly for 4 wk, then a 2-wk rest; repeat 6-wk regimen.

*PEDIATRIC:* Not recommended.

### Pharmacokinetics

| Route | Onset | Peak |
|---|---|---|
| IV | Immediate | 1–2 h |

*Metabolism:* Hepatic; $T_{1/2}$: 6 h

*Distribution:* Crosses placenta; may pass into breast milk

*Excretion:* Urine and bile

### IV facts
**Preparation:** Dilute in 5% Dextrose Injection or 0.9% Sodium Chloride Injection to final concentration of 0.12–1.1 mg/ml. Store diluted drug protected from light; use within 24 h if refrigerated or within 6 h if at room temperature. Store vials at room temperature, protected from light.

**Infusion:** Infuse total dose over 90 min.

### Adverse effects
- CNS: Insomnia, dizziness, asthenia
- GI: *Nausea, vomiting, diarrhea,* constipation, stomatitis, flatulence, dyspepsia
- Respiratory: *Dyspnea,* cough, rhinitis
- Hematologic: **Neutropenia, leukopenia, anemia**
- Dermatologic: *Alopecia,* sweating, flushing, rashes
- Other: Fatigue, malaise, pain, infections, fever, cramping

## ■ Nursing Considerations

### Assessment
- *History:* Allergy to irinotecan, diarrhea, pregnancy, lactation, bone marrow depression
- *Physical:* T; skin lesions, color, turgor; orientation, affect, reflexes; R; abdominal exam, bowel sounds; CBC with differential

### Implementation
- Obtain CBC before each infusion; do not give to patients with a baseline neutrophil count of $<1500$ cells/$mm^2$; consult with physician for reduction in dose or withholding of drug if bone marrow depression becomes evident.
- Monitor infusion site; if extravasation occurs, flush with sterile water and apply ice.
- Monitor for diarrhea; assess hydration and arrange to decrease dose if 4–6 stools/d; omit a dose if 7–9 stools/d; if 10 or more stools/d, consult with physician.
- Protect patient from any exposure to infection.
- Arrange for wig or other appropriate head covering when alopecia occurs.

### Drug-specific teaching points
- This drug can only be given by IV infusion, which will run over 90 min. Mark calendar with days to return for infusion. A blood test will be required before each dose.



i

- The following side effects may occur: increased susceptibility to infection (avoid crowded areas or people with known infections; report any injury); nausea, vomiting (eat small, frequent meals; medication may be ordered); headache; loss of hair (arrange for a wig or other head covering; it is important to protect the head from extremes of temperature); diarrhea.
- Report pain at injection site, any injury or illness, fatigue, severe nausea or vomiting, increased, severe, or bloody diarrhea.

## iron dextran

InFeD
**Pregnancy Category B**

### Drug classes
Iron preparation

### Therapeutic actions
Elevates the serum iron concentration and is then converted to Hgb or trapped in the reticuloendothelial cells for storage and eventual conversion to usable form of iron.

### Indications
- Treatment of iron deficiency anemia only when oral administration of iron is unsatisfactory or impossible
- Unlabeled use—may be required for patients receiving epoetin therapy

### Contraindications/cautions
- Contraindications: allergy to iron dextran, anemias other than iron deficiency anemia, pregnancy.
- Use cautiously with impaired liver function, rheumatoid arthritis, allergies, asthma, lactation.

### Dosage
**Available Forms:** Injection—50 mg/ml

ADULT OR PEDIATRIC

- ***Iron deficiency anemia:*** Administer a 0.5 ml IM or IV test dose before therapy. Base dosage on hematologic response with frequent Hgb determinations:

$$\text{mg iron} = \frac{0.3 \times (\text{weight in lbs}) \times [100 - (\text{hemoglobin in g\%}) \times 100]}{14.8}$$

To determine dose in ml, divide the result by 50. For patients <30 lb (14 kg), give 80% the dose calculated from the formula.
- ***Iron replacement for blood loss:*** Determine dosage by the following formula: replacement iron (in mg) = blood loss (in ml) × Hct
- ***IM:*** Inject only into the upper outer quadrant of the buttocks. Do not exceed: 25 mg/d if < 4.5 kg; 50 mg/d if < 9 kg; 100 mg/d if < 50 kg; or 250 mg/d for all others.

### Pharmacokinetics

| Route | Onset | Peak |
|---|---|---|
| IM | Slow | 1–2 wk |

*Metabolism:* $T_{1/2}$: 6 h
*Distribution:* Crosses placenta; enters breast milk
*Excretion:* Blood loss

### IV facts
**Preparation:** Intermittent IV: Calculate dose from formula. Give individual doses of 2 ml or less per day. Use single dose ampules without preservatives. IV infusion: dilute needed dose in 200–250 ml of Normal Saline.
**Infusion:** Intermittent IV: give undiluted and slowly—1 ml or less/min. IV infusion (not approved by the FDA): infuse over 1–2 h after a test dose of 25 ml.

### Adverse effects
- CNS: Headache, backache, dizziness, malaise, transitory paresthesias
- GI: *Nausea, vomiting*
- CV: Hypotension, chest pain, shock, tachycardia
- Hypersensitivity: Hypersensitivity reactions including fatal **anaphylaxis**; dyspnea, urticaria, rash and itching, arthralgia and myalgia, fever, sweating, purpura
- Local: *Pain, inflammation and sterile abscesses at injection site, brown skin discoloration* (IM use); *lymphadenop-*

*athy, local phlebitis, peripheral vascular flushing* (IV administration)
- Other: *Arthritic reactivation*, fever, shivering, cancer

**Clinically important drug-drug interactions**

• Delayed response to iron dextran therapy in patients taking chloramphenicol.

**Drug-lab test interferences**

• Use caution when interpreting serum iron levels when done within 1–2 wk of iron dextran injection • Serum may be discolored to a brownish color following IV injection • Bone scans using Tc-99m diphosphonate may have abnormal areas following IM injection

## ■ Nursing Considerations

### Assessment

- *History:* Allergy to iron dextran, anemias other than iron deficiency anemia, impaired liver function, rheumatoid arthritis, allergies or asthma, lactation
- *Physical:* Skin lesions, color; T; injection site exam; range of motion, joints; R, adventitious sounds; liver evaluation; CBC, Hgb, Hct, serum ferritin assays, liver function tests

### Implementation

- Ensure that patient does have iron deficiency anemia before treatment.
- Arrange treatment of underlying cause of iron deficiency anemia.
- Give IM injections using the Z-track technique (displace skin laterally before injection) to avoid injection into the tissue and tissue staining. Use a large-gauge needle; if standing, have patient support self on leg not receiving the injection. If lying, have the injection site uppermost.
- Monitor patient for hypersensitivity reactions; test dose is highly recommended. Maintain epinephrine on standby in case severe hypersensitivity reaction occurs.
- Monitor serum ferritin levels periodically; these correlate well with iron stores. Do not give with oral iron preparations.
- Caution patients with rheumatoid arthritis that acute exacerbation of joint pain and swelling may occur; provide appropriate comfort measures.

### Drug-specific teaching points

- Treatment will end if anemia is corrected.
- Have periodic blood tests during therapy to assess drug response and determine appropriate dosage.
- Do not take oral iron products or vitamins with iron added while on this drug.
- The following side effects may occur: pain at injection site, headache, joint and muscle aches, GI upset.
- Report difficulty breathing, pain at injection site, rash, itching.

# Isoetharine

## isoetharine hydrochloride

*(eye soe **eth'** a reen)*

Arm-a-Med Isoetharine HCl, Beta-2, Bronkosol

## isoetharine mesylate

Bronkometer

**Pregnancy Category C**

**Drug classes**

Sympathomimetic
Beta-2 selective adrenergic agonist
Bronchodilator
Antiasthmatic agent

**Therapeutic actions**

In low doses, acts relatively selectively at beta-2 adrenergic receptors to cause bronchodilation; at higher doses, beta-2 selectivity is lost, and the drug acts at beta-1 receptors to cause typical sympathomimetic cardiac effects.

**Indications**

- Prophylaxis and treatment of bronchial asthma and reversible bronchospasm that may occur with bronchitis and emphysema

**Contraindications/cautions**

- Contraindications: hypersensitivity to isoetharine; allergy to sulfites; tachyarrhythmias, tachycardia caused by digitalis intoxication; general anesthesia with halogenated hydrocarbons or cyclopropane (sensitize the myocardium to catecholamines); unstable vasomotor system disorders.

- Use cautiously with hypertension, coronary insufficiency, CAD, history of stroke, COPD patients with degenerative heart disease, hyperthyroidism, history of seizure disorders, psychoneurotic individuals, labor and delivery (may inhibit labor; parenteral use of $\beta_2$-adrenergic agonists can accelerate fetal heart beat, cause hypoglycemia, hypokalemia, and pulmonary edema in the mother and hypoglycemia in the neonate); lactation.

## Dosage

**Available Forms:** Solution for inhalation—0.062%, 0.08%, 0.1%, 0.125%, 0.167%, 0.17%, 0.2%, 0.25%, 1%; aerosol—0.61% or 340 μg/actuation

ADULT

- ***Inhalation, metered-dose inhaler:*** Each actuation of aerosol dispenser delivers 340 μg isoetharine. Dose is 1 or 2 inhalations. More may be required; however, wait 1 full min after the initial dose. Usual interval between treatments is 4 h.
- ***Inhalant solutions:*** Administer from hand bulb nebulizer (3–7 inhalations), with oxygen aerosolization, or using an IPPB device, following manufacturer's instructions.

PEDIATRIC: Dosage not established.

GERIATRIC: Patients >60 y are more likely to develop adverse effects; use with extreme caution.

### Pharmacokinetics

| *Route* | *Onset* | *Duration* |
|---|---|---|
| Inhalation | 5 min | 1–3 h |

*Metabolism:* Tissue

*Distribution:* Crosses placenta; may enter breast milk

*Excretion:* Urine

### Adverse effects

- CNS: *Restlessness, apprehension, anxiety, fear,* CNS stimulation, hyperkinesia, insomnia, tremor, drowsiness, irritability, weakness, vertigo, headache
- GI: *Nausea,* vomiting, heartburn, unusual or bad taste
- CV: *Cardiac arrhythmias, tachycardia, palpitations,* PVCs, anginal pain
- **Respiratory**: *Respiratory difficulties, pulmonary edema, coughing,* bronchospasm, paradoxical airway resistance with repeated, excessive use of inhalation preparations
- **Other**: Sweating, pallor, flushing

### Clinically important drug-drug interactions

- Increased likelihood of cardiac arrhythmias with halogenated hydrocarbon anesthetics (halothane), cyclopropane

## ■ Nursing Considerations

### Assessment

- ***History:*** Hypersensitivity to isoetharine, allergy to sulfites, tachyarrhythmias, general anesthesia with halogenated hydrocarbons or cyclopropane, unstable vasomotor system disorders, hypertension, coronary insufficiency, history of stroke, COPD patients who have developed degenerative heart disease, hyperthyroidism, history of seizure disorders, psychoneuroses
- ***Physical:*** Weight; skin color, temperature, turgor; orientation, reflexes; P, BP; R, adventitious sounds; blood and urine glucose, serum electrolytes, thyroid function tests, ECG

### Implementation

- Use minimal doses for minimal periods of time; drug tolerance can occur with prolonged use.
- Maintain a beta-adrenergic blocker (a cardioselective beta-blocker, such as atenolol, should be used in patients with respiratory distress) on standby in case cardiac arrhythmias occur.
- Do not exceed recommended dosage; give aerosol during second half of inspiration, because the airways are open wider, and the aerosol distribution is more extensive.

### Drug-specific teaching points

- Do not exceed recommended dosage; adverse effects or loss of effectiveness may result. Read the instructions that come with the aerosol product, and ask your health care provider or pharmacist if you have any questions.
- The following side effects may occur: dizziness, drowsiness, fatigue, apprehension (use caution if driving or performing tasks that require alertness); nausea, heartburn, unusual taste (small, frequent meals may help); fast heart rate, anxiety, changes in breathing.
- Report chest pain, dizziness, insomnia, weakness, tremor or irregular heart beat, difficulty breathing, productive cough, failure to respond to usual dosage.

## isoniazid

*(eye soe **nye'** a zid)*

isonicotinic acid hydrazide

INH

Isotamine (CAN), Laniazid, Nydrazid, Rimifon (CAN)

**Pregnancy Category C**

### Drug classes

Antituberculous agent

### Therapeutic actions

Bactericidal: interferes with lipid and nucleic acid biosynthesis in actively growing tubercle bacilli.

### Indications

- Tuberculosis, all forms in which organisms are susceptible
- Prophylaxis in specific patients who are tuberculin reactors or household members of recently diagnosed tuberculars
- Unlabeled use of 300–400 mg/d, increased over 2 wk to 20 mg/kg per day for improvement of severe tremor in patients with multiple sclerosis

### Contraindications/cautions

- Contraindications: allergy to isoniazid, isoniazid-associated hepatic injury or other severe adverse reactions to isoniazid, acute hepatic disease, pregnancy.
- Use cautiously with renal dysfunction, lactation.

### Dosage

**Available Forms:** Tablets—50, 100, 300 mg; syrup—50 mg/5 ml; injection—100 mg/ml

**ADULT**

- *Treatment of active TB:* 5 mg/kg per day (up to 300 mg) PO in a single dose, with other effective agents. "First-line treatment" is considered to be 300 mg INH plus 600 mg rifampin, each given in a single daily oral dose.
- *Prophylaxis for TB:* 300 mg/d PO in a single dose. Concomitant administration of 6–50 mg/d of pyridoxine is recommended for those who are malnourished or predisposed to neuropathy (alcoholics, diabetics).

**PEDIATRIC**

- *Treatment of active TB:* 10–20 mg/kg per day (up to 300–500 mg) PO in a single dose, with other effective agents.
- *Prophylaxis for TB:* 10 mg/kg per day (up to 300 mg) PO in a single dose. Continuous treatment for a sufficient time is needed to prevent relapse.

### Pharmacokinetics

| *Route* | *Onset* | *Peak* | *Duration* |
|---|---|---|---|
| Oral | Varies | 1–2 h | 24 h |

*Metabolism:* Hepatic; $T_{1/2}$: 1–4 h

*Distribution:* Crosses placenta; enters breast milk

*Excretion:* Urine

### Adverse effects

- CNS: *Peripheral neuropathy*, convulsions, toxic encephalopathy, optic neuritis and atrophy, memory impairment, toxic psychosis
- GI: *Nausea, vomiting, epigastric distress,* bilirubinemia, bilirubinuria, *elevated AST,* ALT levels, jaundice, **hepatitis**
- Hematologic: Agranulocytosis, hemolytic or aplastic anemia, thrombocytopenia,

eosinophilia, pyridoxine deficiency, pellagra, hyperglycemia, metabolic acidosis, hypocalcemia, hypophosphatemia due to altered vitamin D metabolism

- **Hypersensitivity**: Fever, skin eruptions, lymphadenopathy, vasculitis
- **Local**: *Local irritation at IM injection site*
- **Other**: Gynecomastia, rheumatic syndrome, systemic lupus erythematous syndrome

### Clinically important drug-drug interactions

• Increased incidence of isoniazid-related hepatitis with alcohol and possibly if taken in high doses with rifampin • Increased serum levels of phenytoin • Increased effectiveness and risk of toxicity of carbamazepine • Risk of high output renal failure in fast INH acetylators with enflurane

### Clinically important drug-food interactions

• Risk of sympathetic-type reactions with tyramine-containing foods and exaggerated response (headache, palpitations, sweating, hypotension, flushing, diarrhea, itching) to histamine-containing food (fish–skipjack, tuna–sauerkraut juice, yeast extracts)

## ■ Nursing Considerations

### Assessment

- *History:* Allergy to isoniazid, isoniazid-associated adverse reactions; acute hepatic disease; renal dysfunction; lactation
- *Physical:* Skin color, lesions; T; orientation, reflexes, peripheral sensitivity, bilateral grip strength; ophthalmologic examination; R, adventitous sounds; liver evaluation; CBC, liver and kidney function tests, blood glucose

### Implementation

- Give on an empty stomach, 1 h before or 2 h after meals; may be given with food if GI upset occurs.
- Give in a single daily dose.
- Decrease tyramine-containing and histamine-containing food in diet.
- Consult with physician and arrange for daily pyridoxine in diabetic, alcoholic, or malnourished patients; also for patients who develop peripheral neuritis.
- Discontinue drug, and consult with physician if signs of hypersensitivity occur.

### Drug-specific teaching points

- Take this drug in a single daily dose. Take on an empty stomach, 1 h before or 2 h after meals. If GI distress occurs, may be taken with food.
- Take this drug regularly; avoid missing doses; do not discontinue without first consulting with your prescriber.
- Do not drink alcohol, or drink as little as possible. There is an increased risk of hepatitis if these two drugs are combined.
- Avoid tyramine-containing foods; consult a dietician to obtain a list of tyramine-containing and histamine-containing foods.
- The following side effects may occur: nausea, vomiting, epigastric distress (take drug with meals); skin rashes or lesions; numbness, tingling, loss of sensation (use caution to prevent injury or burns).
- Have periodic medical check-ups, including an eye examination and blood tests to evaluate the drug effects.
- Report weakness, fatigue, loss of appetite, nausea, vomiting, yellowing of skin or eyes, darkening of the urine, numbness or tingling in hands or feet.

# Isoproterenol

## isoproterenol hydrochloride

*(eye soe proe **ter'** e nole)*

Isuprel, Isuprel Mistometer

## isoproterenol sulfate

Medihaler-Iso

**Pregnancy Category C**

## Drug classes
Sympathomimetic
Beta-1 and beta-2 adrenergic agonist
Bronchodilator
Antiasthmatic agent
Drug used in shock

## Therapeutic actions
Effects are mediated by beta-1 and beta-2 adrenergic receptors; acts on beta-1 receptors in the heart to produce positive chronotropic and positive inotropic effects and to increase automaticity; acts on beta-2 receptors in the bronchi to cause bronchodilation; acts on beta-2 receptors in smooth muscle in the walls of blood vessels in skeletal muscle and splanchnic beds to cause dilation (cardiac stimulation, vasodilation may be adverse effects when drug is used as bronchodilator).

## Indications
- Inhalation: treatment of bronchospasm associated with acute and chronic bronchial asthma, pulmonary emphysema, bronchitis, bronchiectasis
- Injection: management of bronchospasm during anesthesia
- Adjunct in the management of shock (hypoperfusion syndrome) and in the treatment of cardiac standstill or arrest; carotid sinus hypersensitivity; Stokes-Adams syndrome; ventricular tachycardia and ventricular arrhythmias that require increased inotropic activity for therapy
- Sublingual: management of patients with bronchopulmonary disease; Stokes-Adams syndrome and AV heart block
- Rectal: Stokes-Adams syndrome and AV heart block

## Contraindications/cautions
- Contraindications: hypersensitivity to isoproterenol; tachyarrhythmias, tachycardia caused by digitalis intoxication; general anesthesia with halogenated hydrocarbons or cyclopropane (sensitize the myocardium to catecholamines); labor and delivery (may delay second stage of labor; can accelerate fetal heart beat; may cause hypoglycemia, hypokalemia, pulmonary edema in the mother and hypoglycemia in the neonate); lactation.
- Use cautiously with unstable vasomotor system disorders, hypertension, coronary insufficiency, history of stroke, COPD patients with degenerative heart disease, diabetes mellitus, hyperthyroidism, history of seizure disorders, psychoneuroses.

## Dosage
**Available Forms:** Solution for inhalation—0.25%, 0.5%, 1%; aerosol—0.25%, 131 μg/mist, 80 μg/dose; injection—0.2 mg/ml

### ADULT
- ***Injection***
  - *Bronchospasm during anesthesia:* 0.01–0.02 mg of diluted solution IV; repeat when necessary.
  - *Shock:* Dilute to 2 μg/ml and infuse IV at a rate adjusted on the basis of HR, central venous pressure, systemic BP, and urine flow.
  - *Cardiac standstill and arrhythmias:* IV injection: 0.02–0.06 mg of diluted solution. IV infusion: 5 μg/min of diluted solution. IM, SC: 0.2 mg of undiluted 1:5,000 solution. Intracardiac: 0.02 mg of undiluted 1:5,000 solution
- ***Sublingual***
  - *Bronchospasm:* 10 mg average dose SL (15–20 mg may be required). Do not repeat more than every 3 or 4 h or more than tid. Do not exceed a total dose of 60 mg/d.
  - *Heart block, certain ventricular arrhythmias:* Administer glossets sublingually or rectally for maintenance after stabilization with other therapy; 10–30 mg sublingually 4–6×/d to prevent heart block in carotid sinus hypersensitivity; 5–15 mg rectally to treat heart block.
  - *Acute bronchial asthma: Hand bulb nebulizer*: Administer the 1:200 solution in a dosage of 5–15 deep inhalations. If desired, administer the 1:100 solution in 3–7 deep inhalations. If no relief after 5–10 min, repeat doses once more. If acute attack recurs, may repeat treatment up to five times per day. *Metered-dose inhaler*: Start with one inhalation; if no relief after 2–5 min, repeat. *Daily maintenance*: 1–2 inhalations 4–6×/d. Do

not take more than 2 inhalations at a time. Do not take more than 6 inhalations per hour.

– *Bronchospasm in COPD: Hand bulb nebulizer*: 5–15 inhalations using the 1:200 solution. Patients with severe attacks may require 3–7 inhalations using the 1:100 solution. Do not use at less than 3- to 4-h intervals. *Nebulization by compressed air or $O_2$, IPPB*: 0.5 ml of a 1:200 solution is diluted to 2–2.5 ml with appropriate diluent for a concentration of 1:800 to 1:1,000 and delivered over 10–20 min. May repeat up to 5×/d. *Metered-dose inhaler*: 1 or 2 inhalations; repeat at no less than 3- to 4-h intervals.

PEDIATRIC

- ***Nebulization (bronchospasm):*** Administration is similar to that of adults; children's smaller ventilatory exchange capacity provides smaller aerosol intake. Use the 1:200 solution for an acute attack; do not use more than 0.25 ml of the 1:200 solution for each 10- to 15-min programmed treatment.

*GERIATRIC:* Patients >60 y are more likely to experience adverse effects; use with extreme caution.

### Pharmacokinetics

| *Route* | *Onset* | *Duration* |
|---|---|---|
| Inhalation | Rapid | 50–60 min |
| IV | Immediate | 1–2 min |
| PR | Slow | 2–4 h |

*Metabolism:* Tissue; $T_{1/2}$: unknown

*Distribution:* Crosses placenta; enters breast milk

*Excretion:* Urine

### IV facts

**Preparation:** Dilute the 1:5,000 solutions for IV injection or infusion with 5% Dextrose Injection; a convenient dilution is 1 mg isoproterenol (5 ml) in 500 ml diluent (final concentration 1:500,000 or 2 μg/ml).

**Infusion:** Dosage of 5 μg/min is provided by infusing 2.5 ml/min; adjust dosage to keep heart rate <110.

### Adverse effects

- CNS: *Restlessness, apprehension, anxiety, fear,* CNS stimulation, hyperkinesia, insomnia, tremor, drowsiness, irritability, weakness, vertigo, headache
- GI: *Nausea, vomiting, heartburn,* unusual or bad taste, swelling of the parotid glands
- CV: *Cardiac arrhythmias, tachycardia, palpitations,* anginal pain, changes in BP, paradoxical precipitation of Stokes-Adams seizures during normal sinus rhythm or transient heart block
- Respiratory: *Respiratory difficulties,* ***pulmonary edema,*** *coughing, bronchospasm, paradoxical airway resistance with repeated, excessive use*
- Other: *sweating, pallor,* flushing, muscle cramps

## ■ Nursing Considerations

### Assessment

- ***History:*** Hypersensitivity to isoproterenol; tachyarrhythmias; general anesthesia with halogenated hydrocarbons or cyclopropane; unstable vasomotor system disorders; hypertension; coronary artery disease; history of stroke; COPD patients with degenerative heart disease; diabetes mellitus; hyperthyroidism; history of seizure disorders; psychoneurotic individuals; labor and delivery; lactation
- ***Physical:*** Weight; skin color, temperature, turgor; orientation, reflexes; P, BP; R, adventitious sounds; blood and urine glucose, serum electrolytes, thyroid function tests, ECG

### Implementation

- Use minimal doses for minimuml periods; drug tolerance can occur with prolonged use.
- Maintain a beta-adrenergic blocker (a cardioselective beta-blocker, such as atenolol, should be used in patients with respiratory distress) on standby in case cardiac arrhythmias occur.
- Do not exceed recommended dosage of inhalation products; administer pressurized inhalation drug forms during second

half of inspiration, because the airways are open wider and the aerosol distribution is more extensive. If a second inhalation is needed, give at peak effect of previous dose, 3–5 min.

### Drug-specific teaching points

- Do not exceed recommended dosage; adverse effects or loss of effectiveness may result. Read product instructions (respiratory inhalant products), and ask your health care provider or pharmacist if you have any questions. Use inhalator correctly for best results and avoiding adverse effects.
- The following side effects may occur: drowsiness, dizziness, inability to sleep (use caution if driving or performing tasks that require alertness); nausea, vomiting (small, frequent meals may help); anxiety; rapid heart rate.
- Report chest pain, dizziness, insomnia, weakness, tremor or irregular heart beat, failure to respond to usual dosage.

## isosorbide

*(eye soe **sor'** bide)*
Ismotic, Monoket
**Pregnancy Category C**

### Drug classes

Osmotic diuretic

### Therapeutic actions

Elevates the osmolarity of the glomerular filtrate, hindering the reabsorption of water and leading to a loss of water, sodium, and chloride; creates an osmotic gradient in the eye between plasma and ocular fluids, reducing intraocular pressure.

### Indications

- Glaucoma: to interrupt acute attacks; poses less risk of nausea and vomiting than other oral osmotic agents
- Short-term reduction of intraocular pressure prior to and after ocular surgery

### Contraindications/cautions

- Allergy to isosorbide, anuria due to severe renal disease, severe dehydration, pulmonary edema, CHF, diseases associated with salt retention.

### Dosage

**Available Forms:** Solution—100 g/220 ml; tablets—10, 20 mg; ER tablets—60 mg

*ADULT:* PO use only. 1.5 g/kg (range 1–3 mg/kg) bid–qid as needed.

### Pharmacokinetics

| *Route* | *Onset* | *Peak* | *Duration* |
|---|---|---|---|
| Oral | 10–30 min | 1–1 1/2 h | 5–6 h |

*Metabolism:* $T_{1/2}$: 5–9.5 h
*Distribution:* Crosses placenta
*Excretion:* Urine

### Adverse effects

- CNS: *Headache, confusion, disorientation, dizziness,* lightheadedness, syncope, vertigo, irritability
- GI: Nausea, vomiting, GI discomfort, thirst, hiccoughs
- **Hematologic**: Hypernatremia, hyperosmolarity
- Other: Rash

## ■ Nursing Considerations

### Assessment

- *History:* Allergy to isosorbide, anuria due to severe renal disease, severe dehydration, pulmonary edema, CHF, diseases associated with salt retention
- *Physical:* Skin color, edema; orientation, reflexes, muscle strength, pupillary reflexes; pulses, BP, perfusion; R, pattern, adventitious sounds; urinary output patterns; serum electrolytes, urinalysis

### Implementation

- Administer by oral route only; not for injection.
- Pour over cracked ice, and have patient sip drug to improve palatability.
- Monitor urinary output carefully.
- Monitor BP regularly and carefully.

### Drug-specific teaching points

- Pour the drug over cracked ice to make it easier to take.
- The following side effects may occur: increased urination; GI upset (small, fre-

quent meals may help); dry mouth (sucking sugarless lozenges may help); headache, blurred vision, feelings of irritability (use caution when moving around; ask for assistance)
- Report severe headache, confusion, dizziness.

## isosorbide dinitrate

*(eye soe **sor'** bide)*

Dilatrate SR, Isordil, Isordil Tembids, Isordil Titradose, Sorbitrate

**Pregnancy Category C**

### Drug classes
Antianginal agent
Nitrate

### Therapeutic actions
Relaxes vascular smooth muscle with a resultant decrease in venous return and decrease in arterial BP, which reduces left ventricular workload and decreases myocardial oxygen consumption.

### Indications
- Treatment and prevention of angina pectoris

### Contraindications/cautions
- Allergy to nitrates, severe anemia, head trauma, cerebral hemorrhage, hypertrophic cardiomyopathy, pregnancy, lactation.

### Dosage
**Available Forms:** SL tablets—2.5, 5, 10 mg; chewable tablets—5, 10 mg

**ADULT**
- *Angina pectoris:* Starting dose: 2.5–5 mg sublingual, 5-mg chewable tablets, 5- to 20-mg oral tablets or capsules. Maintenance: 10–40 mg q6h oral tablets or capsules; sustained release, initially 40 mg, then 40–80 mg PO q8–12h.
- *Acute prophylaxis:* Initial dosage: 5–10 mg sublingual or chewable tablets q2–3h.

**PEDIATRIC:** Safety and efficicacy not established.

### Pharmacokinetics

| Route | Onset | Duration |
|---|---|---|
| Oral | 15–45 min | 4 h |
| SL | 2–5 min | 1–2 h |

*Metabolism:* Hepatic, $T_{1/2}$: 5 min, then 2–5 h
*Distribution:* May cross placenta; may enter breast milk
*Excretion:* Urine

### Adverse effects
- CNS: *Headache, apprehension, restlessness, weakness,* vertigo, dizziness, faintness
- GI: *Nausea,* vomiting, incontinence of urine and feces, abdominal pain
- CV: *Tachycardia, retrosternal discomfort, palpitations, hypotension,* ***syncope,*** *collapse, postural hypotension, angina*
- Dermatologic: Rash, exfoliative dermatitis, cutaneous vasodilation with flushing
- Other: Muscle twitching, pallor, perspiration, cold sweat

### Clinically important drug-drug interactions
- Increased systolic BP and decreased antianginal effect if taken concurrently with ergot alkaloids

### Drug-lab test interferences
- False report of decreased serum cholesterol if done by the Zlatkis-Zak color reaction

## ■ Nursing Considerations

### Assessment
- *History:* Allergy to nitrates, severe anemia, GI hypermobility, head trauma, cerebral hemorrhage, hypertrophic cardiomyopathy, pregnancy, lactation
- *Physical:* Skin color, temperature, lesions; orientation, reflexes, affect; P, BP, orthostatic BP, baseline ECG, peripheral perfusion; R, adventitious sounds; liver evaluation, normal output; CBC, Hgb

### Implementation
- Give sublingual preparations under the tongue or in the buccal pouch; encourage the patient not to swallow.

- Give chewable tablets slowly, only 5 mg initially because severe hypotension can occur; ensure that patient does not chew or crush sustained-release preparations.
- Give oral preparations on an empty stomach, 1 h before or 2 h after meals; take with meals if severe, uncontrolled headache occurs.
- Maintain life support equipment on standby if overdose occurs or cardiac condition worsens.
- Gradually reduce dose if anginal treatment is being terminated; rapid discontinuation can lead to problems of withdrawal.

### Drug-specific teaching points

- Place sublingual tablets under your tongue or in your cheek; do not chew or swallow the tablet. Take the isosorbide before chest pain begins, when activities or situation may precipitate an attack. Take oral isosorbide dinitrate on an empty stomach, 1 h before or 2 h after meals; do not chew or crush sustained-release preparations.
- The following side effects may occur: dizziness, lightheadedness (may be transient; use care to change positions slowly); headache (lie down in a cool environment, rest; OTC preparations may not help; take drug with meals); flushing of the neck or face (reversible).
- Report blurred vision, persistent or severe headache, skin rash, more frequent or more severe angina attacks, fainting.

## isotretinoin

*(eye so **tret'** i noyn)*

13-*cis*-retinoic acid

vitamin A metabolite

Accutane

**Pregnancy Category X**

### Drug classes

Vitamin metabolite
Acne product

### Therapeutic actions

Decreases sebaceous gland size and inhibits sebaceous gland differentiation, resulting in a reduction in sebum secretion; inhibits follicular keratinization; exact mechanism of action is not known.

### Indications

- Treatment of severe recalcitrant cystic acne unresponsive to conventional treatments
- Unlabeled uses: treatment of cutaneous disorders of keratinization; cutaneous T-cell lymphoma and leukoplakia

### Contraindications/cautions

- Contraindications: allergy to isotretinoin, parabens, or product component; pregnancy (has caused severe fetal malformations and spontaneous abortions); lactation.
- Use cautiously with diabetes mellitus.

### Dosage

**Available Forms:** Capsules—10, 20, 40 mg

Individualize dosage based on side effects and disease response.

***Initial dose:*** 0.5–1 mg/kg per day PO; usual dosage range is 0.5–2 mg/kg per day divided into 2 doses for 15–20 wk. Maximum daily dose: 2 mg/kg. If a second course of therapy is needed, allow a rest period of at least 8 wk between courses.

### Pharmacokinetics

| *Route* | *Onset* | *Peak* | *Duration* |
|---|---|---|---|
| Oral | Varies | 2.9–3.2 h | 6–20 h |

*Metabolism:* Hepatic; $T_{1/2}$: 10–20 h
*Distribution:* Crosses placenta; may enter breast milk
*Excretion:* Urine

### Adverse effects

- CNS: *Lethargy, insomnia, fatigue, headache,* pseudotumor cerebri (papilledema, headache, nausea, vomiting, visual disturbances)
- GI: *Nausea, vomiting, abdominal pain,* anorexia, inflammatory bowel disease

- **Respiratory**: *Epistaxis, dry nose, dry mouth*
- **Hematologic**: *Elevated sedimentation rate, hypertriglyceridemia,* abnormal liver function tests, increased fasting serum glucose
- **GU**: *White cells in the urine, proteinuria, hematuria*
- **MS**: Skeletal hyperostosis, arthralgia, bone and joint pain and stiffness
- **EENT**: *Cheilitis, eye irritation, conjunctivitis,* corneal opacities
- **Dermatologic**: *Skin fragility, dry skin, pruritus, rash,* thinning of hair, peeling of palms and soles, skin infections, photosensitivity, nail brittleness, petechiae

### Clinically important drug-drug interactions

- Increased toxicity when taken with vitamin A; avoid this combination

## ■ Nursing Considerations

### Assessment

- *History:* Allergy to isotretinoin, parabens or product component; diabetes mellitus; pregnancy; lactation
- *Physical:* Skin color, lesions, turgor, texture; joints—range of motion; orientation, reflexes, affect, ophthalmologic exam; mucous membranes, bowel sounds; serum triglycerides, HDL, sedimentation rate, CBC and differential, urinalysis, pregnancy test

### Implementation

- Ensure that patient is not pregnant before therapy; test for pregnancy within 2 wk of beginning therapy. Advise patient to use contraception during treatment and for 1 mo after treatment is discontinued.
- Do not give a second course of therapy within 8 wk of first course.
- Give drug with meals; do not crush capsules.
- Do not give vitamin supplements that contain vitamin A.
- Discontinue drug if signs of papilledema occur; consult with a neurologist for further care.
- Discontinue drug if visual disturbances occur; arrange for an ophthalmologic exam.
- Discontinue drug if abdominal pain, rectal bleeding, or severe diarrhea occurs; consult with physician.
- Monitor triglycerides during therapy; if elevation occurs, institute measures to lower serum triglycerides: reduce weight, reduce dietary fat, exercise, increase intake of insoluble fiber, decrease alcohol consumption.
- Monitor diabetic patients with frequent bood glucose determinations.
- Do not allow blood donation from patients taking isotretinoin due to the teratogenic effects of the drug.

### Drug-specific teaching points

- Take drug with meals; do not crush capsules.
- Transient flare-ups of acne may occur at beginning of therapy.
- Use contraception during treatment and for 1 mo after treatment is discontinued. This drug has been associated with severe birth defects and miscarriages; it is contraindicated in pregnant women. If you think that you have become pregnant, consult your physician immediately.
- Do not donate blood while on this drug because of its potential effects on the fetus of a blood recipient.
- The following side effects may occur: dizziness, lethargy, headache, visual changes (avoid driving or performing tasks that require alertness); sensitivity to the sun (avoid sunlamps, exposure to the sun; use sunscreens, protective clothing); diarrhea, abdominal pain, loss of appetite (take drug with meals); dry mouth (sucking sugarless lozenges may help); eye irritation and redness, inability to wear contact lenses; dry skin, itching, redness.
- Avoid vitamin supplements containing vitamin A; serious toxic effects may occur. Limit your consumption of alcohol. You also may need to limit your intake of fats and increase exercise to limit drug effects on blood triglyceride levels.

- Report headache with nausea and vomiting, severe diarrhea or rectal bleeding, visual difficulties.

## isradipine

*(eyes* ***rad'*** *i peen)*

DynaCirc, DynaCirc CR

**Pregnancy Category C**

### Drug classes

Calcium channel blocker
Antihypertensive

### Therapeutic actions

Inhibits the movement of calcium ions across the membranes of cardiac and arterial muscle cells; calcium is involved in the generation of the action potential in specialized automatic and conducting cells in the heart and in arterial smooth muscle and excitation-contraction coupling in cardiac muscle cells; inhibition of transmembrane calcium flow results in the depression of impulse formation in specialized cardiac pacemaker cells, slowing of the velocity of conduction of the cardiac impulse, the depression of myocardial contractility, and the dilation of coronary arteries and arterioles and peripheral arterioles. These effects lead to decreased cardiac work, cardiac energy consumption, and blood pressure.

### Indications

- Management of hypertension alone or in combination with thiazide-type diuretics

### Contraindications/cautions

- Contraindications: allergy to isradipine; sick sinus syndrome, except in presence of ventricular pacemaker; heart block (second or third degree); IHSS; cardiogenic shock, severe CHF; pregnancy; lactation.
- Use cautiously with hypotension, impaired hepatic or renal function (repeated doses may accumulate).

### Dosage

**Available Forms:** Capsules—2.5, 5 mg

*ADULT:* Initial dose of 2.5 mg PO bid. An antihypertensive effect is usually seen within 2–3h; maximal response may require 2–4 wk. Dosage may be increased in increments of 5 mg/d at 2- to 4-wk intervals. Maximum dose: 20 mg/d. CR: 5 mg PO qd as monotherapy or combined with thiazide diuretic.

### Pharmacokinetics

| *Route* | *Onset* | *Peak* |
|---|---|---|
| Oral | 40 min | 1 1/2 h |

*Metabolism:* Hepatic; $T_{1/2}$: 8 h
*Distribution:* Crosses placenta; enters breast milk
*Excretion:* Urine

### Adverse effects

- CNS: *Dizziness,* vertigo, emotional depression, sleepiness, *headache*
- GI: *Nausea,* constipation
- CV: *Peripheral edema, hypotension,* arrhythmias, bradycardia, **AV heart block, angina, MI, stroke** (increased risk with isradipine than with other calcium channel blockers)
- Other: Muscle fatigue, diaphoresis

### Clinically important drug-drug interactions

• Increased cardiac depression with beta-adrenergic blocking agents • Increased serum levels of digoxin, carbamazepine, prazosin, quinidine • Increased respiratory depression with atracurium, gallamine, metocurine, pancuronium, tubocurarine, vecuronium • Decreased effects with calcium, rifampin

## ■ Nursing Considerations

### Assessment

- *History:* Allergy to isradipine; sick sinus syndrome, heart block; IHSS; cardiogenic shock, severe CHF; hypotension; impaired hepatic or renal function; pregnancy; lactation
- *Physical:* Skin color, edema; orientation, reflexes; P, BP, baseline ECG, peripheral perfusion, auscultation; R, adventitious sounds; liver evaluation, normal output; liver and renal function tests, urinalysis

### Implementation

- Consider increased risk of angina, MI, stroke with use of this drug; select patients carefully.
- Monitor patient carefully (BP, cardiac rhythm, and output) while drug is being titrated to therapeutic dose.
- Monitor BP very carefully with concurrent doses of other antihypertensive drugs.
- Monitor cardiac rhythm regularly during stabilization of dosage and periodically during long-term therapy.
- Monitor patients with renal or hepatic impairment carefully for drug accumulation and adverse reactions.

### Drug-specific teaching points

- The following side effects may occur: nausea, vomiting (small, frequent meals may help); headache (monitor lighting, noise, and temperature; medication may be ordered if severe); dizziness, sleepiness (avoid driving or operating dangerous equipment); emotional depression (should pass when the drug is stopped); constipation (measures may be taken to alleviate this problem).
- Report irregular heart beat, shortness of breath, swelling of the hands or feet, pronounced dizziness, constipation.

## itraconazole

*(eye tra **kon'** a zole)*

Sporanox

**Pregnancy Category C**

### Drug classes

Antifungal

### Therapeutic actions

Binds to sterols in the fungal cell membrane, changing membrane permeability; fungicidal or fungistatic depending on concentration and organism.

### Indications

- Treatment of blastomycosis, histoplasmosis in immunocompromised and nonimmunocompromised patients
- Treatment of aspergillosis in patients intolerant to amphotericin B
- Treatment of onychomycosis due to dermatophytes
- Treatment of fungal infections of the esophagus or mouth
- Unlabeled uses: treatment of superficial and systemic mycoses, fungal keratitis, cutaneous leishmaniasis

### Contraindications/cautions

- Contraindications: hypersensitivity to itraconazole or other azoles, lactation.
- Use cautiously with hepatic impairment.

### Dosage

**Available Forms:** Capsules—100 mg; solution—100 mg/ml

ADULT: 200 mg PO qd. If no obvious improvement, increase dose in 100-mg increments to a maximum of 400 mg qd. Give doses > 200 mg/d in divided doses. Continue treatment for a minimum of 3 mo and until clinical parameters and laboratory tests indicate that the active fungal infection has subsided.

- ***Life-threatening infections:*** Loading dose of 200 mg PO tid for the first 3 d.
- ***Fingernail onychomycosis:*** 200 mg bid PO for 1 wk, followed by 3-wk rest period; repeat.
- ***Oral solution:*** Rinse and hold, swallow solution; tid for 3–5 days

PEDIATRIC: Safety and efficacy not established.

### Pharmacokinetics

| *Route* | *Onset* | *Peak* | *Duration* |
|---|---|---|---|
| Oral | Slow | 4.6 h | 4–6 d |

*Metabolism:* Hepatic; $T_{1/2}$: 21 h, then 64 h
*Distribution:* Crosses placenta; may enter breast milk
*Excretion:* Urine

### Adverse effects

- CNS: *Headache,* dizziness
- GI: *Nausea, vomiting, diarrhea, abdominal pain,* abdominal pain, anorexia
- Other: *Skin rash, edema,* fever, malaise

**Clinically important drug-drug interactions**

• Increased serum levels and therefore therapeutic and toxic effects of cyclosporine, digoxin, oral hypoglycemics, warfarin anticoagulants, terfenadine, phenytoin • Decreased serum levels with $H_2$ antagonists, isoniazid, phenytoin, rifampin • Potential for serious CV events with lovastatin, simvastatin, terfenadine, astemizole, cisapride, triazolam, midazolam; avoid these combintions

## ■ Nursing Considerations

### Assessment

- *History:* Hypersensitivity to itraconazole, hepatic impairment, lactation
- *Physical:* Skin color, lesions; T; orientation, reflexes, affect; bowel sounds; hepatic function tests; culture of area involved

### Implementation

- Culture of infection before beginning therapy; begin treatment before laboratory results are returned.
- Decrease dosage in cases of hepatic failure.
- Give drug with meals to facilitate absorption.
- Monitor hepatic function tests regularly in patients with a history of hepatic dysfunction; discontinue or decrease dosage at signs of increased renal toxicity.
- Discontinue drug at any sign of active liver disease—elevated enzymes, hepatitis.

### Drug-specific teaching points

- Take the full course of drug therapy that has been prescribed. Therapy may need to be long term.
- Take drug with food.
- Adopt hygiene measures to prevent reinfection or spread of infection.
- Have frequent follow-up while you are on this drug. Keep all appointments, which may include blood tests.
- The following side effects may occur: nausea, vomiting, diarrhea (small frequent meals may help); headache (analgesics may be ordered); rash, itching (appropriate medication may help).
- Report unusual fatigue, anorexia, vomiting, jaundice, dark urine, pale stool.

# ivermectin

*(eye ver* ***mek'*** *tin)*

Stromectol

**Pregnancy Category C**

**Drug classes**

Anthelmintic

**Therapeutic actions**

Semisynthetic broad-spectrum antiparasitic agent; binds to chloride channels in nerve and muscle cells, leading to increased cell permeability, hyperpolarization of the nerve or muscle, paralysis and death of the parasite.

**Indications**

- Treatment of intestinal strongyloidiasis caused by the nematode parasite *Strongyloides stercoralis*
- Treatment of onchocerciasis caused by the nematode parasite *Onchocerca volvulus*

**Contraindications/cautions**

- Contraindications: hypersensitivity to any component of the drug; pregnancy (embryotoxic and teratogenic in preclinical studies; avoid use in pregnancy), lactation.
- Use cautiously with ophthalmologic conditions.

### Dosage

Available Forms: Tablets—6 mg

ADULT

- ***Strongyloidosis:*** Single oral dose of 200 μg/kg.
- ***Onchocerciasis:*** Single oral dose of 150 μg/kg; may be retreated in 3–12 mo as needed.

PEDIATRIC: Safety and efficacy for use in children < 33 lbs not established.

**Pharmacokinetics**

| Route | Onset | Peak |
|---|---|---|
| Oral | Gradual | 4 h |

*Metabolism:* Hepatic; $T_{1/2}$: 16 h
*Distribution:* Crosses placenta; passes into breast milk
*Excretion:* Feces

### Adverse effects

*Strongyloidiasis*

- CNS: Dizziness, tremors, somnolence, vertigo
- GI: Diarrhea, nausea, anorexia, constipation, vomiting
- **Dermatologic**: Pruritus, rash, urticaria
- **Other**: Fatigue, abdominal pain

*Onchocerciasis*

- EENT: Limbitis, punctate opacities
- **Dermatologic**: *Mazzotti reaction* (rash, pruitus, fever, edema, lymph node enlargement and tenderness)
- **Other**: Headache, tachycardia, myalgia

## ■ Nursing Considerations

### Assessment

- ***History:*** Allergy to ivermectin; pregnancy, lactation, ophthalmic impairment
- ***Physical:*** T; orientation; skin color, lesions; reflexes, affect; eye exam

### Implementation

- Obtain stool specimens to determine accurate diagnosis and baseline levels of parasites.
- Administer drug with water.
- Perform follow-up stool examinations to determine eradication of parasite; retreatment may be done as early as 3 months if necessary.
- Offer supportive care to patients experience ophthalmic or dermatologic reaction.

### Drug-specific teaching points

- Take this drug with water. Follow-up stool examinations will be needed to ensure that the parasite has been eradicated. Treatment for onchocerciasis will require repeating as it does not kill the adult parasite.
- This drug can cause serious fetal harm; do not take this drug while you are pregnant. Use of a barrier contraceptive is recommended during and for 1 month after therapy with this drug.
- The following side effects may occur: nausea, vomiting (eat small, frequent meals); dizziness (avoid driving or operating dangerous machinery); skin rash and swelling (discuss skin care with health care provider).
- Report fever, pregnancy, severe swelling, visual changes, difficulty breathing.

## kanamycin sulfate

***(kan a mye' sin)***
Anamid (CAN), Kantrex
**Pregnancy Category C**

### Drug classes

Aminoglycoside antibiotic

### Therapeutic actions

Bactericidal: inhibits protein synthesis in strains of gram-negative bacteria; functional integrity of cell membrane appears to be disrupted, causing cell death.

### Indications

- Infections caused by susceptible strains of *E. coli, Proteus, Enterobacter aerogenes, Klebsiella pneumoniae, Serratia marcescens, Acinetobacter*
- Treatment of severe infections due to susceptible strains of staphylococci in patients allergic to other antibiotics
- Suppression of GI bacterial flora (oral, adjunctive therapy)
- Hepatic coma, to reduce ammonia-forming bacteria in the GI tract (oral)

### Contraindications/cautions

- Contraindications: allergy to aminoglycosides; intestinal obstruction, pregnancy, lactation.
- Use cautiously with elderly or any patient with diminished hearing, decreased renal function, dehydration, neuromuscular disorders.

### Dosage

**Available Forms:** Injection—500 mg, 1 g; pediatric injection—75 mg

ADULT OR PEDIATRIC

- ***IM:*** 7.5 mg/kg q12h or 15 mg/kg per day in equally divided doses q6–8h.

Usual duration is 7–10 d. If no effect in 3–5 d, discontinue therapy. *Do not exceed 1.5 g/d.*

- ***IV:*** 15 mg/kg per day divided into 2 to 3 equal doses, administered slowly.
- ***Intraperitoneal:*** 500 mg diluted in 20 ml sterile water instilled into the wound closure.
- ***Aerosol:*** 250 mg bid–qid, nebulized.
- ***Oral***
  - *Suppression of intestinal bacteria:* 1 g every hour for 4 h followed by 1 g q6h for 36–72 h.
  - *Hepatic coma:* 8–12 g/d in divided doses PO.

GERIATRIC OR RENAL FAILURE PATIENTS: Reduce dosage, and carefully monitor serum drug levels and renal function tests. When not possible, reduce frequency of administration. Calculate dosage formula from the following: dosage interval in h serum creatinine (mg/100 ml) × 9.

### Pharmacokinetics

| *Route* | *Onset* | *Peak* |
|---|---|---|
| IM/IV | Rapid | 30–120 min |
| PO | Slow; not absorbed systemically | |

*Metabolism:* $T_{1/2}$: 2–3 h
*Distribution:* Crosses placenta; enters breast milk
*Excretion:* Urine

### IV facts

**Preparation:** Do not mix with other antibacterial agents; administer separately; dilute contents of 500-mg vial with 100–200 ml of Normal Saline or 5% Dextrose in Water; dilute 1 g-vial with 200–400 ml of diluent; vials may darken during storage, does not effect potency.
**Infusion:** Administer dose slowly over 30–60 min (especially important in children).

### Adverse effects

Although oral kanamycin is only negligibly absorbed from the intact GI mucosa, there is a risk of absorption from ulcerated areas or when used as an irrigant or aerosol.

- CNS: *Ototoxicity—tinnitus, dizziness, vertigo, deafness (partially reversible to irreversible),* confusion, disorientation, depression, lethargy, nystagmus, visual disturbances, headache, fever, numbness, tingling, tremor, paresthesias, muscle twitching, convulsions, muscular weakness, neuromuscular blockade, apnea
- GI: *Nausea, vomiting, anorexia, diarrhea,* weight loss, stomatitis, increased salivation, splenomegaly, malabsorption syndrome
- CV: Palpitations, hypotension, hypertension
- **Hematologic**: Leukemoid reaction, agranulocytosis, granulocytosis, leukopenia, leukocytosis, thrombocytopenia, eosinophilia, pancytopenia, anemia, hemolytic anemia, increased or decreased reticulocyte count, electrolyte disturbances
- GU: *Nephrotoxicity*
- **Hypersensitivity**: Purpura, rash, urticaria, exfoliative dermatitis, itching
- **Hepatic**: Hepatic toxicity; hepatomegaly
- **Other**: *Superinfections, pain and irritation at IM injection sites*

### Clinically important drug-drug interactions

• Increased ototoxic and nephrotoxic effects with potent diuretics and other ototoxic and nephrotoxic drugs (cephalosporins, penicillins) • Increased likelihood of neuromuscular blockade if given shortly after general anesthetics, depolarizing and nondepolarizing neuromuscular junction blockers, succinylcholine • Decreased absorption and therapeutic levels of digoxin with kanamycin

## ■ Nursing Considerations

### Assessment

- *History:* Allergy to aminoglycosides; intestinal obstruction, lactation, diminished hearing, decreased renal function, dehydration, neuromuscular disorders
- *Physical:* Site of infection, skin color, lesions; orientation, reflexes, eighth cranial nerve function; P, BP; R, adventitious

sounds; bowel sounds, liver evaluation; urinalysis, BUN, serum creatinine, serum electrolytes, liver function tests, CBC

### Implementation

- Arrange culture and sensitivity tests on infection before beginning therapy.
- Monitor length of treatment: usual duration 7–10 d. If clinical response does not occur within 3–5 d, stop therapy. Prolonged treatment risks increased toxicity. If drug is used longer than 10 d, monitor auditory and renal function daily.
- Give IM dosage by deep IM injection in upper outer quadrant of the gluteal muscle.
- Ensure that patient is well hydrated before and during therapy.

### Drug-specific teaching points

- Complete the full course of drug therapy.
- The following side effects may occur: ringing in the ears, headache, dizziness (reversible; use safety); nausea, vomiting, loss of appetite (small frequent meals, frequent mouth care may help).
- Report severe headache, dizziness, loss of hearing, severe diarrhea.

## ketoconazole

*(kee toe **koe'** na zole)*
Nizoral
**Pregnancy Category C**

### Drug classes

Antifungal

### Therapeutic actions

Impairs the synthesis of ergosterol, the main sterol of fungal cell membranes, allowing increased permeability and leakage of cellular components and causing cell death.

### Indications

- Treatment of systemic fungal infections: candidiasis, chronic mucocutaneous candidiasis, oral thrush, candiduria, blastomycosis, coccidioidomycosis, histoplasmosis, chromomycosis, paracoccidioidomycosis
- Treatment of dermatophytosis (recalcitrant infections not responding to topical or griseofulvin therapy)
- Unlabeled uses: treatment of onychomycosis, pityriasis versicolor, vaginal candidiasis; CNS fungal infections at high doses (800–1,200 mg/d); treatment of advanced prostate cancer at doses of 400 mg q8h
- Topical treatment of tinea corporis and tinea cruris caused by *Trichophyton rubrum, Trichophyton mentagrophytes*, and *Epidermophyton floccosum* and the treatment of tinea versicolor caused by *Malassezia furfur* (topical administration)
- Reduction of scaling due to dandruff (shampoo)
- Orphan drug use: with cyclosporine to diminish cyclosporine-induced nephrotoxicity in organ transplant

### Contraindications/cautions

- Contraindications: allergy to ketoconazole; fungal meningitis; pregnancy; lactation.
- Use cautiously with hepatocellular failure (increased risk of hepatocellular necrosis).

### Dosage

**Available Forms:** Tablets—200 mg; topical cream—2%; shampoo—2%

**ADULT:** 200 mg PO, qd. Up to 400 mg/d in severe infections. Treatment period must be long enough to prevent recurrence, 3 wk–6 mo, depending on infecting organism and site.

**PEDIATRIC:** *>2 y:* 3.3–6.6 mg/kg per day PO as a single dose. Apply topical cream once daily to affected area and surrounding area. Severe cases may be treated twice daily. Continue treatment for at least 2 wk. *<2 y:* Safety and efficacy not established.

***Topical cream:*** Apply once daily to affected area and immediate surrounding area. Severe cases may be treated twice daily. Continue treatment for at least 2 wk.

***Shampoo:*** Moisten hair and scalp thoroughly with water; apply sufficient shampoo to produce a lather; gently massage for 1 min; rinse hair with warm water; repeat, leaving on hair for 3 min. Shampoo twice a week for 4 wk with at least 3 d between shampooing.

**Pharmacokinetics**

| *Route* | *Onset* | *Peak* |
|---|---|---|
| Oral | Varies | 1–4 h |
| Topical | Slow; not appreciably systemically absorbed | |

*Metabolism:* Hepatic; $T_{1/2}$: 8 h
*Distribution:* Crosses placenta; enters breast milk
*Excretion:* Bile

**Adverse effects**

- CNS: Headache, dizziness, somnolence, photophobia
- GI: Hepatotoxicity, *nausea, vomiting,* abdominal pain
- GU: Impotence, oligospermia (with very high doses)
- **Hematologic**: Thrombocytopenia, leudopenia, hemolytic anemia
- **Hypersensitivity**: Urticaria to anaphylaxis
- General: *Pruritus,* fever, chills, gynecomastia
- Local: *Severe irritation, pruritus, stinging* with topical application

**Clinically important drug-drug interactions**

• Decreased blood levels of ketoconazole with rifampin • Increased blood levels of cyclosporine and risk of toxicity • Increased duration of adrenal suppression with methylprednisolone, corticosteroids

## ■ Nursing Considerations

### Assessment

- *History:* Allergy to ketoconazole, fungal meningitis, hepatocellular failure, pregnancy, lactation
- *Physical:* Skin color, lesions; orientation, reflexes, affect; bowel sounds, liver evaluation; liver function tests; CBC and differential; culture of area involved

### Implementation

- Culture fungus prior to therapy; begin treatment before return of laboratory results.
- Maintain epinephrine on standby in case of severe anaphylaxis after first dose.
- Administer oral drug with food to decrease GI upset.
- Do not administer with antacids; ketoconazole requires an acid environment for absorption; if antacids are required, administer at least 2 h apart.
- Continue administration for long-term therapy until infection is eradicated: candidiasis, 1–2 wk; other systemic mycoses, 6 mo; chronic mucocutaneous candidiasis, often requires maintainance therapy; tinea veriscolor, 2 wk of topical application.
- Stop treatment, and consult physician about diagnosis if no improvement is seen within 2 wk of topical application.
- Discontinue topical applications if sensitivity or chemical reaction occurs.
- Administer shampoo as follows: moisten hair and scalp thoroughly with water; apply sufficient shampoo to produce a lather; gently massage for 1 min; rinse hair with warm water; repeat, leaving on hair for 3 min.
- Arrange to monitor hepatic function tests before therapy and monthly or more frequently throughout treatment.

### Drug-specific teaching points

- Take the full course of drug therapy. Long-term use of the drug will be needed; beneficial effects may not be seen for several weeks.
- Take oral drug with meals to decrease GI upset.
- Apply topical drug to affected area and surrounding area.
- If using shampoo, moisten hair and scalp thoroughly with water; apply sufficient shampoo to produce a lather; gently massage for 1 min; rinse hair with warm water; repeat, leaving on hair for 3 min. Shampoo twice a week for 4 wk with at least 3 d between shampooing.
- Use appropriate hygiene measures to prevent reinfection or spread of infection.
- The following side effects may occur: nausea, vomiting, diarrhea (take drug

k

with food); sedation, dizziness, confusion (avoid driving or performing tasks that require alertness); stinging, irritation (local application).
- Do not take antacids with this drug; if they are needed, take this drug at least 2 h after their administration.
- Report skin rash, severe nausea, vomiting, diarrhea, fever, sore throat, unusual bleeding or bruising, yellow skin or eyes, dark urine or pale stools, severe irritation (local application).

# ketoprofen

*(kee toe **proe'** fen)*

Actron caplets, Orudis, Orudis KT, Oruvail (SR)

**Pregnancy Category B**

## Drug classes

NSAID
Non-narcotic analgesic

## Therapeutic actions

Anti-inflammatory and analgesic activity; inhibits prostaglandin and leukotriene synthesis and has antibradykinin and lysosomal membrane-stabilizing actions.

## Indications

- Acute and long-term treatment of signs and symptoms of rheumatoid arthritis and osteoarthritis (capsules or sustained release—Oruvail)
- Relief of mild to moderate pain
- Treatment of dysmenorrhea
- Reduction of fever
- OTC use: temporary relief of minor aches and pains

## Contraindications/cautions

- Contraindications: significant renal impairment, pregnancy, lactation.
- Use cautiously with impaired hearing, allergies, hepatic, CV, and GI conditions

## Dosage

**Available Forms:** Tablets—12.5 mg; capsules—25, 50, 75 mg; ER capsules—100, 150, 200 mg

Do not exceed 300 mg/d.

**ADULT**

- ***Rheumatoid arthritis, osteoarthritis:*** Starting dose: 75 mg tid or 50 mg qid PO. Maintenance dose: 150–300 mg PO in 3 to 4 divided doses. Oruvail, 200 mg PO qd.
- ***Mild to moderate pain, primary dysmenorrhea:*** 25–50 mg PO q6–8h as needed. Do not use Oruvail.
- ***OTC:*** 12.5 mg PO q4–6h; do not exceed 25 mg in 4–6 h or 75 mg in 24 h.

**PEDIATRIC:** Safety and efficacy not established.

**GERIATRIC OR HEPATIC OR RENAL IMPAIRED:** Reduce starting dose by one-half or one-third. Do not use Oruvail.

## Pharmacokinetics

| *Route* | *Onset* | *Peak* |
|---|---|---|
| Oral | 30–60 min | 0.5–2 h |

*Metabolism:* Hepatic; $T_{1/2}$: 2–4 h
*Distribution:* Crosses placenta; enters breast milk
*Excretion:* Urine.

## Adverse effects

*NSAIDs*

- CNS: *Headache, dizziness, somnolence, insomnia,* fatigue, tiredness, dizziness, tinnitus, ophthalmologic effects
- GI: *Nausea, dyspepsia, GI pain,* diarrhea, vomiting, *constipation,* flatulence
- Respiratory: Dyspnea, hemoptysis, pharyngitis, bronchospasm, rhinitis
- Hematologic: Bleeding, platelet inhibition with higher doses, neutropenia, eosinophilia, leukopenia, pancytopenia, thrombocytopenia, agranulocytosis, granulocytopenia, aplastic anemia, decreased Hgb or Hct, bone marrow depression, menorrhagia
- GU: Dysuria, **renal impairment**
- Dermatologic: *Rash*, pruritus, sweating, dry mucous membranes, stomatitis
- Other: Peripheral edema, **anaphylactoid reactions to fatal anaphylactic shock**

## ■ Nursing Considerations

### Assessment

- *History:* Renal impairment, impaired hearing, allergies, hepatic, CV, and GI conditions, lactation
- *Physical:* Skin color and lesions; orientation, reflexes, ophthalmologic and audiometric evaluation, peripheral sensation; P, edema; R, adventitious sounds; liver evaluation; CBC, clotting times, renal and liver function tests; serum electrolytes, stool guaiac

### Implementation

- Administer drug with food or after meals if GI upset occurs.
- Arrange for periodic ophthalmologic examination during long-term therapy.
- Institute emergency procedures if overdose occurs: gastric lavage, induction of emesis, supportive therapy.

### Drug-specific teaching points

- Take drug with food or meals if GI upset occurs; take only the prescribed dosage.
- Dizziness, drowsiness can occur (avoid driving or the use of dangerous machinery).
- Report sore throat, fever, rash, itching, weight gain, swelling in ankles or fingers; changes in vision; black, tarry stools.

## ketorolac tromethamine

*(**kee'** toe role ak)*

Acular (ophthalmic), Toradol

**Pregnancy Category B**

### Drug classes

NSAID

Non-narcotic analgesic

### Therapeutic actions

Anti-inflammatory and analgesic activity; inhibits prostaglandins and leukotriene synthesis.

### Indications

- Short-term management of pain
- Relief of ocular itching due to seasonal conjunctivitis (ophthalmic)

### Contraindications/cautions

- Contraindications: significant renal impairment, pregnancy, lactation; patients wearing soft contact lenses (ophthalmic).
- Use cautiously with impaired hearing, allergies, hepatic, CV, and GI conditions.

### Dosage

**Available Forms:** Ophthalmic solution—0.5%; tablets—10 mg; injection—15, 30 mg/ml

For short-term use only (up to 5 days). Potent NSAID with many adverse affects.

*ADULT:* Initial dosage: 30–60 mg IM, as a loading dose, followed by half of the loading dose q6h as long as needed to control pain. Maximum total dose: 150 mg for the first day and 120 mg qd thereafter.

- ***Oral:*** 10 mg PO q4–6h as needed; maximum daily dose: 40 mg.
- ***Transition from IM to oral:*** Do not exceed total combined dose of 120 mg on day of transition.
- ***Ophthalmic:*** 1 drop (0.25 mg) qid.
- ***IV:*** Single dose of 30mg given over no less than 15 sec.

*PEDIATRIC:* Safety and efficacy not established.

*GERIATRIC:* Use the lower recommended dosage range for patients < 110 lb, older than 65 y, or with reduced renal function.

### Pharmacokinetics

| Route | Onset | Peak | Duration |
|---|---|---|---|
| Oral | Varies | 1/2–1 h | 6 h |
| IM/IV | 30 min | 1–2 h | 6 h |

*Metabolism:* Hepatic; $T_{1/2}$: 2.4–8.6 h

*Distribution:* Crosses placenta; enters breast milk

*Excretion:* Urine

### IV facts

**Preparation:** No further preparation is required.

**Infusion:** Infuse slowly as a bolus over no less than 15 sec.

**Incompatibilities:** Do not mix with morphine, sulfate, meperidine, promethazine or hydroxyzine; a precipitate will form.

k

**Adverse effects**

*NSAIDs*

- CNS: *Headache, dizziness, somnolence, insomnia,* fatigue, tiredness, dizziness, tinnitus, ophthamological effects
- GI: *Nausea, dyspepsia, GI pain,* diarrhea, vomiting, *constipation,* flatulence
- Respiratory: Dyspnea, hemoptysis, pharyngitis, bronchospasm, rhinitis
- Hematologic: Bleeding, platelet inhibition with higher doses, neutropenia, eosinophilia, leukopenia, pancytopenia, thrombocytopenia, agranulocytosis, granulocytopenia, aplastic anemia, decreased Hgb or Hct, bone marrow depression, menorrhagia
- GU: Dysuria, **renal impairment**
- Dermatologic: *Rash,* pruritus, sweating, dry mucous membranes, stomatitis
- Other: Peripheral edema, **anaphylactoid reactions to fatal anaphylactic shock**, *local burning, stinging* (ophthalmic)

## ■ Nursing Considerations

### Assessment

- *History:* Renal impairment; impaired hearing; allergies; hepatic, CV, and GI conditions; lactation
- *Physical:* Skin color and lesions; orientation, reflexes, ophthalmologic and audiometric evaluation, peripheral sensation; P, edema; R, adventitious sounds; liver evaluation; CBC, clotting times, renal and liver function tests; serum electrolytes, stool guaiac

### Implementation

- Maintain emergency equipment on standby at time of initial dose, in case of severe hypersensitivity reaction.
- Protect drug vials from light.
- Administer every 6 h to maintain serum levels and control pain.

### Drug-specific teaching points

- Every effort will be made to administer the drug on time to control pain; dizziness, drowsiness can occur (avoid driving or using dangerous machinery); burning and stinging on application (ophthalmic).
- Report sore throat, fever, rash, itching, weight gain, swelling in ankles or fingers; changes in vision; black, tarry stools.

# labetalol hydrochloride

*(la **bet'** a lol)*

Normodyne, Trandate

**Pregnancy Category C**

**Drug classes**

Alpha/Beta adrenergic blocker

Antihypertensive

**Therapeutic actions**

Competetively blocks $\alpha_1$ and $\beta_1$- and $\beta_2$-adrenergic receptors, and has some sympathomimetic activity at $\beta_2$-receptors. Alpha- and beta-blocking actions contribute to the BP-lowering effect; beta blockade prevents the reflex tachycardia seen with most alpha-blocking drugs and decreases plasma renin activity.

**Indications**

- Hypertension, alone or with other oral drugs, especially diuretics
- Severe hypertension (parenteral preparations)
- Unlabeled uses—control of BP in pheochromocytoma; clonidine withdrawal hypertension

**Contraindications/cautions**

- Contraindications: sinus bradycardia, second or third-degree heart block, cardiogenic shock, CHF, asthma, pregnancy, lactation.
- Use cautiously with diabetes or hypoglycemia (can mask cardiac signs of hypoglycemia), nonallergic bronchospasm (oral drug—IV is absolutely contraindicated), pheochromocytoma (paradoxical increases in BP have occurred).

### Dosage

**Available Forms:** Tablets—100, 200, 300 mg; injection—5 mg/ml

ADULT

- ***Oral:*** Initial dose 100 mg bid. After 2–3 d, using standing BP as indicator, titrate dosage in increments of 100 mg bid q2–3 d. *Maintenance:* 200 to 400 mg bid. Up to 2,400 mg/d may be required; to improve tolerance, divide total daily dose and give tid.

- ***Parenteral (severe hypertension):*** *Repeated IV injection:* 20 mg (0.25 mg/kg) slowly over 2 min. Individualize dosage using supine BP; additional doses of 40 or 80 mg can be given at 10-min intervals until desired BP is achieved or until a 300 mg dose has been injected. *Continuous IV infusion:* Dilute ampule (below), infuse at the rate of 2 mg/min, adjust according to BP response up to 300 mg total dose. Transfer to oral therapy as soon as possible.

PEDIATRIC: Safety and efficacy not established.

### Pharmacokinetics

| *Route* | *Onset* | *Peak* | *Duration* |
|---|---|---|---|
| Oral | Varies | 1–2 h | 8–12 h |
| IV | Immediate | 5 min | 5.5 h |

*Metabolism* : Hepatic, $T_{1/2}$: 6–8 h
*Distribution* : Crosses placenta; enters breast milk
*Excretion* : Urine

### IV facts

**Preparation:** Add 2 mg (2 ampules) to 160 ml of a compatible IV fluid to make a 1 mg/ml solution; infuse at 2 ml/min, or add 200 mg (2 ampules) to 250 mg of IV fluid. Compatible IV fluids include Ringer's, Lactated Ringer's, 0.9% Sodium Chloride, 2.5% Dextrose and 0.45% Sodium Chloride, 5% Dextrose, 5% Dextrose and Ringer's, 5% Dextrose and 5% Lactated Ringer's, and 5% Dextrose and 0.2%, 0.33%, or 0.9% Sodium Chloride. Stable for 24 h in these solutions at concentrations between 1.25 and 3.75 mg/ml.

**Infusion:** Administer infusion at 3 ml/min; inject slowly over 2 min.

**Compatibilities:** Do not dilute drug in 5% Sodium Bicarbonate Injection.

### Adverse effects

- CNS: *Dizziness, vertigo, tinnitus, fatigue,* emotional depression, paresthesias, sleep disturbances, hallucinations, disorientation, memory loss, slurred speech
- GI: *Gastric pain, flatulence, constipation, diarrhea, nausea, vomiting,* anorexia, ischemic colitis, renal and mesenteric arterial thrombosis, retroperitoneal fibrosis, hepatomegaly, acute pancreatitis
- CV: CHF, cardiac arrhythmias, peripheral vascular insufficiency, claudication, cerebrovascular accident, pulmonary edema, hypotension
- **Respiratory**: *Bronchospasm, dyspnea, cough*, bronchial obstruction, nasal stuffiness, rhinitis, pharyngitis
- GU: *Impotence, decreased libido,* Peyronie's disease, dysuria, nocturia, polyuria
- **EENT**: Eye irritation, dry eyes, conjunctivitis, blurred vision
- **Dermatologic**: Rash, pruritus, sweating, dry skin
- **Other**: *Decreased exercise tolerance,* development of antinuclear antibodies, hyperglycemia or hypoglycemia, elevated liver enzymes

### Clinically important drug-drug interactions

• Risk of excessive hypotension with enflurane, halothane, or isoflurane

### Drug-lab test interferences

• Possible falsely elevated urinary catecholamines in lab tests using a trihydroxyindole reaction • Potential for added anithypertensive effects with nitroglycerin

## ■ Nursing Considerations

### Assessment

- *History:* Sinus bradycardia, second or third-degree heart block, cardiogenic shock, CHF, asthma, pregnancy, lactation, diabetes or hypoglycemia, nonallergic bronchospasm, pheochromocytoma
- *Physical:* Weight, skin condition, neurologic status, P, BP, ECG, respiratory

status, kidney and thyroid function, blood and urine glucose

### Implementation

- Do not discontinue drug abruptly after chronic therapy. (Hypersensitivity to catecholamines may have developed, causing exacerbation of angina, MI and ventricular dysrhythmias; taper drug gradually over 2 wk with monitoring.)
- Consult with physician about withdrawing the drug if the patient is to undergo surgery (withdrawal is controversial).
- Keep patient supine during parenteral therapy, and assist initial ambulation.
- Position to decrease effects of edema.
- Provide support and encouragement to deal with drug effects and disease.

### Drug-specific teaching points

- Take drug with meals.
- Do not stop taking unless instructed to do so by a health care provider.
- The following side effects may occur: dizziness, lightheadedness, loss of appetite, nightmares, depression, sexual impotence.
- Report difficulty breathing, night cough, swelling of extremities, slow pulse, confusion, depression, rash, fever, sore throat.

## lactulose

***(lak' tyoo lose)***

*Laxative:* Chronulac, Constilac, Duphalac

*Ammonia-reducing agent:* Cephulac, Cholac, Enulose, Heptalac

**Pregnancy Category C**

### Drug classes

Laxative
Ammonia reduction agent

### Therapeutic actions

The drug passes unchanged into the colon where bacteria break it down to organic acids that increase the osmotic pressure in the colon and slightly acidify the colonic contents, resulting in an increase in stool water content, stool softening, laxative action, and migration of blood ammonia into the colon contents with subsequent trapping and expulsion in the feces.

### Indications

- Treatment of constipation
- Prevention and treatment of portal-systemic encephalopathy

### Contraindications/cautions

- Contraindications: allergy to lactulose, low-galactose diet.
- Use cautiously with diabetes and lactation.

### Dosage

**Available Forms:** Syrup—10 g/15 ml

**ADULT**

- *Laxative:* 15–30 ml/d PO; may be increased to 60 ml/d as needed.
- *Portal-systemic encephalopathy*
- ***Oral:*** 30–45 ml tid or qid. Adjust dosage every day or two to produce 2–3 soft stools/day. 30–45 ml/h may be used if necessary. Return to standard dose as soon as possible.
- ***Rectal:*** 300 ml lactulose mixed with 700 ml water or physiologic saline as a retention enema, retained for 30–60 min. May be repeated q4–6h. Start oral drug as soon as feasible and before stopping enemas.

**PEDIATRIC**

- *Laxative:* Safety and efficacy not established.
- ***Oral:*** Standards not clearly established. Initial dose of 2.5–10 ml/d in divided dose for small children or 40–90 ml/d for older children is suggested. Attempt to produce 2–3 soft stools daily.

### Pharmacokinetics

| *Route* | *Onset* | *Peak* | *Duration* |
|---|---|---|---|
| Oral | Varies | 20 h | 24–48 h |

Very minimally absorbed systemically

### Adverse effects

- GI: *Transient flatulence, distension, intestinal cramps, belching,* diarrhea, nausea
- Hematologic: Acid–base imbalances

## ■ Nursing Considerations

### Assessment

- *History:* Allergy to lactulose, low-galactose diet, diabetes, lactation
- *Physical:* Abdominal exam, bowel sounds, serum electrolytes, serum ammonia levels

### Implementation

- Do not freeze laxative form. Extremely dark or cloudy syrup may be unsafe; do not use.
- Give laxative syrup orally with fruit juice, water or milk to increase palatability.
- Administer retention enema using a rectal balloon catheter. Do not use cleansing enemas containing soap suds or other alkaline agents that counteract the effects of lactulose.
- Do not administer other laxatives while using lactulose.
- Monitor serum ammonia levels.
- Monitor with long-term therapy for potential electrolyte and acid–base imbalances.

### Drug-specific teaching points

- Do not use other laxatives. The drug may be mixed in water, juice, or milk to make it more tolerable.
- The following side effects may occur: abdominal fullness, flatulence, belching.
- Assure ready access to bathroom; bowel movements will be increased to 2–3 per day.
- Report diarrhea, severe belching, abdominal fullness.

## lamivudine

*(lam ah vew' den)*

3TC

Epivir

**Pregnancy Category C**

### Drug classes

Antiviral

### Therapeutic actions

Nucleoside analogue inhibitor of HIV reverse transcriptase via DNA viral chain termination.

### Indications

- Treatment of HIV infection in combination with zidovudine when therapy is warranted based on clinical or immunological evidence of disease progression; this combination has shown evidence of decreased viral load and increased or maintained CD4 cell counts.

### Contraindications/cautions

- Contraindication: life-threatening allergy to any component, pregnancy, lactation.
- Use cautiously with compromised bone marrow, impaired renal function.

### Dosage

**Available Forms:** Tablets—150 mg; oral solution—10 mg/ml

*ADULTS AND CHILDREN 12–16 Y:* 150 mg PO bid in combination with zidovudine.

*PEDIATRIC:* 3 mo–12 y: 4 mg/kg PO bid; up to a maximum of 150 mg bid.

*RENAL FUNCTION IMPAIRED*

| *Creatinine Clearance (ml/min)* | *Dosage* |
|---|---|
| 50 | 150 mg PO bid |
| 30–49 | 150 mg PO qd |
| 15–29 | 150 mg PO first dose and then 100mg PO qd |
| 5–14 | 150 mg PO first dose and then 50 mg PO qd |
| <5 | 50 mg PO first dose and then 25 mg PO qd |

### Pharmacokinetics

| *Route* | *Onset* | *Peak* |
|---|---|---|
| Oral | Slow | 2–4 h |

*Metabolism:* Unknown; $T_{1/2}$: 5–7 h

*Distribution:* Crosses placenta; passes into breast milk

*Excretion:* Urine

### Adverse effects

- CNS: *Headache*, insomnia, myalgia, *asthenia*, malaise, dizziness, parestesia, somnolence
- GI: *Nausea, GI pain, diarrhea*, anorexia, vomiting, dyspepsia, **pancreatitis** (children)

- Hematologic: *Agranulocytopenia*
- Respiratory: *Nasal signs and symptoms, cough*
- Other: *Fever, rash*, taste perversion

**Clinically important drug-drug interactions**

• Increased serum levels and effectiveness of zidovudine • Increased levels of lamivudine taken concurrently with trimethoprim-sulfamethoxazole

## ■ Nursing Considerations

### Assessment

- *History:* Life-threatening allergy to any component, compromised bone marrow, impaired renal function, pregnancy, lactation
- *Physical:* Skin rashes, lesions, texture; T; affect, reflexes, peripheral sensation; bowel sounds, liver evaluation; renal function tests, CBC and differential

### Implementation

- Arrange to monitor hematologic indices every 2 wk during therapy.
- Monitor children for any sign of pancreatitis and discontinue immediately if it occurs.
- Monitor patient for signs of opportunistic infections that will need to be treated appropriately.
- Administer the drug concurrently with zidovudine (AZT).
- Offer support and encouragement to the patient to deal with the diagnosis as well as the effects of drug therapy and the high expense of treatment.

### Drug-specific teaching points

- Take drug as prescribed; take concurrently with zidovudine (AZT).
- These drugs are not a cure for AIDs or ARC; opportunisitic infections may occur and regular medical care should be sought to deal with the disease.
- Arrange for frequent blood tests, needed during the course of treatment; results of blood counts may indicate a need for decreased dosage or discontinuation of the drug for a period of time.
- The following side effects may occur: nausea, loss of appetite, change in taste (small, frequent meals may help); dizziness, loss of feeling (take appropriate precautions); headache, fever, muscle aches (an analgesic may help, consult with your health care provider).
- Lamivudine does not reduce the risk of transmission of HIV to others by sexual contact or blood contamination—use appropriate precautions.
- Report extreme fatigue, lethargy, severe headache, severe nausea, vomiting, difficulty breathing, skin rash.

# lamotrigine

*(la mo' tri geen)*

Lamictal

**Pregnancy Category C**

**Drug classes**

Antiepileptic agent

**Therapeutic actions**

Mechanism not understood; may inhibit voltage-sensitive sodium channels, stabilizing the neuronal membrane and modulating calcium-dependent presynaptic release of excitatory amino acids.

**Indications**

- Adjuvant therapy in the treatment of partial seizures in adults with epilepsy
- Unlabeled use: generalized tonic-clonic, absence, and myoclonic seizures (adults); Lennox-Gastaut syndrome in infants and children

**Contraindications/cautions**

- Contraindicated in lactation.
- Use cautiously with impaired hepatic, renal or cardiac function.

### Dosage

**Available Forms:** Tablets—25, 100, 150, 200 mg

*ADULT*

- ***Patients taking enzyme-inducing antiepiletic drugs:*** 50 mg PO qd for 2 wk; then 100 mg PO qd in 2 divided doses for 2 wks; may increase by 100 mg/d every wk up to a maintenance dose of 300–500 mg/d in 2 divided doses. *If valproic acid is also being taken*: 25 mg PO every other d for 2 wk; then 25 mg PO qd for 2 wk, then may increase by 25–50 mg every 1-2 wk up to a maintenance dose of 100-150 mg/d PO in 2 divided doses.

PEDIATRIC: Not recommended in children <16 yr.

### Pharmacokinetics

| *Route* | *Onset* | *Peak* |
|---|---|---|
| Oral | Rapid | 2–5 h |

*Metabolism:* Hepatic metabolism; $T_{1/2}$: 29 h

*Distribution* : Crosses placenta; may pass into breast milk

*Excretion* : Urine

### Adverse effects

- CNS: *dizziness*, insomnia, headache, somnolence, *ataxia*, diplopia, blurred vision
- GI: *nausea*, vomiting
- **Dermatologic**: *rash:* potentially life threatening, including Stevens-Johnson syndrome and toxic epidermal necrosis with multiorgan failure

### Clinically important drug-drug interactions

• Rapid elimination of lamotrigine with enzyme-inducing antiepiletic agents: carbamazepine, phenytoin, phenobarbital, primidone • Decreased clearance of lamotrigine, requiring a lower dose, if taken with valproic acid

## ■ Nursing Considerations

### Assessment

- *History:* Lactation; impaired hepatic, renal or cardiac function
- *Physical:* Weight; T; skin color, lesions; orientation, affect, reflexes; P, BP, perfusion; bowel sounds, normal output; liver and renal function tests

### Implementation

- Monitor renal and hepatic function before and periodically during therapy; if abnormal, reevaluate therapy.
- Monitor drug doses carefully when starting therapy and with each increase in dose; special care will be needed when changing the dose or frequency of any other antiepiletic.
- Monitor patient for any sign of rash; discontinue lamotrigine immediately if rash appears and be prepared with appropriate life support if needed.
- Taper drug slowly over a 2 wk period when discontinuing.

### Drug-specific teaching points

- Take this drug exactly as prescribed.
- Do not discontinue this drug abruptly or change dosage, except on the advice of your physician.
- The following side effects may occur: dizziness, drowsiness (avoid driving or performing tasks requiring alertness or visual acuity); GI upset (take drug with food or milk, frequent small meals may help); headache (medication can be ordered).
- Wear a medical ID tag to alert emergency medical personnel that you are an epileptic taking antiepileptic medication.
- Notify health care provider immediately if skin rash occurs.
- Report yellowing of skin, abdominal pain, changes in color of urine or stools, fever, sore throat, mouth sores, unusual bleeding or bruising.

## lanisoprazole

*(lan iz **ah'** pray zol)*

Prevacid

**Pregnancy Category B**

### Drug classes

Antisecretory agent

Protein pump inhibitor

### Therapeutic actions
Gastric acid-pump inhibitor: suppresses gastric acid secretion by specific inhibition of the hydrogen/potassium ATPase enzyme system at the secretory surface of the gastric parietal cells; blocks the final step of acid production.

### Indications
- Short-term treatment of active duodenal ulcer
- Short-term treatment of gastroesophageal reflux disease: severe erosive esophagitis; poorly responsive symptomatic gastroesophageal reflux disease
- Treatment of pathological hypersecretory conditions (e.g. Zollinger-Ellison syndrome, multiple adenomas, systemic mastocytosis) — long term therapy
- Maintenance therapy for healing of erosive esophagitis, duodenal ulcers
- Eradication of H pylori infection in patients with active or recurrent duodenal ulcers in combination with clarithromycin and amoxicillin

### Contraindications/cautions
- Contraindications: hypersensitivity to lanisoprazole or any of its components.
- Use cautiously with pregnancy, lactation.

### Dosage
**Available Forms:** SR capsules—15, 30 mg

ADULT
- *Active duodenal ulcer:* 15 mg PO qd before eating for 4 wk. Maintenance: 13 mg PO qd.
- *Duodenal ulcers associated with H pylori:* 30 mg lanisoprazole, 500 mg clarithromycin, 1 g amoxicillin, all give PO bid for 14 days; or 30 mg lanisoprazole and 1 g amoxicillin PO tid for 14 days.
- *Erosive esophagitis or poorly responsive gastroesophageal reflux disease:* 30 mg PO daily before eating for up to 8 wk. An additional 8 wk course may be helpful for patients who do not heal with 8 wk therapy.
- *Maintenance of healing of erosive esophagitis:* 15 mg/d PO.
- *Pathological hypersecretory conditions:* Individualize dosage. Initial dose is 60 mg PO qd. Doses up to 90 mg bid have been used. Administer daily doses of >120 mg in divided doses.

PEDIATRIC: Safety and efficacy not established.

HEPATIC DYSFUNCTION: Consider lowering dose and monitoring patient response.

### Pharmacokinetics
| *Route* | *Onset* | *Peak* |
|---|---|---|
| Oral | Varies | 1.7 h |

*Metabolism:* Hepatic metabolism; $T_{1/2}$: 2 h
*Distribution:* Crosses placenta; may pass into breast milk
*Excretion:* Bile

### Adverse effects
- GI: *Diarrhea, abdominal pain, nausea, vomiting*, constipation, dry mouth, tongue atrophy
- CNS: *Headache, dizziness*, asthenia, vertigo, insomnia, apathy, anxiety, paresthesias, dream abnormalities
- **Respiratory**: *URI symptoms*, cough, epistaxis
- **Dermatological**: Rash, inflammation, urticaria, pruritus, alopecia, dry skin
- **Other**: Cancer in preclinical studies, back pain, fever

### Clinically important drug-drug interactions
• Decreased serum levels if taken concurrently with sucralfate • Decreased serum levels of ketoconazole, theophylline where taken with lanisoprazole

## ■ Nursing Considerations

### Assessment
- *History:* Hypersensitivity to lanisoprazole or any of its components; pregnancy; lactation
- *Physical:* Skin lesions; body temperature; reflexes, affect; urinary output, abdominal exam; respiratory auscultation

### Implementation
- Administer before meals. Caution patient to swallow capsules whole, not to open,

chew or crush. Open capsule and sprinkle granules on apple sauce if patient cannot swallow capsules; for NG tube, mix granules from capsule with apple juice and inject through tube.

- Arrange for further evaluation of patient after 4 wk of therapy for acute gastroreflux disorders. Symptomatic improvement does not rule out gastric cancer, which did occur in preclinical studies.

### Drug-specific teaching points

- Take the drug before meals. Swallow the capsules whole — do not chew, open or crush. If you are unable to swallow capsule, open and sprinkle granules on apple sauce.
- Arrange to have regular medical follow-up while you are on this drug.
- The following side effects may occur: dizziness (avoid driving a car or performing hazardous tasks); headache (medications may be available to help); nausea, vomiting, diarrhea (proper nutrition is important, consult with your dietician to maintain nutrition); symptoms of upper respiratory tract infection, cough (reversible; do not self-medicate, consult with your health care provider if this becomes uncomfortable).
- Report severe headache, worsening of symptoms, fever, chills.

## letrozole

*(le' tro zol)*

Femara

**Pregnancy Category D**

### Drug classes

Antiestrogen

### Therapeutic actions

Inhibits the conversion of androgens to estrogens by the aromatase enzyme system (in postmenopausal women, the aromatase system is the main source of estrogens); reduces estrogen levels in all tissues, peripheral and cancer tissue.

### Indications

- Treatment of advanced breast cancer in postmenopausal women with disease progression following traditional antiestrogen therapy

### Contraindications/cautions

- Contraindications: allergy to letrozole, pregnancy.
- Use cautiously with hepatic impairment, lactation.

### Dosage

**Available Forms:** Tablets—2.5 mg

*ADULT:* 2.5 mg PO qd; continue until tumor progression is evident.

### Pharmacokinetics

| *Route* | *Onset* | *Peak* |
|---|---|---|
| Oral | Varies | 2–6 wks |

*Metabolism:* Hepatic; $T_{1/2}$: 2 d

*Distribution:* Crosses placenta; may pass into breast milk

*Excretion:* Urine

### Adverse effects

- CNS: *Depression,* headache, fatigue
- GI: *Nausea, GI upset,* elevated liver enzymes
- **Hematologic: Thromobcytopenia,** hypercalcemia
- **Dermatologic:** *Alopecia, hot flashes*
- **Other:** Peripheral edema; arthralgia

## ■ Nursing Considerations

### Assessment

- *History:* Allergy to letrozole, hepatic impairment, pregnancy, lactation
- *Physical:* Skin lesions, color, turgor; orientation, affect, reflexes; peripheral pulses, edema; liver function tests, CBC and differential, estrogen receptor evaluation of tumor cells

### Implementation

- Arrange for perodic blood counts during therapy.
- Counsel patient about the need to use contraceptive measures to avoid pregnancy while taking this drug; inform patient that serious fetal harm could occur.

- Provide comfort measures to help patient deal with drug effects: hot flashes (environmental temperature control); headache, depression (monitoring of light and noise); vaginal bleeding (hygiene measures).
- Discontinue drug at signs that tumor is progressing.

### Drug-specific teaching points

- The following side effects may occur: hot flashes (stay in cool temperatures); nausea, GI upset (eat small, frequent meals); headache, lightheadedness (use caution if driving or performing tasks that require alertness).
- This drug can cause serious fetal harm and must not be taken during pregnancy. Contraceptive measures should be used while you are taking this drug. If you become pregnant or decide that you would like to become pregnant, consult with your physician or nurse immediately.
- Report changes in color of urine or stool, increased fatigue, skin rash, fever, chills, severe depression.

## leucovorin calcium

*(loo koe vor' in)*
citrovorum factor, folinic acid
Wellcovorin
**Pregnancy Category C**

### Drug classes
Folic acid derivative

### Therapeutic actions
Active reduced form of folic acid; required for nucleoprotein synthesis and maintenance of normal erythropoiesis.

### Indications
- "Leucovorin rescue"—after high-dose methotrexate therapy in osteosarcoma
- Treatment of megaloblastic anemias due to sprue, nutritional deficiency, pregnancy, and infancy when oral folic acid therapy is not feasible—parenteral form
- With 5-fluorouracil for palliative treatment of metastatic colorectal cancer

### Contraindications/cautions
- Allergy to leucovorin on previous exposure, pernicious anemia or other megaloblastic anemias in which vitamin $B_{12}$ is deficient, lactation

### Dosage
**Available Forms:** Tablets—5, 15, 25 mg; injection—3 mg/ml; powder for injection—50, 100, 350 mg/vial

ADULT

- *Rescue after methotrexate therapy:* Give 12–15 g/$m^2$ PO or parenterally, followed by 10 mg/$m^2$ PO q6h for 72 h. If at 24 h following methotrexate administration, the serum creatinine is 50% greater than the pretreatment level, increase the leucovorin dose to 100 mg/$m^2$ q3h until the serum methotrexate level is $< 5 \times 10^{-8}$ M. For drugs with less affinity for mammalian dihydrofolate reductase, 5 to 15 mg/d has been used.
- *Megaloblastic anemia:* Up to 1 mg/d IM may be used. Do not exceed 1 mg/d.
- *Metastatic colon cancer:* Give 200 mg/$m^2$ by slow IV injection over 3 min, followed by 5-FU 370 mg/$m^2$ IV *or* 20 mg/$m^2$ IV, followed by 5-FU 425 mg/$m^2$ IV. Repeat daily for 5 d; may be repeated at 4-wk intervals.

### Pharmacokinetics

| Route | Onset | Peak | Durations |
|---|---|---|---|
| Oral | 30 min | 2.4 h | 3–6 h |
| IM | Rapid | 52 min | 3–6 h |
| IV | Immediate | 10 min | 3–6 h |

*Metabolism* : Hepatic, $T_{1/2}$: unknown
*Distribution* : Crosses placenta; enters breast milk
*Excretion* : Urine and feces

### IV facts
**Preparation:** Prepare solution by diluting a 50-mg vial of powder with 5 ml Bacteriostatic Water for Injection, which contains benzyl alcohol, and use within 7 d, or reconstitute with Water for Injection, and use immediately. Protect from light.
**Infusion:** Infuse slowly over 3–5 min; not more than 160 mg/min.

### Adverse effects

- **Hypersensitivity:** Allergic reactions
- **Local:** *Pain and discomfort at injection site*

## ■ Nursing Considerations

### Assessment

- ***History:*** Allergy to leucovorin on previous exposure, pernicious anemia or other megaloblastic anemias, lactation
- ***Physical:*** Skin lesions, color; R, adventitious sounds; CBC, Hgb, Hct, serum folate levels

### Implementation

- Do not use benzyl alcohol solutions when giving leucovorin to premature infants; a fatal gasping syndrome has occurred.
- Begin leucovorin rescue within 24 h of methotrexate administration. Arrange for fluid loading and urine alkalinization during this procedure to decrease methotrexate nephrotoxicity.
- Give drug orally unless intolerance to oral route develops due to nausea and vomiting from chemotherapy or clinical condition. Switch to oral drug when feasible.
- Monitor patient for hypersensitivity reactions, especially if drug has been used previously. Maintain supportive equipment and emergency drugs on standby in case of serious allergic response.

### Drug-specific teaching points

- Leucovorin "rescues" normal cells from the effects of chemotherapy and allows them to survive.
- Report rash, difficulty breathing, pain, or discomfort at injection site.

## leuprolide acetate

*(loo **proe'** lide)*

Lupron, Lupron Depot, Lupron Depot-Ped, Lupron Depot—3 Month, Lupron Depot—4 months

**Pregnancy Category X**

### Drug classes

Antineoplastic
Hormone

### Therapeutic actions

An LH-RH agonist that occupies pituitary gonadotropin-releasing hormone receptors and desensitizes them; inhibits gonoadotropin secretion when given continuously.

### Indications

- Advanced prostatic cancer—palliation, alternative to orchiectomy or estrogen therapy
- Endometriosis (depot only)
- Central precocious puberty
- Uterine leiomyomata (depot only)
- Unlabeled uses: treatment of breast, ovarian, and endometrial cancer; infertility; prostatic hypertrophy

### Contraindications/cautions

- Allergy to leuprolide, pregnancy

### Dosage

**Available Forms:** Injection—5 mg/ml; depot—3.75, 7.5 mg/ml; depot-ped—7.5, 11.25, 15 mg; 3-mo depot—11.25, 22.5 mg; 4-mo depot—30 mg

**ADULT**

- ***Advanced prostate cancer:*** 1 mg/d SC; use only the syringes that come with the drug.
- ***Depot:*** 7.5 mg IM monthly (q28–33 d). Do not use needles smaller than 22 gauge.
- ***3-mo depot:*** 22.5 mg IM every 3 mo (84 d).
- ***4-mo depot:*** 30 mg IM every 4 mo.
- ***Central precocious puberty:*** 50 μg/kg per d SC; may be titrated up to 10 μg/kg per d.
- ***Depot:*** 0.3 mg/kg IM monthly every 4 wk.
- ***Endometriosis:*** 3.75 mg as a single monthly IM injection. Continue for 6 mo.
- ***Uterine leiomyomata:*** 3.75 mg as a single monthly injection; continue for 3 mo.

### Adverse effects

- **CNS:** *Dizziness, headache, pain*, paresthesia, blurred vision, lethargy, fatigue, insomnia, memory disorder
- **GI:** GI bleeding, *nausea, vomiting, anorexia*, sour taste, *constipation*

- **CV**: *Peripheral edema, cardiac arrhythmias*, thrombophlebitis, CHF, MI
- **Respiratory**: Difficulty breathing, pleural rub, worsening of pulmonary fibrosis
- **GU**: *Frequency, hematuria*, decrease in size of testes, increased BUN and creatinine
- **Dermatologic**: Skin rash, hair loss, itching, erythema
- **General**: *Hot flashes, sweats*, bone pain
- **Local**: Ecchymosis at injection site

## ■ Nursing Considerations

### Assessment

- ***History:*** Allergy to leuprolide, pregnancy
- ***Physical:*** Skin lesions, color, turgor; testes; injection sites; orientation, affect, reflexes, peripheral sensation; peripheral pulses, edema, P; R, adventitious sounds; serum testosterone and acid phosphatase

### Implementation

- Administer only with the syringes provided with the drug.
- Administer SC; monitor injection sites for bruising and rash; rotate injection sites to decrease local reaction.
- Give depot injection deep into muscle. Prepare a calendar of monthly (28–33 d) return visits for new injection.
- Refrigerate the vials until dispensed; must be stored below 30°C if unrefrigerated.
- Arrange for periodic serum testosterone and acid phosphatase determinations.
- Teach patient and significant other the technique for SC injection, and observe administration before home administration.

### Drug-specific teaching points

- Administer SC only, using the syringes that come with the drug. If depot route is used, prepare calendar for return dates, stressing the importance of receiving the injection each mo.
- Do not stop taking this drug without first consulting the health care provider.
- The following side effects may occur: bone pain, difficulty urinating (usually transient); hot flashes (staying in cool temperatures may help); nausea, vomiting (small, frequent meals may help); dizziness, headache, lightheadedness (use caution when driving or performing tasks that require alertness).
- Report injection site pain, burning, itching, swelling, numbness, tingling, severe GI upset, pronounced hot flashes.

# levamisole hydrochloride

*(lev **am'** ih sole)*

Ergamisol

**Pregnancy Category C**

### Drug classes

Antineoplastic

### Therapeutic actions

Immunomodulator: appears to restore depressed immune function, stimulates formation of antibodies, enhances T cell response, potentiates monocyte and macrophage activity

### Indications

- Adjunctive treatment in combination with fluorouracil after surgical resection in patients with Dukes' stage C colon cancer

### Contraindications/cautions

- Allergy to levamisole or any of its components, pregnancy, lactation

### Dosage

**Available Forms:** Tablets—50 mg

ADULT

- ***Initial therapy:*** 50 mg PO q8h for 3 d starting 7–30 d after surgery with fluorouracil 450 mg/m$^2$ per day IV for 5 d concomitant with a 3-day course of levamisole starting 21–34 d after surgery.
- ***Maintenance therapy:*** 50 mg PO q8h for 3 d every 2 wk with fluorouracil 450 mg/m$^2$ per d IV once a wk beginning 28 d after the start of the 5 d course.

### Pharmacokinetics

| *Route* | *Onset* | *Peak* |
|---|---|---|
| Oral | Varies | 1.5–2 h |

*Metabolism* : Hepatic, $T_{1/2}$: 3–4 h
*Distribution* : Crosses placenta; may enter breast milk
*Excretion* : Urine

### Adverse effects

- CNS: *Taste perversion*, dizziness, headache, paresthesia, somnolence, depression
- GI: *Nausea, diarrhea*, stomatitis, anorexia, abdominal pain, constipation
- **Hematologic:** Bone marrow depression
- **Dermatologic:** Dermatitis, alopecia
- **General:** *Fatigue,* fever, rigors, *arthralgia*, myalgia, infection

### Clinically important drug-drug interactions

• Disulfiram-like reaction possible with alcohol • Increased phenytoin levels and possible toxicity

## ■ Nursing Considerations

### Assessment

- ***History:*** Allergy to levamisole, lactation
- ***Physical:*** T; skin lesions, color; R, adventitious sounds; orientation, reflexes; CBC, Hgb, Hct, liver function tests, electrolytes

### Implementation

- Initiate levamisole therapy no earlier than 7 and no later than 30 d after surgery. Initiate fluorouracil no earlier than 21 d and no later than 35 d after surgery.
- Do not exceed recommended dosage. Monitor CBC before, during, and after therapy. Defer administration of fluorouracil until WBC is $> 3{,}500/mm^3$.
- Advise patient to use birth control; drug causes fetal toxicity.

### Drug-specific teaching points

- Avoid crowds and exposure to infection.
- The following side effects may occur: nausea, vomiting (small, frequent meals may help); diarrhea; skin rash (request medication, avoid exposure to the sun or extremes of temperature).
- Do not become pregnant; use birth control.
- Report fever, chills, muscle aches, extreme vomiting, or diarrhea.

# levodopa

*(lee voe **doe'** pa)*
Dopar, Larodopa
**Pregnancy Category C**

### Drug classes

Antiparkinsonism agent

### Therapeutic actions

Biochemical precursor of the neurotransmitter dopamine, which is deficient in the basal ganglia of parkinsonism patients; unlike dopamine, levodopa penetrates the blood–brain barrier. It is transformed in the brain to dopamine; thus, levodopa is a form of replacement therapy. It is efficacious for 2–5 y in relieving the symptoms of parkinsonism but not drug-induced extrapyramidal disorders.

### Indications

- Treatment of parkinsonism (postencephalitic, arteriosclerotic, and idiopathic types) and symptomatic parkinsonism, following injury to the nervous system by carbon monoxide or manganese intoxication
- Given with carbidopa (Lodosyn; fixed combinations, *Sinemet*), an enzyme inhibitor that decreases the activity of dopa decarboxylase in the periphery, thus reducing blood levels of levodopa and decreasing the intensity and incidence of many of the adverse effects of levodopa
- Unlabeled use: relief of herpes zoster (shingles) pain

### Contraindications/cautions

- Contraindications: hypersensitivity to levodopa; allergy to tartrazine (marketed as Dopar); glaucoma, especially angle-closure glaucoma; history of melanoma; suspicious or undiagnosed skin lesions; lactation.
- Use cautiously with severe CV or pulmonary disease; occlusive cerebrovascular disease; history of MI with residual arrhythmias; bronchial asthma; renal, hepatic, endocrine disease; history of peptic

ulcer; psychiatric patients, especially the depressed or psychotic; pregnancy.

### Dosage

**Available Forms:** Tablets—100, 250, 500 mg; capsules—100, 250, 500 mg

*ADULT:* Individualize dosage. Increase dosage gradually to minimize side effects; titrate dosage carefully to optimize benefits and minimize side effects. Initially, 0.5–1 g PO daily divided into 2 or more doses given with food. Increase gradually in increments not exceeding 0.75 g/d q3–7 d as tolerated. Do not exceed 8 g/d, except for exceptional patients. A significant therapeutic response may not be obtained for 6 mo.

*PEDIATRIC:* Safety for use in children < 12 y not established.

### Pharmacokinetics

| *Route* | *Onset* | *Peak* |
|---|---|---|
| Oral | Varies | 0.5–2 h |

*Metabolism:* Hepatic metabolism, $T_{1/2}$: 1–3 h

*Distribution:* Crosses placenta; enters breast milk

*Excretion:* Urine

### Adverse effects

- CNS: *Adventitious movements, ataxia, increased hand tremor, headache, dizziness, numbness, weakness and faintness*, bruxism, confusion, insomnia, nightmares, hallucinations and delusions, *agitation and anxiety, malaise, fatigue, euphoria*, mental changes (including paranoid ideation), psychotic episodes, depression with or without suicidal tendencies, dementia, bradykinesia (''on-off'' phenomenon), muscle twitching and blepharospasm, diplopia, blurred vision, dilated pupils
- GI: *Anorexia, nausea, vomiting, abdominal pain or distress, dry mouth, dysphagia, dysgeusia*, bitter taste, sialorrhea, trismus, burning sensation of the tongue, diarrhea, constipation, flatulence, weight change, upper GI hemorrhage in patients with history of peptic ulcer
- CV: Cardiac irregularities, palpitations, orthostatic hypotension
- Respiratory: Bizarre breathing patterns
- **Hematologic**: Leukopenia, decreased Hgb and Hct, elevated BUN, SGOT, SGPT, LDH, bilirubin, alkaline phosphatase, protein-bound iodine
- GU: Urinary retention, urinary incontinence
- Dermatologic: Flushing, hot flashes, increased sweating, skin rash

### Clinically important drug-drug interactions

• Increased therapeutic effects and possible hypertensive crisis with MAOIs; withdraw MAOIs at least 14 d before starting levodopa therapy • Decreased efficacy with pyridoxine (vitamin $B_6$) and phenytoin

### Drug-lab test interferences

• May interfere with urine tests for sugar or ketones • False Coombs' test results • False elevations of uric acid when using colorimetric method

## ■ Nursing Considerations

### Assessment

- *History:* Hypersensitivity to levodopa, tartrazine; glaucoma; history of melanoma; suspicious or undiagnosed skin lesions; severe CV or pulmonary disease; occlusive cerebrovascular disease; history of MI with residual arrhythmias; bronchial asthma; renal, hepatic, endocrine disease; history of peptic ulcer; psychiatric disorders; lactation
- *Physical:* Weight; T; skin color, lesions; orientation, affect, reflexes, bilateral grip strength, vision exam; P, BP, orthostatic BP, auscultation; R, depth, adventitious sounds; bowel sounds, normal output, liver evaluation; voiding pattern, normal output, prostate palpation; liver and kidney function tests; CBC with differential

### Implementation

- Arrange to decrease dosage if therapy is interrupted; observe for the development of suicidal tendencies.
- Give with meals if GI upset occurs.
- Ensure that patient voids before receiving dose if urinary retention is a problem.

- Monitor hepatic, renal, hematopoietic, and CV function.
- For patients who take multivitamins provide Larobec, a preparation without pyridoxine.

**Drug-specific teaching points**

- Take this drug exactly as prescribed.
- Do not take multivitamin preparations with pyridoxine. These may prevent any therapeutic effect of levodopa. Notify your health care provider if you need vitamins.
- The following side effects may occur: drowsiness, dizziness, confusion, blurred vision (avoid driving or engaging in activities that require alertness and visual acuity); nausea (take with meals, frequent small meals); dry mouth (sucking sugarless lozenges or ice chips may help); painful or difficult urination (empty bladder before each dose); constipation (maintain adequate fluid intake and exercise regularly, request correctives); dark sweat or urine (not harmful); dizziness or faintness when you get up (change position slowly and use caution when climbing stairs).
- Report fainting, lightheadedness, dizziness; uncontrollable movements of the face, eyelids, mouth, tongue, neck, arms, hands, or legs; mental changes; irregular heartbeat or palpitations; difficult urination; severe or persistent nausea or vomiting.

# levofloxacin

*(lee voe **flox'** a sin)*
Levaquin
**Pregnancy Category C**

## Drug classes
Antibiotic
Flouroquinolone

## Therapeutic actions
Bactericidal; interferes with DNA replication in susceptible gram-negative and gram-positive bacteria, preventing cell reproduction.

## Indications
- Treatment of adults with community-acquired pneumonia, acute maxillary sinusitis
- Treatment of acute exacerbation of chronic bronchitis
- Treatment of uncomplicated skin and skin structure infections
- Treatment of complicated UTIs and acute pyelonephritis

## Contraindications/cautions
- Contraindications: allergy to fluoroquinolones, pregnancy, lactation
- Use cautiously with renal dysfunction, seizures

## Dosage
**Available Forms:** Tablets—250, 500 mg; injection—500 mg; premixed injection—250, 500 mg

ADULT
- ***Pneumonia:*** 500 mg qd PO or IV for 7–14 d.
- ***Sinusitis:*** 500 mg qd PO or IV for 10–14 d.
- ***Chronic bronchitis:*** 500 mg qd PO or IV for 7 d.
- ***Skin infection:*** 500 mg qd PO or IV for 7–10 d.
- ***UTIs, nephritis:*** 250 mg qd PO or IV for 10 d.

PEDIATRIC: Not recommended in children <18 y.

RENAL IMPAIRMENT

| Ccr (ml/min) | Dose |
|---|---|
| 50–80 | No adjustment |
| 20–49 | 500 mg initially, then 250 mg qd |
| 10–19 | 500 mg initially, then 250 mg q48h |

## Pharmacokinetics

| Route | Onset | Peak | Duration |
|---|---|---|---|
| Oral | Varies | 1–2 h | 3–5 h |
| IV | Rapid | End of infusion | 3–5 h |

*Metabolism:* Hepatic; $T_{1/2}$: 4–7 h
*Distribution:* Crosses placenta; passes into breast milk
*Excretion:* Urine

## IV facts
**Preparation:** No further preparation is needed if using the premixed solution;

dilute single-use vials in 50–100 ml D5W.

**Infusion:** Administer slowly over at least 60 min.

### Adverse effects

- CNS: *Headache,* dizziness, *insomnia,* fatigue, somnolence, depression, blurred vision
- GI: *Nausea,* vomiting, dry mouth, *diarrhea,* abdominal pain (occur less with this drug than with oflaxacin)
- **Hematologic**: Elevated BUN, SGOT, SGPT, serum creatinine, and alkaline phosphatase; decreased WBC, neutrophil count, Hct
- Other: Fever, rash

### Clinically important drug-drug interactions

• Decreased therapeutic effect with iron salts, sulcrafate, antacids, zinc, magnesium (separate by at least 2 h) • Increased risk of seizures with NSAIDs; avoid this combination

## ■ Nursing Considerations

### Assessment

- *History:* Allergy to fluoroquinolones, renal dysfunction, seizures, lactation
- *Physical:* Skin color, lesions; T; orientation, reflexes, affect; mucous membranes, bowel sounds; renal and liver function tests

### Implementation

- Arrange for culture and sensitivity tests before beginning therapy.
- Continue therapy as indicated for condition being treated.
- Administer oral drug 1 h before or 2 h after meals with a glass of water; separate oral drug from other cation administration, including antacids, by at least 2 h.
- Ensure that patient is well hydrated during course of therapy.
- Discontinue drug at any sign of hypersensitivity (rash, photophobia) or at complaint of tendon pain, inflammation, or rupture.
- Monitor clinical response; if no improvement is seen or a relapse occurs, repeat culture and sensitivity test.

### Drug-specific teaching points

- Take oral drug on an empty stomach, 1 h before or 2 h after meals. If an antacid is needed, do not take it within 2 h of levofloxacin dose.
- Drink plenty of fluids while you are on this drug.
- The following side effects may occur: nausea, vomiting, abdominal pain (eat small, frequent meals); diarrhea or constipation (consult nurse or physician); drowsiness, blurred vision, dizziness (use caution if driving or operating dangerous equipment) sensitivity to sunlight (avoid exposure, use a sunscreen if necessary).
- Report rash, visual changes, severe GI problems, weakness, tremors.

## levomethadyl acetate hydrochloride

*(lev oh* ***meth'*** *a dil)*

ORLAAM

**Pregnancy Category B**
**C-II controlled substance**

### Drug classes

Narcotic agonist analgesic

### Therapeutic actions

Acts at specific opioid receptors, causing analgesia, respiratory depression, physical depression, euphoria.

### Indications

- Management of opiate dependence

### Contraindications/cautions

- Contraindications: hypersensitivity to narcotics, diarrhea caused by poisoning, acute bronchial asthma, upper airway obstruction, pregnancy.
- Use cautiously with bradycardia, history of seizures, lactation.

### Dosage

**Available Forms:** Solution—10 mg/ml

Must be given in an opiate withdrawal clinic that maintains control over drug delivery.

ADULT

- *Usual induction dose:* 20–40 mg PO, increase in increments of 5–10 mg every 48–72 h as tolerated.
- *Maintenance:* 60–90 mg PO 3 times a wk.
- *Transfer from methadone:* Higher initial doses may be needed.
- *Transfer from levomethadyl to methadone:* Start methadone at 80% of the usual dose, giving the initial methadone dose no sooner than 48 h after the last levomethadyl dose.

PEDIATRIC: Safety and efficacy not established.

### Pharmacokinetics

| *Route* | *Onset* | *Duration* |
|---|---|---|
| PO | Varies | up to 72 h |

*Metabolism* : Plasma, $T_{1/2}$: 15–40 h

*Distribution* : Crosses placenta; enters breast milk

### Adverse effects

- CNS: *Sedation, clamminess, sweating, headache, vertigo, floating feeling, dizziness, lethary, confusion, lightheadedness,* nervousness, unusual dreams, agitation, euphoria, hallucinations, delirium, insomnia, anxiety, fear, disorientation, impaired mental and physical performance, coma, mood changes, weakness, headache, tremor, convulsions
- GI: *Nausea, vomiting,* dry mouth, anorexia, constipation, biliary tract spasm
- CV: Palpitation, increase or decrease in BP, circulatory depression, **cardiac arrest, shock**, arrhythmia, palpitations
- Respiratory: Slow, shallow respiration; apnea; suppression of cough reflex; laryngospasm; bronchospasm
- EENT: Diplopia, blurred vision
- Dermatologic: Rash, hives, pruritus, flushing, warmth, sensitivity to cold
- Other: Physical tolerance and dependence, psychological dependence

### Clinically important drug-drug interactions

- Potentiation of effects with barbiturate anesthetics

### Drug-lab test interferences

- Elevated biliary tract pressure may cause increases in plasma amylase and lipase; determinations of these levels may be unreliable for 24 h after administration of narcotics.

## ■ Nursing Considerations

### Assessment

- *History:* Hypersensitivity to narcotics, physical dependence on a narcotic analgesic, pregnancy, labor, lactation, bronchial asthma, COPD, respiratory depression, anoxia, increased intracranial pressure, acute MI, ventricular failure, coronary insufficiency, hypertension, biliary tract surgery, and renal or hepatic dysfunction
- *Physical:* Orientation, reflexes, bilateral grip strength, affect; pupil size, vision; P, auscultation, BP; R, adventitious sounds; bowel sounds, normal output; liver and kidney function tests

### Implementation

- Give to lactating women 4–6 h before the next feeding to minimize amount in milk.
- Provide narcotic antagonist, and have facilities for assisted or controlled respiration on standby during parenteral administration.
- Caution patient that clinic visits must be kept; use of street drugs can cause serious complications and even death.

### Drug-specific teaching points

- Return to the clinic for scheduled dosing; skipping doses can cause serious side effects. Use of street drugs can cause serious complications.
- The following side effects may occur: dizziness, sedation, drowsiness, impaired visual acuity (ask for assistance to move); nausea, loss of appetite (lying quietly, frequent small meals may help); constipation (request laxative).

- Report severe nausea, vomiting, palpitations, shortness of breath, or difficulty breathing.

## levonorgestrel

*(lee' voe nor jess trel)*

Norplant System

**Pregnancy Category X**

### Drug classes

Hormone
Progestin
Contraceptives

### Therapeutic actions

Synthetic progestational agent. The endogenous female progestin, progesterone, transforms proliferative endometrium into secretory endometrium; inhibits the secretion of pituitary gonadotropins, which prevents follicular maturation and ovulation; and inhibits spontaneous uterine contractions. The primary mechanism by which norgestrel prevents conception is not known, but progestin-only oral contraceptives are known to alter the cervical mucus, exert a progestional effect on the endometrium that interferes with implantation, and in some patients, suppress ovulation.

### Indications

- Prevention of pregnancy

### Contraindications/cautions

- Contraindicatoins: allergy to progestins; thrombophlebitis, thromboembolic disorders, cerebral hemorrhage, or history of these conditions; CAD; hepatic disease, carcinoma of the breast or genital organs, undiagnosed vaginal bleeding, missed abortion; lactation; pregnancy.
- Use cautiously with epilepsy, migraine, asthma, cardiac or renal dysfunction.

### Dosage

**Available Forms:** 6 capsules with 36 mg each

**ADULT:** Six Silastic capsules, each containing 36 mg of levonorgestrel implanted, for a total dose of 216 mg. All 6 capsules should be inserted during the first 7 d of the onset of menses by a health care professional instructed in the insertion technique. Capsules are effective for 5 y. 150-mg 2-rod implant with 3-y duration also available.

**PEDIATRIC:** Safety and efficacy not established.

### Pharmacokinetics

| *Route* | *Onset* | *Peak* |
|---|---|---|
| Implant | Slow | 24 h |

*Metabolism* : Hepatic and cellular, $T_{1/2}$: unknown
*Distribution* : Crosses placenta; enters breast milk
*Excretion* : Urine

### Adverse effects

- CNS: Neuro-ocular lesions, mental depression, migraine, *headache, changes in corneal curvature,* contact lens intolerance
- GI: Gallbladder disease, liver tumors, hepatic lesions, *nausea,* vomiting, *abdominal cramps*, bloating, cholestatic jaundice, *change in appetite*
- CV: Thrombophlebitis, thrombosis, pulmonary embolism, coronary thrombosis, MI, cerebral thrombosis, Raynaud's disease, arterial thromboembolism, renal artery thrombosis, cerebral hemorrhage, hypertension
- GU: *Breakthrough bleeding, spotting, change in menstrual flow, amenorrhea,* changes in cervical erosion and cervical secretions, endocervical hyperplasia, vaginal candidiasis, *vaginitis*
- **Dermatologic**: Rash with or without pruritus, *dermatitis, hirsutism, hypertrichosis, scalp hair loss, acne*, melasma
- **Local**: Pain or itching at insertion site, removal difficulties, infection at insertion site
- **Other**: *Breast tenderness and secretion, enlargement*; fluid retention; edema; *increase in weight; musculoskeletal pain*

**Clinically important drug-drug interactions**
• Pregnancy has occurred when users of levonorgestrel took carbamazepine and phenytoin.

**Drug-lab test interferences**
• Abnormal tests of endocrine function

## ■ Nursing Considerations

### Assessment
• *History:* Allergy to progestins, thrombophlebitis, thromboembolic disorders, cerebral hemorrhage, CAD, hepatic disease, carcinoma of the breast or genital organs, undiagnosed vaginal bleeding, missed abortion, epilepsy, migraine, asthma, cardiac or renal dysfunction, pregnancy, lactation
• *Physical:* Skin color, lesions, turgor; hair; breasts; pelvic exam; insertion site; orientation, affect; ophthalmologic exam; P, auscultation, peripheral perfusion, edema; R, adventitious sounds; liver evaluation; liver and renal function tests, glucose tolerance, Pap smear, pregnancy test

### Implementation
• Arrange for pretreatment and periodic (at least annual) history and physical exam, which should include BP, breasts, abdomen, pelvic organs, and a Pap smear.
• Arrange for insertion of capsules during the first 7 d of the menstrual cycle. Insertion is made in the midportion of the upper arm about 8–10 cm above the elbow crease. Distribution is in a fanlike pattern about 15 degrees apart, for a total area of 75 degrees. Insertion area is closed using a skin closure; cover the area with a dry compress and gauze wrap. Sterile technique should be observed.
• Monitor insertion site for signs of bleeding, infection, and irritation.
• Capsules are removed using a local anesthetic, aseptic technique, and small incision in the area. Remove capsules at the end of 5 y or if the patient desires to become pregnant.

### Drug-specific teaching points
• This drug must be inserted using a local anesthetic; six capsules are inserted into the mid-upper arm, just above the elbow crease. The procedure takes 15–20 min and should not be too uncomfortable. The drug is slowly released from the capsules, and the capsules are effective for 5 y. If you decide to become pregnant before that time, the capsules can be removed in a procedure similar to the insertion. If you keep the capsules in place for 5 y, you can then have them replaced.
• Arrange for annual medical exams, including Pap smear, to monitor the drug's effect on your body.
• The following side effects may occur: sensitivity to light (avoid exposure to the sun, use sunscreen and protective clothing); dizziness, sleeplessness, depression (use caution driving or performing tasks that require alertness); skin rash, skin color changes, loss of hair; fever; nausea; breakthrough bleeding or spotting (may occur in first month; if it continues, consult your health care provider); intolerance to contact lenses due to corneal changes.
• Do not use during pregnancy—serious fetal abnormalities have ocurred. If you think that you are pregnant, consult physician immediately.
• Report pain or swelling and warmth in the calves, acute chest pain or shortness of breath, sudden severe headache or vomiting, dizziness or fainting, visual disturbances, numbness or tingling in the arm or leg, breakthrough bleeding or spotting, pain or irritation at insertion site.

## levorphanol sulfate

*(lee vor' fa nole)*

Levo-Dromoran

**Pregnancy Category C**
**C-II controlled substance**

**Drug classes**
Narcotic agonist analgesic

**Therapeutic actions**
Acts as agonist at specific opioid receptors in the CNS to produce analgesia, euphoria, se-

dation; the receptors are thought to be the same as those mediating the effects of endogenous opioids (enkephalins, endorphins).

## Indications

- Relief of moderate to severe acute and chronic pain
- Preoperative medication to allay apprehension, provide prolonged analgesia, reduce thiopental requirements, and shorten recovery time

## Contraindications/cautions

- Contraindications: hypersensitivity to narcotics, diarrhea caused by poisoning (before toxins are eliminated), pregnancy (neonatal withdrawal), labor or delivery (respiratory depression of neonate—premature infants are especially at risk; may prolong labor), bronchial asthma, acute alcoholism, increased intracranial pressure, respiratory depression, anoxia.
- Use cautiously with COPD, cor pulmonale, acute abdominal conditions, CV disease, supraventricular tachycardias, myxedema, convulsive disorders, delirium tremens, cerebral arteriosclerosis, ulcerative colitis, fever, kyphoscoliosis, Addison's disease, prostatic hypertrophy, urethral stricture, recent GI or GU surgery, toxic psychosis, and renal or hepatic dysfunction.

## Dosage

**Available Forms:** Injection—2 mg/ml; tablets—2 mg

*ADULT:* Average dose is 2 mg PO or SC. Increase to 3 mg if necessary. Has been given by slow IV injection; not recommended.

*GERIATRIC OR IMPAIRED ADULT:* Use caution—respiratory depression may occur; elderly, the very ill, and those with respiratory problems. Reduced dosage may be necessary.

## Pharmacokinetics

| Route | Onset | Peak | Duration |
|---|---|---|---|
| Oral/SC | 30–90 min | 0.5–1 h | 6–8 h |

*Metabolism*: Hepatic, $T_{1/2}$: 12–16 h
*Distribution*: Crosses placenta; enters breast milk
*Excretion*: Urine

## Adverse effects

- CNS: *Lightheadedness, dizziness, sedation,* euphoria, dysphoria, delirium, insomnia, agitation, anxiety, fear, hallucinations, disorientation, drowsiness, lethargy, impaired mental and physical performance, coma, mood changes, weakness, headache, tremor, convulsions, miosis, visual disturbances, suppression of cough reflex
- GI: *Nausea, vomiting,* dry mouth, anorexia, constipation, biliary tract spasm; increased colonic motility in patients with chronic ulcerative colitis
- CV: Facial flushing, peripheral circulatory collapse, tachycardia, bradycardia, arrhythmia, palpitations, chest wall rigidity, hypertension, hypotension, orthostatic hypotension, syncope
- GU: Ureteral spasm, spasm of vesicle sphincters, urinary retention or hesitancy, oliguria, antidiuretic effect, reduced libido or potency
- Dermatologic: Pruritus, urticaria, laryngospasm, bronchospasm, edema, hemorrhagic urticaria (rare)
- Local: Tissue irritation and induration (SC injection)
- **Major hazards: Respiratory depression, apnea, circulatory depression, respiratory arrest, shock, cardiac arrest**
- Other: *Sweating* (more common in ambulatory patients and those without severe pain), physical tolerance and dependence, psychological dependence

## Clinically important drug-drug interactions

- Potentiation of effects of levorphanol when given with barbiturate anesthetics; decrease dose of levorphanol when coadministering.

## Drug-lab test interferences

- Elevated biliary tract pressure may cause increases in plasma amylase and lipase; determinations of these levels may be unreliable for 24 h after administration of narcotics.

## Nursing Considerations

### Assessment

- *History:* Hypersensitivity to narcotics, diarrhea caused by poisoning, labor or delivery, bronchial asthma, acute alcoholism, increased intracranial pressure, respiratory depression, cor pulmonale, acute abdominal conditions, CV disease, myxedema, convulsive disorders, delirium tremens, cerebral arteriosclerosis, ulcerative colitis, fever, kyphoscoliosis, Addison's disease, prostatic hypertrophy, urethral stricture, recent GI or GU surgery, toxic psychosis, renal or hepatic dysfunction
- *Physical:* T; skin color, texture, lesions; orientation, reflexes, pupil size, bilateral grip strength, affect; P, auscultation, BP, orthostatic BP, perfusion; R, adventious sounds; bowel sounds, normal output; frequency and pattern of voiding, normal output; ECG; EEG; thyroid, liver, kidney function tests

### Implementation

- Give to lactating women 4–6 h before the next feeding to minimize the amount in milk.
- Provide narcotic antagonist and have facilities for assisted or controlled respiration on standby during parenteral administration.
- Use caution when injecting SC into chilled areas or in patients with hypotension or in shock; impaired perfusion may delay absorption. With repeated doses, an excessive amount may be absorbed when circulation is restored.
- Reassure about addiction liability; most patients who receive opiates for medical reasons do not develop dependency.

### Drug-specific teaching points

- Take drug exactly as prescribed.
- The following side effects may occur: nausea, loss of appetite (take with food, lie quietly, eat frequent small meals); constipation (laxative may help); dizziness, sedation, drowsiness, impaired visual acuity (avoid driving, performing other tasks that require alertness, visual acuity).
- Do not take leftover medication for other disorders, do not let anyone else take your prescription.
- Report severe nausea, vomiting, constipation, shortness of breath, or difficulty breathing.

## levothyroxine sodium

*(lee voe thye **rox'** een)*

L-thyroxine, $T_4$

Eltroxin, Levo-T, Levothroid, Levoxyl, Synthroid

**Pregnancy Category A**

### Drug classes

Thyroid hormone

### Therapeutic actions

Increases the metabolic rate of body tissues, thereby increasing oxygen consumption; R and heart rate; rate of fat, protein, and carbohydrate metabolism; and growth and maturation.

### Indications

- Replacement therapy in hypothyroidism
- Pituitary TSH suppression in the treatment and prevention of euthyroid goiters and in the management of thyroid cancer
- Thyrotoxicosis in conjunction with antithyroid drugs and to prevent goitrogenesis, hypothyroidism, and thyrotoxicosis during pregnancy
- Treatment of myxedema coma

### Contraindications/cautions

- Contraindications: allergy to active or extraneous constituents of drug, thyrotoxicosis, and acute MI uncomplicated by hypothyroidism.
- Use cautiously with Addison's disease (treat hypoadrenalism with corticosteroids before thyroid therapy) and lactation.

### Dosage

**Available Forms:** Tablets—0.025, 0.05, 0.075, 0.088, 0.1, 0.112, 0.125, 0.137, 0.15, 0.175, 0.2, 0.3 mg; powder for injection—200, 500 μg/vial

0.1 mg equals approximately 65 mg (1 grain) thyroid.

**ADULT**

- *Hypothyroidism:* Initial dose: 0.05 mg PO, with increasing increments of 0.025 mg PO q2–3 wk; maintenance of 0.2 mg/d IV or IM injection can be substituted for the oral dosage form when oral ingestion is not possible.
- *Myxedema coma without severe heart disease:* 0.4 mg IV as initial dose, then 0.1 to 0.2 mg IV as a solution containing 0.1 mg/ml; daily maintenance of 0.05 to 0.1 mg.
- *TSH suppression in thyroid cancer, nodules, and euthyroid goiters:* Larger amounts than used for normal suppression.
- *Thyroid suppression therapy:* 2.6 μg/kg per d PO for 7–10 d.

**PEDIATRIC**

- *Cretinism:* Infants require replacement therapy from birth. Starting dose is 0.025 to 0.05 mg/d PO with 0.05–0.1-mg increments at weekly intervals until the child is euthyroid. Maintenance dose may be as high as 0.3–0.4 mg/d PO.

## Pharmacokinetics

| *Route* | *Onset* | *Peak* |
|---|---|---|
| Oral | Slow | 1–3 wk |
| IV | 6–8 h | 24–48 h |

*Metabolism* : Hepatic, $T_{1/2}$: 6–7 d
*Distribution* : Crosses placenta; enters breast milk
*Excretion* : Bile

### IV facts

**Preparation:** Add 5 ml 0.9% Sodium Chloride Injection, USP or Bacteriostatic Sodium Chloride Injection, USP with benzyl alcohol. Shake the vial to assure complete mixing. Use immediately after reconstitiution. Discard any unused portion.

**Infusion:** Inject directly, each 100 mcg over 1 min.

**Incompatabilities:** Do not mix with any other IV fluids.

## Adverse effects

- Endocrine: Symptoms of hyperthyroidism
- Dermatologic: Allergic skin reactions, partial loss of hair in first few months of therapy in children

## Clinically important drug-drug interactions

• Decreased absorption of oral thyroid preparation with cholestyramine • Increased risk of bleeding with warfarin, dicumarol, anisindione—reduce dosage of anticoagulant when $T_4$ is begun • Decreased effectiveness of digitalis glycosides if taken with thyroid replacement • Decreased theophylline clearance when patient is in hypothyroid state; monitor levels and patient response as euthyroid state is achieved

## ■ Nursing Considerations

### Assessment

- *History:* Allergy to active or extraneous constituents of drug, thyrotoxicosis, acute MI uncomplicated by hypothyroidism, Addison's disease, lactation
- *Physical:* Skin lesions, color, temperature, texture; T; muscle tone, orientation, reflexes; P, auscultation, baseline ECG, BP; R, adventitious sounds; thyroid function tests

### Implementation

- Monitor response carefully at start of therapy, adjust dosage.
- Do not change brands of $T_4$ products, due to bioequivalence problems.
- Do not add IV doses to other IV fluids; full therapeutic effect may not be seen until the second day; use caution in patients with CV disease.
- Administer oral drug as a single daily dose before breakfast.
- Arrange for regular, periodic blood tests of thyroid function.
- Monitor cardiac response.

### Drug-specific teaching points

- Take as a single dose before breakfast.
- This drug replaces an important hormone and will need to be taken for life. Do not discontinue without consulting your health care provider; serious problems can occur.

- Wear a medical ID tag to alert emergency medical personnel that you are on this drug.
- Arrange to have periodic blood tests and medical evaluations. Keep your scheduled appointments.
- Report headache, chest pain, palpitations, fever, weight loss, sleeplessness, nervousness, irritability, unusual sweating, intolerance to heat, diarrhea.

## Lidocaine hydrochloride

### lidocaine HCl in 5% dextrose

### lidocaine HCl without preservatives

***(lye' doe kane)***

*Antiarrhythmic Preparations:* Xylocaine HCl IV for Cardiac Arrhythmias, LidoPen Auto-Injector, Xylocaine HCl IM for Cardiac Arrhythmias

*Local Anesthetic Preparations:* Dilocaine, Duo-Trach Kit, Lidoject, Nervocaine, Xylocaine HCL (injectable)

*Topical for Mucous Membranes:* Anestacon, Xylocaine

*Topical Dermatologic:* Xylocaine

**Pregnancy Category B**

### Drug classes

Antiarrhythmic
Local anesthetic

### Therapeutic actions

Type 1 antiarrhythmic: decreases diastolic depolarization, decreasing automaticity of ventricular cells; increases ventricular fibrillation threshold.

Local anesthetic: blocks the generation and conduction of action potentials in sensory nerves by reducing sodium permeability, reducing height and rate of rise of the action potential, increasing excitation threshold, and slowing conduction velocity.

### Indications

- As antiarrhythmic: Management of acute ventricular arrhythmias during cardiac surgery and MI (IV use). Use IM when IV administration is not possible or when ECG monitoring is not available and the danger of ventricular arrhythmias is great (single-dose IM use, for example, by paramedics in a mobile coronary care unit).
- As anesthetic: Infiltration anesthesia, peripheral and sympathetic nerve blocks, central nerve blocks, spinal and caudal anesthesia, retrobulbar and transtracheal injection; topical anesthetic for skin disorders and accessible mucous membranes

### Contraindications/cautions

- Contraindications: allergy to lidocaine or amide-type local anesthetics, CHF, cardiogenic shock, second- or third-degree heart block (if no artificial pacemaker), Wolff-Parkinson-White syndrome, Stokes-Adams syndrome.
- Use cautiously with hepatic or renal disease, inflammation or sepsis in the region of injection (local anesthetic), labor and delivery (epidural anesthesia may prolong the second stage of labor; monitor for fetal and neonatal CVS and CNS toxicity), and lactation.

### Dosage

**Available Forms:** Direct injection—10, 20 mg/ml; IV injection (admixture) 40, 100, 200 mg/ml; IV infusion—2, 4, 8 mg/ml; topical liquid—2.5%, 5%; topical ointment—2.5%, 5%; topical cream—0.5%; topical gel—0.5%, 2.5%; topical spray—0.5%, 10%, topical solution—2%, 4%; topical jelly—2%; injection—0.5%, 1%, 1.5%, 2%, 4%

**ADULT**

- ***IM:*** Use only the 10% solution for IM injection. 300 mg in deltoid or thigh muscle. Switch to IV lidocaine or oral antiarrhythmic as soon as possible.
- ***IV bolus:*** Use only lidocaine injection labeled for IV use and without preservatives or catecholamines. Give 50 to 100 mg at rate of 20–50 mg/min. One-third to one-half the initial dose may be given

after 5 min if needed. *Do not exceed* 200–300 mg in 1 h.

- ***IV continuous infusion:*** Give 1–4 mg/min. Titrate the dose down as soon as the cardiac rhythm stabilizes.

PEDIATRIC: Safety and efficacy have not been established. American Heart Association recommends bolus of 1 mg/kg IV, followed by 30 $\mu$g/kg per min with caution. The IM auto-injector device is not recommended.

*As local anesthetic:* Preparations containing preservatives should not be used for spinal or epidural anesthesia. Drug concentration and diluent should be appropriate to particular local anesthetic use: 5% solution with glucose is used for spinal anesthesia, 1.5% solution with dextrose for low spinal or "saddle block" anesthesia. Dosage varies with the area to be anesthetized and the reason for the anesthesia; use the lowest dose possible to achieve results. Caution: Use lower concentrations in debilitated, elderly, and pediatric patients.

## Pharmacokinetics

| Route | Onset | Peak | Duration |
|---|---|---|---|
| IM | 5–10 min | 5–15 min | 2 h |
| IV | Immediate | Immediate | 10–20 min |
| Topical | Minimally absorbed systemically | | |

*Metabolism:* Hepatic, $T_{1/2}$: 10 min, then 1.5 to 3 h

*Distribution:* Crosses placenta; enters breast milk

*Excretion:* Urine

### IV facts

**Preparation:** Prepare solution for IV infusion as follows: 1–2 g lidocaine to 1 L 5% Dextrose in Water 0.1%–0.2% solution; 1–2 mg lidocaine/ml. Stable for 24 h after dilution.

**Infusion:** IV bolus: give 50–100 mg at rate of 20–50 mg/min. An infusion rate of 1–4 ml/min will provide 1–4 mg lidocaine/min. Use only preparations of lidocaine specifically labeled for IV infusion.

## Adverse effects

*Lidocaine as Antiarrhythmic—Systemic Administration*

- CNS: *Dizziness/lightheadedness, fatigue, drowsiness*, unconsciousness, tremors, twitching, vision changes, may progress to seizures, convulsions
- GI: *Nausea*, vomiting
- CV: *Cardiac arrhythmias,* cardiac arrest, vasodilation, *hypotension*
- **Respiratory**: Respiratory depression and arrest
- **Hypersensitivity**: Rash, anaphylactoid reactions
- **Other**: Malignant hyperthermia

*Lidocaine as Injectable Local Anesthetic for Epidural or Caudal Anesthesia*

- CNS: *Headache, backache*, septic meningitis, persistent sensory, motor, or autonomic deficit of lower spinal segments, sometimes with incomplete recovery
- CV: *Hypotension* due to sympathetic block
- GU: *Urinary retention, urinary or fecal incontinence*

*Lidocaine as Topical Local Anesthetic*

- **Dermatologic**: Contact dermatitis, urticaria, cutaneous lesions
- **Hypersensitivity**: Anaphylactoid reactions
- **Local**: *Burning, stinging, tenderness, swelling, tissue irritation*, tissue sloughing and necrosis
- **Other**: Methemoglobinemia, seizures

## Clinically important drug-drug interactions

- Increased lidocaine levels with beta-blockers (propranolol, metoprolol, nadolol, pindolol, atenolol), cimetidine, ranitidine
- Prolonged apnea with succinlycholine

## Drug-lab test interferences

- Increased CPK if given IM

## ■ Nursing Considerations

### Assessment

- *History:* Allergy to lidocaine or amide-type local anesthetics, CHF, cardiogenic shock, second or third-degree heart block, Wolff-Parkinson-White syndrome, Stokes-

Adams syndrome, hepatic or renal disease, inflammation or sepsis in region of injection, lactation
- *Physical:* T; skin color, rashes, lesions; orientation, speech, reflexes, sensation and movement (local anesthetic); P, BP, auscultation, continuous ECG monitoring during use as antiarrhythmic, edema; R, adventitious sounds; bowel sounds, liver evaluation; urine output; serum electrolytes, liver and renal function tests

**Implementation**

- Check drug concentration carefully; many concentrations are available.
- Reduce dosage with hepatic or renal failure.
- Continuously monitor response when used as antiarrhythmic or injected as local anesthetic.
- Maintain life-support equipment, and have vasopressors on standby if severe adverse reaction (CNS, CVS, or respiratory) occurs when lidocaine is injected.
- Establish safety precautions if CNS changes occur; have IV diazepam or short-acting barbiturate (thiopental, thiamylal) on standby in case of convulsions.
- Monitor for malignant hyperthermia (jaw muscle spasm, rigidity); have life-support equipment and IV dantrolene on standby.
- Titrate dose to minimum needed for cardiac stability, when using lidocaine as antiarrhythmic, .
- Reduce dosage when treating arrhythmias in CHF, digitalis toxicity with AV block, and geriatric patients.
- Monitor fluid load carefully; more concentrated solutions can be used to treat arrhythmias in patients on fluid restrictions.
- Have patients who have received lidocaine as a spinal anesthetic remain lying flat for 6–12 h afterward, and ensure that they are adequately hydrated to minimize risk of headache.
- Check lidocaine preparation carefully; epinephrine is added to solutions of lidocaine to retard the absorption of the local anesthetic from the injection site. Be sure that such solutions are used *only* to produce local anesthesia. These solutions should be injected cautiously in body areas supplied by end arteries and used cautiously in patients with peripheral vascular disease, hypertension, thyrotoxicosis, or diabetes.
- Use caution to prevent choking. Patient may have difficulty swallowing following use of oral topical anesthetic. Do not give food or drink for 1 h after use of oral anesthetic.
- Treat methemoglobinemia with 1% methylene blue, 0.1 mg/kg, IV over 10 min.
- Apply lidocaine ointments or creams to a gauze or bandage before applying to the skin.
- Monitor for safe and effective serum drug concentrations (antiarrhythmic use; 1–5 $\mu$g/ml).

**Drug-specific teaching points**

- Dosage is changed frequently in response to cardiac rhythm on monitor.
- The following side effects may occur: drowsiness, dizziness, numbness, double vision; nausea, vomiting; stinging, burning, local irritation (local anesthetic).
- Oral lidocaine can cause numbness of the tongue, cheeks, and throat. Do not eat or drink for 1 h after using oral lidocaine to prevent biting cheeks or tongue and choking.
- Report difficulty speaking, "thick" tongue, numbness, tingling, difficulty breathing, pain or numbness at IV site, swelling, or pain at site of local anesthetic use.



## lincomycin hydrochloride

*(lin koe **mye'** sin)*

Lincocin, Lincorex

**Pregnancy Category B**

**Drug classes**

Lincosamide antibiotic

**Therapeutic actions**

Inhibits protein synthesis in susceptible bacteria, causing cell death.

### Indications

- Treatment of some staphylcoccal, streptococcal, and pneumococcal infections resistant to other antibiotics in penicillin-allergic patients or when penicillin is inappropriate. Less toxic antibiotics (erythromycin) should be considered.

### Contraindications/cautions

- Contraindications: allergy to lincomycin, history of asthma or other allergies, and lactation.
- Use cautiously with hepatic or renal dysfunction.

### Dosage

**Available Forms:** Capsules—250, 500 mg; injection—300 mg/ml

ADULT

- ***Oral:*** 500 mg q6–8h, depending on severity of infection.
- ***IM:*** 600 mg q12–24h, depending on severity of infection.
- ***IV:*** 600 mg–1 g q8–12h, up to 8 g/d in severe infections.

PEDIATRIC (> 1 MO)

- ***Oral:*** 30–60 mg/kg per d in 3–4 equally divided doses.
- ***IM:*** 10 mg/kg q12–24h, depending on severity of infection.
- ***IV:*** 10–20 mg/kg per d in divided doses, depending on severity of infection.

NEWBORNS: Not indicated for use in newborns.

GERIATRIC OR RENAL FAILURE PATIENTS: Reduce dose to 25% to 30% of that normally recommended.

### Pharmacokinetics

| *Route* | *Onset* | *Peak* | *Duration* |
|---|---|---|---|
| Oral | Varies | 2–4 h | 6–8 h |
| IM | 20–30 min | 0.5 h | 24 h |
| IV | Immediate | Immediate | 14 h |

*Metabolism* : Hepatic, $T_{1/2}$: 5 h
*Distribution* : Crosses placenta; enters breast milk
*Excretion* : Urine and feces

### IV facts

**Preparation:** Dilute to a concentration of 1 g/100 ml. Severe cardiopulmonary reactions have occurred when given at greater than recommended concentrations and rate. IV administration in 250–500 ml of 5% Dextrose in Water or Normal Saline produces no local irritation or phlebitis. Use with 5% Dextrose in Water or in Saline.

**Infusion:** *Do not* inject as a bolus, infuse over 10–60 min.

**Incompatibilities:** Lincomycin is *not* compatible in solution with novobiocin, kanamycin, or phenytoin sodium.

### Adverse effects

- CNS: Tinnitus, vertigo
- GI: Severe colitis, including **pseudomembranous colitis** (fatal in some instances), *nausea, vomiting, diarrhea, stomatitis, glossitis, pruritus ani*, jaundice, liver function changes
- Hematologic: *Neutropenia,* leukopenia, agranulocytosis, thrombocytopenia, aplastic anemia
- GU: Vaginitis, kidney function changes
- Dermatologic: Skin rashes, urticaria to anaphylactoid reactions, angioneurotic edema
- Local: *Pain following injection*
- Other: Serum sickness

### Clinically important drug-drug interactions

• Increased neuromuscular blockade with neuromuscular blocking agents • Decreased GI absorption with kaolin, aluminum salts, magaldrate

## ■ Nursing Considerations

### Assessment

- *History:* Allergy to lincomycin, history of asthma or other allergies, hepatic or renal dysfunction, lactation
- *Physical:* Site of infection, skin color, lesions; orientation, reflexes, auditory function; BP; R, adventitious sounds; bowel sounds, output, liver evaluation; CBC, renal and liver function tests

### Implementation

- Administer oral drug on an empty stomach, 1 h before or 2–3 h after meals. Give with a full glass of water.

- Culture infection site before therapy.
- Do not use for minor bacterial or viral infections.
- Monitor renal function tests with prolonged therapy.
- Arrange for vancomycin and corticosteroids to be available for serious colitis.

### Drug-specific teaching points

- Take drug on an empty stomach, 1 h before or 2–3 h after meals. Take the drug with a full glass of water.
- Take prescribed course. Do not stop taking without notifying your health care provider.
- The following side effects may occur: nausea, vomiting (small frequent meals may help); superinfections in the mouth, vagina (use frequent hygiene measures,request treatment if severe); rash, flulike sickness (report if severe).
- Report severe or watery diarrhea, inflamed mouth or vagina, skin rash or lesions.

## liothyronine sodium

***(lye' oh thye' roe neen)***

$T_3$, triiodithyronine

Cytomel, Triostat

**Pregnancy Category A**

### Drug classes

Thyroid hormone

### Therapeutic actions

Increases the metabolic rate of body tissues, thereby increasing oxygen consumption; respiratory and heart rate; rate of fat, protein, and carbohydrate metabolism; and growth and maturation.

### Indications

- Replacement therapy in hypothyroidism
- Pituitary TSH suppression in the treatment and prevention of euthyroid goiters and in the management of thyroid cancer
- Thyrotoxicosis in conjunction with antithyroid drugs and to prevent goitrogenesis, hypothyroidism, and thyrotoxicosis during pregnancy
- Synthetic hormone used with patients allergic to desiccated thyroid or thyroid extract derived from pork or beef
- Diagnostic use: $T_3$ suppression test to differentiate suspected hyperthyroidism from euthyroidism
- Orphan drug use—treatment of myxedema coma and precoma

### Contraindications/cautions

- Contraindications: allergy to active or extraneous constituents of drug, thyrotoxicosis, and acute MI uncomplicated by hypothyroidism.
- Use cautiously with Addison's disease (treat hypoadrenalism with corticosteroids before thyroid therapy) and lactation.

### Dosage

**Available Forms:** Tablets—5, 25, 50 μg; injection—10 μg/ml

Drug is given only PO. 25 μg equals approximately 65 mg (1 grain) thyroid.

**ADULT**

- ***Hypothyroidism:*** Initial dosage: 25 μg/d PO. May be increased every 1–2 wk in 12.5- to 25-μg increments. Maintenance: 25 to 75 μg/d.
- ***Myxedema:*** Initial dosage: 5 μg/d PO. Increase in 5- to 10-μg increments every 1–2 wk. Maintenance: 50 to 100 μg/d.
- ***Myxedema coma and precoma:*** 25 to 50 μg IV q4–12h; do not give IM or SC.
- ***Simple goiter:*** Initial dosage: 5 μg/d PO. May be increased by 5- to 10-μg increments every 1–2 wk. Maintenance: 75 μg/d.
- ***$T_3$ suppression test:*** 75 to 100 μg/d PO for 7 d, then repeat I-131 uptake test. I-131 uptake will be unaffected in the hyperthyroid patient but will be decreased by 50% or more in the euthyroid patient.

**PEDIATRIC**

- ***Cretinism:*** Infants require replacement therapy from birth. Starting dose is 5 μg/d PO with 5-μg increments q3–4 d until the desired dosage is reached. Usual maintenance dosage: 20 μg/d PO up to 1 y of age; 50 μg/d for 1–3 y of age. Adult dosage after 3 y.

**GERIATRIC:** Start therapy with 5 μg/d PO. Increase by only 5-μg increments, and monitor patient response.

### Pharmacokinetics

| Route | Onset | Peak | Duration |
|---|---|---|---|
| Oral | Varies | 2-3 d | 3–4 d |
| IV | Rapid | End of infusion | |

*Metabolism* : Hepatic; $T_{1/2}$: 1–2 d
*Distribution* : Does not cross placenta; enters breast milk
*Excretion* : Urine

### IV facts

**Preparation:** No further preparation is needed; refrigerate vials before use; discard unused portions.
**Infusion:** Infuse slowly, each 10 mcg over 1 min. Switch to oral form as soon as possible.

### Adverse effects

- **Dermatologic**: Allergic skin reactions, partial loss of hair in first few months of therapy in children
- **Endocrine**: Mainly symptoms of hyperthyroidism: *palpitations, elevated P pressure, tachycardia, arrhythmias*, angina pectoris, cardiac arrest; tremors, *headache, nervousness, insomnia; nausea,* diarrhea, changes in appetite; weight loss, menstrual irregularities, sweating, heat intolerance, fever

### Clinically important drug-drug interactions

• Decreased absorption of oral thyroid preparation with cholestyramine • Increased risk of bleeding with warfarin or dicumarol—reduce dosage of anticoagulant when $T_4$ is begun • Decreased effectiveness of digitalis glycosides with thyroid replacement • Decreased clearance of theophyllines if patient is in hypothyroid state; monitor response and adjust dosage as patient approaches euthyroid state

## ■ Nursing Considerations

### Assessment

- *History:* Allergy to active or extraneous constituents of drug, thyrotoxicosis, acute MI uncomplicated by hypothyroidism, Addison's disease, lactation
- *Physical:* Skin lesions, color, temperature, texture; T; muscle tone, orientation, reflexes; P, auscultation, baseline ECG, BP; R, adventitious sounds; thyroid function tests

### Implementation

- Monitor patient response carefully at start of therapy, adjust dosage.
- Monitor exchange from one form of thyroid replacement to $T_3$. Discontinue the other medication, then begin this drug at a low dose with gradual increases based on the patient's response.
- Administer as a single daily dose before breakfast.
- Arrange for regular, periodic blood tests of thyroid function.
- Monitor cardiac response.

### Drug-specific teaching points

- Take as a single dose before breakfast.
- This drug replaces an important hormone and will need to be taken for life. Do not discontinue for any reason without consulting your health care provider; serious problems can occur.
- Wear a medical ID tag to alert emergency medical personnel that you are on this drug.
- Nausea and diarrhea may occur (dividing the dose may help).
- Have periodic blood tests and medical evaluations.
- Report headache, chest pain, palpitations, fever, weight loss, sleeplessness, nervousness, irritability, unusual sweating, intolerance to heat, diarrhea.

## liotrix

*(lye' oh trix)*
Thyrolar
**Pregnancy Category A**

### Drug classes

Thyroid hormone (contains synthetic T3 and T4 in a ratio of 1 to 4 by weight)

**Therapeutic actions**

Increases the metabolic rate of body tissues, thereby increasing oxygen consumption; respiratory and heart rate; rate of fat, protein, and carbohydrate metabolism; and growth and maturation.

**Indications**

- Replacement therapy in hypothyroidism
- Pituitary TSH suppression in the treatment and prevention of euthyroid goiters and in the management of thyroid cancer
- Thyrotoxicosis in conjunction with antithyroid drugs and to prevent goitrogenesis, hypothyroidism, and thyrotoxicosis during pregnancy

**Contraindications/cautions**

- Contraindications: allergy to active or extraneous constituents of drug, thyrotoxicosis, and acute MI uncomplicated by hypothyroidism.
- Use cautiously with Addison's disease (hypoadrenalism treatment with corticosteroids before thyroid therapy) and lactation.

## Dosage

**Available Forms:** Tablets—1/4, 1/2, 1, 2, 3 grains

60 mg equals 65 mg (1 grain) thyroid; administered only PO.

ADULT

- *Hypothyroidism:* Initial dosage: 15–30 mg/d PO. Increase gradually every 1–2 wk in 15-mg increments (2 wk in children).
- *Maintenance dose:* 60 to 120 mg/d PO.

PEDIATRIC

- *0–6 Mo:* 25–50 μg/d (8–10 μg/kg/d PO).
- *6–12 Mo:* 50–75 μg/d (6–8 μg/kg/d PO).
- *1–5 Y:* 75–100 μg/d (5–6 μg/kg/d PO).
- *6–12 Y:* 100–150 μg/d (4–5 μg/kg/d PO).
- *>12 Y:* >150 μg/d (2–3 μg/kg/d PO).

**Pharmacokinetics**

| *Route* | *Onset* | *Peak* | *Duration* |
|---|---|---|---|
| Oral | Varies | 2–3 d | 3 d |

*Metabolism* : Hepatic, $T_{1/2}$: 1–6 d
*Distribution* : Does not cross placenta; enters breast milk
*Excretion* : Urine

**Adverse effects**

- **Dermatologic**: Allergic skin reactions, partial hair loss in first few months of therapy in children
- **Endocrine**: Mainly symptoms of hyperthyroidism: *palpitations, elevated pulse pressure, tachycardia, arrhythmias*, angina pectoris, cardiac arrest; tremors, *headache, nervousness, insomnia; nausea,* diarrhea, changes in appetite; weight loss, menstrual irregularities, sweating, heat intolerance, fever

**Clinically important drug-drug interactions**

• Decreased absorption of oral thyroid preparation with cholestyramine • Increased risk of bleeding with warfarin or dicumarol—reduce dosage of anticoagulant when $T_4$ is begun • Decreased effectiveness of digitalis glycosides if taken with thyroid replacement • Decreased clearance of theophyllines in hypothyroid state; monitor response and adjust dosage as patient approaches euthyroid state

## ■ Nursing Considerations

### Assessment

- *History:* Allergy to active or extraneous constituents of drug, thyrotoxicosis, acute MI uncomplicated by hypothyroidism, Addison's disease, lactation
- *Physical:* Skin lesions, color, temperature, texture; T; muscle tone, orientation, reflexes; P, auscultation, baseline ECG, BP; R, adventitious sounds; thyroid function tests

### Implementation

- Monitor response carefully at start of therapy, and adjust dosage.
- Administer as a single daily dose before breakfast.
- Arrange for regular, periodic blood tests of thyroid function.
- Monitor cardiac response.

### Drug-specific teaching points

- Take as a single dose before breakfast.
- This drug replaces an important hormone and will need to be taken for life. Do not discontinue without consulting your health care provider; serious problems can occur.
- Wear a medical ID tag to alert emergency medical personnel that you take this drug.
- Nausea and diarrhea may occur (divide the dose).
- Have periodic blood tests and medical evaluations.
- Report headache, chest pain, palpitations, fever, weight loss, sleeplessness, nervousness, irritability, unusual sweating, intolerance to heat, diarrhea.

## lisinopril

*(lyse **in'** oh pril)*

Prinivil, Zestril

**Pregnancy Category C**

### Drug classes

Antihypertensive

Angiotensin converting enzyme inhibitor (ACE inhibitor)

### Therapeutic actions

Renin, synthesized by the kidneys, is released into the circulation where it acts on a plasma precursor to produce angiotensin I, which is converted by angiotensin-converting enzyme to angiotensin II, a potent vasoconstrictor that also causes release of aldosterone from the adrenals. Lisinopril blocks the conversion of angiotensin I to angiotensin II, leading to decreased BP, decreased aldosterone secretion, a small increase in serum potassium levels, and sodium and fluid loss.

### Indications

- Treatment of hypertension alone or in combination with thiazide-type diuretics
- Adjunctive therapy in CHF for patients unresponsive to diuretics and digitalis
- Treatment of stable patients within 24 h of acute MI to improve survival

### Contraindications/cautions

- Contraindications: allergy to lisinopril or enalapril.
- Use cautiously with impaired renal function, CHF, salt or volume depletion, and lactation.

### Dosage

**Available Forms:** Tablets—2.5, 5, 10, 20, 40 mg

**ADULT**

- ***Patients not taking diuretics:*** Initial dose: 10 mg/d PO. Adjust dosage based on response. Usual range is 20–40 mg/d as a single dose.
- ***Patients taking diuretics:*** Discontinue diuretic for 2–3 d. If it is not possible to discontinue, give initial dose of 5 mg, and monitor for excessive hypotension.
- *CHF:* 5 mg PO qd with diuretics and digitalis. Effective range: 5 to 20 mg/d.
- *Acute MI:* Start within 24 h of MI with 5 mg PO followed in 24 h by 5 mg PO; 10 mg after 48 h, then 10 mg PO qd for 6 wk.

**PEDIATRIC:** Safety and efficacy not established.

**GERIATRIC AND RENAL IMPAIRED:** Excretion is reduced in renal failure. Use smaller initial dose, and titrate upward to a maximum of 40 mg/d PO.

| *Creatinine Clearance (ml/min)* | *Initial Dose* |
|---|---|
| >30 | 10 mg/d |
| ≥10 ≤30 | 5 mg/d (2.5 mg for CHF) |
| <10 | 2.5 mg/d |
| Dialysis | 2.5 mg on dialysis d |

### Pharmacokinetics

| *Route* | *Onset* | *Peak* | *Duration* |
|---|---|---|---|
| Oral | 1 h | 7 h | 24 h |

*Metabolism* : Hepatic, $T_{1/2}$: 12 h

*Distribution* : Crosses placenta; enters breast milk

*Excretion* : Urine

### Adverse effects

- CNS: *Headache, dizziness, insomnia, fatigue*, paresthesias
- GI: *Gastric irritation, nausea, diarrhea*, aphthous ulcers, peptic ulcers, dysgeusia,

cholestatic jaundice, hepatocellular injury, anorexia, constipation
- CV: *Orthostatic hypotension,* tachycardia, angina pectoris, MI, Raynaud's syndrome, CHF, severe hypotension in salt or volume depleted patients
- **Hematologic**: Neutropenia, agranulocytosis, thrombocytopenia, hemolytic anemia, **fatal pancytopenia**
- GU: *Proteinuria*, renal insufficiency, renal failure, polyuria, oliguria, frequency
- **Other**: *Angioedema* (particularly of the face, extremities, lips, tongue, larnyx; death has been reported with **airway obstruction**); *cough,* muscle cramps, impotence

### Clinically important drug-drug interactions

- Decreased antihypertensive effects if taken with indomethacin

## ■ Nursing Considerations

### Assessment

- *History:* Allergy to lisinopril or enalapril, impaired renal function, CHF, salt or volume depletion, lactation
- *Physical:* Skin color, lesions, turgor; T; P, BP, peripheral perfusion; mucous membranes, bowel sounds, liver evaluation; urinalysis, renal and liver function tests, CBC and differential

### Implementation

- Begin drug within 24 h of acute MI; ensure that patient is also receiving standard treatment (thrombolytics, aspirin, beta blockers, etc.).
- Maintain epinephrine on standby in case of angioedema of the face or neck region; if breathing difficulty occurs, consult physician, and administer epinephrine.
- Alert surgeon, and mark patient's chart with notice that lisinopril is being taken. The angiotensin II formation subsequent to compensatory renin release during surgery will be blocked. Hypotension may be reversed with volume expansion.
- Monitor patients on diuretic therapy for excessive hypotension following the first few doses of lisinopril.
- Monitor patients closely in any situation that may lead to a decrease in BP secondary to reduction in fluid volume—excessive perspiration and dehydration, vomiting, diarrhea—because excessive hypotension may occur.
- Arrange for reduced dosage in patients with impaired renal function.

### Drug-specific teaching points

- Take this drug once a day. It may be taken with meals. Do not stop taking without consulting your prescriber.
- The following side effects may occur: GI upset, loss of appetite, change in taste perception (may be transient; take with meals); mouth sores (use frequent mouth care); skin rash; fast heart rate; dizziness, lightheadedness (transient; change position slowly, and limit activities to those that do not require alertness and precision); headache, fatigue, sleeplessness.
- Be careful in situations that may lead to a drop in BP—diarrhea, sweating, vomiting, dehydration. If lightheadedness or dizziness occurs, consult your health care provider.
- Report mouth sores; sore throat; fever; chills; swelling of the hands or feet; irregular heartbeat; chest pains; swelling of the face, eyes, lips, or tongue; and difficulty breathing.

# Lithium

## lithium carbonate

***(lith' ee um)***

Carbolith (CAN), Duralith (CAN), Eskalith, Lithane, Lithizine (CAN), Lithonate, Lithotabs

## lithium citrate

**Pregnancy Category D**

### Drug classes

Antimanic agent

### Therapeutic actions

Mechanism is not known; alters sodium transport in nerve and muscle cells; inhibits release of norepinephrine and dopamine, but not serotonin, from stimulated neurons; slightly increases intraneuronal stores of catecholamines; decreases intraneuronal content of second messengers and may thereby selectively modulate the responsiveness of hyperactive neurons that might contribute to the manic state.

## Indications

- Treatment of manic episodes of manic-depressive illness; maintenance therapy to prevent or diminish frequency and intensity of subsequent manic episodes
- Unlabeled use—improvement of neutrophil counts in patients with cancer chemotherapy-induced neutropenia and in children with chronic neutropenia (doses of 300–1000 mg/d, serum levels of 0.5 and 1.0 mEq/L); prophylaxis of cluster headache and cyclic migraine headache (doses of 600–900 mg/d)

## Contraindications/cautions

- Contraindications: hypersensitivity to tartrazine (marketed as *Lithane*); significant renal or CV disease; severe debilitation, dehydration; sodium depletion, patients on diuretics (lithium decreases sodium reabsorption, and hyponatremia increases lithium retention); pregnancy; lactation.
- Use cautiously with protracted sweating and diarrhea; suicidal or impulsive patients; infection with fever.

## Dosage

**Available Forms:** Capsules—150, 300, 600 mg; tablets—300 mg; SR tablets—300 mg; CR tablets—450 mg; syrup—300 mg/5 ml

Individualize dosage according to serum levels and clinical response.

**ADULT**

- *Acute mania:* 600 mg PO tid or 900 mg slow-release form PO bid to produce effective serum levels between 1 and 1.5 mEq/L. Serum levels should be determined twice wkly in samples drawn immediately before a dose and 8–12 h after the previous dose.
- *Long-term use:* 300 mg PO tid to qid to produce a serum level of 0.6 to 1.2 mEq/L. Serum levels should be determined at least every 2 mo in samples drawn immediately before a dose and 8 to 12 h after the previous dose.
- *Conversion from conventional to slow-release dosage forms:* Give the same total daily dose divided into 2 or 3 doses.

**PEDIATRIC:** Safety and efficacy for children < 12 y not established.

**GERIATRIC AND RENAL IMPAIRED:** Reduced dosage may be necessary. Elderly patients often respond to reduced dosage and may exhibit signs of toxicity at serum levels tolerated by other patients. Plasma half-life is prolonged in renal impairment.

## Pharmacokinetics

| *Route* | *Onset* | *Peak* |
|---|---|---|
| Oral | 5–7 d | 10–21 d |

*Metabolism* : Hepatic, $T_{1/2}$: 17–36 h

*Distribution* : Crosses placenta; enters breast milk

*Excretion* : Urine

Reactions are related to serum lithium levels (toxic lithium levels are close to therapeutic levels: therapeutic levels in acute mania range between 1 and 1.5 mEq/L; therapeutic levels for maintenance are 0.6 to 1.2 mEq/L).

## Adverse effects

*< 1.5 mEq/L*

- CNS: *Lethargy, slurred speech, muscle weakness, fine hand tremor*
- GI: *Nausea, vomiting, diarrhea, thirst*
- GU: *Polyuria*

*1.5–2.0 mEq/L (mild to moderate toxic reactions)*

- CNS: Coarse hand tremor, mental confusion, hyperirritability of muscles, drowsiness, incoordination
- GI: Persistent GI upset, gastritis, salivary gland swelling, abdominal pain, excessive salivation, flatulence, indigestion
- CV: ECG changes

*2.0–2.5 mEq/L (moderate to severe toxic reactions)*

- CNS: Ataxia, giddiness, fasciculations, tinnitus, blurred vision, clonic movements, seizures, stupor, coma
- CV: Serious ECG changes, severe hypotension
- Respiratory: Fatalities secondary to **pulmonary complications**
- GU: Large output of dilute urine

*> 2.5 mEq/L (life-threatening toxicity)*

- General: Complex involvement of multiple organ systems

*Reactions unrelated to serum levels*

- CNS: Headache, worsening of organic brain syndromes, fever, reversible short-term memory impairment, dyspraxia
- GI: Dysgeusia/taste distortion, salty taste; swollen lips; dental caries
- CV: ECG changes; hyperkalemia associated with ECG changes; syncope; tachycardia-bradycardia syndrome; rarely, arrhythmias, CHF, diffuse myocarditis, death
- Dermatologic: Pruritus with or without rash; maculopapular, acneiform, and follicular eruptions; cutaneous ulcers; edema of ankles or wrists
- Endocrine: diffuse nontoxic goiter; hypercalcemia associated with hyperparathyroidism; transient hyperglycemia; irreversible nephrogenic diabetes insipidus, which improves with diuretic therapy; impotence or sexual dysfunction
- Miscellaneous: Weight gain (5–10 kg); chest tightness; reversible respiratory failure; swollen or painful joints, eye irritation, worsening of cataracts, disturbance of visual accommodation

### Clinically important drug-drug interactions

• Increased risk of toxicity with thiazide diuretics due to decreased renal clearance of lithium—reduced lithium dosage may be necessary • Increased plasma lithium levels with indomethacin and some other NSAIDs—phenylbutazone, piroxicam, ibuprofen • Increased CNS toxicity with carbamazepine • Encephalopathic syndrome (weakness, lethargy, fever, tremulousness, confusion, extrapyramidal symptoms, leukocytosis, elevated serum enzymes) with irreversible brain damage when taken with haloperidol • Greater risk of hypothyroidsim with iodide salts • Decreased effectiveness due to increased excretion of lithium with urinary alkalinizers, including antacids, tromethamine

## ■ Nursing Considerations

### Assessment

- *History:* Hypersensitivity to tartrazine; significant renal or CV disease; severe debilitation, dehydration; sodium depletion, patients on diuretics; protracted sweating, diarrhea; suicidal or impulsive patients; infection with fever; pregnancy; lactation
- *Physical:* Weight and T; skin color, lesions; orientation, affect, reflexes; ophthalmic exam; P, BP, R, adventitious sounds; bowel sounds, normal output; normal fluid intake, normal output, voiding pattern; thyroid, renal glomerular and tubular function tests, urinalysis, CBC and differential, baseline ECG

### Implementation

- Give with caution and daily monitoring of serum lithium levels to patients with renal or CV disease, debilitation, or dehydration or life-threatening psychiatric disorders.
- Give drug with food or milk or after meals.
- Monitor clinical status closely, especially during initial stages of therapy; monitor for therapeutic serum levels of 0.6–1.2 mEq/l.
- Individuals vary in their reponse to this drug; some patients may exhibit toxic signs at serum lithium levels considered within the therapeutic range.
- Decrease dosage after the acute manic episode is controlled; lithium tolerance is greater during the acute manic phase and decreases when manic symptoms subside.

- Ensure that patient maintains adequate intake of salt and adequate intake of fluid (2,500–3,000 ml/d).

**Drug-specific teaching points**

- Take this drug exactly as prescribed, after meals or with food or milk.
- Eat a normal diet with normal salt intake; maintain adequate fluid intake (at least 2 1/2 quarts/d).
- Arrange for frequent checkups, including blood tests. Keep all appointments for checkups to receive maximum benefits and minimum risks of toxicity.
- The following side effects may occur: drowsiness, dizziness (avoid driving or performing tasks that require alertness); GI upset (frequent small meals may help); mild thirst, greater than usual urine volume, fine hand tremor (may persist throughout therapy; notify heath care provider if severe).
- Use contraception to avoid pregnancy. If you wish to become pregnant or believe that you have become pregnant, consult your care provider.
- Discontinue drug, and notify care provider if toxicity occurs: diarrhea, vomiting, ataxia, tremor, drowsiness, lack of coordination or muscular weakness.
- Report diarrhea or fever.

# lomefloxacin hydrochloride

*(low ma **flox'** a sin)*

Maxaquin

**Pregnancy Category C**

## Drug classes

Antibiotic
Fluoroquinolone

## Therapeutic actions

Bactericidal: interferes with DNA replication in gram-negative bacteria, preventing cell reproduction and causing cell death.

## Indications

- For the treatment of infections in adults caused by susceptible organisms: lower respiratory tract infections caused by *Haemophilus influenzae, Moraxella catarrhalis*; urinary tract infections due to *Escherichia coli, Klebsiella pneumoniae, Proteus mirabilis, Staphylococcus epidermidis, Enterobacter cloacae, Citrobacter diversus, Pseudomonas aeruginosa*
- Prophylaxis: preoperatively to reduce the incidence of urinary tract infections in early postoperative period in patients undergoing transurethral procedures
- Preoperative prevention of infection in transrectal prostate biopsy

## Contraindications/cautions

- Contraindications: allergy to lomefloxacin, norfloxacin, syphilis, pregnancy, lactation.
- Use cautiously with renal dysfunction and seizures.

## Dosage

**Available Forms:** Tablets—400 mg

*ADULT*

- ***Lower respiratory tract infection:*** 400 mg qd PO for 10 d.
- ***UTIs:*** 400 mg qd PO for 10 d.
- ***Complicated UTIs:*** 400 mg qd PO for 14 d.
- ***Prophylaxis:*** Single dose of 400 mg PO 2–6 h prior to surgery when oral preoperative medication is appropriate.

*PEDIATRIC:* Not recommended for children > 18 y; produced lesions of joint cartilage in immature experimental animals.

*IMPAIRED RENAL FUNCTION:* Creatinine clearance > 10 but < 30 ml/min per 1.73 $m^2$: initial dose of 400 mg followed by 200 mg qd for the rest of the course.

## Pharmacokinetics

| *Route* | *Onset* | *Peak* | *Duration* |
|---|---|---|---|
| Oral | Varies | 1–1.5 h | 8–10 h |

*Metabolism* : Hepatic, $T_{1/2}$: 8 h
*Distribution* : Crosses placenta; enters breast milk
*Excretion* : Urine and feces

## Adverse effects

- CNS: *Headache, dizziness*, insomnia, fatigue, somnolence, depression, blurred vision

- GI: *Nausea, vomiting,* dry mouth, diarrhea, abdominal pain
- **Hematologic**: Elevated BUN, SGOT, SGPT, serum creatinine, and alkaline phosphatase; decreased WBC, neutrophil count, Hct
- Other: Fever, rash, photosensitivity

### Clinically important drug-drug interactions

• Decreased therapetic effect with iron salts • Decreased absorption with antacids • Increased serum levels and toxic effects of theophyllines

## ■ Nursing Considerations

### Assessment

- *History:* Allergy to lomefloxacin, ciprofloxacin, norfloxacin; renal dysfunction; seizures; lactation
- *Physical:* Skin color, lesions; T; orientation, reflexes, affect; mucous membranes, bowel sounds; renal and liver function tests

### Implementation

- Arrange for culture and sensitivity tests before beginning therapy.
- Continue therapy for 2 d after the signs and symptoms of infection have disappeared.
- Give oral drug without regard to meals.
- Ensure that patient is well hydrated.
- Give antacids at least 2 h after dosing.
- Monitor clinical response; if no improvement is seen or a relapse occurs, repeat culture and sensitivity.

### Drug-specific teaching points

- Take oral drug without regard to meals. If an antacid is needed, do not take it within 2 h of lomefloxacin dose.
- Drink plenty of fluids.
- The following side effects may occur: nausea, vomiting, abdominal pain (small, frequent meals may help); drowsiness, blurred vision, dizziness (observe caution if driving or using dangerous equipment).
- Report rash, visual changes, severe GI problems, weakness, tremors.

# lomustine

*(loe **mus'** teen)*

CCNU

CeeNu

**Pregnancy Category D**

### Drug classes

Alkylating agent, nitrosourea
Antineoplastic

### Therapeutic actions

Cytotoxic: exact mechanism of action is not known, but it alkylates DNA and RNA, thus inhibiting DNA, RNA, and protein synthesis.

### Indications

- Palliation with other agents for primary and metastatic brain tumors and Hodgkin's disease

### Contraindications/cautions

- Contraindications: allergy to lomustine, radiation therapy, chemotherapy, hematopoietic depression, pregnancy (teratogenic and embryotoxic in preclinical studies), and lactation.
- Use cautiously with impaired renal or hepatic function.

### Dosage

**Available Forms:** Capsules—10, 40, 100 mg

*ADULT AND PEDIATRIC:* 130 mg/m$^2$ PO as a single dose every 6 wk. Adjustments must be made with bone marrow suppression; initially reduce the dose to 100 mg/m$^2$ PO every 6 wk; do not give a repeat dose until platelets are > 100,000/mm$^3$ and leukocytes are > 4,000/mm$^3$; adjust dosage after initial dose based on hematologic response as follows: Minimum count after prior dose:

| *Leukocytes* | *Platelets* | *Percentage of Prior Dose to Give* |
|---|---|---|
| >4000 | >100,000 | 100 |
| 3000–3999 | 75,000–99,999 | 100 |
| 2000–2999 | 25,000–74,999 | 70 |
| <2000 | <25,000 | 50 |

**Pharmacokinetics**

| *Route* | *Onset* | *Peak* | *Duration* |
|---|---|---|---|
| Oral | 10 min | 3 h | 48 h |

*Metabolism* : Hepatic, $T_{1/2}$: 16 to 72 h
*Distribution* : Crosses placenta; enters breast milk
*Excretion* : Urine

**Adverse effects**
- GI: *Nausea, vomiting,* stomatitis, hepatotoxicity
- **Hematologic:** *Leukopenia; thrombocytopenia; anemia*, delayed for 4 to 6 wk; immunosuppression
- GU: Renal toxicity
- **Other:** Cancer

## ■ Nursing Considerations

### Assessment
- ***History:*** Allergy to lomustine, radiation therapy, chemotherapy, hematopoietic depression, impaired renal or hepatic function, pregnancy, lactation
- ***Physical:*** T; weight; mucous membranes, liver evaluation; CBC, differential; urinalysis, liver and renal function tests

### Implementation
- Arrange for blood tests to evaluate hematopoietic function before therapy and wkly for at least 6 wk there after.
- Do not give full dosage within 2–3 wk after a full course of radiation therapy or chemotherapy due to risk of severe bone marrow depression; reduced dosage may be needed.
- Reduce dosage in patients with depressed bone marrow function.
- Administer tablets on an empty stomach to decrease GI upset; antiemetics may be needed for nausea and vomiting.

### Drug-specific teaching points
- Take this drug on an empty stomach.
- The following side effects may occur: nausea, vomiting, loss of appetite (take on an empty stomach, an antiemetic may be ordered; small frequent meals may help).
- Maintain your fluid intake and nutrition.
- Use birth control; this drug can cause severe birth defects.
- Report unusual bleeding or bruising, fever, chills, sore throat, stomach or flank pain, sores on your mouth or lips, unusual tiredness, confusion.

# loperamide hydrochloride

*(loe **per'** a mide)*

*Prescription:* Imodium

*OTC:* Imodium A-D, Kaopectate II, Maalox Anti-Diarrheal Caplets, Pepto-Bismol

**Pregnancy Category B**

**Drug classes**
Antidiarrheal agent

**Therapeutic actions**
Slows intestinal motility and affects water and electrolyte movement through the bowel by inhibiting peristalsis through direct effects on the circular and longitudinal muscles of the intestinal wall.

**Indications**
- Control and symptomatic relief of acute nonspecific diarrhea and chronic diarrhea associated with inflammatory bowel disease
- Reduction of volume of discharge from ileostomies
- OTC use: control of diarrhea, including traveler's diarrhea

**Contraindications/cautions**
- Contraindications: allergy to loperamide, patients who must avoid constipation, diarrhea associated with organisms that penetrate the intestinal mucosa (*E. coli, Salmonella, Shigella*).
- Use cautiously with hepatic dysfunction, acute ulcerative colitis, pregnancy, and lactation.

### Dosage
**Available Forms:** Tablets—2 mg; capsules—2 mg; liquid—1 mg/5 ml

ADULT

- *Acute diarrhea:* Initial dose of 4 mg PO followed by 2 mg after each unformed stool. Do not exceed 16 mg/d. Clinical improvement is usually seen within 48 h.
- *Chronic diarrhea:* Initial dose of 4 mg PO followed by 2 mg after each unformed stool until diarrhea is controlled. Individualize dose based on patient response. Optimal daily dose is 4–8 mg. If no clinical improvement is seen with dosage of 16 mg/d for 10 d, further treatment will probably not be effective.
- *OTC—traveler's diarrhea:* 4 mg PO after first loose stool, followed by 2 mg after each subsequent stool; do not exceed 8 mg/d for more than 2 d.

PEDIATRIC: Avoid use in children < 2 y, and use extreme caution in younger children. Do not use OTC product with children.

- *Acute diarrhea:* First-day dosage schedule:

| *Age* | *Weight* | *Dose Form* | *Amount* |
|---|---|---|---|
| 2–5 y | 13–20 kg | Liquid | 1 mg tid |
| 5–8 y | 20–30 kg | Liquid or capsule | 2 mg bid |
| 8–12 y | >30 kg | Liquid or capsule | 2 mg tid |

Subsequent doses: Administer 1 mg/10 kg PO only after a loose stool. Do not exceed daily dosage of the recommended dosage for the first day.

- *Chronic diarrhea:* Dosage schedule has not been established.
- *OTC—traveler's diarrhea: 9–11 y:* 2 mg PO after first loose stool followed by 1 mg after each subsequent stool; *6–8 y:* 1 mg PO after first loose stool, followed by 1 mg after each subsequent loose stool—do not exceed 4 mg/d; *< 6 y:* consult with physician; not recommended.

### Pharmacokinetics

| *Route* | *Onset* | *Peak* |
|---|---|---|
| Oral | Varies | 5 h |

*Metabolism* : Hepatic, $T_{1/2}$: 10.8 h
*Distribution* : May cross placenta and enter breast milk
*Excretion* : Urine and feces

### Adverse effects

- CNS: Tiredness, drowsiness, or dizziness
- GI: **Toxic megacolon** (in patients with ulcerative colitis), *abdominal pain, distention or discomfort, constipation, dry mouth, nausea,* vomiting
- Hypersensitivity: Skin rash

## ■ Nursing Considerations

### Assessment

- *History:* Allergy to loperamide, patients who must avoid constipation, diarrhea associated with organisms that penetrate the intestinal mucosa (*E. coli, Salmonella, Shigella*); hepatic dysfunction, acute ulcerative colitis, lactation
- *Physical:* Skin color, lesions; orientation, reflexes; abdominal exam, bowel sounds, liver evaluation; serum electrolytes (with extended use)

### Implementation

- Monitor for response. If improvement is not seen within 48 h, discontinue treatment and notify physician.
- Give drug after each unformed stool. Keep track of amount given to avoid exceeding the recommended daily dosage.
- Have the narcotic antagonist naloxone on standby in case of overdose and CNS depression.

### Drug-specific teaching points

- Take drug as prescribed. Do not exceed prescribed dosage or recommended daily dosage.
- The following side effects may occur: abdominal fullness, nausea, vomiting; dry mouth (suck on sugarless lozenges); dizziness.
- Report abdominal pain or distention, fever, and diarrhea that does not stop after a few days.

# loracarbef

*(lor ah **kar'** bef)*

Lorabid

**Pregnancy Category B**

## Drug classes

Antibiotic

Cephalosporin (second generation)

## Therapeutic actions

Bactericidal: inhibits synthesis of bacterial cell wall, causing cell death.

## Indications

- Pharyngitis/tonsillitis caused by *Streptococcus pyogenes*
- Secondary bacterial infection of acute bronchitis and exacerbation of chronic bronchitis caused by *S. pneumoniae, H. influenzae, M. catarrhalis*
- Pneumonia caused by *S. pneumoniae, H. influenzae*
- Dermatologic infections caused by *Staphylococcus aureus, S. pyogenes*
- Urinary tract infections caused by *E. coli, Staphylococcus saprophyticus*
- Otitis media caused by *S. pneumoniae, H. influenzae, M. catarrhalis, S. pyogenes*

## Contraindications/cautions

- Allergy to cephalosporins or penicillins, renal failure, lactation

## Dosage

**Available Forms:** Capsules—200 mg; powder for suspension—100 mg/5 ml

*ADULT:* 200 to 400 mg PO q12h. Continue treatment for 7 to 14 d, depending on the severity of the infection.

*PEDIATRIC:* 15 to 30 mg/kg per d in divided doses q12h PO. Continue treatment for 7 to 10 d.

*GERIATRIC OR RENAL IMPAIRED:* Creatinine clearance >50 ml/min—use standard dose. Creatinine clearance 10–49 ml/min—use 50% of standard dose.

## Pharmacokinetics

| Route | Peak |
|---|---|
| PO | 90 min |

*Metabolism* : Hepatic, $T_{1/2}$: 60 min

*Distribution* : Crosses the placenta, enters breast milk

*Excretion* : Renal, unchanged

## Adverse effects

- CNS: Headache, dizziness, lethargy, paresthesias
- GI: *Nausea, vomiting, diarrhea, anorexia, abdominal pain, flatulence,* **pseudomembranous colitis**, liver toxicity
- **Hematologic**: Bone marrow depression
- GU: Nephrotoxicity
- Hypersensitivity: *Ranges from rash to fever* to **anaphylaxis;** serum sickness reaction
- Other: *Superinfections*

## Clinically important drug-drug interactions

• Increased nephrotoxicity with aminoglycosides • Increased bleeding effects if taken with oral anticoagulants • Decreased dose of anticoagulant may be needed • Disulfiram-like reaction if alcohol is taken within 72 h after loracarbef administration

## Drug-lab test interferences

• Possibility of false results on tests of urine glucose using Benedict's solution, Fehling's solution, Clinitest tablets, urinary 17-ketosteroids, direct Coombs' test

## ■ Nursing Considerations

### Assessment

- *History:* Penicillin or cephalosporin allergy, pregnancy or lactation
- *Physical:* Kidney function, respiratory status, skin status; culture and sensitivity tests of infected area

### Implementation

- Culture infection before drug therapy.
- Give drug on an empty stomach, 1 h before or 2 h after meals.
- Reconstitute solution by adding 30–60 ml water in two portions to the dry mixture in the 50 or 100-ml bottle, respectively.

- Keep suspension at room temperature after reconstitution, discard after 14 d.
- Stop drug if hypersensitivy reaction occurs.
- Arrange for oral vancomycin for serious colitis that fails to respond to discontinuation.
- Reculture infected area if infection fails to respond.

### Drug-specific teaching points

- Take this drug on an empty stomach, 1 h before or 2 h after meals. Store suspension at room temperature, and discard any unused portions after 14 d.
- Complete the full course of this drug, even if you feel better before the treatment is over.
- This drug is prescribed for this infection; do not self-treat other infections.
- The following side effects may occur: stomach upset, loss of appetite, nausea (take with food); diarrhea, headache, dizziness.
- Report severe diarrhea with blood, pus, or mucus; rash or hives; difficulty breathing; unusual tiredness or fatigue; unusual bleeding or bruising.

## loratidine

*(lor at' a deen)*

Claritin, Claritin Reditabs (rapid dissolution)

**Pregnancy Category C**

### Drug classes

Antihistamine (nonsedating type)

### Therapeutic actions

Competitively blocks the effects of histamine at peripheral $H_1$ receptor sites; has anticholinergic (atropine-like) and antipruritic effects.

### Indications

- Symptomatic relief of perennial and seasonal allergic rhinitis, vasomotor rhinitis, allergic conjunctivitis, and mild, uncomplicated urticaria and angioedema
- Treatment of rhinitis and chronic urticaria in children >6 y
- Amelioraton of allergic reactions to blood or plasma
- Dermatographism
- Adjunctive therapy in anaphylactic reactions

### Contraindications/cautions

- Allergy to any antihistamines; narrow-angle glaucoma, stenosing peptic ulcer, symptomatic prostatic hypertrophy, asthmatic attack, bladder neck obstruction, pyloroduodenal obstruction (avoid use or use with caution, condition may be exacerbated by drug); lactation

### Dosage

**Available Forms:** Tablets—10 mg; syrup—1 mg/ml; Reditabs—10 mg

**Adult and Children > 12 Y:** 10 mg qd PO on an empty stomach.

**Pediatric < 12 Y:** Safety and efficacy not established.

**Geriatric or Hepatic Impairment:** 10 mg PO qod.

### Pharmacokinetics

| *Route* | *Onset* | *Peak* | *Duration* |
|---|---|---|---|
| Oral | 1–3 h | 8–12 h | 24 h |

*Metabolism* : Hepatic, $T_{1/2}$: 8.4 h

*Distribution* : Crosses placenta; enters breast milk

*Excretion* : Urine and feces

### Adverse effects

- CNS: *Headache, nervousness, dizziness,* depression
- GI: *Appetite increase*, nausea, diarrhea, abdominal pain
- CV: Palpitation, edema
- **Respiratory**: Bronchospasm, pharyngitis
- **General**: *Weight gain*
- **Other**: Fever, photosensitivity, rash, myalgia, arthralgia, angioedema

### Clinically important drug-drug interactions

• Additive CNS depressant effects with alcohol or other CNS depressants • Increased and prolonged anticholinergic (drying) effects with MAO inhibitors; avoid this combination.

### Drug-lab test interferences

- False skin testing procedures if done while patient is on antihistamines.

## ■ Nursing Considerations

### Assessment

- *History:* Allergy to any antihistamines; narrow-angle glaucoma, stenosing peptic ulcer, symptomatic prostatic hypertrophy, asthmatic attack, bladder neck obstruction, pyloroduodenal obstruction; lactation
- *Physical:* Skin color, lesions, texture; orientation, reflexes, affect; vision exams; R, adventitious sounds; prostate palpation; serum transaminase levels

### Implementation

- Administer on an empty stomach 1 h before or 2 h after meals.

### Drug-specific teaching points

- Take this drug on an empty stomach 1 h before or 2 h after meals or food.
- The following side effects may occur: dizziness, sedation, drowsiness (use caution if driving or performing tasks that require alertness); headache; thickening of bronchial secretions, dryness of nasal mucosa (use a humidifier).
- Avoid the use of alcohol; serious sedation could occur.
- Report difficulty breathing, hallucinations, tremors, loss of coordination, irregular heartbeat.

## lorazepam

*(lor a' ze pam)*

Apo-Lorazepam (CAN), Ativan, Novolorazem (CAN)

**Pregnancy Category D**
**C-IV controlled substance**

### Drug classes

Benzodiazepine
Antianxiety agent
Sedative/hypnotic

### Therapeutic actions

Exact mechanisms are not understood; acts mainly at subcortical levels of the CNS, leaving the cortex relatively unaffected. Main sites of action may be the limbic system and reticular formation; benzodiazepines potentiate the effects of GABA, an inhibitory neurotransmitter; anxiolytic effects occur at doses well below those necessary to cause sedation and ataxia.

### Indications

- Management of anxiety disorders or for short-term relief of symptoms of anxiety or anxiety associated with depression (oral)
- Preanesthetic medication in adults to produce sedation, relieve anxiety, and decrease recall of events related to surgery (parenteral)
- Unlabeled parenteral use—management of status epilepticus, chemotherapy induced nausea and vomiting, acute alcohol withdrawal

### Contraindications/cautions

- Contraindications: hypersensitivity to benzodiazepines, propylene glycol, polyethylene glycol or benzyl alcohol (parenteral lorazepam); psychoses; acute narrow-angle glaucoma; shock; coma; acute alcoholic intoxication with depression of vital signs; pregnancy (crosses placenta; risk of congenital malformations and neonatal withdrawal syndrome); labor and delivery (''floppy infant'' syndrome); and lactation.
- Use cautiously with impaired liver or kidney function or debilitation.

### Dosage

**Available Forms:** Injection—2, 4 mg/ml; oral solution—2 mg/ml; tablets—0.5, 1, 2 mg

**ADULT**

- ***Oral:*** Usual dose is 2–6 mg/d; range 1–10 mg/d given in divided doses with largest dose hs. Insomnia due to transient stress: 2–4 mg given hs.
- ***IM:*** 0.05 mg/kg up to a maximum of 4 mg administered at least 2 h before operative procedure.
- ***IV:*** Initial dose is 2 mg total or 0.044 mg/kg, whichever is smaller. Do not ex-

ceed this dose in patients older than 50 y. Doses as high as 0.05 mg/kg up to a total of 4 mg may be given 15 to 20 min before the procedure to those benefitted by a greater lack of recall.

*PEDIATRIC:* Drug should not be used in children < 12 y.

*GERIATRIC PATIENTS OR THOSE WITH DEBILITATING DISEASE:* Initially, 1 to 2 mg/d in divided doses. Adjust as needed and tolerated.

**Pharmacokinetics**

| *Route* | *Onset* | *Peak* | *Duration* |
|---|---|---|---|
| Oral | Intermed. | 1–6 h | 12–24 h |
| IM | 15–30 min | 60–90 min | 12-24 h |
| IV | 1–5 min | 10–15 min | 12–24 h |

*Metabolism* : Hepatic, $T_{1/2}$: 10–20 h
*Distribution* : Crosses placenta; enters breast milk
*Excretion* : Urine

**IV facts**

**Preparation:** Dilute lorazepam immediately prior to IV use. For direct IV injection or injection into IV line, dilute with an equal volume of compatible solution (Sterile Water for Injection, Sodium Chloride Injection or 5% Dextrose Injection); do not use if solution is discolored or contains a precipitate. Protect from light; refrigerate.

**Infusion:** Direct inject slowly, or infuse at maximum rate of 2 mg/min.

**Adverse effects**

- CNS: *Transient, mild drowsiness initially; sedation, depression, lethargy, apathy, fatigue, lightheadedness, disorientation, anger, hostility,* episodes of mania and hypomania, *restlessness, confusion, crying,* delirium, *headache,* slurred speech, dysarthria, stupor, rigidity, tremor, dystonia, vertigo, euphoria, nervousness, difficulty concentrating, vivid dreams, psychomotor retardation, extrapyramidal symptoms; *mild paradoxical excitatory reactions during first 2 wk of treatment*
- GI: *Constipation, diarrhea, dry mouth,* salivation, *nausea,* anorexia, vomiting, difficulty in swallowing, gastric disorders, hepatic dysfunction
- CV: Bradycardia, tachycardia, CV collapse, hypertension and hypotension, palpitations, edema
- **Hematologic**: Elevations of blood enzymes: LDH, alkaline phosphatase, SGOT, SGPT; blood dyscrasias: agranulocytosis, leukopenia
- GU: Incontinence, urinary retention, changes in libido, menstrual irregularities
- **EENT**: Visual and auditory disturbances, diplopia, nystagmus, depressed hearing, nasal congestion
- **Dermatologic**: Urticaria, pruritus, skin rash, dermatitis
- **Other**: Hiccups, fever, diaphoresis, paresthesias, muscular disturbances, gynecomastia. *Drug dependence with withdrawal syndrome when drug is discontinued; more common with abrupt discontinuation of higher dosage used for longer than 4 mo.*

**Clinically important drug-drug interactions**

- Increased CNS depression with alcohol
- Decreased effectiveness with theophyllines

## ■ Nursing Considerations

### Assessment

- *History:* Hypersensitivity to benzodiazepines, propylene glycol, polyethylene glycol or benzyl alcohol; psychoses; acute narrow-angle glaucoma; shock; coma; acute alcoholic intoxication with depression of vital signs; pregnancy; lactation; impaired liver or kidney function, debilitation
- *Physical:* Skin color, lesions; T; orientation, reflexes, affect, ophthalmologic exam; P, BP; R, adventitious sounds; liver evaluation, abdominal exam, bowel sounds, normal output; CBC, liver and renal function tests

### Implementation

- Do not administer intra-arterially; arteriospasm, gangrene may result.

- Give IM injections of undiluted drug deep into muscle mass, monitor injection sites.
- Do not use solutions that are discolored or contain a precipitate. Protect drug from light, and refrigerate solution.
- Keep equipment to maintain a patent airway on standby when drug is given IV.
- Reduce dose of narcotic analgesics by at least half in patients who have received parenteral lorazepam.
- Keep patients who have received parenteral doses under close observation, preferably in bed, up to 3 h. Do not permit ambulatory patients to drive following an injection.
- Taper dosage gradually after long-term therapy, especially in epileptic patients.

### Drug-specific teaching points

- Take drug exactly as prescribed; do not stop taking drug (long-term therapy) without consulting health care provider.
- The following side effects may occur: drowsiness, dizziness (may be transient; avoid driving or engaging in dangerous activities); GI upset (take drug with food); nocturnal sleep disturbances for several nights after discontinuing the drug used as a sedative/hypnotic; depression, dreams, emotional upset, crying.
- Report severe dizziness, weakness, drowsiness that persists, rash or skin lesions, palpitations, edema of the extremities; visual changes; difficulty voiding.

## losartan potassium

*(low **sar'** tan)*

Cozaar

**Pregnancy Category D**

### Drug classes

Angiotensin II receptor blocker

### Therapeutic actions

Selectively blocks the binding of angiotensin II to specific tissue receptors found in the vascular smooth muscle and adrenal gland; this action blocks the vasoconstriction effect of the renin-angiotensin system as well as the release of aldosterone leading to decreased blood pressure.

### Indications

- Treatment of hypertension, alone or in combination with other antihypertensive agents

### Contraindications/cautions

- Contraindications: hypersensitivity to losartan, pregnancy (use during the second or third trimester can cause injury or even death to the fetus), lactation.
- Use cautiously with hepatic or renal dysfunction, hypovolemia.

### Dosage

**Available Forms:** Tablets—25, 50 mg

*ADULT:* Starting dose of 50 mg PO qd. Patients on diuretics or hypovolemic may only require 25 mg qd. Dosage ranges from 25–100 mg PO given once or twice a day have been used.

*PEDIATRIC:* Safety and efficacy not established.

### Pharmacokinetics

| *Route* | *Onset* | *Peak* |
|---|---|---|
| Oral | Varies | 1–3 h |

*Metabolism:* Hepatic: $T_{1/2}$: 2 h, then 6–9 h

*Distribution:* Crosses placenta; passes into breast milk

*Excretion:* Feces and urine

### Adverse effects

- CNS: *Headache, dizziness*, syncope, muscle weakness
- CV: Hypotension
- GI: *Diarrhea, abdominal pain, nausea*, constipation, dry mouth, dental pain
- Respiratory: *URI symptoms, cough*, sinus disorders
- Dermatological: Rash, inflammation, urticaria, pruritus, alopecia, dry skin
- Other: Cancer in preclinical studies, back pain, fever, gout

### Clinically important drug-drug interactions

- Decreased serum levels and effectiveness if taken concurrently with phenobarbital

## ■ Nursing Considerations

### Assessment

- *History:* Hypersensitivity to losartan, pregnancy, lactation, hepatic or renal dysfunction, hypovolemia.
- *Physical:* Skin lesions, turgor; T; reflexes, affect; BP; R, respiratory auscultation; liver and kidney function tests

### Implementation

- Administer without regard to meals.
- Assure that patient is not pregnant before beginning therapy, suggest the use of barrier birth control while using losartan; fetal injury and deaths have been reported.
- Find an alternative method of feeding the baby if given to a nursing mother. Depression of the renin-angiotensin system in infants is potentially very dangerous.
- Alert surgeon and mark patient's chart with notice that losartan is being taken. The blockage of the renin-angiotensin system following surgery can produce problems. Hypotension may be reversed with volume expansion.
- Monitor patient closely in any situation that may lead to a decrease in blood pressure secondary to reduction in fluid volume—excessive perspiration, dehydration, vomiting, diarrhea—excessive hypotension can occur.

### Drug-specific teaching points

- Take drug without regard to meals. Do not stop taking this drug without consulting your health care provider.
- Use a barrier method of birth control while on this drug; if you become pregnant or desire to become pregnant, consult with your physician.
- The following side effects may occur: dizziness (avoid driving a car or performing hazardous tasks); headache (request medications); nausea, vomiting, diarrhea (proper nutrition is important, consult with your dietician to maintain nutrition); symptoms of upper respiratory tract infection, cough (do not self-medicate; consult your health care provider if uncomfortable).
- Report fever, chills, dizziness, pregnancy.

# lovastatin

*(loe va **sta'** tin)*

mevinolin

Mevacor

**Pregnancy Category X**

### Drug classes

Antihyperlipidemic
HMG CoA inhibitor

### Therapeutic actions

Inhibits the enzyme that catalyzes the rate-limiting step in the cholesterol synthesis pathway, resulting in a decrease in serum cholesterol, serum LDL's (the lipids associated with the development of coronary artery disease), and either an increase or no change in serum HDL's (the lipids associated with decreased risk of CAD).

### Indications

- Treatment of familial hypercholesterolemia
- Adjunctive treatment of type II hyperlipidemia
- To slow the progression of atherosclerosis in patients with CAD

### Contraindications/cautions

- Contraindications: allergy to lovastatin, fungal byproducts, pregnancy.
- Use cautiously with impaired hepatic function, cataracts, and lactation.

### Dosage

**Available Forms:** Tablets—10, 20, 40 mg

*ADULT:* Initial 20 mg/d PO given in the evening. Maintenance doses range: 20 to 80 mg/d PO. Do not exceed 80 mg/d. Adjust at intervals of 4 wk or more. Patients receiving immunosuppressives should receive a maximum of 20 mg/d PO.

*PEDIATRIC:* Safety and efficacy not established.

### Pharmacokinetics

| *Route* | *Onset* | *Peak* |
|---|---|---|
| Oral | 2 wk | 4–6 wk |

*Metabolism:* Hepatic, $T_{1/2}$: unknown

*Distribution:* Crosses placenta; enters breast milk

*Excretion:* Bile and feces

### Adverse effects

- CNS: *Headache, blurred vision*, dizziness, insomnia, fatigue, muscle cramps, cataracts
- GI: *Flatulence, abdominal pain, cramps, constipation, nausea*, dyspepsia, heartburn
- **Hematologic**: Elevations of creatinine phosphokinase, alkaline phosphatase, and transaminases

### Clinically important drug-drug interactions

- Possibility of severe myopathy or rhabdomyolysis with cyclosporine or gemfibrozil

## ■ Nursing Considerations

### Assessment

- *History:* Allergy to lovastatin, fungal byproducts; impaired hepatic function; cataracts; pregnancy; lactation
- *Physical:* Orientation, affect, ophthalmologic exam; liver evaluation; lipid studies, liver function tests

### Implementation

- Give in the evening; highest rates of cholesterol synthesis are between midnight and 5 AM.
- Arrange for regular check-ups.
- Arrange for periodic ophthalmologic exams to check for cataract development, and liver function studies q 4–6 wk during first 15 mo and then periodically.
- Adminster only when diet restricted in cholesterol and saturated fats fails to lower cholesterol/lipids adequately.

### Drug-specific teaching points

- Take drug in the evening. Continue following a cholesterol-lowering diet while on this medication.
- The following side effects may occur: nausea (small frequent meals may help), headache, muscle and joint aches and pains (may lessen).
- Have periodic ophthalmic exams.
- Report severe GI upset, changes in vision, unusual bleeding or bruising, dark urine, or light colored stools.

# Loxapine

## loxapine hydrochloride

***(lox' a peen)***

*Oral concentrate:* Loxitane-C

*IM injection:* Loxitane

## loxapine succinate

*Oral capsules:* Loxapac (CAN), Loxitane

**Pregnancy Category C**

### Drug classes

Dopaminergic blocking agent
Antipsychotic

### Therapeutic actions

Mechanism of action is not fully understood: antipsychotic drugs block postsynaptic dopamine receptors in the brain, but this may not be necessary and sufficient for antipsychotic activity.

### Indications

- Management of manifestations of psychotic disorders

### Contraindications/cautions

- Contraindications: coma or severe CNS depression; bone marrow depression; blood dyscrasia; circulatory collapse; subcortical brain damage; Parkinson's disease; liver damage; cerebral arteriosclerosis; coronary disease; severe hypotension or hypertension.
- Use cautiously with respiratory disorders ("silent pneumonia"); glaucoma, prostatic hypertrophy; epilepsy or history of epilepsy; breast cancer (elevations in prolactin may stimulate a prolactin-dependent tumor); thyrotoxicosis; peptic ulcer, decreased renal function; myelography within previous 24 h or myelography scheduled within 48 h; exposure to heat or phosphorus insecticides; pregnancy; and lactation.

### Dosage

**Available Forms:** Capsules—5, 10, 25, 50 mg; concentrate—25 mg/ml; injection—50 mg/ml

*ADULT*

- ***Oral:*** Individualize dosage, and administer in divided doses bid to qid, initially 10 mg bid. Severely disturbed patients may need up to 50 mg/d. Increase dosage fairly rapidly over the first 7–10 d until symptoms are controlled. Usual dosage range is 60–100 mg/d; dosage greater than 250 mg/d is not recommended. Maintenance: reduce to minimum effective dose. Usual range is 20–60 mg/d.
- ***IM:*** For prompt control of symptoms in acutely agitated patients, 12.5 to 50 mg q4–6h or longer, depending on response. Once symptoms are controlled (about 5 d), change to oral medication.

*PEDIATRIC:* Not recommended for children < 16 y.

*GERIATRIC:* Use lower doses, and increase dosage more gradually than in younger patients.

### Pharmacokinetics

| *Route* | *Onset* | *Peak* | *Duration* |
|---|---|---|---|
| Oral | 30 min | 1.5–3 h | 12 h |
| IM | Rapid | | |

*Metabolism* : Hepatic, $T_{1/2}$: 19 h
*Distribution* : Not known
*Excretion* : Urine

### Adverse effects

- CNS: *Drowsiness*, insomnia, vertigo, headache, weakness, tremor, ataxia, slurring, cerebral edema, seizures, exacerbation of psychotic symptoms, extrapyramidal syndromes—*pseudoparkinsonism; dystonias; akathisia*, tardive dyskinesias, potentially irreversible, **neuroleptic malignant syndrome**
- CV: Hypotension, orthostatic hypotension, hypertension, tachycardia, bradycardia, cardiac arrest, CHF, cardiomegaly, **refractory arrhythmias** (some fatal), pulmonary edema
- Respiratory: Bronchospasm, laryngospasm, dyspnea; suppression of cough reflex and potential for aspiration
- Hematologic: Eosinophilia, leukopenia, leukocytosis, anemia; aplastic anemia; hemolytic anemia; thrombocytopenic, or nonthrombocytopenic purpura; pancytopenia
- Autonomic: Dry mouth, salivation, nasal congestion, nausea, vomiting, anorexia, fever, pallor, flushed facies, sweating, constipation, paralytic ileus, urinary retention, incontinence, polyuria, enuresis, priapism, ejaculation inhibition, male impotence
- Endocrine: Lactation, breast engorgement, galactorrhea; syndrome of inappropriate ADH secretion; amenorrhea, menstrual irregularities; gynecomastia; changes in libido; hyperglycemia or hypoglycemia; glycosuria; hyponatremia; pituitary tumor with hyperprolactinemia; inhibition of ovulation, infertility, pseudopregnancy; reduced urinary levels of gonadotropins, estrogens, progestins
- Hypersensitivity: Jaundice, urticaria, angioneurotic edema, laryngeal edema, photosensitivity, eczema, asthma, anaphylactoid reactions, exfoliative dermatitis

## ■ Nursing Considerations

### Assessment

- ***History:*** Coma or severe CNS depression; blood dyscrasia; circulatory collapse; subcortical brain damage; Parkinson's disease; liver damage; cerebral arteriosclerosis; coronary disease; severe hypotension or hypertension; respiratory disorders; glaucoma, prostatic hypertrophy; epilepsy; breast cancer; thyrotoxicosis; peptic ulcer, decreased renal function; myelography within previous 24 h or myelography scheduled within 48 h; exposure to heat or phosphorus insecticides; pregnancy
- ***Physical:*** Weight, T; reflexes, orientation, intraocular pressure; P, BP, orthostatic BP; R, adventitious sounds; bowel sounds and normal output, liver evaluation; urinary output, prostate size; CBC, urinalysis, thyroid, liver, and kidney function tests

### Implementation

- Mix the oral concentrate with orange or grapefruit juice shortly before administration.

- Do not give *Loxitane IM* intravenously.
- Arrange for discontinuation if serum creatinine or BUN become abnormal or if WBC count is depressed.
- Monitor elderly patients for dehydration, and institute remedial measures promptly; sedation and decreased sensation of thirst due to CNS effects can lead to severe dehydration.
- Consult physician regarding appropriate warning of patient or patient's guardian about tardive dyskinesias.
- Consult physician about dosage reduction and use of anticholinergic antiparkinsonian drugs (controversial) if extrapyramidal effects occur.

### Drug-specific teaching points

- Take drug exactly as prescribed.
- Avoid driving or engaging in dangerous activities if CNS or vision changes occur.
- Avoid prolonged exposure to sun or use a sunscreen or covering garments.
- Maintain fluid intake, and use precautions against heat stroke in hot weather.
- Report sore throat, fever, unusual bleeding or bruising, rash, weakness, tremors, impaired vision, dark urine, pale stools, and yellowing of the skin or eyes.

## lypressin

*(lye **press'** in)*

8-lysine vasopressin

Diapid

**Pregnancy Category C**

### Drug classes

Hormone

### Therapeutic actions

Synthetic vasopressin analog with antidiuretic hormone activity and relatively little oxytocic or vasopressor activity; promotes resorption of water in the renal tubular epithelium.

### Indications

- Control or prevention of symptoms and complications of neurogenic diabetes insipidus, especially in patients who are unresponsive to other therapy or sensitive to antidiuretic preparations of animal origin

### Contraindications/cautions

- Contraindications: allergy to lypressin or antidiuretic hormone.
- Use cautiously with vascular disease (large doses can cause coronary vasoconstriction) and pregnancy.

### Dosage

**Available Forms:** Nasal spray—0.185 mg/ml

*Nasal spray:* Administer 1–2 sprays to one or both nostrils whenever frequency of urination increases or significant thirst develops. Usual dosage is 1–2 sprays into each nostril qid. An additional hs dose helps to eliminate nocturia not controlled with regular daily dosage. If more drug is needed, decrease the interval between doses, not the number of sprays per dose (more than 2–3 sprays in each nostril is wasteful); drug will not be absorbed and will drain into the nasopharnyx and digestive tract and be digested.

### Pharmacokinetics

| *Route* | *Onset* | *Peak* | *Duration* |
|---|---|---|---|
| Intranasal | Prompt | 30–120 min | 3–8 h |

*Metabolism:* Hepatic and renal, $T_{1/2}$: 15 min

*Distribution:* Crosses placenta; enters breast milk

*Excretion:* Urine

### Adverse effects

- CNS: *Headache*, conjunctivitis, periorbital edema with itching
- GI: Heartburn secondary to excessive intranasal administration with drippage into the pharynx, abdominal cramps, diarrhea
- **Respiratory:** *Rhinorrhea, nasal congestion*, irritation and pruritus of the nasal passages, nasal ulceration, substernal tightness, coughing, transient dyspnea with inadvertent inhalation

**Clinically important drug-drug interactions**

- Possibly increased antidiuretic effect with carbamazepine, chlorpropamide

## ■ Nursing Considerations

### Assessment

- *History:* Allergy to lypression or antidiuretic hormone, vascular disease, pregnancy
- *Physical:* Nasal mucous membranes; P, BP, edema; R, adventitous sounds; bowel sounds, abdominal exam

### Implementation

- Administer intranasally only: Hold bottle upright with patient in a vertical position with head upright; spray only 2 to 3 sprays at any given dose.
- Monitor therapeutic effects with nasal congestion, allergic rhinitis, or upper respiratory infections; larger doses or adjunctive therapy may be needed because of decreased nasal absorption.
- Monitor nasal passages during long-term therapy; inappropriate administration can lead to nasal ulcerations.
- Monitor patients with CV diseases carefully for cardiac reactions.

### Drug-specific teaching points

- Learn proper administration technique for nasal use (see above). Watch patient administer drug, and review administration technique periodically with patient.
- The following side effects may occur: GI cramping, passing of gas, diarrhea; nasal irritation (use proper administration).
- Report drowsiness, listlessness, headache, shortness of breath, heartburn, abdominal cramps, severe nasal congestion or irritation.

# magaldrate

*(mag' al drate)*

hydroxymagnesium aluminate

Isopan, Lowsium, Riopan

**Pregnancy Category C**

**Drug classes**

Antacid

**Therapeutic actions**

Neutralizes or reduces gastric acidity, resulting in an increase in the pH of the stomach and duodenal bulb and inhibiting the proteolytic activity of pepsin; the combination of magnesium (causes diarrhea when administered alone) and aluminum (constipating when administered alone) salts usually minimizes adverse GI effects.

**Indications**

- Symptomatic relief of upset stomach associated with hyperacidity
- Hyperacidity associated with peptic ulcer, gastritis, peptic esophagitis, gastric hyperacidity, and hiatal hernia

**Contraindications/cautions**

- Contraindications: allergy to magnesium or aluminum products.
- Use cautiously with renal insufficiency, gastric outlet obstruction (aluminum salt may inhibit gastric emptying).

### Dosage

**Available Forms:** Suspension—540 mg/5 ml; liquid—540 mg/5 ml

*ADULT:* 480–1,080 mg PO 1 and 3 h after meals and at hs.

**Pharmacokinetics**

| *Route* | *Onset* | *Peak* |
|---|---|---|
| Oral | 30 min | 30–60 min |

Not generally absorbed systemically.

**Adverse effects**

- GI: *Rebound hyperacidity*
- **Metabolic**: Decreased absorption of fluoride and accumulation of aluminum in serum, bone, CNS (aluminum may be neurotoxic), *alkalosis,* hypermagnesemia and toxicity in renal failure patients

**Clinically important drug-drug interactions**

- Do not administer other oral drugs within 1–2 h of antacid administration; change in gastric pH may interfere with absorption of oral drugs • Decreased pharmacologic effect of tetracyclines, penicillamine, nitrofurantoin • Decreased absorption and therapeutic effects of clindamycin and lincomycin

## Nursing Considerations

### Assessment

- *History:* Allergy to magnesium or aluminum products, renal insufficiency, gastric outlet obstruction
- *Physical:* Bone and muscle strength; abdominal exam, bowel sounds; renal function tests, serum magnesium as appropriate

### Implementation

- Do not administer oral drugs within 1–2 h of antacid administration.
- Have patient chew tablets thoroughly before swallowing; follow with a glass of water or milk.
- Give between meals and at hs.
- Monitor patients on long-term therapy for signs of aluminum accumulation: bone pain, muscle weakness, malaise. Discontinue drug as needed.

### Drug-specific teaching points

- Take between meals and at bedtime. If tablets are being used, chew thoroughly before swallowing, and follow with a glass of water.
- Do not take with any other oral medications; absorption of those medications can be inhibited. Take other oral medications at least 1–2 h after aluminum salt.
- Report bone pain, muscle weakness, coffee ground vomitus, black tarry stools, no relief from symptoms being treated.

# Magnesium salts

## magnesium citrate

*(mag **nee'** zhum)*

Citrate of Magnesia

## magnesium hydroxide

Milk of Magnesia

## magnesia

## magnesium oxide

Maox 420, Mag-Ox, Uro-mag

**Pregnancy Category C**

### Drug classes

Antacid
Laxative

### Therapeutic actions

Antacid (magnesium hydroxide, magnesium oxide): neutralizes or reduces gastric acidity, resulting in an increase in the pH of the stomach and duodenal bulb and inhibition of the proteolytic activity of pepsin. Laxative (magnesium citrate, magnesium hydroxide): attracts/retains water in intestinal lumen and distends bowel; causes the duodenal secretion of cholecystokinin, which stimulates fluid secretion and intestinal motility.

### Indications

- Symptomatic relief of upset stomach associated with hyperacidity
- Hyperacidity associated with peptic ulcer, gastritis, peptic esophagitis, gastric hyperacidity, and hiatal hernia
- Prophylaxis of GI bleeding, stress ulcers, aspiration pneumonia
- Short-term relief of constipation; evacuation of the colon for rectal and bowel examination

### Contraindications/cautions

- Contraindication: allergy to magnesium products.
- Use cautiously with renal insufficiency.

### Dosage

**Available Forms:** Tablets—400, 420, 500 mg; capsules—140 mg; liquid—various

**ADULT**

- **Magnesium citrate:** 1 glassful (240 ml) PO as needed.
- **Magnesium hydroxide:** Antacid: 5–15 ml liquid or 650 mg to 1.3 g tablets PO qid (adult and children older than 12 y). Laxative: 15–60 ml PO taken with liquid.

**Magnesium oxide:** Capsules: 280 mg–1.5 g PO taken with water or milk, qid. Tablets: 400–820 mg/d PO.

PEDIATRIC

**Magnesium citrate:** Half the adult dose; repeat as needed.

**Magnesium hydroxide as laxative:** One-fourth to one-half the adult dose, depending on age.

### Pharmacokinetics

| Route | Onset |
|---|---|
| PO | 3–6 h |

Minimally absorbed systemically
*Excretion:* Renal

### Adverse effects

- CNS: Dizziness, fainting, sweating
- GI: *Diarrhea, nausea, perianal irritation*
- **Metabolic**: Hypermagnesemia and toxicity in renal failure patients

### Clinically important drug-drug interactions

- Do not give other oral drugs within 1–2h of antacid administration; change in gastric pH may interfere with absorption
- Decreased pharmacologic effect of tetracyclines, penicillamine, nitrofurantoin

## ■ Nursing Considerations

### Assessment

- *History:* Allergy to magnesium products; renal insufficiency
- *Physical:* Abdominal exam, bowel sounds; renal function tests, serum magnesium

### Implementation

- Do not administer oral drugs within 1–2 h of antacid administration.
- Have patient chew antacid tablets thoroughly before swallowing; follow with a glass of water.
- Give antacid between meals and hs.

### Drug-specific teaching points

- Take antacid between meals and at bedtime. If tablets are being used, chew thoroughly before swallowing, and follow with a glass of water.
- Do not use laxatives with abdominal pain, nausea, or vomiting.
- Refrigerate magnesium citrate solutions to retain potency and increase palatability.
- Do not take with any other oral medications; absorption of those medications can be inhibited. Take other oral medications at least 1–2 h after aluminum salt.
- Diarrhea may occur with antacid therapy.
- The following side effects may occur as a result of laxative therapy: excessive bowel activity, gripping, diarrhea, nausea, dizziness (exercise precaution not to fall).
- Do not use laxatives chronically. Prolonged or excessive use can lead to serious problems. You should increase your intake of water (6–8 glasses/d) and fiber, and exercise regularly.
- Report: Antacid use—diarrhea; coffee ground vomitus; black, tarry stools; no relief from symptoms being treated. Laxative use—rectal bleeding, muscle cramps or pain, weakness, dizziness (not related to abdominal cramps and bowel movement), unrelieved constipation.

m

## magnesium sulfate

*(mag **nee'** zhum)*

epsom salt granules

**Pregnancy Category A**

### Drug classes

Electrolyte
Anticonvulsant
Laxative

### Therapeutic actions

Cofactor of many enzyme systems involved in neurochemical transmission and muscular excitability; prevents or controls convulsions by blocking neuromuscular transmission; attracts/retains water in the intestinal lumen and distends the bowel to promote mass movement and relieve constipation.

## Indications

- Hypomagnesemia, replacement therapy (IV)
- Toxemia/eclampsia/nephritis (IV, IM)
- Short-term treatment of constipation (PO)
- Evacuation of the colon for rectal and bowel examinations (PO)
- Unlabeled use: inhibition of premature labor (parenteral)

## Contraindications/cautions

- Contraindications: allergy to magnesium products; heart block, myocardial damage; abdominal pain, nausea, vomiting or other symptoms of appendicitis; acute surgical abdomen, fecal impaction, intestinal and biliary tract obstruction, hepatitis. Do not give during 2 h preceding delivery because of risk of magnesium toxicity in the neonate.
- Use cautiously with renal insufficiency.

## Dosage

**Available Forms:** Granules—40 mEq/5 g; injection—0.8, 1, 4 mEq/ml

ADULT

- *Hyperalimentation:* 8–24 mEq/d IV.
- *Mild magnesium deficiency:* 1 g IM q6h for four doses (32.5 mEq/24 h).
- *Severe hypomagnesemia:* Up to 2 mEq/kg IM within 4 h or 5 g (40 mEq)/1,000 ml $D_5W$ IV infused over 3 h.
- *Toxemia/eclampsia/nephritis*
  - *IM:* 4–5 g of a 50% solution q4h as necessary.
  - *IV:* 1–4 g of a 10%–20% solution. Do not exceed 1.5 ml/min of a 10% solution.
  - *IV infusion:* 4–5 g in 250 ml of 5% dextrose. Do not exceed 3 ml/min.
- *Laxative:* 10–15 g PO epsom salt in glass of water.

PEDIATRIC

- *Hyperalimentation (infants):* 2–10 mEq/d IV.
- *Anticonvulsant:* 20–40 mg/kg in a 20% solution, IM. Repeat as necessary.
- *Laxative:* 5–10 g PO epsom salt in glass of water.

## Pharmacokinetics

| Route | Onset | Duration |
|---|---|---|
| IV | Immediate | 30 min |
| IM | 60 min | 3–4 h |
| PO | 1–2 h | 3–4 h |

*Metabolism:* $T_{1/2}$: unknown

*Distribution:* Crosses placenta, enters breast milk

*Excretion:* Urine

## IV facts

**Preparation:** Dilute IV infusion to a concentration of 20% or less prior to IV administration; dilute 4–5 g in 250 ml $D_5W$ or Sodium Chloride Solution.

**Infusion:** Do not exceed 1.5 ml of a 10% solution per minute IV or 3 ml/min IV infusion.

## Adverse effects

- CNS: *Weakness, dizziness*, fainting, sweating (PO)
- GI: *Excessive bowel activity, perianal irritation* (PO)
- CV: Palpitations
- **Metabolic:** *Magnesium intoxication* (flushing, sweating, hypotension, depressed relfexes, flaccid paralysis, hypothermia, circulatory collapse, cardiac and CNS depression—parenteral); hypocalcemia with tetany (secondary to treatment of eclampsia—parenteral)

## Clinically important drug-drug interactions

- Potentiation of neuromuscular blockade produced by nondepolarizing neuromuscular relaxants (tubocurarine, atracurium, gallamine, metocurine iodide, pancuronium, vecuronium)

## ■ Nursing Considerations

### Assessment

- *History:* Allergy to magnesium products; renal insufficiency; heart block, myocardial damage; symptoms of appendicitis; acute surgical abdomen, fecal impaction, intestinal and biliary tract obstruction, hepatitis

- *Physical:* Skin color, texture; muscle tone; T; orientation, affect, reflexes, peripheral sensation; P, auscultation, BP, rhythm strip; abdominal exam, bowel sounds; renal function tests, serum magnesium and calcium, liver function tests (oral use)

### Implementation

- Reserve IV use in eclampsia for immediate life threatening situations.
- Give IM route by deep IM injection of the undiluted (50%) solution for adults; dilute to a 20% solution for children.
- Monitor serum magnesium levels during parenteral therapy. Arrange to discontinue administration as soon as levels are within normal limits (1.5–3 mEq/L) and desired clinical response is obtained.
- Monitor knee-jerk reflex before repeated parenteral administration. If knee-jerk reflexes are suppressed, do not administer magnesium because respiratory center failure may occur.
- Give oral magnesium sulfate as a laxative only as a temporary measure. Arrange for dietary measures (fiber, fluids) and exercise, environmental control to return to normal bowel activity.
- Do not give oral magnesium sulfate with abdominal pain, nausea, vomiting.
- Monitor bowel function; if diarrhea and cramping occur, discontinue oral drug.
- Maintain urine output at a level of 100 ml q4h during parenteral administration.

### Drug-specific teaching points

- Use only as a temporary measure to relieve constipation. Do not take if abdominal pain, nausea, or vomiting occur.
- The following side effects may occur: diarrhea (discontinue drug, consult care porvider—oral use).
- Report sweating, flushing, muscle tremors, or twitching, inability to move extremities.

## mannitol

*(man' i tole)*

Osmitrol, Resectisol (urinary irrigant)

**Pregnancy Category C**

### Drug classes

Osmotic diuretic
Diagnostic agent
Urinary irrigant

### Therapeutic actions

Elevates the osmolarity of the glomerular filtrate, thereby hindering the reabsorption of water and leading to a loss of water, sodium, chloride (used for diagnosis of glomerular filtration rate); creates an osmotic gradient in the eye between plasma and ocular fluids, thereby reducing intraocular pressure; creates an osmotic effect, leading to decreased swelling in post-transurethral prostatic resection.

### Indications

- Prevention and treatment of the oliguric phase of renal failure
- Reduction of intracranial pressure and treatment of cerebral edema; of elevated intraocular pressure when the pressure cannot be lowered by other means
- Promotion of the urinary excretion of toxic substances
- Measurement of glomerular filtration rate (diagnostic use)
- Irrigant in transurethral prostatic resection or other transurethral procedures

### Contraindications/cautions

- Anuria due to severe renal disease, pulmonary congestion, active intracranial bleeding (except during craniotomy), dehydration, renal disease, CHF

### Dosage

**Available Forms:** Injection—5%, 10%, 15%, 20%, 25%; solution—5 g/100 ml

*ADULT:* IV infusion only; individualize concentration and rate of administration. Dosage is 50–200 g/d. Adjust dosage to maintain urine flow of 30–50 ml/h.

- *Prevention of oliguria:* 50–100 g IV as a 5%–25% solution.
- *Treatment of oliguria:* 50–100 g IV of a 15%–25% solution.
- *Reduction of intracranial pressure and brain mass:* 1.5–2 g/kg IV as a 15%–25% solution over 30–60 min. Evidence of reduced pressure should be seen in 15 min.
- *Reduction of intraocular pressure:* Infuse 1.5–2 g/kg IV as a 25% solution,

m

20% solution, or 15% solution over 30 min. If used preoperatively, use 1–1 1/2 h before surgery.

- *Adjunctive therapy to promote diuresis in intoxications:* Maximum of 200 g IV of mannitol with other fluids and electrolytes.
- *Measurement of glomerular filtration rate:* Dilute 100 ml of a 20% solution with 180 ml of sodium chloride injection. Infuse this 280 ml of 7.2% solution IV at a rate of 20 ml/min. Collect urine with a catheter for the specified time for measurement of mannitol excreted in mg/min. Draw blood at the start and at the end of the time for measurement of mannitol in mg/ml plasma.
- *Test dose of mannitol:* 0.2 g/kg IV (about 60 ml of a 25% solution, 75 ml of a 20% solution, or 100 ml of a 15% solution) in 3–5 min to produce a urine flow of 30–50 ml/h. If urine flow does not increase, repeat dose. If no response to second dose, reevaluate patient situation.

*Urologic irrigation:* Add contents of two 50-ml vials (25%) to 900 ml sterile water for injection; irrigate as needed.

PEDIATRIC: Dosage for children <12 y not established.

### Pharmacokinetics

| *Route* | *Onset* | *Peak* | *Duration* |
|---|---|---|---|
| IV | 30–60 min | 1 h | 6–8 h |
| Irrigant | Rapid | Rapid | Short |

*Metabolism:* $T_{1/2}$: 15–100 min
*Distribution:* Crosses placenta; may enter breast milk
*Excretion:* Urine

### IV facts

**Preparation:** Prepare as listed (above).
**Infusion:** Infuse at rates listed (above).

### Adverse effects

- CNS: *Dizziness,* headache, blurred vision, convulsion
- GI: *Nausea, anorexia, dry mouth, thirst*
- CV: Hypotension, hypertension, edema, thrombophlebitis, tachycardia, chest pain
- **Respiratory**: Pulmonary congestion, rhinitis
- **Hematologic**: Fluid and electrolyte imbalances
- GU: *Diuresis,* urinary retention
- **Dermatologic**: Uriticaria, skin necrosis

## Nursing Considerations

### Assessment

- *History:* Pulmonary congestion, active intracranial bleeding, dehydration, renal disease, CHF
- *Physical:* Skin color, lesions, edema, hydration; orientation, reflexes, muscle strength, pupils; pulses, BP, perfusion; R, pattern, adventitious sounds; urinary output patterns; CBC, serum electrolytes, urinalysis, renal function tests

### Implementation

- Do not give electrolyte-free mannitol with blood. If blood must be given, add at least 20 mEq of sodium chloride to each liter of mannitol solution.
- Do not expose solutions to low temperatures; crystallization may occur. If crystals are seen, warm the bottle in a hot water bath, then cool to body temperature before administering.
- Make sure the infusion set contains a filter if giving concentrated mannitol.
- Monitor serum electrolytes periodically with prolonged therapy.

### Drug-specific teaching points

- The following side effects may occur: increased urination; GI upset (small, frequent meals may help); dry mouth (sugarless lozenges to suck may help); headache, blurred vision (use caution when moving, ask for assistance).
- Report difficulty breathing, pain at the IV site, chest pain.

# maprotiline hydrochloride

*(ma **proe'** ti leen)*
Ludiomil
**Pregnancy Category B**

**Drug classes**
Antidepressant

**Therapeutic actions**
Mechanism of action unknown; appears to act similarly to TCAs; the TCAs act to inhibit the presynaptic reuptake of the neurotransmitters norepinephrine and serotonin; anticholinergic at CNS and peripheral receptors; sedating; the relation of these effects to clinical efficacy is unknown.

**Indications**
- Relief of symptoms of depression (endogenous depression most responsive)
- Treatment of depression in patients with manic-depressive illness
- Treatment of anxiety associated with depression

**Contraindications/cautions**
- Contraindications: hypersensitivity to any tricyclic drug, concomitant therapy with an MAO inhibitor, recent MI, myelography within previous 24 h or scheduled within 48 h, pregnancy (limb reduction abnormalities reported), lactation.
- Use cautiously with EST; preexisting CV disorders (increased risk of serious CVS toxicity); angle-closure glaucoma, increased intraocular pressure, urinary retention, ureteral or urethral spasm; seizure disorders (lower seizure threshold); hyperthyroidism (predisposes to CVS toxicity, including cardiac arrhythmias); impaired hepatic, renal function; psychiatric patients (schizophrenics or paranoids may worsen); manic-depressives (may shift to hypomanic or manic phase); elective surgery (discontinue as long as possible before surgery).

**Dosage**
**Available Forms:** Tablets—25, 50, 75 mg
ADULT
- *Mild to moderate depression:* Initially, 75 mg/d PO in outpatients. Maintain initial dosage for 2 wk due to long drug half-life. Dosage may then be increased gradually in 25-mg increments. Most patients respond to 150 mg/d, but some may require 225 mg/d.
- *More severe depression:* Initially, 100–150 mg/d PO in hospitalized patients. If needed, may gradually increase to 300 mg/d.
- *Maintenance:* Reduce dosage to lowest effective level, usually 75–150 mg/d PO.

PEDIATRIC: Not recommended in children <18 y.

GERIATRIC: Give lower doses to patients older than 60 y; use 50–75 mg/d PO for maintenance.

**Pharmacokinetics**

| Route | Onset | Peak | Duration |
|---|---|---|---|
| Oral | Slow | 2–4 h | 2–4 wk |

*Metabolism:* Hepatic, $T_{1/2}$: 51 h
*Distribution:* Crosses placenta; enters breast milk
*Excretion:* Urine and feces

**Adverse effects**
- CNS: *Sedation and anticholinergic (atropine-like) effects; confusion* (especially in elderly), *disturbed concentration*, hallucinations, disorientation, decreased memory, feelings of unreality, delusions, anxiety, nervousness, restlessness, agitation, panic, insomnia, nightmares, hypomania, mania, exacerbation of psychosis, drowsiness, weakness, fatigue, headache, numbness, tingling, paresthesias of extremities, incoordination, motor hyperactivity, akathisia, ataxia, tremors, peripheral neuropathy, extrapyramidal symptoms, *seizures*, speech blockage, dysarthria, tinnitus, altered EEG
- GI: *Dry mouth, constipation,* paralytic ileus, *nausea*, vomiting, anorexia, epigastric distress, diarrhea, flatulence, dysphagia, peculiar taste, increased salivation, stomatitis, glossitis, parotid swelling, abdominal cramps, black tongue, hepatitis, jaundice (rare), elevated transaminase, altered alkaline phosphatase
- CV: *Orthostatic hypotension,* hypertension, syncope, tachycardia, palpitations, MI, arrhythmias, heart block, precipitation of CHF, stroke

m

- **Hematologic**: Bone marrow depression, eosinophila, purpura, thrombocytopenia, leukopenia
- GU: Urinary retention, delayed micturition, dilation of the urinary tract, gynecomastia, testicular swelling; breast enlargement, menstrual irregularity and galactorrhea; increased or decreased libido; impotence
- **Hypersensitivity**: Skin rash, pruritus, vasculitis, petechiae, photosensitization, edema
- **Endocrine**: Elevated or depressed blood sugar, elevated prolactin levels, inappropriate ADH secretion
- **Withdrawal**: Symptoms with abrupt discontinuation of prolonged therapy: nausea, headache, vertigo, nightmares, malaise
- **Other**: Nasal congestion, excessive appetite, weight gain or loss; sweating (paradoxical effect in a drug with prominent anticholinergic effects), alopecia, lacrimation, hyperthermia, flushing, chills

## ■ Nursing Considerations

### Assessment

- *History:* Hypersensitivity to any tricyclic drug; concomitant therapy with an MAO inhibitor; recent MI; myelography within previous 24 h or scheduled within 48 h; lactation; EST; preexisting CV disorders; angle-closure glaucoma, increased intraocular pressure, urinary retention, ureteral or urethral spasm; seizure disorders; hyperthyroidism; impaired hepatic, renal function; psychiatric problems; manic-depressive patients; elective surgery
- *Physical:* Weight; T; skin color, lesions; orientation, affect, reflexes, vision and hearing; P, BP, orthostatic BP, perfusion; bowel sounds, normal output, liver evaluation; urine flow, normal output; usual sexual function, frequency of menses, breast and scrotal examination; liver function tests, urinalysis, CBC, ECG

### Implementation

- Limit drug access to depressed and potentially suicidal patients.
- Expect clinical response in 3–7 d up to 2–3 wk (the latter is more usual).
- Give major portion of dose at hs if drowsiness, severe anticholinergic effects occur.
- Reduce dosage with minor side effects; discontinue drug if serious side effects occur.
- Arrange for CBC if patient develops fever, sore throat, or signs of infection.

### Drug-specific teaching points

- Take drug exactly as prescribed, and do not to stop taking this drug without consulting your care provider.
- Avoid alcohol, sleep-inducing drugs, OTC drugs.
- Avoid prolonged exposure to sunlight or sunlamps, use sunscreen or protective garments if exposure is unavoidable.
- The following side effects may occur: headache, dizziness, drowsiness, weakness, blurred vision (reversible; use caution if severe, avoid driving or performing tasks that require alertness); nausea, vomiting, loss of appetite, dry mouth (small frequent meals, frequent mouth care, sucking sugarless candies may help); nightmares, inability to concentrate, confusion; changes in sexual function.
- Report dry mouth, difficulty in urination, excessive sedation

# mebendazole

*(me **ben'** da zole)*

Vermox

**Pregnancy Category C**

### Drug classes

Anthelmintic

### Therapeutic actions

Irreversibly blocks glucose uptake by susceptible helminths, depleting glycogen stores needed for survival and reproduction of the helminths, causing death.

### Indications

- Treatment of *Trichuris trichiura* (whipworm), *Enterobius vermicularis* (pinworm), *Ascaris lumbricoides* (roundworm), *Ancylostoma duodenale* (common hookworm), *Necator americanus* (American hookworm)

**Contraindications/cautions**

- Allergy to mebendazole, pregnancy (embryotoxic and teratogenic; avoid use, especially during first trimester), lactation.

**Dosage**

**Available Forms:** Chewable tablets—100 mg

**ADULT**

- ***Trichuriasis, ascariasis, hookworm infections:*** 1 tablet PO morning and evening on 3 consecutive d.
- ***Enterobiasis:*** 1 tablet PO. If not cured 3 wk after treatment, a second treatment course is advised.

**PEDIATRIC:** Safety and efficacy for use in children <2 y not established.

**Pharmacokinetics**

| Route | Onset | Peak |
|---|---|---|
| Oral | Slow | 2–4 h |

*Metabolism:* Hepatic, $T_{1/2}$: 2 1/2–9 h
*Distribution:* Crosses placenta; may enter breast milk
*Excretion:* Feces and urine

**Adverse effects**

- GI: *Transient abdominal pain, diarrhea*
- General: Fever

## ■ Nursing Considerations

**Assessment**

- ***History:*** Allergy to mebendazole, pregnancy, lactation
- ***Physical:*** T; bowel sounds, output

**Implementation**

- Culture for ova and parasites.
- Administer drug with food; tablets may be chewed, swallowed whole, or crushed and mixed with food.
- Arrange for second course of treatment if patient is not cured 3 wk after treatment.
- Treat all family members for pinworm infestation.
- Disinfect toilet facilities after patient use (pinworms).
- Arrange for daily laundry of bed linens, towels, nightclothes, and undergarments (pinworms).

**Drug-specific teaching points**

- Chew or swallow whole or crushed and mixed with food.
- Pinworms are easily transmitted; all family members should be treated for complete eradication.
- Use strict handwashing and hygiene measures. Launder undergarments, bedlinens, nightclothes daily. Disinfect toilet facilities daily and bathroom floors periodically (pinworms).
- The following side effects may occur: nausea, abdominal pain, diarrhea (small, frequent meals may help).
- Report fever, return of symptoms, severe diarrhea.

# mecamylamine hydrochloride

***(mek a mill' a meen)***

Inversine

**Pregnancy Category C**

**Drug classes**

Antihypertensive
Ganglionic blocker

**Therapeutic actions**

Occupies cholinergic receptors of autonomic postganglionic neurons, blocking the effects of acetylcholine released from preganglionic nerve terminals, decreasing the effects of the sympathetic (and parasympathetic) nervous systems on effector organs; reduces sympathetic tone on the vasculature, causing vasodilation and decreased BP; decreases sympathetic impulses to the heart; and decreases the release of catecholamines from the adrenal medulla.

**Indications**

- Moderately severe to severe hypertension
- Uncomplicated malignant hypertension

## Contraindications/cautions

- Contraindications: hypersensitivity to mecamylamine; coronary insufficiency, recent MI; uncooperative patients; uremia; chronic pyelonephritis when patient is receiving antibiotics and sulfonamides; glaucoma; organic pyloric stenosis; lactation.
- Use cautiously with prostatic hypertrophy, bladder neck obstruction, urethral stricture (urinary retention, may be more serious with these disorders); cerebral or renal insufficiency; high ambient temperature, fever, infection, hemorrhage, surgery, vigorous exercise, salt depletion resulting from diminished intake or increased excretion due to diarrhea, vomiting, sweating or diuretics; pregnancy.

### Dosage

**Available Forms:** Tablets—2.5 mg

*ADULT:* Initially 2.5 mg PO bid. Adjust dosage in increments of 2.5 mg in intervals of at least 2 d until desired BP response occurs (dosage below that causing signs of mild postural hypotension). Average total daily dosage is 25 mg, usually in three divided doses. Partial tolerance may develop, necessitating increased dosage. With other antihypertensives, reduce both the dosage of the other agents and mecamylamine; exception: give thiazides at usual dosage while decreasing mecamylamine by at least 50%.

## Pharmacokinetics

| *Route* | *Onset* | *Peak* | *Duration* |
|---|---|---|---|
| Oral | 1/2–2 h | 3–5 h | 6–12 h |

*Metabolism:* $T_{1/2}$: 4–6 h

*Distribution:* Crosses placenta; enters breast milk

*Excretion:* Urine

## Adverse effects

- CNS: Syncope, paresthesia, *weakness, fatigue, sedation,* dilated pupils and blurred vision, tremor, choreiform movements, mental aberrations, convulsions
- GI: *Anorexia, dry mouth, glossitis, nausea,* vomiting, constipation and ileus
- CV: *Orthostatic hypotension* and dizziness
- Respiratory: Interstitial pulmonary edema and fibrosis
- GU: *Decreased libido, impotence, urinary retention*

## ■ Nursing Considerations

### Assessment

- ***History:*** Hypersensitivity to mecamylamine; coronary insufficiency, recent MI; uremia; chronic pyelonephritis; glaucoma; organic pyloric stenosis; prostatic hypertrophy, bladder neck obstruction, urethral stricture; cerebral or renal insufficiency; high ambient temperature, fever, infection, hemorrhage, surgery, vigorous exercise, salt depletion, vomiting, sweating, or diuretics; lactation
- ***Physical:*** T; orientation, affect, reflexes; ophthalmic exam, including tonometry; P, BP, orthostatic BP, supine BP, perfusion, edema, auscultation; bowel sounds, normal output; normal urinary output, voiding pattern, prostate palpation; renal, hepatic function tests

### Implementation

- Give after meals for more gradual absorption and smoother control of BP; timing of doses with regard to meals should be consistent.
- Consider giving larger doses at noontime and in the evening rather than in the morning; the response is greater in the morning. The morning dose should be relatively small or omitted, based on BP response, and symptoms of faintness, lightheadedness.
- Determine the initial and maintenance dosage by BP readings in the erect position at the time of maximal drug effect and by other signs and symptoms of orthostatic hypotension.
- Discontinue drug gradually, concurrently replace with another antihypertensive drug. Abrupt discontinuation in patients with malignant hypertension may cause return of hypertension and fatal CVAs or acute CHF.
- Decrease dosage with fever, infection, salt depletion, that decrease drug requirements.

- Monitor patient for orthostatic hypotension: most marked in the morning, accentuated by hot weather, alcohol, exercise.
- Ensure adequate salt intake; use caution where increased sodium loss exists.
- Monitor bowel function carefully; paralytic ileus has occurred. Prevent constipation by giving pilocarpine or neostigmine with each dose. Treat constipation with Milk of Magnesia or similar laxative; do not use bulk laxatives.
- Discontinue drug immediately, and arrange for remedial steps at the first signs of paralytic ileus: frequent loose bowel movements with abdominal distention and decreased borborygmi.

### Drug-specific teaching points

- Take after meals and in a consistent relation to meals. Do not stop taking without consulting your health care provider.
- Learn, alone or with a significant other, to monitor your BP frequently to ensure safe, effective therapy (may be given instructions to reduce or omit a dose if readings fall below a designated level or if faintness or lightheadedness occurs).
- Ensure an adequate intake of salt, especially in hot weather, during exercise, or if sweating excessively.
- The following side effects may occur: dizziness, weakness (most likely on changing position, in the early morning, after exercise, in hot weather, and with alcohol consumption; some tolerance to drug may occur; avoid driving or engaging in tasks that require alertness, and change position slowly; use caution in climbing stairs); blurred vision, dilated pupils, sensitivity to bright light (revised eyeglass prescription, wearing sunglasses may help); constipation (request a laxative or GI stimulant); dry mouth (sucking sugarless lozenges, ice chips may help); GI upset (frequent, small meals may help); impotence, decreased libido.
- Report tremor, seizure, frequent dizziness or fainting, severe or persistent constipation, or frequent loose stools with abdominal distention.

## mechlorethamine hydrochloride

*(me klor eth' a meen)*

$HN_2$, nitrogen mustard

Mustargen

**Pregnancy Category D**

### Drug classes

Alkylating agent
Nitrogen mustard
Antineoplastic

### Therapeutic actions

Cytotoxic: reacts chemically with DNA, RNA, other proteins to prevent replication and function of susceptible cells, causing cell death; cell cycle nonspecific.

### Indications

- Palliative treatment of Hodgkin's disease, lymphosarcoma, chronic myelocytic or chronic lymphocytic leukemia, polycythemia vera, mycosis fungoides, bronchogenic carcinoma (IV use)
- Palliative treatment of effusion secondary to metastatic carcinoma (intrapleural, intraperitoneal, intrapericardial use)
- Unlabeled use: topical treatment of cutaneous mycosis fungoides

### Contraindications/cautions

- Contraindications: allergy to mechlorethamine, infectious disease, pregnancy, lactation.
- Use cautiously with amyloidosis, hematopoietic depression, chronic lymphatic leukemia, concomitant steroid therapy.

### Dosage

**Available Forms:** Powder for injection—10 mg

Individualize dosage based on hematologic profile and response.

*ADULT:* Usual dose: total of 0.4 mg/kg IV for each course of therapy as a single dose *or* in 2 to 4 divided doses of 0.1–0.2 mg/kg per day. Give at night in case sedation is required for side effects. Interval between courses of therapy is usually 3–6 wk.

- ***Intracavitary administration:*** Dose and preparation vary considerably

m

with cavity and disease being treated: consult manufacturer's label.

### Pharmacokinetics

| *Route* | *Onset* | *Peak* | *Duration* |
|---|---|---|---|
| IV | Immediate | Seconds | Minutes |

*Metabolism:* $T_{1/2}$: minutes
*Distribution:* Crosses placenta; may enter breast milk
*Excretion:* Urine

### IV facts

**Preparations:** Reconstitute vial with 10 ml of Sterile Water for Injection or Sodium Chloride Injection; resultant solution contains 1 mg/ml of mechlorethamine HCl. Prepare solution immediately before use; decomposes on standing.

**Infusion:** Inject into tubing of a flowing IV infusion over 3–5 min.

### Adverse effects

- CNS: *Weakness, vertigo,* tinnitus, diminished hearing
- Local: *Vesicant thrombosis, thrombophlebitis,* tissue necrosis if extravasation occurs
- GI: *Nausea, vomiting, anorexia,* diarrhea, jaundice
- **Hematologic:** *Bone marrow depression,* immunosuppression, hyperuricemia
- GU: *Impaired fertility*
- **Dermatologic:** Maculopapular skin rash, alopecia (infrequently)

## ■ Nursing Considerations

### Assessment

- ***History:*** Allergy to mechlorethamine, infectious disease, amyloidosis, hematopoietic depression, chronic lymphatic leukemia, concomitant steroid therapy, pregnancy, lactation
- ***Physical:*** T; weight; skin color, lesions; injection site; orientation, reflexes, hearing evaluation; CBC, differential, uric acid

### Implementation

- Arrange for blood tests to evaluate hematopoietic function before and during therapy.
- Use caution when preparing drug for administration; use rubber gloves for handling drug; drug is highly toxic and a vesicant. Avoid inhalation of dust or vapors and contact with skin or mucous membranes (especially the eyes). If eye contact occurs, immediately irrigate with copious amount of ophthalmic irrigating solution, and obtain an ophthalmologic consultation. If skin contact occurs, irrigate with copious amount of water for 15 min, followed by application of 2% sodium thiosulfate.
- *Use caution when determining correct amount of drug for injection.* The margin of safety is very small; double check dosage before administration.
- Monitor injection site for any sign of extravasation. Painful inflammation and induration or sloughing of skin may occur. If leakage is noted, promptly infiltrate with sterile isotonic sodium thiosulfate (1/6 molar), and apply an ice compress for 6–12 h. Notify physician.
- Consult physician for premedication with antiemetics or sedatives to prevent severe nausea and vomiting. Giving at night may help alleviate the problem.
- Ensure that patient is well hydrated before treatment.
- Monitor uric acid levels; ensure adequate fluid intake, and prepare for appropriate treatment if hyperuricemia occurs.

### Drug-specific teaching points

- This drug must be given IV or directly into a body cavity.
- The following side effects may occur: nausea, vomiting, loss of appetite (use antiemetic or sedative at night; maintain fluid intake and nutrition); weakness, dizziness, ringing in the ears or loss of hearing (use special precautions to avoid injury); infertility, from irregular menses to complete amenorrhea; men may stop producing sperm (may be irreversible).

- Use birth control. This drug cannot be taken during pregnancy; serious fetal effects can occur. If you think you are pregnant or wish to become pregnant, consult your prescriber.
- Report pain, burning at IV site, severe GI distress, sore throat, rash, joint pain.

## meclizine hydrochloride

***(mek' li zeen)***

Bonamine (CAN), Bonine, Dizmiss

*Oral prescription tablets:*
Antivert, Antrizine, Ru-Vert M, Meni-D

**Pregnancy Category B**

### Drug classes

Antiemetic
Anti-motion sickness agent
Antihistamine
Anticholinergic

### Therapeutic actions

Reduces sensitivity of the labyrinthine apparatus; probably acts at least partly by blocking cholinergic synapses in the vomiting center, which receives input from the chemoreceptor trigger zone and from peripheral nerve pathways; peripheral anticholinergic effects may contribute to efficacy.

### Indications

- Prevention and treatment of nausea, vomiting, motion sickness
- "Possibly effective" for the management of vertigo associated with diseases affecting the vestibular system

### Contraindications/cautions

- Contraindications: allergy to meclizine or cyclizine, pregnancy.
- Use cautiously with lactation, narrow-angle glaucoma, stenosing peptic ulcer, symptomatic prostatic hypertrophy, bronchial asthma, bladder neck obstruction, pyloroduodenal obstruction, cardiac arrhythmias, postoperative state (hypotensive effects may be confusing and dangerous).

### Dosage

**Available Forms:** Tablets—12.5, 25, 50 mg; chewable tablets—25 mg; capsules—25 mg

ADULT

- ***Motion sickness:*** 25–50 mg PO 1 h prior to travel. May repeat dose every 24 h for the duration of the journey.
- ***Vertigo:*** 25–100 mg PO daily in divided doses.

PEDIATRIC: Not recommended for use in children younger than 12 y.

GERIATRIC: More likely to cause dizziness, sedation, syncope, toxic confusional states and hypotension in elderly patients; use with caution.

### Pharmacokinetics

| *Route* | *Onset* | *Peak* | *Duration* |
|---|---|---|---|
| Oral | 1 h | 1–2 h | 12–24 h |

*Metabolism:* $T_{1/2}$: 6 h
*Distribution:* Crosses placenta; may enter breast milk
*Excretion:* Feces

m

### Adverse effects

- CNS: *Drowsiness, confusion,* euphoria, nervousness, restlessness, insomnia and excitement, convulsions, vertigo, tinnitus, blurred vision, diplopia, auditory and visual hallucinations
- GI: *Dry mouth, anorexia, nausea,* vomiting, diarrhea or constipation
- CV: Hypotension, palpitations, tachycardia
- Respiratory: **Respiratory depression, death** (overdose, especially in young children), dry nose and throat
- GU: *Urinary frequency, difficult urination,* urinary retention
- Dermatologic: Urticaria, drug rash

## ■ Nursing Considerations

### Assessment

- ***History:*** Allergy to meclizine or cyclizine, pregnancy, narrow-angle glaucoma, stenosing peptic ulcer, symptomatic prostatic hypertrophy, bronchial asthma, bladder neck obstruction, pyloroduodenal obstruction, cardiac arrhythmias, postoperative patients, lactation

- *Physical:* Skin color, lesions, texture; orientation, reflexes, affect; ophthalmic exam; P, BP; R, adventitious sounds; bowel sounds, normal output, status of mucous membranes; prostate palpation, normal output

### Implementation

- Monitor I&O, and take appropriate measures with urinary retention.

### Drug-specific teaching points

- Take as prescribed. Avoid excessive dosage. Chew the chewable tablets carefully before swallowing.
- Anti-motion sickness drugs work best if used prophylactically.
- The following side effects may occur: dizziness, sedation, drowsiness (use caution driving or performing tasks that require alertness); epigastric distress, diarrhea, or constipation (take with food ); dry mouth (frequent mouth care, sucking sugarless lozenges may help); dryness of nasal mucosa (try another motion sickness, antivertigo remedy).
- Avoid alcohol; serious sedation could occur.
- Report difficulty breathing, hallucinations, tremors, loss of coordination, visual disturbances, irregular heartbeat.

## meclofenamate sodium

*(me kloe fen **am'** ate)*

**Pregnancy Category C**

### Drug classes

Nonsteroidal anti-inflammatory drug (NSAID)

### Therapeutic actions

Anti-inflammatory, analgesic, and antipyretic activities related to inhibition of prostaglandin synthesis; exact mechanisms of action are not known.

### Indications

- Acute and chronic rheumatoid arthritis and osteoarthritis (not recommended as initial therapy due to adverse GI effects: severe diarrhea)
- Relief of mild to moderate pain
- Treatment of idiopathic heavy menstrual blood loss
- Treatment of primary dysmenorrhea

### Contraindications/cautions

- Contraindications: pregnancy and lactation.
- Use cautiously with allergies, renal, hepatic, CV, and GI dysfunction.

### Dosage

**Available Forms:** 50, 100 mg

ADULT

- *Rheumatoid arthritis:* Usual dosage 200–400 mg/d PO in 3 to 4 equal doses. Initiate therapy with a lower dose, and increase as needed. Do not exceed 400 mg/d. 2–3 wk may be needed to achieve optimum therapeutic effect.
- *Mild to moderate pain:* 50 mg PO q4–6h. Doses of 100 mg may be required for optimal pain relief. Do not exceed 400 mg/d.
- *Excessive menstrual blood loss and primary dysmenorrhea:* 100 mg PO tid for up to 6 d, starting at the onset of menstrual flow.

PEDIATRIC: Safety and efficacy in children younger than 14 y not established.

### Pharmacokinetics

| *Route* | *Onset* | *Peak* |
|---|---|---|
| Oral | Varies | 30–60 min |

*Metabolism:* Hepatic, $T_{1/2}$: 2–4 h
*Distribution:* Crosses placenta; enters breast milk
*Excretion:* Urine

### Adverse effects

*NSAIDs*

- CNS: *Headache, dizziness, somnolence, insomnia,* fatigue, tiredness, dizziness, tinnitus, ophthalmologic effects

- GI: *Nausea, dyspepsia, GI pain,* diarrhea, vomiting, *constipation*, flatulence
- **Respiratory**: Dyspnea, hemoptysis, pharyngitis, bronchospasm, rhinitis
- GU: Dysuria, renal impairment
- **Hematologic**: Bleeding, platelet inhibition with higher doses, neutropenia, eosinophilia, leukopenia, pancytopenia, thrombocytopenia, agranulocytosis, granulocytopenia, aplastic anemia, decreased hemoglobin or Hct, bone marrow depression, mennorhagia
- **Dermatologic**: *Rash*, pruritus, sweating, dry mucous membranes, stomatitis
- **Other**: Peripheral edema, **anaphylactoid reactions to fatal anaphylactic shock**

## ■ Nursing Considerations

### Assessment

- *History:* Renal, hepatic, CV, and GI conditions, pregnancy, lactation
- *Physical:* Skin color and lesions; orientation, reflexes, ophthalmologic and audiometric evaluation, peripheral sensation; P, edema; R, adventitious sounds; liver evaluation; CBC, clotting times, renal and liver function tests; serum electrolytes, stool guaiac.

### Implementation

- Give with milk or food to decrease GI upset.
- Arrange for periodic ophthalmologic examination during long-term therapy.
- Institute emergency procedures if overdose occurs: gastric lavage, induction of emesis, supportive therapy.

### Drug-specific teaching points

- Take drug with food; take only the prescribed dosage.
- Dizziness, drowsiness can occur (avoid driving or the use of dangerous machinery).
- Report sore throat, fever, rash, itching, weight gain, swelling in ankles or fingers; changes in vision; black, tarry stools; severe diarrhea.

# medroxyprogesterone acetate

*(me **drox'** ee proe **jess'** te rone)*

*Oral:* Amen, Curretab, Cycrin, Provera

*Parenteral, antineoplastic:* Depo-Provera

**Pregnancy Category X**

### Drug classes

Hormone
Progestin
Antineoplastic

### Therapeutic actions

Progesterone derivative; endogenous progesterone transforms proliferative endometrium into secretory endometrium; inhibits the secretion of pituitary gonadotropins, which prevents follicular maturation and ovulation; inhibits spontaneous uterine contraction.

### Indications

- Treatment of secondary amenorrhea (oral)
- Abnormal uterine bleeding due to hormonal imbalance in the absence of organic pathology (oral)
- Adjunctive therapy and palliation of inoperable, recurrent, and metastatic endometrial carcinoma or renal carcinoma (parenteral)
- Unlabeled use for depot form: long-acting contraceptive, treatment of breast cancer

### Contraindications/cautions

- Contraindications: allergy to progestins; thrombophlebitis, thromboembolic disorders, cerebral hemorrhage or history of these conditions; hepatic disease, carcinoma of the breast or genital organs, undiagnosed vaginal bleeding, missed abortion; pregnancy (fetal abnormalities, including masculinization of the female fetus have been reported); lactation.
- Use cautiously with epilepsy, migraine, asthma, cardiac or renal dysfunction.

### Dosage

**Available Forms:** Tablets—2.5, 5, 10 mg; injection—150, 400 mg/ml

*ADULT*

- *Secondary amenorrhea:* 5–10 mg/d PO for 5–10 d. A dose for inducing an optimum secretory transformation of an endometrium that has been primed with exogenous or endogenous estrogen is 10 mg/d for 10 d. Start therapy at any time; withdrawal bleeding usually occurs 3–7 d after therapy ends.
- *Abnormal uterine bleeding:* 5–10 mg/d PO for 5–10 d, beginning on the 16th or 21st day of the menstrual cycle. To produce an optimum secretory transformation of an endometrium that has been primed with estrogen, give 10 mg/d PO for 10 d, beginning on the 16th day of the cycle. Withdrawal bleeding usually occurs 3–7 d after discontinuing therapy. If bleeding is controlled, administer two subsequent cycles.
- *Endometrial or renal carcinoma:* 400–1,000 mg/wk IM. If improvement occurs within a few weeks or months and the disease appears stabilized, it may be possible to maintain improvement with as little as 400 mg/mo IM.

### Pharmacokinetics

| *Route* | *Onset* | *Peak* |
|---|---|---|
| Oral | Slow | Unknown |
| IM | Weeks | Months |

*Metabolism:* Hepatic, $T_{1/2}$: unknown
*Distribution:* Crosses placenta; enters breast milk
*Excretion:* Unknown

### Adverse effects

- CNS: Sudden, partial, or complete loss of vision; proptosis, diplopia, migraine, precipitation of acute intermittent porphyria, mental depression, pyrexia, insomnia, somnolence
- GI: Cholestatic jaundice, nausea
- CV: Thrombophlebitis, cerebrovascular disorders, retinal thrombosis, pulmonary embolism, thromboembolic and thrombotic disease, increased BP
- GU: *Breakthrough bleeding, spotting, change in menstrual flow, amenorrhea,* changes in cervical erosion and cervical secretions, breast tenderness and secretion
- Dermatologic: *Rash with or without pruritus, acne,* melasma or chloasma, alopecia, hirsutism, photosensitivity
- General: *Fluid retention, edema, increase or decrease in weight*
- Other: Decreased glucose tolerance

### Drug-lab test interferences

- Inaccurate tests of hepatic and endocrine function

## ■ Nursing Considerations

### Assessment

- *History:* Allergy to progestins; thrombophlebitis, thromboembolic disorders, cerebral hemorrhage; hepatic disease, carcinoma of the breast or genital organs, undiagnosed vaginal bleeding, missed abortion; epilepsy, migraine, asthma, cardiac or renal dysfunction; pregnancy; lactation
- *Physical:* Skin color, lesions, turgor; hair; breasts; pelvic exam; orientation, affect; ophthalmologic exam; P, auscultation, peripheral perfusion, edema; R, adventitious sounds; liver evaluation; liver and renal function tests, glucose tolerance, Pap smear

### Implementation

- Arrange for pretreatment and periodic (at least annual) history and physical, which should include BP, breasts, abdomen, pelvic organs and a Pap smear.
- Alert patient before therapy to prevent pregnancy and to have frequent medical follow-ups.
- Discontinue medication and consult physician if sudden partial or complete loss of vision occurs; if papilledema or retinal vascular lesions are present discontinue drug.
- Discontinue medication and consult physician at the first sign of thromboembolic disease (leg pain, swelling, peripheral perfusion changes, shortness of breath).

**Drug-specific teaching points**

- Prepare a calendar, marking drug days (PO drug).
- The following side effects may occur: sensitivity to light (avoid exposure to the sun; use sunscreen and protective clothing); dizziness, sleeplessness, depression (use caution driving or performing tasks that require alertness); skin rash, color changes, loss of hair; fever; nausea.
- This drug should not be taken during pregnancy due to risk of serious fetal abnormalities
- Report pain or swelling and warmth in the calves, acute chest pain or shortness of breath, sudden severe headache or vomiting, dizziness or fainting, visual disturbances, numbness or tingling in the arm or leg.

## mefenamic acid

*(me fe **nam'** ik)*

Ponstan (CAN), Ponstel

**Pregnancy Category C**

### Drug classes

Nonsteroidal anti-inflammatory drug (NSAID)

Analgesic (non-narcotic)

### Therapeutic actions

Anti-inflammatory, analgesic, and antipyretic activities related to inhibition of prostaglandin synthesis; exact mechanisms of action are not known.

### Indications

- Relief of moderate pain when therapy will not exceed 1 wk
- Treatment of primary dysmenorrhea

### Contraindications/cautions

- Contraindications: pregnancy, lactation.
- Use cautiously with allergies; renal, hepatic, cardiovascular, and GI conditions.

### Dosage

**Available Forms:** Capsules—250 mg

ADULT

- *Acute pain:* Initially 500 mg PO followed by 250 mg q6h as needed. Do not exceed 1 wk of therapy.
- *Primary dysmenorrhea:* Initially 500 mg PO then 250 mg q6h starting with the onset of bleeding. Can be initiated at start of menses and should not be necessary for longer than 2–3 d.

*PEDIATRIC:* Safety and efficacy for children younger than 14 y not established; use adult dosage for children older than 14 y.

### Pharmacokinetics

| *Route* | *Onset* | *Peak* | *Duration* |
|---|---|---|---|
| Oral | Varies | 2–4 h | 6 h |

*Metabolism:* Hepatic, $T_{1/2}$: 2–4 h

*Distribution:* Crosses placenta; enters breast milk

*Excretion:* Urine and feces

### Adverse effects

*NSAIDs*

- CNS: *Headache, dizziness, somnolence, insomnia,* fatigue, tiredness, dizziness, tinnitus, ophthalmologic effects
- GI: *Nausea, dyspepsia, GI pain,* diarrhea, vomiting, *constipation*, flatulence
- Respiratory: Dyspnea, hemoptysis, pharyngitis, bronchospasm, rhinitis
- Hematologic: Bleeding, platelet inhibition with higher doses, neutropenia, eosinophilia, leukopenia, pancytopenia, thrombocytopenia, agranulocytosis, granulocytopenia, aplastic anemia, decreased Hgb or Hct, bone marrow depression, menorrhagia
- GU: Dysuria, **renal impairment**
- Dermatologic: *Rash,* pruritus, sweating, dry mucous membranes, stomatitis
- Other: Peripheral edema, anaphylactoid reactions to fatal anaphylactic shock

### Drug-lab test interferences

- False-positive reaction for urinary bile using the diazo tablet test

## ■ Nursing Considerations

### Assessment

- *History:* Allergies; renal, hepatic, CV, GI conditions; pregnancy; lactation
- *Physical:* Skin color and lesions; orientation, reflexes, ophthalmologic and audiometric evaluation, peripheral sensa-

tion; P, edema; R, adventitious sounds; liver evaluation; CBC, clotting times, renal and liver function tests; serum electrolytes, stool guaiac

### Implementation

- Give with milk or food to decrease GI upset.
- Arrange for periodic ophthalmologic examination during long-term therapy.
- Institute emergency procedures if overdose occurs: gastric lavage, induction of emesis, supportive therapy.

### Drug-specific teaching points

- Take drug with food; take only the prescribed dosage; do not take the drug longer than 1 wk.
- Dizziness, drowsiness can occur (avoid driving or the use of dangerous machinery).
- Discontinue drug and consult care provider if rash, diarrhea, or digestive problems occur.
- Report sore throat, fever, rash, itching, weight gain, swelling in ankles or fingers; changes in vision; black, tarry stools; severe diarrhea.

## mefloquine hydrochloride

*(me' floe kwin)*

Lariam, Mephaquin

**Pregnancy Category C**

### Drug classes

Antimalarial

### Therapeutic actions

Acts as a blood schizonticide; exact mechanism of action is not known, but may act by raising intravesicular pH in parasite acid vesicles, causing death; is structurally related to quinine.

### Indications

- Treatment of acute malaria infections
- Prophylaxis of *Plasmodium falciparum* and *Plasmodium vivax* malaria infections, including prophylaxis of chloroquine-resistant *P. falciparum*. Recommended by the CDC for use in travel to areas of risk where chloroquine-resistant *P. falciparum* exists.

### Contraindications/cautions

- Contraindications: allergy to mefloquine or related compounds; life threatening or overwhelming infection with *P. falciparum* (IV malarial drug should be used for treatment; mefloquine may be given orally following completion of the IV treatment); pregnancy (teratogenic and embryotoxic effects; women should avoid travel to malaria-endemic areas during pregnancy and use contraceptive methods during and 2 mo before and after such travel).
- Use caution in lactation.

### Dosage

**Available Forms:** Tablets—250 mg

**ADULT**

- ***Treatment of mild to moderate malaria:*** 5 tablets (1,250 mg) PO as a single dose. Do not give on an empty stomach. Give with at least 240 mg (8 oz) water.
- ***Prophylaxis:*** 250 mg PO once weekly for 4 wk, then 250 mg PO every other week. CDC recommends a single dose taken weekly starting 1 wk before travel and for 4 wk after leaving the area. For prolonged stays in endemic area, take weekly for 4 wk, then every other week until the traveler has taken three doses after return to a malaria-free area. Do not give on an empty stomach. Give with at least 240 mg (8 oz) water.

**PEDIATRIC**

- ***Prophylaxis:*** Starting 1 wk before travel and continued weekly during travel and for 4 wk after leaving such areas: 15–19 kg: 1/4 tablet PO. 20–30 kg: 1/2 tablet PO. 31–45 kg: 3/4 tablet PO. > 45 kg: 1 tablet PO.

### Pharmacokinetics

| Route | Onset | Peak |
|---|---|---|
| Oral | Varies | Days |

*Metabolism:* Hepatic, $T_{1/2}$: 13–24 d
*Distribution:* Crosses placenta; may enter breast milk
*Excretion:* Unknown

**Adverse effects**

*Prophylaxis*

- CNS: Dizziness, encephalopathy, syncope
- GI: *Vomiting*
- **Hematologic**: Elevations of transaminases, leukocytosis, thrombocytopenia

*Treatment*

- CNS: *Dizziness, myalgia, headache*, fatigue, tinnitus, vertigo, visual disturbances, psychotic manifestations, hallucinations, confusion, anxiety, depression, convulsions, ocular lesions
- GI: *Nausea, vomiting, diarrhea,* abdominal pain, anorexia
- CV: Bradycardia
- **Dermatologic**: Rash, loss of hair, pruritus
- **Hematologic**: Decreased Hct, elevation of transaminases, leukopenia, thrombocytopenia
- Other: *Fever*

**Clinically important drug-drug interactions**

• Increased risk of convulsions with chloroquine • Increased risk of cardiac toxicity and convulsions with quinine, quinidine; delay mefloquine for at least 12 h after the last dose of quinine or quinidine

## ■ Nursing Considerations

### Assessment

- *History:* Allergy to mefloquine or related compounds; life threatening or overwhelming infection with *P. falciparum*; lactation
- *Physical:* Skin lesions; T; reflexes, affect, ophthalmic exam; P; CBC, Hct, transaminase levels

### Implementation

- Obtain cultures to determine sensitivity to mefloquine in acute treatment.
- Arrange for subsequent treatment with an 8-aminoquinolone (primaquine) for patients with acute *P. vivax* infection; mefloquine does not eliminate the exoerythrocytic parasites, relapse may occur.
- Do not give on an empty stomach; always administer with at least 8 oz (240 ml) of water.
- Give prophylactic drug 1 wk prior to departure to endemic area; prepare a calendar for the patient noting weekly drug days: the same day each wk for 4 wk and every other week until traveler has taken three doses after return to malaria-free area.
- Arrange for periodic ophthalmic examinations with long-term therapy.

### Drug-specific teaching points

- Take the drug weekly, on the same day of the week, for 4 wk, beginning 1 wk before traveling to an endemic area. If staying in the area longer, the drug should be taken every other week; continue the drug for three doses after returning to a malaria-free area (prophylaxis). Mark a calendar for the patient with these dates. Treatment consists of 5 tablets taken as one dose. Do not take on an empty stomach. Always take the drug with at least 8 oz of water.
- Periodic physical exams, including ophthalmic exams are needed if drug is taken for a prolonged period.
- The following side effects may occur: dizziness, visual disturbances (avoid driving or performing hazardous tasks); headache, fatigue, joint pain (request medication); nausea, vomiting, diarrhea (proper nutrition is important).
- This drug should be avoided during pregnancy. Use contraception before, during, and for 2 mo after travel to a malaria-endemic area.
- Report anxiety, depression, restlessness, confusion, palpitations.



## megestrol acetate

*(me **jess'** trole)*

Megace

**Pregnancy Category X**

**Drug classes**

Hormone
Progestin
Antineoplastic

## Therapeutic actions

Synthetic progestational agent; mechanism of antineoplastic activity is unknown but may be due to a pituitary-mediated antileutinizing effect.

## Indications

- Palliation of advanced carcinoma of the breast or endometrium; not for use instead of surgery, radiation, or chemotherapy
- Orphan drug use: appetite stimulant in HIV-related cachexia

## Contraindications/cautions

- Contraindications: allergy to progestins; thrombophlebitis, thromboembolic disorders, cerebral hemorrhage or history of these conditions; hepatic disease, carcinoma of the breast or genital organs, undiagnosed vaginal bleeding, missed abortion; pregnancy (masculinization of female fetus); lactation.
- Use cautiously with epilepsy, migraine, asthma, cardiac or renal dysfunction.

## Dosage

**Available Forms:** Tablets—20, 40 mg; suspension—40 mg/ml

### Adult

- *Breast cancer:* 160 mg/d PO (40 mg qid).
- *Endometrial cancer:* 40–320 mg/d PO in divided doses.
- *Cachexia:* 80 mg PO 4 ×/d.

## Pharmacokinetics

| Route | Onset | Peak |
|---|---|---|
| Oral | Slow | Weeks |

*Metabolism:* Hepatic, $T_{1/2}$: unknown
*Distribution:* Crosses placenta; enters breast milk
*Excretion:* Urine

## Adverse effects

- CNS: Sudden, partial, or complete loss of vision; proptosis; diplopia; migraine; precipitation of acute intermittent porphyria; mental depression; pyrexia; insomnia; somnolence
- GI: Cholestatic jaundice, nausea
- CV: Thrombophlebitis, cerebrovascular disorders, retinal thrombosis, pulmonary embolism, thromboembolic and thrombotic disease, increased BP
- GU: *Breakthrough bleeding, spotting, change in menstrual flow, amenorrhea*, changes in cervical erosion and cervical secretions, breast tenderness and secretion
- **Dermatologic**: *Rash with or without pruritus, acne*, melasma or chloasma, alopecia, hirsutism, photosensitivity
- **General**: *Fluid retention, edema, increase in weight*
- **Other**: Decreased glucose tolerance

## Drug-lab test interferences

- Inaccurate tests of hepatic and endocrine function

## ■ Nursing Considerations

### Assessment

- ***History:*** Allergy to progestins; thrombophlebitis, thromboembolic disorders, cerebral hemorrhage; hepatic disease, carcinoma of the breast or genital organs, undiagnosed vaginal bleeding, missed abortion; epilepsy, migraine, asthma, cardiac or renal dysfunction; pregnancy; lactation
- ***Physical:*** Skin color, lesions, turgor; hair; breasts; pelvic exam; orientation, affect; ophthalmologic exam; P, auscultation, peripheral perfusion, edema; R, adventitious sounds; liver evaluation; liver and renal function tests, glucose tolerance, Pap smear

### Implementation

- Discontinue drug and consult physician at signs of thromboembolic disease: leg pain, swelling, peripheral perfusion changes, shortness of breath.

### Drug-specific teaching points

- The following side effects may occur: sensitivity to light (avoid exposure to the sun; use sunscreen and protective clothing); dizziness, sleeplessness, depression (use caution if driving or performing tasks that require alertness); skin rash, color changes, loss of hair; fever; nausea.

- This drug causes serious fetal abnormalities or fetal death; avoid pregnancy.
- Report pain or swelling and warmth in the calves, acute chest pain or shortness of breath, sudden severe headache or vomiting, dizziness or fainting, numbness or tingling in the arm or leg.

## melphalan

*(mel' fa lan)*

L-Pam, L-Phenylalanine Mustard, L-Sarcolysin

Alkeran

**Pregnancy Category D**

### Drug classes

Alkylating agent
Nitrogen mustard
Antineoplastic

### Therapeutic actions

Cytotoxic: alkylates cellular DNA, thus interfering with the replication of susceptible cells, causing cell death.

### Indications

- Palliation of multiple myeloma, nonresectable epthelial ovarian carcinoma; use IV when oral therapy is not possible

### Contraindications/cautions

- Allergy to melphalan or chlorambucil, radiation therapy, chemotherapy, pregnancy (potentially mutagenic and teratogenic; avoid use in the first trimester), lactation.

### Dosage

**Available Forms:** Tablets—2 mg; powder for injection—50 mg

Individualize dosage based on hematologic profile and response.

**ADULT**

- ***Multiple myeloma:*** 6 mg/d PO. After 2–3 wk, stop drug for up to 4 wk, and monitor blood counts. When blood counts are rising, institute maintenance dose of 2 mg/d PO. Response may occur gradually over many months (many alternative regimens, some including predinisone, are used).
- ***Epithelial ovarian carcinoma:*** 0.2 mg/kg per day PO for 5 d as a single course. Repeat courses every 4–5 wk, depending on hematologic response.
- ***IV:*** 16 mg/m$^2$ administered as a single infusion over 15–20 min; administered at 2-wk intervals for 4 doses, then at 4-wk intervals

### Pharmacokinetics

| *Route* | *Onset* | *Peak* |
|---|---|---|
| Oral | Varies | 2 h |
| IV | Rapid | 1 h |

*Metabolism:* $T_{1/2}$: 90 min
*Distribution:* Crosses placenta; enters breast milk
*Excretion:* Urine

### IV facts

**Preparation:** Reconstitute with 10 ml of supplied diluent, and shake vigorously until a clear solution is obtained; this provides 5 mg/ml solution. Immediately dilute in 0.9% Sodium Chloride Injection to a dilution of $< 0.45$ mg/ml. Complete infusion within 60 min of reconstitution. Protect from light. Dispense in glass containers. Do not refrigerate reconstituted solution.

**Infusion:** Administer dilute product over a minimum of 15 min; complete within 60 min of reconstitution.

### Adverse effects

- GI: *Nausea, vomiting,* oral ulceration
- Respiratory: Bronchopulmonary dysplasia, **pulmonary fibrosis**
- Hematologic: *Bone marrow depression*, hyperuricemia
- Dermatologic: Maculopapular skin rash, urticaria, *alopecia*
- Other: *Amenorrhea,* cancer, acute leukemia

### Drug-lab test interferences

- Increased urinary 5-hydroxyindole acetic acid levels (5-HIAA) due to tumor cell destruction



m

## Nursing Considerations

### Assessment

- *History:* Allergy to melphalan or chlorambucil, radiation therapy, chemotherapy, pregnancy, lactation
- *Physical:* T; weight; skin color, lesions; R, adventitious sounds; liver evaluation; CBC, differential, hemoglobin, uric acid, renal function tests

### Implementation

- Arrange for blood tests to evaluate hematopoietic function before therapy and weekly during therapy.
- Do not give full dosage until 4 wk after a full course of radiation therapy or chemotherapy due to risk of severe bone marrow depression.
- Reduce dosage in patients with impaired renal function.
- Ensure that patient is well hydrated before treatment.
- Monitor uric acid levels; ensure adequate fluid intake, and prepare for appropriate treatment if hyperuricemia occurs.
- Divide single daily dose if nausea and vomiting occur with single dose.

### Drug-specific teaching points

- Take drug once a day. If nausea and vomiting occur, consult with care provider about dividing the dose.
- The following side effects may occur: nausea, vomiting, loss of appetite (divided dose, small frequent meals may help; maintain fluid intake and nutrition; drink at least 10–12 glasses of fluid each day); skin rash, loss of hair (obtain a wig if hair loss occurs; head should be covered at extremes of temperature).
- This drug causes severe birth defects; use birth control.
- Report unusual bleeding or bruising, fever, chills, sore throat, cough, shortness of breath, black, tarry stools, flank or stomach pain, joint pain.

## menotropins

*(men oh **troe'** pins)*

Pergonal, Humegon

**Pregnancy Category C**

### Drug classes

Hormone

Fertility drug

### Therapeutic actions

A purified preparation of human gonadotropins; in women, produces ovarian follicular growth; when followed by administration of HCG, produces ovulation; used with HCG for at least 3 mo to induce spermatogenesis in men with primary or secondary pituitary hypofunction who have previously achieved adequate masculinization with HCG administration.

### Indications

- Women: Given with HCG sequentially to induce ovulation and pregnancy in anovulatory infertile patients without primary ovarian failure. Used with HCG to stimulate multiple follicles for in vitro fertilization programs.
- Men: With concomitant HCG therapy to stimulate spermatogenesis in men with primary hypogonadotropic hypogonadism due to a congenital factor or prepubertal hypophysectomy and in men with secondary hypogonadotropic hypogonadism due to hypophysectomy, craniopharyngioma, cerebral aneurysm, or chromophobe adenoma.

### Contraindications/cautions

- Known sensitivity to menotropins; high gonadotropin levels, indicating primary ovarian failure; overt thyroid or adrenal dysfunction, abnormal bleeding of undetermined origin, ovarian cysts or enlargement not due to polycystic ovary syndrome, intracranial lesion, such as pituitary tumor, pregnancy (women); normal gonadotropin levels, indicating pituitary function; elevated gonadotropin levels, indicating primary testicular failure; infertility disorders other than hypogonadotropin hypogonadism (men).

### Dosage

**Available Forms:** Powder for injection—75 IU FSH/75 IU LH, 150 IU FSH/150 IU LH

***Women:*** To achieve ovulation, HCG must be given following menotropins when clinical assessment indicates sufficient follicular maturation as indicated by urinary excretion of estrogens; initial dose is 5 IU FSH/75 IU LH/d IM for 9–12 d. Follow administration with 10,000 IU HCG 1 d after the last dose of menotropins. Do not administer for longer than 12 d. Treat until estrogen levels are normal or slightly higher than normal. When urinary estrogen excretion is < 100 μg/24 h, and urinary estriol excretion is < 50 μg/24 h prior to HCG administration, there is less risk of ovarian overstimulation. Do not administer if urinary excretion exceeds these values. Couple should engage in intercourse daily beginning on the day prior to the HCG administration and until ovulation occurs. If there is evidence of ovulation but pregnancy does not occur, repeat regimen for at least 2 more courses before increasing dose to 150 IU FSH/150 IU LH/d IM for 9–12 d followed by 10,000 IU HCG 1 d after the last dose of menotropins. If there is evidence of ovulation but pregnancy does not occur, repeat this regimen twice more. Larger doses are not recommended.

*MEN:* Pretreat with HCG (5,000 IU three times per week) until serum testosterone levels are within a normal range and masculinization has occurred. Pretreatment may take 4–6 mo. Then give 1 amp (75 IU FSH/75 IU LH) menotropins IM 3× per wk and HCG 2,000 IU twice a wk. Continue for a minimum of 4 mo. If increased spermatogenesis has not occurred at the end of 4 mo, continue treatment with 1 amp menotropins three times per week or 2 amps (dose of 150 IU FSH/150 IU LH) menotropins three times per week with the HCG dose unchanged.

### Pharmacokinetics

| *Route* | *Onset* | *Peak* | *Duration* |
|---|---|---|---|
| IM | Slow | Weeks | Months |

*Metabolism:* $T_{1/2}$: unknown
*Distribution:* Crosses placenta
*Excretion:* Urine

### Adverse effects

*Women*

- CV: Arterial thromboembolism
- GU: *Ovarian enlargement,* hyperstimulation syndrome, hemoperitoneum
- **Hypersensitivity:** Hypersensitivity reactions
- Other: *Febrile reactions;* birth defects in resulting pregnancies, *multiple pregnancies*

*Men*

- Endocrine: Gynecomastia

## ■ Nursing Considerations

### Assessment

- ***History:*** Sensitivity to menotropins; high gonadotropin levels; overt thyroid or adrenal dysfunction, abnormal bleeding of undetermined origin, ovarian cysts or enlargement not due to polycystic ovary syndrome, intracranial lesion (women); normal gonadotropin levels; elevated gonadotropin levels; infertility disorders other than hypogonadotropin hypogonadism (men)
- ***Physical:*** T; masculinization (men); abdominal exam, pelvic exam; testicular exam; serum gonadotropin levels; 24 h urinary estrogens and estriol excretion (women); serum testosterone levels (men)

m

### Implementation

- Dissolve contents of 1 amp in 1–2 ml of Sterile Saline. Administer IM immediately. Discard any unused portion.
- Store ampules at room temperature or in refrigerator; do not freeze.
- Monitor women at least every other day during treatment and for 2 wk after treatment for any sign of ovarian enlargement.
- Discontinue drug at any sign of ovarian overstimulation, and arrange to have patient admitted to the hospital for observation and supportive measures. Do not attempt to remove ascitic fluid because of the risk of injury to the ovaries. Have the patient refrain from intercourse if ovarian enlargement occurs.
- Provide women with calendar of treatment days and explanations about what signs of estrogen and progesterone activity to watch for. Caution patient that 24-h urine collections will be needed periodi-

cally, that HCG also must be given to induce ovulation, and that daily intercourse should begin 1 d prior to HCG administration and until ovulation occurs.

- Alert patient to risks and hazards of multiple births.
- Provide support and encouragement to the male patient, explaining the need for long-term treatment, regular sperm counts, and masculinizing effects of HCG.

### Drug-specific teaching points

- Prepare a calendar showing the treatment schedule; drug can only be given IM and must be used with HCG to achieve the desired effects.
- Have intercourse daily beginning on the day prior to HCG therapy until ovulation occurs.
- The following may occur: breast enlargement (men); ovarian enlargement, abdominal discomfort, fever, multiple births (women).
- Report pain at injection site, severe abdominal or lower back pain, fever, fluid in the abdomen.

## meperidine hydrochloride

*(me **per'** i deen)*

pethidine

Demer-Idine (CAN), Demerol HCl

**Pregnancy Category C**
**C-II controlled substance**

### Drug classes

Narcotic agonist analgesic

### Therapeutic actions

Acts as agonist at specific opioid receptors in the CNS to produce analgesia, euphoria, sedation; the receptors mediating these effects are thought to be the same as those mediating the effects of endogenous opioids (enkephalins, endorphins).

### Indications

- Relief of moderate to severe pain (oral, parenteral)
- Preoperative medication, support of anesthesia, and obstetric analgesia (parenteral)

### Contraindications/cautions

- Contraindications: hypersensitivity to narcotics, diarrhea caused by poisoning (before toxins are eliminated), bronchial asthma, COPD, cor pulmonale, respiratory depression, anoxia, kyphoscoliosis, acute alcoholism, increased intracranial pressure, pregnancy.
- Use cautiously with acute abdominal conditions, CV disease, supraventricular tachycardias, myxedema, convulsive disorders, delirium tremens, cerebral arteriosclerosis, ulcerative colitis, fever, Addison's disease, prostatic hypertrophy, urethral stricture, recent GI or GU surgery, toxic psychosis, labor or delivery (narcotics given to the mother can cause respiratory depression of neonate; premature infants are especially at risk), renal or hepatic dysfunction.

### Dosage

**Available Forms:** Tablets—50, 100 mg; syrup—50 mg/ml; injection—10, 25, 50, 75, 100 mg/ml

**ADULT**

- ***Relief of pain:*** Individualize dosage; 50–150 mg IM, SC, or PO q3–4h as necessary. Diluted solution may be given by slow IV injection. IM route is preferred for repeated injections.
- ***Preoperative medication:*** 50–100 mg IM or SC, 30–90 min before beginning anesthesia.
- ***Support of anesthesia:*** Dilute to 10 mg/ml, and give repeated doses by slow IV injection, or dilute to 1 mg/ml and infuse continuously. Individualize dosage.
- ***Obstetric analgesia:*** When pains become regular 50–100 mg IM or SC; repeat q1–3h.

**PEDIATRIC:** Contraindicated in premature infants.

- ***Relief of pain:*** 0.5–0.8 mg/lb (1–1.8 mg/kg) IM, SC, or PO up to adult dose q3–4h as necessary.
- ***Preoperative medication:*** 0.5–1 mg/lb (1–2 mg/kg) IM or SC, up to adult

dose, 30–90 min before beginning anesthesia.

GERIATRIC OR IMPAIRED ADULT: Use caution; respiratory depression may occur in elderly, the very ill, those with respiratory problems. Reduced dosage may be necessary.

### Pharmacokinetics

| Route | Onset | Peak | Duration |
|---|---|---|---|
| Oral | 15 min | 60 min | 2–4 h |
| IM, SC | 10–15 min | 30–60 min | 2–4 h |
| IV | Immediate | 5–7 min | 2–4 h |

*Metabolism:* Hepatic, $T_{1/2}$: 3–8 h
*Distribution:* Crosses placenta; enters breast milk
*Excretion:* Urine

### IV facts

**Preparation:** Dilute parenteral solution prior to IV injection using 5% Dextrose and Lactated Ringer's; Dextrose-Saline combinations; 2.5%, 5%, or 10% Dextrose in Water, Ringer's, or Lactated Ringer's; 0.45% or 0.9% Sodium Chloride; 1/6 Molar Sodium Lactate.

**Infusion:** Administer by slow IV injection over 4–5 min or by continuous infusion when diluted to 1 mg/ml.

**Incompatibilities:** Do *not* mix meperidine solutions with solutions of barbiturates, aminophylline, heparin, morphine sulfate, methicillin, phenytoin, sodium bicarbonate, iodide, sulfadiazine, sulfisoxazole.

### Adverse effects

- CNS: *Lightheadedness, dizziness, sedation,* euphoria, dysphoria, delirium, insomnia, agitation, anxiety, fear, hallucinations, disorientation, drowsiness, lethargy, impaired mental and physical performance, coma, mood changes, weakness, headache, tremor, convulsions, miosis, visual disturbances, suppression of cough reflex
- GI: *Nausea, vomiting,* dry mouth, anorexia, constipation, biliary tract spasm, increased colonic motility in patients with chronic ulcerative colitis
- CV: Facial flushing, peripheral circulatory collapse, tachycardia, bradycardia, arrhythmia, palpitations, chest wall rigidity, hypertension, hypotension, orthostatic hypotension, syncope
- GU: Ureteral spasm, spasm of vesical sphincters, urinary retention or hesitancy, oliguria, antidiuretic effect, reduced libido or potency
- Dermatologic: Pruritus, urticaria, laryngospasm, bronchospasm, edema
- Local: tissue irritation and induration (SC injection)
- Major hazards: **Respiratory depression, apnea, circulatory depression, respiratory arrest, shock, cardiac arrest**
- Other: *Sweating,* physical tolerance and dependence, psychological dependence

### Clinically important drug-drug interactions

• Potentiation of effects with barbiturate anesthetics; decrease dose of meperidine when coadministering • Severe and sometimes fatal reactions (resembling narcotic overdose; characterized by convulsions, hypertension, hyperpyrexia) when given to patients receiving or who have recently received MAOIs; do not give meperidine to patients on MAOIs. • Increased likelihood of respiratory depression, hypotension, profound sedation, or coma with phenothiazines

### Drug-lab test interferences

• Elevated biliary tract pressure may cause increases in plasma amylase, lipase; determinations of these levels may be unreliable for 24 h after administration of narcotics.

## ■ Nursing Considerations

### Assessment

- *History:* Hypersensitivity to narcotics, diarrhea caused by poisoning, bronchial asthma, COPD, cor pulmonale, respiratory depression, anoxia, kyphoscoliosis, acute alcoholism, increased intracranial pressure; acute abdominal conditions, CV disease, supraventricular tachycardias, myxedema, convulsive disorders, delir-

m

ium tremens, cerebral arteriosclerosis, ulcerative colitis, fever, Addison's disease, prostatic hypertrophy, urethral stricture, recent GI or GU surgery, toxic psychosis, renal or hepatic dysfunction, pregnancy
- *Physical:* T; skin color, texture, lesions; orientation, reflexes, bilateral grip strength, affect, pupil size; P, auscultation, BP, orthostatic BP, perfusion; R, adventitious sounds; bowel sounds, normal output; frequency and pattern of voiding, normal output; ECG; EEG; thyroid, liver, kidney function tests

### Implementation
- Administer to lactating women 4–6 h before the next feeding to minimize the amount in milk.
- Provide narcotic antagonist, facilities for assisted or controlled respiration on standby during parenteral administration.
- Use caution when injecting SC into chilled areas or in patients with hypotension or in shock; impaired perfusion may delay absorption; with repeated doses, an excessive amount may be absorbed when circulation is restored.
- Reduce dosage of meperidine by 25%–50% in patients receiving phenothiazines or other tranquilizers.
- Give each dose of the oral syrup in half glass of water. If taken undiluted, it may exert a slight local anesthetic effect on mucous membranes.
- Reassure patient about addiction liability; most patients who receive opiates for medical reasons do not develop dependence syndromes.

### Drug-specific teaching points
- Take drug exactly as prescribed.
- Avoid alcohol, antihistamines, sedatives, tranquilizers, OTC drugs.
- The following side effects may occur: nausea, loss of appetite (take with food and lie quietly, eating frequent small meals may help); constipation (request a laxative); dizziness, sedation, drowsiness, impaired visual acuity (avoid driving, performing other tasks that require alertness, visual acuity).
- Do not take leftover medication for other disorders, and do not let anyone else take this prescription.
- Report severe nausea, vomiting, constipation, shortness of breath, or difficulty breathing.

## mephentermine sulfate

*(me **fen'** ter meen)*

Wyamine

**Pregnancy Category D**

### Drug classes
Sympathomimetic

### Therapeutic actions
Sympathomimetic amine that acts directly and indirectly (causes norepinephrine release); increases cardiac output, increases peripheral resistance.

### Indications
- Treatment of hypotension secondary to ganglionic blockade, spinal anesthesia
- Emergency maintenance of BP until blood or blood substitute is available

### Contraindications/cautions
- Contraindications: hypotension induced by chlorpromazine (drug interaction will potentiate hypotension); use of MAO inhibitors.
- Use cautiously with CV disease, chronic illness, pregnancy, lactation.

### Dosage
**Available Forms:** Injection—15, 30 mg/ml

**Adult**
- *Prevention of hypotension attendant to spinal anesthesia:* 30–45 mg IM, 10–20 min prior to procedure.
- *Hypotension following spinal anesthesia:* 30–45 mg IV as a single injection. Repeat doses of 30 mg as necessary.
- *Hypotension following spinal anesthesia in obstetric patients:* Initial dose of 15 mg IV; repeat as needed.
- *Treatment of shock following hemorrhage:* Continuous IV infusion of 0.1%

solution in 5% dextrose in water just until blood replacement can be achieved.

### Pharmacokinetics

| *Route* | *Onset* | *Peak* | *Duration* |
|---|---|---|---|
| IM | 10–15 min | 30–60 min | 1–2 h |
| IV | Immediate | 15–30 min | |

*Metabolism:* Hepatic, $T_{1/2}$: 15–20 min
*Distribution:* Crosses placenta; may enter breast milk
*Excretion:* Urine

### IV facts

**Preparation:** Prepare 0.1% solution by adding 10 or 20 ml mephentermine, 30 mg/ml, to 250 or 500 ml of 5% Dextrose in Water, respectively.
**Infusion:** Administer as a single IV injection, each 30 mg over 1 min, or by continuous infusion of 0.1% solution; regulate dose based on BP response.

### Adverse effects

- CNS: *Anxiety,* fear, hallucinations
- CV: *BP changes,* arrhythmias (most likely with heart disease)

### Clinically important drug-drug interactions

• Decreased effects of guanethidine with mephentermine • Severe and sometimes fatal reactions (including hypertensive crisis and intracranial hemorrhage) with MAOIs, furazolidone • Increased likelihood of serious arrhythmias with halogenated hydrocarbon anesthetics

## ■ Nursing Considerations

### Assessment

- *History:* Hypotension induced by chlorpromazine; use of MAOIs, CV disease, chronic illness, pregnancy, lactation
- *Physical:* T; skin color, texture, lesions; orientation; P, auscultation, BP, orthostatic BP, perfusion; R, adventious sounds; liver, kidney function tests

### Implementation

- Monitor BP continously during and after administration.
- Arrange for immediate replacement with blood or blood products if used in emergency situation for shock.

### Drug-specific teaching points

Drug teaching should be incorporated into total teaching plan of patient receiving spinal anesthesia.

- Drug may produce a feeling of anxiety.
- Report difficulty breathing, numbness of tingling, palpitations.

# mephenytoin

*(me **fen'** i toyn)*
Mesantoin
**Pregnancy Category C**

### Drug classes

Antiepileptic agent
Hydantoin

### Therapeutic actions

Has antiepileptic activity without causing general CNS depression; stabilizes neuronal membranes and prevents hyperexcitability caused by excessive stimulation; limits the spread of seizure activity from an active focus.

### Indications

- Control of grand mal (tonic-clonic), psychomotor, focal, and Jacksonian seizures in patients refractory to less toxic antiepileptic drugs

### Contraindications/cautions

- Contraindications: hypersensitivity to hydantoins; pregnancy; lactation; hepatic abnormalities; hematologic disorders.
- Use cautiously with acute intermittent porphyria; hypotension, severe myocardial insufficiency; diabetes mellitus, hyperglycemia.

### Dosage

**Available Forms:** Tablets—100 mg
*ADULT:* Start with 50–100 mg/d PO during the first wk. Thereafter increase the daily dose by 50–100 mg at weekly intervals. No dose should be increased until it

has been taken for at least 1 wk. Average dose ranges from 200–600 mg/d PO. Up to 800 mg/d may be needed for full seizure control.

- *Replacement therapy:* 50–100 mg/d PO during the first wk. Gradually increase (above), while decreasing the dose of discontinued drug, over 3–6 wk. If patient is also receiving phenobarbital, continue until the transition is completed, then gradually withdraw phenobarbital.

*PEDIATRIC:* Usual dose is 100–400 mg/d PO.

*GERIATRIC AND HEPATIC IMPAIRMENT:* Use caution and monitor for early signs of toxicity; mephenytoin is metabolized in the liver.

## Pharmacokinetics

| *Route* | *Onset* | *Peak* | *Duration* |
|---|---|---|---|
| Oral | 30 min | 1–3 h | 24–48 h |

*Metabolism:* Hepatic, $T_{1/2}$: 144 h
*Distribution:* Crosses placenta; enters breast milk
*Excretion:* Urine

## Adverse effects

- CNS: *Nystagmus, ataxia, dysarthria, slurred speech, mental confusion, dizziness, drowsiness, insomnia, transient nervousness, motor twitchings, fatigue, irritability, depression, numbness, tremor, headache*, photophobia, diplopia, conjunctivitis
- GI: *Nausea*, vomiting, diarrhea, constipation, *gingival hyperplasia*, toxic hepatitis, **liver damage**, sometimes fatal; hypersensitivity reactions with hepatic involvement, including hepatocellular degeneration and fatal **hepatocellular necrosis**
- Respiratory: Pulmonary fibrosis, acute pneumonitis
- Hematologic: **Hematopoietic complications**, sometimes fatal: thrombocytopenia, leukopenia, granulocytopenia, agranulocytosis, pancytopenia; macrocytosis and megaloblastic anemia that usually respond to folic acid therapy; eosinophilia, monocytosis, leukocytosis, simple anemia, hemolytic anemia, aplastic anemia, hyperglycemia
- GU: Nephrosis
- Dermatologic: Scarlatiniform, morbilliform, maculopapular, urticarial and nonspecific rashes; also serious and sometimes fatal **dermatologic reactions**: bullous, exfoliative, or purpuric dermatitis, lupus erythematosus, and Stevens-Johnson syndrome; toxic epidermal necrolysis, hirsutism, alopecia, coarsening of the facial features, enlargement of the lips, Peyronie's disease
- Other: lymph node hyperplasia, sometimes progressing to frank malignant lymphoma; monoclonal gammopathy and multiple myeloma (prolonged therapy); polyarthropathy; osteomalacia; weight gain; chest pain; periarteritis nodosa

## Clinically important drug-drug interactions

• Increased effects with: chloramphenicol, cimetidine, disulfiram, isoniazid, phenacemide, phenylbutazone, sulfonamides, trimethoprim • Complex interactions and effects when hydantoins and valproic acid are given together: toxicity with apparently normal serum ethotoin levels; decreased plasma levels of valproic acid; breakthrough seizures when the two drugs are given together • Decreased effects with antineoplastics, diazoxide, folic acid, rifampin, theophyllines • Increased effects and toxicity when primidone, oxyphenbutazone, fluconazole, amiodarone are given with hydantoins • Increased hepatotoxicity with acetaminophen • Decreased effects of the following drugs with hydantoins: corticosteroids, cyclosporine, dicumarol, disopyramide, doxycycline, estrogens, levodopa, methadone, metyrapone, mexiletine, oral contraceptives, quinestrol, carbamazepine

## Drug-lab test interferences

• Interference with the metyrapone and the 1-mg dexamethasone tests; avoid hydantoins for at least 7 d prior to metyrapone testing

## ■ Nursing Considerations

### Assessment

- ***History:*** Hypersensitivity to hydantoins; hepatic abnormalities; hematologic disorders; acute intermittent porphyria; hypotension, severe myocardial insufficiency; diabetes mellitus, hyperglycemia; pregnancy; lactation
- ***Physical:*** T; skin color, lesions; lymph node palpation; orientation, affect, reflexes, vision exam; P, BP; R, adventitious sounds; bowel sounds, normal output, liver evaluation; periodontal exam; liver function tests, urinalysis, CBC and differential, blood proteins, blood and urine glucose, EEG and ECG

### Implementation

- Give with food to enhance absorption and reduce GI upset.
- Reduce dosage, discontinue mephenytoin, or substitute other antiepileptic medication gradually; abrupt discontinuation may precipitate status epilepticus.
- Mephenytoin is ineffective in controlling absence (petit mal) seizures; patients with combined seizures will need other medication for their absence seizures.
- Discontinue drug if skin rash, depression of blood count, enlarged lymph nodes, hypersensitivity reaction, signs of liver damage, or Peyronie's disease (induration of the corpora cavernosa of the penis) occurs; arrange to institute another antiepileptic drug promptly.
- Monitor CBC and differential before therapy is instituted, at 2 wk, 4 wk, and monthly thereafter for the first year, then every 3 mo. If neutrophils drop to between 2,500 and 1,600/mm$^3$, counts should be made every 2 wk. If neutrophils drop to $<$ 1,600/mm$^3$, discontinue drug.
- Monitor hepatic function periodically during chronic therapy.
- Have lymph node enlargement occurring during therapy evaluated carefully, lymphadenopathy simulates Hodgkin's disease; lymph node hyperplasia may progress to lymphoma.
- Arrange dental instruction in oral hygiene techniques for long-term patients to prevent gum hyperplasia.
- Arrange counseling for childbearing age women who need chronic maintenance therapy with antiepileptic drugs and who wish to become pregnant.

### Drug-specific teaching points

- Take this drug exactly as prescribed, with food to enhance absorption and reduce GI upset. Do not discontinue abruptly or change dosage, except on the advice of your health care provider.
- Be especially careful not to miss a dose if you are on once-a-day therapy.
- Maintain good oral hygiene (regular brushing and flossing) to prevent gum disease; have frequent dental checkups to prevent serious gum disease.
- Have frequent checkups to monitor drug response. Keep all appointments.
- The following side effects may occur: drowsiness, dizziness, confusion, blurred vision (avoid driving or performing other tasks requiring alertness or visual acuity); GI upset (take with food, frequent, small meals may help).
- Wear a medical alert tag so that emergency medical personnel will know that you are an epileptic taking antiepileptic medication.
- Report skin rash, severe nausea or vomiting, drowsiness, slurred speech, impaired coordination (ataxia), swollen glands, bleeding, swollen or tender gums, yellowish discoloration of the skin or eyes, joint pain, unexplained fever, sore throat, unusual bleeding or bruising, persistent headache, malaise, any indication of an infection or bleeding tendency, abnormal erection, pregnancy.

m

## mephobarbital

*(me foe* ***bar'*** *bi tal)*
Mebaral
**Pregnancy Category D**
**C-IV controlled substance**

### Drug classes

Barbiturate
Sedative/hypnotic
Antiepileptic agent

## Therapeutic actions

General CNS depressant; barbiturates inhibit impulse conduction in the ascending RAS, depress the cerebral cortex, alter cerebellar function, depress motor output, and can produce excitation (especially with subanesthetic doses in the presence of pain), sedation, hypnosis, anesthesia, and deep coma.

## Indications

- Sedative for the relief of anxiety, tension, and apprehension
- Antiepileptic for the treatment of grand mal and petit mal epilepsy

## Contraindications/cautions

- Contraindications: hypersensitivity to barbiturates; manifest or latent porphyria; marked liver impairment; nephritis; severe respiratory distress; previous addiction to sedative/hypnotic drugs; pregnancy.
- Use cautiously with acute or chronic pain (may cause paradoxical excitement or mask important symptoms); seizure disorders (abrupt discontinuation of daily doses can result in status epilepticus); lactation (secreted in breast milk; caused drowsiness in nursing infants); fever, hyperthyroidism, diabetes mellitus, severe anemia, pulmonary or cardiac disease, status asthmaticus, shock, uremia; impaired liver or kidney function, debilitation.

## Dosage

**Available Forms:** Tablets—32, 50, 100 mg

***Adult***

- ***Daytime sedation:*** 32–100 mg PO tid–qid. Optimum dose is 50 mg tid–qid PO.
- ***Epilepsy:*** Average dose is 400–600 mg/d PO. Start treatment with a low dose and gradually increase over 4–5 d until optimum dosage is reached. Give hs if seizures occur at night, during the day if attacks are diurnal. May be given with phenobarbital or with phenytoin; decrease dose of mephobarbital and phenobarbital to about half that when drug is used alone. Decrease dose of phenytoin, but not mephobarbital, when phenytoin is given with mephobarbital. Satisfactory results have been obtained with an average daily dose of 230 mg phenytoin and 600 mg mephobarbital.

***Pediatric:*** Use caution: barbiturates may produce irritability, excitability, inappropriate tearfulness, and aggression. Base dosage on body weight, age (see Appendix C), and response.

- ***Sedative:*** 16–32 mg PO tid–qid.
- ***Epilepsy***
  - *<5 Y:* 16–32 mg tid–qid PO.
  - *>5 Y:* 32–64 mg tid–quid PO.

***Geriatric Patients or Those With Debilitating Disease:*** Reduce dosage and monitor closely; may produce excitement, depression, confusion.

## Pharmacokinetics

| Route | Onset | Peak | Duration |
|---|---|---|---|
| Oral | 30–60 min | 3–4 h | 10–16 h |

*Metabolism:* Hepatic, $T_{1/2}$: 11–67 h
*Distribution:* Crosses placenta; enters breast milk
*Excretion:* Urine

## Adverse effects

- CNS: *Somnolence, agitation, confusion, hyperkinesia, ataxia, vertigo, CNS depression, nightmares, lethargy, residual sedation (hangover), paradoxical excitement, nervousness, psychiatric disturbance, hallucinations, insomnia, anxiety, dizziness, thinking abnormality*
- GI: *Nausea, vomiting, constipation, diarrhea, epigastric pain*
- CV: *Bradycardia, hypotension, syncope*
- Respiratory: *Hypoventilation, apnea, respiratory depression,* laryngospasm, bronchospasm, **circulatory collapse**
- Hypersensitivity: Skin rashes, angioneurotic edema, serum sickness, morbiliform rash, urticaria; rarely, exfoliative dermatitis, **Stevens-Johnson syndrome, sometimes fatal**

- **Other**: Tolerance, psychological and physical dependence; **withdrawal syndrome**

**Clinically important drug-drug interactions**
• Increased CNS depression with alcohol • Increased risk of nephrotoxicity with methoxyflurane • Decreased effects of the following with barbiturates: theophyllines, oral anticoagulants, beta-blockers, doxycycline, griseofulvin corticosteroids, oral contraceptives and estrogens, metronidazole, phenylbutazones, quinidine, carbamazepine

## ■ Nursing Considerations

### Assessment

- *History:* Hypersensitivity to barbiturates, manifest or latent porphyria; marked liver impairment, nephritis, severe respiratory distress; previous addiction to sedative-hypnotic drugs, acute or chronic pain, seizure disorders, fever, hyperthyroidism, diabetes mellitus, severe anemia, pulmonary or cardiac disease, shock, uremia, debilitation, pregnancy, lactation
- *Physical:* Weight; T; skin color, lesions; orientation, affect, reflexes; P, BP, orthostatic BP; R, adventitious sounds; bowel sounds, normal output, liver evaluation; liver and kidney function tests, blood and urine glucose, BUN

### Implementation

- Monitor patient responses, blood levels when above interacting drugs are given with mephobarbital; suggest alternate contraception to women on oral contraceptives.
- Provide resuscitative facilities on standby in case of respiratory depression, hypersensitivity reaction.
- Taper dosage gradually after repeated use, especially in epileptic patients. When changing antiepileptic medications, taper dosage of discontinued drug while replacement drug dosage is increased.

### Drug-specific teaching points

- Take this drug exactly as prescribed; do not reduce the dosage or discontinue this drug (when used for epilesy) without consulting care provider; the abrupt discontinuation of the drug could result in a serious increase in seizures.
- This drug is habit forming.
- Avoid alcohol, sleep-inducing, or OTC drugs because these could cause dangerous effects.
- Change birth control method from oral contraception while on mephobarbital; avoid becoming pregnant.
- The following side effects may occur: drowsiness, dizziness, "hangover," impaired thinking (may be transient; avoid driving or engaging in dangerous activities); GI upset (taking the drug with food may help); dreams, nightmares, difficulty concentrating, fatigue, nervousness (reversible).
- Wear a medical ID tag to alert emergency medical personnel that you are an epileptic taking this medication.
- Report severe dizziness, weakness, drowsiness that persists, rash or skin lesions, fever, sore throat, mouth sores, easy bruising or bleeding, nosebleed, petechiae, pregnancy.

## meprobamate

*(me proe **ba'** mate)*

Apo-Meprobamate (CAN), Equanil, Miltown, Neo-Tran (CAN), Novomepro (CAN)

**Pregnancy Category D**
**C-IV controlled substance**

**Drug classes**
Antianxiety agent

**Therapeutic actions**
Has effects at many sites in the CNS, including the thalamus and limbic system; inhibits multineuronal spinal reflexes; is mildly tranquilizing; has some anticonvulsant and central skeletal muscle relaxing properties.

**Indications**

- Management of anxiety disorders for the short-term relief of the symptoms of anxiety (anxiety or tension associated with the stress of everyday life usually does not require treatment with anxiolytic drugs); effectiveness for longer than 4 mo not established.

### Contraindications/cautions

- Contraindications: hypersensitivity to meprobamate or to related drugs, such as carisoprodol; acute intermittent porphyria; hepatic or renal impairment; pregnancy; lactation.
- Use cautiously with epilepsy (drug may precipitate seizures).

### Dosage

**Available Forms:** Tablets—200, 400, 600 mg; SR capsules—200, 400 mg

*ADULT:* 1,200–1,600 mg/d PO in 3 to 4 divided doses. *Sustained release:* 400–800 mg PO in the morning and at hs. Do not exceed 2,400 mg/d.

*PEDIATRIC*

- *6–12 Y:* 100–200 mg PO bid–tid. *Sustained release:* 200 mg PO in the morning and hs.
- *<6 Y:* Safety and efficacy not established.

*GERIATRIC:* Use lowest effective dose to avoid oversedation.

### Pharmacokinetics

| *Route* | *Onset* | *Peak* |
|---|---|---|
| Oral | Varies | 1–3 h |

*Metabolism:* Hepatic, $T_{1/2}$: 6–17 h
*Distribution:* Crosses placenta; enters breast milk
*Excretion:* Urine

### Adverse effects

- CNS: *Drowsiness, ataxia, dizziness, slurred speech, headache, vertigo, weakness, impairment of visual accommodation,* euphoria, overstimulation, paradoxical excitement, paresthesias
- GI: *Nausea, vomiting, diarrhea*
- CV: *Palpitations, tachycardia,* various arrhythmias, syncope, **hypotensive crisis**
- Hematologic: Agranulocytosis, aplastic anemia; thrombocytopenic purpura; exacerbation of porphyric symptoms
- Hypersensitivity: Allergic or idiosyncratic reactions (usually seen between first and fourth doses in patients without previous drug exposure): *itchy, urticarial or erythematous maculopapular rash;* leukopenia, acute nonthromobocytopenic purpura, petechiae, ecchymoses, eosinophilia, peripheral edema, adenopathy, fever, fixed drug eruption; hyperpyrexia, chills, angioneurotic edema, bronchospasm, oliguria, anuria, anaphylaxis, erythema multiforme, exfoliative dermatitis, stomatitis, proctitis; Stevens-Johnson syndrome, bullous dermatitis
- Other: Physical, psychological dependence; withdrawal reaction

### Clinically important drug-drug interactions

- Additive CNS depression with alcohol

## ■ Nursing Considerations

### Assessment

- *History:* Hypersensitivity to meprobamate or to related drugs; acute intermittent porphyria; hepatic or renal impairment; epilepsy; pregnancy; lactation
- *Physical:* T; skin color, lesions; orientation, affect, reflexes, vision exam; P, BP; R, adventitious sounds; bowel sounds, normal output, liver evaluation; liver and kidney function tests, CBC and differential, EEG and ECG

### Implementation

- Supervise dose and amount for patients who are addiction prone or alcoholic.
- Dispense least amount of drug feasible to patients who are depressed or suicidal.
- Caution patient not to crush or chew sustained-release capsules.
- Withdraw gradually over 2 wk if patient has been maintained on high doses for weeks or months.
- Withdraw drug if allergic or idiosyncratic reactions occur.
- Provide epinephrine, antihistamines, corticosteroids, life support equipment on standby in case allergic or idiosyncratic reaction occurs.

### Drug-specific teaching points

- Take this drug exactly as prescribed. This drug may not be effective after several months of therapy; continue to see your health care provider. Do not crush or chew sustained-release capsules.

- Avoid alcohol, sleep-inducing, or OTC drugs; these could cause dangerous effects.
- The following side effects may occur: drowsiness, dizziness, lightheadedness, blurred vision (avoid driving or performing other tasks requiring alertness or visual acuity); GI upset (frequent, small meals may help).
- Use birth control while on this drug; do not take this drug during pregnancy. Consult your physician immediately if you decide to become pregnant or find that you are pregnant.
- Report skin rash, sore throat, fever.

# mercaptopurine

*(mer kap toe **pyoor'** een)*

6-mercaptopurine, 6-MP

Purinethol

**Pregnancy Category D**

## Drug classes

Antimetabolite
Antineoplastic

## Therapeutic actions

Tumor-inhibiting properties, probably due to interference with purine nucleotide synthesis and hence with RNA and DNA synthesis, leading to cell death.

## Indications

- Remission induction, remission consolidation, and maintenance therapy of acute leukemia (lymphatic, myelogenous and acute myelomonocytic)

## Contraindications/cautions

- Contraindications: allergy to mercaptopurine, prior resistance to mercaptopurine (cross-resistance with thioguanine is frequent), hematopoietic depression, pregnancy, lactation.
- Use cautiously with impaired renal function (slower elimination and greater accumulation; reduce dosage).

## Dosage

**Available Forms:** Tablets—50 mg

**ADULT AND PEDIATRIC**

- ***Induction therapy:*** Usual initial dose is 2.5 mg/kg per day PO (about 100–200 mg in adults, 50 mg in the average 5-year-old). Continue daily for several weeks. After 4 wk, if no clinical improvement or toxicity, increase to 5 mg/kg per day.
- ***Maintenance therapy after complete hematologic remission:*** 1.5–2.5 mg/kg per day PO as a single daily dose. Often effective in children with acute lymphatic leukemia, especially in combination with methotrexate. Effectiveness in adults has not been noted.

## Pharmacokinetics

| *Route* | *Onset* | *Peak* |
|---|---|---|
| Oral | Varies | 2 h |

*Metabolism:* Hepatic, $T_{1/2}$: 20–50 min
*Distribution:* Crosses placenta; enters breast milk
*Excretion:* Urine

## Adverse effects

- **GI:** Hepatotoxicity; oral lesions—resemble thrush; nausea; vomiting; anorexia
- **Hematologic:** *Bone marrow depression, immunosuppression, hyperuricemia* as consequence of antineoplastic effect and cell lysis
- **Other:** Drug fever, cancer, chromosomal aberrations

## Clinically important drug-drug interactions

• Increased risk of severe toxicity with allopurinol; reduce mercaptopurine to one-third to one-fourth the usual dose • Decreased or reversed actions of nondepolarizing neuromuscular relaxants (atracurium, gallamine, metocurine iodide, pancuronium, tubocurarine, vecuronium)

## ■ Nursing Considerations

### Assessment

- ***History:*** Allergy to mercaptopurine; prior resistance to mercaptopurine; hemato-

m

poietic depression; impaired renal function; pregnancy; lactation
- *Physical:* T; mucous membranes, liver evaluation, abdominal exam; CBC, differential, Hgb, platelet counts; renal and liver function tests; urinalysis; serum uric acid

### Implementation
- Evaluate hematopoietic status before and frequently during therapy.
- Ensure that patient is well hydrated before and during therapy to minimize adverse effects of hyperuricemia.
- Administer as a single daily dose.

### Drug-specific teaching points
- Drink adequate fluids; drink at least 8–10 glasses of fluid each day.
- The following side effects may occur: mouth sores (frequent mouth care will be needed); miscarriages (use birth control).
- Have frequent, regular medical follow-ups, including blood tests to follow the drug effects.
- Report fever, chills, sore throat, unusual bleeding or bruising, yellow discoloration of the skin or eyes, abdominal pain, flank pain, joint pain, fever, weakness, diarrhea.

## meropenem

*(mare oh **pen'** ehm)*

Merrem IV

**Pregnancy Category B**

### Drug classes
Antibiotic (carbapenem)

### Therapeutic actions
Bactericidal: inhibits synthesis of bacterial cell wall and causes cell death in susceptible cells.

### Indications
- Susceptible intra-abdominal infections caused by viridans group streptococci, *E. coli, K. pneumoniae, P. aeruginosa, B. fragilis, B. thetaiotaomicron,* and *Peptostreptococci* s sp.
- Bacterial meningitis caused by *S. pneumoniae, H. influenzae, N. meningitidis*

### Contraindications/cautions
- Contraindications: allergy to cephalosporins, penicillins, beta lactams; renal failure; lactation
- Use cautiously with CNS disorders, seizures, renal or hepatic impairment, pregnancy

### Dosage
**Available Forms:** Powder for injection—500 mg, 1 g

*ADULT:* 1 g IV q8h.

*PEDIATRIC*
- *<3 Mo:* Not recommended.
- *>3 Mo*
  - ***Intra-abdominal infections:*** <50 kg: 20 mg/kg IV q8h. >50 kg: 1 g IV q8h.
  - ***Meningitis:*** <50 kg: 40 mg/kg IV q8h. >50 kg: 2 g IV q8h.

*GERIATRIC OR IMPAIRED RENAL FUNCTION*

| *Ccr (ml/min)* | *Dose* |
|---|---|
| 26–50 | 1 g IV q12h |
| 10–25 | 500 mg IV q12h |
| <10 | 500 mg IV q24h |

### Pharmacokinetics

| *Route* | *Onset* | *Peak* | *Duration* |
|---|---|---|---|
| IV | Immediate | 5 min | 10–12 h |

*Metabolism:* $T_{1/2}$: 0.8–1.1 h

*Distribution:* Crosses placenta; passes into breast milk

*Excretion:* Renal—unchanged

### IV facts
**Preparation:** Dilute in 0.9% Sodium Chloride Injection; 5% or 10% Dextrose Injection; Dextrose in Sodium Chloride, Potassium Chloride, Sodium Bicarbonate, Normosol-M, Ringer's Lactate; Mannitol Injection; Ringer's Injection; Ringer's Lactate Injection; Sodium Lactate Injection 1/6N; Sodium Bicarbonate or Sterile Water for Injection. Store at room temperature; stability in each solution varies—consult manufacturer's instructions if not used immediately.

**Infusion:** Infuse over 15–30 min or give by direct IV injection over 3–5 min.

**Incompatibilities:** Do not mix in solution with other drugs.

**Adverse effects**

- CNS: *Headache,* dizziness, lethargy, paresthesias
- GI: *Nausea, vomiting, diarrhea, anorexia, abdominal pain, flatulence,* **pseudomembranous colitis,** liver toxicity
- Other: *Superinfections, pain,* abscess (redness, tenderness, heat, tissue sloughing), inflammation at injection site, *phlebitis, rash*

## ■ Nursing Considerations

### Assessment

- *History:* Allergy to cephalosporins, penicillins, beta lactams; renal failure; CNS disorders, seizures, renal or hepatic impairment; pregnancy, lactation
- *Physical:* Orientation, affect; skin color, lesions; culture site of infection; R, adventitious sounds; bowel sounds, abdominal exam; renal and liver function tests

### Implementation

- Culture infected area and arrange for sensitivity tests before beginning therapy.
- Monitor for occurence of superinfections and arrange treatment as appropriate.
- Discontinue drug at any sign of colitis and arrange for appropirate supportive treatment.

### Drug-specific teaching points

- This drug can only be given IV.
- The following side effects may occur: stomach upset, loss of appetite, nausea (take drug with food); diarrhea (stay near bathroom); headache, dizziness.
- Report severe diarrhea, difficulty breathing, unusual tiredness or fatigue, pain at injection site.

# mesalamine

*(me sal' a meen)*

5-aminosalicylic acid, 5-ASA

Asacol (oral), Rowasa, Pentasa

**Pregnancy Category B**

**Drug classes**

Anti-inflammatory agent

**Therapeutic actions**

Mechanism of action is unknown; thought to be a direct, local anti-inflammatory effect in the colon where mesalamine blocks cyclooxygenase and inhibits prostaglandin production in the colon.

**Indications**

- Treatment of active mild to moderate distal ulcerative colitis, proctosigmoiditis, or proctitis

**Contraindications/cautions**

- Contraindications: hypersensitivity to mesalamine, salicylates, any component of the formulation.
- Use cautiously with renal impairment, pregnancy, lactation.

### Dosage

**Available Forms:** DR tablets—400 mg; CR capsules—250 mg; suppositories—500 mg; rectal suspension—4 g/60 ml

ADULT

- ***Suspension enema:*** 60 ml U in one rectal instillation (4 g) once a day, preferably at hs, and retained for approximately 8 h. Usual course of therapy is 3–6 wk. Effects may be seen within 3–21 d.
- ***Rectal suppository:*** 500 mg (1 suppository) bid. Retain suppository for 1–3 h or more. Usual course is 3–6 wk.
- ***Oral:*** 800 mg PO tid for 6 wk.

PEDIATRIC: Safety and efficacy not established.

**Pharmacokinetics**

| Route | Onset | Peak |
|---|---|---|
| Oral | Varies | 3–6 h |
| Rectal | Slow | 3–6 h |

*Metabolism:* $T_{1/2}$: 5–10 h
*Distribution:* Unknown
*Excretion:* Feces

**Adverse effects**

- CNS: *Headache, fatigue, malaise,* dizziness, asthenia, insomnia

m

- GI: *Abdominal pain, cramps, discomfort; gas; flatulence; nausea*; diarrhea, bloating, hemmorhoids, rectal pain, constipation
- GU: UTI, urinary burning
- Other: *Flulike symptoms, fever, cold*, rash, back pain, hair loss, peripheral edema

## ■ Nursing Considerations

### Assessment

- ***History:*** Hypersensitivity to mesalamine, salicylates, any component of the formulation; renal impairment; lactation
- ***Physical:*** T, hair status; reflexes, affect; abdominal exam, rectal exam; urinary output; renal function tests

### Implementation

- Administer enemas as follows: Shake bottle well to ensure suspension is homogenous. Remove protective applicator sheath; hold bottle at the neck to ensure that none of the dose is lost. Have patient lie on the left side (to facilitate migration of drug into the sigmoid colon) with the lower leg extended and the upper leg flexed forward. Knee-chest position can be used if more acceptable to the patient. Gently insert the application tip into the rectum pointing toward the umbilicus; steadily squeeze the bottle to discharge the medication. Patient must retain medication for approximately 8 h.
- Administer rectal suppository as follows: remove the foil wrapper; avoid excessive handling (suppository will melt at body temperature); insert completely into the rectum with pointed end first; have patient retain for 3 h or more.
- Caution patient not to chew tablet; swallow whole. Notify physician if intact tablets are found in the stool.
- Monitor patients with renal impairment for possible adverse effects.

### Drug-specific teaching points

- This drug is given as a suspension enema, so the medication must be retained for approximately 8 h; it is best given at hs to facilitate the retention; the effects of the drug are usually seen within 3–21 d, but a full course of therapy is about 6 wk. (Review administration with patient and significant other.)
- Administer rectal suppository as follows: remove the foil wrapper; avoid excessive handling (suppository will melt at body temperature); insert completely into the rectum with pointed end first; retain for 3 h or more.
- Do not chew oral tablets; swallow whole. If intact tablets are seen in the stool, notify physician.
- The following side effects may occur: abdominal cramping, discomfort, pain, gas (relax; maintain the position used for insertion to relieve pressure on the abdomen); headache, fatigue, fever, flulike symptoms (request medication); hair loss (usually mild and transient).
- Report difficulty breathing, rash, severe abdominal pain, fever, headache.

# mesna

***(mes' na)***

Mesnex

**Pregnancy Category B**

### Drug classes

Antidote

Cytoprotective agent

### Therapeutic actions

Reacts chemically with the urotoxic ifosfamide metabolites to inhibit hemorrhagic cystitis induced by ifosfamide.

### Indications

- Prophylactic agent to reduce the incidence of ifosfamide-induced hemorrhagic cystitis
- Orphan drug use: reduction of the incidence of cyclophosphamide-induced hemorrhagic cystitis

### Contraindications/cautions

- Hypersensitivity to mesna or thiol compounds, pregnancy, lactation.

### Dosage

**Available Forms:** Injection—100 mg/ml

*ADULT/PEDIATRIC:* Dosage is equal to 20% of the ifosfamide dose, given as a single bolus IV injection at the time of ifosfamide injection and at 4 and 8 h after each dose (eg, 1.2 g/m$^2$ ifosfamide: mesna 240 mg/m$^2$ at time of dose, at 4 h, and at 8 h). Repeat each day that ifosfamide is given; if ifosfamide dose is adjusted, adjust mesna dose accordingly.

### Pharmacokinetics

| Route | Onset | Duration |
|---|---|---|
| IV | Rapid | Hours |

*Metabolism:* $T_{1/2}$: 0.36–1.7 h
*Distribution:* Crosses placenta; may enter breast milk
*Excretion:* Urine

### IV facts

**Preparation:** Dilute by adding the contents of a mesna ampule to obtain a final concentration of 20 mg mesna/ml fluid to 5% Dextrose Injection, 5% Dextrose and Sodium Chloride Injection, 0.9% Sodium Chloride Injection or Lactated Ringer's Injection. Refrigerate for use within 6 h of dilution; discard any unused drug in the ampule after opening.
**Infusion:** Administer as an IV bolus over 1 min; administer at same rate as ifosfamide if given together.
**Incompatibilities:** Do not mix with cisplatin.

### Adverse effects

- GI: *Nausea, vomiting, diarrhea*

### Drug-lab test interferences

- False-positive test for urinary ketones

## ■ Nursing Considerations

### Assessment

- *History:* Hypersensitivity to mesna, thiol compounds, pregnancy, lactation
- *Physical:* T; skin color, texture, lesions; orientation, frequency and pattern of voiding, normal output; kidney function tests

### Implementation

- Prepare within 6 h of use; discard any unused drug in the ampule.
- Record timing of ifosfamide administration accurately to determine timing of mesna dose.
- Monitor for signs of bladder hemorrhage.

### Drug-specific teaching points

- This drug will be given IV to help prevent some of the side effects of chemotherapy.

## mesoridazine besylate

*(mez oh **rid'** a zeen)*
Serentil
**Pregnancy Category C**

### Drug classes

Phenothiazine (piperidine)
Dopaminergic blocking agent
Antipsychotic
Antianxiety agent

### Therapeutic actions

Mechanism not fully understood: antipsychotic drugs block postsynaptic dopamine receptors in the brain, depressing the RAS, including the parts of the brain involved with wakefulness and emesis; anticholinergic, antihistaminic ($H_1$), and alpha-adrenergic blocking activity also may contribute to some of its therapeutic (and adverse) actions.

### Indications

- Schizophrenia: reduces severity of symptoms
- Behavioral problems in mental deficiency and chronic brain syndrome: reduces hyperactivity and uncooperativeness
- Alcoholism: ameliorate anxiety, depression, nausea in acute and chronic alcoholics
- Psychoneurotic manifestations: reduces symptoms of anxiety and tension

### Contraindications/cautions

- Contraindications: coma or severe CNS depression; bone marrow depression; blood dyscrasia; circulatory collapse; subcortical brain damage; Parkinson's dis-

m

ease; liver damage; cerebral arteriosclerosis; coronary disease; severe hypotension or hypertension.

- Use cautiously with respiratory disorder ("silent pneumonia"); glaucoma, prostatic hypertrophy, epilepsy or history of epilepsy, breast cancer, thyrotoxicosis, peptic ulcer, decreased renal function, myelography within previous 24 h or scheduled within 48 h, exposure to heat or phosphorous insecticides; pregnancy; lactation; children <12 y, especially those with chickenpox, CNS infections (children are especially susceptible to dystonias that may confound the diagnosis of Reye's syndrome).

## Dosage

**Available Forms:** Tablets—10, 25, 50, 100 mg; concentrate—25 mg/ml; injection—25 mg/ml

Full clinical effects may require 6 wk–6 mo of therapy.

**ADULT**

- ***Schizophrenia:*** Initial dosage 50 mg PO tid (optimal total dosage range 100–400 mg/d).
- ***Behavior problems in mental deficiency:*** Initial dosage 25 mg PO (optimal total dosage range 75–300 mg/d).
- ***Alcoholism:*** Initial dosage 25 mg PO bid (optimal total dosage range 50–200 mg/d).
- ***Psychoneurotic manifestations:*** Initial dosage 10 mg PO tid (optimal total dosage range 30–150 mg/d).
  - ***IM administration:*** Initial dose 25 mg; may repeat in 30–60 min if necessary (optimum dosage range 25–500 mg/d).

**PEDIATRIC:** Generally not recommended for children <12 y.

**GERIATRIC:** Use lower doses, and increase dosage more gradually than in younger patients.

## Pharmacokinetics

| *Route* | *Onset* | *Peak* | *Duration* |
|---|---|---|---|
| Oral | Varies | 2–4 h | 4–6 h |
| IM | Rapid | 30 min | 6–8 h |

*Metabolism:* Hepatic, $T_{1/2}$: 24–48 h

*Distribution:* Crosses placenta; enters breast milk

*Excretion:* Renal and bile

## Adverse effects

### *Antipsychotic Drugs*

- CNS: *Drowsiness*, insomnia, vertigo, headache, weakness, tremor, ataxia, slurring, cerebral edema, seizures, exacerbation of psychotic symptoms, extrapyramidal syndromes—*pseudoparkinsonism; dystonias; akathisia,* tardive dyskinesias, potentially irreversible (no known treatment), neuroleptic malignant syndrome (NMS)
- CV: Hypotension, orthostatic hypotension, hypertension, tachycardia, bradycardia, cardiac arrest, CHF, cardiomegaly, **refractory arrhythmias**, pulmonary edema
- Respiratory: Bronchospasm, laryngospasm, dyspnea, suppression of cough reflex and potential for aspiration
- Hematologic: Eosinophilia, leukopenia, leukocytosis, anemia; aplastic anemia; hemolytic anemia; thrombocytopenic or nonthrombocytopenic purpura; pancytopenia
- Hypersensitivity: Jaundice, urticaria, angioneurotic edema, laryngeal edema, photosensitivity, eczema, asthma, anaphylactoid reactions, exfoliative dermatitis
- Endocrine: Lactation, breast engorgement in females, galactorrhea; SIADH; amenorrhea, menstrual irregularities; gynecomastia; changes in libido; hyperglycemia or hypoglycemia; glycosuria; hyponatremia; pituitary tumor with hyperprolactinemia; inhibition of ovulation, infertility, pseudopregnancy; reduced urinary levels of gonadotropins, estrogens, progestins
- Autonomic: Dry mouth, salivation, nasal congestion, nausea, vomiting, anorexia, fever, pallor, flushed facies, sweating, constipation, paralytic ileus, urinary retention, incontinence, polyuria, enuresis, priapism, ejaculation inhibition, male impotence

**Clinically important drug-drug interactions**
• Additive CNS depression with alcohol • Additive anticholinergic effects and possibly decreased antipsychotic efficacy with anticholinergic drugs • Increased likelihood of seizures with metrizamide (contrast agent used in myelography) • Decreased antihypertensive effect of guanethidine with antipsychotic drugs

**Drug-lab test interferences**
• False-positive pregnancy tests (less likely if serum test is used) • Increase in PBI, not attributable to an increase in thyroxine

## ■ Nursing Considerations

### Assessment

- *History:* Coma or severe CNS depression, bone marrow depression, circulatory collapse, subcortical brain damage, Parkinson's disease, liver damage, cerebral arteriosclerosis, coronary disease, severe hypotension or hypertension, respiratory disorders, glaucoma, prostatic hypertrophy, epilepsy, breast cancer, thyrotoxicosis, peptic ulcer, decreased renal function, myelography within previous 24 h or scheduled within 48 h, exposure to heat or phosphorous insecticides, lactation, children younger than 12
- *Physical:* Weight, T; reflexes, orientation, intraocular pressure; P, BP, orthostatic BP; R, adventitious sounds; bowel sounds and normal output, liver evaluation; urinary output, prostate size; CBC, urinalysis, thyroid, liver and kidney function tests

### Implementation

- Do not change dosage in chronic therapy more often than weekly; drug requires 4–7 d to achieve steady state plasma levels.
- Avoid skin contact with oral solution; contact dermatitis has occurred.
- Discontinue drug if serum creatinine, BUN become abnormal or if WBC count is depressed.
- Monitor elderly patients for dehydration, and institute remedial measures promptly; sedation and decreased sensation related to CNS effects of drug can lead to severe dehydration.
- Consult physician regarding appropriate warning of patient or patient's guardian about tardive dyskinesias.
- Consult physician about dosage reduction; use of anticholinergic antiparkinsonian drugs (controversial) if extrapyramidal effects occur.

### Drug-specific teaching points

- Take drug exactly as prescribed.
- Avoid skin contact with drug solutions.
- Avoid driving or engaging in other dangerous activities if CNS, vision changes occur.
- Avoid prolonged exposure to sun or use a sunscreen or covering garments.
- Maintain fluid intake and use precautions against heatstroke in hot weather.
- Report sore throat, fever, unusual bleeding or bruising, rash, weakness, tremors, impaired vision, dark colored urine (pink or reddish brown urine), pale stools, yellow of the skin or eyes.

# metaproterenol sulfate

*(met a proe **ter'** e nole)*
Alupent, Metaprel
**Pregnancy Category C**

**Drug classes**
Sympathomimetic
Beta-2 selective adrenergic agonist
Bronchodilator
Antiasthmatic agent

**Therapeutic actions**
In low doses, acts relatively selectively at $\beta_2$ adrenergic receptors to cause bronchodilation; at higher doses, $\beta_2$ selectivity is lost and the drug also acts at $\beta_1$ receptors to cause typical sympathomimetic cardiac effects.

**Indications**
- Prophylaxis and treatment of bronchial asthma and reversible bronchospasm that may occur with bronchitis and emphysema

**Contraindications/cautions**
- Contraindications: hypersensitivity to metaproterenol; tachyarrhythmias, tachycardia

caused by digitalis intoxication; general anesthesia with halogenated hydrocarbons or cyclopropane, which sensitize the myocardium to catecholamines.

- Use cautiously with unstable vasomotor system disorders; hypertension; CAD; history of stroke; COPD patients who have developed degenerative heart disease; hyperthyroidism; history of seizure disorders; psychoneurotic individuals; pregnancy; labor and delivery (may inhibit labor; parenteral use of $\beta_2$-adrenergic agonists can accelerate fetal heart beat, cause hypoglycemia, hypokalemia, and pulmonary edema in the mother and hypoglycemia in the neonate); lactation.

### Dosage

**Available Forms:** Tablets—10, 20 mg; syrup—10 mg/5 ml; aerosal—75, 150 mg; solution for injection—0.4%, 0.6%, 5%

ADULT

- ***Oral:*** 20 mg tid or qid.
- ***Inhalation—metered dose inhaler:*** Each actuation of aerosol dispenser delivers 0.65 micronized metaproterenol powder: 2–3 inhalations q3–4h. Do not exceed 12 inhalations/d.
- ***Inhalant solutions:*** Administer tid–qid from hand bulb nebulizer or using an IPPB device, following manufacturer's instructions.

PEDIATRIC

- ***Oral***
- *9 Y or 60 LBS:* 20 mg tid or qid.
- ***Oral***
- *6–9 Y OR <60 LBS:* 10 mg tid or qid.
- *<6 Y:* Doses of 1.3–2.6 mg/kg/d in divided doses of syrup have been well tolerated.
- ***Inhalation***
- *>12 Y:* Same as adult.
- *<12 Y:* Not recommended.

GERIATRIC: Patients > 60 y are more likely to develop adverse effects, use extreme caution.

### Pharmacokinetics

| Route | Onset | Peak | Duration |
|---|---|---|---|
| PO | 15 min | 1 h | 4 h |
| Inhal. | 1–4 min | 1 h | 3–4 h |

*Metabolism:* Liver and tissue; T1/2: unknown

*Excretion:* Bile and feces

### Adverse effects

- CNS: *Restlessness, apprehension, anxiety, fear, CNS stimulation*, hyperkinesia, insomnia, tremor, drowsiness, irritability, weakness, vertigo, headache
- GI: *Nausea, vomiting, heartburn*, unusual or bad taste
- CV: *Cardiac arrhythmias, tachycardia*, palpitations, PVC's (rare), anginal pain—less likely with bronchodilator doses of this drug than with bronchodilator doses of a non-selective beta-agonist (isoproterenol), changes in BP
- **Respiratory**: Respiratory difficulties, pulmonary edema, coughing, bronchospasm, paradoxical airway resistance with repeated, excessive use of inhalation preparations
- Other: *Sweating, pallor, flushing*

## ■ Nursing Considerations

### Assessment

- ***History:*** Hypersensitivity to metaproterenol; tachyarrhythmias; general anesthesia with halogenated hydrocarbons or cyclopropane; unstable vasomotor system disorders; hypertension; CAD; stroke; COPD patients who have developed degenerative heart disease; hyperthyroidism; seizure disorders; psychoneuroses; pregnancy; labor; lactation.
- ***Physical:*** Weight, skin color, temperature, turgor; orientation, reflexes; P, BP; R, adventitious sounds; blood and urine glucose, serum electrolytes, thyroid function tests, ECG

### Implementation

- Use minimal doses for minimal periods of time–drug tolerance can occur with prolonged use.
- Maintain a beta-adrenergic blocker (a cardioselective beta blocker such as atenolol should be used in patients with respiratory distress) on standby in case cardiac arrhythmias occur.

- Do not exceed recommended dosage. Administer aerosol during second half of inspiration, when airways are wider and distribution is more extensive.
- Consult manufacturer's instructions for use of aerosal delivery equipment; specifics of administration vary with each product.

### Drug-specific teaching points

- Do not exceed recommended dosage; adverse effects or loss of effectiveness may result. Read product instructions and ask your health care provider or pharmacist if you have any questions.
- The following side effects may occur: nausea, vomiting, change in taste (small, frequent meals may help); dizziness, drowsiness, fatigue, weakness (use caution if driving or performing tasks that require alertness); irritability, apprehension, sweating, flushing.
- Report chest pain, dizziness, insomnia, weakness, tremor or irregular heart beat, difficulty breathing, productive cough, failure to respond to usual dosage.

## metaraminol bitartrate

*(met a **ram'** i nole)*

Aramine

**Pregnancy Category D**

### Drug classes

Sympathomimetic
Alpha adrenergic agonist
Vasopressor
Shock, agent used in

### Therapeutic actions

Vasopressor without cardiac stimulation; effects are mediated by alpha adrenergic receptors in the vasculature; potent vasoconstrictor.

### Indications

- Prevention and treatment of acute hypotension with spinal anesthesia
- Adjunctive treatment of hypotension due to hemorrhage, drug reactions, surgical complications, shock associated with brain damage due to trauma or tumor
- "Probably effective" as adjunct in treatment of hypotension due to cardiogenic or septicemic shock

### Contraindications/cautions

- Contraindications: cyclopropane or halothane anesthesia (cardiac arrhythmias); hypovolemia (not a substitute for restoration of fluids, plasma, electrolytes, which should be replaced promptly when loss has occurred).
- Use cautiously with hyperthyroidism, severe hypertension, heart disease, diabetes mellitus, cirrhosis (restore electrolytes lost in drug-induced diuresis), malaria, pregnancy, lactation.

### Dosage

**Available Forms:** Injection—10 mg/ml

Individualize dosage on the basis of response. At least 10 min should be allowed between successive doses so that effects of previous dose are fully apparent.

*ADULT*

- ***IM or SC (prevention of hypotension):*** 2–10 mg.
- ***IV infusion (adjunctive therapy of hypotension):*** 15–100 mg in 250 or 500 ml Sodium Chloride Injection or 5% Dextrose Injection. Adjust rate of infusion to maintain desired BP. Adjust drug concentration on the basis of the patient's need for fluid. Concentrations of 150–500 mg/500 ml of infusion fluid have been used.
- ***Direct IV injection (severe shock):*** 0.5–5 mg, followed by infusion of 15–100 mg in 250 or 500 ml IV fluid.

*PEDIATRIC:* 0.01 mg/kg as a single dose or a solution of 1 mg/25 ml in dextrose or saline.

### Pharmacokinetics

| *Route* | *Onset* | *Duration* |
|---|---|---|
| SC | 5–20 min | 1 h |
| IM | 10 min | 1 h |
| IV | 1–2 min | 15–20 min |

*Metabolism:* Tissue; $T_{1/2}$: unknown

## IV facts

**Preparation:** Dilute 15–100 mg in 250 or 500 ml Sodium Chloride Injection or 5% Dextrose Injection for continuous infusion. Direct injection can be given undiluted, but follow with infusion of 15–100 mg in 250 or 500 ml of IV fluid. Use diluted solutions within 24 h.

**Infusion:** Inject each 5 mg over 1 min; rate of infusion is determined by response to drug; use slowest rate possible to maintain BP.

**Compatibilities:** Compatible with Sodium Chloride Injection, 5% Dextrose Injection, Ringer's Injection, Lactated Ringer's Injection, 6% Dextran in Saline, Normosol-R, Normosol-M in $D_5W$.

### Adverse effects

- CNS: *Headache, flushing*, sweating, tremors, dizziness, apprehension
- CV: *Sinus or ventricular tachycardia, other arrhythmias* (especially in MI patients), cardiac arrest, palpitation, hypertension; hypotension upon withdrawal
- GI: Nausea
- Local: Abscess formation, tissue necrosis, sloughing at injection site

### Clinically important drug-drug interactions

- Increased hypertensive effects with TCAs (imipramine), MAO inhibitors; guanethidine, methyldopa, furazoladine.

## ■ Nursing Considerations

### Assessment

- *History:* Cyclopropane or halothane anesthesia; hypovolemia; hyperthyroidism; severe hypertension; heart disease; diabetes mellitus; cirrhosis; malaria; pregnancy; lactation
- *Physical:* Weight, skin color, temperature, turgor; injection sites; orientation, reflexes, affect; P, BP; R, adventitious sounds; liver palpation; urine output; serum electrolytes, thyroid and liver function tests, blood and urine glucose, ECG

### Implementation

- Give IV infusions into a large vein, preferably of the antecubital fossa, to prevent extravasation.
- Do not infuse into veins of the ankle or dorsum of the hand with peripheral vascular disease, diabetes mellitus, or hypercoagulability states.
- Monitor BP frequently; avoid excessive BP response—rapidly induced hypertensive responses have been reported to cause pulmonary edema, arrhythmias, cardiac arrest.
- Provide phentolamine on standby in case extravasation occurs (5–10 mg phentolamine in 10–15 ml saline should be used to infiltrate the affected area).

### Drug-specific teaching points

- Since metaraminol is used mainly during anesthesia or acute emergency states, patient teaching will relate mainly to anesthesia, the procedure, and monitors rather than specifically to therapy with metaraminol. Patient should be told the following:
- This drug may cause dizziness, apprehension, sweating, flushing.
- Report any pain at the injection site.

# metformin

*(met fore' min)*

Glucophage

**Pregnancy Category C**

### Drug classes

Antidiabetic agent

### Therapeutic actions

Exact mechanism is not understood; possibly increases peripheral utilization of glucose, increases production of insulin, decreases hepatic glucose production and alters intestinal absorption of glucose.

### Indications

- Adjunct to diet to lower blood glucose with non-insulin-dependent diabetes mellitus (type II)

### Contraindications/cautions

- Allergy to metformin; diabetes complicated by fever, severe infections, severe trauma, major surgery, ketosis, acidosis, coma (use insulin); type I or juvenile diabetes, serious hepatic impairment, serious renal impairment, uremia, thyroid or endocrine impairment, glycosuria, hyperglycemia associated with primary renal disease; ; labor and delivery— if metformin is used during pregnancy, discontinue drug at least 1 mo before delivery; lactation, safety not established.

### Dosage

**Available Forms:** Tablets—500, 850 mg

*ADULT:* 500–850 mg/d PO in divided doses to a maximum of 3000 mg/d. Dose should be titrated based on response and blood glucose level.

*PEDIATRIC:* Safety and efficacy not established.

*GERIATRIC AND RENAL IMPAIRED:* Smaller doses may be necessary; monitor closely and titrate slowly

### Pharmacokinetics

| *Route* | *Peak* | *Duration* |
|---|---|---|
| Oral | 2–2.5 h | 10–16h |

*Metabolism:* Hepatic metabolism; $T_{1/2}$: 6.2 and 17.6 hours

*Distribution* : Crosses placenta; passes into breast milk

*Excretion* : Urine

### Adverse effects

- GI: *anorexia, nausea*, vomiting, *epigastric discomfort, heartburn, diarrhea*
- Endocrine: *hypoglycemia,* ***lactic acidosis***
- Hypersensitivity: *allergic skin reactions*, eczema, pruritus, erythema, urticaria

### Clinically important drug-drug interactions

• Increased risk of hypoglycemia with cimetidine • Increased risk of lactic acidosis with glucocorticoids or ethanol

## ■ Nursing Considerations

### Assessment

- ***History:*** Allergy to metformin; diabetes complicated by fever, severe infections, severe trauma, major surgery, ketosis, acidosis, coma; type I or juvenile diabetes, serious hepatic or renal impairment, uremia, thyroid or endocrine impairment, glycosuria, hyperglycemia associated with primary renal disease.
- ***Physical:*** Skin color, lesions; T, orientation, reflexes, peripheral sensation; R, adventitious sounds; liver evaluation, bowel sounds; urinalysis, BUN, serum creatinine, liver function tests, blood glucose, CBC.

### Implementation

- Monitor urine and serum glucose levels frequently to determine effectiveness of drug and dosage.
- Arrange for transfer to insulin therapy during periods of high stress (infections, surgery, trauma).
- Use IV glucose if severe hypoglycemia occurs as a result of overdose.



### Drug-specific teaching points

- Do not discontinue this medication without consulting your physician.
- Monitor urine or blood for glucose and ketones as prescribed.
- Do not use this drug during pregnancy.
- Avoid the use of alcohol while on this drug.
- Report fever, sore throat, unusual bleeding or bruising, skin rash, dark urine, light-colored stools, hypo- or hyperglycemic reactions.

## methadone hydrochloride

***(meth' a done)***

Dolophine

**Pregnancy Category C**

**C-II controlled substance**

## Drug Classes

Narcotic agonist analgesic

## Therapeutic actions

Acts as agonist at specific opioid receptors in the CNS to produce analgesia, euphoria, sedation; the receptors mediating these effects are thought to be the same as those mediating the effects of endogenous opioids (enkephalins, endorphins); when used in approved methadone maintenance programs, can substitute for heroin, other illicit narcotics in patients who want to terminate a drug use.

## Indications

- Relief of severe pain
- Detoxification and temporary maintenance treatment of narcotic addiction (ineffective for relief of general anxiety)

## Contraindications/cautions

- Contraindications: hypersensitivity to narcotics, diarrhea caused by poisoning (before toxins are eliminated), bronchial asthma, COPD, cor pulmonale, respiratory depression, anoxia, kyphoscoliosis, acute alcoholism, increased intracranial pressure.
- Use cautiously with acute abdominal conditions, CV disease, supraventricular tachycardias, myxedema, convulsive disorders, delirium tremens, cerebral arteriosclerosis, ulcerative colitis, fever, Addison's disease, prostatic hypertrophy, urethral stricture, recent GI or GU surgery, toxic psychosis, pregnancy prior to labor (crosses placenta; neonatal withdrawal observed in infants born to drug-using mothers; safety for use in pregnancy before labor not established), labor or delivery (administration of narcotics to mother can cause respiratory depression of neonate—risk greatest for prematures), renal or hepatic dysfunction, lactation.

## Dosage

**Available Forms:** Tablets—5, 10 mg; oral solution—5 mg/5 ml, 10 mg/5 ml, 10 mg/10 ml; oral concentrate—10 mg/ml; injection—10 mg/ml; dispersible tablets—40 mg

Oral methadone is approximately 1/2 as potent as parenteral methadone.

**ADULT**

- ***Relief of pain:*** 2.5–10 mg IM, SC or PO q3–4 h as necessary. IM route is preferred to SC for repeated doses. Individualize dosage: patients with excessively severe pain and those who have become tolerant to the analgesic effect of narcotics may need higher dosage.
- ***Detoxification:*** Initially, 15–20 mg PO or parenteral–PO preferred. Increase dose to suppress withdrawal signs. 40 mg/d in single or divided doses is usually an adeqate stabilizing dose for those physically dependent on high doses. Continue stabilizing doses for 2–3 d, then gradually decrease dosage every d or every 2 d. A daily reduction of 20% of the total dose may be tolerated. Provide sufficient dosage to keep withdrawal symptoms at tolerable level. Treatment should not exceed 21 d and may not be repeated earlier than 4 wk after completion of previous course. Detoxification treatment continued longer than 21 d becomes maintenance treatment, which may be undertaken only by approved programs (addicts hospitalized for other medical conditions may receive methadone maintenance treatment).
- ***Maintenance treatment:*** For patients who are heavy heroin users up until hospital admission, initial dose of 20 mg q4-8 h or 40 mg in a single dose PO. For patients with little or no narcotic tolerance, half this dose may suffice. Dosage should suppress withdrawal symptoms but not produce acute narcotic effects of sedation, respiratory depression. Give additional 10 mg doses if needed to suppress withdrawal syndrome. Adjust dosage, up to 120 mg/d.

**PEDIATRIC:** Not recommended for relief of pain in children due to insufficient documentation.

**GERIATRIC OR IMPAIRED ADULT:** Use caution–respiratory depression may occur in the elderly, the very ill, those with respiratory problems. Reduced dosage may be necessary.

### Pharmacokinetics

| *Route* | *Onset* | *Peak* | *Duration* |
|---|---|---|---|
| PO | 30–60 min | 90–120 min | 4–12 h |
| IM | 10–20 min | 1–2 h | 4–6 h |
| SC | 10–20 min | 1–2 h | 4–6 h |

*Metabolism:* Liver; $T_{1/2}$: 25 h
*Distribution:* Crosses placenta and enters breast milk
*Excretion:* Bile and feces

### Adverse effects

- CNS: *Lightheadedness, dizziness, sedation,* euphoria, dysphoria, delirium, insomnia, agitation, anxiety, fear, hallucinations, disorientation, drowsiness, lethargy, impaired mental and physical performance, coma, mood changes, weakness, headache, tremor, convulsions, miosis, visual disturbances, suppression of cough reflex
- GI: *Nausea, vomiting,* dry mouth, anorexia, constipation, biliary tract spasm; increased colonic motility in patients with chronic ulcerative colitis
- CV: Facial flushing, peripheral circulatory collapse, arrhythmia, palpitations, chest wall rigidity, hypertension, hypotension, orthostatic hypotension, syncope
- GU: Ureteral spasm, spasm of vesical sphincters, urinary retention or hesitancy, oliguria, antidiuretic effect, reduced libido or potency
- Dermatologic: Pruritus, urticaria, laryngospasm, bronchospasm, edema, hemorrhagic urticaria (rare)
- Local: Tissue irritation and induration (SC injection)
- Other: Sweating (more common in ambulatory patients and those without severe pain),physical tolerance and dependence, psychological dependence
- Major hazards: **Respiratory depression, apnea, circulatory depression, respiratory arrest, shock, cardiac arrest**

### Clinically important drug-drug interactions

• Potentiation of effects of levorphanol with barbiturate anesthetics–decrease dose of meperidine when coadministering • Decreased effectiveness of methadone with hydantoins, rifampin, urinary acidifiers (ammonium chloride, potassium acid phosphate, sodium acid phosphate) • Increased effects and toxicity of methadone with cimetidine, ranitidine

### Drug-lab test interferences

• Elevated biliary tract pressure (narcotic effect) may cause increases in plasma amylase, lipase; determinations of these levels may be unreliable for 24 h after administration of narcotics.

## ■ Nursing Considerations

### Assessment

- *History:* Hypersensitivity to narcotics, diarrhea caused by poisoning, bronchial asthma, COPD, cor pulmonale, respiratory depression, kyphoscoliosis, acute alcoholism, increased intracranial pressure; acute abdominal conditions, CV disease, supraventricular tachycardias, myxedema, convulsive disorders, delirium tremens, cerebral arteriosclerosis, ulcerative colitis, fever, Addison's disease, prostatic hypertrophy, urethral stricture, recent GI or GU surgery, toxic psychosis; pregnancy; labor; lactation.
- *Physical:* T; skin color, texture, lesions; orientation, reflexes, bilateral grip strength, affect, pupil size; pulse, auscultation, BP, orthostatic BP, perfusion; R, adventious sounds; bowel sounds, normal output; frequency and pattern of voiding, normal output; ECG; EEG; thyroid, liver, kidney function tests.

### Implementation

- Give to nursing women 4–6 h before the next feeding to minimize the amount in milk.
- Provide narcotic antagonist, facilities for assisted or controlled respiration on standby during parenteral administration.
- Use caution when injecting SC into chilled areas or in patients with hypotension or in shock—impaired perfusion may delay absorption; with repeated

m

doses, an excessive amount may be absorbed when circulation is restored.

### Drug-specific teaching points

- Take drug exactly as prescribed.
- Avoid alcohol.
- The following side effects may occur: nausea, loss of appetite (take with food, lie quietly, eat frequent small meals); constipation (laxative may help); dizziness, sedation, drowsiness, impaired visual acuity (avoid driving, performing other tasks that require alertness, visual acuity).
- Do not take leftover medication for other disorders; do not let anyone else take the prescription.
- Report severe nausea, vomiting, constipation, shortness of breath or difficulty breathing.

# methazolamide

*(meth a zoe' la mide)*

Neptazane

**Pregnancy Category C**

### Drug classes

Carbonic anhydrase inhibitor
Antiglaucoma agent
Diuretic
Sulfonamide, nonbacteriostatic

### Therapeutic actions

Inhibits the enzyme carbonic anhydrase, thereby: decreasing aqueous humor formation and hence decreasing intraocular pressure; decreasing hydrogen ion secretion by renal tubule cells and hence increasing sodium, potassium, bicarbonate, and water excretion by the kidney.

### Indications

- Adjunctive treatment of chronic open-angle glaucoma, secondary glaucoma
- Preoperative use in acute angle-closure glaucoma where delay of surgery is desired to lower intraocular pressure
- Unlabeled uses: treatment of hyperkalemia and hypokalemia periodic paralysis

### Contraindications/cautions

- Contraindications: allergy to dichlorphenamide, sulfonamides.
- Use cautiously with renal or liver disease; adrenocortical insufficiency; respiratory acidosis; COPD; chronic noncongestive angle-closure glaucoma; decreased sodium, potassium; hyperchloremic acidosis; pregnancy; lactation.

### Dosage

**Available Forms:** Tablets—25, 50 mg

*ADULT:* 50–100 mg PO bid or tid. Most effective if taken with other miotics.

### Pharmacokinetics

| *Route* | *Onset* | *Peak* | *Duration* |
|---|---|---|---|
| PO | 2–4 h | 6–8 h | 10–18 h |

*Metabolism:* Liver, $T_{1/2}$: 14 h
*Distribution:* Crosses placenta and enters breast milk
*Excretion:* Urine

### Adverse effects

- CNS: *Photophobia,* weakness, fatigue, nervousness, sedation, drowsiness, dizziness, depression, tremor, ataxia, headache, paresthesias, convulsions, flaccid paralysis, transient myopia
- GI: *Anorexia, nausea, vomiting, constipation,* melena, hepatic insufficiency
- **Hematologic**: Bone marrow depression
- GU: Hematuria, glycosuria, urinary frequency, renal colic, renal calculi, crystalluria, polyuria
- **Dermatologic**: Urticaria, pruritis, rash, *photosensitivity*, erythema multiforme
- **Other**: Weight loss, fever, acidosis

### Clinically important drug-drug interactions

- Increased risk of salicylate toxicity, due to metabolic acidosis with salicylates.

### Drug-lab test interferences

- False-positive results on tests for urinary protein.

## ■ Nursing Considerations

### Assessment

- *History:* Allergy to dichlorphenamide, sulfonamides; renal or liver disease; adrenocortical insufficiency; respiratory acidosis; COPD; chronic noncongestive angle-closure glaucoma; pregnancy; lactation.

- *Physical:* Skin color and lesions; T; weight; orientation, reflexes, muscle strength, ocular pressure; R, pattern, adventitious sounds; liver evaluation and bowel sounds; CBC, serum electrolytes, liver and renal function tests, urinalysis.

### Implementation
- Administer with food if GI upset occurs; provide small, frequent meals.

### Drug-specific teaching points
- Have periodic checks of intraocular pressure.
- Sensitivity to sun: use sunscreen or wear protective clothing.
- Report loss or gain of more than 3 lbs/d, unusual bleeding or bruising, dizziness, muscle cramps or weakness, skin rash.

## methdilazine hydrochloride

*(meth dill' a zeen)*

Dilosyn (CAN), Tacaryl

**Pregnancy Category C**

### Drug classes
Phenothiazine
Dopaminergic blocking agent
Antihistamine

### Therapeutic actions
Selectively blocks $H_1$ receptors, thereby diminishing the effects of histamine on cells of the upper respiratory tract and eyes and decreasing the sneezing, mucus production, itching, and tearing that accompany allergic reactions in sensitized people exposed to antigens.

### Indications
- Symptomatic relief of symptoms associated with perennial and seasonal allergic rhinitis, vasomotor rhinitis, allergic conjunctivitis
- Mild, uncomplicated urticaria and angioedema
- Amelioration of allergic reactions to blood or plasma
- Dermatographism, adjunctive therapy (with epinephrine and other measures) in anaphylactic reactions

### Contraindications/cautions
- Contraindications: hypersensitivity to antihistamines or phenothiazines, coma or severe CNS depression; bone marrow depression; vomiting of unknown cause; concomitant therapy with MAO inhibitors; lactation (lactation may be inhibited; may be secreted in breast milk; higher risk of adverse effects in newborns and prematures).
- Use cautiously with lower respiratory tract disorders (may thicken secretions and impair expectoration); glaucoma, prostatic hypertrophy (anticholinergic effects may exacerbate glaucoma and urinary retention); CV disease or hypertension; breast cancer (elevations in prolactin may stimulatea prolactin-dependent tumor); thyrotoxicosis (severe neurotoxicity); peptic ulcer; decreased renal function; pregnancy; lactation; children <12 y of age, especially those with chicken pox, CNS infections (children are susceptible to dystonias that may confound the diagnosis of Reye's syndrome); the elderly (likely to cause dizziness, sedation, syncope, toxic confusional states, hypotension, and extrapyramidal effects).

m

### Dosage
**Available Forms:** Chewable tablets—4 mg; tablets—8 mg

**ADULT:** 8 mg PO bid–qid.

**PEDIATRIC <3 Y:** 4 mg PO bid–qid.

**GERIATRIC:** Use special cautiously, elderly are more susceptible to adverse effects, reduced dosage may be needed.

### Pharmacokinetics

| *Route* | *Onset* | *Peak* | *Duration* |
|---|---|---|---|
| PO | 15–30 min | 1–2 h | 4–6 h |

*Metabolism:* Liver; $T_{1/2}$: 18 h

*Distribution:* Crosses placenta and enters breast milk

*Excretion:* Urine

### Adverse effects

- CNS: *Dizziness, drowsiness, poor coordination, confusion, restlessness, excitation,* convulsions, tremors, headache, blurred vision, diplopia, vertigo, tinnitus
- GI: *Epigastric distress*, nausea, vomiting, diarrhea, constipation
- CV: Hypotension, palpitations, bradycardia, tachycardia, extrasystoles
- **Respiratory**: *Thickening of bronchial secretions*; chest tightness; dry mouth, nose and throat; respiratory depression; suppression of cough reflex, potential for aspiration
- **Hematologic**: Hemolytic anemia, hypoplastic anemia, thrombocytopenia, leukopenia, agranulocytosis, pancytopenia
- GU: *Urinary frequency, dysuria*, urinary retention, decreased libido, impotence
- **Dermatologic**: Uritcaria, rash, photosensitivity, chills
- **Other**: Tingling, heaviness and wetness of the hands

### Clinically important drug-drug interactions

• Additive anticholinergic effects with anticholinergics. Increased likelihood of seizures with metrizamide (contrast agent used in myelography) • Decreased antihypertensive effect of guanethidine

## ■ Nursing Considerations

### Assessment

- *History:* Hypersensitivity to antihistamines or phenothiazines, coma or severe CNS depression; bone marrow depression; vomiting of unknown cause; concomitant therapy with MAO inhibitors; lactation; lower respiratory tract disorders ; glaucoma, prostatic hypertrophy; CV disease or hypertension; breast cancer; thyrotoxicosis; peptic ulcer; chicken pox, CNS infections; pregnancy; lactation
- *Physical:* Weight, T; reflexes, orientation, intraocular pressure; P, BP, orthostatic BP; R, adventitious sounds; bowel sounds and normal output, liver evaluation; urinary output, prostate size; CBC, urinalysis, thyroid, liver and kidney function tests

### Implementation

- Monitor for adverse anticholinergic responses and provide supportive care.

### Drug-specific teaching points

- Take this drug exactly as prescribed.
- Avoid skin contact with drug solutions.
- Avoid driving or engaging in other dangerous activities if CNS, vision changes occur.
- Avoid prolonged exposure to sun or use a sunscreen or covering garments.
- Maintain fluid intake and use precautions against heatstroke in hot weather.
- Report sore throat, fever, unusual bleeding or bruising, rash, weakness, tremors, impaired vision, dark-colored urine, pale stools, yellowing of the skin or eyes.

# Methenamine

## methenamine

*(meth **en'** a meen)*

## methenamine hippurate

Hiprex, Hip-Rex (CAN), Urex

## methenamine mandelate

Sterine (CAN)

**Pregnancy Category C**

### Drug classes

Urinary tract anti-infective
Antibacterial

### Therapeutic actions

Hydrolyzed in acid urine to ammonia and formaldehyde, which is bactericidal; the hippurate and mandelate salts help to maintain an acid urine.

### Indications

- Suppression or elimination of bacteriuria associated with pyelonephritis, cystitis, chronic urinary tract infections, residual urine (accompanying some neurologic disorders), and in anatomic abnormalities or the urinary tract

### Contraindications/cautions

- Contraindications: allergy to methenamine, tartrazine (in methenamine hippurate marketed as *Hiprex*), aspirin (associated with tartrazine allergy), pregnancy, lactation.
- Use cautiously with hepatic or renal dysfunction; gout (causes urate crystals to precipitate in urine).

### Dosage

**Available Forms:** Tablets—0.5, 1 g; suspension—0.5 g/5 ml

*ADULT*

**Methenamine:** 1 g qid PO.

**Methenamine hippurate:** 1 g bid PO.

**Methenamine mandelate:** 1 g qid PO after meals and at hs.

*PEDIATRIC*

**Methenamine**

- *6–12 Y:* 500 mg qid PO.
- *<6 Y:* 50 mg/kg/d PO divided into 3 doses.

**Methenamine hippurate**

- *6–12 Y:* 0.5–1 g bid PO.
- *>12 Y:* 1 g bid PO.

**Methenamine mandelate**

- *6–12 Y:* 0.5 gm qid PO.
- *<6 Y:* 0.25 g/14 kg qid PO.

### Pharmacokinetics

| *Route* | *Onset* | *Peak* |
|---|---|---|
| Oral | Rapid | 2–3 h |

*Metabolism:* Hepatic, $T_{1/2}$: 3–6 h
*Distribution:* Crosses placenta; enters breast milk
*Excretion:* Urine

### Adverse effects

- GI: *Nausea, abdominal cramps, vomiting, diarrhea,* anorexia, stomatitis
- GU: *Bladder irritation, dysuria,* proteinuria, hematuria, frequency, urgency, cystalluria
- **Dermatologic**: pruritus, urticaria, erythematous eruptions
- **Other**: Headache, dyspnea, generalized edema, elevated serum transaminase (with hippurate salt)

### Drug-lab test interferences

• False increase in 17-hydroxycorticosteroids, catecholamines • False decrease in 5-hydroxyindoleacetic acid • Inaccurate measurement of urine estriol levels by acid hydrolysis procedures during pregnancy

## ■ Nursing Considerations

### Assessment

- *History:* Allergy to methenamine, tartrazine, aspirin; renal or hepatic dysfunction; dehydration; gout; lactation
- *Physical:* Skin color, lesions; hydration; ear lobes—tophi; joints; liver evaluation; urinalysis, liver function tests; serum uric acid

### Implementation

- Arrange for culture and sensitivity tests before and during therapy.
- Administer drug with food or milk to prevent GI upset; give drug around the clock for best effects.
- Ensure avoidance of foods or medications that alkalinize the urine (see Appendix T).
- Ensure adequate hydration for patient.
- Monitor clinical response; if no improvement is seen or a relapse occurs, repeat urine culture and sensitivity tests.
- Monitor liver function tests with methenamine hippurate.

### Drug-specific teaching points

- Take drug with food. Complete the full course of therapy to resolve the infection. Take this drug at regular intervals around the clock; develop a schedule with the help of your nurse or pharmacist.
- Avoid alkalinizing foods: citrus fruits, milk products; or alkalinizing medications (sodium bicarbonate).
- Review other medications with your care provider.
- Drink plenty of fluids.
- The following side effects may occur: nausea, vomiting, abdominal pain

m

(small, frequent meals may help); diarrhea; painful urination, frequency, blood in urine (drink plenty of fluids).
- Report rash, painful urination, severe GI upset.

## methicillin sodium

*(meth i **sill'** in)*
Staphcillin
**Pregnancy Category B**

### Drug classes
Antibiotic
Penicillinase-resistant pencillin

### Therapeutic actions
Bactericidal: inhibits cell wall synthesis of sensitive organisms, causing cell death.

### Indications
- Infections due to penicillinase-producing staphylococci
- Initiation of treatment in any infection suspected to be staphylococcal

### Contraindications/cautions
- Contraindications: allergies to penicillins, cephalosporins, or other allergens.
- Use cautiously with renal disorders, pregnancy, lactation (may cause diarrhea or candidiasis in the infant).

### Dosage
**Available Forms:** Powder for injection—1, 4, 6, 10 g

Maximum recommended dosage: 4 g/d.

**ADULT:** 4–12 g/d IM or IV in divided doses q4–6h.

**PEDIATRIC:** 100–300 mg/kg per d IM or IV in divided doses q4–6h. Reduced dosage is necessary in newborn and premature babies. See manufacturer's instructions.

**GERIATRIC OR RENAL IMPAIRED:** If creatinine clearance $< 10$ ml/min, do not exceed 2 g q2h IM or IV.

### Pharmacokinetics

| Route | Onset | Peak | Duration |
|---|---|---|---|
| IM | Rapid | 30–60 min | 4 h |
| IV | Immediate | 15 min | 2 h |

*Metabolism:* Hepatic, $T_{1/2}$: 20–30 min
*Distribution:* Crosses placenta; enters breast milk
*Excretion:* Urine and feces

### IV facts
**Preparation:** Reconstitute in 50 ml of Sodium Chloride Injection. Dilute each ml of reconstituted solution with 20–25 ml Sodium Chloride Injection or Sterile Water for Injection. Further dilute reconstituted IV infusion solution with compatible IV solution: 0.9% Sodium Chloride Injection, 5% Dextrose in Water or in Normal Saline, 10% D-Fructose in Water or in Normal Saline, M/6 Sodium Lactate Solution, Lactated Ringer's Injection, Lactated Potassic Saline Injection, 5% Plasma Hydrolysate in Water, 10% Invert Sugar in Water or in Normal Saline, 10% Invert Sugar plus 0.3% Potassium Chloride in Water, Travert 10% Electrolyte 1, 2, or 3.

**Infusion:** Administer at rate of 10 ml/min.

**Incompatibilities:** Do not mix other agents with methicillin; give separately.

### Adverse effects
- CNS: Lethargy, hallucinations, seizures
- GI: *Glossitis, stomatitis, gastritis, sore mouth,* furry tongue, black "hairy" tongue, *nausea, vomiting, diarrhea,* abdominal pain, bloody diarrhea, enterocolitis, pseudomembranous colitis, nonspecific hepatitis
- **Hematologic**: Anemia, thrombocytopenia, leukopenia, neutropenia, prolonged bleeding time
- GU: Nephritis (more common than with other penicillins)
- **Hypersensitivity reactions**: *Rash, fever, wheezing,* anaphylaxis
- **Local**: Pain, phlebitis, thrombosis at injection site
- **Other**: *Superinfections*—oral and rectal moniliasis, vaginitis

### Clinically important drug-drug interactions
- Decreased effectiveness with tetracyclines
- Inactivation of parenteral aminoglyco-

sides: amikacin, gentamicin, kanamycin, neomycin, metilmicin, streptomycin, tobramycin

**Drug-lab test interferences**
• Monitor for false-positive Coombs' test with IV use.

## ■ Nursing Considerations

### Assessment
• *History:* Allergies to penicillins, cephalosporins, or other allergens; renal disorders; lactation.
• *Physical:* Culture infected area; skin color, lesion; R, adventitious sounds; bowel sounds; CBC, liver and renal function tests, serum electrolytes, Hct, urinalysis.

### Implementation
• Culture infection before treatment; reculture if response is not as expected.
• Administer by IV and IM routes only.
• Reconstitute powder with Sterile Water for Injection or Sodium Chloride Injection.
• Dilute for IM injection as follows: 1-g vial, 1.5 ml of diluent; 4-g vial, 5.7 ml of diluent; 6-g vial, 8.6 ml of diluent. Each ml of reconstituted solution contains 500 mg of methicillin.
• Date reconstituted solution; stable for 8 h except for 2 mg/ml solutions in 10% Invert Sugar in Normal Saline (4-h stability).
• Give IM by deep intragluteal injection to avoid irritation.
• Give IV slowly to avoid irritation to the vein.
• Arrange to continue treatment for 48–72 h after patient is asymptomatic.
• Do not give IM injections repeatedly in the same site; atrophy can occur. Monitor injection sites.

### Drug-specific teaching points
• This drug can only be given by injection.
• Upset stomach, nausea, diarrhea, mouth sores, pain or discomfort at injection sites may occur.
• Report difficulty breathing, rashes, severe diarrhea, severe pain at injection site, mouth sores.

# methimazole

*(meth **im'** a zole)*

Tapazole

**Pregnancy Category D**

**Drug classes**
Antithyroid agent

**Therapeutic actions**
Inhibits the synthesis of thyroid hormones.

**Indications**
• Hyperthyroidism

**Contraindications/cautions**
• Allergy to antithyroid products, pregnancy (use only if absolutely necessary and when mother has been informed about potential harm to the fetus; if an antithyroid agent is required, propylthiouracil is the drug of choice), lactation.

### Dosage
**Available Forms:** Tablets—5, 10 mg

Administer only PO, usually in three equal doses q8h.

ADULT: *Initial dose:* 15 mg/d PO up to 30–60 mg/d in severe cases. *Maintenance dose:* 5–15 mg/d PO.

PEDIATRIC: *Initial dose:* 0.4 mg/kg per day PO. *Maintenance:* approximately half the initial dose; actual dose is determined by the patient's response, or initial dose 0.5–0.7 mg/kg per day or 15–20 mg/m$^2$ per day PO in three divided doses. *Maximum dose:* 30 mg/24 h.

**Pharmacokinetics**

| *Route* | *Onset* | *Peak* | *Duration* |
|---|---|---|---|
| Oral | 30–40 min | 60 min | 2–4 h |

*Metabolism:* $T_{1/2}$: 6–13 h
*Distribution:* Crosses placenta; enters breast milk
*Excretion:* Urine

**Adverse effects**
• CNS: *Paresthesias, neuritis,* vertigo, drowsiness, neuropathies, depression, headache
• GI: *Nausea,* vomiting, epigastric distress, loss of taste, sialadenopathy, jaundice, hepatitis



m

- Hematologic: *Agranulocytosis, granulocytopenia, thrombocytopenia, hypoprothrombinemia, bleeding,* vasculitis, periarteritis
- GU: Nephritis
- Dermatologic: *Skin rash,* urticaria, pruritus, skin pigmentation, exfoliative dermatitis, lupuslike syndrome, loss of hair
- Other: Arthralgia, myalgia, edema, lymphadenopathy, drug fever

### Clinically important drug-drug interactions

• Increased theophylline clearance and decreased effectiveness if given to hyperthyroid patients; clearance will change as patient approaches euthyroid state • Altered effects of oral anticoagulants with methimazole • Increased therapeutic effects and toxicity of digitalis glycosides, metroprolol, propranolol when hyperthyroid patients become euthyroid

## ■ Nursing Considerations

### Assessment

- *History:* Allergy to antithyroid poroducts, pregnancy, lactation
- *Physical:* Skin color, lesions, pigmentation; orientation, reflexes, affect; liver evaluation; CBC, differential, prothrombin time, liver and renal function tests

### Implementation

- Give drug in 3 equally divided doses at 8-h intervals; try to schedule to allow patient to sleep at his or her regular time.
- Obtain regular, periodic blood tests to monitor bone marrow depression and bleeding tendencies.
- Advise medical/surgical personnel that patient is taking this drug, thereby increasing the risk of bleeding problems.

### Drug-specific teaching points

- Take this drug around the clock at 8-h intervals. Establish a schedule that fits your routine with the aid of your health care provider.
- This drug will need to be taken for a prolonged period to achieve the desired effects.
- The following side effects may occur: dizziness, weakness, vertigo, drowsiness (use caution driving or operating dangerous machinery); nausea, vomiting, loss of appetite (small, frequent meals may help); rash, itching.
- Report fever, sore throat, unusual bleeding or bruising, headache, general malaise.

# methocarbamol

*(meth oh **kar'** ba mole)*

Robaxin

**Pregnancy Category C**

### Drug classes

Skeletal muscle relaxant, centrally acting

### Therapeutic actions

Precise mechanism of action not known but may be due to general CNS depression; does not directly relax tense skeletal muscles or directly affect the motor end plate or motor nerves.

### Indications

- Relief of discomfort associated with acute, painful musculoskeletal conditions, as an adjunct to rest, physical therapy, and other measures
- May have a beneficial role in the control of neuromuscular manifestations of tetanus

### Contraindications/cautions

- Contraindications: hypersensitivity to methocarbamol; known or suspected renal pathology (parenteral methocarbamol is contraindicated because of presence of polyethylene glycol 300 in vehicle).
- Use cautiously with epilepsy, pregnancy, lactation.

### Dosage

**Available Forms:** Tablets—500, 750 mg; injection—100 mg/ml

**ADULT**

- *Parenteral:* IV and IM use only. Do not use SC. Do not exceed total dosage of 3

g/d for more than 3 consecutive d, except in the treatment of tetanus. Repeat treatment after a lapse of 48 h if condition persists. Injection need not be repeated, because tablets will sustain the relief.
- ***IV:*** Administer undiluted at a maximum rate of 3 ml/min.

• ***Tetanus:*** Give 1–2 g directly IV and add 1–2 g to IV infusion bottle so that initial dose is 3 g. Repeat q6h until conditions allow for insertion of nasogastric tube and administration of crushed tablets suspended in water or saline. Total daily oral doses up to 24 g may be required.
- ***IM:*** Do not give more than 5 ml at any gluteal injection site. Repeat q8h if needed.
- ***Oral:*** Initially, 1.5 g qid PO. For the first 48–72 h, 6 g/d or up to 8 g/d is recommended. Maintenance: 1 g qid or 750 mg q4h IV or 1.5 g bid–tid for total dosage of 4 g/d.

PEDIATRIC

• ***Tetanus:*** A minimum initial dose of 15 mg/kg IV by direct IV injection or IV infusion. Repeat q6h as needed.

### Pharmacokinetics

| *Route* | *Onset* | *Peak* |
|---|---|---|
| Oral | 30 min | 2 h |
| IM/IV | Rapid | Unknown |

*Metabolism:* Hepatic, $T_{1/2}$: 1–2 h
*Distribution:* Crosses placenta; may enter breast milk
*Excretion:* Urine and feces

### IV facts

**Preparation:** Administer undiluted. May be added to IV drip of Sodium Chloride Injection or 5% Dextrose Injection; do not dilute one vial given as a single dose to more than 250 ml for IV infusion.
**Infusion:** Inject directly 1 or 2 g into IV tubing at maximum rate of 3 ml/min; may add 1–2 g to infusion for a total of 3 g.

### Adverse effects

*Parenteral*

- CNS: *Syncope, dizziness, lightheadedness, vertigo, headache, mild muscular incoordination,* convulsions during IV administration, blurred vision
- GI: GI upset, metallic taste
- CV: *Hypotension*
- Dermatologic: *Urticaria,* pruritus, rash, flushing
- Local: Sloughing or pain at injection site
- Other: Nasal congestion

*Oral*

- CNS: *Lightheadedness, dizziness, drowsiness,* headache, fever, blurred vision
- GI: *Nausea*
- Dermatologic: *Urticaria,* pruritus, rash
- Other: Conjuctivitis with nasal congestion

### Drug-lab test interferences

• May cause interference with color reactions in tests for 5-HIAA and vanilylmandelic acid

## ■ Nursing Considerations

### Assessment

- ***History:*** Hypersensistivity to methocarbamol; known or suspected renal pathology, epilepsy (use caution with parenteral administration)
- ***Physical:*** T; skin color, lesions; nasal mucous membranes, conjunctival exam; orientation, affect, vision exam, reflexes; P, BP; bowel sounds, normal output; urinalysis, renal function tests

m

### Implementation

- Ensure patient is recumbent during IV injection and for at least 15 min thereafter.
- Administer IV slowly to minimize risk of CVS reactions, seizures.
- Monitor IV injection sites carefully to prevent extravasation; solution is hypertonic; can cause sloughing of tissue.
- Ensure that patients receiving methocarbamol for tetanus receive other appropriate care—debridement of wound, penicillin, tetanus antitoxin, tracheotomy, attention to fluid/electrolyte balance.
- Provide epinephrine, injectable steroids, or injectable antihistamines on standby in case syncope, hypotension occur with IV administration.
- Patient's urine may darken on standing.

### Drug-specific teaching points

- Take this drug exactly as prescribed. Do not take a higher dosage than prescribed, and do not take it longer than prescribed.
- Avoid alcohol, sleep-inducing, or OTC drugs; these could cause dangerous effects.
- Your urine may darken to a brown, black, or green color on standing.
- The following side effects may occur: drowsiness, dizziness, blurred vision (avoid driving or engaging in activities that require alertness); nausea (take with food, eat frequent, small meals).
- Report skin rash, itching, fever, or nasal congestion.

## methotrexate

*(meth oh **trex'** ate)*

amethopterin, MTX

Folex PFS, Rheumatrex, Rheumatrex Dose Pak (treatment of psoriasis or rheumatoid arthritis)

**Pregnancy Category X**

### Drug classes

Antimetabolite
Antineoplastic
Antirheumatic

### Therapeutic actions

Inhibits folic acid reductase, leading to inhibition of DNA synthesis and inhibition of cellular replication; selectively affects the most rapidly dividing cells (neoplastic and psoriatic cells).

### Indications

- Treatment of gestational choriocarcinoma, chorioadenoma destruens, hydatidiform mole
- Treatment and prophylaxis of meningeal leukemia
- Symptomatic control of severe, recalcitrant, disabling psoriasis
- Management of severe, active, classical, or definite rheumatoid arthritis
- Unlabeled uses: high-dose regimen followed by leucovorin rescue for adjuvant therapy of nonmetastatic osteosarcoma (orphan drug designation); to reduce corticosteriod requirements in patients with severe corticosteroid-dependent asthma
- Orphan drug use: treatment of juvenile rheumatoid arthritis

### Contraindications/cautions

- Contraindications: allergy to methotrexate, lactation, proriasis with renal or hepatic disorders, pregnancy or childbearing age.
- Use cautiously with hematopoietic depression; leukopenia, thrombocytopenia, anemia, severe hepatic or renal disease, infection, peptic ulcer, ulcerative colitis, debility.

### Dosage

**Available Forms:** Tablets—2.5 mg; powder for injection—20 mg/vial; injection—25 mg/ml; 2.5 mg/ml

ADULT

- ***Choriocarcinoma and other trophoblastic diseases:*** 15–30 mg PO or IM daily for a 5-d course. Repeat courses 3 to 5×, with rest periods of 1 wk or more between courses until toxic symptoms subside. Continue 1–2 courses of methotrexate after chorionic gonadotropin hormone levels are normal.
- ***Leukemia:*** Induction: 3.3 mg/m$^2$ of methorexate PO or IM with 60 mg/m$^2$ of prednisone daily for 4–6 wk. Maintenance: 30 mg/m$^2$ methotrexate PO or IM twice weekly or 2.5 mg/m$^2$ IV every 14 d. If relapse occurs, return to induction doses.
- ***Meningeal leukemia:*** Give methotrexate intrathecally in cases of lymphocytic leukemia as prophylaxis. 12 mg/m$^2$ intrathecally at intervals of 2–5 d and repeat until cell count of CSF is normal.
- ***Lymphomas:*** Burkitt's tumor, Stages I and II: 10–25 mg/d PO for 4–8 d. In stage III, combine with other neoplastic drugs. All usually require several courses of therapy with 7- to 10-d rest periods between doses.
- ***Mycosis fungoides:*** 2.5–10 mg/d PO for weeks or months or 50 mg IM once weekly or 25 mg IM twice weekly.

- *Osteosarcoma:* Starting dose is 12 g/m$^2$ or up to 15 g/m$^2$ PO, IM or IV to give a peak serum concentration of 1,000 $\mu$mol. Must be used as part of a cytotoxic regimen with leucovorin rescue.
- *Severe psoriasis:* 10–25 mg/wk PO, IM, or IV as a single weekly dose. Do not exceed 50 mg/wk or 2.5 mg PO at 12-h intervals for 3 doses or at 8-h intervals for 4 doses each wk. Do not exceed 30 mg/wk. Alternatively, 2.5 mg/d PO for 5 d followed by at least 2 d rest. Do not exceed 6.25 mg/d. After optimal clinical response is achieved, reduce dosage to lowest possible with longest rest periods and consider return to conventional, topical therapy.
- *Severe rheumatoid arthritis:* Starting dose: single doses of 7.5 mg/wk PO or divided dosage of 2.5 mg PO at 12-h intervals for 3 doses given as a course once weekly. Dosage may be gradually increased, based on response. Do not exceed 20 mg/wk. Therapeutic response usually begins within 3–6 wk, and improvement may continue for another 12 wk. Improvement may be maintained for up to 2 y with continued therapy.

### Pharmacokinetics

| *Route* | *Onset* | *Peak* |
|---|---|---|
| Oral | Varies | 1–4 h |
| IM/IV | Rapid | 1/2–2 h |

*Metabolism:* $T_{1/2}$: 2–4 h
*Distribution:* Crosses placenta; enters breast milk
*Excretion:* Urine

### IV facts

**Preparation:** Reconstitute 20- and 50-mg vials with an appropriate sterile preservative free medium, 5% Dextrose Solution or Sodium Chloride Injection to a concentration no greater than 25 mg/ml; reconstitute 1-g vial with 19.4 ml to a concentration of 50 mg/ml.

**Infusion:** Administer diluted drug by direct IV injection at a rate of not more than 10 mg/min.

### Adverse effects

- CNS: Headache, drowsiness, blurred vision, aphasia, hemiparesis, paresis, seizures, *fatigue, malaise, dizziness*
- GI: *Ulcerative stomatitis*, gingivitis, pharyngitis, anorexia, *nausea,* vomiting, diarrhea, hematemesis, melena, GI ulceration and bleeding, enteritis, **hepatic toxicity**
- Respiratory: Interstitial pneumonitis, chronic interstitial obstructive pulmonary disease
- Hematologic: *Bone marrow depression, increased susceptibility to infection*
- GU: Renal failure, *effects on fertility* (defective oogenesis, defective spermatogenesis, transient oligospermia, menstrual dysfunction, infertility, abortion, fetal defects)
- Dermatologic: *Erythematous rashes*, pruritus, urticaria, photosensitivity, depigmentation, *alopecia*, ecchymosis, telangiectasia, ance, furunculosi
- Hypersensitivity: **Anaphylaxis, sudden death**
- Other: *Chills and fever*, metabolic changes (diabetes, osteoporosis), cancer

### Clinically important drug-drug interactions

• Increased risk of toxicity with salicylates, phenytoin, probenecid, sulfonamides • Decreased serum levels and therapeutic effects of digoxin

## ■ Nursing Considerations

### Assessment

- *History:* Allergy to methotrexate, hematopoietic depression, severe hepatic or renal disease, infection, peptic ulcer, ulcerative colitis, debility, psorosis, pregnancy, lactation
- *Physical:* Weight; T; skin lesions, color; hair; vision, speech, orientation, reflexes, sensation; R, adventitious sounds; mucous membranes, liver evaluation, abdominal exam; CBC, differential; renal and liver function tests; urinalysis, blood and urine glucose, glucose tolerance test, chest x-ray



m

### Implementation

- Arrange for tests to evaluate CBC, urinalysis, renal and liver function tests, chest x-ray before therapy, during therapy, and for several weeks after therapy.
- Reduce dosage or discontinue if renal failure occurs.
- Reconstitute powder for intrathecal us with preservative free sterile Sodium Chloride Injection; intended for one dose only; discard remainder. The solution for injection contains benzyl alcohol and should *not* be given intrathecally.
- Arrange to have leucovorin readily available as antidote for methotrexate overdose or when large doses are used. In general, doses of leucovorin (calcium leucovorin) should equal or be higher than doses of methotrexate and should be given within the first hour. Up to 75 mg IV within 12 h, followed by 12 mg IM q6h for 4 doses. For average doses of methotrexate that cause adverse effects, give 6–12 mg leucovorin IM, q6h for 4 doses or 10 mg/m$^2$ PO followed by 10 mg/m$^2$ q6h for 72 h.
- Arrange for an antiemetic if nausea and vomiting are severe.
- Arrange for adequate hydration during therapy to reduce the risk of hyperuricemia.
- Do not administer any other medications containing alcohol.

### Drug-specific teaching points

- Prepare a calendar of treatment days.
- The following side effects may occur: nausea, vomiting (request medication; small, frequent meals may help); numbness, tingling, dizziness, drowsiness, blurred vision, difficulty speaking (drug effects; seek dosage adjustment; avoid driving or operating dangerous machinery): mouth sores (frequent mouth care is needed); infertility; loss of hair (obtain a wig or other suitable head covering; keep the head covered at extremes of temperature); skin rash, sensitivity to sun and ultraviolet light (avoid sun; use a sunscreen and protective clothing).
- This drug may cause birth defects or miscarriages. Use birth control while on this drug and for 8 wk thereafter.
- Avoid alcohol; serious side effects may occur.
- Arrange for frequent, regular medical follow-up, including blood tests to follow the drug's effects.
- Report black, tarry stools; fever; chills; sore throat; unusual bleeding or bruising; cough or shortness of breath; darkened or bloody urine; abdominal, flank, or joint pain; yellow color to the skin or eyes; mouth sores.

## methotrimeprazine hydrochloride

*(meth oh trye **mep'** ra zeen)*

Levoprome, Nozinan (CAN)

**Pregnancy Category C**

### Drug classes

Analgesic (non-narcotic)
Phenothiazine

### Therapeutic actions

CNS depressant; suppresses sensory impulses; reduces motor activity; produces sedation and tranquilization; raises pain threshold; produces amnesia. Also has antihistaminic, anticholinergic, antiadrenergic activity.

### Indications

- Relief of moderate to marked pain in nonambulatory patients
- Obstetric analgesia and sedation where respiratory depression is to be avoided
- Preanesthetic for producing sedation, somnolence, relief of apprehension and anxiety

### Contraindications/cautions

- Contraindications: hypersensitivity to phenothiazines, sulfites; coma; severe myocardial, hepatic or renal disease; hypotension.
- Use cautiously with heart disease, pregnancy prior to labor, lactation.

### Dosage

**Available Forms:** Injection—20 mg/ml

For IM use only. Do *not* give SC or IV. Do *not* administer for longer than 30 d, unless narcotic analgesics are contraindicated or patient has terminal illness.

ADULT

- *Analgesia:* 10–20 mg IM q4–6h as required (range, 5–40 mg q1–24h)
- *Obstetric analgesia:* During labor, an initial dose of 15–20 mg PO. May be repeated or adjusted as needed.
- *Preanesthetic medication:* 2–20 mg IM 45 min–3 h before surgery; 10 mg is often satisfactory. 15–20 mg IM may be given for more sedation. Atropine sulfate or scopolamine HBr may be used concurrently in lower than usual doses.
- *Postoperative analgesia:* 2.5–7.5 mg IM in the immediate postoperative period. Supplement q4–6h as needed.

PEDIATRIC < 12 Y: Not recommended.

GERIATRIC: Initial dose of 5–10 mg IM; gradually increase subsequent doses if needed and tolerated.

### Pharmacokinetics

| *Route* | *Onset* | *Peak* | *Duration* |
|---|---|---|---|
| IM | 20 min | 30–90 min | 4 h |

*Metabolism:* Hepatic, $T_{1/2}$: 15–30 h

*Distribution:* Crosses placenta; enters breast milk

*Excretion:* Urine

### Adverse effects

- CNS: *Weakness,* disorientation, dizziness, excessive sedation, slurring of speech
- GI: Abdominal discomfort, nausea, vomiting, *dry mouth,* jaundice
- CV: *Orthostatic hypotension, fainting, syncope*
- GU: Difficult urination, uterine inertia
- **Local**: Local inflammation, swelling, pain at injection site
- **Other**: Nasal congestion, agranulocytosis, chills

### Clinically important drug-drug interactions

• Additive anticholinergic effects and possibly decreased antipsychotic efficacy with anticholinergic drugs • Increased likelihood of seizures with metrizamide (contrast agent used in myelography)

### Drug-lab test interferences

• False-positive pregnancy tests (less likely if serum test is used) • Increase in PBI, not attributable to an increase in thyroxine

## ■ Nursing Considerations

### Assessment

- *History:* Hypersensitivity to phenothiazines, sulfites; coma; severe myocardial, hepatic, renal or heart disease; hypotension; lactation
- *Physical:* Weight, T; reflexes, orientation, intraocular pressure; P, BP, orthostatic BP; R, adventitious sounds; bowel sounds and normal output, liver evaluation; urinary output, prostate size; CBC, urinalysis, thyroid, liver and kidney function tests

### Implementation

- Do not mix drugs other than atropine or scopolamine in the same syringe with methotrimeprazine.
- Rotate IM injection sites.
- Keep patient supine for about 6–12 h after injection to prevent severe hypotension, syncope; tolerance to hypotensive effects usually occurs with repeated administration but may be lost if dosage is interrupted for several days.
- Provide methoxamine, phenylephrine on standby in case severe hypotension occurs. Do not give epinephrine; paradoxical hypotension may occur.

### Drug-specific teaching points

- The following side effects may occur: dizziness, sedation, drowsiness (remain supine for 12 h after the injection; request assistance if you need to sit or stand); nausea, vomiting (frequent, small meals may help).
- Report severe nausea, vomiting, urinary difficulty, yellowing of the skin or eyes, pain at injection site.

m

## methoxsalen

***(meth ox' a len)***

8-MOP

Oxsoralen (topical), Uvadex

**Pregnancy Category C**

### Drug classes
Psoralen

### Therapeutic actions
Strong photosensitizing effect on epidermal cells, combined with ultraviolet light (UVA) produces an inflammatory reaction that produces an increased synthesis of melanin, increased number of melanocytes.

### Indications
- Repigmentation of vitiliginous skin
- Symptomatic treatment of severe disabling psoriasis that is refractory to other forms of therapy
- Unlabeled use: with UVA for the treatment of mycosis fungoides
- Orphan drug use: with UVA photopheresis to treat diffuse systemic sclerosis; prevention of acute rejection of cardiac allografts

### Contraindications/cautions
- Contraindications: allergies to psoralens, sensitivity to sun, diseases associated with photosensitivity, squamous cell carcinoma, cataracts, pregnancy.
- Use cautiously with hepatic dysfunction, chronic infection, GI diseases, immunosuppression, CV disease, lactation.

### Dosage
**Available Forms:** Capsules—10 mg; lotion—1%

#### ADULT
- ***Oral:*** < 30 kg, 10 mg; 30–50 kg, 20 mg; 51–65 kg, 30 mg; 66–80 kg, 40 mg; 81–90 kg, 50 mg; 91–115 kg, 60 mg; > 115 kg, 70 mg. Give 90–120 min before exposure to UV light, 2 to 3 ×/wk.
- ***Topical:*** Apply lotion to skin 1–2 h before exposure to UV light.

### Pharmacokinetics

| *Route* | *Peak* | *Duration* |
|---|---|---|
| PO | 2 h | 8–10 h |
| Topical | Slow | 8–10 h |

*Metabolism:* Hepatic, $T_{1/2}$: 45–125 min
*Distribution:* Crosses placenta; may enter breast milk
*Excretion:* Urine

### Adverse effects
- CNS: Nervousness, depression, headache, dizziness, malaise
- GI: *Nausea*
- **Dermatologic**: *Burns,* hypopigmentation, vesicultion and bullae formation, rash, urticaria, skin carcinoma

## ■ Nursing Considerations

### Assessment
- ***History:*** Allergies to psoralens, sensitivity to sun, diseases associated with photosensitivity, squamous cell carcinoma, cataracts, use of drugs known to cause photosensitivity, pregnancy, hepatic dysfunction, chronic infection, GI diseases, immunosuppression, CV disease, lactation
- ***Physical:*** Culture infected area; skin color, lesion; orientation, reflexes

### Implementation
- Store in light-resistant containers.
- Administer oral drug with food or meals to reduce GI upset.
- Apply topical drug to small areas; protect borders of lesion with petrolatum and sunscreen to prevent hypopigmentation.
- Use finger cot or rubber glove to apply lotion.
- This drug is given in combination with ultraviolet light; should only be applied by experienced physician.
- Do not give topical methoxsalen for self-administration.

### Drug-specific teaching points
- This drug is given in conjunction with ultraviolet light treatments; timing of drug use is important.
- Take oral drug consistently with food or meals.
- Do not expose yourself to additional ultraviolet light (use sunscreen if outdoors).
- Upset stomach, skin rash, and burning may occur.

- Report new psoratic lesions, burning, dizziness.

# methscopolamine bromide

*(meth skoe **pol'** a meen)*
Pamine
**Pregnancy Category C**

## Drug classes
Anticholinergic
Antimuscarinic agent
Parasympatholytic
Antispasmodic

## Therapeutic actions
Competitively blocks the effects of acetylcholine at muscarinic cholinergic receptors that mediate the effects of parasympathetic postganglionic impulses, relaxing the GI tract and inhibiting gastric acid secretion.

## Indications
- Adjunctive therapy in the treatment of peptic ulcer

## Contraindications/cautions
- Contraindications: glaucoma; adhesions between iris and lens, stenosing peptic ulcer, pyloroduodenal obstruction, paralytic ileus, intestinal atony, severe ulcerative colitis, toxic megacolon, symptomatic prostatic hypertrophy, bladder neck obstruction, bronchial asthma, COPD, cardiac arrhythmias, myocardial ischemia; sensitivity to anticholinergic drugs; bromides, tartrazine (tartrazine sensitivity is more common with allergy to aspirin), impaired metabolic, liver or kidney function, myasthenia gravis.
- Use cautiously with Down's syndrome, brain damage, spasticity, hypertension, hyperthyroidism, pregnancy, lactation.

## Dosage
**Available Forms:** Tablets—2.5 mg
**ADULT:** 2.5 mg PO 30 min before meals and 2.5–5 mg at hs.
**PEDIATRIC:** Safety and efficacy not established.

## Pharmacokinetics

| *Route* | *Onset* | *Duration* |
|---|---|---|
| Oral | 1 h | 4–6 h |

*Metabolism:* Hepatic, $T_{1/2}$: 2–3 h
*Distribution:* Crosses placenta; may enter breast milk
*Excretion:* Urine and bile

## Adverse effects
- CNS: *Blurred vision*, mydriasis, cycloplegia, photophobia, increased intraocular pressure
- GI: *Dry mouth, altered taste perception, nausea, vomiting, dysphagia,* heartburn, constipation, bloated feeling, paralytic ileus, gastroesophageal reflux
- CV: Palpitations, tachycardia
- GU: *Urinary hesitancy and retention;* impotence
- Local: *Irritation at site of IM injection*
- Other: Decreased sweating and predisposition to heat prostration, suppression of lactation, nasal congestion

## Clinically important drug-drug interactions
- Decreased antipsychotic effectiveness of haloperidol with anticholinergic drugs

## ■ Nursing Considerations

### Assessment
- *History:* Glaucoma, adhesions between iris and lens, stenosing peptic ulcer, pyloroduodenal obstruction, paralytic ileus, intestinal atony, severe ulcerative colitis, toxic megacolon, symptomatic prostatic hypertrophy, bladder neck obstruction, bronchial asthma, COPD, cardiac arrhythmias, myocardial ischemia; sensitivity to anticholinergic drugs; bromides, tartrazine, impaired metabolic, liver or kidney function, myasthenia gravis, Down's syndrome, brain damage, spasticity, hypertension, hyperthyroidism, pregnancy, lactation
- *Physical:* Bowel sounds, normal output; urinary output, prostate palpation; R ad-

m

ventitious sounds; P, B; intraocular pressure, vision; bilateral grip strength, reflexes; liver palpation, liver and renal function tests; skin color, lesions, texture

### Implementation

- Ensure adequate hydration; provide environmental control (temperature) to prevent hyperpyrexia.
- Encourage patient to void before each dose of medication if urinary retention becomes a problem.

### Drug-specific teaching points

- Take drug exactly as prescribed.
- Avoid hot environments (you will be heat intolerant, and dangerous reactions may occur).
- The following side effects may occur: constipation (ensure adequate fluid intake, proper diet); dry mouth (sugarless lozenges, frequent mouth care may help; may lessen); blurred vision, sensitivity to light (avoid tasks that require acute vision; wear sunglasses when in bright light); impotence (reversible); difficulty in urination (empty bladder immediately before taking dose).
- Report skin rash, flushing, eye pain, difficulty breathing, tremors, loss of coordination, irregular heartbeat, palpitations, headache, abdominal distention, hallucinations, severe or persistent dry mouth, difficulty swallowing, difficulty in urination, severe constipation, sensitivity to light.

## methsuximide

*(meth **sux'** i mide)*

Celontin Kapseals

**Pregnancy Category C**

### Drug classes

Antiepileptic agent
Succinimide

### Therapeutic actions

Suppresses the paroxysmal three-cycle-per-second spike and wave EEG pattern associated with lapses of consciousness in absence (petit mal) seizures; reduces frequency of attacks; mechanism of action not understood.

### Indications

- Control of absence (petit mal) seizures when refractory to other drugs

### Contraindications/cautions

- Contraindications: hypersensitivity to succinimides.
- Use cautiously with hepatic, renal abnormalities; pregnancy (there is an association between antiepileptic drugs in epileptic women and elevated risk of birth defects in their children; therapy for major seizures should continue; the effect of seizures on fetus is unknown); lactation.

### Dosage

**Available Forms:** Capsules—500 mg

Determine optimal dosage by trial.

*ADULT:* Suggested schedule is 300 mg/d PO for the first week. If required, increase at weekly intervals by increments of 300 mg/d for 3 wk, up to a dosage of 1.2 g/d. Individualize therapy according to response. May be given with other antiepileptic drugs when other forms of epilepsy coexist with absence (petit mal) seizures.

*PEDIATRIC:* 150 mg half-strength capsules aid pediatric administration; determine dosage by trial.

### Pharmacokinetics

| Route | Onset | Peak |
|---|---|---|
| Oral | Rapid | 1–4 h |

*Metabolism:* Hepatic, $T_{1/2}$: 2.6–4 h

*Distribution:* Crosses placenta; may enter breast milk

*Excretion:* Urine

### Adverse effects

*Succinimides*

- CNS: *Drowsiness, ataxia, dizziness,* irritability, nervousness, headache, blurred vision, myopia, photophobia, hiccups, euphoria, dreamlike state, lethargy, hyperactivity, fatigue, insomnia, confusion, instability, mental slowness, depression, hypochondriacal behavior, sleep disturbances
- GI: *Nausea, vomiting, vague gastric upset, epigastric and abdominal pain,*

cramps, anorexia, diarrhea, contipation, weight loss, swelling of tongue, gum hypertrophy
- **Hematologic**: Eosinophilia, granulocytopenia, leukopenia, agranulocytosis, aplastic anemia, monocytosis, **pancytopenia**
- **Dermatologic**: Pruritus, urticaria, Stevens-Johnson syndrome, pruritic erythematous rashes, skin eruptions, erythema multiforme, systemic lupus erythematosus, alopecia, hirsutism
- **Other**: Periorbital edema, hyperemia, muscle weakness, abnormal liver and kidney function tests, vaginal bleeding

### Clinically important drug-drug interactions
- Decreased serum levels and therapeutic effects of primidone

## ■ Nursing Considerations

### Assessment
- *History:* Hypersensitivity to succinimides; hepatic, renal abnormalities; pregnancy; lactation
- *Physical:* Skin color, lesions; orientation, affect, reflexes, bilateral grip strength, vision exam; bowel sounds, normal output, liver evaluation; liver and kidney function tests, urinalysis, CBC with differential, EEG

### Implementation
- Reduce dosage, discontinue, or substitute other antiepileptic medication gradually; abrupt discontinuation may precipitate absence (petit mal) seizures.
- Monitor CBC and differential before therapy and frequently during therapy.
- Discontinue drug if skin rash, depression of blood count, or unusual depression, aggressiveness, or behavioral alterations occur.

### Drug-specific teaching points
- Take this drug exactly as prescribed; do not discontinue abruptly or change dosage, except on the advice of your physician.
- Avoid alcohol, sleep-inducing, or OTC drugs. These could cause dangerous effects. If you need one of these preparations, consult your health care provider.
- Have frequent check-ups to monitor drug response.
- The following side effects may occur: drowsiness, dizziness, confusion, blurred vision (avoid driving a car or performing other tasks requiring alertness or visual acuity); GI upset (take with food or milk, eat frequent, small meals).
- Wear a medical ID tag to alert emergency medical personnel that you are an epileptic taking antiepileptic medication.
- Report skin rash, joint pain, unexplained fever, sore throat, unusual bleeding or bruising, drowsiness, dizziness, blurred vision, pregnancy.

# methyclothiazide

*(meth i kloe **thye'** a zide)*

Aquatensen, Duretic (CAN), Enduron

**Pregnancy Category C**

### Drug classes
Thiazide diuretic

### Therapeutic actions
Inhibits reabsorption of sodium and chloride in distal renal tubule, thereby increasing excretion of sodium, chloride, and water by the kidney.

### Indications
- Adjunctive therapy in edema associated with CHF, cirrhosis, corticosteroid and estrogen therapy, renal dysfunction
- Hypertension, as sole therapy or in combination with other antihypertensives
- Unlabeled use: diabetes insipidus, especially nephrogenic diabetes insipidus

### Contraindications/cautions
- Contraindications: hypersensitivity to thiazides, pregnancy.
- Use cautiously with fluid or electrolyte imbalances, renal or liver disease, gout, SLE, glucose tolerance abnormalities, hyperparathyroidism, manic-depressive disorders, lactation.

### Dosage

**Available Forms:** Tablets—2.5, 5 mg

*ADULT*

- *Edema:* 2.5–10 mg qd PO. Maximum single dose is 10 mg.
- *Hypertension:* 2.5–5 mg qd PO. If BP is not controlled by 5 mg qd within 8–12 wk, another antihypertensive may be needed.

### Pharmacokinetics

| *Route* | *Onset* | *Peak* | *Duration* |
|---|---|---|---|
| Oral | 2 h | 6 h | 24 h |

*Metabolism:* $T_{1/2}$: unknown

*Distribution:* Crosses placenta; enters breast milk

*Excretion:* Urine

### Adverse effects

- CNS: *Dizziness, vertigo,* paresthesias, weakness, headache, drowsiness, fatigue, leukopenia, thrombocytopenia, agranulocytosis, aplastic anemia, neutropenia
- GI: *Nausea, anorexia, vomiting, dry mouth,* diarrhea, constipation, jaundice, hepatitis
- CV: Orthostatic hypotension, venous thrombosis, volume depletion, cardiac arrhythmias, chest pain
- GU: *polyuria, nocturia,* impotence, loss of libido
- Dermatologic: Photosensitivity, rash, purpura, exfoliative dermatitis, hives
- Other: Muscle cramp

### Clinically important drug-drug interactions

• Risk of hyperglycemia with diazoxide • Decreased absorption with cholestyramine, colestipol • Increased risk of digitalis glycoside toxicity if hypokalemia occurs • Increased risk of lithium toxicity when taken with thiazides • Increased fasting blood glucose leading to need to adjust dosage of antidiabetic agents

### Drug-lab test interferences

• Decreased PBI levels without clinical signs of thyroid disturbances

## ■ Nursing Considerations

### Assessment

- *History:* Fluid or electrolyte imbalances, renal or liver disease, gout, SLE, glucose tolerance abnormalities, hyperparathyroidism, manic-depressive disorders, pregnancy, lactation
- *Physical:* Skin color and lesions; orientation, reflexes, muscle strength; pulses, BP, orthostatic BP, perfusion, edema, baseline ECG; R, adventitious sounds; liver evaluation, bowel sounds; CBC, serum electrolytes, blood glucose, liver and renal function tests, serum uric acid, urinalysis

### Implementation

- Give with food or milk if GI upset occurs.
- Administer early in the day so increased urination will not disturb sleep.
- Measure and record regular body weights to monitor fluid changes.

### Drug-specific teaching points

- Take drug early in day so sleep will not be disturbed by increased urination.
- Weigh yourself daily, and record weight on a calendar.
- Protect skin from exposure to sun or bright lights (sensitivity may occur).
- Increased urination will occur.
- Use caution if dizziness, drowsiness, feeling faint occur.
- Report rapid weight change, swelling in ankles or fingers, unusual bleeding or bruising, muscle cramps.

# Methyldopa

## methyldopate hydrochloride

*(meth ill* ***doe'*** *pa)*

Aldomet, Dopamet (CAN), Medimet (CAN), Novomedopa (CAN)

**Pregnancy Category C**

### Drug classes

Antihypertensive

Sympatholytic, centrally acting

### Therapeutic actions

Mechanism of action not conclusively demonstrated; probably due to drug's metabolism to alpha-methyl norepinephrine, which lowers arterial blood pressure by stimulating central (CNS) $alpha_2$-adrenergic receptors, which in turn decreases sympathetic outflow from the CNS.

### Indications

- Hypertension
- Acute hypertensive crises (IV methyldopate); not drug of choice because of slow onset of action

### Contraindications/cautions

- Contraindications: hypersensitivity to methyldopa, active hepatic disease, previous methyldopa therapy associated with liver disorders.
- Use cautiously with previous liver disease, renal failure, dialysis, bilateral cerebrovascular disease, pregnancy, lactation.

### Dosage

**Available Forms:** Tablets—125, 250, 500 mg; oral suspension—50 mg; injection—50 mg/ml

ADULT

- ***Oral therapy (methyldopa):*** Initial therapy: 250 mg bid–tid in the first 48 h. Adjust dosage at minimum intervals of at least 2 d until response is adequate. Increase dosage in the evening to minimize sedation. Maintenance: 500 mg–3 g/d in 2 to 4 doses. Usually given in 2 doses; some patients may be controlled with a single hs dose.
- ***Concomitant therapy:*** With antihypertensives other than thiazides, limit initial dosage to 500 mg/d in divided doses. When added to a thiazide, dosage of thiazide need not be changed.
- ***IV therapy (methyldopate):*** 250–500 mg q6h as required (maximum 1 g q6h). Switch to oral therapy as soon as control is attained, use the dosage schedule used for parenteral therapy.

PEDIATRIC

- ***Oral therapy (methyldopa):*** Individualize dosage; initial dosage is based on 10 mg/kg per day in 2 to 4 doses. Maximum dosage is 65 mg/kg per day or 3 g/d, whichever is less.
- ***IV therapy (methyldopate):*** 20–40 mg/kg per day in divided doses q6h. Maximum dosage is 65 mg/kg or 3 g/d, whichever is less.

GERIATRIC OR IMPAIRED RENAL FUNCTION: Reduce dosage. Drug is largely excreted by the kidneys.

### Pharmacokinetics

| *Route* | *Onset* | *Peak* | *Duration* |
|---|---|---|---|
| Oral | Varies | 2–4 h | 24–48 h |
| IV | 4–6 h | Unknown | 10–16 h |

*Metabolism:* Hepatic, $T_{1/2}$: 1.7 h
*Distribution:* Crosses placenta; enters breast milk
*Excretion:* Urine

### IV facts

**Preparation:** Add the dose to 100 ml of 5% Dextrose, or give in 5% Dextrose in Water in a concentration of 10 mg/ml.
**Infusion:** Administer over 30–60 min.

m

### Adverse effects

- CNS: *Sedation, headache, asthenia, weakness* (usually early and transient), dizziness, lightheadedness, symptoms of cerebrovascular insufficiency, paresthesias, parkinsonism, Bell's palsy, decreased mental acuity, involuntary choreoathetotic movements, psychic disturbances
- GI: *Nausea, vomiting, distention, constipation*, flatus, diarrhea, colitis, dry mouth, sore or "black" tongue, pancreatitis, sialadenitis, abnormal liver function tests, jaundice, hepatitis, **fatal hepatic necrosis**
- CV: *Bradycardia*, prolonged carotid sinus hypersensitivity, aggravation of angina pectoris, paradoxical pressor response, pericarditis, **myocarditis** (fatal), orthostatic hypotension, edema
- Hematologic: Positive Coombs' test, hemolytic anemia, bone marrow depression, leukopenia, granulocytopenia, thrombocytopenia, positive tests for anti-

nuclear antibody, LE cells, and rheumatoid factor
- **Dermatologic**: Rash as in eczema or lichenoid eruption, toxic epidermal necrolysis fever, lupuslike syndrome
- **Endocrine**: Breast enlargement, gynecomastia, lactation, hyperprolactinemia, amenorrhea, galactorrhea, impotence, failure to ejaculate, decreased libido
- **Other**: Nasal stuffiness, mild arthralgia, myalgia, septic shocklike syndrome

### Clinically important drug-drug interactions

• Potentiation of the pressor effects of sympathomimetic amines • Increased hypotension with levodopa • Risk of hypotension during surgery with central anesthetics; monitor patient carefully

### Drug-lab test interferences

• Methyldopa may interfere with tests for urinary uric acid, serum creatinine, SGOT, urinary catecholamines

## ■ Nursing Considerations

### Assessment

- *History:* Hypersensitivity to methyldopa; hepatic disease; previous methyldopa therapy associated with liver disorders; renal failure; dialysis; bilateral cerebrovascular disease; lactation
- *Physical:* Weight; body temperature; skin color, lesions; mucous membranes color, lesions; orientation, affect, reflexes; P, BP, orthostatic BP, perfusion, edema, auscultation; bowel sounds, normal output, liver evaluation; breast exam; liver and kidney function tests, urinalysis, CBC and differential, direct Coombs' test

### Implementation

- Administer IV slowly; monitor injection site.
- Monitor hepatic function, especially in the first 6–12 wk of therapy or if unexplained fever appears. Discontinue drug if fever, abnormalities in liver function tests, or jaundice occur. Ensure that methyldopa is not reinstituted in such patients.
- Monitor blood counts periodically to detect hemolytic anemia; a direct Coombs' test before therapy and 6 and 12 mo later may be helpful. Discontinue drug if Coombs' positive hemolytic anemia occurs. If hemolytic anemia is related to methyldopa, ensure that drug is not reinstituted.
- Discontinue therapy if involuntary choreoathetotic movements occur.
- Discontinue if edema progresses or signs of CHF occur.
- Add a thiazide to drug regimen or increase dosage if methyldopa tolerance occurs (second and third mo of therapy).
- Monitor BP carefully when discontinuing methyldopa; drug has short duration of action, and hypertension usually returns within 48 h.

### Drug-specific teaching points

- Take this drug exactly as prescribed; it is important that you not miss doses.
- The following side effects may occur: drowsiness, dizziness, lightheadedness, headache, weakness (often transient; avoid driving or engaging in tasks that require alertness); GI upset (frequent, small meals may help); dreams, nightmares, memory impairment (reversible); dizziness, lightheadedness when you get up (get up slowly; use caution when climbing stairs); urine that darkens on standing (expected effect); impotence, failure of ejaculation, decreased libido; breast enlargement, sore breasts.
- Report unexplained, prolonged general tiredness; yellowing of the skin or eyes; fever; bruising; skin rash.

## methylene blue

***(meth' i leen)***
Urolene Blue
**Pregnancy Category C**

### Drug classes

Urinary tract anti-infective
Antidote

### Therapeutic actions

Oxidation-reduction agent that converts the ferrous iron of reduced Hgb to the ferric form, producing methemoglobin; weak germicide in lower doses; tissue staining.

### Indications

- Treatment of cyanide poisoning and drug-induced methemoglobinemia
- GU antiseptic for cystitis and urethritis
- Unlabeled uses: delineation of body structures and fistulas through dye effect; diagnosis/confirmation of rupture of amniotic membranes

### Contraindications/cautions

- Contraindications: allergy to methylene blue, renal insufficiency, intraspinal injections.
- Use cautiously with G6PD deficiency; anemias; CV deficiencies.

### Dosage

**Available Forms:** Tablets—65 mg; injection—10 mg/ml

ADULT

- ***Oral:*** 65–130 mg tid with a full glass of water.
- ***IV:*** 1–2 mg/kg (0.1–0.2 ml/kg) injected over several minutes.

### Pharmacokinetics

| *Route* | *Onset* | *Peak* |
|---|---|---|
| Oral | Varies | Unknown |
| IV | Immediate | End of infusion |

*Metabolism:* Tissue, $T_{1/2}$: unknown
*Excretion:* Urine, bile, and feces

### IV facts

**Preparation:** No preparation required.
**Infusion:** Inject directly IV or into tubing of actively running IV; inject slowly over several minutes.

### Adverse effects

- CNS: Dizziness, headache, mental confusion, sweating
- GI: *Nausea*, vomiting, diarrhea, abdominal pain, *blue-green stool*
- CV: Precordial pain
- GU: *Discolored urine* (blue-green); bladder irritation
- Other: Necrotic abscess (SC injection); fetal anemia and distress (amniotic injection); neural damage, paralysis (intrathecal injection); *skin stained blue*

## ■ Nursing Considerations

### Assessment

- ***History:*** Allergy to methylene blue, renal insufficiency, presence of G6PD deficiency; anemias; CV deficiencies
- ***Physical:*** Skin color, lesions; urinary output, bladder palpation; abdominal exam, normal output; CBC with differential

### Implementation

- Give oral drug after meals with a full glass of water.
- Give IV slowly over several minutes; avoid exceeding recommended dosage.
- Use care to avoid SC injection; monitor intrathecal sites used for diagnostic injection for necrosis and damage.
- Contact with skin will dye the skin blue; stain may be removed by hypochlorite solution.
- Monitor CBC for signs of marked anemia.

### Drug-specific teaching points

- Take drug after meals with a full glass of water.
- Avoid bubble baths, excessive ingestion of citrus juice, and sexual contacts if bladder infection or urethritis is being treated.
- The following side effects may occur: urine or stool discolored blue-green; abdominal pain, nausea, vomiting (small frequent meals may help).
- Report difficulty breathing, severe nausea or vomiting, fatigue.



## methylergonovine maleate

*(meth ill er goe **noe'** veen)*
Methergine
**Pregnancy Category C**

### Drug classes

Oxytocic

### Therapeutic actions

A partial agonist or antagonist at alpha receptors; as a result, it increases the strength, duration, and frequency of uterine contractions.

### Indications

- Routine management after delivery of the placenta
- Treatment of postpartum atony and hemorrhage; subinvolution of the uterus
- Uterine stimulation during the second stage of labor following the delivery of the anterior shoulder, under strict medical supervision

### Contraindications/cautions

- Contraindications: allergy to methylergonovine, hypertension, toxemia, lactation.
- Use cautiously with sepsis, obliterative vascular disease, hepatic or renal impairment, pregnancy.

### Dosage

**Available Forms:** Tablets—0.2 mg; injection—0.2 mg/ml

ADULT

- ***IM:*** 0.2 mg after delivery of the placenta, after delivery of the anterior shoulder, during puerperium. May be repeated q2–4 h.
- ***IV:*** Same dosage as IM; infuse slowly over at least 60 sec. Monitor BP very carefully as severe hypertensive reaction can occur.
- ***Oral:*** 0.2 mg tid or qid daily in the puerperium for up to 1 wk.

### Pharmacokinetics

| *Route* | *Onset* | *Peak* | *Duration* |
|---|---|---|---|
| Oral | 5–10 min | 30–60 min | 3 h |
| IM | 2–5 min | 30 min | 3 h |
| IV | Immediate | 2–3 min | 1–3 h |

*Metabolism:* Hepatic, $T_{1/2}$: 30 min

*Distribution:* Crosses placenta; enters breast milk

*Excretion:* Urine

### IV facts

**Preparation:** No additional preparation required.

**Infusion:** Inject directly IV or into tubing of running IV; inject very slowly, over no less than 60 sec; rapid infusion can result in sudden hypertension or cerebral events.

### Adverse effects

- CNS: *Dizziness, headache*, tinnitus, diaphoresis
- GI: *Nausea*, vomiting
- CV: *Transient hypertension*, palpitations, chest pain, dyspnea

## ■ Nursing Considerations

### Assessment

- ***History:*** Allergy to methylergonovine, hypertension, toxemia, sepsis, obliterative vascular disease, hepatic or renal impairment, lactation
- ***Physical:*** Uterine tone, vaginal bleeding; orientation, reflexes, affect; P, BP, edema; CBC, renal and liver function tests

### Implementation

- Administer by IM injection or orally unless emergency requires IV use. Complications are more frequent with IV use.
- Monitor postpartum women for BP changes and amount and character of vaginal bleeding.
- Discontinue if signs of toxicity occur.
- Avoid prolonged use of the drug.

### Drug-specific teaching points

The patient receiving a parenteral oxytocic is usually receiving it as part of an immediate medical situation, and the drug teaching should be incorporated into the teaching about delivery. The patient needs to know the name of the drug and what she can expect once it is administered.

- This drug should not be needed for longer than 1 wk.
- The following side effects may occur: nausea, vomiting, dizziness, headache, ringing in the ears (short time use may make it tolerable).
- Report difficulty breathing, headache, numb or cold extremities, severe abdominal cramping.

# methylphenidate hydrochloride

*(meth ill **fen'i** date)*

Ritalin, Ritalin SR

**Pregnancy Category C**
**C-II controlled substance**

## Drug classes
Central nervous system stimulant

## Therapeutic actions
Mild cortical stimulant with CNS actions similar to those of the amphetamines; efficacy in hyperkinetic syndrome, attention-deficit disorders in children appears paradoxical and is not understood.

## Indications
- Narcolepsy
- Attention-deficit disorders, hyperkinetic syndrome, minimal brain dysfunction in children or adults with a behavioral syndrome characterized by the following symptoms: moderate to severe distractibility, short attention span, hyperactivity, emotional lability and impulsivity, not secondary to environmental factors or psychiatric disorders
- Unlabeled use: treatment of depression in the elderly, cancer and stroke patients; anesthesia-related hiccups

## Contraindications/cautions
- Contraindicated in the presence of hypersensitivity to methylphenidate; marked anxiety, tension, and agitation; glaucoma; motor tics, family history or diagnosis of Gilles de la Tourette's syndrome; severe depression of endogenous or exogenous origin; normal fatigue states.
- Use caution in the presence of seizure disorders; hypertension; drug dependence, alcoholism; emotional instability; lactation.

## Dosage
**Available Forms:** Tablets—5, 10, 20 mg; SR tablets—20 mg

*ADULT:* Individualize dosage. Give orally in divided doses bid–tid, preferably 30–45 min before meals; dosage ranges from 10–60 mg/d PO. If insomnia is a problem, drug should be taken before 6 PM. Timed-release tablets have a duration of 8 h and may be used when timing and dosage are titrated to the 8-h regimen.

*PEDIATRIC:* Start with small oral doses (5 mg PO before breakfast and lunch with gradual increments of 5–10 mg weekly). Daily dosage > 60 mg not recommended. Discontinue use after 1 mo if no improvement. Discontinue periodically to assess condition; usually discontinued after puberty.

## Pharmacokinetics

| *Route* | *Onset* | *Peak* | *Duration* |
|---|---|---|---|
| Oral | Varies | 1–3 h | 4–6 h |

*Metabolism:* Hepatic, $T_{1/2}$: 1–3 h
*Distribution:* Crosses placenta; enters breast milk
*Excretion:* Urine

## Adverse effects
- CNS: *Nervousness, insomnia,* dizziness, headache, dyskinesia, chorea, drowsiness, Gilles de la Tourette's syndrome, toxic psychosis, blurred vision, accommodation difficulties
- GI: *Anorexia, nausea, abdominal pain,* weight loss
- CV: *Increased or decreased pulse and BP; tachycardia,* angina, cardiac arrhythmias, palpitations
- Hematologic: Leukopenia, anemia
- Dermatologic: Skin rash, urticaria, fever, arthralgia, exfoliative dermatitis, erythema multiforme with necrotizing vasculitis and thrombocytopenic purpura, loss of scalp hair
- Other: Tolerance, psychological dependence, abnormal behavior with abuse

## Clinically important drug-drug interactions
• Decreased effects of guanethidine; avoid this combination • Increased effects and toxicity of methylphenidate with MAOIs • Increased serum leels of phenytoin, TCAs with methyphenidate; monitor for toxicity

### Drug-lab test interferences

• Methylphenidate may increase the urinary excretion of epinephrine

## ■ Nursing Considerations

### Assessment

- *History:* Hypersensitivity to methylphenidate; marked anxiety, tension and agitation; glaucoma; motor tics, Gilles de la Tourette's syndrome; severe depression; normal fatigue state; seizure disorders; hypertension; drug dependence, alcoholism, emotional instability
- *Physical:* Weight; T; skin color, lesions; orientation, affect, ophthalmic exam (tonometry); P, BP, auscultation; R, adventitious sounds; bowel sounds, normal output; CBC with differential, platelet count, baseline ECG

### Implementation

- Ensure proper diagnosis before administering to children for behavioral syndromes; drug should not be used until other causes/concomitants of abnormal behavior (learning disability, EEG abnormalities, neurologic deficits) are ruled out.
- Interrupt drug dosage periodically in children to determine if symptoms warrant continued drug therapy.
- Monitor growth of children on long-term methylphenidate therapy.
- Ensure that timed-release tablets are swallowed whole, not chewed or crushed.
- Dispense the least feasible dose to minimize risk of overdosage.
- Give before 6 PM to prevent insomnia.
- Monitor CBC, platelet counts periodically in patients on long-term therapy.
- Monitor BP frequently early in treatment.

### Drug-specific teaching points

- Take this drug exactly as prescribed. Timed-release tablets must be swallowed whole, not chewed or crushed.
- Take drug before 6 PM to avoid nighttime sleep disturbance.
- Avoid alcohol and OTC drugs, including nose drops, cold remedies; some OTC drugs could cause dangerous effects.
- The following side effects may occur: nervousness, restlessness, dizziness, insomnia, impaired thinking (may lessen; avoid driving or engaging in activities that require alertness); headache, loss of appetite, dry mouth.
- Report nervousness, insomnia, palpitations, vomiting, skin rash, fever.

# Methylprednisolones

## methylprednisolone

*(meth ill pred **niss'** oh lone)*

*Oral:* Medrol

## methylprednisolone acetate

*IM, intra-articular, soft-tissue injection, retention enema, topical dermatologic ointment:* Dep Medalone, Depoject, Depo-Medrol, Depo-pred, Duralone, Medralone, M-Prednisol

## methylprednisolone sodium succinate

*IV, IM injection:* Solu-Medrol

**Pregnancy Category C**

### Drug classes

Corticosteroid
Glucocorticoid
Hormone

### Therapeutic actions

Enters target cells and binds to intracellular corticosteroid receptors, initiating many complex reactions that are responsible for its anti-inflammatory and immunosuppressive effects.

### Indications

*Systemic Administration*

- Hypercalcemia associated with cancer
- Short-term management of various inflammatory and allergic disorders, such as rheumatoid arthritis, collagen diseases (SLE), dermatologic diseases (pemphigus), status asthmaticus, and autoimmune disorders
- Hematologic disorders: thrombocytopenia purpura, erythroblastopenia

- Ulcerative colitis, acute exacerbations of mutiple sclerosis and palliation in some leukemias and lymphomas
- Trichinosis with neurologic or myocardial involvement
- Unlabeled use: septic shock

*Intra-articular or Soft-Tissue Administration*

- Arthritis, psoriatic plaques

## Contraindications/cautions

- Contraindications: infections, especially tuberculosis, fungal infections, amebiasis, vaccinia and varicella, and antibiotic-resistant infections; lactation; allergy to tartrazine or aspirin in products labeled *Medrol*.
- Use cautiously with kidney or liver disease, hypothyroidism, ulcerative colitis with impending perforation, diverticulitis, active or latent peptic ulcer, inflammatory bowel disease, CHF, hypertension, thromboembolic disorders, osteoporosis, convulsive disorders, diabetes mellitus.

## Dosage

**Available Forms:** Tablets—2, 4, 8, 16, 24, 32 mg; powder for injection—40, 125, 500 mg/ml, 1, 2 g/vial; injection—20, 40, 80 mg

**ADULT**

- *Systemic administration:* Individualize dosage, depending on severity and response. Give daily dose before 9 AM to minimize adrenal suppression. For maintenance, reduce initial dose in small increments at intervals until the lowest satisfactory clinical dose is reached. If long-term therapy is needed, consider alternate-day therapy with a short-acting corticosteroid. After long-term therapy, withdraw drug slowly to prevent adrenal insufficiency.

– ***Oral (methylprednisolone, oral):*** 4–48 mg/d. Alternate-day therapy: twice the usual dose every other morning.

– ***IM (methylprednisolone acetate):*** As temporary substitute for oral therapy, give total daily dose as a single IM injection.

- *Adrenogenital syndrome:* 40 mg every 2 wk PO or IM.
- *Rheumatoid arthritis:* 40–120 mg once a week PO or IM.
- *Dermatologic lesions:* 40–120 mg weekly for 1–4 wk PO or IM; in severe dermatitis, 80–120 mg as a single dose.
- *Seborrheic dermatitis:* 80 mg once a week PO or IM.
- *Asthma, allergic rhinitis:* 80–120 mg PO or IM.

– ***IV, IM (methylprednisolone sodium succinate):*** 10–40 mg IV administered over 1 to several min. Give subsequent doses IV or IM. *Caution:* Rapid IV administration of large doses (more than 0.5–1.0 g in less than 10–120 min) has caused serious cardiac complications.

**PEDIATRIC:** Individualize dosage on the basis of severity and response rather than by formulae that correct doses for age or weight. Carefully observe growth and development in infants and children on prolonged therapy. Not less than 0.5 mg/kg per 24 h. High-dose therapy: 30 mg/kg IV infused over 10–20 min; may repeat q4–6h, but not beyond 48–72 h.

**ADULT/PEDIATRIC**

- ***Intra-articular, intralesional (methylprednisolone acetate):*** 4–80 mg intra-articular, soft tissue; 20–60 mg intralesional (depending on joint or soft-tissue injection site).

## Pharmacokinetics

| *Route* | *Onset* | *Peak* | *Duration* |
|---|---|---|---|
| Oral | Varies | 1–2 h | 1.2–1.5 d |
| IV | Rapid | Rapid | Unknown |
| IM | Rapid | 4–8 d | 1–5 wk |

*Metabolism:* Hepatic, $T_{1/2}$: 78–188 min
*Distribution:* Crosses placenta; enters breast milk
*Excretion:* Urine

## IV facts

**Preparation:** No additional preparation in required.
**Infusion:** Inject directly into vein or into tubing of running IV; administer slowly, over 1–20 min to reduce cardiac effects.

m

### Adverse effects

Effects depend on dose, route and duration of therapy. The following effects occur more often with systemically administered steroid than those locally administered

- CNS: *Vertigo, headache*, paresthesias, insomnia, convulsions, psychosis, cataracts, increased intraocular pressure, glaucoma
- GI: Peptic or esophageal ulcer, pancreatitis, abdominal distention, nausea, vomiting, *increased appetite, weight gain*
- CV: Hypotension, shock, hypertension and CHF secondary to fluid retention, thromboembolism, thrombophlebitis, fat embolism, cardiac arrhythmias
- **MS**: Muscle weakness, steroid myopathy, loss of muscle mass, osteoporosis, spontaneous fractures
- **Endocrine**: Amenorrhea, irregular menses, growth retardation, decreased carbohydrate tolerance, diabetes mellitus, cushingoid state (long-term effect), increased blood sugar, increased serum cholesterol, decreased $T_3$ and $T_4$ levels, hypothalamic-pituitary-adrenal (HPA) suppression with systemic therapy longer than 5 d
- **Electrolyte imbalance**: *$Na^+$ and fluid retention*, hypokalemia, hypocalcemia
- **Hypersensitivity or anaphylactoid reactions:**
- Other: *Immunosuppression, aggravation, or masking of infections; impaired wound healing*; thin, fragile skin; petechiae, ecchymoses, purpura, striae; subcutaneous fat atrophy
- **The following effects are related to various local routes of steroid administration:**
- **Intra-articular**: Osteonecrosis, tendon rupture, infection
- **Intralesional therapy:**: Blindness—face and head

Systemic absorption can lead to HPA suppression, growth retardation in children, and other systemic adverse effects. Children may be at special risk of systemic absorption because of their larger skin surface area to body weight ratio.

### Clinically important drug-drug interactions

• Increased therapeutic and toxic effects with erythromycin, ketoconazole, troleandomycin • Risk of severe deterioration of muscle strength when given to myasthenia gravis patients who are receiving ambenonium, edrophonium, neostigmine, pyridostigmine • Decreased steroid blood levels with barbiturates, phenytoin, rifampin • Decreased effectiveness of salicylates

### Drug-lab test interferences

• False-negative nitroblue-tetrazolium test for bacterial infection • Suppression of skin test reactions

## ■ Nursing Considerations

### Assessment

- ***History:*** Infections; kidney or liver disease, hypothyroidism, ulcerative colitis, diverticulitis, active or latent peptic ulcer, inflammatory bowel disease, CHF, hypertension, thromboembolic disorders, osteoporosis, convulsive disorders, diabetes mellitus; pregnancy; lactation
- ***Physical:*** Weight, T, reflexes and grip strength, affect and orientation, P, BP, peripheral perfusion, peripheral perfusion, prominence of superficial veins, R and adventitious sounds, serum electrolytes, blood glucose

### Implementation

***Systemic (Oral and Parenteral) Administration***

- Use caution with the 24-mg tablets marketed as Medrol; these contain tartrazine, which may cause allergic reactions, especially in people who are allergic to aspirin.
- Give daily dose before 9 AM to mimic normal peak corticosteroid blood levels.
- Increase dosage when patient is subject to stress.
- Taper doses when discontinuing high-dose or long-term therapy.

- Do not give live virus vaccines with immunosuppressive doses of corticosteroids.

### Drug-specific teaching points

*Systemic (Oral and Parenteral) Administration*

- Do not to stop taking the drug (oral) without consulting your health-care provider.
- Avoid exposure to infections.
- Report unusual weight gain, swelling of the extremities, muscle weakness, black or tarry stools, fever, prolonged sore throat, colds or other infections, worsening of disorder.

*Intra-articular Therapy*

- Do not overuse the joint after therapy, even if the pain is gone.

## methysergide maleate

*(meth i ser' jide)*

Sansert

**Pregnancy Category X**

### Drug classes

Antimigraine agent
Semisynthetic ergot derivative

### Therapeutic actions

Mechanism of action unknown; inhibits the effects of serotonin; serotonin may be involved in vascular headaches and may be a "headache substance," lowering pain threshold during headaches; methysergide also inhibits histamine release from mast cells and stabilizes platelets against serotonin release.

### Indications

- Prevention or reduction in intensity and frequency of vascular headaches in specific patients: patients suffering from one or more severe vascular headaches per week, from vascular headaches that are so severe that preventive measures are necessary
- Prophylaxis of vascular headache; not for management of acute attacks

### Contraindications/cautions

- Allergy to ergot preparations, tartrazine (more likely in patients with aspirin sensitivity) in 2-mg tablets marketed as Sansert; peripheral vascular disease, severe arteriosclerosis, severe hypertension, coronary artery disease, phlebitis or cellulitis of the lower limbs, pulmonary disease, collagen disease, fibrotic processes, impaired liver or renal function, valvular heart disease, debilitated states, serious infection, pregnancy, lactation.

### Dosage

**Available Forms:** Tablets—2 mg

*ADULT:* 4–8 mg/d PO, taken with meals. There must be a 3- to 4-wk drug free interval after every 6-mo course of treatment. If efficacy has not been demonstrated after a 3-wk trial period, benefit is unlikely to occur.

*PEDIATRIC:* Not recommended for children.

### Pharmacokinetics

| *Route* | *Onset* | *Peak* |
|---|---|---|
| Oral | Varies | 1–2 d |

*Metabolism:* Hepatic, $T_{1/2}$: 10 h

*Distribution:* Crosses placenta; enters breast milk

*Excretion:* Urine

### Adverse effects

- CNS: *Insomnia, drowsiness, mild euphoria, dizziness,* ataxia, weakness, lightheadedness, hyperesthesia, hallucinatory experiences
- GI: *Nausea, vomiting, diarrhea, heartburn,* abdominal pain
- CV: *Vascular insufficiency of lower limbs, intense vasoconstriction* (chest pain; abdominal pain; cold, numb, painful extremities), postural hypotension
- **Hematologic**: Neutropenia, eosinophilia
- **Dermatologic**: *Facial flushing,* telangiectasia, rashes, hair loss, peripheral edema, dependent edema
- **Other**: Arthralgia, myalgia, weight gain; retroperitoneal fibrosis, pleuropulmonary fibrosis and fibrotic thickening of cardiac valves with long-term therapy

**Clinically important drug-drug interactions**
- Increased risk of peripheral ischemia with beta-blockers

## ■ Nursing Considerations

### Assessment
- *History:* Allergy to ergot preparations, tartrazine; peripheral vascular disease, severe arteriosclerosis, severe hypertension, coronary artery disease, phlebitis or cellulitis of the lower limbs, pulmonary disease, collagen disease, fibrotic processes, impaired liver or renal function, valvular heart disease, debilitated states, serious infection; pregnancy; lactation
- *Physical:* Skin color, edema, lesions; weight; T; orientation, gait, reflexes, affect; P, BP, peripheral perfusion, auscultation; R, adventitious sounds; liver evaluation, bowel sounds; CBC, liver and renal function tests

### Implementation
- Do not give continuously for longer than 6 mo; ensure a drug free interval for 3–4 wk after each 6-mo course.
- Reduce dosage gradually during the last 2–3 wk of treatment to avoid "headache rebound."
- Give with food to prevent GI upset.

### Drug-specific teaching points
- Take drug with meals to prevent GI upset. Drug is meant to prevent migraines, not as treatment of acute attacks. Drug is given in treatment courses of 6 mo; a 3- to 4-wk drug-free interval is necessary between treatment courses.
- The following side effects may occur: weight gain (monitor caloric intake); drowsiness, dizziness, weakness, lightheadedness (use caution if driving or operating dangerous machinery); diarrhea; nausea, vomiting, heartburn (may lessen).
- This drug should not be taken during pregnancy. If you become pregnant or desire to become pregnant, consult with your physician. Contraception is recommended while using this drug.
- Report cold, numb, painful extremities, leg cramps when walking, girdle, flank or chest pain, painful urination, shortness of breath.

# ☆ metoclopramide

*(met oh kloe **pra'** mide)*

Maxeran (CAN), Maxolon, Octamide PFS, Reglan

**Pregnancy Category B**

**Drug classes**

GI stimulant
Antiemetic
Dopaminergic blocking agent

**Therapeutic actions**

Stimulates motility of upper GI tract without stimulating gastric, biliary, or pancreatic secretions; appears to sensitize tissues to action of acetylcholine; relaxes pyloric sphincter, which, when combined with effects on motility, accelerates gastric emptying and intestinal transit; little effect on gallbladder or colon motility; increases lower esophageal sphincter pressure; has sedative properties; induces release of prolactin.

**Indications**
- Relief of symptoms of acute and recurrent diabetic gastroparesis
- Short-term therapy (4–12 wk) for adults with symptomatic gastroesophageal reflux who fail to respond to conventional therapy
- Prevention of nausea and vomiting associated with emetogenic cancer chemotherapy (parenteral)
- Prophylaxis of postoperative nausea and vomiting when nasogastric suction is undesirable
- Facilitation of small bowel intubation when tube does not pass the pylorus with conventional maneuvers (single-dose parenteral use)
- Stimulation of gastric emptying and intestinal transit of barium when delayed emptying interferes with radiologic exam of the stomach or small intestine (single dose parenteral use)
- Unlabeled uses: improvement of lactation (doses of 30–45 mg/d); treatment of

nausea and vomiting of a variety of etiologies: emesis during pregnancy and labor, gastric ulcer, anorexia nervosa

### Contraindications/cautions

- Contraindications: allergy to metoclopramide; GI hemorrhage, mechanical obstruction or perforation; pheochromocytoma (may cause hypertensive crisis); epilepsy.
- Use cautiously with previously detected breast cancer (one-third of such tumors are prolactin-dependent); lactation.

### Dosage

**Available Forms:** Tablets—5, 10 mg; syrup—5 mg/5 ml; injection—5 mg/ml

ADULT

- ***Relief of symptoms of gastroparesis:*** 10 mg PO 30 min before each meal and hs for 2–8 wk. If symptoms are severe, initiate therapy with IM or IV administration for up to 10 d until symptoms subside.
- ***Symptomatic gastroesophageal reflux:*** 10–15 mg PO up to 4× a day 30 min before meals and hs. If symptoms occur only at certain times or in relation to specific stimuli, single doses of 20 mg may be preferable; guide therapy by endoscopic results. Do not use longer than 12 wk.
- ***Prevention of postoperative nausea and vomiting:*** 10–20 mg IM at the end of surgery.
- ***Prevention of chemotherapy-induced emesis:*** Dilute and give by IV infusion over not less than 15 min. Give first dose 1/2 h before chemotherapy; repeat q2h for 2 doses, then q3h for 3 doses. The initial 2 doses should be 2 mg/kg for highly emetogenic drugs (cisplatin, dacarbazine); 1 mg/kg may suffice for other chemotherapeutic agents.
- ***Facilitation of small bowel intubation, gastric emptying:*** 10 mg (2 ml) by direct IV injection over 1–2 min.

PEDIATRIC

- ***Facilitation of intubation, gastric emptying:*** *6–14 y:* 2.5–5 mg by direct IV injection over 1–2 min. *< 6 y:* 0.1 mg/kg by direct IV injection over 1–2 min.

### Pharmacokinetics

| Route | Onset | Peak | Duration |
|---|---|---|---|
| Oral | 30–60 min | 60–90 min | 1–2 h |
| IM | 10–15 min | 60–90 min | 1–2 h |
| IV | 1–3 min | 60–90 min | 1–2 h |

*Metabolism:* Hepatic, $T_{1/2}$: 5–6 h

*Distribution:* Crosses placenta; enters breast milk

*Excretion:* Urine

### IV facts

**Preparation:** Dilute dose in 50 ml of a parenteral solution (Dextrose 5% in Water, Sodium Chloride Injection, Dextrose 5% in 0.45% Sodium Chloride, Ringer's Injection, or Lactated Ringer's Injection). May be stored for up to 48 h if protected from light or up to 24 h under normal light.

**Infusion:** Give direct IV doses slowly (over 1–2 min); give infusions over at least 15 min.

**Incompatabilities:** Do not mix with solutions containing cephalothin, chloramphenicol, sodium bicarbonate.

### Adverse effects

- CNS: *Restlessness, drowsiness, fatigue, lassitude*, insomnia, *extrapyramidal reactions, parkinsonism-like reactions*, akathisia, dystonia, myoclonus, dizziness, anxiety
- GI: *Nausea, diarrhea*
- CV: Transient hypertension

### Clinically important drug-drug interactions

• Decreased absorption of digoxin from the stomach • Increased toxic and immunosuppressive effects of cyclosporine

## ■ Nursing Considerations

### Assessment

- *History:* Allergy to metoclopramide, GI hemorrhage, mechanical obstruction or perforation, pheochromocytoma, epilepsy, lactation, previously detected breast cancer

m

- *Physical:* Orientation, reflexes, affect; P, BP; bowel sounds, normal output; EEG

### Implementation

- Monitor BP carefully during IV administration.
- Monitor for extrapyramidal reactions, and consult physician if they occur.
- Monitor diabetic patients, arrange for alteration in insulin dose or timing if diabetic control is compromised by alterations in timing of food absorption.
- Provide diphenhydramine injection on standby in case extrapyramidal reactions occur (50 mg IM).
- Provide phentolamine on standby in case of hypertensive crisis (most likely to occur with undiagnosed pheochromocytoma).

### Drug-specific teaching points

- Take this drug exactly as prescribed.
- Do not use alcohol, sleep remedies, sedatives; serious sedation could occur.
- The following side effects may occur: drowsiness, dizziness (do not drive or perform other tasks that require alertness); restlessness, anxiety, depression, headache, insomnia (reversible); nausea, diarrhea.
- Report involuntary movement of the face, eyes, or limbs, severe depression, severe diarrhea.

## metolazone

*(me **tole'** a zone)*

Mykrox, Zaroxolyn

**Pregnancy Category B**

### Drug classes

Thiazide-like diuretic

### Therapeutic actions

Inhibits reabsorption of sodium and chloride in distal renal tubule, increasing excretion of sodium, chloride, and water by the kidney.

### Indications

- Adjunctive therapy in edema associated with CHF, cirrhosis, corticosteroid and estrogen therapy, renal dysfunction
- Hypertension, as sole therapy or in combination with other antihypertensives
- Unlabeled uses: calcium nephrolithiasis alone or with amiloride or allopurinol to prevent recurrences in hypercalciuric or normal calciuric patients; diabetes insipidus, especially nephrogenic diabetes insipidus

### Contraindications/cautions

- Contraindications: hypersensitivity to thiazides, hepatic coma, fluid or electrolyte imbalances, renal or liver disease.
- Use cautiously with gout, SLE, glucose tolerance abnormalities, hyperparathyroidism, manic-depressive disorders, lactation.

### Dosage

**Available Forms:** Zaroxolyn—2.5, 5, 10 mg; Mykrox—0.5 mg

ADULT

- *Zaroxolyn*
- ***Hypertension:*** 2.5–5 mg qd PO.
- ***Edema of renal disease:*** 5–20 mg qd PO.
- ***Edema of CHF:*** 5–10 mg qd PO.
- ***Calcium nephrolithiasis:*** 2.5–10 mg/d PO.
- *Mykrox*
- ***Mild to moderate hypertension:*** 0.5 mg qd PO taken as a single dose early in the morning. May be increased to 1 mg qd; do not exceed 1 mg/d. If switching from Zaroxolyn to Mykrox, determine the dose by titration starting at 0.5 mg qd and increasing to 1 mg qd.

PEDIATRIC: Not recommended.

### Pharmacokinetics

| Brand | Onset | Peak | Duration |
|---|---|---|---|
| Mykrox | 20–30 min | 2–4 h | 12–24 h |
| Zaroxolyn | 1 h | 2 h | 12–24 h |

*Metabolism:* Hepatic, $T_{1/2}$: 14 h (Mykrox), unknown (Zaroxolyn)

*Distribution:* Crosses placenta; enters breast milk

*Excretion:* Urine

**Adverse effects**

- CNS: *Dizziness, vertigo,* paresthesias, weakness, *headache*, drowsiness, *fatigue*
- GI: *Nausea, anorexia, vomiting, dry mouth, diarrhea, constipation*, jaundice, hepatitis, pancreatitis
- CV: Orthostatic hypotension, venous thrombosis, volume depletion, cardiac arrhythmias, chest pain
- Hematologic: Leukopenia, thrombocytopenia, agranulocytosis, aplastic anemia, neutropenia, fluid and electrolyte imbalances
- GU: *Polyuria, nocturia, impotence*, loss of libido
- Dermatologic: Photosensitivity, rash, purpura, exfoliative dermatitis
- Other: Muscle cramps and muscle spasms, fever, hives, gouty attacks, flushing

**Clinically important drug-drug interactions**

• Increased thiazide effects and chance of acute hyperglycemia with diazoxide • Decreased absorption with cholestyramine, colestipol • Increased risk of cardiac glycoside toxicity if hypokalemia occurs • Increased risk of lithium toxicity • Increased dosage of antidiabetic agents may be needed • Increased risk of hyperglycemia if taken concurrently with diazoxide

**Drug-lab test interferences**

• Decreased PBI levels without clinical signs of thyroid disturbances

## ■ Nursing Considerations

### Assessment

- *History:* Fluid or electrolyte imbalances, renal or liver disease, gout, SLE, glucose tolerance abnormalities, hyperparathyroidism, manic-depressive disorders, hepatic coma or precoma, lactation
- *Physical:* Skin color and lesions; orientation, reflexes, muscle strength; pulses, BP, orthostatic BP, perfusion, edema, baseline ECG; R, adventitious sounds; liver evaluation, bowel sounds; CBC, serum electrolytes, blood glucose, liver and renal function tests, serum uric acid, urinalysis

### Implementation

- Withdraw drug 2–3 d before elective surgery; if emergency surgery is indicated, reduce dosage of preanesthetic or anesthetic agents.
- Administer with food or milk if GI upset occurs.
- Measure and record body weights to monitor fluid changes.

### Drug-specific teaching points

- Take drug early in the day so sleep will not be disturbed by increased urination.
- Weigh yourself daily, and record weights.
- Protect skin from exposure to the sun or bright lights.
- The following side effects may occur: increased urination; dizziness, drowsiness, feeling faint (use caution; avoid driving or operating dangerous machinery); headache.
- Report rapid weight change, swelling in ankles or fingers, unusual bleeding or bruising, muscle cramps.



## metoprolol tartrate

*(me toe' proe lole)*

Betaloc (CAN), Lopresor (CAN), Lopressor, Toprol XL

**Pregnancy Category B**

**Drug classes**

Beta-1 selective adrenergic blocker
Antihypertensive

**Therapeutic actions**

Competitively blocks beta-adrenergic receptors in the heart and juxtaglomerular apparatus, decreasing the influence of the sympathetic nervous system on these tissues and the excitability of the heart, decreasing cardiac output and the release of renin, and lowering BP; acts in the CNS to reduce sympathetic outflow and vasoconstrictor tone.

**Indications**

- Hypertension, alone or with other drugs, especially diuretics

- Prevention of reinfarction in MI patients who are hemodynamically stable or within 3–10 d of the acute MI
- Treatment of angina pectoris

## Contraindications/cautions

- Contraindications: sinus bradycardia (HR < 45 beats/min), second or third-degree heart block (PR interval > 0.24 sec), cardiogenic shock, CHF, systolic BP < 100 mm Hg; lactation.
- Use cautiously with diabetes or thyrotoxicosis; asthma or COPD; pregnancy.

## Dosage

**Available Forms:** Tablets—50, 100 mg; ER tablets—50, 100, 200 mg; injection—1 mg/ml

**ADULT**

- *Hypertension:* Initially 100 mg/d PO in single or divided doses; gradually increase dosage at weekly intervals. Usual maintenance dose is 100–450 mg/d.
- ***Angina pectoris:*** Initially 100 mg/d PO in 2 divided doses; may be increased gradually, effective range 100–400 mg/d.
- ***MI, early treatment:*** Three IV bolus doses of 5 mg each at 2-min intervals with careful monitoring. If these are tolerated, give 50 mg PO 15 min after the last IV dose and q6h for 48 h. Thereafter, give a maintenance dosage of 100 mg PO bid. Reduce initial PO doses to 25 mg, or discontinue in patients who do not tolerate the IV doses.
- ***MI, late treatment:*** 100 mg PO bid as soon as possible after infarct, continuing for at least 3 mo and possibly for 1–3 y.
- *Hypertension:*
  - ***Extended-release tablets:*** 50–100 mg/d PO as one dose.
- ***Angina:*** 100 mg/d PO as a single dose.

**PEDIATRIC:** Safety and efficacy not established.

## Pharmacokinetics

| *Route* | *Onset* | *Peak* | *Duration* |
|---|---|---|---|
| Oral | 15 min | 90 min | 15–19 h |
| IV | Immediate | 60–90 min | 15–19 h |

*Metabolism:* Hepatic, $T_{1/2}$: 3–4 h
*Distribution:* Crosses placenta; enters breast milk
*Excretion:* Urine

### IV facts

**Preparation:** No additional preparation is required.
**Infusion:** Inject directly into vein or into tubing of running IV over 1 min. Inject as a bolus; monitor carefully; wait 2 min between doses; do not give if bradycardia of <45 beats/min, heart block, systolic pressure <100 mm Hg.

## Adverse effects

- CNS: Dizziness, vertigo, tinnitus, fatigue, emotional depression, paresthesias, sleep disturbances, hallucinations, disorientation, memory loss, slurred speech
- GI: *Gastric pain, flatulence, constipation, diarrhea, nausea, vomiting,* anorexia, ischemic colitis, renal and mesenteric arterial thrombosis, retroperitoneal fibrosis, hepatomegaly, acute pancreatitis
- CV: *CHF, cardiac arrhythmias,* peripheral vascular insufficiency, claudication, CVA, pulmonary edema, hypotension
- **Respiratory**: Bronchospasm, dyspnea, cough, bronchial obstruction, nasal stuffiness, rhinitis, pharyngitis
- GU: *Impotence, decreased libido*, Peyronie's disease, dysuria, nocturia, frequent urination
- **MS**: Joint pain, arthralgia, muscle cramp
- **EENT**: Eye irritation, dry eyes, conjunctivitis, blurred vision
- **Dermatologic**: Rash, pruritus, sweating, dry skin
- **Allergic**: Pharyngitis, erythematous rash, fever, sore throat, laryngospasm
- **Other**: *Decreased exercise tolerance, development of antinuclear antibodies (ANA)*, hyperglycemia or hypoglycemia, elevated serum transaminase, alkaline phosphatase

## Clinically important drug-drug interactions

- Increased effects of metoprolol with verapamil, cimetidine, methimazole, propylthiouracil • Increased effects of both drugs if metoprolol is taken with hydralazine • Increased serum levels and toxicity of IV lidocaine, if given concurrently • Increased risk of postural hypotension with prazosin • Decreased antihypertensive effects if taken with NSAIDs, clonidine, rifampin. Decreased therapeutic effects with barbiturates • Hypertension followed by severe bradycardia if given concurrently with epinephrine

**Drug-lab test interferences**

• Possible false results with glucose or insulin tolerance tests (oral)

## ■ Nursing Considerations

### Assessment

- *History:* Sinus bradycardia (HR < 45 beats/min), second or third-degree heart block (PR interval > 0.24 sec), cardiogenic shock, CHF, systolic BP < 100 mg Hg; diabetes or thyrotoxicosis; asthma or COPD; lactation
- *Physical:* Weight, skin condition, neurologic status, P, BP, ECG, respiratory status, kidney and thyroid function, blood and urine glucose

### Implementation

- Do not discontinue drug abruptly after chronic therapy (hypersensitivity to catecholamines may have developed, causing exacerbation of angina, MI, and ventricular dysrhythmias). Taper drug gradually over 2 wk with monitoring.
- Consult physician about withdrawing drug if patient is to undergo surgery (controversial).
- Give oral drug with food to facilitate absorption.
- Provide continual cardiac monitoring for patients receiving IV metoprolol.

### Drug-specific teaching points

- Do not stop taking this drug unless instructed to do so by a health care provider.
- The following side effects may occur: dizziness, drowsiness, lightheadedness, blurred vision (avoid driving or dangerous activities); nausea, loss of appetite (small, frequent meals may help); nightmares, depression (discuss change of medication); sexual impotence.
- Report difficulty breathing, night cough, swelling of extremities, slow pulse, confusion, depression, rash, fever, sore throat

# metronidazole

*(me troe **ni'** da zole)*

Apo-Metronidazole (CAN), Flagyl, MetroGel, Metro I.V., Neo-Tric (CAN), Noritate, Novonidazol (CAN), PMS-Metronidazole (CAN), Protostat, Trikacide (CAN)

**Pregnancy Category B**

**Drug classes**

Antibiotic
Antibacterial
Amebicide
Antiprotozoal

**Therapeutic actions**

Bactericidal: inhibits DNA synthesis in specific (obligate) anaerobes, causing cell death; antiprotozoal-trichomonacidal, amebicidal: biochemical mechanism of action is not known.

**Indications**

- Acute infection with susceptible anaerobic bacteria
- Acute intestinal amebiasis
- Amebic liver abscess
- Trichomoniasis (acute and partners of patients with acute infection)
- Preoperative, intraoperative, postoperative prophylaxis for patients undergoing colorectal surgery
- Topical application in the treatment of inflammatory papules, pustules, and erythema of rosacea
- Unlabeled uses: prophylaxis for patients undergoing gynecologic, abdominal surgery; hepatic encephalopathy; Crohn's disease; antibiotic-associated pseudomembranous colitis; treatment of *Gardnerella vaginalis*, giardiasis (use recommended by the CDC)

**Contraindications/cautions**

- Contraindications: hypersensitivity to metronidazole; pregnancy (do not use for trichomoniasis in first trimester).

m

- Use cautiously with CNS diseases, hepatic disease, candidiasis (moniliasis), blood dyscrasias, lactation.

## Dosage

**Available Forms:** Tablets—250, 500 mg; powder for injection—500 mg; injection—500 mg/100 ml

### Adult

- ***Anaerobic bacterial infection:*** 15 mg/kg IV infused over 1 h; then 7.5 mg/kg infused over 1 h q6h for 7–10 d, not to exceed 4 g/d.
- ***Amebiasis:*** 750 mg/tid PO for 5–10 d. (In amebic dysentary, combine with iodoquinol 650 mg PO tid for 20 d).
- ***Trichomoniasis:*** 2 g PO in one day (1-d treatment) *or* 250 mg tid PO for 7 d.
- ***Prophylaxis:*** 15 mg/kg infused IV over 30–60 min and completed about 1 h before surgery. Then 7.5 mg/kg infused over 30–60 min at 6- to 12-h intervals after initial dose during the day of surgery only.
- ***Gardnerella vaginalis***: 500 mg bid PO for 7 d.
- ***Giardiasis:*** 250 mg tid PO for 7 d.
- ***Antibiotic-associated pseudomembranous colitis:*** 1–2 g/d PO for 7–10 d.
- ***Treatment of inflammatory papules, pustules, and erythema of rosacea (MetroGel):*** Apply and rub in a thin film twice daily, morning and evening, to entire affected areas after washing; results should be seen within 3 wk; treatment through 9 wk has been effective.

### Pediatric

- ***Anaerobic bacterial infection:*** Not recommended.
- ***Amebiasis:*** 35–50 mg/kg per day PO in three doses for 10 d.

## Pharmacokinetics

| Route | Onset | Peak |
|---|---|---|
| Oral | Varies | 1–2 h |
| IV | Rapid | 1–2 h |
| Topical | Not generally absorbed systemically | |

*Metabolism:* Hepatic, $T_{1/2}$: 6–8 h
*Distribution:* Crosses placenta; enters breast milk
*Excretion:* Urine and feces

## IV facts

**Preparation:** Reconstitute by adding 4.4 ml of Sterile Water for Injection, Bacteriostatic Water for Injection, 0.9% Sodium Chloride Injection, Bacteriostatic 0.9% Sodium Chloride Injection to the vial and mix thoroughly. Resultant volume is 5 ml with a concentration of 100 mg/ml. Solution should be clear to pale yellow to yellow-green; do not use if cloudy or if containing precipitates; use within 24 h; protect from light. Add reconstituted solution to glass or plastic container containing 0.9% Sodium Chloride Injection, 5% Dextrose Injection or Lactated Ringer's; discontinue other solutions while running metronidazole.

**Infusion:** Prior to administration, add 5 mEq Sodium Bicarbonate Injection for each 500 mg used, mix thoroughly. Do not refrigerate neutralized solution. Do not administer solution that has not been neutralized. Infuse over 1 h.

## Adverse effects

- CNS: *Headache, dizziness, ataxia,* vertigo, incoordination, insomnia, seizures, peripheral neuropathy, fatigue
- GI: *Unpleasant metallic taste, anorexia, nausea, vomiting, diarrhea*, GI upset, cramps
- GU: Dysuria, incontinence, *darkening of the urine*
- **Local**: Thrombophlebitis (IV); *redness, burning, dryness, and skin irritation* (topical)
- **Other**: Severe disulfiramlike interaction with alcohol, candidiasis (superinfection)

## Clinically important drug-drug interactions

- Decreased effectiveness with barbiturates
- Disulfiram-like reaction (flushing, tachycardia, nausea, vomiting) with alcohol
- Psychosis if taken with disulfiram

• Increased bleeding tendencies with oral anticoagulants

**Drug-lab test interferences**

• Falsely low (or zero) values in SGOT (AST), SGPT (ALT), LDH, triglycerides, hexokinase glucose tests

## ■ Nursing Considerations

### Assessment

- *History:* CNS or hepatic disease; candidiasis (moniliasis); blood dyscrasias; pregnancy; lactation
- *Physical:* Reflexes, affect; skin lesions, color (with topical application); abdominal exam, liver palpation; urinalysis, CBC, liver function tests

### Implementation

- Avoid use unless necessary. Metronidazole is carcinogenic in some rodents.
- Administer oral doses with food.
- Apply topically (MetroGel) after cleansing the area. Advise patient that cosmetics may be used over the area after application.
- Reduce dosage in hepatic disease.

### Drug-specific teaching points

- Take full course of drug therapy; take the drug with food if GI upset occurs.
- The following side effects may occur: dry mouth with strange metallic taste (frequent mouth care, sucking sugarless candies may help); nausea, vomiting, diarrhea (small, frequent meals may help).
- Do not drink alcohol (beverages or preparations containing alcohol, cough syrups); severe reactions may occur.
- Be aware that your urine may appear dark; this is expected.
- Refrain from sexual intercourse unless partner wears a condom during treatment for trichomoniasis.
- Report severe GI upset, dizziness, unusual fatigue or weakness, fever, chills.

*Topical Application*

- Apply the topical preparation by cleansing the area and then rubbing a thin film into the affected area. Avoid contact with the eyes. Cosmetics may be applied to the area after application.

# metyrosine

*(me tye' roe seen)*

Demser

**Pregnancy Category C**

**Drug classes**

Enzyme inhibitor

**Therapeutic actions**

Blocks the enzyme tyrosine hydroxylase; inhibits the conversion of tyrosine to DOPA, which is the first step in the synthesis of catecholamines. In patients with pheochromocytoma, this reduces catecholamine synthesis, substantially reducing hypertensive attacks and associated symptoms.

**Indications**

- Preoperative preparation for surgery for pheochromocytoma
- Management of pheochromocytoma when surgery is contraindicated
- Chronic treatment for malignant pheochromocytoma

**Contraindications/cautions**

- Contraindication: hypersensitivity to metyrosine.
- Use cautiously with pregnancy, lactation.

### Dosage

**Available Forms:** Capsules—250 mg

**ADULTS AND CHILDREN > 12 Y:** Initial dose of 250 mg PO qid; may be increased by 250–500 mg qd to a maximum of 4 g/d.

• *Preoperative:* 2–3 g/d PO for 5–7 d.

**PEDIATRIC < 12 Y:** Not recommended.

**Pharmacokinetics**

| *Route* | *Onset* | *Peak* | *Duration* |
|---|---|---|---|
| Oral | Slow | 2–3 d | 3–4 d |

*Metabolism:* Hepatic, $T_{1/2}$: 3.4–3.7 h
*Distribution:* Crosses placenta; may enter breast milk
*Excretion:* Urine and feces

**Adverse effects**

- CNS: *Sedation,* drooling, tremor, speech difficulty, depression, hallucinations
- GI: *Diarrhea,* dry mouth, nausea, vomiting, abdominal pain

m

- GU: Impotence, failure of ejaculation, dysuria, hematuria, crystalluria
- Other: Nasal congestion, breast swelling

## ■ Nursing Considerations

### Assessment

- *History:* Hypersensitivity to metyrsoine, pregnancy, lactation
- *Physical:* Orientation, affect, reflexes; bowel sounds, normal output; urinalysis

### Implementation

- Ensure a very liberal intake of fluids.
- Use antidiarrheals if diarrhea is severe.
- Monitor urine for changes associated with drug; less likely when fluids are encouraged.

### Drug-specific teaching points

- Drink plenty of fluids.
- Avoid alcohol, sleep-inducing, or OTC drugs. These could cause dangerous effects.
- The following side effects may occur: drowsiness, dizziness, blurred vision (avoid driving or engaging in activities that require alertness); nausea, dry mouth (good mouth care, taking with food, and frequent, small meals may help); diarrhea (medication may be ordered if severe).
- Report drooling, speech difficulty, tremors, disorientation, severe diarrhea, painful urination.

## mexiletine HCl

*(mex **ill'** i teen)*

Mexitil

**Pregnancy Category C**

### Drug classes

Antiarrhythmic

### Therapeutic actions

Type 1 antiarrhythmic: decreases automaticity of ventricular cells by membrane stabilization.

### Indications

- Treatment of documented life-threatening ventricular arrhythmias (use with lesser arrhythmias is not recommended)
- Unlabeled uses: prophylactic use to decrease arrhythmias in acute phase of acute MI (mortality may not be affected); reduction of pain, dysesthesia, and paresthesia associated with diabetic neuropathy

### Contraindications/cautions

- Contraindications: allergy to mexiletine, CHF, cardiogenic shock, hypotension, second or third-degree heart block (without artificial pacemaker), lactation.
- Use cautiously with hepatic disease, seizure disorders, pregnancy.

### Dosage

**Available Forms:** Capsules—150, 200, 250 mg

ADULT: 200 mg q8h PO. Increase in 50- to 100-mg increments every 2–3 d until desired antiarrhythmic effect is obtained. Maximum dose: 1,200 mg/d PO. Rapid control: 400 mg loading dose, then 200 mg q8h PO.

- ***Transferring from other antiarrhythmics:*** *Lidocaine:* Stop the lidocaine with the first dose of mexiletine; leave IV line open until adequate arrhythmia suppression is assured. *Quinidine sulfate:* Initial dose of 200 mg 6–12 h PO after the last dose of quinidine. *Procainamide:* Initial dose of 200 mg 3–6 h PO after the last dose of procainamide. *Disopyramide:* 200 mg 6–12 h PO after the last dose of disopyramide. *Tocainide:* 200 mg 8–12 h PO after the last dose of tocainide.

PEDIATRIC: Safety and efficacy not established.

### Pharmacokinetics

| Route | Onset | Peak |
|---|---|---|
| Oral | Varies | 2–3 h |

*Metabolism:* Hepatic, $T_{1/2}$: 10–12 h
*Distribution:* Crosses placenta; enters breast milk
*Excretion:* Urine

### Adverse effects

- CNS: *Dizziness/lightheadedness, headache,* fatigue, drowsiness, *tremors, coordination difficulties, visual disturbances,* numbness, nervousness, *sleep difficulties*
- GI: *Nausea, vomiting, heart burn,* abdominal pain, diarrhea, liver injury
- CV: *Cardiac arrhythmias, chest pain*
- **Respiratory**: *Dyspnea*
- **Hematologic**: Positive ANA, thrombocytopenia, leukopenia
- Other: *Rash*

### Clinically important drug-drug interactions

• Decreased mexiletine levels with phenytoins • Increased theophylline levels and toxicity with mexiletine

## ■ Nursing Considerations

### Assessment

- *History:* Allergy to mexiletine, CHF, cardiogenic shock, hypotension, second or third-degree heart block, hepatic disease, seizure disorders, lactation
- *Physical:* Weight; orientation, reflexes; P, BP, auscultation, ECG, edema; R, adventitious sounds; bowel sounds, liver evaluation; urinalysis, urine pH, CBC, electrolytes, liver and renal function tests

### Implementation

- Monitor patient response carefully, especially when beginning therapy.
- Reduce dosage with hepatic failure.
- Monitor for safe and effective serum levels (0.5–2 μg/ml).

### Drug-specific teaching points

- Take with food to reduce GI problems.
- Frequent monitoring of cardiac rhythm is necessary.
- The following side effects may occur: drowsiness, dizziness, numbness, visual disturbances (avoid driving or working with dangerous machinery); nausea, vomiting, heartburn (small, frequent meals may help); diarrhea; headache; sleep disturbances.
- Do not stop taking this drug without checking with your health care provider.
- Return for regular follow-ups to check your heart rhythm; and have blood tests.
- Do not change your diet. Maintain acidity level in urine. Discuss dietary change with your health care provider.
- Report fever, chills, sore throat, excessive GI discomfort, chest pain, excessive tremors, numbness, lack of coordination, headache, sleep disturbances.

## mezlocillin sodium

*(mez loe **sill'** in)*
Mezlin
**Pregnancy Category B**

### Drug classes

Antibiotic
Penicillin

### Therapeutic actions

Bactericidal: inhibits synthesis of cell wall in sensitive organisms, causing cell death.

### Indications

- Lower respiratory tract infections caused by *Haemophilus influenzae; Klebsiella,* including *Klebsiella pneumoniae; Proteus mirabilis; Pseudomonas* species, including *Pseudomonas aeruginosa; Escherichia coli; Bacteroides* species, including *Bacteroides fragilis*
- Intra-abdominal infections caused by *E. coli, P. mirabilis, Klebsiella, Pseudomonas, Streptococcus faecalis, Bacteroides, Peptococcus, Peptostreptococcus*
- UTIs caused by *E. coli, Proteus mirabilis, Proteus, Morganella morganii, Klebsiella, Enterobacter, Serratia, Pseudomonas, S. faecalis*
- Gynecologic infections caused by *Neisseria gonorrhoeae, Peptococcus, Peptostreptococcus, Bacteroides, E. coli, P. mirabilis, Klebsiella, Enterobacter*
- Skin and skin-structure infections caused by *S. faecalis, E. coli, P. mirabilis, Proteus, Proteus vulgaris, Providencia rettgeri, Klebsiella, Enterobacter, Pseudomonas, Peptococcus, Bacteroides*

m

- Septicemia caused by *E. coli, Klebsiella, Enterobacter, Pseudomonas, Bacteroides, Peptococcus*
- Infections caused by *Streptococcus*
- Severe life threatening infections caused by *P. aeruginosa,* in combination with an aminoglycoside antibiotic
- Prophylaxis to decrease the incidence of infections in patients undergoing "dirty" surgical procedures

### Contraindications/cautions

- Contraindications: allergies to penicillins, cephalosporins, or other allergens.
- Use cautiously with renal disorders; lactation (may cause diarrhea or candidiasis in the infant).

### Dosage

**Available Forms:** Powder for injection—1, 2, 3, 4, 20 g

Do not exceed 24 g/d.

*ADULT:* 200–300 mg/kg per day IV or IM, given in 4 to 6 divided doses, up to 350 mg/kg per day in severe cases.

- *Gonococcal urethritis:* 1–2 g IV or IM with 1 g probenecid PO.

*PEDIATRIC*

- *>1 MO, UP TO 12 Y:* 50 mg/kg q4h, IM or by IV infusion over 30 min.
- *<2000 G BODY WEIGHT OR <7 D:* 75 mg/kg q12h.
- *7 D:* 75 mg/kg q8h.
- *>2000 G BODY WEIGHT OR <7 D:* 75 mg/kg q12h.
- *>7 D:* 75 mg/kg q6h.

*GERIATRIC OR RENAL INSUFFICIENCY*

| *Creatinine Clearance (ml/min)* | *Dosage--UTIs* | *Systemic Infection* |
|---|---|---|
| >30 | Usual dosage | Usual dosage |
| 10–30 | 1.5 g q6–8h | 3 g q8h |
| <10 | 1.5 g q8h | 2 g q8h |

### Pharmacokinetics

| *Route* | *Onset* | *Peak* |
|---|---|---|
| IM | Rapid | 45 min |
| IV | Immediate | 5 min |

*Metabolism:* Hepatic, $T_{1/2}$: 50–55 min

*Distribution:* Crosses placenta; enters breast milk

*Excretion:* Urine and bile

### IV facts

**Preparation:** Reconstitute each gram of mezlocillin for IV use by vigorous shaking with 10 ml of Sterile Water for Injection, 5% Dextrose Injection, 0.9% Sodium Chloride Injection. Date reconstituted solution; reconstituted solution is stable for 24–48 h at room temperature, up to 7 d if refrigerated, depending on concentration and diluent—see manufacturer's instructions. Product may darken during storage. If precipitation occurs while refrigerated, warm solution to 37°C, and shake well.

**Infusion:** Direct injection—administer as slowly as possible (3–5 min) to avoid vein irritation. Infusion should be run over a 30-min period. Discontinue any other IV solution running in the same line while mezlocillin is being administered.

**Compatabilities:** Compatible diluents include Sterile Water for Injection, 0.9% Sodium Chloride Injection, 5% Dextrose Injection, 5% Dextrose in 0.225% or 0.45% Sodium Chloride, Lactated Ringer's Injection, 5% Dextrose in Electrolyte #75 Injection, Ringer's Injection, 10% Dextrose Injection, 5% Fructose Injection.

### Adverse effects

- CNS: Lethargy, hallucinations, seizures
- GI: *Glossitis, stomatitis, gastritis, sore mouth*, furry tongue, black "hairy" tongue, *nausea, vomiting, diarrhea,* abdominal pain, bloody diarrhea, enterocolitis, pseudomembranous colitis, nonspecific hepatitis
- **Hematologic**: Anemia, thrombocytopenia, leukopenia, neutropenia, prolonged bleeding time
- GU: Nephritis—oliguria, proteinuria, hematuria, casts, azotemia, pyuria
- **Hypersensitivity reactions**: *Rash, fever, wheezing,* anaphylaxis

- Local: *Pain, phlebitis,* thrombosis at injection site
- Other: *Superinfections,* vaginitis, sodium overload leading to CHF

**Clinically important drug-drug interactions**
- Decreased effectiveness with tetracyclines
- Inactivation of parenteral aminoglycosides (amikacin, gentamicin, kanamycin, neomycin, metilmicin, streptomycin, tobramycin)

**Drug-lab test interferences**
- False-positive Coombs' test with IV use; false-positive urine protein tests if using sulfosalicylic acid and boiling test, acetic acid test, biuret reaction, nitric acid test

## ■ Nursing Considerations

### Assessment
- *History:* Allergies to penicillins, cephalosporins, or other allergens; renal disorders, lactation
- *Physical:* Culture infected area; skin color, lesion; R, adventitious sounds; bowel sounds; CBC, liver and renal function tests, serum electrolytes, Hct, urinalysis

### Implementation
- Culture infection before treatment; reculture if response is not as expected.
- Administer by IV and IM routes only.
- Reconstitute each gram of mezlocillin for IM use by vigorous shaking with 3–4 ml Sterile Water for Injection, 0.5% or 1.0% Lidocaine HCl without epinephrine. Do not exceed 2 g per injection. Inject deep into a large muscle, such as upper outer quadrant of the buttock; slow injection (12–15 sec) will minimize the pain of injection.
- Carefully check IV site for signs of thrombosis or local drug reaction.
- Do not give IM injections repeatedly in the same site; atrophy can occur. Monitor injection sites.

### Drug-specific teaching points
- This drug can only be given IV or IM.
- Upset stomach, nausea, diarrhea, mouth sores, pain, or discomfort at injection sites may occur.
- Report difficulty breathing, rashes, severe diarrhea, severe pain at injection site, mouth sores.

# mibefradil dihydrochloride

*(ma **bif'** ri dil)*

Posicor

**Pregnancy Category C**

**Drug classes**

Antianginal agent
Antihypertensive
Calcium channel blocker

**Therapeutic actions**

Inhibits the movement of calcium ions across the membranes of cardiac and arterial muscle cells, both high voltage channels, L-type, and low voltage channels, T-type; inhibition of transmembrane calcium flow results in the depression of impulse formation in specialized cardiac pacemaker cells, in slowing of the velocity of conduction of the cardiac impulse, and in the depression of myocardial contractility, as well as in the dilation of coronary arteries and arterioles and peripheral arterioles; these effects in turn lead to decreased cardiac work, decreased cardiac energy consumption, and, in patients with vasospastic (Prinzmetal's) angina, increased delivery of oxygen to cardiac cells as well as lower blood pressure. Mibefradil does not cause reflex tachycardia (often seen with other calcium channel blockers).

**Indications**
- Treatment of hypertension as a single agent or in combination with other antihypertensives
- Treatment of chronic, stable angina pectoris, alone or in combination with other antianginal agents

**Contraindications/cautions**
- Contraindications: allergy to mibefradil, sick sinus syndrome, heart block (second or third degree), pregnancy, lactation
- Use cautiously with hypotension, history of serious ventricular arrhythmias, un-

compensated CHF, congenital QT interval prolongation, hepatic failure.

### Dosage

**Available Forms:** Tablets—50, 100 mg

ADULT

- *Hypertension:* 50 mg PO qd; titrate to 100 mg PO qd over a 2-wk period.
- *Chronic stable angina:* 50 mg PO qd as an initial dose; titrate to 100 mg PO qd based on patient response.

PEDIATRIC: Safety and efficacy not established.

## Pharmacokinetics

| Route | Onset | Peak |
|---|---|---|
| Oral | Varies | 1–2 h |

*Metabolism:* Hepatic; $T_{1/2}$: 17–25 h

*Distribution:* Crosses placenta; passes into breast milk

*Excretion:* Bile and urine

## Adverse effects

- CNS: *dizziness, lightheadedness, nervousness, headache, asthenia,* fatigue
- GI: *Nausea,* hepatic injury, *constipation*
- CV: *Peripheral edema,* hypotension, arrhythmias, *bradycardia, AV block,* **ventricular tachycardia, asystole, suppression of sinus node activity**
- Dermatologic: *Rash*

## Clinically important drug-drug interactions

• Possibility of severe toxicity with terfenadine, astemizole, cisapride; avoid these combinations • Increased serum levels of cyclosporine and metoprolol with mibefradil; monitor patients closely for any sign of toxicity and adjust dosage accordingly • Risk of heart block and serious adverse effects with any drug that decreases heart rate (beta blockers, digitalis, calcium channel blockers, etc.) • Risk of statin-induced rhabdomyolysis in conjunction with simvastatin, lovastatin, other HMG CoA inhibitors

## ■ Nursing Considerations

### Assessment

- *History:* Allergy to mibefradil, sick sinus syndrome, heart block (second or third degree), hypotension, history of serious ventricular arrhythmias, uncompensated CHF, congenital QT interval prolongation, hepatic impairment, pregnancy, lactation.
- *Physical:* Skin lesions, color, edema; P, BP, baseline ECG, peripheral perfusion, auscultation, R, adventitious sounds; liver evaluation, GI normal output; liver function tests, renal function tests.

### Implementation

- Monitor patient carefully (BP, cardiac rhythm and output) while drug is being titrated to therapeutic dose; dosage may be increased more rapidly in hospitalized patients under close supervision.
- Monitor BP very carefully if patient is on concurrent doses of other antihypertensives or antianginal drugs.
- Monitor heart rate for any sign of bradycardia if patient has received any other drugs that might decrease heart rate.
- Administer with food if GI upset is bothersome.

### Drug-specific teaching points

- Take this drug exactly as prescribed; take with food if GI upset occurs.
- The following side effects may occur: nausea, vomiting (eat small, frequent meals); headache (monitor lighting, noise and temperature; medication may be ordered if severe); dizziness, shakiness (avoid driving or operating dangerous machinery).
- Report irregular heart beat, shortness of breath, swelling of the hands or feet, pronounced dizziness, constipation, unusual bleeding or bruising.

# Miconazole

## miconazole

*(mi **kon'** a zole)*

*Parenteral:* Monistat I.V.

## miconazole nitrate

*Vaginal suppositories, topical:* Micatin, Monistat 3, Monistat 7, Monistat-Derm, Monistat Dual Pak

**Pregnancy Category B**

**Drug classes**
Antifungal

**Therapeutic actions**
Fungicidal: alters fungal cell membrane permeability, causing cell death; also may alter fungal cell DNA and RNA metabolism or cause accumulation of toxic peroxides intracellularly.

**Indications**
- Treatment of severe systemic fungal infections: coccidioidomycosis, candidiasis, cryptococcosis, petriellidiosis, paracoccidioidomycosis, chronic mucocutaneous candidiasis (parenteral)
- Fungal meningitis or fungal urinary bladder infections (intrathecal, bladder instillation)
- Local treatment of vulvovaginal candidiasis (moniliasis; vaginal suppositories)
- Tinea pedis, tinea cruris, tinea corporis caused by *Trichophyton rubrum, Trichophyton mentagrophytes, Epidermophyton floccosum;* cutaneous candidiasis (moniliasis), tinea versicolor (topical administration)

**Contraindications/cautions**
- Contraindications: allergy to miconazole or components used in preparation.
- Use cautiously with pregnancy, lactation.

**Dosage**
**Available Forms:** Vaginal suppositories—100, 200 mg; topical cream—2%; vaginal cream—2%; topical powder 2%, topical spray—2%

*ADULT:* Daily dosage for parenteral administration may be divided into 3 infusions. Recommended dosage varies with organism involved:

| *Organism* | *Total Daily Dosage Range* | *Duration (wk)* |
|---|---|---|
| Coccidioidomycosis | 1800–3600 mg | 3 to >20 |
| Cryptococcosis | 1200–2400 mg | 3 to >12 |
| Petriellidiosis | 600–3000 mg | 5 to >20 |
| Candidiasis | 600–1800 mg | 1 to >20 |
| Paracoccidioidomycosis | 200–1200 mg | 2 to >16 |

- *Intrathecal administration:* 20 mg/dose administered undiluted as an adjunct to IV treatment. Alternate injections between lumbar, cervical, and cisternal punctures q3–7 d.
- *Bladder instillation:* 200 mg diluted solution for urinary bladder mycoses.
- *Vaginal suppositories:* Monistat 3: Insert 1 suppository intravaginally once daily hs for 3 d. Monistat 7: one applicator cream or 1 suppository in the vagina daily hs for 7 d. Repeat course if necessary.
- *Topical:* Cream and lotion: Cover affected areas bid, morning and evening. Powder: Spray or sprinkle powder liberally over affected area in the morning and evening.

*PEDIATRIC*
- *Parenteral:* 20–40 mg/kg IV as a total dose. Do not exceed 15 mg/kg per dose.
- *Topical:* Not recommended for children younger than 2 y.

**Pharmacokinetics**

| *Route* | *Onset* | *Peak* |
|---|---|---|
| IV | Rapid | Unknown |

*Metabolism:* Hepatic, $T_{1/2}$: 21–24 h
*Distribution:* Crosses placenta; may enter breast milk
*Excretion:* Urine and feces

**IV facts**
**Preparation:** Dilute in at least 200 ml of fluid, preferably 0.9% Sodium Chloride or 5% Dextrose Solution.
**Infusion:** Administer initial IV dose of 200 mg with physician in attendance, monitoring patient response. Infuse IV over 30–60 min; avoid rapid infusion; transient tachycardia or arrhythmias may occur.

**Adverse effects**
*Systemic Administration*
- GI: *Nausea, vomiting*, diarhea, anorexia
- Dermatologic: *Phlebitis, pruritus, rash*, flushes
- Hematologic: Decreased Hct, thrombocytopenia, aggregation of erythrocytes or

m

rouleau formation, hyperlipemia (associated with vehicle used), Cremophor EL (PEG 40, castor oil)
- **Other:** *Febrile reactions*, drowsiness, anaphylactoid reactions

*Vaginal Suppositories*
- **Local:** *Irritation*, sensitization or vulvovaginal burning, pelvic cramps
- **Other:** Skin rash, headache

*Topical Application*
- **Local:** *Irritation, burning, maceration*, allergic contact dermatitis

## ■ Nursing Considerations

### Assessment
- ***History:*** Allergy to miconazole or components used in preparation, lactation
- ***Physical:*** Skin color, lesions, area around lesions; T; orientation, affect; CBC and differential, serum sodium; serum Hgb and lipids (IV administration); culture of area involved

### Implementation
- Culture fungus involved before therapy.
- Continue IV treatments until clinical and laboratory tests no longer indicate presence of active fungal infection; length of treatment varies with causative organism.
- Alternate intrathecal injections between lumbar, cervical, and cisternal sites every 3–7 d.
- Insert vaginal suppositories high into the vagina; have patient remain recumbent for 10–15 min after insertion; provide sanitary napkin to protect clothing from stains.
- Monitor response; if none is noted, arrange for further cultures to determine causative organism.
- Apply lotion to intertriginous areas if topical application is required; if cream is used, apply sparingly to avoid maceration of the area.
- Ensure patient receives the full course of therapy to eradicate the fungus and to prevent recurrence.
- Discontinue topical or vaginal administration if rash or sensitivity occurs.

### Drug-specific teaching points
- Take the full course of drug therapy even if symptoms improve. Continue during menstrual period if vaginal route is being used. Long-term use will be needed; beneficial effects may not be seen for several weeks. Vaginal suppositories should be inserted high into the vagina.
- Use hygiene measures to prevent reinfection or spread of infection.
- This drug is for the fungus being treated; do not self-medicate other problems with this drug.
- Refrain from sexual intercourse, or advise partner to use a condom to avoid reinfection; use a sanitary napkin to prevent staining of clothing (vaginal use)
- The following side effects may occur: nausea, vomiting, diarrhea (request medication to help this problem); local use: irritation, burning, stinging.
- Report local irritation, burning (topical application); rash, irritation, pelvic pain (vaginal use); drowsiness, difficulty breathing, rash, nausea (parenteral administration).

# midodrine hydrochloride

***(mid' oh dryn)***
ProAmatine
**Pregnancy Category C**

### Drug classes
Antihypotensive

### Therapeutic actions
Activates alpha receptors in the arteriolar and venous vasculature, producing an increase in vascular tone and elevation of BP.

### Indications
- Treatment of symptomatic orthostatic hypotension in patients whose lives are considerably impaired by the disorder and who do not respond to other therapy
- Unlabeled use: management of urinary incontinence at doses of 2.5–5 mg bid–tid

### Contraindications/cautions

- Contraindications: severe CAD, acute renal disease; urinary retention; pheochromocytoma; thyrotoxicosis; persistent or excessive supine hypertension
- Use cautiously with renal or hepatic impairment, lactation, pregnancy, visual problems

### Dosage

**Available Forms:** Tablets—2.5, 5 mg

*ADULT:* 10 mg PO tid during daytime hours when upright.

*PEDIATRIC:* Safety and efficacy not established.

*RENAL IMPAIRMENT:* Starting dose of 2.5 mg PO tid.

### Pharmacokinetics

| Route | Onset | Peak |
|---|---|---|
| Oral | Rapid | 30 min |

*Metabolism:* Hepatic and tissue; $T_{1/2}$: 25 min

*Distribution:* Crosses placenta; may pass into breast milk

*Excretion:* Urine

### Adverse effects

- CNS: Headache, *paresthesias, pain,* dizziness, vertigo, visual field changes
- CV: *Supine hypertension, bradycardia*
- Dermatologic: *Piloerection, pruritus,* rash
- Other: *Dysuria, chills*

### Clinically important drug-drug interactions

- Increased effects and toxicity of cardiac glycosides, beta blockers, alpha adrenergic agents, steroids (fludrocortisone) with midodrine; monitor patient carefully and adjust dosage as needed

## ■ Nursing Considerations

### Assessment

- *History:* Severe CAD, acute renal disease; urinary retention; pheochromocytoma; thyrotoxicosis; persistent or excessive supine hypertension; renal or hepatic impairment, lactation, pregnancy; visual problems
- *Physical:* T; orientation, visual field checks; skin color, lesions, temperature; BP—sitting, standing, supine, P; renal and hepatic function tests

### Implementation

- Establish baseline hepatic and renal function and evaluate periodically during therapy.
- Monitor BP carefully, especially if used with any agent that causes vasoconstriction; give only to patients who are up and about—do not give to bedridden patients or before bed.
- Monitor heart rate when beginning therapy. Bradycardia is common as therapy bgins; persistent bradycardia should be evaluated and drug discontinued.
- Monitor patients with known visual problems or who are taking fludrocortisone for any change in visual fields. Discontinue drug and consult physician if changes occur.
- Encourage patient to take drug after voiding if urinary retention is a problem

m

### Drug-specific teaching points

- Take this drug during the day when you will be up and around. Do not take it before bed or lying down.
- Empty your bladder before taking this drug if urinary retention has been a problem.
- Return for regular medical evaluation of your BP and response to this drug.
- The following side effects may occur: numbness or tingling in the extremities (avoid injury); slow heart rate; rash, "goose bumps."
- Report changes in vision, pounding in the head when lying down, very slow heart rate, difficulty urinating.

## mifepristone

*(miff eh* ***prist'*** *own)*

RU-486, Mifegyne

**Pregnancy Category C**

**Drug classes**
Abortifacient

**Therapeutic actions**
Acts as an antagonist of progesterone sites in the endometrium, allowing protaglandins to stimulate uterine contractions, causing implanted trophoblast to separate from the placental wall; may also decrease placental viability and accelerate degenerative changes resulting in sloughing of the endometrium.

**Indications**
- Termination of pregnancy through 49 d gestational age; most effective when combined with a prostaglandin

**Contraindications/cautions**
- Contraindications: allergy to prostaglandin preparations; acute PID; active cardiac, hepatic, pulmonary, renal disease
- Use cautiously with history of asthma; anemia; jaundice; diabetes; epilepsy; scarred uterus; cervicitis, infected endocervical lesions, acute vaginitis

**Dosage**
**Available Forms:** Tablets—25 mg
*ADULT:* 25 mg PO bid for 4 d or 50 mg PO tid for 4 d; one-time dose of 600 mg PO has been used with success.

**Pharmacokinetics**

| *Route* | *Onset* | *Peak* |
|---|---|---|
| Oral | Rapid | 1–3 h |

*Metabolism:* Tissue; $T_{1/2}$: 20–54 h
*Distribution:* Crosses placenta; passes into breast milk
*Excretion:* Urine

**Adverse effects**
- CNS: *Headache*
- GI: *Vomiting, diarrhea, nausea, abdominal pain*
- GU: Heavy uterine bleeding, endometritis, uterine/vaginal pain

## ■ Nursing Considerations

**Assessment**
- *History:* Allergy to prostaglandin preparations; acute PID; active cardiac, hepatic, pulmonary, renal disease; history of asthma; hypotension; hypertension; CV, adrenal, renal or hepatic disease; anemia; jaundice; diabetes; epilepsy; scarred uterus; cervicitis, infected endocervical lesions, acute vaginitis
- *Physical:* T; BP, P, auscultation; bowel sounds, liver evaluation; vaginal discharge, pelvic exam, uterine tone; liver and renal function tests, WBC, urinalysis, CBC

**Implementation**
- Provide appropriate referrals and counseling for abortion.
- Alert patient that menses usually begins within 5 d of treatment and lasts for 1–2 wk.
- Arrange to follow drug within 48 h with a prostaglandin (Cytotec).
- Ensure that abortion is complete or that other measures are used to complete the abortion if drug effects are not sufficient.
- Prepare for D & C if heavy bleeding does not resolve.
- Provide analgesic and antiemetic agents as needed to increase comfort.

**Drug-specific teaching points**
Teaching about mifepristone should be incorporated into the total teaching plan for the patient undergoing an abortion; specific information that should be included follows:
- Menses begin within 5 d of treatment and will last 1–2 wk.
- The following side effects may occur: nausea, vomiting, diarrhea (medication may be ordered); uterine/vaginal pain, headache (an analgesic may be ordered).
- Report severe pain; persistent, heavy bleeding; extreme fatigue, dizziness on arising.

## miglitol

***(mig' lah tall)***
Glyset
**Pregnancy Category B**

**Drug classes**
Antidiabetic agent

**Therapeutic actions**
An alpha-glucosidase inhibitor that delays the digestion of ingested carbohydrates, leading to a smaller rise in blood glucose following meals and a decrease in glycosylated hemoglobin; does not enhance insulin secretion and so its effects are additive to those of the sulfonylureas in controlling blood glucose.

**Indications**
- Adjunct to diet to lower blood glucose in patients with non-insulin-dependent diabetes mellitus (Type II) whose hyperglycemia cannot be managed by diet alone
- Combination therapy with a sulfonylurea to enhance glycemic control in those patients who do not receive adequate control with diet and either drug

**Contraindications/cautions**
- Contraindications: hypersensitivity to the drug; diabetic ketoacidosis; cirrhosis; inflammatory bowel disease; intestinal obstruction or predisposition to intestinal obstruction; Type I diabetes; conditions that would deteriorate with increased gas in the bowel.
- Use cautiously with renal impairment, pregnancy, lactation.

**Dosage**
**Available Forms:** Tablets—25, 50, 100 mg
*ADULT:* Initial dose: 25 mg PO tid at the first bite of each meal; may start at 25 mg PO qd if severe GI effects are seen. Maintenance: 50 mg PO tid at first bite of each meal. Maximum dose: 100 mg PO tid.
- ***Combination with a sulfonylurea:*** Blood glucose may be much lower; monitor closely and adjust dosages of each drug accordingly.

*PEDIATRIC:* Safety and efficacy not established.

**Pharmacokinetics**

| *Route* | *Onset* | *Peak* |
|---|---|---|
| Oral | Rapid | 2–3 h |

*Metabolism:* Not metabolized; $T_{1/2}$: 2 h
*Distribution:* Very little
*Excretion:* Urine

**Adverse effects**
- GI: *Abdominal pain, flatulence, diarrhea,* anorexia, nausea, vomiting
- **Endocrine:** *Hypoglycemia* (taken in combination with other antidiabetic drugs)
- **Dermatologic:** Rash

## ■ Nursing Considerations

### Assessment
- *History:* Hypersensitivity to the drug; diabetic ketoacidosis; cirrhosis; inflammatory bowel disease; intestinal obstruction or predisposition to intestinal obstruction; Type I diabetes; conditions that would deteriorate with increased gas in the bowel; renal impairment; pregnancy; lactation.
- *Physical:* Skin color, lesions; T; orientation, reflexes, peripheral sensation; R, adventitious sounds; liver evaluation, bowel sounds; urinalysis, BUN, blood glucose.

m

### Implementation
- Administer drug 3 X/d with the first bite of each meal.
- Monitor urine and serum glucose levels frequently to determine effectiveness of drug and dosage being used.
- Inform patient of likelihood of abdominal pain and flatulence.
- Arrange for consult with dietician to establish weight loss program and dietary control as appropriate.
- Arrange for thorough diabetic teaching program to include diesease, dietary control, exercise, signs and symptoms of hypo- and hyperglycemia, avoidance of infection, hygiene.

### Drug-specific teaching points
- Do not discontinue this medication without consulting your care provider.
- Take this drug three times a day with the first bite of each meal.
- Monitor urine or blood for glucose and ketones as prescribed.

- Continue diet and exercise program established for control of diabetes.
- The following side effects may occur: abdominal pain, flatulence, bloating.
- Report fever, sore throat, unusual bleeding or bruising, severe abdominal pain.

# milrinone lactate

***(mill' ri none)***

Primacor

**Pregnancy Category C**

## Drug classes

Cardiotonic agent

## Therapeutic actions

Increases force of contraction of ventricles (positive inotropic effect); causes vasodilation by a direct relaxant effect on vascular smooth muscle.

## Indications

- CHF: short-term IV management of those patients who are receiving digitalis and diuretics

## Contraindications/cautions

- Contraindications: allergy to milrinone or bisulfites; severe aortic or pulmonic valvular disease.
- Use cautiously with the elderly, pregnancy.

## Dosage

**Available Forms:** Injection—1 mg/ml; premixed injection—200 μg/ml

*ADULT:* Loading dose: 50 μg/kg IV bolus, given over 10 min. Maintenance infusion: 0.375–0.75 μg/kg per minute. Do not exceed a total of 1.13 mg/kg per day.

*PEDIATRIC:* Not recommended.

*GERIATRIC OR RENAL IMPAIRMENT:* Creatinine clearance: 5 (0.2 μg/kg per min IV), 10 (0.23 μg/kg per min IV), 20 (0.28 μg/kg per min IV); 30 (0.3 μg/kg per min IV); 40 (0.38 μg/kg per min IV); 50 (0.43 μg/kg per min IV). Do not exceed 1.13 mg/kg per day.

## Pharmacokinetics

| *Route* | *Onset* | *Peak* | *Duration* |
|---|---|---|---|
| IV | Immediate | 5–15 min | 8 h |

*Metabolism:* Hepatic, $T_{1/2}$: 2.3–2.5 h

*Distribution:* Crosses placenta; may enter breast milk

*Excretion:* Urine

## IV facts

**Preparation:** Add diluent of 0.45% or 0.9% Sodium Chloride Injection, USP or 5% Dextrose Injection, USP. Add 180 ml per 20-mg vial to prepare solution of 100 μg/ml$^2$; 113 ml per 20-mg vial to prepare a solution of 150 μg/ml$^2$; add 80 ml diluent to 20-mg vial to prepare solution of 200 μg/ml$^2$.

**Infusion:** Administer while carefully monitoring patient's hemodynamic and clinical response; see manufacturer's insert for detailed guidelines.

**Incompatibilities:** Do not mix directly with furosemide.

## Adverse effects

- CV: *Ventricular arrhythmias*, hypotension, supraventricular arrhythmias, chest pain, angina, death
- Hematologic: Thrombocytopenia, hypokalemia

## Clinically important drug-drug interactions

- Precipitate formation in solution if given in the same IV line with furosemide

# ■ Nursing Considerations

## Assessment

- ***History:*** Allergy to milrinone or bisulfites, severe aortic or pulmonic valvular disease, lactation
- ***Physical:*** Weight, orientation, P, BP, cardiac auscultation, peripheral pulses and perfusion, R, adventitious sounds, serum electrolyte levels, platelet count, ECG

## Implementation

- Monitor cardiac rhythm continually.
- Monitor BP and P and reduce dose if marked decreases occur.

- Monitor intake and output and electrolyte levels.

### Drug-specific teaching points

- You will need frequent BP and P and heart activity monitoring during therapy.
- You may experience increased voiding; appropriate bathroom arrangements will be made.
- Report pain at IV injection site, numbness or tingling, shortness of breath, chest pain.

## minocycline hydrochloride

*(mi noe sye' kleen)*

Minocin

**Pregnancy Category D**

### Drug classes

Antibiotic

Tetracycline

### Therapeutic actions

Bacteriostatic: inhibits protein synthesis of susceptible bacteria, causing cell death.

### Indications

- Infections caused by rickettsiae; *Mycoplasma pneumoniae;* agents of psittacosis, ornithosis, lymphogranuloma venereum and granuloma inguinale; *Borrelia recurrentis; Hemophilus ducreyi; Pasteurella pestis; Pasteurella tularensis; Bartonella bacilliformis; Bacteroides; Vibrio comma; Vibrio fetus; Brucella; E. coli; Enterobacter aerogenes; Shigella; Acinetobacter calcoaceticus; H. influenzae; Klebsiella; Diplococcus pneumoniae; S. aureus*
- When penicillin is contraindicated, infections caused by *N. gonorrhoeae, Treponema pallidum, Treponema pertenue, Listeria monocytogenes, Clostridium, Bacillus anthracis*. As an adjunct to amebicides in acute intestinal amebiasis
- *Oral* tetracyclines are indicated for treatment of acne, uncomplicated urethral, endocervical, or rectal infections in adults caused by *Chlamydia trachomatis*
- *Oral* minocycline is indicated in treatment of asymptomatic carriers of *Neisseria meningitidis* (not useful for treating the infection); infections caused by *Mycobacterium marinum*; uncomplicated urethral, endocervical, or rectal infections caused by *Ureaplasma urealyticum*; uncomplicated gonococcal urethritis in men due to *N. gonorrhoeae*
- Unlabeled use: alternative to sulfonamides in the treatment of nocardiosis

### Contraindications/cautions

- Contraindication: allergy to tetracylines.
- Use cautiously with renal or hepatic dysfunction, pregnancy, lactation.

### Dosage

**Available Forms:** Capsules—50, 100 mg; tablets—50, 100 mg; oral suspension—50 mg/5 ml; powder for injection—100 mg

**ADULT:** 200 mg followed by 100 mg q12h IV. Do not exceed 400 mg/d. Or 200 mg initially, followed by 100 mg q12h PO. May be given as 100–200 mg initially and then 50 mg qid PO.

- *Syphilis:* Usual PO dose for 10–15 d.
- *Urethral, endocervical, rectal infections:* 100 mg bid PO for 7 d.
- *Gonococcal urethritis in men:* 100 mg bid PO for 5 d.
- *Gonorrhea:* 200 mg PO followed by 100 mg q12h for 4 d.
- *Meningococcal carrier state:* 100 mg q12h PO for 5 d.

**PEDIATRIC >8 Y:** 4 mg/kg IV followed by 2 mg/kg q12h IV or PO.

**GERIATRIC OR RENAL FAILURE PATIENTS:** IV doses of minocycline are not as toxic as other tetracyclines in these patients.

### Pharmacokinetics

| Route | Onset | Peak |
|---|---|---|
| Oral | Rapid | 2–3 h |
| IV | Immediate | End of infusion |

*Metabolism:* Hepatic, $T_{1/2}$: 11–26 h

*Distribution:* Crosses placenta; enters breast milk

*Excretion:* Urine and feces

### IV facts

**Preparation:** Dissolve powder and then further dilute to 500–1,000 ml with Sodium Chloride Injection, Dextrose Injection, Dextrose and Sodium Chloride

Injection, Ringer's Injection, or Lactated Ringer's Injection; administer immediately.

**Infusion:** Infuse slowly over 5–10 min; discard any diluted solution not used within 24 h.

**Incompatibilities:** Avoid solutions with calcium; a precipitate may form.

### Adverse effects

- GI: Fatty liver, liver failure, *anorexia, nausea, vomiting, diarrhea, glossitis,* dysphagia, enterocolitis, esophageal ulcer
- Hematologic: Hemolytic anemia, thrombocytopenia, neutropenia, eosinophilia, leukocytosis, leukopenia
- Dermatologic: *Phototoxic reactions, rash,* exfoliative dermatitis (more frequent, more severe with this tetracycline than with any others)
- Dental: *Discoloring and inadequate calcification of primary teeth of fetus if used by pregnant women; discoloring and inadequate calcification of permanent teeth if used during period of dental development*
- Local: Local irritation at injection site
- Other: Superinfections, nephrogenic diabetes insipidus syndrome

### Clinically important drug-drug interactions

• Decreased absorption of minocycline with antacids, iron, alkali • Increased digoxin toxicity • Increased nephrotoxicity with methoxyflurane • Decreased activity of penicillin

### Clinically important drug-food interactions

• Decreased absorption of minocycline if taken with food, dairy products

## ■ Nursing Considerations

### Assessment

- *History:* Allergy to tetracylines, renal or hepatic dysfunction, pregnancy, lactation
- *Physical:* Skin status, orientation and reflexes, R and sounds, GI function and liver evaluation, urinalysis and BUN, liver and renal function tests; culture infected area

### Implementation

- Administer oral medication without regard to food or meals; if GI upset occurs, give with meals.

### Drug-specific teaching points

- Take drug throughout the day for best results.
- Take with meals if GI upset occurs.
- The following side effects may occur: sensitivity to sunlight (wear protective clothing, use sunscreen); diarrhea, nausea (take with meals, small, frequent meals may help).
- Report rash, itching; difficulty breathing; dark urine or light-colored stools; severe cramps, watery diarrhea.

## minoxidil

*(mi **nox'** i dill)*

*Oral:* Loniten

*Topical:* Rogaine, Rogaine Extra Strength

**Pregnancy Category C**

### Drug classes

Antihypertensive
Vasodilator

### Therapeutic actions

Acts directly on vascular smooth muscle to cause vasodilation, reducing elevated systolic and diastolic BP; does not interfere with CV reflexes; does not usually cause orthostatic hypotension but does cause reflex tachycardia and renin release, leading to sodium and water retention; mechanism in stimulating hair growth is not known, possibly related to arterial dilation.

### Indications

- Severe hypertension that is symptomatic or associated with target organ damage and is not manageable with maximum therapeutic doses of a diuretic plus two other antihypertensive drugs; use in milder hypertension not recommended
- Alopecia areata and male pattern alopecia—topical use when compounded as a 1%–5% lotion or 1% ointment

## Contraindications/cautions

- Contraindications: hypersensitivity to minoxidil or any component of the topical preparation (topical); pheochromocytoma (may stimulate release of catecholamines from tumor); acute MI; dissecting aortic aneurysm; lactation.
- Use cautiously with malignant hypertension; CHF (use diuretic); angina pectoris (use a beta-blocker); pregnancy.

## Dosage

**Available Forms:** Tablets—2.5, 10 mg; topical 2%, 5%

*ADULT:* Initial dosage is 5 mg/d PO as a single dose. Daily dosage can be increased to 10, 20, then 40 mg in single or divided doses. Effective range is usally 10–40 mg/d PO. Maximum dosage is 100 mg/d. Magnitude of within-day fluctuation in BP is directly proportional to extent of BP reduction. If supine diastolic BP has been reduced less than 30 mm Hg, administer the drug only once a day. If reduced more than 30 mm Hg, divide the daily dosage into two equal parts. Dosage adjustment should normally be at least 3 d (q6h with careful monitoring).

- *Concomitant therapy: Diuretics:* Use minoxidil with a diuretic in patients relying on renal function for maintaining salt and water balance; the following diuretic dosages have been used when starting minoxidil therapy: hydrochlorothiazide, 50 mg bid; chlorthalidone, 50–100 mg qd; furosemide, 40 mg bid. If excessive salt and water retention result in weight gain > 5 lb, change diuretic therapy to furosemide; if patient already takes furosemide, increase dosage. *Beta-adrenergic blockers or other sympatholytics:* The following dosages are recommended when starting minoxidil therapy: propranolol, 80–160 mg/d; other beta-blockers, dosage equivalent to the above, methyldopa 250–750 mg bid (start methyldopa at least 24 h before minoxidil); clonidine, 0.1–0.2 mg bid.

– ***Topical:*** Apply 1 ml to the total affected areas of the scalp twice daily. The total daily dosage should not exceed 2 ml. Twice daily appliation for > 4 mo may be required before evidence of hair regrowth is observed. Once hair growth is realized, twice daily application is necessary for continued and additional hair regrowth. Balding process reported to return to untreated state 3–4 mo after cessation of the drug.

*PEDIATRIC:* Experience is limited, particularly in infants; use recommendations as a guide; careful titration is necessary. *≤12 y:* As adult. *< 12 y:* Initial dosage is 0.2 mg/kg per day PO as a single dose. May increase 50%–100% increments until optimum BP control is achieved. Effective range is usually 0.25–1 mg/kg per day; maximum dosage is 50 mg daily. Experience in children is limited; monitor carefully.

*GERIATRIC OR IMPAIRED RENAL FUNCTION:* Smaller doses may be required; closely supervise to prevent cardiac failure or exacerbation of renal failure.

## Pharmacokinetics

| *Route* | *Onset* | *Peak* | *Duration* |
|---|---|---|---|
| Oral | 30 min | 2–3 h | 75 h |
| Topical | Not generally absorbed systemically | | |

*Metabolism:* Hepatic, $T_{1/2}$: 4.2 h
*Distribution:* Crosses placenta; enters breast milk
*Excretion:* Urine

## Adverse effects

- CNS: Fatigue, headache
- GI: Nausea, vomiting
- CV: Tachycardia (unless given with beta-adrenergic blocker or other sympatholytic drug), pericardial effusion and tamponade; *changes in direction and magnitude of T-waves*; cardiac necrotic lesions (reported in patients with known ischemic heart disease, but risk of minoxidil-associated cardiac damage cannot be excluded)
- **Respiratory**: *bronchitis, upper respiratory infection, sinusitis* (topical use)

- **Hematologic**: Initial decrease in Hct, Hgb, RBC count
- **Dermatologic**: *Temporary edema, hypertrichosis* (elongation, thickening, and enhanced pigmentation of fine body hair occurring within 3–6 wk of starting therapy; usually first noticed on temples, between eyebrows and extending to other parts of face, back, arms, legs, scalp); rashes including bullous eruptions; Stevens-Johnson syndrome; darkening of the skin
- **Local**: *Irritant dermatitis, allergic contact dermatitis, eczema, pruritus, dry skin/scalp, flaking, alopecia* (topical use)

## ■ Nursing Considerations

### Assessment

- ***History:*** Hypersensitivity to minoxidil or any component of the topical preparation; pheochromocytoma; acute MI, dissecting aortic aneurysm; malignant hypertension; CHF; angina pectoris; lactation
- ***Physical:*** Skin color, lesions, hair, scalp; P, BP, orthostatic BP, supine BP, perfusion, edema, auscultation; bowel sounds, normal output; CBC with differential, kidney function tests, urinalysis, ECG

### Implementation

- Apply topical preparation to affected area; if fingers are used to facilitate drug application, wash hands thoroughly afterward.
- Do not apply other topical agents, including topical corticosteroids, retinoids, and petrolatum or agents known to enhance cutaneous drug absorption.
- Do not apply topical preparation to open lesions or breaks in the skin, which could increase risk of systemic absorption.
- Arrange to withdraw drug gradually, especially from children; rapid withdrawal may cause a sudden increase in BP (rebound hypertension has been reported in children, even with gradual withdrawal; use caution and monitor BP closely when withdrawing from children).
- Arrange for echocardiographic evaluation of possible pericardial effusion; more vigorous diuretic therapy, dialysis, other treatment (including minoxidil withdrawal) may be required.

### Drug-specific teaching points

***Oral***

- Take this drug exactly as prescribed. Take all other medications that have been prescribed. Do not discontinue any drug or reduce the dosage without consulting your health care provider.
- The following side effects may occur: enhanced growth and darkening of fine body and face hair (do not discontinue medication without consulting care provider); GI upset (frequent small meals may help).
- Report increased heart rate of $\leq$ 20 beats per minute over normal (your normal heart rate is ____ beats per minute); rapid weight gain of more than 5 lb; unusual swelling of the extremities, face, or abdomen; difficulty breathing, especially when lying down; new or aggravated symptoms of angina (chest, arm, or shoulder pain); severe indigestion; dizziness, lightheadedness, or fainting.

***Topical***

- Apply the prescribed amount to affected area twice a day. If using the fingers to facilitate application, wash hands thoroughly after application. It may take 4 mo or longer for any noticeable hair regrowth to appear. Response to this drug is very individual. If no response is seen within 4 mo, consult with your care provider about efficacy of continued use.
- Do not apply more frequent or larger applications. This will not speed up or increase hair growth but may increase side effects.
- If one or two daily applications are missed, restart twice-daily applications, and return to usual schedule. Do not attempt to make up missed applications.
- Do not apply any other topical medication to the area while you are using this drug.

- Do not apply to any sunburned, broken skin or open lesions; this increases the risk of systemic effects. Do not apply to any part of the body other than the scalp.
- Twice daily use of the drug will be necessary to retain or continue the hair regrowth.

## mirtazapine

*(mer **tah'** zah peen)*

Remeron

**Pregnancy Category B**

### Drug classes

Antidepressant (tetracyclic)

### Therapeutic actions

Mechanism of action unknown; appears to act similarly to TCAs, which inhibit the presynaptic reuptake of the neurotransmitters norepinephrine and serotonin; anticholinergic at CNS and peripheral receptors; sedating; relation of these effects to clinical efficacy is unknown.

### Indications

- Relief of symptoms of depression (endogenous depression most responsive)

### Contraindications/cautions

- Contraindications: hypersensitivity to any tricyclic or tetracyclic drug; comcomitant therapy with an MAOI; recent MI; myelography within previous 24 h or scheduled within 48 h; pregnancy (limb reduction abnormalities reported): lactation
- Use cautiously with ET; preexisting CV disorders, eg, severe coronary heart disease, progressive heart failure, angina pectoris, paroxysmal tachycardia (possible increased risk of serious CVS toxicity with TCAs); angle-closure glaucoma, increased intraocular pressure, urinary retention, ureteral or urethral spasm; seizure disorders (TCAs lower the seizure threshold); hyperthyroidism (predisposes to CVS toxicity, including cardiac arrhythmias); impaired hepatic, renal function; psychiatric patients (schizophrenic or paranoid patients may exhibit a worsening of psychosis with TCAs); manic-depressive patients (may shift to hypomanic or manic phase); elective surgery (TCAs should be discontinued as long as possible before surgery)

### Dosage

**Available Forms:** Tablets—15, 30 mg

*ADULT:* Initial dose: 15 mg PO qd, as a single dose in evening. Continue treatment for up to 6 mo for acute episodes.

- *Switching from MAOI:* Allow at least 14 d between discontinuation of MAOI and beginning of mirtazapine therapy. Allow 14 d after stopping mirtazapine before starting MAOI.

*PEDIATRIC:* Not recommended in children $<$18 y.

*GERIATRIC:* Give lower doses to patients $>$60 y.

### Pharmacokinetics

| *Route* | *Onset* | *Peak* | *Duration* |
|---|---|---|---|
| Oral | Slow | 2–4 h | 2–4 wk |

*Metabolism:* Hepatic; $T_{1/2}$: 20–40 h

*Distribution:* Crosses placenta; passes into breast milk

*Excretion:* Urine and feces

### Adverse effects

- CNS: *Sedation and anticholinergic (atropine-like) effects; confusion* (especially in elderly), *disturbed concentration,* hallucinations, disorientation, decreased memory, feelings of unreality, delusions, anxiety, nervousness, restlessness, agitation, panic, insomnia, nightmares, hypomania, mania, eacerbation of psychosis, drowsiness, weakness, fatigue, headache, numbness, agitation (less likely with this drug than with other antidepressants)
- GI: *Dry mouth, constipation,* paralytic ileus, *nausea* (less likely with this drug than with other antidepressants), vomiting, anorexia, epigastric distress, diarrhea, flatulence, dysphagia, peculiar taste, increased salivation, stomatitits,

glossitis, parotid swelling, abdominal cramps, black tongue, liver enzyme elevations
- **CV**: Orthostatic hypotension, hypertension, syncope, tachycardia, palpitations, MI, arrhythmias, heart block, precipitation of CHF, stroke
- **Hematologic**: *Agranulocytosis, neutropenia*
- **GU**: Urinary retention, delayed micturition, dilation of urinary tract, gynecomastia, testicular swelling in men; breast enlargement, menstrual irregularity, galactorrhea in women; increased or decreased libido; impotence
- **Endocrine**: Elevated or depressed blood sugar; elevated prolactin levels; inappropriate ADH secretion
- **Hypersensitivity**: Skin rash, pruritus, vasculitis, petechiae, photosensitization, edema

## ■ Nursing Considerations

### Assessment
- *History:* Hypersensitivity to any antidepresssant; concomitant therapy with MAOI; recent MI; myelography within previous 24 h or scheduled within 48 h; lactation; ET; preexisting CV disorders; angle-closure glaucoma; increasd intraocular pressure, urinary retention, ureteral or urethral spasm; seizure disorders; hyperthyroidism; impaired hepatic, renal function; psychiatric problems; manic-depressive patients; elective surgery
- *Physical:* Body weight; T; skin color, lesions; orientation, affect, reflexes, vision and hearing; P, BP, orthostatic BP, perfusion; bowel sounds, normal output, liver evaluation; urine flow, normal output; usual sexual function, frequency of menses, breast and scrotal examination; liver function tests, urinalysis, CBC, ECG

### Implementation
- Ensure that depressed and potentially suicidal patients have access only to limited quantities of the drug.
- Expect clinical response in 3–7 d up to 2–3 wk (latter is more usual).
- Arrange for CBC if patient develops fever, sore throat, or other sign of infection during therapy.
- Establish safety precautions if CNS changes occur (siderails, accompany patient when ambulating, etc.).

### Drug-specific teaching points
- Take this drug exactly as prescribed; do not stop taking the drug abruptly or without consulting your physician or nurse.
- Avoid using alcohol, other sleep-inducing drugs, OTC drugs while on this drug.
- Avoid prolonged exposure to sunlight or sunlamps; use a sunscreen or protective garments if long exposure to sunlight is unavoidable.
- The following side effects may occur: headache, dizziness, drowsiness, weakness, blurred vision (reversible; avoid driving or performing tasks that require alertness); nausea, vomiting, loss of appetite, dry mouth (eat small, frequent meals; frequent mouth care and sucking on sugarless candies may help); nightmares, inability to concentrate, confusion; changes in sexual function.
- Report fever, flulike illness, any infection, dry mouth, difficulty urinating, excessive sedation.

# misoprostol

*(mye soe **prost'** ole)*
Cytotec
**Pregnancy Category X**

### Drug classes
Prostaglandin

### Therapeutic actions
A synthetic prostaglandin $E_1$ analog; inhibits gastric acid secretion and increases bicarbonate and mucus production, protecting the lining of the stomach.

### Indications
- Prevention of NSAID (including aspirin)-induced gastric ulcers in patients at high risk of complications from a gastric ulcer

(elderly, patients with concomitant debilitating disease, history of ulcers)
- Unlabeled use: appears effective in treating duodenal ulcers in those patients unresponsive to $H_2$ antagonists

### Contraindications/cautions
- History of allergy to prostaglandins; pregnancy (abortifacient; advise women of childbearing age in written and oral form of use, have a negative serum pregnancy test within 2 wk prior to therapy, provice contraceptives, and begin therapy on the second or third day of the next normal menstrual period); lactation.

### Dosage
**Available Forms:** Tablets—100, 200 μg
*ADULT:* 200 μg four times daily PO with food. If this dose cannot be tolerated, 100 μg can be used. Take misoprostol for the duration of the NSAID therapy. Take the last dose of the day hs.
*PEDIATRIC:* Safety and efficacy in children <18 y not established.
*GERIATRIC OR RENAL IMPAIRED:* Adjustment in dosage is usually not necessary, but dosage can be reduced if 200-μg PO dose cannot be tolerated.

### Pharmacokinetics

| Route | Onset | Peak |
|---|---|---|
| Oral | Rapid | 12–15 min |

*Metabolism:* Hepatic, $T_{1/2}$: 20–40 min
*Distribution:* Crosses placenta; enters breast milk
*Excretion:* Urine

### Adverse effects
- GI: *Nausea, diarrhea, abdominal pain, flatulence,* vomiting, dyspepsia, constipation
- GU: *Miscarriage,* excessive bleeding, death; *spotting, cramping,* hypermenorrhea, menstrual disorders, dysmenorrhea
- Other: Headache

## ■ Nursing Considerations

### Assessment
- *History:* Allergy to prostaglandins, pregnancy, lactation
- *Physical:* Abdominal exam, normal output; urinary output

### Implementation
- Give to patients at high risk for developing NSAID-induced gastric ulcers; give for the full term of the NSAID use.
- Arrange for serum pregnancy test for any woman of childbearing age; must have a negative test within 2 wk of beginning therapy.
- Arrange for oral and written explanation of the risks to pregnancy; appropriate contraceptive measures must be taken; begin therapy on the second or third day of a normal menstrual period.

### Drug-specific teaching points
- Take this drug four times a day, with meals and at bedtime. Continue to take your NSAID while on this drug. Take the drug exactly as prescribed. Do not give this drug to anyone else.
- The following side effects may occur: abdominal pain, nausea, diarrhea, flatulence (take with meals); menstrual cramping, abnormal menstrual periods, spotting, even in postmenopausal women (request analgesics); headache.
- This drug can cause miscarriage, and is often associated with dangerous bleeding. Do not take if pregnant; do not become pregnant while taking this medication. If pregnancy occurs, discontinue drug, and consult physician immediately.
- Report severe diarrhea, spotting or menstrual pain, severe menstrual bleeding, pregnancy.

## mitomycin

*(mye toe **mye'** sin)*
mitomycin-C, MTC
Mutamycin
**Pregnancy Category D**

### Drug classes
Antibiotic
Antineoplastic

m

### Therapeutic actions

Cytotoxic: inhibits DNA synthesis and cellular RNA and protein synthesis in susceptible cells, causing cell death.

### Indications

- Disseminated adenocarcinoma of the stomach or pancreas; part of combination therapy or as palliative measure when other modalities fail
- Unlabeled use: superficial bladder cancer (intravesical route)

### Contraindications/cautions

- Allergy to mitomycin; thrombocytopenia, coagulation disorders, or increase in bleeding tendencies, impaired renal function (creatinine > 17 mg%); myelosuppression; pregnancy; lactation.

### Dosage

**Available Forms:** Powder for injection—5, 20, 40 mg

**ADULT:** *After hematologic recovery from previous chemotherapy, use either of the following schedules at 6 to 8-wk intervals:* 20 mg/m² IV as a single dose or 2 mg/m² per day IV for 5 d followed by a drug-free interval of 2 d, and then by 2 mg/m² per day for 5 d (total of 20 mg/m² for 10 d). Reevaluate patient for hematologic response between courses of therapy; adjust dose accordingly:

| *Leukocytes* | *Platelets* | *% of Prior Dose to Be Given* |
|---|---|---|
| >4000 | >100,000 | 100 |
| 3000–3999 | 75,000–99,999 | 100 |
| 2000–2999 | 25,000–74,999 | 70 |
| <2000 | <25,000 | 50 |

Do not repeat dosage until leukocyte count has returned to 3,000/mm³ and platelet count to 75,000/mm³.

### Pharmacokinetics

| *Route* | *Onset* | *Peak* |
|---|---|---|
| IV | Slow | Unknown |

*Metabolism:* Hepatic, $T_{1/2}$: 17 min
*Distribution:* Crosses placenta; enters breast milk
*Excretion:* Urine

### IV facts

**Preparation:** Reconstitute 5 to 20-mg vial with 10 or 40 ml of Sterile Water for Injection, respectively; if product does not dissolve immediately, allow to stand at room temperature until solution is obtained. This solution is stable for 14 d if refrigerated, 7 d at room temperature; further dilution in various IV fluids reduces stability—check manufacturer's insert.

**Infusion:** Infuse slowly over 5–10 min; monitor injection site to avoid local reaction.

### Adverse effects

- CNS: Headache, blurred vision, confusion, drowsiness, syncope, fatigue
- GI: *Anorexia, nausea, vomiting,* diarrhea, hematemesis, stomatitis
- Respiratory: **Pulmonary toxicity**
- Hematologic: *Bone marrow toxicity,* microangiopathic hemolytic anemia (a syndrome of anemia, thrombocytopenia, renal failure, hypertension)
- GU: Renal toxicity
- Other: *Fever,* cancer in preclinical studies, *cellulitis at injection site, alopecia*

## ■ Nursing Considerations

### Assessment

- *History:* Allergy to mitomycin; thrombocytopenia, coagulation disorders or increase in bleeding tendencies, impaired renal function; myelosuppression; pregnancy; lactation
- *Physical:* T; skin color, lesions; weight; hair; local injection site; orientation, reflexes; R, adventitious sounds; mucus membranes; CBC, clotting tests, renal function tests

### Implementation

- Do not give IM or SC due to severe local reaction and tissue necrosis.

- Monitor injection site for extravasation: reports of burning or stinging; discontinue infusion immediately and restart in another vein.
- Monitor response frequently at beginning of therapy (CBC, renal function tests, pulmonary exam); adverse effects may require a decreased dose or discontinuation of drug; consult with physician.

### Drug-specific teaching points

- Prepare a calendar with return dates for drug therapy; this drug can only be given IV.
- The following side effects may occur: rash, skin lesions, loss of hair (obtain a wig; skin care may help); loss of appetite, nausea, mouth sores (frequent mouth care, small frequent meals may help; maintain good nutrition; consult a dietician; request an antiemetic); drowsiness, dizziness, syncope, headache (use caution driving or operating dangerous machinery; take special precautions to prevent injuries).
- Have regular medical follow-ups, including blood tests to monitor drug's effects.
- Report difficulty breathing, sudden weight gain, swelling, burning or pain at injection site, unusual bleeding or bruising.

## mitotane

*(mye' toe tane)*

o, p' - DDD

Lysodren

**Pregnancy Category C**

### Drug classes

Antineoplastic
Adrenal cytotoxic drug

### Therapeutic actions

Acts by unknown mechanism to reduce plasma and urinary levels of adrenocorticosteroids; selectively cytotoxic to normal and neoplastic adrenal cortical cells.

### Indications

- Treatment of inoperable adrenal cortical carcinoma, functional (hormone-secreting) and nonfunctional

### Contraindications/cautions

- Contraindications: allergy to mitotane, lactation.
- Use cautiously with impaired liver function, pregnancy.

### Dosage

**Available Forms:** Tablets—500 mg

ADULT: Institute therapy in a hospital. Start at 2–6 g/d PO in divided doses tid or qid. Increase dose incrementally to 9–10 g/d. If severe side effects occur, reduce to maximum tolerated dose (2–16 g/d), usually 9–10 g/d. Continue therapy as long as benefits are observed. If no clinical benefits are seen after 3 mo, consider the case a clinical failure.

### Pharmacokinetics

| Route | Onset | Peak | Duration |
|---|---|---|---|
| Oral | Slow | Varies | 10 wk |

*Metabolism:* Hepatic, $T_{1/2}$: 18–159 d
*Distribution:* Crosses placenta; may enter breast milk
*Excretion:* Urine and bile

### Adverse effects

- CNS: *Depression, sedation, lethargy, vertigo, dizziness*, visual blurring, diplopia, lens opacity, toxic retinopathy, brain damage and possible behavioral and neurologic changes (therapy longer than 2 y)
- GI: *Nausea, vomiting, diarrhea, anorexia*
- CV: Hypertension, orthostatic hypotension, flushing
- GU: Hematuria, hemorrhagic cystitis, proteinuria
- Endocrine: *Adrenal insufficiency*
- Other: *Rash*, fever, generalized aching

### Drug-lab test interferences

- Decreased levels of PBI, urinary 17-hydroxycorticsteroids

## ■ Nursing Considerations

### Assessment
- ***History:*** Allergy to mitotane; impaired liver function; lactation
- ***Physical:*** Weight, skin integrity; orientation, affect, vestibular nerve function, ophthalmologic exam; BP, P, orthostatic BP; bowel sounds, output; liver and renal function tests, urinalysis, plasma cortisol, serum electrolytes

### Implementation
- Large metastatic tumor masses are usually removed surgically before therapy to minimize risk of tumor infarction and hemorrhage.
- Administer cautiously with impaired liver function; drug metabolism may be impaired, and drug may accumulate to toxic levels if usual dosage is continued.
- Monitor for adrenal insufficiency; adrenal steroid replacement therapy may be necessary.

### Drug-specific teaching points
- Have frequent follow-ups and monitoring.
- Use contraceptives during therapy; this drug can cause birth defects or fetal death.
- The following side effects may occur: dizziness, drowsiness, tiredness (avoid driving or performing hazardous tasks); nausea, vomiting, diarrhea (small, frequent meals, proper nutrition may help); aching muscles, fever (request medication).
- Report severe nausea, vomiting, loss of appetite, diarrhea, aching muscles, muscle twitching, fever, flushing, emotional depression, rash or darkening of skin.

# mitoxantrone hydrochloride

*(mye toe **zan'** trone)*

Novantrone

**Pregnancy Category D**

### Drug classes
Antineoplastic

### Therapeutic actions
Cytotoxic; cell cycle nonspecific, appears to be DNA reactive, causing the death of both proliferating and nonproliferting cells.

### Indications
- As part of combination therapy in the treatment of ANLL in adults, including myelogenous, promyelocytic, monocytic and erythroid acute leukemias
- Treatment of bone pain in patients with advanced prostatic cancer, in combination with steroids
- Unlabeled uses: treatment of breast cancer, refractory lymphomas

### Contraindications/cautions
- Contraindications: hypersensitivity to mitoxantrone
- Use cautiously with bone marrow suppression, CHF, pregnancy, lactation

### Dosage
**Available Forms:** Injection—2 mg

ADULT
- ***Combination therapy:*** For induction, 12 $mg/m^2$ per day on days 1–3, with 100 $mg/m^2$ of cytosine arabinoside for 7 d given as a continuous infusion on days 1–7. If remission does not occur a second series can be used, with mitoxantrone given for 2 d and cytosine arabinoside for 5 d.
- ***Consolidation therapy:*** Mitoxantrone 12 $mg/m^2$ IV for days 1 and 2, and cytosine arabinoside 100 $mg/m^2$ given as a continuous 24-h infusion on days 1–5; given 6 wk after induction therapy if needed. Severe myelosuppression may occur.

PEDIATRIC: Safety and efficacy not established.

### Pharmacokinetics

| *Route* | *Onset* | *Duration* |
|---|---|---|
| IV | Rapid | 2–3 d |

*Metabolism:* Hepatic, $T_{1/2}$: 5.8 d
*Distribution:* Crosses placenta; may enter breast milk
*Excretion:* Bile and urine

### IV facts
**Preparation:** Dilute solution to at least 50 ml in either 0.9% Sodium Chloride In-

jection or 5% Dextrose Injection; may be further diluted in Dextrose 5% in Water, Normal Saline, or Dextrose 5% in Normal Saline if needed. Inject this solution into tubing of a freely running IV of 0.9% Sodium Chloride Injection or 5% Dextrose Injection over period of at least 3 min. Use immediately after dilution and discard any leftover solution immediately. Wear gloves and goggles and avoid any contact with skin or mucous membranes.

**Infusion:** Inject slowly over at least 3 min.

**Compatibilities:** *Do not mix in solution with heparin*; a precipitate may form. Do not mix in solution with any other drug; studies are not yet available regarding the safety of such mixtures.

### Adverse effects

- CNS: Headache, seizures,
- GI: *Nausea, vomiting, diarrhea,* abdominal pain, mucositis, GI bleeding, jaundice
- CV: **CHF,** arrhythmias, chest pain
- Hematologic: **Bone marrow depression,** *infections of all kinds, hyperuricemia*
- Pulmonary: *Cough,* dyspnea
- Other: *Fever, alopecia, cancer in laboratory animals*

## ■ Nursing Considerations

### Assessment

- *History:* Hypersensitivity to mitoxantrone, bone marrow depression; CHF; pregnancy, lactation
- *Physical:* Neurologic status, T; P, BP, auscultation, peripheral perfusion; R, adventitious sounds; abdominal exam, mucous membranes; liver function tests, CBC with differential

### Implementation

- Follow CBC and liver function tests carefully before and frequently during therapy; dose adjustment may be needed if myelosuppression becomes severe.
- Monitor patient for hyperuricemia, which frequently occurs as a result of rapid tumor lysis; monitor serum uric acid levels and arrange for appropriate treatment as needed.
- Handle drug with great care; the use of gloves, gowns, and goggles is recommended; if drug comes in contact with skin, wash immediately with warm water; clean spills with calcium hypochlorite solution.
- Monitor IV site for signs of extravasation; if extravasation occurs, stop administration and restart at another site immediately.
- Monitor BP, P, cardiac output regularly during administration; supportive care for CHF should be started at the first sign of failure.
- Protect patient from exposure to infection; monitor occurrence of infection at any site and arrange for appropriate treatment.

### Drug-specific teaching points

- This drug will need to be given IV for 3 d in conunction with cytosine therapy; mark calendar with days of treatment. Regular blood tests will be needed to evaluate the effects of this treatment.
- The following side effects may occur: nausea, vomiting (may be severe; antiemetics may be helpful; eat small, frequent meals); increased susceptibility to infection (avoid crowds and exposure to disease); loss of hair (obtain a wig; it is important to keep the head covered in extremes of temperature); blue-green color of the urine (may last for 24 h after treatment is finished; the whites of the eyes may also be tinted blue for a time; this is expected and will pass).
- Report severe nausea and vomiting; fever, chills, sore throat; unusual bleeding or bruising; fluid retention or swelling; severe joint pain.

## moexipril

*(mox **ex'** ah pril)*

Univasc

**Pregnancy Category D, second and third trimesters**

**Pregnancy Category C, first trimester**

## Drug classes

Antihypertensive
Angiotensin converting enzyme inhibitor (ACE inhibitor)

## Therapeutic actions

Renin, synthesized by the kidneys, is released into the circulation where it acts on a plasma precursor to produce angiotensin I, which is converted by angiotensin converting enzyme to angiotensin II, a potent vasoconstrictor that also causes release of aldosterone from the adrenals. Both of these actions increase BP; moexipril blocks the conversion of angiotensin I to angiotensin II, leading to decreased BP, decreased aldosterone secretion, a small increase in serum potassium levels, and sodium and fluid loss; increased prostaglandin synthesis may also be involved in the antihypertensive action.

## Indications

- Treatment of hypertension, alone or in combination with thiazide-type diuretics

## Contraindications/cautions

- Contraindications: allergy to ACE inhibitors; impaired renal function; CHF; salt or volume depletion, lactation.

## Dosage

**Available Forms:** Tablets—7.5, 15 mg

**ADULT:** Not receiving diuretics: initially, 7.5 mg PO qd, given 1h before a meal; maintenance–7.5–30 mg PO qd or in 1–2 divided doses given 1h before meals. Receiving diuretics: discontinue diuretic for 2–3 days before beginning moexipril; follow dosage listed above, if BP is not controlled, diuretic therapy may be added. If diuretic cannot be stopped, start moexipril therapy with 3.75 mg and monitor for symptomatic hypotension.

**PEDIATRIC:** Safety and efficacy not established.

**GERIATRIC AND RENAL IMPAIRED:** Excretion is reduced in renal failure; use with caution, if Ccr $\geq$ 40 ml/min/1.73 m$^2$ start with 3.75 mg PO qd, titrate up to a maximum of 15 mg/day.

## Pharmacokinetics

| Route | Onset | Peak | Duration |
|---|---|---|---|
| PO | 1 h | 3–4 h | 24 h |

*Metabolism* : $T_{1/2}$: 2–9 h
*Distribution* : Crosses placenta; passes into breast milk
*Excretion* : Urine

## Adverse effects

- CV: *Tachycardia,* angina pectoris, **myocardial infarction,** Raynaud's syndrome, CHF, hypotension in salt- or volume-depleted patients
- GI: *Gastric irritation, aphthous ulcers, peptic ulcers, diarrhea, dysgeusia,* cholestatic jaundice, hepatocellular injury, anorexia, constipation
- **Hematologic**: Neutropenia, agranulocytosis, thrombocytopenia, hemolytic anemia, **fatal pancytopenia**
- GU: *Proteinuria,* renal insufficiency, renal failure, polyuria, oliguria, urinary frequency
- **Skin**: *Rash, pruritus, flushing,* scalded mouth sensation, exfoliative dermatitis, photosensitivity, alopecia
- **Other**: *Cough,* malaise, dry mouth, lymphadenopathy, *flulike syndrome, dizziness*

## Clinically important drug-drug interactions

• Increased risk of hyperkalemia with K supplements, K sparing diuretics, salt substitutes • Risk of excessive hypotension with diuretics • Risk of abnormal response with lithium

## Drug-lab test interferences

- False-positive test for urine acetone

# ■ Nursing Considerations

## Assessment

- ***History:*** Allergy to ACE inhibitors; impaired renal function; CHF; salt or volume depletion; pregnancy; lactation
- ***Physical:*** Skin color, lesions, turgor; T; P, BP, peripheral perfusion; mucous membranes, bowel sounds, liver evalua-

tion; urinalysis, renal and liver function tests, CBC and differential

### Implementation

- Alert surgeon and mark patient's chart with notice that moexipril is being taken; the angiotensin II formation subsequent to compensatory renin release during surgery will be blocked; hypotension may be reversed with volume expansion.
- Monitor patient closely for a falll in BP secondary to reduction in fluid volume from excessive perspiration and dehydration, vomiting, or diarrhea; excessive hypotension may occur. Monitor K levels carefully in patients receiving K supplements, using K-sparing diuretics or salt substitutes.
- Reduce dosage in patients with impaired renal function.
- Monitor for excessive hypotension with any diuretic therapy.

### Drug-specific teaching points

- Do not stop taking this drug without consulting your physician.
- The following side effects may occur: GI upset, diarrhea, loss of appetite, change in taste perception; mouth sores (frequent mouth care may help); skin rash; fast heart rate; dizziness, lightheadedness (transient; change position slowly and limit activities to those that do not require alertness and precision).
- Be careful in any situation that may lead to a drop in blood pressure (diarrhea, sweating, vomiting, dehydration); if lightheadedness or dizziness occurs, consult your health care provider.
- Report mouth sores; sore throat, fever, chills; swelling of the hands or feet; irregular heartbeat, chest pains; swelling of the face, eyes, lips, tongue; difficulty breathing; leg cramps.

## molindone hydrochloride

*(moe **lin'** done)*

Moban

**Pregnancy Category C**

### Drug classes

Dopaminergic blocking agent
Antipsychotic

### Therapeutic actions

Mechanism of action not fully understood: antipsychotic drugs block postsynaptic dopamine receptors in the brain, but this may not be necessary and sufficient for antipsychotic activity; clinically resembles the piperazine phenothiazines (fluphenazine).

### Indications

- Management of manifestations of psychotic disorders

### Contraindications/cautions

- Contraindications: coma or severe CNS depression, bone marrow depression, blood dyscrasia, circulatory collapse, subcortical brain damage, Parkinson's disease, liver damage, cerebral arteriosclerosis, coronary disease, severe hypotension or hypertension.
- Use cautiously with respiratory disorders ("silent pneumonia"); glaucoma, prostatic hypertrophy; epilepsy or history of epilepsy (drug lowers seizure threshold); breast cancer (elevations in prolactin may stimulate a prolactin-dependent tumor); thyrotoxicosis; peptic ulcer, decreased renal function; exposure to heat or phosphorous insecticides; pregnancy; lactation; children <12 y, especially those with chickenpox, CNS infections (children are especially susceptible to dystonias that may confound the diagnosis of Reye's syndrome).

### Dosage

**Available Forms:** Tablets—5, 10, 25, 50, 100 mg; concentrate—20 mg/ml

**Adult:** Initially 50–75 mg/d PO increased to 100 mg/d in 3–4 d. Individualize dosage; severe symptoms may require up to 225 mg/d. *Maintenance therapy:* mild symptoms, 5–15 mg PO tid–qid; moderate symptoms, 10–25 mg PO tid–qid; severe symptoms, 225 mg/d.

**Pediatric:** Not recommended for children <12 y.

**Geriatric:** Use lower doses and increase dosage more gradually than in younger patients.

m

## Pharmacokinetics

| Route | Onset | Peak | Duration |
|---|---|---|---|
| Oral | Varies | 1 1/2 h | 24–36 h |

*Metabolism:* Hepatic, $T_{1/2}$: 1.5 h
*Distribution:* Crosses placenta; enters breast milk
*Excretion:* Urine and feces

## Adverse effects

*Antipsychotic Drugs*

- CNS: *Drowsiness*, insomnia, vertigo, headache, weakness, tremor, ataxia, slurring, cerebral edema, seizures, exacerbation of psychotic symptoms, extrapyramidal syndromes—*pseudoparkinsonism; dystonias; akathisia*, tardive dyskinesias, potentially irreversible (no known treatment), **NMS**—extrapyramidal symptoms, hyperthermia, autonomic disturbances (rare, but 20% fatal)
- CV: Hypotension, orthostatic hypotension, hypertension, tachycardia, bradycardia, cardiac arrest, CHF, cardiomegaly, **refractory arrhythmias**, pulmonary edema
- Respiratory: Bronchospasm, laryngospasm, dyspnea; suppression of cough reflex and potential for aspiration (sudden death related to **asphyxia** or **cardiac arrest**)
- Hematologic: Eosinophilia, leukopenia, leukocytosis, anemia; aplastic anemia; hemolytic anemia; thrombocytopenic or nonthrombocytopenic purpura
- Hypersensitivity: Jaundice, urticaria, angioneurotic edema, laryngeal edema, eczema, asthma, anaphylactoid reactions, exfoliative dermatitis
- Endocrine: Lactation, breast engorgement, galactorrhea; SIADH; amenorrhea, menstrual irregularities; gynecomastia; changes in libido; hyperglycemia or hypoglycemia; glycosuria; hyponatremia; pituitary tumor with hyperprolactinemia; inhibition of ovulation, infertility, pseudopregnancy; reduced urinary levels of gonadotropins, estrogens, progestins
- Autonomic: Dry mouth, salivation, nasal congestion, nausea, vomiting, anorexia, fever, pallor, flushed facies, sweating, constipation, paralytic ileus, urinary retention, incontinence, polyuria, enuresis, priapism, ejaculation inhibition, male impotence

## Clinically important drug-drug interactions

• Decreased absorption of oral phenytoin, tetracycline

## Drug-lab test interferences

• False-positive pregnancy tests (less likely if serum test is used) • Increase in PBI, not attributable to an increase in thyroxine

## ■ Nursing Considerations

### Assessment

- *History:* Coma or severe CNS depression; bone marrow depression; circulatory collapse; subcortical brain damage; Parkinson's disease; liver damage; cerebral arteriosclerosis; coronary disease; severe hypotension or hypertension; respiratory disorders; glaucoma, prostatic hypertrophy; epilepsy; breast cancer; thyrotoxicosis; peptic ulcer, decreased renal function; exposure to heat or phosphorous insecticides; pregnancy; lactation; children $< 12$ y
- *Physical:* Weight, T; reflexes, orientation, intraocular pressure; P, BP, orthostatic BP; R, adventitious sounds; bowel sounds and normal output, liver evaluation; urinary output, prostate size; CBC, urinalysis, thyroid, liver and kidney function tests

### Implementation

- Discontinue drug if serum creatinine, BUN become abnormal or if WBC count is depressed.
- Monitor elderly for dehydration, and institute remedial measures promptly; sedation and decreased sensation of thirst related to CNS effects can lead to severe dehydration.
- Consult physician regarding appropriate warning of patient or patient's guardian about tardive dyskinesias.

- Consult physician about dosage reduction, use of anticholinergic antiparkinsonian drugs (controversial) if extrapyramidal effects occur.

### Drug-specific teaching points

- Take drug exactly as prescribed.
- Avoid driving or engaging in other dangerous activities if CNS, vision changes occur.
- Maintain fluid intake, and use precautions against heatstroke in hot weather.
- Report sore throat, fever, unusual bleeding or bruising, rash, weakness, tremors, impaired vision, dark urine (pink or reddish brown urine is to be expected), pale stools, yellowing of the skin or eyes.

## monoctanoin

*(mon ok ta **no'** in)*
Moctanin
**Pregnancy Category C**

### Drug classes

Gallstone solubilizing agent

### Therapeutic actions

An esterified glycerol that solubilizes cholesterol gallstones in the biliary tract.

### Indications

- Dissolution of cholesterol gallstones retained in the biliary tract following cholecystectomy when other means of stone removal have failed or are contraindicated
- Orphan drug use: dissolution of cholesterol gallstones retained in the common bile duct

### Contraindications/cautions

- Allergy to monoctanoin; hepatic dysfunction, clinical jaundice, biliary tract infection; recent duodenal ulcer; recent jejunitis; pregnancy; lactation.

### Dosage

**Available Forms:** Infusion—120 ml

**ADULT:** 3–5 ml/h on a 24-h basis at a pressure of 10 cm $H_2O$ as a continuous perfusion through a catheter inserted directly into the common bile duct. Therapy is continued for 7–21 d.

**PEDIATRIC:** Safety and efficacy not established.

### Pharmacokinetics

Metabolized to fatty acids and glycerol, which are absorbed into the portal vein. Not absorbed systemically.

### Adverse effects

- GI: *GI pain/discomfort, nausea, vomiting, diarrhea*, anorexia, indigestion, burning, gastric, duodenal and bile duct irritation
- **Hematologic**: Leukopenia, metabolic acidosis
- **Other**: *Fever*, pruritus, fatigue/lethargy

## ■ Nursing Considerations

### Assessment

- *History:* Allergy to monoctanoin; hepatic dysfunction, clinical jaundice, biliary tract infection; recent duodenal ulcer; recent jejunitis; pregnancy; lactation
- *Physical:* T; liver evaluation, abdominal exam; liver function tests, CBC

m

### Implementation

- Do not administer IV or IM.
- Administer drug as a continuous perfusion through a catheter inserted directly into the common bile duct using a perfusion pump that does not exceed perfusion pressure of 15 cm $H_2O$. Administration may be interrupted during meals.
- Warm monoctanoin to 60–80°F before perfusion.
- Continue administration for 7–21 d if periodic x-rays show response to therapy.
- Discontinue drug and consult with physician if fever, chills, leukocytosis, upper right quadrant pain, or jaundice occurs.
- Arrange for periodic, regular monitoring of liver function tests.
- Schedule periodic oral cholecystograms or ultrasonograms to evaluate drug effectiveness.
- Arrange for outpatients to have the use of battery-operated infusion pumps and home follow-up.

### Drug-specific teaching points

- This drug should be continually perfused through an infusion pump. Infusion can be interrupted during meals.
- This drug may dissolve your gallstones. It does not "cure" the underlying problem. In many cases the stones can recur; medical follow-up is important.
- Obtain periodic x-rays or ultrasound tests of your gallbladder. Obtain periodic blood tests to evaluate drug response.
- Abdominal pain/discomfort and GI upset may occur; small, frequent meals may help.
- Report fever, chills, upper right quadrant pain, yellowing of skin or eyes, rapid, difficult breathing.

## moricizine hydrochloride

*(mor i' siz een)*

Ethmozine

**Pregnancy Category B**

### Drug classes

Antiarrhythmic

### Therapeutic actions

Type I antiarrhythmic with potent local anesthetic acitivity; decreases diastolic depolarization, decreasing automaticity of ventricular cells; increases ventricular fibrillation threshold.

### Indications

- Treatment of documented ventricular arrhythmias, such as sustained ventricular tachycardias, that are deemed to be life threatening; because of proarrhythmic effects, reserve use for patients in whom the benefit outweighs the risk

### Contraindications/cautions

- Contraindications: hypersensitivity to moricizine; preexisiting second or third-degree AV block; right bundle branch block when associated with left hemiblock (unless a pacemaker is present), cardiogenic shock, CHF; pregnancy; lactation.
- Use cautiously with sick sinus syndrome, hepatic or renal impairment.

### Dosage

**Available Forms:** Tablets—200, 250, 300 mg

*ADULT:* 600–900 mg/d PO, given q8h in three equally divided doses. Adjust dosage within this range in increments of 150 mg/d at 3-d intervals until the desired effect is seen. Patients with good response may be retained on the same dosage at q12h intervals instead of q8h if this is more convenient. Patients with malignant arrhythmias who respond well may be maintained on long-term therapy.

- ***Transfer from another antiarrhythmic:*** Withdraw previous antiarrhythmic for 1–2 half-lives before starting moricizine therapy. Hospitalize patients in whom withdrawal may precipitate serious arrhythmias. Transferring from quinidine, disopyramide, start moricizine 6–12 h after last dose; procainamide, start moricizine 3–6 h after last dose; encainide, propafenone, tocainide, mexiletine, start moricizine 8–12 h after last dose.

*PEDIATRIC:* Safety and efficacy not established for children <18 y.

*GERIATRIC OR HEPATIC IMPAIRED:* Start < 600 mg/d, and monitor closely, including measurement of ECG intervals, before adjusting dosage.

### Pharmacokinetics

| *Route* | *Onset* | *Peak* | *Duration* |
|---|---|---|---|
| Oral | 2 h | 1/2–2 h | 10–24 h |

*Metabolism:* Hepatic, $T_{1/2}$: 1.5–3.5 h
*Distribution:* Crosses placenta; enters breast milk
*Excretion:* Urine

### Adverse effects

- CNS: *Headache, dizziness, fatigue, hypoesthesias, asthenia, nervousness, sleep disorders,* tremor, anxiety, depression, euphoria, confusion, seizure, nystagmus, ataxia, loss of memory
- GI: *Nausea, vomiting, diarrhea, abdominal pain, dyspepsia,* flatulence, anorexia, bitter taste, ileus

- CV: *Arrhythmias, palpitations, ventricular tachycardia, CHF,* ***death*** (up to 5% occurence), *conduction defects, heart block, hypotension,* ***cardiac arrest****, MI*
- GU: Urinary retention, dysuria, urinary incontinence, kidney pain, impotence
- Respiratory: *Dyspnea,* hyperventilation, apnea, asthma, pharyngitis, cough, sinusitis
- Other: Sweating, muscle pain, dry mouth, blurred vision, fever

**Clinically important drug-drug interactions**

• Increased serum levels of moricizine with cimetidine • Increased risk of heart block with digoxin, propranolol • Decreased serum levels and therapeutic effects of theophylline

## ■ Nursing Considerations

### Assessment

- *History:* Hypersensitivity to moricizine; preexisiting second or third-degree AV block; right bundle branch block associated with left hemiblock; cardiogenic shock, CHF; sick sinus syndrome; hepatic or renal impairment; lactation
- *Physical:* T; reflexes, affect; BP, P, ECG including interval monitoring, exercise testing; R, auscultation; abdominal exam, normal output; urinary output; liver and renal function tests, serum electrolytes

### Implementation

- Administer only to patients with life threatening arrhythmias who do not respond to conventional therapy and in whom the benefits outweigh the risks.
- Correct electrolyte disturbances (hypokalemia, hyperkalemia, hypomagnesemia), which may alter the effects of class I antiarrhythmics, before therapy.
- Patient should be hospitalized and monitored continually during start of therapy.
- Reduce dosage for patients with hepatic failure.
- Maintain life support equipment and vasopressor agents on standby in case of severe reactions or generation of arrhythmias.
- Administer with food if severe GI upset occurs; food delays but does not change peak serum levels.
- Frequently monitor heart rhythm, including ECG intervals during long-term therapy.

### Drug-specific teaching points

- Take drug exactly as prescribed. Arrange schedule to decrease interruptions in your day.
- Frequent monitoring will be necessary to determine the drug effects on your heart and to determine the dosage needed. Keep appointments for these tests, which may include Holter monitoring, stress tests.
- The following side effects may occur: arrhythmias or abnormal heart rhythm (hospitalization is required to start drug therapy and to monitor drug response until dosage is determined and stabilized); dizziness, headache, fatigue, nervousness (avoid driving or performing hazardous tasks); nausea, vomiting, diarrhea (eat small, frequent meals; maintain proper nutrition); cough, difficulty breathing, sweating.
- Report palpitations, lethargy, vomiting, difficulty breathing, edema of the extremities, chest pain.

m

## morphine sulfate

***(mor' feen)***

*Immediate-release tablets:* MSIR

*Timed-release:* Kadian, MS Contin, MS Contin II, Roxanol SR, Oramorph

*Oral solution:* Roxanol Rescudose

*Rectal suppositories:* RMS, MS/S, Roxanol

*Injection:* Astramorph PF, Duramorph, Epimorph (CAN)

*Concentrate for microinfusion devices for intraspinal use:* Infumorph

*Oral solution:* MS/L, MS/L concentrate, OMS concentrate

**Pregnancy Category C**

**C-II controlled substance**

**Drug classes**
Narcotic agonist analgesic

**Therapeutic actions**
Principal opium alkaloid; acts as agonist at specific opioid receptors in the CNS to produce analgesia, euphoria, sedation; the receptors mediating these effects are thought to be the same as those mediating the effects of endogenous opioids (enkephalins, endorphins).

**Indications**
- Relief of moderate to severe acute and chronic pain
- Preoperative medication to sedate and allay apprehension, facilitate induction of anesthesia, and reduce anesthetic dosage
- Analgesic adjunct during anesthesia
- Component of most preparations that are referred to as Brompton's Cocktail or Mixture, an oral alcoholic solution that is used for chronic severe pain, especially in terminal cancer patients
- Intraspinal use with microinfusion devices for the relief of intractable pain
- Unlabeled use: dyspnea associated with acute left ventricular failure and pulmonary edema

**Contraindications/cautions**
- Contraindications: hypersensitivity to narcotics; diarrhea caused by poisoning until toxins are eliminated; during labor or delivery of a premature infant (may cross immature blood–brain barrier more readily); after biliary tract surgery or following surgical anastomosis; pregnancy; labor (respiratory depression in neonate, may prolong labor).
- Use cautiously with head injury and increased intracranial pressure; acute asthma, COPD, cor pulmonale, preexisting respiratory depression, hypoxia, hypercapnia (may decrease respiratory drive and increase airway resistance); lactation (wait 4–6 h after administration to nurse the baby); acute abdominal conditions, CV disease, supraventricular tachycardias, myxedema, convulsive disorders, acute alcoholism, delirium tremens, cerebral arteriosclerosis, ulcerative colitis, fever, kyphoscoliosis, Addison's disease, prostatic hypertrophy, urethral stricture, recent GI or GU surgery, toxic psychosis, renal or hepatic dysfunction.

**Dosage**
**Available Forms:** Injection—0.5, 1, 2, 3, 4, 5, 8, 10, 15 mg/ml; tablets—15, 30 mg; CR tablets—15, 20, 50, 60, 100, 200 mg; SR tablets—30, 60, 100 mg; solution—20 mg/ml; oral solution—10, 100 mg/5 ml; suppositories—5, 10, 20, 30 mg

ADULT
- ***Oral:*** 1/3 to 1/6 as effective as parenteral administration because of first-pass metabolism; 10–30 mg q4h PO. *Controlled-release:* 30 mg q8–12h PO or as directed by physician; Kadian: 20–100 mg PO qd–24-h release system
- ***SC/IM:*** 10 mg (5–20 mg)/70 kg q4h or as directed by physician.
- ***IV:*** 2.5–15 mg/70 kg in 4–5 ml Water for Injection administered over 4–5 min, or as directed by physician. *Continuous IV infusion:* 0.1–1 mg/ml in 5% Dextrose in Water by controlled infusion device.
- ***Rectal:*** 10–20 mg q4h or as directed by physician.
- ***Epidural:*** Initial injection of 5 mg in the lumbar region may provide pain relief for up to 24 h. If adequate pain relief is not achieved within 1 h, incremental doses of 1–2 mg may be given at intervals sufficient to assess effectiveness, up to 10 mg/24 h. For continuous infusion, initial dose of 2–4 mg/24 h is recommended. Further doses of 1–2 mg may be given if pain relief is not achieved initially.
- ***Intrathecal:*** Dosage is usually 1/10 that of epidural dosage; a single injection of 0.2–1 mg may provide satisfactory pain relief for up to 24 h. Do not inject more than 2 ml of the 5 mg/10 ml ampule or more than 1 ml of the 10 mg/10 ml ampule. Use only in the lumbar area. Repeated intrathecal injections are not recommended; use other routes if pain recurs.

PEDIATRIC: Do not use in premature infants.
- ***SC/IM:*** 0.1–0.2 mg/kg (up to 15 mg) q4h or as directed by physician.

GERIATRIC OR IMPAIRED ADULT: Use caution. Respiratory depression may occur in the elderly, the very ill, those with respiratory problems. Reduced dosage may be necessary.

- ***Epidural:*** Use extreme caution; injection of <5 mg in the lumbar region may provide adequate pain relief for up to 24 h.
- ***Intrathecal:*** Use lower dosages than recommended for adults above.

### Pharmacokinetics

| Route | Onset | Peak | Duration |
|---|---|---|---|
| Oral | Varies | 60 min | 5–7 h |
| tPR | Rapid | 20–60 min | 5–7 h |
| SC | Rapid | 50–90 min | 5–7 h |
| IM | Rapid | 30–60 min | 5–6 h |
| IV | Immediate | 20 min | 5–6 h |

*Metabolism:* Hepatic; $T_{1/2}$: 1.5–2 h
*Distribution:* Crosses placenta; enters breast milk
*Excretion:* Urine and bile

### IV facts

**Preparation:** No further preparation needed for direct injection; prepare infusion by adding 0.1–1 mg/ml to 5% Dextrose in Water.

**Infusion:** Inject slowly directly IV or into tubing of running IV, each 15 mg over 4–5 min; monitor by controlled infusion device to maintain pain control.

### Adverse effects

- CNS: *Lightheadedness, dizziness, sedation,* euphoria, dysphoria, delirium, insomnia, agitation, anxiety, fear, hallucinations, disorientation, drowsiness, lethargy, impaired mental and physical performance, coma, mood changes, weakness, headache, tremor, convulsions, miosis, visual disturbances, suppression of cough reflex
- GI: *Nausea, vomiting,* dry mouth, anorexia, constipation, biliary tract spasm; increased colonic motility in patients with chronic ulcerative colitis
- CV: Facial flushing, peripheral circulatory collapse, tachycardia, bradycardia, arrhythmia, palpitations, chest wall rigidity, hypertension, hypotension, orthostatic hypotension, syncope
- GU: Ureteral spasm, spasm of vesical sphincters, urinary retention or hesitancy, oliguria, antidiuretic effect, reduced libido or potency
- Dermatologic: Pruritus, urticaria, laryngospasm, bronchospasm, edema
- Local: Tissue irritation and induration (SC injection)
- Major hazards: **Respiratory depression, apnea, circulatory depression, respiratory arrest, shock, cardiac arrest**
- Other: *Sweating,* physical tolerance and dependence, psychological dependence

### Clinically important drug-drug interactions

- Increased likelihood of respiratory depression, hypotension, profound sedation or coma in patients receiving barbiturate general anesthetics

### Drug-lab test interferences

- Elevated biliary tract pressure (an effect of narcotics) may cause increases in plasma amylase, lipase; determinations of these levels may be unreliable for 24 h

## ■ Nursing Considerations

### Assessment

- *History:* Hypersensitivity to narcotics; diarrhea cuased by poisoning; labor or delivery of a premature infant; biliary tract surgery or surgical anastomosis; head injury and increased intracranial pressure; acute asthma, COPD, cor pulmonale, preexisting respiratory depression; acute abdominal conditions, CV disease, supraventricular tachycardias, myxedema, convulsive disorders, acute alcoholism, delirium tremens, cerebral arteriosclerosis, ulcerative colitis, fever, kyphoscoliosis, Addison's disease, prostatic hyperetrophy, urethral stricture, recent GI or GU surgery, toxic psychosis, renal or hepatic dysfunction; pregnancy; lactation
- *Physical:* T; skin color, texture, lesions; orientation, reflexes, bilateral grip

m

strength, affect; P, auscultation, BP, orthostatic BP, perfusion; R, adventitious sounds; bowel sounds, normal output; urinary frequency, voiding pattern, normal output; ECG; EEG; thyroid, liver, kidney function tests

### Implementation

- Caution patient not to chew or crush controlled-release preparations.
- Dilute and administer slowly IV to minimize likelihood of adverse effects.
- Direct patient to lie down during IV administation.
- Provide narcotic antagonist, facilities for assisted or controlled respiration on standby during IV administration.
- Use caution when injecting SC or IM into chilled areas or in patients with hypotension or in shock; impaired perfusion may delay absorption; with repeated doses, an excessive amount may be absorbed when circulation is restored.
- Reassure patient about addiction liability; most patients who receive opiates for medical reasons do not develop dependence syndromes.

### Drug-specific teaching points

- Take this drug exactly as prescribed. Avoid alcohol, antihistamines, sedatives, tranquilizers, OTC drugs.
- The following side effects may occur: nausea, loss of appetite (take with food, lie quietly); constipation (use laxative); dizziness, sedation, drowsiness, impaired visual acuity (avoid driving or performing tasks that require alertness and visual acuity).
- Do not take leftover medication for other disorders, and do not let anyone else take your prescription.
- Report severe nausea, vomiting, constipation, shortness of breath or difficulty breathing, skin rash.

## muromonab-CD3

*(mew **ro'** mon ab)*

Orthoclone OKT3

**Pregnancy Category C**

### Drug classes

Immunosuppressant

### Therapeutic actions

A murine monoclonal antibody to the antigen of human T cells; functions as an immunosuppressant by enabling T cells.

### Indications

- Acute allograft rejection in renal transplant patients
- Treatment of steroid-resistant acute allograft rejection in cardiac and hepatic transplant patients

### Contraindications/cautions

- Contraindications: allergy to muromonab or any murine product, fluid overload as evidenced by chest x-ray, or > 3% weight gain in 1 wk.
- Use cautiously with fever (use antipyretics to decrease fever before therapy); previous administration of muromonab-CD3 (antibodies frequently develop, risks serious reactions on repeat administration); pregnancy.

### Dosage

**Available Forms:** Injection—5 mg/5 ml

Give only as an IV bolus in < 1 min. Do not infuse or give by any other route.

*ADULT:* 5 mg/d for 10–14 d. Begin treatment once acute renal rejection is diagnosed. It is strongly recommended that methylprednisolone sodium succinate 1 mg/kg IV be given prior to muromonab-CD3 and IV hydrocortisone sodium succinate 100 mg be given 30 min after muromonab-CD3 administration.

*PEDIATRIC:* Safety and efficacy not established.

### Pharmacokinetics

| Route | Onset | Peak | Duration |
|---|---|---|---|
| IV | Minutes | 2–7 d | 7 d |

*Metabolism:* Tissue, $T_{1/2}$: 47–100 h

*Distribution:* Crosses placenta

### IV facts

**Preparation:** Draw solution into a syringe through a low protein-binding 0.2- or 0.22-$\mu$m filter. Discard filter and attach needle for IV bolus injection.

Solution may develop fine translucent particles that do not affect its potency. Refrigerate solution; do not freeze or shake.

**Infusion:** Administer as an IV bolus over < 1 min. Do not give as an IV infusion or with other drug solutions.

**Incompatabilities:** Do not mix with any other drug solution; do not infuse simultaneously with any other drug.

### Adverse effects

- CNS: Malaise, *tremors*
- GI: *Vomiting, nausea, diarrhea*
- General: *Fever, chills*
- Respiratory: **Acute pulmonary edema,** *dyspnea, chest pain*, wheezing
- Other: Lymphomas, *increased susceptibility to infection,* **cytokine release syndrome** ("flu" to shock)

### Clinically important drug-drug interactions

• Reduce dosage of other immunosuppressive agents; severe immunosuppression can lead to increased susceptibility to infection and increased risk of lymphomas; other immunosuppressives can be restarted about 3 d prior to cessation of muromonab • Risk of encephalopathy and CNS effects with indomethacin

## ■ Nursing Considerations

### Assessment

- *History:* Allergy to muromonab or any murine product; fluid overload; fever; previous administration of muromonab-CD3; pregnancy; lactation
- *Physical:* T, weight; P, BP; R, adventitious sounds; chest x-ray, CBC

### Implementation

- Obtain chest x-ray within 24 h of therapy to ensure chest is clear.
- Arrange for antipyretics (acetaminophen) if patient is febrile before therapy.
- Monitor WBC levels and circulating T cells periodically during therapy.
- Monitor patient very closely after first dose; acetaminophen prn should be ordered to cover febrile reactions; cooling blanket may be needed in severe cases. Equipment for intubation and respiratory support should be on standby for severe pulmonary reactions.

### Drug-specific teaching points

- There is often a severe reaction to the first dose, including high fever and chills, difficulty breathing, and chest congestion (you will be closely watched, and comfort measures will be given).
- Avoid infection; people may wear masks and rubber gloves when caring for you; visitors may be limited.
- Report chest pain, difficulty breathing, nausea, chills.

## mycophenolate mofetil

*(my coe **fin'** oh late)*

CellCept

**Pregnancy Category C**

### Drug classes

Immunosuppressant

### Therapeutic actions

Immunosuppressant; inhibits T-lymphocyte activation; exact mechanism of action unknown, but binds to intracellular protein, which may prevent the generation of nuclear factor of activated T cells, and suppresses the immune activation and response of T cells; inhibits proliferative responses of T and B cells

### Indications

- Prophylaxis of organ rejection in patients receiving allogeneic renal and heart transplants; intended to be used concomitantly with corticosteroids and cyclosporine

### Contraindications/cautions

- Contraindications: allergy to mycophenolate, pregnancy, lactation.
- Use cautiously with impaired renal function.

### Dosage

**Available Forms:** Capsules—250 mg

*ADULT:* 1 g bid PO starting within 72 h of transplant.

*PEDIATRIC:* Safety and efficacy not established.

*SEVERELY RENAL IMPAIRED:* Avoid doses >1 g/d. Monitor patient carefully for adverse response.

### Pharmacokinetics

| *Route* | *Onset* | *Peak* |
|---|---|---|
| Oral | Varies | 45–60 min |

*Metabolism:* Hepatic; $T_{1/2}$: 17.9 h
*Distribution:* Crosses placenta; enters breast milk
*Excretion:* Urine

### Adverse effects

- CNS: *Tremor, headache, insomnia,* paresthesias
- GI: **Hepatotoxicity,** *constipation, diarrhea, nausea, vomiting,* anorexia
- Hematologic: Leukopenia, *anemia,* hyperjalemia, hypokalemia, hyperglycemia
- GU: *Renal dysfunction,* nephrotoxicity, *UTI,* oliguria
- Other: Abdominal pain, pain, fever, asthenia, back pain, ascites, neoplasms, *infection*

### Clinically important drug-drug interactions

• Decreased levels and effectiveness with cholestyramine • Decreased levels and effectiveness of theophylline, phenytoin

## ■ Nursing Considerations

### Assessment

- *History:* Allergy to mycophenolate, pregnancy, lactation, renal function
- *Physical:* T; skin color, lesions; BP, peripheral perfusion; liver evaluation, bowel sounds, gum evaluation; renal and liver function tests, CBC

### Implementation

- Monitor renal and liver function before and periodically during therapy; marked decreases in function may require dosage change or discontinuation of therapy.
- Protect patient from exposure to infections and maintain sterile technique for invasive procedures.

### Drug-specific teaching points

- Avoid infection while on this drug; avoid crowds or people with infections. Notify your physician immediately if you injure yourself.
- The following side effects may occur: nausea, vomiting (take drug with food); diarrhea; headache (request analgesics).
- This drug should not be taken during pregnancy. If you think you are pregnant or you want to become pregnant, discuss this with your physician.
- Have periodic blood tests to monitor your response to the drug and its effects.
- Do not discontinue this drug without your physician's advice.
- Report unusual bleeding or bruising, fever, sore throat, mouth sores, tiredness.

## nabumetone

*(nah **byew'** meh tone)*

Relafen

**Pregnancy Category B**

### Drug classes

Nonsteroidal anti-inflammatory drug (NSAID)
Analgesic (non-narcotic)

### Therapeutic actions

Analgesic, anti-inflammatory, and antipyretic activities largely related to inhibition of prostaglandin synthesis; exact mechanisms of action are not known.

### Indications

- Acute and chronic treatment of signs and symptoms of rheumatoid arthritis and osteoarthritis

### Contraindications/cautions

- Contraindications: significant renal impairment, pregnancy, lactation.
- Use cautiously with impaired hearing; allergies; hepatic, CV, and GI conditions

### Dosage

**Available Forms:** Tablets—500, 750 mg

***Adult:*** 1,000 mg PO as a single dose with or without food. 1,500–2,000 mg/d have been used. May be given in divided doses.

***Pediatric:*** Safety and efficacy have not been established.

### Pharmacokinetics

| *Route* | *Onset* | *Peak* |
|---|---|---|
| Oral | 30 min | 30–60 min |

*Metabolism:* Hepatic, $T_{1/2}$: 22.5–30 h

*Distribution:* Crosses placenta; enters breast milk

*Excretion:* Urine.

### Adverse effects

*NSAIDs*

- CNS: *Headache, dizziness, somnolence, insomnia*, fatigue, tiredness, dizziness, tinnitus, ophthamological effects
- GI: *Nausea, dyspepsia, GI pain,* diarrhea, vomiting, *constipation*, flatulence
- Respiratory: Dyspnea, hemoptysis, pharyngitis, bronchospasm, rhinitis
- Hematologic: Bleeding, platelet inhibition with higher doses, neutropenia, eosinophilia, leukopenia, pancytopenia, thrombocytopenia, agranulocytosis, granulocytopenia, aplastic anemia, decreased Hgb or Hct, bone marrow depression, mennorhagia
- GU: Dysuria, **renal impairment**
- Dermatologic: *Rash*, pruritus, sweating, dry mucous membranes, stomatitis
- Other: Peripheral edema, **anaphylactoid reactions to fatal anaphylactic shock**

## ■ Nursing Considerations

### Assessment

- ***History:*** Renal impairment; impaired hearing; allergies; hepatic, CV, and GI conditions; lactation
- ***Physical:*** Skin color and lesions; orientation, reflexes, ophthalmological and audiometric evaluation, peripheral sensation; P, edema; R, adventitious sounds; liver evaluation; CBC, clotting times, renal and liver function tests; serum electrolytes, stool guaiac

### Implementation

- Administer drug with food or after meals if GI upset occurs.
- Arrange for periodic ophthalmologic examination during long-term therapy.
- Institute emergency procedures if overdose occurs: gastric lavage, induction of emesis, supportive therapy.

### Drug-specific teaching points

- Take drug with food or meals if GI upset occurs; take only the prescribed dosage.
- Dizziness, drowsiness can occur (avoid driving or the use of dangerous machinery).
- Report sore throat, fever, rash, itching, weight gain, swelling in ankles or fingers; changes in vision; black, tarry stools.

## nadolol

*(nay **doe'** lol)*

Corgard

**Pregnancy Category C**

n

### Drug classes

Beta adrenergic blocker (nonselective)

Antianginal agent

Antihypertensive

### Therapeutic actions

Competitively blocks beta-adrenergic receptors in the heart and juxtaglomerular apparatus, decreasing the influence of the sympathetic nervous system on these tissues and decreasing the excitability of the heart, cardiac output, oxygen consumption, and the release of renin, and lowering BP.

### Indications

- Hypertension alone or with other drugs, especially diuretics
- Long-term management of angina pectoris caused by atherosclerosis
- Unlabeled uses: treatment of ventricular arrhythmias, migraines, lithium induced tremors, aggressive behavior, essential tremors, rebleeding from esophageal var-

ices, reduction of intraocular pressure, situational anxiety

## Contraindications/cautions

- Contraindicated in the presence of sinus bradycardia (HR < 45 beats/min), second- or third-degree heart block (PR interval > 0.24 sec), cardiogenic shock, CHF, asthma, COPD, pregnancy, lactation.
- Use caution in the presence of diabetes or thyrotoxicosis.

## Dosage

**Available Forms:** Tablets—20, 40, 80, 120, 160 mg

**ADULT**

- *Hypertension:* Initially 40 mg PO qd; gradually increase dosage in 40- to 80-mg increments until optimum response is achieved. Usual maintenance dose is 40–80 mg/d; up to 320 mg qd may be needed.
- *Angina:* Initially 40 mg PO qd; gradually increase dosage in 40- to 80-mg increments at 3- to 7-d intervals until optimum response is achieved or heart rate markedly decreases. Usual maintenance dose is 40–80 mg qd; up to 240 mg/d may be needed. Safety and efficacy of larger doses not established. To discontinue, reduce dosage gradually over 1- to 2-wk period.

**PEDIATRIC:** Safety and efficacy not established.

**GERIATRIC OR RENAL FAILURE:**

| *Creatinine Clearance (ml/min)* | *Dosage Intervals (h)* |
|---|---|
| >50 | 24 |
| 31–50 | 24–36 |
| 10–30 | 24–48 |
| <10 | 40–60 |

## Pharmacokinetics

| *Route* | *Onset* | *Peak* | *Duration* |
|---|---|---|---|
| Oral | Varies | 2–4 h | 17–24 h |

*Metabolism:* $T_{1/2}$: 20–24 h
*Distribution:* Crosses placenta; enters breast milk
*Excretion:* Urine

## Adverse effects

- CNS: Dizziness, vertigo, tinnitus, fatigue, emotional depression, paresthesias, sleep disturbances, hallucinations, disorientation, memory loss, slurred speech
- GI: *Gastric pain, flatulence, constipation, diarrhea, nausea, vomiting,* anorexia, ischemic colitis, renal and mesenteric arterial thrombosis, retroperitoneal fibrosis, hepatomegaly, acute pancreatitis
- CV: *CHF, cardiac arrhythmias,* peripheral vascular insufficiency, claudication, CVA, pulmonary edema, hypotension
- **Respiratory**: Bronchospasm, dyspnea, cough, bronchial obstruction, nasal stuffiness, rhinitis, pharyngitis (less likely than with propranolol)
- GU: *Impotence, decreased libido,* Peyronie's disease, dysuria, nocturia, frequency
- **MS**: Joint pain, arthralgia, muscle cramp
- **EENT**: Eye irritation, dry eyes, conjunctivitis, blurred vision
- **Dermatologic**: Rash, pruritus, sweating, dry skin
- **Allergic reactions**: Pharyngitis, erythematous rash, fever, sore throat, laryngospasm, respiratory distress
- **Other**: *Decreased exercise tolerance, development of antinuclear antibodies,* hyperglycemia or hypoglycemia, elevated serum transaminase, alkaline

## Clinically important drug-drug interactions

• Increased effects with verapamil • Increased serum levels and toxicity of IV lidocaine, aminophylline • Increased risk of postural hypotension with prazosin • Increased risk of peripheral ischemia with ergotamine, methysergide, dihydroergotamine • Decreased antihypertensive effects with NSAIDs, clonidine • Hypertension followed by severe bradycardia with epinephrine

## Drug-lab test interferences

• Possible false results with glucose or insulin tolerance tests

## ■ Nursing Considerations

### Assessment

- *History:* Sinus bradycardia, second- or third-degree heart block, cardiogenic shock, CHF, asthma, COPD; diabetes or thyrotoxicosis; pregnancy; lactation
- *Physical:* Weight, skin condition, neurologic status, P, BP, ECG, respiratory status, kidney and thyroid function, blood and urine glucose

### Implementation

- Do not discontinue drug abruptly after chronic therapy (hypersensitivity to catecholamines may have developed, causing exacerbation of angina, MI, and ventricular dysrhythmias). Taper drug gradually over 2 wk with monitoring.
- Consult with physician about withdrawing drug if patient is to undergo surgery (controversial).

### Drug-specific teaching points

- Do not stop taking unless instructed to do so by a health care provider.
- Avoid driving or dangerous activities if CNS effects occur.
- Report difficulty breathing, night cough, swelling of extremities, slow pulse, confusion, depression, rash, fever, sore throat.

# nafarelin acetate

***(naf' a re lin)***

Synarel

**Pregnancy Category X**

### Drug classes

GnRH (gonadotropic releasing hormone)
Hormone

### Therapeutic actions

A potent agonistic analog of gonadotropic-releasing hormone (GnRH) which is released from the hypothalamus to stimulate LH and FSH release from the pituitary; these hormones are responsible for regulating reproductive status. Repeated dosing abolishes the stimulatory effect on the pituitary gland, leading to decreased secretion of gonadal steroids by about 4 wk; consequently, tissues and functions that depend on gonadal steroids for their maintenance become quiescent.

### Indications

- Treatment of endometriosis, including pain relief and reduction of endometriotic lesions
- Treatment of central precocious puberty in children of both sexes

### Contraindications/cautions

- Known sensitivity to GnRH, GnRH-agonist analogs, excipients in the product; undiagnosed abnormal genital bleeding; pregnancy; lactation (potential androgenic effects on the fetus).

### Dosage

**Available Forms:** Nasal solution—2 mg/ml

*ADULT*

- *Endometriosis:* 400 μg/d. One spray (200 μg) into one nostril in the morning and one spray into the other nostril in the evening. Start treatment between days 2 and 4 of the menstrual cycle. 800-μg dose may administered as one spray into each nostril in the morning (a total of two sprays) and again in the evening for patients with persistent regular menstruation after months of treatment. Treatment for 6 mo is recommended. Retreatment is not recommended because safety has not been established.

*PEDIATRIC*

- *Central precocious puberty:* 1,600 μg/d. Two sprays (400 μg) in each nostril in the morning and two sprays in each nostril in the evening; may be increased to 1,800 μg/d. Continue until resumption of puberty is desired.

### Pharmacokinetics

| Route | Onset | Peak |
|---|---|---|
| Nasal | Rapid | 4 wk |

*Metabolism:* $T_{1/2}$: 85.5 h
*Distribution:* Crosses placenta; enters breast milk
*Excretion:* Urine

### Adverse effects
- CNS: Dizziness, headache, sleep disorders, fatigue, tremor
- GI: Hepatic dysfunction
- GU: Fluid retention
- **Endocrine**: *Androgenic effects* (acne, edema, mild hirsutism, decrease in breast size, deepening of the voice, oily skin or hair, weight gain, clitoral hypertrophy or testicular atrophy), *hypoestrogenic effects* (flushing, sweating, vaginitis, nervousness, emotional lability)
- **Local**: *Nasal irritation*
- **Other**: With prolonged therapy, bone density loss has been noted

## ■ Nursing Considerations

### Assessment
- *History:* Sensitivity to GnRH, GnRH-agonist analogs, excipients in the product; undiagnosed abnormal genital bleeding; pregnancy; lactation
- *Physical:* Weight; hair distribution pattern; skin color, texture, lesions; breast exam; nasal mucosa; orientation, affect, reflexes; P, auscultation, BP, peripheral edema; liver evaluation; bone density studies in long-term therapy

### Implementation
- Ensure that patient is not pregnant before therapy; begin therapy for endometriosis during menstrual period, days 2–4.
- Store drug upright; protect from exposure to light.
- Arrange for bone density studies before therapy if retreatment is suggested because of return of endometriosis.
- Ensure patient has enough of the drug to prevent interruption of therapy.
- Caution patient that androgenic effects may not be reversible when the drug is withdrawn.
- Monitor nasal mucosa for signs of erosion during course of therapy.
- Provide topical decongestant to be used at least 30 min after dosing with nafarelin.

### Drug-specific teaching points
- Use this drug without interruption; be sure that you have enough on hand to prevent interruption. Store the drug upright. Protect the bottle from exposure to light.
- Regular menstruation should cease within 4–6 wk of therapy. Breakthrough bleeding or ovulation may still occur.
- The following side effects may occur: masculinizing effects (acne, hair growth, deepening of voice, oily skin or hair; may not be reversible); low estrogen effects (flushing, sweating, vaginal irritation, nervousness); nasal irritation.
- Consult with your nurse or physician if you need a topical nasal decongestant; a decongestant should be used at least 30 min after nafarelin use.
- This drug is contraindicated during pregnancy; use a nonhormonal form of birth control during therapy. If you become pregnant, discontinue the drug and consult with your physician immediately.
- Report abnormal growth of facial hair, deepening of the voice, unusual bleeding or bruising, fever, chills, sore throat, vaginal itching or irritation; nasal irritation, burning.

# nafcillin sodium

*(naf **sill'in**)*

Nafcil, Nallpen, Unipen

**Pregnancy Category B**

### Drug classes
Antibiotic

Penicillinase-resistant pencillin

### Therapeutic actions
Bactericidal: inhibits cell wall synthesis of sensitive organisms, causing cell death

### Indications
- Infections due to penicillinase-producing staphylococci
- Infections caused by group A beta-hemolytic streptococci, *Streptococcus viridans*

### Contraindications/cautions
- Contraindications: allergies to penicillins, cephalosporins, or other allergens.

- Use cautiously with renal disorders, pregnancy, lactation (may cause diarrhea or candidiasis in infant).

## Dosage

**Available Forms:** Tablets—500 mg; capsules—250 mg; powder for injection—500 mg; 1, 2 g

### Adult

- ***IV:*** 500–1,000 mg q4h for short-term (24–48 h) therapy only, especially in the elderly
- ***IM:*** 500 mg q6h (q4h in severe infections).
- ***PO:*** 250–500 mg q4–6h, up to 1 g q4–6h in severe infections.

### Pediatric

- ***IM:*** 25 mg/kg bid; newborns, 10 mg/kg bid.
- ***PO***
  - *Staphylococcal infections:* 50 mg/kg per day in four divided doses; newborns, 10 mg/kg tid–qid.
  - *Scarlet fever, pneumonia:* 25 mg/kg per day in four divided doses.
  - *Streptococcal pharyngitis:* 250 mg tid (penicillin G is preferred).

## Pharmacokinetics

| *Route* | *Onset* | *Peak* | *Duration* |
|---|---|---|---|
| Oral | Varies | 60 min | 4 h |
| IM | Rapid | 3–90 min | 4–6 h |
| IV | Immediate | 15 min | 4 h |

*Metabolism:* Hepatic, $T_{1/2}$: 1 h
*Distribution:* Crosses placenta; enters breast milk
*Excretion:* Urine and bile

## IV facts

**Preparation:** Dilute solution for IV use in 15–30 ml Sodium Chloride Injection or Sterile Water for Injection; dilute reconstituted solution with compatible IV solution: 0.9% Sodium Chloride Injection, Sterile Water for Injection, 5% Dextrose in Water or in 0.4% Sodium Chloride Solution, M/6 Sodium Lactate Solution, or Ringer's Solution. Solutions at concentrations of 2–40 mg/ml are stable for 24 h at room temperature or 4 d refrigerated; discard solution after this time.

**Infusion:** Infuse slowly, each 500 mg over 5–10 min.

**Incompatibilities:** Do not mix in the same IV solution as other antibiotics.

## Adverse effects

- CNS: Lethargy, hallucinations, seizures
- GI: *Glossitis, stomatitis, gastritis, sore mouth*, furry tongue, black "hairy" tongue, *nausea, vomiting, diarrhea,* abdominal pain, bloody diarrhea, enterocolitis, pseudomembranous colitis, nonspecific hepatitis
- **Hematologic**: Anemia, thrombocytopenia, leukopenia, neutropenia, prolonged bleeding time (more common than with other penicillinase-resistant penicillins)
- GU: Nephritis—oliguria, proteinuria, hematuria, casts, azotemia, pyuria
- **Hypersensitivity reactions**: *Rash, fever, wheezing,* anaphylaxis
- **Local**: *Pain, phlebitis*, thrombosis at injection site
- **Other**: *Superinfections*—oral and rectal moniliasis, vaginitis

## Clinically important drug-drug interactions

- Decreased effectiveness with tetracyclines
- Inactivation of parenteral aminoglycosides: amikacin, gentamicin, kanamycin, neomycin, metilmicin, streptomycin, tobramycin

## Drug-lab test interferences

- False-positive Coombs' test with IV use.

## ■ Nursing Considerations

### Assessment

- *History:* Allergies to penicillins, cephalosporins, or other allergens; renal disorders; pregnancy; lactation
- *Physical:* Culture infection; skin color, lesions; R, adventitious sounds; bowel sounds: CBC, liver and renal function tests, serum electrolytes, Hct, urinalysis

### Implementation

- Culture infection before treatment; reculture if response is not as expected.

n

- Continue therapy for at least 2 d after signs of infection have disappeared, usually 7–10 d.
- Reconstitute powder for IM use with Sterile or Bacteriostatic Water for Injection or Sodium Chloride Injection. Administer by deep intragluteal injection. Reconstituted solution is stable for 7 d if refrigerated or 3 d at room temperature.
- Do not give IM injections repeatedly in the same site; atrophy can occur; monitor injection sites.
- Administer oral drug on an empty stomach, 1 h before or 2 h after meals, with a full glass of water. Do not administer with fruit juices or soft drinks.

### Drug-specific teaching points

- Take oral drug on an empty stomach with a full glass of water; take the full course of drug therapy.
- Avoid self-treating other infections with this antibiotic because it is specific to the infection being treated.
- Nausea, vomiting, diarrhea, mouth sores, pain at injection sites may occur.
- Report difficulty breathing, rashes, severe diarrhea, severe pain at injection site, mouth sores, unusual bleeding or bruising.

## nalbuphine hydrochloride

*(nal' byoo feen)*

Nubain

**Pregnancy Category C**

### Drug classes

Narcotic agonist-antagonist analgesic

### Therapeutic actions

Nalbuphine acts as an agonist at specific opioid receptors in the CNS to produce analgesia, sedation but also acts to cause hallucinations and is an antagonist at $\mu$ receptors.

### Indications

- Relief of moderate to severe pain
- Preoperative analgesia, as a supplement to surgical anesthesia, and for obstetric analgesia during labor and delivery

### Contraindications/cautions

- Contraindications: hypersensitivity to nalbuphine, sulfites; lactation.
- Use cautiously with emotionally unstable patients or those with a history of narcotic abuse; pregnancy prior to labor (neonatal withdrawal may occur if mothers used drug during pregnancy), labor or delivery (use with caution during delivery of premature infants who are especially sensitive to respiratory depressant effects of narcotics), bronchial asthma, COPD, respiratory depression, anoxia, increased intracranial pressure, acute MI when nausea and vomiting are present, biliary tract surgery (may cause spasm of the sphincter of Oddi).

### Dosage

**Available Forms:** Injection—10 mg/ml, 20 mg/ml

*ADULT:* Usual dose is 10 mg/70 kg, SC, IM, or IV q 3–6 h as necessary. Individualize dosage. In nontolerant patients, the recommended single maximum dose is 20 mg, with a maximum total daily dose of 160 mg. Patients dependent on narcotics may experience withdrawal symptoms with administration of nalbuphine; control by small increments of morphine by slow IV administration until relief occurs. If the previous narcotic was morphine, meperidine, codeine, or another narcotic with similar duration of activity, administer 1/4 the anticipated nalbuphine dose initially, and observe for signs of withdrawal. If no untoward symptoms occur, progressively increase doses until analgesia is obtained.

*PEDIATRIC < 18 Y:* Not recommended.

*GERIATRIC OR RENAL OR HEPATIC IMPAIRMENT:* Reduce dosage.

### Pharmacokinetics

| Route | Onset | Peak | Duration |
|---|---|---|---|
| IV | 2–3 min | 15–20 min | 3–6 h |
| SC/IM | < 15 min | 30–60 min | 3–6 h |

*Metabolism:* Hepatic, $T_{1/2}$: 5 h

*Distribution:* Crosses placenta; enters breast milk

*Excretion:* Urine

### IV facts

**Preparation:** No additional preparation is required.

**Infusion:** Administer by direct injection or into the tubing of a running IV, each 10 mg over 3–5 min.

### Adverse effects

- CNS: *Sedation, clamminess, sweating, headache,* nervousness, restlessness, depression, crying, confusion, faintness, hostility, unusual dreams, hallucinations, euphoria, dysphoria, unreality, *dizziness, vertigo,* floating feeling, feeling of heaviness, numbness, tingling, flushing, warmth, blurred vision
- GI: Nausea, vomiting, cramps, dyspepsia, bitter taste, *dry mouth*
- CV: Hypotension, hypertension, bradycardia, tachycardia
- **Respiratory**: Respiratory depression, dyspnea, asthma
- GU: Urinary urgency
- **Dermatologic**: Itching, burning, urticaria

### Clinically important drug-drug interactions

- Potentiation of effects with other barbiturate anesthetics.

## ■ Nursing Considerations

### Assessment

- *History:* Hypersensitivity to nalbuphine, sulfites; lactation; emotional instability or history of narcotic abuse; pregnancy; bronchial asthma, COPD, respiratory depression, anoxia, increased intracranial pressure, MI, biliary tract surgery
- *Physical:* Orientation, reflexes, bilateral grip strength, affect; pupil size, vision; pulse, auscultation, BP; R, adventitious sounds; bowel sounds, normal output; urine output; liver, kidney function tests

### Implementation

- Taper dosage when discontinuing after prolonged use to avoid withdrawal symptoms.
- Provide narcotic antagonist, facilities for assisted or controlled respiration on standby in case of respiratory depression.
- Reassure patient about addiction liability; most patients who receive opiates for medical reasons do not develop dependence syndromes.

### Drug-specific teaching points

- The following side effects may occur: dizziness, sedation, drowsiness, impaired visual acuity (avoid driving, performing tasks that require alertness); nausea, loss of appetite (lying quietly, eating frequent, small meals may help).
- Report severe nausea, vomiting, palpitations, shortness of breath, or difficulty breathing.

## nalidixic acid

*(nal i **dix'** ik)*

NegGram

**Pregnancy Category C**

### Drug classes

Urinary tract anti-infective

Antibacterial

### Therapeutic actions

Bactericidal; interferes with DNA and RNA synthesis in susceptible gram-negative bacteria, causing cell death.

### Indications

- Urinary tract infections caused by susceptible gram-negative bacteria, including *Proteus* strains, *Klebsiella* species, *Enterobacter* species, *Escherichia coli*

### Contraindications/cautions

- Contraindications: allergy to nalidixic acid, seizures, epilepsy, pregnancy, lactation.
- Use cautiously with G-6-PD deficiency, renal or liver dysfunction, cerebral arteriosclerosis.

### Dosage

**Available Forms:** Caplets—250, 500 mg; 7000 g; suspension—250 mg/5ml

**ADULT:** Initial therapy, 1 g PO qid for 1–2 wk. For prolonged therapy, total dose may be reduced to 2 g/d.

**PEDIATRIC < 12 Y:** Exact dosage is based on weight; total daily dose for initial therapy, 55 mg/kg per day PO divided into four equal doses. For prolonged therapy, may be reduced to 33 mg/kg per day. Not recommended for children <3 mo.

### Pharmacokinetics

| *Route* | *Onset* | *Peak* |
|---|---|---|
| Oral | Varies | 1–2 h |

*Metabolism:* Hepatic, $T_{1/2}$: 1–2.5 h
*Distribution:* Crosses placenta; enters breast milk
*Excretion:* Urine

### Adverse effects
- CNS: *Drowsiness, weakness, headache, dizziness, vertigo*, visual disturbances
- GI: *Abdominal pain, nausea, vomiting, diarrhea*
- **Hematologic**: Thrombocytopenia, leukopenia, hemolytic anemia
- **Dermatologic**: Photosensitivity reactions
- **Hypersensitivity**: Rash, pruritus, urticaria, angioedema, eosinophilia, arthralgia

### Clinically important drug-drug interactions
• Increased risk of bleeding if given with oral anticoagulants

### Drug-lab test interferences
• False-positive urinary glucose results when using Benedict's reagent, Fehling's reagent, Clinitest tablets • False elevations of urinary 17-keto and ketogenic steroids when assay uses m-dinitrobenzene

## ■ Nursing Considerations

### Assessment
- *History:* Allergy to nalidixic acid, seizures, epilepsy, G-6-PD deficiency, renal or liver dysfunction, cerebral arteriosclerosis, pregnancy, lactation
- *Physical:* Skin color, lesions; joints; orientation, reflexes; CBC, liver and renal function tests

### Implementation
- Arrange for culture and sensitivity tests.
- Give with food if GI upset occurs.
- Obtain periodic blood counts, renal and liver function tests during prolonged therapy.
- Monitor clinical response; if no improvement is seen or a relapse occurs, send urine for repeat culture and sensitivity.

### Drug-specific teaching points
- Take drug with food. Complete the full course of therapy to ensure resolution of the infection.
- The following side effects may occur: nausea, vomiting, abdominal pain (small, frequent meals may help); diarrhea; sensitivity to sunlight (wear protective clothing, and use sunscreen); drowsiness, blurring of vision, dizziness (observe caution if driving or using dangerous equipment).
- Report severe rash, visual changes, weakness, tremors.

# nalmefene hydrochloride

***(nal' me feen)***
Revex
**Pregnancy Category B**

### Drug classes
Narcotic antagonist

### Therapeutic actions
Pure opiate antagonist; prevents or blocks the effects of opioids, including respiratory depression, sedation and hypotension.

### Indications
- Complete or partial reversal of opioid drug effects, including respiratory depression, induced by either natural or synthetic opioids
- Management of known or suspected opioid overdose

### Contraindications/cautions
- Contraindications: allergy to narcotic antagonists, pregnancy.
- Use cautiously with narcotic addiction (may produce withdrawal), liver or renal impairment, lactation.

### Dosage

**Available Forms:** Injection—100 μg/ml, 1 mg/ml

*ADULT:* Titrate dose to reverse the undesired effects of opioids; once reversal has been achieved, no further administration is required.

- ***Postoperative use:*** Use 100 μg/ml strength (blue label) IV, repeat at 2—5 min intervals until reversal is achieved, then stop administration:

| Body Weight (kg) | Nalmefene (ml of 100 μg/ml solution) |
|---|---|
| 50 | 0.125 |
| 60 | 0.15 |
| 70 | 0.175 |
| 80 | 0.2 |
| 90 | 0.225 |
| 100 | 0.25 |

- ***Management of known or suspected overdose:*** Use 1 mg/ml strength (green label); initial dose of 0.5 mg/70 kg IV; if needed, a second dose of 1 mg/70 kg IV is given 2–5 min later; maximum effective dose is 1.5 mg/70 kg.
- ***Suspected opioid dependency:*** Challenge dose of 0.1 mg/70 kg IV; if no evidence of withdrawal within 2 min, proceed as above.
- ***Loss of IV access:*** Single 1-mg dose IM or SC should be effective within 5–15 min.

*PEDIATRIC:* Safety has not been established in children <18 years.

*GERIATRIC OR RENAL IMPAIRED:* Slowly administer incremental doses over 60 sec to minimize side effects.

### Pharmacokinetics

| Route | Onset | Peak |
|---|---|---|
| IV | Immediate | 15 min |
| SC/IM | 5–15 min | 1–3 hrs |

*Metabolism:* Hepatic; $T_{1/2}$: 10.8 hrs

*Distribution:* Crosses placenta; enters breast milk

*Excretion:* Urine

### IV facts

**Preparation:** No further preparation is required; assure that correct concentration is being used for indication: blue label—postoperative reversal; green label—overdose.

**Infusion:** Inject initial dose directly into line of running IV over 15–30 sec or directly into vein in emergency situations; titrate subsequent doses based on patient response.

### Adverse effects

- CNS: *Difficulty sleeping, anxiety, nervousness, headache, low energy*, increased energy, irritability, dizziness
- GI: Hepatocellular injury, *abdominal pain/cramps, nausea, vomiting*, loss of appetite, diarrhea, constipation
- CV: Hypertension, hypotension, arrhythmias
- Other: *Chills*, fever, pharyngitis, pruritus

## ■ Nursing Considerations

### Assessment

- *History:* Allergy to narcotic antagonists, pregnancy, narcotic addiction, liver or renal impairment, lactation
- *Physical:* Sweating; skin lesions, color; reflexes, affect, orientation, muscle strength; P, BP, edema, baseline ECG, renal and liver function tests

### Implementation

- Administer challenge test in situations of suspected or known opioid dependency.
- Check vial carefully to assure use of correct concentration for indication: blue label–postoperative reversal of effects; green label–overdose.
- Monitor patient carefully during treatment; discontinue drug as soon as reversal is achieved.
- The effects of the drug may continue for several days becasuse of the long half-life of nalmefene.
- Do not use opioid drugs for analgesia, cough and cold; do not use opioid antidiarrheal preparations; patient will not have a response to these drugs for an

n

extended period of time–use a nonopioid preparation if possible.

### Drug-specific teaching points

- This drug blocks the effects of narcotics and other opiates.
- The following side effects may occur for several days: drowsiness, dizziness, blurred vision, anxiety (avoid driving or operating dangerous machinery); nausea, vomiting; headache.
- Report unusual bleeding or bruising; dark, tarry stools; yellowing of eyes or skin; dizziness; headache; palpitations.

## naloxone hydrochloride

*(nal* ***ox'*** *one)*

Narcan

**Pregnancy Category B**

### Drug classes

Narcotic antagonist
Diagnostic agent

### Therapeutic actions

Pure narcotic antagonist; reverses the effects of opioids, including respiratory depression, sedation, hypotension; can reverse the psychotomimetic and dysphoric effects of narcotic agonist-antagonists, such as pentazocine.

### Indications

- Complete or partial reversal of narcotic depression, including respiratory depression induced by opioids, including natural and synthetic narcotics, propoxyphene, methadone, nalbuphine, butorphanol, pentazocine
- Diagnosis of suspected acute opioid overdosage
- Unlabeled uses: improvement of circulation in refractory shock, reversal of alcoholic coma, dementia of Alzheimer or schizophrenic type

### Contraindications/cautions

- Contraindicatiopns: allergy to narcotic antagonists.
- Use cautiously with narcotic addiction, CV disorders, pregnancy, lactation.

### Dosage

**Available Forms:** Injection—0.4, 1 mg/ml; neonatal injection—0.02 mg/ml

IV administration is recommended in emergencies when rapid onset of action is required.

#### Adult

- *Narcotic overdose:* Initial dose of 0.4–2 mg, IV. Additional doses may be repeated at 2 to 3-min intervals. If no response after 10 mg, question the diagnosis. IM or SC routes may be used if IV route is unavailable.
- ***Postoperative narcotic depression:*** Titrate dose to patient's response. Initial dose of 0.1–0.2 mg IV at 2–3 min intervals until desired degree of reversal. Repeat doses may be needed within 1 to 2-h intervals, depending on amount and type of narcotic. Supplemental IM doses produce a longer lasting effect.

#### Pediatric

- *Narcotic overdose:* Initial dose is 0.01 mg/kg IV. Subsequent dose of 0.1 mg/kg may be administered if needed. May be given IM or SC in divided doses.
- ***Postoperative narcotic depression:*** For the initial reversal of respiratory depression, inject in increments of 0.005–0.01 mg IV at 2- to 3-min intervals to the desired degree of reversal.

#### Neonates

- *Narcotic-induced depression:* Initial dose if 0.01 mg/kg IV, SC, IM. May be repeated as indicated in the adult guidelines.

### Pharmacokinetics

| Route | Onset | Duration |
|---|---|---|
| IV | 2 min | 4–6 h |
| IM/SC | 3–5 min | 4–6 h |

*Metabolism:* Hepatic, $T_{1/2}$: 30–81 min
*Distribution:* Crosses placenta; enters breast milk
*Excretion:* Urine

### IV facts

**Preparation:** Dilute in Normal Saline or 5% Dextrose Solutions for IV infusions. The addition of 2 mg in 500 ml of solution provides a concentration of 0.004 mg/ml; titrate rate by response. Use di-

luted mixture within 24 h. After that time, discard any remaining solution.
**Infusion:** Inject directly, each 0.4 mg over 15 sec, or titrate rate of infusion based on response.
**Incompatibilities:** Do not mix naloxone with preparations containing bisulfite, metabisulfite, high molecular weight anions, alkaline pH solutions.

### Adverse effects
- CNS: Reversal of analgesia and excitement (postoperative use)
- CV: *Hypotension, hypertension*, ventricular tachycardia and fibrillation, pulmonary edema (postoperative use)
- **Acute narcotic abstinence syndrome**: *nausea, vomiting, sweating, tachycardia, increased BP, tremulousness*

## ■ Nursing Considerations
### Assessment
- *History:* Allergy to narcotic antagonists; narcotic addiction; CV disorders; lactation
- *Physical:* Sweating; reflexes, pupil size; P, BP; R, adventitious sounds

### Implementation
- Monitor patient continuously after use of naloxone; repeat doses may be necessary, depending on duration of narcotic and time of last dose.
- Maintain open airway, and provide artificial ventilation, cardiac massage, vasopressor agents if needed to counteract acute narcotic overdosage.

### Drug-specific teaching points
- Report sweating, feelings of tremulousness.

## naltrexone hydrochloride

*(nal **trex'** one)*
ReVia
**Pregnancy Category C**

### Drug classes
Narcotic antagonist

### Therapeutic actions
Pure opiate antagonist; markedly attenuates or completely, reversibly blocks the subjective effects of IV opioids, including those with mixed narcotic agonist-antagonist properties.

### Indications
- Adjunct to treatment of alcohol or narcotic dependence as part of a comprehensive treatment program
- Unlabeled uses: treatment of postconcussional syndrome unresponsive to other treatments; eating disorders

### Contraindications/cautions
- Contraindications: allergy to narcotic antagonists, pregnancy.
- Use cautiously with narcotic addiction (may produce withdrawal symptoms; do not administer unless patient has been opioid free for 7–10 d); opioid withdrawal; acute hepatitis, liver failure; lactation; depression, suicidal tendencies.

### Dosage
**Available Forms:** Tablets—50 mg
ADULT: Give naloxone challenge before use except in patients showing clinical signs of opioid withdrawal.
- ***IV:*** Draw 2 ampules of naloxone, 2 ml into a syringe. Inject 0.5 ml. Leave needle in vein, and observe for 30 sec. If no signs of withdrawal occur, inject remaining 1.5 ml, and observe for 20 min for signs and symptoms of withdrawal (stuffiness or running nose, tearing, yawning, sweating, tremor, vomiting, piloerection, feeling of temperature change, joint or bone and muscle pain, abdominal cramps, skin crawling).
- ***SC:*** Administer 2 ml, and observe for signs and symptoms of withdrawal for 45 min. If any of the signs and symptoms of withdrawal occur or if there is any doubt that the patient is opioid free, do not administer naltrexone. Confirmatory rechallenge can be done within 24 h. Inject 4 ml IV, and observe for signs and symptoms of withdrawal. Repeat until no signs and symptoms are seen and patient is no longer at risk.

– *Naltrexone maintenance: Alcoholism*: 50 mg PO per day. *Narcotic dependence*: Initial dose of 25 mg PO. Observe for 1 h; if no signs or symptoms are seen, complete dose with 25 mg. Usual maintenance dose is 50 mg/24 h PO. Flexible dosing schedule can be used with 100 mg every other day or 150 mg every third day, and so forth.

*PEDIATRIC:* Safety has not been established in children < 18 y.

### Pharmacokinetics

| *Route* | *Onset* | *Peak* | *Duration* |
|---|---|---|---|
| Oral | 15–30 min | 60 min | 24–72 h |

*Metabolism:* Hepatic, $T_{1/2}$: 3.9–12.9 h
*Distribution:* Crosses placenta; enters breast milk
*Excretion:* Urine

### Adverse effects

- CNS: *Difficulty sleeping, anxiety, nervousness, headache, low energy*, increased energy, irritability, dizziness, blurred vision, burning, light sensitivity
- GI: Hepatocellular injury, *abdominal pain/cramps, nausea, vomiting*, , loss of appetite, diarrhea, constipation
- CV: Phlebitis, edema, increased BP, nonspecific ECG changes
- **Respiratory**: Nasal congestion, rhinorrhea, sneezing, sore throat, excess mucus or phlegm, sinus trouble, epistaxis
- GU: *Delayed ejaculation, decreased potency*, increased frequency/discomfort voiding
- **Dermatologic**: *Skin rash*, itching, oily skin, pruritus, acne
- **Other**: *Chills, increased thirst*, increased appetite, weight change, yawning, swollen glands, *joint and muscle pain*

## ■ Nursing Considerations

### Assessment

- *History:* Allergy to narcotic antagonists; narcotic addiction; opioid withdrawal; acute hepatitis, liver failure; lactation; depression, suicidal tendencies
- *Physical:* Sweating; skin lesions, color; reflexes, affect, orientation, muscle strength; P, BP, edema, baseline ECG; R, adventitious sounds; liver evaluation; urine screen for opioids, liver function tests

### Implementation

- Do not use until patient has been opioid free for 7–10 d; check urine opioid levels.
- Do not administer until patient has passed a naloxone challenge.
- Initiate treatment slowly, and monitor until patient has been given naltrexone in the full daily dose with no signs and symptoms of withdrawal.
- Obtain periodic liver function tests during therapy; discontinue therapy at sign of increasing liver dysfunction.
- Do not use opioid drugs for analgesia, cough, and cold; do not use opioid antidiarrheal preparations; patient will not respond; use a nonopioid preparation.
- Assure that patient is actively participating in a comprehensive treatment program.

### Drug-specific teaching points

- This drug will help facilitate abstinence from alcohol.
- This drug blocks the effects of narcotics and other opiates.
- Wear a medical ID tag to alert emergency medical personnel that you are taking this drug.
- Small doses of heroin or other opiate drugs will not have an effect. Self-administration of large doses of heroin or other narcotics can overcome the blockade effect but may cause death, serious injury or coma.
- The following side effects may occur: drowsiness, dizziness, blurred vision, anxiety (avoid driving or operating dangerous machinery); diarrhea, nausea, vomiting; decreased sexual function.
- Report unusual bleeding or bruising; dark, tarry stools; yellowing of eyes or skin; running nose; tearing; sweating; chills; joint or muscle pain.

## Nandrolone

### nandrolone decanoate

*(nan' droe lone)*

Androlone-D, Deca-Durabolin, Hybolin Decanoate, Neo-Durabolic

### nandrolone phenpropionate

Durabolin, Hybolin Improved

**Pregnancy Category X**
**C-III controlled substance**

### Drug classes
Anabolic steroid
Hormone

### Therapeutic actions
Testosterone analogue; promotes body tissue-building processes and reverses catabolic or tissue-depleting processes; increases Hgb and red cell mass.

### Indications
- Nandrolone decanoate: Management of anemia related to renal insufficiency
- Nandrolone phenpropionate: Control of metastatic breast cancer

### Contraindications/cautions
- Known sensitivity to nandrolone or anabolic steroids; prostate or breast cancer in males; benign prostatic hypertrophy; breast cancer (females); pituitary insufficiency; MI (contraindicated because of effects on cholesterol); nephrosis; liver disease; hypercalcemia; pregnancy; lactation.

### Dosage
**Available Forms:** Injection—25, 50, 100, 200 mg/ml

Administer by deep IM injection; therapy should be intermittent.

**ADULT**
- *Anemia of renal insufficiency (nandrolone decanoate): Women:* 50–100 mg/wk IM; *men:* 100–200 mg/wk IM; *children (2–13 y):* 25–50 mg IM every 3–4 wk.
- *Control of metastatic breast cancer (nandrolone phenpropionate):* 50–100 mg/wk IM based on therapeutic response.

**INFANTS:** Contraindicated: risk of serious disruption of growth and development.

### Pharmacokinetics

| *Route* | *Onset* | *Peak* |
|---|---|---|
| IM | Slow | Unknown |

*Metabolism:* Hepatic, $T_{1/2}$: unknown
*Distribution:* Crosses placenta; enters breast milk
*Excretion:* Unknown

### Adverse effects
- CNS: *Excitation, insomnia,* chills, toxic confusion
- GI: Hepatotoxicity, peliosis, hepatitis with life threatening **liver failure** or **intra-abdominal hemorrhage**; liver cell tumors, sometimes malignant and fatal, *nausea, vomiting, diarrhea, abdominal fullness, loss of appetite, burning of tongue*
- Hematologic: *Blood lipid changes* (increased risk of atherosclerosis); iron-deficiency anemia, hypercalcemia, altered serum cholesterol levels; *retention of sodium, chloride, water,* potassium, phosphates and calcium
- GU: Increased risk of prostatic hypertrophy, carcinoma in geriatric patients
- Endocrine: *Virilization, prepubertal males*, phallic enlargement, hirsutism, increased skin pigmentation; *postpubertal males*, inhibition of testicular function, gynecomastia, testicular atrophy, priapism, baldness, epidiymitis, change in libido; *females*, hirsutism, hoarseness, deepening of the voice, clitoral enlargement, menstrual irregularities, baldness; decreased glucose tolerance
- Other: *Acne,* premature closure of the epiphyses

**Clinically important drug-drug interactions**

• Potentiation of oral anticoagulants with anabolic steroids • Decreased need for insulin, oral hypoglycemica agents with anabolic steroids

**Drug-lab test interferences**

• Altered glucose tolerance tests • Decrease in thyroid function tests, which may persist for 2–3 wk after stopping therapy • Increased creatinine, creatinine clearance, which may last for 2 wk after therapy

## ■ Nursing Considerations

### Assessment

- *History:* Sensitivity to nandrolone or anabolic steroids; prostate or breast cancer in males; benign prostatic hypertrophy; breast cancer in females; pituitary insufficiency; MI; nephrosis; liver disease; hypercalcemia; pregnancy; lactation
- *Physical:* Skin color, texture; hair distribution pattern; affect, orientation; abdominal exam, liver evaluation; serum electrolytes, serum cholesterol levels, glucose tolerance tests, thyroid function tests, long-bone x-ray (in children)

### Implementation

- Inject nandrolone deeply into gluteal muscle.
- Intermittent administration decreases adverse effects.
- Monitor effect on children with long-bone x-rays every 3–6 mo; discontinue drug well before the bone age reaches the norm for the patient's chronologic age.
- Monitor patient for edema; arrange for diuretic therapy.
- Monitor liver function, serum electrolytes, and consult with physician for appropriate corrective measures.
- Measure cholesterol levels periodically with high risk for CAD.
- Monitor diabetic patients closely as glucose tolerance may change; adjustments may be needed in insulin, oral hypoglycemic dosage, and diet.

### Drug-specific teaching points

- This drug can only be given IM; mark calendar indicating days to return for injection.
- The following side effects may occur: nausea, vomiting, diarrhea, burning of the tongue (small, frequent meals); body hair growth, baldness, deepening of the voice, loss of libido, impotence; (most effects are reversible); excitation, confusion, insomnia (avoid driving, performing tasks that require alertness); swelling of the ankles, fingers (request medication).
- Diabetic patients—monitor urine sugar closely because glucose tolerance may change. Report any abnormalities to physician, so corrective action can be taken.
- Report ankle swelling, skin color changes, severe nausea, vomiting, hoarseness, body hair growth, deepening of the voice, acne, menstrual irregularities (women).

# Naproxen

## naproxen

*(na **prox'** en)*

Apo-Naproxen (CAN), EC—Naprosyn, Naprelan, Napron X, Naprosyn, Naproxen, Naxen (CAN), Novonaprox (CAN)

## naproxen sodium

Aleve, Anaprox, Anaprox DS

**Pregnancy Category B**

**Drug classes**

Nonsteroidal anti-inflammatory drug (NSAID)
Analgesic (non-narcotic)

**Therapeutic actions**

Analgesic, anti-inflammatory, and antipyretic activities largely related to inhibition of prostaglandin synthesis; exact mechanisms of action are not known.

**Indications**

- Mild to moderate pain
- Treatment of primary dysmenorrhea, rheumatoid arthritis, osteoarthritis, ankylosing spondylitis, tendinitis, bursitis, acute gout
- OTC use: temporary relief of minor aches and pains associated with the common cold, headache, toothache, muscular

aches, backache, minor pain of arthritis, pain of menstrual cramps, reduction of fever
- Treatment of juvenile arthritis (naproxen only)

## Contraindications/cautions

- Contraindications: allergy to naproxen, salicylates, other NSAIDs; pregnancy; lactation.
- Use cautiously with asthma, chronic urticaria, CV dysfunction; hypertension; GI bleeding; peptic ulcer; impaired hepatic or renal function.

## Dosage

**Available Forms:** Tablets—200, 250, 375, 500 mg; DR tablets—375, 500 mg; CR tablets—375, 500 mg; suspension—125 mg/5 ml

Do not exceed 1,250 mg/d (1,375 mg/d naproxen sodium).

**ADULT**

- ***Rheumatoid arthritis/osteoarthritis, ankylosing spondylitis:***
  - **Naproxen:** 250–500 mg bid, PO. May increase to 1.5 g/d for a limited period.
  - **Delayed release (EC-Naprosyn):** 375–500 mg PO bid.
  - **Controlled release (Naprelan):** 750–1000 mg PO qd.
  - **Naproxen sodium:** 275–550 mg bid PO. May increase to 1.65 g/d for a limited period.
- ***Acute gout***
  - **Naproxen:** 750 mg PO followed by 250 mg q8h until the attack subsides.
  - **Controlled release (Naprelan):** 1000–1500 mg PO qd.
  - **Naproxen sodium:** 825 mg PO followed by 275 mg q8h until the attack subsides.
- ***Mild to moderate pain***
  - **Naproxen:** 500 mg PO followed by 250 mg q6–8h. *Note:* Naproxen sodium is used more often than naproxen as an analgesic because it is absorbed more quickly.
  - **Controlled release (Naprelan):** 1000 mg PO qd.
  - **Naproxen sodium:** 550 mg PO followed by 275 mg q6–8h.
- *OTC:* 200 mg PO q8–12h with a full glass of liquid while symptoms persist. Do not exceed 600 mg in 24 h.

**PEDIATRIC**

- ***Juvenile arthritis***
  - **Naproxen:** Total daily dose of 10 mg/kg PO in 2 divided doses. Suspension, 13 kg, 2.5 ml bid; 25 kg, 5 ml bid; 38 kg, 7.5 ml bid.
  - **Naproxen sodium:** Safety and efficacy not established.
- *OTC:* Do not give to children < 12 y unless under advice of physician.

**GERIATRIC:** Do not take > 200 mg q12h PO.

## Pharmacokinetics

| *Drug* | *Onset* | *Peak* | *Duration* |
|---|---|---|---|
| Naproxen | 1 h | 2–4 h | up to 7 h |
| Naproxen sodium | 1 h | 1–2 h | up to 7 h |

*Metabolism:* Hepatic, $T_{1/2}$: 12–15 h
*Distribution:* Crosses placenta; enters breast milk
*Excretion:* Urine

## Adverse effects

*NSAIDs*

- CNS: *Headache, dizziness, somnolence, insomnia*, fatigue, tiredness, dizziness, tinnitus, ophthalmologic effects
- GI: *Nausea, dyspepsia, GI pain,* diarrhea, vomiting, *constipation*, flatulence
- **Respiratory**: Dyspnea, hemoptysis, pharyngitis, bronchospasm, rhinitis
- **Hematologic**: Bleeding, platelet inhibition with higher doses, neutropenia, eosinophilia, leukopenia, pancytopenia, thrombocytopenia, agranulocytosis, granulocytopenia, aplastic anemia, decreased Hgb or Hct, bone marrow depression, mennorhagia
- GU: Dysuria, renal impairment, including renal failure, interstitial nephritis, hematuria
- **Dermatologic**: *Rash*, pruritus, sweating, dry mucous membranes, stomatitis

- Other: Peripheral edema, **anaphylactoid reactions to fatal anaphylactic shock**

### Clinically important drug-drug interactions

- Increased serum lithium levels and risk of toxicity with naproxen.

### Drug-lab test interferences

- Falsely increased values for urinary 17-ketogenic steroids; discontinue naproxen therapy for 72 h before adrenal function tests • Inaccurate measurement of urinary 5-hydroxy indoleacetic acid

## ■ Nursing Considerations

### Assessment

- *History:* Allergy to naproxen, salicylates, other NSAIDs; asthma, chronic urticaria, CV dysfunction; hypertension; GI bleeding; peptic ulcer; impaired hepatic or renal function; pregnancy; lactation
- *Physical:* Skin color and lesions; orientation, reflexes, ophthalmologic and audiometric evaluation, peripheral sensation; P, edema; R, adventitious sounds; liver evaluation; CBC, clotting times, renal and liver function tests; serum electrolytes, stool guaiac

### Implementation

- Give with food or after meals if GI upset occurs.
- Arrange for periodic ophthalmologic examination during long-term therapy.
- Institute emergency procedures if overdose occurs: gastric lavage, induction of emesis, supportive therapy.

### Drug-specific teaching points

- Take drug with food or meals if GI upset occurs; take only the prescribed dosage.
- Dizziness, drowsiness can occur (avoid driving or the use of dangerous machinery).
- Report sore throat; fever; rash; itching; weight gain; swelling in ankles or fingers; changes in vision; black, tarry stools.

# nedocromil sodium

*(nee **doc'** ro mill)*

Tilade

**Pregnancy Category B**

### Drug classes

Antiasthmatic agent
Antiallergic agent

### Therapeutic actions

Inhibits the mediators of a variety of inflammatory cells, including eosinophils, neutrophils, macrophages, mast cells; decreases the release of histamine and blocks the overall inflammatory reaction.

### Indications

- Maintenance therapy in the management of patients with mild to moderate bronchial asthma

### Contraindications/cautions

- Allergy to nedocromil or any other ingredients in the preparation, pregnancy, lactation.

### Dosage

**Available Forms:** Aerosol—1.75 mg/actuation

**ADULTS, CHILDREN > 12 Y:** 2 inhalations qid at regular intervals to provide 14 mg/d; to lower dose, first reduce to tid inhalations (10.5 mg/d), then after several weeks to bid (7 mg/d).

### Pharmacokinetics

| Route | Onset | Peak | Duration |
|---|---|---|---|
| Inhal. | Rapid | 28 min | 10–12 h |

*Metabolism:* Hepatic, $T_{1/2}$: 3.3 h
*Distribution:* Crosses placenta; may enter breast milk
*Excretion:* Urine

### Adverse effects

- CNS: Dizziness, *headache*, fatigue, lacrimation
- GI: *Nausea,* vomiting, dyspepsia, diarrhea, *unpleasant taste*
- Respiratory: *Cough, pharyngitis, rhinitis, URI*, increased sputum, dyspnea, bronchitis

## ■ Nursing Considerations

### Assessment

- *History:* Allergy to nedocromil, lactation
- *Physical:* Skin color, lesions; orientation; R, auscultation, patency of nasal passages; abdominal exam, normal output; kidney and liver function tests, urinalysis

### Implementation

- Do not use during acute bronchospasm; begin therapy when acute episode has subsided and patient can inhale adequately.
- Continue treatment; nedocromil must be taken continuously, even during periods with no asthmatic attacks.
- Use caution if cough or bronchospasm occurs after inhalation; this may (rarely) preclude continuation of treatment.
- Administer corticosteroids concomitantly.

### Drug-specific teaching points

- Take drug at regular intervals, even during periods with no asthmatic attacks. Do not use during acute bronchospasm.
- Take the drug according to guidelines in manufacturer's insert; the effect of the drug depends on contact with the lungs; therefore you must follow the manufacturer's directions.
- Do not discontinue drug abruptly except on advice of your health care provider
- The following side effects may occur: dizziness, drowsiness, fatigue (avoid driving or operating dangerous machinery); headache (if severe, request analgesics); coughing, running nose.
- Report coughing, wheezing, dizziness.

# nefazodone hydrochloride

*(ne **faz'** oh don)*

Serzone

**Pregnancy Category C**

### Drug classes

Antidepressant
Reuptake inhibitor

### Therapeutic actions

Acts as an antidepressant by inhibiting CNS neuronal uptake of serotonin and norepinephrine; also thought to antagonize $\alpha_1$-adrenergic receptors.

### Indications

- Treatment of depression

### Contraindications/cautions

- Contraindication: pregnancy, allergy to nefazodone.
- Use cautiously with CV or cerebrovascular disorders, dehydration, hypovolemia, mania, hypomania, suicidal patients, hepatic cirrhosis, EST, debilitation, lactation.

### Dosage

**Available Forms:** Tablets—100, 150, 200, 250 mg

*ADULT:* 200 mg PO in 2 divided doses; increase at 1 wk intervals in increments of 100–200 mg/d; usual range is 300–600 mg/d.

*PEDIATRIC:* Not recommended in children <18 yr.

*GERIATRIC OR DEBILITATED:* Initially 100 mg/d in 2 divided doses.

### Pharmacokinetics

| *Route* | *Onset* | *Peak* |
|---|---|---|
| Oral | Slow | 2d |

*Metabolism:* Hepatic metabolism; $T_{1/2}$: 2–3 days

*Distribution:* Crosses placenta; passes into breast milk

*Excretion:* Urine and feces

### Adverse effects

- CNS: *headache, nervousness, insomnia, drowsiness, anxiety, tremor, dizziness, lightheadedness,* agitation, sedation, abnormal gait, confusion
- GI: *nausea, vomiting, diarrhea, dry mouth, anorexia, dyspepsia, constipation, taste changes,* flatulence, gastroenteritis, dysphagia, gingivitis
- CV: *postural hypotension*
- Dermatologic: *sweating, rash, pruritus,* acne, alopecia, contact dermatitis

### Clinically important drug-drug interactions

- Increased risk of severe toxic effects with MAOIs, astemizole, terfenadine; avoid these combinations • Risk of increased depression with general anesthetics

## Nursing Considerations

### Assessment

- *History:* Pregnancy, CV or cerebrovascular disorders, dehydration, hypovolemia, mania, hypomania, suicidal patients, hepatic cirrhosis, EST, debilitation, lactation.
- *Physical:* Weight, T, skin rash, lesions; reflexes, affect; bowel sounds, liver evaluation; P, BP, peripheral perfusion; urinary output, renal function; renal and liver function tests

### Implementation

- Give lower doses or less frequently in the elderly or debilitated.
- Establish suicide precautions for severely depressed patients. Limit number of capsules dispensed.
- Ensure that patient is well hydrated while on this therapy; monitor for postural hypotension.
- Ensure at least 14 days elapse between discontinuing MAO inhibitor and starting nefazodone; at least 7 days between stopping nefazodone and starting MAO inhibitor.

### Drug-specific teaching points

- Take this drug exactly as prescribed; do not increase dosage or combine with other drugs without consulting prescriber; several weeks may be needed to see full effects.
- The following side effects may occur: dizziness, drowsiness, nervousness, insomnia (avoid driving or performing hazardous tasks, change positions slowly, take care in conditions of extremes of temperature); nausea, vomiting, weight loss (small, frequent meals; if weight loss becomes marked, consult with your heath care provider).
- Report changes in stool or urine; chest pain, dizziness, vision changes

# nelfinavir mesylate

*(nell **fin'** a veer)*
Viracept
**Pregnancy Category B**

### Drug classes

Antiviral

### Therapeutic actions

Inhibitor of the HIV-1 protease; prevents viral cleavage resulting in the production of immature, non-infectious virus. Though no controlled trials of the effectiveness of nelfinavir exists, studies may indicate effectiveness in combination with nucleoside analogs.

### Indications

- Treatment of HIV infection when antiretroviral therapy is warranted in combination with nucleoside analogs.

### Contraindications/cautions

- Contraindications: life-threatening allergy to any component.
- Use cautiously with renal and hepatic impairment, hemophilia, pregnancy, lactation.

### Dosage

**Available Forms:** Tablets—250 mg; powder—50 mg/g

***ADULTS AND CHILDREN >13 Y:*** 750 mg PO tid in combination with nucleoside analogs.

***PEDIATRIC***

- *2–13 y:* 20–30 mg/kg/dose PO tid.
- *<2 y:* Not recommeded.

### Pharmacokinetics

| *Route* | *Onset* | *Peak* |
|---|---|---|
| Oral | Slow | 2–4 h |

*Metabolism:* Hepatic; $T_{1/2}$: 3.5–5 h
*Distribution:* May cross placenta; may pass into breast milk
*Excretion:* Feces

### Adverse effects

- CNS: Anxiety, depression, insomnia, myalgia, dizziness, paresthesia, seizures, suicide ideation

- GI: *Diarrhea, nausea, GI pain,* anorexia, vomiting, dyspepsia, liver enzyme elevations
- **Respiratory**: Dyspnea, pharyngitis, rhinitis, sinusitis
- **Dermatologic**: Dermatitis, folliculitis, fungal dermatitis, rash, sweating, urticaria
- **Other**: Eye disorders, sexual dysfunction

### Clinically important drug-drug interactions

• Decreased effectiveness with rifabutin, phenobarbital, phenytoin, dexamthasone, carbamazepine • Risk of severe toxic effects and life-threatening arrhythmias with terfenadine, astemizole, cisapride, rifampin, triazolam, midazolam; avoid these combinations • Possible loss of effectiveness of oral contraceptives with nelfinavir; recommend use of barrier contraceptives

## ■ Nursing Considerations

### Assessment

- ***History:*** Life-threatening allergy to any component, impaired hepatic or renal function, pregnancy, lactation, hemophilia
- ***Physical:*** T; affect, reflexes, peripheral sensation; R, adventitious sounds; bowel sounds, liver evaluation; liver and renal function tests

### Implementation

- Administer with meals or a light snack; powder may be mixed with a small amount of non-acidic food or beverage; use within 6 h of mixing.
- Monitor patient for signs of opportunistic infections that will need to be treated appropriately.
- Administer the drug concurrently with nucleoside analogs.
- Arrange for loperamide to control diarrhea if it occurs.
- Recommend the use of barrier contraceptives while on this drug.

### Drug-specific teaching points

- Take drug exactly as prescribed; take missed doses as soon as possible and return to normal schedule; do not double up skipped doses; take with meals or a light snack; powder may be mixed with water, milk or formula; use within 6 h of mixing; take in combination with nucleoside analogs.
- These drugs are not a cure for AIDS or ARC; opportunistic infections may occur and regular medical care should be sought to deal with the disease.
- The long-term effects of this drug are not yet known.
- The following side effects may occur: nausea, loss of appetite, diarrhea (eat small, frequent meals; medication is available to control diarrhea); dizziness, loss of feeling (take appropriate precautions).
- This drug combination does not reduce the risk of transmission of HIV to others by sexual contact or blood contamination; use appropriate precautions.
- Use of barrier contraceptives; this drug may block the effectveness of oral contraceptives.
- Report extreme fatigue, lethargy, severe headache, severe nausea, vomiting, difficulty breathing, skin rash, changes in color of urine or stool.

## neomycin sulfate

*(nee o **mye'** sin)*

*Systemic:* Mycifradin Sulfate

*Topical dermatologic preparations:* Mycifradin (CAN), Myciguent, Neocin (CAN)

**Pregnancy Category C**

### Drug classes

Aminoglycoside

### Therapeutic actions

Bactericidal: inhibits protein synthesis in susceptible strains of gram-negative bacteria; functional integrity of bacterial cell membrane appears to be disrupted, causing cell death

### Indications

- Preoperative suppression of GI bacterial flora (oral)

- Hepatic coma to reduce ammonia-forming bacteria in the GI tract (oral)
- Infection prophylaxis in minor skin wounds and treatment of superficial skin infections due to susceptible organisms (topical dermatologic preparations)
- Unlabeled oral use: lowering of plasma lipids (LDL cholesterol)

## Contraindications/cautions

- Contraindications: allergy to aminoglycosides, intestinal obstruction, pregnancy, lactation.
- Use cautiously with the elderly or with any patient with diminished hearing, decreased renal function, dehydration, neuromuscular disorders (myasthenia gravis, parkinsonism, infant botulism).

## Dosage

**Available Forms:** Tablets—500 mg; oral solution—125 mg/5 ml; ointment/cream—3.5 mg

ADULT

- ***IM:*** 15 mg/kg per day in divided doses q6h. 300 mg q6h for four doses, then 300 mg q12h yields blood concentrations of 12–30 μg/ml in 48–72 h. Do not exceed 1 g/d. Do not continue therapy for more than 10 d.
- ***Oral*** Preoperative preparation for elective colorectal surgery: see manufacturer's recommendations for a complex 3-d regimen that includes oral erythromycin, magnesium sulfate, enemas, and dietary restrictions.
  - *Hepatic coma:* 4–12 g/d in divided doses for 5–6 d, as adjunct to protein-free diet and supportive therapy, including transfusions, as needed.
- ***Topical dermatologic:*** Apply to affected area one to five times daily, except burns affecting more than 20% of the body surface should be treated once daily.

PEDIATRIC

- *IM:* Do not use in infants and children.
- *Oral:* Hepatic coma: 50–100 mg/kg per day in divided doses for 5–6 d, as adjunct to protein-free diet and supportive therapy including transfusions, as needed.

GERIATRIC OR RENAL FAILURE PATIENTS: Reduce dosage and carefully monitor serum drug levels and renal function tests throughout treatment. If this is not possible, reduce frequency of administration.

## Pharmacokinetics

| Route | Onset | Peak |
|---|---|---|
| Oral | Varies | 1–4 h |
| IM | Rapid | 1/2–1 h |
| Topical | Not generally absorbed systemically. | |

*Metabolism:* $T_{1/2}$: 3 h

*Distribution:* Crosses placenta; enters breast milk

*Excretion:* Feces and urine (IM)

## Adverse effects

While limited absorption occurs across the intact GI mucosa, the risk of absorption from ulcerated area requires consideration of all side effects with oral and parenteral therapy. These side effects also should be considered with dermatologic applications to ulcerated, burned skin or large skin areas where absorption is possible.

- CNS: Ototoxicity—*tinnitus, dizziness*, vertigo, deafness (partially reversible to irreversible), vestibular paralysis, confusion, disorientation, depression, lethargy, nystagmus, visual disturbances, headache, *numbness, tingling*, tremor, paresthesias, muscle twitching, convulsions
- GI: Hepatic toxicity, *nausea, vomiting, anorexia,* weight loss, stomatitis, increased salivation
- CV: Palpitations, hypotension, hypertension
- **Hematologic**: *Leukemoid reaction,* agranulocytosis, granulocytosis, leukopenia, leukocytosis, thrombocytopenia, eosinophilia, pancytopenia, anemia, hemolytic anemia, increased or decreased reticulocyte count, electrolyte disturbances
- GU: *Nephrotoxicity*
- **Hypersensitivity**: Hypersensitivity reactions: *purpura, rash*, urticaria, exfoliative dermatitis, itching

- Local: *Pain, irritation, arachnoiditis at IM injection sites*
- Other: Fever, apnea, splenomegaly, joint pain, *superinfections*

### Clinically important drug-drug interactions

• Increased ototoxic, nephrotoxic, neurotoxic effects with other aminoglycosides, cephalothin, potent diuretics • Increased neuromuscular blockade and muscular paralysis with anesthetics, nondepolarizing neuromuscular blocking drugs, succinylcholine, citrate-anticoagulated blood • Potential inactivation of both drugs if mixed with beta-lactam-type antibiotics • Increased bactericidal effect with penicillins, cephalopsorins, carbenicillin, ticarcillin • Decreased absorption and therapeutic effects of digoxin

### Drug-lab test interferences

• Falsely low serum aminoglycoside levels with penicillin or cephalosporin therapy; these antibiotics can inactivate aminoglycosides after the blood sample is drawn.

## ■ Nursing Considerations

### Assessment

- *History:* Allergy to aminoglycosides; intestinal obstruction, diminished hearing, decreased renal function, dehydration, neuromuscular disorders; pregnancy, lactation
- *Physical:* Renal function, eighth cranial nerve function, state of hydration, CBC, skin color and lesions, orientation and affect, reflexes, bilateral grip strength, body weight, bowel sounds

### Implementation

- Arrange culture and sensitivity tests of infection before beginning therapy.
- Administer parenteral preparation only by deep IM injection. Prepare solution by adding 2 ml Sodium Chloride Injection to 500-mg vial. Store unreconstituted solution at room temperature; refrigerate reconstituted solution; protect from light and use within 1 wk.
- Ensure that the patient is well hydrated.

### Drug-specific teaching points

- Report hearing changes, dizziness, severe diarrhea.

## neostigmine methylsulfate

*(nee oh **stig'** meen)*

Prostigmin

**Pregnancy Category C**

### Drug classes

Cholinesterase inhibitors
Parasympathomimetic
Urinary tract agent
Antimyasthenic agent
Antidote

### Therapeutic actions

Increases the concentration of acetylcholine at the sites of cholinergic transmission, and prolongs and exaggerates the effects of acetylcholine by reversibly inhibiting the enzyme acetylcholinesterase, causing parasympathomimetic effects and facilitating transmission at the skeletal neuromuscular junction; also has direct cholinomimetic activity on skeletal muscle; may have direct cholinomimetic activity on neurons in autonomic ganglia and the CNS.

### Indications

- Prevention and treatment of postoperative distention and urinary retention (neostigmine methylsulfate)
- Symptomatic control of myasthenia gravis
- Diagnosis of myasthenia gravis (edrophonium preferred)
- Antidote for nondepolarizing neuromuscular junction blockers (tubocurarine) after surgery

### Contraindications/cautions

- Contraindications: hypersensitivity to anticholinesterases; adverse reactions to bromides (neostigmine bromide); intestinal or urogenital tract obstruction, peritonitis; pregnancy (may stimulate uterus and induce premature labor); lactation.

- Use cautiously with asthma, peptic ulcer, bradycardia, cardiac arrhythmias, recent coronary occlusion, vagotonia, hyperthyroidism, epilepsy.

## Dosage

**Available Forms:** Tablets—15 mg; injection—0.25, 0.5, 1, 2.5 mg

### ADULT

- *Prevention of postoperative distention and urinary retention:* 1 ml of the 1:4,000 solution (0.25 mg) neostigmine methylsulfate SC or IM as soon as possible after operation. Repeat q4–6h for 2–3 d.
- *Treatment of postoperative distention:* 1 ml of the 1:2,000 solution (0.5 mg) neostigmine methylsulfate SC or IM, as required.
- *Treatment of urinary retention:* 1 ml of the 1:2,000 solution (0.5 mg) neostigmine methylsulfate SC or IM. If urination does not occur within 1 h, catheterize the patient. After the bladder is emptied, continue 0.5 mg injections q3h for at least 5 injections.
- *Symptomatic control of myasthenia gravis:* 1 ml of the 1:2,000 solution (0.5 mg) SC or IM. Individualize subsequent doses.
- *Diagnosis of myasthenia gravis:* 0.022 mg/kg IM.
- *Antidote for nondepolarizing neuromuscular blockers:* Give atropine sulfate 0.6–1.2 mg IV several min before slow IV injection of neostigmine 0.5–2 mg. Repeat as required. Total dose should usually not exceed 5 mg.

### PEDIATRIC

- *Prevention, treatment of postoperative retention, and so forth:* Safety and efficacy not established.
- *Symptomatic control of myasthenia gravis:* 0.01–0.04 mg/kg per dose IM, IV, or SC q2–3h as needed.
- *Diagnosis of myasthenia gravis:* 0.04 mg/kg IM.
- *As antidote for nondepolarizing neuromuscular blocker:* Give 0.008–0.025 mg/kg atropine sulfate IV several min before slow IV injection of neostigmine 0.07–0.08 mg/kg.

## Pharmacokinetics

| Route | Onset | Peak | Duration |
|---|---|---|---|
| SC/IM | 20–30 min | 20–30 min | 2.5–4 h |
| IV | 10–30 min | 20–30 min | 2.5–4 h |

*Metabolism:* Hepatic, $T_{1/2}$: 47–60 min
*Distribution:* May cross placenta or enter breast milk
*Excretion:* Urine

### IV facts

**Preparation:** No further preparation is required.
**Infusion:** Inject slowly directly into vein or into tubing of running IV, each 0.5 mg over 1 min.

## Adverse effects

- CNS: Convulsions, dysarthria, dysphonia, drowsiness, dizziness, headache, loss of consciousness
- GI: *Salivation, dysphagia, nausea, vomiting, increased peristalsis, abdominal cramps,* flatulence, diarrhea
- CV: *Cardiac arrhythmias,* cardiac arrest; decreased cardiac output leading to hypotension, syncope
- Respiratory: *Increased pharyngeal and tracheobronchial secretions,* laryngospasm, bronchospasm, bronchiolar constriction, dyspnea, respiratory muscle paralysis, central respiratory paralysis
- GU: *Urinary frequency and incontinence,* urinary urgency
- EENT: *Lacrimation, miosis,* spasm of accommodation, diplopia, conjunctival hyperemia
- Dermatologic: Diaphoresis, flushing, skin rash, urticaria, anaphylaxis
- Peripheral: Skeletal muscle weakness, fasciculations, muscle cramps, arthralgia
- Local: Thrombophlebitis after IV use

## Clinically important drug-drug interactions

• Decreased neuromuscular blockade of succinylcholine • Decreased effects and possible muscular depression with corticosteroids

## Nursing Considerations

### Assessment

- *History:* Hypersensitivity to anticholinesterases; adverse reactions to bromides; intestinal or urogenital tract obstruction, peritonitis; asthma, peptic ulcer, cardiac arrhythmias, recent coronary occlusion, vagotonia, hyperthyroidism, epilepsy; lactation
- *Physical:* Skin color, texture, lesions; reflexes, bilateral grip strength; P, auscultation, BP; R, adventious sounds; salivation, bowel sounds, normal output; frequency, voiding pattern, normal output; EEG, thyroid tests

### Implementation

- Administer IV slowly.
- Overdosage with anticholinesterase drugs can cause muscle weakness (cholinergic crisis) that is difficult to differentiate from myasthenic weakness. The administration of atropine may mask the parasympathetic effects of anticholinesterase overdose and further confound the diagnosis.
- Maintain atropine sulfate on standby as an antidote and antagonist in case of cholinergic crisis or hypersensitivity reaction.
- Discontinue drug, and consult physician if excessive salivation, emesis, frequent urination, or diarrhea occur.
- Decrease dosage if excessive sweating, nausea occur.

### Drug-specific teaching points

- Take this drug exactly as prescribed; patient and a significant other should receive extensive teaching about the effects of the drug, the signs and symptoms of myasthenia gravis, the fact that muscle weakness may be related both to drug overdosage and to exacerbation of the disease, and that it is important to report muscle weakness promptly to the nurse or physician so that proper evaluation can be made.
- The following side effects may occur: blurred vision, difficulty with far vision, difficulty with dark adaptation (use caution while driving, especially at night, or performing hazardous tasks in reduced light); increased urinary frequency, abdominal cramps; sweating (avoid hot or excessively humid environments).
- Report muscle weakness, nausea, vomiting, diarrhea, severe abdominal pain, excessive sweating, excessive salivation, frequent urination, urinary urgency, irregular heartbeat, difficulty in breathing.

## netilmicin sulfate

*(ne til **mye'** sin)*

Netromycin

**Pregnancy Category C**

### Drug classes

Aminoglycoside

Antibiotic

### Therapeutic actions

Bactericidal: inhibits protein synthesis in strains of gram-negative bacteria; mechanism of lethal action not fully understood, but functional integrity of cell membrane appears to be disrupted, leading to cell death.

### Indications

- Short-term treatment of serious infections caused by susceptible strains of *E. coli, Klebsiella pneumoniae, Pseudomonas aeruginosa, Enterobacter* species, *Proteus mirabilis,* indole-positive *Proteus* species, *Serratia, Citrobacter* species, *Staphylococcus aureus*
- Treatment of staphylococcal infections when other antibiotics are ineffective or contraindicated
- Treatment of staphylococcal infections or infections of which the cause is unknown, before antibiotic susceptibility studies can be completed (often given in conjunction with a penicillin or cephalosporin)

### Contraindications/cautions

- Contraindications: allergy to aminoglycosides, intestinal obstruction (oral), lactation.
- Use cautiously with the elderly or any patient with diminished hearing, decreased renal function, dehydration, neuromuscular disorders (myasthenia gravis, parkinsonism, infant botulism).

### Dosage

**Available Forms:** Injection—100 mg/ml IM or IV (dosage is the same).

ADULT

- *Complicated UTIs:* 1.5–2 mg/kg q12h.
- *Systemic infections:* 1.3–2.2 mg/kg q8h or 2–3.25 mg/kg q12h.

PEDIATRIC (6 WK–12 Y): 1.8–2.7 mg/kg q8h or 2.7–4 mg/kg q12h.

NEONATES: 2–3.25 mg/kg q12h.

GERIATRIC OR RENAL FAILURE PATIENTS: Reduce dosage, and carefully monitor serum drug levels and renal function tests throughout treatment. Manufacturer suggests three ways to adjust dosage based on serum creatinine or creatinine clearance; see package insert.

### Pharmacokinetics

| Route | Onset | Peak |
|---|---|---|
| IM | Rapid | 30–60 min |
| IV | Immediate | End of infusion |

*Metabolism:* Hepatic, $T_{1/2}$: 2–2.5 h
*Distribution:* Crosses placenta; enters breast milk
*Excretion:* Urine

#### IV facts

**Preparation:** Dilute with 50–200 ml of solution. Stable when stored in glass in concentrations of 2.1–3 mg/ml for up to 72 h at room temperature or refrigerated. Discard after that time.
**Infusion:** Infuse over 1/2–2 h.
**Compatibilities:** Compatible with Sterile Water for Injection; 0.9% Sodium Chloride Injection alone or with 5% Dextrose; 5% or 10% Dextrose Injection in Water; 5% Dextrose with Electrolyte 48 or 75; Ringer's and Lactated Ringer's; Lactated Ringer's and 5% Dextrose Injecton; Plasma-Lyte 56 or 148 Injection with 5% Dextrose; 10% Travert with Electrolyte 2 or 3 Injection; Isolyte E, M, or P with 5% Dextrose Injection; 10% Dextran 40 or 6% Dextran 75 in 5% Dextrose Injection; Plasma-Lyte M Injection with 5% Dextrose; Ionosol B in D5W; Normosol-R; Plasma-Lyte 148 Injection; 10% Fructose Injection; Electrolyte 3 with 10% Invert Sugar Injection; Normosol-M or R in D5W, Isolyte H or S with 5% Dextrose; Isolyte S; Plasma-Lyte 148 Injection in Water; Normosol-R pH 7.4.

### Adverse effects

- CNS: Ototoxicity—*tinnitus, dizziness,*, vertigo, deafness (partially reversible to irreversible), vestibular paralysis, confusion, disorientation, depression, lethargy, nystagmus, visual disturbances, headache, *numbness, tingling*, tremor, paresthesias, muscle twitching, convulsions, muscular weakness, neuromuscular blockade
- GI: Hepatic toxicity, *nausea, vomiting, anorexia,* weight loss, stomatitis
- CV: Palpitations, hypotension, hypertension
- **Hematologic:** *Leukemoid reaction,* agranulocytosis, granulocytosis, leukopenia, leukocytosis, thrombocytopenia, eosinophilia, pancytopenia, anemia, hemolytic anemia, changed reticulocyte count, electrolyte disturbances
- GU: *Nephrotoxicity*
- **Hypersensitivity:** *Purpura, rash,* urticaria, exfoliative dermatitis, itching
- **Local:** *Pain, irritation, arachnoiditis at IM injection sites*
- **Other:** Fever, apnea, splenomegaly, joint pain, *superinfections*

### Clinically important drug-drug interactions

• Increased ototoxic, nephrotoxic, neurotoxic effects with other aminoglycosides, cephalothin, potent diuretics • Increased neuromuscular blockade and muscular paralysis with anesthetics, nondepolarizing neuromuscular blocking drugs, succinylcholine, citrate-anticoagulated blood • Potential inactivation of both drugs if mixed with beta-lactam-type antibiotics. Increased bactericidal effect with penicillins, cephalopsorins, carbenicillin, ticarcillin

## ■ Nursing Considerations

### Assessment

- *History:* Allergy to aminoglycosides; intestinal obstruction (oral); pregnancy;

lactation; diminished hearing; decreased renal function, dehydration, neuromuscular disorders
- *Physical:* Weight, renal function, eighth cranial nerve function, state of hydration, hepatic function, CBC, skin color and lesions, orientation and affect, reflexes, bilateral grip strength, bowel sounds

### Implementation
- Arrange culture and sensitivity tests of infection before beginning therapy.
- Limit duration of treatment to short term to reduce the risk of toxicity; usual duration of treatment is 7–14 d.
- Give IM dose by deep IM injection.
- Ensure that patient is well hydrated before and during therapy.

### Drug-specific teaching points
- The following side effects may occur: nausea, loss of appetite (small, frequent meals may help); diarrhea; superinfections in mouth, vagina (request treatment).
- Report any hearing changes, dizziness, lesions in mouth, vaginal itching.

## nevirapine

*(neh veer' ah pine)*
Vistide
**Pregnancy Category C**

### Drug classes
Antiviral

### Therapeutic actions
Antiretroviral activity; binds directly to HIV-1 reverse transcriptase and blocks the replication of HIV by changing the structure of the HIV enzyme.

### Indications
- Treatment of HIV-1–infected adults who have experienced clinical and/or immunologic deterioration; used in combination with nucleoside analogues

### Contraindications/cautions
- Contraindications: allergy to nevirapine; pregnancy, lactation
- Use cautiously with renal or hepatic impairment, rash

### Dosage
**Available Forms:** Tablets—200 mg
*ADULT:* 200 mg PO qd for 14 d; if no rash appears, then 200 mg PO bid.
*PEDIATRIC:* Safety and efficacy not established in children <12 y.

### Pharmacokinetics

| *Route* | *Onset* | *Peak* |
|---|---|---|
| PO | Rapid | 4 h |

*Metabolism:* Hepatic; $T_{1/2}$: 45 h, then 25–30 h
*Distribution:* Crosses placenta; passes into breast milk
*Excretion:* Urine

### Adverse effects
- CNS: *Headache*
- GI: *Nausea, vomiting, diarrhea,* dry mouth, **liver dysfunction**
- Dermatologic: **Rash** (may be life threatening)
- Other: Infection, chills, fever

### Clinically important drug-drug interactions
- Avoid concurrent use with protease inhibitors, oral contraceptives (metabolism is increased and effectiveness decreased) • Significant decrease in serum indinavir levels with nevirapine—avoid this combination; if combination is necessary, increase indinavir to 1000 mg q8h with nevirapine 200 mg bid; carefully monitor effectiveness of indinavir if starting or stopping nevirapine

## ■ Nursing Considerations

### Assessment
- *History:* Allergy to nevirapine; renal or hepatic dysfunction, pregnancy, lactation, rash
- *Physical:* T; orientation, reflexes; peripheral perfusion; urinary output; skin color, perfusion, hydration; hepatic and renal function tests

## Implementation

- Monitor renal and hepatic function tests before and during treatment. Discontinue drug at any sign of hepatic dysfunction.
- Do not administer if severe rash occurs, especially accompanied by fever, blistering, lesion, swelling, general malaise; discontinue if rash recurs on rechallenge.

## Drug-specific teaching points

- Take this drug exactly as prescribed; do not double up missed doses.
- Use some method of barrier birth control (not oral contraceptives) while on this medication. Severe birth defects can occur, and this drug causes loss of effectiveness of oral contraceptives.
- This drug does not cure HIV infection. Follow routine preventive measures and continue any other medication that has been prescribed.
- The following side effects may occur: nausea, vomiting, loss of appetite, diarrhea, headache, fever.
- Report rash, any lesions or blistering, changes in color of stool or urine, fever, muscle or joint pain.

# niacin

***(nye' ah sin)***

Niaspan

**Pregnancy Category C**

### Drug classes

Antihyperlipidemic
Vitamin

### Therapeutic actions

May partially inhibit the release of free fatty acids from adipose tissue and increase lipoprotein activity, which could increase the rate of triglyceride removal from plasma; these actions reduce the total LDL and triglycerides and increase HDL. Niacin also decreases serum levels of apo B and lipoprotein A.

### Indications

- Adjunct to diet in primary hypercholesterolemia and mixed dyslipidemia to reduce elevated cholesterol, LDL cholesterol, apolipoprotein B and triglycerides
- Combined with a bile acid sequestrant to reduce elevated total cholesterol and LDL cholesterol in primary hypercholesterolemia when diet and diet plus monotherapy have been inadequate
- Adjunct in patients with very high serum triglycerides who are at risk for pancreatitis
- Reduction of the risk of recurrent MI in patients with a history of MI and hypercholesterolemia
- Combined with a bile sequestrant to slow the progression or promote regression of atherosclerosis in patients with CAD and hypercholesteremia

### Contraindications/cautions

- Contraindications: hepatic dysfunction, active peptic ulcer disease, arterial bleeding, lactation.
- Use cautiously with history of jaundice, hepatobiliary disease, peptic ulcer, high alcohol consumption, renal dysfunction, unstable angina, gout, recent surgery, pregnancy.

## Dosage

**Available Forms:** ER tablets—375, 500, 750, 1,000 mg

***Adult and Pediatric < 16 Y:*** 375 mg PO qd for the 1st wk, then 500 mg PO qd for 2nd wk, then 750 mg PO qd for 3rd wk, then 1 g PO qd for wks 4–7. May increase by 500 mg every 4 wk until adequate response is reached. Do not exceed 2 g/d.

***Pediatric < 16 Y:*** Safety and efficacy not established.

### Pharmacokinetics

| *Route* | *Onset* | *Peak* |
|---|---|---|
| Oral | Rapid | 45 min |

*Metabolism:* Hepatic: $T_{1/2}$: unknown
*Distribution:* Crosses placenta, enters breast milk
*Excretion:* Urine

### Adverse effects

- CNS: *Headache,* anxiety
- GI: *GI upset,* peptic ulcer, abnormal liver function tests
- CV: Arrhythmias, hypotension

- **Hematologic**: Hyperurcemia
- **Dermatologic**: *Flushing,* acanthosis nigricans, dry skin
- **Other**: Glucose intolerance

### Clinically important drug-drug interactions

• Increased risk of rhabdomyolysis with HMG-CoA inhibitors • Increased effectiveness of antihypertensives, vasoactive drugs • Increased risk of bleeding with anticoagulants; monitor PT and platelet counts and adjust dose accordingly • Decreased absorption with bile acid sequestrants; separate doses by at least 4–6 h

## ■ Nursing Considerations

### Assessment

- *History:* Hepatic dysfunction, active peptic ulcer disease, arterial bleeding, lactation, hepatobiliary disease, peptic ulcer; high alcohol consumption, renal dysfunction, unstable angina, gout, recent surgery, pregnancy
- *Physical:* Skin lesions, color, temperature; orientation, affect, reflexes; P, auscultation, baseline ECG, BP; liver evaluation; lipid studies, liver function tests

### Implementation

- Administer drug at bedtime to minimize effects of flushing.
- Administer bile sequestrants at least 4–6 h apart from niacin.
- Consult with dietician regarding low-cholesterol diets.
- Arrange for regular follow-up during long-term therapy.

### Drug-specific teaching points

- Take drug at bedtime. The dose will change each week until the desired response is achieved.
- Take your bile acid sequestrant (if appropriate) 4–6 hours apart from niacin; avoid alcohol while on this drug.
- The following side effects may occur: nausea, heartburn, loss of appetite (eat small, frequent meals); headache (may lessen over time; if bothersome, consult with your nurse or physician); skin rash, flushing (take drug at bedtime).
- Report unusual bleeding or bruising, palpitations, fainting, rash, fever.

# nicardipine hydrochloride

*(nye **kar'** de peen)*

Cardene, Cardene SR, Cardene IV

**Pregnancy Category C**

### Drug classes

Calcium channel blocker
Antianginal agent
Antihypertensive

### Therapeutic actions

Inhibits the movement of calcium ions across the membranes of cardiac and arterial muscle cells; calcium is involved in the generation of the action potential in specialized automatic and conducting cells in the heart, in arterial smooth muscle, and in excitation-contraction coupling in cardiac muscle cells. Inhibition of calcium flow results in the depression of impulse formation in specialized cardiac pacemaker cells, in slowing of the velocity of conduction of the cardiac impulse, in the depression of myocardial contractility, and in the dilation of coronary arteries and arterioles and peripheral arterioles; these effects lead to decreased cardiac work, decreased cardiac energy consumption, and increased delivery of oxygen to myocardial cells.

### Indications

- Chronic stable (effort-associated) angina. Use alone or with beta-blockers.
- Management of essential hypertension alone or with other antihypertensives (immediate release and sustained release)
- Short-term treatment of hypertension when oral use is not feasible (IV)

### Contraindications/cautions

- Contraindications: allergy to nicardipine, pregnancy, lactation.
- Use cautiously with impaired hepatic or renal function, sick sinus syndrome, heart block (second or third-degree).

n

## Dosage

**Available Forms:** Capsules—20, 30 mg; SR capsules—30, 45, 60 mg; injection—2.5 mg/ml

ADULT

- *Angina:* Immediate release only. Individualize dosage. Usual initial dose is 20 mg tid PO. Range 20–40 mg tid PO. Allow at least 3 d before increasing dosage to ensure steady-state plasma levels.
- *Hypertension:* Immediate release. *Initial dose:* 20 mg tid PO. Range 20–40 mg tid. The maximum BP-lowering effect occurs in 1–2 h. Adjust dosage based on BP response, allow at least 3 d before increasing dosage. *Sustained release:* Initial dose is 30 mg bid PO. *Range:* 30–60 mg bid.

PEDIATRIC: Safety and efficacy not established.

GERIATRIC OR RENAL OR HEPATIC IMPAIRMENT

- *Renal impairment:* Titrate dose beginning with 20 mg tid PO (immediate release).
- *Hepatic impairment:* Starting dose 20 mg bid PO (immediate release) with individual titration.

## Pharmacokinetics

| *Route* | *Onset* | *Peak* |
|---|---|---|
| Oral | 20 min | 0.5–2 h |

*Metabolism:* Hepatic, $T_{1/2}$: 2–4 h
*Distribution:* Crosses placenta; enters breast milk
*Excretion:* Urine

### IV facts

**Preparation:** Dilute each amp with 240 ml of solution; store at room temperature; protect from light; stable for 24 h.

**Infusion:** Slow IV infusion, 1.2–2.2 mg/hr based on patient response.

**Compatibilities:** Dextrose 5% Injection, Dextrose 5% and Sodium Chloride 0.45% or 0.9% Injection; Dextrose 5% with Potassium; 0.45% or 0.9% Sodium Chloride. Do not mix with 5% Sodium Bicarbonate or Lactated Ringer's.

## Adverse effects

- CNS: *Dizziness, lightheadedness, headache, asthenia,* fatigue
- GI: *Nausea,* hepatic injury
- CV: *Peripheral edema, angina,* hypotension, arrhythmias, *bradycardia, AV block,* asystole
- Dermatologic: *Flushing,* rash

## Clinically important drug-drug interactions

- Increased serum levels and toxicity of cyclosporine

## ■ Nursing Considerations

### Assessment

- *History:* Allergy to nicardipine, impaired hepatic or renal function, sick sinus syndrome, heart block (second or third degree), pregnancy, lactation
- *Physical:* Skin lesions, color, edema; P, BP, baseline ECG, peripheral perfusion, auscultation; R, adventitious sounds; liver evaluation, normal GI output; liver and renal function tests, urinalysis

### Implementation

- Monitor patient carefully (BP, cardiac rhythm, and output) while drug is being titrated to therapeutic dose; dosage may be increased more rapidly in hospitalized patients under close supervision.
- Monitor BP very carefully with concurrent doses of nitrates.
- Monitor cardiac rhythm regularly during stabilization of dosage and long-term therapy.
- Provide small, frequent meals if GI upset occurs.

### Drug-specific teaching points

- The following side effects may occur: nausea, vomiting (small, frequent meals may help); headache (monitor lighting, noise, and temperature; request medication if severe).
- Report irregular heart beat, shortness of breath, swelling of the hands or feet, pronounced dizziness, constipation.

# nicotine polacrilex

*(nik' oh teen)*
nicotine resin complex
Nicorette, Nicorette DS
**Pregnancy Category X**

## Drug classes
Smoking deterrent

## Therapeutic actions
Acts as an agonist at nicotinic receptors in the peripheral and CNS; produces behavioral stimulation and depression, cardiac acceleration, peripheral vasoconstriction, and elevated BP.

## Indications
- Temporary aid to the cigarette smoker seeking to give up smoking while in a behavioral modification program under medical supervision

## Contraindications/cautions
- Contraindications: allergy to nicotine or resin used; nonsmoker; post-MI period; arrhythmias; angina pectoris; active TMJ disease; pregnancy; lactation.
- Use cautiously with hyperthyroidism, pheochromocytoma, Type II diabetes (releases catecholamines from the adrenal medulla); hypertension, peptic ulcer disease.

## Dosage
**Available Forms:** Chewing gum—2,4 mg/square

**ADULT:**
- *Chewing gum:* Have patient chew one piece of gum whenever the urge to smoke occurs. Chew each piece slowly and intermittently for about 30 min to promote even, slow, buccal absorption of nicotine. Patients often require 10 pieces/d during the first month. Do not exceed 30 pieces/d (2 mg) or 20 pieces/d (4 mg). Therapy may be effective for up to 3 mo; 4–6 mo for complete cessation has been used. Should not be used for longer than 6 mo.

**PEDIATRIC:** Safety and efficacy in children and adolescents who smoke have not been established.

## Pharmacokinetics

| Route | Onset | Peak |
|---|---|---|
| Oral | Slow | 15–30 min |

*Metabolism:* Hepatic, $T_{1/2}$: 30–120 min
*Distribution:* Crosses placenta; enters breast milk
*Excretion:* Urine

## Adverse effects
- CNS: Dizziness, lightheadedness
- GI: *Mouth or throat soreness; hiccoughs, nausea, vomiting,* nonspecific GI distress, excessive salivation
- **Local:** Mechanical effects of chewing gum—traumatic injury to oral mucosa or teeth, *jaw ache,* eructation secondary to air swallowing

## Clinically important drug-drug interactions
• Increased circulating levels of cortisol, catecholamines with nicotine use, smoking—dosage of adrenergic agonists, adrenergic blockers may need to adjusted according to nicotine, smoking status of patient • Smoking increases metabolism and lowers blood levels of caffeine, theophylline, imipramine, pentazocine; decreases effects of furosemide, propranolol • Cessation of smoking may decrease absorption of glutethimide, decrease metabolism of propoxyphene

## ■ Nursing Considerations

### Assessment
- ***History:*** Allergy to nicotine or resin used; nonsmoker; post-MI period; arrhythmias; angina pectoris; active TMJ disease; hyperthyroidism, pheochromocytoma, type II diabetes; hypertension, peptic ulcer disease; pregnancy; lactation
- ***Physical:*** Jaw strength, symmetry; orientation, affect; P, auscultation, BP; oral mucous membranes, abdominal exam; thyroid function tests

### Implementation
- Review mechanics of chewing gum with patient; patient must chew the gum slowly and intermittently to promote

even, slow absorption of nicotine; discard chewed gum in wrapper to prevent access by children or pets.

- Arrange to withdraw or taper use of gum in abstainers at 3 mo; effectiveness after that time has not been established, and patients may be using gum as substitute source for nicotine dependence.

### Drug-specific teaching points

- Chew one piece of gum every time you have the desire to smoke. Chew slowly and intermittently for about 30 min; do not chew more than 30 pieces of gum each day. Discard chewed gum in wrapper to prevent access by children or pets.
- Abstain from smoking.
- The following side effects may occur: dizziness, headache, lightheadedness (use caution driving or performing tasks that require alertness); nausea, vomiting, increased burping; jaw muscle ache (modify chewing technique).
- Report nausea and vomiting, increased salivation, diarrhea, cold sweat, headache, disturbances in hearing or vision, chest pain, palpitations.
- Do not offer to nonsmokers; serious reactions can occur if used by nonsmokers.

## nicotine transdermal

***(nik' oh teen)***

Habitrol, Nicoderm, Nicoderm CQ, Nicotrol, Nicotrol NS, ProStep

**Pregnancy Category X**

### Drug classes

Smoking deterrent

### Therapeutic actions

Nicotine acts at nicotinic receptors in the peripheral and CNS; produces behavioral stimulation and depression, cardiac acceleration, peripheral vasoconstriction, and elevated BP.

### Indications

- Temporary aid to the cigarette smoker seeking to give up smoking while in a behavioral modification program under medical supervision
- Unlabeled use: improvement of symptoms of Gilles de la Tourette's syndrome

### Contraindications/cautions

- Contraindications: allergy to nicotine; nonsmokers; post-MI period; arrhythmias; angina pectoris; pregnancy; lactation
- Use cautiously with hyperthyroidism, pheochromocytoma, Type II diabetes (releases catecholamines from the adrenal medulla); hypertension, peptic ulcer disease.

### Dosage

**Available Forms:** Transdermal system—7, 14, 21 mg/d, 5, 10, 15 mg/d, 11, 22 mg/d; nasal spray—0.5 mg/actuation

**ADULT**

- *Topical:* Apply system, 5–22 mg, once every 24 h. Dosage is based on response and stage of withdrawal *Habitrol, Nicoderm*: 21 mg/d for first 6 wk; 14 mg/d for next 2 wk; 7 mg/d for next 2 wk. *Nicotrol*: 15 mg/d for first 6 wk; 10 mg/d for next 2 wk; 5 mg/d for last 2 wk. *ProStep*: 22 mg/d for 4–6 wk; 11 mg/d for 2–4 wk.
- *Nasal spray:* 1 mg (2 sprays, 1 in each nostril), 1–2 doses/h to a maximum of 5 doses/h or 40 doses/d. Do not use > 3 mo.

**PEDIATRIC:** Safety and efficacy in children and adolescents who smoke have not been established.

### Pharmacokinetics

| Route | Onset | Peak | Duration |
|---|---|---|---|
| Dermal | 1–2 h | 4–6 min | 4–24 h |
| Nasal | immed | 5–10 min | – |

*Metabolism:* Hepatic, $T_{1/2}$: 3–4 h
*Distribution:* Crosses placenta; enters breast milk
*Excretion:* Urine

### Adverse effects

- CNS: *Headache, insomnia,* abnormal dreams, dizziness, lightheadedness, sweating
- GI: Diarrhea, constipation, nausea, dyspepsia, abdominal pain, dry mouth

- **Respiratory**: Cough, pharyngitis, sinusitis
- **Local**: *Erythema, burning, pruritus* at site of patch, local edema
- **Other**: Back ache, chest pain, asthenia, dysmenorrhea

### Clinically important drug-drug interactions

• Increased circulating levels of cortisol, catecholamines with nicotine use; smoking dosage of adrenergic agonists, adrenergic blockers may need to be adjusted according to nicotine, smoking status of patient • Smoking increases metabolism and lowers blood levels of caffeine, theophylline, imipramine, pentazocine; decreases effects of furosemide, propranolol • Cessation of smoking may decrease absorption of glutethimide, decrease metabolism of propoxyphene

## ■ Nursing Considerations

### Assessment

- *History:* Allergy to nicotine; nonsmoker; post-MI period; arrhythmias; angina pectoris; hyperthyroidism, pheochromocytoma, type II diabetes; hypertension, peptic ulcer disease; pregnancy; lactation
- *Physical:* Jaw strength, symmetry; orientation, affect; P, auscultation, BP; oral mucous membranes, abdominal exam; thyroid function tests

### Implementation

- Protect systems from heat; slight discoloration of system is not significant.
- Apply system to nonhairy, clean, dry skin site on upper body or upper outer arm; use only when the pouch is intact; use immediately after removal from pouch; use each system only once.
- Wash hands thoroughly after application; do not touch eyes.
- Wrap used system in foil pouch of newly applied system; fold over and dispose of immediately to prevent access by pets or children.
- Apply new system after 24 h; do not reuse same site for at least 1 wk. *Nicotrol*: apply a new system each day after waking, and remove at bedtime.
- Ensure that patient has stopped smoking; if the patient is unable to stop smoking within the first 4 wk of therapy, drug therapy should be stopped.
- Encourage patients who have been unsuccessful at any dose to take a "therapy holiday" before trying again; counseling should explore factors contributing to their failure and other means of success.

### Drug-specific teaching points

- Protect systems from heat; slight discoloration of system is not significant.
- Apply system to nonhairy, clean, dry skin site on upper body or upper outer arm; use only when the pouch is intact; use immediately after removal from pouch; use each system only once.
- Wash hands thoroughly after application; do not touch eyes. Wrap used system in foil pouch of newly applied system; fold over and dispose of immediately to prevent access by pets or children.
- Apply new system after 24 h; do not reuse same site for at least 1 wk. *Nicotrol*: apply a new system each day after waking, and remove at bedtime.
- Do not exceed 5 doses/h of nasal spray or 40 doses/d. Do not use > 3 mo.
- Abstain from smoking.
- The following side effects may occur: dizziness, headache, lightheadedness (use caution driving or performing tasks that require alertness); nausea, vomiting, constipation or diarrhea (small, frequent meals, regular mouth care may help); skin redness, swelling at application site (good skin care, switching sites daily may help).
- Report nausea and vomiting, diarrhea, cold sweat, chest pain, palpitations, burning or swelling at application site.

## nifedipine

*(nye **fed'** i peen)*

Adalat, Adalat CC, Procardia, Procardia XL

**Pregnancy Category C**

**Drug classes**
Calcium channel blocker
Antianginal agent
Antihypertensive

**Therapeutic actions**
Inhibits the movement of calcium ions across the membranes of cardiac and arterial muscle cells; inhibition of transmembrane calcium flow results in the depression of impulse formation in specialized cardiac pacemaker cells, in slowing of the velocity of conduction of the cardiac impulse, in the depression of myocardial contractility, and in the dilation of coronary arteries and arterioles and peripheral arterioles; these effects lead to decreased cardiac work, decreased cardiac energy consumption, and increased delivery of oxygen to myocardial cells.

**Indications**
- Angina pectoris due to coronary artery spasm (Prinzmetal's variant angina)
- Chronic stable angina (effort-associated angina)
- Treatment of hypertension (sustained-release preparation only)
- Orphan drug use: treatment of interstitial cystitis

**Contraindications/cautions**
- Contraindications: allergy to nifedipine, pregnancy.
- Use cautiously with lactation.

**Dosage**
**Available Forms:** SR tablets—30, 60, 90 mg; capsules—10, 20 mg
*ADULT:* 10 mg tid PO initial dose. Maintenance range: 10–20 mg tid. Higher doses (20–30 mg tid–qid) may be required, depending on patient response. Titrate over 7–14 d. More than 180 mg/d is not recommended.
- ***Sustained release:*** 30–60 mg PO once daily. Titrate over 7–14 d.

**Pharmacokinetics**

| *Route* | *Onset* | *Peak* |
|---|---|---|
| Oral | 20 min | 30 min |
| SR | 20 min | 6 h |

*Metabolism:* Hepatic, $T_{1/2}$: 2–5 h
*Distribution:* Crosses placenta; enters breast milk
*Excretion:* Urine and feces

**Adverse effects**
- CNS: *Dizziness, lightheadedness, headache, asthenia,* fatigue, *nervousness,* sleep disturbances, blurred vision
- GI: *Nausea, diarrhea, constipation,* cramps, flatulence, hepatic injury
- CV: *Peripheral edema, angina,* hypotension, arrhythmias, *bradycardia, AV block,* asystole
- Dermatologic: *Flushing, rash,* dermatitis, pruritis, urticaria
- Other: *Nasal congestion, cough,* fever, chills, shortness of breath, muscle cramps, joint stiffness, sexual difficulties

**Clinically important drug-drug interactions**
- Increased effects with cimetidine, ranitidine

## ■ Nursing Considerations

### Assessment
- ***History:*** Allergy to nifedipine; pregnancy; lactation
- ***Physical:*** Skin lesions, color, edema; orientation, reflexes; P, BP, baseline ECG,peripheral perfusion, auscultation; R, adventitious sounds; liver evaluation, normal GI output; liver function tests

### Implementation
- Monitor patient carefully (BP, cardiac rhythm, and output) while drug is being titrated to therapeutic dose; the dosage may be increased more rapidly in hospitalized patients under close supervision. *Do not exceed 30 mg/dose.*
- Ensure that patients do not chew or divide sustained-release tablets.
- Taper dosage of beta-blockers before nifedipine therapy.
- Protect drug from light and moisture.

### Drug-specific teaching points
- Do not chew or divide sustained-release tablets. Swallow whole.

- The following side effects may occur: nausea, vomiting (small, frequent meals may help); dizziness, lightheadedness, vertigo (avoid driving, operating dangerous machinery; take special precautions to avoid falling); muscle cramps, joint stiffness, sweating, sexual difficulties (reversible).
- Report irregular heart beat, shortness of breath, swelling of the hands or feet, pronounced dizziness, constipation.

## nilutamide

*(nah **loo'** ta mide)*

Anandron (CAN), Nilandron

**Pregnancy Category C**

### Drug classes
Antiandrogen

### Therapeutic actions
Nonsteroidal agent; exerts potent antiandrogenic activity by inhibiting androgen uptake or inhibiting nuclear binding of androgen in target tissues.

### Indications
- Treatment of metastatic prostatic carcinoma (stage D2) in combination with surgical castration

### Contraindications/cautions
- Contraindications: hypersensitivity to nilutamide or any component of preparation; severe hepatic impairment; severe respiratory insufficiency
- Use cautiously with impaired liver function; Asian patients (adverse effects more pronounced); pregnancy, lactation

### Dosage
**Available Forms:** Tablets—50 mg; tablets (CAN) 50, 100 mg

**ADULT:** 300 mg PO qd for 30 d beginning day of or day following surgery; 150 mg PO qd after initial 30-d period.

**PEDIATRIC:** Safety and efficacy not established.

### Pharmacokinetics

| *Route* | *Onset* | *Peak* | *Duration* |
|---|---|---|---|
| Oral | Rapid | Days | Weeks |

*Metabolism:* Hepatic and tissue; $T_{1/2}$: days

*Distribution:* Crosses placenta; may pass into breast milk

*Excretion:* Urine

### Adverse effects
- CNS: Dizziness, headache, insomnia, asthenia, *impaired adaptation to dark or light,*, abnormal vision, hyperesthesia
- GI: *GI upset,* constipation, anorexia
- CV: Hypertension, peripheral edema
- Respiratory: **Interstitial pneumonia,** dyspnea
- Hematologic: Elevated AST, ALT
- GU: *Impotence, loss of libido,* UTIs, **liver failure**
- Endocrine: *Gynecomastia, hot flashes*
- Other: *Flulike syndrome,* pain

### Clinically important drug-drug interactions
- Antabuse-type reaction with alcohol; avoid this combination

## ■ Nursing Considerations

### Assessment
- ***History:*** Hypersensitivity to nilutamide or any component of preparation; severe hepatic impairment, severe respiratory insufficiency; pregnancy, lactation; date of surgical castration
- ***Physical:*** Skin color, lesions; reflexes, affect, vision exam; urinary output; bowel sounds, liver evaluation; R, adventitious sounds; CBC, Hct, electrolytes, liver function tests, chest x-ray

### Implementation
- Arrange for baseline and periodic monitoring of liver function tests during therapy; discontinue drug and notify physician if transaminases exceed 2–3 X normal.
- Monitor for baseline respiratory function, including chest x-ray; discontinue if any sign of interstitial pneumonia occurs.

- Begin drug on the day of or the day after surgical castration; do not interrupt therapy.
- Offer support and encouragement to deal with diagnosis, change in self-concept, and alteration in sexual functioning.

### Drug-specific teaching points

- Take this drug exactly as prescribed. Do not interrupt dosing or stop taking the medication without consulting your health care provider. Note that the dosage will be changed after 30 d of treatment.
- Periodic blood tests will need to be done to monitor the drug effects. It is important that you keep these appointments.
- The following side effects may occur: dizziness, drowsiness (avoid driving or performing hazardous tasks); loss of ability to accomodate to light and dark (avoid night driivng and take special care in low-light or changing-light situations); impotence, loss of libido (drug effects; consult with your nurse or physician if bothersome or if you desire to talk about them); alcohol intolerance (do not drink alcohol while on this drug; serious reactions could occur).
- Report change in stool or urine color, yellow skin, difficult or painful breathing, cough, chest pain, difficulty voiding.

## nimodipine

*(nye **moe'** di peen)*

Nimotop

**Pregnancy Category C**

### Drug classes

Calcium channel blocker

### Therapeutic actions

Inhibits the movement of calcium ions across the membranes of cardiac and arterial muscle cells; inhibition of transmembrane calcium flow results in the depression of impulse formation in specialized cardiac pacemaker cells, in slowing of the velocity of conduction of the cardiac impulse, in the depression of myocardial contractility, and in the dilation of coronary arteries and arterioles and peripheral arterioles.

### Indications

- Improvement of neurologic deficits due to spasm following subarachnoid hemorrhage (SAH) from ruptured congenital intracranial aneurysms in patients who are in good neurologic condition postictus (Hunt and Hess Grades I–III)
- Unlabeled uses: treatment of common and classic migraines and chronic cluster headaches

### Contraindications/cautions

- Allergy to nimodipine, impaired hepatic function, pregnancy (teratogenic), lactation.

### Dosage

**Available Forms:** Capsules, liquid—40 mg

*ADULT:* Begin therapy within 96 h of the SAH. 60 mg q4h PO for 21 consecutive d.

*PEDIATRIC:* Safety and efficacy not established.

### Pharmacokinetics

| *Route* | *Onset* | *Peak* |
|---|---|---|
| Oral | Unknown | > 60 min |

*Metabolism:* Hepatic, $T_{1/2}$: 1–2 h

*Distribution:* Crosses placenta; enters breast milk

*Excretion:* Urine

### Adverse effects

- CNS: Dizziness, lightheadedness, *headache*, asthenia, fatigue
- GI: *Diarrhea,* nausea, hepatic injury
- CV: Peripheral edema, angina, *hypotension*, **arrhythmias**, bradycardia, AV block, asystole
- Dermatologic: Flushing, *rash*

## ■ Nursing Considerations

### Assessment

- *History:* Allergy to nimodipine, impaired hepatic function, pregnancy, lactation
- *Physical:* Skin lesions, color, edema; reflexes, affect, complete neurologic exam; P, BP, baseline ECG, peripheral perfusion, auscultation; R, adventitious sounds; liver

evaluation, normal output; liver function tests, urinalysis

### Implementation

- Begin therapy within 96 h of subarachnoid hemorrhage.
- Administer PO. If patient is unable to swallow capsule, make a hole in both ends of the capsule with an 18-gauge needle, and extract the contents into a syringe. Empty the contents into the patient's in-situ nasogastric tube, and wash down the tube with 30 ml of normal saline.
- Monitor neurologic effects closely to determine progress and patient response.

### Drug-specific teaching points

- Take drug for 21 consecutive d.
- The following side effects may occur: nausea, diarrhea (small, frequent meals may help); headache (monitor lighting, noise, and temperature; request medication if severe).
- Report irregular heart beat, shortness of breath, swelling of the hands or feet, pronounced dizziness, constipation.

## nisoldipine

*(nye **sole'** di peen)*

Sular

**Pregnancy Category C**

### Drug classes

Calcium channel blocker
Antihypertensive

### Therapeutic actions

Inhibits the movement of calcium ions across the membranes of cardiac and arterial muscle cells; inhibits transmembrane calcium flow, which results in the depression of impulse formation in specialized cardiac pacemaker cells, slowing of the velocity of conduction of the cardiac impulse, depression of myocardial contractility, and dilation of coronary arteries and arterioles and peripheral arterioles; these effects in turn lead to decreased cardiac work, decreased cardiac energy consumption.

### Indications

- Essential hypertension, alone or in combination with other antihypertensives

### Contraindications/cautions

- Contraindications: allergy to nisoldipine, impaired hepatic or renal function, sick sinus syndrome, CHF, heart block (second or third-degree).
- Use cautiously with MI or severe CAD (increased severity of disease has occurred), lactation.

### Dosage

**Available Forms:** ER tablets—10, 20, 30, 40 mg

*ADULT:* Initial dose of 20 mg PO qd; increase in weekly increments of 10 mg/wk until BP control is achieved. Usual maintenance dose is 20–40 mg PO qd. Maximum dose 60 mg/d.

*PEDIATRIC:* Safety and efficacy not established.

*GERIATRIC OR HEPATIC IMPAIRMENT:* Monitor BP very carefully. Lower starting doses and lower maintenance doses are recommended.

### Pharmacokinetics

| *Route* | *Onset* | *Peak* | *Duration* |
|---|---|---|---|
| Oral | Slow | 6–12 h | 24 h |

*Metabolism:* Hepatic; $T_{1/2}$: 7–12 hr
*Distribution:* Crosses placenta; may enter breast milk
*Excretion:* Urine

### Adverse effects

- CNS: *Dizziness, lightheadedness, headache*, asthenia, *fatigue, lethargy*
- GI: *Nausea*, abdominal discomfort
- CV: *Peripheral edema*, arrhythmias, **MI, increased angina**
- Dermatologic: *Flushing*, rash

### Clinically important drug-drug interactions

• Possible increased serum levels and toxicity of cyclosporine • Possible increased serum levels and toxocity with cimetidine

## ■ Nursing Considerations

### Assessment

- *History:* Allergy to nisoldipine, impaired hepatic or renal function, sick sinus syn-

n

drome, heart block (second or third-degree), lactation, CHF, CAD

- *Physical:* Skin lesions, color, edema; P, BP; baseline ECG, peripheral perfusion, auscultation, R, adventitious sounds; liver evaluation, GI normal output; liver function tests, renal function tests, urinalysis

### Implementation

- Monitor patient carefully (BP, cardiac rhythm and output) while drug is being titrated to therapeutic dose; dosage may be increased more rapidly in hospitalized patients under close supervision.
- Monitor BP very carefully if patient is on concurrent doses of nitrates or other antihypertensives.
- Monitor cardiac rhythm regularly during stabilization of dosage and periodically during long-term therapy.
- Administer drug without regard to meals.

### Drug-specific teaching points

- Take this drug with meals if upset stomach occurs; do not take with high-fat meals or grapefruit juice.
- Swallow tablet whole; do not chew or crush.
- The following side effects may occur: nausea, vomiting (small, frequent meals may help); headache (monitor lighting, noise and temperature; request medication if severe).
- Report irregular heart beat, shortness of breath, swelling of the hands or feet, pronounced dizziness, constipation, chest pain.

## Nitrofurantoin

### nitrofurantoin

*(nye troe fyoor **an'** toyn)*

Furadantin, Nephronex (CAN), Novofuran (CAN)

### nitrofurantoin macrocrystals

Macrodantin, Macrobid

**Pregnancy Category B**

### Drug classes

Urinary tract anti-infective
Antibacterial

### Therapeutic actions

Bacteriostatic in low concentrations, possibly by interfering with bacterial carbohydrate metabolism; bactericidal in high concentrations, possibly by disrupting bacterial cell wall formation, causing cell death.

### Indications

- Treatment of urinary tract infections caused by susceptible strains of *E. coli, S. aureus, Klebsiella, Enterobacter, Proteus*

### Contraindications/cautions

- Contraindications: allergy to nitrofurantoin, renal dysfunction, pregnancy, lactation.
- Use cautiously with G-6-PD deficiency, anemia, diabetes.

### Dosage

**Available Forms:** Capsules—25, 50, 100 mg; oral suspension—25 mg/5ml

**ADULT:** 50–100 mg PO qid for 10–14 d. Do not exceed 400 mg/d.

- ***Chronic suppressive therapy:*** 50–100 mg PO at bedtime.

**PEDIATRIC:** Not recommended in children < 1 mo. 5–7 mg/kg per day in 4 divided doses PO.

- ***Chronic suppressive therapy:*** As low as 1 mg/kg per day PO in 1 to 2 doses.

### Pharmacokinetics

| *Route* | *Onset* | *Peak* |
|---|---|---|
| Oral | Rapid | 30 min |

*Metabolism:* Hepatic, $T_{1/2}$: 20–60 min
*Distribution:* Crosses placenta; enters breast milk
*Excretion:* Urine

### Adverse effects

- CNS: Peripheral neuropathy, headache, dizziness, nystagmus, drowsiness, vertigo
- GI: *Nausea, abdominal cramps, vomiting, diarrhea, anorexia*, parotitis, pancreatitis, **hepatotoxicity**
- Respiratory: **Pulmonary hypersensitivity**

- **Hematologic**: Hemolytic anemia in G-6-PD deficiency; granulocytopenia, agranulocytosis, leukopenia, thrombocytopenia, eosinophilia, megaloblastic anemia
- **Dermatologic**: Exfoliative dermatitis, Stevens-Johnson syndrome, alopecia, pruritus, urticartia, angioedema
- **Other**: Superinfections of the GU tract, hypotension, muscular aches; *brown-rust urine*

### Clinically important drug-drug interactions

- Delayed or decreased absorption with magnesium trisilicate, magaldrate

### Drug-lab test interferences

- False elevations of serum glucose, bilirubin, alkaline phosphatase, BUN, urinary creatinine • False-positive urine glucose when using Benedict's reagent.

## ■ Nursing Considerations

### Assessment

- *History:* Allergy to nitrofurantoin, renal dysfunction, G-6-PD deficiency, anemia, diabetes, pregnancy, lactation
- *Physical:* Skin color, lesions; orientation, reflexes; R, adventitious sounds; liver evaluation; CBC; liver and kidney function tests; serum electrolytes; blood, urine glucose

### Implementation

- Arrange for culture and sensitivity tests before and during therapy.
- Give with food or milk to prevent GI upset.
- Continue drug for at least 3 d after a sterile urine specimen is obtained.
- Monitor clinical response; if no improvement is seen or a relapse occurs, send urine for repeat culture and sensitivity.
- Monitor pulmonary function carefully; reactions can occur within hours or weeks of nitrofurantoin therapy.
- Arrange for periodic CBC and liver function tests during long-term therapy.

### Drug-specific teaching points

- Take drug with food or milk. Complete the full course of drug therapy to ensure a resolution of the infection. Take this drug at regular intervals around the clock; consult your nurse or pharmacist to set up a convenient schedule.
- The following side effects may occur: nausea, vomiting, abdominal pain (small, frequent meals may help); diarrhea; drowsiness, blurring of vision, dizziness (observe caution driving or using dangerous equipment); brown or yellow-rust urine (expected effect).
- Report fever, chills, cough, chest pain, difficulty breathing, rash, numbness or tingling of the fingers or toes.

# Nitroglycerin

## nitroglycerin, intravenous

*(nye troe **gli'** ser in)*

Nitro-Bid IV, Tridil

## nitroglycerin, sublingual

Nitrostat

## nitroglycerin, sustained release

Nitroglyn, Nitrong, Nitro-Time

## nitroglycerin, topical

Nitrobid, Nitrol, Nitrong, Nitrostat

## nitroglycerin, transdermal

Nitro-Dur, Nitrodisc, Transderm-Nitro, Nitro-Derm

## nitroglycerin, translingual

Nitrolingual

## nitroglycerin, transmucosal

Nitrogard

**Pregnancy Category C**

**Drug classes**

Antianginal agent
Nitrate

**Therapeutic actions**

Relaxes vascular smooth muscle with a resultant decrease in venous return and decrease in arterial BP, which reduces left ventricular workload and decreases myocardial oxygen consumption.

**Indications**

- Acute angina: sublingual, translingual preparations
- Prophylaxis of angina: oral sustained release, sublingual, topical, transdermal, translingual, transmucosal preparations
- Angina unresponsive to recommended doses of organic nitrates or $\beta$ -blockers (IV preparations)
- Perioperative hypertension (IV preparations)
- CHF associated with acute MI (IV preparations)
- To produce controlled hypertension during surgery (IV preparations)
- Unlabeled uses: reduction of cardiac workload in acute MI and in CHF (sublingual, topical); adjunctive treatment of Raynaud's disease (topical)

**Contraindications/cautions**

- Contraindications: allergy to nitrates, severe anemia, early MI, head trauma, cerebral hemorrhage, hypertrophic cardiomyopathy, pregnancy, lactation.
- Use cautiously with hepatic or renal disease, hypotension or hypovolemia, increased intracranial pressure, constrictive pericarditis, pericardial tamponade, low ventricular filling pressure or low PCWP.

**Dosage**

**Available Forms:** Injection—0.5, 5 mg/ml; injection solution—25, 50, 100, 200 mg; sublingual tablets—0.15, 0.3, 0.4, 0.6 mg; translingual spray—0.4 mg/spray; transmucosal tablets—1, 2, 3 mg; transmucosal SR tablets—2.6, 6.5, 9 mg; transmucosal SR capsules—2.5, 6.5, 9, 13 mg; transdermal—0.1, 0.2, 0.3, 0.4, 0.6, 0.8 mg/hr; topical ointment—2%

ADULT

- ***Intravenous:*** *Initial:* 5 $\mu$g/min delivered through an infusion pump. Increase by 5-$\mu$g increments every 3–5 min as needed. If no response at 20 $\mu$g, increase increments to 10–20 $\mu$g. Once a partial BP response is obtained, reduce dose and lengthen dosage intervals; continually monitor response and titrate carefully.
- ***Sublingual***
  - *Acute attack:* Dissolve 1 tablet under tongue or in buccal pouch at first sign of anginal attack; repeat every 5 min until relief is obtained. Do not take more than 3 tablets/15 min. If pain continues or increases, patient should call physician or go to hospital.
  - *Prophylaxis:* Use 5–10 min before activities that might precipitate an attack.
- ***Sustained release (oral):*** *Initial:* 2.5–2.6 mg tid or qid. Titrate upward by 2.5- or 2.6-mg increments until side effects limit the dose. Doses as high as 26 mg given 4 × daily have been used.
- ***Topical:*** *Initial dose:* 1/2 in q8h. Increase by 1/2 in to achieve desired results. Usual dose is 1–2 in q8h; up to 4–5 in q4h have been used. 1 inch 15 mg nitroglycerin.
- ***Transdermal:*** Apply one pad each day. Titrate to higher doses by using pads that deliver more drug or by applying more than one pad.
- ***Translingual:*** Spray preparation delivers 0.4 mg/metered dose. At onset of attack, 1–2 metered doses into oral mucosa; no more than 3 doses/15 min should be used. If pain persists, seek medical attention. May be used prophylactically 5–10 min prior to activity that might precipitate an attack.
- ***Transmucosal:*** 1 mg q3–5h during waking hours. Place tablet between lip and gum above incisors, or between cheek and gum.

PEDIATRIC: Safety and efficacy not established.

**Pharmacokinetics**

| *Route* | *Onset* | *Duration* |
|---|---|---|
| IV | 1–2 min | 3–5 min |
| Sublingual | 1–3 min | 30–60 min |
| TL spray | 2 min | 30–60 min |
| Trans/tablet | 1–2 min | 3–5 min |
| Oral, SR | 20–45 min | 3–8 h |
| Topical ointment | 30–60 min | 2–12 h |
| Transdermal | 30–60 min | 24 h |

*Metabolism:* Hepatic, $T_{1/2}$: 47–100 h
*Distribution:* Crosses placenta; enters breast milk
*Excretion:* Urine

**IV facts**

**Preparations:** Dilute in 5% Dextrose Injection or 0.9% Sodium Chloride Injection. Do not mix with other drugs; check the manufacturer's instructions carefully because products vary considerably in concentration and volume per vial. Use only with glass IV bottles and the administration sets provided. Protect from light and extremes of temperature.
**Infusion:** Do not give by IV push; regulate rate based on patient response.

**Adverse effects**

- CNS: Headache, apprehension, restlessness, weakness, vertigo, dizziness, faintness
- GI: Nausea, vomiting, incontinence of urine and feces, abdominal pain
- CV: Tachycardia, retrosternal discomfort, palpitations, **hypotension**, syncope, collapse, postural hypotension, angina
- Dermatologic: Rash, exfoliative dermatitis, cutaneous vasodilation with flushing, pallor, perspiration, cold sweat, contact dermatitis—transdermal preparations, topical allergic reactions—topical nitroglycerin ointment
- Local: Local burning sensation at the point of dissolution (sublingual)
- Other: Ethanol intoxication with high dose IV use (alcohol in diluent)

**Clinically important drug-drug interactions**

• Increased risk of hypertension and decreased antianginal effect with ergot alkaloids • Decreased pharmacologic effects of heparin

**Drug-lab test interferences**

• False report of decreased serum cholesterol if done by the Zlatkis-Zak color reaction

## ■ Nursing Considerations

### Assessment

- *History:* Allergy to nitrates, severe anemia, early MI, head trauma, cerebral hemorrhage, hypertrophic cardiomyopathy, hepatic or renal disease, hypotension or hypovolemia, increased intracranial pressure, constrictive pericarditis, pericardial tamponade, low ventricular filling pressure or low PCWP, pregnancy, lactation
- *Physical:* Skin color, temperature, lesions; orientation, reflexes, affect; P, BP, orthostatic BP, baseline ECG, peripheral perfusion; R, adventitious sounds; liver evaluation, normal output; liver and renal function tests (IV); CBC, Hgb

### Implementation

- Give sublingual preparations under the tongue or in the buccal pouch. Encourage patient not to swallow. Ask patient if the tablet "fizzles" or burns. Always check the expiration date on the bottle; store at room temperature, protected from light. Discard unused drug 6 mo after bottle is opened (conventional tablets); stabilized tablets (*Nitrostat*) are less subject to loss of potency.
- Give sustained-release preparations with water; warn the patient not to chew the tablets or capsules; do not crush these preparations.
- Administer topical ointment by applying the ointment over a 6 × 6 inch area in a thin, uniform layer using the applicator. Cover area with plastic wrap held in place by adhesive tape. Rotate sites of application to decrease the chance of inflammation and sensitization; close tube tightly when finished.
- Administer transdermal systems to skin site free of hair and not subject to much

movement. Shave areas that have a lot of hair. Do not apply to distal extremities. Change sites slightly to decrease the chance of local irritation and sensitization. Remove transdermal system before attempting defibrillation or cardioversion.
- Administer transmucosal tablets by placing them between the lip and gum above the incisors or between the cheek and gum. Encourage patient not to swallow and not to chew the tablet.
- Administer the translingual spray directly onto the oral mucosa; preparation is not to be inhaled.
- Arrange to withdraw drug gradually. 4–6 wk is the recommended withdrawal period for the transdermal preparations.

### Drug-specific teaching points

- Place sublingual tablets under your tongue or in your cheek; do not chew or swallow the tablet; the tablet should burn or "fizzle" under the tongue. Take the nitroglycerin before chest pain begins, when you anticipate that your activities or situation may precipitate an attack. Do not buy large quantities; this drug does not store well. Keep the drug in a dark, dry place, in a dark-colored glass bottle with a tight lid; do not combine with other drugs. You may repeat your dose every 5 min for a total of _____ tablets. If the pain is still not relieved, go to an emergency room.
- Do not chew or crush the timed-release preparations; take on an empty stomach.
- Spread a thin layer of topical ointment on the skin using the applicator. Do not rub or massage the area. Cover with plastic wrap held in place with adhesive tape. Wash your hands after application. Keep the tube tightly closed. Rotate the sites frequently to prevent local irritation.
- Use transdermal systems, you may need to shave an area for application. Apply to a slightly different area each day. Use care if changing brands; each system has a different concentration.
- Place transmucosal tablets these between the lip and gum or between the gum and cheek. Do not chew; try not to swallow.
- Spray translingual spray directly onto oral mucous membranes; do not inhale. Use 5–10 min before activities that you anticipate will precipitate an attack.
- The following side effects may occur: dizziness, lightheadedness (may be transient; change positions slowly); headache (lie down in a cool environment and rest; OTC preparations may not help); flushing of the neck or face (transient).
- Report blurred vision, persistent or severe headache, skin rash, more frequent or more severe angina attacks, fainting.

## nitroprusside sodium

*(nye troe **pruss'** ide)*

Nitropress

**Pregnancy Category C**

### Drug classes

Antihypertensive
Vasodilator

### Therapeutic actions

Acts directly on vascular smooth muscle to cause vasodilation (arterial and venous) and reduce BP. Mechanism involves interference with calcium influx and intracellular activation of calcium. CV reflexes are not inhibited and reflex tachycardia, increased renin release occur.

### Indications

- Hypertensive crises for immediate reduction of BP
- Controlled hypotension during anesthesia to reduce bleeding in surgical procedures
- Acute CHF
- Unlabeled use: acute MI, with dopamine; left ventricular failure, with $O_2$, morphine, loop diuretic

### Contraindications/cautions

- Contraindications: treatment of compensatory hypertension; to produce controlled hypotension during surgery with known inadequate cerebral circulation; emergency use in moribund patients.
- Use cautiously with hepatic, renal insufficiency (drug decomposes by cyanide, which is metabolized by the liver and kid-

neys to thiocyanate ion); hypothyroidism (thiocyanate inhibits the uptake and binding of iodine); pregnancy; lactation.

### Dosage

**Available Forms:** Powder for injection—50 mg/vial

Administer only by continuous IV infusion with Sterile 5% Dextrose in Water.

*ADULT AND PEDIATRIC:* In patients not receiving antihypertensive medication, the average dose is 3 μg/kg per minute (range 0.5–10.0 μg/kg per minute). At this rate, diastolic BP is usually lowered by 30%–40% below pretreatment diastolic levels. Use smaller doses in patients on antihypertensive medication. Do not exceed infusion rate of 10 μg/kg per minute. If this rate of infusion does not reduce BP within 10 min, discontinue administration.

*GERIATRIC OR RENAL IMPAIRED:* Use with caution and in initial low dosage. The elderly may be more sensitive to the hypotensive effects.

### Pharmacokinetics

| *Route* | *Onset* | *Duration* |
|---|---|---|
| IV | 1–2 min | 1–10 min |

*Metabolism:* Hepatic, $T_{1/2}$: 2 min

*Distribution:* Crosses placenta; may enter breast milk

*Excretion:* Urine

### IV facts

**Preparation:** Dissolve the contents of the 50-mg vial in 2–3 ml of 5% Dextrose in Water. Dilute the prepared stock solution in 250–1,000 ml of 5% Dextrose in Water, and promptly wrap container in aluminum foil or other opaque material to protect from light; the administration set tubing does not need to be covered. Observe solution for color changes. The freshly prepared solution has a faint brown tint; discard it if it is highly colored (blue, green, or dark red). If properly protected from light, reconstituted solution is stable for 24 h. Do not use the infusion fluid for administration of any other drugs.

**Infusion:** Infuse slowly to reduce likelihood of adverse effects; use an infusion pump, micro-drip regulator, or similar device to allow precise control of flow rate; carefully monitor BP and regulate dose based on response.

**Incompatibilities:** Do not mix in solution with any other drugs.

### Adverse effects

- CNS: *Apprehension, headache, restlessness, muscle twitching,* dizziness
- GI: *Nausea, vomiting, abdominal pain*
- CV: *Restrosternal pressure, palpitations,* bradycardia, tachycardia, ECG changes
- **Hematologic**: Methemoglobinemia, antiplatelet effects
- **Dermatologic**: *Diaphoresis,* flushing
- **Endocrine**: Hypothyroidism
- **Local**: Irritation at injection site
- **Cyanide toxicity**: Increasing tolerance to drug and metabolic acidosis are early signs, followed by dyspnea, headache, vomiting, dizziness, ataxia, loss of consciousness, imperceptible pulse, absent reflexes, widely dilated pupils, pink color, distant heart sounds, shallow breathing (seen in overdose)

n

## ■ Nursing Considerations

### Assessment

- ***History:*** Hepatic or renal insufficiency, hypothyroidism, pregnancy, lactation
- ***Physical:*** Reflexes, affect, orientation, pupil size; BP, P, orthostatic BP, supine BP, perfusion, edema, auscultation; R, adventitious sounds; renal, liver and thyroid function tests, blood acid–base balance

### Implementation

- Monitor injection site carefully to prevent extravasation.
- Do not allow BP to drop too rapidly; do not lower systolic BP below 60 mm Hg.
- Provide amyl nitrate inhalation, materials to make 3% sodium nitrite solution, sodium thiosulfate on standby in case overdose of nitroprusside; depletion of patient's body stores of sulfur occur, leading to cyanide toxicity.

- Monitor blood acid–base balance (metabolic acidosis is early sign of cyanide toxicity), serum thiocyanate levels daily during prolonged therapy, especially in patients with renal impairment.

**Drug-specific teaching points**
- Anticipate frequent monitoring of BP, blood tests, checks of IV dosage and rate.
- Report pain at injection site, chest pain.

## nizatidine

*(ni za' ti deen)*
Axid AR, Axid Pulvules
**Pregnancy Category C**

### Drug classes
Histamine$_2$ ($H_2$) antagonist

### Therapeutic actions
Inhibits the action of histamine at the histamine $H_2$ receptors of the parietal cells of the stomach, inhibiting basal gastric acid secretion and gastric acid secretion that is stimulated by food, caffeine, insulin, histamine, cholinergic agonists, gastrin and pentagastrin. Total pepsin output also is reduced.

### Indications
- Short-term and maintenance treatment of duodenal ulcer
- Short-term treatment of benign gastric ulcer
- Gastroesophageal reflux disease
- Prevention of heartburn, acid indigesion, and sour stomach brought on by eating (OTC)

### Contraindications/cautions
- Contraindications: allergy to nizatidine, lactation.
- Use cautiously with impaired renal or hepatic function, pregnancy.

### Dosage
**Available Forms:** Capsules—150, 300 mg; OTC tablets—75 mg

**ADULT**
- *Active duodenal ulcer:* 300 mg PO qd at hs. 150 mg PO bid may be used.
- *Maintenance of healed duodenal ulcer:* 150 mg PO qd at hs.
- *GERD:* 150 mg PO bid.
- *Benign gastric ulcer:* 150 mg PO bid or 300 mg qd.
- *Prevention of heartburn, acid indigestion:* 75 mg PO 1/2–1 h before food or beverages that cause the problem, taken with water.

**PEDIATRIC:** Safety and efficacy not established.

**GERIATRIC OR RENAL IMPAIRED:** *Creatinine clearance 20–50 ml/min:* 150 mg/d PO for active ulcer; 150 mg every other day for maintenance. *Creatinine clearance < 20 ml/min:* 150 mg PO every other day for active ulcer; 150 mg PO every 3 d for maintenance.

### Pharmacokinetics

| Route | Onset | Peak |
|---|---|---|
| Oral | Varies | 1/2–3 h |

*Metabolism:* Hepatic, $T_{1/2}$: 1–2 h
*Distribution:* Crosses placenta; enters breast milk
*Excretion:* Urine

### Adverse effects
- CNS: *Dizziness, somnolence, headache, confusion, hallucinations*, peripheral neuropathy; symptoms of brainstem dysfunction (dysarthria, ataxia, diplopia)
- GI: *Diarrhea*, hepatitis, pancreatitis, hepatic fibrosis
- CV: Cardiac arrhythmias, **cardiac arrest**
- Hematologic: Neutropenia, agranulocytosis, increases in plasma creatinine, serum transaminase
- Other: *Impotence*, gynecomastia, rash, arthralgia, myalgia

### Clinically important drug-drug interactions
- Increased serum salicylate levels with aspirin

### Drug-lab test interferences
- False-positive tests for urobilinogen

## Nursing Considerations

### Assessment

- *History:* Allergy to nizatidine, impaired renal or hepatic function, pregnancy, lactation
- *Physical:* Skin lesions; orientation, affect; P, baseline ECG; liver evaluation, abdominal exam, normal output; CBC, liver and renal function tests

### Implementation

- Administer drug at bedtime.
- Decrease doses in renal and liver dysfunction.
- Prepare liquid by mixing 150 or 300 mg in apple juice, *Gatorade, Ocean Spray*; stable for 48 h refrigerated or at room temperature.
- Arrange for regular follow-up, including blood tests to evaluate effects.

### Drug-specific teaching points

- Take OTC drug 1/2–1 h before the food or beverage that causes the problem; take with water.
- Take drug at bedtime. Therapy may continue for 4–6 wk or longer.
- Take antacids exactly as prescribed, being careful of the times of administration. Do not take OTC drugs, and avoid alcohol. Many OTC drugs contain ingredients that might interfere with this drug's effectiveness.
- Tell all physicians, nurses, or dentists that you are taking this drug. Dosage and timing of all your medications must be coordinated. If anything changes the drugs that you are taking, consult with your nurse or physician.
- Have regular medical follow-ups to evaluate drug response.
- Report sore throat, fever, unusual bruising or bleeding, tarry stools, confusion, hallucinations, dizziness, muscle or joint pain.

## norepinephrine bitartrate

*(nor ep i **nef** rin)*

levarterenol

Levophed

**Pregnancy Category D**

### Drug classes

Sympathomimetic
Alpha adrenergic agonist
Beta-1 selective adrenergic blocker
Cardiac stimulant
Vasopressor

### Therapeutic actions

Vasopressor and cardiac stimulant; effects are mediated by alpha or beta-1 adrenergic receptors in target organs; potent vasoconstrictor (alpha effect) acting in arterial and venous beds; potent positive inotropic agent (beta-1 effect), increasing the force of myocardial contraction and increasing coronary blood flow.

### Indications

- Restoration of BP in controlling certain acute hypotensive states (pheochromocytomectomy, sympathectomy, poliomyelitis, spinal anesthesia, MI, septicemia, blood transfusion, and drug reactions)
- Adjunct in the treatment of cardiac arrest and profound hypotension

### Contraindications/cautions

- Hypovolemia (not a substitute for restoration of fluids, plasma, electrolytes, and should not be used in the presence of blood volume deficits except as an emergency measure to maintain coronary and cerebral perfusion until blood volume replacement can be effected; if administered continuously to maintain BP in the presence of hypovolemia, perfusion of vital organs may be severely compromised and tissue hypoxia may result); general anesthesia with halogenated hydrocarbons or cyclopropane, profound hypoxia or hypercarbia, mesenteric or peripheral vascular thrombosis (risk of extending the infarct); pregnancy.

### Dosage

**Available Forms:** Injection—1 mg/ml

Individualize infusion rate based on response.

**ADULT**

- ***Restoration of BP in acute hypotensive states:*** Add 4 ml of the solution (1 mg/ml) to 1,000 ml of 5% Dextrose Solution for a concentration of 4 $\mu g$ base/ml. Initially give 2–3 ml (8–12 $\mu g$

base) per minute, IV. Adjust flow to establish and maintain a low normal BP (usually 80–100 mm Hg systolic) sufficient to maintain circulation to vital organs; average maintenance rate of infusion is 2–4 μg/min. Occasionally enormous daily doses are necessary (68 mg base/d). Continue the infusion until adequate BP and tissue perfusion are maintained without therapy. Treatment may be required up to 6 d (vascular collapse due to acute MI). Reduce infusion gradually.

- ***Adjunct in cardiac arrest:*** Administer IV during cardiac resuscitation to restore and maintian BP after effective heartbeat and ventilation established.

### Pharmacokinetics

| *Route* | *Onset* | *Duration* |
|---|---|---|
| IV | Rapid | 1–2 min |

*Metabolism:* Neural, $T_{1/2}$: unknown
*Distribution:* Crosses placenta
*Excretion:* Urine

### IV facts

**Preparation:** Dilute drug in 5% Dextrose Solution in Distilled Water or 5% Dextrose in Saline Solution; these dextrose solutions protect against oxidation. Do not administer in saline solution alone.

**Infusion:** Infusion rate is determined by response with constant BP monitoring; check manufacturer's insert for detailed guidelines.

### Adverse effects

- CNS: *Headache*
- CV: *Bradycardia*, hypertension

### Clinically important drug-drug interactions

• Increased hypertensive effects with TCAs (imipramine), guanethidine or reserpine, furazolidone, methyldopa • Decreased vasopressor effects with phenothiazines

## ■ Nursing Considerations

### Assessment

- ***History:*** Hypovolemia, general anesthesia with halogenated hydrocarbons or cyclopropane, profound hypoxia or hypercarbia, mesenteric or peripheral vascular thrombosis, lactation
- ***Physical:*** Weight; skin color, temperature, turgor; P, BP; R, adventitious sounds; urine output; serum electrolytes, ECG

### Implementation

- Give whole blood or plasma separately, if indicated.
- Administer IV infusions into a large vein, preferably the antecubital fossa, to prevent extravasation.
- Do not infuse into femoral vein in elderly patients or those suffering from occlusive vascular disease (atherosclerosis, arteriosclerosis, diabetic endarteritis, Buerger's disease); occlusive vascular disease is more likely to occur in lower extremity.
- Avoid catheter tie-in technique, if possible, because stasis around tubing may lead to high local concentrations of drug.
- Monitor BP every 2 min from the start of infusion until desired BP is achieved, then monitor every 5 min if infusion is continued.
- Monitor infusion site for extravasation.
- Provide phentolamine on standby in case extravasation occurs (5–10 mg phentolamine in 10–15 ml saline should be used to infiltrate the affected area).
- Do not use drug solutions that are pink or brown; drug solutions should be clear and colorless.

### Drug-specific teaching points

Because norepinephrine is used only in acute emergency situations, patient teaching will depend on patient's awareness and will relate mainly to patient's status, monitors rather than specifically to therapy with norepinephrine.

## norethindrone acetate

*(nor eth **in'** drone)*

Aygestin

**Pregnancy Category X**

### Drug classes
Hormone
Progestin

### Therapeutic actions
Progesterone derivative. Progesterone transforms proliferative endometrium into secretory endometrium; inhibits the secretion of pituitary gonadotropins, which prevents follicular maturation and ovulation; and inhibits spontaneous uterine contraction. Progestins have varying profiles of estrogenic, antiestrogenic, anabolic, and androgenic activity.

### Indications
- Treatment of amenorrhea; abnormal uterine bleeding due to hormonal imbalance
- Treatment of endometriosis
- Component of some oral contraceptive preparations

### Contraindications/cautions
- Contraindications: allergy to progestins; thrombophlebitis, thromboembolic disorders, cerebral hemorrhage or history of these conditions; hepatic disease, carcinoma of the breast or genital organs, undiagnosed vaginal bleeding, missed abortion; pregnancy; lactation.
- Use cautiously with epilepsy, migraine, asthma, cardiac or renal dysfunction.

## Dosage
**Available Forms:** Tablets—5 mg
Administer PO only

*ADULT*
- ***Amenorrhea; abnormal uterine bleeding:*** 2.5–10 mg PO starting with day 5 of the menstrual cycle and ending on day 25.
- ***Endometriosis:*** 5 mg/d PO for 2 wk. Increase in increments of 2.5 mg/d every 2 wk until 15 mg/d is reached. May be maintained for 6–9 mo or until breakthrough bleeding demands temporary termination.

### Pharmacokinetics

| Route | Onset |
|---|---|
| Oral | Varies |

*Metabolism:* Hepatic, $T_{1/2}$: unknown
*Distribution:* Crosses placenta; enters breast milk
*Excretion:* Urine and feces

### Adverse effects
- CNS: Sudden, partial or complete loss of vision, proptosis, diplopia, migraine, precipitation of acute intermittent porphyria, mental depression, pyrexia, insomnia, somnolence
- GI: Cholestatic jaundice, nausea
- CV: Thrombophlebitis, cerebrovascular disorders, retinal thrombosis, pulmonary embolism, thromboembolic and thrombotic disease, increased blood pressure
- GU: *Breakthrough bleeding, spotting, change in menstrual flow, amenorrhea*, changes in cervical erosion and cervical secretions, breast tenderness and secretion
- **Dermatologic:** *Rash with or without pruritus, acne*, melasma or chloasma, alopecia, hirsutism, photosensitivity
- **General:** *Fluid retention, edema, increase in weight*
- **Other:** Decreased glucose tolerance

### Clinically important drug-drug interactions
- Inaccurate tests of hepatic and endocrine function.

## ■ Nursing Considerations

### Assessment
- ***History:*** Allergy to progestins; thrombophlebitis, thromboembolic disorders, cerebral hemorrhage; hepatic disease, carcinoma of the breast or genital organs, undiagnosed vaginal bleeding, missed abortion; pregnancy; lactation; epilepsy, migraine, asthma, cardiac or renal dysfunction
- ***Physical:*** Skin color, lesions, turgor; hair; breasts; pelvic exam; orientation, affect; ophthalmologic exam; P, auscultation, peripheral perfusion, edema; R, adventitious sounds; liver evaluation; liver and renal function tests, glucose tolerance, Pap smear

n

### Implementation

- Arrange for pretreatment and periodic (at least annual) history and physical, including BP, breasts, abdomen, pelvic organs, and a Pap smear.
- Warn patient prior to therapy to prevent pregnancy and to obtain frequent medical follow-ups.
- Use caution when administering drug to ensure preparation ordered is the one being used; norethindrone acetate is approximately twice as potent as norethindrone.
- Discontinue medication and consult physician if sudden partial or complete loss of vision occurs; if papilledema or retinal vascular lesions are present, discontinue drug.
- Discontinue medication and consult physician at sign of thromboembolic disease: leg pain, swelling, peripheral perfusion changes, shortness of breath.

### Drug-specific teaching points

- Take drugs in accordance with marked calendar.
- The following side effects may occur: sensitivity to light (avoid exposure to the sun; use sunscreen and protective clothing); dizziness, sleeplessness, depression (use caution driving or performing tasks that require alertness); skin rash, color changes, loss of hair; fever; nausea.
- Avoid pregnancy: serious fetal abnormalities or fetal death could occur.
- Report pain or swelling and warmth in the calves, acute chest pain or shortness of breath, sudden severe headache or vomiting, dizziness or fainting, numbness or tingling in the arm or leg.

## norfloxacin

*(nor **flox'** a sin)*
Noroxin
**Pregnancy Category C**

### Drug classes

Urinary tract anti-infective
Antibiotic
Fluoroquinolone

### Therapeutic actions

Bactericidal; interferes with DNA replication in susceptible gram-negative bacteria, leading to cell death.

### Indications

- For the treatment of adults with urinary tract infections caused by susceptible gram-negative bacteria, including *E. coli, Proteus mirabilis, K. pneumoniae, Enterobacter cloacae, Proteus vulgaris, Providencia rettgeri, Morganella morganii, Proteus aeruginosa, Citrobacter freundii, S. aureus, Staphylococcus epidermidis,* group D streptococci
- Uncomplicated urethral and cervical gonorrhea caused by *Neisseria gonorrhoeae*.
- Prostatitis caused by *E. Coli*

### Contraindications/cautions

- Contraindications: allergy to norfloxacin, nalidixic acid or cinoxacin; pregnancy; lactation.
- Use cautiously with renal dysfunction, seizures.

### Dosage

**Available Forms:** Tablets—400 mg

*ADULT*

- ***Uncomplicated urinary tract infections:*** 400 mg q12h PO for 7–10 d. Maximum dose of 800 mg/d.
- ***Complicated urinary tract infections:*** 400 mg q12h PO for 10–21 d. Maximum dose of 800 mg/d.
- ***Uncomplicated sexually transmitted disease:*** 800 mg PO as a single dose.
- ***Prostatitis:*** Prostatitis: 400mg q 12 hr PO for 28 d.

*PEDIATRIC:* Not recommended; produced lesions of joint cartilage in immature experimental animals.

*GERIATRIC OR IMPAIRED RENAL FUNCTION:* *Creatinine clearance* $<$ *30 ml/min/1.73* $m^2$: 400 mg/d, PO for 7–10 d.

### Pharmacokinetics

| *Route* | *Onset* | *Peak* |
|---|---|---|
| Oral | Varies | 2–3 h |

*Metabolism:* Hepatic, $T_{1/2}$: 3–4.5 h
*Distribution:* Crosses placenta; enters breast milk
*Excretion:* Urine

### Adverse effects

- CNS: *Headache*, dizziness, insomnia, fatigue, somnolence, depression, blurred vision
- GI: *Nausea*, vomiting, dry mouth, diarrhea, abdominal pain, dyspepsia, flatulence, constipation, heartburn
- **Hematologic**: Elevated BUN, SGOT, SGPT, serum creatinine and alkaline phosphatase; decreased WBC, neutrophil count, Hct
- Other: Fever, rash

### Clinically important drug-drug interactions

• Decreased therapeutic effect with iron salts, sulcrafate • Decreased absorption with antacids • Increased serum levels and toxic effects of theophyllines

## ■ Nursing Considerations

### Assessment

- *History:* Allergy to norfloxacin, nalidixic acid or cinoxacin; renal dysfunction; seizures; pregnancy; lactation
- *Physical:* Skin color, lesions; T; orientation, reflexes, affect; mucous membranes, bowel sounds; renal and liver function tests

### Implementation

- Arrange for culture and sensitivity tests before therapy.
- Administer drug 1 h before or 2 h after meals with a glass of water.
- Ensure that patient is well hydrated.
- Administer antacids at least 2 h after dosing.
- Monitor clinical response; if no improvement is seen or a relapse occurs, send urine for repeat culture and sensitivity.

### Drug-specific teaching points

- Take drug on an empty stomach, 1 h before or 2 h after meals. If an antacid is needed, do not take it within 2 h of norfloxacin dose.
- Drink plenty of fluids.
- The following side effects may occur: nausea, vomiting, abdominal pain (small, frequent meals may help); diarrhea or constipation; drowsiness, blurring of vision, dizziness (observe caution driving or using dangerous equipment).
- Report rash, visual changes, severe GI problems, weakness, tremors.

## norgestrel

*(nor jess' trel)*

Ovrette

**Pregnancy Category X**

### Drug classes

Hormone
Progestin
Oral contraceptive

### Therapeutic actions

Progestational agent; the endogenous female progestin, progesterone, transforms proliferative endometrium into secretory endometrium; inhibits the secretion of pituitary gonadotropins, which prevents follicular maturation and ovulation; and inhibits spontaneous uterine contractions. The primary mechanism by which norgestrel prevents conception is not known, but progestin-only oral contraceptives alter the cervical mucus, exert a progestional effect on the endometrium that interferes with implantation, and in some patients, suppress ovulation.

### Indications

- Prevention of pregnancy using oral contraceptives; somewhat less efficacious (3 pregnancies per 100 woman years) than the combined estrogen/progestin oral contraceptives (about 1 pregnancy per 100 woman years, depending on formulation)

### Contraindications/cautions

- Contraindications: allergy to progestins, tartrazine; thrombophlebitis, thromboembolic disorders, cerebral hemorrhage or history of these conditions; CAD; hepatic disease, carcinoma of the breast or genital organs, undiagnosed vaginal bleeding, missed abortion; as a diagnostic

n

test for pregnancy; pregnancy (fetal abnormalities: masculinization of the female fetus, congenital heart defects, and limb reduction defects); lactation.
- Use cautiously with epilepsy, migraine, asthma, cardiac or renal dysfunction.

### Dosage

**Available Forms:** Tablets—0.075 mg

*ADULT:* Administer daily, starting on the first day of menstruation. Take one tablet, PO, at the same time each day, every day of the year. *Missed dose:* 1 tablet—take as soon as remembered, then take the next tablet at regular time; 2 consecutive tablets—take 1 of the missed tablets, discard the other, and take daily tablet at usual time; 3 consecutive tablets—discontinue immediately.

### Pharmacokinetics

| *Route* | *Onset* |
|---|---|
| Oral | Varies |

*Metabolism:* Hepatic, $T_{1/2}$: unknown
*Distribution:* Crosses placenta; enters breast milk
*Excretion:* Urine

### Adverse effects

- CNS: Neuro-ocular lesions, mental depression, migraine, *changes in corneal curvature,* contact lens intolerance
- GI: Gallbladder disease, liver tumors, hepatic lesions, *nausea, vomiting*, abdominal cramps, bloating, cholestatic jaundice
- CV: *Thrombophlebitis, thrombosis*, **pulmonary embolism**, coronary thrombosis, MI, cerebral thrombosis, Raynaud's disease, arterial thromboembolism, renal artery thrombosis, cerebral hemorrhage, hypertension
- GU: *Breakthrough bleeding, spotting, change in menstrual flow, amenorrhea,* changes in cervical erosion and cervical secretions, endocervical hyperplasia, vaginal candidiasis
- Dermatologic: Rash with or without pruritus, acne, melasma
- Other: *Breast tenderness and secretion, enlargement*; fluid retention, edema, increase or decrease in weight

## ■ Nursing Considerations

### Assessment

- ***History:*** Allergy to progestins, tartrazine; thrombophlebitis, thromboembolic disorders, cerebral hemorrhage; CAD; hepatic disease, carcinoma of the breast or genital organs, undiagnosed vaginal bleeding, missed abortion; epilepsy, migraine, asthma, cardiac or renal dysfunction; pregnancy; lactation
- ***Physical:*** Skin color, lesions, turgor; hair; breasts; pelvic exam; orientation, affect; ophthalmologic exam; P, auscultation, peripheral perfusion, edema; R, adventitious sounds; liver evaluation; liver and renal function tests, glucose tolerance, Pap smear, pregnancy test

### Implementation

- Arrange for pretreatment and periodic (at least annual) history and physical, including BP, breasts, abdomen, pelvic organs and a Pap smear.
- Discontinue medication and consult physician if sudden partial or complete loss of vision occur; if papilledema or retinal vascular lesions are present on exam, discontinue.
- Discontinue medication and consult physician at any sign of thromboembolic disease: leg pain, swelling, peripheral perfusion changes, shortness of breath.

### Drug-specific teaching points

- Take exactly as prescribed at intervals not exceeding 24 h. Take at bedtime or with a meal to establish a routine; medication must be taken daily for prevention of pregnancy; if you miss one tablet, take as soon as remembered, then take the next tablet at regular time. If you miss two consecutive tablets, take 1 of the missed tablets, discard the other, and take daily tablet at usual time. If you miss three consecutive tablets, discontinue immediately, and use another method of birth control until your cycle starts again. It is a good idea to use an additional method of birth control if any tablets are missed.

- Discontinue drug and consult your care provider if you decide to become pregnant. It may be suggested that you use a nonhormonal birth control for a few months before becoming pregnant.
- The following side effects may occur: sensitivity to light (avoid exposure to the sun; use sunscreen and protective clothing); dizziness, sleeplessness, depression (use caution driving or performing tasks that require alertness); skin rash, skin color changes, loss of hair; fever; nausea; breakthrough bleeding or spotting (transient); intolerance to contact lenses due to corneal changes.
- Do not take this drug during pregnancy; serious fetal abnormalities have been reported. If you think that you are pregnant consult physician immediately.
- Tell your nurse, physician, or dentist that you take this drug. If other medications are prescribed, they may decrease the effectiveness of oral contraceptives and an additional method of birth control may be needed.
- Report pain or swelling and warmth in the calves, acute chest pain or shortness of breath, sudden severe headache or vomiting, dizziness or fainting, visual disturbances, numbness or tingling in the arm or leg, breakthrough bleeding or spotting that lasts into the second month of therapy.

## nortriptyline hydrochloride

*(nor **trip'** ti leen)*

Aventyl, Pamelor

**Pregnancy Category C**

### Drug classes

Tricyclic antidepressant (TCA) (secondary amine)

### Therapeutic actions

Mechanism of action unknown; the TCAs are structurally related to the phenothiazine antipsychotic drugs (eg, chlorpromazine), but inhibit the presynaptic reuptake of the neurotransmitters norepinephrine and serotonin; anticholinergic at CNS and peripheral receptors; sedating; the relationship of these effects to clinical efficacy is unknown.

### Indications

- Relief of symptoms of depression (endogenous depression most responsive)
- Unlabeled uses: treatment of panic disorders (25–75 mg/d), premenstrual depression (50–125 mg/d), dermatologic disorders (75 mg/d)

### Contraindications/cautions

- Contraindications: hypersensitivity to any tricyclic drug; concomitant therapy with an MAO inhibitor; recent MI; myelography within previous 24 h or scheduled within 48 h; pregnancy (limb reduction abnormalities); lactation.
- Use cautiously with EST (increased hazard with TCAs); preexisting CV disorders (possibly increased risk of serious CVS toxicity); angle-closure glaucoma, increased intraocular pressure, urinary retention, ureteral or urethral spasm (anticholinergic effects may exacerbate these conditions); seizure disorders; hyperthyroidism (predisposes to CVS toxicity, including cardiac arrhythmias); impaired hepatic, renal function; psychiatric patients (schizophrenics or paranoids may exhibit a worsening of psychosis); manic-depressive patients (may shift to hypomanic or manic phase); elective surgery (discontinued as long as possible before surgery).

### Dosage

**Available Forms:** Capsules—10, 25, 50, 75 mg; solution—10 mg/5ml

*ADULT:* 25 mg tid–qid PO. Begin with low dosage and gradually increase as required and tolerated. Doses > 150 mg/d are not recommended.

*PEDIATRIC, ADOLESCENTS:* 30–50 mg/d PO in divided doses. Not recommended for use in children younger than 12 y.

*GERIATRIC:* 30–50 mg/d PO in divided doses.

n

### Pharmacokinetics

| Route | Onset | Peak | Duration |
|---|---|---|---|
| Oral | Varies | 2–4 h | 2–4 wk |

*Metabolism:* Hepatic, $T_{1/2}$: 18–28 h
*Distribution:* Crosses placenta; enters breast milk
*Excretion:* Urine

### Adverse effects

- **CNS**: *Sedation and anticholinergic (atropine-like) effects* (dry mouth, blurred vision, disturbance of accommodation for near vision, mydriasis, increased intraocular pressure), *confusion* (especially in elderly), *disturbed concentration*, hallucinations, disorientation, decreased memory, feelings of unreality, delusions, anxiety, nervousness, restlessness, agitation, panic, insomnia, nightmares, hypomania, mania, exacerbation of psychosis, drowsiness, weakness, fatigue, headache, numbness, tingling, paresthesias of extremities, incoordination, motor hyperactivity, akathisia, ataxia, tremors, peripheral neuropathy, extrapyramidal symptoms, *seizures*, speech blockage, dysarthria
- **GI**: *Dry mouth, constipation*, paralytic ileus, *nausea*, vomiting, anorexia, epigastric distress, diarrhea, flatulence, dysphagia, peculiar taste, increased salivation, stomatitis, glossitis, parotid swelling, abdominal cramps, black tongue, hepatitis; elevated transaminase, altered alkaline phosphatase
- **CV**: *Orthostatic hypotension*, hypertension, syncope, tachycardia, palpitations, MI, arrhythmias, heart block, precipitation of CHF, stroke
- **Hematologic**: Bone marrow depression, including agranulocytosis; eosinophila; purpura; thrombocytopenia; leukopenia
- **GU**: Urinary retention, delayed micturition, dilation of the urinary tract, gynecomastia, testicular swelling; breast enlargement, menstrual irregularity and galactorrhea; increased or decreased libido; impotence
- **Hypersensitivity**: Skin rash, pruritus, vasculitis, petechiae, photosensitization, edema (generalized, facial, tongue), drug fever
- **Endocrine**: Elevated or depressed blood sugar; elevated prolactin levels; inappropriate ADH secretion
- **Withdrawal**: Symptoms with abrupt discontinuation of prolonged therapy: nausea, headache, vertigo, nightmares, malaise
- **Other**: Nasal congestion, excessive appetite, weight gain or loss; sweating, alopecia, lacrimation, hyperthermia, flushing, chills

### Clinically important drug-drug interactions

• Increased TCA levels and pharmacologic (especially anticholinergic) effects with cimetidine, fluoxetine, ranitidine • Increased half-life and therefore increased bleeding with dicumarol • Altered response, including dysrhythmias and hypertension with sympathomimetics • Risk of severe hypertension with clonidine • Hyperpyretic crises, severe convulsions, hypertensive episodes and deaths when MAO inhibitors are given with TCAs • Decreased hypotensive activity of guanethidine

*Note:* MAOIs and tricyclic antidepressants have been used successfully in some patients resistant to therapy with single agents; however, case reports indicate that the combination can cause serious and potentially fatal adverse effects.

## ■ Nursing Considerations

### Assessment

- *History:* Hypersensitivity to any tricyclic drug; concomitant therapy with an MAO inhibitor; recent MI; myelography within previous 24 h or scheduled within 48 h; pregnancy; lactation; EST; preexisting CV disorders; angle-closure glaucoma, increased intraocular pressure, urinary retention, ureteral or urethral spasm; seizure disorders; hyperthyroidism; impaired hepatic, renal function; psychiatric patients; manic-depressive patients; elective surgery
- *Physical:* Weight; T; skin color, lesions; orientation, affect, reflexes, vision and

hearing; P, BP, orthostatic BP, perfusion; bowel sounds, normal output, liver evaluation; urine flow, normal output; usual sexual function, frequency of menses, breast and scrotal examination; liver function tests, urinalysis, CBC, ECG

### Implementation

- Limit drug access to depressed and potentially suicidal patients.
- Give major portion of dose hs if drowsiness, severe anticholinergic effects occur.
- Reduce dosage if minor side effects develop; discontinue if serious side effects occur.
- Arrange for CBC if patient develops fever, sore throat, or other sign of infection.

### Drug-specific teaching points

- Take drug exactly as prescribed; do not stop taking this drug abruptly or without consulting your care provider.
- Avoid alcohol, other sleep-inducing, OTC drugs.
- Avoid prolonged exposure to sunlight or sunlamps; use a sunscreen or protective garments if possible.
- The following side effects may occur: headache, dizziness, drowsiness, weakness, blurred vision (reversible; use safety measures if severe; avoid driving or performing tasks that require alertness); nausea, vomiting, loss of appetite, dry mouth (small, frequent meals, frequent mouth care and sucking sugarless candies may help); nightmares, inability to concentrate, confusion; changes in sexual function.
- Report dry mouth, difficulty in urination, excessive sedation.

## nystatin

*(nye **stat'** in)*

*Oral, oral suspensions, oral troche:* Mycostatin, Nadostine (CAN), Nilstat, Nystex

*Vaginal preparations:* Mycostatin

*Topical application:* Mycostatin, Nadostine (CAN), Nilstat, Nystex

**Pregnancy Category A**

### Drug classes

Antifungal

### Therapeutic actions

Fungicidal and fungistatic: binds to sterols in the cell membrane of the fungus with a resultant change in membrane permeability, allowing leakage of intracellular components and causing cell death.

### Indications

- Treatment of intestinal candidiasis (oral)
- Treatment of oral candidiasis (oral suspension, troche)
- Local treatment of vaginal candidiasis (moniliasis; vaginal)
- Treatment of cutaneous or mucocutaneous mycotic infections caused by *Candida albicans* and other *Candida* species (topical applications)

### Contraindications/cautions

- Allergy to nystatin or components used in preparation.

### Dosage

**Available Forms:** Tablets—500,000 units; oral suspension—100,000 U/ml; troche—200,000 units; vaginal tablets—100,000 units; topical cream, ointment, powder—100,000 U/g

***Oral:*** 500,000–1,000,000 U tid. Continue for at least 48 h after clinical cure.

***Oral Suspension:*** 400,000–600,000 U qid (1/2 of dose in each side of mouth, retaining the drug as long as possible before swallowing). *Troche:* Dissolve 1–2 tablets in mouth 4–5 times/day for up to 14 days. *Infants:* 200,000 U qid (100,000 in each side of mouth).

- *Premature and low-birth-weight infants:* 100,000 U qid.

***Vaginal preparations:*** 1 tablet (100,000 U) intravaginally qd for 2 wk.

***Topical***

- *Vaginal preparations:* Apply to affected area two to three times per day until healing is complete. For fungal infections of the feet, dust powder on feet and in shoes and socks.

### Pharmacokinetics

Not generally absorbed systemically. Excreted unchanged in the feces after oral use.

**Adverse effects**

***Oral Doses***

- GI: *Diarrhea, GI distress, nausea,* vomiting

***Oral Suspension***

- GI: *Nausea, vomiting, diarrhea,* GI distress

***Vaginal***

- Local: *Irritation, vulvovaginal burning*

***Topical***

- Local: *Local irritation*

## ■ Nursing Considerations

### Assessment

- ***History:*** Allergy to nystatin or components used in preparation
- ***Physical:*** Skin color, lesions, area around lesions; bowel sounds; culture of area involved

### Implementation

- Culture fungus before therapy.
- Have patient retain oral suspension in mouth as long as possible before swallowing. Paint suspension on each side of the mouth. Continue local treatment for at least 48 h after clinical improvement is noted.
- Prepare nystatin in the form of frozen flavored popsicles to improve oral retention of the drug for local application.
- Administer nystatin troche orally for the treatment of oral candidiasis; have patient dissolve 1–2 tablets in mouth.
- Insert vaginal suppositories high into the vagina. Have patient remain recumbent for 10–15 min after insertion. Provide sanitary napkin to protect clothing from stains.
- Cleanse affected area before topical application, unless otherwise indicated.
- Monitor response to drug therapy. If no response is noted, arrange for further cultures to determine causative organism.
- Ensure that patient receives the full course of therapy to eradicate the fungus and to prevent recurrence.
- Discontinue topical or vaginal administration if rash or sensitivity occurs.

### Drug-specific teaching points

- Take the full course of drug therapy even if symptoms improve. Continue during menstrual period if vaginal route is being used. Long-term use of the drug may be needed; beneficial effects may not be seen for several weeks. Vaginal suppositories should be inserted high into the vagina.
- Use appropriate hygiene measures to prevent reinfection or spread of infection.
- This drug is for the fungus being treated; do not self-medicate other problems.
- Refrain from sexual intercourse or advise partner to use a condom to avoid reinfection; use a sanitary napkin to prevent staining of clothing with vaginal use.
- The following side effects may occur: nausea, vomiting, diarrhea (oral use); irritation, burning, stinging (local use).
- Report worsening of condition; local irritation, burning (topical application); rash, irritation, pelvic pain (vaginal use); nausea, GI distress (oral administration).

# octreotide acetate

*(ok trye' oh tide)*

Sandostatin

**Pregnancy Category B**

**Drug classes**

Hormone

**Therapeutic actions**

Mimics the natural hormone somatostatin; suppresses secretion of serotonin, gastrin, vasoactive intestinal peptide, insulin, glucagon, secretin, motilin, and pancreatic polypeptide; also suppresses growth hormone and decreases splanchnic blood flow.

**Indications**

- Symptomatic treatment of patients with metastatic carcinoid tumors to suppress or inhibit the associated severe diarrhea and flushing episodes
- Treatment of the profuse watery diarrhea associated with vasoactive intestinal polypeptide tumors (VIPomas)

- Reduction of growth hormone blood levels in patients with acromegaly not responsive to other treatment

## Contraindications/cautions

- Contraindications: hypersensitivity to octreotide or any of its components.
- Use cautiously with renal impairment, thyroid disease, diabetes mellitus, pregnancy, lactation.

## Dosage

**Available Forms:** Injection—0.05, 0.1, 0.2, 0.5, 1 mg/ml

*ADULT:* SC injection is the route of choice. Initial dose is 50 $\mu$g SC qd or bid; the number of injections is increased based on response, usually 2 to 3 ×/d. IV bolus injections have been used in emergency situations—not recommended.

- ***Carcinoid tumors:*** First 2 wk of therapy: 100–600 $\mu$g/d SC in 2 to 4 divided doses (mean daily dosage 300 $\mu$g).
- ***VIPomas:*** 200–300 $\mu$g SC in 2 to 4 divided doses during initial 2 wk of therapy to control symptoms. Range: 150–750 $\mu$g SC; doses above 450 $\mu$g are usually not required.
- ***Acromegaly:*** 50 $\mu$g tid SC, titrated up to 100–500$\mu$g tid. Withdraw for 4 wks once yearly.

*PEDIATRIC:* Safety and efficacy not established.

*GERIATRIC OR RENAL IMPAIRED:* Half-life may be prolonged; adjust dose.

## Pharmacokinetics

| *Route* | *Onset* | *Peak* |
|---|---|---|
| SC | Rapid | 15 min |

*Metabolism:* Hepatic, $T_{1/2}$: 1.5 h
*Distribution:* Crosses placenta; may enter breast milk
*Excretion:* Urine

## Adverse effects

- CNS: *Headache, dizziness, lightheadedness*, fatigue, anxiety, convulsions, depression, drowsiness, vertigo, hyperesthesia, irritability, forgetfulness, malaise, nervousness, visual disturbances
- GI: *Nausea, vomiting, diarrhea, abdominal pain, loose stools,* fat malabsorption, constipation, flatulence, hepatitis, rectal spasm, GI bleeding, heartburn, cholelithiasis, dry mouth, burning mouth
- CV: Shortness of breath, hypertension, thrombophlebitis, ischemia, CHF, palpitations
- **Respiratory:** Rhinorrhea
- **MS:** Asthenia/weakness, leg cramps, muscle pain
- **Dermatologic:** *Flushing*, edema, hair loss, thinning of skin, skin flaking, bruising, pruritus, rash
- **Endocrine:** *Hyperglycemia, hypoglycemia*, galactorrhea, clinical hypothyroidism
- **Local:** *Injection site pain*

## ■ Nursing Considerations

### Assessment

- ***History:*** Hypersensitivity to octreotide or any of its components; renal impairment; thyroid disease, diabetes mellitus; lactation
- ***Physical:*** Skin lesions, hair; reflexes, affect; BP, P, orthostatic BP; abdominal exam, liver evaluation, mucous membranes; renal and thyroid function tests, blood glucose, electrolytes

### Implementation

- Administer by SC injection; avoid multiple injections in the same site within short periods of time.
- Monitor patients with renal function impairment closely; reduced dosage may be necessary.
- Store ampules in the refrigerator; may be at room temperature on day of use. Do not use if particulates or discoloration are observed.
- Monitor patient closely for endocrine reactions: blood glucose alterations, thyroid hormone changes, growth hormone level.
- Arrange for baseline and periodic gall bladder ultrasound to pick up cholelithiasis.
- Monitor blood glucose, especially at start of therapy, to detect hypoglycemia or hyperglycemia. Diabetic patients will require close monitoring.

- Arrange to withdraw the drug for 4 weeks once yearly in treating acromegaly.

### Drug-specific teaching points

- This drug must be injected. You and a significant other can be instructed in the procedure of SC injections. Review technique and process periodically. Do not use the same site for repeated injections; rotate injection sites. Dosage will be adjusted based on your response.
- The following side effects may occur: headache, dizziness, lightheadedness, fatigue (avoid driving or performing tasks that require alertness); nausea, diarrhea, abdominal pain (small, frequent meals may help; maintain nutrition); flushing, dry skin, flaking of skin (skin care may prevent breakdown); pain at the injection site.
- Arrange for periodic medical exams, including blood tests and gall bladder tests.
- Report sweating, dizziness, severe abdominal pain, fatigue, fever, chills, infection, or severe pain at injection sites.

## ofloxacin

*(oe **flox'** a sin)*

Floxin, Ocuflox

**Pregnancy Category C**

### Drug classes

Antibiotic

Fluoroquinolone

### Therapeutic actions

Bactericidal; interferes with DNA replication in susceptible gram-negative bacteria, preventing cell reproduction.

### Indications

- Lower respiratory tract infections caused by *Haemophilus influenzae, Streptococcus pneumoniae*
- Acute, uncomplicated urethral and cervical gonorrhea due to *Neisseria gonorrhoeae*, nongonococcal urethritis, and cervicitis due to *Chlamydia trachomatis*, mixed infections due to both
- Skin and skin-structure infections due to *Staphylococcus aureus, Staphylococcus pyogenes, Proteus mirabilis*
- Urinary tract infections due to *Citrobacter diversus, Enterobacter aerogenes, Escherichia coli, Klebsiella pneumoniae, Pseudomonas aeruginosa*
- Primary treatment of PID (oral)
- Prostatitis due to *E. coli*
- Treatment of ocular infections caused by susceptible organisms
- Orphan drug use: treatment of bacterial corneal ulcers

### Contraindications/cautions

- Contraindications: allergy to fluoroquinolones, pregnancy, lactation.
- Use cautiously with renal dysfunction, seizures.

### Dosage

**Available Forms:** Ophthalmic solution—3 mg/ml; tablets—200, 300, 400 mg; injection—200, 400 mg

**ADULT**

- ***Uncomplicated urinary tract infections:*** 200 mg q12h PO or IV for 3 d.
- ***Complicated urinary tract infections:*** 200 mg bid PO or IV for 10 d.
- ***Lower respiratory tract infections:*** 400 mg q12h PO or IV for 10 d.
- ***Mild to moderate skin infections:*** 400 mg q12h PO or IV for 10 d.
- ***Prostatitis:*** 300 mg q12h PO or IV for 6 weeks.
- ***Acute, uncomplicated gonorrhea:*** 400 mg PO or IV as a single dose.
- ***Cervicitis, urethritis:*** 300 mg q12h PO or IV for 7 d.

**PEDIATRIC:** Not recommended; produced lesions of joint cartilage in immature experimental animals.

**GERIATRIC OR IMPAIRED RENAL FUNCTION:** Ccr 10–50 ml/min, use a 24-h interval and adjust dosage; Ccr $<$ 10 ml/min, use a 2-h interval and half the recommended dose.

### Pharmacokinetics

| Route | Onset | Peak | Duration |
|---|---|---|---|
| Oral | Varies | 1–2 h | 9 h |
| IV | 10 min | 30 min | 9 h |

*Metabolism:* Hepatic, $T_{1/2}$: 5–10 h

*Distribution:* Crosses placenta; enters breast milk

*Excretion:* Urine and bile

### IV facts

**Preparation:** Dilute the single-dose vial to a final concentration of 4 mg/ml using 0.9% NaCl Injection, 5% Dextrose Injection, 5% Dextrose/0.9% Sodium Chloride; 5% Dextrose in Lactated Ringer's; 5% Sodium Bicarbonate; Plasma-Lyte 56 in 5% Dextrose; 5% Dextrose, 0.45% Sodium Chloride and 0.15% Potassium Chloride; Sodium Lactate (M/6); Water for Injection. Premixed bottles require no further dilution. Discard any unused portion.

**Infusion:** Administer slowly over 60 min.

### Adverse effects

- CNS: *Headache*, dizziness, *insomnia*, fatigue, somnolence, depression, blurred vision
- GI: *Nausea*, vomiting, dry mouth, *diarrhea*, abdominal pain
- Hematologic: Elevated BUN, SGOT, SGPT, serum creatinine and alkaline phosphatase; decreased WBC, neutrophil count, Hct
- Other: Fever, rash

### Clinically important drug-drug interactions

• Decreased therapeutic effect with iron salts, sulcrafate • Decreased absorption with antacids

## ■ Nursing Considerations

### Assessment

- *History:* Allergy to fluoroquinolones, renal dysfunction, seizures, lactation
- *Physical:* Skin color, lesions; T; orientation, reflexes, affect; mucous membranes, bowel sounds; renal and liver function tests

### Implementation

- Arrange for culture and sensitivity tests before beginning therapy.
- Continue therapy for 2 d after the signs of infection have disappeared.
- Administer oral drug 1 h before or 2 h after meals with a glass of water.
- Ensure that patient is well hydrated.
- Administer antacids at least 2 h after dosing.
- Monitor clinical response; if no improvement is seen or a relapse occurs, repeat culture and sensitivity.

### Drug-specific teaching points

- Take oral drug on an empty stomach, 1 h before or 2 h after meals. If an antacid is needed, do not take it within 2 h of ofloxacin dose.
- Drink plenty of fluids.
- The following side effects may occur: nausea, vomiting, abdominal pain (small, frequent meals may help); diarrhea or constipation; drowsiness, blurring of vision, dizziness (observe caution if driving or using dangerous equipment).
- Report rash, visual changes, severe GI problems, weakness, tremors.

## olanzapine

*(oh **lan'** za peen)*

Zyprexa

**Pregnancy Category C**

### Drug classes

Antipsychotic

Dopaminergic blocking agent

### Therapeutic actions

Mechanism of action not fully understood; blocks dopamine receptors in the brain, depresses the RAS; blocks serotonin receptor sites; anticholinergic, antihistaminic ($H_1$) and alpha-adrenergic blocking activity may contribute to some of its therapeutic (and adverse) actions; produces fewer extrapyramidal effects than most antipsychotics.

### Indications

- Management of manifestations of schizophrenia and psychotic disorders

### Contraindications/cautions

- Contraindications: allergy to olanzapine, myeloproliferative disorders, severe CNS depression, comatose states, history of seizure disorders, lactation

- Use cautiously with CV or cerebrovascular disease, dehydration, seizure disorders, Alzheimer's disease, prostate enlargement, narrow-angle glaucoma, history of paralytic ileus or breast cancer, elderly or debilitated ptients, pregnancy

### Dosage

**Available Forms:** Tablets—5, 7.5, 10 mg

*ADULTS:* Initially, 5–10 mg PO qd, increase to 10 mg PO qd within several days; may be increased by 5 mg/d at 1-wk intervals to achieve desired effect. Do not exceed 20 mg/d.

*PEDIATRIC:* Safety and efficacy not established in children <18 y.

### Pharmacokinetics

| *Route* | *Onset* | *Peak* | *Duration* |
|---|---|---|---|
| Oral | Varies | 6 h | Weeks |

*Metabolism:* Hepatic; $T_{1/2}$: 30 h

*Distribution:* Crosses placenta; passes into breast milk

*Excretion:* Urine and feces

### Adverse effects

- CNS: *Somnolence, dizziness,* nervousness, headache, akathisia, pesonality disorders, tardive dyskinesia, **neuroleptic malignant syndrome**
- GI: *Constipation,* abdominal pain
- CV: *Postural hypotension,* peripheral edema, tachycardia
- Respiratory: Cough, pharyngitis
- Other: *Fever,* weight gain, joint pain

### Clinically important drug-drug interactions

• Increased risk of orthostatic hypotension with antihypertensives, alcohol, benzodiazepines; avoid use of alcohol and use caution with antihypertensives • Increased risk of seizures with anticholinergics, CNS drugs • May decrease effectiveness of levodopa, dopamine agonists • Decreased effectiveness with rifampin, omeprazole, carbamazepine, smoking • Increased risk of toxicity with fluvoxamine

## ■ Nursing Considerations

### Assessment

- ***History:*** Allergy to olanzapine, myeloproliferative disorders, severe CNS depression, comatose states, history of seizure disorders, lactation; CV or cerebrovascular disease, dehydration, Alzheimer's disease, prostate enlargement, narrow-angle glaucoma, history of paralytic ileus or breast cancer, elderly or debilitated patients, pregnancy
- ***Physical:*** T, weight; reflexes, orientation, intraocular pressure, ophthalmologic exam; P, BP, orthostatic BP, ECG; R, adventitious sounds; bowel sounds, normal output, liver evaluation; prostate palpation, normal urine output; CBC, urinalysis, liver and renal function tests

### Implementation

- Do not dispense more than 1-wk supply at a time.
- Monitor for the many possible drug–drug interactions before beginning therapy.
- Monitor elderly patients for dehydration and institute remedial measures promptly; sedation and decreased sensation of thirst related to CNS effects of drug can lead to dehydration.
- Encourage patient to void before taking the drug to help decrease anticholinergic effects of urinary retention.
- Monitor for elevations of temperature and differentiate between infection and neuroleptic malignant syndrome.
- Monitor for postural hypotension and provide appropriate safety measures as needed.

### Drug-specific teaching points

- Take this drug exactly as prescribed; do not change dose without consulting your health care provider.
- The following side effects may occur: drowsiness, dizziness, sedation, seizures (avoid driving, operating machinery, or performing tasks that require concentration); dizziness, faintness on arising (change positions slowly, use caution); increased salivation (if bothersome, con-

tact your nurse or physician); constipation (consult with your nurse of physician for appropriate relief measures); fast heart rate (rest and take your time if this occurs).

- This drug cannot be taken during pregnancy. If you think you are pregnant or wish to become pregnant, contact your nurse or physician.
- Report lethargy, weakness, fever, sore throat, malaise, mouth ulcers, and flulike symptoms.

## olsalazine sodium

*(ole **sal'** a zeen)*

Dipentum

**Pregnancy Category C**

### Drug classes

Anti-inflammatory agent

### Therapeutic actions

Mechanism of action is unknown; thought to be a direct, local anti-inflammatory effect in the colon where olsalazine is converted to mesalamine (5-ASA), which blocks cyclooxygenase and inhibits prostaglandin production in the colon.

### Indications

- Maintenance of remission of ulcerative colitis in patients intolerant of sulfasalazine

### Contraindications/cautions

- Contraindications: hypersensitivity to salicylates, pregnancy (fetal abnormalities).
- Use caution in the presence of lactation.

### Dosage

**Available Forms:** Capsules—250 mg

*ADULT:* 1 g/d PO in two divided doses.

*PEDIATRIC:* Safety and efficacy not established.

### Pharmacokinetics

| *Route* | *Onset* | *Peak* |
|---|---|---|
| Oral | Varies | 60 min |

*Metabolism:* Hepatic, $T_{1/2}$: 0.9 h

*Distribution:* Crosses placenta; may enter breast milk

*Excretion:* Feces and urine

### Adverse effects

- CNS: *Headache, fatigue, malaise, depression,* dizziness, asthenia, insomnia
- GI: *Abdominal pain, cramps, discomfort; gas; flatulence; nausea; diarrhea, dyspepsia,* bloating, hemmorhoids, rectal pain, constipation
- Other: *Flulike symptoms,rash,* fever, cold, rash, back pain, hair loss, peripheral edema, *arthralgia*

### ■ Nursing Considerations

#### Assessment

- ***History:*** Hypersensitivity to salicylates, pregnancy, lactation
- ***Physical:*** T, hair status; reflexes, affect; abdominal and rectal exam; urinary output, renal function tests

#### Implementation

- Administer with meals in evenly divided doses.
- Monitor patients with renal impairment for possible adverse effects.

#### Drug-specific teaching points

- Take the drug with meals in evenly divided doses.
- The following side effects may occur: abdominal cramping, discomfort, pain, diarrhea (take with meals); headache, fatigue, fever, flulike symptoms (request medications); skin rash, itching (skin care may help).
- Report severe diarrhea, malaise, fatigue, fever, blood in the stool.

O

## omeprazole

*(oh **me'** pray zol)*

Prilosec

**Pregnancy Category C**

### Drug classes

Antisecretory agent

### Therapeutic actions

Gastric acid-pump inhibitor: suppresses gastric acid secretion by specific inhibition of the hydrogen/potassium ATPase enzyme system at the secretory surface of the gastric parietal cells; blocks the final step of acid production.

### Indications

- Short-term treatment of active duodenal ulcer
- First-line therapy in treatment of heartburn or symptoms of gastroesophageal reflux disease (GERD)
- Short-term treatment of active benign gastric ulcer
- GERD, severe erosive esophagitis, poorly responsive symptomatic GERD
- Treatment of pathologic hypersecretory conditions ( Zollinger-Ellison syndrome, multiple adenomas, systemic mastocytosis) (long-term therapy)
- Unlabeled use: eradication of *H. pylori* with amoxicillin

### Contraindications/cautions

- Contraindications: hypersensitivity to omeprazole or its components.
- Use cautiously with pregnancy, lactation.

### Dosage

**Available Forms:** DR capsules—10, 20 mg

**ADULT**

- ***Active duodenal ulcer:*** 20 mg PO qd for 4–8 wk. Should not be used for maintenance therapy.
- ***Active gastric ulcer:*** 40 mg PO qd for 4–8 wk.
- ***Severe erosive esophagitis or poorly responsive GERD:*** 20 mg PO daily for 4–8 wk. Do not use as maintenance therapy. Do not use >8 wk.
- ***Pathologic hypersecretory conditions:*** Individualize dosage. Initial dose is 60 mg PO qd. Doses up to 120 mg tid have been used. Administer daily doses of > 80 mg in divided doses.

**PEDIATRIC:** Safety and efficacy not established.

### Pharmacokinetics

| *Route* | *Onset* | *Peak* |
|---|---|---|
| Oral | Varies | 0.5–3.5 h |

*Metabolism:* Hepatic, $T_{1/2}$: 0.5–1 h
*Distribution:* Crosses placenta; may enter breast milk
*Excretion:* Urine and bile

### Adverse effects

- CNS: *Headache, dizziness*, asthenia, vertigo, insomnia, apathy, anxiety, paresthesias, dream abnormalities
- GI: *Diarrhea, abdominal pain, nausea, vomiting*, constipation, dry mouth, tongue atrophy
- **Respiratory**: *URI symptoms,* cough, epistaxis
- **Dermatologic**: Rash, inflammation, urticaria, pruritus, alopecia, dry skin
- **Other**: Cancer in preclinical studies, back pain, fever

### Clinically important drug-drug interactions

- Increased serum levels and potential increase in toxicity of benzodiazepines

## ■ Nursing Considerations

### Assessment

- ***History:*** Hypersensitivity to omeprazole or any of its components, pregnancy, lactation
- ***Physical:*** Skin lesions; T; reflexes, affect; urinary output, abdominal exam; respiratory auscultation

### Implementation

- Administer before meals. Caution patient to swallow capsules whole, not to open, chew, or crush.
- Arrange for further evaluation of patient after 8 wk of therapy for gastroreflux disorders; not intended for maintenance therapy. Symptomatic improvement does not rule out gastric cancer, which did occur in preclinical studies.
- Administer antacids with omeprazole, if needed.

### Drug-specific teaching points

- Take the drug before meals. Swallow the capsules whole; do not chew, open, or crush. This drug will need to be taken for up to 8 wk (short-term therapy) or for a prolonged period (> 5 y in some cases).
- Have regular medical follow-ups.
- The following side effects may occur: dizziness (avoid driving or performing hazardous tasks); headache (request medications); nausea, vomiting, diarrhea (maintain proper nutrition); symptoms of upper respiratory tract infection, cough (do not self-medicate; consult with your health care provider if uncomfortable).
- Report severe headache, worsening of symptoms, fever, chills.

## ondansetron hydrochloride

*(on **dan'** sah tron)*

Zofran

**Pregnancy Category B**

### Drug classes

Antiemetic

### Therapeutic actions

Blocks specific receptor sites (5-$HT_3$), which are associated with nausea and vomiting in the CTZ (chemoreceptor trigger zone) centrally and at specific sites peripherally. It is not known whether its antiemetic actions are from actions at the central, peripheral, or combined sites.

### Indications

- Treatment of nausea and vomiting associated with emetogenic cancer chemotherapy (parenteral and oral)
- Treatment of postoperative nausea and vomiting—to prevent further episodes or, when postoperative nausea and vomiting must be avoided (oral), prophylactically (parenteral)
- Treatment of nausea and vomiting associated with radiotherapy.

### Contraindications/cautions

- Contraindication: allergy to ondansetron.
- Use cautiously with pregnancy, lactation.

### Dosage

**Available Forms:** Tablets—4, 8 mg; injection—2 mg/ml, 32 mg/50 ml

**ADULT**

- *Antiemetic*
  - ***Parenteral:*** Three 0.15 mg/kg doses IV: first dose is given over 15 min, beginning 20 min before the chemotherapy; subsequent doses are given at 4 and 8 h, or a single 32-mg dose infused over 30 min beginning 30 min before the start of the chemotherapy.
  - ***Oral:*** 8 mg PO tid; administer the first dose 30 min before beginning the chemotherapy at 4 and 8 h; continue q8h for 1–2 d after the chemotherapy treatment; for radiotherapy, administer 1–2h before radiation.
- ***Prevention of postoperative nausea and vomiting:*** 4 mg undiluted IV, preferably over 3–5 min, or as a single IM dose: 16 mg PO 1h before anesthesia.

**PEDIATRIC**

- *Antiemetic*
  - *4–18 Y:* IV dose same as adult.
  - *<3 Y:* Safety and efficacy not established.
  - *4–12 y:* 4 mg PO tid, using same schedule as adults.
- *Prevention of postoperative nausea and vomiting:* Safety and efficacy not established.

**HEPATIC IMPAIRMENT:** Do not exceed 8 mg PO; maximum daily dose of 8 mg IV.

### Pharmacokinetics

| Route | Onset | Peak |
|---|---|---|
| Oral | 30–60 min | 1.7–2.2 h |
| IV | Immediate | Immediate |

*Metabolism:* Hepatic, $T_{1/2}$: 3.5–6 h

*Distribution:* Crosses placenta; may enter breast milk

*Excretion:* Urine

### IV facts

**Preparation:** Dilute in 50 ml of 5% Dextrose Injection or 0.9% Sodium Chloride Injection; stable for 48 h at room temperature after dilution.

**Infusion:** Infuse slowly over 15 min diluted or 2–5 min undiluted.

**Compatibilities:** May be diluted with 0.9% Sodium Chloride Injection, 5% Dextrose Injection, 5% Dextrose and 0.9% Sodium Chloride injection; 5% Dextrose and 0.45% Sodium Chloride Injection; 3% Sodium Chloride Injection; do not mix with alkaline solutions.

### Adverse effects

- CNS: *Headache, dizziness,* drowsiness, shivers, malaise, fatigue, weakness, *myalgia*
- GI: Abdominal pain, constipation
- CV: Chest pain, hypotension
- GU: Urinary retention
- Dermatologic: Pruritis
- Local: Pain at injection site

### Clinically important drug-food interactions

- Increased extent of absorption if taken orally with food

## ■ Nursing Considerations

### Assessment

- ***History:*** Allergy to ondansetron, pregnancy, lactation, nausea and vomiting
- ***Physical:*** Skin color and texture; orientation, reflexes, bilateral grip strength, affect; P, BP; abdominal exam; urinary output

### Implementation

- Ensure that the timing of drug doses corresponds to that of the chemotherapy or radiation.
- Administer oral drug for 1–2 d following completion of chemotherapy or radiation.

### Drug-specific teaching points

- Take oral drug for 1–2 d following chemotherapy or radiation therapy to maximize prevention of nausea and vomiting. Take the drug every 8 h around the clock for best results.
- The following side effects may occur: weakness, dizziness (change postion slowly to avoid injury); dizziness, drowsiness (do not drive or perform tasks that require alertness).
- Report continued nausea and vomiting, pain at injection site, chest pain, palpitations.

# opium preparations

*(oh' pee um)*

Camphorated tincture of opium

Paregoric

**Pregnancy Category C**

**C-III controlled substance**

### Drug classes

Narcotic agonist analgesic

Antidiarrheal agent

### Therapeutic actions

Activity is primarily due to morphine content; acts as agonist at specific opioid receptors in the CNS to produce analgesia, euphoria, sedation; the receptors mediating these effects are thought to be the same as those mediating the effects of endogenous opioids (enkephalins, endorphins); inhibits peristalsis and diarrhea by producing spasm of GI tract smooth muscle.

### Indications

- Antidiarrheal
- Disorders requiring the analgesic, sedative/hypnotic narcotic, or opiate effect is needed
- For relief of severe pain in place of morphine (not a drug of choice)

### Contraindications/cautions

- Contraindications: hypersensitivity to narcotics, diarrhea caused by poisoning (before toxins are eliminated), pregnancy, labor or delivery (narcotics given to mother can cause respiratory depression of neonate; prematures are at special risk; may prolong labor), bronchial asthma, COPD, cor pulmonale, respiratory depression, anoxia, kyphoscoliosis, acute alcoholism, increased intracranial pressure.
- Use cautiously with acute abdominal conditions, CV disease, supraventricular tachycardias, myxedema, convulsive disorders, delirium tremens, cerebral arteriosclerosis, ulcerative colitis, fever, Addison's disease, prostatic hypertrophy, urethral stricture, recent GI or GU sur-

gery, toxic psychosis, renal or hepatic dysfunction.

### Dosage

**Available Forms:** Liquid—2 mg/5 ml

ADULT

- *Paregoric:* 5–10 ml PO qd–qid (5 ml is equivalent to 2 mg morphine).

PEDIATRIC: Contraindicated in premature infants.

- *Paregoric:* 0.25–0.5 ml/kg PO qd–qid.

GERIATRIC OR IMPAIRED ADULT: Use caution; respiratory depression may occur in elderly, the very ill, those with respiratory problems: reduced dosage may be necessary.

### Pharmacokinetics

| Route | Onset | Peak | Duration |
|---|---|---|---|
| Oral | Varies | 0.5–1 | 3–7 h |

*Metabolism:* Hepatic, $T_{1/2}$: 1.5–2 h
*Distribution:* Crosses placenta; enters breast milk
*Excretion:* Urine

### Adverse effects

- CNS: *Lightheadedness, dizziness, sedation,* euphoria, dysphoria, delirium, insomnia, agitation, anxiety, fear, hallucinations, disorientation, drowsiness, lethargy, impaired mental and physical performance, coma, mood changes, weakness, headache, tremor, convulsions, miosis, visual disturbances
- GI: *Nausea, vomiting, sweating,* dry mouth, anorexia, constipation, biliary tract spasm; increased colonic motility with chronic ulcerative colitis
- CV: Facial flushing, peripheral circulatory collapse, tachycardia, bradycardia, arrhythmia, palpitations, chest wall rigidity, hypertension, hypotension, orthostatic hypotension, syncope, circulatory depression, shock, cardiac arrest
- Respiratory: Suppression of cough reflex, respiratory depression, apnea, **respiratory arrest**, laryngospasm, bronchospasm
- GU: Ureteral spasm, spasm of vesical sphincters, urinary retention or hesitancy, oliguria, antidiuretic effect, reduced libido or potency
- **Dermatologic:** Pruritus, urticaria, edema, hemorrhagic urticaria (rare)
- **Other:** Physical tolerance and dependence, psychological dependence

### Clinically important drug-drug interactions

- Increased likelihood of respiratory depression, hypotension, profound sedation or coma with barbiturate general anesthetics.

### Drug-lab test interferences

- Elevated biliary tract pressure may cause increases in plasma amylase, lipase; determinations 24 h after administration

## ■ Nursing Considerations

### Assessment

- *History:* Hypersensitivity to narcotics, diarrhea caused by poisoning, bronchial asthma, COPD, cor pulmonale, respiratory depression, kyphoscoliosis, acute alcoholism, increased intracranial pressure,acute abdominal conditions, CV disease, supraventricular tachycardias, myxedema, convulsive disorders, delirium tremens, cerebral arteriosclerosis, ulcerative colitis, fever, Addison's disease, prostatic hypertrophy, urethral stricture, recent GI or GU surgery, toxic psychosis, renal or hepatic dysfunction
- *Physical:* T; skin color, texture, lesions; orientation, reflexes, bilateral grip strength, affect, pupil size; P, auscultation, BP, orthostatic BP, perfusion; R, adventious sounds; bowel sounds, normal output; frequency and pattern of voiding, normal output; thyroid, liver, kidney function tests

### Implementation

- Give to lactating women 4–6 h before the next feeding to minimize the amount in milk.
- Reassure patient about addiction liability; most patients who receive opiates for medical reasons do not develop dependence syndromes.

### Drug-specific teaching points

- Take this drug exactly as prescribed.
- The following side effects may occur: nausea, loss of appetite (take with food

O

and lie quietly, eating frequent, small meals may help); constipation (a laxative may help); dizziness, sedation, drowsiness, impaired visual acuity (avoid driving, performing other tasks that require alertness, visual acuity)

- Do not take leftover medication for other disorders, and do not to let anyone else take the prescription.
- Report severe nausea, vomiting, constipation, shortness of breath, or difficulty breathing.

## oprelvelkin

*(op **rahl'** vel kin)*

recombinant human interleukin-11

Neumega

**Pregnancy Category C**

### Drug classes

Interleukin

### Therapeutic actions

Human interleukin produced by *E. coli* bacteria; an endogenous hematopoietic growth factor with various effects on hematopoietic systems; regulates megakaryocytopoiesis and thrombopoiesis, early and mature hematocyte cells; also has effects on the cardiac, hepatic, GI, respiratory, CNS, and immune systems.

### Indications

- Prevention of severe thrombocytopenia and reduction of platelet transfusions following myelosuppressive chemotherapy in patients with nonmyeloid malignancies at high risk to develop severe thrombocytopenia

### Contraindications/cautions

- Contraindications: hypersensitivity to oprelvelkin or *E. coli*—produced products; pregnancy, lactation.
- Use cautiously with renal, liver, cardiac, respiratory, or CNS impairment.

### Dosage

**Available Forms:** Powder for injection—5 mg/single-dose vial

**ADULT:** 25–75 μg/kg/d SC staring 1 d after chemotherapy and continuing for 14–21 d following chemotherapy until the platelet count has reached >100,000/μL.

**PEDIATRIC:** Safety not established.

### Pharmacokinetics

| *Route* | *Onset* | *Peak* |
|---|---|---|
| SC | Slow | NA |

*Metabolism:* Tissue; $T_{1/2}$: Unknown

*Distribution:* Crosses placenta; passes into breast milk

*Excretion:* Unknown

### Adverse effects

- CNS: *Mental status changes, dizziness,* sensory dysfunction, syncope, headache
- CV: Tachycardia, atrial arrhythmias, hypertension
- **Respiratory**: *Respiratory difficulties, dyspnea,* pulmonary edema, cough
- **General**: *Fever, chills, pain, fatigue, weakness, malaise, edema,* infections
- **Other**: Rash, purpura

## ■ Nursing Considerations

### Assessment

- ***History:*** Hypersensitivity to oprelvelkin or *E. coli.*—produced products, lactation, pregnancy
- ***Physical:*** Body weight; skin color, temperature, turgor; orientation, reflexes, affect; P, BP; CBC, platelet count

### Implementation

- Monitor platelet count before chemotherapy and several times each week during therapy; if platelet count is <50,000/μL, more frequent monitoring will be necessary.
- Protect patient from invasive procedures and injury during therapy.
- Advise patient to use birth control methods during drug use; if patient is nursing a baby, help her select another method of feeding.
- Establish safety precautions if CNS changes occur.
- Provide comfort measures if flulike syndrome or headache occurs.

### Drug-specific teaching points

- This drug can be given only by injection; you will need to have frequent blood tests while it is being given.
- This drug is given for 14 to 21 days to decrease the effects that chemotherapy will have on your blood and blood-clotting activity.
- Avoid situations that might expose you to any injury while you are on this drug.
- The following side effects may occur: fever, chills, rash, fluid retention, difficulty breathing, nausea, vomiting, diarrhea.
- Report chest pain, dizziness, weakness, irregular heart beat, difficulty breathing, swelling, fever, malaise, fatigue, changes in stool or urine color.

## orphenadrine citrate

*(or **fen'** a dreen)*

Banflex, Flexoject, Norflex

**Pregnancy Category C**

### Drug classes

Skeletal muscle relaxant, centrally acting

### Therapeutic actions

Precise mechanisms not known; acts in the CNS; does not directly relax tense skeletal muscles; does not directly affect the motor endplate or motor nerves.

### Indications

- Relief of discomfort associated with acute, painful musculoskeletal conditions, as an adjunct to rest, physical therapy and other measures
- Unlabeled use: 100 mg at hs for the treatment of quinidine-resistant leg cramps

### Contraindications/cautions

- Contraindications: hypersensistivity to orphenadrine; glaucoma, pyloric, or duodenal obstruction; stenosing peptic ulcers; achalasia; cardiospasm (megaesophagus); prostatic hypertrophy; obstruction of bladder neck; myasthenia gravis; lactation.
- Use cautiously with cardiac decompensation, coronary insufficiency, cardiac arrhythmias, hepatic or renal dysfunction, pregnancy.

### Dosage

**Available Forms:** Injection—30 mg/ml

*ADULT:* 60 mg IV or IM. May repeat q12h. Inject IV over 5 min.

*PEDIATRIC:* Safety and efficacy not established; not recommended.

*GERIATRIC:* Use caution and regulate dosage carefully; patients older than 60 y frequently develop increased sensitivity to adverse CNS effects of anticholinergic drugs.

### Pharmacokinetics

| *Route* | *Onset* | *Peak* | *Duration* |
|---|---|---|---|
| IM/IV | Rapid | 2 h | 4–6 h |

*Metabolism:* Hepatic, $T_{1/2}$: 14 h

*Distribution:* Crosses placenta; enters breast milk

*Excretion:* Urine and feces

### IV facts

**Preparation:** No further preparation is required.

**Infusion:** Administer slowly IV, each 60 mg over 5 min.

### Adverse effects

- CNS: *Weakness, headache, dizziness, confusion* (especially in elderly), hallucinations, drowsiness, memory loss, psychosis, agitation, nervousness, delusions, delirium, paranoia, euphoria, depression, paresthesia, blurred vision, pupil dilation, increased intraocular tension
- GI: *Dry mouth, gastric irritation, vomiting, nausea, constipation*, dilation of the colon, paralytic ileus
- CV: *Tachycardia*, palpitation, transient syncope, hypotension, orthostatic hypotension
- GU: *Urinary hesitancy and retention*, dysuria, difficulty achieving or maintaining an erection
- **Dermatologic**: Urticaria, other dermatoses

O

- General: *Flushing, decreased sweating*, elevated temperature, muscle weakness, cramping

### Clinically important drug-drug interactions

• Additive anticholinergic effects with other anticholinergic drugs • Additive adverse CNS effects with phenothiazines • Possible masking of the development of persistent extrapyramidal symptoms, tardive dyskinesia in long-term therapy with phenothiazines, haloperidol • Decreased antipsychotic efficacy of phenothiazines, haloperidol

## ■ Nursing Considerations

### Assessment

- *History:* Hypersensitivity to orphenadrine; glaucoma, pyloric, or duodenal obstruction; stenosing peptic ulcers; achalasia; cardiospasm; prostatic hypertrophy; obstruction of bladder neck; myasthenia gravis; cardiac, hepatic or renal dysfunction; lactation
- *Physical:* Weight; T; skin color, lesions; orientation, affect, reflexes, bilateral grip strength, vision exam with tonometry; P, BP, orthostatic BP, auscultation; bowel sounds, normal output, liver evaluation; prostate palpation, normal output, voiding pattern; urinalysis, CBC with differential, liver and renal function tests, ECG

### Implementation

- Ensure that patient is supine during IV injection and for at least 15 min thereafter; assist patient from the supine position after treatment.
- Decrease or discontinue drug temporarily if dry mouth is so severe that swallowing or speaking becomes difficult.
- Give with caution, reduce dosage in hot weather; drug interferes with sweating and body's ability to thermoregulate in hot environments.
- Arrange for analgesics if headache occurs (adjunct for relief of muscle spasm).

### Drug-specific teaching points

- The following side effects may occur: drowsiness, dizziness, blurred vision (avoid driving or engaging in activities that require alertness and visual acuity); dry mouth (sucking on sugarless lozenges or ice chips may help); nausea (frequent, small meals may help); difficulty urinating (be sure that you empty the bladder just before taking the medication); constipation (increase fluid and fiber intake and exercise regularly); headache (request medication).
- Report dry mouth, difficult urination, constipation, headache, or GI upset that persists; skin rash or itching; rapid heart rate or palpitations; mental confusion; eye pain; fever; sore throat; bruising.

# oxacillin sodium

*(ox a **sill'in**)*

Bactocill, Prostaphilin

**Pregnancy Category B**

### Drug classes

Antibiotic

Penicillinase-resistant pencillin

### Therapeutic actions

Bactericidal: inhibits cell wall synthesis of sensitive organisms, causing cell death.

### Indications

- Infections due to penicillinase-producing staphylococci
- Infections caused by streptococci

### Contraindications/cautions

- Contraindications: allergies to penicillins, cephalosporins, or other allergens.
- Use cautiously with renal disorders, pregnancy, lactation (may cause diarrhea or candidiasis in infants).

### Dosage

**Available Forms:** Powder for injection—250, 500 mg; 1, 2, 4 g

Maximum recommended dosage is 6 g/d.

**ADULT**

- ***PO:*** 500 mg q4–6h PO for at least 5 d. Follow-up therapy after parenteral oxacillin in severe infections: 1 g q4–6h PO for up to 1–2 wk.

- ***Parenteral:*** 250–500 mg q4–6h IM or IV. Up to 1 g q4–6h in severe infections.

*PEDIATRIC (<40 KG)*

- ***PO:*** 50 mg/kg per day in equally divided doses q6h for at least 5 d. Follow-up therapy after parenteral oxacillin for severe infections: 100 mg/kg per day in equally divided doses q4–6h for 1–2 wk.
- ***Parenteral:*** 50 mg/kg per day IM or IV in equally divided doses q6h. Up to 100 mg/kg per day in equally divided doses q4–6h in severe infections.

*PREMATURES AND NEONATES:* 25 mg/kg per day IM or IV.

### Pharmacokinetics

| *Route* | *Onset* | *Peak* | *Duration* |
|---|---|---|---|
| Oral | Varies | 30–60 min | 4 h |
| IM | Rapid | 30–120 min | 4–6 h |
| IV | Rapid | 15 min | Length of infusion |

*Metabolism:* Hepatic, $T_{1/2}$: 0.5–1 h
*Distribution:* Crosses placenta; enters breast milk
*Excretion:* Urine and bile

### IV facts

**Preparation:** Dilute for direct IV administration to a maximum concentration of 1 g/10 ml using Sodium Chloride Injection or Sterile Water for Injection. For IV infusion: reconstituted solution may be diluted with compatible IV solution: 0.9% Sodium Chloride Injection, 5% Dextrose in Water or in Normal Saline, 10% D-Fructose in Water or in Normal Saline, Lactated Ringer's Solution, Lactated Potassic Saline Injections, 10% Invert Sugar in Water or in Normal Saline, 10% Invert Sugar plus 0.3% Potassium Chloride in Water, Travert 10% Electrolyte 1, 2, or 3. 0.5–40 mg/ml solutions are stable for up to 6h at room temperature. Discard after that time.
**Infusion:** Give by direct administration slowly to avoid vein irritation, each 1 g over 10 min; infusion—over up to 6 h.
**Incompatibilities:** *Do not* mix in the same IV solution as other antibiotics.

### Adverse effects

- CNS: Lethargy, hallucinations, seizures
- GI: *Glossitis, stomatitis, gastritis, sore mouth*, furry tongue, black "hairy" tongue, *nausea, vomiting, diarrhea,* abdominal pain, bloody diarrhea, enterocolitis, pseudomembranous colitis, nonspecific hepatitis
- **Hematologic**: Anemia, thrombocytopenia, leukopenia, neutropenia, prolonged bleeding time (more common than with other penicillinase-resistant penicillins)
- GU: Nephritis—oliguria, proteinuria, hematuria, casts, azotemia, pyuria
- **Hypersensitivity reactions**: *Rash, fever, wheezing,* anaphylaxis
- **Local**: *Pain, phlebitis*, thrombosis at injection site
- **Other**: *Superinfections*, sodium overload leading to CHF

### Clinically important drug-drug interactions

- Decreased effectiveness with tetracyclines
- Inactivation of aminoglycosides in parenteral solutions with oxacillin.

### Drug-lab test interferences

- False-positive Coombs' test with IV oxacillin

O

## ■ Nursing Considerations

### Assessment

- *History:* Allergies to penicillins, cephalosporins, or other allergens; renal disorders; pregnancy; lactation
- *Physical:* Culture infection; skin color, lesions; R, adventitious sounds; bowel sounds: CBC, liver and renal function tests, serum electrolytes, Hct, urinalysis

### Implementation

- Culture infection before treatment; reculture if response is not as expected.
- Continue therapy for at least 2 d after infection has disappeared, usually 7–10 d.
- Reconstitute for IM use to a dilution of 250 mg/1.5 ml using Sterile Water for Injection or Sodium Chloride Injection. Discard after 3 d at room temperature or after 7 d if refrigerated.

- Maintain epinephrine, IV fluids, vasopressors, bronchodilators, oxygen, and emergency equipment on standby in case of serious hypersensitivity reaction.

### Drug-specific teaching points

- The following side effects may occur: upset stomach, nausea, diarrhea (small, frequent meals may help), mouth sores (frequent mouth care may help), pain or discomfort at the injections site.
- Report difficulty breathing, rashes, severe diarrhea, severe pain at injection site, mouth sores.

## oxamniquine

*(ox **am'** ni kwin)*

Vansil

**Pregnancy Category C**

### Drug classes

Anthelmintic

### Therapeutic actions

Antischistosomal versus *Schistosoma mansoni*; causes worms to move from mesentery to liver where tissue reactions trap male worms; female worms move back, but cease to lay eggs; mechanism of action not fully understood.

### Indications

- Treatment of all stages of *S. mansoni* infection
- Unlabeled use: concurrent low-dose administration with praziquantel as a single-dose treatment of neurocysticercosis

### Contraindications/cautions

- Allergy to oxamniquine, seizures, pregnancy, lactation.

### Dosage

**Available Forms:** Capsules—250 mg

*ADULT:* 12–15 mg/kg PO as a single dose.

*PEDIATRIC (< 30 KG):* 20 mg/kg PO, in two divided doses of 10 mg/kg PO with 2–8 h between doses.

### Pharmacokinetics

| *Route* | *Onset* | *Peak* |
|---|---|---|
| Oral | Varies | 1–1 1/2 h |

*Metabolism:* Hepatic, $T_{1/2}$: 1–2.5 h

*Distribution:* Crosses placenta; may enter breast milk

*Excretion:* Urine

### Adverse effects

- CNS: *Drowsiness, dizziness, headache,* epileptiform convulsions
- GI: *Nausea*, vomiting, abdominal discomfort, loss of appetite
- **Dermatologic**: Urticaria

### ■ Nursing Considerations

#### Assessment

- *History:* Allergy to oxamniquine, seizures, pregnancy, lactation
- *Physical:* Skin color, lesions; orientation, reflexes

#### Implementation

- Culture for ova.
- Administer drug with food to improve tolerance.

#### Drug-specific teaching points

- Take drug with meals to avoid GI upset.
- The following side effects may occur: nausea, abdominal pain, GI upset (small, frequent meals); drowsiness, dizziness (use caution driving or operating dangerous equipment).
- Report rash, severe abdominal pain, marked weakness, dizziness.

## oxandrolone

*(ox **an'** droh lone)*

Oxandrin

**Pregnancy Category X**

### Drug classes

Anabolic steroid

Hormone

### Therapeutic actions

Testosterone analog with androgenic and anabolic activity; promotes body tissue-building processes and reverses catabolic or tissue-depleting processes; increases Hgb and red cell mass.

### Indications

- Adjunctive therapy to promote weight gain after weight loss following extensive surgery, chronic infections, trauma
- Offset protein catabolism associated with prolonged use of corticosteroids
- Relief of bone pain accompanying osteoporosis
- Unlabeled use: alcoholic hepatitis
- Orphan drug uses: short stature associated with Turner syndrome, HIV wasting syndrome, and HIV-associated muscle weakness

### Contraindications/cautions

- Known sensitivity to anabolic steroids; prostate, breast cancer; benign prostatic hypertrophy; pituitary insufficiency; MI (contraindicated because of effects on cholesterol); nephrosis; liver disease; hypercalcemia; pregnancy, lactation.

### Dosage

**Available Forms:** Tablets—2.5 mg

ADULT: *2.5 mg PO bid–qid:* up to 20 mg has been used to achieve the desired effect; 2–4 wk is needed to evaluate response.

PEDIATRIC: Total daily dose of < 0.1 mg/kg or < 0.045 mg/lb PO, may be repeated intermittently.

### Pharmacokinetics

| Route | Onset |
|---|---|
| Oral | Slow |

*Metabolism:* Hepatic, $T_{1/2}$: 9 h

*Distribution:* Crosses placenta; enters breast milk

*Excretion:* Urine

### Adverse effects

- CNS: *Excitation, insomnia,* chills, toxic confusion
- GI: Hepatotoxicity, peliosis, **hepatitis** with life threatening liver failure or intra-abdominal hemorrhage; **liver cell tumors**, sometimes malignant and fatal, *nausea, vomiting, diarrhea, abdominal fullness, loss of appetite, burning of tongue*
- Hematologic: *Blood lipid changes*; iron deficiency anemia, hypercalcemia, altered serum cholesterol levels; *retention of sodium, chloride, water,* potassium, phosphates and calcium
- GU: Possible increased risk of prostatic hypertrophy, carcinoma in geriatric patients
- Endocrine: *Virilization: prepubertal males*—phallic enlargement, hirsutism, increased skin pigmentation; *postpubertal males*—inhibition of testicular function, gynecomastia, testicular atrophy, priapism, baldness, epidiymitis, change in libido; *females*—hirsutism, hoarseness, deepening of the voice, clitoral enlargement, menstrual irregularities, baldness; decreased glucose tolerance
- Other: *Acne,* premature closure of the epiphyses

### Clinically important drug-drug interactions

• Potentiation of oral anticoagulants with anabolic steroids • Decreased need for insulin, oral hypoglycemica agents with anabolic steroids

### Drug-lab test interferences

• Altered glucose tolerance tests • Decrease in thyroid function tests (may persist for 2–3 wk after stopping therapy) • Increased creatinine, creatinine clearance, which may last for 2 wk after therapy

## ■ Nursing Considerations

### Assessment

- *History:* Sensitivity to anabolic steroids; prostate or breast cancer; benign prostatic hypertrophy; pituitary insufficiency; MI; nephrosis; liver disease; hypercalcemia; pregnancy; lactation
- *Physical:* Skin color, texture; hair distribution pattern; affect, orientation; abdominal exam, liver evaluation; serum electrolytes and cholesterol levels, glucose tolerance tests, thyroid function tests, long bone x-ray (in children)

### Implementation

- Administer with food if GI upset or nausea occurs.
- Monitor effect on children with long-bone x-rays every 3–6 mo; discontinue drug well before the bone age reaches the norm for the patient's chronologic age because effects may continue for 6 mo after therapy.
- Monitor patient for occurrence of edema; arrange for diuretic therapy.
- Monitor liver function, serum electrolytes periodically and consult with physician for corrective measures.
- Measure cholesterol levels periodically in patients who are at high risk for CAD.
- Monitor diabetic patients closely because glucose tolerance may change. Adjustments may be needed in insulin, oral hypoglycemic dosage, and diet.

### Drug-specific teaching points

- Take drug with food if nausea or GI upset occur.
- The following side effects may occur: nausea, vomiting, diarrhea, burning of the tongue (eat small, frequent meals); body hair growth, baldness, deepening of the voice, loss of libido, impotence (most reversible); excitation, confusion, insomnia (avoid driving, performing tasks that require alertness); swelling of the ankles, fingers (request medication).
- Diabetic patients need to monitor urine or blood sugar closely because glucose tolerance may change; report any abnormalities to physician for corrective action.
- These drugs do not enhance athletic ability but do have serious effects. They should not be used for increasing muscle strength.
- Report ankle swelling, skin color changes, severe nausea, vomiting, hoarseness, body hair growth, deepening of the voice, acne, menstrual irregularities.

## oxaprozin

*(oks a* ***pro'*** *zin)*

Daypro

**Pregnancy Category C**

### Drug classes

Analgesic (non-narcotic)
Antipyretic
Nonsteroidal anti-inflammatory drug (NSAID)

### Therapeutic actions

Inhibits prostaglandin synthetase to cause antipyretic and anti-inflammatory effects; the exact mechnanism of action is not known.

### Indications

- Acute or long-term use in the management of signs and symptoms of osteoarthritis and rheumatoid arthritis

### Contraindications/cautions

- Contraindications: significant renal impairment, pregnancy, lactation.
- Use cautiously with impaired hearing, allergies, hepatic, CV, and GI conditions.

### Dosage

**Available Forms:** Caplets—600 mg

Titrate to the lowest effective dose to minimize side effects. Maximum daily dose: 1,800 mg or 26 mg/kg, whichever is lower.

**ADULT**

- ***Osteoarthritis:*** 1,200 mg PO qd; use initial dose of 600 mg with low body weight or milder disease.
- ***Rheumatoid arthritis:*** 1,200 mg PO qd.

**PEDIATRIC:** Safety and efficacy not established.

### Pharmacokinetics

| *Route* | *Onset* | *Peak* | *Duration* |
|---|---|---|---|
| Oral | Varies | 3–5 h | 24–36 h |

*Metabolism:* Hepatic, $T_{1/2}$: 42–50 h
*Distribution:* Crosses placenta; enters breast milk
*Excretion:* Urine and feces

### Adverse effects

- CNS: Dizziness, somnolence, insomnia, fatigue, tiredness, dizziness, tinnitus, ophthalmologic effects
- GI: *Nausea, dyspepsia,* GI pain, *diarrhea*, vomiting, *constipation*, flatulence

- **Hematologic**: Bleeding, platelet inhibition with higher doses
- GU: Dysuria, renal impairment
- **Dermatologic**: Rash, pruritus, sweating, dry mucous membranes, stomatitis
- **Other**: Peripheral edema, **anaphylactoid reactions** to fatal anaphylactic shock

## ■ Nursing Considerations

### Assessment

- *History:* Renal impairment, impaired hearing, allergies, hepatic, CV, and GI conditions, lactation
- *Physical:* Skin—color and lesions; orientation, reflexes, ophthalmologic and audiometric evaluation, peripheral sensation; P, edema; R, adventitious sounds; liver evaluation; CBC, clotting times, renal and liver function tests; serum electrolytes, stool guaiac

### Implementation

- Administer drug with food or after meals if GI upset occurs.
- Arrange for periodic ophthalmologic examination during long-term therapy.
- Institute emergency procedures if overdose occurs (gastric lavage, induction of emesis, supportive therapy).

### Drug-specific teaching points

- Take drug with food or meals if GI upset occurs.
- Dizziness, drowsiness can occur (avoid driving or the use of dangerous machinery).
- Report sore throat, fever, rash, itching, weight gain, swelling in ankles or fingers, changes in vision, black, tarry stools.

## oxazepam

*(ox **a'** ze pam)*

Apo-Oxazepam (CAN), Novoxapam (CAN), Ox-Pam(CAN), Serax, Zapex (CAN)

**Pregnancy Category D**
**C-IV controlled substance**

### Drug classes

Benzodiazepine
Antianxiety agent

### Therapeutic actions

Exact mechanisms not understood; acts mainly at subcortical levels of the CNS, leaving the cortex relatively unaffected; main sites of action may be the limbic system and reticular formation; benzodiazepines potentiate the effects of GABA, an inhibitory neurotransmitter; anxiolytic effects occur at doses well below those necessary to cause sedation, ataxia.

### Indications

- Management of anxiety disorders or for short-term relief of symptoms of anxiety; anxiety associated with depression also is responsive
- Management of anxiety, tension, agitation, and irritability in older patients
- Alcoholics with acute tremulousness, inebriation, or anxiety associated with alcohol withdrawal

### Contraindications/cautions

- Contraindications: hypersensitivity to benzodiazepines, tartrazine (in the tablets); psychoses; acute narrow-angle glaucoma; shock; coma; acute alcoholic intoxication with depression of vital signs; pregnancy (risk of congenital malformations, neonatal withdrawal syndrome); labor and delivery ("floppy infant" syndrome); lactation (may cause infants to become lethargic and lose weight).
- Use cautiously with impaired liver or kidney function, debilitation.

### Dosage

**Available Forms:** Capsules—10, 15, 30 mg; tablets—15 mg

Increase dosage gradually to avoid adverse effects.

*ADULT:* 10–15 mg PO or up to 30 mg, PO tid–qid, depending on severity of symptoms of anxiety. The higher dosage range is recommended in alcoholics.

*PEDIATRIC 6–12 Y:* Dosage not established.

O

*Geriatric Patients or Those With Debilitating Disease:* Initially 10 mg PO tid. Gradually increase to 15 mg PO tid–qid if needed and tolerated.

**Pharmacokinetics**

| *Route* | *Onset* | *Peak* |
|---|---|---|
| Oral | Slow | 2–4 h |

*Metabolism:* Hepatic, $T_{1/2}$: 5–20 h
*Distribution:* Crosses placenta; enters breast milk
*Excretion:* Urine

**Adverse effects**

- CNS: *Transient, mild drowsiness* (initially), *sedation, depression, lethargy, apathy, fatigue, lightheadedness, disorientation*, restlessness, confusion, crying, delirium, headache, slurred speech, dysarthria, stupor, rigidity, tremor, dystonia, vertigo, euphoria, nervousness, difficulty in concentration, vivid dreams, psychomotor retardation, extrapyramidal symptoms, mild paradoxical excitatory reactions during first 2 wk of treatment, visual and auditory disturbances, diplopia, nystagmus, depressed hearing
- GI: *Constipation, diarrhea, dry mouth*, salivation, nausea, anorexia, vomiting, difficulty in swallowing, gastric disorders
- CV: Bradycardia, tachycardia, **CV collapse**, hypertension and hypotension, palpitations, edema
- Hematologic: Elevations of blood enzymes, hepatic dysfunction, blood dyscrasias: agranulocytosis, leukopenia
- GU: *Incontinence, urinary retention*, changes in libido, menstrual irregularities
- Dermatologic: Urticaria, pruritus, skin rash, dermatitis
- Other: *Nasal congestion, hiccups, fever, diaphoresis*, paresthesias, muscular disturbances, gynecomastia, drug dependence with withdrawal syndrome when drug is discontinued: more common with abrupt discontinuation of higher dosage used for longer than 4 mo

**Clinically important drug-drug interactions**

- Increased CNS depression with alcohol
- Decreased sedation when given to heavy smokers of cigarettes or if taken concurrently with theophyllines

## ■ Nursing Considerations

### Assessment

- *History:* Hypersensitivity to benzodiazepines, tartrazine; psychoses; acute narrow-angle glaucoma; shock; coma; acute alcoholic intoxication; pregnancy; labor and delivery; lactation; impaired liver or kidney function, debilitation
- *Physical:* Skin color, lesions; T; orientation, reflexes, affect, ophthalmologic exam; P, BP; R, adventitious sounds; liver evaluation, abdominal exam, bowel sounds, normal output; CBC, liver and renal function tests.

### Implementation

- Taper dosage gradually after long-term therapy, especially in epileptics.

### Drug-specific teaching points

- Take this drug exactly as prescribed; do not stop taking drug (long-term therapy) without consulting health care provider.
- The following side effects may occur: drowsiness, dizziness (may lessen; avoid driving or engaging in other dangerous activities); GI upset (take with food); depression, dreams, emotional upset, crying.
- Report severe dizziness, weakness, drowsiness that persists, palpitations, swelling of the extremities, visual changes, difficulty voiding, rash or skin lesion.

## oxtriphylline

*(ox* ***trye'*** *fi lin)*
choline theophyllinate
Choledyl SA
**Pregnancy Category C**

## Drug classes
Bronchodilator
Xanthine

## Therapeutic actions
Oxtriphylline, the choline salt of theophylline, is 64% theophylline; it relaxes bronchial smooth muscle, causing bronchodilation and increasing vital capacity, which has been impaired by bronchospasm and air trapping; actions may be mediated by inhibition of phosphodiesterase, which increases the concentration of cyclic adenosine monophosphate (cAMP).

## Indications
- Symptomatic relief or prevention of bronchial asthma and reversible bronchospasm associated with chronic bronchitis and emphysema

## Contraindications/cautions
- Contraindications: hypersensitivity to any xanthine, peptic ulcer, active gastritis.
- Use cautiously with cardiac arrhythmias, acute myocardial injury, CHF, cor pulmonale, severe hypertension, severe hypoxemia, renal or hepatic disease, hyperthyroidism, alcoholism, labor, pregnancy (tachycardia, jitteriness, and withdrawal apnea observed in neonates), lactation.

## Dosage
**Available Forms:** Tablets—100, 200 mg; SA tablets—400, 600 mg; syrup—50 mg/5 ml; elixir—100 mg/5 ml

Individualize dosage, basing adjustments on clinical responses with monitoring of serum theophylline levels, if possible, to maintain levels in the therapeutic range of 10–20 μg/ml. Base dosage on lean body mass.

***Adult:*** 4.7 mg/kg PO q8h. Sustained release, 400–600 mg PO q12h.

***Pediatric:*** Use in children < 6 mo not recommended. Use of timed-release products in children < 6 y not recommended. Children are very sensitive to CNS stimulant action of theophylline. Use caution in younger children who cannot complain of minor side effects.

- *9–16 Y:* 4.7 mg/kg PO q6h.
- *1–9 Y:* 6.2 mg/kg PO q6h.

## Pharmacokinetics

| *Route* | *Onset* | *Peak* |
|---|---|---|
| Oral | Rapid | 2 h |

*Metabolism:* Hepatic, $T_{1/2}$: 3–15 h
*Distribution:* Crosses placenta; enters breast milk
*Excretion:* Urine

## Adverse effects
- CNS: *Irritability (especially children); restlessness,* dizziness, muscle twitching, convulsions, severe depression, stammering speech; abnormal behavior characterized by withdrawal, mutism and unresponsiveness alternating with hyperactive periods
- GI: *Loss of appetite*, hematemesis, epigastric pain, gastroesophageal reflux
- CV: Palpitations, sinus tachycardia, ventricular tachycardia, **life threatening ventricular arrhythmias**, circulatory failure
- Respiratory: Tachypnea, respiratory arrest
- GU: Proteinuria, increased excretion of renal tubular cells and RBCs; diuresis, urinary retention with prostate enlargement
- Other: Fever, flushing, hyperglycemia, SIADH, rash, increased SGOT
- Serum theophylline levels <20 μg/ml: Adverse effects uncommon.
- Serum theophylline levels >20–25 μg/ml: Nausea, vomiting, diarrhea, headache, insomnia, irritability (75% of patients)
- Serum theophylline levels >30–35 μg/ml: Hyperglycemia, hypotension, cardiac arrhythmias, tachycardia (>10 μg/ml in premature newborns); **seizures, brain damage, death**

## Clinically important drug-drug interactions
• Increased effects and toxicity with cimetidine, erythromycin, troleandomycin, ciprofloxacin, norfloxacin, enoxacin, pefloxacin, oral contraceptives, ticlopidine, rifampin • Increased serum levels and risk of toxicity in hypothyroid patients; de-

creased drug levels in hyperthyroid; monitor patients on thioamines, thyroid hormones for changes in serum levels as patients become euthyroid • Increased cardiac toxicity with halothane • Decreased effects in cigarette smokers (1–2 packs/d) • Decreased effects with barbiturates • Decreased effects of phenytoins, benzodiazepines, nondepolarizing neuromuscular blockers, and theophylline preparations • Mutually antagonistic effects of beta-blockers and theophylline preparations

**Clinically important drug-food interactions**

• Elimination of theophylline is increased by a low-carbohydrate, high-protein diet and by charcoal broiled beef • Elimination of theophylline is decreased by a high-carbohydrate, low-protein diet • Food may alter bioavailability, absorption of timed-release preparations; these may rapidly release their contents in the presence of food and cause toxicity; timed-release forms should be taken on an empty stomach

**Drug-lab test interferences**

• Interference with spectrophotometric determinations of serum theophylline levels by furosemide, phenylbutazone, probenecid, theobromine; coffee, tea, cola beverages, chocolate, acetaminophen, which cause falsely high values • Alteration in assays of uric acid, urinary catecholamines, plasma free fatty acids by theophylline preparations

## ■ Nursing Considerations

### Assessment

- *History:* Hypersensitivity to any xanthine, peptic ulcer, active gastritis, cardiac disorders, cor pulmonale, severe hypertension, severe hypoxemia, renal or hepatic disease, hyperthyroidism, alcoholism, pregnancy, lactation
- *Physical:* Bowel sounds, normal output; P, auscultation, BP, perfusion, ECG; R, adventitious sounds; urinary frequency, voiding, normal output pattern, urinalysis; liver palpation; liver, renal, thyroid function tests; skin color, texture, lesions; reflexes, bilateral grip strength, affect, EEG

### Implementation

- Caution patient not to chew or crush enteric-coated timed-release preparations.
- Give immediate-release, liquid dosage forms with food if GI effects occur.
- Do not give timed-release preparations with food; these should be given on an empty stomach, 1 h before or 2 h after meals.
- Monitor results of serum theophylline level determinations carefully, and arrange for reduced dosage if serum levels exceed therapeutic range of 10–20 $\mu$g/ml.
- Monitor patient carefully for clinical signs of adverse effects, particularly if serum theophylline levels are not available.
- Maintain diazepam on standby to treat seizures.

### Drug-specific teaching points

- Take this drug exactly as prescribed; if a timed-release product is prescribed, take this drug on an empty stomach, 1 h before or 2 h after meals; it may be necessary to take this drug around the clock for adequate control of asthma attacks.
- Do not chew or crush timed-release preparations.
- Avoid excessive intake of coffee, tea, cocoa, cola beverages, chocolate.
- Smoking cigarettes or other tobacco products may markedly influence theophylline effects; it is better not to smoke while using this drug. Notify the care provider if smoking habits change.
- Frequent blood tests may be necessary to monitor drug effect and ensure safe and effective dosage.
- The following side effects may occur: nausea, loss of appetite (take with food—applies only to immediate-release or liquid dosage forms); difficulty sleeping, depression, emotional lability (reversible).
- Report nausea, vomiting, severe GI pain, restlessness, convulsions, irregular heartbeat.

# oxybutynin chloride

*(ox i **byoo'** ti nin)*

Ditropan

**Pregnancy Category B**

**Drug classes**

Urinary antispasmodic

**Therapeutic actions**

Acts directly to relax smooth muscle and inhibits the effects of acetylcholine at muscarinic receptors; reported to be less potent an anticholinergic than atropine but more potent as antispasmodic and devoid of antinicotinic activity at skeletal neuromuscular junctions or autonomic ganglia.

**Indications**

- Relief of symptoms of bladder instability associated with voiding in patients with uninhibited neurogenic and reflex neurogenic bladder

**Contraindications/cautions**

- Contraindications: allergy to oxybutynin, pyloric or duodenal obstruction, obstructive intestinal lesions or ileus, intestinal atony, megacolon, colitis, obstructive uropathies, glaucoma, myasthenia gravis, CV instability in acute hemorrhage.
- Use cautiously with hepatic, renal impairment; pregnancy; lactation.

**Dosage**

**Available Forms:** Tablets—5 mg; syrup—5 mg/5 ml

*ADULT:* 5 mg PO bid or tid. Maximum dose is 5 mg qid.

*PEDIATRIC (>5 Y):* 5 mg PO bid. Maximum dose is 5 mg tid.

**Pharmacokinetics**

| *Route* | *Onset* | *Peak* | *Duration* |
|---|---|---|---|
| Oral | 30–60 min | 3–6 h | 6–10 h |

*Metabolism:* Hepatic, $T_{1/2}$: unknown

*Distribution:* Crosses placenta; may enter breast milk

*Excretion:* Urine

**Adverse effects**

- CNS: *Drowsiness, dizziness, blurred vision,* dilatation of the pupil, cycloplegia, increased ocular tension, weakness
- GI: *Dry mouth, nausea*, vomiting, constipation, bloated feeling
- CV: Tachycardia, palpitations
- GU: *Urinary hesitancy*, retention, impotence
- Hypersensitivity: Allergic reactions including urticaria, dermal effect
- Other: *Decreased sweating*, heat prostration in high environmental temperatures secondary to loss of sweating

**Clinically important drug-drug interactions**

• Decreased effectiveness of phenothiazines with oxybutynin • Decreased effectiveness of haloperidol and development of tardive dyskinesia

## ■ Nursing Considerations

### Assessment

- *History:* Allergy to oxybutynin, intestinal obstructions or lesions, intestinal atony, obstructive uropathies, glaucoma, myasthenia gravis, CV instability in acute hemorrhage, hepatic or renal impairment, pregnancy
- *Physical:* Skin color, lesions; T; orientation, affect, reflexes, ophthalmic exam, ocular pressure measurement; P, rhythm, BP; bowel sounds, liver evaluation; renal and liver function tests, cystometry

### Implementation

- Arrange for cystometry and other diagnostic tests before and during treatment.
- Arrange for ophthalmic exam before therapy and during therapy.

### Drug-specific teaching points

- Take this drug as prescribed.
- Periodic bladder exams will be needed during this treatment to evaluate therapeutic response.
- The following side effects may occur: dry mouth, GI upset (sucking on sugarless lozenges and frequent mouth care may help); drowsiness, blurred vision (avoid driving or performing tasks that require alertness); decreased sweating (avoid high temperatures; serious complications can occur because you will be heat intolerant).
- Report blurred vision, fever, skin rash, nausea, vomiting.

O

# oxycodone hydrochloride

*(ox i **koe'** done)*

OxyContin II, OxyIR, Roxicodone, Supeudol (CAN)

**Pregnancy Category C**
**C-II controlled substance**

## Drug classes

Narcotic agonist analgesic

## Therapeutic actions

Acts as agonist at specific opioid receptors in the CNS to produce analgesia, euphoria, sedation; the receptors mediating these effects are thought to be the same as those mediating the effects of endogenous opioids (enkephalins, endorphins).

## Indications

- Relief of moderate to moderately severe pain

## Contraindications/cautions

- Contraindications: hypersensitivity to narcotics, diarrhea caused by poisoning (before toxins are eliminated); pregnancy (readily crosses placenta; neonatal withdrawal); labor or delivery (narcotics given to the mother can cause respiratory depression in neonate; premature infants are at special risk; may prolong labor); bronchial asthma, COPD, cor pulmonale, respiratory depression, anoxia, kyphoscoliosis, acute alcoholism, increased intracranial pressure, lactation.
- Use cautiously with acute abdominal conditions, CV disease, supraventricular tachycardias, myxedema, convulsive disorders, delirium tremens, cerebral arteriosclerosis, ulcerative colitis, fever, Addison's disease, prostatic hypertrophy, urethral stricture, recent GI or GU surgery, toxic psychosis, renal or hepatic dysfunction.

## Dosage

**Available Forms:** Tablets—5 mg; IR capsules—5 mg; oral solution—5 mg/5 ml

Individualize dosage.

*ADULT:* 5 mg or 5 ml PO q6h as needed.

- **Controlled release (OxyContin):** 10–20 mg PO q12h.
- **Immediate release (OxyIR):** 5 mg PO to cover breakthrough pain.

*PEDIATRIC:* Not recommended.

*GERIATRIC OR IMPAIRED ADULT:* Use caution. Respiratory depression may occur in elderly, the very ill, those with respiratory problems.

## Pharmacokinetics

| *Route* | *Onset* | *Peak* | *Duration* |
|---|---|---|---|
| Oral | 15–30 min | 1 h | 4–6 h |

*Metabolism:* Hepatic, $T_{1/2}$: unknown
*Distribution:* Crosses placenta; enters breast milk
*Excretion:* Urine

## Adverse effects

- CNS: *Lightheadedness, dizziness, sedation,* euphoria, dysphoria, delirium, insomnia, agitation, anxiety, fear, hallucinations, disorientation, drowsiness, lethargy, impaired mental and physical performance, coma, mood changes, weakness, headache, tremor, convulsions, miosis, visual disturbances
- GI: *Nausea, vomiting, sweating* (more common in ambulatory patients and those without severe pain), dry mouth, anorexia, constipation, biliary tract spasm; increased colonic motility in patients with chronic ulcerative colitis
- CV: Facial flushing, peripheral circulatory collapse, tachycardia, bradycardia, arrhythmia, palpitations, chest wall rigidity, hypertension, hypotension, orthostatic hypotension, syncope, circulatory depression, shock, cardiac arrest
- **Respiratory**: Suppression of cough reflex, respiratory depression, apnea, respiratory arrest, laryngospasm, bronchospasm
- GU: Ureteral spasm, spasm of vesical sphincters, urinary retention or hesitancy, oliguria, antidiuretic effect, reduced libido or potency
- **Dermatologic**: Pruritus, urticaria, edema, hemorrhagic urticaria (rare)

- **Other**: Physical tolerance and dependence, psychological dependence

### Clinically important drug-drug interactions

• Increased likelihood of respiratory depression, hypotension, profound sedation or coma in patients receiving barbiturate general anesthetics

### Drug-lab test interferences

• Elevated biliary tract pressure may cause increases in plasma amylase, lipase; determinations for 24 h after administration

## ■ Nursing Considerations

### Assessment

- *History:* Hypersensitivity to narcotics, diarrhea caused by poisoning, pregnancy, labor or delivery, bronchial asthma, COPD, cor pulmonale, respiratory depression, kyphoscoliosis, acute alcoholism, increased intracranial pressure, acute abdominal conditions, CV disease, myxedema, convulsive disorders, cerebral arteriosclerosis, ulcerative colitis, fever, Addison's disease, prostatic hypertrophy, urethral stricture, recent GI or GU surgery, toxic psychosis, renal or hepatic dysfunction
- *Physical:* T; skin color, texture, lesions; orientation, reflexes, bilateral grip strength, affect, pupil size; P, auscultation, BP, orthostatic BP, perfusion; R, adventious sounds; bowel sounds, normal output; frequency and pattern of voiding, normal output; ECG; EEG; thyroid, liver, kidney function tests

### Implementation

- Administer to nursing women 4–6 h before the next feeding to minimize amount in milk.
- Do not crush or allow patient to chew controlled-release preparations.
- Administer immediate-release preparations to cover breakthrough pain.
- Provide narcotic antagonist, facilities for assisted or controlled respiration on standby during parenteral administration.
- Reassure patient about addiction liability; most patients who receive opiates for medical reasons do not develop dependence syndromes.

### Drug-specific teaching points

- Take drug exactly as prescribed. Do not crush or chew controlled-release preparations.
- The following side effects may occur: nausea, loss of appetite (take with food, lie quietly, eat frequent, small meals); constipation (use a laxative); dizziness, sedation, drowsiness, impaired visual acuity (avoid driving, performing other tasks that require alertness, visual acuity).
- Do not take any leftover medication for other disorders, and do not let anyone else take the prescription.
- Report severe nausea, vomiting, constipation, shortness of breath, or difficulty breathing.

## oxymetazoline

*(ox i met **az'** oh leen)*

Afrin, Allerest 12-hour Nasal, Dristan Long Lasting, Duramist Plus, Genasal, Neo-Synephrine, Nostrilla, Sinex Long Lasting, Twice-A-Day Nasal

**Pregnancy Category C**

### Drug classes

Nasal decongestant

### Therapeutic actions

Acts directly on alpha receptors to produce vasoconstriction of arterioles in nasal passages, which produces a decongestant response; no effect on beta receptors.

### Indications

- Symptomatic relief of nasal and nasopharyngeal mucosal congestion due to colds, hay fever, or other respiratory allergies (topical)

### Contraindications/cautions

- Contraindications: allergy to oxymetalozine, angle-closure glaucoma, anesthesia with cyclopropane or halothane, thyrotoxicosis, diabetes, hypertension, CV

O

disorders, women in labor whose BP > 130/80.
- Use cautiously with angina, arrhythmias, prostatic hypertrophy, unstable vasomotor syndrome, lactation.

### Dosage

**Available Forms:** Nasal spray—0.05%; nasal drops—0.025%

*ADULT:* 2–3 sprays or 2–3 drops of 0.05% solution in each nostril bid, morning and evening or q10–12h.

*PEDIATRIC:*
- *>6 Y:* Adult dosage.
- *2–5 y:* 2–3 drops of 0.025% solution in each nostril twice daily, morning and evening.

### Pharmacokinetics

| Route | Onset | Duration |
|---|---|---|
| Nasal | 5–10 min | 6–10 h |

*Metabolism:* Hepatic, $T_{1/2}$: unknown
*Distribution:* Crosses placenta; may enter breast milk
*Excretion:* Urine

### Adverse effects

Systemic effects are less likely with topical administration than with systemic administration, but because systemic absorption can take place, the systemic effects should be considered:
- CNS: *Fear, anxiety, tenseness, restlessness, headache, lightheadedness, dizziness*, drowsiness, tremor, insomnia, hallucinations, psychological disturbances, convulsions, CNS depression, weakness, blurred vision, ocular irritation, tearing, photophobia, symptoms of paranoid schizophrenia
- GI: *Nausea*, vomiting, anorexia
- CV: Arrhythmias, hypertension resulting in intracranial hemorrhage, CV collapse with hypotension, palpitations, tachycardia, precordial pain in patients with ischemic heart disease
- GU: Constriction of renal blood vessels, *dysuria, vesical sphincter spasm* resulting in difficult and painful urination, urinary retention with prostatism
- Local: *Rebound congestion* with topical nasal application
- Other: *Pallor*, respiratory difficulty, orofacial dystonia, sweating

### Clinically important drug-drug interactions

• Severe hypertension with MAO-inhibitors, TCAs, furazolidone • Additive effects and increased risk of toxicity if taken with urinary alkalinizers • Decreased vasopressor response with reserpine, methyldopa, urinary acidifiers • Decreased hypotensive action of guanethidine

## ■ Nursing Considerations

### Assessment

- *History:* Allergy to oxymetazoline; angle-closure glaucoma; anesthesia with cyclopropane or halothane; thyrotoxicosis, diabetes, hypertension, CV disorders; prostatic hypertrophy, unstable vasomotor syndrome; lactation
- *Physical:* Skin color, temperature; orientation, reflexes, peripheral sensation, vision; P, BP, auscultation, peripheral perfusion; R, adventitious sounds; urinary output pattern, bladder percussion, prostate palpation; nasal mucous membrance evaluation

### Implementation

- Monitor CV effects carefully; patients with hypertension may experience changes in BP because of the additional vasoconstriction. If a nasal decongestant is needed, pseudoephedrine is the drug of choice.

### Drug-specific teaching points

- Do not exceed recommended dose. Demonstrate proper administration technique for topical nasal application. Avoid prolonged use because underlying medical problems can be disguised.
- The following side effects may occur: dizziness, weakness, restlessness, lightheadedness, tremor (avoid driving or operating dangerous equipment); urinary retention (void before taking drug).
- Rebound congestion may occur when this drug is stopped; drink plenty of fluids, use

a humidifier, and avoid smoke-filled areas to help decrease problems.
- Report nervousness, palpitations, sleeplessness, sweating.

## oxymetholone

*(ox i* ***meth'*** *oh lone)*

Anadrol-50, Anapolon 50 (CAN)

**Pregnancy Category X**
**C-III controlled substance**

### Drug classes
Anabolic steroid
Hormone

### Therapeutic actions
Testosterone analog with androgenic and anabolic activity; promotes body tissue-building processes and reverses catabolic or tissue-depleting processes; increases Hgb and red cell mass.

### Indications
- Anemias caused by deficient red cell production
- Acquired or congenital aplastic anemia
- Myelofibrosis and hypoplastic anemias due to myelotoxic drugs

### Contraindications/cautions
- Known sensitivity to oxymetholone or anabolic steroids, prostate or breast cancer; benign prostatic hypertrophy, pituitary insufficiency, MI, nephrosis, liver disease, hypercalcemia, pregnancy, lactation.

### Dosage
**Available Forms:** Tablets—50 mg

**ADULTS:** 1–5 mg/kg per day PO. Usual effective dose is 1–2 mg/kg per day. Give for a minimum trial of 3–6 mo. Following remission, patients may be maintained without the drug or on a lower daily dose. Continuous therapy is usually needed in cases of congenital aplastic anemia.

**PEDIATRIC:** Long-term therapy is contraindicated due to risk of serious disruption of growth and development; weigh benefits and risks.

### Pharmacokinetics

| Route | Onset |
|---|---|
| Oral | Rapid |

*Metabolism:* Hepatic, $T_{1/2}$: 9 h
*Distribution:* Crosses placenta; enters breast milk
*Excretion:* Urine

### Adverse effects
- CNS: *Excitation, insomnia,* chills, toxic confusion
- GI: Hepatotoxicity, peliosis, **hepatitis** with life-threatening liver failure or intra-abdominal hemorrhage; liver cell tumors, sometimes malignant and fatal, *nausea, vomiting, diarrhea, abdominal fullness, loss of appetite, burning of tongue*
- Hematologic: *Blood lipid changes:* decreased HDL and sometimes increased LDL; iron deficiency anemia, hypercalcemia, altered serum cholesterol levels; *retention of sodium, chloride, water,* potassium, phosphates and calcium
- GU: Possible increased risk of prostatic hypertrophy, carcinoma in geriatric patients
- Endocrine: *Virilization: prepubertal males*—phallic enlargement, hirsutism, increased skin pigmentation; *postpubertal males*—inhibition of testicular function, gynecomastia, testicular atrophy, priapism, baldness, epidiymitis, change in libido; *females*—hirsutism, hoarseness, deepening of the voice, clitoral enlargement, menstrual irregularities, baldness; decreased glucose tolerance
- Other: *Acne,* premature closure of the epiphyses

### Clinically important drug-drug interactions
• Potentiation of oral anticoagulants with anabolic steroids • Decreased need for insulin, oral hypoglycemica agents

### Drug-lab test interferences
• Altered glucose tolerance tests • Decrease in thyroid function tests, which may persist for 2–3 wk after therapy • Increased creatinine, creatinine clearance, which may last for 2 wk after therapy

## Nursing Considerations

### Assessment

- *History:* Known sensitivity to oxymetholone or anabolic steroids; prostate or breast cancer; benign prostatic hypertrophy; pituitary insufficiency; MI; nephrosis; liver disease; hypercalcemia; pregnancy; lactation
- *Physical:* Skin color, texture; hair distribution pattern; affect, orientation; abdominal exam, liver evaluation; serum electrolytes and cholesterol levels, glucose tolerance tests, thyroid function tests, long bone x-ray (in children)

### Implementation

- Administer with food if GI upset or nausea occurs.
- Monitor effect on children with long-bone x-rays every 3–6 mo; discontinue drug well before the bone age reaches the norm for the patient's chronologic age because effects may continue for 6 mo after therapy.
- Monitor for occurrence of edema; arrange for diuretic therapy as needed.
- Monitor liver function, serum electrolytes during therapy, and consult with physician for corrective measures.
- Measure cholesterol levels in patients who are at high risk for CAD.
- Monitor diabetic patients closely because glucose tolerance may change. Adjust insulin, oral hypoglycemic dosage, and diet.

### Drug-specific teaching points

- Take with food if nausea or GI upset occurs.
- The following side effects may occur: nausea, vomiting, diarrhea, burning of the tongue (small, frequent meals may help); body hair growth, baldness, deepening of the voice, loss of libido, impotence (most reversible); excitation, confusion, insomnia (avoid driving, performing tasks that require alertness); swelling of the ankles, fingers (request medication).
- Diabetic patients need to monitor urine sugar closely as glucose tolerance may change; report any abnormalities to physician, so corrective action can be taken.
- These drugs do not enhance athletic ability but do have serious effects and should not be used for increasing muscle strength.
- Report ankle swelling, skin color changes, severe nausea, vomiting, hoarseness, body hair growth, deepening of the voice, acne, menstrual irregularities in women.

# oxymorphone hydrochloride

*(ox i **mor'** fone)*

Numorphan

**Pregnancy Category C**
**C-II controlled substance**

### Drug classes

Narcotic agonist analgesic

### Therapeutic actions

Acts as agonist at specific opioid receptors in the CNS to produce analgesia, euphoria, sedation; the receptors mediating these effects are thought to be the same as those mediating the effects of endogenous opioids (enkephalins, endorphins).

### Indications

- Relief of moderate to moderately severe pain
- Parenterally for preoperative medication, support of anesthesia, obstetric analgesia
- For relief of anxiety with dyspnea associated with acute left ventricular failure and pulmonary edema

### Contraindications/cautions

- Contraindications: hypersensitivity to narcotics, diarrhea caused by poisoning (before toxins are eliminated), pregnancy (readily crosses placenta; neonatal withdrawal), labor or delivery (narcotics given to the mother can cause respiratory depression of neonate; premature infants are at special risk; may prolong labor), bronchial asthma, COPD, cor pulmonale, respiratory depression, anoxia, kyphoscoliosis, acute alcoholism, increased intracranial pressure, lactation.
- Use cautiously with acute abdominal conditions, CV disease, supraventricular

tachycardias, myxedema, convulsive disorders, delirium tremens, cerebral arteriosclerosis, ulcerative colitis, fever, Addison's disease, prostatic hypertrophy, urethral stricture, recent GI or GU surgery, toxic psychosis, renal or hepatic dysfunction

### Dosage

**Available Forms:** Injection—1, 1.5 mg/ml; suppositories—5 mg

**ADULT**

- ***IV:*** Initially 0.5 mg.
- ***SC or IM:*** Initially 1–1.5 mg q4–6h as needed. For analgesia during labor, 0.5–1 mg IM.
- ***Rectal suppositories:*** 5 mg q4–6h. After initial dosage, cautiously increase dose in nondebilitated patients until pain relief is obtained.

**PEDIATRIC:** Safety and efficacy not established for children < 12 y.

**GERIATRIC OR IMPAIRED ADULT:** Use caution; respiratory depression may occur in elderly, the very ill, those with respiratory problems.

### Pharmacokinetics

| *Route* | *Onset* | *Peak* | *Duration* |
|---|---|---|---|
| IV | 5–10 min | 1/2–1 h | 3–6 h |
| IM/SC | 10–15 min | 1/2–1 h | 3–6 h |
| PR | 15–30 min | 1–1 1/2 h | 3–6 h |

*Metabolism:* Hepatic, $T_{1/2}$: 2.6–4 h

*Distribution:* Crosses placenta; enters breast milk

*Excretion:* Urine

### IV facts

**Preparation:** No further preparation needed.

**Infusion:** Inject slowly over 5 min directly into vein or into tubing of running IV.

### Adverse effects

- CNS: *Lightheadedness, dizziness, sedation,* euphoria, dysphoria, delirium, insomnia, agitation, anxiety, fear, hallucinations, disorientation, drowsiness, lethargy, impaired mental and physical performance, coma, mood changes, weakness, headache, tremor, convulsions, miosis, visual disturbances
- GI: *Nausea, vomiting, sweating* (more common in ambulatory patients and those without severe pain), dry mouth, anorexia, constipation, biliary tract spasm; increased colonic motility in patients with chronic ulcerative colitis
- CV: Facial flushing, peripheral circulatory collapse, tachycardia, bradycardia, arrhythmia, palpitations, chest wall rigidity, hypertension, hypotension, orthostatic hypotension, syncope, circulatory depression, shock, cardiac arrest
- Respiratory: Suppression of cough reflex, respiratory depression, apnea, respiratory arrest, laryngospasm, bronchospasm
- GU: Ureteral spasm, spasm of vesical sphincters, urinary retention or hesitancy, oliguria, antidiuretic effect, reduced libido or potency
- Dermatologic: Pruritus, urticaria, edema, hemorrhagic urticaria (rare)
- Local: Pain at injection site, tissue irritation and induration (SC injection)
- Other: Physical tolerance and dependence, psychological dependence

O

### Clinically important drug-drug interactions

- Increased likelihood of respiratory depression, hypotension, profound sedation or coma in patients receiving barbiturate general anesthetics

### Drug-lab test interferences

- Elevated biliary tract pressure may cause increases in plasma amylase, lipase; determinations for 24 h after administration of narcotics

## ■ Nursing Considerations

### Assessment

- *History:* Hypersensitivity to narcotics, diarrhea caused by poisoning, pregnancy; labor or delivery; bronchial asthma, COPD, cor pulmonale, respiratory depression, kyphoscoliosis, acute alcoholism, increased intracranial pressure, acute abdominal conditions, CV disease, myxedema, convulsive disorders, delirium tremens, cerebral arteriosclerosis, ulcerative colitis, fever, Addison's disease, prostatic hypertrophy, urethral stricture, recent GI or GU surgery, toxic psychosis, renal or hepatic dysfunction

- *Physical:* T; skin color, texture, lesions; orientation, reflexes, bilateral grip strength, affect, pupil size; P, auscultation, BP, orthostatic BP, perfusion; R, adventious sounds; bowel sounds, normal output; frequency and pattern of voiding, normal output; ECG; EEG; thyroid, liver, kidney function tests

### Implementation

- Give to women lactating 4–6 h before the next feeding to minimize amount in milk.
- Refrigerate rectal suppositories.
- Provide narcotic antagonist, facilities for assisted or controlled respiration on standby during parenteral administration.
- Use caution when injecting SC into chilled areas or in patients with hypotension or in shock; impaired perfusion may delay absorption; with repeated doses, an excessive amount may be absorbed when circulation is restored.
- Reassure patient about addiction liability; most patients who receive opiates for medical reasons do not develop dependence syndromes.

### Drug-specific teaching points

- Take drug exactly as prescribed.
- The following side effects may occur: nausea, loss of appetite (take drug with food and lie quietly, eating frequent small meals may help); constipation (use a laxative); dizziness, sedation, drowsiness, impaired visual acuity (avoid driving, performing other tasks that require alertness, visual acuity).
- Do not take leftover medication for other disorders, and do not let anyone else take the prescription.
- Report severe nausea, vomiting, constipation, shortness of breath or difficulty breathing.

## oxyphencyclimine hydrochloride

*(oks' ee fen cy' kli meen)*

Daricon

**Pregnancy Category C**

### Drug classes

Antispasmodic
Anticholinergic
Antimuscarinic agent
Parasympatholytic

### Therapeutic actions

Direct GI smooth muscle relaxant; competitively blocks the effects of acetylcholine at muscarinic cholinergic receptors that mediate the effects of parasympathetic postganglionic impulses, thus relaxing the GI tract.

### Indications

- Treatment of functional bowel/irritable bowel syndrome (irritable colon, spastic colon, mucous colitis)
- Adjunctive treatment of peptic ulcer

### Contraindications/cautions

- Contraindications: glaucoma; adhesions between iris and lens; stenosing peptic ulcer, pyloroduodenal obstruction, paralytic ileus, intestinal atony, severe ulcerative colitis, toxic megacolon; symptomatic prostatic hypertrophy, bladder neck obstruction; bronchial asthma, COPD; cardiac arrhythmias, tachycardia, myocardial ischemia; impaired metabolic, liver or kidney function; myasthenia gravis; lactation
- Use cautiously with Down's syndrome, brain damage, spasticity, hypertension, hyperthyroidism.

### Dosage

**Available Forms:** Tablets—10 mg

*ADULT:* 5–10 mg PO bid–tid, in the morning and at hs.

*PEDIATRIC:* Not recommended for children < 12 y.

### Pharmacokinetics

| *Route* | *Onset* | *Duration* |
|---|---|---|
| Oral | 1–2 h | > 12 h |

*Metabolism:* Hepatic, $T_{1/2}$: 9–10 h
*Distribution:* Crosses placenta; enters breast milk
*Excretion:* Urine and feces

### Adverse effects

- CNS: *Blurred vision*, mydriasis, cycloplegia, photophobia, increased intraocular pressure
- GI: *Dry mouth, altered taste perception, nausea, vomiting, dysphagia*, heartburn, constipation, bloated feeling, paralytic ileus, gastroesophageal reflux
- CV: Palpitations, tachycardia
- GU: *Urinary hesitancy and retention*, impotence
- Other: Decreased sweating and predisposition to heat prostration, suppression of lactation

### Clinically important drug-drug interactions

• Decreased antipsychotic effect of haloperidol • Decreased effectiveness of phenothiazines but increased incidence of paralytic ileus

## ■ Nursing Considerations

### Assessment

- *History:* Glaucoma; adhesions between iris and lens; stenosing peptic ulcer; pyloroduodenal obstruction; intestinal atony; severe ulcerative colitis; symptomatic prostatic hypertrophy; bladder neck obstruction; bronchial asthma; COPD; cardiac arrhythmias; myocardial ischemia; impaired metabolic, liver, or kidney function; myasthenia gravis; Down syndrome; brain damage; spasticity; hypertension; hyperthyroidism; lactation
- *Physical:* Bowel sounds, normal output; normal urinary output, prostate palpation; R, adventitious sounds; P, BP; intraocular pressure, vision; bilateral grip strength, reflexes; liver palpation, liver and renal function tests; skin color, lesions, texture

### Implementation

- Encourage voiding before each dose if urinary retention is a problem.

### Drug-specific teaching points

- Take drug exactly as prescribed.
- Avoid hot environments (you will be heat intolerant, and dangerous reactions may occur).
- The following side effects may occur: constipation (adequate fluid intake, proper diet); dry mouth (sugarless lozenges, frequent mouth care may help; may lessen); blurred vision, sensitivity to light (avoid tasks that require acute vision; wear sunglasses); impotence (reversible); difficulty in urination (empty bladder immediately before each dose).
- Report skin rash, flushing, eye pain, difficulty breathing, tremors, loss of coordination, irregular heartbeat, palpitations, headache, abdominal distention, hallucinations, severe or persistent dry mouth, difficulty swallowing, difficulty in urination, severe constipation, sensitivity to light.

## oxytetracycline

*(ox i tet ra sye' kleen)*

Terramycin, Terramycin IM

**Pregnancy Category D**

O

### Drug classes

Antibiotic
Tetracycline antibiotic

### Therapeutic actions

Bacteriostatic: inhibits protein synthesis of susceptible bacteria, causing cell death.

### Indications

- Infections caused by rickettsiae; *Mycoplasma pneumoniae;* agents of psittacosis, ornithosis, lymphogranuloma venereum and granuloma inguinale; *Borrelia recurrentis; Hemophilus ducreyi; Pasteurella pestis; Pasteurella tularensis; Bartonella bacilliformis; Bacteroides; Vibrio comma; Vibrio fetus; Brucella; E. coli; E. aerogenes; Shigella; Acinetobacter calcoaceticus; H. influenzae; Klebsiella; Streptococcus pneumoniae; S. aureus*

- When penicillin is contraindicated, infections caused by *N. gonorrhoeae, Treponema pallidum, Treponema pertenue, Listeria monocytogenes, Clostridium, Bacillus anthracis, Fusobacterium fusiforme, Actinomyces, Neisseria meningitidis*
- As an adjunct to amebicides in acute intestinal amebiasis

## Contraindications/cautions

- Allergy to tetracylines, renal or hepatic dysfunction, pregnancy, lactation.

## Dosage

**Available Forms:** Capsules—250 mg; injection—50, 125 mg/ml

*Adult:* 250 mg qd or 300 mg in divided doses q8–12h IM. 250–500 mg q12h IV. *Do not exceed 500 mg q6h.* 1–2 g/d PO in 2 to 4 equal doses up to 500 mg qid PO.

*Pediatric >8 y:* 15–25 mg/kg per day IM. May be given in single dose of up to 250 mg, or divided into equal doses q8–12h. 12 mg/kg per day divided into 2 doses IV. Up to 10–20 mg/kg per day IV in severe cases. 25–50 mg/kg per day in 2–4 equal doses PO.

*Geriatric or Renal Failure Patients:* IV and IM doses of tetracyclines have been associated with severe hepatic failure and death with renal dysfunction. Lower than normal doses are required, and serum levels should be checked regularly.

## Pharmacokinetics

| Route | Onset | Peak |
|---|---|---|
| Oral | Varies | 2–4 h |
| IM | Rapid | 2–4 h |
| IV | Immediate | Minutes |

*Metabolism:* Hepatic, $T_{1/2}$: 6–12 h
*Distribution:* Crosses placenta; enters breast milk
*Excretion:* Urine

### IV facts

**Preparation:** Dissolve powder in 10 ml of Sterile Water for Injection or 5% Dextrose Injection. Dilute further with at least 100 ml of Ringer's Solution, Isotonic Sodium Chloride Solution, or 5% Dextrose in Water.

**Infusion:** Administer slowly over 30–60 min.

## Adverse effects

- GI: Fatty liver, liver failure, *anorexia, nausea, vomiting, diarrhea, glossitis,* dysphagia, enterocolitis, esophageal ulcer
- Hematologic: Hemolytic anemia, thrombocytopenia, neutropenia, eosinophilia, leukocytosis, leukopenia
- Dermatologic: *Phototoxic reactions, rash,* exfoliative dermatitis (more frequent and more severe with this tetracycline)
- Dental: *Discoloring and inadequate calcification of primary teeth of fetus if used by pregnant women; discoloring and inadequate calcification of permanent teeth if used during period of dental development*
- Local: Local irritation at injection site
- Other: Superinfections, nephrogenic diabetes insipidus syndrome

## Clinically important drug-drug interactions

• Decreased absorption with antacids, iron, alkali, food, dairy products, urine alkalinizers • Increased digoxin toxicity • Increased nephrotoxicity with methoxyflurane • Decreased activity of penicillins

## ■ Nursing Considerations

### Assessment

- *History:* Allergy to tetracylines, renal or hepatic dysfunction, pregnancy, lactation
- *Physical:* Skin status, orientation and reflexes, R, sounds, GI function and liver evaluation, urinalysis and BUN, liver and renal function tests; culture infection before therapy

### Implementation

- Administer oral medication without regard to food or meals; if GI upset occurs, give with meals.

### Drug-specific teaching points

- Take drug throughout the day.
- Take with meals if GI upset occurs.

- Sensitivity to sunlight may occur (wear protective clothing, and use a sunscreen).
- Report rash, itching; difficulty breathing; dark urine or light-colored stools; severe cramps, watery diarrhea.

## oxytocin

*(ox i **toe'** sin)*

*Parenteral:* Pitocin, Syntocinon

*Nasal spray:* Syntocinon

**Pregnancy Category C**

### Drug classes

Oxytocic
Hormone

### Therapeutic actions

Synthetic form of an endogenous hormone produced in the hypothalamus and stored in the posterior pituitary; stimulates the uterus, especially the gravid uterus just before parturition, and causes myoepithelium of the lacteal glands to contract, which results in milk ejection in lactating women.

### Indications

- Antepartum: to initate or improve uterine contractions to achieve early vaginal delivery; stimulation or reinforcement of labor in selected cases of uterine inertia; management of inevitable or incomplete abortion; second trimester abortion (parenteral)
- Postpartum: to produce uterine contractions during the third stage of labor and to control postpartum bleeding or hemorrhage (parenteral)
- To stimulate initial milk let-down (nasal)
- Unlabeled use: antepartum fetal heart rate testing (oxytocin challenge test), treatment of breast engorgement

### Contraindications/cautions

- Significant cephalopelvic disproportion, unfavorable fetal positions or presentations, obstetric emergencies that favor surgical intervention, prolonged use in severe toxemia, uterine inertia, hypertonic uterine patterns, induction or augmentation of labor when vaginal delivery is contraindicated, previous cesarean section, pregnancy (nasal).

### Dosage

**Available Forms:** Injection—10 U/ml; nasal spray—40 U/ml

Adjust dosage based on uterine response.

**ADULT**

- *Induction or stimulation of labor:* Initial dose of no more than 1–2 mU/min (0.001–0.002 U/min) by IV infusion through an infusion pump. Increase the dose in increments of no more than 1–2 mU/min at 15 to 30-min intervals until a contraction pattern similar to normal labor is established. Do not exceed 20 mU/min. Discontinue in event of uterine hyperactivity, fetal distress.
- *Control of postpartum uterine bleeding*
  - ***IV drip:*** Add 10–40 U to 1,000 ml of a nonhydrating diluent, run at a rate to control uterine atony.
  - ***IM:*** Administer 10 U after delivery of the placenta.
- *Treatment of incomplete or inevitable abortion:* IV infusion of 10 U of oxytocin with 500 ml physiologic saline solution or 5% dextrose in physiologic saline infused at a rate of 10–20 mU (20–40 drops)/min.
- *Initial milk let-down:* One spray into one or both nostrils 2–3 min before nursing or pumping of breasts.



### Pharmacokinetics

| *Route* | *Onset* | *Duration* |
|---|---|---|
| IV | Immediate | 60 min |
| IM | 3–5 min | 2–3 h |
| Nasal | Varies | 20 min |

*Metabolism:* Hepatic, $T_{1/2}$: 1–6 min
*Distribution:* Crosses placenta; enters breast milk
*Excretion:* Urine

### IV facts

**Preparation:** Add 1 ml (10 U) to 1,000 ml of 0.9% Aqueous Sodium Chloride or other IV fluid; the resulting solution will contain 10 mU/ml (0.01 U/ml).

**Infusion:** Infuse constant infusion pump to ensure accurate control of rate;

rate determined by uterine response; begin with 1–2 ml/min and increase at 15–30-min intervals.

**Compatibilities:** Compatible at a concentration of 5 U/L in Dextrose–Ringer's combinations; Dextrose–Lactated Ringer's combinations; Dextrose–Saline combinations; Dextrose 2%, 5%, and 10% in Water; Fructose 10% in Water; Ringer's Injection; Lactated Ringer's Injection; Sodium Chloride 0.45% and 0.9% Injection; and 1/6 M Sodium Lactate.

## Adverse effects

- GI: *Nausea, vomiting*
- CV: *Cardiac arrhythmias*, PVCs, hypertension, subarachnoid hemorrhage
- GU: Postpartum hemorrhage, uterine rupture, pelvic hematoma, *uterine hypertonicity*, spasm, tetanic contraction, rupture of the uterus with excessive dosage or hypersensitivity
- Hypersensitivity: **Anaphylactic reaction**
- Fetal effects: *Fetal bradycardia,* neonatal jaundice, low Apgar scores
- Other: Maternal and fetal deaths when used to induce labor or in first or second stages of labor; fatal afibrinogenemia; **severe water intoxication** with convulsions and coma, **maternal death** (associated with slow oxytocin infusion over 24 h; oxytocin has antidiuretic effects)

## ■ Nursing Considerations

### Assessment

- *History:* Significant cephalopelvic disproportion, unfavorable fetal positions or presentations, severe toxemia, uterine inertia, hypertonic uterine patterns, previous cesarean section
- *Physical:* Fetal heart rate (continuous monitoring is recommended); fetal positions; fetal-pelvic proportions; uterine tone; timing and rate of contractions; breast exam; orientation, reflexes; P, BP, edema; R, adventitious sounds; CBC, bleeding studies, urinary output

### Implementation

- Ensure fetal position and size and absence of complications that are contraindicated with oxytocin before therapy.
- Give nasal preparation by having patient hold the squeeze bottle upright; patient should be sitting, not lying down. If preferred, the solution can be instilled in drop form by inverting the squeeze bottle and exerting gentle pressure to allow drop formation.
- Ensure continuous observation of patient receiving IV oxytocin for induction or stimulation of labor; fetal monitoring is preferred. A physician should be immediately available to deal with complications if they arise.
- Regulate rate of oxytocin delivery to establish uterine contractions that are similar to normal labor; monitor rate and strength of contractions; discontinue drug and notify physician at any sign of uterine hyperactivity or spasm.
- Monitor maternal BP during oxytocin administration, discontinue drug and notify physician with any sign of hypertensive emergency.
- Monitor neonate for the occurrence of jaundice.

### Drug-specific teaching points

The patient receiving parenteral oxytocin is usually receiving it as part of an immediate medical situation, and the drug teaching should be incorporated into the teaching about the procedure, labor, or complication of delivery that is involved. The patient needs to know the name of the drug and what she can expect once it is administered.

- Initial milk let-down: Administer one spray into one or both nostrils 2–3 min before nursing or pumping the breasts to initiate milk let-down. Proper administration is important; hold the bottle upright and squeeze into nostril while sitting up, not lying down.
- Report sores in the nostrils, palpitations, unusual bleeding or bruising.

## paclitaxel

*(pass leh* ***tax'*** *ell)*

Taxol

**Pregnancy Category D**

### Drug classes
Antineoplastic

### Therapeutic actions
Inhibits the normal dynamic reorganization of the microtubule network that is essential for dividing cells; leads to cell death in rapidly dividing cells.

### Indications
- Treatment of metastatic carcinoma of the ovary after failure of first-line or subsequent therapy
- Treatment of breast cancer after failure of combination therapy
- Second-line treatment of AIDS-related Kaposi's sarcoma
- Unlabeled uses: treatment of advanced head and neck cancer, previously untreated extensive-stage small-cell lung cancer, adenocarcinoma of the upper GI stract, hormone-refractory prostate cancer, advanced non–small-cell lung cancer, leukemias

### Contraindications/cautions
- Contraindications: hypersensitivity to paclitaxel or drug formulated with polyoxethylated castor oil, bone marrow depression, severe neurologic toxicity, lactation, pregnancy.
- Use cautiously with cardiac conduction defects, severe hepatic impairment.

### Dosage
**Available Forms:** Injection—30 mg/5 ml

ADULT

- *Ovarian cancer:* 135 mg/m$^2$ IV over 24 h every 3 wk. Do not repeat until neutrophil count is at least 1,500 cells/mm$^2$ and platelet count is at least 100,000 cells/mm$^2$.
- *Breast cancer:* 175 mg/m$^2$ IV over 3 h every 3 wk after failure of chemotherapy.
- *AIDS-related Kaposi's sarcoma:* 135 mg/m$^2$ IV over 3 h every 3 wk *or* 100 mg/m$^2$ IV over 3 h every 2 wk.

PEDIATRIC: Safety and efficacy not established.

### Pharmacokinetics

| Route | Onset | Duration |
|---|---|---|
| IV | Rapid | 6–12 h |

*Metabolism:* Hepatic, $T_{1/2}$: 5.3–17.4 h
*Distribution:* Crosses placenta; enters breast milk
*Excretion:* Bile

### IV facts
**Preparation:** Use extreme caution when handling drug; dilute prior to infusion in 0.9% Sodium Chloride, 5% Dextrose Injection, 5% Dextrose and 0.9% Sodium Chloride Injection, 5% Dextrose in Ringer's Injection to a concentration of 0.3–1.2 mg/ml; stable at room temperature for 24 h. Refrigerate unopened vials; avoid use of PVC infusion bags and tubing.

**Infusion:** Administer over 24 h through an in-line filter not greater than 0.22 μm.

### Adverse effects
- CNS: Peripheral sensory neuropathy, mild to severe
- GI: *Nausea, vomiting,* mucositis, anorexia, elevated liver enzymes
- CV: Bradycardia, hypotension, severe CV events
- Hematologic: **Bone marrow depression, *infection***
- Other: *Hypersensitivity reactions, myalgia, arthralgia, alopecia*

### Clinically important drug-drug interactions
• Increased myelosuppression with cisplatin • Decreased paclitaxel effects with ketoconazole

## ■ Nursing Considerations

### Assessment
- *History:* Hypersensitivity to paclitaxel, castor oil; bone marrow depression; car-

P

diac conduction defects; severe hepatic impairment; pregnancy; lactation

- *Physical:* Neurologic status, T; P, BP, peripheral perfusion; skin color, texture, hair distribution; abdominal exam, mucous membranes; kidney and liver function tests, CBC

### Implementation

- Do not administer drug unless blood counts are within acceptable parameters.
- Handle drug with great care; gloves are recommended. If drug comes in contact with skin, wash immediately with soap and water.
- Premedicate with one of the following drugs to prevent severe hypersensitivity reactions: oral dexamethasone 20 mg, 12 h and 6 h before paclitaxel, 10 mg if AIDS-related Kaposi's sarcoma; diphenhydramine 50 mg IV 30–60 min before paclitaxel; or cimetidine 300 mg IV 30–60 min before paclitaxel.
- Monitor BP and pulse during administration.
- Obtain blood counts before and at least monthly during treatment.
- Monitor patient's neurologic status frequently during treatment.

### Drug-specific teaching points

- This drug will need to be given over a 24-h period once every 3 wk. Mark a calendar noting drug days.
- Have regular blood tests and neurologic exams while receiving this drug.
- The following side effects may occur: nausea and vomiting (if severe, request antiemetics; small frequent meals also may help); weakness, lethargy (frequent rest periods will help); increased susceptibility to infection (avoid crowds and exposure to diseases); numbness and tingling in the fingers or toes (avoid injury to these areas; use care with tasks requiring precision); loss of hair (obtain a wig or other head covering; keep the head covered at extremes of temperature).
- Report severe nausea and vomiting; fever, chills, sore throat; unusual bleeding or bruising; numbness or tingling in your fingers or toes; chest pain.

## pamidronate disodium

*(pah **mih'** dro nate)*

Aredia

**Pregnancy Category C**

### Drug classes

Calcium regulator

### Therapeutic actions

Slows normal and abnormal bone resorption without inhibiting bone formation and mineralization.

### Indications

- Treatment of hypercalcemia of malignancy
- Unlabeled uses: postmenopausal osteoporosis, hyperparathyroidism, prostatic carcinoma, mutiple myeloma, immobilization-related hypercalcemia to prevent fractures and bone pain
- Treatment of moderate to severe Paget's disease
- Treatment of osteolytic lesions in breast cancer patients receiving chemotherapy and hormonal therapy
- Treatment of osteolytic bone lesions of multiple myeloma

### Contraindications/cautions

- Contraindications:allergy to pamidronate disodium or biphosphates.
- Use cautiously with renal failure, enterocolitis, pregnancy, lactation.

### Dosage

**Available Forms:** Powder for injection—30, 60, 90 mg

**ADULT**

- *Hypercalcemia:* 60–90 mg IV given over 24 h.
- *Paget's disease:* 30 mg/d IV as a 4-h infusion on 3 consecutive d.
- *Osteolytic bone lesions:* 90 mg IV as a 4-h infusion on a monthly basis.

**PEDIATRIC:** Safety and efficacy not established.

### Pharmacokinetics

| Route | Onset | Duration |
|---|---|---|
| IV | Rapid | 72 h |

*Metabolism:* Hepatic, $T_{1/2}$: 1.6 h, then 27.3 h
*Distribution:* Crosses placenta; may enter breast milk
*Excretion:* Urine

### IV facts

**Preparation:** Reconstitute by adding 10 ml Sterile Water for Injection to each vial; resulting solution contains 30 mg/10 ml; allow drug to dissolve. May be further diluted in 1,000 ml sterile 0.45% or 0.9% Sodium Chloride or 5% Dextrose Injection; stable for 24 h at room temperature.

**Infusion:** Infuse over 24 h (90-mg dose); over 4 h (30–60-mg dose).

**Incompatibilities:** Do not mix with calcium-containing infusions, such as Ringer's; give in a single IV infusion and keep line separate from all other drugs.

### Adverse effects

- GI: *Nausea, diarrhea*
- MS: *Increased or recurrent bone pain* at pagetic sites, focal osteomalacia

## ■ Nursing Considerations

### Assessment

- ***History:*** Allergy to pamidronate disodium or any biphosphates, renal failure, enterocolitis, lactation
- ***Physical:*** Skin lesions, color, temperature; muscle tone, bone pain; bowel sounds; urinalysis, serum calcium

### Implementation

- Provide saline hydration before administration.
- Monitor serum calcium levels before, during, and after therapy. Consider retreatment if hypercalcemia recurs, but allow at least 7 wk between treatments.
- Do not give foods high in calcium, vitamins with mineral supplements, or antacids high in metals within 2 h of dosing.
- Maintain adequate nutrition, particularly intake of calcium and vitamin D.
- Monitor patients with renal impairment carefully; arrange for reduction of dosage if glomerular filtration rate is reduced.
- Maintain calcium on standby in case hypocalcemic tetany develops.

### Drug-specific teaching points

- Do not take foods high in calcium, antacids, or vitamins with minerals within 2 h of taking this drug.
- The following side effects may occur: nausea, diarrhea; recurrent bone pain.
- Report twitching, muscle spasms, dark urine, severe diarrhea.

# Pancreatic enzymes

## pancrelipase

*(pan kre **li'** pase)*

*Prescription products:* Cotazym, Cotazym-S, Iliozyme, Ku-Zyme HP Capsules, Pancrease Capsules, Protilase, Ultrase MT, Viokase, Zymase

## pancreatin

Creon Capsules, Donnazyme

*OTC products:* Pancrezyme 4X, 4X and 8X Pancreatin

**Pregnancy Category C**

### Drug classes

Digestive enzyme

### Therapeutic actions

Replacement of pancreatic enzymes: helps to digest and absorb fat, proteins, and carbohydrates.

### Indications

- Replacement therapy in patients with deficient exocrine pancreatic secretions, cystic fibrosis, chronic pancreatitis, postpancreatectomy, ductal obstructions, pancreatic insufficiency, steatorrhea or malabsorption syndrome, and postgastrectomy
- Presumptive test for pancreatic function
- Treatment of steatorrhea due to exocrine pancreatic enzyme deficiency in cystic fibrosis and chronic pancreatitis (Cotazym)

## Contraindications/cautions

- Contraindications: allergy to any component, pork products.
- Use cautiously with pregnancy, lactation.

## Dosage

**Available Forms:** Pancrelipase capsules—4000, 5000, 8000, 12,000, 16,000, 20,000, 24,000 U; powder—16,800 U; Pancreatin tablets—250, 500, 2400, 7200 mg

**ADULT**

- *Pancrelipase*
  - *Capsules and tablets:* 4,000–48,000 U PO with each meal and with snacks, usually 1–3 capsules or tablets before or with meals and snacks. May be increased to 8 tablets in severe cases. Patients with pancreatectomy or obstruction, 8,000–16,000 U PO lipase at 2-h intervals, may be increased to 64,000–88,000 U.
  - *Powder:* 0.7 g PO with meals.
- *Pancreatin*
  - *Capsules and tablets:* 1–2 PO with meals or snacks.

**PEDIATRIC**

- *6 Mo–1 Y:* 2,000 U lipase PO per meal.
- *1–6 Y:* 4,000–8,000 U PO lipase with each meal and 4,000 U with snacks.
- *7–12 Y:* 4,000–12,000 U PO lipase with each meal and with snacks.

## Pharmacokinetics

Not known.

## Adverse effects

- GI: *Nausea, abdominal cramps, diarrhea*
- GU: Hyperuricosuria, hyperuricemia with extremely high doses
- Hypersensitivity: Asthma with inhalation of fine-powder concentrates in sensitized individuals

## ■ Nursing Considerations

### Assessment

- *History:* Allergy to any component, pork products; pregnancy; lactation
- *Physical:* R, adventitious sounds; abdominal exam, bowel sounds; pancreatic function tests

### Implementation

- Administer before or with meals and snacks.
- Avoid inhaling or spilling powder on hands because it may irritate skin or mucous membranes.
- Do not crush or let patient chew the enteric-coated capsules; drug will not survive acid environment of the stomach.

### Drug-specific teaching points

- Take drug before or with meals and snacks.
- Do not crush or chew the enteric-coated capsules; swallow whole.
- Do not inhale powder dosage forms; severe reaction can occur.
- The following side effects may occur: abdominal discomfort, diarrhea.
- Report joint pain, swelling, soreness; difficulty breathing; GI upset.

# paraldehyde

*(par* ***al'*** *de hyde)*

Paral

**Pregnancy Category C**
**C-IV controlled substance**

## Drug classes

Sedative/hypnotic (nonbarbiturate)

## Therapeutic actions

Hypnotic that produces nonspecific, reversible depression of the CNS.

## Indications

- Oral, rectal: sedative and hypnotic; quiets the patient and produces sleep in delirium tremens and other psychiatric states characterized by excitement

## Contraindications/cautions

- Contraindications: hypersensitivity to paraldehyde, gastroenteritis.
- Use cautiously with bronchopulmonary disease, hepatic insufficiency, pregnancy, lactation.

## Dosage

**Available Forms:** Liquid—1 g/ml

All doses expressed in volume refer to the 1 g/ml solution of paraldehyde that is commercially available.

*ADULT*

- *Oral:* 4–8 ml in milk or iced fruit juice to mask the taste and odor. For hypnosis, 10–30 ml; for sedation, 5–10 ml; for delirium tremens, 10–35 ml.
- *Rectal:* Dissolve in oil as a retention enema; mix 10–20 ml, as appropriate, with 1 or 2 parts of olive oil or isotonic sodium chloride solution. *For hypnosis:* 10–30 ml of the 1 g/ml solution diluted as described above. *For sedation:* 5–10 ml of the 1 g/ml solution.

*PEDIATRIC*

- *Hypnosis:* Give 0.3 ml/kg or 12 ml/m$^2$ of the 1-g/ml solution PO or rectally.
- *Sedation:* Give 0.15 ml/kg or 6 ml/m$^2$ PO, rectally, or IM.

## Pharmacokinetics

| *Route* | *Onset* | *Peak* | *Duration* |
|---|---|---|---|
| Oral | 10–15 min | 30–60 min | 8–12 h |
| PR | Slow | 2 1/2 h | 8–12 h |

*Metabolism:* Hepatic, $T_{1/2}$: 3.4–9.8 h
*Distribution:* Crosses placenta; may enter breast milk
*Excretion:* Lungs and bile

## Adverse effects

- **GI**: *GI upset, irritation of the mucous membranes,* esophagitis, gastritis, proctitis, hepatitis, *strong, unpleasant breath for up to 24 h after ingestion*
- **CV**: Unusually slow heart beat, right heart edema, dilation, and failure
- **Respiratory**: Shortness of breath, troubled breathing, coughing
- **Hematologic**: *Metabolic acidosis,* particularly with high dosage or addiction
- **Dermatologic**: Skin rash, redness
- **Local**: Swelling or pain at injection site (thrombophlebitis), severe and permanent nerve damage, including paralysis, particularly of the sciatic nerve, when injected too close to a nerve trunk
- **Other**: *Addiction resembling alcoholism,* with withdrawal syndrome characterized by delirium tremens, hallucinations (prolonged use)

## ■ Nursing Considerations

### Assessment

- *History:* Hypersensitivity to paraldehyde, bronchopulmonary disease, hepatic insufficiency, gastroenteritis, lactation
- *Physical:* Skin injection site; orientation, reflexes; P, BP, perfusion; R, depth, adventitious sounds; bowel sounds, liver evaluation; liver function tests

### Implementation

- Dilute before oral or rectal use, as described in dosage section.
- Give with food or mix with milk or iced fruit juice to improve taste and reduce GI upset when administering drug orally.
- Do not let paraldehyde contact plastic surfaces (eg, syringes, glasses, spoons); paraldehyde reacts with plastic.
- Discard unused paraldehyde after opening bottle; paraldehyde decomposes to acetaldehyde if exposed to light and air.
- Do not use drug solutions that are brownish or have a sharp odor of acetic acid (vinegar).
- Keep away from heat, open flame, or sparks.
- Liquefy drug solution that has solidified due to exposure to temperatures less than 12°C or 54°F.
- Do not store in direct sunlight or expose to temperatures > 25°C (77°F).
- Taper drug to withdraw after chronic use.

### Drug-specific teaching points

- Take this drug exactly as directed, diluted in iced fruit juice or milk.
- Do not let this drug contact plastic; avoid plastic glasses, spoons, and so forth.
- Do not use if liquid is brownish or has a strong odor of vinegar.
- Discard any unused drug.
- The following side effects may occur: drowsiness (use caution and avoid driving or performing other tasks that require

alertness); GI upset (take drug with food or with milk or iced juices); strong, unpleasant-smelling breath for up to 24 h after you have taken this drug (you may be unaware of this).
- Report yellowing of the skin or eyes, pale stools, bloody stools.

## paromomycin sulfate

*(par oh moe **mye'** sin)*

Humatin

**Pregnancy Category C**

### Drug classes
Amebicide
Antibiotic/antibacterial
Cesticide

### Therapeutic actions
Bactericidal: inhibits bacterial protein synthesis, effective against *Shigella* and *Salmonella*, amebicidal, cesticidal.

### Indications
- Acute or chronic intestinal amebiasis (not indicated in extraintestinal amebiasis because it is poorly absorbed)
- Adjunctive use in hepatic coma (reduces population of ammonia-forming intestinal bacteria)
- Unlabeled uses: tapeworm (cestode) infestations and *Dientamoeba fragilis* infections

### Contraindications/cautions
- Contraindications: allergy to paromomycin, intestinal obstruction.
- Use cautiously with pregnancy, lactation.

### Dosage
**Available Forms:** Capsules—250 mg

Absorption is very poor; nearly 100% is excreted unchanged in the stool.

**ADULT**
- ***Intestinal amebiasis:*** 25–35 mg/kg per day PO in 3 divided doses for 5–10 d.
- ***Hepatic coma:*** 4 g/d PO in divided doses for 5–6 d.
- ***Fish, beef, pork, dog tapeworm:*** 1 g q15 min PO for four doses.
- ***Dwarf tapeworm:*** 45 mg/kg per day PO in one dose for 5–7 d.
- ***Dientamoeba fragilis:*** 25–30 mg/kg per day PO in three doses for 7 d.

**PEDIATRIC**
- ***Intestinal amebiasis:*** 25–35 mg/kg per day PO, in 3 divided doses for 5–10 d.
- ***Fish, beef, pork, dog tapeworm:*** 11 mg/kg PO q15 min for four doses.
- ***Dwarf tapeworm:*** 45 mg/kg per day PO in one dose for 5–7 d.

### Pharmacokinetics
Not generally absorbed systemically.

### Adverse effects
- CNS: Vertigo, headache, change in hearing, ringing in the ears
- GI: *Nausea, abdominal cramps, diarrhea*, heartburn, vomiting
- GU: BUN increase, decrease in urinary output, hematuria
- Other: *Superinfections*

### Clinically important drug-drug interactions
• Increased or decreased bioavailability of digoxin • Increased neuromuscular blockade with succinylcholine; delay administration of paromomycin as long as possible after recovery of spontaneous respirations after use of succinylcholine

## ■ Nursing Considerations

### Assessment
- *History:* Allergy to paromomycin, renal failure, intestinal obstruction, lactation
- *Physical:* Reflexes, eighth cranial nerve function; bowel sounds; BUN, urinalysis

### Implementation
- Administer drug with meals.

### Drug-specific teaching points
- Take drug three times a day with meals; small, frequent meals will help if stomach upset occurs.
- The following side effects may occur: nausea, vomiting, diarrhea.
- Report ringing in the ears, dizziness, skin rash, fever, severe GI upset.

# paroxetine

*(pah rox' a teen)*
Paxil
**Pregnancy Category B**

## Drug classes
Antidepressant

## Therapeutic actions
Potentiates serotonergic activity in the CNS, resulting in antidepressant effect.

## Indications
- Treatment of depression
- Treatment of obsessive-compulsive disorders
- Treatment of panic disorders
- Unlabeled uses: treatment of diabetic neuropathy, headaches, premature ejaculation

## Contraindications/cautions
- Contraindications: MAO inhibitor use.
- Use cautiously with renal or hepatic impairment, the elderly, pregnancy, lactation, suicidal patients.

## Dosage
**Available Forms:** Tablets—10, 20, 30, 40 mg

ADULT
- *Depression:* 20 mg/d PO as a single daily dose. *Range:* 20–50 mg/d.
- *Obsessive-compulsive disorder:* 40 mg/d PO as a single dose, may increase in 10-mg/d increments; do not exceed 60 mg/d.
- *Panic disorder:* 40 mg PO qd.
- *Switching to or from an MAO inhibitor:* At least 14 d should elapse between discontinuation of MAO inhibitor and initiation of paroxetine therapy; similarly, allow 14 d between discontinuing paroxetine and beginning MAO inhibitor.

PEDIATRIC: Safety and efficacy not established.

GERIATRIC, RENAL, OR HEPATIC IMPAIRMENT: 10 mg/d PO. Do not exceed 40 mg/d.

## Pharmacokinetics

| Route | Onset |
|---|---|
| Oral | Slow |

*Metabolism:* Hepatic, $T_{1/2}$: 1 h
*Distribution:* Crosses placenta; enters breast milk
*Excretion:* Urine

## Adverse effects
- CNS: *Somnolence, dizziness, insomnia, tremor, nervousness, headache,* anxiety, paresthesia, blurred vision
- GI: *Nausea, dry mouth, constipation, diarrhea,* anorexia, flatulence, vomiting
- CV: Palpitations, vasodilation, postural hypotension, hypertension
- **Respiratory**: Yawns, pharyngitis, cough
- GU: *Ejaculatory disorders, male genital disorders,* urinary frequency
- **Dermatologic**: *Sweating,* skin rash, redness
- General: *Headache, asthenia*

## Clinically important drug-drug interactions
• Increased paroxetine levels and toxicity with cimetidine, MAOIs • Decreased therapeutic effects of phenytoin, digoxin • Decreased effectiveness of paroxetine with phenobarbital, phenytoin • Increased serum levels and possible toxicity of procyclidine, tryptophane, warfarin

P

## ■ Nursing Considerations

### Assessment
- *History:* Hypersensitivity to paroxetine, lactation, renal or hepatic impairment, seizure disorder
- *Physical:* Orientation, reflexes; P, BP, perfusion; R, adventitious sounds; bowel sounds, normal output; urinary output; liver evaluation; liver and renal function tests

### Implementation
- Administer once a day in the morning.
- Encourage patient to continue use for 1–4 wk to ensure adequate levels to affect depression.
- Limit amount of drug given to potentially suicidal patients.

- Advise patient to avoid use if pregnant or lactating.

### Drug-specific teaching points

- Take this drug exactly as directed and as long as directed.
- The following side effects may occur: drowsiness, dizziness, tremor (use caution and avoid driving or performing other tasks that require alertness); GI upset (small, frequent meals, frequent mouth care may help); alterations in sexual function.
- This drug should not be taken during pregnancy or when nursing a baby.
- Report severe nausea, vomiting; palpitations; blurred vision; excessive sweating.

## pegasparagase

*(peg ass **par'** a gase)*

PEG-L

Oncaspar

**Pregnancy Category C**

### Drug classes

Antineoplastic

### Therapeutic actions

Formulation of L-asparaginase, an enzyme that hydrolyzes the amino acid asparagine, which is needed by some malignant cells (but not normal cells) for protein synthesis; thus, it inhibits malignant cell proliferation by interrupting protein synthesis; maximal effect in $G_1$ phase of the cell cycle; causes less frequent and less severe hypersensitivity reactions than asparaginase.

### Indications

- Acute lymphocytic leukemia (ALL) in patients hypersensitive to native forms of L-asparaginase
- Orphan drug use: ALL

### Contraindications/cautions

- Allergy to asparaginase, severe response to asparaginase, pancreatitis or history of pancreatitis, immunosuppression, pregnancy, lactation

### Dosage

**Available Forms:** Injection—75 IU/ml

*ADULTS AND CHILDREN > 1 Y:* 2500 IU/$m^2$ IM (preferred) or IV every 14 d.

*PEDIATRIC (BSA < 0.6 $M^2$):* 82.5 IU/kg IM or IV every 14 d.

### Pharmacokinetics

| Route | Onset |
|---|---|
| IM | Varies |
| IV | 30–40 min |

*Metabolism:* $T_{1/2}$: 5 d

*Distribution:* Crosses placenta; enters breast milk

*Excretion:* Small amount in urine

### IV facts

**Preparation:** No further preparation necessary. Single-use vial; discard any extra.

**Infusion:** Infuse over not less than 30 min into an already running IV infusion of Sodium Chloride Injection or 5% Dextrose Injection.

### Adverse effects

- CNS: CNS depression
- GI: Hepatotoxicity, **pancreatitis** (sometimes fatal), *nausea, vomiting, anorexia*, abdominal cramps, pancreatitis
- Hematologic: Bleeding problems, hyperurecemia, **bone marrow depression**
- GU: Uric acid nephropathy; **renal toxicity**
- Hypersensitivity: *Skin rashes, urticaria, arthralgia,* respiratory distress to anaphylaxis
- Endocrine: Hyperglycemia—glucosuria, polyuria, hypoglycemia
- Other: Chills, fever, weight loss, **fatal hyperthermia**

### Clinically important drug-drug interactions

• Diminished or decreased effect of methotrexate on malignant cells with or immediately following asparaginase • Increased toxicity of anticoagulants, immunosuppressives

**Drug-lab test interferences**
- Inaccurate interpretation of thyroid-function tests in patients taking asparaginase because of decreased serum levels of thyroxine-binding globulin; levels usually return to pretreatment levels within 4 wk of the last dose of asparaginase

## ■ Nursing Considerations

### Assessment
- *History:* Allergy to asparaginase, pancreatitis, impaired hepatic function, bone marrow depression, lactation
- *Physical:* Weight; T; skin color, lesions; orientation, reflexes; liver evaluation, abdominal exam; CBC, blood sugar, liver, andrenal function tests, serum amylase, clotting time, urinalysis, serum uric acid levels

### Implementation
- Arrange for laboratory tests (CBC, serum amylase, blood glucose, liver function tests, uric acid) before and frequently during therapy.
- Administer IM if at all possible; reserve IV use for extreme situations.
- Monitor for signs of hypersensitivity (eg, rash, difficulty breathing). If these occur, discontinue drug and consult with physician.
- Maintain life support equipment for dealing with anaphylaxis on standby anytime the drug is used.
- Monitor for pancreatitis; if serum amylase levels rise, discontinue drug and consult with physician.
- Monitor for hyperglycemia; reaction may resemble hyperosmolar nonketotic hyperglycemia. If present, discontinue drug, and be prepared for use of IV fluids and insulin.

### Drug-specific teaching points
- Prepare a calendar for patients who need to return for treatment and additional courses of therapy. Drug can be given only in the hospital under the direct supervision of physician.
- The following side effects may occur: loss of appetite, nausea, vomiting (frequent mouth care, small, frequent meals may help; maintain good nutrition; an antiemetic also may be ordered); fatigue, confusion, agitation, hallucinations, depression (use special precautions to avoid injury).
- Have regular blood tests to monitor the drug's effects.
- Report fever, chills, sore throat; unusual bleeding or bruising; yellow skin or eyes; light-colored stools, dark urine; thirst, frequent urination.

## pemoline

*(pem' oh leen)*
Cylert
**Pregnancy Category B**
**C-IV controlled substance**

**Drug classes**
Central nervous system stimulant

**Therapeutic actions**
CNS actions similar to those of the amphetamines and methylphenidate but has minimal sympathomimetic effects; may act through dopaminergic mechanisms; efficacy in hyperkinetic syndrome, attention-deficit disorders in children appears paradoxical and is not understood.

**Indications**
- Attention-deficit disorders, hyperkinetic syndrome, minimal brain dysfunction in children with behavioral syndrome characterized by the following symptoms: moderate to severe distractibility, short attention span, hyperactivity, emotional lability and impulsivity not secondary to environmental factors or psychiatric disorders (part of treatment program)
- Unlabeled use: narcolepsy and excessive daytime sleepiness at doses of 50–200 mg/d

**Contraindications/cautions**
- Contraindications: hypersensitivity to pemoline, impaired hepatic function.
- Use cautiously with impaired renal function, psychosis in children, epilepsy, drug dependence, alcoholism, emotional instability, lactation.

### Dosage
**Available Forms:** Tablets—18.75, 37.5, 75 mg; chewable tablets—37.5 mg

ADULT/PEDIATRIC >6 Y: Administer as a single oral dose each morning. Recommended starting dose is 37.5 mg/d PO. Gradually increase at 1-wk intervals using increments of 18.75 mg until desired response is obtained. Mean effective dose range is 56.25–75 mg/d. Do not exceed 112.5 mg/d.

*Narcolepsy:* 50–200 mg PO in two divided doses daily.

PEDIATRIC: Not recommended in children <6 y.

### Pharmacokinetics

| *Route* | *Onset* | *Peak* |
|---|---|---|
| Oral | Gradual | 2–4 h |

*Metabolism:* Hepatic, $T_{1/2}$: 12 h
*Distribution:* Crosses placenta; may enter breast milk
*Excretion:* Urine

### Adverse effects

- CNS: *Insomnia, anorexia with weight loss* (most common), dyskinetic movements of tongue, lips, face, and extremities; Gilles de la Tourette's syndrome; nystagmus; oculogyric crisis; convulsive seizures; increased irritability; mild depression; dizziness; headache; drowsiness; hallucinations
- GI: *Stomach ache*, nausea, hepatitis; elevations of SGOT, SGPT, LDH; jaundice
- Dermatologic: Skin rashes
- Other: Aplastic anemia; tolerance, psychological or physical dependence

## ■ Nursing Considerations

### Assessment

- *History:* Hypersensitivity to pemoline; impaired hepatic or renal function, psychosis in children, epilepsy; drug dependence, alcoholism, emotional instability; lactation
- *Physical:* Body weight; T; skin color, lesions; orientation, affect, reflexes; P, BP, auscultation; R, adventitious sounds; bowel sounds, normal output; CBC with differential, liver and kidney function tests, baseline ECG

### Implementation

- Ensure proper diagnosis before administering to children for behavioral syndromes: drug should not be used until other causes/concomitants of abnormal behavior (learning disability, EEG abnormalities, neurologic deficits) are ruled out.
- Interrupt drug dosage periodically in children to determine if symptoms warrant continued drug therapy.
- Monitor growth of children on long-term pemoline therapy.
- Dispense the smallest feasible amount of drug to minimize risk of overdosage.
- Give drug in the morning to prevent insomnia.
- Monitor liver function tests during long-term therapy.

### Drug-specific teaching points

- Take this drug exactly as prescribed.
- The following side effects may occur: insomnia, nervousness, restlessness, dizziness, impaired thinking (may lessen after a few days; avoid driving or engaging in activities that require alertness); diarrhea; headache, loss of appetite, weight loss.
- Report insomnia, abnormal body movements, skin rash, severe diarrhea, pale stools, yellowing of the skin or eyes.

## penbutolol sulfate

*(pen **byoo'** toe lole)*

Levatol

**Pregnancy Category C**

### Drug classes

Beta adrenergic blocker
Antihypertensive

### Therapeutic actions

Competitively blocks beta-adrenergic receptors in the heart and juxtaglomerular apparatus, reducing the influence of the sympathetic nervous system on these tissues; decreasing the excitability of the heart, cardiac output, and release of renin; and lowering BP.

### Indications
- Treatment of mild to moderate hypertension

### Contraindications/cautions
- Contraindications: sinus bradycardia, second- or third-degree heart block, cardiogenic shock, CHF, pregnancy, lactation.
- Use cautiously with renal failure, diabetes or thyrotoxicosis, asthma, COPD, impaired hepatic function.

### Dosage
**Available Forms:** Tablets—20 mg

**ADULT:** *Usual starting dose, maintenance dose, and dose used in combination with other antihypertensives:* 20 mg PO qd. Doses of 40–80 mg qd have been used but with no additional antihypertensive effect.

**PEDIATRIC:** Safety and efficacy not established.

### Pharmacokinetics

| Route | Onset | Peak | Duration |
|---|---|---|---|
| Oral | Varies | 2–3 h | 20 h |

*Metabolism:* Hepatic, $T_{1/2}$: 5 h
*Distribution:* Crosses placenta; enters breast milk
*Excretion:* Urine

### Adverse effects
- CNS: Dizziness, vertigo, tinnitus, fatigue, emotional depression, paresthesias, sleep disturbances, hallucinations, disorientation, memory loss, slurred speech
- GI: *Gastric pain, flatulence, constipation, diarrhea, nausea, vomiting,* anorexia, ischemic colitis, renal and mesenteric arterial thrombosis, retroperitoneal fibrosis, hepatomegaly, acute pancreatitis
- CV: *Bradycardia, CHF, cardiac arrhythmias, sinoartial or AV nodal block, tachycardia,* peripheral vascular insufficiency, claudication, CVA, pulmonary edema, hypotension
- **Respiratory:** Bronchospasm, dyspnea, cough, bronchial obstruction, nasal stuffiness, rhinitis, pharyngitis (less likely than with propranolol)
- GU: *Impotence, decreased libido,* Peyronie's disease, dysuria, nocturia, frequent urination
- **MS:** Joint pain, arthralgia, muscle cramp
- **EENT:** Eye irritation, dry eyes, conjunctivitis, blurred vision
- **Dermatologic:** Rash, pruritus, sweating, dry skin
- **Allergic reactions:** Pharyngitis, erythematous rash, fever, sore throat, laryngospasm, respiratory distress
- **Other:** *Decreased exercise tolerance, development of antinuclear antibodies (ANA),* hyperglycemia or hypoglycemia, elevated serum transaminase, alkaline phosphatase, and LDH

### Clinically important drug-drug interactions
• Increased effects with verapamil • Decreased effects with epinephrine • Increased risk of peripheral ischemia, even gangrene, with ergot alkaloids (dihydroergotamine, methysergide, ergotamine) • Prolonged hypoglycemic effects of insulin • Increased "first-dose response" to prazosin • Paradoxical hypertension when clonidine is given with beta-blockers; increased rebound hypertension when clonidine is discontinued in patients on beta-blockers • Decreased hypertensive effect if given with NSAIDs (piroxicam, indomethacin, ibuprofen) • Decreased bronchodilator effects of theophylline and decreased bronchial and cardiac effects of sympathomimetics with penbutolol

### Drug-lab test interferences
• Possible false results with glucose or insulin tolerance tests

## ■ Nursing Considerations

### Assessment
- *History:* Sinus bradycardia, heart block, cardiogenic shock, CHF, renal failure, diabetes or thyrotoxicosis, asthma or COPD, impaired hepatic function, lactation
- *Physical:* Weight, skin condition, neurologic status, P, BP, ECG, respiratory

status, kidney and thyroid function, blood and urine glucose

### Implementation

- Give drug once a day. Monitor response and maintain at lowest possible dose.
- Do not discontinue drug abruptly after chronic therapy (hypersensitivity to catecholamines may have developed, causing exacerbation of angina, MI, and ventricular dysrhythmias; taper drug gradually over 2 wk with monitoring).
- Consult with physician about withdrawing drug if patient is to undergo surgery (withdrawal is controversial).

### Drug-specific teaching points

- Do not stop taking this drug unless instructed to do so by a health care provider.
- Avoid driving or dangerous activities if dizziness, drowsiness occur.
- Report difficulty breathing, night cough, swelling of extremities, slow pulse, confusion, depression, rash, fever, sore throat.

# penicillamine

*(pen i* ***sill'*** *a meen)*

Cuprimine, Depen

**Pregnancy Category C**

## Drug classes

Chelating agent
Antirheumatic

## Therapeutic actions

Chelating agent that removes excessive copper in Wilson's disease; exact mechanism of action as antirheumatoid agent is not known, but penicillamine lowers IgM rheumatoid factor; reduces excessive cystine excretion by disulfide interchange with cystine, resulting in a substance more soluble than cystine that is readily excreted.

## Indications

- Rheumatoid arthritis: severe active disease in patients in whom other therapies have failed
- Wilson's disease
- Cystinuria when conventional measures are inadequate to control stone formation
- Unlabeled uses: primary biliary cirrhosis, scleroderma

## Contraindications/cautions

- Contraindications: allergy to penicillamine, penicillin; history of penicillamine-related aplastic anemia or agranulocytosis; renal insufficiency; pregnancy (teratogenic).
- Use cautiously with lactation.

### Dosage

**Available Forms:** Capsules—125, 250 mg; titratable tablets—250 mg

*Warning:* interruptions of daily therapy of Wilson's disease or cystinuria for even a few days have been followed by sensitivity reactions when the drug is reinstituted.

**ADULT**

- ***Wilson's disease:*** Base dosage on urinary copper excretion. Suggested initial dosage is 1 g/d PO given in divided doses qid. Up to 2 g/d may be needed.
- ***Rheumatoid arthritis (2–3 mo may be required for a clinical response):*** *Initial therapy:* a single daily dose of 125–250 mg PO. Thereafter increase dose at 1- to 3-mo intervals by 125 or 250 mg/d based on patient response, tolerance, and toxicity. Continue increases at 2- to 3-mo intervals. Doses of 1,000–1,500 mg/d for 3–4 mo with no improvement indicate that patient will not respond. *Maintenance:* many patients respond to 500–750 mg/d PO. Dosage above 1 g/d is unusual. *Exacerbations:* some patients experience exacerbation of disease activity that can subside in 12 wk. Treatment with NSAIDs is usually sufficient for control. Increase maintenance dose only if flare fails to subside within the 12-wk time period. *Duration of therapy:* after 6 mo of remission, attempt a gradual, stepwise dosage reduction in decrements of 125–250 mg/d at 3-mo intervals.
- ***Cystinuria:*** Usual dosage is 2 g/d (range 1–4 g/d) PO in divided doses qid, with the last dose hs. Initiate dosage with 250 mg/d and increase gradually. Individualize dosage to limit cystine excretion to 100–200 mg/d in those with no

history of stones, and to <100 mg/d in those with a history of stones.

**PEDIATRIC**

- ***Wilson's disease:*** Base dosage on urinary copper excretion. Suggested intial dosage is 1 g/d PO given in divided doses qid. Up to 2 g/d may be needed.
- ***Rheumatoid arthritis:*** Efficacy in juvenile rheumatoid arthritis has not been established.
- ***Cystinuria:*** 30 mg/kg per day PO in divided doses qid with the last dose hs. Consider patient's age, size, and rate of growth in determining dosage.

### Pharmacokinetics

| *Route* | *Onset* | *Peak* |
|---|---|---|
| Oral | Varies | 1–3 h |

*Metabolism:* Hepatic, $T_{1/2}$: 1.7–3.2 h
*Distribution:* Crosses placenta; enters breast milk
*Excretion:* Urine

### Adverse effects

- CNS: Tinnitus, reversible optic neuritis, **myasthenic syndrome** (sometimes fatal)
- GI: *Anorexia, epigastric pain, nausea, vomiting, diarrhea, altered taste perception*, intrahepatic cholestasis and toxic hepatitis, *oral ulcerations*, cheilosis, glossitis, colitis
- Hematologic: *Bone marrow depression*—leukopenia, thrombocytopenia, thrombocytic thrombocytopenic purpura, hemolytic anemia, red cell aplasia, monocytosis, leukocytosis, eosinophilia—fatalities from thrombocytopenia, agranulocytosis, and aplastic anemia
- GU: *Proteinuria*, hematuria, which may progress to nephrotic syndrome
- Hypersensitivity: Allergic reactions: *generalized pruritus*, lupus erythematosus-like syndrome, pemphigoid-type reactions, drug eruptions, uritcaria and exfoliative dermatitis, migratory polyarthralgia, **polymyositis**, Goodpasture's syndrome, alveolitis, obliterative bronchiolitis

### Clinically important drug-drug interactions

- Decreased absorption with iron salts, antacids, food • Decreased serum levels of digoxin

## ■ Nursing Considerations

### Assessment

- ***History:*** Allergy to penicillamine, penicillin; history of penicillamine related aplastic anemia or agranulocytosis; renal insufficiency; pregnancy; lactation
- ***Physical:*** Skin color, lesions; T; orientation, reflexes, ophthalmologic evaluation, audiometric evaluation, peripheral sensation; R, adventitious sounds; liver evaluation, bowel sounds, mucous membranes; CBC, clotting times, urinalysis, renal and liver function tests, x-ray for renal stones

### Implementation

- Use caution when administering this drug due to potential serious side effects.
- Arrange for monitoring of urinalysis, CBC before and every 2 wk during the first 6 mo of therapy and monthly thereafter; also monitor liver function tests and x-ray for renal stones before and periodically during therapy.
- Discontinue therapy if drug fever occurs—briefly in Wilson's disease and cystinuria, permanently in rheumatoid arthritis—and switch to another therapy.
- Consult physician about the advisability of decreasing dosage to 250 mg/d when surgery is contemplated; wound healing may be delayed by the effects on collagen and elastin.
- Administer drug on an empty stomach, 1 h before or 2 h after meals and at least 1 h apart from any other drug, food, or milk.
- Administer drug for Wilson's disease on an empty stomach, 30–60 min before meals and hs, at least 2 h after the evening meal.
- Administer drug for cystinuria in four equal doses; if this is not possible, give

p

the larger dose hs; the bedtime dose is of utmost importance.

- Ensure that patient with cystinuria drinks 1 pint of fluid hs and another pint once during night; the greater the fluid intake, the lower the dose of penicillamine required.
- Arrange for nutritional consultation; pyridoxine supplements may be needed; ensure that multivitamin preparations do not contain copper for patients with Wilson's disease; iron deficiency may occur; if iron supplements are used, ensure that they are given with at least a 2-h interval between iron and penicillamine; hypogeusia (loss of taste) may lead to anorexia or inappropriate eating habits.

### Drug-specific teaching points

- Take drug on an empty stomach 1 h before or 2 h after meals and at least 1 h apart from any other drug, food, or milk. Wilson's disease: take 30–60 min before meals and at bedtime. Cystinuria: be sure to take the bedtime dose; drink one pint of fluid at bedtime and one pint of fluid during the night; drink copious amounts of fluid during the day.
- The following side effects may occur: nausea, GI upset, vomiting (take drug with food); diarrhea; rash, delays in healing (use good skin care; avoid injury); mouth sores, loss of taste perception (frequent mouth care will help; taste perception usually returns within 2–3 mo).
- This drug is not to be used during pregnancy; if you become pregnant or want to become pregnant, consult your physician.
- Report skin rash, unusual bruising or bleeding, sore throat, difficulty breathing, cough or wheezing, fever, chills.
- Keep this drug and all medications out of the reach of children; this drug can be very dangerous for children.

## penicillin G benzathine

*(pen i **sill'** in)*

Bicillin L-A, Permapen

**Pregnancy Category B**

### Drug classes

Antibiotic
Penicillin antibiotic

### Therapeutic actions

Bactericidal: inhibits synthesis of cell wall of sensitive organisms, causing cell death.

### Indications

- Severe infections caused by sensitive organisms (streptococci)
- Treatment of syphilis, neurosyphilis, congenital syphilis, yaws, uncomplicated erysipeloid infection

### Contraindications/cautions

- Contraindications: allergies to penicillins, cephalosporins, or other allergens.
- Use cautiously with renal disorders, pregnancy, lactation (may cause diarrhea or candidiasis in the infant).

### Dosage

**Available Forms:** Injection—300,000, 600,000, 1,200,000, 2,400,000 U/dose.

**ADULT**

- *Streptococcal infections (including otitis media, URIs of mild to moderate severity):* A single injection of 1.2 million U IM.
- *Early syphilis:* 2.4 million U IM in a single dose.
- *Congenital syphilis:* 50,000 U/kg IM in a single dose.
- *Syphilis lasting >1 y:* 7.2 million U given as 2.4 million U IM weekly for 3 wk.
- *Yaws:* 1.2 million U IM as a single dose.
- *Erysipeloid:* 1.2 million U IM as a single dose.

**PEDIATRIC**

- *Streptococcal infections (including otitis media, URIs of mild to moderate severity):* A single injection of 900,000–1.2 million U IM in older children. A single injection of 300,000–600,000 U IM for children under 60 lb.

**NEONATES:** 50,000 U/kg IM as a single injection.

### Pharmacokinetics

| *Route* | *Onset* | *Peak* | *Duration* |
|---|---|---|---|
| IM | Slow | 12–24 h | Days |

*Metabolism:* Hepatic, $T_{1/2}$: 30–60 min
*Distribution:* Crosses placenta; enters breast milk
*Excretion:* Urine

**Adverse effects**

- CNS: Lethargy, hallucinations, seizures
- GI: *Glossitis, stomatitis, gastritis, sore mouth,* furry tongue, black "hairy" tongue, *nausea, vomiting, diarrhea,* abdominal pain, bloody diarrhea, enterocolitis, pseudomembranous colitis, nonspecific hepatitis
- **Hematologic**: Anemia, thrombocytopenia, leukopenia, neutropenia, prolonged bleeding time (more common than with other penicillinase-resistant penicillins)
- GU: Nephritis
- **Hypersensitivity reactions**: *Rash, fever, wheezing,* anaphylaxis
- Local: *Pain, phlebitis*, thrombosis at injection site, Jarisch-Herxheimer reaction when used to treat syphilis
- Other: *Superinfection,* sodium overload, leading to CHF

**Clinically important drug-drug interactions**

• Decreased effectiveness of penicillin G benzathine with tetracyclines • Inactivation of parenteral aminoglycosides (amikacin, gentamicin, kanamycin, neomycin, metilmicin, streptomycin, tobramycin)

## ■ Nursing Considerations

### Assessment

- *History:* Allergies to penicillins, cephalosporins, other allergens, renal disorders, pregnancy, lactation
- *Physical:* Culture infection; skin color, lesions; R, adventitious sounds; bowel sounds: CBC, liver and renal function tests, serum electrolytes, Hct, urinalysis

### Implementation

- Culture infection before beginning treatment; reculture if response is not as expected.
- Give by IM route only.
- Continue therapy for at least 2 d after infection has disappeared, usually 7–10 d.
- Give IM injection in upper outer quadrant of the buttock. In infants and small children, the midlateral aspect of the thigh may be preferred.

### Drug-specific teaching points

- You will need to receive a full course of drug therapy.
- The following side effects may occur: nausea, vomiting, diarrhea, mouth sores, pain at injection sites.
- Report difficulty breathing, rashes, severe diarrhea, severe pain at injection site, mouth sores, unusual bleeding or bruising.

# Penicillin G potassium

## penicillin G (aqueous)

*(pen i **sill'** in)*

Falapen (CAN), Megacillin (CAN), Pfizerpen

## penicillin G sodium

Crystapen (CAN)

**Drug classes**

Antibiotic
Penicillin antibiotic

**Therapeutic actions**

Bactericidal: inhibits synthesis of cell wall of sensitive organisms, causing cell death.

**Indications**

- Treatment of severe infections caused by sensitive organisms—streptococci, pneumococci, staphylococci, *Neisseria gonorrhoeae, Treponema pallidum,* meningococci, *Actinomyces israelii, Clostridium perfringens* and *tetani, Leptotrichia buccalis* (Vincent's disease), *Spirillum minus* or *Streptobacillus moniliformis, Listeria monocytogenes, Pasteurella multocida, Erysipelothrix insidiosa, Escherichia coli, Enterobacter aerogenes, Alcaligenes faecalis, Salmonella, Shigella, Proteus mirabilis, Corynebacterium diphtheriae, Bacillus anthracis*

P

- Treatment of syphilis, gonococcal infections
- Unlabeled use: treatment of Lyme disease

### Contraindications/cautions

- Contraindications: allergy to penicillins, cephalosporins, other allergens.
- Use cautiously with renal disease, pregnancy, lactation (may cause diarrhea or candidiasis in the infant).

### Dosage

**Available Forms:** Injection—1, 2, 3 million U/50 ml; powder for injection—5, 10, 20 million U/vial

ADULT

- *Meningococcal meningitis:* 1–2 million U q2h IM or by continuous IV infusion of 20–30 million U/d.
- *Actinomycosis:* 1–6 million U/d IM or IV for cervicofacial cases. 10–20 million U/d IM or IV for thoracic and abdominal diseases.
- *Clostridial infections:* 20 million U/d IM or IV with antitoxin therapy.
- *Fusospirochetal infections (Vincent's disease):* 5–10 million U/d IM or IV *or* 200,000–500,000 U q6–8h PO for milder infections.
- *Rat-bite fever:* 12–15 million U/d IM or IV for 3–4 wk.
- *Listeria infections:* 15–20 million U/d IM or IV for 2 or 4 wk (meningitis or endocarditis, respectively).
- *Pasteurella infections:* 4–6 million U/d IM or IV for 2 wk.
- *Erysipeloid endocarditis:* 12–20 million U/d IM or IV for 4–6 wk.
- *Gram-negative bacillary bacteremia:* 20–30 million U/d IM or IV.
- *Diphtheria (adjunctive therapy with antitoxin to prevent carrier state):* 2–3 million U/d IM or IV in divided doses for 10–12 d.
- *Anthrax:* Minimum of 5 million U/d IM or IV in divided doses.
- *Pneumococcal infections:* 5–24 million U/d in divided doses.
- *Syphilis:* 12–24 million U/d IV for 10 d followed by benzathine penicillin G 2.4 million U IM weekly for 3 wk.
- *Gonorrhea:* 10 million U/d IV until improvement occurs, followed by amoxicillin or ampicillin 500 mg qid PO for 7 d.

PEDIATRIC

- *Meningitis:* 100,000–250,000 U/kg per day IM or IV in divided doses q4h.
- *Listeria infections: Neonates:* 500,000–1 million U/d IM or IV.
- *Infants born to mothers with gonococcal infections:* 50,000 U in a single IM or IV injection to full-term infants. 20,000 U to low–birth-weight infants.

### Pharmacokinetics

| Route | Onset | Peak |
|---|---|---|
| IM/IV | Rapid | 1/4–1/2 h |

*Metabolism:* Hepatic, $T_{1/2}$: 30–60 min
*Distribution:* Crosses placenta; enters breast milk
*Excretion:* Urine

### IV facts

**Preparation:** Prepare solution using Sterile Water for Injection, Isotonic Sodium Chloride Injection, or Dextrose Injection. Do not use with carbohydrate solutions at alkaline pH; do not refrigerate powder; sterile solution is stable for 1 wk refrigerated. IV solutions are stable at 24 h at room temperature. Discard solution after 24 h.

**Infusion:** Administer doses of 10–20 million U by slow infusion.

### Adverse effects

- CNS: Lethargy, hallucinations, seizures
- GI: *Glossitis, stomatitis, gastritis, sore mouth*, furry tongue, black "hairy" tongue, *nausea, vomiting, diarrhea,* abdominal pain, bloody diarrhea, enterocolitis, pseudomembranous colitis, nonspecific hepatitis
- Hematologic: Anemia, thrombocytopenia, leukopenia, neutropenia, prolonged bleeding time
- GU: Nephritis—oliguria, proteinuria, hematuria, casts, azotemia, pyuria
- **Hypersensitivity reactions:** *Rash, fever, wheezing,* anaphylaxis

- **Local:** *Pain, phlebitis,* thrombosis at injection site, Jarisch-Herxheimer reaction when used to treat syphilis
- **Other:** *Superinfections,* sodium overload, leading to CHF

### Clinically important drug-drug interactions

• Decreased effectiveness of penicillin G with tetracyclines • Inactivation of parenteral aminoglycosides (amikacin, gentamicin, kanamycin, neomycin, metilmicin, streptomycin, tobramycin)

### Drug-lab test interferences

- False-positive Coombs' test (IV)

## ■ Nursing Considerations

### Assessment

- *History:* Allergy to penicillins, cephalosporins, other allergens, renal disease, lactation
- *Physical:* Culture infection; skin rashes, lesions; R, adventitious sounds; bowel sounds, normal output; CBC, liver and renal function tests, serum electrolytes, Hct, urinalysis; skin test with benzylpenicyllolyl-polylysine if hypersensitivity reactions to penicillin have occurred

### Implementation

- Culture infection before beginning treatment; reculture if response is not as expected.
- Use the smallest dose possible for IM injection to avoid pain and discomfort.
- Continue treatment for 48–72 h beyond time that the patient is asymptomatic.
- Monitor serum electrolytes and cardiac status if penicillin G is given by IV infusion. Sodium or potassium preparations have been associated with severe electrolyte imbalances.
- Explain the reason for parenteral administration; offer support and encouragement to deal with therapy.
- Maintain epinephrine, IV fluids, vasopressors, bronchodilators, oxygen, and emergency equipment on standby in case of serious hypersensitivity reaction.
- Arrange for the use of corticosteroids, antihistamines for skin reactions.

### Drug-specific teaching points

- This drug must be given by injection.
- The following side effects may occur: upset stomach, nausea, vomiting (small, frequent meals may help); sore mouth (frequent mouth care may help); diarrhea; pain or discomfort at the injection site.
- Report unusual bleeding, sore throat, rash, hives, fever, severe diarrhea, difficulty breathing.

## penicillin G procaine

*(pen i **sill'** in)*

penicillin G procaine, aqueous, APPG

Ayercillin (CAN), Crysticillin-AS, Wycillin

**Pregnancy Category B**

### Drug classes

Antibiotic

Penicillin, long-acting, parenteral

### Therapeutic actions

Bactericidal: inhibits cell wall synthesis of sensitive organisms, causing cell death.

### Indications

- Treatment of moderately severe infections caused by sensitive organisms—streptococci, pneumococci, staphylococci, meningococci, *A. israelii, C. perfringens* and *tetani, L. buccalis* (Vincent's disease), *S. minus* or *S. moniliformis, L. monocytogenes, P. multocida, E. insidiosa, E. coli, E. aerogenes, A. faecalis, Salmonella, Shigella, P. mirabilis, C. diphtheriae, B. anthracis*
- Treatment of specific sexually transmitted diseases

### Contraindications/cautions

- Contraindications: allergies to penicillins, cephalosporins, procaine, or other allergens.

- Use cautiously with renal disorders, pregnancy, lactation (may cause diarrhea or candidiasis in the infant).

### Dosage

**Available Forms:** 300,000, 500,000, 600,000, 1,200,000, 2,400,000 U/dose

**ADULT**

- *Moderately severe infections caused by sensitive strains of streptococci, pneumococci, staphylococci:* Minimum of 600,000–1.2 million U/d IM.
- *Bacterial endocarditis (group A streptococci):* 600,000–1.2 million U/d IM.
- *Fusospirochetal infections:* 600,000–1.2 million U/d IM.
- *Rat-bite fever:* 600,000–1.2 million U/d IM.
- *Erysipeloid:* 600,000–1.2 million U/d IM.
- *Diphtheria:* 300,000–600,000 U/d IM with antitoxin.
- *Diphtheria carrier state:* 300,000 U/d IM for 10 d.
- *Anthrax:* 600,000–1.2 million U/d IM.
- *Syphilis (negative spinal fluid):* 600,000 U/d IM for 8 d.
- *Late syphilis:* 600,000 U/d for 10–15 d.
- *Neurosyphilis:* 2–4 million U/d IM with 500 mg probenecid PO qid for 10 d, followed by 2.4 million U IM benzathine penicillin G weekly for three doses.
- *Uncomplicated gonococcal infections:* 4.8 million U IM in divided doses at two sites together with 1 g probenecid.

**PEDIATRIC**

- *Congenital syphilis:* Patients weighing $<$ 70 lb: 50,000 U/kg per day IM for 10–14 d.
- *Neurosyphilis:* Infants 50,000 U/kg per day IM for at least 10 d.

### Pharmacokinetics

| *Route* | *Onset* | *Peak* | *Duration* |
|---|---|---|---|
| IM | Varies | 4 h | 15–20 h |

*Metabolism:* Hepatic, $T_{1/2}$: 30–60 min
*Distribution:* Crosses placenta; enters breast milk
*Excretion:* Urine

### Adverse effects

- CNS: Lethargy, hallucinations, seizures
- GI: *Glossitis, stomatitis, gastritis, sore mouth*, furry tongue, black "hairy" tongue, *nausea, vomiting, diarrhea,* abdominal pain, bloody diarrhea, enterocolitis, pseudomembranous colitis, nonspecific hepatitis
- **Hematologic**: Anemia, thrombocytopenia, leukopenia, neutropenia, prolonged bleeding time
- GU: Nephritis—oliguria, proteinuria, hematuria, casts, azotemia, pyuria
- **Hypersensitivity reactions**: *Rash, fever, wheezing,* anaphylaxis
- Local: *Pain, phlebitis*, thrombosis at injection site, Jarisch-Herxheimer reaction when used to treat syphilis
- Other: *Superinfections,* sodium overload, leading to CHF

### Clinically important drug-drug interactions

• Decreased effectiveness of penicillin G procaine with tetracyclines • Inactivation of parenteral aminoglycosides (amikacin, gentamicin, kanamycin, neomycin, metilmicin, streptomycin, tobramycin)

## ■ Nursing Considerations

### Assessment

- *History:* Allergies to penicillins, cephalosporins, procaine, other allergens, renal disorders, pregnancy, lactation
- *Physical:* Culture infection; skin color, lesions; R, adventitious sounds; bowel sounds: CBC, liver and renal function tests, serum electrolytes, Hct, urinalysis

### Implementation

- Culture infection before beginning treatment; reculture if response is not as expected.
- Administer by IM route only.
- Continue therapy for at least 2 d after infection has disappeared, usually 7–10 d.
- Administer IM injection in upper outer quadrant of the buttock. In infants and small children, the midlateral aspect of the thigh may be preferred.

### Drug-specific teaching points

- This drug can be given only by IM injection.
- The following side effects may occur: nausea, vomiting, diarrhea, mouth sores, pain at injection sites.
- Report difficulty breathing, rashes, severe diarrhea, severe pain at injection site, mouth sores, unusual bleeding or bruising.

## penicillin V

*(pen i **sill'** in)*

pencillin V potassium

Beepen VK, Betapen VK, Nadopen-V (CAN), Novopen VK (CAN), Penbec-V (CAN), Pen-Vee-K, Robicillin VK, V-Cillin K, Veetids

**Pregnancy Category B**

### Drug classes

Antibiotic
Penicillin (acid stable)

### Therapeutic actions

Bactericidal: inhibits cell wall synthesis of sensitive organisms, causing cell death.

### Indications

- Mild to moderately severe infections caused by sensitive organisms—streptococci, pneumococci, staphylococci, fusospirochetes
- Prophylaxis against bacterial endocarditis in patients with valvular heart disease undergoing dental or upper respiratory tract surgery
- Unlabeled uses: prophylactic treatment of children with sickle cell anemia, mild to moderate anaerobic infections, Lyme disease

### Contraindications/cautions

- Contraindications: allergies to penicillins, cephalosporins, or other allergens.
- Use cautiously with renal disorders, pregnancy, lactation (may cause diarrhea or candidiasis in the infant).

### Dosage

**Available Forms:** Tablets—125, 250, 500 mg; powder for oral solution—125, 250 mg/5 ml

**ADULT**

- *Fusospirochetal infections:* 250–500 mg q6–8h PO.
- *Streptococcal infections (including otitis media, URIs of mild to moderate severity, scarlet fever, erysipelas):* 125–250 mg q6–8h PO for 10 d.
- *Pneumococcal infections:* 250–500 mg q6h PO until afebrile for 48h.
- *Staphylococcal infections of skin and soft tissues:* 250–500 mg q6–8h PO.
- *Prophylaxis against bacterial endocarditis, dental or upper respiratory procedures:* 2 g PO 1/2–1 h before the procedure, then 500 mg q6h for eight doses.
- *Alternate prophylaxis:* 1 million U penicillin G IM mixed with 600,000 U procaine penicillin G 1/2–1 h before the procedure, then 500 mg pencillin V PO q6h for 8-h doses.
- *Lyme disease:* 250–500 mg PO qid for 10–20 d.

**PEDIATRIC**

- *<12 y:* 25–50 mg/kg per day PO given q6–8 h. Calculate doses according to weight.
- *Prophylaxis against bacterial endocarditis, dental or upper respiratory procedures: Children >60 lb*: 2 g PO 1/2–1 h before the procedure, then 500 mg q6h for eight doses. *Children <60 lb*: 1 g PO 1/2–1 h before the procedure, then 250 mg q6h for eight doses.
- *Alternate prophylaxis: < 30 kg*: 30,000 U penicillin G/kg IM mixed with 600,000 U procaine penicillin G 1/2–1 h before the procedure and then 250 mg penicillin V PO q6h for eight doses.
- *Sickle cell anemia:* 125 mg PO bid.
- *Lyme disease:* 50 mg/kg per day PO in four divided doses for 10–20 d

### Pharmacokinetics

| Route | Onset | Peak |
|---|---|---|
| Oral | Varies | 60 min |

*Metabolism:* Hepatic, $T_{1/2}$: 30–60 min
*Distribution:* Crosses placenta; enters breast milk
*Excretion:* Urine

**Adverse effects**

- CNS: Lethargy, hallucinations, seizures
- GI: *Glossitis, stomatitis, gastritis, sore mouth,* furry tongue, black "hairy" tongue, *nausea, vomiting, diarrhea,* abdominal pain, bloody diarrhea, enterocolitis, pseudomembranous colitis, nonspecific hepatitis
- **Hematologic**: Anemia, thrombocytopenia, leukopenia, neutropenia, prolonged bleeding time
- GU: Nephritis—oliguria, proteinuria, hematuria, casts, azotemia, pyuria
- **Hypersensitivity reactions**: *Rash, fever, wheezing,* anaphylaxis (sometimes fatal)
- **Other**: *Superinfections*, sodium overload leading to CHF; potassium poisoning—hyperreflexia, coma, cardiac arrhythmias, cardiac arrest (potassium preparations)

**Clinically important drug-drug interactions**

- Decreased effectiveness with tetracyclines

## ■ Nursing Considerations

### Assessment

- *History:* Allergies to penicillins, cephalosporins, or other allergens; renal disorders; pregnancy; lactation
- *Physical:* Culture infection; skin color, lesions; R, adventitious sounds; bowel sounds: CBC, liver and renal function tests, serum electrolytes, Hct, urinalysis

### Implementation

- Culture infection before beginning treatment; reculture if response is not as expected.
- Continue therapy for at least 2 d after infection has disappeared, usually 7–10 d.
- Administer drug on an empty stomach, 1 h before or 2 h after meals, with a full glass of water.
- Do not administer oral drug with milk, fruit juices, or soft drinks; a full glass of water is preferred; this oral penicillin is less affected by food than other penicillins.

### Drug-specific teaching points

- Take drug on an empty stomach with a full glass of water.
- Avoid self-treating other infections with this antibiotic because it is specific for the infection being treated.
- The following side effects may occur: nausea, vomiting, diarrhea, mouth sores.
- Report difficulty breathing, rashes, severe diarrhea, mouth sores, unusual bleeding or bruising.

# pentamidine isethionate

*(pen ta' ma deen)*
*Parenteral:* Pentam 300
*Inhalation:* NebuPent
**Pregnancy Category C**

**Drug classes**
Antiprotozoal

**Therapeutic actions**
Antiprotozoal acitivity in susceptible *Pneumocystis carinii* infections; mechanism of action is not fully understood, but the drug interferes with nuclear metabolism and inhibits the synthesis of DNA, RNA, phospholipids, and proteins, which leads to cell death.

**Indications**

- Treatment of *P. carinii* pneumonia, especially in patients unresponsive to therapy with the less toxic trimethoprim/sulfamethoxazole combination (injection)
- Prevention of *P. carinii* pneumonia in high-risk, HIV-infected patients (inhalation)
- Unlabeled use (injection): treatment of trypanosomiasis, visceral leishmaniasis

**Contraindications/cautions**

- If the diagnosis of *P. carinii* pneumonia has been confirmed, there are no absolute contraindications to the use of this drug.

- Contraindications: history of anaphylactic reaction to inhaled or parenteral pentamidine isethionate (inhalation therapy); pregnancy; lactation.
- Use cautiously with hypotension, hypertension, hypoglycemia, hyperglycemia, hypocalcemia, leukopenia, thrombocytopenia, anemia, hepatic or renal dysfunction.

## Dosage

**Available Forms:** Injection—300 mg/vial; aerosol—300 mg

*ADULT AND PEDIATRIC*

- ***Parenteral:*** 4 mg/kg once a day for 14 d by deep IM injection or IV infusion over 60 min.
- ***Inhalation:*** 300 mg once every 4 wk administered through the Respirgard II nebulizer.

## Pharmacokinetics

| *Route* | *Onset* |
|---|---|
| IM | Slow |
| Inhalation | Rapid |

*Metabolism:* $T_{1/2}$: 6.4–9.4 h
*Distribution:* Crosses placenta; enters breast milk
*Excretion:* Urine

### IV facts

**Preparation:** Prepare solution by dissolving contents of 1 vial in 3–5 ml of Sterile Water for Injection or 5% Dextrose Injection. Dilute the calculated dose further in 50–250 ml of 5% Dextrose solution; solutions of 1 and 2.5 mg/ml in 5% Dextrose are stable at room temperature for up to 24 h. Protect from light.
**Infusion:** Infuse the diluted solution over 60 min.

## Adverse effects

*Parenteral*

- GI: *Nausea, anorexia*
- CV: *Hypotension,* tachycardia
- Hematologic: *Leukopenia, hypoglycemia,* thrombocytopenia, hypocalcemia, elevated liver function tests
- GU: *Elevated serum creatinine,* acute renal failure
- Local: *Pain, abscess at injection site*
- Other: Stevens-Johnson syndrome, *fever, rash,* deaths due to severe hypotension, hypoglycemia and cardiac arrhythmias

*Inhalation*

- CNS: *Fatigue, dizziness,* headache, tremors, confusion, anxiety, memory loss, seizure, insomnia, drowsiness
- GI: *Metallic taste to mouth, anorexia, nausea, vomiting,* gingivitis, dyspepsia, oral ulcer, gastritis, hypersalivation, dry mouth, melena, colitis, abdominal pain
- CV: Tachycardia, hypotension, hypertension, palpitations, syncope, vasodilatation
- Respiratory: *Shortness of breath, cough, pharyngitis, congestion, bronchospasm,* rhinitis, laryngitis, laryngospasm, hyperventilation, pneumothorax
- Other: *Rash, night sweats, chill*

## ■ Nursing Considerations

### Assessment

- ***History:*** History of anaphylactic reaction to inhaled or parenteral pentamidine isethionate, hypotension, hypertension, hypoglycemia, hyperglycemia, hypocalcemia, leukopenia, thrombocytopenia, anemia, hepatic or renal dysfunction, pregnancy, lactation
- ***Physical:*** Skin lesions, color; T; reflexes, affect (inhalation); BP, P, baseline ECG; BUN, serum creatinine, blood glucose, CBC, platelet count, liver function tests, serum calcium

P

### Implementation

- Monitor patient closely during administration; fatalities have been reported.
- Arrange for the following tests to be performed before, during, and after therapy: daily BUN, daily serum creatinine, daily blood glucose; regular CBC, platelet counts, liver function tests, serum calcium; periodic ECG.
- Position patient in supine position before parenteral administration to protect patient if BP changes occur.
- Reconstitute for inhalation: Dissolve contents of 1 vial in 6 ml of Sterile Water for Injection. Use only sterile water. Sa-

line cannot be used, precipitates will form. Place entire solution in nebulizer reservoir. Solution is stable for 48 h in original vial at room temperature if protected from light. Do not mix with other drugs.

- Administer inhalation using the *Respirgard II* nebulizer. Deliver the dose until the chamber is empty (30–45 min).
- For IM use: Prepare IM solution by dissolving contents of 1-g vial in 3 ml of Sterile Water for Injection; protect from light. Discard any unused portions. Inject deeply into large muscle group. Inspect injection site regularly; rotate injection sites.
- Instruct patient and significant other in the reconstitution of inhalation solutions and administration for outpatient use.

### Drug-specific teaching points

- Parenteral drug can be given only IV or IM and must be given every day. Inhalation drug must be given using the *Respirgard II* nebulizer. Prepare the solution as instructed by your nurse, using only Sterile Water for Injection. Protect the medication from exposure to light. Use freshly reconstituted solution. The drug must be used once every 4 wk. Prepare a calendar with drug days marked as a reminder. Do not mix any other drugs in the nebulizer.
- Have frequent blood tests and BP checks because this drug may cause many changes in your body.
- You may feel weak and dizzy with sudden position changes; take care to change position slowly.
- If using the inhalation, metallic taste and GI upsets may occur. Small, frequent meals and mouth care may help.
- Report pain at injection site, confusion, hallucinations, unusual bleeding or bruising, weakness, fatigue.

# Pentazocine

## pentazocine lactate

*(pen **taz'** oh seen)*

*Parenteral:* Talwin

## pentazocine hydrochloride with naloxone hydrochloride, 0.5 mg

*Oral:* Talwin NX

**Pregnancy Category C**
**C-IV controlled substance**

### Drug classes

Narcotic agonist-antagonist analgesic

### Therapeutic actions

Pentazocine acts as an agonist at specific (kappa) opioid receptors in the CNS to produce analgesia, sedation; acts as an agonist at *sigma* opioid receptors to cause dysphoria, hallucinations; acts at *mu* opioid receptors to antagonize the analgesic and euphoric activities of some other narcotic analgesics. Has lower abuse potential than morphine, other pure narcotic agonists; the oral preparation contains the opioid antagonist, naloxone, which has poor bioavailability when given orally and does not interfere with the analgesic effects of pentazocine but serves as a deterrent to the unintended IV injection of solutions made from the oral tablets.

### Indications

- Relief of moderate to severe pain (oral)
- Preanesthetic medication and as supplement to surgical anesthesia (parenteral)

### Contraindications/cautions

- Contraindications: hypersensitivity to narcotics, to naloxone (oral form); pregnancy (neonatal withdrawal); labor or delivery (narcotics given to the mother can cause neonatal respiratory depression; premature infants are especially at risk; may prolong labor); lactation.
- Use cautiously with physical dependence on a narcotic analgesic (can precipitate a withdrawal syndrome); bronchial asthma, COPD, cor pulmonale, respiratory depression, anoxia, increased intracranial pressure; acute MI with hypertension, left ventricular failure or nausea and vomiting; renal or hepatic dysfunction.

### Dosage

**Available Forms:** Injection—30 mg/ml; tablets—50 mg

**ADULT**

- *Oral:* Initially, 50 mg q3–4h. Increase to 100 mg if necessary. Do not exceed a total dose of 600 mg/24 h.
- *Parenteral:* 30 mg IM, SC, or IV. May repeat q3–4h. Doses > 30 mg IV or 60 mg IM or SC are not recommended. Do not exceed 360 mg/24 h. Give SC only when necessary; repeat injections should be given IM.
- – *Patients in labor:* A single 30-mg IM dose is most common. A 20-mg IV dose given 2–3× at 2- to 3-h intervals relieves pain when contractions become regular.

**PEDIATRIC (<2 Y):** Not recommended.

**GERIATRIC OR IMPAIRED ADULT:** Use caution; respiratory depression may occur in elderly, very ill, those with respiratory problems. Reduced dosage may be necessary.

### Pharmacokinetics

| *Route* | *Onset* | *Peak* | *Duration* |
|---|---|---|---|
| Oral, IM, SC | 15–30 min | 1–3 h | 3 h |
| IV | 2–3 min | 15 min | 1 h |

*Metabolism:* Hepatic, $T_{1/2}$: 2–3 h

*Distribution:* Crosses placenta; enters breast milk

*Excretion:* Urine and feces

### IV facts

**Preparation:** No further preparation is required.

**Infusion:** Inject directly into vein or into tubing of actively running IV; infuse slowly, each 5 mg over 1 min.

**Incompatibilities:** Do not mix in same syringe as barbiturates; precipitate will form.

### Adverse effects

- CNS: *Lightheadedness, dizziness, sedation, euphoria,* dysphoria, delirium, insomnia, agitation, anxiety, fear, hallucinations, disorientation, drowsiness, lethargy, impaired mental and physical performance, coma, mood changes, weakness, headache, tremor, convulsions, miosis, visual disturbances
- GI: *Nausea, vomiting, sweating* (more common in ambulatory patients and those without severe pain), dry mouth, anorexia, constipation, biliary tract spasm; increased colonic motility in patients with chronic ulcerative colitis
- CV: Facial flushing, peripheral circulatory collapse, tachycardia, bradycardia, arrhythmia, palpitations, chest wall rigidity, hypertension, hypotension, orthostatic hypotension, syncope, circulatory depression, shock, cardiac arrest
- **Respiratory**: Suppression of cough reflex, respiratory depression, apnea, respiratory arrest, laryngospasm, bronchospasm
- GU: Ureteral spasm, spasm of vesical sphincters, urinary retention or hesitancy, oliguria, antidiuretic effect, reduced libido or potency
- **Dermatologic**: Pruritus, urticaria, edema
- **Local**: Pain at injection site, tissue irritation and induration (SC injection)
- **Other**: Physical tolerance and dependence, psychological dependence (the oral form has especially been abused in combination with tripelennamine—"Ts and Blues"—with serious and fatal consequences; the addition of naloxone to the oral formulation may decrease this abuse)

### Clinically important drug-drug interactions

• Increased likelihood of respiratory depression, hypotension, profound sedation, or coma with barbiturate general anesthetics • Precipitation of withdrawal syndrome in patients previously given other narcotic analgesics, including morphine, methadone (note that this applies to the parenteral preparation without naloxone and to the oral preparation that includes naloxone).

## ■ Nursing Considerations

### Assessment

- *History:* Hypersensitivity to narcotics, to naloxone (oral form); physical depen-

dence on a narcotic analgesic; pregnancy; labor or delivery; lactation; respiratory disease; anoxia; increased intracranial pressure; acute MI; renal or hepatic dysfunction.
- *Physical:* T; skin color, texture, lesions; orientation, reflexes, bilateral grip strength, affect, pupil size; P, auscultation, BP, orthostatic BP, perfusion; R, adventitious sounds; bowel sounds, normal output; frequency and pattern of voiding, normal output; liver, kidney function tests, CBC with differential.

### Implementation
- Do not mix parenteral pentazocine in same syringe as barbiturates; precipitate will form.
- Provide narcotic antagonist, facilities for assisted or controlled respiration on standby during parenteral administration.
- Use caution when injecting SC into chilled areas or in patients with hypotension or in shock; impaired perfusion may delay absorption; with repeated doses, an excessive amount may be absorbed when circulation is restored.
- Withdraw drug gradually if it has been given for 4–5 d, especially to emotionally unstable patients or those with a history of drug abuse; a withdrawal syndrome sometimes occurs in these circumstances.
- Reassure patient about addiction liability; most patients who receive opiates for medical reasons do not develop dependence syndromes.

### Drug-specific teaching points
- Take drug exactly as prescribed.
- Avoid alcohol, antihistamines, sedatives, tranquilizers, OTC drugs while taking this drug.
- The following side effects may occur: nausea, loss of appetite (take drug with food, lie quietly, eat frequent small meals); constipation (a laxative may help); dizziness, sedation, drowsiness, impaired visual acuity (avoid driving or performing other tasks that require alertness, visual acuity).
- Do not take any leftover medication for other disorders, and do not let anyone else take the prescription.
- Report severe nausea, vomiting, constipation, shortness of breath or difficulty breathing.

## ☆ pentobarbital

*(pen toe **bar'** bi tal)*

pentobarbital sodium

Nembutal Sodium, Novopentobarb (CAN)

**Pregnancy Category D**
**C-II controlled substance**

### Drug classes
Barbiturate
Sedative/hypnotic
Hypnotic
Anticonvulsant

### Therapeutic actions
General CNS depressant; barbiturates inhibit impulse conduction in the ascending RAS, depress the cerebral cortex, alter cerebellar function, depress motor output, and can produce excitation, sedation, hypnosis, anesthesia, and deep coma; at anesthetic doses, has anticonvulsant activity.

### Indications
- Sedative or hypnotic for short-term treatment of insomnia (appears to lose effectiveness for sleep induction and maintenance after 2 wk; oral)
- Preanesthetic medication (oral)
- Sedation when oral or parenteral administration may be undesirable (rectal)
- Hypnotic for short-term treatment of insomnia (rectal)
- Sedative (parenteral)
- Anticonvulsant, in anesthetic doses, for emergency control of certain acute convulsive episodes (eg, status epilepticus, eclampsia, meningitis, tetanus, toxic reactions to strychnine or local anesthetics; parenteral)

### Contraindications/cautions
- Contraindications: hypersensitivity to barbiturates, manifest or latent porphyria, marked liver impairment, nephritis, severe respiratory distress, previous addiction to sedative- hypnotic drugs, preg-

nancy (fetal damage, neonatal withdrawal syndrome), lactation.

- Use cautiously with acute or chronic pain (paradoxical excitement or masking of important symptoms); seizure disorders (abrupt discontinuation of daily doses can result in status epilepticus); fever, hyperthyroidism, diabetes mellitus, severe anemia, pulmonary or cardiac disease, status asthmaticus, shock, uremia.

## Dosage

**Available Forms:** Capsules—50, 100 mg; suppositories—30, 60, 120, 200 mg; injection—50 mg/ml

ADULT

- ***Oral***
- *Daytime sedation:* 20 mg tid–qid.
- *Hypnotic:* 100 mg hs.
- ***Rectal:*** 120–200 mg.
- ***IV***
- *Parenteral:* Use only when other routes are not feasible or prompt action is imperative. Give by slow IV injection, 50 mg/min. Initial dose is 100 mg in a 70-kg adult. Wait at least 1 min for full effect. Base dosage on response. Additional small increments may be given up to a total of 200–500 mg. Minimize dosage in convulsive states to avoid compounding the depression that may follow convulsions.
- ***IM:*** Inject deeply into a muscle mass. Usual adult dose is 150–200 mg. Do not exceed a volume of 5 ml at any site due to tissue irritation.

PEDIATRIC: Use caution: barbiturates may produce irritability, aggression, inappropriate tearfulness.

- ***Oral***
- *Preoperative sedation:* 2–6 mg/kg per day (maximum: 100 mg), depending on age, weight, degree of sedation desired.
- *Hypnotic:* Base dosage on age and weight.
- ***Rectal:*** Do not divide suppositories.
- *12–14 Y: (80–110 lb)* 60 or 120 mg.
- *5–12 Y: (40–80 lb)* 60 mg.
- *1–4 Y: (20–40 lb)* 30 or 60 mg.
- *2 Mo–1 Y: (10–20 lb)* 30 mg.
- ***IV***
- *Parenteral:* Reduce initial adult dosage on basis of age, weight, and patient's condition.
- ***IM:*** Dosage frequently ranges from 25 to 80 mg or 2–6 mg/kg.

GERIATRIC PATIENTS OR THOSE WITH DEBILITATING DISEASE: Reduce dosage and monitor closely. May produce excitement, depression, confusion.

## Pharmacokinetics

| *Route* | *Onset* | *Duration* |
|---|---|---|
| Oral | 10–15 min | 3–4 h |
| IM/IV | Rapid | 2–3 h |

*Metabolism:* Hepatic, $T_{1/2}$: 15–20 h

*Distribution:* Crosses placenta; enters breast milk

*Excretion:* Urine

### IV facts

**Preparation:** No further preparation is required.

**Infusion:** Infuse slowly, each 50 mg over 1 min; monitor patient response to dosage.

## Adverse effects

- CNS: *Somnolence, agitation, confusion, hyperkinesia, ataxia, vertigo, CNS depression, nightmares, lethargy, residual sedation (hangover), paradoxical excitement, nervousness, psychiatric disturbance, hallucinations, insomnia, anxiety, dizziness, thinking abnormality*
- GI: *Nausea, vomiting, constipation, diarrhea, epigastric pain*
- CV: *Bradycardia, hypotension, syncope*
- Respiratory: *Hypoventilation, apnea, respiratory depression,* laryngospasm, bronchospasm, circulatory collapse
- Hypersensitivity: Skin rashes, angioneurotic edema, serum sickness, morbiliform rash, urticaria; rarely, exfoliative dermatitis, **Stevens-Johnson syndrome** (sometimes fatal)
- Local: *Pain, tissue necrosis at injection site,* gangrene; arterial spasm with inadvertent intra-arterial injection; throm-

p

bophlebitis; permanent neurologic deficit if injected near a nerve
- Other: Tolerance, psychological and physical dependence; **withdrawal syndrome** (sometimes fatal)

### Clinically important drug-drug interactions

• Increased CNS depression with alcohol • Increased nephrotoxicity with methoxyflurane • Decreased effects of the following drugs: oral anticoagulants, corticosteroids, oral contraceptives and estrogens, beta-adrenergic blockers (especially propranolol, metoprolol), theophylline, metronidazole, doxycycline, griseofulvin, phenylbutazones, quinidine

## ■ Nursing Considerations

### Assessment

- *History:* Hypersensitivity to barbiturates, manifest or latent porphyria, marked liver impairment, nephritis, severe respiratory distress, previous addiction to sedative-hypnotic drugs, acute or chronic pain, seizure disorders, pregnancy, lactation, fever, hyperthyroidism, diabetes mellitus, severe anemia, pulmonary or cardiac disease, shock, uremia
- *Physical:* Weight; T; skin color, lesions, injection site; orientation, affect, reflexes; P, BP, orthostatic BP; R, adventitious sounds; bowel sounds, normal output, liver evaluation; liver and kidney function tests, blood and urine glucose, BUN

### Implementation

- Do not administer intra-arterially; may produce arteriospasm, thrombosis, gangrene.
- Administer IV doses slowly.
- Administer IM doses deep in a muscle mass.
- Do not use parenteral form if solution is discolored or contains a precipitate.
- Monitor injection sites carefully for irritation, extravasation (IV use); solutions are alkaline and very irritating to the tissues.
- Monitor P, BP, respiration carefully during IV administration.
- Taper dosage gradually after repeated use, especially in epileptic patients.

### Drug-specific teaching points

- This drug will make you drowsy and less anxious.
- Do not try to get up after you have received this drug (request assistance to sit up or move about).

*Outpatients*

- Take this drug exactly as prescribed. This drug is habit-forming; its effectiveness in facilitating sleep disappears after a short time. Do not take this drug longer than 2 wk (for insomnia) and do not increase the dosage without consulting your physician. If the drug appears to be ineffective, consult your health care provider.
- Avoid alcohol, sleep-inducing, or OTC drugs. These could cause dangerous effects.
- Avoid becoming pregnant while you are taking this drug. Use other methods of contraception in place of oral contraceptives, which may lose their effectiveness with this drug.
- The following side effects may occur: drowsiness, dizziness, "hangover," impaired thinking (may lessen after a few days; avoid driving or engaging in activities that require alertness); GI upset (take drug with food); dreams, nightmares, difficulty concentrating, fatigue, nervousness (reversible).
- Report severe dizziness, weakness, drowsiness that persists, rash or skin lesions, pregnancy.

# pentosan polysulfate sodium

*(pen **toe'** san)*

Elmiron

**Pregnancy Category B**

### Drug classes

Bladder protectant

### Therapeutic actions

Low-molecular-weight heparin-like compound with both anticoagulant and fibrinoloytic effects; adheres to the bladder wall mucosal membrane, acting as a buffer to control cell permeability, preventing irritating solutes in the urine from reaching the cells.

### Indications

- Relief of bladder pain or discomfort associated with interstitial cystitis

### Contraindications/cautions

- Contraindications: bleeding conditions or situations associated with increased risk of bleeding (surgery, anticoagulation, hemophilia, etc.); history of heparin-induced thrombocytopenia
- Use cautiously with any hepatic insufficiency, splenic disorders, pregnancy, lactation

### Dosage

**Available Forms:** Capsules—100 mg

*ADULT:* 100 mg PO tid, on an empty stomach, 1 h before or 2 h after meals.

*PEDIATRIC < 16 Y:* Not recommended.

### Pharmacokinetics

| Route | Onset | Peak |
|---|---|---|
| Oral | 30–60 min | 1–2 h |

*Metabolism:* Hepatic; $T_{1/2}$: 1–2 h

*Distribution:* Crosses placenta; may pass into breast milk

*Excretion:* Urine

### Adverse effects

- CNS: *Headache,* dizziness
- GI: Abdominal pain, GI disturbances, liver function abnormalities
- Hematologic: **Hemorrhage,** increased bleeding times
- Dermatologic: *Alopecia,* rash

### Clinically important drug-drug interactions

- Increased risk of bleeding with coumarin anticoagulants, heparin, t-PA, streptokinase, aspirin, NSAIDs

## ■ Nursing Considerations

### Assessment

- ***History:*** Bleeding conditions or situations associated with increased risk of bleeding; heparin-induced thrombocytopenia; hepatic insufficiency, splenic disorders, pregnancy, lactation
- ***Physical:*** Skin lesions, color, hair distribution; orientation, affect, reflexes; liver function tests; bleeding times

### Implementation

- Establish presence of interstitial cystitis with cytoscopy, cytology, and/or biopsy results.
- Obtain baseline bleeding time before beginning therapy; monitor periodically.
- Administer drug on an empty stomach, 1 h before or 2 h after meals.
- Arrange for wig or other appropriate head covering if alopecia occurs.

### Drug-specific teaching points

- Take this drug on an empty stomach, 1 h before or 2 h after meals.
- The following side effects may occur: GI upset, abdominal pain (eat small, frequent meals); headache (medication may be ordered); loss of hair (arrange for wig or other head covering; it is important to protect the head from extremes of temperature); increased bleeding tendencies (avoid injury—use an electric razor, avoid contact sports, etc.).
- Avoid the use of OTC medications; many of these contain ingredients that may interact with this drug. If you feel you need one of these preparations, consult your health care provider.
- Report bleeding, bruising, changes in color of urine or stool, yellowing of eyes or skin, increased pain or discomfort.

## pentostatin

***(pen' toe stah tin)***

2′-doxycoformycin, DCF

Nipent

**Pregnancy Category D**

### Drug classes
Antineoplastic
Antibiotic

### Therapeutic actions
Potent inhibitor of the enzyme ADA, which has its greatest activity in the T cells and B cells of the immune system; presence of pentostatin leads to cell toxicity and death; exact mechanism of action in hairy cell leukemia is not understood.

### Indications
- Single agent for the treatment of adult patients with alpha-interferon-refractory hairy cell leukemia
- Orphan drug use: treatment of chronic lymphocytic leukemia

### Contraindications/cautions
- Contraindications: hypersensitivity to pentostatin, pregnancy, lactation.
- Use cautiously with myelosuppression, renal failure.

### Dosage
**Available Forms:** Powder for injection—10 mg/vial

*ADULT:* 4 mg/m$^2$ IV every other week. Hydrate with 500–1,000 ml 5% Dextrose in 0.5% Normal Saline before administration, and give an additional 500 ml 5% Dextrose after pentostatin.

*PEDIATRIC:* Safety and efficacy not established.

*GERIATRIC OR RENAL IMPAIRED:* Decrease dose and monitor patient carefully. 2 mg/m$^2$ IV may be sufficient.

### Pharmacokinetics

| Route | Onset | Peak |
|---|---|---|
| IV | Rapid | 11 min |

*Metabolism:* Hepatic, $T_{1/2}$: 5.7 h
*Distribution:* Crosses placenta; enters breast milk
*Excretion:* Urine

### IV facts
**Preparation:** Transfer 5 ml Sterile Water for Injection to the vial containing pentostatin; mix thoroughly to obtain a solution of 2 mg/ml; may dilute further in 25 or 50 ml of 5% Dextrose Injection or 0.9% Sodium Chloride Injection; results in a solution of 0.33 or 0.18 mg/ml respectively. Stable at room temperature for up to 8 h; discard after that time.

**Infusion:** Administer by bolus injection over 1 min, or slowly infuse more dilute solution over 20–30 min.

### Adverse effects
- CNS: *Headache,* tremor, anxiety, confusion, depression, insomnia, nervousness
- GI: *Nausea, vomiting, anorexia, diarrhea*, constipation, flatulence, stomatitis
- CV: Angina, chest pain, arrhythmia
- Respiratory: *Cough, URI, lung disorders*, dyspnea, epistaxis, pneumonia, **fatal pulmonary toxicity**
- Hematologic: *Leukopenia, anemia, thrombocytopenia*, petechiae, ecchymosis
- Dermatologic: *Rash*, urticaria, eczema, pruritus, seborrhea, sweating
- General: *Fever, infection, fatigue, pain, allergic reaction, fever*, **death**, sepsis

### Clinically important drug-drug interactions
• Increased incidence of severe skin rashes with allopurinol • Fatal pulmonary toxicity with fludarabine • Increased risk of toxicity and side effects of pentostatin and vidarabine if taken concurrently

## ■ Nursing Considerations

### Assessment
- *History:* Hypersensitivity to pentostatin, pregnancy, lactation, myelosuppression, renal failure
- *Physical:* T; skin color, temperature; orientation, reflexes; P, BP; liver evalution, bowel sounds; R, adventitious sounds; urinary output; liver and renal function tests; CBC with differential

### Implementation
- Monitor laboratory tests for renal function, myelosuppression before and frequently during therapy.

- Hold drug and notify physician in cases of active infection, neutrophil count < 200 cells/mm$^3$, severe CNS toxicity, severe rash, signs of pulmonary toxicity, elevated creatinine.
- Wear protective clothing and gloves while preparing drug; arrange for proper disposal of chemotherapeutic agent.
- Hydrate patient with 500–1,000 ml of 5% Dextrose in 0.5 Normal Saline prior to drug administration; infuse an additional 500 ml of 5% Dextrose after administration.

### Drug-specific teaching points

- This drug can only be given IV and only every other week. Mark calendar with days to return for drug therapy.
- Have frequent blood tests and monitoring to determine your body's response to this drug. Frequent monitoring will be used to determine the timing of the next dose if adverse effects occur.
- The following side effects may occur: nausea, vomiting (request medication; frequent mouth care may also help); dizziness, nervousness, confusion (avoid driving or operating dangerous machinery); increased susceptibility to infection (avoid crowded areas and infections); headache, muscle aches and pains (request medication).
- Report bleeding, bruising, fatigue, abscesses, severe nausea or vomiting, difficulty breathing, hallucinations, severe headache, swelling.

## pentoxifylline

*(pen tox i' fi leen)*

Trental

**Pregnancy Category C**

### Drug classes

Hemorheologic agent
Xanthine

### Therapeutic actions

Reduces RBC aggregation and local hyperviscosity, decreases platelet aggregation, decreases fibrinogen concentration in the blood; precise mechanism of action is not known.

### Indications

- Intermittent claudication
- Unlabeled use: cerebrovascular insufficiency, to improve psychopathologic symptoms, diabetic vascular disease

### Contraindications/cautions

- Contraindications: allergy to pentoxifylline or methylxanthines (eg, caffeine, theophylline; drug is a dimethylxanthine derivative), lactation.
- Use cautiously with pregnancy.

### Dosage

**Available Forms:** CR tablets—400 mg

*ADULT:* 400 mg tid PO with meals. Decrease to 400 mg bid if adverse side effects occur. Continue for at least 8 wk.

*PEDIATRIC:* Safety and efficacy not established.

### Pharmacokinetics

| *Route* | *Onset* | *Peak* |
|---|---|---|
| Oral | Varies | 60 min |

*Metabolism:* Hepatic, $T_{1/2}$: 0.4–1.6 h

*Distribution:* Crosses placenta; enters breast milk

*Excretion:* Urine

### Adverse effects

- CNS: *Dizziness, headache*, tremor, anxiety, confusion
- GI: *Dyspepsia, nausea*, vomiting
- CV: Angina, chest pain, arrhythmia, hypotension, dyspnea
- **Hematologic**: Pancytopenia, purpura, thrombocytopenia
- **Dermatologic**: Brittle fingernails, pruritus, rash, urticaria

### Clinically important drug-drug interactions

- Increased therapeutic and toxic effects of theophylline when combined; monitor closely and adjust dosage as needed

## Nursing Considerations

### Assessment

- *History:* Allergy to pentoxifylline or methylxanthines, pregnancy, lactation
- *Physical:* Skin color, temperature; orientation, reflexes; P, BP, peripheral perfusion; CBC

### Implementation

- Monitor patient for angina, arrhythmias.
- Administer drug with meals.

### Drug-specific teaching points

- Take drug with meals.
- This drug helps the signs and symptoms of claudication, but additional therapy is needed.
- Dizziness may occur as a result of therapy; avoid driving and operating dangerous machinery; take precautions to prevent injury.
- Report chest pain, flushing, loss of consciousness, twitching, numbness and tingling.

# pergolide mesylate

*(per' go lide)*
Permax
**Pregnancy Category B**

## Drug classes

Antiparkinsonism agent

## Therapeutic actions

Potent dopamine receptor agonist; inhibits the secretion of prolactin, causes a transient rise in growth hormone and decrease in luteinizing hormone; directly stimulates postsynaptic dopamine receptors in the nigrostriatal system.

## Indications

- Adjunctive treatment to levodopa-carbidopa in the management of the signs and symptoms of Parkinson's disease

## Contraindications/cautions

- Contraindications: hypersensitivity to pergolide or ergot derivatives, lactation (suppression of prolactin may inhibit nursing).
- Use cautiously with cardiac dysrhythmias, hallucinations, confusion, dyskinesias, pregnancy.

### Dosage

**Available Forms:** Tablets—0.05, 0.25, 1 mg

*ADULT:* Initiate with a daily dose of 0.05 mg PO for the first 2 d. Gradually increase dosage by 0.1 or 0.15 mg/d every third day over the next 12 d of therapy. May then be increased by 0.25 mg/d every third day until an optimal therapeutic dosage is achieved. *Usual dose:* 3 mg given in three equally divided doses per day.

*PEDIATRIC:* Safety and efficacy not established.

## Pharmacokinetics

| *Route* | *Onset* | *Peak* |
|---|---|---|
| Oral | Varies | 2 h |

*Metabolism:* Hepatic, $T_{1/2}$: 8–12 h
*Distribution:* May cross placenta; may enter breast milk
*Excretion:* Urine and lungs

## Adverse effects

- CNS: *Dyskinesias, dizziness, hallucinations, dystonias, confusion, somnolence, insomnia, anxiety, tremor*, fatigue, anxiety, convulsions, depression, drowsiness, vertigo, hyperesthesia, irritability, nervousness, visual disturbances
- GI: *Nausea, constipation, diarrhea, dyspepsia*, anorexia, dry mouth, vomiting
- CV: *Postural hypotension, vasodilation*, palpitation, hypotension, syncope, hypertension, arrhythmia
- Respiratory: *Rhinitis, dyspnea*, epistaxis, hiccups
- GU: Urinary frequency, urinary tract infection, hematuria
- Dermatologic: Rash, sweating
- General: *Pain, abdominal pain, headache, asthenia*, chest pain, neck pain, chills, *peripheral edema*, edema, weight gain, anemia

## ■ Nursing Considerations

### Assessment

- *History:* Hypersensitivity to pergolide or ergot derivatives, cardiac dysrhythmias, hallucinations, confusion, dyskinesias, lactation
- *Physical:* Reflexes, affect; BP, P, peripheral perfusion; abdominal exam, normal output; auscultation, R; urinary output

### Implementation

- Administer with extreme caution to patients with a history of cardiac arrhythmias, hallucinations, confusion, or dyskinesias.
- Monitor patient while titrating drug to establish therapeutic dosage. Dosage of levodopa/carbidopa may require adjustment to balance therapeutic effects.

### Drug-specific teaching points

- Take this drug with your levodopa/carbidopa. The dosage will need to be adjusted carefully over the next few weeks to get the best effect for you. Keep appointments to have this dosage evaluated. Instruct a family member or significant other about this medication, because confusion and hallucinations are common effects; you may not be able to remember or follow instructions.
- The following side effects may occur: dizziness, confusion, shaking (avoid driving or performing hazardous tasks; change position slowly; use caution when climbing stairs); nausea, diarrhea, constipation (proper nutrition is important); pain, swelling (generalized pain and discomfort may occur); running nose (common problem; do not self-medicate).
- Report hallucinations, palpitations, tingling in the arms or legs, chest pain.

## perphenazine

*(per **fen'** a zeen)*

Apo-Perphenazine (CAN), Phenazine (CAN), Trilafon

**Pregnancy Category C**

### Drug classes

Phenothiazine (piperazine)
Dopaminergic blocking agent
Antipsychotic
Antiemetic

### Therapeutic actions

Mechanism of action not fully understood: antipsychotic drugs block postsynaptic dopamine receptors in the brain, but this may not be necessary and sufficient for antipsychotic activity; depresses the RAS, including the parts of the brain involved with wakefulness and emesis; anticholinergic, antihistaminic ($H_1$), and alpha-adrenergic blocking activity also may contribute to some of its therapeutic (and adverse) actions.

### Indications

- Management of manifestations of psychotic disorders
- Control of severe nausea and vomiting, intractable hiccups

### Contraindications/cautions

- Contraindications: coma or severe CNS depression, bone marrow depression, blood dyscrasia, circulatory collapse, subcortical brain damage, Parkinson's disease, liver damage, cerebral arteriosclerosis, coronary disease, severe hypotension or hypertension.
- Use cautiously with respiratory disorders ("silent pneumonia" may develop); glaucoma, prostatic hypertrophy; epilepsy or history of epilepsy; breast cancer; thyrotoxicosis; peptic ulcer, decreased renal function; myelography within previous 24 h or scheduled within 48 h; exposure to heat or phosphorous insecticides; pregnancy; lactation; children younger than 12 y, especially those with chickenpox, CNS infections (children are especially susceptible to dystonias that may confound the diagnosis of Reye's syndrome).

### Dosage

**Available Forms:** Tablets—2, 4, 8, 16 mg; concentrate—16 mg/5 ml; injection—5 mg/ml

Full clinical antipsychotic effects may require 6 wk–6 mo of therapy.

p

ADULT

- ***Moderately disturbed nonhospitalized patients:*** 4–8 mg PO tid; reduce as soon as possible to minimum effective dosage.
- *Hospitalized patients:* 8–16 mg PO bid–qid. Avoid dosages > 64 mg/d.

– *IM:* Initial dose 5–10 mg q6h. Total dosage should not exceed 15 mg/d in ambulatory, 30 mg/d in hospitalized patients. Switch to oral dosage as soon as possible.

- *Antiemetic:* 8–16 mg/d PO in divided doses (occasionally 24 mg may be needed); 5–10 mg IM for rapid control of vomiting; 5 mg IV in divided doses by slow infusion of dilute solutions. Give IV only when necessary to control severe vomiting.

PEDIATRIC: Not recommended for children < 12 y; children > 12 y may receive lowest adult dosage.

GERIATRIC OR DEBILITATED: Use lower doses (one-third to one-half adult dose), and increase dosage more gradually than in younger patients.

## Pharmacokinetics

| *Route* | *Onset* | *Peak* | *Duration* |
|---|---|---|---|
| Oral | Varies | Unknown | |
| IM/IV | 5–10 min | 1–2 h | 6 h |

*Metabolism:* Hepatic, $T_{1/2}$: unknown
*Distribution:* Crosses placenta; enters breast milk
*Excretion:* Urine

### IV facts

**Preparation:** Dilute drug to 0.5 mg/ml.

**Infusion:** Give by either fractional injection or slow drip infusion. When giving as divided doses, give no more than 1 mg/injection at not less than 1- to 2-min intervals. Do not exceed 5 mg total dose; hypotensive and extrapyramidal effects may occur.

## Adverse effects

- CNS: *Drowsiness*, insomnia, vertigo, headache, weakness, tremor, ataxia, slurring, cerebral edema, seizures, exacerbation of psychotic symptoms, extrapyramidal syndromes—*pseudoparkinsonism; dystonias; akathisia*, tardive dyskinesias, potentially irreversible (no known treatment), **neuroleptic malignant syndrome**
- CV: Hypotension, orthostatic hypotension, hypertension, tachycardia, bradycardia, cardiac arrest, CHF, cardiomegaly, **refractory arrhythmias** (some fatal), pulmonary edema
- Respiratory: Bronchospasm, laryngospasm, dyspnea; suppression of cough reflex and potential for aspiration (**sudden death related to asphyxia** or cardiac arrest has been reported)
- Hematologic: Eosinophilia, leukopenia, leukocytosis, anemia; aplastic anemia; hemolytic anemia; thrombocytopenic or nonthrombocytopenic purpura; pancytopenia
- EENT: Glaucoma, *photophobia, blurred vision*, miosis, mydriasis, deposits in the cornea and lens (opacities), pigmentary retinopathy
- Hypersensitivity: Jaundice, urticaria, angioneurotic edema, laryngeal edema, photosensitivity, eczema, asthma, anaphylactoid reactions, exfoliative dermatitis
- Endocrine: Lactation, breast engorgement, galactorrhea; syndrome of inappropriate ADH secretion (SIADH); amenorrhea, menstrual irregularities; gynecomastia; changes in libido; hyperglycemia or hypoglycemia; glycosuria; hyponatremia; pituitary tumor with hyperprolactinemia; inhibition of ovulation, infertility, pseudopregnancy; reduced urinary levels of gonadotropins, estrogens, progestins
- Autonomic: Dry mouth, salivation, nasal congestion, nausea, vomiting, anorexia, fever, pallor, flushed facies, sweating, constipation, paralytic ileus, urinary retention, incontinence, polyuria, enuresis, priapism, ejaculation inhibition, male impotence
- Other: *urine discolored pink to red-brown*

### Clinically important drug-drug interactions

• Additive CNS depression with alcohol • Additive anticholinergic effects and possibly decreased antipsychotic efficacy with anticholinergic drugs • Increased likelihood of seizures with metrizamide (contrast agent used in myelography) • Increased chance of severe neuromuscular excitation and hypotension with barbiturate anesthetics (methohexital, thiamylal, phenobarbital, thiopental) • Decreased antihypertensive effect of guanethidine when taken with antipsychotics

### Drug-lab test interferences

• False-positive pregnancy tests (less likely if serum test is used) • Increase in protein-bound iodine, not attributable to an increase in thyroxine

## ■ Nursing Considerations

### Assessment

- *History:* Coma or severe CNS depression; bone marrow depression; circulatory collapse; subcortical brain damage; Parkinson's disease; liver damage; cerebral arteriosclerosis; coronary disease; severe hypotension or hypertension; respiratory disorders; glaucoma, prostatic hypertrophy; epilepsy; breast cancer; thyrotoxicosis; peptic ulcer, decreased renal function; myelography within previous 24 h or myelography scheduled within 48 h; exposure to heat or phosphorus insecticides; pregnancy; children younger than 12 y
- *Physical:* Weight, T; reflexes, orientation, intraocular pressure; P, BP, orthostatic BP; R, adventitious sounds; bowel sounds and normal output, liver evaluation; urinary output, prostate size; CBC, urinalysis, thyroid, liver, and kidney function tests

### Implementation

- Dilute oral concentrate *only* with water, saline, 7-Up, homogenized milk, carbonated orange drink, and pineapple, apricot, prune, orange, V-8, tomato, and grapefruit juices; use 60 ml of diluent for each 16 mg (5 ml) of concentrate.
- Do *not* mix with beverages that contain caffeine (coffee, cola), tannics (tea), or pectinates (apple juice); physical incompatibility may result.
- Give IM injections only to seated or recumbent patients, and observe for adverse effects for a brief period afterward.
- Monitor pulse and BP continuously during IV administration.
- Do not change dosage in chronic therapy more often than weekly; drug requires 4–7 d to achieve steady-state plasma levels.
- Avoid skin contact with oral solution; contact dermatitis has occurred.
- Discontine drug if serum creatinine, BUN become abnormal or if WBC count is depressed.
- Monitor elderly patients for dehydration, and institute remedial measures promptly; sedation and decreased sensation of thirst related to CNS effects of drug can lead to severe dehydration.
- Consult physician regarding appropriate warning of patient or patient's guardian about tardive dyskinesias.
- Consult physician about dosage reduction, use of anticholinergic antiparkinsonian drugs (controversial) if extrapyramidal effects occur.

### Drug-specific teaching points

- Take drug exactly as prescribed.
- Avoid skin contact with drug solutions.
- Avoid driving or engaging in other dangerous activities if CNS, vision changes occur.
- Avoid prolonged exposure to sun; use a sunscreen or covering garments.
- Maintain fluid intake, and use precautions against heat stroke in hot weather.
- Report sore throat, fever, unusual bleeding or bruising, rash, weakness, tremors, impaired vision, dark urine (pink or reddish brown urine is expected), pale stools, yellowing of the skin or eyes.

## phenazopyridine hydrochloride

*(fen az oh* ***peer'*** *i deen)*

phenylazo-diaminopyridine hydrochloride

Azo-Standard, Baridium, Phenazo (CAN), Prodium, Pyridate, Pyridium, Urogesic

**Pregnancy Category B**

### Drug classes
Urinary analgesic

### Therapeutic actions
An azo dye that is excreted in the urine and exerts a direct topical analgesic effect on urinary tract mucosa; exact mechanism of action is not understood.

### Indications
- Symptomatic relief of pain, urgency, burning, frequency, and discomfort related to irritation of the lower urinary tract mucosa caused by infection, trauma, surgery, endoscopic procedures, passage of sounds or catheters

### Contraindications/cautions
- Contraindications: allergy to phenazopyridine, renal insufficiency.
- Use cautiously with pregnancy, lactation.

### Dosage
**Available Forms:** Tablets—95, 100, 200 mg

**Adult:** 200 mg PO tid after meals. Do not exceed 2 d if used with antibacterial agent.

**Pediatric**
- *6–12 Y:* 12 mg/kg/d or 350 mg/m$^2$/d divided into 3 doses PO.

### Pharmacokinetics

| Route | Onset |
|---|---|
| Oral | Rapid |

*Metabolism:* Hepatic, $T_{1/2}$: unknown

*Distribution:* Crosses placenta; may enter breast milk

*Excretion:* Urine

### Adverse effects
- CNS: *Headache*
- GI: *GI disturbances*
- **Hematologic**: Methemoglobinemia, hemolytic anemia
- **Dermatologic**: *Rash*, yellowish tinge to skin or sclera
- **Other**: Renal and hepatic toxicity, cancer, *yellow-orange discoloration of urine*

### Drug-lab test interferences
- Interference with colorimetric laboratory test procedures

## ■ Nursing Considerations

### Assessment
- *History:* Allergy to phenazopyridine, renal insufficiency, pregnancy
- *Physical:* Skin color, lesions; urinary output; normal GI output, bowel sounds, liver palpation; urinalysis, renal and liver function tests, CBC

### Implementation
- Give after meals to avoid GI upset.
- Do not give longer than 2 d if being given with antibacterial agent for treatment of UTI.
- Alert patient that urine may be reddish-orange and may stain fabric.
- Discontinue drug if skin or sclera become yellowish, a sign of drug accumulation.

### Drug-specific teaching points
- Take drug after meals to avoid GI upset.
- Urine may be reddish-orange (normal effect; urine may stain fabric).
- Report yellowish stain to skin or eyes, headache, unusual bleeding or bruising, fever, sore throat.

## phenelzine sulfate

*(fen' el zeen)*

Nardil

**Pregnancy Category C**

### Drug classes
Antidepressant

Monoamine oxidase inhibitor (MAO Inhibitor)

### Therapeutic actions
Irreversibly inhibits MAO, an enzyme that breaks down biogenic amines, such as epinephrine, norepinephrine, and serotonin, thus allowing these biogenic amines to accumulate in neuronal storage sites. According to the "biogenic amine hypothesis," this accumulation of amines is responsible for the clinical efficacy of MAOIs as antidepressants.

## Indications

- Treatment of patients with depression characterized as "atypical," "nonendogenous," or "neurotic"; patients who are unresponsive to other antidepressive therapy; and patients in whom other antidepressive therapy is contraindicated

## Contraindications/cautions

- Contraindications: hypersensitivity to any MAOI, pheochromocytoma, CHF, history of liver disease or abnormal liver function tests, severe renal impairment, confirmed or suspected cerebrovascular defect, CV disease, hypertension, history of headache, myelography within previous 24 h or scheduled within 48 h.
- Use cautiously with seizure disorders; hyperthyroidism; impaired hepatic, renal function; psychiatric patients (agitated or schizophrenic patients may show excessive stimulation; manic-depressive patients may shift to hypomanic or manic phase); patients scheduled for elective surgery; pregnancy; lactation.

## Dosage

**Available Forms:** Tablets—15 mg

*ADULT:* Initially, 15 mg PO tid. Increase dosage to at least 60 mg/d at a fairly rapid pace consistent with patient tolerance. Many patients require therapy at 60 mg/d for at least 4 wk before response. Some patients may require 90 mg/d. After maximum benefit is achieved, reduce dosage slowly over several weeks. Maintenance may be 15 mg/d or every other day.

*PEDIATRIC:* Not recommended for children <16 y.

*GERIATRIC:* Patients >60 y are more prone to develop adverse effects; adjust dosage accordingly.

## Pharmacokinetics

| *Route* | *Onset* | *Duration* |
|---|---|---|
| Oral | Slow | 48–96 h |

*Metabolism:* Hepatic, $T_{1/2}$: unknown

*Distribution:* Crosses placenta; enters breast milk

*Excretion:* Urine

## Adverse effects

- CNS: *Dizziness, vertigo, headache, overactivity, hyperreflexia, tremors, muscle twitching, mania, hypomania, jitteriness, confusion, memory impairment, insomnia, weakness, fatigue, drowsiness, restlessness, overstimulation, increased anxiety, agitation, blurred vision, sweating,* akathisa, ataxia, coma, euphoria, neuritis, repetitious babbling, chills, glaucoma, nystagmus
- GI: *Constipation, diarrhea, nausea, abdominal pain, edema, dry mouth, anorexia, weight changes*
- CV: **Hypertensive crises** (sometimes fatal, sometimes with intracranial bleeding, usually attributable to ingestion of contraindicated food or drink containing tyramine; see "Drug-Food Interactions" below; symptoms include some or all of the following: occipital headache, which may radiate frontally; palpitations; neck stiffness or soreness; nausea; vomiting; sweating; dilated pupils; photophobia; tachycardia or bradycardia; chest pain); *orthostatic hypotension, sometimes associated with falling; disturbed cardiac rate and rhythm,* palpitations, tachycardia
- GU: Dysuria, incontinence, urinary retention, sexual disturbances
- Dermatologic: Minor skin reactions, spider telangiectases, photosensitivity
- Other: Hematologic changes, black tongue, hypernatremia

## Clinically important drug-drug interactions

- Increased sympathomimetic effects (hypertensive crisis) with sympathomimetic drugs (norepinephrine, epinephrine, dopamine, dobutamine, levodopa, ephedrine), amphetamines, other anorexiants, local anesthetic solutions containing sympathomimetics • Hypertensive crisis, coma, severe convulsions with TCAs (eg, imipramine, desipramine). Note: MAOIs and TCAs have been used successfully in some patients resistant to therapy with single agents;



p

however, case reports indicate that the combination can cause serious and potentially fatal adverse effects. • Additive hypoglycemic effect with insulin, oral sulfonylureas • Increased risk of adverse interaction with meperidine

### Clinically important drug-food interactions

• Tyraminie (and other pressor amines) contained in foods are normally broken down by MAO enzymes in the GI tract; in the presence of MAOIs, these vasopressors may be absorbed in high concentrations; in addition, tyramine releases accumulated norepinephrine from nerve terminals; thus, hypertensive crisis may occur when the following foods that contain tyramine or other vasopressors are ingested by a patient on an MAOI: dairy products (blue, camembert, cheddar, mozzarella, parmesan, romano, roquefort, Stilton cheeses; sour cream; yogurt); meats, fish (liver, pickled herring, fermented sausages—bologna, pepperoni, salami; caviar; dried fish; other fermented or spoiled meat or fish); undistilled beverages (imported beer, ale; red wine, especially Chianti; sherry; coffee, tea, colas containing caffeine; chocolate drinks); fruit/vegetables (avocado, fava beans, figs, raisins, bananas, yeast extracts, soy sauce, chocolate)

## ■ Nursing Considerations

### Assessment

- *History:* Hypersensitivity to any MAOI; pheochromocytoma, CHF; abnormal liver function tests; severe renal impairment; cerebrovascular defect; CV disease, hypertension; history of headache; myelography within previous 24 h or scheduled within 48 h; seizure disorders; hyperthyroidism; impaired hepatic, renal function; psychiatric patients; elective surgery; lactation
- *Physical:* Weight; T; skin color, lesions; orientation, affect, reflexes, vision; P, BP, orthostatic BP, auscultation, perfusion; bowel sounds, normal output, liver evaluation; urine flow, normal output; thyroid palpation; liver, kidney and thyroid function tests, urinalysis, CBC, ECG, EEG

### Implementation

- Limit amount of drug that is available to suicidal patients.
- Monitor BP and orthostatic BP carefully; arrange for more gradual increase in dosage in patients who show tendency for hypotension.
- Have periodic liver function tests during therapy; discontine drug at first sign of hepatic dysfunction or jaundice.
- Discontinue drug and monitor BP carefully if patient reports unusual or severe headache.
- Provide phentolamine or another $\alpha$-adrenergic blocking drug on standby in case hypertensive crisis occurs.
- Provide diet that is low in tyramine-containing foods

### Drug-specific teaching points

- Take drug exactly as prescribed. Do not stop taking this drug abruptly or without consulting your health care provider.
- Avoid ingestion of tyramine-containing foods while you are taking this drug and for 2 wk afterward (patient and significant other should receive a list of such foods).
- Avoid alcohol; other sleep-inducing drugs; all OTC drugs, including nose drops, cold, and hay fever remedies; and appetite suppressants. Many of these contain substances that could cause serious or even life-threatening problems.
- The following side effects may occur: dizziness, weakness or fainting when arising from a horizontal or sitting position (transient; change position slowly); drowsiness, blurred vision (reversible; if severe, avoid driving or performing tasks that require alertness); nausea, vomiting, loss of appetite (small, frequent meals, frequent mouth care may help); memory changes, irritability, emotional changes, nervousness (reversible).
- Report headache, skin rash, darkening of the urine, pale stools, yellowing of the eyes or skin, fever, chills, sore throat, any other unusual symptoms.

# Phenobarbital

## phenobarbital

*(fee noe **bar'** bi tal)*

*Oral preparations:* Gardenal (CAN), Solfoton

## phenobarbital sodium

*Parenteral:* Luminal Sodium

**Pregnancy Category D**
**C-IV controlled substance**

### Drug classes

Barbiturate (long acting)
Sedative
Hypnotic
Anticonvulsant
Antiepileptic agent

### Therapeutic actions

General CNS depressant; barbiturates inhibit impulse conduction in the ascending RAS, depress the cerebral cortex, alter cerebellar function, depress motor output, and can produce excitation, sedation, hypnosis, anesthesia and deep coma; at subhypnotic doses, has anticonvulsant activity, making it suitable for long-term use as an antiepileptic.

### Indications

- Sedative (oral or parenteral)
- Hyponotic, short-term (up to 2 wk) treatment of insomnia (oral or parenteral)
- Long-term treatment of generalized tonic-clonic and cortical focal seizures (oral)
- Emergency control of certain acute convulsive episodes (e.g., those associated with status epilepticus, eclampsia, meningitis, tetanus and toxic reactions to strychnine or local anesthetics; oral)
- Preanesthetic (parenteral)
- Anticonvulsant treatment of generalized tonic-clonic and cortical focal seizures (parenteral)
- Emergency control of acute convulsions (tetanus, eclampsia, epilepticus; parenteral)

### Contraindications/cautions

- Contraindications: hypersensitivity to barbiturates, manifest or latent porphyria; marked liver impairment; nephritis; severe respiratory distress; previous addiction to sedative-hypnotic drugs (may be ineffective and may contribute to further addiction); pregnancy (fetal damage, neonatal withdrawal syndrome).
- Use cautiously with acute or chronic pain (drug may cause paradoxical excitement or mask important symptoms); seizure disorders (abrupt discontinuation of daily doses can result in status epilepticus); lactation (secreted in breast milk; drowsiness in nursing infants); fever, hyperthyroidism, diabetes mellitus, severe anemia, pulmonary or cardiac disease, status asthmaticus, shock, uremia; impaired liver or kidney function, debilitation.

### Dosage

**Available Forms:** Tablets—15, 16, 30, 60, 100 mg; capsules—16 mg; elixir—15, 20 mg/5 ml; injection—30, 60, 65, 130 mg/ml

**ADULT**

- ***Oral***
- *Sedation:* 30–120 mg/d in two to three divided doses.
- *Hypnotic:* 100–200 mg.
- *Anticonvulsant:* 60–100 mg/d.
- ***Parenteral (IM or IV)***
- *Sedation:* 30–120 mg/d IM or IV in two to three divided doses.
- *Preoperative sedation:* 100–200 mg IM, 60–90 min before surgery.
- *Hypnotic:* 100–320 mg IM or IV.
- *Acute convulsions:* 200–320 mg IM or IV repeated in 6 h if necessary.

**PEDIATRIC**

- ***Oral***
- *Sedation:* 8–32 mg/d.
- *Hypnotic:* Determine dosage using age and weight charts.
- *Anticonvulsant:* 3–6 mg/kg per day.
- ***Parenteral***
- *Preoperative sedation:* 1–3 mg/kg IM or IV.
- *Anticonvulsant:* 4–6 mg/kg per day for 7–10 d to a blood level of 10–15 μg/ml *or* 10–15 mg/kg per day IV or IM.

– *Status epilepticus:* 15–20 mg/kg IV over 10–15 min.

GERIATRIC PATIENTS OR THOSE WITH DEBILITATING DISEASE, RENAL OR HEPATIC IMPAIRMENT: Reduce dosage and monitor closely—may produce excitement, depression, confusion.

### Pharmacokinetics

| *Route* | *Onset* | *Duration* |
|---|---|---|
| Oral | 30–60 min | 10–16 h |
| IM, SC | 10–30 min | 4–6 h |
| IV | 5 min | 4–6 h |

*Metabolism:* Hepatic, $T_{1/2}$: 79 h
*Distribution:* Crosses placenta; enters breast milk
*Excretion:* Urine

### IV facts

**Preparation:** No further preparation is needed.
**Infusion:** Infuse very slowly, each 60 mg over 1 min, directly IV or into tubing or running IV; inject partial dose and observe for response before continuing.

### Adverse effects

- CNS: *Somnolence, agitation, confusion, hyperkinesia, ataxia, vertigo, CNS depression, nightmares, lethargy, residual sedation (hangover), paradoxical excitement, nervousness, psychiatric disturbance, hallucinations, insomnia, anxiety, dizziness, thinking abnormality*
- GI: *Nausea, vomiting, constipation, diarrhea, epigastric pain*
- CV: *Bradycardia, hypotension, syncope*
- Respiratory: *Hypoventilation, apnea, respiratory depression,* laryngospasm, bronchospasm, circulatory collapse
- Hypersensitivity: Skin rashes, angioneurotic edema, serum sickness, morbiliform rash, urticaria; rarely, exfoliative dermatitis, **Stevens-Johnson syndrome**
- Local: *Pain, tissue necrosis at injection site,* gangrene; arterial spasm with inadvertent intra-arterial injection; thrombophlebitis; permanent neurologic deficit if injected near a nerve
- Other: Tolerance, psychological and physical dependence, **withdrawal syndrome**

### Clinically important drug-drug interactions

• Increased serum levels and therapeutic and toxic effects with valproic acid • Increased CNS depression with alcohol • Increased risk of nephrotoxicity with methoxyflurane • Increased risk of neuromuscular excitation and hypotension with barbiturate anesthetics • Decreased effects of the following drugs: theophyllines, oral anticoagulants, beta-blockers, doxycycline, griseofulvin corticosteroids, oral contraceptives and estrogens, metronidazole, phenylbutazones, quinidine

## ■ Nursing Considerations

### Assessment

- *History:* Hypersensitivity to barbiturates, manifest or latent porphyria; marked liver impairment; nephritis; severe respiratory distress; previous addiction to sedative-hypnotic drugs; pregnancy; acute or chronic pain; seizure disorders; lactation, fever; hyperthyroidism; diabetes mellitus; severe anemia; cardiac disease; shock; uremia; impaired liver or kidney function; debilitation
- *Physical:* Weight; T; skin color, lesions; orientation, affect, reflexes; P, BP, orthostatic BP; R, adventitious sounds; bowel sounds, normal output, liver evaluation; liver and kidney function tests, blood and urine glucose, BUN

### Implementation

- Monitor patient responses, blood levels (as appropriate) if any of the above interacting drugs are given with phenobarbital; suggest alternative means of contraception to women on oral contraceptives.
- Do not administer intra-arterially; may produce arteriospasm, thrombosis, gangrene.
- Administer IV doses slowly.
- Administer IM doses deep in a large muscle mass (gluteus maximus, vastus later-

alis) or other areas where there is little risk of encountering a nerve trunk or major artery.

- Monitor injection sites carefully for irritation, extravasation (IV use). Solutions are alkaline and very irritating to the tissues.
- Monitor P, BP, respiration carefully during IV administration.
- Arrange for periodic laboratory tests of hematopoietic, renal, and hepatic systems during long-term therapy.
- Taper dosage gradually after repeated use, especially in epileptic patients. When changing from one antiepileptic drug to another, taper dosage of the drug being discontinued while increasing the dosage of the replacement drug.

### Drug-specific teaching points

- This drug will make you drowsy and less anxious; do not try to get up after you have received this drug (request assistance to sit up or move around).
- Take this drug exactly as prescribed; this drug is habit forming; its effectiveness in facilitating sleep disappears after a short time.
- Do not take this drug longer than 2 wk (for insomnia), and do not increase the dosage without consulting the prescriber.
- Do not reduce the dosage or discontinue this drug (when used for epilepsy); abrupt discontinuation could result in a serious increase in seizures.
- The following side effects may occur: drowsiness, dizziness, "hangover," impaired thinking (may lessen after a few days; avoid driving or engaging in dangerous activities); GI upset (take drug with food); dreams, nightmares, difficulty concentrating, fatigue, nervousness (reversible).
- Wear a medical alert tag so that emergency medical personnel will know you are an epileptic taking this medication.
- Avoid pregnancy while taking this drug; use a means of contraception other than oral contraceptives.
- Report severe dizziness, weakness, drowsiness that persists, rash or skin lesions, fever, sore throat, mouth sores, easy bruising or bleeding, nosebleed, petechiae, pregnancy.

## phenoxybenzamine hydrochloride

*(fen ox ee **ben'** za meen)*

Dibenzyline

**Pregnancy Category C**

### Drug classes

Alpha adrenergic blocker

### Therapeutic actions

Irreversibly blocks postsynaptic alpha$_1$-adrenergic receptors, decreasing sympathetic tone on the vasculature, dilating blood vessels, and lowering arterial BP (no longer used to treat essential hypertension because it also blocks presynaptic alpha$_2$-adrenergic receptors that are believed to mediate a feedback inhibition of further norepinephrine release; this accentuates the reflex tachycardia caused by the lowering of BP); produces a "chemical sympathectomy."

### Indications

- Pheochromocytoma to control episodes of hypertension and sweating (concomitant treatment with a beta-adrenergic blocker may be necessary to control excessive tachycardia)
- Unlabeled use: micturition disorders resulting from neurogenic bladder, functional outlet obstruction, partial prostatic obstruction

### Contraindications/cautions

- Contraindications: hypersensitivity to phenoxybenzamine or related drugs, MI, evidence of CAD.
- Use cautiously with pregnancy, lactation.

### Dosage

**Available Forms:** Capsules—10 mg

*ADULT:* Give small initial doses and increase gradually until desired effects are obtained or side effects become troublesome. Initially, give 10 mg PO bid. Increase dosage every other day until an optimal dosage is obtained. Usual dosage range is 20–40 mg PO bid–tid.

p

*PEDIATRIC:* 1–2 mg/kg per day divided every 6–8 h PO.

**Pharmacokinetics**

| *Route* | *Onset* | *Peak* | *Duration* |
|---|---|---|---|
| Oral | 2 h | 4–6 h | 3–4 d |

*Metabolism:* Hepatic, $T_{1/2}$: 24 h
*Distribution:* Crosses placenta; may enter breast milk
*Excretion:* Urine and bile

**Adverse effects**
- CNS: *Miosis*, drowsiness, fatigue
- GI: GI upset
- CV: *Postural hypotension, tachycardia*
- Respiratory: *Nasal congestion*
- GU: *Inhibition of ejaculation*

## ■ Nursing Considerations

### Assessment
- ***History:*** Hypersensitivity to phenoxybenzamine or related drugs, evidence of CAD, lactation
- ***Physical:*** Orientation, affect, reflexes; ophthalmologic exam; P, BP, orthostatic BP, supine BP, perfusion, edema, auscultation; bowel sounds, normal output

### Implementation
- Monitor BP response, heart rate carefully.

### Drug-specific teaching points
- Take this drug exactly as prescribed. Do not stop taking this drug without consulting your nurse or physician.
- Do not ingest alcohol.
- The following side effects may occur: dizziness when you change position (change position slowly; use caution when exercising, climbing stairs); drowsiness, fatigue (avoid driving or performing tasks that require alertness); GI upset (frequent, small meals may help); nasal stuffiness (do not use nose drops or cold remedies); constricted pupils and difficulty with far vision (avoid tasks that require visual acuity); inhibition of ejaculation (diminishes with time).
- Report increased heart rate; rapid weight gain; unusual swelling of the extremities; difficulty in breathing, especially when lying down; new or aggravated symptoms of angina (chest, arm, or shoulder pain); severe indigestion; dizziness, lightheadedness, or fainting.

# phensuximide

*(fen **sux'** i mide)*
Milontin Kapseals
**Pregnancy Category C**

**Drug classes**
Antiepileptic agent
Succinimide

**Therapeutic actions**
Suppresses the paroxysmal three cycle per second spike and wave EEG pattern associated with lapses of consciousness in absence (petit mal) seizures; reduces frequency of attacks; mechanism of action not understood, but may act in inhibitory neuronal systems that are important in the generation of the three per second rhythm.

**Indications**
- Control of absence (petit mal) seizures when refractory to other drugs

**Contraindications/cautions**
- Contraindications: hypersensitivity to succinimides.
- Use cautiously with hepatic, renal abnormalities, acute intermittent porphyria, pregnancy (association between use of antiepileptic drugs by women with epilepsy and an elevated incidence of birth defects in children born to these women; however, antiepileptic therapy should not be discontinued in pregnant women who are receiving such therapy to prevent major seizures; the effect of even minor seizures on the developing fetus is unknown, and this should be considered when deciding whether to continue antiepileptic therapy in pregnant women), lactation.

### Dosage
**Available Forms:** Capsules—500 mg
*ADULT AND PEDIATRIC:* Administer 500–1,000 mg PO bid–tid. The total dosage may

vary between 1 and 3 g/d (average, 1.5 g/d). May be administered with other antiepileptic drugs when other forms of epilepsy coexist with absence (petit mal) seizures.

### Pharmacokinetics

| *Route* | *Onset* | *Peak* |
|---|---|---|
| Oral | Varies | 1–4 h |

*Metabolism:* Hepatic, $T_{1/2}$: 4 h
*Distribution:* Crosses placenta; enters breast milk
*Excretion:* Urine and bile

### Adverse effects

*Succinimides*

- CNS: *Drowsiness, ataxia, dizziness*, irritability, nervousness, headache, blurred vision, myopia, photophobia, hiccups, euphoria, dreamlike state, lethargy, hyperactivity, fatigue, insomnia, increased frequency of grand mal seizures may occur when used alone; in some patients with mixed types of epilepsy, confusion, instability, mental slowness, depression, hypochondriacal behavior, sleep disturbances, night terrors, aggressiveness, inability to concentrate
- GI: *Nausea, vomiting, vague gastric upset, epigastric and abdominal pain*, cramps, anorexia, diarrhea, constipation, weight loss, swelling of tongue, gum hypertrophy
- Hematologic: Eosinophilia, granulocytopenia, leukopenia, agranulocytosis, aplastic anemia, monocytosis, **pancytopenia**
- Dermatologic: Pruritus, urticaria, Stevens-Johnson syndrome, pruritic erythematous rashes, skin eruptions, erythema multiforme, systemic lupus erythmatosus, alopecia, hirsutism
- Other: Periorbital edema, hyperemia, muscle weakness, abnormal liver and kidney function tests, vaginal bleeding, *discoloration of urine* (pink, red, or brown; not harmful)

### Clinically important drug-drug interactions

- Decreased serum levels and therapeutic effects of primidone

## ■ Nursing Considerations

### Assessment

- *History:* Hypersensitivity to succinimides; hepatic, renal abnormalities; acute intermittent porphyria; pregnancy; lactation
- *Physical:* Skin color, lesions; orientation, affect, reflexes, bilateral grip strength, vision exam; bowel sounds, normal output, liver evaluation; liver and kidney function tests, urinalysis, CBC with differential, EEG

### Implementation

- Reduce dosage, discontinue phensuximide, or substitute other antiepileptic medication gradually; abrupt discontinuation may precipitate absence (petit mal) status.
- Monitor CBC and differential before and frequently during therapy.
- Discontinue drug if skin rash, depression of blood count, or unusual depression, aggressiveness, or behavioral alterations occur.

### Drug-specific teaching points

- Take this drug exactly as prescribed; do not discontinue this drug abruptly or change dosage, except on the advice of your prescriber.
- Arrange for frequent checkups to monitor your response to this drug.
- The following side effects may occur: drowsiness, dizziness, confusion, blurred vision (avoid driving or performing other tasks requiring alertness or visual acuity); GI upset (take drug with food or milk, eat frequent, small meals).
- Wear a medical alert tag at all times so that emergency medical personnel will know that you are an epileptic taking antiepileptic medication.
- Report skin rash, joint pain, unexplained fever, sore throat, unusual bleeding or

p

bruising, drowsiness, dizziness, blurred vision, pregnancy.

## phentolamine mesylate

*(fen **tole'** a meen)*

Regitine, Rogitine (CAN)

**Pregnancy Category C**

### Drug classes

Alpha adrenergic blocker
Diagnostic agent

### Therapeutic actions

Competitively blocks postsynaptic $alpha_1$-adrenergic receptors, decreasing sympathetic tone on the vasculature, dilating blood vessels, and lowering arterial BP (no longer used to treat essential hypertension because it also blocks presynaptic $alpha_2$-adrenergic receptors that are believed to mediate a feedback inhibition of further norepinephrine release; this accentuates the reflex tachycardia caused by the lowering of BP); use of phentolamine injection as a test for pheochromocytoma depends on the premise that a greater BP reduction will occur with pheochromocytoma than with other etiologies of hypertension.

### Indications

- Pheochromocytoma—prevention or control of hypertensive episodes that may occur as a result of stress or manipulation during preoperative preparation and surgical excision
- Pharmacologic test for pheochromocytoma (urinary assays of catecholamines, other biochemical tests have largely supplanted the phentolamine test)
- Prevention and treatment of dermal necrosis and sloughing following IV administration or extravasation of norepinephrine or dopamine
- Unlabeled use: treatment of hypertensive crises secondary to MAOI/sympathomimetic amine interactions, or secondary to rebound hypertension on withdrawal of clonidine, propranolol, or other antihypertensive drugs

### Contraindications/cautions

- Contraindications: hypersensitivity to phentolamine or related drugs, evidence of CAD.
- Use cautiously with pregnancy.

### Dosage

**Available Forms:** Injection—5 mg/vial

**ADULT**

- ***Prevention or control of hypertensive episodes in pheochromocytoma:*** For use in preoperative reduction of elevated BP, inject 5 mg IV or IM 1–2 h before surgery. Repeat if necessary. Administer 5 mg IV during surgery as indicated to control paroxysms of hypertension, tachycardia, respiratory depression, convulsions.
- ***Prevention and treatment of dermal necrosis following IV administration or extravasation of norepinephrine:*** For prevention, add 10 mg to each liter of solution containing norepinephrine. The pressor effect of norepinephrine is not affected. For treatment, inject 5–10 mg in 10 ml saline into the area of extravasation within 12 h.
- ***Diagnosis of pheochromocytoma:*** See manufacturer's recommendations. This test should be used only to confirm evidence and after the risks have been carefully considered.

**PEDIATRIC**

- ***Prevention or control of hypertensive episodes in pheochromocytoma:*** For use in preoperative reduction of elevated BP, inject 1 mg IV or IM 1–2 h before surgery. Repeat if necessary. Administer 1 mg IV during surgery as indicated to control of paroxysms of hypertension, tachycardia, respiratory depression, convulsions.

### Pharmacokinetics

| *Route* | *Onset* | *Peak* | *Duration* |
|---|---|---|---|
| IM | Rapid | 20 min | 30–45 min |
| IV | Immediate | 2 min | 15–30 min |

*Metabolism* : Unknown
*Distribution* : Unknown
*Excretion* : Kidneys

### IV facts

**Preparation:** No further preparation is required.

**Infusion:** Inject slowly directly into vein or into tubing of actively running IV, each 5 mg over 1 min.

### Adverse effects

- CNS: *Weakness, dizziness*
- GI: *Nausea*, vomiting, diarrhea
- CV: *Acute and prolonged hypotensive episodes*, orthostatic hypotension, MI, cerebrovascular spasm, cerebrovascular occlusion, *tachycardia, arrhythmias*
- Other: Flushing, nasal stuffiness

### Clinically important drug-drug interactions

- Decreased vasoconstrictor and hypertensive effects of epinephrine, ephedrine

## ■ Nursing Considerations

### Assessment

- *History:* Hypersensitivity to phentolamine or related drugs, evidence of CAD
- *Physical:* Orientation, affect, reflexes; ophthalmologic exam; P, BP, orthostatic BP, supine BP, perfusion, edema, auscultation; bowel sounds, normal output

### Implementation

- Monitor BP response, heart rate carefully.

### Drug-specific teaching points

- Report dizziness, palpitations.

## phenylephrine hydrochloride

*(fen ill ef' rin)*

*Parenteral:* Neo-Synephrine

*Topical OTC Nasal Decongestants:* Alconefrin, Allerest Nasal, Coricidin, Duration Mild, Neo-Synephrine, Nostril, Rhinall, Sinarest Nasal

*Ophthalmic preparations (0.12% solutions are OTC):* AK-Dilate, AK-Nefrin, Mydfrin, Neo-Synephrine

**Pregnancy Category C**

### Drug classes

Sympathomimetic amine
Alpha adrenergic agonist
Vasopressor
Nasal decongestant
Ophthalmic vasoconstrictor/mydriatic

### Therapeutic actions

Powerful postsynaptic alpha-adrenergic receptor stimulant that causes vasoconstriction and increased systolic and diastolic BP with little effect on the beta receptors of the heart. Topical application causes vasoconstriction of the mucous membranes, which in turn relieves pressure and promotes drainage of the nasal passages. Topical ophthalmic application causes contraction of the dilator muscles of the pupil (mydriasis), vasoconstriction, and increased outflow of aqueous humor.

### Indications

- Treatment of vascular failure in shock, shocklike states, drug-induced hypotension, or hypersensitivity (parenteral)
- To overcome paroxysmal supraventricular tachycardia (parenteral)
- To prolong spinal anesthesia (parenteral)
- Vasoconstrictor in regional anesthesia (parenteral)
- To maintain an adequate level of BP during spinal and inhalation anesthesia (parenteral)
- Symptomatic relief of nasal and nasopharyngeal mucosal congestion due to the common cold, hay fever, or other respiratory allergies (topical)
- Adjunctive therapy of middle ear infections by decreasing congestion around the eustachian ostia (topical)
- 10% solution: decongestant and vasoconstrictor and for pupil dilation in uveitis, wide-angle glaucoma and surgery (ophthalmic solution)
- 2.5% solution: decongestant and vasoconstrictor and for pupil dilation in uveitis, open-angle glaucoma in conjunction with miotics, refraction, ophthalmoscopic examination, diagnostic procedures, and before intraocular surgery (ophthalmic solution)

p

- 0.12% solution: decongestant to provide temporary relief of minor eye irritations caused by hay fever, colds, dust, wind, smog, or hard contact lenses (ophthalmic solution)

**Contraindications/cautions**

- Contraindications: hypersensitivity to phenylephrine; severe hypertension, ventricular tachycardia; narrow-angle glaucoma; pregnancy.
- Use cautiously with thyrotoxicosis, diabetes, hypertension, CV disorders; prostatic hypertrophy, unstable vasomotor syndrome; lactation.

## Dosage

**Available Forms:** Nasal solution—0.125%, 0.16%, 0.25%, 0.5%, 1%; ophthalmic solution—0.12%, 2.5%, 10%; injection—10 mg/ml

Parenteral preparations may be given IM, SC, by slow IV injection, or as a continuous IV infusion of dilute solutions; for supraventricular tachycardia and emergency use, give by direct IV injection.

### Adult

- *Mild to moderate hypotension (adjust dosage on basis of BP response):* 1–10 mg SC or IM; do not exceed an initial dose of 5 mg. A 5-mg IM dose should raise BP for 1–2 h.
  - ***IV:*** 0.1–0.5 mg. Do not exceed initial dose of 5 mg. Do not repeat more often than q10–15 min. 5 mg IV should raise the pressure for 15 min.
- *Severe hypotension and shock:* Continuous infusion: add 10 mg to 500 ml of Dextrose Injection or Sodium Chloride Injection. Start infusion at 100–180 μg/min (based on a drop factor of 20 drops/ml; this would be 100–180 drops/min). When BP is stabilized, maintain at 40–60 μg/min. If prompt vasopressor response is not obtained, add 10-mg increments to infusion bottle.
- *Spinal anesthesia:* 2–3 mg SC or IM 3–4 min before injection of spinal anesthetic.
- *Hypotensive emergencies during anesthesia:* Give 0.2 mg IV. Do not exceed 0.5 mg/dose.
- *Prolongation of spinal anesthesia:* Addition of 2–5 mg to the anesthetic solution increases the duration of motor block by as much as 50%.
- *Vasoconstrictor for regional anesthesia:* 1:20,000 concentration (add 1 mg of phenylephrine to every 20 ml of local anesthetic solution).
- *Paroxysmal supraventricular tachycardia:* Rapid IV injection (within 20–30 sec) is recommended. Do not exceed an initial dose of 0.5 mg. Subsequent doses should not exceed the preceding dose by more than 0.1–0.2 mg and should never exceed 1 mg.
- *Nasal decongestant:* 1–2 sprays of the 0.25% solution in each nostril q3–4h. In severe cases, the 0.5% or 1% solutions may be needed.
- *Vasoconstriction and pupil dilation:* 1 drop of 2.5% or 10% solution on the upper limbus. May be repeated in 1 h. Precede instillation with a local anesthetic to prevent tearing and dilution of the drug solution.
- *Uveitis to prevent posterior synechiae:* 1 drop of the 2.5% or 10% solution on the surface of the cornea with atropine.
- *Glaucoma:* 1 drop of 10% solution on the upper surface of the cornea repeated as often as necessary and in conjunction with miotics in patients with wide-angle glaucoma.
- *Intraocular surgery:* 2.5% or 10% solution may be instilled in the eye 30–60 min before the operation.
- *Refraction:* 1 drop of a cycloplegic drug followed in 5 min by 1 drop of phenylephrine 2.5% solution and in 10 min by another drop of the cycloplegic.
- *Ophthalmoscopic exam:* 1 drop of 2.5% phenylephrine solution in each eye. Mydriasis is produced in 15–30 min and lasts for 1–3 h.
- *Minor eye irritation:* 1–2 drops of the 0.12% solution in eye bid to qid as needed.

### Pediatric

- *Hypotension during spinal anesthesia:* 0.5–1 mg/25 lb SC or IM.

- *Nasal decongestion*
  - *>6 Y:* 1–2 sprays of the 0.25% solution in each nostril q3–4h.
- *Nasal decongestion*
  - *Infants:* 1 drop of the 0.125%–0.2% solution in each nostril q2–4h.
- *Refraction:* 1 drop of atropine sulfate 1% in each eye. Follow in 10–15 min with 1 drop of phenylephrine 2.5% solution and in 5–10 min with a second drop of atropine. Eyes will be ready for refraction in 1–2 h.

*GERIATRIC:* These patients are more likely to experience adverse reactions; use with caution.

## Pharmacokinetics

| *Route* | *Onset* | *Duration* |
|---|---|---|
| IV | Immediate | 15–20 min |
| IM/SC | 10–15 min | 30–120 min |

Topical generally not absorbed systemically.
*Metabolism:* Hepatic and tissue, $T_{1/2}$: 47–100 h
*Distribution:* Crosses placenta; enters breast milk

## IV facts

**Preparation:** Inject directly for emergency use; dilute phenylephrine 1 mg/L is compatible with Dextrose-Ringer's combinations; Dextrose-Lactated Ringer's combinations; Dextrose-Saline combinations; Dextrose 2 1/2%, 5%, and 10% in Water; Ringer's Injection; Lactated Ringer's Injection; 0.45% and 0.9% Sodium Chloride Injection; 1/6 M Sodium Lactate Injection.

**Infusion:** Give single dose over 20–30 sec to 1 min. Determine actual rate of continuous infusion using an infusion pump by patient response.

## Adverse effects

Less likely with topical administration.
*Systemic Administration*

- CNS: *Fear, anxiety, tenseness, restlessness, headache, lightheadedness, dizziness*, drowsiness, tremor, insomnia, hallucinations, psychological disturbances, convulsions, CNS depression, weakness, blurred vision, ocular irritation, tearing, photophobia, symptoms of paranoid schizophrenia
- CV: Cardiac arrhythmias
- GI: *Nausea*, vomiting, anorexia
- GU: Constriction of renal blood vessels and *decreased urine formation* (initial parenteral administration), *dysuria, vesical sphincter spasm* resulting in difficult and painful urination, urinary retention in males with prostatism
- Local: Necrosis and sloughing if extravasation occurs with IV use
- Other: *Pallor*, respiratory difficulty, orofacial dystonia, sweating

*Nasal Solution*

- EENT: *Blurred vision*, ocular irritation, tearing, photophobia
- Local: *Rebound congestion, local burning and stinging,* sneezing, dryness, contact dermatitis

*Ophthalmic Solutions*

- CNS: *Headache, browache, blurred vision*, photophobia, difficulty with night vision, photophobia, *pigmentary (adrenochrome) deposits in the cornea*, conjunctiva, or lids if applied to damaged cornea
- Local: *Transitory stinging on initial instillation*
- Other: Rebound miosis, decreased mydriatic response in older patients; significant BP elevation in compromised elderly patients with cardiac problems

## Clinically important drug-drug interactions

• Severe headache, hypertension, hyperpyrexia, possibly resulting in hypertensive crisis with MAO inhibitors (isocarboxazid, pargyline, phenelzine, tranylcypromine. *Do not* administer sympathomimetic amines to patients on MAOIs • Increased sympathomimetic effects with TCAs (eg, imipramine) • Excessive hypertension with furazolidone • Decreased antihypertensive effect of guanethidine, methyldopa • Potential for serious arrhythmias with halogenated hydrocarbon anesthetics

p

## ■ Nursing Considerations

### Assessment

- ***History:*** Hypersensitivity to phenylephrine; severe hypertension, ventricular tachycardia; narrow-angle glaucoma; thyrotoxicosis; diabetes, CV disorders; prostatic hypertrophy; unstable vasomotor syndrome; pregnancy; lactation
- ***Physical:*** Skin color, temperature; orientation, reflexes, affect, peripheral sensation, vision, pupils; BP, P, auscultation, peripheral perfusion; R, adventitious sounds; urinary output, bladder percussion, prostate palpation; ECG

### Implementation

- Protect parenteral solution from light; do not administer unless solution is clear; discard unused portion.
- Maintain an alpha-adrenergic blocking agent on standby in case of severe reaction or overdose.
- Infiltrate area of extravasation with phentolamine (5–10 mg in 10–15 ml of saline), using a fine hypodermic needle; usually effective if area is infiltrated within 12 h of extravasation.
- Monitor P, BP continuously during parenteral administration.
- Do not administer ophthalmic solution that has turned brown or contains precipitates; prevent prolonged exposure to air and light.
- Administer ophthalmic solution as follows: have patient lie down or tilt head backward and look at ceiling. Hold dropper above eye; drop medicine inside lower lid while patient is looking up. Do not touch dropper to eye, fingers, or any surface. Have patient keep eye open and avoid blinking for at least 30 sec. Apply gentle pressure with fingers to inside corner of the eye for about 1 min. Caution patient not to close eyes tightly and not to blink more often than usual.
- Do not administer other eye drops for at least 5 min after phenylephrine.
- Do not administer nasal decongestant for longer than 3–5 d.
- Do not administer ophthalmic solution for longer than 72 h.
- Monitor BP and cardiac response regularly in patients with any CV disorders.
- Use topical anesthetics if ophthalmic preparations are painful and burning.
- Monitor CV effects carefully; patients with hypertension who take this drug may experience changes in BP because of the additional vasoconstriction. If a nasal decongestant is needed, pseudoephedrine is the drug of choice.

### Drug-specific teaching points

- Do not exceed recommended dose. Demonstrate proper administration technique for topical nasal and ophthalmic preparations.
- Avoid prolonged use, because underlying medical problems can be disguised. Limit is 3–5 d for nasal decongestant, 72 h for ophthalmic preparations.
- The following side effects may occur: dizziness, drowsiness, fatigue, apprehension (use caution if driving or performing tasks that require alertness); *nasal solution*, burning or stinging when first used (transient); *ophthalmic solution*, slight stinging when first used (usually transient); blurring of vision.
- Report nervousness, palpitations, sleeplessness, sweating; *ophthalmic solution*, severe eye pain, vision changes, floating spots, eye redness or sensitivity to light, headache.

## phenytoin

***(fen' i toe in)***

phenytoin sodium

diphenylhydantoin

Dilantin-125, Dilantin Infetab, Dilantin Kapseals

**Pregnancy Category D**

### Drug classes

Antiepileptic agent
Hydantoin

### Therapeutic actions

Has antiepileptic activity without causing general CNS depression; stabilizes neuronal membranes and prevents hyperexcitability caused by excessive stimulation; limits the spread of seizure activity from an active focus; also effective in treating cardiac arrhythmias, especially those induced by digitalis; antiarrhythmic properties are very similar to those of lidocaine; both are Class IB antiarrhythmics.

### Indications

- Control of grand mal (tonic-clonic) and psychomotor seizures
- Prevention and treatment of seizures occurring during or following neurosurgery
- Control of status epilepticus of the grand mal type (parenteral administration)
- Unlabeled uses: antiarrhythmic, particularly in digitalis-induced arrhythmias (IV preparations); treatment of trigeminal neuralgia (tic douloureux)

### Contraindications/cautions

- Contraindications: hypersensitivity to hydantoins, sinus bradycardia, sinoatrial block, Stokes-Adams syndrome, pregnancy (data suggest an association between antiepileptic drug use and an elevated incidence of birth defects; however, do not discontinue antiepileptic therapy in pregnant women who are receiving such therapy to prevent major seizures; this is likely to precipitate status epilepticus, with attendant hypoxia and risk to both mother and fetus), lactation.
- Use cautiously with acute intermittent porphyria, hypotension, severe myocardial insufficiency, diabetes mellitus, hyperglycemia.

### Dosage

**Available Forms:** Chewable tablets—50 mg; oral suspension—125 mg/5 ml; capsules—30, 100 mg; injection—50 mg/ml

**ADULT**

**Phenytoin sodium, parenteral**

- *Status epilepticus:* 10–15 mg/kg by slow IV. Maintenance: 100 mg PO or IV q6–8h. Higher doses may be required. Dosage also may be calculated on the basis of 10–15 mg/kg administered in divided doses of 5–10 mg/kg. Do not exceed an infusion rate of 50 mg/min. Follow each IV injection with an injection of sterile saline through the same needle or IV catheter to avoid local venous irritation by the alkaline solution. Continuous IV infusion is not recommended.
- *Neurosurgery (prophylaxis):* 100–200 mg IM q4h during surgery and the postoperative period (IM route is not recommended because of erratic absorption, pain and muscle damage at the injection site).
- *IM therapy in a patient previously stabilized on oral dosage:* Increase dosage by 50% over oral dosage. When returning to oral dosage, decrease dose by 50% of the original oral dose for 1 wk to prevent excessive plasma levels due to continued absorption from IM tissue sites.

**Phenytoin and phenytoin sodium, oral**

Individualize dosage. Determine serum levels for optimal dosage adjustments. The clinically effective serum level is usually between 10 and 20 μg/ml.

- *Loading dose (hospitalized patients without renal or liver disease):* Initially, 1 g of phenytoin capsules (phenytoin sodium, prompt) is divided into 3 doses (400 mg, 300 mg, 300 mg) and given q2h. Normal maintenance dosage is then instituted 24 h after the loading dose with frequent serum determinations.
- *No previous treatment:* Start with 100 mg tid PO. Satisfactory maintenance dosage is usually 300–400 mg/d. An increase to 600 mg/d may be necessary.
- *Single daily dosage (phenytoin sodium, extended):* If seizure control is established with divided doses of 3 100-mg extended phenytoin sodium capsules per day, once-a-day dosage with 300 mg PO may be considered.

**PEDIATRIC**

**Phenytoin sodium, parenteral**

- *Status epilepticus:* Administer phenytoin IV. Determine dosage according to weight in proportion to dose for a 150 lb (70 kg) adult (see adult dosage above; see Appendix C for calculation of pediatric doses). Pediatric dosage may be calculated on the basis of 250 mg/m$^2$. Dosage for infants and children also may be calculated on the basis of 10–15 mg/kg, given in divided doses of 5–10 mg/kg.

p

For neonates, 15–20 mg/kg in divided doses of 5–10 mg/kg is recommended.

**Phenytoin and phenytoin sodium, oral**

– *Children not previously treated:* Initially, 5 mg/kg per day in 2–3 equally divided doses. Subsequent dosage should be individualized to a maximum of 300 mg/d. Daily maintenance dosage is 4–8 mg/kg. Children >6 y may require the minimum adult dose of 300 mg/d.

GERIATRIC AND HEPATIC IMPAIRMENT: Use caution and monitor for early signs of toxicity; phenytoin is metabolized in the liver.

### Pharmacokinetics

| *Route* | *Onset* | *Peak* | *Duration* |
|---|---|---|---|
| Oral | Slow | 2–12 h | 6–12 h |
| IV | 1–2 h | Rapid | 12–24 h |

*Metabolism:* Hepatic, $T_{1/2}$: 6–24 h
*Distribution:* Crosses placenta; enters breast milk
*Excretion:* Urine

### IV facts

**Preparation:** Administration by IV infusion is not recommended because of low solubility of drug and likelihood of precipitation; however, this may be feasible if proper precautions are observed. Use suitable vehicle of 0.9% Sodium Chloride or Lactated Ringer's Injection, appropriate concentration; prepare immediately before administration, and use an inline filter.

**Infusion:** Infuse slowly in small increments, each 25–50 mg over 1–5 min; infuse flush immediately after drug to reduce the risk of damage to vein and tissues.

### Adverse effects

Some adverse effects are related to plasma concentrations, as follows:

| | |
|---|---|
| 5–10 μg/ml | Some therapeutic effects |
| 10–20 μg/ml | Usual therapeutic range |
| >20 μg/ml | Far-lateral nystagmus risk |
| >30 μg/ml | Ataxia is usually seen |
| >40 μg/ml | Significantly diminished mental capacity |

- CNS: *Nystagmus, ataxia, dysarthria, slurred speech, mental confusion, dizziness, drowsiness, insomnia, transient nervousness, motor twitchings, fatigue, irritability, depression, numbness, tremor, headache*, photophobia, diplopia, conjunctivitis
- GI: *Nausea*, vomiting, diarrhea, constipation, *gingival hyperplasia*, toxic hepatitis, **liver damage,** sometimes fatal; hypersensitivity reactions with hepatic involvement, including hepatocellular degeneration and fatal hepatocellular necrosis
- Respiratory: Pulmonary fibrosis, acute pneumonitis
- Hematologic: **Hematopoietic complications,** sometimes fatal: thrombocytopenia, leukopenia, granulocytopenia, agranulocytosis, pancytopenia; macrocytosis and megaloblastic anemia that usually respond to folic acid therapy; eosinophilia, monocytosis, leukocytosis, simple anemia, hemolytic anemia, aplastic anemia, hyperglycemia
- GU: Nephrosis
- Dermatologic: Dermatologic reactions, scarlatiniform, morbilliform, maculopapular, urticarial and nonspecific rashes; serious and sometimes fatal dermatologic reactions—**bullous, exfoliative, or purpuric dermatitis, lupus erythematosus, and Stevens-Johnson syndrome;** toxic epidermal necrolysis, hirsutism, alopecia, coarsening of the facial features, enlargement of the lips, Peyronie's disease
- Other: Lymph node hyperplasia, sometimes progressing to frank malignant lymphoma, monoclonal gammopathy and multiple myeloma (prolonged therapy), polyarthropathy, osteomalacia, weight gain, chest pain, periarteritis nodosa
- IV use complications: Hypotension, transient hyperkinesia, drowsiness, nystagmus, circumoral tingling, vertigo, nausea, cardiovascular collapse, CNS depression

### Clinically important drug-drug interactions

• Increased pharmacologic effects with chloramphenicol, cimetidine, disulfiram, isoniazid, phenacemide, phenylbutazone, sulfonamides, trimethoprim • Complex interactions and effects when phenytoin and valproic acid are given together; phenytoin toxicity with apparently normal serum phenytoin levels; decreased plasma levels of valproic acid; breakthrough seizures when the two drugs are given together • Decreased pharmacologic effects with antineoplastics, diazoxide, folic acid, sucralfate, rifampin, theophylline (applies only to oral hydantoins, absorption of which is decreased) • Increased pharmacologic effects and toxicity with primidone, oxyphenbutazone, amiodarone, chloramphenicol, fluconazole, isoniazid • Increased hepatotoxicity with acetaminophen • Decreased pharmacologic effects of the following: corticosteroids, cyclosporine, dicumarol, disopyramide, doxycycline, estrogens, furosemide, levodopa, methadone, metyrapone, mexiletine, oral contraceptives, quinidine, atracurium, gallamine triethiodide, metocurine, pancuronium, tubocurarine, vecuronium, carbamazepine, diazoxide • Severe hypotension and bradycardia when IV phenytoin is given with dopamine

**Drug-lab test interferences**

- Interference with the metyrapone and the 1 mg dexamethasone tests for at least 7 d

## ■ Nursing Considerations

### Assessment

- *History:* Hypersensitivity to hydantoins; sinus bradycardia, AV heart block, Stokes-Adams syndrome, acute intermittent porphyria, hypotension, severe myocardial insufficiency, diabetes mellitus, hyperglycemia, pregnancy, lactation
- *Physical:* T; skin color, lesions; lymph node palpation; orientation, affect, reflexes, vision exam; P, BP; R, adventitious sounds; bowel sounds, normal output, liver evaluation; periodontal exam; liver function tests, urinalysis, CBC and differential, blood proteins, blood and urine glucose, EEG and ECG

### Implementation

- Use only clear parenteral solutions; a faint yellow color may develop, but this has no effect on potency. If the solution is refrigerated or frozen, a precipitate might form, but this will dissolve if the solution is allowed to stand at room temperature. Do not use solutions that have haziness or a precipitate.
- Administer IV slowly to prevent severe hypotension; the margin of safety betwen full therapeutic and toxic doses is small. Continually monitor patient's cardiac rhythm and check BP frequently and regularly during IV infusion. Suggest use of fosphenytoin sodium if IV route is needed.
- Monitor injection sites carefully; drug solutions are very alkaline and irritating.
- Monitor for therapeutic serum levels of 10–20 $\mu$g/ml.
- Give oral drug with food to enhance absorption and to reduce GI upset.
- Recommend that the oral phenytoin prescription be filled with the same brand each time; differences in bioavailability have been documented.
- Suggest that adult patients who are controlled with 300-mg extended phenytoin capsules try once-a-day dosage to increase compliance and convenience.
- Reduce dosage, discontinue phenytoin, or substitute other antiepileptic medication gradually; abrupt discontinuation may precipitate status epilepticus.
- Phenytoin is ineffective in controlling absence (petit mal) seizures. Patients with combined seizures will need other medication for their absence seizures.
- Discontinue drug if skin rash, depression of blood count, enlarged lymph nodes, hypersensitivity reaction, signs of liver damage, or Peyronie's disease (induration of the corpora cavernosa of the penis) occurs. Institute another antiepileptic drug promptly.
- Monitor hepatic function periodically during chronic therapy; monitor blood counts, urinalysis monthly.
- Monitor blood or urine sugar of patients with diabetes mellitus regularly. Adjustment of dosage of hypoglycemic drug may be necessary because antiepileptic drug may inhibit insulin release and induce hyperglycemia.
- Have lymph node enlargement occurring during therapy evaluated carefully.

Lymphadenopathy that simulates Hodgkin's disease has occurred. Lymph node hyperplasia may progress to lymphoma.
- Monitor blood proteins to detect early malfunction of the immune system (eg, multiple myeloma).
- Arrange dental instruction in proper oral hygiene technique for long-term patients to prevent development of gum hyperplasia.

### Drug-specific teaching points

- Take this drug exactly as prescribed, with food to enhance absorption and reduce GI upset; be especially careful not to miss a dose if you are on once-a-day therapy.
- Do not discontinue this drug abruptly or change dosage, except on the advice of your prescriber.
- Maintain good oral hygiene (regular brushing and flossing) to prevent gum disease; arrange frequent dental checkups to prevent serious gum disease.
- Arrange for frequent checkups to monitor your response to this drug.
- Monitor your blood or urine sugar regularly, and report any abnormality to your nurse or physician if you are a diabetic.
- This drug is not recommended for use during pregnancy. It is advisable to use some form of contraception other than birth control pills.
- The following side effects may occur: drowsiness, dizziness, confusion, blurred vision (avoid driving or performing other tasks requiring alertness or visual acuity); GI upset (take drug with food, eat frequent, small meals).
- Wear a medical alert tag so that any emergency medical personnel will know that you are an epileptic taking antiepileptic medication.
- Report skin rash, severe nausea or vomiting, drowsiness, slurred speech, impaired coordination (ataxia), swollen glands, bleeding, swollen or tender gums, yellowish discoloration of the skin or eyes, joint pain, unexplained fever, sore throat, unusual bleeding or bruising, persistent headache, malaise, any indication of an infection or bleeding tendency, abnormal erection, pregnancy.

## pimozide

*(pi' moe zyde)*
Orap
**Pregnancy Category C**

### Drug classes

Diphenylbutylpiperdine
Antipsychotic

### Therapeutic actions

Blocks CNS dopaminergic receptors with no effect on the norephinephrine receptors.

### Indications

- Suppression of severely compromising motor and phonic tics in patients with Gilles de la Tourette's syndrome who have failed to respond adequately to standard treatment

### Contraindications/cautions

- Contraindications: simple tics or tics not associated with Tourette's syndrome, drug-induced motor tics, congenital long Q-T intervals, history of cardiac arrhythmias, severe toxic CNS depression, comatose states, hypersensitivity to pimozide, lactation.
- Use cautiously with pregnancy, hepatic or renal impairment, hypokalemia.

### Dosage

**Available Forms:** Tablets—2 mg
*ADULT:* 1–2 mg/d PO in divided doses; increase every other day to maintenance of not more than 10 mg/d.
*PEDIATRIC < 12 Y):* Not recommended.

### Pharmacokinetics

| *Route* | *Onset* | *Peak* |
|---|---|---|
| Oral | Varies | 6–8 h |

*Metabolism:* Hepatic, $T_{1/2}$: 55 h
*Distribution:* Crosses placenta; may enter breast milk
*Excretion:* Urine

**Adverse effects**

- CNS: *Lightheadedness, dizziness, sedation,* extrapyramidal effects, persistent tardive dyskinesia, neuroleptic malignant syndrome, *headache, visual disturbances*
- GI: Nausea, vomiting, dry mouth, anorexia, constipation, diarrhea, belching
- CV: Prolonged Q-T intervals, cardiac arrhythmias, hypotension, postural hypotension
- GU: Impotence, nocturia, urinary frequency
- **Dermatologic**: Rash, sweating, skin irritation
- **Other**: Weight change, periorbital edema

## ■ Nursing Considerations

### Assessment

- *History:* Simple tics or tics not associated with Tourette's syndrome, congenital long Q-T intervals, history of cardiac arrhythmias, severe toxic CNS depression, hypersensitivity to pimozide, lactation, hepatic or renal impairment, hypokalemia
- *Physical:* T; skin color, texture, lesions; orientation, reflexes, affect, orientation; pulse, auscultation, BP, orthostatic BP, perfusion; bowel sounds, normal output; frequency and pattern of voiding, normal output; liver, kidney function tests, electrolytes, ECG

### Implementation

- Monitor serum potassium; correct any deficiencies before administration.
- Obtain baseline ECG and Q-T interval measurement before and periodically during treatment.
- Increase dosage very slowly every other day; monitor ECG during treatment.
- Caution patient about the development of tardive dyskinesia, extrapyramidal effects; support patient if these occur; consider the use of antiparkinsonian drugs if needed.
- Do not stop drug suddenly, withdraw gradually to decrease adverse effects.

### Drug-specific teaching points

- Take drug exactly as prescribed; do not stop drug suddenly; take only the prescribed dose; sudden deaths have occurred with overdose.
- The following may be experienced while taking this drug: nausea, loss of appetite (take drug with food; lie quietly; eat frequent, small meals); dizziness, sedation, drowsiness, impaired visual acuity (avoid driving or performing other tasks that require alertness, visual acuity); restlessness, drooling, lack of coordination (request medication; the drug may need to be stopped); headache (request medication).
- Report shortness of breath or difficulty breathing, drooling, inability to walk, palpitation, feeling faint, "blacking out."

# pindolol

*(pin' doe lole)*
Visken
**Pregnancy Category B**

**Drug classes**

Beta adrenergic blocker (nonselective)
Antihypertensive

**Therapeutic actions**

Competitively blocks beta-adrenergic receptors, but also has some intrinsic sympathomimetic activity; however, the mechanism by which it lowers BP is unclear, because it only slightly decreases resting cardiac output and inconsistently affects plasma renin levels.

**Indications**

- Management of hypertension, alone or with other drugs, especially diuretics
- Unlabeled uses: treatment of ventricular arrhythmias, antipschotic-induced akathisia, situational anxiety

**Contraindications/cautions**

- Contraindications: sinus bradycardia, second- or third-degree heart block, cardiogenic shock, CHF, pregnancy (embryotoxic in preclinical studies), lactation.
- Use cautiously with diabetes or thyrotoxicosis.

P

### Dosage

**Available Forms:** Tablets—5, 10 mg

*ADULT:* Initially 5 mg PO bid. Ajdust dose as necessary in increments of 10 mg/d at 3- to 4-wk intervals to a maximum of 60 mg/d. Usual maintenance dose is 5 mg tid.

*PEDIATRIC:* Safety and efficacy not established.

### Pharmacokinetics

| Route | Onset |
|---|---|
| Oral | Varies |

*Metabolism:* Hepatic, $T_{1/2}$: 3–4 h

*Distribution:* Crosses placenta; enters breast milk

*Excretion:* Urine

### Adverse effects

- CNS: Dizziness, vertigo, tinnitus, fatigue, emotional depression, paresthesias, sleep disturbances, hallucinations, disorientation, memory loss, slurred speech
- GI: *Gastric pain, flatulence, constipation, diarrhea, nausea, vomiting,* anorexia, ischemic colitis, renal and mesenteric arterial thrombosis, retroperitoneal fibrosis, hepatomegaly, acute pancreatitis
- CV: *Bradycardia, CHF, cardiac arrhythmias, sinoatrial or AV nodal block, tachycardia,* peripheral vascular insufficiency, claudication, CVA, pulmonary edema, hypotension
- **Respiratory**: Bronchospasm, dyspnea, cough, bronchial obstruction, nasal stuffiness, rhinitis, pharyngitis (less likely than with propranolol)
- GU: *Impotence, decreased libido*, Peyronie's disease, dysuria, nocturia, frequency
- **MS**: Joint pain, arthralgia, muscle cramp
- **EENT**: Eye irritation, dry eyes, conjunctivitis, blurred vision
- **Dermatologic**: Rash, pruritus, sweating, dry skin
- **Allergic reactions**: Pharyngitis, erythematous rash, fever, sore throat, laryngospasm, respiratory distress
- **Other**: *Decreased exercise tolerance, development of ANAs,* hyperglycemia or hypoglycemia, elevated serum transaminase, alkaline phosphatase, and LDH

### Clinically important drug-drug interactions

• Increased effects with verapamil • Decreased effects with indomethacin, ibuprofen, piroxicam, sulindac • Prolonged hypoglycemic effects of insulin • Peripheral ischemia possible if pindolol combined with ergot alkaloids • Initial hypertensive episode followed by bradycardia with epinephrine • Increased "first-dose response" to prazosin • Increased serum levels and toxic effects with lidocaine • Paradoxical hypertension when clonidine is given with beta-blockers; increased rebound hypertension when clonidine is discontinued in patients on beta-blockers • Decreased bronchodilator effects of theophyllines

### Drug-lab test interferences

• Possible false results with glucose or insulin tolerance tests.

## ■ Nursing Considerations

### Assessment

- *History:* Sinus bradycardia, second- or third-degree heart block, cardiogenic shock, CHF, pregnancy, lactation, diabetes, thyrotoxicosis
- *Physical:* Weight, skin condition, neurologic status, P, BP, ECG, respiratory status, kidney and thyroid function, blood and urine glucose

### Implementation

- Do not discontinue drug abruptly after chronic therapy (hypersensitivity to catecholamines may have developed, causing exacerbation of angina, MI, and ventricular dysrhythmias). Taper drug gradually over 2 wk with monitoring.
- Consult with physician about withdrawing drug if patient is to undergo surgery (withdrawal is controversial).

### Drug-specific teaching points

- Do not stop taking this drug unless instructed to do so by a health care provider.

- Avoid driving or dangerous activities if CNS effects occur.
- Report difficulty breathing, night cough, swelling of extremities, slow pulse, confusion, depression, rash, fever, sore throat.

## piperacillin sodium

*(pi **per'** a sill in)*
Pipracil
**Pregnancy Category B**

### Drug classes
Antibiotic
Penicillin with extended spectrum

### Therapeutic actions
Bactericidal: inhibits synthesis of cell wall of sensitive organisms, causing cell death.

### Indications
- Treatment of mixed infections and presumptive therapy prior to identification of organisms
- Lower respiratory tract infections caused by *Haemophilus influenzae, Klebsiella, Pseudomonas aeruginosa, Serratia, E. coli, Bacteroides, Enterobacter*
- Intra-abdominal infections caused by *E. coli, P. aeruginosa, Clostridium, Bacteroides* species, including *Bacteroides fragilis*
- UTIs caused by *E. coli, Proteus* species, including *Proteus mirabilis, Klebsiella, P. aeruginosa,* enterococci
- Gynecologic infections caused by *Neisseria gonorrhoeae, Bacteroides,* enterococci, anaerobic cocci
- Skin and skin-structure infections caused by *E. coli, P. mirabilis,* indole-positive *Proteus, P. aeruginosa, Klebsiella, Enterobacter, Bacteroides, Serratia, Acinetobacter*
- Bone and joint infections caused by *P. aeruginosa, Bacteroides,* enterococci, anaerobic cocci
- Septicemia caused by *E. coli, Klebsiella, Enterobacter, Serratia, P. mirabilis, Streptococcus pneumoniae, P. aeruginosa, Bacteroides,* enterococci, anaerobic cocci
- Infections caused by *Streptococcus* (narrower spectrum antibiotic usually used)
- Prophylaxis in abdominal surgery

### Contraindications/cautions
- Contraindications: allergies to penicillins, cephalosporins, procaine, or other allergens.
- Use cautiously with pregnancy, lactation (may cause diarrhea or candidiasis in the infant).

### Dosage
**Available Forms:** Powder for injection—2, 3, 4 g

*ADULT:* 3–4 g q4–6h IV or IM. Do not exceed 24 g/d.

| *Surgery* | *First Dose* | *Second Dose* | *Third Dose* |
|---|---|---|---|
| Intra-abdominal | 2 g IV just before surgery | 2 g during surgery | 2 g q6h, no longer than 24 h |
| Vaginal hysterectomy | 2 g IV just before surgery | 2 g at 6 h | 2 g at 12 h |
| Cesarean section | 2 g IV after cord is clamped | 2 g at 4 h | 2 g at 8 h |
| Abdominal hysterectomy | 2 g IV just before surgery | 2 g in recovery room | 2 g after 6 h |

*PEDIATRIC:* Dosage not established for children <12 y.

*GERIATRIC OR RENAL INSUFFICIENCY:*

| *Creatinine Clearance (ml/min)* | *Dosage, UTIs* | *Systemic Infection* |
|---|---|---|
| >40 | Usual dosage | Usual dosage |
| 20–40 | 3 g q8h | 4 g q8h |
| <20 | 3 g q12h | 4 g q12h |

### Pharmacokinetics

| *Route* | *Onset* | *Peak* |
|---|---|---|
| IV | Rapid | End of infusion |
| IM | Rapid | 30–60 min |

*Metabolism:* Hepatic, $T_{1/2}$: 0.7–1.3 h
*Distribution:* Crosses placenta; enters breast milk
*Excretion:* Urine

## IV facts

**Preparation:** Reconstitute each gram for IV use with 5 ml of Bacteriostatic Water for Injection, Bacteriostatic Sodium Chloride Injection, Bacteriostatic or Sterile Water for Injection, Dextrose 5% in Water, 0.9% Sodium Chloride, Dextrose 5% and 0.9% Sodium Chloride, Lactated Ringer's Injection, Dextran 6% in 0.9% Sodium Chloride, Ringer's Injection; stable for 24 h at room temperature, up to 7 d if refrigerated.

**Infusion:** Direct injection: Administer as slowly as possible (3–5 min) to avoid vein irritation. Infusion should be run over 20–30 min.

**Incompatibilities:** Do not mix in solution with aminoglycoside solution; **do not mix** in the same IV solution as other antibiotics.

### Adverse effects

- CNS: Lethargy, hallucinations, seizures
- GI: *Glossitis, stomatitis, gastritis, sore mouth*, furry tongue, black "hairy" tongue, *nausea, vomiting, diarrhea,* abdominal pain, bloody diarrhea, enterocolitis, pseudomembranous colitis, nonspecific hepatitis
- **Hematologic**: Anemia, thrombocytopenia, leukopenia, neutropenia, prolonged bleeding time
- GU: Nephritis
- **Hypersensitivity reactions**: *Rash, fever, wheezing,* anaphylaxis
- **Other**: *Superinfections*, sodium overload—CHF
- **Local**: *Pain, phlebitis*, thrombosis at injection site

### Clinically important drug-drug interactions

- Decreased effectiveness with tetracyclines
- Inactivation of parenteral aminoglycosides (amikacin, gentamicin, kanamycin, neomycin, metilmicin, streptomycin, tobramycin)

### Drug-lab test interferences

- False-positive Coombs' test with IV piperacillin.

## ■ Nursing Considerations

### Assessment

- *History:* Allergies to penicillins, cephalosporins, procaine, or other allergens; pregnancy; lactation
- *Physical:* Culture infection; skin color, lesions; R, adventitious sounds; bowel sounds: CBC, liver and renal function tests, serum electrolytes, Hct, urinalysis

### Implementation

- Culture infection before beginning treatment; reculture if response is not as expected.
- Continue therapy for at least 2 d after signs of infection have disappeared, usually 7–10 d.
- Administer by IM or IV routes only.
- Reconstitute each gram for IM use with 2 ml Sterile or Bacteriostatic Water for Injection, 0.5% or 1.0% lidocaine HCl without epinephrine, Bacteriostatic Sodium Chloride Injection, Sodium Chloride Injection. Do not exceed 2 g per injection. Inject deep into a large muscle, such as upper outer quadrant of the buttock. Do not inject into lower or mid-third of upper arm.
- Carefully check IV site for signs of thrombosis or drug reaction.
- Do not give IM injections repeatedly in the same site, atrophy can occur; monitor injection sites.
- Maintain epinephrine, IV fluids, vasopressors, bronchodilators, oxygen, and emergency equipment on standby in case of serious hypersensitivity reaction.

### Drug-specific teaching points

- This drug must be given by injection.
- The following side effects may occur: upset stomach, nausea, diarrhea (small, frequent meals may help), mouth sores (frequent mouth care may help), pain or discomfort at the injection site.
- Report difficulty breathing, rashes, severe diarrhea, severe pain at injection site, mouth sores.

# pirbuterol acetate

*(peer **byoo'** ter ole)*

Maxair

**Pregnancy Category C**

## Drug classes

Sympathomimetic
Beta-2 selective adrenergic agonist
Bronchodilator
Antiasthmatic agent

## Therapeutic actions

Relatively selective beta-adrenergic stimulator; acts at beta$_2$-adrenergic receptors to cause bronchodilation (and vasodilation); at higher doses, beta$_2$-selectivity is lost, and the drug also acts at beta$_1$ receptors to cause typical sympathomimetic cardiac effects.

## Indications

- Prophylaxis and treatment of reversible bronchospasm, including asthma

## Contraindications/cautions

- Contraindications: hypersensitivity to pirbuterol, tachyarrhythmias, general anesthesia with halogenated hydrocarbons or cyclopropane, unstable vasomotor system disorders, hypertension.
- Use cautiously with coronary insufficiency, history of stroke, COPD patients who have developed degenerative heart disease, hyperthyroidism, history of seizure disorders, psychoneurotic individuals, pregnancy, lactation.

## Dosage

**Available Forms:** Aerosol—0.2 mg/actuation

*ADULT:* 2 inhalations (0.4 mg) repeated q4–6h. One inhalation (0.2 mg) may be sufficient. Do not exceed a total daily dose of 12 inhalations.

*PEDIATRIC*

- *> 12 Y:* Same as adult; safety and efficacy in children < 12 y not established.

## Pharmacokinetics

| *Route* | *Onset* | *Duration* |
|---|---|---|
| Inhalation | 5 min | 5 h |

*Metabolism:* Hepatic and tissue, $T_{1/2}$: unknown

*Distribution:* Crosses placenta; may enter breast milk

*Excretion:* Urine

## Adverse effects

- CNS: *Restlessness, apprehension*, anxiety, fear, CNS stimulation, hyperkinesia, *insomnia,* tremor, drowsiness, *irritability,* weakness, vertigo, headache
- GI: *Nausea,* vomiting, heartburn, unusual or bad taste
- CV: Cardiac arrhythmias, tachycardia, palpitations, PVCs (rare), anginal pain (less likely with this drug than with bronchodilator doses of a nonselective beta-agonist; ie, isoproterenol), changes in BP, sweating, pallor, flushing
- **Respiratory**: Respiratory difficulties, pulmonary edema, coughing, bronchospasm, paradoxical airway resistance with repeated, excessive use of inhalation preparations
- **Hypersensitivity**: Immediate hypersensitivity (allergic) reactions

## Clinically important drug-drug interactions

- Increased sympathomimetic effects when given with other sympathomimetic drugs

## ■ Nursing Considerations

### Assessment

- *History:* Hypersensitivity to pirbuterol, tachyarrhythmias, general anesthesia with halogenated hydrocarbons or cyclopropane, unstable vasomotor system disorders, hypertension, coronary insufficiency, history of stroke, COPD, hyperthyroidism, seizure disorders, psychoneurotic individuals, pregnancy, lactation
- *Physical:* Weight, skin color, temperature, turgor; orientation, reflexes, affect; P, BP; R, adventitious sounds; blood and urine glucose, serum electrolytes, thyroid and liver function tests, ECG, CBC

### Implementation

- Use smallest dose for least time; drug tolerance can occur with prolonged use.

- Maintain a beta-adrenergic blocker (a cardioselective beta-blocker, such as atenolol should be used in patients with respiratory distress) on standby in case cardiac arrhythmias occur.
- Do not exceed recommended dosage; administer during second half of inspiration, as the airways are wider and distribution is more extensive.

### Drug-specific teaching points

- Do not exceed recommended dosage; adverse effects or loss of effectiveness may result. Read product instructions and ask your health care provider or pharmacist if you have any questions.
- The following side effects may occur: drowsiness, dizziness, fatigue, apprehension (use caution if driving or performing tasks that require alertness); nausea, heartburn, change in taste (small, frequent meals may help); sweating, flushing, rapid heart rate.
- Report chest pain, dizziness, insomnia, weakness, tremor or irregular heart beat, difficulty breathing, productive cough, failure to respond to usual dosage.

## piroxicam

*(peer **ox'** i kam)*

Apo-Piroxicam (CAN), Feldene, Novo-Pirocam (CAN)

**Pregnancy Category B**

### Drug classes

Nonsteroidal anti-inflammatory drug (NSAID) (oxicam derivative)

### Therapeutic actions

Anti-inflammatory, analgesic, and antipyretic activities related to inhibition of prostaglandin synthesis; exact mechanisms of action are not known.

### Indications

- Relief of the signs and symptoms of acute and chronic rheumatoid arthritis and osteoarthritis

### Contraindications/cautions

- Contraindications: pregnancy, lactation.
- Use cautiously with allergies, renal, hepatic, cardiovascular, GI conditions.

### Dosage

**Available Forms:** Capsules—10, 20 mg

*ADULT:* Single daily dose of 20 mg PO. Dose may be divided. Steady-state blood levels are not achieved for 7–12 d. Therapeutic response occurs early but progresses over several weeks; do not evaluate for 2 wk.

*PEDIATRIC:* Safety and efficacy not established.

### Pharmacokinetics

| Route | Onset | Peak |
|---|---|---|
| Oral | 1 h | 3–5 h |

*Metabolism:* Hepatic, $T_{1/2}$: 30–86 h

*Distribution:* Crosses placenta; enters breast milk

*Excretion:* Urine

### Adverse effects

*NSAIDs*

- CNS: *Headache, dizziness, somnolence, insomnia*, fatigue, tiredness, dizziness, tinnitus, ophthalmologic effects
- GI: *Nausea, dyspepsia, GI pain,* diarrhea, vomiting, *constipation*, flatulence
- Respiratory: Dyspnea, hemoptysis, pharyngitis, **bronchospasm**, rhinitis
- Hematologic: Bleeding, platelet inhibition with higher doses, neutropenia, eosinophilia, leukopenia, pancytopenia, thrombocytopenia, agranulocytosis, granulocytopenia, aplastic anemia, decreased Hgb or Hct, bone marrow depression, mennorhagia
- GU: Dysuria, renal impairment
- Dermatologic: *Rash*, pruritus, sweating, dry mucous membranes, stomatitis
- Other: Peripheral edema, **anaphylactoid reactions to fatal anaphylactic shock**

### Clinically important drug-drug interactions

• Increased serum lithium levels and risk of toxicity • Decreased antihypertensive effects of beta-blockers • Decreased therapeutic effects with cholestyramine

## ■ Nursing Considerations

### Assessment

- *History:* Allergies; renal, hepatic, CV, and GI conditions; history of ulcers; pregnancy; lactation
- *Physical:* Skin color and lesions; orientation, reflexes, ophthalmologic and audiometric evaluation, peripheral sensation; P, edema; R, adventitious sounds; liver evaluation; CBC, clotting times, renal and liver function tests; serum electrolytes, stool guaiac

### Implementation

- Give drug with food or milk if GI upset occurs.
- Arrange for periodic ophthalmologic examination during long-term therapy.
- Institute emergency procedures if overdose occurs (gastric lavage, induction of emesis, supportive therapy).

### Drug-specific teaching points

- Take drug with food or meals if GI upset occurs.
- The following side effects may occur: dizziness, drowsiness can occur (avoid driving or using dangerous machinery).
- Report sore throat, fever, rash, itching, weight gain, swelling in ankles or fingers, changes in vision, black, tarry stools.

## plasma protein fraction

Plasmanate, Plasma-Plex, Plasmatein, Protenate

**Pregnancy Category C**

### Drug classes

Blood product
Plasma protein

### Therapeutic actions

Maintains plasma colloid osmotic pressure and carries intermediate metabolites in the transport and exchange of tissue products; important in the maintenance of normal blood volume.

### Indications

- Supportive treatment of shock due to burns, trauma, surgery, and infections
- Hypoproteinemia—nephrotic syndrome, hepatic cirrhosis, toxemia of pregnancy, postoperative patients, tuberculous patients, premature infants
- Acute liver failure
- Sequestration of protein-rich fluids
- Hyperbilirubinemia and erythroblastosis fetalis as an adjunct to exchange transfusions

### Contraindications/cautions

- Contraindications: allergy to albumin, severe anemia, cardiac failure, normal or increased intravascular volume, current use of cardiopulmonary bypass.
- Use cautiously with hepatic or renal failure, pregnancy.

### Dosage

**Available Forms:** Injection—5%

Administer by IV infusion only. Contains 130–160 mEq sodium/L. Do not give more than 250 g in 48 h; if it seems that more is required, patient probably needs whole blood or plasma.

**ADULT**

- *Hypovolemic shock:* 250–500 ml as an initial dose. Do not exceed 10 ml/min. Adjust dose based on patient response.
- *Hypoproteinemia:* Daily doses of 1,000–1,500 ml are appropriate. Do not exceed 5–8 ml/min. Adjust infusion rate based on patient response.

**PEDIATRIC**

- *Hypovolemic shock:* Infuse a dose of 20–30 ml/kg at a rate not to exceed 10 ml/min. Dose may be repeated depending on patient's response.

### Pharmacokinetics

| *Route* | |
|---|---|
| IV | Stays in the intravascular space |

*Metabolism:* $T_{1/2}$: unknown
*Excretion:* Unknown

### IV facts

**Preparation:** No further preparation required; store at room temperature; discard within 4 h of entering a bottle; store at room temperature; do not use if there is sediment in the bottle.

**Infusion:** Regulate base on patient response. Do not exceed 10 ml/min.

p

**Incompatibilities:** Administer in combination with or through the same administration set as the usual IV solutions of saline or carbohydrates. Do not use with alcohol or protein hydrolysates; precipitates may form.

### Adverse effects

- CV: *Hypotension,* CHF, pulmonary edema following rapid infusion
- **Hypersensitivity reactions**: Fever, chills, changes in BP, flushing, nausea, vomiting, changes in respiration, rashes

## ■ Nursing Considerations

### Assessment

- *History:* Allergy to albumin, severe anemia, cardiac failure, normal or increased intravascular volume, current use of cardiopulmonary bypass, renal or hepatic failure
- *Physical:* Skin color, lesions; T; P, BP, peripheral perfusion; R, adventitious sounds; liver and renal function tests, Hct, serum electrolytes

### Implementation

- Administer by IV infusion only.
- Administer without regard to blood group or type.
- Consider the need for whole blood based on the patient's clinical condition; this infusion only provides symptomatic relief of the patient's hypoproteinemia.
- Monitor BP during infusion; discontinue if hypotension occurs.
- Stop infusion if headache, flushing, fever, changes in BP occur. Arrange to treat reaction with antihistamines. If a plasma protein is still needed, try material from a different lot number.
- Monitor patient's clinical response and adjust infusion rate accordingly.

### Drug-specific teaching points

- Rate will be adjusted based on your response, so constant monitoring is necessary.
- Report headache, nausea, vomiting, difficulty breathing, back pain.

# plicamycin

*(plye kay* ***mye'*** *sin)*
mithramycin
Mithracin
**Pregnancy Category X**

### Drug classes

Antibiotic
Antineoplastic

### Therapeutic actions

Tumoricidal: binds to DNA and inhibits DNA-dependent and DNA-directed RNA synthesis. Exhibits a calcium-lowering effect, acts on osteoclasts, and blocks the action of parathyroid hormone.

### Indications

- Malignant testicular tumors not amenable to successful treatment by surgery or radiation
- Hypercalcemia and hypercalciuria not responsive to other treatments in symptomatic patients with advanced neoplasms

### Contraindications/cautions

- Contraindications: allergy to plicamycin, bone marrow suppression, thrombocytopenia, thrombocytopathy, coagulation disorders or increased susceptibility to bleeding, electrolyte imbalance, pregnancy, lactation.
- Use cautiously with hepatic or renal impairment.

### Dosage

**Available Forms:** Powder for injection—2500 $\mu$g/vial

**ADULT**

- *Testicular tumors:* 25–30 $\mu$g/kg per day IV for 8–10 d unless limited by toxicity. Do not exceed 30 $\mu$g/d. Do not use course of therapy longer than 10 d. If tumor masses remain unchanged after 3–4 wk, additional courses of therapy at monthly intervals may be prescribed.
- *Hypercalcemia, hypercalciuria:* 25 $\mu$g/kg per day IV for 3–4 d. May be

repeated at 1-wk intervals until the desired effect is reached. Serum calcium may be maintained with single, weekly doses or 2–3 doses/wk.

### Pharmacokinetics

| *Route* | *Onset* | *Peak* |
|---|---|---|
| IV | Rapid | 4 h |

*Metabolism:* Hepatic, $T_{1/2}$: unknown
*Distribution:* Crosses placenta; enters breast milk
*Excretion:* Urine

### IV facts

**Preparation:** Reconstitute with 4.9 ml Sterile Water for Injection to prepare a solution of 500 mg plicamycin/ml. Prepare fresh solutions each day of therapy; dilute daily dose in 1 L of 5% Dextrose Injection or Sodium Chloride Injection.
**Infusion:** Administer by slow infusion over 4–6 h.

### Adverse effects

- CNS: Drowsiness, weakness, lethargy, malaise, headache, depression
- GI: *Anorexia, nausea, vomiting, diarrhea, stomatitis*, hepatic impairment
- Hematologic: Hemorrhagic syndrome—**epistaxis to severe bleeding and death**; depression of platelet count, WBC count, Hgb, and prothrombin content; elevated clotting time and bleeding time, abnormal clot retraction; *electrolyte abnormalities—decreased serum calcium, phosphorus, and potassium*
- GU: Renal impairment
- Local: *Cellulitis, local reaction at injection site*
- Other: Fever, phlebitis, facial flushing, skin rash

## ■ Nursing Considerations

### Assessment

- *History:* Allergy to plicamycin, bone marrow suppression, thrombocytopenia, thrombocytopathy, coagulation disorders, electrolyte imbalance, hepatic or renal impairment, pregnancy, lactation
- *Physical:* T; skin color, lesions; weight; orientation, reflexes, affect; mucous membranes, abdominal exam; CBC, platelet count, coagulation studies, renal and liver function tests, serum electrolytes, urinalysis

### Implementation

- Do not administer IM or SC as severe local reaction and tissue necrosis occurs.
- Base daily dose on body weight, using ideal weight if patient has abnormal fluid retention.
- Monitor injection site for extravasation: reports of burning or stinging. Discontinue infusion immediately, and restart in another vein. Apply moderate heat to the extravasation area.
- Monitor patient's response to therapy frequently at beginning of therapy and for several days following the last dose: monitor platelet count, PT, and bleeding time; discontinue drug, and consult with physician if significant prolongation of PT or bleeding times or thrombocytopenia occurs.
- Advise patients to avoid pregnancy while on this drug; serious fetal defects could occur; suggest contraceptive use.

### Drug-specific teaching points

- This drug must be given by injection. Prepare a calendar of return dates for additional drug therapy.
- The following side effects may occur: loss of appetite, nausea, vomiting, mouth sores (frequent mouth care, small, frequent meals may help; maintain good nutrition; an antiemetic also may be ordered); drowsiness, fatigue, lethargy, weakness (use caution if driving or operating dangerous machinery; use caution to avoid injury); serious fetal deformities if used during pregnancy (use contraceptive measures).
- Have regular blood tests to monitor the drug's effects.
- Report severe GI upset, diarrhea, vomiting, burning or pain at injection site, unusual bleeding or bruising, fever, chills, sore throat, pregnancy.

## polymyxin B sulfate

*(pol i* ***mix'*** *in)*

*Parenteral:*

*Ophthalmic:* Polymyxin B Sulfate Sterile Ophthalmic

**Pregnancy Category B**

### Drug classes
Antibiotic

### Therapeutic actions
Bactericidal: has surfactant (detergent) activity that allows it to penetrate and disrupt the cell membranes of susceptible gram-negative bacteria, causing cell death; not effective against *Proteus* species.

### Indications
- Acute infections caused by susceptible strains of *P. aeruginosa, H. influenzae, E. coli, E. aerogenes, Klebsiella pneumoniae* when less toxic drugs are ineffective or contraindicated
- Infections of the eye caused by susceptible strains of *P. aeruginosa* (ophthalmic preparations)
- Meningeal infections caused by *P. aeruginosa* (intrathecal)

### Contraindications/cautions
- Contraindications: allergy to polymyxins (polymyxin B, colistin, colistimethate).
- Use cautiously with renal disease, pregnancy, lactation.

### Dosage
**Available Forms:** Injection—500,000 U/vial; ophthalmic solution—500,000 U

ADULTS AND PEDIATRIC
- ***IV:*** 15,000–25,000 U/kg per day may be given q12h. Do not exceed 25,000 U/d.
- ***IM:*** 25,000–30,000 U/kg per day divided and given at 4- to 6-h intervals.
- ***Intrathecal:*** 50,000 U once daily for 3–4 d; then 50,000 U every other day for at least 2 wk after cultures of CSF are negative, and glucose content is normal.
- ***Ophthalmic:*** 1–2 drops in infected eye bid–q4h or as often as needed.

INFANTS
- ***IV:*** Up to 40,000 U/kg per day.
- ***IM:*** Up to 40,000 U/kg per day; doses as high as 45,000 U/kg per day have been used in cases of sepsis caused by *P. aeruginosa.*
- ***Intrathecal (<2 y):*** 20,000 U once daily for 3–4 d or 25,000 U once every other day. Continue with 25,000 U once every other day for at least 2 wk after cultures of CSF are negative and glucose content is normal.

GERIATRIC OR RENAL FAILURE: Reduce dosage from the recommended dose, and follow renal function tests during therapy.

### Pharmacokinetics

| *Route* | *Onset* | *Peak* |
|---|---|---|
| IV | Rapid | Unknown |
| IM | Gradual | 2 h |

*Metabolism:* $T_{1/2}$: 4.3–6 h
*Distribution:* Does not cross placenta
*Excretion:* Urine

### IV facts
**Preparation:** Dissolve 500,000 U in 300–500 ml of 5% Dextrose in Water. Dissolve 500,000 U in 2 ml sterile distilled water or Sodium Chloride Injection, or 1% procaine hydrochloride solution; refrigerate and discard any unused portion after 72 h.

**Infusion:** Administer by continuous IV drip using an infusion pump.

### Adverse effects
- CNS: Neurotoxicity—*facial flushing, dizziness, ataxia, drowsiness*, paresthesias
- Respiratory: Apnea (high dosage)
- GU: *Nephrotoxicity*
- Dermatologic: Rash, urticaria
- Local: *Pain at IM injection site; thrombophlebitis at IV injection sites; irritation, burning, stinging, itching, blurring of vision* (ophthalmic preparations)
- Other: Drug fever, superinfections

### Clinically important drug-drug interactions
- Increased neuromuscular blockade, apnea, and muscular paralysis when given

with nondepolarizing neuromuscular blocking drugs

## ■ Nursing Considerations

### Assessment

- *History:* Allergy to polymyxins, renal disease, lactation
- *Physical:* Site of infection, skin color, lesions; orientation, reflexes, speech; R; urinary output; urinalysis, serum creatinine, renal function tests

### Implementation

- Store drug solutions in refrigerator, and discard any unused portion after 72 h.
- For intrathecal use: Dissolve 500,000 U in 10 ml sterile physiologic saline for a concentration of 50,000 U/ml.
- For ophthalmic use: Reconstitute powder with 20–50 ml of diluent.
- Culture infection before beginning therapy.
- Monitor renal function tests during therapy.

### Drug-specific teaching points

- Administer ophthalmic preparation as follows: tilt head back; place medication into eyelid and close eyes; gently hold the inner corner of the eye for 1 min. Do not touch dropper to the eye.
- The following side effects may occur: vertigo, dizziness, drowsiness, slurring of speech (avoid driving or using hazardous equipment); numbness, tingling of the tongue, extremities (decrease the dosage); superinfections (frequent hygiene measures will help; request medications); burning, stinging, blurring of vision (ophthalmic; transient).
- Report difficulty breathing, rash or skin lesions, pain at injection site or IV site, change in urinary voiding patterns, fever, flulike symptoms, changes in vision, severe stinging or itching (ophthalmic).

## polythiazide

*(pol i* ***thye'*** *a zide)*

Renese

**Pregnancy Category C**

### Drug classes

Thiazide diuretic

### Therapeutic actions

Inhibits reabsorption of sodium and chloride in distal renal tubule, thereby increasing excretion of sodium, chloride, and water by the kidney.

### Indications

- Adjunctive therapy in edema associated with CHF, cirrhosis, corticosteroid and estrogen therapy, renal dysfunction
- Hypertension, as sole therapy or in combination with other antihypertensives
- Unlabeled use: diabetes insipidus, especially nephrogenic diabetes insipidus

### Contraindications/cautions

- Contraindications: fluid or electrolyte imbalances, pregnancy, lactation.
- Use cautiously with renal or liver disease, gout, SLE, glucose tolerance abnormalities, hyperparathyroidism, manic-depressive disorders.

### Dosage

**Available Forms:** Tablets—1, 2, 4 mg

ADULT

- *Edema:* 1–4 mg qd PO.
- *Hypertension:* 2–4 mg qd PO.

PEDIATRIC: Safety and efficacy not established.

### Pharmacokinetics

| Route | Onset | Peak | Duration |
|---|---|---|---|
| Oral | 2 h | 6 h | 24–48 h |

*Metabolism:* $T_{1/2}$: 25.7 h

*Distribution:* Crosses placenta; enters breast milk

*Excretion:* Urine

### Adverse effects

- CNS: *Dizziness, vertigo,* paresthesias, weakness, headache, drowsiness, fatigue, leukopenia, thrombocytopenia, agranulocytosis, aplastic anemia, neutropenia
- GI: *Nausea, anorexia, vomiting, dry mouth*, diarrhea, constipation, jaundice, hepatitis, pancreatitis
- CV: Orthostatic hypotension, venous thrombosis, volume depletion, cardiac arrhythmias, chest pain

p

- GU: *Polyuria, nocturia,* impotence, loss of libido
- **Dermatologic**: Photosensitivity, rash, purpura, exfoliative dermatitis, hives
- **Other**: Muscle cramps and muscle spasms, fever, gouty attacks, flushing, weight loss, rhinorrhea

### Clinically important drug-drug interactions

• Risk of hyperglycemia with diazoxide • Decreased absorption with cholestyramine, colestipol • Increased risk of digitalis glycoside toxicity if hypokalemia occurs • Increased risk of lithium toxicity with thiazides • Increased fasting blood glucose leading to need to adjust dosage of antidiabetic agents.

### Drug-lab test interferences

• Monitor for decreased PBI levels without clinical signs of thyroid disturbances.

## ■ Nursing Considerations

### Assessment

- *History:* Electrolyte imbalances, renal or liver disease, gout, SLE, glucose tolerance abnormalities, hyperparathyroidism, manic-depressive disorders, pregnancy, lactation
- *Physical:* Skin color, lesions; orientation, reflexes, muscle strength; pulses, BP, orthostatic BP, perfusion, edema, baseline ECG; R, adventitious sounds; liver evaluation, bowel sounds; CBC, serum electrolytes, blood glucose, liver and renal function tests, serum uric acid, urinalysis

### Implementation

- Administer with food or milk if GI upset occurs.
- Administer early in the day so increased urination will not disturb sleep.
- Measure and record regular body weights to monitor fluid changes.

### Drug-specific teaching points

- Take drug early in the day so sleep will not be disturbed by increased urination.
- Weigh yourself daily and record weights.
- Protect skin from exposure to sun or bright lights
- Increased urination will occur.
- Use caution if dizziness, drowsiness, feeling faint occur.
- Report rapid weight gain or loss, swelling in ankles or fingers, unusual bleding or bruising, muscle cramps.

# porfimer sodium

***(poor' fa mer)***

Photofrin

**Pregnancy Category C**

### Drug classes

Antineoplastic

### Therapeutic actions

Photosensitizing agent; cytotoxic and antitumor activity when combined with laser light to cause tumor destruction; porfimer is cleared from tissues within 72 h of injection but retained in tumor cells, which are then exposed to laser light, initiating radical formation and cell death leading to decreased tumor size.

### Indications

- Photodynamic therapy for palliation of patients with completely or partially obstructing esophageal cancer who cannot be satisfactorily treated with laser therapy alone

### Contraindications/cautions

- Contraindications: hypersensitivity to porphyrins; existing tracheoesophageal or bronchoesophageal fistula; tumors eroding a blood vessel; pregnancy; lactation

### Dosage

**Available Forms:** Cake or powder for injection—75 mg

Part of a two-stage treatment; IV infusion is followed in 40–50 h and again in 96–120 h by laser light treatment.

*ADULT:* 2 mg/kg given as a slow, single IV injection over 3–5 min.

*PEDIATRIC:* Not recommended.

### Pharmacokinetics

| *Route* | *Onset* | *Peak* |
|---|---|---|
| IV | Slow | 48 h |

*Metabolism:* Cellular; $T_{1/2}$: 250 h
*Distribution:* Crosses placenta; may enter breast milk
*Excretion:* Dispersed at the cellular level

**IV facts**

**Preparation:** Reconstitute each vial with 31.8 ml of either 5% Dextrose Injection or 0.9% Sodium Chloride Injection, resulting in a final concentration of 2.5 mg/ml and a pH of 7–8. Shake well until dissolved; do not mix with any other drugs in solution; protect from light; use immediately.
**Infusion:** Inject slowly over 3–5 min.
**Compatibilities:** Do not mix in solution with any other drugs.

### Adverse effects

- CNS: *Insomnia,* anorexia, anxiety, confusion
- GI: *Nausea, constipation, dysphagia, abdominal pain, vomiting*
- CV: Chest pain, hypotension, hypertension, arrhythmias
- Respiratory: **Pleural effusion,** *dyspnea, pneumonia, pharyngitis,* coughing, **fistula**
- Other: *Fever, pain, chest pain*

### Clinically important drug-drug interactions

- Increased photosensitizing effect with tetracyclines, sulfonamides, phenothiazines, sulfonylureas, thiazide diuretics, griseofulvin, which antagonize adenosine's activity

## ■ Nursing Considerations

### Assessment

- *History:* Hypersensitivity to porphyrins; existing tracheoesophageal or bronchoesophageal fistula; tumors eroding a blood vessel; pregnancy; lactation
- *Physical:* T; orientation, affect; BP, P, auscultation; R, adventitious sounds

### Implementation

- Ensure that patient does not have a tracheoesophageal or bronchoesophageal fistula before administering porfimer.
- Schedule administration to coincide with laser treatment at appropriate times (40–50 h and 96–120 h after injection).
- A minimum of 30 days must elapse before treatment is repeated; treatment may be repeated up to three times.
- Avoid extravasation; if it occurs, protect area from exposure to light.
- Avoid contact with any spilled drug; wipe up spills with a damp cloth, using rubber gloves and eye protection; dispose of as contaminated material.
- Protect patient from exposure to light; protect eyes and cover skin for 30 d after treatment. Sunscreens are of no value.
- Provide burn therapy for patients exposed to bright light during photosensitization period.

### Drug-specific teaching points

- This drug will be given IV and will be followed by laser light therapy.
- Avoid any exposure to sunlight or bright indoor light (examination lamps, dentist's lights, unshaded light bulbs) for 30 days after use of this drug. Cover skin and use protective eyewear. You will be extremely sensitive to light, and exposure could cause burns, blistering, and severe damage.
- The following side effects may occur: feelings of anxiety, insomnia; GI disturbances; fever.
- Report chest pain, increased difficulty swallowing, difficulty breathing, skin or eye damage from light exposure.

P

# Potassium salts

## potassium acetate

## potassium chloride

*(po **tass'** ee um)*

*Oral:* Cena-K, Gen-K, Kaochlor, Kaon-Cl, Kay Ciel, K-Dur 10, K-Dur 20, K-Lor, Klor-Con, Klorvess, Klotrix, K-Lyte/Cl, Kolyum. Potasalan, Rum-K, Slow-K, Ten K

*Injection:* Potassium Chloride

*(continues)*

## potassium gluconate

Kaon, K-G Elixir, Kolyum, Tri-K, Twin-K

**Pregnancy Category C**

### Drug classes

Electrolyte

### Therapeutic actions

Principal intracellular cation of most body tissues, participates in a number of physiologic processes—maintaining intracellular tonicity, transmission of nerve impulses, contraction of cardiac, skeletal and smooth muscle, maintenance of normal renal function; also plays a role in carbohydrate metabolism and various enzymatic reactions.

### Indications

- Prevention and correction of potassium deficiency; when associated with alkalosis, use potassium chloride; when associated with acidosis, use potassium acetate, bicarbonate, citrate, or gluconate
- Treatment of cardiac arrhythmias due to cardiac glycosides (IV)

### Contraindications/cautions

- Contraindications: allergy to tartrazine, aspirin (tartrazine is found in some preparations marketed as Kaon-Cl, Klor-Con); severe renal impairment with oliguria, anuria, azotemia; untreated Addison's disease; hyperkalemia; adynamia episodica hereditaria; acute dehydration; heat cramps; GI disorders that delay passage in the GI tract.
- Use cautiously with cardiac disorders, especially if treated with digitalis, pregpancy, lactation.

### Dosage

**Available Forms:** Liquids—20, 30, 40, 45 mEq/15 ml; powders—15, 20, 25 mEq/packet; effervescent tablets—20, 25, 50 mEq; CR tablets—6, 7, 8, 10, 20 mEq; CR capsules—8, 10 mEq; tablets—500, 595 mg; injection—2, 4, 10, 20, 30, 40, 60, 90 mEq

Individualize dosage based on patient response using serial ECG and electrolyte determinations in severe cases.

ADULT

- *Prevention of hypokalemia:* 16–24 mEq/d PO.
- *Treatment of potassium depletion:* 40–100 mEq/d PO.
- *IV infusion:* Do not administer undiluted. Dilute in dextrose solution to 40–80 mEq/L. Use the following as a guide to administration:

| *Serum $K^+$ in mEq/L* | *Maximum Infusion Rate* | *Maximum Concentration* | *Maximum 24-h Dose* |
|---|---|---|---|
| >2.6 | 10 mEq/h | 40 mEq/L | 200 mEq |
| <2.0 | 40 mEq/h | 80 mEq/L | 400 mEq |

PEDIATRIC: Replacement: 3 mEq/Kg/d or 40 mg/m$^2$/d PO or IV.

GERIATRIC AND RENAL IMPAIRED: Carefully monitor serum potassium concentration and reduce dosage appropriately.

### Pharmacokinetics

| *Route* | *Onset* | *Peak* |
|---|---|---|
| Oral | Slow | 1–2 h |
| IV | Rapid | |

*Metabolism:* Cellular, $T_{1/2}$: unknown
*Distribution:* Crosses placenta; enters breast milk
*Excretion:* Urine

### IV facts

**Preparation:** Do not administer undiluted potassium IV; dilute in dextrose solution to 40–80 mEq/L; in critical states, potassium chloride can be administered in saline.

**Infusion:** Adjust dosage based on patient response at a maximum of 10 mEq/l.

### Adverse effects

- **GI:** *Nausea, vomiting, diarrhea, abdominal discomfort,* GI obstruction, GI bleeding, GI ulceration or perforation
- **Hematologic:** Hyperkalemia—increased serum $K^+$, ECG changes (peaking of T

waves, loss of P waves, depression of ST segment, prolongation of QT interval)
- **Dermatologic**: Skin rash
- **Local**: Tissue sloughing, local necrosis, local phlebitis, and venospasm with injection

### Clinically important drug-drug interactions

• Increased risk of hyperkalemia with potassium-sparing diuretics, salt substitutes using potassium

## ■ Nursing Considerations

### Assessment

- *History:* Allergy to tartrazine, aspirin; severe renal impairment; untreated Addison's disease; hyperkalemia; adynamia episodica hereditaria; acute dehydration; heat cramps, GI disorders that cause delay in passage in the GI tract, cardiac disorders, lactation
- *Physical:* Skin color, lesions, turgor; injection sites; P, baseline ECG; bowel sounds, abdominal exam; urinary output; serum electrolytes, serum bicarbonate

### Implementation

- Arrange for serial serum potassium levels before and during therapy.
- Administer liquid form to any patient with delayed GI emptying.
- Administer oral drug after meals or with food and a full glass of water to decrease GI upset.
- Caution patient not to chew or crush tablets; have patient swallow tablet whole.
- Mix or dissolve oral liquids, soluble powders, and effervescent tablets completely in 3–8 oz of cold water, juice, or other suitable beverage, and have patient drink it slowly.
- Arrange for further dilution or dose reduction if GI effects are severe.
- Agitate prepared IV solution to prevent "layering" of potassium; do not add potassium to an IV bottle in the hanging position.
- Monitor IV injection sites regularly for necrosis, tissue sloughing, phlebitis.
- Monitor cardiac rhythm carefully during IV administration.
- Caution patient that expended wax matrix capsules will be found in the stool.
- Caution patient not to use salt substitutes.

### Drug-specific teaching points

- Take drug after meals or with food and a full glass of water to decrease GI upset. Do not chew or crush tablets, swallow tablets whole. Mix or dissolve oral liquids, soluble powders, and effervescent tablets completely in 3–8 oz of cold water, juice, or other suitable beverage, and drink it slowly. Take the drug as prescribed; do not take more than prescribed.
- The following side effects may occur: nausea, vomiting, diarrhea (taking the drugs with meals, diluting them further may help).
- Do not use salt substitutes.
- You may find wax matrix capsules in the stool. The wax matrix is not absorbed in the GI tract.
- Have periodic blood tests and medical evaluation.
- Report tingling of the hands or feet, unusual tiredness or weakness, feeling of heaviness in the legs, severe nausea, vomiting, abdominal pain, black or tarry stools, pain at IV injection site.

p

## pralidoxime chloride

*(pra li **dox'** eem)*

PAM

Protopam Chloride

**Pregnancy Category C**

### Drug classes

Antidote

### Therapeutic actions

Reactivates cholinesterase (mainly outside the CNS) inactivated by phosphorylation due to organophosphate pesticide or related compound.

## Indications

- Antidote in poisoning due to organophosphate pesticides and chemicals with anticholinesterase activity
- IM use as an adjunct to atropine in poisoning by nerve agents having anticholinesterase activity (autoinjector)
- Control of overdosage by anticholinesterase drugs used to treat myasthenia gravis

## Contraindications/cautions

- Contraindications: allergy to any component of drug.
- Use cautiously with impaired renal function, myasthenia gravis, pregnancy, lactation.

## Dosage

**Available Forms:** Injection—600 mg, 1 g

### Adult

- ***Organophosphate poisoning:*** In absence of cyanosis, give atropine 2–4 mg IV. If cyanosis is present, give 2–4 mg atropine IM while improving ventilation; repeat every 5–10 min until signs of atropine toxicity appear. Maintain atropinization for at least 48 h. *Give pralidoxime concomitantly:* inject an initial dose of 1–2 g pralidoxime IV, preferably as a 15- to 30-min infusion in 100 ml of saline. After 1 h, give a second dose of 1–2 g IV if muscle weakness is not relieved. Give additional doses cautiously. If IV administration is not feasible or if pulmonary edema is present, give IM or SC.
- ***Anticholinesterase overdosage (eg, neostigmine, pyridostigmine, ambenonium):*** 1–2 g IV followed by increments of 250 mg q5 min.
- ***Exposure to nerve agents:*** Administer atropine and pralidoxime as soon as possible after exposure. Use the autoinjectors, giving the atropine first; repeat after 15 min. If symptoms exist after an additional 15 min, repeat injections. If symptoms persist after third set of injections, seek medical help.

### Pediatric

- ***Organophosphate poisoning:*** 20–40 mg/kg IV per dose given as above.

## Pharmacokinetics

| *Route* | *Onset* | *Peak* |
|---|---|---|
| IV | Rapid | 5–15 min |
| IM | Rapid | 10–20 min |

*Metabolism:* Hepatic, $T_{1/2}$: 0.8–2.7 h
*Distribution:* May cross placenta or enter breast milk
*Excretion:* Urine

## IV facts

**Preparation:** Dilute in 1–2 g pralidoxime in 100 ml saline.
**Infusion:** Administer over 15–30 min.

## Adverse effects

- CNS: *Dizziness, blurred vision, diplopia,* impaired accommodation, *headache*, drowsiness, nausea
- CV: Tachycardia
- **Respiratory**: Hyperventilation
- **Hematologic**: *Transient SGOT, SGPT, CPK elevations*
- **Local**: *Mild to moderate pain at the injection site* 40–60 min after IM injection
- **Other**: Muscular weakness

## ■ Nursing Considerations

### Assessment

- ***History:*** Allergy to any component of drug; impaired renal function; myasthenia gravis; lactation
- ***Physical:*** Reflexes, orientation, vision exam, muscle strength; P, auscultation, baseline ECG; liver evaluation; renal and liver function tests

### Implementation

- Remove secretions, maintain patent airway, and provide artificial ventilation as needed for acute organophosphate poisoning; then begin drug therapy.
- Institute treatment as soon as possible after exposure to the poison.
- Remove clothing; thoroughly wash hair and skin with sodium bicarbonate or alcohol as soon as possible after dermal exposure to organophosphate poisoning.
- Use IV sodium thiopental or diazepam if convulsions interfere with respiration after organophosphate poisoning.

- Administer by slow IV infusion; tachycardia, laryngospasm, muscle rigidity have occurred with rapid injection.

### Drug-specific teaching points

- Discomfort may be experienced at IM injection site. If you receive the autoinjector, you need to understand the indications and proper use of the mechanism, review the signs, and symptoms of poisoning.
- Report blurred or double vision, dizziness, nausea.

## pramipexole

*(pram ah **pex'** ole)*
Mirapex

### Drug classes

Antiparkinsonism agent
Dopamine receptor agonist

### Therapeutic actions

Stimulates dopamine receptors in the striatum, leading to decrease in parkinsonian symptoms thought to be related to low dopamine levels.

### Indications

- Treatment of the signs and symptoms of idiopathic Parkinson's disease

### Contraindications/cautions

- Contraindications: hypersensitivity to pramipexole.
- Use cautiously with symptomatic hypotension, impaired renal function, pregnancy, lactation.

### Dosage

**Available Forms:** Tablets—0.125, 0.25, 1, 1.5 mg

*ADULT:* Increase dosage gradually from a starting dose of 0.125 mg PO tid; wk 2—0.25 mg PO tid; wk 3—0.5 mg PO tid; wk 4—0.75 mg PO tid; wk 5—1 mg PO tid; wk 6—1.25 mg PO tid; wk 7—1.5 mg PO tid. If used in combination with levodopa, consider a reduction of dose.

*PEDIATRIC:* Safety and efficacy not established.

*RENAL IMPAIRMENT*

| Ccr | Dose |
|---|---|
| >60 | 0.125 mg PO tid starting dose to maximum of 1.5 mg PO tid |
| 35–59 | 0.125 mg PO bid starting dose to maximum of 1.5 mg PO bid |
| 15–34 | 0.125 mg PO qd starting dose to maximum of 1.5 mg PO qd |

### Pharmacokinetics

| Route | Onset | Peak |
|---|---|---|
| Oral | Varies | 2 h |

*Metabolism:* Hepatic; $T_{1/2}$:8 h
*Distribution:* May cross placenta; may pass into breast milk
*Excretion:* Urine

### Adverse effects

- CNS: *Headache, dizziness, insomnia, somnolence,* hallucinations, confusion, amnesia
- GI: *Nausea, constipation,* anorexia, dysphagia
- CV: Orthostatic hypotension, hypertension, arrhythmia, palpitations, hypotension, tachycardia
- Other: Peripheral edema, decreased weight, *asthenia,* fever

### Clinically important drug-drug interactions

• Increase in levodopa levels and effects if combined • Increase in levels with cimetidine, ranitidine, diltiazem, triamterene, verapamil, quinidine, quinine • Decreased effectiveness with dopamine antagonists

## ■ Nursing Considerations

### Assessment

- ***History:*** Hypersensitivity to pramipexole, symptomatic hypotension, impaired renal function, pregnancy, lactation
- ***Physical:*** Reflexes, affect; T, BP, P, peripheral perfusion; abdominal exam,



p

normal output; auscultation, R; urinary output, renal function tests

### Implementation

- Administer with extreme caution to patients with a history of hypotension, hallucinations, confusion, or dyskinesias.
- Administer with food if GI upset becomes a problem.
- Do not discontinue abruptly; taper gradually over at least 1 wk.
- Monitor patient while titrating drug to establish therapeutic dosage. Dosage of levodopa/carbidopa may need to be reduced accordingly to balance therapeutic effects.
- Provide safety precautions as needed if hallucinations occur (more common with elderly).

### Drug-specific teaching points

- Take this drug exactly as prescribed, three times/d, with breakfast and lunch. Continue to take your levodopa/carbidopa if prescribed. The dosage of the levodopa may need to be decreased after a few days of therapy. The dosage of pramipexole will be slowly increased over a 7-wk period. Write your dose down and follow this pattern.
- Do not stop taking this drug without consulting your nurse or physician; serious side effects could occur. The drug should be tapered over at least 1 wk.
- The following side effects may occur: dizziness, lightheadedness, insomnia (avoid driving or operating dangerous machinery); nausea (take drug with meals); edema; weight loss; low blood pressure (change positions slowly; use caution in extremes of heat or exertion); hallucinations (safety precautions may be necessary).
- Avoid becoming pregnant while on this drug; use of barrier contraceptives is advised. If you think you are pregnant, notify your health care provider.
- Report severe nausea, severe swelling, sweating, hallucinations, dizziness, fainting.

## pravastatin

*(prah va **sta'** tin)*

Pravachol

**Pregnancy Category X**

### Drug classes

Antihyperlipidemic
HMG CoA inhibitor

### Therapeutic actions

A fungal metabolite that inhibits the enzyme HMG CoA that catalyzes the first step in the cholesterol synthesis pathway, resulting in a decrease in serum cholesterol, serum LDLs (associated with increased risk of CAD), and either an increase or no change in serum HDLs (associated with decreased risk of CAD).

### Indications

- Prevention of first MI and reduction of death from CV disease in patients at risk of first MI
- Adjunct to diet in the treatment of elevated total cholesterol and LDL cholesterol with primary hypercholesterolemia (types IIa and IIb) in patients unresponsive to dietary restriction of saturated fat and cholesterol and other nonpharmacologic measures
- Slow the progression of coronary atherosclerosis in patients with clinically evident CAD to reduce the risk of acute coronary events

### Contraindications/cautions

- Contraindications: allergy to pravastatin, fungal byproducts, pregnancy, lactation.
- Use cautiously with impaired hepatic function, cataracts, alcoholism.

### Dosage

**Available Forms:** Tablets—10, 20, 40 mg

*ADULT:* Initially, 10–20 mg/d PO administered hs. Maintenance doses range from 10–40 mg/d PO in single hs dose.

- *Concomitant immunosuppressive therapy:* 10 mg PO qd to a maximum of 20 mg/d.

*PEDIATRIC:* Safety and efficacy not established.

*GERIATRIC:* 10 mg PO once daily at bedtime.

### Pharmacokinetics

| *Route* | *Onset* | *Peak* |
|---|---|---|
| Oral | Slow | 1–1 1/2 h |

*Metabolism:* Hepatic, $T_{1/2}$: 1.8 h
*Distribution:* Crosses placenta; enters breast milk
*Excretion:* Urine and feces

**Adverse effects**
- CNS: *Headache, blurred vision*, dizziness, insomnia, fatigue, muscle cramps, cataracts
- GI: *Flatulence, abdominal pain, cramps, constipation, nausea, vomiting*, heartburn
- **Hematologic**: Elevations of CPK, alkaline phosphatase, and transaminases

**Clinically important drug-drug interactions**
• Possible severe myopathy or rhabdomyolysis with cyclosporine, erythromycin, gemfibrozil, niacin • Possible increased digoxin, warfarin levels if combined; monitor patient and decrease dosage as needed • Increased pravastatin levels with itraconazole; avoid this combination

## ■ Nursing Considerations

### Assessment
- ***History:*** Allergy to pravastatin, fungal byproducts; impaired hepatic function; cataracts; pregnancy; lactation
- ***Physical:*** Orientation, affect, ophthalmologic exam; liver evaluation; lipid studies, liver function tests

### Implementation
- Administer drug hs; highest rates of cholesterol synthesis are between midnight and 5 AM.
- Arrange for periodic ophthalmologic exam to check for cataract development; monitor liver function.

### Drug-specific teaching points
- Take drug at bedtime.
- The following side effects may occur: nausea (small, frequent meals may help); headache, muscle and joint aches and pains (may lessen); sensitivity to sunlight (use sunblock and wear protective clothing).
- Have periodic ophthalmic exams while you are on this drug.
- Report severe GI upset, changes in vision, unusual bleeding or bruising, dark urine or light colored stools, muscle pain or weakness.

## praziquantel

*(pray zi **kwon'** tel)*
Biltricide
**Pregnancy Category B**

**Drug classes**
Anthelmintic

**Therapeutic actions**
Increases cell membrane permeability in susceptible worms, resulting in a loss of intracellular calcium, massive contractions, and paralysis of the worm's musculature; also causes a disintegration of the schistosome's tegument.

**Indications**
- Infections caused by *Schistosoma mekongi, Schistosoma japonicum, Schistosoma mansoni, Schistosoma haematobium,* liver flukes
- Orphan drug use: treatment of neurocysticercosis

**Contraindications/cautions**
- Allergy to praziquantel; pregnancy (abortifacient in some high-dose preclinical studies); lactation (secreted in breast milk; avoid nursing on treatment day and for 72 h thereafter); ocular cysticercosis (irreparable lesions can occur).

P

### Dosage
**Available Forms:** Tablets—600 mg
*ADULT AND PEDIATRIC (>4 Y)*
- ***Schistosomiasis:*** Three doses of 20 mg/kg PO as a 1-d treatment, with intervals of 4–6 h between doses.
- ***Clonorchiasis and opisthorchiasis:*** Three doses of 25 mg/kg PO as a 1-d treatment.

*PEDIATRIC (<4 Y):* Safety not established.

**Pharmacokinetics**

| Route | Onset | Peak |
|---|---|---|
| Oral | Varies | 1–3 h |

*Metabolism:* Hepatic, $T_{1/2}$: 0.8–1.5 h
*Distribution:* Crosses placenta; enters breast milk
*Excretion:* Urine

### Adverse effects

- CNS: Malaise, headache, dizziness
- GI: Abdominal discomfort, slight increase in liver enzymes
- Other: Fever, urticaria

## ■ Nursing Considerations

### Assessment

- *History:* Allergy to praziquantel, pregnancy, lactation
- *Physical:* Skin color, lesions; orientation, reflexes; liver function tests

### Implementation

- Culture urine or feces for ova.
- Do not administer with ocular cysticercosis.
- Do not administer on an outpatient basis with cerebral cysticercosis; consult with physician regarding hospital admission.
- Administer drug with food; have patient swallow the tablets unchewed with some liquid. If the patient keeps the tablets in the mouth, a bitter taste may result that could cause gagging or vomiting.

### Drug-specific teaching points

- Tablets should be swallowed unchewed during meals, with a small amount of liquid. Do not hold the tablet in your mouth; it has a bitter taste that could cause gagging or vomiting.
- The following side effects may occur: nausea, abdominal pain, GI upset (small, frequent meals may help); drowsiness, dizziness (use caution when driving or operating dangerous equipment).
- Report rash, severe abdominal pain, marked weakness, dizziness.

## prazosin hydrochloride

***(pra' zoe sin)***

Apo-Prazo (CAN), Minipress, Novo-Prazin (CAN), Nu-Prazo (CAN)

**Pregnancy Category C**

### Drug classes

Antihypertensive
Alpha adrenergic blocker

### Therapeutic actions

Selectively blocks postsynaptic $alpha_1$-adrenergic receptors, decreasing sympathetic tone on the vasculature, dilating arterioles and veins, and lowering supine and standing BP; unlike conventional alpha-adrenergic blocking agents (eg, phentolamine), it does not also block $alpha_2$ presynaptic receptors, so it does not cause reflex tachycardia.

### Indications

- Treatment of hypertension, alone or in combination with other agents
- Unlabeled uses: refractory CHF, management of Raynaud's vasospasm, treatment of prostatic outflow obstruction

### Contraindications/cautions

- Contraindications: hypersensitivity to prazosin, lactation.
- Use cautiously with CHF, renal failure, pregnancy.

### Dosage

**Available Forms:** Capsules—1, 2, 5 mg
*ADULT:* First dose may cause syncope with sudden loss of consciousness. First dose should be limited to 1 mg PO and given hs. Initial dosage is 1 mg PO bid–tid. Increase dosage to a total of 20 mg/d given in divided doses. When increasing dosage, give the first dose of each increment hs. Maintenance dosages most commonly range from 6–15 mg/d given in divided doses.

- *Concomitant therapy:* When adding a diuretic or other antihypertensive drug, reduce dosage to 1–2 mg PO tid and then retitrate.

*PEDIATRIC:* 0.5–7 mg PO tid.

### Pharmacokinetics

| *Route* | *Onset* | *Peak* |
|---|---|---|
| Oral | Varies | 1–3 h |

*Metabolism:* Hepatic, $T_{1/2}$: 2–3 h
*Distribution:* Crosses placenta; may enter breast milk
*Excretion:* Bile/feces, urine

### Adverse effects

- CNS: *Dizziness, headache, drowsiness, lack of energy, weakness,* nervousness, vertigo, depression, paresthesia
- GI: *Nausea,* vomiting, diarrhea, constipation, abdominal discomfort or pain
- CV: *Palpitations,* sodium and water retention, increased plasma volume, edema, dyspnea, syncope, tachycardia, orthostatic hypotension
- GU: Urinary frequency, incontinence, impotence, priapism
- EENT: Blurred vision, reddened sclera, epistaxis, tinnitus, dry mouth, nasal congestion
- Dermatologic: Rash, pruritus, alopecia, lichen planus
- Other: Diaphoresis, lupus erythematosus

### Clinically important drug-drug interactions

- Severity and duration of hypotension following first dose of prazosin may be greater in patients receiving beta-adrenergic blocking drugs (eg, propranolol), verapamil; first dose of prazosin should be only 0.5 mg or less

## ■ Nursing Considerations

### Assessment

- ***History:*** Hypersensitivity to prazosin, CHF, renal failure, lactation
- ***Physical:*** Weight; skin color, lesions; orientation, affect, reflexes; ophthalmologic exam; P, BP, orthostatic BP, supine BP, perfusion, edema, auscultation; R, adventitious sounds; status of nasal mucous membranes; bowel sounds, normal output; voiding pattern, normal output; kidney function tests, urinalysis

### Implementation

- Administer, or have patient take, first dose just before bedtime to lessen likelihood of first dose effect (syncope)—believed due to excessive postural hypotension.
- Have patient lie down and treat supportively if syncope occurs; condition is self-limiting.
- Monitor for orthostatic hypotension, which is most marked in the morning and is accentuated by hot weather, alcohol, exercise.
- Monitor edema, weight in patients with incipient cardiac decompensation, and add a thiazide diuretic to the drug regimen if sodium and fluid retention, signs of impending CHF occur.

### Drug-specific teaching points

- Take this drug exactly as prescribed. Take the first dose just before bedtime. Do not drive or operate machinery for 4 h after the first dose.
- The following side effects may occur: dizziness, weakness (more likely when changing position, in the early morning, after exercise, in hot weather, and with alcohol; some tolerance may occur; avoid driving or engaging in tasks that require alertness; change position slowly, and use caution when climbing stairs; lie down for a while if dizziness persists); GI upset (frequent, small meals may help); impotence; dry mouth (sucking on sugarless lozenges, ice chips may help); stuffy nose. Most effects are transient.
- Report frequent dizziness or faintness.

P

# Prednisolone

## prednisolone

*(pred **niss'** oh lone)*

*Oral:* Delta-Cortef, Novoprednisolone (CAN), Prelone

## prednisolone acetate

*IM, ophthalmic solution:* Articulose, Econopred, Key-Pred, Pred-Forte, Pred Mild, and others

*(continues)*

## prednisolone acetate and sodium phosphate IM, intra-articular, prednisolone sodium phosphate

*IV, IM, intra-articular injection, ophthalmic solution:* AK-Pred, Hydeltrasol, Hydrocortone, Inflamase, Key-Pred

## prednisolone tebutate

*Intra-articular, intralesional injection:* Hydeltra, Hydeltrasol, Prednisol TBA

**Pregnancy Category C**

### Drug classes

Corticosteroid (intermediate acting)
Glucocorticoid
Hormone

### Therapeutic actions

Enters target cells and binds to intracellular corticosteroid receptors, thereby initiating many complex reactions that are responsible for its anti-inflammatory and immunosuppressive effects.

### Indications

- Hypercalcemia associated with cancer (systemic)
- Short-term management of various inflammatory and allergic disorders, such as rheumatoid arthritis, collagen diseases (eg, SLE), dermatologic diseases (eg, pemphigus), status asthmaticus, and autoimmune disorders (systemic)
- Hematologic disorders: thrombocytopenia purpura, erythroblastopenia (systemic)
- Ulcerative colitis, acute exacerbations of mutiple sclerosis and palliation in some leukemias and lymphomas (systemic)
- Trichinosis with neurologic or myocardial involvement (systemic)
- Arthritis, psoriatic plaques (intra-articular, soft tissue administration)
- Inflammation of the lid, conjunctiva, cornea, and globe (ophthalmic)
- Prednisolone has weaker mineralocortiocoid activity than hydrocortisone and is not used as physiologic replacement therapy (ophthalmic)

### Contraindications/cautions

- Contraindications: infections, especially tuberculosis, fungal infectons, amebiasis, vaccinia and varicella, and antibiotic-resistant infections; lactation.
- Use cautiously with kidney or liver disease, hypothyroidism, ulcerative colitis with impending perforation, diverticulitis, active or latent peptic ulcer, inflammatory bowel disease, CHF, hypertension, thromboembolic disorders, osteoporosis, convulsive disorders, diabetes mellitus, pregnancy.

*Ophthalmic Preparations*

- Contraindications: acute superficial herpes simplex keratitis; fungal infections of ocular structures; vaccinia, varicella, and other viral diseases of the cornea and conjunctiva; ocular tuberculosis.

### Dosage

**Available Forms:** Tablets— 5 mg; oral syrup—15 mg/5 ml; injection—20, 25, 50 mg/ml; ophthalmic suspension—0.12%, 0.125%, 1%

*ADULT:* Individualize dosage, depending on severity of condition and patient's response. Administer daily dose before 9 AM to minimize adrenal suppression. If long-term therapy is needed, consider alternate-day therapy. After long-term therapy, withdraw drug slowly to avoid adrenal insufficiency. Maintenance therapy: reduce initial dose in small increments at intervals until the lowest dose that maintains satisfactory clinical response is reached.

*PEDIATRIC:* Individualize dosage depending on severity of condition and patient's response rather than by strict adherence to formulae that correct adult doses for age or weight. Carefully observe growth and development in infants and children on prolonged therapy.

***Oral (prednisolone):*** 5–60 mg/d. Acute exacerbations of multiple sclerosis: 200 mg/d for 1 wk, followed by 80 mg every other day for 1 mo.

***IM (prednisolone acetate):*** 4–60 mg/d. Acute exacerbations of multiple sclerosis: 200 mg/d for 1 wk followed by 80 mg every other day for 1 mo.

***IM, IV (prednisolone sodium phosphate):*** Initial dosage, 4–60 mg/day. Acute exacerbations of multiple sclerosis: 200 mg/d for 1 wk followed by 80 mg every other day for 1 mo.

***IM (prednisolone acetate and sodium phosphate):*** Initial dose 0.25–1.0 ml. Repeat within several days, up to 3–4 wk or more often as necessary.

***Intra-articular, intralesional (dose will vary with joint or soft tissue site to be injected)***

- *Prednisolone acetate:* 5–100 mg.
- *Prednisolone acetate and sodium phosphate:* 0.25–0.5 ml.
- *Prednisolone sodium phosphate:* 2–30 mg.
- *Prednisolone tebutate:* 4–30 mg.

***Ophthalmic (prednisolone acetate suspension; prednisolone sodium phosphate solution):*** 1–2 drops into the conjunctival sac every hour during the day and every 2 h during the night. After a favorable response, reduce dose to 1 drop q4h and then 1 drop tid or qid.

## Pharmacokinetics

| *Route* | *Onset* | *Peak* | *Duration* |
|---|---|---|---|
| Oral | Varies | 1–2 h | 1–1 1/2 d |

*Metabolism:* Hepatic, $T_{1/2}$: 3.5 h
*Distribution:* Crosses placenta; enters breast milk
*Excretion:* Urine

## IV facts

**Preparation:** May be given undiluted or added to $D_5W$ or Normal Saline solution; use within 24 h if diluted.

**Infusion:** Infuse slowly, each 10 mg over 1 min—slower if discomfort at the injection site.

**Compatibilities:** Do not mix in solution with other drugs.

## Adverse effects

Effects depend on dose, route, and duration of therapy. The following are primarily associated with systemic absorption.

- CNS: *Vertigo, headache,* paresthesias, insomnia, convulsions, psychosis, cataracts, increased intraocular pressure, glaucoma (long-term therapy)
- GI: Peptic or esophageal ulcer, pancreatitis, abdominal distention, nausea, vomiting, *increased appetite, weight gain* (long-term therapy)
- CV: Hypotension, shock, hypertension and CHF secondary to fluid retention, thromboembolism, thrombophlebitis, fat embolism, cardiac arrhythmias
- MS: Muscle weakness, steroid myopathy, loss of muscle mass, osteoporosis, spontaneous fractures (long-term therapy)
- **Hypersensitivity**: Hypersensitivity or anaphylactoid reactions
- Endocrine: Amenorrhea, irregular menses, growth retardation, decreased carbohydrate tolerance, diabetes mellitus, cushingoid state (long-term effect), increased blood sugar, increased serum cholesterol, decreased $T_3$ and $T_4$ levels, hypothalamic-pituitary-adrenal (HPA) suppression with systemic therapy longer than 5 d
- Electrolyte imbalance: *$Na^+$ and fluid retention*, hypokalemia, hypocalcemia
- Other: *Immunosuppression, aggravation, or masking of infections; impaired wound healing*; thin, fragile skin; petechiae, ecchymoses, purpura, striae; subcutaneous fat atrophy
- The following effects are related to various local routes of steroid administration:

*Intra-articular*

- Local: Osteonecrosis, tendon, rupture, infection

*Intralesional (Face and Head)*

- Local: Blindness (rare)

*Ophthalmic Solutions, Ointments*

- Local: Infections, especially fungal; glaucoma, cataracts with long-term therapy
- Other: Systemic absorption and adverse effects (see above) with prolonged use

P

## Clinically important drug-drug interactions

• Increased therapeutic and toxic effects of prednisolone with troleandomycin, ketoconazole • Increased therapeutic and toxic effects of estrogens, including oral contraceptives • Risk of severe deterioration of muscle strength in myasthenia gravis patients who also are receiving ambenonium, edrophonium, neostigmine, pyridostigmine • Decreased steroid blood levels with barbiturates, phenytoin, rifampin • Decreased effectiveness of salicylates

## Drug-lab test interferences

• False-negative nitroblue-tetrazolium test for bacterial infection • Suppression of skin test reactions

## ■ Nursing Considerations

### Assessment

- *History:* Infections; kidney or liver disease; hypothyroidism; ulcerative colitis with impending perforation; diverticulitis; active or latent peptic ulcer; inflammatory bowel disease; CHF; hypertension; thromboembolic disorders; osteoporosis; convulsive disorders; diabetes mellitus; pregnancy; lactation. Ophthalmic: acute superficial herpes simplex keratitis; fungal infections of ocular structures; vaccinia, varicella, and other viral diseases of the cornea and conjunctiva; ocular tuberculosis
- *Physical:* Weight, T, reflexes and grip strength, affect and orientation, P, BP, peripheral perfusion, prominence of superficial veins, R, adventitious sounds, serum electrolytes, blood glucose

### Implementation

- Administer once-a-day doses before 9 AM to mimic normal peak corticosteroid blood levels.
- Increase dosage when patient is subject to stress.
- Taper doses when discontinuing high-dose or long-term therapy.
- Do not give live virus vaccines with immunosuppressive doses of corticosteroids.

### Drug-specific teaching points

*Systemic*

- Do not stop taking the drug without consulting your health care provider.
- Avoid exposure to infections.
- Report unusual weight gain, swelling of the extremities, muscle weakness, black or tarry stools, fever, prolonged sore throat, colds or other infections, worsening of the disorder for which the drug is being taken.

*Intra-articular Administration*

- Do not overuse joint after therapy, even if pain is gone.

*Ophthalmic Preparations*

- Learn the proper administration technique: Lie down or tilt head backward, and look at ceiling. Drop suspension inside lower eyelid while looking up. After instilling eye drops, release lower lid, but do not blink for at least 30 sec; apply gentle pressure to the inside corner of the eye for 1 min. Do not close eyes tightly, and try not to blink more often than usual. Do not touch dropper to eye, fingers, or any surface. Wait at least 5 min before using any other eye preparations.
- Eyes may be sensitive to bright light; sunglasses may help.
- Report worsening of the condition, pain, itching, swelling of the eye, failure of the condition to improve after 1 wk.

# prednisone

***(pred' ni sone)***

Apo-Prednisone (CAN), Deltasone, Liquid Pred, Meticorten, Novoprednisone (CAN), Orasone, Prednicen-M, Prednisone-Intensol, Winpred (CAN), Winpred (CAN)

**Pregnancy Category C**

## Drug classes

Corticosteroid (intermediate acting)
Glucocorticoid
Hormone

## Therapeutic actions

Enters target cells and binds to intracellular corticosteroid receptors, thereby initiating many complex reactions that are responsible for its anti-inflammatory and immunosuppressive effects.

## Indications

- Replacement therapy in adrenal cortical insufficiency
- Hypercalcemia associated with cancer
- Short-term management of various inflammatory and allergic disorders, such as rheumatoid arthritis, collagen diseases (eg, SLE), dermatologic diseases (eg, pemphigus), status asthmaticus, and autoimmune disorders
- Hematologic disorders: thrombocytopenia purpura, erythroblastopenia
- Ulcerative colitis, acute exacerbations of multiple sclerosis and palliation in some leukemias and lymphomas
- Trichinosis with neurologic or myocardial involvement

## Contraindications/cautions

- Contraindications: infections, especially tuberculosis, fungal infections, amebiasis, vaccinia and varicella, and antibiotic-resistant infections; lactation.
- Use cautiously with kidney or liver disease, hypothyroidism, ulcerative colitis with impending perforation, diverticulitis, active or latent peptic ulcer, inflammatory bowel disease, CHF, hypertension, thromboembolic disorders, osteoporosis, convulsive disorders, diabetes mellitus; hepatic disease; pregnancy (monitor infants for adrenal insufficiency).

## Dosage

**Available Forms:** Tablets—1, 2.5, 5, 10, 20, 50 mg; oral solution—5 mg/5 ml, 5 mg/ml; syrup—5 mg/ml

*ADULT:* Individualize dosage depending on severity of condition and patient's response. Administer daily dose before 9 AM to minimize adrenal suppression. If long-term therapy is needed, consider alternate-day therapy. After long-term therapy, withdraw drug slowly to avoid adrenal insufficiency. Initial dose: 5–60 mg/d PO. Maintenance therapy: reduce initial dose in small increments at intervals until lowest dose that maintains satisfactory clinical response is reached.

*PEDIATRIC*

- ***Physiologic replacement:*** 0.1–0.15 mg/kg per day PO or 4–5 mg/m$^2$ per day PO in equal divided doses q12h.
- ***Other indications:*** Individualize dosage depending on severity of condition and patient's response rather than by strict adherence to formulae that correct adult doses for age or body weight. Carefully observe growth and development in infants and children on prolonged therapy.

## Pharmacokinetics

| *Route* | *Onset* | *Peak* | *Duration* |
|---|---|---|---|
| Oral | Varies | 1–2 h | 1–1 1/2 d |

*Metabolism:* Hepatic, $T_{1/2}$: 3.5 h
*Distribution:* Crosses placenta; enters breast milk
*Excretion:* Urine

## Adverse effects

- CNS: *Vertigo, headache*, paresthesias, insomnia, convulsions, psychosis, cataracts, increased intraocular pressure, glaucoma (long-term therapy)
- GI: Peptic or esophageal ulcer, pancreatitis, abdominal distention, nausea, vomiting, *increased appetite, weight gain* (long-term therapy)
- CV: Hypotension, shock, hypertension and CHF secondary to fluid retention, thromboembolism, thrombophlebitis, fat embolism, cardiac arrhythmias
- MS: Muscle weakness, steroid myopathy, loss of muscle mass, osteoporosis, spontaneous fractures (long-term therapy)
- **Hypersensitivity**: Hypersensitivity or anaphylactoid reactions
- **Endocrine**: Amenorrhea, irregular menses, growth retardation, decreased carbohydrate tolerance, diabetes mellitus, cushingoid state (long-term effect), increased blood sugar, increased serum cholesterol, decreased $T_3$ and $T_4$ levels, HPA suppression with systemic therapy longer than 5 d
- **Electrolyte imbalance**: *$Na^+$ and fluid retention*, hypokalemia, hypocalcemia

P

- Other: *Immunosuppression, aggravation, or masking of infections; impaired wound healing*; thin, fragile skin; petechiae, ecchymoses, purpura, striae; subcutaneous fat atrophy

**Clinically important drug-drug interactions**
• Increased therapeutic and toxic effects with troleandomycin, ketoconazole • Increased therapeutic and toxic effects of estrogens, including oral contraceptives • Risk of severe deterioration of muscle strength in myasthenia gravis patients who also are receiving ambenonium, edrophonium, neostigmine, pyridostigmine • Decreased steroid blood levels with barbiturates, phenytoin, rifampin • Decreased effectiveness of salicylates

**Drug-lab test interferences**
• False-negative nitroblue-tetrazolium test for bacterial infection • Suppression of skin test reactions

## ■ Nursing Considerations

### Assessment

- *History:* Infections; kidney or liver disease, hypothyroidism, ulcerative colitis with impending perforation, diverticulitis, active or latent peptic ulcer, inflammatory bowel disease, CHF, hypertension, thromboembolic disorders, osteoporosis, convulsive disorders, diabetes mellitus; hepatic disease; lactation
- *Physical:* Weight, T, reflexes and grip strength, affect and orientation, P, BP, peripheral perfusion, prominence of superficial veins, R, adventitious sounds, serum electrolytes, blood glucose

### Implementation

- Administer once-a-day doses before 9 AM to mimic normal peak corticosteroid blood levels.
- Increase dosage when patient is subject to stress.
- Taper doses when discontinuing high-dose or long-term therapy.
- Do not give live virus vaccines with immunosuppressive doses of corticosteroids.

### Drug-specific teaching points

- Do not stop taking the drug without consulting your health care provider.
- Avoid exposure to infections.
- Report unusual weight gain, swelling of the extremities, muscle weakness, black or tarry stools, fever, prolonged sore throat, colds or other infections, worsening of the disorder for which the drug is being taken.

# primaquine phosphate

*(prim' a kween)*
**Pregnancy Category C**

**Drug classes**
Antimalarial
8-aminoquinoline

**Therapeutic actions**
Disrupts the parasite's mitochondria, creating a major disruption in the metabolic processes; some gametocytes and exoerythrocytic forms are destroyed, and others are rendered incapable of undergoing division; by eliminating exoerythrocytic forms, primaquine prevents development of erythrocytic forms responsible for relapses in vivax malaria.

**Indications**
- Radical cure of vivax malaria
- Prevention of relapse in vivax malaria or following the termination of chloroquine phosphate suppressive therapy in an area where vivax malaria is endemic

**Contraindications/cautions**
- Contraindications: allergy to primaquine; the acutely ill suffering from systemic disease with hematologic depression.
- Use cautiously with pregnancy.

### Dosage

**Available Forms:** Tablets—26.3 mg; powder—5, 25, 100, 500 g
Patients should receive a course of chloroquine phosphate to eliminate erythrocytic forms of the parasite.

*ADULT:* Begin treatment during the last 2 wk of, or following, a course of suppression with chloroquine or a comparable drug; 26.3 mg (15 mg base)/d PO for 14 d.
*PEDIATRIC:* 0.5 mg/kg per day PO ( 0.3 mg base/kg per day) for 14 d. Maximum 15 mg base/dose.

### Pharmacokinetics

| Route | Onset | Peak |
|---|---|---|
| Oral | Varies | 1–3 h |

*Metabolism:* Hepatic, $T_{1/2}$: 4 h
*Distribution:* Crosses placenta; may enter breast milk
*Excretion:* Urine

### Adverse effects

- GI: *Nausea, vomiting, epigastric distress*, abdominal cramps
- **Hematologic**: Leukopenia, hemolytic anemia in patients with G-6-PD deficiency, methhemoglobinemia in NADH methemoglobin reductase deficient individuals

### Clinically important drug-drug interactions

• Increased toxicity with quinacrine • Increased risk of bone marrow depression with hemolytic drugs or drugs that cause bone marrow depression

## ■ Nursing Considerations

### Assessment

- *History:* Allergy to primaquine; acutely ill suffering from systemic disease with hematologic depression
- *Physical:* Abdominal exam; CBC, hemoglobin, G-6-PD in deficient patients

### Implementation

- Administer with food if GI upset occurs.
- Administer with chloroquine phosphate.
- Schedule doses for weekly same-day therapy on a calendar.
- Arrange for CBC and Hgb determinations before and periodically during therapy.

### Drug-specific teaching points

- Take full course of drug therapy as prescribed.
- Take drug with food if GI upset occurs.
- Mark your calendar with the drug days for once-a-week therapy.
- This drug may cause stomach pain, loss of appetite, nausea, vomiting, or abdominal cramps; report severe problems.
- Have regular blood tests to evaluate drug effects.
- Report darkening of the urine, severe abdominal cramps, GI distress, persistent nausea, vomiting.

## primidone

*(pri' mi done)*

Apo-Primidone (CAN), Mysoline, Primaclone (CAN)

**Pregnancy Category D**

### Drug classes

Antiepileptic agent

### Therapeutic actions

Mechanism of action not understood; primidone and its two metabolites, phenobarbital and phenylethylmalonamide, all have antiepileptic activity.

### Indications

- Control of grand mal, psychomotor, or focal epileptic seizures, either alone or with other antiepileptics; may control grand mal seizures refractory to other antiepileptics
- Unlabeled use: treatment of benign familial tremor (essential tremor)—750 mg/d

### Contraindications/cautions

- Contraindications: hypersensitivity to phenobarbital, porphyria, lactation (somnolence and drowsiness may occur in nursing newborns).
- Use cautiously with pregnancy (association between use of antiepileptic drugs and an elevated incidence of birth defects; however, do not discontinue antiepileptic therapy in pregnant women who are receiving such therapy to prevent major seizures; discontinuing medication is likely

p

to precipitate status epilepticus, with attendant hypoxia and risk to both mother and fetus; to prevent neonatal hemorrhage, primidone should be given with prophylactic vitamin $K_1$ therapy for 1 mo prior to and during delivery).

### Dosage

**Available Forms:** Tablets—50, 250 mg; oral suspension—250 mg/5 ml

ADULT

- ***Regimen for patients who have received no previous therapy:*** Days 1–3, 100–125 mg PO hs; days 4–6, 100–125 mg bid; days 7–9, 100–125 mg tid; day 10–maintenance, 250 mg tid. The usual maintenance dosage is 250 mg tid–qid. If required, increase dosage to 250 mg five to six times daily, but do not exceed dosage of 500 mg qid (2 g/d).
- ***Regimen for patients already receiving other antiepileptic drugs:*** Start primidone at 100–125 mg PO hs. Gradually increase to maintenance level as the other drug is gradually decreased. Continue this regimen until satisfactory dosage level is achieved for the combination, or the other medication is completely withdrawn. When use of primidone alone is desired, the transition should not be completed in less than 2 wk.

PEDIATRIC

- *CHILDREN > 8 Y: Regimen for patients who have received no previous therapy:* Days 1–3, 100–125 mg PO hs; days 4–6, 100–125 mg bid; days 7–9, 100–125 mg tid; day 10–maintenance, 250 mg tid. The usual maintenance dosage is 250 mg tid–qid. If required, increase dosage to 250 mg five to six times daily, but do not exceed dosage of 500 mg qid (2 g/d).
- *CHILDREN < 8 Y: Regimen for patients who have received no previous therapy:* Days 1–3, 50 mg PO at bedtime; days 4–6, 50 mg bid; days 7–9, 100 mg bid; day 10–maintenance, 125–250 mg tid. The usual maintenance dosage is 125–250 mg tid or 10–25 mg/kg per day in divided doses.

### Pharmacokinetics

| Route | Onset | Peak |
|---|---|---|
| Oral | Varies | 3–7 h |

*Metabolism:* Hepatic, $T_{1/2}$: 3–24 h
*Distribution:* Crosses placenta; enters breast milk
*Excretion:* Urine

### Adverse effects

- CNS: *Ataxia, vertigo, fatigue, hyperirritability*, emotional disturbances, nystagmus, diplopia, drowsiness, personality deterioration with mood changes and paranoia
- GI: *Nausea, anorexia*, vomiting
- **Hematologic**: Megaloblastic anemia that responds to folic acid therapy
- GU: Sexual impotence
- **Other**: Morbiliform skin eruptions

### Clinically important drug-drug interactions

• Toxicity with phenytoins • Increased CNS effects, impaired hand-eye coordination, and death may occur with acute alcohol ingestion • Decreased serum concentrations of primidone and increased serum concentrations of carbamazepine if taken concurrently • Decreased serum concentrations with acetazolamide • Increased levels with isoniazid, nicotinamide, succinimides

## ■ Nursing Considerations

### Assessment

- ***History:*** Hypersensitivity to phenobarbital, porphyria, pregnancy, lactation
- ***Physical:*** Skin color, lesions; orientation, affect, reflexes, vision exam; bowel sounds, normal output; CBC and a sequential multiple analysis-12 (SMA-12), EEG

### Implementation

- Reduce dosage, discontinue primidone, or substitute other antiepileptic medication gradually; abrupt discontinuation may precipitate status epilepticus.
- Arrange for patient to have CBC and SMA-12 test every 6 mo during therapy.

- Arrange for folic acid therapy if megaloblastic anemia occurs; primidone does not need to be discontinued.
- Obtain counseling for women of childbearing age who wish to become pregnant.
- Evaluate for therapeutic serum levels: 5–12 μg/ml for primidone.

### Drug-specific teaching points

- Take this drug exactly as prescribed; do not discontinue this drug abruptly or change dosage, except on the advice of your prescriber.
- Arrange for frequent checkups, including blood tests, to monitor your response to this drug. Keep all appointments for checkups.
- Use contraception at all times. If you wish to become pregnant while you are taking this drug, you should consult your physician.
- The following side effects may occur: drowsiness, dizziness, muscular incoordination (transient; avoid driving or performing other tasks requiring alertness); vision changes (avoid performing tasks that require visual acuity); GI upset (take drug with food or milk, eat frequent, small meals).
- Wear a medical alert tag at all times so that emergency medical personnel will know that you are an epileptic taking antiepileptic medication.
- Report skin rash, joint pain, unexplained fever, pregnancy.

## probenecid

*(proe **ben'** e sid)*

Benemid (CAN), Benuryl (CAN), Probalan

**Pregnancy Category C**

### Drug classes

Uricosuric agent
Antigout agent

### Therapeutic actions

Inhibits the renal tubular reabsorption of urate, increasing the urinary excretion of uric acid, decreasing serum uric acid levels, retarding urate deposition, and promoting resorption of urate deposits; also inhibits the renal tubular reabsorption of most penicillins and cephalosporins.

### Indications

- Treatment of hyperuricemia associated with gout and gouty arthritis
- Adjuvant to therapy with penicillins or cephalosporins, for elevation and prolongation of plasma levels of the antibiotic

### Contraindications/cautions

- Contraindications: allergy to probenecid, blood dyscrasias, uric acid kidney stones, acute gouty attack, pregnancy.
- Use cautiously with peptic ulcer, acute intermittent porphyria, G-6-PD deficiency, chronic renal insufficiency, lactation.

### Dosage

**Available Forms:** Tablets—0.5 g

*ADULT*

- *Gout:* 0.25 g PO bid for 1 wk; then 0.5 g PO bid. Maintenance: continue dosage that maintains the normal serum uric acid levels. When no attacks occur for 6 mo or more, decrease the daily dosage by 0.5 g every 6 mo.
- ***Penicillin or cephalosporin therapy:*** 2 g/d PO in divided doses.
- ***Gonorrhea treatment:*** Single 1-g dose PO 1/2 h before penicillin administration.

*PEDIATRIC*

- ***Penicillin or cephalosporin therapy:*** *2–14 y:* 25 mg/kg PO initial dose, then 40 mg/kg per day divided in four doses. Children weighing 50 kg: adult dosage. Do not use in children <2 y.
- ***Gonorrhea treatment:*** Children weighing < 45 kg: 23 mg/kg PO in one single dose 1/2 h before penicillin administration.

*GERIATRIC OR RENAL IMPAIRED:* 1 g/d PO may be adequate. Daily dosage may be increased by 0.5 g every 4 wk. Probenecid may not be effective in chronic renal insufficiency when glomerular filtration rate < 30 ml/min.

### Pharmacokinetics

| Route | Onset | Peak |
|---|---|---|
| Oral | Varies | 2–4 h |

P

*Metabolism:* Hepatic, $T_{1/2}$: 5–8 h
*Distribution:* Crosses placenta; may enter breast milk
*Excretion:* Urine

### Adverse effects

- CNS: *Headache*
- GI: *Nausea, vomiting, anorexia*, sore gums
- **Hematologic**: Anemia, hemolytic anemia
- GU: *Urinary frequency,* exacerbation of gout and uric acid stones
- **Hypersensitivity**: Reactions including anaphylaxis, dermatitis, pruritus, fever
- **Other**: Blushing, dizziness

### Clinically important drug-drug interactions

• Decreased effectiveness wiith salicylates • Decreased renal excretion and increased serum levels of methotrexate, dyphylline • Increased pharmacologic effects of thiopental, acyclovir, allopurinol, benzodiazepines, clofibrate, dapsone, NSAIDs, sulfonamides, zidovudine, rifampin

### Drug-lab test interferences

• False-positive test for urine glucose if using Benedict's test, Clinitest (use Clinistix) • Falsely high determination of theophylline levels • Inhibited excretion of urinary 17-ketosteroids, phenolsulfonphthalein, sulfobromophthalein

## ■ Nursing Considerations

### Assessment

- ***History:*** Allergy to probenecid, blood dyscrasias, uric acid kidney stones, acute gouty attack, peptic ulcer, acute intermittent porphyria, G-6-PD deficiency, chronic renal insufficiency, pregnancy, lactation
- ***Physical:*** Skin lesions, color; reflexes, gait; liver evaluation, normal output, gums; urinary output; CBC, renal and liver function tests, urinalysis

### Implementation

- Administer drug with meals or antacids if GI upset occurs.
- Force fluids—2.5 to 3 L/d—to decrease the risk of renal stone development.
- Check urine alkalinity; urates crystallize in acid urine; sodium bicarbonate or potassium citrate may be ordered to alkalinize urine.
- Arrange for regular medical follow-up and blood tests.
- Double-check any analgesics ordered for pain; salicylates should be avoided.

### Drug-specific teaching points

- Take the drug with meals or antacids if GI upset occurs.
- The following side effects may occur: headache (monitor lighting, temperature, noise; consult with nurse or physician if severe); dizziness (change position slowly; avoid driving or operating dangerous machinery); exacerbation of gouty attack or renal stones (drink plenty of fluids—2.5–3 L/d); nausea, vomiting, loss of appetite (take drug with meals or request antacids).
- Report flank pain, dark urine or blood in urine, acute gout attack, unusual fatigue or lethargy, unusual bleeding or bruising.

## procainamide HCl

*(proe kane a' mide)*
Pronestyl, Pronestyl SR
**Pregnancy Category C**

### Drug classes

Antiarrhythmic

### Therapeutic actions

Type 1A antiarrhythmic: decreases rate of diastolic depolarization (decreases automaticity) in ventricles, decreases the rate of rise and height of the action potential, increases fibrillation threshold.

### Indications

- Treatment of documented ventricular arrhythmias that are judged to be life-threatening

### Contraindications/cautions

- Contraindications: allergy to procaine, procainamide, or similar drugs; tartrazine sensitivity (tablets marketed as *Pro-*

*nestyl* contain tartrazine); second- or third-degree heart block (unless electrical pacemaker operative); SLE; torsade de pointes; pregnancy; lactation.
- Use cautiously with myasthenia gravis, hepatic or renal disease.

## Dosage

**Available Forms:** Tablets—250, 375, 500 mg; capsules—250, 375, 500 mg; SR tablets—250, 500, 750 mg; injection—100, 500 mg/ml

*ADULT*

- ***Oral:*** 50 mg/kg per day PO in divided doses q3h. Maintenance dose of 50 mg/kg per day (sustained release) in divided doses q6h, starting 2–3 h after last dose of standard oral preparation.

| *Body Weight* | *Standard Preparation* | *Sustained-Release Preparation* |
|---|---|---|
| <55 kg | 250 mg q3h | 500 mg q6h |
| 55–90 kg | 375 mg q3h | 750 mg q6h |
| >90 kg | 500 mg q3h | 1000 mg q6h |

- ***IM administration:*** 0.5–1.0 g q4–8h until oral therapy can be started.
- ***Direct IV injection:*** Dilute in 5% Dextrose Injection. Give 100 mg q5min at a rate not to exceed 25–50 mg/min (maximum dose 1 g).
- ***IV infusion:*** 500–600 mg over 25–30 min, then 2–6 mg/min. Monitor very closely.

*PEDIATRIC:*

- ***Oral:*** 15–50 mg/kg per day divided every 3–6 h; maximum, 4 g/d.
- ***IM:*** 20–30 mg/kg per day divided every 4—6 h; maximum 4 g/d.
- ***IV:*** Loading dose, 3–6 mg/kg per dose over 5 min; maintenance, 20–80 mg/kg per minute per continuous infusion; maximum, 100 mg/dose or 2 g/d.

## Pharmacokinetics

| *Route* | *Onset* | *Peak* | *Duration* |
|---|---|---|---|
| Oral | 30 min | 60–90 min | 3–4 h |
| IV | Immediate | 20–60 min | 3–4 h |
| IM | 10–30 min | 15–60 min | 3–4 h |

*Metabolism:* Hepatic, $T_{1/2}$: 2.5–4.7 h
*Distribution:* Crosses placenta; enters breast milk
*Excretion:* Urine

### IV facts

**Preparation:** Dilute the 100 or 500 mg/ml dose in 5% Dextrose in Water.
**Infusion:** Slowly inject directly into vein or into tubing of actively running IV, 100 mg q5 min, not faster than 25–50 mg/min; maintenance doses should be given by continual IV infusion with a pump to maintain rate—first 500–600 mg over 25–30 min, then 2–6 mg/min.

## Adverse effects

- CNS: Mental depression, giddiness, convulsions, confusion, psychosis
- GI: *Anorexia, nausea,* vomiting, bitter taste, diarrhea
- CV: *Hypotension*, cardiac conduction disturbances
- **Hematologic**: Granulocytopenia
- Dermatologic: *Rash,* pruritus, urticaria
- Other: Lupus syndrome, fever, chills

## Clinically important drug-drug interactions

- Increased levels with cimetidine, trimethoprim, amiodarone; monitor for toxicity

## ■ Nursing Considerations

P

### Assessment

- *History:* Allergy to procaine, procainamide, or similar drugs; tartrazine sensitivity; second- or third-degree heart block (unless electrical pacemaker operative); myasthenia gravis; hepatic or renal disease; SLE; torsade de pointes; pregnancy; lactation
- *Physical:* Weight, skin color, lesions; bilateral grip strength; P, BP, auscultation, ECG, edema; bowel sounds, liver evaluation; urinalysis, renal and liver function tests, complete blood count

### Implementation

- Monitor patient response carefully, especially when beginning therapy.

- Reduce dosage in patients under 120 lb.
- Reduce dosage in patients with hepatic or renal failure.
- Dosage adjustment may be necessary when procainamide is given with other antiarrhythmics, antihypertensives, cimetidine, or alcohol.
- Check to see that patients with supraventricular tachyarrhythmias have been digitalized before giving procainamide.
- Differentiate the sustained-release (SR) form from the regular preparation.
- Monitor cardiac rhythm and BP frequently if IV route is used.
- Arrange for periodic ECG monitoring and determination of ANA titers when on long-term therapy.
- Arrange for frequent monitoring of blood counts.
- Give dosages at evenly spaced intervals, around the clock; determine a schedule that will minimize sleep interruption.
- Evaluate for safe and effective serum drug levels: 4–8 $\mu$g/ml.

### Drug-specific teaching points

- Take this drug at evenly spaced intervals, around the clock. Do not double up doses; do not skip doses; take exactly as prescribed. You may need an alarm clock to wake you up to take the drug. The best schedule for you will be determined to decrease sleep interruption as much as possible. *Do not* chew the sustained-release tablets.
- You will require frequent monitoring of cardiac rhythm.
- The following side effects may occur: nausea, loss of appetite, vomiting (small, frequent meals may help); small wax cores may be passed in the stool (from sustained-release tablet); rash (use careful skin care).
- Do not stop taking this drug for any reason without checking with your health care provider.
- Return for regular follow-up visits to check your heart rhythm and blood counts.
- Report joint pain, stiffness; sore mouth, throat, gums; fever, chills; cold or flulike syndromes; extensive rash, sensitivity to the sun.

## procarbazine hydrochloride

*(proe **kar'** ba zeen)*

N-methylhydrazine, MIH

Matulane, Natulan (CAN)

**Pregnancy Category D**

### Drug classes

Antineoplastic

### Therapeutic actions

Cytotoxic: inhibits DNA, RNA, and protein synthesis, causing cell death, but the exact mechanism of action is not fully understood.

### Indications

- In combination with other antineoplastics for treatment of stage III and IV Hodgkin's disease (part of the MOPP—nitrogen mustard, vincristine, procarbazine, prednisone—therapy)

### Contraindications/cautions

- Contraindications: allergy to procarbazine, irradiation, other chemotherapy, leukopenia, thrombocytopenia, anemia, inadequate bone marrow reserve (by bone marrow aspiration), pregnancy (teratogenic); lactation.
- Use cautiously with impaired hepatic or renal function.

### Dosage

**Available Forms:** Capsules—50 mg

*ADULT:* Base dosage on actual body weight: use estimated dry weight if patient is obese or if fluid gain is marked. 2–4 mg/kg per day PO for the first wk in single or divided doses. Maintain at 4–6 mg/kg per day PO until maximum response is obtained or WBC falls below 4,000/mm$^3$ or platelets fall below 100,000/mm$^3$. If hematologic toxicity occurs, discontinue drug until satisfactory recovery is made, then resume treatment at 1–2 mg/kg per day. When maximum response is obtained, maintain dose at 1–2 mg/kg per day.

*PEDIATRIC:* Dosage regimen not established. As a general guide, give 50 mg/d PO for the first week; maintain daily dose at 100 mg/m$^2$ until hematologic toxicity occurs (see above). Discontinue drug, and when possible resume treatment with 50 mg/d.

### Pharmacokinetics

| *Route* | *Onset* | *Peak* |
|---|---|---|
| Oral | Rapid | 30–90 min |

*Metabolism:* Hepatic, $T_{1/2}$: 10–60 min
*Distribution:* Crosses placenta; enters breast milk
*Excretion:* Urine

### Adverse effects

- CNS: Paresthesias, neuropathies, headache, *dizziness,* depression, apprehension, nervousness, insomnia, nightmares, hallucinations, falling, weakness, fatigue, lethargy, *drowsiness, unsteadiness*, ataxia, foot drop, decreased reflexes, tremors, coma, confusion, convulsions
- GI: Stomatitis, anorexia, *nausea, vomiting*, diarrhea, constipation, dry mouth, dysphagia
- **Hematologic:** *Bone marrow depression*, bleeding tendencies
- GU: Hematuria, urinary frequency, nocturia
- **Dermatologic:** Dermatitis, pruritus, herpes, hyperpigmentation, flushing, alopecia
- **Other:** Fever, chills, malaise, myalgia, arthralgia, pain, sweating, edema, cough, pneumonitis symptoms, cancer

### Clinically important drug-drug interactions

• Disulfiram-like reaction with alcohol • Decreased serum levels and therapeutic actions of digoxin • Risk of increased BP reaction with levodopa, sympathomimetics • Severe toxic reactions possible with TCAs, narcotics

### Clinically important drug-food interactions

• Possible severe hypertensive reaction, even fatal hypertensive crisis, with foods high in tyramine (Appendix T)

## ■ Nursing Considerations

### Assessment

- ***History:*** Allergy to procarbazine, irradiation, chemotherapy, leukopenia, thrombocytopenia, anemia, inadequate bone marrow reserve, impaired hepatic or renal function, pregnancy, lactation
- ***Physical:*** Weight; T; skin color, lesions; hair; reflexes, orientation, affect, gait; mucous membranes, abdominal exam; CBC, renal and liver function tests, urinalysis

### Implementation

- Arrange for laboratory tests (Hgb, Hct, WBC, differential, reticulocytes, platelets) before and every 3–4 d during therapy.
- Arrange for baseline and weekly repeat of urinalysis, transaminase, alkaline phosphatase, BUN.
- Discontinue drug therapy, and consult with physician if any of the following occur: CNS signs or symptoms, leukopenia (WBC $< 4{,}000/mm^3$), platelets $< 100{,}000/mm^3$, stomatitis, hypersensitivity reaction, bleeding tendencies, diarrhea.

### Drug-specific teaching points

- Prepare a calendar noting return for specific treatment days, diagnostic tests, and additional courses of drug therapy.
- The following side effects may occur: loss of appetite, nausea, vomiting, mouth sores (frequent mouth care, small frequent meals may help; maintain good nutrition; request an antiemetic); constipation or diarrhea (a bowel program may be established); disorientation, dizziness, headache (take special precautions to avoid injury); rash, loss of hair (reversible; obtain a wig or other suitable head covering before hair loss occurs; keep head covered in extremes of temperature).
- Have regular blood tests to monitor the drug's effects.
- Avoid alcoholic beverages or products containing alcohol; severe reactions can occur.

p

- Avoid foods high in tyramine (a list will be provided by the dietician); severe reactions can occur.
- Use contraception (both men and women); serious fetal harm can occur.
- Report fever, chills, sore throat, unusual bleeding or bruising, vomiting of blood, black or tarry stools, cough, shortness of breath, thick bronchial secretions, pregnancy.

## Prochlorperazine

### prochlorperazine

*(proe klor* ***per'*** *a zeen)*

*Rectal suppositories:* Compazine

### prochlorperazine edisylate

*Oral syrup, injection:* Compazine

### prochlorperazine maleate

*Oral tablets and sustained-release capsules:* Compazine, PMS-Prochlorperazine (CAN), Stemetil (CAN)

**Pregnancy Category C**

### Drug classes

Phenothiazine (piperazine)
Dopaminergic blocking agent
Antipsychotic
Antiemetic
Antianxiety agent

### Therapeutic actions

Mechanism of action not fully understood: antipsychotic drugs block postsynaptic dopamine receptors in the brain, but this may not be necessary and sufficient for antipsychotic activity; depresses the RAS, including the parts of the brain involved with wakefulness and emesis; anticholinergic, antihistaminic ($H_1$), and alpha-adrenergic blocking activity also may contribute to some of its therapeutic (and adverse) actions.

### Indications

- Management of manifestations of psychotic disorders
- Control of severe nausea and vomiting
- Short-term treatment of nonpsychotic anxiety (not drug of choice)

### Contraindications/cautions

- Contraindications: coma or severe CNS depression, bone marrow depression, blood dyscrasia, circulatory collapse, subcortical brain damage, Parkinson's disease, liver damage, cerebral arteriosclerosis, coronary disease, severe hypotension or hypertension.
- Use cautiously with respiratory disorders, glaucoma, prostatic hypertrophy, epilepsy, breast cancer (elevations in prolactin may stimulate a prolactin-dependent tumor), thyrotoxicosis, peptic ulcer, decreased renal function, myelography within previous 24 h or scheduled within 48 h, exposure to heat or phosphorous insecticides, pregnancy, lactation, children younger 12 y, especially those with chickenpox, CNS infections (children are especially susceptible to dystonias that may confound the diagnosis of Reye's syndrome).

## Dosage

**Available Forms:** Tablets—5, 10, 25 mg; SR capsules—10, 15, 30 mg; syrup—5 mg/5 ml; injection—5 mg/ml; suppositories—2.5, 5, 25 mg

*ADULT*

- ***Psychiatry:*** Initially, 5–10 mg PO tid or qid. Gradually increase dosage every 2–3 d as necessary up to 50–75 mg/d for mild or moderate disturbances, 100–150 mg/d for more severe disturbances. For immediate control of severely disturbed adults, 10–20 mg IM repeated q2–4h (every hour for resistant cases); switch to oral therapy as soon as possible.
- ***Antiemetic:*** *Control of severe nausea and vomiting:* 5–10 mg PO tid–qid; 15 mg (sustained-release) on arising; 10 mg (sustained-release) q12h; 25 mg rectally bid; or 5–10 mg IM initially, repeated q3–4h up to 40 mg/d.
- ***Surgery, to control nausea, vomiting:*** 5–10 mg IM 1–2 h before anes-

thesia or during and after surgery (may repeat once in 30 min); 5–10 mg IV 15 min before anesthesia or during and after surgery (may repeat once); or as IV infusion, 20 mg/L of isotonic solution added to infusion 15–30 min before anesthesia.

*PEDIATRIC:* Generally not recommended for children under 20 lb (9.1 kg) or younger than 2 y; do not use in pediatric surgery.

- *CHILDREN 2–12 Y:* 2.5 mg PO or rectally bid–tid. Do not give more than 10 mg on first day. Increase dosage according to patient response; total daily dose usually does not exceed 20 mg (2–5 y) or 25 mg (6–12 y).
- *CHILDREN <12 Y:* 0.13 mg/kg by deep IM injection. Switch to oral dosage as soon possible (usually after one dose).
- *Antiemetic: Control of severe nausea/vomiting in children >20 lb or >2 y:* Oral or rectal administration: 9.1–13.2 kg, 2.5 mg qd–bid, not to exceed 7.5 mg/d.
- *13.6–17.7 kg:* 2.5 mg bid–tid, not to exceed 10 mg/d.
- *18.2–38.6 kg:* 2.5 mg tid or 5 mg bid, not to exceed 15 mg/d.

– ***IM:*** 18.2–38.6 kg: IM 0.132 mg/kg (usually only one dose).

## Pharmacokinetics

| *Route* | *Onset* | *Duration* |
|---|---|---|
| Oral | 30–40 min | 3–4 h (10–12 SR) |
| PR | 60–90 min | 3–4 h |
| IM | 10–20 min | 3–4 h |
| IV | Immediate | 3–4 h |

*Metabolism:* Hepatic, $T_{1/2}$: unknown
*Distribution:* Crosses placenta; enters breast milk
*Excretion:* Urine

## IV facts

**Preparation:** Dilute 20 mg in not less than 1 L of isotonic solution.
**Infusion:** Inject 5–10 mg directly IV 15–30 min before induction (may be repeated once), or infuse dilute solution 15–30 min before induction; do not exceed 5 mg/ml per minute.

## Adverse effects

***Antipsychotic Drugs***

- CNS: *Drowsiness*, insomnia, vertigo, headache, weakness, tremor, ataxia, slurring, cerebral edema, seizures, exacerbation of psychotic symptoms, extrapyramidal syndromes—*pseudoparkinsonism; dystonias; akathisia*, tardive dyskinesias, potentially irreversible; **neuroleptic malignant syndrome**
- CV: Hypotension, orthostatic hypotension, hypertension, tachycardia, bradycardia, cardiac arrest, CHF, cardiomegaly, **refractory arrhythmias** (some fatal), pulmonary edema
- Respiratory: Bronchospasm, laryngospasm, dyspnea; suppression of cough reflex and potential for aspiration
- Hematologic: Eosinophilia, leukopenia, leukocytosis, anemia; aplastic anemia; hemolytic anemia; thrombocytopenic or nonthrombocytopenic purpura; pancytopenia
- Hypersensitivity: Jaundice, urticaria, angioneurotic edema, laryngeal edema, photosensitivity, eczema, asthma, anaphylactoid reactions, exfoliative dermatitis
- EENT: Glaucoma, *photophobia, blurred vision*, miosis, mydriasis, deposits in the cornea and lens (opacities), pigmentary retinopathy
- Endocrine: Lactation, breast engorgement, galactorrhea; SIADH; amenorrhea, menstrual irregularities; gynecomastia; changes in libido; hyperglycemia or hypoglycemia; glycosuria; hyponatremia; pituitary tumor with hyperprolactinemia; inhibition of ovulation, infertility, pseudopregnancy; reduced urinary levels of gonadotropins, estrogens, progestins
- Autonomic: Dry mouth, salivation, nasal congestion, nausea, vomiting, anorexia, fever, pallor, flushed facies, sweating, constipation, paralytic ileus, urinary retention, incontinence, polyuria, enuresis,

P

priapism, ejaculation inhibition, male impotence
- **Other:** *Urine discolored pink to red-brown*

### Clinically important drug-drug interactions

• Additive CNS depression with alcohol • Additive anticholinergic effects and possibly decreased antipsychotic efficacy with anticholinergic drugs • Increased likelihood of seizures with metrizamide • Increased chance of severe neuromuscular excitation and hypotension with barbiturate anesthetics (methohexital, thiamylal, phenobarbital, thiopental) • Decreased antihypertensive effect of guanethidine

### Drug-lab test interferences

• False-positive pregnancy tests (less likely if serum test is used) • Increase in PBI, not attributable to an increase in thyroxine

## ■ Nursing Considerations

### Assessment

- *History:* Coma or severe CNS depression; bone marrow depression; circulatory collapse; subcortical brain damage; Parkinson's disease; liver damage; cerebral arteriosclerosis; coronary disease; severe hypotension or hypertension; respiratory disorders; glaucoma, prostatic hypertrophy; epilepsy; breast cancer; thyrotoxicosis; peptic ulcer, decreased renal function; myelography within previous 24 h or scheduled within 48 h; exposure to heat or phosphorous insecticides; pregnancy; lactation; children younger than 12 y
- *Physical:* Weight, T; reflexes, orientation, intraocular pressure; P, BP, orthostatic BP; R, adventitious sounds; bowel sounds and normal output; liver evaluation; urinary output, prostate size; CBC; urinalysis; thyroid, liver, and kidney function tests

### Implementation

- Do not change brand names of oral preparations; bioavailability differences have been documented.
- Do not allow patient to crush or chew sustained-release capsules.
- Do not administer SC because of local irritation.
- Give IM injections deeply into the upper outer quadrant of the buttock.
- Avoid skin contact with oral solution; contact dermatitis has occurred.
- Discontinue drug if serum creatinine, BUN become abnormal or if WBC count is depressed.
- Monitor elderly patients for dehydration, and institute remedial measures promptly; sedation and decreased sensation of thirst related to CNS effects of drug can lead to severe dehydration.
- Consult physician regarding appropriate warning of patient or patient's guardian about tardive dyskinesias.
- Consult physician about dosage reduction, use of anticholinergic antiparkinsonian drugs (controversial) if extrapyramidal effects occur.

### Drug-specific teaching points

- Take drug exactly as prescribed.
- Do not crush or chew sustained-release capsules.
- Avoid skin contact with drug solutions.
- Avoid driving or engaging in other dangerous activities if CNS, vision changes occur.
- Avoid prolonged exposure to sun, or use a sunscreen or covering garments.
- Maintain fluid intake, and use precautions against heatstroke in hot weather.
- Report sore throat, fever, unusual bleeding or bruising, rash, weakness, tremors, impaired vision, dark urine (expect pink or reddish-brown urine), pale stools, yellowing of the skin or eyes.

# procyclidine

*(proe sye' kli deen)*

Kemadrin, PMS Procyclidine (CAN), Procyclid (CAN)

**Pregnancy Category C**

### Drug classes

Antiparkinsonism drug (anticholinergic type)

### Therapeutic actions

Has anticholinergic activity in the CNS that is believed to help normalize the hypothesized imbalance of cholinergic/dopaminergic neurotransmission created by the loss of dopaminergic neurons in the basal ganglia of the brain in parkinsonism; reduces severity of rigidity and reduces the akinesia and tremor that characterize parkinsonism; less effective overall than levodopa; peripheral anticholinergic effects suppress secondary symptoms of parkinsonism, such as drooling.

### Indications

- Treatment of parkinsonism (postencephalitic, arteriosclerotic, and idiopathic types), alone or with other drugs in more severe cases
- Relief of symptoms of extrapyramidal dysfunction that accompany phenothiazine and reserpine therapy
- Control of sialorrhea resulting from neuroleptic medication

### Contraindications/cautions

- Contraindications: hypersensitivity to procyclidine; glaucoma, especially angle-closure glaucoma; pyloric or duodenal obstruction; stenosing peptic ulcers; achalasia (megaesophagus); prostatic hypertrophy or bladder neck obstructions; myasthenia gravis; lactation.
- Use cautiously with tachycardia, cardiac arrhythmias, hypertension, hypotension, hepatic or renal dysfunction, alcoholism, chronic illness, people who work in hot environments, pregnancy.

### Dosage

**Available Forms:** Tablets—5 mg

ADULT

- *Parkinsonism not previously treated:* Initially 2.5 mg PO tid after meals. If well tolerated, gradually increase dose to 5 mg tid and as needed before retiring.
- *Transferring from other therapy:* Substitute 2.5 mg PO tid for all or part of the original drug, then increase procyclidine while withdrawing other drug.
- *Drug-induced extrapyramidal symptoms:* Initially 2.5 mg PO tid. Increase by 2.5-mg increments until symptomatic relief is obtained. In most cases, results will be obtained with 10–20 mg/d.

PEDIATRIC: Safety and efficacy not established.

GERIATRIC PATIENTS: Strict dosage regulation may be necessary. Patients older than 60 y often develop increased sensitivity to the CNS effects of anticholinergic drugs.

### Pharmacokinetics

| *Route* | *Onset* | *Peak* |
|---|---|---|
| Oral | Varies | 1.1–2 h |

*Metabolism:* Hepatic, $T_{1/2}$: 11.5–12.6 h

*Distribution:* Crosses placenta; enters breast milk

*Excretion:* Urine

### Adverse effects

*Peripheral Anticholinergic Effects*

- CNS: *Blurred vision, mydriasis*, diplopia, increased intraocular tension, angle-closure glaucoma
- GI: *Dry mouth, constipation*, dilation of the colon, paralytic ileus
- CV: Tachycardia, palpitations
- GU: *Urinary retention*, urinary hesitancy, dysuria, difficulty achieving or maintaining an erection
- General: *Flushing, decreased sweating*, elevated temperature
- CNS (some of these are characteristic of centrally acting anticholinergic drugs): *Disorientation, confusion*, memory loss, hallucinations, psychoses, agitation, nervousness, delusions, delirium, paranoia, euphoria, excitement, *lightheadedness, dizziness*, depression, drowsiness, weakness, giddiness, paresthesia, heaviness of the limbs, numbness of fingers
- GI: Acute suppurative parotitis, nausea, vomting, epigastric distress
- CV: Hypotension, orthostatic hypotension
- Dermatologic: Skin rash, urticaria, other dermatoses
- Other: Muscular weakness, muscular cramping

p

**Clinically important drug-drug interactions**

• Paralytic ileus, sometimes fatal, with phenothiazines • Additive adverse CNS effects, toxic psychosis, with other drugs that have central (CNS) anticholinergic properties, phenothiazines • Possible masking of the development of persistent extrapyramidal symptoms, tardive dyskinesia, in long-term therapy with phenothiazines, haloperidol • Decreased therapeutic efficacy of phenothiazines and haloperidol, possibly due to central antagonism

## ■ Nursing Considerations

### Assessment

- *History:* Hypersensitivity to procyclidine; glaucoma; pyloric or duodenal obstruction; stenosing peptic ulcers; achalasia; prostatic hypertrophy or bladder neck obstructions; myasthenia gravis; cardiac arrhythmias; hypertension, hypotension; hepatic or renal dysfunction; alcoholism; chronic illness; people who work in hot environment; pregnancy; lactation
- *Physical:* Weight; T; skin color, lesions; orientation, affect, reflexes, bilateral grip strength; visual exam including tonometry; P, BP, orthostatic BP, auscultation; bowel sounds, normal output, liver evaluation; urinary output, voiding pattern, prostate palpation; liver and kidney function tests

### Implementation

- Decrease dosage or discontinue drug temporarily if dry mouth is so severe that swallowing or speaking becomes difficult.
- Give with caution, and reduce dosage in hot weather; drug interferes with sweating and ability of body to maintain body heat equilibrium; anhidrosis and fatal hyperthermia have occurred.
- Give with meals if GI upset occurs; give before meals to patients bothered by dry mouth; give after meals if drooling is a problem or if drug causes nausea.
- Have patient void before receiving each dose if urinary retention is a problem.

### Drug-specific teaching points

- Take this drug exactly as prescribed.
- The following side effects may occur: drowsiness, dizziness, confusion, blurred vision (avoid driving or engaging in activities that require alertness and visual acuity); nausea (eat frequent, small meals); dry mouth (suck sugarless lozenges or ice chips); painful or difficult urination (empty the bladder immediately before each dose); constipation (if maintaining adequate fluid intake, exercising regularly do not help, consult your nurse or physician); use caution in hot weather (you are more susceptible to heat prostration).
- Report difficult or painful urination, constipation, rapid or pounding heartbeat, confusion, eye pain or rash.

# Progesterone

## progesterone in oil

*(proe **jess'** ter one)*

*Parenteral:* Progestilin (CAN)

*Intrauterine system:* Progestasert

*Vaginal gel:* Crinone

## progesterone aqueous

## progesterone powder

**Pregnancy Category X**

**Drug classes**

Hormone
Progestin

**Therapeutic actions**

Endogenous female progestational substance; transforms proliferative endometrium into secretory endometrium; inhibits the secretion of pituitary gonadotropins, which prevents follicular maturation and ovulation; inhibits spontaneous uterine contractions; may have some estrogenic, anabolic, or androgenic activity.

## Indications

- Treatment of primary and secondary amenorrhea
- Treatment of functional uterine bleeding
- Contraception in parous and nulliparous women (intrauterine system)
- Infertility, as part of assisted reproductive technology for infertile women—gel
- Unlabeled uses: treatment of premenstrual syndrome, prevention of premature labor and habitual abortion in the first trimester, treatment of menorrhagia (intrauterine system)

## Contraindications/cautions

- Contraindications: allergy to progestins, thrombophlebitis, thromboembolic disorders, cerebral hemorrhage or history of these conditions, hepatic disease, carcinoma of the breast or genital organs, undiagnosed vaginal bleeding, missed abortion, diagnostic test for pregnancy, pregnancy (fetal abnormalities, including masculinization of the female fetus have occurred), lactation; PID, venereal disease, postpartum endometritis, pelvic surgery, uterine or cervical carcinoma (intrauterine system).
- Use cautiously with epilepsy, migraine, asthma, cardiac or renal dysfunction.

## Dosage

**Available Forms:** Injection—50 mg/ml; powder—1, 10, 25, 100 g; vaginal gel—90 mg (8%)

Administer parenteral preparation by IM route only.

### Adult

- *Amenorrhea:* 5–10 mg/d IM for 6–8 consecutive d. Expect withdrawal bleeding 48–72 h after the last injection. Spontaneous normal cycles may follow.
- *Functional uterine bleeding:* 5–10 mg/d IM for six doses. Bleeding should cease within 6 d. If estrogen is being given, begin progesterone after 2 wk of estrogen therapy. Discontinue injections when menstrual flow begins.
- *Contraception:* Insert a single intrauterine system into the uterine cavity. Contraceptive effectiveness is retained for 1 y. The system must be replaced 1 y after insertion.
- *Infertility:* 90 mg vaginally qd in women requiring progesterone supplementation; 90 mg vaginally bid for replacement—continue for 10–12 wk into pregnancy if it occurs.

## Pharmacokinetics

| *Route* | *Onset* | *Peak* | *Duration* |
|---|---|---|---|
| IM | Varies | Unknown | |
| Vaginal gel | Slow | Unknown | 25–50 h |

*Metabolism:* Hepatic, $T_{1/2}$: 5 min
*Distribution:* Crosses placenta; enters breast milk
*Excretion:* Urine

## Adverse effects

*Parenteral*

- CNS: Sudden, partial or complete loss of vision, proptosis, diplopia, migraine, precipitation of acute intermittent porphyria, mental depression, pyrexia, insomnia, somnolence, *dizziness*
- GI: Cholestatic jaundice, nausea
- CV: Thrombophlebitis, cerebrovascular disorders, retinal thrombosis, pulmonary embolism
- GU: *Breakthrough bleeding, spotting, change in menstrual flow, amenorrhea, changes in cervical erosion and cervical secretions, breast tenderness* and secretion, transient increase in sodium and chloride excretion
- Dermatologic: Rash with or without pruritus, acne, melasma or chloasma, alopecia, hirsutism, *photosensitivity*
- General: Fluid retention, edema, *change in weight*, effects similar to those seen with oral contraceptives

*Effects of Oral Contraceptives*

- GI: Hepatic adenoma
- CV: Increased BP, **thromboembolic and thrombotic disease**
- Endocrine: Decreased glucose tolerance

*Intrauterine System*

- CV: Bradycardia and syncope related to insertional pain
- GU: Endometritis, spontaneous abortion, septic abortion, septicemia, perforation of

P

the uterus and cervix, pelvic infection, cervical erosion, vaginitis, leukorrhea, amenorrhea, uterine embedment, *complete or partial expulsion of the device*

*Vaginal Gel*

- CNS: *Somnolence, headache,* nervousness, depression
- GI: *Constipation,* nausea, diarrhea
- General: *Breast enlargement,* nocturia, perineal pain

**Drug-lab test interferences**

- Inaccurate tests of hepatic and endocrine function

## ■ Nursing Considerations

### Assessment

- ***History:*** Allergy to progestins, thrombophlebitis, thromboembolic disorders, cerebral hemorrhage, hepatic disease, carcinoma of the breast or genital organs, undiagnosed vaginal bleeding, missed abortion, epilepsy, migraine, asthma, cardiac or renal dysfunction, PID, venereal disease, postpartum endometritis, pelvic surgery, uterine or cervical carcinoma, pregnancy, lactation
- ***Physical:*** Skin color, lesions, turgor; hair; breasts; pelvic exam; orientation, affect; ophthalmologic exam; P, auscultation, peripheral perfusion, edema; R, adventitious sounds; liver evaluation; liver and renal function tests, glucose tolerance; Pap smear

### Implementation

- Arrange for pretreatment and periodic (at least annual) history and physical, including BP, breasts, abdomen, pelvic organs, and a Pap smear.
- Arrange for insertion of intrauterine system during or immediately after menstrual period to ensure that the patient is not pregnant; arrange to have patient reexamined after first month menses to ensure that system has not been expelled.
- Caution patient before therapy of the need to prevent pregnancy during treatment and to obtain frequent medical follow-up.
- Administer parenteral preparations by IM injection only.
- Discontinue medication and consult physician if sudden partial or complete loss of vision occur; discontinue if papilledema or retinal vascular lesions are present on exam.
- Discontinue medication and consult physician at the first sign of thromboembolic disease: leg pain, swelling, peripheral perfusion changes, shortness of breath.

### Drug-specific teaching points

- This drug can be given IM; it will be given daily for the specified number of days, or inserted vaginally and can remain for 1 y (as appropriate), or inserted vaginally using the applicator system 1 to 2 times/d.
- If used for fertility program, continue vaginal gel 10–12 wk into pregnancy until placental autonomy is achieved.
- The following side effects may occur: sensitivity to light (avoid exposure to the sun; use sunscreen and protective clothing); dizziness, sleeplessness, depression (use caution if driving or performing tasks that require alertness); skin rash, skin color changes, loss of hair; fever; nausea.
- This drug should not be taken during pregnancy (except vaginal gel); serious fetal abnormalities have been reported. If you may be pregnant, consult physician immediately.
- Report pain or swelling and warmth in the calves, acute chest pain or shortness of breath, sudden severe headache or vomiting, dizziness or fainting, visual disturbances, numbness or tingling in the arm or leg.

*Intrauterine System*

- Report excessive bleeding, severe cramping, abnormal vaginal discharge, fever or flulike symptoms.

*Vaginal Gel*

- Report severe headache, abnormal vaginal bleeding or discharge, acute calf or chest pain, fever.

## promazine hydrochloride

***(proe' ma zeen)***

Prozine-50, Sparine

**Pregnancy Category C**

### Drug classes
Phenothiazine (aliphatic)
Dopaminergic blocking agent
Antipsychotic

### Therapeutic actions
Mechanism of action not fully understood: antipsychotic drugs block postsynaptic dopamine receptors in the brain, but this may not be necessary and sufficient for antipsychotic activity; depresses the RAS, including the parts of the brain involved with wakefulness and emesis; anticholinergic, antihistaminic ($H_1$), and alpha-adrenergic blocking activity also may contribute to some of its therapeutic (and adverse) actions.

### Indications
- Management of manifestations of psychotic disorders

### Contraindications/cautions
- Contraindications: coma or severe CNS depression, bone marrow depression, blood dyscrasia, circulatory collapse, subcortical brain damage, Parkinson's disease, liver damage, cerebral arteriosclerosis, coronary disease, severe hypotension or hypertension.
- Use cautiously with respiratory disorders, glaucoma, prostatic hypertrophy, epilepsy or history of epilepsy, breast cancer, thyrotoxicosis, allergy to aspirin (the oral 25-mg tablets and the syrup contain tartrazine; allergy to aspirin may indicate allergy to tartrazine), peptic ulcer, decreased renal function, myelography within previous 24 h or scheduled within 48 h, exposure to heat or phosphorous insecticides, pregnancy, lactation, children younger than 12 y, especially those with chickenpox, CNS infections (children are especially susceptible to dystonias that may confound the diagnosis of Reye's syndrome).

### Dosage
**Available Forms:** Tablets—25, 50, 100 mg; injection—25, 50 mg/ml
Full clinical effects may require 6 wk–6 mo of therapy.

*ADULT:* Dosage varies with severity of condition.
- ***Severely agitated patients:*** 50–150 mg IM. Repeat if necessary in 30 min (up to 300 mg total dose). *After control is obtained, change to oral (or IM) maintenance dosage:* 10–200 mg PO or IM q4–6h. Do not exceed 1,000 mg/d, because higher doses are not more effective. IV use not recommended; drug is very irritating to vein and tissues.

*PEDIATRIC*
*CHILDREN > 12 Y: Acute episodes of psychotic chronic disease:* 10–25 mg PO or IM q4–6h. Generally not recommended for children <12 y.
*GERIATRIC:* Use lower doses and increase dosage more gradually than in younger patients.

### Pharmacokinetics

| Route | Onset | Duration |
|---|---|---|
| Oral | 30 min | 4–6 h |
| IM | 15–30 min | |

*Metabolism:* Hepatic, $T_{1/2}$: unknown
*Distribution:* Crosses placenta; enters breast milk
*Excretion:* Urine

### Adverse effects
*Antipsychotic Drugs*
- CNS: *Drowsiness*, insomnia, vertigo, headache, weakness, tremor, ataxia, slurring, cerebral edema, seizures, exacerbation of psychotic symptoms, extrapyramidal syndromes—*pseudoparkinsonism; dystonias; akathisia*, tardive dyskinesias, potentially irreversible (no known treatment), **neuroleptic malignant syndrome**
- CV: Hypotension, orthostatic hypotension, hypertension, tachycardia, bradycardia, cardiac arrest, CHF, cardiomegaly, **refractory arrhythmias** (some fatal), pulmonary edema
- Respiratory: Bronchospasm, laryngospasm, dyspnea; suppression of cough reflex and potential for aspiration
- Hematologic: Eosinophilia, leukopenia, leukocytosis, anemia; aplastic anemia;

p

hemolytic anemia; thrombocytopenic or nonthrombocytopenic purpura; pancytopenia

- EENT: Glaucoma, *photophobia, blurred vision*, miosis, mydriasis, deposits in the cornea and lens (opacities), pigmentary retinopathy
- **Hypersensitivity**: Jaundice, urticaria, angioneurotic edema, laryngeal edema, photosensitivity, eczema, asthma, anaphylactoid reactions, exfoliative dermatitis
- **Endocrine**: Lactation, breast engorgement, galactorrhea; SIADH; amenorrhea, menstrual irregularities; gynecomastia; changes in libido; hyperglycemia or hypoglycemia; glycosuria; hyponatremia; pituitary tumor with hyperprolactinemia; inhibition of ovulation, infertility, pseudopregnancy; reduced urinary levels of gonadotropins, estrogens, progestins
- **Autonomic**: Dry mouth, salivation, nasal congestion, nausea, vomiting, anorexia, fever, pallor, flushed facies, sweating, constipation, paralytic ileus, urinary retention, incontinence, polyuria, enuresis, priapism, ejaculation inhibition, male impotence
- **Other**: *Urine discolored pink to red-brown*

### Clinically important drug-drug interactions

• Additive CNS depression with alcohol • Additive anticholinergic effects and possibly decreased antipsychotic efficacy with anticholinergic drugs • Increased likelihood of seizures with metrizamide • Increased chance of severe neuromuscular excitation and hypotension with barbiturate anesthetics (methohexital, thiamylal, phenobarbital, thiopental) • Decreased antihypertensive effect of guanethidine with antipsychotic drugs

### Drug-lab test interferences

• False-positive pregnancy tests • Increase in protein-bound iodine, not attributable to an increase in thyroxine

## ■ Nursing Considerations

### Assessment

- *History:* Severe CNS depression, blood dyscrasia, circulatory collapse, subcortical brain damage, Parkinson's disease, liver damage, cerebral arteriosclerosis, coronary disease, severe hypotension or hypertension, respiratory disorders, glaucoma, prostatic hypertrophy, epilepsy, breast cancer, thyrotoxicosis, allergy to aspirin or tartrazine, peptic ulcer, decreased renal function, myelography within previous 24 h or scheduled within 48 h, exposure to heat or phosphorous insecticides, pregnancy, lactation, children <12 y
- *Physical:* Weight, T; reflexes, orientation; intraocular pressure; P, BP, orthostatic BP; R, adventitious sounds; bowel sounds and normal output, liver evaluation; urinary output, prostate size; CBC; urinalysis; thyroid, liver, and kidney function tests

### Implementation

- Do not change dosage in chronic therapy more often than weekly; drug requires 4–7 d to achieve steady-state plasma levels.
- Reserve parenteral administration for bed ridden patients. If IM injections are given to ambulatory patients, provide proper precautions to prevent orthostatic hypotension.
- Give IM injections deeply into large muscle mass (gluteal region is preferred).
- Reduce initial dose to 50 mg in patients who are acutely inebriated (to avoid additive depressant effects with alcohol).
- Use the syrup for oral administration to patients who refuse the tablets; syrup may be diluted in citrus or chocolate-flavored drinks.
- Avoid skin contact with oral solution; contact dermatitis has occurred.
- Discontinue drug if serum creatinine, BUN become abnormal or if WBC count is depressed.
- Monitor elderly patients for dehydration, and institute remedial measures

promptly; sedation and decreased sensation of thirst related to CNS effects can lead to severe dehydration.
- Consult physician regarding appropriate warning of patient or patient's guardian about tardive dyskinesias.
- Consult physician about dosage reduction, use of anticholinergic antiparkinsonian drugs (controversial) if extrapyramidal effects occur.

**Drug-specific teaching points**
- Take drug exactly as prescribed.
- Avoid skin contact with drug solutions.
- Avoid driving or engaging in other dangerous activities if CNS, vision changes occur.
- Avoid prolonged exposure to sun or use a sunscreen or covering garments.
- Maintain fluid intake, and use precautions against heatstroke in hot weather.
- Report sore throat, fever, unusual bleeding or bruising, rash, weakness, tremors, impaired vision, dark urine (expect pink or reddish-brown urine), pale stools, yellowing of the skin or eyes.

## promethazine hydrochloride

*(proe **meth'** a zeen)*

Anergan, Histanil (CAN), Pentazine, Phenazine, Phenergan, Phenoject-50, PMS-Promethazine (CAN), Pro-50, Prorex

**Pregnancy Category C**

### Drug classes
Phenothiazine
Dopaminergic blocking agent
Antihistamine
Antiemetic
Anti-motion sickness agent
Sedative/hypnotic

### Therapeutic actions
Selectively blocks $H_1$ receptors, diminishing the effects of histamine on cells of the upper respiratory tract and eyes and decreasing the sneezing, mucus production, itching, and tearing that accompany allergic reactions in sensitized people exposed to antigens; blocks cholinergic receptors in the vomiting center that are believed to mediate the nausea and vomiting caused by gastric irritation, by input from the vestibular apparatus (motion sickness, nausea associated with vestibular neuritis), and by input from the chemoreceptor trigger zone (drug- and radiation-induced emesis); depresses the RAS, including the parts of the brain involved with wakefulness.

### Indications
- Symptomatic relief of perennial and seasonal allergic rhinitis, vasomotor rhinitis, allergic conjunctivitis; mild, uncomplicated urticaria and angioedema; amelioration of allergic reactions to blood or plasma; dermatographism, adjunctive therapy (with epinephrine and other measures) in anaphylactic reactions
- Treatment and prevention of motion sickness; prevention and control of nausea and vomiting associated with anesthesia and surgery
- Preoperative, postoperative, or obstetric sedation
- Adjunct to analgesics to control postoperative pain
- Adjunctive IV therapy with reduced amounts of meperidine or other narcotic analgesics in special surgical situations, such as repeated bronchoscopy, ophthalmic surgery, or in poor-risk patients

### Contraindications/cautions
- Contraindications: hypersensitivity to antihistamines or phenothiazines, coma or severe CNS depression, bone marrow depression, vomiting of unknown cause, concomitant therapy with MAOIs, lactation (lactation may be inhibited).
- Use cautiously with lower respiratory tract disorders (may cause thickening of secretions and impair expectoration), glaucoma, prostatic hypertrophy, CV disease or hypertension, breast cancer, thyrotoxicosis, pregnancy (jaundice and extrapyramidal effects in infants; drug may inhibit platelet aggregation in neonate if taken by mother within 2 wk of delivery), children (antihistamine overdosage may cause hallucinations, convulsions, and death), a child with a history of sleep

apnea, a family history of SIDS, or Reye's syndrome (may mask the symptoms of Reye's syndrome and contribute to its development), the elderly (more likely to cause dizziness, sedation, syncope, toxic confusional states, hypotension, and extrapyramidal effects).

## Dosage

**Available Forms:** Tablets—12.5, 25, 50 mg; syrup—6.25, 25 mg/5 ml; suppositories—12.5, 25, 50 mg; injection—25, 50 mg/ml

**ADULT**

- *Allergy:* Average dose is 25 mg PO or by rectal suppository, preferably hs. If necessary, 12.5 mg PO before meals and hs; 25 mg IM or IV for serious reactions. May repeat within 2 h if necessary.
- *Motion sickness:* 25 mg PO bid. Initial dose should be scheduled 1/2–1 h before travel; repeat in 8–12 h if necessary. Thereafter, give 25 mg on arising and before evening meal.
- *Nausea and vomiting:* 25 mg PO; repeat doses of 12.5–25.0 mg as needed, q4–6h. Give rectally or parenterally if oral dosage is not tolerated. 12.5–25.0 mg IM or IV, not to be repeated more frequently than q4–6h.
- *Sedation:* 25–50 mg PO, IM, or IV.
- *Preoperative use:* 50 mg PO the night before, or 50 mg with an equal dose of meperidine and the required amount of belladonna alkaloid.
- *Postoperative sedation and adjunctive use with analgesics:* 25–50 mg PO, IM, or IV.
- *Labor:* 50 mg IM or IV in early stages. When labor is established, 25–75 mg with a reduced dose of narcotic. May repeat once or twice at 4-h intervals. Maximum dose within 24 h is 100 mg.

**PEDIATRIC**

- *Allergy:* 25 mg PO hs or 6.25–12.5 mg tid.
- *Motion sickness:* 12.5–25.0 mg PO or rectally bid.
- *Nausea and vomiting:* 1 mg/kg PO q4–6h as needed.
- *Sedation:* 12.5–50.0 mg PO or rectally.
- *Preoperative use:* 1 mg/kg PO in combination with an equal dose of meperidine and the required amount of an atropine-like drug.
- *Postoperative sedation and adjunctive use with analgesics:* 12.5–50.0 mg PO.

## Pharmacokinetics

| Route | Onset | Duration |
|---|---|---|
| Oral | 20 min | 12 h |
| IM | 20 min | 12 h |
| IV | 3–5 min | 12 h |

*Metabolism:* Hepatic, $T_{1/2}$: unknown
*Distribution:* Crosses placenta; enters breast milk
*Excretion:* Urine

## IV facts

**Preparation:** Dilute to a concentration no greater than 25 mg/ml.
**Infusion:** Infuse no faster than 25 mg/min.

## Adverse effects

- **CNS:** *Dizziness, drowsiness, poor coordination, confusion, restlessness, excitation,* convulsions, tremors, headache, blurred vision, diplopia, vertigo, tinnitus
- **GI:** *Epigastric distress*, nausea, vomiting, diarrhea, constipation
- **CV:** Hypotension, palpitations, bradycardia, tachycardia, extrasystoles
- **Respiratory:** *Thickening of bronchial secretions;* chest tightness; dry mouth, nose, and throat; respiratory depression; suppression of cough reflex, potential for aspiration
- **Hematologic:** Hemolytic anemia, hypoplastic anemia, thrombocytopenia, leukopenia, agranulocytosis, pancytopenia
- **GU:** *Urinary frequency, dysuria*, urinary retention, decreased libido, impotence
- **Dermatologic:** Urticaria, rash, photosensitivity, chills
- **Other:** Tingling, heaviness and wetness of the hands

**Clinically important drug-drug interactions**
• Additive anticholinergic effects with anticholinergic drugs • Increased frequency and severity of neuromuscular excitation and hypotension with methohexital, thiamylal, phenobarbital anesthetic, thiopental • Enhanced CNS depression with alcohol

## ■ Nursing Considerations

### Assessment

- *History:* Hypersensitivity to antihistamines or phenothiazines, severe CNS depression, bone marrow depression, vomiting of unknown cause, concomitant therapy with MAO inhibitors, lactation, lower respiratory tract disorders, glaucoma, prostatic hypertrophy,CV disease or hypertension, breast cancer, thyrotoxicosis, pregnancy, history of sleep apnea or a family history of SIDS, child with Reye's syndrome
- *Physical:* Weight, T; reflexes, orientation, intraocular pressure; P, BP, orthostatic BP; R, adventitious sounds; bowel sounds and normal output, liver evaluation; urinary output, prostate size; CBC; urinalysis; thyroid, liver, and kidney function tests

### Implementation

- Do not give tablets, rectal suppositories to children <2 y.
- Give IM injections deep into muscle.
- Do not administer SC; tissue necrosis may occur.
- Do not administer intra-arterially; arteriospasm and gangrene of the limb may result.
- Reduce dosage of barbiturates given concurrently with promethazine by at least half; arrange for dosage reduction of narcotic analgesics given concomitantly by one-fourth to one-half.

### Drug-specific teaching points

- Take drug exactly as prescribed
- Avoid using alcohol.
- Avoid driving or engaging in other dangerous activities if CNS, vision changes occur.
- Avoid prolonged exposure to sun, or use a sunscreen or covering garments.
- Maintain fluid intake, and use precautions against heat stroke in hot weather.
- Report sore throat, fever, unusual bleeding or bruising, rash, weakness, tremors, impaired vision, dark urine, pale stools, yellowing of the skin or eyes.

# propafenone hydrochloride

*(proe **paf'** a non)*

Rythmol

**Pregnancy Category C**

**Drug classes**
Antiarrhythmic

**Therapeutic actions**
Class 1C antiarrhythmic: local anesthetic effects with a direct membrane stablizing action on the myocardial membranes; refractory period is prolonged with a reduction of spontaneous automaticity and depressed trigger activity.

**Indications**

- Treatment of documented life-threatening ventricular arrhythmias; reserve use for those patients in whom the benefits outweigh the risks
- In patients without structural heart disease, for prolongation of the time to recurrence of paroxysmal atrial fibrillation/flutter and paroxysmal supraventricular tachycardia associated with disabling symptoms
- Unlabeled uses; treatment of supraventricular tachycardias, including atrial fibrillation associated with Wolff-Parkinson-White syndrome

**Contraindications/cautions**

- Contraindications: hypersensitivity to propafenone, uncontrolled CHF, cardiogenic shock, cardiac conduction disturbances in the absence of an artificial pacemaker, bradycardia, marked hypotension, bronchospastic disorders, manifest electrolyte imbalance, pregnancy (teratogenic in preclinical studies), lactation.
- Use cautiously with hepatic, renal dysfunction.

### Dosage

**Available Forms:** Tablets—150, 225, 300 mg

p

*ADULT:* Initially titrate on the basis of response and tolerance. Initiate with 150 mg PO q8h (450 mg/d). Dosage may be increased at a minimum of 3- to 4-d intervals to 225 mg PO q8h (675 mg/d) and if necessary, to 300 mg PO q8h (900 mg/d). Do not exceed 900 mg/d. Decrease dosage with significant widening of the QRS complex or with AV block.

*PEDIATRIC:* Safety and efficacy not established.

*GERIATRIC:* Use with caution; increase dose more gradually during the initial phase of treatment.

### Pharmacokinetics

| *Route* | *Onset* | *Peak* |
|---|---|---|
| Oral | Varies | 3 1/2 h |

*Metabolism:* Hepatic, $T_{1/2}$: 2–10 h
*Distribution:* Crosses placenta; enters breast milk
*Excretion:* Urine

### Adverse effects

- CNS: *Dizziness, headache, weakness, blurred vision,* abnormal dreams, speech or vision disturbances, coma, confusion, depression, memory loss, numbness, paresthesias, psychosis/mania, seizures, tinnitus, vertigo
- GI: *Unusual taste, nausea, vomiting, constipation,* dyspepsia, cholestasis, gastroenteritis, hepatitis
- CV: *First-degree AV block, intraventricular conduction disturbances,* CHF, atrial flutter, AV dissociation, cardiac arrest, sick sinus syndrome, sinus pause, sinus arrest, supraventricular tachycardia
- **Hematologic**: Agranulocytosis, anemia, granulocytopenia, leukopenia, purpura, thrombocytopenia, positive ANA
- **MS**: Muscle weakness, leg cramps, muscle pain
- **Dermatologic**: Alopecia, pruritus

### Clinically important drug-drug interactions

• Increased serum levels of propafenone and risk of increased toxicity with quinidine, cimetidine, beta-blockers • Increased serum levels of digoxin, warfarin

## ■ Nursing Considerations

### Assessment

- *History:* Hypersensitivity to propafenone, uncontrolled CHF, cardiogenic shock, cardiac conduction disturbances in the absence of an artificial pacemaker, bradycardia, marked hypotension, bronchospastic disorders, manifest electrolyte imbalance, hepatic or renal dysfunction, pregnancy, lactation
- *Physical:* Reflexes, affect; BP, P, ECG, peripheral perfusion, auscultation; abdomen, normal function; renal and liver function tests; CBC, Hct, electrolytes; ANA

### Implementation

- Monitor patient response carefully, especially when beginning therapy. Increase dosage at minimum of 3- to 4-d intervals only.
- Reduce dosage with renal or liver dysfunction and with marked previous myocardial damage.
- Increase dosage slowly in patients with renal, liver, or myocardial dysfunction.
- Arrange for periodic ECG monitoring to monitor effects on cardiac conduction.

### Drug-specific teaching points

- Take the drug every 8 h around the clock; determine with nurse a schedule that will interrupt sleep the least.
- Frequent monitoring of ECG will be necessary to adjust dosage or determine effects of drug on cardiac conduction.
- The following side effects may occur: dizziness, headache (avoid driving or performing hazardous tasks); headache, weakness (request medications; rest periods may help); nausea, vomiting, unusual taste (maintain proper nutrition; take drug with meals); constipation.
- Do not stop taking this drug for any reason without checking with your health care provider.
- Report swelling of the extremities, difficulty breathing, fainting, palpitations, vision changes, chest pain.

# propantheline bromide

*(proe **pan'** the leen)*

Pro-Banthine

**Pregnancy Category C**

## Drug classes

Anticholinergic
Antimuscarinic agent
Parasympatholytic
Antispasmodic

## Therapeutic actions

Competitively blocks the effects of acetylcholine at muscarinic cholinergic receptors that mediate the effects of parasympathetic postganglionic impulses, relaxing the GI tract and inhibiting gastric acid secretion.

## Indications

- Adjunctive therapy in the treatment of peptic ulcer
- Unlabeled uses: antisecretory and antispasmodic effects

## Contraindications/cautions

- Contraindications: glaucoma, adhesions between iris and lens, stenosing peptic ulcer, pyloroduodenal obstruction, paralytic ileus, intestinal atony, severe ulcerative colitis, toxic megacolon, symptomatic prostatic hypertrophy, bladder neck obstruction, bronchial asthma, COPD, cardiac arrhythmias, tachycardia, myocardial ischemia, sensitivity to anticholinergic drugs or bromides, impaired metabolic, liver or kidney function, myasthenia gravis, lactation.
- Use cautiously with pregnancy, Down syndrome, brain damage, spasticity, hypertension, hyperthyroidism.

## Dosage

**Available Forms:** Tablets—7.5, 15 mg

**ADULT:** 15 mg PO 1/2 h before meals and hs.

- ***Mild symptoms or person of small stature:*** 7.5 mg PO tid.

**PEDIATRIC**

- ***Peptic ulcer:*** Safety and efficacy not established.
- ***Antisecretory:*** 1.5 mg/kg per day PO divided into doses tid–qid.
- ***Antispasmodic:*** 2–3 mg/kg per day PO in divided doses q4–6h and hs.

**GERIATRIC:** 7.5 mg PO tid.

## Pharmacokinetics

| Route | Onset | Peak | Duration |
|---|---|---|---|
| Oral | 30–60 min | 2–6 h | 6 h |

*Metabolism:* Hepatic, $T_{1/2}$: 3–4 h
*Distribution:* Crosses placenta; enters breast milk
*Excretion:* Urine

## Adverse effects

- CNS: *Blurred vision*, mydriasis, cycloplegia, photophobia, increased intraocular pressure
- GI: *Dry mouth, altered taste perception, nausea, vomiting, dysphagia*, heartburn, constipation, bloated feeling, paralytic ileus, gastroesophageal reflux
- CV: Palpitations, tachycardia
- GU: *Urinary hesitancy and retention*; impotence
- Local: *Irritation at site of IM injection*
- Other: Decreased sweating and predisposition to heat prostration, suppression of lactation, nasal congestion

## Clinically important drug-drug interactions

• Decreased antipsychotic effectiveness of haloperidol • Decreased pharmacologic/therapeutic effects of phenothiazines

## ■ Nursing Considerations

### Assessment

- ***History:*** Adhesions between iris and lens, stenosing peptic ulcer, pyloroduodenal obstruction, intestinal atony, severe ulcerative colitis, symptomatic prostatic hypertrophy, bladder neck obstruction, bronchial asthma, COPD, cardiac arrhythmias, myocardial ischemia, sensitivity to anticholinergic drugs; bromides, impaired metabolic, liver or kidney function, myasthenia gravis, lactation, Down's syndrome, brain damage, spasticity, hypertension, hyperthyroidism
- ***Physical:*** Bowel sounds, normal output; urinary output, prostate palpation; R, ad-

ventitious sounds; pulse, BP; intraocular pressure, vision exam; bilateral grip strength, reflexes; liver palpation, liver and renal function tests.

### Implementation

- Ensure adequate hydration; provide environmental control (temperature) to prevent hyperpyrexia.
- Have patient void before each dose of medication if urinary retention becomes a problem.

### Drug-specific teaching points

- Take drug exactly as prescribed.
- Avoid hot environments (you will be heat intolerant, and dangerous reactions may occur).
- The following side effects may occur: constipation (ensure adequate fluid intake, proper diet); dry mouth (sugarless lozenges, frequent mouth care may help; may lessen); blurred vision, sensitivity to light (reversible; avoid tasks that require acute vision; wear sunglasses when in bright light); impotence (reversible); difficulty urinating (empty the bladder immediately before taking drug).
- Report skin rash, flushing, eye pain, difficulty breathing, tremors, loss of coordination, irregular heartbeat, palpitations, headache, abdominal distention, hallucinations, severe or persistent dry mouth, difficulty swallowing, difficulty in urination, severe constipation, sensitivity to light.

## Propoxyphene

### propoxyphene hydrochloride

*(proe **pox'** i feen)*

dextropropoxyphene

Darvon, Dolene

### propoxyphene napsylate

Darvocet-N, Darvon-N,

**Pregnancy Category C**
**C-IV controlled substance**

### Drug classes

Narcotic agonist analgesic

### Therapeutic actions

Acts as agonist at specific opioid receptors in the CNS to produce analgesia, euphoria, sedation; the receptors mediating these effects are thought to be the same as those mediating the effects of endogenous opioids (enkephalins, endorphins).

### Indidications

- Relief of mild to moderate pain

### Contraindications/cautions

- Contraindications: hypersensitivity to narcotics, pregnancy (neonatal withdrawal has occurred; neonatal safety not established), labor or delivery (especially when delivery of a premature infant is expected; narcotics given to mother can cause respiratory depression of neonate; may prolong labor), lactation.
- Use cautiously with renal or hepatic dysfunction, emotional depression.

### Dosage

**Available Forms:** Capsules—65 mg; tablets—100 mg

*ADULT*

- **Propoxyphene hydrochloride:** 65 mg PO q4h as needed. Do not exceed 390 mg/d.
- **Propoxyphene napsylate:** 100 mg PO q4h as needed. Do not exceed 600 mg/d.

*PEDIATRIC:* Not recommended.

*GERIATRIC OR IMPAIRED ADULT:* Use caution; reduced dosage may be necessary.

### Pharmacokinetics

| *Route* | *Onset* | *Peak* |
|---|---|---|
| Oral | Varies | 2–2 1/2 h |

*Metabolism:* Hepatic, $T_{1/2}$: 6–12 h
*Distribution:* Crosses placenta; enters breast milk
*Excretion:* Urine

### Adverse effects

- CNS: *Dizziness, sedation*, lightheadedness, headache, weakness, euphoria, dysphoria, minor visual disturbances
- GI: *Nausea, vomiting*, constipation, abdominal pain, liver dysfunction

- **Dermatologic**: Skin rashes
- **Other**: Tolerance and dependence, psychological dependence

### Clinically important drug-drug interactions

• Increased likelihood of respiratory depression, hypotension, profound sedation, or coma with barbiturate general anesthetics • Increased serum levels and toxicity of carbamazepine • Decreased absorption and serum levels with charcoal

## ■ Nursing Considerations

### Assessment

- *History:* Hypersensitivity to narcotics, pregnancy, lactation, renal or hepatic dysfunction, emotional depression
- *Physical:* Skin color, texture, lesions; orientation, reflexes, affect; bowel sounds, normal output; liver, kidney function tests

### Implementation

- Administer to lactating women 4–6 h before the next feeding to minimize the amount in milk.
- Limit amount of drug dispensed to depressed, emotionally labile, or potentially suicidal patients; propoxyphene intake alone or with other CNS depressants has been associated with deaths.
- Provide narcotic antagonist, facilities for assisted or controlled respiration on standby in case respiratory depression occurs.
- Give drug with milk or food if GI upset occurs.
- Reassure patient about addiction liability; most patients who receive opiates for medical reasons do not develop dependence syndromes.

### Drug-specific teaching points

- Take drug exactly as prescribed.
- The following side effects may occur: nausea, loss of appetite (take drug with food, eat frequent, small meals); constipation (request laxative); dizziness, sedation, drowsiness, impaired visual acuity (avoid driving or performing other tasks that require alertness, visual acuity).
- Do not take leftover medication for other disorders, and do not let anyone else take the prescription.
- Report severe nausea, vomiting, constipation, shortness of breath or difficulty breathing.

# propranolol hydrochloride

*(proe **pran'** oh lole)*

Apo-Propranolol (CAN), Inderal, Inderal LA, Novopranol (CAN), PMS-Propranolol (CAN)

**Pregnancy Category C**

### Drug classes

Beta adrenergic blocker (nonselective)
Antianginal agent
Antiarrhythmic
Antihypertensive

### Therapeutic actions

Competitively blocks beta-adrenergic receptors in the heart and juxtoglomerular apparatus, decreasing the influence of the sympathetic nervous system on these tissues, the excitablity of the heart, cardiac workload and oxygen consumption, and the release of renin and lowering BP; has membrane-stabilizing (local anesthetic) effects that contribute to its antiarrhythmic action; acts in the CNS to reduce sympathetic outflow and vasoconstrictor tone. The mechanism by which it prevents migraine headaches is unknown.

### Indications

- Hypertension alone or with other drugs, especially diuretics
- Angina pectoris caused by coronary atherosclerosis
- IHSS to manage associated stress-induced angina, palpitations, and syncope
- Cardiac arrhythmias, especially supraventricular tachycardia, and ventricular tachycardias induced by digitalis or catecholamines
- Prevention of reinfarction in clinically stable patients 1–4 wk after MI

- Pheochromocytoma, an adjunctive therapy after treatment with an alpha-adrenergic blocker to manage tachycardia before or during surgery or if the pheochromocytoma is inoperable.
- Prophylaxis for migraine headache
- Management of acute situational stress reaction (stage fright)
- Treatment of essential tremor, familial or hereditary
- Unlabeled uses: recurrent GI bleeding in cirrhotic patients, schizophrenia, tardive dyskinesia, acute panic symptoms, vaginal contraceptive

### Contraindications/cautions

- Contraindications: allergy to beta-blocking agents, sinus bradycardia, second- or third-degree heart block, cardiogenic shock, CHF, bronchial asthma, bronchospasm, COPD, pregnancy (neonatal bradycardia, hypoglycemia, and apnea, and low birth weight with chronic use during pregnancy), lactation.
- Use cautiously with hypoglycemia and diabetes, thyrotoxicosis, hepatic dysfunction.

### Dosage

**Available Forms:** Tablets—10, 20, 40, 60, 80, 90 mg; SR capsules—60, 80, 120, 160 mg; injection—1 mg/ml

**ADULT**

- ***Oral***
- *Hypertension:* 40 mg regular propranolol bid *or* 80 mg sustained-release (SR) qd initially; usual maintenance dose, 120–240 mg/d given bid or tid *or* 120–160 mg SR qd (maximum dose, 640 mg/d).
- *Angina:* 10–20 mg tid or qid *or* 80 mg SR qd initially; gradually increase dosage at 3- to 7-d intervals; usual maintenance dose, 160 mg/d (maximum dose, 320 mg/d).
- *IHSS:* 20–40 mg tid or qid *or* 80–160 mg SR qd.
- *Arrhythmias:* 10–30 mg tid or qid.
- *MI:* 180–240 mg/d given tid or qid (maximum dose, 240 mg/d).
- *Pheochromocytoma:* Preoperatively, 60 mg/d for 3 d in divided doses; inoperable tumor, 30 mg/d in divided doses.
- *Migraine:* 80 mg/d qd (SR) or in divided doses; usual maintenance dose, 160–240 mg/d.
- *Essential tremor:* 40 mg bid; usual maintenance dose, 120 mg/d.
- *Situational anxiety:* 40 mg, timing based on the usual onset of action.
- ***Parenteral***
- *Life-threatening arrhythmias:* 1–3 mg IV with careful monitoring, not to exceed 1 mg/min; may give second dose in 2 min, but then do not repeat for 4 h. (*Note:* IV dosage is *markedly* less than oral because of "first pass effect" with oral propranolol).

**PEDIATRIC:** Safety and efficacy not established.

### Pharmacokinetics

| *Route* | *Onset* | *Peak* | *Duration* |
|---|---|---|---|
| Oral | 20–30 min | 60–90 min | 6–12 h |
| IV | Immediate | 1 min | 4–6 h |

*Metabolism:* Hepatic, $T_{1/2}$: 3–5 h
*Distribution:* Crosses placenta; enters breast milk
*Excretion:* Urine

### IV facts

**Preparation:** No further preparation is needed.

**Infusion:** Inject directly IV or into tubing of running IV; do not exceed 1 mg/min.

### Adverse effects

- CNS: Dizziness, vertigo, tinnitus, *fatigue*, emotional depression, paresthesias, sleep disturbances, hallucinations, disorientation, memory loss, slurred speech
- GI: *Gastric pain, flatulence, constipation, diarrhea, nausea, vomiting,* anorexia, ischemic colitis, renal and mesenteric arterial thrombosis, retroperitoneal fibrosis, hepatomegaly, acute pancreatitis

- **CV**: *Bradycardia, CHF, cardiac arrhythmias, sinoartial or AV nodal block,* peripheral vascular insufficiency, claudication, CVA, pulmonary edema, hypotension
- **Respiratory**: Bronchospasm, dyspnea, cough, bronchial obstruction, nasal stuffiness, rhinitis, pharyngitis
- **GU**: *Impotence, decreased libido*, Peyronie's disease, dysuria, nocturia, frequency
- **MS**: Joint pain, arthralgia, muscle cramp
- **EENT**: Eye irritation, dry eyes, conjunctivitis, blurred vision
- **Dermatologic**: Rash, pruritus, sweating, dry skin
- **Allergic reactions**: Pharyngitis, erythematous rash, fever, sore throat, laryngospasm, respiratory distress
- **Other**: *Decreased exercise tolerance, development of ANAs*, hyperglycemia or hypoglycemia, elevated serum transaminase, alkaline phosphatase, and LDH

### Clinically important drug-drug interactions

• Increased effects with verapamil • Decreased effects with indomethacin, ibuprofen, piroxicam, sulindac, barbiturates • Prolonged hypoglycemic effects of insulin • Peripheral ischemia possible with ergot alkaloids • Initial hypertensive episode followed by bradycardia with epinephrine • Increased "first-dose response" to prazosin • Increased serum levels and toxic effects with lidocaine, cimetidine • Increased serum levels of propranolol and phenothiazines, hydralazine if the two drugs are taken concurrently • Paradoxical hypertension when clonidine is given with beta-blockers; increased rebound hypertension when clonidine is discontinued in patients on beta-blockers • Decreased serum levels and therapeutic effects with methimazole, propylthiouracil • Decreased bronchodilator effects of theophyllines • Decreased antihypertensive effects with NSAIDs (ie, ibuprofen, indomethacin, piroxicam, sulindac), rifampin

### Drug-lab test interferences

• Interference with glucose or insulin tolerance tests, glaucoma screening tests

## ■ Nursing Considerations

### Assessment

- *History:* Allergy to beta-blocking agents, sinus bradycardia, second- or third-degree heart block, cardiogenic shock, CHF, bronchial asthma, bronchospasm, COPD, hypoglycemia and diabetes, thyrotoxicosis, hepatic dysfunction, pregnancy, lactation
- *Physical:* Weight, skin color, lesions, edema, temperature; reflexes, affect, vision, hearing, orientation; BP, P, ECG, peripheral perfusion; R, auscultation; bowel sounds, normal output, liver evaluation; bladder palpation; liver and thyroid function tests; blood and urine glucose

### Implementation

- Do not discontinue drug abruptly after chronic therapy (hypersensitivity to catecholamines may have developed, causing exacerbation of angina, MI, and ventricular dysrhythmias). Taper drug gradually over 2 wk with monitoring.
- Ensure that alpha-adrenergic blocker has been given before giving propranolol when treating patients with pheochromocytoma; endogenous catecholamines secreted by the tumor can cause severe hypertension if vascular beta receptors are blocked without concomitant alpha blockade.
- Consult with physician about withdrawing drug if patient is to undergo surgery (withdrawal is controversial).
- Provide continuous cardiac and regular BP monitoring with IV form.
- Give oral drug with food to facilitate absorption.

### Drug-specific teaching points

- Take this drug with meals. Do not discontinue the medication abruptly; abrupt discontinuation can cause a worsening of your disorder.

p

- The following side effects may occur: dizziness, drowsiness, light-headedness, blurred vision (avoid driving or performing hazardous tasks); nausea, loss of appetite (frequent, small meals may help); nightmares, depression (request change of your medication); sexual impotence.
- Report difficulty breathing, night cough, swelling of extremities, slow pulse, confusion, depression, rash, fever, sore throat.
- For diabetic patients: The normal signs of hypoglycemia (sweating, tachycardia) may be blocked by this drug; monitor your blood/urine glucose carefully; eat regular meals and take your diabetic medication regularly.

## propylthiouracil

*(proe pill thye oh* ***yoor'*** *a sill)*

PTU

Propyl-Thyracil (CAN)

**Pregnancy Category D**

### Drug classes
Antithyroid agent

### Therapeutic actions
Inhibits the synthesis of thyroid hormones; partially inhibits the peripheral conversion of $T_4$ to $T_3$, the more potent form of thyroid hormone.

### Indications
- Hyperthyroidism

### Contraindications/cautions
- Contraindications: allergy to antithyroid poroducts, pregnancy (can induce hypothyroidism or cretinism in the fetus; use only if absolutely necessary and when mother has been informed about potential harm to the fetus; if antithyroid drug is needed, this is the drug of choice).
- Use cautiously with lactation (if antithyroid drug is needed, this is the drug of choice).

### Dosage
**Available Forms:** Tablets—50 mg

Administered only PO usually in three equal doses q8h.

**ADULT:** *Initial:* 300 mg/d PO, up to 400–900 mg/d in severe cases. Maintenance, 100–150 mg/d.

**PEDIATRIC**
- *6–10 Y: Initial:* 50–150 mg/d PO.
- *>10 Y: Initial:* 150–300 mg/d PO. Maintenance is determined by the needs of the patient.

### Pharmacokinetics

| *Route* | *Onset* |
|---|---|
| Oral | Varies |

*Metabolism:* Hepatic, $T_{1/2}$: 1–2 h

*Distribution:* Crosses placenta; enters breast milk

*Excretion:* Urine

### Adverse effects
- CNS: *Paresthesias, neuritis, vertigo, drowsiness,* neuropathies, depression, headache
- GI: *Nausea, vomiting, epigastric distress,* loss of taste, jaundice, hepatitis
- CV: Vasculitis, periarteritis
- **Hematologic: Agranulocytosis, granulocytopenia, thrombocytopenia, hypoprothrombinemia, bleeding**
- GU: Nephritis
- Dermatologic: *Skin rash, urticaria,* pruritus, skin pigmentation, exfoliative dermatitis, lupus-like syndrome, loss of hair
- Other: Arthralgia, myalgia, edema, lymphadenopathy, drug fever

### Clinically important drug-drug interactions
• Increased risk of bleeding with oral anticoagulants • Alterations in theophylline, metoprolol, propranolol, digitalis glycoside clearance, serum levels and effects as patient moves from hyperthyroid state to euthryoid state

## ■ Nursing Considerations

### Assessment
- *History:* Allergy to antithyroid poroducts, pregnancy, lactation
- *Physical:* Skin color, lesions, pigmentation; orientation, reflexes, affect; liver

evaluation; CBC, differential, PT time; liver and renal function tests

### Implementation

- Administer drug in 3 equally divided doses at 8-h intervals; schedule to maintain patient's sleep pattern.
- Arrange for regular, periodic blood tests to monitor bone marrow depression and bleeding tendencies.
- Advise medical personnel doing surgical procedures that this patient is using this drug and is at greater risk for bleeding problems.

### Drug-specific teaching points

- Take around the clock at 8-h intervals.
- This drug must be taken for a prolonged period to achieve the desired effects.
- The following side effects may occur: dizziness, weakness, vertigo, drowsiness (use caution if operating a car or dangerous machinery); nausea, vomiting, loss of appetite (small, frequent meals may help); rash, itching.
- Report fever, sore throat, unusual bleeding or bruising, headache, general malaise.

## protamine sulfate

***(proe' ta meen)***

**Pregnancy Category C**

### Drug classes

Heparin antagonist

### Therapeutic actions

Strongly basic proteins found in salmon sperm; protamines form stable salts with heparin, which results in the immediate loss of anticoagulant activity; administered when heparin has not been given; protamine has anticoagulant activity.

### Indications

- Heparin overdose

### Contraindications/cautions

- Allergy to protamine sulfate or fish products, pregnancy, lactation.

### Dosage

**Available Forms:** Injection—10 mg/ml

Dosage is determined by the amount of heparin in the body and the time that has elapsed since the heparin was given; the longer the interval, the smaller the dose required.

***ADULT AND PEDIATRIC:*** 1 mg IV neutralizes 90 USP U of heparin derived from lung tissue or 115 USP U of heparin derived from intestinal mucosa.

### Pharmacokinetics

| *Route* | *Onset* | *Duration* |
|---|---|---|
| IV | 5 min | 2 h |

*Metabolism:* Degraded in body, $T_{1/2}$: unknown

*Distribution:* Crosses placenta; may enter breast milk

### IV facts

**Preparation:** Administer injection undiluted; if dilution is necessary, use 5% Dextrose in Water or Saline; refrigerate any diluted solution. Do not store diluted solution; no preservatives are added. Reconstitute powder for injection with 5 ml Bacteriostatic Water for Injection with benzyl alcohol added to the 50-mg vial (25 ml to the 250-mg vial); stable at room temperature for 72 h.

**Infusion:** Administer very slowly IV over at least 10 min; do not exceed 50 mg in any 10-min period; do not give more than 100 mg over a short period of time.

**Incompatibilities:** Do not mix in lines with incompatible antibiotics, including many penicillins and cephalosporins.

### Adverse effects

- GI: *Nausea/vomiting*
- CV: *Hypotension*
- Hypersensitivity: Anaphylactoid reactions—dyspnea, flushing, hypotension, bradycardia, **anaphylaxis** (sometimes fatal)

## ■ Nursing Considerations

### Assessment

- *History:* Allergy to protamine sulfate or fish products, pregnancy, lactation

p

- *Physical:* Skin color, temperature; orientation, reflexes; P, BP, auscultation, peripheral perfusion; R, adventitous sounds; plasma thrombin time

### Implementation

- Maintain emergency equipment for resuscitation and treatment of shock on standby in case of anaphylactoid reaction.
- Monitor coagulation studies to adjust dosage, and screen for heparin "rebound" and response to drug.

### Drug-specific teaching points

- Report shortness of breath, difficulty breathing, flushing, feeling of warmth, dizziness, lack or orientation, numbness, tingling.

## protriptyline hydrochloride

*(proe **trip'** ti leen)*

Triptil (CAN), Vivactil

**Pregnancy Category C**

### Drug classes

Tricyclic antidepressant (TCA) (secondary amine)

### Therapeutic actions

Mechanism of action unknown; the TCAs are structurally related to the phenothiazine antipsychotic drugs (eg, chlorpromazine), but in contrast to the phenothiazines, TCAs inhibit the presynaptic reuptake of the neurotransmitters norepinephrine and serotonin; anticholinergic at CNS and peripheral receptors; the relation of these effects to clinical efficacy is unknown.

### Indications

- Relief of symptoms of depression (endogenous depression most responsive; unlike other TCAs, protriptyline is "activating" and may be useful in withdrawn and anergic patients)
- Unlabeled use: treatment of obstructive sleep apnea

### Contraindications/cautions

- Contraindications: hypersensitivity to any tricyclic drug, concomitant therapy with an MAOI, recent MI, myelography within previous 24 h or scheduled within 48 h, pregnancy (limb reduction abnormalities), lactation.
- Use cautiously with EST; preexisting CV disorders (eg, severe coronary heart disease, progressive heart failure, angina pectoris, paroxysmal tachycardia); angle-closure glaucoma, increased intraocular pressure, urinary retention, ureteral or urethral spasm; seizure disorders (TCAs lower the seizure threshold); hyperthyroidism (predisposes to CVS toxicity, including cardiac arrhythmias); impaired hepatic, renal function; psychiatric patients (schizophrenic or paranoid patients may exhibit a worsening of psychosis); manic-depressive patients (may shift to hypomanic or manic phase); elective surgery (TCAs should be discontinued as long as possible before surgery).

### Dosage

**Available Forms:** Tablets—5, 10 mg

*ADULT:* 15–40 mg/d PO in 3–4 divided doses initially. May gradually increase to 60 mg/d if necessary. Do not exceed 60 mg/d. Make increases in dosage in the morning dose.

*PEDIATRIC:* Not recommended.

*GERIATRIC AND ADOLESCENTS:* Initially 5 mg tid PO. Increase gradually if necessary. Monitor CV system closely if dose exceeds 20 mg/d.

### Pharmacokinetics

| Route | Onset | Peak |
|---|---|---|
| Oral | Slow | 24–30 h |

*Metabolism:* Hepatic, $T_{1/2}$: 67–89 h

*Distribution:* Crosses placenta; enters breast milk

*Excretion:* Urine

### Adverse effects

- CNS: *Sedation and anticholinergic (atropine-like) effects*—dry mouth, blurred vision, disturbance of accommodation for near vision, mydriasis, increased intraocular pressure, *confusion* (especially in elderly), *disturbed concentration*, hallucinations, disorientation, decreased memory, feelings of unreality, delusions, anxiety, nervousness, restlessness, agitation, panic, insomnia, nightmares, hypomania, mania, exacerbation of psychosis, drowsiness, weakness, fatigue, headache, numbness, tingling, paresthesias of extremities, incoordination, motor hyperactivity, akathisia, ataxia, tremors, peripheral neuropathy, extrapyramidal symptoms, *seizures*, speech blockage, dysarthria, tinnitus, altered EEG

- GI: *Dry mouth, constipation*, paralytic ileus, *nausea*, vomiting, anorexia, epigastric distress, diarrhea, flatulence, dysphagia, peculiar taste, increased salivation, stomatitis, glossitis, parotid swelling, abdominal cramps, black tongue
- CV: *Orthostatic hypotension*, hypertension, syncope, tachycardia, palpitations, MI, arrhythmias, heart block, precipitation of CHF, stroke
- **Hematologic**: Bone marrow depression, including agranulocytosis; eosinophila; purpura; thrombocytopenia; leukopenia
- GU: Urinary retention, delayed micturition, dilation of the urinary tract, gynecomastia, testicular swelling; breast enlargement, menstrual irregularity and galactorrhea; increased or decreased libido; impotence
- **Hypersensitivity**: Skin rash, pruritus, vasculitis, petechiae, photosensitization, edema (generalized or of face and tongue), drug fever
- **Endocrine**: Elevated or depressed blood sugar; elevated prolactin levels; inappropriate ADH secretion
- **Withdrawal**: Symptoms with abrupt discontinuation of prolonged therapy: nausea, headache, vertigo, nightmares, malaise
- **Other**: Nasal congestion, excessive appetite, weight change, sweating, alopecia, lacrimation, hyperthermia, flushing, chills

### Clinically important drug-drug interactions

• Increased TCA levels and pharmacologic effects with cimetidine, fluoxetine, ranitidine • Increased half-life and therefore increased bleeding with dicumarol • Altered response, including dysrhythmias and hypertension with sympathomimetics • Risk of severe hypertension with clonidine • Hyperpyretic crises, severe convulsions, hypertensive episodes, and deaths with MAO inhibitors • Decreased hypotensive activity of guanethidine

## ■ Nursing Considerations

### Assessment

- *History:* Hypersensitivity to any tricyclic drug; concomitant therapy with an MAOI; recent MI; myelography within previous 24 h or scheduled within 48 h; pregnancy; lactation; EST; preexisting CV disorders; angle-closure glaucoma, increased intraocular pressure, urinary retention, ureteral or urethral spasm; seizure disorders; hyperthyroidism; impaired hepatic, renal function; psychiatric patients; manic-depressive patients; elective surgery
- *Physical:* Weight; T; skin color, lesions; orientation, affect, reflexes, vision and hearing; P, BP, orthostatic BP, perfusion; bowel sounds, normal output, liver evaluation; urine flow, normal output; usual sexual function, frequency of menses, breast and scrotal examination; liver function tests, urinalysis, CBC, ECG

p

### Implementation

- Limit drug access for depressed and potentially suicidal patients.
- Reduce dosage if minor side effects develop; discontinue if serious side effects occur.
- Arrange for CBC if patient develops fever, sore throat, or other sign of infection.

### Drug-specific teaching points

- Take drug exactly as prescribed; do not stop taking this drug abruptly or without consulting the physician or nurse.
- Avoid alcohol, other sleep-inducing drugs, OTC drugs.
- Avoid prolonged exposure to sunlight or sunlamps; use a sunscreen or protective garments.

- The following side effects may occur: headache, dizziness, drowsiness, weakness, blurred vision (reversible; take safety measures if severe; avoid driving or performing tasks that require alertness); nausea, vomiting, loss of appetite, dry mouth (small, frequent meals, frequent mouth care and sucking sugarless candies may help); nightmares, inability to concentrate, confusion; changes in sexual function.
- Report dry mouth, difficulty in urination, excessive sedation.

# Pseudoephedrine

## pseudoephedrine hydrochloride

*(soo dow e **fed'** rin)*

d-isoephedrine hydrochloride

Cenafed, Decofed, Dorcol Pediatric Formula, Eltor (CAN), Halofed, Pediacare, Robidrine (CAN), Sudafed

## pseudoephedrine sulfate

Afrin (prescription drug)

**Pregnancy Category C**

### Drug classes

Nasal decongestant
Sympathomimetic amine

### Therapeutic actions

Effects are mediated by alpha-adrenergic receptors; causes vasoconstriction in mucous membranes of nasal passages, resulting in their shrinkage, which promotes drainage and improves ventilation.

### Indications

- Temporary relief of nasal congestion caused by the common cold, hay fever, other respiratory allergies
- Nasal congestion associated with sinusitis
- Promotes nasal or sinus drainage
- Relief of eustachian tube congestion

### Contraindications/cautions

- Contraindications: allergy or idiosyncrasy to sympathomimetic amines, severe hypertension and coronary artery disease, lactation, pregnancy.
- Use cautiously with hyperthyroidism, diabetes mellitus, arteriosclerosis, ischemic heart disease, increased intraocular pressure, prostatic hypertrophy.

### Dosage

**Available Forms:** Tablets—30, 60 mg; ER tablets—120 mg; capsules—60 mg; TR capsules—120 mg; liquid—15, 30 mg/5 ml; drops—7.5 mg/0.8 ml

*ADULT:* 60 mg q4–6h PO (sustained-release, q12h); do not exceed 240 mg in 24 h.

*PEDIATRIC:*

- *6–12 Y:* 30 mg q4–6h PO; do not exceed 120 mg in 24 h.
- *2–5 Y:* 15 mg as syrup q4–6h PO; do not exceed 60 mg in 24 h.
- *1–2 Y:* 7 drops (0.02 ml.kg) q4–6h PO; up to four doses per day.
- *3–12 Mo:* 3 drops/kg q4–6h PO, up to four doses per day.

*GERIATRIC:* These patients are more likely to experience adverse reactions; use with caution.

### Pharmacokinetics

| *Route* | *Onset* | *Duration* |
|---|---|---|
| Oral | 30 min | 4–6 h |

*Metabolism:* Hepatic, $T_{1/2}$: 7 h
*Distribution:* Crosses placenta; enters breast milk
*Excretion:* Urine

### Adverse effects

- CNS: *Fear, anxiety, tenseness, restlessness, headache, light-headedness, dizziness, drowsiness, tremors,* insomnia, hallucinations, psychological disturbances, prolonged psychosis, convulsions, CNS depression, weakness, blurred vision, ocular irritation, tearing, photophobia, orofacial dystonia
- GI: *Nausea/vomiting*, anorexia

- **CV:** *Hypertension, arrhythmias,* CV collapse with hypotension, palpitations, tachycardia, precordial pain
- **Respiratory:** Respiratory difficulty
- **GU:** Dysuria
- **Dermatologic:** *Pallor,* sweating

**Clinically important drug-drug interactions**

• Increased hypertension with MAOIs, guanethidine, furazoladine • Increased duration of action with urinary alkalinizers (potassium citrate, sodium citrate, sodium lactate, tromethamine, sodium acetate, sodium bicaronate) • Decreased therapeutic effects and increased elimination of pseudoephedrine with urinary acidifiers (ammonium chloride, sodium acid phosphate, potassium phosphate) • Decreased antihypertensive effects of methyldopa

## ■ Nursing Considerations

### Assessment

- *History:* Allergy or idiosyncrasy to sympathomimetic amines, severe hypertension and CAD, hyperthyroidism, diabetes mellitus, arteriosclerosis, increased intraocular pressure, prostatic hypertrophy, pregnancy, lactation
- *Physical:* Skin color, temperature; reflexes, affect, orientation, peripheral sensation, vision; BP, P, auscultation; R, adventitious sounds; urinary output, bladder percussion, prostate palpation

### Implementation

- Administer cautiously to patients with CV disease, diabetes mellitus, hyperthyroidism, increased intraocular pressure, hypertension, and to patients >60 y who may have increased sensitivity to sympathomimetic amines.
- Avoid prolonged use; underlying medical problems may be causing the congestion.
- Monitor CV effect carefully; hypertensive patients who take this drug may experience changes in BP because of the additional vasoconstriction. However, if a nasal decongestant is needed, pseudoephedrine is the drug of choice.

### Drug-specific teaching points

- Do not exceed the recommended daily dose; serious overdosage can occur. Use caution when using more than one OTC preparation because many of these drugs contain pseudoephedrine, and unintentional overdose may occur.
- Avoid prolonged use because underlying medical problems can be disguised.
- The following side effects may occur: dizziness, weakness, restlessness, lightheadedness, tremors (avoid driving or performing hazardous tasks).
- Report palpitations, nervousness, sleeplessness, sweating.

## pyrantel pamoate

*(pi* ***ran'*** *tel)*

Antiminth, Combantrin (CAN), Pin-Rid, Pin-X, Reese's Pinworm

**Pregnancy Category C**

**Drug classes**

Anthelmintic

**Therapeutic actions**

A depolarizing neuromuscular blocking agent that causes spastic paralysis of *Enterobius vermicularis* and *Ascaris lumbricoides.*

**Indications**

- Treatment of enterobiasis (pinworm infection)
- Treatment of ascariasis (roundworm infection)

**Contraindications/cautions**

- Allergy to pyrantel pamoate, pregnancy, lactation, hepatic disease.

### Dosage

**Available Forms:** Capsules—180 mg; oral suspension—50 mg; liquid—50 mg

**ADULT:** 11 mg/kg (5 mg/lb) PO as a single oral dose. Maximum total dose of 1 g.

**PEDIATRIC:** Safety and efficacy not established for children <2 y.

P

### Pharmacokinetics

| *Route* | *Onset* | *Peak* |
|---|---|---|
| Oral | Slow | 1–3 h |

*Metabolism:* Hepatic, $T_{1/2}$: 47–100 h
*Distribution:* Crosses placenta; may enter breast milk
*Excretion:* Feces and urine

### Adverse effects

- CNS: Headache, dizziness, drowsiness, insomnia
- GI: *Anorexia, nausea, vomiting, abdominal cramps, diarrhea*, gastralgia, tenesmus, transient elevation of SGOT
- Dermatologic: Rash

### Clinically important drug-drug interactions

- Pyrantel and piperazine are antagonistic in *Ascaris;* avoid concomitant use

## ■ Nursing Considerations

### Assessment

- *History:* Allergy to pyrantel pamoate, pregnancy, lactation
- *Physical:* Skin color, lesions; orientation, affect; bowel sounds; SGOT levels

### Implementation

- Culture for ova and parasites.
- Administer drug with fruit juice or milk; ensure that entire dose is taken at once.
- Treat all family members (pinworm infestations).
- Disinfect toilet facilities after patient use (pinworms).
- Launder bed linens, towels, nightclothes, and undergarments (pinworms) daily.

### Drug-specific teaching points

- Take the entire dose at once. Drug may be taken with fruit juice or milk.
- Pinworms are easily transmitted; all family members should be treated for complete eradication.
- Strict handwashing and hygiene measures are important. Launder undergarments, bed linens, nightclothes daily; disinfect toilet facilities daily and bathroom floors periodically (pinworm).
- The following side effects may occur: nausea, abdominal pain, diarrhea (small, frequent meals may help); drowsiness, dizziness, insomnia (avoid driving and using dangerous machinery).
- Report skin rash, joint pain, severe GI upset, severe headache, dizziness.

# pyrazinamide

*(peer a* ***zin'*** *a mide)*
PMS-Pyrazinamide (CAN), Tebrazid (CAN)
**Pregnancy Category C**

### Drug classes

Antituberculous drug ("second-line")

### Therapeutic actions

Bacteriostatic or bacteriocidal against *Mycobacterium tuberculosis*; mechanism of action is unknown.

### Indications

- Initial treatment of active TB in adults and children when combined with other antituberculous agents.
- Treatment of active TB after treatment failure with primary drugs

### Contraindications/cautions

- Contraindications: allergy to pyrazinamide, acute hepatic disease, pregnancy, lactation.
- Use cautiously with gout, diabetes mellitus, acute intermittent porphyria.

### Dosage

**Available Forms:** Tablets—500 mg
**ADULT AND PEDIATRIC:** 15–30 mg/kg per day PO, given once a day; do not exceed 3 g/d. Always use with up to 4 other antituberculous agents; administer for the first 2 mo of a 6-mo treatment program. 50–70 mg/kg PO twice weekly may increase compliance and is being studied as an alternate dosing schedule.

### Pharmacokinetics

| *Route* | *Onset* | *Peak* |
|---|---|---|
| Oral | Rapid | 2 h |

*Metabolism:* Hepatic, $T_{1/2}$: 9–10 h
*Distribution:* Crosses placenta; enters breast milk
*Excretion:* Urine

**Adverse effects**
- GI: *Hepatotoxicity, nausea, vomiting,* diarrhea
- **Hematologic**: Sideroblastic anemia, adverse effects on clotting mechanism or vascular integrity
- **Dermatologic**: Rashes, photosensitivity
- **Other**: Active gout

**Drug-lab test interferences**
- False readings on Acetest, Ketostix urine tests

## ■ Nursing Considerations

### Assessment
- ***History:*** Allergy to pyrazinamide, acute hepatic disease, gout, diabetes mellitus, acute intermittent porphyria, pregnancy, lactation
- ***Physical:*** Skin color, lesions; joint status; T; liver evaluation; liver function tests, serum and urine uric acid levels, blood and urine glucose, CBC

### Implementation
- Administer only in conjunction with other antituberculous agents.
- Administer once a day.
- Arrange for follow-up of liver function tests (AST, ALT) prior to and every 2–4 wk during therapy.
- Discontinue drug if liver damage or hyperuricemia in conjunction with acute gouty arthritis occurs.

### Drug-specific teaching points
- Take this drug once a day; it will need to be taken with your other TB drugs.
- Take this drug regularly; avoid missing doses. Do not discontinue this drug without first consulting your prescriber.
- The following side effects may occur: loss of appetite, nausea, vomiting (take drug with food); skin rash, sensitivity to sunlight (avoid exposure to the sun).
- Have regular, periodic medical checkups, including blood tests to evaluate the drug effects.
- Report fever, malaise, loss of appetite, nausea, vomiting, darkened urine, yellowing of skin and eyes, severe pain in great toe, instep, ankle, heel, knee, or wrist.

# pyridostigmine bromide

*(peer id oh* ***stig'*** *meen)*
Mestinon, Regonol
**Pregnancy Category C**

**Drug classes**
Cholinesterase inhibitor
Antimyasthenic agent
Antidote

**Therapeutic actions**
Increases the concentration of acetylcholine at the sites of cholinergic transmission and prolongs and exaggerates the effects of acetylcholine by reversibly inhibiting the enzyme acetylcholinesterase, thus facilitating transmission at the skeletal neuromuscular junction.

**Indications**
- Treatment of myasthenia gravis
- Antidote for nondepolarizing neuromuscular junction blockers (eg, tubocurarine) after surgery (parenteral)

**Contraindications/cautions**
- Contraindications: hypersensitivity to anticholinesterases; adverse reactions to bromides; intestinal or urogenital tract obstruction, peritonitis, lactation.
- Use cautiously with asthma, peptic ulcer, bradycardia, cardiac arrhythmias, recent coronary occlusion, vagotonia, hyperthyroidism, epilepsy, pregnancy (given IV near term, drug may stimulate uterus and induce premature labor).

### Dosage
**Available Forms:** Tablets—60 mg; SR tablets—180 mg; syrup—60 mg/5 ml; injection—5 mg/ml

p

**ADULT**

***Symptomatic control of myasthenia gravis***

- *Oral:* Average dose is 600 mg given over 24 h; range, 60–1,500 mg, spaced to provide maximum relief. Sustained-release tablets, average dose is 180–540 mg qd or bid. Individualize dosage, allowing at least 6 h between doses. Optimum control may require supplementation with the more rapidly acting syrup or regular tablets.

***To supplement oral dosage preoperatively and postoperatively, during labor, during myasthenic crisis, etc.***

- *Parenteral:* Give 1/30 the oral dose IM or very slowly IV. May be given 1 h before second stage of labor is complete (enables patient to have adequate strength and protects neonate in immediate postnatal period).

*Antidote for nondepolarizing neuromuscular blockers*

- Give atropine sulfate 0.6–1.2 mg IV immediately before slow IV injection of pyridostigmine 0.1–0.25 mg/kg. 10–20 mg pyridostigmine usually suffices. Full recovery usually occurs within 15 min but may take 30 min.

**PEDIATRIC**

***Symptomatic control of myasthenia gravis***

- *Oral:* 7 mg/kg per day divided into five or six doses.

***Neonates of myasthenic mothers who have difficulty swallowing, sucking, breathing***

- *Parenteral:* 0.05–0.15 mg/kg IM. Change to syrup as soon as possible.

## Pharmacokinetics

| *Route* | *Onset* | *Duration* |
|---|---|---|
| Oral | 35–45 min | 3–6 h |
| IM | 15 min | 3–6 h |
| IV | 5 min | 3–6 h |

*Metabolism:* Hepatic and tissue, $T_{1/2}$: 1.9–3.7 h
*Distribution:* Crosses placenta; enters breast milk
*Excretion:* Urine

## IV facts

**Preparation:** No further preparation is required.
**Infusion:** Infuse very slowly, each 0.5 mg over 1 min for myasthenia gravis, each 5 mg over 1 min as a muscle relaxant agonist, directly into vein or into tubing of actively running IV of D5W, 0.9% Sodium Chloride, Lactated Ringer's, or D5/Lactated Ringer's.

## Adverse effects

*Parasympathomimetic Effects*

- GI: *Salivation, dysphagia, nausea, vomiting, increased peristalsis, abdominal cramps,* flatulence, diarrhea
- CV: *Bradycardia, cardiac arrhythmias,* AV block and nodal rhythm, cardiac arrest, decreased cardiac output leading to hypotension, syncope
- **Respiratory**: *Increased pharyngeal and tracheobronchial secretions*, laryngospasm, bronchospasm, bronchiolar constriction, dyspnea
- GU: *Urinary frequency and incontinence*, urinary urgency
- EENT: *Lacrimation, miosis,* spasm of accommodation, diplopia, conjunctival hyperemia
- Dermatologic: Diaphoresis, flushing

*Skeletal Muscle Effects*

- CNS: Convulsions, dysarthria, dysphonia, drowsiness, dizziness, headache, loss of consciousness
- **Respiratory**: Respiratory muscle paralysis, central respiratory paralysis
- Dermatologic: Skin rash, urticaria, anaphylaxis
- Peripheral: Skeletal muscle weakness, fasciculations, muscle cramps, arthralgia
- Local: Thrombophlebitis after IV use

## Clinically important drug-drug interactions

- Decreased effectiveness with profound muscular depression with corticosteroids
- Increased and prolonged neuromuscular blockade with succinylcholine

## ■ Nursing Considerations

### Assessment

- *History:* Hypersensitivity to anticholinesterases; adverse reactions to bromides; intestinal or urogenital tract obstruction, peritonitis, lactation, asthma, peptic ulcer, cardiac arrhythmias, recent coronary occlusion, vagotonia, hyperthyroidism, epilepsy, pregnancy
- *Physical:* Bowel sounds, normal output; urinary frequency, voiding pattern, normal output; R, adventitious sounds; P, auscultation, BP; reflexes, bilateral grip strength, ECG; thyroid function tests; skin color, texture, lesions

### Implementation

- Administer IV slowly.
- Overdosage with anticholinesterase drugs can cause muscle weakness (cholinergic crisis) that is difficult to differentiate from myasthenic weakness; administration of atropine may mask the parasympathetic effects of anticholinesterase overdose and further confound the diagnosis.
- Maintain atropine sulfate on standby as an antidote and antagonist to pyridostigmine in case of cholinergic crisis or unusual sensitivity to pyridostigmine.
- Discontinue drug and consult physician if excessive salivation, emesis, frequent urination, or diarrhea occurs.
- Decrease dosage of drug if excessive sweating, nausea occur.

### Drug-specific teaching points

- Take drug exactly as prescribed (patient and significant other should be taught about drug effects, signs and symptoms of myasthenia gravis, the fact that muscle weakness may be related both to drug overdosage and to exacerbation of the disease, and the importance of reporting muscle weakness promptly to the nurse or physician for proper evaluation).
- The following side effects may occur: blurred vision, difficulty with far vision, difficulty with dark adaptation (use caution while driving, especially at night, or performing hazardous tasks in reduced light); increased urinary frequency, abdominal cramps; sweating (avoid hot or excessively humid environments).
- Report muscle weakness, nausea, vomiting, diarrhea, severe abdominal pain, excessive sweating, excessive salivation, frequent urination, urinary urgency, irregular heartbeat, difficulty in breathing.

## pyrimethamine

*(peer i **meth'** a meen)*

Daraprim

**Pregnancy Category C**

### Drug classes

Antimalarial

Folic acid antagonist

### Therapeutic actions

Folic acid antagonist: selectively inhibits plasmodial dihydrofolate reductase, which is important to cellular biosynthesis of purines, pyrimidines, and certain amino acids; highly selective against plasmodia and *Toxoplasma gondii.*

### Indications

- Chemoprophylaxis of malaria due to susceptible strains of plasmodia; fast-acting schizonticides are preferable for treatment of acute attacks, but concurrent use of pyrimethamine will initiate transmission control and suppressive cure
- Treatment of toxoplasmosis with concurrent use of a sulfonamide

### Contraindications/cautions

- Contraindications: allergy to pyrimethamine, G-6-PD deficiency (may cause hemolytic anemia).
- Use cautiously with pregnancy (teratogenic in preclinical studies), lactation.

### Dosage

**Available Forms:** Tablets—25 mg

*ADULT AND PEDIATRIC > 10 Y*

- ***Chemoprophylaxis of malaria:*** 25 mg PO once weekly for at least 6–10 wk.
- ***With fast-acting schizonticides for treatment of acute attack:*** 25 mg/d PO for 2 d.

p

- *Toxoplasmosis:* Initially 50–75 mg/d PO with 1–4 g of a sulfapyrimidine; continue for 1–3 wk. Dosage of each drug may then be decreased by half and continued for an additional 4–5 wk.

PEDIATRIC

- ***Chemoprophylaxis of malaria:*** *4–10 y*: 12.5 mg PO once weekly for 6–10 wk. *<4 y*: 6.25 mg PO once weekly for 6–10 wk.
- ***With fast-acting schizonticides for treatment of acute attacks:*** *4–10 y*: 25 mg/d PO for 2 d.
- *Toxoplasmosis:* 1 mg/kg per day PO divided into two equal daily doses. After 2–4 d, reduce to half and continue for approximately 1 mo.

### Pharmacokinetics

| *Route* | *Onset* | *Peak* |
|---|---|---|
| Oral | Varies | 2–6 h |

*Metabolism:* Hepatic, $T_{1/2}$: 4 d
*Distribution:* crosses placenta; enters breast milk
*Excretion:* urine

### Adverse effects

- **GI**: *Anorexia, vomiting*, atrophic glossitis
- **Hematologic**: *Megaloblastic anemia, leukopenia, thrombocytopenia, pancytopenia*, folic acid deficiency with large doses used to treat toxoplasmosis, hemolytic anemia in patients with G-6-PD deficiency

## ■ Nursing Considerations

### Assessment

- ***History:*** Allergy to pyrimethamine, G-6-PD deficiency, pregnancy, lactation
- ***Physical:*** Abdominal exam, mucous membranes; CBC, Hgb, G-6-PD in deficient patients

### Implementation

- Administer with food if GI upset occurs.
- Schedule dosages for weekly same-day therapy on a calendar.
- Obtain CBC and Hgb determinations before and semiweekly during therapy.
- Decrease dosage or discontinue drug if signs of folic acid deficiency develop; leucovorin may be given in a dose of 3–9 mg/d IM for 3 d to return depressed platelet or WBC counts to safe levels.

### Drug-specific teaching points

- Take full course of drug therapy as prescribed; take with food or meals if GI upset occurs.
- Mark your calendar for once-a-week drug therapy.
- The following side effects may occur: stomach pain, loss of appetite, nausea, vomiting or abdominal cramps.
- Have regular blood tests to evaluate drug effects.
- Report darkening of the urine, severe abdominal cramps, GI distress, persistent nausea, vomiting.

## quazepam

***(kwa' ze pam)***

Doral

**Pregnancy Category X**
**C-IV controlled substance**

### Drug classes

Benzodiazepine
Sedative/hypnotic

### Therapeutic actions

Exact mechanisms of action not understood; acts mainly at subcortical levels of the CNS, leaving the cortex relatively unaffected; main sites of action may be the limbic system and mesencephalic reticular formation; benzodiazepines potentiate the effects of GABA, an inhibitory neurotransmitter.

### Indications

- Insomnia characterized by difficulty in falling asleep, frequent nocturnal awakenings, or early morning awakening
- Recurring insomnia or poor sleeping habits
- Acute or chronic medical situations requiring restful sleep

## Contraindications/cautions

- Contraindications: hypersensitivity to benzodiazepines, psychoses, acute narrow-angle glaucoma, shock, coma, acute alcoholic intoxication with depression of vital signs, pregnancy (congenital malformations, neonatal withdrawal syndrome), labor and delivery ("floppy infant" syndrome), lactation (infants become lethargic and lose weight).
- Use cautiously with impaired liver or kidney function, debilitation, depression, suicidal tendencies.

### Dosage

**Available Forms:** Tablets—7.5, 15 mg

*ADULT:* Initially 15 mg PO until desired response is seen. May reduce to 7.5 mg in some patients.

*PEDIATRIC:* Not for use in children < 18 y.

*GERIATRIC PATIENTS OR THOSE WITH DEBILITATING DISEASE:* Attempt to reduce nightly dosage after the first one or two nights of therapy.

## Pharmacokinetics

| Route | Onset | Peak |
|---|---|---|
| Oral | Varies | 2 h |

*Metabolism:* Hepatic, $T_{1/2}$: 39 h

*Distribution:* Crosses placenta; enters breast milk

*Excretion:* Urine

## Adverse effects

- CNS: *Transient, mild drowsiness initially; sedation; depression; lethargy; apathy; fatigue; lightheadedness; disorientation; restlessness; confusion*; crying; delirium; headache; slurred speech; dysarthria; stupor; rigidity; tremor; dystonia; vertigo; euphoria; nervousness; difficulty in concentration; vivid dreams; psychomotor retardation; extrapyramidal symptoms; *mild paradoxical excitatory reactions during first 2 wk of treatment* (especially in psychiatric patients, aggressive children, and with high dosage); visual and auditory disturbances; diplopia; nystagmus; depressed hearing; nasal congestion
- GI: *Constipation, diarrhea,* dry mouth, salivation, nausea, anorexia, vomiting, difficulty in swallowing, gastric disorders, elevations of blood enzymes, hepatic dysfunction, jaundice
- CV: *Bradycardia, tachycardia*, CV collapse, hypertension and hypotension, palpitations, edema
- **Hematologic**: Decreased Hct (primarily with long-term therapy), blood dyscrasias (agranulocytosis, leukopenia, neutropenia)
- GU: *Incontinence, urinary retention, changes in libido*, menstrual irregularities
- **Dermatologic**: Urticaria, pruritus, skin rash, dermatitis
- **Other**: Hiccups, fever, diaphoresis, paresthesias, muscular disturbances, gynecomastia
- **Dependence**: *Drug dependence with withdrawal syndrome* when drug is discontinued (more common with abrupt discontinuation of higher dosage used for longer than 4 mo)

## Clinically important drug-drug interactions

• Increased CNS depression with alcohol, omeprazole • Increased pharmacologic effects with cimetidine, disulfiram, oral contraceptives • Decreased sedative effects with theophylline, aminophylline, dyphylline, oxitriphylline

## ■ Nursing Considerations

### Assessment

- *History:* Hypersensitivity to benzodiazepines, psychoses, acute narrow-angle glaucoma, shock, coma, acute alcoholic intoxication, pregnancy, labor and delivery, lactation, impaired liver or kidney function, debilitation, depression, suicidal tendencies
- *Physical:* Skin color, lesions; T; orientation, reflexes, affect, ophthalmologic exam; P, BP; R, adventitious sounds; liver evaluation, abdominal exam, bowel sounds, normal output; CBC, liver and renal function tests

### Implementation

- Monitor liver and kidney function, CBC during long-term therapy.

q

- Taper dosage gradually after long-term therapy, especially in epileptics.

### Drug-specific teaching points

- Take drug exactly as prescribed.
- Do not stop taking this drug (long-term therapy) without consulting your health care provider.
- The following side effects may occur: drowsiness, dizziness (may lessen; avoid driving or engaging in other dangerous activities); GI upset (take with water); depression, dreams, emotional upset, crying; nocturnal sleep may be disturbed for several nights after discontinuing the drug.
- Report severe dizziness, weakness, drowsiness that persists, rash or skin lesions, palpitations, swelling of the extremities, visual changes, difficulty voiding.

## quetiapine fumarate

*(kwe **tie'** ah pine)*

Seroquel

**Pregnancy Category C**

### Drug classes

Dibenzothiazepine
Antipsychotic

### Therapeutic actions

Mechanism of action not fully understood: blocks dopamine and serotonin receptors in the brain; also acts as a receptor antagonist at histamine and adrenergic receptor sites (which may contribute to the adverse effects of orthostatic hypotension and somnolence).

### Indications

- Treatment of the manifestations of psychotic disorders in patients >18 y

### Contraindications/cautions

- Contraindications: coma or severe CNS depression, allergy to quetiapine, lactation, pregnancy.
- Use cautiously with cardiovascular disease, hypotension, hepatic dysfunction, seizures, exposure to extreme heat, autonomic instability, tardive dyskinesia, dehydration, thyroid disease, suicidal tendencies.

### Dosage

**Available Forms:** Tablets—25, 100, 200 mg

*Adult:* 25 mg PO bid. Increase in increments of 25–50 mg 2–3×/d on the 2nd and 3rd days; dosage range by day 4: 300–400 mg/d in 2–3 divided doses. Further increases can be made at 2-day intervals. Maximum dose: 800 mg/d.

*Pediatric:* Not recommended for children <18 yr old.

*Geriatric, Hepatic Impairment, or Debilitated:* Use lower doses and increase dosage more gradually than in other patients.

### Pharmacokinetics

| Route | Onset | Peak | Duration |
|---|---|---|---|
| Oral | Varies | 2–4 h | 8–10 h |

*Metaolism:* Hepatic; $T_{1/2}$: 6 h

*Distribution:* Crosses placenta; enters breast milk

*Excretion:* Urine

### Adverse effects

- CNS: *Drowsiness,* insomnia, vertigo, headache, weakness, tremor, tardive dyskinesias, **NMS**
- CV: Hypotension, *orthostatic hypotension,* syncope
- Hematologic: Increased SGPT, total cholesterol and triglycerides
- Autonomic: Dry mouth, salivation, nasal congesion, nausea, vomiting, anorexia, fever, pallor, flushed facies, sweating, constipation

### Clinically important drug-drug interactions

• CNS effects potentiated by alcohol, CNS depressants • Effects decreased with phenytoin, thioridazine, carbamazepine, phenobarbital, rifampin, glucocorticoids; monitor patient closely and adjust dosages appropriately when these drugs are added to or discontinued from regimen • Increased effects of antihypertensives, lorazepam • Decreased effects of levodopa, dopamine antagonists • Potential for heat stroke and intolerance with drugs that affect temperature regulation (anticholinergics); use extreme caution and monitor patient closely

## ■ Nursing Considerations

### Assessment

- *History:* Coma or severe CNS depression; allergy to quetiapine, lactation, pregnancy, cardiovascular disease, hypotension, hepatic dysfunction, seizures, exposure to extreme heat, autonomic instability, tardive dyskinesia, dehydration, thyroid disease, suicidal tendencies
- *Physical:* Body weight, T; reflexes, orientation, intraocular pressure; P, BP, orthostatic BP; R, adventitious sounds; CBC, urinalysis, thyoid, liver, and kidney function tests

### Implementation

- Administer small quantity to any patient with suicidal ideation.
- Monitor elderly patients for dehydration and institute remedial measures promptly; sedation and decreased sensation of thirst related to CNS effects of drug can lead to severe dehydration.
- Monitor patient closely in any setting that would promote overheating.
- Consult physician about dosage reduction and use of anticholinergic antiparkinsonian drugs (controversial) if extrapyramidal effects occur.

### Drug-specific teaching points

- Take this drug exactly as prescribed.
- The following side effects may occur: dizziness, drowsiness, syncope (avoid driving or engaging in other dangerous activities); dry mouth, nausea, loss of appetite (frequent mouth care, small, frequent meals, and increased fluid intake may help).
- Maintain fluid intake and use precautions against heat stroke in hot weather.
- Report sore throat, fever, unusual bleeding or bruising, rash, weakness, tremors, dark-colored urine, pale stools, yellowing of the skin or eyes.

# quinapril hydrochloride

***(kwin'** ah pril)*

Accupril

**Pregnancy Category D**

### Drug classes

Antihypertensive

Angiotensin converting enzyme inhibitor (ACE inhibitor)

### Therapeutic actions

Quinapril blocks ACE from coverting angiotensin I to angiotensin II, a powerful vasoconstrictor, leading to decreased BP, decreased aldosterone secretion, a small increase in serum potassium levels, and sodium and fluid loss; increased prostaglandin synthesis also may be involved in the antihypertensive action.

### Indications

- Treatment of hypertension alone or in combination with thiazide-type diuretics
- Adjunctive therapy in the management of CHF when added to regimen of digitalis and diuretics

### Contraindications/cautions

- Contraindications: allergy to quinapril or other ACE inhibitors.
- Use cautiously with impaired renal function, CHF, salt/volume depletion, lactation.

q

### Dosage

**Available Forms:** Tablets—5, 10, 20, 40 mg

ADULT

- *Hypertension:* Initial dose 10 mg PO qd. Maintenance dose, 20–80 mg/d PO as a single dose or two divided doses. Patients on diuretics should discontinue the diuretic 2–3 d before beginning benazepril therapy. If BP is not controlled, add diuretic slowly. If diuretic cannot be discontinued, begin quinapril therapy with 5 mg.
- *CHF:* Initial dose 5 mg PO bid. Dose may be increased as needed to relieve symptoms, 10-20 mg PO bid usual range.

PEDIATRIC: Safety and efficacy not established.

GERIATRIC OR RENAL IMPAIRED: Initial dose, 10 mg with Ccr > 60 ml/min, 5 mg with Ccr 30–60 ml/min, 2.5 mg with Ccr 10–30 ml/min.

### Pharmacokinetics

| Route | Onset | Peak | Duration |
|---|---|---|---|
| Oral | 1 h | 1 h | 24 h |

*Metabolism:* Hepatic, $T_{1/2}$: 2 h
*Distribution:* Crosses placenta; enters breast milk
*Excretion:* Urine and feces

### Adverse effects

- GI: *Nausea*, abdominal pain, vomiting, dairrhea
- CV: Angina pectoris, orthostatic hypotension in salt/volume depleted patients, palpitations
- Respiratory: *Cough,* asthma, bronchitis, dyspnea, sinusitis
- Dermatologic: Rash, pruritus, diaphoresis, flushing
- Other: Angioedema, asthenia, myalgia, arthralgia

## ■ Nursing Considerations

### Assessment

- *History:* Allergy to quinapril, other ACE inhibitors; impaired renal function; CHF; salt/volume depletion; lactation
- *Physical:* Skin color, lesions, turgor; T; P, BP, peripheral perfusion; mucous membranes, bowel sounds, liver evaluation; urinalysis, renal and liver function tests, CBC and differential

### Implementation

- Alert surgeon and mark patient's chart with notice that quinapril is being taken; the angiotensin II formation subsequent to compensatory renin release during surgery will be blocked; hypotension may be reversed with volume expansion.
- Monitor patient closely in any situation that may lead to a fall in BP secondary to reduction in fluid volume (excessive perspiration and dehydration, vomiting, diarrhea) because excessive hypotension may occur.

### Drug-specific teaching points

- Do not stop taking the medication without consulting your physician.
- The following side effects may occur: GI upset, loss of appetite (transient); lightheadedness (usually transient; change position slowly and limit activities to those that do not require alertness and precision); dry cough (not harmful).
- Be careful in any situation that may lead to a drop in BP (diarrhea, sweating, vomiting, dehydration); if lightheadedness or dizziness should occur, consult your care provider.
- Report mouth sores; sore throat, fever, chills; swelling of the hands, feet; irregular heartbeat, chest pains; swelling of the face, eyes, lips, tongue; difficulty breathing; persistent cough.

## quinethazone

*(kwin eth' a zone)*
Aquamox (CAN), Hydromox
**Pregnancy Category C**

### Drug classes

Thiazide-like diuretic

### Therapeutic actions

Inhibits reabsorption of sodium and chloride in distal renal tubule, increasing excretion of sodium, chloride, and water by the kidney.

### Indications

- Adjunctive therapy in edema associated with CHF, cirrhosis, corticosteroid and estrogen therapy, renal dysfunction
- Hypertension, as sole therapy or in combination with other antihypertensives
- Unlabeled use: diabetes insipidus, especially nephrogenic diabetes insipidus

### Contraindications/cautions

- Contraindications: fluid or electrolyte imbalances, pregnancy, lactation.
- Use cautiously with renal or liver disease, gout, SLE, glucose tolerance abnormalities, hyperparathyroidism, manic-depressive disorders.

### Dosage

**Available Forms:** Tablets—50 mg
**ADULT:** 50–100 mg qd PO. 150–200 mg/d may be needed.

*PEDIATRIC:* Safety and efficacy not established.

### Pharmacokinetics

| *Route* | *Onset* | *Peak* | *Duration* |
|---|---|---|---|
| Oral | 2 h | 6 h | 18–24 h |

*Metabolism:* Hepatic, $T_{1/2}$: unknown
*Distribution:* Crosses placenta; enters breast milk
*Excretion:* Urine

### Adverse effects

- CNS: *Dizziness, vertigo,* paresthesias, weakness, headache, drowsiness, fatigue, leukopenia, thrombocytopenia, agranulocytosis, aplastic anemia, neutropenia
- GI: *Nausea, anorexia, vomiting, dry mouth*, diarrhea, constipation, jaundice, hepatitis, pancreatitis
- CV: Orthostatic hypotension, venous thrombosis, volume depletion, cardiac arrhythmias, chest pain
- GU: *Polyuria, nocturia,* impotence, loss of libido
- Dermatologic: Photosensitivity, rash, purpura, exfoliative dermatitis, hives
- Other: Muscle cramps and muscle spasms, fever, gouty attacks, flushing, weight loss, rhinorrhea

### Clinically important drug-drug interactions

• Risk of hyperglycemia with diazoxide • Decreased absorption with cholestyramine, colestipol • Increased risk of digitalis glycoside toxicity if hypokalemia occurs • Increased risk of lithium toxicity when taken with thiazides • Increased fasting blood glucose, leading to need to adjust dosage of antidiabetic agents.

### Drug-lab test interferences

• Decreased PBI levels without clinical signs of thyroid disturbances

## ■ Nursing Considerations

### Assessment

- *History:* Fluid or electrolyte imbalances, renal or liver disease, gout, SLE, glucose tolerance abnormalities, hyperparathyroidism, manic-depressive disorders, pregnancy, lactation
- *Physical:* Orientation, reflexes, muscle strength; pulses, BP, orthostatic BP, perfusion, edema, baseline ECG; R, adventitious sounds; liver evaluation, bowel sounds; CBC, serum electrolytes, blood glucose; liver and renal function tests; serum uric acid, urinalysis

### Implementation

- Withdraw drug 2–3 d before elective surgery; reduce dosage of preanesthetic and anesthetic agents if emergency surgery is indicated.
- Give with food or milk if GI upset occurs.
- Mark calendars or use other reminders of alternate or 3- to 5-d/wk drug therapy.
- Measure and record regular body weights to monitor fluid changes.

### Drug-specific teaching points

- Take drug early in the day so sleep will not be disturbed by increased urination.
- Weigh yourself daily, and record weights.
- Protect skin from exposure to sun or bright lights.
- Increased urination will occur.
- Use caution if dizziness, drowsiness, feeling faint occur.
- Report rapid weight gain or loss, swelling in ankles or fingers, unusual bleeding or bruising, muscle cramps.

q

# Quinidine

## quinidine

***(kwin' i deen)***

## quinidine gluconate (contains 62% anhydrous quinidine alkaloid)

Quinaglute Dura-Tabs, Quinate (CAN)

*(continues)*

## quinidine polygalacturonate (contains 60% anhydrous quinidine alkaloid)

Cardioquin

## quinidine sulfate (contains 83% anhydrous quinidine alkaloid)

Novoquindin (CAN), Quinidex Extentabs, Quinora

**Pregnancy Category C**

### Drug classes

Antiarrhythmic

### Therapeutic actions

Type 1A antiarrhythmic: decreases automaticity in ventricles, decreases height and rate of rise of action potential, decreases conduction velocity, increases fibrillation threshold.

### Indications

- Treatment of atrial arrhythmias, paroxysmal or chronic ventricular tachycardia without heart block
- Maintenance therapy after electrocardioversion of atrial fibrillation or atrial flutter
- Treatment of life-threatening *P. falciperum* infections or when IV therapy (quinidine gluconate) is indicated

### Contraindications/cautions

- Contraindications: allergy or idiosyncrasy to quinidine, second or third-degree heart block, myasthenia gravis, pregnancy (neonatal thrombocytopenia), lactation.
- Use cautiously with renal disease, especially renal tubular acidosis, CHF, hepatic insufficiency.

### Dosage

**Available Forms:** Tablets—200, 275, 300 mg; SR tablets—300, 324 mg; injection—80 mg/ml

*ADULT:* Administer a test dose of one tablet PO or 200 mg IM to test for idiosyncratic reaction. 200–300 mg tid or qid PO or 300–600 mg q8h or q12h if sustained-release form is used.

- ***Paroxysmal supraventricular arrhythmias:*** 400–600 mg PO q2–3h until paroxysm is terminated.
- ***IM:*** Acute tachycardia: 600 mg IM quinidine gluconate, followed by 400 mg every 2 h until rhythm is stable.
- ***IV:*** 330 mg quinidine gluconate injected slowly IV at rate of 1 ml/min of diluted solution (10 ml of quinidine gluconate injection diluted to 50 ml with 5% glucose).

*PEDIATRIC:* Safety and efficacy not established.

### Pharmacokinetics

| *Route* | *Onset* | *Duration* |
|---|---|---|
| Oral | 1–3 h | 6–8 h |
| IM | 30–90 min | 6–8 h |
| IV | Rapid | 6–8 h |

*Metabolism:* Hepatic, $T_{1/2}$: 6–7 h
*Distribution:* Crosses placenta; enters breast milk
*Excretion:* Urine and feces

### IV facts

**Preparation:** Dilute 800 mg quinidine gluconate in 50 ml 5% Dextrose Injection.
**Infusion:** Inject slowly at rate of 1 ml/min.

### Adverse effects

- CNS: Vision changes (photophobia, blurring, loss of night vision, diplopia)
- GI: *Nausea, vomiting, diarrhea*, liver toxicity
- CV: *Cardiac arrhythmias*, cardiac conduction disturbances, including heart block, hypotension
- **Hematologic**: Hemolytic anemia, hypoprothrombinemia, thrombocytopenic purpura, agranulocytosis, lupus erythematosus (resolves after withdrawal)
- **Hypersensitivity**: Rash, flushing, urticaria, angioedema, respiratory arrest

• Other: *Cinchonism* (tinnitus, headache, nausea, dizziness, fever, tremor, visual disturbances)

### Clinically important drug-drug interactions

• Increased effects and increased risk of toxicity with cimetidine, amiodarone, verapamil • Increased cardiac depressant effects with sodium bicarbonate, antacids • Decreased levels with phenobarbital, hydantoins, rifampin • Increased neuromuscular blocking effects of depolarizing and nondepolarizing neuromuscular blocking agents, succinylcholine • Increased digoxin and digitoxin levels and toxicity • Increased effect of oral anticoagulants and bleeding

### Drug-lab test interferences

• Quinidine serum levels are inaccurate if the patient is also taking triamterene

## ■ Nursing Considerations

### Assessment

- *History:* Allergy or idiosyncrasy to quinidine, second or third-degree heart block, myasthenia gravis, renal disease, CHF, hepatic insufficiency, pregnancy, lactation
- *Physical:* Skin color, lesions; orientation, cranial nerves, reflexes, bilateral grip strength; P, BP, auscultation, ECG, edema; bowel sounds, liver evaluation; urinalysis, renal and liver function tests; CBC

### Implementation

- Monitor response carefully, especially when beginning therapy.
- Reduce dosage in patients with hepatic or renal failure.
- Reduced dosage with digoxin, digitoxin; adjust dosage if phenobarbital, hydantoin, or rifampin is added or discontinued.
- Check to see that patients with atrial flutter or fibrillation have been digitalized before starting quinidine.
- Differentiate the sustained-release form from the regular.
- Monitor cardiac rhythm carefully, and frequently monitor BP if given IV or IM.
- Arrange for periodic ECG monitoring when on long-term therapy.
- Monitor blood counts, liver function tests frequently during long-term therapy.
- Evaluate for safe and effective serum drug levels: 2–6 $\mu$g/ml.

### Drug-specific teaching points

- Take this drug exactly as prescribed. *Do not chew* the sustained-release tablets. If GI upset occurs, take drug with food.
- Frequent monitoring of cardiac rhythm, blood tests will be needed.
- The following side effects may occur: nausea, loss of appetite, vomiting (eat small, frequent meals); dizziness, lightheadedness, vision changes (do not drive or operate dangerous machinery); rash (use skin care).
- Wear a medical alert tag stating that you are on this drug.
- Return for regular follow-ups to check your heart rhythm and blood counts.
- Report sore mouth, throat, or gums, fever, chills, cold or flulike syndromes, ringing in the ears, severe vision disturbances, headache, unusual bleeding or bruising.

## quinine sulfate

***(kwi' nine)***

**Pregnancy Category X**

### Drug classes

Antimalarial

### Therapeutic actions

Believed to act by entering plasmodial DNA molecules, reducing effectiveness of DNA as template; also affects many enzyme systems of the plasmodia, depresses oxygen uptake and carbohydrate metabolism (antimalarial).

### Indications

- Treatment of chloroquine-resistant falciparum malaria as an adjunct with pyri-

q

methamine and sulfadiazine or tetracycline

### Contraindications/cautions

- Contraindications: allergy to quinine, G-6-PD deficiency, optic neuritis, tinnitus, history of blackwater fever, pregnancy, lactation.
- Use cautiously with cardiac arrhythmias.

### Dosage

**Available Forms:** Capsules—200, 260, 325 mg; tablets—260 mg

**ADULT**

- ***Chloroquine resistant malaria:*** 650 mg q8h PO for 5–7 d.
- ***Chloroquine sensitive malaria:*** 600 mg q8h PO for 5–7 d.

**PEDIATRIC**

- ***Chloroquine resistant malaria:*** 25 mg/kg per day given q8h PO for 5–7 d.
- ***Chloroquine sensitive malaria:*** 10 mg/kg PO q8h for 5–7 d.

### Pharmacokinetics

| Route | Onset | Peak |
|---|---|---|
| Oral | Varies | 1–3 h |

*Metabolism:* Hepatic, $T_{1/2}$: 4–5 h
*Distribution:* Crosses placenta; enters breast milk
*Excretion:* Urine

### Adverse effects

- **CNS**: *Visual disturbances*, including disturbed color vision and perception, photophobia, blurred vision with scotomata, night blindness, amblyopia, diplopia, diminished visual fields, mydriasis, optic atrophy; tinnitus, deafness, vertigo; headache; fever; apprehension, restlessness, confusion; syncope, excitement; delirium; hypothermia; convulsions
- **GI**: *Nausea, vomiting,* epigastric pain, hepatitis, diarrhea
- **Hematologic**: **Acute hemolysis, hemolytic anemia, thrombocytopenia purpura, agranulocytosis, hypoprothrombinemia**
- **Hypersensitivity**: Cutaneous rashes, pruritus, flushing, sweating, facial edema, asthmatic symptoms
- **Other**: *Cinchonism* (tinnitus, headache, nausea, slightly disturbed vision, GI upset, nervousness, CV effects), anginal symptoms

### Clinically important drug-drug interactions

• Increased serum levels of digoxin and digitoxin with quinidine, possible interaction with quinine • Increased effectiveness of neuromuscular blocking agents, succinylcholine, and possible respiratory difficulties • Increased anticoagulant effect of warfarin, other oral anticoagulants

### Drug-lab test interferences

• Interference with results of 17-hydroxycorticosteroid determinations • Falsely elevated levels of 17 ketogenic steroids using the Zimmerman method

## ■ Nursing Considerations

### Assessment

- *History:* Allergy to quinine, G-6-PD deficiency, optic neuritis, tinnitus, history of blackwater fever, cardiac arrhythmias, pregnancy, lactation
- *Physical:* Skin color, lesions; T; orientation, affect, reflexes, ophthalmic examination, audiologic examination; P, rhythm; liver evaluation; CBC, differential; PT; G-6-PD in appropriate patients

### Implementation

- Give with food or meals to decrease GI upset.
- Administer with pyrimethamine and sulfadiazine or tetracycline.
- Discontinue at any sign of hypersensitivity or cinchonism.
- Monitor CBC and differential periodically.

### Drug-specific teaching points

- Take drug with food or meals to decrease GI upset.
- The following side effects may occur: dizziness, fainting, confusion, restlessness, blurred vision (use caution driving or performing tasks that require alertness); diarrhea, nausea, stomach cramps, vomiting (take with food or meals); blurred

vision; decreased hearing; ringing in the ears.
- This drug should not be taken during pregnancy; serious birth defects may occur. If you think you are pregnant or are trying to become pregnant, consult your health care provider.
- Report severe ringing in the ears, headache, marked changes in vision, unusual bleeding or bruising, marked loss of hearing, fever, chills.

## raloxifene hydrochloride

*(rah **lox'** i feen)*

Evista

**Pregnancy Category X**

### Drug classes
Estrogen receptor modulator

### Therapeutic actions
Increases bone mineral density without stimulating endometrium in women; modulates effects of endogenous estrogen at specific receptor sites.

### Indications
- Prevention of osteoporosis in postmenopausal women

### Contraindications/cautions
- Contraindications: allergy to raloxifene, pregnancy, lactation.
- Use cautiously with history of smoking, venous thrombosis.

### Dosage
**Available Forms:** Tablets—60 mg

*ADULT:* 60 mg PO qd.

### Pharmacokinetics

| *Route* | *Onset* | *Peak* |
|---|---|---|
| Oral | Varies | 4–7 h |

*Metabolism:* Hepatic; $T_{1/2}$: 27.7 h

*Distribution:* Crosses placenta; passes into breast milk

*Excretion:* Feces

### Adverse effects
- CNS: Depression, lightheadedness, dizziness, headache, corneal opacity, decreased visual acuity, retinopathy
- GI: *Nausea, vomiting,* food distaste
- CV: **Venous thromboembolism**
- GU: Vaginal bleeding, vaginal discharge, pruritus vulvae
- Dermatologic: *Hot flashes, skin rash*
- Other: Peripheral edema

### Clinically important drug-drug interactions
- Increased risk of bleeding with oral anticoagulants

## ■ Nursing Considerations

### Assessment
- *History:* Allergy to raloxifene, pregnancy, lactation, smoking, history of venous thrombosis
- *Physical:* Skin lesions, color, turgor; pelvic exm; orientation, affect, reflexes; peripheral pulses, edema; liver function tests, CBC and differential, bone density

### Implementation
- Administer qd without regard to food.
- Arrange for periodic blood counts during therapy.
- Monitor patient for possible long-term effects, including cancers, thromboses associated with other drugs in this class.
- Counsel patient about the need to use contraceptive measures to avoid pregnancy while taking this drug; inform patient that serious fetal harm could occur.
- Provide comfort measures to help patient deal with drug effects: hot flashes (environmental temperature control); headache, depression (monitoring of light and noise); vaginal bleeding (hygiene measures).

### Drug-specific teaching points
- Take this drug as prescribed.
- The following side effects may occur: bone pain; hot flashes (staying in cool temperatures may help); nausea, vomiting (eat small, frequent meals); weight gain; dizziness, headache, lightheaded-

r

ness (use caution if driving or performing tasks that require alertness).
- This drug can cause serious fetal harm and must not be taken during pregnancy. Contraceptive measures should be used while you are taking this drug. If you become pregnant or would like to become pregnant, consult with your physician immediately.
- Report marked weakness, sleepiness, mental confusion, pain or swelling of the legs, shortness of breath, blurred vision.

## ramipril

*(ra **mi'** prill)*

Altace

**Pregnancy Category C**

### Drug classes

Antihypertensive
Angiotensin-converting enzyme (ACE) inhibitor

### Therapeutic actions

Ramipril blocks ACE from converting angiotensin I to angiotensin II, a powerful vasoconstrictor, leading to decreased BP, decreased aldosterone secretion, a small increase in serum potassium levels, and sodium and fluid loss; increased prostaglandin synthesis also may be involved in the antihypertensive action.

### Indications

- Treatment of hypertension alone or in combination with thiazide-type diuretics
- Treatment of CHF in stable patients in the first few days after MI

### Contraindications/cautions

- Contraindications: allergy to ramipril, pregnancy (embryocidal in preclinical studies).
- Use cautiously with impaired renal function, CHF, salt/volume depletion, lactation.

### Dosage

**Available Forms:** Capsules—1.25, 2.5, 5, 10 mg

**ADULT**

- *Hypertension:* Initial dose 2.5 mg PO qd. Adjust dose according to BP response, usually 2.5–20 mg/d as a single dose or in 2 equally divided doses. Discontinue diuretic 2–3 d before beginning therapy; if not possible, administer initial dose of 1.25 mg.
- *CHF:* Initial dose 2.5 mg PO bid; if patient becomes hypotensive, 1.25 mg PO bid may be used while titrating up to target dose of 5 mg PO bid.

**PEDIATRIC:** Safety and efficacy not established.

**GERIATRIC AND RENAL IMPAIRED:** Excretion is reduced in renal failure; use smaller initial dose, 1.25 mg PO qd in patients with Ccr < 40 ml/min; dosage may be titrated upward until pressure is controlled or a maximum of 5 mg/d.

### Pharmacokinetics

| *Route* | *Onset* | *Peak* | *Duration* |
|---|---|---|---|
| Oral | 1–2 h | 1–4 h | 24 h |

*Metabolism:* Hepatic, $T_{1/2}$: 13–17 h
*Distribution:* Crosses placenta; enters breast milk
*Excretion:* Urine and feces

### Adverse effects

- GI: *Gastric irritation, aphthous ulcers, peptic ulcers, dysgeusia*, cholestatic jaundice, hepatocellular injury, anorexia, constipation
- CV: *Tachycardia*, angina pectoris, MI, Raynaud's syndrome, CHF, hypotension in salt/volume depleted patients
- **Hematologic**: Neutropenia, agranulocytosis, thrombocytopenia, hemolytic anemia, fatal pancytopenia
- GU: *Proteinuria*, renal insufficiency, renal failure, polyuria, oliguria, urinary frequency
- **Dermatologic**: *Rash, pruritus,* pemphigoid-like reaction, scalded mouth sensation, exfoliative dermatitis, photosensitivity, alopecia
- **Other**: *Cough,* malaise, dry mouth, lymphadenopathy

**Clinically important drug-drug interactions**

- Decreased absorption may occur with food

**Drug-lab test interferences**

- False-positive test for urine acetone.

## ■ Nursing Considerations

### Assessment

- *History:* Allergy to ramipril, impaired renal function, CHF, salt/volume depletion, pregnancy, lactation
- *Physical:* Skin color, lesions, turgor; T; P, BP, peripheral perfusion; mucous membranes, bowel sounds, liver evaluation; urinalysis, renal and liver function tests, CBC and differential

### Implementation

- Administer 1 h before or 2 h after meals.
- Discontinue diuretic for 2–3 d before beginning therapy, if possible, to avoid severe hypotensive effect.
- Open capsules and sprinkle contents over a small amount of applesauce or mix in applesauce or water if patient has difficulty swallowing capsules. Mixture is stable for 24 h at room temperature and 48 h if refrigerated.
- Alert surgeon and mark chart that ramipril is being used; the angiotensin II formation subsequent to compensatory renin release during surgery will be blocked; hypotension may be reversed with volume expansion.
- Monitor patient closely for falling BP secondary to reduction in fluid volume (excessive perspiration and dehydration, vomiting, diarrhea) because excessive hypotension may occur.
- Reduce dosage in patients with impaired renal function.

### Drug-specific teaching points

- Take drug 1 h before meals. Do not stop taking without consulting your prescriber.
- The following side effects may occur: GI upset, loss of appetite, change in taste perception (transient; mouth sores (frequent mouth care may help); skin rash; fast heart rate; dizziness, lightheadedness (transient; change position slowly, and limit your activities to those that do not require alertness and precision).
- Be careful in any situation that may lead to a drop in BP (diarrhea, sweating, vomiting, dehydration); if lightheadedness or dizziness should occur, consult your nurse or physician.
- Report mouth sores; sore throat, fever, chills; swelling of the hands, feet; irregular heartbeat, chest pains; swelling of the face, eyes, lips, tongue, difficulty in breathing.

# ranitidine

*(ra **nye'** te deen)*

Zantac, Zantac EFFERdose, Zantac GELdose, Zantac 75

**Pregnancy Category B**

**Drug classes**

Histamine$_2$ ($H_2$) antagonist

**Therapeutic actions**

Competitively inhibits the action of histamine at the histamine$_2$ ($H_2$) receptors of the parietal cells of the stomach, inhibiting basal gastric acid secretion and gastric acid secretion that is stimulated by food, insulin, histamine, cholinergic agonists, gastrin, and pentagastrin.

**Indications**

- Short-term treatment of active duodenal ulcer
- Maintenance therapy for duodenal ulcer at reduced dosage
- Short-term treatment of active, benign gastric ulcer
- Short-term treatment of gastroesophageal reflux disease
- Pathologic hypersecretory conditions (eg, Zollinger-Ellison syndrome)
- Treatment of erosive esophagitis
- Treatment of heartburn, acid indigestion, sour stomach

**Contraindications/cautions**

- Contraindications: allergy to ranitidine, lactation.
- Use cautiously with impaired renal or hepatic function.

### Dosage

**Available Forms:** Tablets—75, 150, 300 mg; effervescent tablets and granules—150 mg; capsules—150, 300 mg; syrup—15 mg/ml; injection—0.5, 25 mg/ml

ADULT

- *Active duodenal ulcer:* 150 mg bid PO for 4–8 wk. Alternatively, 300 mg PO once daily hs *or* 50 mg IM or IV q6–8h *or* by intermittent IV infusion, diluted to 100 ml and infused over 15–20 min. Do not exceed 400 mg/d.
- *Maintenance therapy, duodenal ulcer:* 150 mg PO hs.
- *Active gastric ulcer:* 150 mg bid PO *or* 50 mg IM or IV q6–8h.
- *Pathologic hypersecretory syndrome:* 150 mg bid PO. Individualize dose with patient's response. *Do not exceed 6 g/d.*
- *Gastroesophageal reflux disease, esophagitis, benign gastric ulcer:* 150 mg bid PO.
- *Treatment of heartburn, acid indigestion:* 75 mg PO as needed.

PEDIATRIC: Safety and efficacy not established.

GERIATRIC OR IMPAIRED RENAL FUNCTION: Ccr < 50 ml/min, accumulation may occur; use lowest dose possible, 150 mg q24h PO *or* 50 mg IM or IV q18–24 h. Dosing may be increased to q12h if patient tolerates it and blood levels are monitored.

### Pharmacokinetics

| Route | Onset | Peak | Duration |
|---|---|---|---|
| Oral | Varies | 1–3 h | 8–12 h |
| IM | Rapid | 15 min | 8–12 h |
| IV | Immediate | 5–10 min | 8–12 h |

*Metabolism:* Hepatic, $T_{1/2}$: 2–3 h
*Distribution:* Crosses placenta; enters breast milk
*Excretion:* Urine

### IV facts

**Preparation:** For IV injection, dilute 50 mg in 0.9% Sodium Chloride Injection, 5% or 10% Dextrose Injection, Lactated Ringer's Solution, 5% Sodium Bicarbonate Injection to a volume of 20 ml; solution is stable for 48 h at room temperature. For intermittent IV, use as follows: dilute 50 mg in 100 ml of 5% Dextrose Injection or other compatible solution

**Infusion:** Inject over 5 min or more; for intermittent infusion, infuse over 15–20 min; continuous infusion, 6.25 mg/h

### Adverse effects

- CNS: *Headache*, malaise, dizziness, somnolence, insomnia, vertigo
- GI: *Constipation, diarrhea, nausea, vomiting, abdominal pain*, hepatitis, increased SGPT levels
- CV: Tachycardia, bradycardia, PVCs (rapid IV administration)
- **Hematologic:** Leukopenia, granulocytopenia, thrombocytopenia, pancytopenia
- GU: Gynecomastia, impotence or loss of libido
- **Dermatologic:** *Rash*, alopecia
- **Local:** *Pain at IM site, local burning or itching at IV site*
- **Other:** Arthralgias

### Clinically important drug-drug interactions

• Increased effects of warfarin, TCAs • Decreased effectiveness of diazepam • Decreased clearance and possible increased toxicity of lidocaine, nifedipine

## ■ Nursing Considerations

### Assessment

- *History:* Allergy to ranitidine, impaired renal or hepatic function, lactation
- *Physical:* Skin lesions; orientation, affect; pulse, baseline ECG; liver evaluation, abdominal exam, normal output; CBC, liver and renal function tests

### Implementation

- Administer oral drug with meals and at bedtime.
- Decrease doses in renal and liver failure.
- Provide concurrent antacid therapy to relieve pain.
- Administer IM dose undiluted, deep into large muscle group.
- Arrange for regular follow-up, including blood tests, to evaluate effects.

### Drug-specific teaching points

- Take drug with meals and at bedtime. Therapy may continue for 4–6 wk or longer.
- If you also are on an antacid, take it exactly as prescribed, being careful of the times of administration.
- Have regular medical follow-up to evaluate your response.
- The following side effects may occur: constipation or diarrhea (request aid from your health care provider); nausea, vomiting (take drug with meals); enlargement of breasts, impotence or loss of libido (reversible); headache (monitor lights, temperature, noise levels).
- Report sore throat, fever, unusual bruising or bleeding, tarry stools, confusion, hallucinations, dizziness, severe headache, muscle or joint pain.

## remifentanil hydrochloride

*(reh ma **fen'** ta nil)*

Ultiva

**Pregnancy Category C**

### Drug classes

Narcotic agonist analgesic

### Therapeutic actions

Acts at specific opioid receptors, causing analgesia, respiratory depression, physical depression, euphoria.

### Indications

- Analgesic adjunct to induce and maintain balanced general anesthesia for inpatient or outpatient procedures and for maintenance of analgesia in immediate postoperative period
- Analgesic component of monitored anesthesia care

### Contraindications/cautions

- Contraindications: known sensitivity to remifentanil and fentanyl analogs, epidural or intrathecal administration, pregnancy
- Use cautiously with obesity, hepatic disease, elderly patients, lactation, labor and delivery

### Dosage

**Available Forms:** Powder for injection—3, 5, 10-ml vials

Individualize dosage; monitor vital signs routinely.

**ADULT**

- ***Adjunct to general anesthetic:*** Induction: 0.5–1.0 mcg/kg/min IV. Maintenance: 0.25–0.4 mcg/kg/min IV depending on general anesthetic being used and patient response. Postoperative analgesia: 0.1 mcg/kg/min IV.
- ***Monitored anesthesia care:***
  - *Single IV injection:* 1 mcg/kg/min IV over 30–60 sec starting 90 sec before local anesthetic.
  - *Continuous IV infusion:* 0.1 mcg/kg/min IV starting 5 min before local anesthetic; then 0.05 mcg/kg/min after local anesthetic.

**PEDIATRIC (2–12 Y):** Use adult dosage with constant monitoring of patient response.

### Pharmacokinetics

| Route | Onset | Duration |
|---|---|---|
| IV | Immediate | 5 min |

*Metabolism:* Tissue; $T_{1/2}$: 3–10 min

*Distribution:* Crosses placenta; passes into breast milk

### IV facts

**Preparation:** Reconstitute and dilute to concentration of 20–250 mcg/ml in Sterile Water for Injection, 5% Dextrose Injection, 5% Dextrose and 0.9% Sodium Chloride Injection, 0.9% Sodium Chloride Injection or 0.45% Sodium Chloride Injection. Stable for 24 h at room temperature.

**Infusion:** Administer slowly at prescribed rates using an infusion device; clear all IV tubing at end of administration.

**Compatibility:** Compatible with propofol when administered in same running IV set.

### Adverse effects

- CNS: Sedation, clamminess, sweating, *headache,* vertigo, floating feeling, dizziness, lethargy, confusion, lightheadedness, nervousness, unusual dreams, agitation, euphoria, hallucinations, delirium, insomnia
- GI: *Nausea, vomiting,* dry mouth, anorexia, constipation
- CV: Hypotension, circulatory depression, **cardiac arrest, shock,** bradycardia
- **Respiratory**: Slow, shallow respiration, apnea, suppression of cough reflex
- **Dermatologic**: Rash, hives, *pruritus, sweating,* flushing, warmth, sensitivity to cold
- **Local**: Phlebitis following IV injection, pain at injection site

## ■ Nursing Considerations

### Assessment

- ***History:*** Hypersensitivity to fentanyl or narcotics, pregnancy, labor, lactation, hepatic dysfunction, obesity
- ***Physical:*** Orientation, reflexes, bilateral grip strength, affect; pupil size, vision; P, auscultation, BP; R, adventitious sounds; bowel sounds, normal output; liver function tests

### Implementation

- Do not administer with epidural or intrathecal anesthesia; presence of glycine in preparation is contraindicated.
- Administer to breastfeeding women 4–6 h before the next scheduled feeding to minimize the amount in milk.
- Provide narcotic antagonist, facilities for assited or controlled respiration on standby during administration.
- Institute safety precautions (siderails, assistance with ambulation, etc.) if CNS, vision, vestibular effects occur.
- Provide environmental control (temperature, lighting) if sweating, visual difficulties occur.
- Provide non-drug measures (backrubs, positioning, etc.) to alleviate pain.

### Drug-specific teaching points

Incorporate teaching about drug into preoperative or postoperative teaching program.

- The following side effects may occur: dizziness, sedation, drowsiness, impaired visual acuity (ask for assistance if you need to move); nausea, loss of appetite (lie quietly; eat small, frequent meals); constipation (notify your nurse or physician; if severe, a laxative may help).
- Report severe nausea, vomiting, palpitations, shortness of breath or difficulty breathing, severe headache.

## reteplase

***(ret' ah place)***

r-PA

Retevase

**Pregnancy Category C**

### Drug classes

Thrombolytic enzyme

### Therapeutic actions

Human tissue enzyme produced by recombinant DNA techniques; converts plasminogen to the enzyme plasmin (fibrinolysin), which degrades fibrin clots; lyses thrombi and emboli; is most active at site of clot and causes little systemic fibrinolysis.

### Indications

- Treatment of coronary artery thrombosis associated with acute MI

### Contraindications/cautions

- Contraindications: allergy to TPA; active internal bleeding; recent (within 2 mo) CVA; intracranial or intraspinal surgery or neoplasm; recent major surgery, obstetrical delivery, organ biopsy, or rupture of noncompressible blood vessel; recent serious GI bleed; recent serious trauma, including CPR; SBE; hemostatic defects; cerebrovascular disease; early-onset, insulin-dependent diabetes; septic thrombosis; severe uncontrolled hypertension

- Use cautiously with liver disease, old age (>75 y) (risk of bleeding may be increased)

### Dosage

**Available Forms:** Powder for injection—10.8 IU

**ADULT**

– *Acute MI:* 10 U + 10 U double-bolus IV injection, each over 2 min; second bolus is given 30 min after start of first.

### Pharmacokinetics

| Route | Onset | Peak |
|---|---|---|
| IV | Immediate | End of infusion |

*Metabolism:* None; $T_{1/2}$: 13–16 min
*Distribution:* Crosses placenta
*Excretion:* Cleared by liver and kidneys

### IV facts

**Preparation:** Reconstitute with Sterile Water for Injection (no preservatives) for immediate use; stable for 4 h after reconstitution. Slight foaming may occur with reconstititon; allowing vial to stand undisturbed for several minutes will allow bubbles to dissipate. Protect from light.

**Infusion:** Infuse each bolus over 2 min into a running IV line in which no other medications are running.

**Incompatibilities:** Do not mix in the same line with heparin. If heparin has run through the line being used, flush with Normal Saline or 5% Dextrose solution before and after reteplase infusion; do not add any other medications to the solution.

### Adverse effects

- CV: Cardiac arrhythmias with coronary reperfusion, hypotension
- Hematologic: **Bleeding**—especially at venous or arterial access sites, GI bleeding, intracranial hemorrhage
- Other: Urticaria, nausea, vomiting, fever

### Clinically important drug-drug interactions

- Increased risk of hemorrhage with heparin or oral anticoagulants, aspirin, dipyridamole, abciximab

## ■ Nursing Considerations

### Assessment

- *History:* Allergy to TPA, active internal bleeding, recent (within 2 mo) obstetrical delivery, organ biopsy, or rupture of noncompressible blood vessel, recent serious GI bleed, recent serious trauma (including CPR), SBE, hemostatic defects, cerebrovascular disease, early-onset insulin-dependent diabetes, septic thrombosis, severe uncontrolled hypertension, liver disease
- *Physical:* Skin color, temperature, lesions; orientation, reflexes; P, BP, peripheral perfusion, baseline ECG; R, adventitious sounds; liver evaluation, Hct, platelet count, thrombin time, APTT, PT

### Implementation

- Discontinue concurrent heparin and reteplase if serious bleeding occurs.
- Arrange for regular monitoring of coagulation studies.
- Apply pressure and/or pressure dressings to control superficial bleeding (at invaded or disturbed areas).
- Avoid any arterial invasive procedures during therapy.
- Arrange for typing and cross-matching of blood in case serious blood loss occurs and whole blood transfusions are required.
- Instititute treatment within 6 h of onset of symptoms for evolving MI.

### Drug-specific teaching points

- This drug can only be given IV; you will need to be closely monitored during treatment.
- Report difficulty breathing, dizziness, disorientation, headache, numbness, tingling.

r

## ribavirin

*(rye ba **vye'** rin)*
Virazole
**Pregnancy Category X**

### Drug classes
Antiviral

### Therapeutic actions
Antiviral activity against respiratory syncytial virus (RSV), influenza virus, and herpes simplex virus; mechnanism of action is not known.

### Indications
- Carefully selected hospitalized infants and children with RSV infection of lower respiratory tract
- Orphan drug use: treatment of hemorrhagic fever with renal syndrome
- Unlabeled use for aerosol: treatment of some influenza A and B infections
- Unlabeled uses of oral preparation: treatment of some viral diseases, including acute and chronic hepatitis, herpes genitalis, measles, Lassa fever, hemorrhagic fever with renal syndrome

### Contraindications/cautions
- Allergy to drug product, COPD, pregnancy (causes fetal damage), lactation.

### Dosage
**Available Forms:** Powder for aerosol reconstitution—6 g/100 ml vial

For use only with small-particle aerosol generator. Check operating instructions carefully.

**ADULT OR PEDIATRIC:** Dilute to 20 mg/ml and deliver for 12–18 h/d for at least 3 but not more than 7 d.

### Pharmacokinetics

| *Route* | *Onset* | *Peak* |
|---|---|---|
| Aerosol | Slow | 60–90 min |

*Metabolism:* Cellular, $T_{1/2}$: 9.5 h

*Distribution:* Crosses placenta; enters breast milk

*Excretion:* Urine and feces

### Adverse effects
- CV: Cardiac arrest, hypotension
- Respiratory: *Deteriorating respiratory function*, pneuomothorax, apnea, bacterial pneumonia
- Hematologic: Anemia
- Dermatologic: Skin rash
- Other: Conjuctivitis

### Clinically important drug-drug interactions
- Increased likelihood of digitalis toxicity

## ■ Nursing Considerations

### Assessment
- *History:* Allergy to drug product, COPD, pregnancy, lactation
- *Physical:* Skin rashes, lesions; P, BP, auscultation; R, adventitious sounds; Hct

### Implementation
- Ensure proper use of small-particle aerosol generator; check operating instructions carefully.
- Ensure that water used as diluent contains no other substance.
- Replace solution in the unit every 24 h.
- Store reconstituted solution at room temperature.
- Do not use with infants requiring ventilatory assistance.
- Monitor respiratory status frequently.
- Monitor BP, P frequently.

### Drug-specific teaching points
- Explain the use of small-particle aerosol generator to patient or family.
- Report any of the following: dizziness, confusion, shortness of breath.

## rifabutin

*(rif ah **byou'** tin)*

Mycobutin

**Pregnancy Category B**

### Drug classes
Antituberculous drug (“first-line”)

Antibiotic

### Therapeutic actions
Inhibits DNA-dependent RNA polymerase activity in susceptible strains of *Escherichia coli, Bacillus subtilis*

### Indications
- Prevention of disseminated *Mycobactrium avium* complex (MAC) disease in patients with advanced HIV infection

### Contraindications/cautions

- Contraindications: allergy to rifabutin or rifampin, lactation, active tuberculosis.
- Use cautiously with pregnancy.

### Dosage

**Available Forms:** Capsules—150 mg

*ADULT:* 300 mg PO qd; doses of 150 mg PO bid may be used in patients intolerant to the GI effects.

*PEDIATRIC:* Safety and efficacy not established.

### Pharmacokinetics

| *Route* | *Onset* | *Peak* |
|---|---|---|
| Oral | Varies | 3.3–4 h |

*Metabolism:* Hepatic, $T_{1/2}$: 45 h

*Distribution:* Crosses placenta; enters breast milk

*Excretion:* Urine

### Adverse effects

- GI: Heartburn, epigastric distress, *anorexia, nausea,* vomiting, gas, cramps, diarrhea, taste perversion, abdominal pain
- **Hematologic:** *Eosinophilia, thrombocytopenia, transient leukopenia*, hemolytic anemia, decreased Hgb, hemolysis
- GU: Discolored urine
- **Other:** Pain in extremities, fever, rash, myalgia, asthenia, yellow color to body fluids

### Clinically important drug-drug interactions

- Decreased plasma levels of zidovudine

### Clinically important drug-food interactions

- Decreased rate of absorption if taken with high-fat meals; extent of absorption not changed

## ■ Nursing Considerations

### Assessment

- *History:* Allergy to rifabutin or rifampin, lactation, active TB, pregnancy
- *Physical:* Skin color, lesions; T; abdominal exam; urinalysis; CBC

### Implementation

- Administer on an empty stomach, 1 h before or 2 h after meals; may be given with food if GI upset is severe.
- Administer in a single daily dose; may be divided into two equal doses if GI effects cannot be tolerated.
- Prepare patient for the reddish-orange coloring of body fluids (urine, sweat, sputum, tears, feces, saliva); soft contact lenses may be permanently stained; advise patient not to wear them during therapy.
- Arrange for follow-up evaluation of hematologic profile.

### Drug-specific teaching points

- Take drug in a single daily dose. Take on an empty stomach, 1 h before or 2 h after meals.
- Take this drug regularly; avoid missing any doses; *do not* discontinue this drug without first consulting your health care provider.
- The following side effects may occur: reddish-orange coloring of body fluids (tears, sweat, saliva, urine, feces, sputum; stain will wash out of clothing, but soft contact lenses may be permanently stained; do not wear them); nausea, vomiting, epigastric distress (drug dosage may need to be divided).
- Have periodic medical checkups, including blood tests, to evaluate drug effects.
- Report fever, chills, muscle and bone pain, excessive tiredness or weakness, loss of appetite, nausea, vomiting, yellowing of eyes.



## rifampin

*(rif' am pin)*

Rifadin, Rimactane, Rofact (CAN)

**Pregnancy Category C**

### Drug classes

Antituberculous drug (''first-line'')

Antibiotic

## Therapeutic actions

Inhibits DNA-dependent RNA polymerase activity in susceptible bacterial cells.

## Indications

- Treatment of pulmonary TB in conjunction with at least one other effective antituberculous drug
- Neisseria meningitidis carriers, for asymptomatic carriers to eliminate meningococci from nasopharynx; not for treatment of meningitis
- Unlabeled uses: infections caused by *Staphylococcus aureus* and *Staphylococcus epidermis*, usually in combination therapy; gram-negative bacteremia in infancy; Legionella (*Legionella pneumophilia)*, not responsive to erythromycin; leprosy (in combination with dapsone); prophylaxis of meningitis due to *Haemophilus influenzae*

## Contraindications/cautions

- Contraindications: allergy to any rifamycin, acute hepatic disease, lactation.
- Use cautiously with pregnancy (teratogenic effects have been reported in preclinical studies; safest antituberculous regimen for use in pregnancy is considered to be rifampin, isoniazid, and ethambutol).

## Dosage

**Available Forms:** Capsules—150, 300 mg; powder for injection—600 mg

*ADULT*

- ***Pulmonary TB:*** 600 mg in a single daily dose PO or IV (used in conjunction with other antituberculous drugs). Continue therapy until bacterial conversion and maximal improvement occur.
- ***Meningococcal carriers:*** 600 mg PO or IV once daily for 4 consecutive d.

*PEDIATRIC (> 5 Y)*

- ***Pulmonary TB:*** 10–20 mg/kg per day PO or IV not to exceed 600 mg/d.
- ***Meningococcal carriers:*** 10–20 mg/kg PO or IV once daily for 4 consecutive d, not to exceed 600 mg/d.

## Pharmacokinetics

| *Route* | *Onset* | *Peak* |
|---|---|---|
| Oral | Varies | 1–4 h |
| IV | Rapid | End of infusion |

*Metabolism:* Hepatic, $T_{1/2}$: 3–5.1 h

*Distribution:* Crosses placenta; enters breast milk

*Excretion:* Feces and urine

## IV facts

**Preparation:** Reconstitute by transferring 10 ml Sterile Water for Injection to vial containing 600 mg rifampin; swirl gently. Resultant fluid contains 60 mg/ml; stable at room temperature. Further mix with 500–100 ml of Dextrose 5% or Sterile Saline.

**Infusion:** Infuse over 30–180 min, depending on volume.

## Adverse effects

- CNS: *Headache, drowsiness, fatigue, dizziness*, inability to concentrate, mental confusion, generalized numbness, ataxia, muscle weakness, visual disturbances, exudative conjunctivitis
- GI: *Heartburn, epigastric distress,* anorexia, nausea, vomiting, gas, cramps, diarrhea, pseudomembranous colitis, pancreatitis, *elevations of liver enzymes,* hepatitis
- **Hematologic**: *Eosinophilia, thrombocytopenia, transient leukopenia*, hemolytic anemia, decreased Hgb, hemolysis
- GU: Hemoglobinuria, hematuria, renal insufficiency, acute renal failure, menstrual disturbances
- **Dermatologic**: *Rash*, pruritus, urticaria, pemphigoid reaction, flushing, reddish-orange discoloration of body fluids—tears, saliva, urine, sweat, sputum
- **Other**: Pain in extremities, osteomalacia, myopathy, fever, *"flulike" syndrome*

## Clinically important drug-drug interactions

• Increased incidence of rifampin-related hepatitis with isoniazid • Decreased effectiveness of rifampin with p-aminosalicyclic acid, ketoconazole; give the drugs at least 8–12 h apart • Decreased effectiveness of metoprolol, propranolol, quinidine, corticosteroids, oral contraceptives, methadone, oral anticoagulants, oral sulfonylureas, digitoxin, theophyllines, phenytoin, cyclosporine, ketoconazole, verapamil

**Drug-lab test interferences**
• Rifampin inhibits the standard assays for serum folate and vitamin $B_{12}$

## ■ Nursing Considerations

### Assessment
- *History:* Allergy to any rifamycin, acute hepatic disease, pregnancy, lactation
- *Physical:* Skin color, lesions; T; gait, muscle strength; orientation, reflexes, ophthalmologic examination; liver evaluation; CBC, liver and renal function tests, urinalysis

### Implementation
- Administer on an empty stomach, 1 h before or 2 h after meals.
- Administer in a single daily dose.
- Consult pharmacist for rifampin suspension for patients unable to swallow capsules.
- Prepare patient for the reddish-orange coloring of body fluids (urine, sweat, sputum, tears, feces, saliva); soft contact lenses may be permanently stained; advise patients not to wear them during therapy.
- Arrange for follow-up of liver and renal function tests, CBC, ophthalmologic examinations.

### Drug-specific teaching points
- Take drug in a single daily dose. Take on an empty stomach, 1 h before or 2 h after meals.
- Take this drug regularly; avoid missing any doses; *do not* discontinue this drug without first consulting your physician.
- The following side effects may occur: reddish-orange coloring of body fluids (tears, sweat, saliva, urine, feces, sputum; stain will wash out of clothing, but soft contact lenses may be permanently stained; do not wear them); nausea, vomiting, epigastric distress; skin rashes or lesions; numbness, tingling, drowsiness, fatigue (use caution if driving or operating dangerous machinery; use precautions to avoid injury).
- Have periodic medical checkups, including an eye examination and blood tests, to evaluate the drug effects.
- Report fever, chills, muscle and bone pain, excessive tiredness or weakness, loss of appetite, nausea, vomiting, yellowing of skin or eyes, unusual bleeding or bruising, skin rash or itching.

# riluzole

***(rill' you zohl)***

Rilutek

**Pregnancy Category C**

**Drug classes**
ALS agent

**Therapeutic actions**
Inhibits glutamate release presynaptically, possibly blocks sodium channels and postsynaptic receptors; this blockage of glutamate accumulation may prevent excessive neural excitement that leads to neuronal injury and death.

**Indications**
- Treatment of ALS; extends survival time or time to tracheostomy

**Contraindications/cautions**
- As no other drug is available for treatment of this progressive and fatal disease, there are no real contraindications to its use.

### Dosage
**Available Forms:** Tablets—50 mg

*ADULT:* 50 mg PO q12h.

*PEDIATRIC:* Safety and efficacy not established.

**Pharmacokinetics**

| *Route* | *Onset* | *Duration* |
|---|---|---|
| PO | Slow | 3–5 d |

*Metabolism:* Hepatic; $T_{1/2}$: 12 h
*Distribution:* Crosses placenta; enters breast milk
*Excretion:* Urine and feces

### Adverse effects

- CNS: Increased asthenia and spasticity
- GI: *Nausea, vomiting*
- Metabolic: Increased aminotransferase activity

## ■ Nursing Considerations

### Assessment

- ***History:*** Hypersensitivity to riluzole; pregnancy; lactation
- ***Physical:*** Orientation, reflexes, bilateral grip strength, muscle strength; abdominal exam; liver function tests

### Implementation

- Administer on an empty stomach, 1 h before or 2 h after meals; protect drug from bright light.
- Monitor disease progression and provide supportive therapy as needed; riluzole has been shown to slow disease progression, but does not stop or cure it.
- Incorporate extensive teaching into patient care plan as to potential benefits and risks associated with use of a drug that has been available only for a short time.

### Drug-specific teaching points

- This drug has been available for only a short time, and long-term effects are not known; it has been shown to slow the rate of progression of ALS, but does not cure the disease.
- Take at the same time each day, on an empty stomach, 1 h before or 2 h after meals.
- Protect drug from bright light.
- Possible adverse effects include nausea and vomiting, increased spasticity, dizziness.
- Report fever, severe nausea, vomiting, changes in color of urine or stool, changes in disease symptoms.

## rimantadine HCl

*(ri **man'** ta deen)*

Flumadine

**Pregnancy Category C**

### Drug classes

Antiviral

### Therapeutic actions

Synthetic antiviral agent that inhibits viral replication, possibly by preventing the uncoating of the virus.

### Indications

- Prophylaxis and treatment of illness caused by influenza A virus in adults
- Prophylaxis against influenza A virus in children

### Contraindications/cautions

- Allergy to amantadine, rimantadine; lactation.
- Use cautiously with seizures, liver or renal disease, pregnancy.

### Dosage

**Available Forms:** Tablets—100 mg; syrup—50 mg/5 ml

**ADULT AND PEDIATRIC > 10 Y**

- ***Prophylaxis:*** 100 mg/d PO bid.
- ***Treatment:*** Same dose as above; start treatment as soon after exposure as possible, continuing for 7 d.
- ***Patients with renal/hepatic disease:*** Dose of 100 mg PO qd is recommended.

**PEDIATRIC**

- ***Prophylaxis for < 10 y:*** 5 mg/kg PO qd; do not exceed 150 mg/d.

### Pharmacokinetics

| Route | Onset | Peak |
|---|---|---|
| Oral | Slow | 6 h |

*Metabolism:* $T_{1/2}$: 25.4 h

*Distribution:* Crosses placenta; enters breast milk

*Excretion:* Unchanged in the urine

### Adverse effects

- CNS: *Lightheadedness, dizziness, insomnia,* confusion, irritability, ataxia, psychosis, depression, hallucinations
- GI: *Nausea*, anorexia, constipation, dry mouth
- CV: CHF, orthostatic hypotension, dyspnea
- GU: Urinary retention

### Clinically important drug-drug interactions

• Decreased effectiveness with acetaminophen, aspirin • Increased serum levels and effects with cimetidine

## ■ Nursing Considerations

### Assessment

- *History:* Allergy to amantadine, rimantidine; seizures; liver or renal disease; lactation
- *Physical:* Orientation, vision, speech, reflexes; BP, orthostatic BP, P, auscultation, perfusion, edema; R, adventitious sounds; urinary output; BUN, creatinine clearance

### Implementation

- Administer full course of drug to achieve the beneficial antiviral effects.

### Drug-specific teaching points

- The following side effects may occur: drowsiness, blurred vision (use caution in driving or using dangerous equipment); dizziness, lightheadedness (avoid sudden position changes); irritability or mood changes (common; if severe, request a drug change).
- Report swelling of the fingers or ankles, shortness of breath, difficulty urinating, tremors, slurred speech, difficulty walking.

## risperidone

*(ris* ***peer'*** *i dohn)*

Risperdal

**Pregnancy Category C**

### Drug classes

Antipsychotic
Benzisoxazole

### Therapeutic actions

Mechanism of action not fully understood: blocks dopamine and serotonin receptors in the brain, depresses the RAS; anticholinergic, antihistaminic, and alpha-adrenergic blocking activity may contribute to some of its therapeutic and adverse actions.

### Indications

- Management of the manifestations of psychotic disorders

### Contraindications/cautions

- Contraindications: allergy to risperidone, lactation.
- Use cautiously with cardiovascular disease, pregnancy, renal or hepatic impairment, hypotension.

### Dosage

**Available Forms:** Tablets—1, 2, 3, 4 mg; oral solution—1 mg/ml

**ADULT:** *Initially:* 1 mg PO bid; then gradually increase with daily dosage increments of 1 mg/d on the second and third days to a target dose of 3 mg PO bid by the third day. *Reinitiation of treatment:* Follow initial dosage guidelines, using extreme care due to increased risk of severe adverse effects with reexposure. *Switching from other antipsychotics:* minimize the overlap period and discontinue other antipsychotic before beginning risperidone therapy.

**PEDIATRIC:** Safety and efficacy not established.

**GERIATRIC OR RENAL/HEPATIC IMPAIRED:** Initial dose of 0.5 mg PO bid; monitor patient for adverse effects and response.

### Pharmacokinetics

| *Route* | *Onset* | *Peak* | *Duration* |
|---|---|---|---|
| Oral | Varies | 3–17 h | weeks |

*Metabolism:* Hepatic, $T_{1/2}$: 20 h
*Distribution:* Crosses placenta; enters breast milk
*Excretion:* Urine and feces

### Adverse effects

- CNS: *Insomnia, anxiety, agitation, headache,* somnolence, aggression. dizziness, **tardive dyskinesias**
- GI: *Nausea, vomiting, constipation,* abdominal discomfort, dry mouth, increased saliva
- CV: Orthostatic hypotension, arrhythmias

- **Respiratory**: Rhinitis, coughing, sinusitis, pharyngitis, dyspnea
- **Dermatologic**: Rash, dry skin, seborrhea, photosensitivity
- **Other**: Chest pain, arthralgia, back pain, fever, **neuroleptic malignant syndrome**

### Clinically important drug-drug interactions

• Increased therapeutic and toxic effects with clozapine • Decreased therapeutic effect with carbamazepine • Decreased effectiveness of levodopa

## ■ Nursing Considerations

### Assessment

- *History:* Allergy to risperidone, lactation, CV disease, pregnancy, renal or hepatic impairment, hypotension
- *Physical:* T, weight; reflexes, orientation; P, BP, orthostatic BP; R, adventitious sounds; bowel sounds, normal output, liver evaluation; CBC, urinalysis, liver and kidney function tests

### Implementation

- Maintain seizure precautions, especially when initiating therapy and increasing dosage.
- Mix oral solution with 3–4 oz. of water, coffee, orange juice, or low-fat milk. Do *not* mix with cola or tea.
- Monitor T. If fever occurs, rule out underlying infection, and consult physician for appropriate comfort measures.
- Advise patient to use contraception during drug therapy.
- Follow guidelines for discontinuation or reinstitution of the drug carefully.

### Drug-specific teaching points

- Dosage will be increased gradually to achieve most effective dose. Do not take more than your prescribed dosage. Do not make up missed doses; contact your health care provider if this occurs. Do not stop taking this drug suddenly; gradual reduction of dosage is needed to prevent side effects.
- Mix oral solution in 3–4 oz. of water, coffee, orange juice, or low-fat milk. Do not mix with cola or tea.
- The following side effects may occur: drowsiness, dizziness, sedation, seizures (avoid driving, operating machinery, or performing tasks that require concentration); dizziness, faintness on arising (change positions slowly; use caution); increased salivation (reversible; constipation; sensitivity to the sun (use a sunscreen or protective clothing).
- This drug cannot be taken during pregnancy. If you think you are pregnant or wish to become pregnant, contact your health care provider.
- Report lethargy, weakness, fever, sore throat, malaise, mouth ulcers, palpitations.

# ritodrine hydrochloride

*(ri' toe dreen)*

Yutopar

**Pregnancy Category B**

### Drug classes

Sympathomimetic

Beta-2 selective adrenergic agonist

Tocolytic drug (uterine relaxant): In low doses, acts relatively selectively to

### Indications

- Management of preterm labor in selected patients ≤20 wk gestation

### Contraindications/cautions

- Contraindications: hypersensitivity to ritodrine or components of preparation (injection contains sodium metabisulfite; some patients are allergic to sulfites); pregnancies of shorter duration than 20 wk; antepartum hemorrhage; eclampsia and severe preeclampsia; intrauterine fetal death; chorioamnionitis; maternal cardiac disease; pulmonary hypertension; maternal hyperthyroidism; uncontrolled maternal diabetes mellitus; preexisting maternal medical conditions that would be seriously affected by a beta-adrenergic agonist, such as hypovolemia, cardiac arrhythmias associated with tachycardia or digitalis toxicity, uncontrolled hypertension, pheochromocytoma, bronchial asthma already treated by betamimetics or steroids.

## Dosage

**Available Forms:** Injection—10, 15 mg/ml; injection in 5% Dextrose—0.3 mg/ml

Individualize dosage by balancing uterine response and unwanted effects. The following is a guide to safe and effective dosage.

***IV:*** 0.05 mg/min IV initially (0.33 ml/min or 20 drops/min using a microdrip chamber at the recommended dilution; see below). Gradually increase by 0.05 mg/min (10 drops/min) every 10 min until desired result is attained. Usual effective dosage is between 0.15 and 0.35 mg/min (30–70 drops/min) continued for at least 12 h after uterine contractions cease.

## Pharmacokinetics

| *Route* | *Onset* | *Peak* |
|---|---|---|
| Oral | Varies | 30–60 min |
| IV | Rapid | |

*Metabolism:* Hepatic, $T_{1/2}$: 1.7–2.6 h

*Distribution:* Crosses placenta; enters breast milk

*Excretion:* Urine

## IV facts

**Preparation:** Empty the contents of three ampuls (50 mg/ampul; total of 150 mg) into 500 ml of compatible IV diluent to make a solution of 0.3 mg/ml concentration. Compatible diluents are 0.9% Sodium Chloride Solution, 5% Dextrose Solution; 10% Dextran 40 in 0.9% Sodium Chloride Solution, 10% Invert Sugar Solution, Ringer's Solution, Hartmann's Solution. Store at room temperature; protect from excessive heat. Do not use after 48 h. Do not use IV solution that is discolored or contains precipitate or particulate matter.

**Infusion:** Use a controlled infusion device to administer IV infusions; an IV microdrip chamber (60 drops/ml) can provide a convenient range of infusion rates.

## Adverse effects

*Maternal Effects*

- CNS: *Headache, weakness, tremor*, nervousness, restlessness, emotional upset, anxiety, malaise
- GI: *Nausea, vomiting*, ileus, constipation, diarrhea
- CV: *Increase in heart rate, increase in systolic BP, decrease in diastolic BP, palpitations*, chest pain, supraventricular tachycardia, sinus bradycardia with withdrawal of drug
- Respiratory: Dyspnea, hyperventilation, **postpartum pulmonary edema** (sometimes fatal)
- Hypersensitivity: Anaphylactic shock, rash
- Other: *Erythema*, transient elevation blood glucose, hypokalemia

*Fetal Effects*

- GI: Ileus
- CV: *Fetal heart rate increase*, hypotension in neonates whose mothers were given other beta-adrenergic agonists
- Hematologic: Hypoglycemia, hypocalcemia in neonates whose mothers were given other beta-adrenergic agonists

## Clinically important drug-drug interactions

• Increased sympathomimetic effects with other sympathomimetic drugs • Decreased therapeutic effects with beta-adrenergic blockers • Potentially fatal pulmonary edema with corticosteroids

## ■ Nursing Considerations

### Assessment

- *History:* Hypersensitivity to ritodrine or components of preparation, pregnancy, antepartum hemorrhage, eclampsia and severe preeclampsia, intrauterine fetal death, chorioamnionitis, maternal cardiac disease, pulmonary hypertension, maternal hyperthyroidism, uncontrolled maternal diabetes mellitus, hypovolemia, cardiac arrhythmias, uncontrolled hypertension, pheochromocytoma, bronchial

r

asthma already treated by betamimetics or steroids
- *Physical:* Maternal and fetal heart rate, maternal BP and R, plasma glucose and electrolytes (potassium)

## Implementation
- Monitor maternal P, R closely; persistent maternal P > 140 beats/min or persistent tachypnea (R > 20/min) may be signs of impending pulmonary edema.
- Avoid fluid overload; serial hemograms may indicate state of hydration.
- Maintain patient in left lateral position during the infusion to minimize hypotension.

## Drug-specific teaching points
- Report chest pain, dizziness, insomnia, weakness, tremor or irregular heart beat.

# ritonavir

*(ri **ton'** ah ver)*

Norvir

**Pregnancy Category B**

## Drug classes
Antiviral

## Therapeutic actions
Antiviral activity; inhibits HIV protease activity, leading to decrease in production of HIV particles.

## Indications
- Treatment of HIV infection, alone or in combination with nucleoside analog

## Contraindications/cautions
- Contraindication: allergy to ritonavir
- Use cautiously with pregnancy, hepatic impairment, lactation

## Dosage
**Available Forms:** Capsules—100 mg; oral solution—80 mg/ml

*ADULT AND PEDIATRIC >2 Y:* 600 mg PO bid with food. Capsule and syrup form available.

*PEDIATRIC:* Safety and efficacy not established in children <2 y.

## Pharmacokinetics

| Route | Onset | Peak |
|---|---|---|
| Oral | Rapid | 2–4 h |

*Metabolism:* Hepatic; $T_{1/2}$: 6–8 h

*Distribution:* Crosses placenta; may pass into breast milk

*Excretion:* Feces and urine

## Adverse effects
- CNS: *Asthenia, peripheral and circumoral paresthesias,* anxiety, dreams, headache, dizziness, hallucinations, personality changes
- GI: *Nausea, vomiting, diarrhea, anorexia, abdominal pain, taste perversion,* dry mouth, hepatitis, liver dysfunction, dehydration
- CV: Hemorrhage, hypotension, syncope, tachycardia
- **Respiratory**: Apnea, dyspnea, cough, rhinitis
- GU: Dysuria, hematuria, nocturia, pyelonephritis
- **Dermatologic**: Acne, dry skin, contact dermatitis, rash
- **Other**: Hypothermia, chills, back pain, chest pain, edema, cachexia

## Clinically important drug-drug interactions
• Potentially large increase in serum concentration of amiodarone, astemizole, bepridil, bupropion, cisapride, cloxapine, encainide, flecainide, meperidine, piroxicam, propafenone, propoxyphene, quinidine, rifabutin, terfenadine; potential for serious arrhythmias, seizure, and fatal reactions; *do not administer ritonavir with any of these drugs* • Potentially large increases in serum concentration of following sedative/hypnotics: alprazolam, clorazepam, diazepam, estazolam, flurazepam, midazolam, triazolam, zolpidem; extreme sedation and respiratory depression could occur; *do not administer ritonavir with any of these drugs*

## Clinically important drug-food interactions
• Absorption increased by presence of food; taking drug with food is strongly recommended

## ■ Nursing Considerations

### Assessment

- *History:* Allergy to ritonavir, hepatic dysfunction, pregnancy, lactation
- *Physical:* T; orientation, reflexes; BP, P, peripheral perfusion; R, adventitious sounds; bowel sounds; skin color, perfusion; liver function tests

### Implementation

- Capsules should be stored in refrigerator; solution may be refrigerated or left at room temperature if used within 30 d; protect from light and extreme heat.
- Administer with meals or food to increase absorption.
- Carefully screen drug history to avoid potentially dangerous drug–drug interactions.

### Drug-specific teaching points

- Take this drug with meals or food; store capsules in refrigerator. Taste of solution may be improved if mixed with chocolate milk, Ensure, or Advera 1 h before taking.
- Take the full course of therapy as prescribed; do not double up doses if one is missed; do not change dosage without consulting you physician.
- This drug does not cure HIV infection; long-term effects are not yet known; continue to take precautions as the risk of transmission is not reduced by this drug.
- Do not take any other drugs, prescription or OTC, without consulting your health care provider; this drug interacts with many other drugs and serious problems can occur.
- The following side effects may occur: nausea, vomiting, loss of appetite, diarrhea, abdominal pain, headache, dizziness, numbness, tingling.
- Report severe diarrhea, severe nausea, personality changes, changes in color of urine or stool, fever, chills.

# ropinirole hydrochloride

*(row **pin'** ah roll)*

Requip

**Pregnancy Category C**

### Drug classes

Antiparkinsonism agent
Dopamine receptor agonist

### Therapeutic actions

Acts as a non-ergot dopamine agonist acting directly on postsynaptic dopamine receptors of neurons in the brain, mimicking the effects of the neurotransmitter dopamine, which is thought to be deficient in parkinsonism.

### Indications

- Treatment of idiopathic Parkinson's disease in the early stages as well as in the late stages when used in combination with levodopa

### Contraindications/cautions

- Contraindications: hypersensitivity to ropinirole, severe ischemic heart disease or peripheral vascular disease, pregnancy, lactation.
- Use cautiously with dyskinesia, orthostatic hypotension, hepatic or renal impairment.

### Dosage

**Available Forms:** Tablets—0.25, 0.5, 1, 2, 5 mg

**ADULT:** Initially 0.25 mg PO tid for 1st wk; 0.5 mg PO tid for 2nd wk; 0.75 mg PO tid for 3rd wk; 1 mg PO tid for 4th wk. May increase by 1.5 mg/d at 1-wk intervals to 9 mg/d, then by up to 3 mg/d at 1-wk intervals to a maximum dose of 24 mg/d.

**PEDIATRIC:** Safety and efficacy not established.

**GERIATRIC:** Elderly are at higher risk for development of hallucinations; monitor closely and adjust dosage more slowly.

### Pharmacokinetics

| *Route* | *Onset* | *Peak* | *Duration* |
|---|---|---|---|
| Oral | Varies | 1–2 h | 8 h |

*Metabolism:* Hepatic; $T_{1/2}$: 6 h
*Distribution:* Crosses placenta; enters breast milk
*Excretion:* Urine

### Adverse effects

- CNS: *Dizziness, somnolence, insomnia, hypo- or hyperkinesia,* syncope, asthenia, confusion, hallucinations (more common in the elderly), abnormal vision, tremor, anxiety, paresthesias, aggravated parkinsonism
- GI: *Nausea, constipation*
- CV: *Postural hypotension,* edema
- Other: Fatigue, infections, sweating, pharyngitis, pain, arthralgia

### Clinically important drug-drug interactions

• Increased effects of levodopa; consider decreasing levodopa dose • Increased CNS depression with alcohol, CNS depressants • Monitor and adjust ropinirole dose if estrogen is added to or discontinued from regimen • Increased effects with ciprofloxacin

## ■ Nursing Considerations

### Assessment

- ***History:*** Hypersensitivity to ropinirole, severe ischemic heart disease or peripheral vascular disease, pregnancy, lactation, dyskinesia, orthostatic hypotension, hepatic or renal impairment
- ***Physical:*** Skin temperature, color, lesions; orientation, affect, reflexes, bilateral grip strength; vision exam including visual fields; P, BP, orthostatic BP, auscultation; liver evaluation; liver and kidney function tests

### Implementation

- Administer drug with food if GI upset becomes a problem.
- Monitor patient for orthostatic hypotension and establish safety precautions if necessary (siderails, accompanying patient, etc.).
- Withdraw gradually over 1 wk to avoid serious adverse effects.
- Monitor patient carefully and titrate dose more slowly if patient has hypotension or dyskinesias.
- Monitor elderly patients for the development of hallucinations; provide appropriate safety measures as needed.
- Start titration of drug over again if drug has been discontinued and is being restarted.
- Monitor hepatic and renal function periodically during therapy.

### Drug-specific teaching points

- Take this drug exactly as prescribed; take with food if GI upset occurs. Dosage will change gradually over several weeks.
- Do not discontinue this drug without first consulting with your nurse or physician; drug must be stopped gradually to prevent serious adverse effects.
- The following side effects may occur: drowsiness, dizziness, confusion (avoid driving or engaging in activities that require alertness); nausea (take drug with meals; eat small, frequent meals); dizziness or faintness when you get up (change position slowly, exercise caution when climbing stairs); headache, nasal stuffiness (inform your nurse or physician; it may be possible to have a medication for these).
- Report fainting, lightheadedness, dizziness; black, tarry stools; hallucinations.

# saliva substitute

*(sa **lie'** vah)*

Entertainer's Secret, Moi-Stir, Mouthkote, Optimoist, Salivart, Salix

**Pregnancy Category Unknown**

### Drug classes

Saliva substitute

### Therapeutic actions

Contains electrolytes and carboxymethylcellulose as a thickening agent to serve as a substitute for saliva in dry mouth syndromes.

### Indications

- Management of dry mouth and throat in xerostomia caused by stroke, medications, radiation therapy, chemotherapy, other illnesses

#### Contraindications/cautions

- Contraindications: hypersensitivity to carboxymethylcellulose, parabens, components of the preparation.
- Use cautiously with renal failure, CHF, hypertension.

### Dosage

**Available Forms:** Solution; lozenges

*ADULT:* Spray or apply to oral mucosa.

*PEDIATRIC:* Safety and efficacy not established.

#### Pharmacokinetics

Not generally absorbed systemically. Electrolytes may be absorbed and dealt with in normal electrolyte pathways.

#### Adverse effects

- Other: Excessive absorption of electrolytes (elevated magnesium, sodium, potassium)

## ■ Nursing Considerations

### Assessment

- *History:* Allergy to carboxymethylcellulose, parabens, CHF, hypertension, renal failure
- *Physical:* BP, P, auscultation, edema; renal function tests; mucosa evaluation

### Implementation

- Give for dry mouth and throat.
- Have patient try to swish saliva substitute around mouth following application.
- Monitor patient while eating; swallowing may be impaired and additional therapy required.

### Drug-specific teaching points

- Apply the drug as instructed; swish it around in your mouth after application.
- Use as needed for dry mouth and throat.
- Take care when eating because swallowing may be difficult; additional therapy may be needed.
- Report swelling, headache, irregular heart beat, leg cramps, failure to relieve discomfort of dry mouth and throat.

## salmeterol

*(sal **mee'** ter ol)*

Serevent

**Pregnancy Category C**

#### Drug classes

Beta-2 selective adrenergic agonist

Antiasthmatic agent

#### Therapeutic actions

Long-acting agonist that binds to $beta_2$ receptors in the lungs, causing bronchodilitation; also inhibits the release of inflammatory mediators in the lung, blocking swelling and inflammation.

#### Indications

- Prevention of and maintenance therapy for bronchospasm in select patients with asthma, reversible obstructive airway disease, and exercise-induced asthma

#### Contraindications/cautions

- Contraindications: hypersensitivity to salmeterol, acute asthma attack, worsening or deteriorating asthma (life-threatening), acute airway obstruction.
- Use cautiously with pregnancy, lactation.

### Dosage

**Available Forms:** Aerosol—25 $\mu$g/actuation

*ADULT:* 2 puffs q12h using pressurized metered-dose inhaler, which delivers 25 $\mu$g; 2 puffs 30–60 min before exertion for exercise-induced asthma. Do not exceed 4 puffs/d.

*PEDIATRIC:* Safety and efficacy not established.

#### Pharmacokinetics

| *Route* | *Onset* | *Peak* | *Duration* |
|---|---|---|---|
| Inhalation | 13–20 m | 3–4 h | 7.5–17 h |

*Metabolism:* Hepatic, $T_{1/2}$: unknown

*Distribution:* Crosses placenta; may enter breast milk

*Excretion:* Feces

**Adverse effects**
- CNS: *Headache, tremor*
- CV: *Tachycardia, palpitations*, hypertension
- **Respiratory**: Worsening of asthma, difficulty breathing, bronchospasm

## ■ Nursing Considerations

### Assessment
- ***History:*** Allergy to salmeterol, pregnancy, acute asthma attack, worsening asthma, lactation
- ***Physical:*** R, adventitious sounds; P, BP, EKG; orientation, reflexes; liver function tests

### Implementation
- Ensure that drug is not used to treat acute asthma or with worsening or deteriorating asthma (risk of death).
- Instruct in the proper use of metered inhaler.
- Monitor use of inhaler; use of more than 4 puffs/d may worsen asthma, obtain evaluation by physician.
- Have patients who experience exercise-induced asthma use it 30–60 min before activity.
- Arrange for periodic evaluation of respiratory condition.

### Drug-specific teaching points
- Use the pressurized metered-dose inhaler as instructed. Use only twice a day. If drug is to be used periodically for exercise-induced asthma, use 30–60 min before activity.
- Obtain periodic evaluations of your respiratory problem.
- The following side effects may occur: headache (request analgesics); tremors (use care in performing dangerous tasks); fast heart, palpitations (monitor activity; rest frequently).
- Report severe headache, irregular heart beat, worsening of asthma, difficulty breathing.

# salsalate

***(sal' sa late)***

salicylsalicylic acid

Amigesic, Argesic, Artha-G, Disalcid, Mono-Gesic, Salflex, Salsitab

**Pregnancy Category C**

**Drug classes**
Antipyretic
Analgesic (non-narcotic)
Anti-inflammatory agent
Antirheumatic
Salicylate
Nonsteroidal anti-inflammatory drug (NSAID)

**Therapeutic actions**
Analgesic and antirheumatic effects are attributable to the ability to inhibit the synthesis of prostaglandins, important mediators of inflammation; antipyretic effects are not fully understood, but salicylates probably act in the thermoregulatory center of the hypothalamus to block the effects of endogenous pyrogen by inhibiting the synthesis of the prostaglandin intermediary; after absorption, this drug is hydrolyzed into two molecules of salicylic acid; insoluble in gastric secretions, it is not absorbed in the stomach, but in the small intestine; reported to cause fewer GI adverse effects than aspirin.

**Indications**
- Relief of mild to moderate pain
- Reduction of fever
- Relief of symptoms of various inflammatory conditions—rheumatic fever, rheumatoid arthritis, osteoarthritis

**Contraindications/cautions**
- Allergy to salicylates or NSAIDs, bleeding disorders, impaired hepatic or renal function, GI ulceration (less of a problem than with others), lactation, pregnancy.

### Dosage
**Available Forms:** Capsules—500 mg; tablets—750 mg

*ADULT:* 3,000 mg/d PO given in divided doses.

*PEDIATRIC:* Safety and efficacy not established.

### Pharmacokinetics

| Route | Onset | Peak | Duration |
|---|---|---|---|
| Oral | 10–30 min | 1–3 h | 3–6 h |

*Metabolism:* Hepatic, $T_{1/2}$: 2–3 h (15–30 h with large doses over extended periods)
*Distribution:* Crosses placenta; enters breast milk
*Excretion:* Urine

### Adverse effects

*NSAIDs*

- CNS: *Headache, dizziness, somnolence, insomnia*, fatigue, tiredness, dizziness, tinnitus, ophthalmologic effects
- GI: *Nausea, dyspepsia, GI pain,* diarrhea, vomiting, *constipation*, flatulence
- **Respiratory**: Dyspnea, hemoptysis, pharyngitis, bronchospasm, rhinitis
- **Hematologic**: Bleeding, platelet inhibition with higher doses, neutropenia, eosinophilia, leukopenia, pancytopenia, thrombocytopenia, agranulocytosis, granulocytopenia, aplastic anemia, decreased Hgb or Hct, bone marrow depression, menorrhagia
- GU: Dysuria, renal impairment
- **Dermatologic**: *Rash*, pruritus, sweating, dry mucous membranes, stomatitis
- **Salicylism**: Dizziness, tinnitus, difficulty hearing, nausea, vomiting, diarrhea, mental confusion, lassitude (dose related)
- **Acute salicylate toxicity**: Respiratory alkalosis, hyperpnea, tachypnea, hemorrhage, excitement, confusion, asterixis, pulmonary edema, convulsions, tetany, metabolic acidosis, fever, coma, CV collapse, renal and respiratory failure
- **Other**: Peripheral edema, anaphylactoid reactions to fatal anaphylactic shock

### Clinically important drug-drug interactions

• Increased risk of GI ulceration with corticosteroids • Increased risk of salicylate toxicity with carbonic anhydrase inhibitors • Increased toxicity of carbonic anhydrase inhibitors, valproic acid • Decreased serum salicylate levels with corticosteroids, antacids, urine alkalinizers (sodium acetate, sodium bicarbonate, sodium citrate, sodium lactate, tromethamine) • Increased methotrexate levels and toxicity • Greater glucose-lowering effect of sulfonylureas, insulin with large doses of salicylates • Decreased uricosuric effect of probenecid, sulfinpyrazone • Decreased diuretic effect of spironolactone

### Drug-lab test interferences

• Decreased serum PBI • False-negative readings for urine glucose by glucose oxidase method and copper reduction method • Interference with urine 5-HIAA determinations by fluorescent methods but not by nitrosonaphthol colorimetric method • Interference with urinary ketone determination by ferric chloride method • Falsely elevated urine VMA levels with most tests; false decrease in VMA using the Pisano method

## ■ Nursing Considerations

### Assessment

- ***History:*** Allergy to salicylates or NSAIDs, bleeding disorders, impaired hepatic or renal function, GI ulceration, lactation, pregnancy
- ***Physical:*** Skin color and lesions; eighth cranial nerve function, orientation, reflexes, affect; P, BP, perfusion; R, adventitious sounds; liver evaluation and bowel sounds; CBC, urinalysis, stool guiaiac, renal and liver function tests



### Implementation

- Administer drug with food or after meals if GI upset occurs.
- Administer drug with a full glass of water to reduce risk of tablet/capsule lodging in the esophagus.
- Institute emergency procedures if overdose occurs: gastric lavage, induction of emesis, activated charcoal, supportive therapy.
- Provide further comfort measures to reduce pain, fever, and inflammation.

### Drug-specific teaching points

- Take the drug with food or after meals if GI upset occurs.
- Report ringing in the ears, dizziness, confusion, abdominal pain, rapid or difficult breathing, nausea, vomiting.

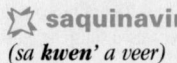

## Saquinavir

### saquinavir

*(sa **kwen'** a veer)*

Fortovase

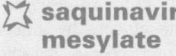

### saquinavir mesylate

Invirase

**Pregnancy Category B**

### Drug classes

Antiviral

### Therapeutic actions

Protease inhibitor which in combination with nucleoside analogues is effective in HIV infections with changes in surrogate markers.

### Indications

- Treatment of HIV infection in combination with other antiretroviral agents

### Contraindications/cautions

- Contraindications: life-threatening allergy to any component.
- Use cautiously with hepatic impairment, pregnancy, lactation.

### Dosage

**Available Forms:** Invirase: capsules—200 mg; Fortovase: soft gel capsules—200 mg

***Adults and Children*** $> 16$ ***Y:*** Invirase: 600 mg PO tid in combination with zidovudine or zalcitabine. Fortovase: 1.2 g tid PO with meals or up to 2 h after meals.

***Pediatric*** $< 16$ ***Y:*** Safety and efficacy not established.

***Hepatic Impaired:*** Reduce dose and monitor hepatic function tests.

### Pharmacokinetics

| Route | Onset | Peak |
|---|---|---|
| Oral | Slow | Unknown |

*Metabolism:* hepatic; $T_{1/2}$: unknown

*Distribution:* may cross placenta; may pass into breast milk

*Excretion:* feces

### Adverse effects

- CNS: *Headache,* insomnia, myalgia, *asthenia,* malaise, dizziness, paresthesia
- GI: *Nausea, GI pain, diarrhea,* anorexia, vomiting, dyspepsia
- Other: *Asthenia, elevated CPK*

### Clinically important drug-drug interactions

- Decreased effectiveness with rifampin, rifabutin, phenobarbital, phenytoin, dexamthasone, carbamazepine

## ■ Nursing Considerations

### Assessment

- ***History:*** Life-threatening allergy to any component, impaired hepatic function, pregnancy, lactation
- ***Physical:*** T; affect, reflexes, peripheral sensation; bowel sounds, liver evaluation; liver function tests, CPK levels

### Implementation

- Administer within 2 hours after a full meal.
- Monitor patient for signs of opportunistic infections that will need to be treated appropriately.
- Administer the drug concurrently with zidovudine (AZT) or zalcitabine.
- Offer support and encouragement to the patient to deal with the diagnosis as well as the effects of drug therapy and the high expense of treatment.

### Drug-specific teaching points

- Take drug as prescribed; take within 2 hours of a full meal; take concurrently with zidovudine (AZT) or zalcitabine.
- These drugs are not a cure for AIDs or ARC; opportunistic infections may occur and regular medical care should be sought to deal with the disease.

- The long-term effects of this drug are not yet known.
- The following side effects may occur: nausea, loss of appetite, change in taste (small, frequent meals may help); dizziness, loss of feeling (take appropriate precautions).
- This drug combination does not reduce the risk of transmission of HIV to others by sexual contact or blood contamination—use appropriate precautions.
- Report extreme fatigue, lethargy, severe headache, severe nausea, vomiting, difficulty breathing, skin rash, changes in color of urine or stool.

## sargramostim

*(sar* ***gram'*** *oh stim)*

granulocyte macrophage colony–stimulating factor, GM-CSF

Leukine

**Pregnancy Category C**

### Drug classes

Colony stimulating factor

### Therapeutic actions

Human GM-CSF produced by recombinant DNA technology; increases the proliferation and differentiation of hematopoietic progenitor cells; can activate mature granulocytes and macrophages.

### Indications

- Myeloid reconstitution after autologous bone marrow transplantation
- Treatment of neutropenia associated with bone marrow transplantation failure or engraftment delay
- Induction chemotherapy in AML to shorten neutrophil recovery time
- Acceleration of myeloid recovery in patients with non-Hodgkin's lymphoma
- Mobilization and following transplantation of autologous peripheral blood product collection (PBPC) by leukapheresis
- Unlabeled uses: treatment of myelodysplastic syndrome, decreases nadir of leukopenia related to myelosuppression of chemotherapy, corrects neutropenia in aplastic anemia patients, decreases transplant-associated organ system damage, promotes early grafting

### Contraindications/cautions

- Contraindications: hypersensitivity to yeast products, excessive leukemic myeloid blasts in bone marrow or peripheral blood, pregnancy.
- Use cautiously with renal or hepatic failure, lactation.

### Dosage

**Available Forms:** Powder for injection—250, 500 μg

**ADULT**

- *Myeloid reconstitution after autologous bone marrow transplantation:* 250 μg/m²/d for 21 d as a 2-h IV infusion beginning 2–4 h after the autologous bone marrow infusion and not less than 24 h after the last dose of chemotherapy.
- *Bone marrow transplantation failure or engraftment delay:* 250 μg/m²/d for 14 d as a 2-h IV infusion; can be repeated after 7 d off therapy.
- *Neutrophil recovery following chemotherapy in AML:* 250 mcg/m²/d IV over 4 h starting on day 11 or 4 d after chemotherapy induction.
- *Mobilization of PBPC:* 250 mcg/m²/d IV over 24 h or SC qd; continue throughout harvesting.
- *Post-PBPC transplant:* 250 mcg/m²/d IV over 24 h or SC qd.

**PEDIATRIC:** Safety and efficacy not established.

### Pharmacokinetics

| *Route* | *Peak* | *Duration* |
|---|---|---|
| IV | 2 h | 6 h |

*Metabolism:* Unknown, $T_{1/2}$: 12–17 min, then 2 h

*Distribution:* Crosses placenta; may enter breast milk

### IV facts

**Preparation:** Reconstitute with 1 ml Sterile Water for Injection; gently swirl contents to avoid foaming; do not shake, and avoid excessive agitation. Resulting

S

solution should be clear, colorless, and isontonic. Do not reenter vial; discard any unused portion. Dilute in 0.9% Sodium Chloirde Injection; administer within 6 h; refrigerate until ready to use.

**Infusion:** Infuse over 2 h; do not use an in-line membrane filter; do not mix with any other medication or in any other diluent.

**Compatabilities:** Do not mix with any solution other than 0.9% Sodium Chloride or add to any other medications.

### Adverse effects

- CNS: Headache, *fever*, generalized weakness, fatigue, *malaise, asthenia*
- GI: *Nausea, vomiting*, stomatitis, anorexia, *diarrhea*, constipation
- CV: Edema
- **Dermatologic**: *Alopecia*, rash, mucositis
- **Other**: *Bone pain*, generalized pain, sore throat, cough

## ■ Nursing Considerations

### Assessment

- *History:* Hypersensitivity to yeast products, pregnancy, lactation, excessive leukemic myeloid blasts in bone marrow or peripheral blood, pregnancy, renal or hepatic failure
- *Physical:* Skin color, lesions, hair; T; abdominal exam, status of mucous membranes; CBC, platelets

### Implementation

- Obtain CBC and platelet count prior to and twice weekly during therapy.
- Administer no less than 24 h after cytotoxic chemotherapy and within 2–4 h of bone marrow infusion.
- Administer daily as a 2-h infusion for 14–21 d.
- Store in refrigerator; allow to warm to room temperature before use; if vial is at room temperature for > 6 h, discard. Use each vial for one dose; do not reenter the vial; discard any unused drug.
- Do not shake vial before use.

### Drug-specific teaching points

- This drug must be given daily IV for as long as needed.
- Avoid exposure to infection (avoid crowds, visitors with infections).
- The following side effects may occur: nausea and vomiting (eat small, frequent meals); loss of hair (obtain appropriate head covering; cover head in temperature extremes); fever (request medication).
- Frequent blood tests will be needed to evaluate drug effects.
- Report fever, chills, sore throat, weakness, pain or swelling at injection site, difficulty breathing, chills.

## scopolamine hydrobromide

*(skoe **pol'** a meen)*

hyoscine HBr

*Parenteral:* Scopolamine HBr

*Transdermal system:* Transderm-Scop

*Ophthalmic solution:* Isopto Hyoscine Ophthalmic

**Pregnancy Category C**

### Drug classes

Anticholinergic
Antimuscarinic agent
Parasympatholytic
Anti-motion sickness agent
Colony stimulating factor
Belladonna alkaloid

### Therapeutic actions

Mechanism of action as antimotion sickness drug not understood; antiemetic action may be mediated by interference with cholinergic impulses to the vomiting center (CTZ); has sedative and amnesia-inducing properties; blocks the effects of acetylcholine at muscarinic cholinergic receptors that mediate the effects of parasympathetic postganglionic impulses, thus depressing salivary and bronchial secretions, inhibiting vagal influences on the heart, relaxing the GI and GU tracts, inhibiting gastric acid secretion, relaxing the pupil of the eye (mydriatic effect), and preventing accommodation for near vision (cycloplegic effect).

### Indications

- Prevention and control of nausea and vomiting due to motion sickness (oral, transdermal, parenteral preparations)
- Adjunctive therapy with antacids and $H_2$ antihistamines in peptic ulcer supportive treatment of functional GI disorders (diarrhea, pylorospasm, hypermotility, irritable bowel syndrome, spastic colon, acute enterocolitis, pancreatitis, infant colic)
- Treatment of biliary colic with narcotic analgesic
- Relief of urinary frequency and urgency, nocturnal enuresis, and ureteral colic (in conjunction with a narcotic analgesic)
- Suppression of vagally mediated bradycardia
- Preanesthetic medication to control bronchial, nasal, pharyngeal, and salivary secretions; prevent bronchospasm and laryngospasm; block cardiac vagal inhibitory reflexes during induction of anesthesia and intubation; produce sedation
- Induction of obstetric amnesia with analgesics calming delirium

*Ophthalmic Solution*

- Diagnostically to produce mydriasis and cycloplegia
- Preoperative and postoperative states in the treatment of iridocyclitis

### Contraindications/cautions

- Contraindications: hypersensitivity to anticholinergic drugs; glaucoma; adhesions between iris and lens; stenosing peptic ulcer, pyloroduodenal obstruction, paralytic ileus, intestinal atony, severe ulcerative colitis, toxic megacolon, symptomatic prostatic hypertrophy, bladder neck obstruction, bronchial asthma, COPD, cardiac arrhythmias, tachycardia, myocardial ischemia; impaired metabolic, liver or kidney function (increased likelihood of adverse CNS effects); myasthenia gravis, pregnancy (causes respiratory depression in neonates, contributes to neonatal hemorrhage); lactation.
- Use cautiously with Down's syndrome, brain damage, spasticity, hypertension, hyperthyroidism; glaucoma or tendency to glaucoma (ophthalmic solution).

### Dosage

**Available Forms:** Injection—0.3, 0.4, 0.86, 1 mg/ml; transdermal system—1.5 mg; ophthalmic solution—0.25%

**ADULT**

- ***Transdermal***
- *Motion sickness:* Apply one transdermal system to the postauricular skin at least 4 h before antiemetic effect is required. Scopolamine 0.5 mg will be delivered over 3 d. If continued effect is needed, replace system every 3 d.
- ***Parenteral:*** 0.32–0.65 mg SC or IM. May give IV after dilution in Sterile Water for Injection.
- ***Ophthalmic solution***
- *Refraction:* Instill 1–2 drops into the eye(s) 1 h before refracting.
- *Uveitis:* Instill 1–2 drops into the eye(s) up to 3× daily.

**PEDIATRIC:** Do not use oral scopolamine in children <6 y unless directed by physician. Do not use transdermal system in children.

- ***Parenteral:*** 0.006 mg/kg SC, IM, or IM; maximum dose is 0.3 mg.

**GERIATRIC:** More likely to cause serious adverse reactions, especially CNS reactions.

### Pharmacokinetics

| *Route* | *Onset* | *Peak* | *Duration* |
|---|---|---|---|
| IM, SC | 30 min | 60 min | 4–6 h |
| IV | 10 min | 60 min | 2–4 h |
| Transdermal | 4–5 h | | 72 h |
| Opthalmologic | 10–20 min | 30–45 min | Days |

*Metabolism:* Hepatic, $T_{1/2}$: 8 h
*Distribution:* Crosses placenta; enters breast milk
*Excretion:* Urine

### IV facts

**Preparation:** Dilute in Sterile Water for Injection.
**Infusion:** Inject directly into vein or into tubing of actively running IV; inject slowly over 5–10 min.

**Adverse effects**

- CNS: *Pupil dilation, photophobia, blurred vision, headache, drowsiness,* dizziness, mental confusion, excitement, restlessness, hallucinations, delirium in the presence of pain
- GI: *Dry mouth, constipation,* paralytic ileus, altered taste perception, nausea, vomiting, dysphagia, heartburn
- CV: Palpitations, tachycardia
- GU: *Urinary hesitancy and retention,* impotence
- **Hypersensitivity**: Anaphylaxis, urticaria, other dermatologic effects
- **Other**: Suppression of lactation, flushing, fever, *nasal congestion, decreased sweating*

**Clinically important drug-drug interactions**

• Decreased antipsychotic effectiveness of haloperidol • Decreased effectiveness of phenothiazines, but increased incidence of paralytic ileus

## ■ Nursing Considerations

### Assessment

- *History:* Hypersensitivity to anticholinergic drugs; glaucoma; adhesions between iris and lens; stenosing peptic ulcer, pyloroduodenal obstruction, intestinal atony, severe ulcerative colitis, symptomatic prostatic hypertrophy, bladder neck obstruction, bronchial asthma, COPD, cardiac arrhythmias, myocardial ischemia; impaired metabolic, liver or kidney function; myasthenia gravis; Down syndrome, brain damage, spasticity; hypertension, hyperthyroidism; pregnancy; lactation
- *Physical:* Skin color, lesions, texture; T; orientation, reflexes, bilateral grip strength; affect; ophthalmic exam; P, BP; R, adventitious sounds; bowel sounds, normal output; urinary output, prostate palpation; liver and kidney function tests, ECG

### Implementation

- Ensure adequate hydration; provide environmental control (temperature) to prevent hyperpyrexia.

### Drug-specific teaching points

- Take as prescribed, 30 min before meals. Avoid excessive dosage.
- Avoid hot environments. You will be heat intolerant, and dangerous reactions may occur.
- The following side effects may occur: dizziness, sedation, drowsiness (use caution driving or performing tasks that require alertness); constipation (ensure adequate fluid intake, proper diet); dry mouth (sugarless lozenges, frequent mouth care may help; may lessen); blurred vision, sensitivity to light (reversible, avoid tasks that require acute vision; wear sunglasses); impotence (reversible); difficulty urinating (empty bladder before taking drug).
- Avoid alcohol; serious sedation could occur.
- Report skin rash, flushing, eye pain, difficulty breathing, tremors, loss of coordination, irregular heartbeat, abdominal distention, hallucinations, severe or persistent dry mouth, difficulty urinating, constipation, sensitivity to light.

## secobarbital

*(see koe **bar'** bi tal)*

secobarbital sodium

Novosecobarb (CAN), Seconal Sodium

**Pregnancy Category D**

**C-II controlled substance**

**Drug classes**

Barbiturate (short-acting)
Sedative/hypnotic
Anticonvulsant

**Therapeutic actions**

General CNS depressant; barbiturates inhibit impulse conduction in the ascending RAS, depress the cerebral cortex, alter cerebellar function, depress motor output, and can produce excitation (especially with subanesthetic doses in the presence of pain), sedation, hypnosis, anesthesia, and deep coma; at anesthetic doses, has anticonvulsant activity.

**Indications**

- Intermittent use as a sedative, hypnotic, or preanesthetic medication
- In anesthetic doses for the emergency control of convulsive seizures associated with tetanus

**Contraindications/cautions**

- Contraindications: hypersensitivity to barbiturates; manifest or latent porphyria; marked liver impairment; nephritis; severe respiratory distress, respiratory disease with dyspnea, obstruction, or cor pulmonale; previous addiction to sedative-hypnotic drugs (drug may be ineffective, and use may contribute to further addiction); pregnancy (readily crosses placenta and has caused fetal damage, neonatal withdrawal syndrome).
- Use cautiously with acute or chronic pain (drug may cause paradoxical excitement or mask important symptoms); seizure disorders (abrupt discontinuation of daily doses can result in status epilepticus); lactation (has caused drowsiness in nursing infants); fever, hyperthyroidism, diabetes mellitus, severe anemia, pulmonary or cardiac disease, status asthmaticus, shock, uremia; impaired liver or kidney function, debilitation.

**Dosage**

**Available Forms:** Injection—50 mg/ml

ADULT: Adjust dosage on basis of age, weight, condition.

- ***IM:*** Inject deeply into large muscle mass. Do not give more than 250 mg (5 ml) in one injection. *Bedtime hypnotic:* 100–200 mg. *Dentistry (as sedative):* Usual dose is 2.2 mg/kg (1 mg/lb), maximum 100 mg, 10–15 min before the procedure. 1.1–1.6 mg/kg may suffice.
- ***IV:*** Restrict this route to when other routes are not feasible or when a rapid effect is imperative. *Anesthetic:* To provide basal hypnosis for general, spinal, or regional anesthesia. To facilitate intubation, administer at a rate ≥50 mg/15 sec. Discontinue administration as soon as desired degree of hypnosis is attained. Do not exceed 250 mg. If hypnosis is inadequate after 250 mg, add a small dose of meperidine. *Dentistry, patients who are to receive nerve blocks:* 100–150 mg IV. Patient will awaken in 15 min and can be discharged in 30 min if accompanied. *Convulsions in tetanus:* Initial dose of 5.5 mg/kg (2.5 mg/lb) IV. Repeat q3–4h as needed. Rate of administration should not exceed 50 mg/15 min.

PEDIATRIC: Use caution: barbiturates may produce irritability, excitability, inappropriate tearfulness, and aggression.

- ***Rectal (injectable solution):*** Prior to ENT procedures. Dilute with lukewarm tap water to a concentration of 1%–1.5% and administer after a cleansing enema. *<40 kg (88lb):* 5 mg/kg (2.3 mg/lb). *>40 kg:* 4 mg/kg (1.8 mg/lb). Hypnosis should follow in 15–20 min.
- ***Parenteral***
  - *IM:* 4–5 mg/kg to provide basal hypnosis. *Dentistry (as sedative):* Usual dose is 2.2 mg/kg (1 mg/lb) IM, maximum 100 mg, 10–15 min before the procedure. 1.1–1.6 mg/kg may suffice.

GERIATRIC PATIENTS OR THOSE WITH DEBILITATING DISEASE: Reduce dosage and monitor closely. May produce excitement, depression, confusion.

**Pharmacokinetics**

| *Route* | *Onset* | *Peak* | *Duration* |
|---|---|---|---|
| IV | Immediate | 1–3 min | 15 min |
| IM | Rapid | 7–10 min | 1–4 h |

*Metabolism:* Hepatic, $T_{1/2}$: 15–40 h

*Distribution:* Crosses placenta; enters breast milk

*Excretion:* Urine

**IV facts**

**Preparation:** No further preparation required; refrigerate; protect from light; do not use if solution contains precipitate.

**Infusion:** Infuse slowly over time periods listed for each use.

S

**Adverse effects**

- CNS: *Somnolence, agitation, confusion, hyperkinesia, ataxia, vertigo, CNS depression, nightmares, lethargy, residual sedation (hangover), paradoxical excitement, nervousness, psychiatric disturbance, hallucinations, insomnia, anxiety, dizziness, thinking abnormality*
- GI: *Nausea, vomiting, constipation, diarrhea, epigastric pain*
- CV: *Bradycardia, hypotension, syncope*
- Respiratory: *Hypoventilation, apnea, respiratory depression,* laryngospasm, bronchospasm, circulatory collapse
- Hypersensitivity: Skin rashes, angioneurotic edema, serum sickness, morbiliform rash, urticaria; rarely, exfoliative dermatitis, Stevens-Johnson syndrome, sometimes fatal
- Local: *Pain, tissue necrosis at injection site,* gangrene; arterial spasm with inadvertent intra-arterial injection; thrombophlebitis; permanent neurologic deficit if injected near a nerve
- Other: Tolerance, psychological and physical dependence; **withdrawal syndrome**

**Clinically important drug-drug interactions**

• Increased CNS depression with alcohol • Increased renal toxicity with methoxyflurane • Decreased effects of oral anticoagulants, corticosteroids, oral contraceptives and estrogens, metronidazole, metoprolol, propranolol, doxycycline, oxyphenbutazone, phenylbutazone, quinidine with barbiturates • Decreased theophylline serum levels and effectiveness secondary to increased clearance

## ■ Nursing Considerations

### Assessment

- *History:* Hpersensitivity to barbiturates; manifest or latent porphyria; marked liver impairment; nephritis; severe respiratory distress; previous addiction to sedative-hypnotic drugs; pregnancy; acute or chronic pain; seizure disorders; lactation; fever, hyperthyroidism, diabetes mellitus, severe anemia, pulmonary or cardiac disease, shock, uremia; impaired liver or kidney function, debilitation
- *Physical:* Weight; T; skin color, lesions; orientation, affect, reflexes; P, BP, orthostatic BP; R, adventitious sounds; bowel sounds, normal output, liver evaluation; liver and kidney function tests, blood and urine glucose, BUN

### Implementation

- Monitor patient responses, blood levels with the above interacting drugs; suggest alternatives to oral contraceptives.
- Do not administer intra-arterially; may produce arteriospasm, thrombosis, gangrene.
- Administer IV doses slowly.
- Give IM doses deep in a muscle mass.
- Do not use discolored parenteral solutions or those that contain a precipitate.
- Remain with children who have received secobarbital rectally.
- Monitor injection sites carefully for irritation, extravasation (IV use); solutions are alkaline and very irritating to the tissues.
- Monitor P, BP, respiration carefully during IV administration.
- Taper dosage gradually after repeated use, especially in epileptics.

### Drug-specific teaching points

- This drug will make you drowsy (or induce sleep) and less anxious.
- Try not to get up after you have received this drug (request assistance if you must sit up or move about).

# sertraline hydrochloride

*(sir' trah leen)*

Zoloft

**Pregnancy Category B**

**Drug classes**

Antidepressant

Selective serotinin reuptake inhibitor (SSRI)

### Therapeutic actions

Acts as an antidepressant by inhibiting CNS neuronal uptake of serotonin; blocks uptake of serotonin with little effect on norepinephrine, muscarinic, histaminergic, and alpha$_1$-adrenergic or dopaminergic receptors.

### Indications

- Treatment of depression
- Treatment of obsessive-compulsive disorders

### Contraindications/cautions

- Contraindications: hypersensitivity to sertraline; pregnancy.
- Use cautiously with impaired hepatic or renal function, lactation.

### Dosage

**Available Forms:** Talbets—50, 100 mg; capsules—25, 50, (CAN) 100 mg

**ADULT:** Administer once a day, morning or evening. 50 mg PO qd; may be increased to up to 200 mg/d; dosage increases should not occur at intervals < 1 wk. Efficacy for up to 16 wk; further study is needed to determine dosage for extended use.

**PEDIATRIC:** Safety and efficacy not established.

**GERIATRIC OR RENAL IMPAIRED:** Give a lower dose. Use response as dosage guide.

### Pharmacokinetics

| Route | Onset | Peak |
|---|---|---|
| Oral | Slow | 4 1/2–8.4 h |

*Metabolism:* Hepatic, $T_{1/2}$: 26 h
*Distribution:* Crosses placenta; may enter breast milk
*Excretion:* Urine and feces

### Adverse effects

- CNS: *Headache, nervousness, drowsiness, anxiety, tremor, dizziness, insomnia* lightheadedness, agitation, sedation, abnormal gait, convulsions, *vision changes, fatigue*
- GI: *Nausea,* vomiting, *diarrhea, dry mouth,* anorexia, dyspepsia, constipation, taste changes, flatulence, gastroenteritis, dysphagia, gingivitis
- CV: Hot flashes, palpitations, chest pain
- **Respiratory:** Upper respiratory infections, pharyngitis, cough, dyspnea, bronchitis, *rhinitis*
- GU: *Painful menstruation,* sexual dysfunction, frequency, cystitis, impotence, urgency, vaginitis
- **Dermatologic:** *Sweating,* rash, pruritus, acne, contact dermatitis
- **Other:** Hot flashes, fever, back pain, thirst

### Clinically important drug-drug interactions

• Serious, sometimes fatal, reactions with MAO inhibitors • Increased serum levels of sertraline with cimetidine • Risk of serious cardiac arrhythmia with astemizole, terfenadine

### Clinically important drug-food interactions

- Increased rate of absorption with food

## ■ Nursing Considerations

### Assessment

- *History:* Hypersensitivity to sertraline, impaired hepatic or renal function, lactation, pregnancy
- *Physical:* Weight; T; skin rash, lesions; reflexes, affect; bowel sounds, liver evaluation; P, peripheral perfusion; urinary output, renal and liver function tests

### Implementation

- Lower dose in elderly patients and with hepatic or renal impairment.
- Establish suicide precautions for severely depressed patients. Limit number of capsules given at any time.
- Give drug once a day, morning or evening.
- Increase dosage at intervals of not less than 1 wk.
- Counsel patient to use nonhormonal contraceptives; pregnancy should be avoided due to risk to fetus.

### Drug-specific teaching points

- Take this drug once a day, at the same time, morning or evening; do not exceed the prescribed dose.

S

- The following side effects may occur: dizziness, drowsiness, nervousness, insomnia (avoid driving or performing hazardous tasks); nausea, vomiting (eat small frequent meals); dry mouth (sucking sugarless lozenges and frequent mouth care may help); excessive sweating (monitor temperature; avoid overheating).
- Do not take this drug during pregnancy. If you think that you are pregnant or wish to become pregnant, consult with your physician.
- Report rash, mania, seizures, edema, difficulty breathing.

## sibutramine hydrochloride

*(sih **bu'** trah meen)*

Meridia

**Pregnancy Category B**

### Drug classes

Reuptake inhibitor
Weight loss agent

### Therapeutic actions

Inhibits the reuptake of various neurotransmitters, including monoamine, norepinephrine, 5-HT and possibly dopamine; these effects act to suppress the appetite and decrease depression; is nonsedating, nonanticholineric and has no central depressant effects.

### Indications

- Treatment of obesity
- Unlabeled use: treatment of depression

### Contraindications/cautions

- Contraindications: hypersensitivity to sibutramine; pregnancy.
- Use cautiously with impaired hepatic function, hypertension, arrhythmias.

### Dosage

**Available Forms:** Tablets—5, 10, 15 mg

*ADULT:* Initial dose 5 mg PO qd; may increase to up to 20 mg PO qd as tolerated. Must be used in conjunction with a weight loss diet and exercise program.

*PEDIATRIC:* Safety and efficacy not established.

### Pharmacokinetics

| *Route* | *Onset* | *Peak* |
|---|---|---|
| Oral | NA | NA |

*Metabolism:* Hepatic; $T_{1/2}$: unknown
*Distribution:* Crosses placenta; may enter breast milk
*Excretion:* Urine and feces

### Adverse effects

- CNS: *Headache, nervousness, sleep difficulties*
- GI: *Dry mouth,* nausea, anorexia
- CV: Hypertension, tachycardia, arrhythmias
- **Dermatologic:** *Rash, dry skin*

## ■ Nursing Considerations

### Assessment

- ***History:*** Hypersensitivity to sibutramine; impaired hepatic or renal function; lactation; pregnancy, hypertension, arrhythmias
- ***Physical:*** Weight, T; skin rash, lesions; reflexes, affect; liver evaluation; P, BP, ECG, peripheral perfusion; renal and liver function test

### Implementation

- Ensure that patient is participating in a weight loss diet and exercise program.
- Establish suicide precautions for severely depressed patients. Dispense only a small number of capsules at a time to these patients.
- Administer drug once a day, in the morning or in the evening.
- Increase dosage at intervals of not less than 1 wk.
- Provide sugarless lozenges, frequent mouth care if dry mouth is a problem.
- Counsel patient about the use of nonhormonal contraceptives while on this drug; pregnancy should be avoided because of the possible risk to the fetus.

### Drug-specific teaching points

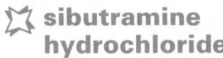

- Take this drug once a day, at the same time each day, in the morning or in the evening; do not exceed the prescribed dose.

- The following side effects may occur: dizziness, drowsiness, nervousness, insomnia (avoid driving or performing hazardous tasks); dry mouth (sucking sugarless lozenges and frequent mouth care may help); dry skin, rash (provide skin care as recommended).
- Do not take this drug during pregnancy. If you think that you are pregnant or wish to become pregnant, consult with your physician.
- Report rash, mania, seizures, edema, difficulty breathing, palpitations.

## simethicone

*(sigh **meth'** ih kohn)*

Flatulex, Gas Relief, Gas-X, Major-Con, Mylanta Gas, Mylicon, Oval (CAN), Phazyme, Phazyme 55 (CAN)

**Pregnancy Category Unknown**

### Drug classes
Antiflatulent

### Therapeutic actions
Defoaming action disperses and prevents the formation of mucus surrounded gas pockets in the GI tract; changes the surface tension of gas bubbles in the stomach and small intestine, enabling the bubbles to coalesce, freeing gas to be more easily freed by belching or flatus.

### Indications
- Relief of symptoms and pressure of excess gas in the digestive tract; postoperative gaseous distention and pain, use in endoscopic examination; air swallowing; functional dyspepsia; spastic or irritable colon; diverticulosis
- Unlabeled use: treatment of colic in infants

### Contraindications/cautions
- Allergy to components of the product.

### Dosage
**Available Forms:** Chewable tablets—40, 80, 125 mg; tablets—60, 95 mg; capsules—125 mg; drops—40 mg/0.6ml

**ADULT**
- ***Capsules:*** 125 mg PO qid, after each meal and hs.
- ***Tablets:*** 40–125 mg PO qid, after each meal and hs.
- ***Drops:*** 40–80 mg PO qid up to 500 mg/d, after each meal and hs.

**PEDIATRIC**
- *<2 Y:* 20 mg PO qid after each meal and hs; up to 240 mg/d.
- *2–12 Y:* 40 mg PO qid after each meal and hs.

### Pharmacokinetics
Not absorbed systemically; excreted unchanged in the feces.

### Adverse effects
- GI: Nausea, vomiting, *diarrhea,* constipation, belching, passing of flatus

## ■ Nursing Considerations

### Assessment
- *History:* Hypersensitivity to simethicone
- *Physical:* Bowel sounds, normal output

### Implementation
- Give after each meal and at hs.
- Shake drops thoroughly before each use.
- Add drops to 30 ml cool water, infant formula, or other liquid to ease administration to infants.
- Ensure chewable tablets are chewed thoroughly before swallowing.

### Drug-specific teaching points
- Take this drug after each meal and at bedtime; chew chewable tablets thoroughly before swallowing; shake drops bottle thoroughly before administration. Parents may want to add drops to 30 ml cool water, infant formula, or other liquid to ease administration.
- You may experience increased belching and passing of flatus as gas disperses.
- Report extreme abdominal pain, worsening of condition being treated, vomiting.

# simvastatin

*(sim va **stab' tin**)*

Zocor

**Pregnancy Category X**

## Drug classes

Antihyperlipidemic
HMG CoA inhibitor

## Therapeutic actions

Inhibits HMG co-enzyme A, the enzyme that catalyzes the first step in the cholesterol synthesis pathway, resulting in a decrease in serum cholesterol, serum LDLs (increased risk of CAD), and either an increase or no change in serum HDLs (decreased risk of CAD).

## Indications

- Adjunct to diet in the treatment of elevated total cholestrol and LDL cholesterol with primary hypercholesterolemia (types IIa and IIb) in those unresponsive to dietary restriction of saturated fat and cholesterol and other nonpharmacologic measures
- Reduce the risk of MI in patients with coronary heart disease and hypercholesterolemia

## Contraindications/cautions

- Contraindications: allergy to simvastatin, fungal byproducts, pregnancy, lactation.
- Use cautiously with impaired hepatic function, cataracts.

## Dosage

**Available Forms:** Tablets—5, 10, 20, 40 mg

**ADULT:** Initially, 5–10 mg PO qd once daily, evening. Maximum dose, 40 mg/d. Adjust at 4-wk intervals.

**PEDIATRIC:** Safety and efficacy not established.

**GERIATRIC:** Starting dose, 5 mg/d PO; increase dose slowly, monitoring response.

## Pharmacokinetics

| Route | Onset | Peak |
|---|---|---|
| Oral | Slow | 1.3–2.4 h |

*Metabolism:* Hepatic, $T_{1/2}$: 3 h

*Distribution:* Crosses placenta; enters breast milk

*Excretion:* Urine and feces

## Adverse effects

- CNS: *Headache*, asthenia, sleep disturbances
- GI: *Flatulence, abdominal pain, cramps, constipation, nausea*, dyspepsia, heartburn

## Clinically important drug-drug interactions

• Possible severe myopathy or rhabdomyolysis with gemfibrozil, cyclosporine, erythromycin, niacin • Increased bleeding effects with warfarin

## ■ Nursing Considerations

### Assessment

- *History:* Allergy to simvastatin, fungal byproducts; impaired hepatic function; pregnancy; lactation
- *Physical:* Orientation, affect; liver evaluation, abdominal exam; lipid studies, liver function tests

### Implementation

- Ensure that patient has tried a cholesterol-lowering diet regimen for 3–6 mo before beginning therapy.
- Give in the evening; highest rates of cholesterol synthesis are between midnight and 5 AM.
- Arrange for regular follow-up during long-term therapy. Consider reducing dose if cholesterol falls below target.

### Drug-specific teaching points

- Take drug in the evening.
- The following side effects may occur: nausea (eat small, frequent meals may help); headache, muscle and joint aches and pains (may lessen); sensitivity to light (use a suncreen and wear protective clothing).
- Have periodic blood tests.
- Report severe GI upset, changes in vision, unusual bleeding or bruising, dark urine or light-colored stools.

## sodium bicarbonate

*Parenteral:* Neut
*Prescription and OTC preparations:* Bell/ans
**Pregnancy Category C**

### Drug classes
Electrolyte
Systemic alkalinizer
Urinary alkalinizer
Antacid

### Therapeutic actions
Increases plasma bicarbonate; buffers excess hydrogen ion concentration; raises blood pH; reverses the clinical manifestations of acidosis; increases the excretion of free base in the urine, effectively raising the urinary pH; neutralizes or reduces gastric acidity, resulting in an increase in the gastric pH, which inhibits the proteolytic activity of pepsin.

### Indications
- Treatment of metabolic acidosis, with measures to control the cause of the acidosis
- Adjunctive treatment in severe diarrhea with accompanying loss of bicarbonate
- Treatment of certain drug intoxications, hemolytic reactions that require alkalinization of the urine; prevention of methotrexate nephrotoxicity by alkalinization of the urine
- Minimization of uric acid crystalluria in gout, with uricosuric agents
- Minimization of sulfonamide crystalluria
- Symptomatic relief of upset stomach from hyperacidity associated with peptic ulcer, gastritis, peptic esophagitis, gastric hyperacidity, hiatal hernia (oral)
- Prophylaxis of GI bleeding, stress ulcers, aspiration pneumonia (oral)

### Contraindications/cautions
- Contraindications: allergy to components of preparations; low serum chloride (secondary to vomiting, continuous GI suction, diuretics associated with hypochloremic alkalosis); metabolic and respiratory alkalosis; hypocalcemia (alkalosis may precipitate tetany).
- Use cautiously with impaired renal function, CHF, edematous or sodium-retaining states, oliguria or anuria, potassium depletion (may predispose to metabolic alkalosis), pregnancy.

### Dosage
**Available Forms:** Injection—0.5, 0.6, 0.9, 1.0 mEq/ml; neutralizing additive solution—0.48, 0.5 mEq/ml; tablets—325, 520, 650 mg

**ADULT**
- *Urinary alkalinization:* 325 mg–2 g qid PO. Maximum daily dose, 16 g in patients <60 y, 8 g in patients >60 y.
- *Antacid:* 0.3–2 g qd to qid PO. Usually 1 and 3 h after meals and hs.
- *Cardiac arrest:* Adjust dosage based on arterial blood pH, $PaCO_2$, and calculation of base deficit; initial dose, 1 mEq/kg IV followed by 0.5 mEq/kg every 10 min during arrest.
- *Metabolic acidosis:* Initially 2–5 mEq/kg over 4–8 h IV. May be added to IV fluids, with rate and dosage determined by arterial blood gases and estimation of base deficit.

**PEDIATRIC**
- *NEONATES AND CHILDREN <2 Y:* Use caution and slow administration to prevent hypernatremia, decrease in CSF pressure, and possible intracranial hemorrhage.
- *Cardiac arrest, infants up to 2 y:* 4.2% solution IV at a rate not to exceed 8 mEq/kg per day. Initially 1–2 mEq/kg given over 1–2 min followed by 1 mEq/kg every 10 min during arrest.
- *Metabolic acidosis:* Older children: follow adult recommendation. Younger children: use caution, and base dosage on blood gases and calculation of base deficit.

**GERIATRIC AND RENAL IMPAIRED:** Reduce dosage and carefully monitor base deficit and clinical response.

### Pharmacokinetics

| Route | Onset | Peak | Duration |
|---|---|---|---|
| Oral | Rapid | 30 min | 1–3 h |
| IV | Immediate | Rapid | |

S

*Metabolism:* $T_{1/2}$: unknown
*Distribution:* Crosses placenta; enters breast milk
*Excretion:* Urine

### IV facts

**Preparation:** Direct IV push requires no further preparation; continuous infusion may be diluted in saline, dextrose, and dextrose/saline solutions.

**Infusion:** Administer by IV direct injection slowly; continuous infusion should be regulated with close monitoring of electrolytes and response, 2–5 mEq/kg over 4–8 h.

**Compatibilities:** Avoid solutions containing calcium; precipitation may occur.

### Adverse effects

- GI: Gastric rupture following ingestion
- Hematologic: *Systemic alkalosis* (headache, nausea, irritability, weakness, tetany, confusion), hypokalemia secondary to intracellular shifting of potassium
- Local: Chemical cellulitis, tissue necrosis, ulceration and sloughing at the site of infiltration (parenteral)

### Clinically important drug-drug interactions

• Increased pharmacologic effects of anorexiants, sympathomimetics with oral sodium bicarbonate • Increased half-lives and duration of effects of amphetamines, ephedrine, pseudoephedrine due to alkalinization of urine • Decreased pharmacologic effects of lithium, salicylates, sulfonylureas, demeclocycline, doxycycline, methacycline, and other tetracyclines

## ■ Nursing Considerations

### Assessment

- *History:* Allergy to components of preparations; low serum chloride; metabolic and respiratory alkalosis; hypocalcemia; impaired renal function; CHF, edematous, or sodium-retaining states; oliguria or anuria; potassium depletion; pregnancy
- *Physical:* Skin color, turgor; injection sites; P, rhythm, peripheral edema; bowel sounds, abdominal exam; urinary output; serum electrolytes, serum bicarbonate, arterial blood gases, urinalysis, renal function tests

### Implementation

- Monitor arterial blood gases, and calculate base deficit when administering parenteral sodium bicarbonate. Adjust dosage based on response. Administer slowly, and do not attempt complete correction within the first 24 h; risk of systemic alkalosis is increased.
- Give parenteral preparations by IV route.
- Check serum potassium levels before IV administration; risk of metabolic acidosis is increased in states of hypokalemia, requiring reduction of sodium bicarbonate. Monitor IV injection sites carefully; if infiltration occurs, promptly elevate the site, apply warm soaks, and if needed, arrange for the local injection of lidocaine or hyaluronidase to prevent sloughing.
- Have patient chew oral tablets thoroughly before swallowing, and follow them with a full glass of water.
- Do not give oral sodium bicarbonate within 1–2 h of other oral drugs to reduce risk of drug-drug interactions.
- Monitor cardiac rhythm carefully during IV administration.

### Drug-specific teaching points

- Chew oral tablets thoroughly, and follow with a full glass of water. Do not take within 1–2 h of any other drugs to decrease risk of drug interactions.
- Have periodic blood tests and medical evaluations.
- Report irritability, headache, tremors, confusion, swelling of extremities, difficulty breathing, black or tarry stools, pain at IV injection site (parenteral form).

## sodium chloride

***(klor' ide)***

*Parenteral:* Sodium Chloride Injection (various)

*Prescription and OTC oral preparations:* Sodium Chloride Tablets

**Pregnancy Category C**

### Drug classes
Electrolyte

### Therapeutic actions
Sodium chloride is the principal salt involved in the maintenance of plasma tonicity; important for maintaining plasma volume, promoting membrane stability and electrolyte balance.

### Indications
- Treatment of hyponatremia
- Dilution and reconstitution of parenteral drugs
- Hydration and replacement of fluid loss

### Contraindications/cautions
- Contraindications: hypernatremia, fluid retention, pregnancy, any condition when increased sodium or chloride could be detrimental.
- Use cautiously with impaired renal function, CHF, edematous or sodium-retaining states, lactation, surgical patients.

### Dosage
**Available Forms:** Tablets—650 mg; 1, 2.25 g; injections—various preparations

ADULT
- ***Oral:*** 1–2 g PO tid.
- ***IV:*** Isotonic (replacement) 1 L administered over 1 h; hypotonic (0.45%; hydration) 1–2 L over 1–2 h; hypertonic (3–5%; treatment of hyponatremia) 100 ml over 1 h.

PEDIATRIC: Safety and efficacy not determined; replacement must be monitored closely and based on clinical response.

GERIATRIC AND RENAL IMPAIRED: Reduce dosage, and carefully monitor base deficit and clinical response.

### Pharmacokinetics

| Route | Onset | Peak |
|---|---|---|
| Oral | Unknown | |
| IV | Immediate | End of infusion |

*Metabolism:* $T_{1/2}$: unknown
*Distribution:* Crosses placenta; enters breast milk
*Excretion:* Urine

### IV facts
**Preparation:** Concentrated sodium chloride must be further diluted before use; other preparations may be given as provided; change infusion q24h; use only if solution is clear.

**Infusion:** Administer by IV direct injection slowly; continuous infusion should be regulated with close monitoring of electrolytes and response.

### Adverse effects
- GI: Anorexia, nausea, abdominal distention
- Hematologic: Hypernatremia, fluid overload
- Local: Chemical cellulitis, tissue necrosis, ulceration and sloughing at the site of infiltration, pain at site of injection (parenteral)

## ■ Nursing Considerations

### Assessment
- *History:* Hypernatremia, fluid retention, pregnancy, impaired renal function, CHF, edematous or sodium-retaining states, lactation, surgical patients
- *Physical:* Skin color, turgor; injection sites; P, rhythm, peripheral edema; bowel sounds, abdominal exam; urinary output; serum electrolytes, urinalysis, renal function tests

### Implementation
- Monitor serum electrolytes carefully before and during administration. Administer slowly. Rapid infusion can result in pain and irritation at injection site.
- Give parenteral preparations by IV route.
- Monitor IV injection sites carefully; if infiltration occurs, promptly elevate the site, apply warm soaks, and if needed, arrange for the local injection of lidocaine or hyaluronidase to prevent sloughing.
- Monitor surgical patients for postoperative salt intolerance (weakness, dehydration, disorientation, nausea, distention, oliguria); if this occurs, discontinue infusion and provide supportive measures.

S

- Assess patients taking oral tablets for actual salt loss; excessive use of these tablets can cause hypernatremia.

### Drug-specific teaching points

- Take these tablets only as prescribed.
- Have periodic blood tests and medical evaluations.
- Report irritability, confusion, tremors, swelling of extremities, difficulty breathing, black or tarry stools.

# sodium fluoride

*(flor' ide)*

Fluor-A-Day (CAN), Fluoritab, Fluotic (CAN), Flura, Flura-Loz, Fluro-Drops, Karidium, Luride Lozi Tablets, PDF (CAN), Pediaflor, Pedident (CAN), Pharmaflur, Phos-Flur

**Pregnancy Category C**

### Drug classes

Mineral

### Therapeutic actions

Acts systemically before tooth eruption and topically after tooth eruption to increase tooth resistance to acid dissolution and promote remineralization of teeth and inhibit caries formation by microbes.

### Indications

- Prevention of dental caries
- Unlabeled use: prevention of osteoporosis

### Contraindications/cautions

- Contraindicated in areas where fluoride content of drinking water exceeds 0.7 ppm, with low sodium or sodium-free diets, hypersensitivity to fluoride.
- Use cautiously with pregnancy, lactation.

### Dosage

**Available Forms:** Chewable tablets—0.5, 1 mg; tablets—1 mg; drops—0.125, 0.25, 0.5 mg/ml; lozenges—1 mg; solution—0.2 mg/ml

**ADULT:** Up to 60 mg/d PO with calcium supplements, estrogen, vitamin D to prevent osteoporosis.

- *Rinse:* 10 ml; swish around teeth and spit out.

**PEDIATRIC:** Dosage refers to daily dose.

- ***Fluoride content of drinking water < 0.3 ppm:*** <2 y: 0.25 mg PO; 2–3 y: 0.5 mg PO; 3–12 y: 1 mg PO.
- ***Fluoride content of drinking water 0.3–0.7 ppm:*** <2 y: 0.125 mg PO; 2–3 y: 0.25 mg PO; 3–14 y: 0.25–0.75 mg PO.
- ***Topical rinse:*** 6–12 y: 5–10 ml/d; > 2 y: 10 ml; swish around teeth and spit out.

### Pharmacokinetics

| Route | Onset | Peak |
|---|---|---|
| Oral | Unknown | |

*Metabolism:* $T_{1/2}$: unknown

*Distribution:* Crosses placenta; enters breast milk

*Excretion:* Urine, sweat glands, feces

### Adverse effects

- Dermatologic: Eczema, atopic dermatitis, urticaria, rash
- Other: Gastric distress, headache, weakness, staining of teeth (with rinse)

### Clinically important drug-food interactions

- Milk, dairy products may decrease absorption; avoid simultaneous use

## ■ Nursing Considerations

### Assessment

- *History:* Fluoride content of drinking water, low sodium or sodium-free diets, hypersensitivity to fluoride, pregnancy, lactation
- *Physical:* Skin color, turgor; state of teeth and gums

### Implementation

- Do not give with milk or dairy products.
- Tablets may be chewed, swallowed whole, added to drinking water or juice.
- Give drops undiluted, or with fluids, food.
- Ensure that patient has brushed and flossed teeth before the use of rinse and that patient expectorates fluid; it should not be swallowed.

- Monitor teeth, and arrange for dental consultation if mottling of teeth occurs.
- Monitor patient for signs of overdose (salivation, nausea, abdominal pain, vomiting, diarrhea, irritability, convulsions, respiratory arrest); forced diuresis, gastric lavage, supportive measures may be required.

### Drug-specific teaching points

- Take this drug as prescribed; chew tablets, swallow whole, or add to drinking water or fruit juice.
- Dilute drops in fluids, food, or take undiluted.
- Brush and floss before use of rinse; swish around mouth and spit out liquid; do not eat, drink, or rinse out mouth for 30 min after use.
- Avoid simultaneous use of milk or diary products and this drug.
- Arrange to have regular dental exams.
- Report increased salivation, nausea, abdominal pain, diarrhea, irritability, mottling of teeth

## sodium hyaluronate

*(hye al you **ron'** ate)*

Hyalgan

**Pregnancy Category Unknown**

### Drug classes

Hyaluronic acid derivative

### Therapeutic actions

Made of hylans, a natural complex sugar acting as a polymer for joint fluids, having elastic and viscous properties; derived from chicken combs.

### Indications

- Treatment of pain in osteoarthritis of the knee in patients who have failed to respond adequately to conservative therapy and simple analgesics.

### Contraindications/cautions

- Contraindications: hypersensitivity to any component of the drug or chicken products; infection of the knee, skin or surrounding area.
- Use cautiously with pregnancy, lactation (no data are available), edema or lymphostasis of the leg, concomitant use of quaternary ammonium salt skin disinfectants.

### Dosage

**Available Forms:** Injection—20 mg/2 ml

*ADULT:* 2 ml by intra-articular injection 1 X/wk for 5 wks; no data are available on repeat treatment cycles.

### Pharmacokinetics

Degraded in the synovium after injection; not absorbed systemically.

### Adverse effects

- Local: Inflammation and edema at site of injection, *injection site pain,* local bruising

### Clinically important drug-drug interactions

- Do not inject local anesthetic at same site and time

## ■ Nursing Considerations

### Assessment

- *History:* Hypersensitivity to any component of the drug or chicken products; infection of the knee or surrounding area, pregancy, lactation, edema or lymphostasis.
- *Physical:* T; knee exam and evaluation including range of motion

### Implementation

- Use strict aseptic technique; do not use if seal is broken; each vial is for one use only, discard after use.
- Do not administer to any other joint; do not administer into severely inflamed knee.
- Do not inject any other medication or anesthetic into knee injected with sodium hyaluronate; do not use skin disinfectants containing quaternary ammonium salts.
- Remove any synovial fluid or effusion before injecting into knee.

S

### Drug-specific teaching points

- Little is known about the long-term effects of this drug; it will need to be injected into your knee once a week for 5 weeks.
- Avoid strenuous activities and prolonged weight bearing following injection.
- Some swelling and discomfort may occur following injection; this should resolve quickly.
- Report increased swelling, redness, heat in knee; fever; worsening of knee pain.

## sodium polystyrene sulfonate

*(pol ee **stye'** reen)*

Kayexalate, SPS

**Pregnancy Category C**

### Drug classes

Potassium-removing resin

### Therapeutic actions

An ion exchange resin that releases sodium ions in exchange for potassium ions as it passes along the intestine after oral administration or is retained in the colon after enema, thus reducing elevated serum potassium levels; action is limited and unpredictable.

### Indications

- Treatment of hyperkalemia

### Contraindications/cautions

- Severe hypertension, severe CHF, marked edema (risk of sodium overload).

### Dosage

**Available Forms:** Suspension—15 g/60 ml; powder 4.1 mEq/g

**ADULT**

- ***Oral:*** 15–60 g/d, best given as 15 g 1 to 4 times qd. May be given as suspension with water or syrup (20–100 ml). Often given with sorbitol to combat constipation. May be introduced into stomach via nasogastric tube.
- ***Enema:*** 30–50 g q6h given in appropriate vehicle and retained for 30–60 min.

**PEDIATRIC:** Give lower doses, using the exchange ratio of 1 mEq potassium/g resin as the basis for calculation.

### Pharmacokinetics

| Route | Onset |
|---|---|
| Oral | 2–12 h |
| Rectal | Very long |

*Excretion:* Through the feces or expelled as enema

### Adverse effects

- GI: *Constipation*, fecal impaction, *gastric irritation, anorexia, nausea, vomiting*
- Hematologic: *Hypokalemia*, electrolyte abnormalities (particularly decrease in calcium and magnesium)

### Clinically important drug-drug interactions

- Risk of metabolic alkalosis with nonabsorbable cation-donating antacids

## ■ Nursing Considerations

### Assessment

- ***History:*** Severe hypertension, severe CHF, marked edema
- ***Physical:*** Orientation, reflexes; P, auscultation, BP, baseline ECG, peripheral edema; bowel sounds, abdominal exam; serum electrolytes

### Implementation

- Administer resin through plastic stomach tube, or mixed with a diet appropriate for renal failure.
- Give powder form of resin in an oral suspension with a syrup base to increase palatability.
- Administer as an enema after first giving a cleansing enema; insert a soft, large rubber tube into the rectum for a distance of about 20 cm; with the tip well into the sigmoid colon, tape into place. Suspend the resin in 100 ml sorbitol or 20% Dextrose in Water at body temperature, introduce by gravity, keeping the particles in suspension by stirring. Flush with 50–100 ml fluid and clamp the tube, leaving it in place. If back leakage occurs, elevate hips or have patient assume the knee-chest position. Retain sus-

pension for at least 30–60 min, several hours is preferable, then irrigate the colon with a non–sodium-containing solution at body temperature; 2 qt of solution may be necessary to remove the resin. Drain the return constantly through a Y-tube connection.
- Prepare fresh suspensions for each dose. Do not store beyond 24 h. Do not heat suspensions; this may alter the exchange properties.
- Monitor patient and consider use of other measures (IV calcium, sodium bicarbonate, or glucose and insulin) in cases of severe hyperkalemia, with rapid tissue breakdown: burns, renal failure.
- Monitor serum electrolytes (potassium, sodium, calcium, magnesium) regularly, and arrange to counteract disturbances.
- Arrange for treatment of constipation with 10–20 ml of 70% sorbitol q2h or as needed to produce two watery stools per day. Establish a bowel training program.

### Drug-specific teaching points

- This drug is often used in emergencies. Drug instruction should be incorporated within general emergency instructions.
- The following side effects may occur: GI upset, constipation.
- Frequent blood tests will be necessary to monitor drug effect.
- Report confusion, irregular heartbeats, constipation, severe GI upset.

## sodium thiosalicylate

*(theye o sall **i'** sill ayte)*

Rexolate

**Pregnancy Category C**

### Drug classes

Antipyretic
Analgesic (non-narcotic)
Anti-inflammatory agent
Antirheumatic
Salicylate
Nonsteroidal anti-inflammatory drug (NSAID)

### Therapeutic actions

Analgesic and antirheumatic effects are attributable to the ability to inhibit the synthesis of prostaglandins, important mediators of inflammation; antipyretic effects are not fully understood, but salicylates probably act in the thermoregulatory center of the hypothalamus to block the effects of endogenous pyrogen by inhibiting the synthesis of the prostaglandin intermediary.

### Indications

- Active gout
- Muscular pain and musculoskeletal disturbances
- Rheumatic fever

### Contraindications/cautions

- Contraindications: chickenpox or viral infection in children.
- Use cautiously with allergy to salicylates or NSAIDs, bleeding disorders, impaired hepatic or renal function, GI ulceration (less of a problem with this salicylate than with some others); pregnancy, lactation.

### Dosage

**Available Forms:** Injection—50 mg/ml

**ADULT**

- *Acute gout:* 100 mg q3–4h IM for 2 d, then 100 mg/d IM.
- *Muscular pain and musculoskeletal disturbances:* 50–100 mg/d or on alternate days IM.
- *Rheumatic fever:* 100–150 mg q4–6h IM for 3 d, then reduce to 100 mg bid. Continue until patient is asymptomatic.

**PEDIATRIC:** Dosage schedule not established.

### Pharmacokinetics

| Route | Onset | Peak |
|---|---|---|
| IM | Immediate | 15–100 min |

*Metabolism:* Hepatic, $T_{1/2}$: 2–18 h
*Distribution:* Crosses placenta; enters breast milk
*Excretion:* Urine

### Adverse effects

*NSAIDs*

- CNS: *Headache, dizziness, somnolence, insomnia*, fatigue, tiredness, dizziness, tinnitus, ophthalmologic effects
- GI: *Nausea, dyspepsia, GI pain,* diarrhea, vomiting, *constipation*, flatulence

- **Respiratory:** Dyspnea, hemoptysis, pharyngitis, bronchospasm, rhinitis
- **Hematologic**: Bleeding, platelet inhibition with higher doses, neutropenia, eosinophilia, leukopenia, pancytopenia, thrombocytopenia, agranulocytosis, granulocytopenia, aplastic anemia, decreased Hgb or Hct, bone marrow depression, mennorhagia
- **GU**: Dysuria, renal impairment
- **Dermatologic**: *Rash*, pruritus, sweating, dry mucous membranes, stomatitis
- **Other**: Peripheral edema, anaphylactoid reactions to fatal anaphylactic shock; salicylism: dizziness, tinnitus, difficulty hearing, nausea, vomiting, diarrhea, mental confusion, lassitude (dose related); acute salicylate toxicity (respiratory alkalosis, hyperpnea, tachypnea, hemmorhage, excitement, confusion, asterixis, pulmonary edema, convulsions, tetany, metabolic acidosis, fever, coma, CV collapse, renal and respiratory failure; dose related: 20–25 g in adults)

### Clinically important drug-drug interactions

• Increased risk of GI ulceration with corticosteroids • Increased risk of salicylate toxicity with carbonic anhydrase inhibitors • Increased toxicity of carbonic anhydrase inhibitors, valproic acid • Decreased serum salicylate levels with corticosteroids, antacids, urine alkalinizers (sodium acetate, sodium bicarbonate, sodium citrate, sodium lactate, tromethamine) • Increased methotrexate levels and toxicity • Greater glucose-lowering effect of sulfonylureas, insulin with large doses of salicylates • Decreased uricosuric effect of probenecid, sulfinpyrazone • Decreased diuretic effect of spironolactone

### Drug-lab test interferences

• Decreased serum PBI • False-negative readings for urine glucose by glucose oxidase method and copper reduction method • Interference with urine 5-HIAA determinations by fluorescent methods but not by nitrosonaphthol colorimetric method • Interference with urinary ketone determination by ferric chloride method • Falsely elevated urine VMA levels with most tests; false decrease in VMA using the Pisano method

## ■ Nursing Considerations

### Assessment

- ***History:*** Allergy to salicylates or NSAIDs, bleeding disorders, impaired hepatic or renal function, GI ulceration; lactation; pregnancy; chickenpox or viral infection
- ***Physical:*** Skin color and lesions; eighth cranial nerve function, orientation, reflexes, affect; P, BP, perfusion; R, adventitious sounds; liver evaluation and bowel sounds; CBC, urinalysis, stool guiaiac; renal and liver function tests.

### Implementation

- Administer by IM injection.
- Avoid use with sodium restrictions.
- Institute emergency procedures if overdose occurs: gastric lavage, induction of emesis, activated charcoal, supportive therapy.

### Drug-specific teaching points

- Report ringing in the ears, dizziness, confusion, abdominal pain, rapid or difficult breathing, nausea, vomiting.

## somatrem

***(soe' ma trem)***

Protropin

**Pregnancy Category C**

### Drug classes

Hormone

### Therapeutic actions

Artificial hormone with identical amino acid sequence of pituitary-derived human growth hormone plus one additional amino acid; therapeutically equivalent to human somatotropin; withdrawn from the market because of microbial impurities; stimulates skeletal (linear) growth, growth of internal organs, protein synthesis, many other metabolic processes required for normal growth.

### Indications
- Long-term treatment of children with growth failure due to lack of adequate endogenous growth hormone secretion
- Treatment of growth failure associated with renal insufficiency
- Orphan drug use: treatment of short stature associated with Turner's syndrome

### Contraindications/cautions
- Known sensitivity to somatrem, benzyl alcohol, closed epiphyses, underlying cranial lesions.

### Dosage
**Available Forms:** Powder for injection—5, 10 mg/vial

*ADULT/PEDIATRIC:* Individualize dosage based on response. Up to 0.1 mg/kg IM given 3×/wk is recommended. Do not exceed this dosage.

### Pharmacokinetics

| Route | Onset | Peak |
|---|---|---|
| IM | Varies | Days to weeks |

*Metabolism:* Hepatic, $T_{1/2}$: 20–30 min
*Excretion:* Urine

### Adverse effects
- Hematologic: *Development of antibodies to growth hormone*
- Endocrine: Hypothyroidism, insulin resistance

## ■ Nursing Considerations

### Assessment
- *History:* Sensitivity to somatrem, benzyl alcohol, closed epiphyses, underlying cranial lesions
- *Physical:* Height; weight; thryoid function tests, glucose tolerance tests, growth hormone levels

### Implementation
- Reconstitute each 5-mg vial for administration to adults or older children with 1–5 ml of Bacteriostatic Water for Injection (Benzyl Alcohol Preserved) only.
- Reconstitute drug for use in newborns with plain Water for Injection without benzyl alcohol. Benzyl alcohol has been associated with severe toxicity in newborns. Use only one dose per vial and discard the unused portion.
- Prepare the solution by injecting the diluent into the vial, aiming the stream of liquid against the glass wall. Swirl the product vial with a gentle rotary motion until the contents are completely dissolved. *Do not shake*. After reconstitution, contents should be clear without particulate matter. Use a needle that is long enough (at least 1 in) to ensure injection deep into the muscle layer.
- Refrigerate vials; reconstituted vials should be used within 7 d; do not freeze drug.
- Arrange for periodic testing of glucose tolerance, thyroid function, and growth hormone antibodies. Arrange for treatment indicated by test results.

### Drug-specific teaching points
- This drug must be given IM three times per week.
- You may experience sudden growth; increase in appetite; a decrease in thyroid function (request replacement hormone).
- Report lack of growth, increased hunger, thirst, increased and frequent voiding, fatigue, dry skin, intolerance to cold.

## somatropin

*(soe ma **troe'** pin)*

Biotropin, Genotropin, Humatrope, Nutropin, Norditropin, Saizen, Serostim

**Pregnancy Category C**

### Drug classes
Hormone

### Therapeutic actions
Hormone of recombinant DNA origin; contains the identical amino acid sequence of pituitary-derived human growth hormone; equivalent to human somatotropin from

S

cadaver sources; withdrawn from the market because of microbial impurities; stimulates skeletal (linear) growth, growth of internal organs, protein synthesis, many other metabolic processes required for normal growth.

## Indications

- Long-term treatment of children with growth failure due to lack of adequate endogenous growth hormone secretion (all except Serostim)
- Treatment of children with growth failure associated with chronic renal failure, chronic renal insuffiency, up to the time of renal transplantation
- Treatment of girls suffering from Turner's syndrome (Nutropin)
- Treatment of AIDS wasting and cachexia (Serostim)
- Somatropin deficiency syndrome—replacement of endogenous somatropin (Humatrope)
- Orphan drug uses:treatment of short children due to intrauterine growth retardation

## Contraindications/cautions

- Known sensitivity to somatropin, benzyl alcohol, glycerin (Humatrope), closed epiphyses, underlying cranial lesions.

## Dosage

**Available Forms:** Powder for injection—varies for each brand name

Individualize dosage based on response.

- *ADULT AND PEDIATRIC*

*Genotropin:* 0.16–0.24 mg/kg/wk SC divided into 6–7 injections

*Serostim:* >55 kg–6 mg SC qd; 45–55 kg–5 mg SC qd; 35–45 kg–4 mg SC qd

- *ADULT*

*Humatrope:* <0.006 mg/kg/d SC; may increase to 0.0125 mg/kg/d

- *PEDIATRIC*

*Humatrope:* 0.18 mg/kg/wk SC or IM divided into doses given 3×/wk or 6×/wk

*Nutropin:* GH deficiency—0.3 mg/kg/wk SC; chronic renal insufficiency—0.35 mg/kg/wk SC; Turner syndrome—≤0.375 mg/kg/wk SC divided into 3–7 injections

*Saizen:* 0.06 mg/kg SC or IM 3×/wk

*Norditropin:* 0.024–0.034 mg/kg SC, 6–7×/wk

## Pharmacokinetics

| Route | Onset | Peak |
|---|---|---|
| IM/SC | Varies | 3–7 1/2 h |

*Metabolism:* Hepatic, $T_{1/2}$: 15–50 min

*Distribution:* Crosses placenta; enters breast milk

*Excretion:* Urine and feces

## Adverse effects

- **Hematologic:** *Development of antibodies to growth hormone* (not as likely as with somatrem)
- **Endocrine:** Hypothyroidism, insulin resistance
- **Other:** Swelling, joint pain, muscle pain

## ■ Nursing Considerations

### Assessment

- ***History:*** Known sensitivity to somatropin, closed epiphyses, underlying cranial lesions
- ***Physical:*** Height; weight; thyroid function tests, glucose tolerance tests, growth hormone levels

### Implementation

- Administer drug IM or SC.
- Divide total dose into smaller increments given 6–7×/wk for smaller patients unable to tolerate injections.
- Reconstitute drug carefully following manufacturer's instructions; do not shake; do not inject if solution is cloudy or contains particulate matter.
- Refrigerate vials; reconstituted vials should be used within 7 d; do not freeze drug.
- Arrange for periodic testing of glucose tolerance, thyroid function, and growth hormone antibodies. Arrange for treatment indicated by test results.

### Drug-specific teaching points

- This drug must be given IM or SC three times per week. Drug can be given in six to seven smaller doses if needed.

- You may experience sudden growth, increase in appetite, decrease in thyroid function (request replacement hormone).
- Report lack of growth, increased hunger, thirst, increased and frequent voiding, fatigue, dry skin, intolerance to cold.

# sotalol hydrochloride

*(soh' tal lole)*

Betapace

**Pregnancy Category B**

### Drug classes

Beta-1 selective adrenergic blocker
Antiarrhythmic

### Therapeutic actions

Blocks beta-adrenergic receptors of the sympathetic nervous system in the heart and juxtaglomerular apparatus (kidney), thus decreasing the excitability of the heart, decreasing cardiac output and oxygen consumption.

### Indications

- Treatment of life-threatening ventricular arrhythmias; because of proarrhythmic effects, use for less than life-threatening arrhythmias, even symptomatic ones, is not recommended.

### Contraindications/cautions

- Contraindications: sinus bradycardia (HR < 45 beats/min), second or third-degree heart block (PR interval > 0.24 sec), cardiogenic shock, CHF, asthma, COPD, lactation.
- Use cautiously with diabetes or thyrotoxicosis, hepatic or renal impairment.

### Dosage

**Available Forms:** Tablets—80, 120, 160, 240 mg

**ADULT:** Initial dose, 80 mg PO bid. Adjust gradually, evey 2–3 d, until appropriate response occurs; may require 240–320 mg/d.

**PEDIATRIC:** Safety and efficacy not established.

**GERIATRIC OR RENAL IMPAIRED**

| *Creatinine Clearance (ml/min)* | *Dosing Intervals* |
|---|---|
| >60 | 12 h |
| 30–60 | 24 h |
| 10–30 | 36 to 48 h |
| <10 | Individualize dose based on response |

### Pharmacokinetics

| *Route* | *Onset* | *Peak* |
|---|---|---|
| Oral | Varies | 3–4 h |

*Metabolism:* $T_{1/2}$: 12 h
*Distribution:* Crosses placenta; enters breast milk
*Excretion:* Urine

### Adverse effects

- CNS: Dizziness, vertigo, tinnitus, fatigue, emotional depression, paresthesias, sleep disturbances, hallucinations, disorientation, memory loss, slurred speech
- GI: *Gastric pain, flatulence, constipation, diarrhea, nausea, vomiting,* anorexia
- CV: *CHF, cardiac arrhythmias, SA or AV nodal block,* peripheral vascular insufficiency, claudication, CVA, pulmonary edema, hypotension
- Respiratory: Bronchospasm, dyspnea, cough, bronchial obstruction, nasal stuffiness, rhinitis
- GU: *Impotence, decreased libido,* Peyronie's disease, dysuria, nocturia, frequent urination
- MS: Joint pain, arthralgia, muscle cramp
- EENT: Eye irritation, dry eyes, conjunctivitis, blurred vision
- Dermatologic: Rash, pruritus, sweating, dry skin
- Allergic reactions: Pharyngitis, erythematous rash, fever, sore throat, **laryngospasm, respiratory distress**
- Other: *Decreased exercise tolerance, development of antinuclear antibodies,* hyperglycemia or hypoglycemia, elevated serum transaminase

S

### Clinically important drug-drug interactions

• Possible increased effects with verapamil • Increased risk of postural hypotension with prazosin • Possible increased BP lowering effects with aspirin, bismuth subsalicylate, magnesium salicylate, sulfinpyrazone, oral contraceptives • Decreased antihypertensive effects with NSAIDs, clonidine • Possible increased hypoglycemic effect of insulin

### Drug-lab test interferences

• Possible false results with glucose or insulin tolerance tests (oral)

## ■ Nursing Considerations

### Assessment

- *History:* Sinus bradycardia, second or third-degree heart block, cardiogenic shock, CHF, asthma, COPD, pregnancy, lactation, diabetes or thyrotoxicosis
- *Physical:* Weight, skin condition, neurologic status, P, BP, ECG, respiratory status, kidney and thyroid function, blood and urine glucose

### Implementation

- This drug may be given with meals.
- Do not give unless patient is unresponsive to other antiarrhythmics and has a life-threatening ventricular arrhythmia. Monitor patient response carefully; proarrhythmic effect can be pronounced.
- Do not discontinue drug abruptly after chronic therapy. Taper drug gradually over 2 wk with monitoring (abrupt withdrawal may cause serious beta-adrenergic rebound effects).
- Discontinue other antiarrhythmics gradually, allowing for two to three plasma half-lives of the drug before starting sotalol. After discontinuing amiodarone, do not start sotalol until QT interval is normalized.
- Consult with physician about withdrawing drug if patient is to undergo surgery (withdrawal is controversial).

### Drug-specific teaching points

- Take drug with meals.
- Do not stop taking unless told to do so by a health care provider.
- Avoid driving or dangerous activities if dizziness, weakness occur.
- The following side effects may occur: dizziness, lightheadedness, loss of appetite, nightmares, depression, sexual impotence.
- Report difficulty breathing, night cough, swelling of extremities, slow pulse, confusion, depression, rash, fever, sore throat.

## sparfloxacin

*(spar **flox'** a sin)*

Zagam

**Pregnancy Category C**

### Drug classes

Antibiotic

Fluoroquinolone

### Therapeutic actions

Bactericidal; interferes with DNA replication in susceptible gram-negative bacteria, preventing cell reproduction.

### Indications

- Treatment of adults with community-acquired pneumonia caused by *chlamydia pneumoniae, H influenza, H parainfluenza, Moraxella catarrhalis, mycoplama pneumonia, staphyloccoccus aureus, S. pneumonia*
- Treatment of acute exacerbation of chronic bronchitis caused by *H. influenza, Moraxella catarrhalis, C. pneumoniae, enterobacter streptococcus pneumoniae, H. parainfluenza klebsiella*

### Contraindications/cautions

- Contraindications: allergy to fluoroquinolones, pregnancy, lactation, known QT prolongation
- Use cautiously with renal dysfunction, seizures

### Dosage

**Available Forms:** Tablets—200 mg

*ADULT:* 400 mg PO on first day, followed by 200 mg PO qd.

*PEDIATRIC:* Not recommended—produced lesions of joint cartilage in immature experimental animals.

*GERIATRIC OR IMPAIRED RENAL FUNCTION:* 400 mg PO on first day, then 200 mg PO q 48 h for a total of 9 days

**Pharmacokinetics**

| *Route* | *Onset* | *Peak* | *Duration* |
|---|---|---|---|
| Oral | Slow | 4–6 h | 8–12 h |

*Metabolism:* Hepatic; $T_{1/2}$: 16–20 h
*Distribution:* Crosses placenta; passes into breast milk
*Excretion:* Urine and bile

**Adverse effects**
- CNS: *Headache, dizziness, insomnia,* fatigue, somnolence, depression, blurred vision
- GI: *Nausea,* vomiting, dry mouth, *diarrhea,* abdominal pain
- **Hematologic**: Elevated BUN, SGOT, SGPT, serum creatinine and alkaline phosphatase; decreased WBC, neutrophil count, Hct
- Other: Fever, rash, photosensitivity

**Clinically important drug-drug interactions**
• Decreased therapeutic effect with iron salts, sulcrafate • Decreased absorption with antacids

## ■ Nursing Considerations

### Assessment
- *History:* Allergy to fluoroquinolones; renal dysfunction; seizures; lactation
- *Physical:* Skin color, lesions; T; orientation, reflexes, affect; mucous membranes, bowel sounds; renal and liver function tests

### Implementation
- Arrange for culture and sensitivity tests before beginning therapy.
- Continue therapy for 2 d after signs and symptoms of infection have disappeared.
- Administer oral drug 1 h before or 2 h after meals with glass of water.
- Ensure that patient is well hydrated during course of therapy.
- Administer antacids (if needed) at least 2 h after dosing.
- Monitor clinical response; if no improvement is seen or a relapse occurs, repeat culture and sensitivity.

### Drug-specific teaching points
- If an antacid is needed, do not take it within 2 h of sparfloxacin dose.
- Drink plenty of fluids while you are on this drug.
- The following side effects may occur: nausea, vomiting, abdominal pain (eat small, frequent meals; take drug with food); diarrhea or constipation (consult nurse or physician); drowsiness, blurred vision, dizziness (use caution if driving or operating dangerous equipment).
- Report rash, visual changes, severe GI problems, weakness, tremors.

# spectinomycin hydrochloride

*(spek ti noe **mye'** sin)*
Trobicin
**Pregnancy Category B**

**Drug classes**
Antibiotic

**Therapeutic actions**
Bactericidal: inhibits protein synthesis of susceptible strains of *Neisseria gonorrhoeae*, causing cell death.

**Indications**
- Acute gonococcal urethritis and proctitis in males
- Acute gonococcal cervicitis and proctitis in females
- *Not effective* in treating syphilis or pharyngeal infections caused by *N. gonorrhoeae*

**Contraindications/cautions**
- Contraindications: allergy to spectinomycin, lactation.
- Use cautiously with pregnancy (safety not established; yet drug is recommended for penicillin or probenecid allergic pregnant women with gonococcal infections).

### Dosage

**Available Forms:** Powder for injection—400 mg

*ADULT:* 2 g IM. In geographic areas where antibiotic resistance is prevalent, 4 g IM divided between two gluteal injection sites is preferred.

*CDC recommended treatment for gonorrhea*

- *Penicillin-allergic patients or penicillinase-producing N. gonorrhoeae*: 2 g IM. < 45 kg: 40 mg/kg IM.
- *Penicillinase-producing N. gonorrhoeae*: 2 g IM. < 45 kg: 40 mg/kg IM.
- *Gonococcal infections in pregnancy:* 2 g IM.

*PEDIATRIC:* Not recommended.

### Pharmacokinetics

| Route | Onset | Peak |
|---|---|---|
| IM | Varies | 1 h |

*Metabolism:* $T_{1/2}$: 1.5–2.8 h
*Distribution:* Crosses placenta; enters breast milk
*Excretion:* Urine

### Adverse effects

- CNS: *Dizziness, chills,* fever, insomnia
- Hematologic: Decreased Hct, Hgb, creatinine clearance, increased alkaline phosphatase, BUN, SGPT
- GU: *Decreased urine output without documented renal toxicity*
- Dermatologic: Urticaria
- Local: *Soreness at injection site*

## ■ Nursing Considerations

### Assessment

- ***History:*** Allergy to spectinomycin, pregnancy, lactation
- ***Physical:*** Site of infection, skin color, lesions; orientation, reflexes; R, adventitious sounds; CBC, liver and renal function tests

### Implementation

- Administer only IM; administer deep into upper outer quadrant of the gluteus to decrease discomfort.
- Reconstitute with Bacteriostatic Water for Injection with 0.9% benzyl alcohol: 3.2 ml diluent for 2-g vial, 6.2 ml diluent for 4-g vial. Stable for 24 h after being reconstituted.
- Culture infection before therapy.
- Monitor for development of resistant strains on prolonged therapy.
- Monitor blood counts, renal and liver function tests on long-term therapy.

### Drug-specific teaching points

- This drug is given only in the IM form.
- Report worsening of infection, dark urine, yellowing of the skin or eyes, skin rash or itching.

## spironolactone

*(speer on oh **lak'** tone)*

Aldactone

**Pregnancy Category D**

### Drug classes

Potassium-sparing diuretic
Aldosterone antagonist

### Therapeutic actions

Competitively blocks the effects of aldosterone in the renal tubule, causing loss of sodium and water and retention of potassium.

### Indications

- Primary hyperaldosteronism, diagnosis, maintenance
- Adjunctive therapy in edema associated with CHF, nephrotic syndrome, hepatic cirrhosis
- Treatment of hypokalemia or prevention of hypokalemia in patients who would be at high risk if hypokalemia occurred: digitalized patients, patients with cardiac arrhythmias
- Essential hypertension, usually in combination with other drugs
- Unlabeled uses: treatment of hirsutism due to its antiandrogenic properties, palliation of symptoms of PMS syndrome, treatment of familial male precocious puberty, short-term treatment of acne vulgaris

## Contraindications/cautions

- Contraindications: allergy to spironolactone, hyperkalemia, renal disease, lactation.
- Use cautiously with pregnancy.

## Dosage

**Available Forms:** Tablets—25, 50, 100 mg

### ADULT

- *Edema:* 100–200 mg/d PO in single or divided doses. Adjust to patient's response. Alternate-day or intermittent-day therapy may be the most effective treatment.
- *Diagnosis of hyperaldosteronism:* 400 mg/d PO for 3–4 wk (long test). Correction of hypokalemia and hypertension are presumptive evidence of primary hyperaldosteronism 400 mg/d PO for 4 d (short test). If serum $K^+$ increases but decreases when drug is stopped, presumptive diagnosis can be made.
- *Maintenance therapy for hyperaldosteronism:* 100–400 mg/d PO.
- *Essential hypertension:* 50–100 mg/d PO. May be combined with other diuretics.
- *Hypokalemia:* 25–100 mg/d PO.

### PEDIATRIC

- *Edema:* 3.3 mg/kg/d PO adjusted to patient's response.

## Pharmacokinetics

| Route | Onset | Peak | Duration |
|---|---|---|---|
| Oral | 24–48 h | 48–72 h | 48–72 h |

*Metabolism:* Hepatic, $T_{1/2}$: 20 h
*Distribution:* Crosses placenta; enters breast milk
*Excretion:* Urine

## Adverse effects

- CNS: *Dizziness, headache, drowsiness,* fatigue, ataxia, confusion
- GI: *Cramping, diarrhea,* dry mouth, thirst
- **Hematologic:** Hyperkalemia, hyponatremia
- GU: Impotence, irregular menses, amenorrhea, postmenopausal bleeding
- Dermatologic: *Rash,* urticaria
- Other: Carcinogenic in animals, *deepening of the voice, hirsutism, gynecomastia*

## Clinically important drug-drug interactions

• Increased hyperkalemia with potassium supplements, diets rich in potassium • Decreased diuretic effect with salicylates

## Drug-lab test interferences

• Interference with radioimmunoassay for digoxin; false increase in serum digoxin levels

## ■ Nursing Considerations

### Assessment

- *History:* Allergy to spironolactone, hyperkalemia, renal disease, pregnancy, lactation
- *Physical:* Skin color, lesions, edema; orientation, reflexes, muscle strength; P, baseline ECG, BP; R, pattern, adventitious sounds; liver evaluation, bowel sounds; urinary output patterns, menstrual cycle; CBC, serum electrolytes, renal function tests, urinalysis

### Implementation

- Mark calendars of edema outpatients as reminders of alternative day or 3- to 5-d/wk therapy.
- Give daily doses early so that increased urination does not interfere with sleep.
- Make suspension as follows: tablets may be pulverized and given in cherry syrup for young children. This suspension is stable for 1 mo if refrigerated.
- Measure and record regular weight to monitor mobilization of edema fluid.
- Avoid giving food rich in potassium.
- Arrange for regular evaluation of serum electrolytes, BUN.

### Drug-specific teaching points

- Record alternate-day therapy on a calendar, or prepare dated envelopes. Take the drug early because of increased urination.
- Weigh yourself on a regular basis, at the same time and in the same clothing, and record the weight on your calendar.

S

- Avoid foods that are rich in potassium (fruits, Sanka).
- The following side effects may occur: increased volume and frequency of urination; dizziness, confusion, feeling faint on arising, drowsiness (avoid rapid position changes, hazardous activities: driving, using alcohol); increased thirst (sucking on sugarless lozenges may help; use frequent mouth care); changes in menstrual cycle, deepening of the voice, impotence, enlargement of the breasts can occur (reversible).
- Report weight change of more than 3 lb in one day, swelling in your ankles or fingers, dizziness, trembling, numbness, fatigue, enlargement of breasts, deepening of voice, impotence, muscle weakness or cramps.

## stanozolol

*(stan **oh'** zoe lole)*

Winstrol

**Pregnancy Category X**
**C-III controlled substance**

### Drug classes

Anabolic steroid
Hormone

### Therapeutic actions

Synthetic testosterone analog with strong anabolic activity and weak androgenic activity; promotes body tissue-building processes and reverses catabolic or tissue-depleting processes; increases Hgb and red cell mass.

### Indications

- Prophylactic use to decrease frequency and severity of hereditary angioedema attacks

### Contraindications/cautions

- Known sensitivity to anabolic steroids; prostate or breast cancer in males, benign prostatic hypertrophy, breast cancer in females, pituitary insufficiency, MI (effects on cholesterol), nephrosis, liver disease, hypercalcemia, pregnancy (masculinization of fetus), lactation.

### Dosage

**Available Forms:** Tablets—2 mg

*ADULT:* Initially, 2 mg PO tid. After favorable response in terms of prevention of attacks, decrease dosage to 2 mg/d over 2–3 mo.

*PEDIATRIC:* Long-term therapy is contraindicated because of possibility of serious disruption of growth and development; weigh benefits and risks.

### Pharmacokinetics

| *Route* | *Onset* |
|---|---|
| Oral | Rapid |

*Metabolism:* Hepatic, $T_{1/2}$: unknown
*Distribution:* Crosses placenta; enters breast milk
*Excretion:* Urine

### Adverse effects

- CNS: *Excitation, insomnia,* chills, toxic confusion
- GI: Hepatotoxicity, peliosis, **hepatitis with life-threatening liver failure or intra-abdominal hemorrhage**; liver cell tumors, sometimes malignant and fatal, *nausea, vomiting, diarrhea, abdominal fullness, loss of appetite, burning of tongue*
- Hematologic: *Blood lipid changes*—decreased HDL and sometimes increased LDL; iron deficiency anemia, hypercalcemia, altered serum cholesterol levels; *retention of sodium, chloride, water,* potassium, phosphates and calcium
- GU: Increased risk of prostatic hypertrophy, carcinoma in geriatric patients
- Endocrine: *Virilization: prepubertal males*—phallic enlargement, hirsutism, increased skin pigmentation; *postpubertal males*—inhibition of testicular function, gynecomastia, testicular atrophy, priapism, baldness, epididymitis, change in libido; *females*—hirsutism, hoarseness, deepening of the voice, clitoral enlargement, menstrual irregularities, baldness; decreased glucose tolerance

- Other: *Acne,* premature closure of the epiphyses

### Clinically important drug-drug interactions

• Potentiation of oral anticoagulants • Decreased need for insulin, oral hypoglycemic agents

### Drug-lab test interferences

• Altered glucose tolerance tests • Decrease in thyroid function tests, an effect that may persist for 2–3 wk after therapy • Increased creatinine, creatinine clearance, which may last for 2 wk after therapy

## ■ Nursing Considerations

### Assessment

- *History:* Known sensitivity to anabolic steroids, prostate or breast cancer, benign prostatic hypertrophy, pituitary insufficiency, MI, nephrosis, liver disease, hypercalcemia, pregnancy, lactation
- *Physical:* Skin color, texture; hair distribution pattern; affect, orientation; abdominal exam, liver evaluation; serum electrolytes, serum cholesterol levels, glucose tolerance tests, thyroid function tests, long-bone x-ray (in children)

### Implementation

- Administer with food if GI upset or nausea occurs.
- Monitor patient for attacks in stressful or traumatic situations; dosage may need to be increased.
- Monitor effect on children with long-bone x-rays every 3–6 mo during therapy; discontinue well before the bone age reaches the norm for the patient's chronologic age because effects may continue for 6 mo after therapy.
- Monitor patient for edema; provide diuretic therapy.
- Arrange to monitor liver function, serum electrolytes, and consult with physician for corrective measures.
- Measure cholesterol levels of patients at high risk for CAD.
- Monitor diabetic patients closely because glucose tolerance may change. Adjust insulin, oral hypoglycemic dosage, and diet.

### Drug-specific teaching points

- Take with food if nausea or GI upset occurs.
- The following side effects may occur: nausea, vomiting, diarrhea, burning of the tongue (eat small, frequent meals); body hair growth, baldness, deepening of the voice, loss of libido, impotence (most reversible); excitation, confusion, insomnia (avoid driving, performing tasks that require alertness); swelling of the ankles, fingers (request medication).
- Diabetic patients need to monitor urine sugar closely as glucose tolerance may change; report any abnormalities to physician, and take corrective action.
- These drugs do not enhance athletic ability but do have serious effects. Do not use for increasing muscle strength.
- Report ankle swelling, skin color changes, severe nausea, vomiting, hoarseness, body hair growth, deepening of the voice, acne, menstrual irregularities in women.

## stavudine

*(stay vew' den)*

Zerit

**Pregnancy Category C**

### Drug classes

Antiviral

### Therapeutic actions

Inhibits replication of some retroviruses, including HIV, HTLV III, LAV, ARV.

### Indications

- Treatment of adults with advanced HIV infection who are intolerant to approved therapies with proven clinical benefit or who have experienced significant clinical or immunologic deterioration while receiving these therapies or for whom these therapies are contraindicated

### Contraindications/cautions

- Contraindications: life-threatening allergy to any component, pregnancy, lactation.

S

- Use cautiously with compromised bone marrow, impaired renal or hepatic function.

## Dosage

**Available Forms:** Powder for oral solution—1 mg/ml; capsules—15, 20, 30, 40 mg

*ADULT:* 40 mg q12h PO without regard to meals; > 60 kg: 40mg bid; < 60 kg: 30 mg bid.

*PEDIATRIC:* Safety and efficacy not established.

*GERIATRIC OR RENAL IMPAIRED*

| *Creatinine Clearance (ml/min)* | *>60 kg* | *<60 kg* |
|---|---|---|
| > 50 | 40 mg q12h | 30 mg q12h |
| 26–50 | 20 mg q12h | 15 mg q12h |
| 10–25 | 20 mg/d | 15 mg/d |

### Pharmacokinetics

| *Route* | *Onset* | *Peak* |
|---|---|---|
| Oral | Varies | 1/2–1 1/2 h |

*Metabolism:* Hepatic, $T_{1/2}$: 30–60 min
*Distribution* : Crosses placenta; may enter breast milk
*Excretion:* Urine

### Adverse effects

- CNS: *Headache*, insomnia, myalgia, *asthenia*, malaise, dizziness, paresthesia, somnolence
- GI: *Nausea, GI pain, diarrhea*, anorexia, vomiting, dyspepsia
- Hematologic: *Agranulocytopenia*, severe anemia requiring transfusions
- Other: *Fever*, diaphoresis, dyspnea, *rash*, taste perversion

## ■ Nursing Considerations

### Assessment

- *History:* Life-threatening allergy to any component, compromised bone marrow, impaired renal or hepatic function, pregnancy, lactation
- *Physical:* Skin rashes, lesions, texture; T; affect, reflexes, peripheral sensation; bowel sounds, liver evaluation; renal and hepatic function tests, CBC and differential

### Implementation

- Monitor hematologic indices every 2 wk during therapy.
- Give every 12 h, around the clock; schedule dose so it will not interrupt sleep.

### Drug-specific teaching points

- Take drug every 12 h. Do not share this drug; take exactly as prescribed. Reconstitute powder with 202 ml purified water
- Stavudine is not a cure for AIDS; opportunisitc infections may occur; regular medical care should be sought to deal with the disease.
- Frequent blood tests are needed; results may indicate a need to decrease or discontinue drug for a period of time.
- The following side effects may occur: nausea, loss of appetite, change in taste (eat small, frequent meals); dizziness, loss of feeling (take precautions); headache, fever, muscle aches.
- Stavudine does not reduce the risk of transmission of HIV to others by sexual contact or blood contamination; use appropriate precautions.
- Report extreme fatigue, lethargy, severe headache, severe nausea, vomiting, difficulty breathing, skin rash.

# streptokinase

*(strep toe **kin'** ase)*
Streptase, Kabikinase
**Pregnancy Category C**

### Drug classes

Thrombolytic agent

### Therapeutic actions

Enzyme isolated from streptococcal bacteria; converts endogenous plasminogen to the enzyme plasmin (fibrinolysin) which degrades fibrin clots, fibrinogen, and other plasma proteins; lyses thrombi and emboli.

### Indications
- Coronary artery thrombosis, IV or intracoronary use within 6 h of onset of symptoms of coronary occlusion
- Pulmonary embolism—for lysis of diagnosed embolus to restore blood flow
- Deep venous thrombosis of the deep veins
- Arterial thrombosis and embolism not originating on the left side of the heart
- Occluded AV cannulae

### Contraindications/cautions
- Contraindications: allergy to streptokinase (Note: most patients have been exposed to streptococci and to streptokinase and therefore have developed resistance to the drug; however, allergic reactions are relatively rare), active internal bleeding, recent (within 2 mo) CVA, intracranial or intraspinal surgery, intracranial neoplasm, recent major surgery, obstetric delivery, organ biopsy, or rupture of a noncompressible blood vessel.
- Use cautiously with recent serious GI bleed, recent serious trauma, including CPR; severe hypertension; SBE; hemostatic defects; cerebrovascular disease; diabetic hemorrhagic retinopathy; septic thrombosis; pregnancy; lactation.

### Dosage
**Available Forms:** Powder for injection—250,000, 750,000, 1,500,000 IU/vial

**ADULT**
- ***Lysis of coronary artery thrombi:*** Bolus dose of 20,000 IU directly into the coronary artery. Maintenance dose of 2,000 IU/min for 60 min for a total dose of 140,000 IU *or* 1,500,000 IU administered over 60 min in an infusion of the 1,500,000-U vial diluted to a total volume of 45 ml.
- ***Deep vein thrombosis, pulmonary or arterial embolism, arterial thrombosis:*** Loading dose of 250,000 IU infused into a peripheral vein over 30 min. Maintenance dose, 100,000 IU/h for 24–72 h depending on the response and area treated. After treatment with streptokinase, treat with continuous infusion heparin, beginning after thrombin time decreases to less than twice the control value.
- ***AV cannula occlusion:*** Slowly instill 250,000 IU in 2 ml IV solution into the occluded cannula; clamp the cannula for 2 h; then aspirate the catheter and flush with saline.

**PEDIATRIC:** Safety and efficacy not established.

### Pharmacokinetics
| *Route* | *Onset* | *Peak* |
|---|---|---|
| IV | Immediate | 30–60 min |

*Metabolism:* $T_{1/2}$: 23 min
*Distribution:* Crosses placenta; may enter breast milk
*Excretion:* Unknown

### IV facts
**Preparation:** Reconstitute vial with 5 ml of Sterile Water for Injection or 5% Dextrose Injection; direct diluent at side of the vial, not directly into the streptokinase. Avoid shaking during reconstitution; gently roll or tilt vial to reconstitute. Further dilute the reconstituted solutions slowly to a total of 45 ml. Solution may be filtered through 0.22 or 0.45 filter. Do not add other medications to reconstituted solutions. Discard solutions that contain large amounts of flocculation. Refrigerate reconstituted solution; discard reconstituted solution after 24 h. Reconstitute the contents of 250,000-IU vial with 2 ml Sodium Chloride or 5% Dextrose Injection for use in AV cannulae.

**Infusion:** Administer as indicated for each specific problem being treated (see Dosage section).

### Adverse effects
- CNS: Headache
- CV: Angioneurotic edema, arrhythmias (with intracoronary artery infusion)
- **Respiratory: Breathing difficulty, bronchospasm**
- **Hematologic:** *Bleeding (minor or surface* to major internal bleeding)

S

- **Dermatologic:** Skin rash, urticaria, itching, flushing
- **Other:** Musculoskeletal pain, *fever*

### Clinically important drug-drug interactions

- Increased risk of hemorrhage with heparin or oral anticoagulants, aspirin, indomethacin, phenylbutazone

### Drug-lab test interferences

- Marked decrease in plasminogen, fibrinogen • Increases in thrombin time (TT), activated partial thromboplastin (APTT), prothrombin time (PT)

## ■ Nursing Considerations

### Assessment

- *History:* Allergy to streptokinase; active internal bleeding, recent CVA; intracranial or intraspinal surgery; intracranial neoplasm; recent major surgery; obstetric delivery; organ biopsy; or rupture of a noncompressible blood vesse; recent serious GI bleed; recent serious trauma; severe hypertension; SBE; hemostatic defects; cerebrovascular disease; diabetic hemorrhagic retinopathy; septic thrombosis; pregnancy; lactation
- *Physical:* Skin color, temperature, lesions; T; orientation, reflexes; P, BP, peripheral perfusion, baseline ECG; R, adventitous sounds; liver evaluation; Hct, platelet count, TT, APTT, PT

### Implementation

- Discontinue heparin, unless ordered specifically for coronary artery infusion.
- Arrange for regular monitoring of coagulation studies.
- Apply pressure or pressure dressings to control superficial bleeding (at invaded or disturbed areas).
- Avoid any arterial invasive procedures.
- Arrange for typing and cross-matching of blood if serious blood loss occurs and whole blood transfusions are required.
- Institute treatment within 2–6 h of onset of symptoms for evolving MI; within 7 d of other thrombotic event.
- Monitor cardiac rhythm continually during coronary artery infusion.

### Drug-specific teaching points

- You will need frequent blood tests and IV injections.
- Report rash, difficulty breathing, dizziness, disorientation, numbness, tingling.

# streptozocin

*(strep toe **zoe'** sin)*

Zanosar

**Pregnancy Category C**

### Drug classes

Alkylating agent, nitrosourea
Antineoplastic

### Therapeutic actions

Cytotoxic: inhibits DNA synthesis, leading to cell death partially through the production of intrastrand cross-links in DNA; cell cycle nonspecific.

### Indications

- Metastatic islet cell carcinoma of the pancreas

### Contraindications/cautions

- Contraindications: allergy to streptozocin; hematopoietic depression; pregnancy (teratogenic and embryotoxic); lactation.
- Use cautiously with impaired renal or hepatic function.

### Dosage

**Available Forms:** Powder for injection—100 mg/ml

Two dosage schedules have been used.

**ADULT:** *Daily schedule:* 500 mg/m$^2$ of body surface area IV for 5 consecutive d every 6 wk. *Weekly schedule:* Initial dose of 1,000 mg/m$^2$ of body surface area IV at weekly intervals for the first 2 wk. Increase subsequent doses if response and toxicity do not occur, but *do not exceed 1,500 mg/m$^2$ of body surface area.*

### Pharmacokinetics

| Route | Onset | Duration |
|---|---|---|
| IV | Varies | 24 h |

*Metabolism:* Hepatic, $T_{1/2}$: 35 min
*Distribution:* Crosses placenta; enters breast milk
*Excretion:* Urine

### IV facts

**Preparation:** Reconstitute with 9.5 ml of Dextrose Injection or 0.9% Sodium Chloride Injection. The resultant pale gold solution contains 100 mg/ml streptozocin. Dilute further with diluents listed above, if needed. Refrigerate vials and protect from light; once reconstituted, use within 12 h.
**Infusion:** Infuse slowly over 5–15 min.

### Adverse effects

- CNS: Lethargy, confusion, depression
- GI: *Nausea, vomiting,* diarrhea, *hepatotoxicity*
- **Hematologic**: Hematologic toxicity, glucose intolerance
- GU: *Renal toxicity*
- **Other**: Infertility, cancer

## ■ Nursing Considerations

### Assessment

- ***History:*** Allergy to streptozocin, hematopoietic depression, impaired renal or hepatic function, pregnancy, lactation
- ***Physical:*** Weight; orientation, affect; liver evaluation; CBC, differential; urinalysis; blood glucose, serum electrolytes, liver and renal function tests

### Implementation

- Arrange for blood and urine tests to evaluate renal function before therapy and weekly during therapy. Monitor liver function tests and CBC.
- Reduce dosage or discontinue if renal toxicity occurs—proteinuria, elevated BUN, plasma creatinine, serum electrolytes.
- Use special precautions when handling the streptozocin; contact with the skin poses a carcinogenic hazard to the area exposed. Wear rubber gloves; if powder or solution comes in contact with the skin, wash immediately with soap and water.
- Administer IV only; intra-arterial administration causes more rapid toxic renal effects.
- Arrange for pretherapy medicating with antiemetic, if needed, to decrease the severity of nausea and vomiting.
- Monitor urine output and perform frequent urinalysis for any sign of renal failure.

### Drug-specific teaching points

- This drug can only be given IV. Prepare a calendar with the course of treatment.
- The following side effects may occur: nausea, vomiting, loss of appetite (request an antiemetic; eat small frequent meals); confusion, depression, lethargy.
- This drug can cause severe birth defects. Use birth control with this drug.
- Arrange to have regular medical follow-ups, including blood and urine tests to evaluate drug effects and to determine next dose.
- Report unusual bleeding or bruising, fever, chills, sore throat, stomach or flank pain, changes in urinary output, confusion, depression.

# succimer

***(sux' i mer)***
Chemet
**Pregnancy Category C**

### Drug classes

Antidote
Chelating agents

### Therapeutic actions

Forms water-soluble chelates with lead, leading to increased urinary excretion of lead.

### Indications

- Treatment of lead poisoning in children with blood levels > 45 $\mu$g/dl (not for prophylactic use)
- Unlabeled uses: treatment of other heavy metal poisonings (mercury, arsenic)

### Contraindications/cautions

- Contraindications: allergy to succimer, pregnancy (teratogenic and embryotoxic), lactation.
- Use cautiously with impaired renal or hepatic function.

### Dosage

**Available Forms:** Capsules—100 mg

*PEDIATRIC:* Starting dose of 10 mg/kg or 350 mg/$m^2$ q8h PO for 5 d; reduce dosage to 10 mg/kg or 350 mg/$m^2$ q12h PO for 2 wk (therapy runs for 19 d).

### Pharmacokinetics

| *Route* | *Onset* | *Peak* |
|---|---|---|
| Oral | Varies | 1–2 h |

*Metabolism:* Hepatic, $T_{1/2}$: 2 d

*Distribution:* Crosses placenta; may enter breast milk

*Excretion:* Feces and urine

### Adverse effects

- CNS: Drowsiness, dizziness, sleepiness, otitis media, watery eyes
- GI: *Nausea, vomiting*, diarrhea, metal taste in mouth, loss of appetite
- GU: Decreased urination, voiding difficulty
- Dermatologic: Papular rash, herpetic rash, mucocutaneous eruptions, pruritus
- General: *Back, stomach, flank, head, rib pain*, chills, fever, flulike symptoms

### Clinically important drug-drug interactions

- High risk of toxicity with other chelating agents (EDTA)

### Drug-lab test interferences

- False-positive tests of urine ketones using *Ketostix* • False decrease in serum uric acid, CPK

## ■ Nursing Considerations

### Assessment

- ***History:*** Allergy to succimer, lactation, pregnancy, renal or hepatic impairment
- ***Physical:*** Weight; orientation, affect; liver evaluation; urinalysis; liver and renal function tests; serum lead levels

### Implementation

- Test serum blood levels before therapy.
- Identify the source of lead and facilitate its removal; succimer is not prophylactic to prevent lead poisoning.
- Ensure that patient continues therapy for full 19 d.
- For children unable to swallow capsules: separate capsules and give medicated beads on a small amount of soft food or by spoon followed by fruit drink.

### Drug-specific teaching points

- For children unable to swallow capsules: separate capsules and give medicated beads on a small amount of soft food or by spoon followed by fruit drink.
- Ensure child maintains good fluid intake.
- The following side effects may occur: nausea, vomiting, loss of appetite (eat small, frequent meals); abdominal, back, rib, flank pain (request medications).
- Report rash, difficulty breathing, difficulty walking, tremors.

## sucralfate

*(soo **kral'** fate)*

Carafate, Sulcrate (CAN)

**Pregnancy Category B**

### Drug classes

Antipeptic agent

### Therapeutic actions

Forms an ulcer-adherent complex at duodenal ulcer sites, protecting the ulcer against acid, pepsin, and bile salts, thereby promoting ulcer healing; also inhibits pepsin activity in gastric juices.

### Indications

- Short-term treatment of duodenal ulcers, up to 8 wk
- Maintenance therapy for duodenal ulcer at reduced dosage after healing
- Unlabeled uses: accelerates healing of gastric ulcers, treatment of NSAID or aspirin-induced GI symptoms and GI damage, prevention of stress ulcers in critically ill patients

- Orphan drug use: treatment of oral and esophageal ulcers due to radiation, chemotherapy, and sclerotherapy

### Contraindications/cautions

- Allergy to sucralfate, chronic renal failure/dialysis (buildup of aluminum may occur with aluminum-containing products), pregnancy, lactation.

### Dosage

**Available Forms:** Tablets—1 g; suspension—1 g/10ml

**ADULT**

- *Active duodenal ulcer:* 1 g PO qid on an empty stomach (1 h before meals and at hs). Continue treatment for 4–8 wk.
- *Maintenance:* 1 g PO bid.

**PEDIATRIC:** Safety and efficacy not established.

### Pharmacokinetics

| *Route* | *Onset* | *Duration* |
|---|---|---|
| Oral | 30 min | 5 h |

*Metabolism:* Hepatic, $T_{1/2}$: 6–20 h
*Distribution:* Crosses placenta; may enter breast milk
*Excretion:* Feces

### Adverse effects

- CNS: Dizziness, sleeplessness, vertigo
- GI: *Constipation*, diarrhea, nausea, indigestion, gastric discomfort, dry mouth
- Dermatologic: Rash, pruritus
- Other: Back pain

### Clinically important drug-drug interactions

• Decreased serum levels and effectiveness of phenytoin, ciprofloxacin, norfloxacin, penicillamine; separate administration by 2 h • Risk of aluminum toxicity with aluminum-containing antacids

## ■ Nursing Considerations

### Assessment

- *History:* Allergy to sucralfate, chronic renal failure/dialysis, pregnancy, lactation
- *Physical:* Skin color, lesions; reflexes, orientation; mucous membranes, normal output

### Implementation

- Give drug on an empty stomach, 1 h before or 2 h after meals and hs.
- Monitor pain; use antacids to relieve pain.
- Administer antacids between doses of sucralfate, not within 1/2 h before or after sucralfate doses.

### Drug-specific teaching points

- Take the drug on an empty stomach, 1 h before or 2 h after meals and at bedtime.
- If you are also taking antacids for pain relief; do not take antacids 1/2 h before or after taking sucralfate.
- The following side effects may occur: dizziness, vertigo (avoid driving or operating dangerous machinery); indigestion, nausea (eat small, frequent meals); dry mouth (frequent mouth care, sucking on sugarless candies may help); constipation (request aid).
- Report severe gastric pain.

## sufentanil citrate

*(soo **fen'** ta nil)*
Sufenta

**Pregnancy Category C**
**C-II controlled substance**

### Drug classes

Narcotic agonist analgesic

### Therapeutic actions

Acts at specific opioid receptors, causing analgesia, respiratory depression, physical depression, euphoria.

### Indications

- Analgesic adjunct to maintain balanced general anesthesia
- Primary anesthetic with 100% oxygen to induce and maintain anesthesia in major surgical procedures

### Contraindications/cautions

- Contraindications: known sensitivity to sufentanil, pregnancy.
- Use cautiously with obesity, hepatic disease, head injury, diabetes, arrhythmias, lactation, severe debilitation.

### Dosage

**Available Forms:** Injection—50 μg/ml

Individualize dosage; monitor vital signs routinely.

#### ADULT

- *Adjunct to general anesthesia:* 2–8 μg/kg IV initially; 25–50 μg for maintenance.
- *With oxygen for anesthesia:* 8–30 μg/kg IV initially; supplement with doses of 25–50 μg IV.

#### PEDIATRIC (2–12 Y)

- *With oxygen for anesthesia:* 10–25 μg/kg IV initially; supplement with doses of 25–50 μg IV.

### Pharmacokinetics

| *Route* | *Onset* | *Duration* |
|---|---|---|
| IV | Immediate | 5 min |

*Metabolism:* Hepatic, $T_{1/2}$: 2.7 h

*Distribution:* Crosses placenta; enters breast milk

#### IV facts

**Preparation:** Protect vials from light.

**Infusion:** Give slowly over 1–2 min by direct injection or into running IV tubing.

### Adverse effects

- CNS: *Sedation, clamminess, sweating, headache, vertigo, floating feeling, dizziness, lethary, confusion, lightheadedness,* nervousness, unusual dreams, agitation, euphoria, hallucinations, delirium, insomnia, anxiety, fear, disorientation, impaired mental and physical performance, coma, mood changes, weakness, headache, tremor, convulsions
- GI: *Nausea, vomiting,* dry mouth, anorexia, constipation, biliary tract spasm
- CV: Palpitation, change in BP, circulatory depression, **cardiac arrest**, **shock**, tachycardia, bradycardia, arrhythmia, palpitations
- Respiratory: Slow, shallow respiration, apnea, suppression of cough reflex, laryngospasm, bronchospasm
- GU: Ureteral spasm, spasm of vesical sphincters, urinary retention or hesitancy, oliguria, antidiuretic effect, reduced libido or potency
- EENT: Diplopia, blurred vision
- Dermatologic: Rash, hives, pruritus, flushing, warmth, sensitivity to cold
- Local: Phlebitis following IV injection, pain at injection site
- Other: Physical tolerance and dependence, psychological dependence, local skin irritation with transdermal system

### Clinically important drug-drug interactions

- Potentiation of effects with barbiturate anesthetics

### Drug-lab test interferences

- Elevated biliary tract pressure may cause increases in plasma amylase, lipase; determinations of these levels may be unreliable for 24 h after administration of narcotics

## ■ Nursing Considerations

### Assessment

- *History:* Hypersensitivity to sufentanil or narcotics, physical dependence on a narcotic analgesic, pregnancy, lactation, COPD, increased intracranial pressure, acute MI, biliary tract surgery, renal or hepatic dysfunction
- *Physical:* Orientation, reflexes, bilateral grip strength, affect; pupil size, vision; pulse, auscultation, BP; R, adventitious sounds; bowel sounds, normal output; liver and kidney function tests

### Implementation

- Give to lactating women 4–6 h before the next feeding to minimize the amount in milk.
- Provide narcotic antagonist, facilities for assisted or controlled respiration on standby during parenteral administration.

### Drug-specific teaching points

- Incorporate teaching about drug into preoperative or postoperative teaching program.
- The following side effects may occur: dizziness, sedation, drowsiness, impaired visual acuity (ask for assistance to move);

nausea, loss of appetite (lie quietly, eat frequent, small meals); constipation (use a laxative).

- Report severe nausea, vomiting, palpitations, shortness of breath or difficulty breathing.

## sulfadiazine

*(sul fa* ***dye'*** *a zeen)*

**Pregnancy Category C**

**Pregnancy Category D (labor & delivery)**

### Drug classes
Antibiotic
Sulfonamide

### Therapeutic actions
Bacteriostatic: competitively antagonizes para-aminobenzoic acid (PABA), an essential component of folic acid synthesis in gram-negative and gram-positive bacteria; prevents cell replication.

### Indications
- Treatment of acute infections caused by susceptible organisms: urinary tract infections, chancroid, inclusion conjunctivitis, trachoma, nocardiosis, toxoplasmosis (with pyrimethamine), malaria (as adjunctive therapy for chloroquine-resistant strains of *P. falciparum*), acute otitis media (due to *H. influenzae* when used with penicillin or erythromycin), *H. influenzae* meningitis (as adjunctive therapy with parenteral streptomycin), meningococcal meningitis, rheumatic fever

### Contraindications/cautions
- Contraindications: allergy to sulfonamides, sulfonylureas, thiazides; pregnancy (teratogenic may cause kernicterus); lactation (risk of kernicterus, diarrhea, rash).
- Use cautiously with impaired renal or hepatic function, G-6-PD deficiency, porphyria.

### Dosage
**Available Forms:** Tablets—500 mg

*ADULT:* Loading dose, 2–4 g PO. Maintenance: 2–4 g/d PO in 4 to 6 divided doses.

- ***Prevention of recurrent attacks of rheumatic fever (not for initial therapy of streptococcal infections):*** >30 kg: 1 g/d PO. <30 kg: 0.5 g/d PO.

*PEDIATRIC*

- *>2 Mo:* Initial dose, 75 mg/kg PO. Maintenance dose, 120–150 mg/kg per day PO in 4–6 divided doses with a maximum dose of 6 g/d. Maximum dose, 6 g/d.
- *<2 Mo: Not recommended except to treat congenital toxoplasmosis:* Loading dose, 75–100 mg/kg PO. Maintenance dose, 100–150 mg/kg per day in four divided doses.
- *3–4 Wk:* 25 mg/kg PO per dose 4×/d.
- *>2 Mo:* 25–50 mg/kg PO per dose qid.

### Pharmacokinetics

| Route | Onset | Peak |
|---|---|---|
| Oral | Varies | 3–6 h |

*Metabolism:* Hepatic, $T_{1/2}$: unknown
*Distribution:* Crosses placenta; enters breast milk
*Excretion:* Urine

### Adverse effects
- CNS: *Headache*, peripheral neuropathy, mental depression, convulsions, ataxia, hallucinations, tinnitus, vertigo, insomnia, hearing loss, drowsiness, transient lesions of posterior spinal column, transverse myelitis
- GI: *Nausea, emesis, abdominal pains*, diarrhea, bloody diarrhea, anorexia, pancreatitis, stomatitis, impaired folic acid absorption, hepatitis, hepatocellular necrosis
- **Hematologic**: *Agranulocytosis,* aplastic anemia, thrombocytopenia, leukopenia, hemolytic anemia, hypoprothrombinemia, methemoglobinemia, megaloblastic anemia
- GU: *Crystalluria, hematuria,* proteinuria, nephrotic syndrome, toxic nephrosis

S

with oliguria and anuria, oligospermia, infertility
- **Dermatologic:** *Photosensitivity,* cyanosis, petechiae, alopecia
- **Hypersensitivity:** Stevens-Johnson syndrome, generalized skin eruptions, epidermal necrolysis, urticaria, serum sickness, pruritus, exfoliative dermatitis, anaphylactoid reactions, periorbital edema, conjunctival and scleral redness, photosensitization, arthralgia, allergic myocarditis, transient pulmonary changes with eosinophilia, decreased pulmonary function
- **Other:** Drug fever, chills, periarteritis nodosum

### Clinically important drug-drug interactions

• Increased risk of hypoglycemia when tolbutamide, tolazamide, glyburide, glipizide, acetohexamide, chlorpropamide are taken concurrently • Increased risk of phenytoin toxicity with sulfonamides • Risk of hemorrhage when combined with oral anticoagulants • Increased risk of nephrotoxicity with cyclosporine

### Drug-lab test interferences

• False-positive urinary glucose tests using Benedict's method

## ■ Nursing Considerations

### Assessment

- *History:* Allergy to sulfonamides, sulfonylureas, thiazides; pregnancy, lactation; impaired renal or hepatic function; G-6-PD deficiency
- *Physical:* T; skin color, lesions; culture of infected site; orientation, reflexes, affect, peripheral sensation; R, adventitious sounds; mucous membranes, bowel sounds, liver evaluation; liver and renal function tests, CBC and differential, urinalysis

### Implementation

- Arrange for culture and sensitivity tests of infection before therapy; repeat cultures if response is not as expected.
- Administer drug on an empty stomach, 1 h before or 2 h after meals, with a full glass of water.
- Ensure adequate fluid intake; sulfadiazine is very insoluble and may cause crystalluria if high concentrations occur in the urine; alkalinization of the urine may be necessary.
- Discontinue drug immediately if hypersensitivity reaction occurs.

### Drug-specific teaching points

- Complete full course of therapy.
- Take the drug on an empty stomach, 1 h before or 2 h after meals, with a full glass of water.
- Drink eight glasses of water per day.
- This drug is specific to this disease; do not self-treat any other infection.
- The following side effects may occur: sensitivity to sunlight (use sunscreens; wear protective clothing); dizziness, drowsiness, difficulty walking, loss of sensation (avoid driving or performing tasks that require alertness); nausea, vomiting, diarrhea; loss of fertility.
- Report blood in the urine, rash, ringing in the ears, difficulty breathing, fever, sore throat, chills.

# sulfamethizole

*(sul fa **meth'** i zole)*

Thiosulfil Forte

**Pregnancy Category C**

**Pregnancy Category D (at term)**

### Drug classes

Antibiotic
Sulfonamide

### Therapeutic actions

Bacteriostatic: competitively antagonizes PABA, an essential component of folic acid synthesis in susceptible gram-negative and gram-positive bacteria, preventing cell replication.

### Indications

- Treatment of urinary tract infections caused by susceptible organisms

### Contraindications/cautions

- Contraindications: allergy to sulfonamides, sulfonylureas, thiazides; pregnancy (teratogenic may cause kernicterus); lactation (risk of kernicterus, diarrhea, rash).
- Use cautiously with impaired renal or hepatic function, G-6-PD deficiency, porphyria.

### Dosage

**Available Forms:** Tablets—500 mg

*Adult:* 0.5–1 g tid–qid PO.

*Pediatric (> 2 Mo):* 30–45 mg/kg per day PO in 4 divided doses.

### Pharmacokinetics

| *Route* | *Onset* | *Peak* |
|---|---|---|
| Oral | Varies | 3–6 h |

*Metabolism:* Hepatic, $T_{1/2}$: unknown

*Distribution:* Crosses placenta; enters breast milk

*Excretion:* Urine

### Adverse effects

- CNS: *Headache*, peripheral neuropathy, mental depression, convulsions, ataxia, hallucinations, tinnitus, vertigo, insomnia, hearing loss, drowsiness, transient lesions of posterior spinal column, transverse myelitis
- GI: *Nausea, emesis, abdominal pains*, diarrhea, bloody diarrhea, anorexia, pancreatitis, stomatitis, impaired folic acid absorption, hepatitis, hepatocellular necrosis
- **Hematologic:** *Agranulocytosis,* aplastic anemia, thrombocytopenia, leukopenia, hemolytic anemia, hypoprothrombinemia, methemoglobinemia, megaloblastic anemia
- GU: *Crystalluria, hematuria,* proteinuria, nephrotic syndrome, toxic nephrosis with oliguria and anuria, oligospermia, infertility
- **Dermatologic:** *Photosensitivity,* cyanosis, petechiae, alopecia
- **Hypersensitivity:** Stevens-Johnson syndrome, generalized skin eruptions, epidermal necrolysis, urticaria, serum sickness, pruritus, exfoliative dermatitis, anaphylactoid reactions, periorbital edema, conjunctival and scleral redness, photosensitization, arthralgia, allergic myocarditis, transient pulmonary changes with eosinophilia, decreased pulmonary function
- **Other:** Drug fever, chills, periarteritis nodosum

### Clinically important drug-drug interactions

• Increased risk of hypoglycemia with tolbutamide, tolazamide, glyburide, glipizide, acetohexamide, chlorpropamide • Increased risk of phenytoin toxicity • Risk of hemorrhage with oral anticoagulants

### Drug-lab test interferences

• Possible false-positive urinary glucose tests using Benedict's method

## ■ Nursing Considerations

### Assessment

- *History:* Allergy to sulfonamides, sulfonylureas, thiazides; pregnancy; lactation; impaired renal or hepatic function; G-6-PD deficiency
- *Physical:* T; skin color, lesions; culture of infected site; orientation, reflexes, affect, peripheral sensation; R, adventitious sounds; mucous membranes, bowel sounds, liver evaluation; liver and renal function tests, CBC and differential, urinalysis

### Implementation

- Arrange for culture and sensitivity tests of infection before therapy; repeat cultures if response is not as expected.
- Administer drug on an empty stomach, 1 h before or 2 h after meals, with a full glass of water.
- Ensure adequate fluid intake; sulfamethizole is very insoluble and may cause crystalluria if high concentrations occur in the urine; alkalinization of the urine may be necessary.

- Discontinue drug immediately if hypersensitivity reaction occurs.

### Drug-specific teaching points

- Complete full course of therapy.
- Take the drug on an empty stomach, 1 h before or 2 h after meals, with a full glass of water.
- Drink eight glasses of water per day.
- This drug is specific to this disease; do not self-treat any other infection.
- The following side effects may occur: sensitivity to sunlight (use sunscreens, wear protective clothing); dizziness, drowsiness, difficulty walking, loss of sensation (avoid driving or performing tasks that require alertness); nausea, vomiting, diarrhea; loss of fertility.
- Report blood in the urine, rash, ringing in the ears, difficulty breathing, fever, sore throat, chills.

## sulfamethoxazole

*(sul fa meth* ***ox'*** *a zole)*

Gantanol

**Pregnancy Category C**

**Pregnancy Category D (at term)**

### Drug classes

Antibiotic
Sulfonamide

### Therapeutic actions

Bacteriostatic: competitively antagonizes PABA, an essential component of folic acid synthesis in susceptible gram-negative and gram-positive bacteria, preventing cell replication.

### Indications

- Treatment of acute infections caused by susceptible organisms: urinary tract infections, chancroid, inclusion conjunctivitis, trachoma, nocardiosis, toxoplasmosis (with pyrimethamine), malaria (as adjunctive therapy for chloroquine-resistant strains of *P. falciparum*), acute otitis media (due to *H. influenzae* when used with penicillin or erythromycin)
- Meningococcal meningitis

### Contraindications/cautions

- Contraindications: allergy to sulfonamides, sulfonylureas, thiazides; pregnancy (teratogenic; may cause kernicterus); lactation (risk of kernicterus, diarrhea, rash).
- Use cautiously with impaired renal or hepatic function, G-6-PD deficiency, porphyria.

### Dosage

**Available Forms:** Tablets—500 mg

*ADULT*

- *Mild to moderate infections:* Loading dose, 2 g PO. Maintenance dose, 1 g PO morning and evening.
- *Severe infections:* 2 g PO initially, then 1 g tid PO.

*PEDIATRIC (> 2 MO):* 50–60 mg/kg PO followed by 25–30 mg/kg morning and evening. Do not exceed 75 mg/kg per day *or* 50–60 mg/kg per day divided q12h, not to exceed 3 g/d.

### Pharmacokinetics

| *Route* | *Onset* | *Peak* |
|---|---|---|
| Oral | 30–60 min | 2 h |

*Metabolism:* Hepatic, $T_{1/2}$: 7–12 h
*Distribution:* Crosses placenta; enters breast milk
*Excretion:* Urine

### Adverse effects

- CNS: *Headache*, peripheral neuropathy, mental depression, convulsions, ataxia, hallucinations, tinnitus, vertigo, insomnia, hearing loss, drowsiness, transient lesions of posterior spinal column, transverse myelitis
- GI: *Nausea, emesis, abdominal pains*, diarrhea, bloody diarrhea, anorexia, pancreatitis, stomatitis, impaired folic acid absorption, hepatitis, hepatocellular necrosis
- **Hematologic**: *Agranulocytosis,* aplastic anemia, thrombocytopenia, leukopenia, hemolytic anemia, hypoprothrombine-

mia, methemoglobinemia, megaloblastic anemia
- GU: *Crystalluria, hematuria,* proteinuria, nephrotic syndrome, toxic nephrosis with oliguria and anuria, oligospermia, infertility
- Dermatologic: *Photosensitivity,* cyanosis, petechiae, alopecia
- **Hypersensitivity:** Stevens-Johnson syndrome, generalized skin eruptions, epidermal necrolysis, urticaria, serum sickness, pruritus, exfoliative dermatitis, anaphylactoid reactions, periorbital edema, conjunctival and scleral redness, photosensitization, arthralgia, allergic myocarditis, transient pulmonary changes with eosinophilia, decreased pulmonary function
- Other: Drug fever, chills, periarteritis nodosum

### Clinically important drug-drug interactions

• Increased risk of hypoglycemia with tolbutamide, tolazamide, glyburide, glipizide, acetohexamide, chlorpropamide • Decreased immunosuppressive effect of cyclosporine and increased risk of nephrotoxicity • Risk of hemorrhage with oral anticoagulant

### Drug-lab test interferences

• Possible false-positive urinary glucose tests using Benedict's method

## ■ Nursing Considerations

### Assessment

- *History:* Allergy to sulfonamides, sulfonylureas, thiazides; pregnancy; lactation; impaired renal or hepatic function; G-6-PD deficiency; porphyria
- *Physical:* T; skin color, lesions; culture of infected site; orientation, reflexes, affect, peripheral sensation; R, adventitious sounds; mucous membranes, bowel sounds, liver evaluation; liver and renal function tests, CBC and differential, urinalysis

### Implementation

- Arrange for culture and sensitivity tests of infection before therapy; repeat cultures if response is not as expected.
- Administer drug on an empty stomach, 1 h before or 2 h after meals, with a full glass of water.
- Ensure adequate fluid intake; sulfamethoxazole is very insoluble and may cause crystalluria if high concentrations occur in the urine; alkalinization of the urine may be necessary.
- Discontinue drug immediately if hypersensitivity reaction occurs.

### Drug-specific teaching points

- Complete full course of therapy.
- Take the drug on an empty stomach, 1 h before or 2 h after meals, with a full glass of water.
- Drink 8 glasses of water per day.
- This drug is specific to this disease; do not self-treat any other infection.
- The following side effects may occur: sensitivity to sunlight (use sunscreens, wear protective clothing); dizziness, drowsiness, difficulty walking, loss of sensation (avoid driving or performing tasks that require alertness); nausea, vomiting, diarrhea; loss of fertility.
- Report blood in the urine, rash, ringing in the ears, difficulty breathing, fever, sore throat, chills.

## sulfasalazine

*(sul fa **sal'** a zeen)*

Azulfidine, Azulfidine En-Tabs

**Pregnancy Category C**

**Pregnancy Category D (at term)**

### Drug classes

Antibiotic
Sulfonamide

### Therapeutic actions

Bacteriostatic: competitively antagonizes PABA, an essential component of folic acid synthesis in susceptible gram-negative and gram-positive bacteria; one-third of the oral dose is absorbed from the small intestine; remaining two-thirds passes into the colon where it is split into 5-aminosalicylic acid and sulfapyridine; most of the sulfapyridine is absorbed; the 5-aminosalicylic acid acts locally as an anti-inflammatory agent.

### Indications

- Treatment of ulcerative colitis
- Treatment of rheumatoid arthritis in patients intolerant or unresponsive to other anti-inflammatories (delayed-release)
- Unlabeled uses: collagenous colitis, Crohn's disease, ankylosing, spondylitis, psoratic arthritis

### Contraindications/cautions

- Contraindications: allergy to sulfonamides, sulfonylureas, thiazides; pregnancy (teratogenic may cause kernicterus); lactation (risk of kernicterus, diarrhea, rash).
- Use cautiously with impaired renal or hepatic function, G-6-PD deficiency, porphyria.

### Dosage

**Available Forms:** Tablets—500 mg

Administer around the clock; dosage intervals should not exceed 8 h. Give after meals.

*ADULT:* Initial therapy, 3–4 g/d PO in evenly divided doses. Initial doses of 1–2 g/d PO may lessen adverse GI effects. Doses > 4 g/d increase risk of toxicity. Maintenance, 2 g/d PO in evenly spaced doses (500 mg qid).

*PEDIATRIC (>2 Y):* Initial therapy, 40–60 mg/kg/24 h PO in 4 to 6 divided doses. Maintenance therapy, 20–30 mg/kg/24 h PO in 4 equally divided doses. Maximum dosage, 2 g/d.

### Pharmacokinetics

| *Route* | *Onset* | *Peak* |
|---|---|---|
| Oral | Varies | 1 1/2–6 h, 6–24 h metabolite |

*Metabolism:* Hepatic, $T_{1/2}$: 5–10 h

*Distribution:* Crosses placenta; enters breast milk

*Excretion:* Urine

### Adverse effects

- **CNS**: Headache, peripheral neuropathy, mental depression, convulsions, ataxia, hallucinations, tinnitus, vertigo, insomnia, hearing loss, drowsiness, transient lesions of posterior spinal column, transverse myelitis
- **GI**: *Nausea, emesis, abdominal pains,* diarrhea, bloody diarrhea, anorexia, pancreatitis, stomatitis, impaired folic acid absorption, hepatitis, hepatocellular necrosis
- **Hematologic**: Agranulocytosis, aplastic anemia, thrombocytopenia, leukopenia, hemolytic anemia, hypoprothrombinemia, methemoglobinemia, megaloblastic anemia
- **GU**: *Crystalluria, hematuria,* proteinuria, nephrotic syndrome, toxic nephrosis with oliguria and anuria, oligospermia, infertility
- **Dermatologic**: Photosensitivity, cyanosis, petechiae, alopecia
- **Hypersensitivity**: Stevens-Johnson syndrome, generalized skin eruptions, epidermal necrolysis, urticaria, serum sickness, pruritus, exfoliative dermatitis, anaphylactoid reactions, periorbital edema, conjunctival and scleral redness, photosensitization, arthralgia, allergic myocarditis, transient pulmonary changes with eosinophilia, decreased pulmonary function
- **Other**: Drug fever, chills, periarteritis nodosum

### Clinically important drug-drug interactions

• Decreased absorption of digoxin with lessened therapeutic effect; monitor patient, space doses > 2 h apart • Increased risk of folate deficiency, monitor for signs of folate deficiency

### Drug-lab test interferences

• Possible false-positive urinary glucose tests using Benedict's method

## ■ Nursing Considerations

### Assessment

- *History:* Allergy to sulfonamides, sulfonylureas, thiazides; pregnancy; lactation;

impaired renal or hepatic function; G-6-PD deficiency; porphyria
- *Physical:* T; skin color, lesions; culture of infected site; orientation, reflexes, affect, peripheral sensation; R, adventitious sounds; mucous membranes, bowel sounds, liver evaluation; liver and renal function tests, CBC and differential, urinalysis

### Implementation
- Administer drug after meals or with food to prevent GI upset. Administer the drug around the clock.
- Ensure adequate fluid intake; sulfasalazine is very insoluble and may cause crystalluria if high concentrations occur in the urine; alkalinization of the urine may be necessary.
- Discontinue drug immediately if hypersensitivity reaction occurs.

### Drug-specific teaching points
- Complete full course of therapy.
- Take the drug with food or meals to decrease GI upset.
- Drink 8 glasses of water per day.
- The following side effects may occur: sensitivity to sunlight (use sunscreens, wear protective clothing); dizziness, drowsiness, difficulty walking, loss of sensation (avoid driving or performing tasks that require alertness); nausea, vomiting, diarrhea; loss of fertility; yellow-orange urine
- Report blood in the urine, rash, ringing in the ears, difficulty breathing, fever, sore throat, chills.

## sulfinpyrazone

*(sul fin **peer'** a zone)*

Anturan (CAN), Anturane

**Pregnancy Category C**

### Drug classes
Uricosuric agent
Antigout agent
Antiplatelet agent

### Therapeutic actions
Inhibits the renal tubular reabsorption of uric acid, increasing the urinary excretion of uric acid, decreasing serum uric acid levels, retarding urate deposition, and promoting the resorption of urate deposits. Inhibits prostaglandin synthesis, which prevents platelet aggregation, but lacks analgesic and anti-inflammatory activity.

### Indications
- Chronic gouty arthritis
- Intermittent gouty arthritis
- Unlabeled uses: post-MI therapy to decrease incidence of sudden death; in rheumatic mitral stenosis to decrease the frequency of systemic embolism

### Contraindications/cautions
- Contraindications: allergy to sulfinpyrazone, phenylbutazone, or other pyrazoles; blood dyscrasias; peptic ulcer or symptoms of GI inflammation.
- Use cautiously with renal failure, pregnancy, lactation.

### Dosage
**Available Forms:** Tablets—100 mg; capsules—200 mg

ADULT
- *Gout:* 200–400 mg/d PO in 2 divided doses with meals or milk, gradually increase to maintenance dose over 1 wk. Maintenance, 400 mg/d PO in 2 divided doses. May increase to 800 mg/d or reduce to 200 mg/d. Regulate dose by monitoring serum uric acid levels.
- *Inhibition of platelet aggregation:* 200 mg PO tid or qid.

PEDIATRIC: Safety and efficacy not established.

### Pharmacokinetics
| Route | Onset | Peak | Duration |
|---|---|---|---|
| Oral | Varies | 1–2 h | 4–6 h |

*Metabolism:* $T_{1/2}$: 2.2–4 h
*Distribution:* Crosses placenta; may enter breast milk
*Excretion:* Urine

### Adverse effects
- GI: *Upper GI disturbances*
- **Hematologic: Blood dyscrasias**

- GU: Exacerbation of gout and uric acid stones, renal failure
- **Dermatologic**: Rash

### Clinically important drug-drug interactions

- Decreased effectiveness with salicylates
- Increased pharmacologic effects of tolbutamide, glyburide, warfarin • Increased risk of hepatotoxicity with acetaminophen

## ■ Nursing Considerations

### Assessment

- *History:* Allergy to sulfinpyrazone, phenylbutazone, or other pyrazoles; blood dyscrasias; peptic ulcer or symptoms of GI inflammation; renal failure; pregnancy; lactation
- *Physical:* Skin lesions, color; liver evaluation, normal output, gums; urinary output; CBC, renal and liver function tests, urinalysis

### Implementation

- Administer drug with meals or antacids to prevent GI upset.
- Force fluids (2.5 to 3 L/d) to decrease the risk of renal stone development.
- Check urine alkalinity (urates crystallize in acid urine) use sodium bicarbonate or potassium citrate to alkalinize urine.
- Arrange for regular medical follow-ups and blood tests.
- Double-check any analgesics ordered for pain; avoid salicylates, acetaminophen.

### Drug-specific teaching points

- Take the drug with meals or antacids to prevent GI upset.
- The following side effects may occur: exacerbation of gouty attack or renal stones (drink plenty of fluids, 2.5–3 L/d); nausea, vomiting, loss of appetite (take with meals, use antacids).
- Avoid the use of aspirin and aspirin-containing products; serious toxic effects could occur
- Report flank pain, dark urine or blood in urine, acute gout attack, unusual fatigue or lethargy, unusual bleeding or bruising.

# sulfisoxazole

*(sul fi **sox'** a zole)*

Novosoxazole (CAN)

**Pregnancy Category C**

**Pregnancy Category D (at term)**

### Drug classes

Antibiotic
Sulfonamide

### Therapeutic actions

Bacteriostatic: competitively antagonizes PABA, an essential component of folic acid synthesis in susceptible gram-negative and gram-positive bacteria, preventing cell replication.

### Indications

- Treatment of acute infections caused by susceptible organisms: urinary tract infections, chancroid, inclusion conjunctivitis, trachoma, nocardiosis, toxoplasmosis (with pyrimethamine), malaria (as adjunctive therapy for chloroquine-resistant strains of *P. falciparum*), acute otitis media (due to *H. influenzae* when used with penicillin or erythromycin), *H. influenzae* meningitis (as adjunctive therapy with parenteral streptomycin), meningicoccal meningitis
- Conjunctivitis, corneal ulcer, superficial ocular infections due to susceptible microorganisms
- CDC recommended for treatment of sexually transmitted diseases
- Unlabeled use: chemoprophylaxis for recurrent otitis media

### Contraindications/cautions

- Contraindications: allergy to sulfonamides, sulfonylureas, thiazides; pregnancy (teratogenic may cause kernicterus); lactation (risk of kernicterus, diarrhea, rash).
- Use cautiously with impaired renal or hepatic function, G-6-PD deficiency, porphyria.

### Dosage

**Available Forms:** Tablets—500 mg

**ADULT**

- ***Oral:*** Loading dose, 2–4 g PO. Maintenance dose, 4–8 g/d PO in 4 to 6 divided doses.
- *CDC recommended treatment of sexually transmitted diseases—lymphogranuloma venereum:* As an alternative regimen to doxycycline, 500 mg PO qid for 21 d.
- *Treatment of uncomplicated urethral, endocervical, or rectal* Chlamydia trachomatis *infections:* As an alternative regimen to doxycycline or tetracycline (if erythromycin is not tolerated), 500 mg PO qid for 10 d.

**PEDIATRIC (>2 MO)**

- *Oral:* Initial dose, 75 mg/kg PO. Maintenance dose, 120–150 mg/kg per day PO in 4–6 divided doses with a maximum dose of 6 g/d.

## Pharmacokinetics

| *Route* | *Onset* | *Peak* |
|---|---|---|
| Oral | Varies | 2–4 h |

*Metabolism:* Hepatic, $T_{1/2}$: 4.5–7.8 h
*Distribution:* Crosses placenta; enters breast milk
*Excretion:* Urine

## Adverse effects

*Systemic*

- CNS: *Headache,* peripheral neuropathy, mental depression, convulsions, ataxia, hallucinations, tinnitus, vertigo, insomnia, hearing loss, drowsiness, transient lesions of posterior spinal column, transverse myelitis
- GI: *Nausea, emesis, abdominal pains,* diarrhea, bloody diarrhea, anorexia, pancreatitis, stomatitis, impaired folic acid absorption, hepatitis, hepatocellular necrosis
- **Hematologic**: *Agranulocytosis,* aplastic anemia, thrombocytopenia, leukopenia, hemolytic anemia, hypoprothrombinemia, methemoglobinemia, megaloblastic anemia
- GU: *Crystalluria, hematuria,* proteinuria, nephrotic syndrome, toxic nephrosis with oliguria and anuria, oligospermia, infertility
- **Dermatologic**: *Photosensitivity,* cyanosis, petechiae, alopecia
- **Hypersensitivity**: Stevens-Johnson syndrome, generalized skin eruptions, epidermal necrolysis, urticaria, serum sickness, pruritus, exfoliative dermatitis, anaphylactoid reactions, periorbital edema, conjunctival and scleral redness, photosensitization, arthralgia, allergic myocarditis, transient pulmonary changes with eosinophilia, decreased pulmonary function
- **Other**: Drug fever, chills, periarteritis nodosum

## Clinically important drug-drug interactions

• Increased risk of hypoglycemia with tolbutamide, tolazamide, glyburide, glipizide, acetohexamide, chlorpropamide • Increased risk of nephrotoxicity with cyclosporine

## Drug-lab test interferences

• False-positive urinary glucose tests using Benedict's method • False-positive results with Urobilistix test and sulfosalicylic acid tests for urinary protein

## ■ Nursing Considerations

### Assessment

- *History:* Allergy to sulfonamides, sulfonylureas, thiazides; impaired renal or hepatic function; G-6-PD deficiency; porphyria; pregnancy; lactation
- *Physical:* T; skin color, lesions; culture of infection; orientation, reflexes, affect, peripheral sensation; R, adventitious sounds; mucous membranes, bowel sounds, liver evaluation; liver and renal function tests, CBC and differential, urinalysis

### Implementation

- Arrange for culture and sensitivity tests of infection before therapy; repeat cultures if response is not as expected.
- Administer oral drug on an empty stomach, 1 h before or 2 h after meals, with a full glass of water.

S

- Discontinue drug immediately if hypersensitivity reaction occurs.
- Monitor CBC, differential, urinalysis before and periodically during therapy.

### Drug-specific teaching points

- Complete full course of therapy
- Take the drug on an empty stomach, 1 h before or 2 h after meals, with a full glass of water.
- This drug is specific to this disease. Do not self-treat any other infection.
- The following side effects may occur: sensitivity to sunlight (use sunscreens, wear protective clothing); dizziness, drowsiness, difficulty walking, loss of sensation (avoid driving or performing tasks that require alertness); nausea, vomiting, diarrhea; loss of fertility.
- Report blood in the urine; rash; ringing in the ears; difficulty breathing; fever; sore throat; chills.

## sulindac

*(sul **in'** dak)*

Clinoril

**Pregnancy Category B**

### Drug classes

Nonsteroidal anti-inflammatory drug (NSAID)

### Therapeutic actions

Anti-inflammatory, analgesic, and antipyretic activities largely related to inhibition of prostaglandin synthesis; exact mechanisms of action are not known.

### Indications

- Acute or long-term use to relieve signs and symptoms of osteoarthritis, rheumatoid arthritis, ankylosing spondylitis, acute painful shoulder (acute subacromial bursitis/supraspinatus tendinitis), acute gouty arthritis

### Contraindications/cautions

- Contraindications: pregnancy, lactation.
- Use cautiously with allergies, renal, hepatic, CV, and GI conditions.

### Dosage

**Available Forms:** Tablets—150, 200 mg

Do not exceed 400 mg/d.

**ADULT**

- ***Rheumatoid arthritis/osteoarthritis, ankylosing spondylitis:*** Initial dose of 150 mg bid PO. Individualize dosage.
- ***Acute painful shoulder, acute gouty arthritis:*** 200 mg bid PO. After adequate response, reduce dosage. Acute painful shoulder usually requires 7–14 d of therapy. Acute gouty arthritis, 7 d.

***PEDIATRIC:*** Safety and efficacy not established.

### Pharmacokinetics

| *Route* | *Onset* | *Peak* | *Duration* |
|---|---|---|---|
| Oral | Varies | 2–4 h | 10–12 h |

*Metabolism:* Hepatic, $T_{1/2}$: 8–10 h

*Distribution:* Crosses placenta; enters breast milk

*Excretion:* Urine and feces

### Adverse effects

*NSAIDs*

- CNS: *Headache, dizziness, somnolence, insomnia*, fatigue, tiredness, dizziness, tinnitus, ophthamological effects
- GI: *Nausea, dyspepsia, GI pain,* diarrhea, vomiting, *constipation*, flatulence
- **Respiratory**: Dyspnea, hemoptysis, pharyngitis, bronchospasm, rhinitis
- **Hematologic**: Bleeding, platelet inhibition with higher doses, neutropenia, eosinophilia, leukopenia, pancytopenia, thrombocytopenia, agranulocytosis, granulocytopenia, aplastic anemia, decreased Hgb or Hct, bone marrow depression, mennorhagia
- GU: Dysuria, renal impairment
- **Dermatologic**: *Rash*, pruritus, sweating, dry mucous membranes, stomatitis
- **Other**: Peripheral edema, anaphylactoid reactions to fatal anaphylactic shock

### Clinically important drug-drug interactions

• Increased serum lithium levels and risk of toxicity. • Decreased antihypertensive effects of beta-blockers • Decreased therapeutic effects of bumetanide, furosemide, ethacrynic acid

### Clinically important drug-food interactions

- Decreased rate but not extent of absorption when taken with food

## ■ Nursing Considerations

### Assessment

- *History:* Allergies, renal, hepatic, CV, and GI conditions; pregnancy; lactation
- *Physical:* Skin color and lesions; orientation, reflexes, ophthalmologic and audiometric evaluation, peripheral sensation; P, edema; R, adventitious sounds; liver evaluation; CBC, clotting times, renal and liver function tests; serum electrolytes, stool guaiac

### Implementation

- Give with food or milk if GI upset occurs.
- Arrange for periodic ophthalmologic examination during long-term therapy.
- Institute emergency procedures if overdose occurs: gastric lavage, induction of emesis, supportive therapy.

### Drug-specific teaching points

- Take with food or meals if GI upset occurs.
- Take only the prescribed dosage.
- Dizziness, drowsiness can occur (avoid driving or the use of dangerous machinery).
- Report sore throat, fever, rash, itching, weight gain, swelling in ankles or fingers; changes in vision; black, tarry stools.

## sumatriptan succinate

*(sew mah* ***trip'*** *tan)*

Imitrex

**Pregnancy Category C**

### Drug classes

Antimigraine agent
Serotonin selective agonist

### Therapeutic actions

Binds to serotonin receptors to cause vascular constrictive effects on cranial bood vessels, causing the relief of migraine in selective patients.

### Indications

- Treatment of acute migraine attacks with or without aura
- Acute treatment of cluster headaches (SC)

### Contraindications/cautions

- Contraindications: allergy to sumatriptan, active CAD, uncontrolled hypertension, hemiplegic migraine, pregnancy.
- Use cautiously with the elderly, lactation.

### Dosage

**Available Forms:** Tablets—25, 50 mg, (CAN) 100 mg; injection—12 mg/ml; nasal spray—5, 20 mg

*ADULT:* 6 mg SC with a maximum of 12 mg/24 h; two 6-mg injections separated by at least 1 h; 25 mg PO with fluids, may repeat in 2 h: maximum daily dose 300mg. 5–20 mg/d nasal spray with a maximum daily dose of 2 uses or 40 mg

*PEDIATRIC:* Safety and efficacy not established.

### Pharmacokinetics

| *Route* | *Onset* | *Peak* |
|---|---|---|
| SC | Varies | 5–20 min |
| Oral | 1–1.5 h | 2–4 h |

*Metabolism:* Hepatic, $T_{1/2}$: 115 min
*Distribution:* Crosses placenta; may enter breast milk
*Excretion:* Urine

S

### Adverse effects

- CNS: *Dizziness, vertigo,* headache, anxiety, malaise/fatigue, *weakness, myalgia*
- GI: Abdominal discomfort, dysphagia
- CV: *Blood pressure alterations, tightness or pressure in chest*
- Local: *Injection site discomfort*
- Other: *Tingling, warm/hot sensations, burning sensation, feeling of heaviness, pressure sensation, numbness, feeling of tightness*, feeling strange, cold sensation
- **Nasal spray:** GI—bad taste, nausea

**Clinically important drug-drug interactions**

• Prolonged vasoactive reactions with ergot-containing drugs • Increased serum levels and toxicity of sumatripton with MAOIs; avoid this combination and for 2 wks after MAOI discontinuation

## ■ Nursing Considerations

### Assessment

- *History:* Allergy to sumatriptan, active CAD, uncontrolled hypertension, hemiplegic migraine, pregnancy, lactation
- *Physical:* Skin color and lesions; orientation, reflexes, peripheral sensation; P, BP; renal and liver function tests

### Implementation

- Administer to relieve acute migraine, not as a prophylactic measure.
- Administer as SC injection just below the skin as soon as possible after symptoms begin.
- Repeat injection only after 1 h if relief is not obtained; only two injections may be given each 24 h.
- Administer PO with fluids; may repeat in 2 h if no relief.
- Monitor BP of patients with possible CAD; discontinue at any sign of angina, prolonged high BP.

### Drug-specific teaching points

- Learn to use the autoinjector; injection may be repeated only after 1 h if relief is not obtained; do not administer more than two injections in 24 h.
- Inject just below the skin as soon as possible after onset of migraine; this drug is for an acute attack only, not for use to prevent attacks.
- Take oral drug with fluids, may be repeated in 2 h if no relief or return of headache.
- This drug should not be taken during pregnancy; if you suspect that you are pregnant, contact physician and refrain from using drug.
- The following side effects may occur: dizziness, drowsiness (avoid driving or the use of dangerous machinery); numbness, tingling, feelings of tightness or pressure.
- Contact physician immediately if you experience severe or continuous chest pain or pressure.
- Report feelings of heat, flushing, tiredness, feelings of sickness, swelling of lips or eyelids.

# tacrine hydrochloride

*(tay' krin)*

tetrahydroaminoacridine, THA

Cognex

**Pregnancy Category C**

**Drug classes**

Cholinesterase inhibitor
Alzheimer's drug

**Therapeutic actions**

Centrally acting reversible cholinesterase inhibitor, leading to elevated acetylcholine levels in the cortex, which slows the neuronal degradation that occurs in Alzheimer's disease.

**Indications**

- Treatment of mild to moderate dementia of the Alzheimer's type

**Contraindications/cautions**

- Contraindications: allergy to tacrine or acridine derivatives, previous tacrine-associated jaundice, pregnancy.
- Use cautiously with renal or hepatic disease; bladder obstruction; seizure conditions; sick sinus syndrome; GI bleeding; anesthesia.

### Dosage

**Available Forms:** Capsules—10, 20, 30, 40 mg

*ADULT:* 10 mg PO qid; maintain this dose for 6 wk with regular monitoring of transaminase levels; after 6 wk, increase dose to 20 mg PO qid; if patient is tolerant to drug and transaminase levels are WNL, increase at 6-wk intervals at 10-mg increases to a total of 120–160 mg/d.

*PEDIATRIC:* Safety and efficacy not established.

**Pharmacokinetics**

| *Route* | *Onset* | *Peak* |
|---|---|---|
| Oral | Varies | 1–2 h |

*Metabolism:* Hepatic, $T_{1/2}$: 2–4 h
*Distribution:* Crosses placenta; may enter breast milk
*Excretion:* Urine

**Adverse effects**

- CNS: *Headache, fatigue, dizziness, confusion,* ataxia, insomnia, somnolence, tremor, agitation, depression, anxiety, abnormal thinking
- GI: *Nausea, vomiting, diarrhea, dyspepsia, anorexia, abdominal pain*, flatulence, constipation, **hepatotoxicity**
- Respiratory: *Rhinitis*, upper respiratory infections, coughing
- GU: Urinary frequency, urinary tract infections
- Dermatologic: *Skin rash*, flushing, purpura

**Clinically important drug-drug interactions**

- Increased effects and risk of toxicity of theophylline, cholinesterase inhibitors
- Decreased effects of anticholinergics
- Increased effects with cimetidine

**Clinically important drug-food interactions**

- Decreased absorption and serum levels of tacrine if taken with food

## ■ Nursing Considerations

### Assessment

- *History:* Allergy to tacrine or acridine derivatives, previous tacrine-associated jaundice; pregnancy; renal or hepatic disease; bladder obstruction; seizure conditions; sick sinus syndrome; GI bleed; anesthesia
- *Physical:* Orientation, affect, reflexes; BP, P; R, adventitious sounds; urinary output; abdominal exam; renal and liver function tests; serum transaminase levels

### Implementation

- Arrange for regular transaminase level determination before and during therapy.
- Use with great care in patients with any history of hepatic dysfunction.
- Administer around the clock at regular intervals for best results.
- Administer on an empty stomach, 1 h before or 2 h after meals.
- Administer with meals only if severe GI upset occurs.
- Decrease dose and slowly discontinue drug if side effects become severe.
- Notify surgeons that patient is on tacrine; exaggerated muscle relaxation may occur if succinylcholine-type drugs are used.
- Do not suddenly discontinue high doses of drug.
- Monitor for any signs of neurologic change or deterioration; drug does not stop the disease but slows the degeneration.

### Drug-specific teaching points

- Take drug exactly as prescribed, around the clock. Work with your nurse to establish a schedule that is least disruptive. Do not take more than the prescribed dose.
- Take drug on an empty stomach, 1 h before or 2 h after meals. If severe GI upset occurs, drug may be taken with meals.
- This drug does not cure the disease but is thought to slow down the degeneration associated with the disease.
- Arrange for regular blood tests and follow-up visits while adjusting to this drug.
- The following side effects may occur: nausea, vomiting (small, frequent meals may help); dizziness, confusion, lightheadedness (use caution if driving or performing tasks that require alertness).
- Report nausea, vomiting, changes in stool or urine color, diarrhea, rash, changes in neurologic functioning, yellowing of eyes or skin.

## tacrolimus

*(tack row' lim us)*
FK506
Prograf
**Pregnancy Category C**

t

### Drug classes
Immunosuppressant

### Therapeutic actions
Immunosuppressant; inhibits T-lymphocyte activation; exact mechanism of action not known but binds to intracellular protein, which may prevent the generation of nuclear factor of activated T cells and suppresses the immune activation and response of T cells.

### Indications
- Prophylaxis for organ rejection in liver transplants in conjunction with adrenal corticosteroids
- Unlabeled use: prophylaxis in kidney, bone marrow, cardiac, pancreas, pancreatic island cell, and small bowel transplantation; treatment of autoimmune disease; recalcitrant psoriasis

### Contraindications/cautions
- Contraindications: allergy to tacrolimus, hypersensitibity to HCO-60 polyoxyl 60 hydrogenated castor oil, pregnancy, lactation.
- Use cautiously with impaired renal function, hypokalemia, malabsorption.

### Dosage
**Available Forms:** Capsules—1, 5 mg; injection—5 mg/ml

ADULT

- ***Oral:*** 0.15–0.3 mg/kg per day; administer inital dose no sooner than 6 h after transplant; divide into two doses given q12h. If transferring from IV, give first dose 8–12 h after discontinuing IV infusion. Titrate dose based on clinical assessment of rejection tolerance of drug.
- ***Parenteral:*** Patients unable to take capsules; 0.05–0.1 mg/kg per day as continuous IV infusion begun no sooner than 6 h after transplant. Switch to oral drug as soon as possible.

PEDIATRIC: Children require the larger dose; begin treatment at higher end of recommended adult dose.

### Pharmacokinetics

| *Route* | *Onset* | *Peak* |
|---|---|---|
| Oral | Varies | 1 1/2–3 1/2 h |
| IV | Rapid | 1–2 h |

*Metabolism:* Hepatic, $T_{1/2}$: 5.7 h then 11.7 h
*Distribution:* Crosses placenta; enters breast milk
*Excretion:* Bile and urine

### IV facts
**Preparation:** Dilute IV solution immediately before use; use 0.9% Sodium Chloride Injection or 5% Dextrose Injection to a concentration of 0.004 and 0.02 mg/ml. Do not store in a PVC container; discard after 24 h.
**Infusion:** Give by continuous IV infusion using an infusion pump.

### Adverse effects
- CNS: *Tremor*, *headache, insomnia*, paresthesias
- GI: **Hepatotoxicity**, *constipation, diarrhea, nausea, vomiting*, anorexia
- CV: Hypertension
- Hematologic: Leukopenia, anemia, hyperkalemia, hypokalemia, hyperglycemia
- GU: *Renal dysfunction*, nephrotoxicity, UTI, oliguria
- Other: Abdominal pain, pain, fever, asthenia, back pain, ascites, neoplasias

### Clinically important drug-drug interactions
• Increased risk of nephrotoxicity with other nephrotoxic agents (erythromycin) • Risk of severe myopathy or rhabdomyolysis with lovastatin • Increased risk of toxicity with diltiazem, metoclopramide, nicardipine, cimetidine, clarithromycin, calcium channel-blockers • Decreased therapeutic effect with carbamazeine, phenobarbital, phenytoin, rifamycins

## ■ Nursing Considerations

### Assessment
- *History:* Allergy to tacrolimus or polyoxyethylated castor oil, impaired renal function, malabsorption, lactation

- *Physical:* T; skin color, lesions; BP, peripheral perfusion; liver evaluation, bowel sounds, gum evaluation; renal and liver function tests, CBC

### Implementation

- Use parenteral administration only if patient is unable to take the oral solution; transfer to oral solution as soon as possible.
- Monitor renal and liver function tests before and periodically during therapy; marked decreases in function may require dosage changes or discontinuation.
- Monitor liver function and hematologic tests to determine titration dosage.

### Drug-specific teaching points

- Avoid infections; avoid crowds or people with infections. Notify your health care provider at once if you injure yourself.
- The following side effects may occur: nausea, vomiting (take drug with food); diarrhea; headache (request analgesics).
- This drug should not be taken during pregnancy. If you think that you are pregnant or you want to become pregnant, discuss this with your prescriber.
- Arrange to have periodic blood tests to monitor drug response and effects.
- Do not discontinue without your prescriber's advice.
- Report unusual bleeding or bruising, fever, sore throat, mouth sores, tiredness.

## tamoxifen citrate

*(ta* ***mox'*** *i fen)*

Alpha-Tamoxifen (CAN), Apo-Tamoxifen (CAN), Nolvadex, Novo-Tamoxifen (CAN), Tamofen (CAN), Tamone (CAN), Tamoplex (CAN)

**Pregnancy Category D**

### Drug classes

Antiestrogen

### Therapeutic actions

Potent antiestrogenic effects: competes with estrogen for binding sites in target tissues, such as the breast.

### Indications

- Adjunct with cytotoxic chemotherapy following radical or modified radical mastectomy to delay recurrence of surgically curable breast cancer in postmenopausal women or women >50 y with positive axillary nodes
- Treatment of advanced, metastatic breast cancer in women and men; alternative to oophorectomy or ovarian radiation in premenopausal women
- Unlabeled uses: treatment of mastalgia; useful for decreasing size and pain of gynecomastia; preventive therapy for women at high risk of breast cancer; treatment of pancreatic, endometrial, and hepatocellular carcinoma

### Contraindications/cautions

- Allergy to tamoxifen, pregnancy, lactation.

### Dosage

**Available Forms:** Tablets—10, 20 mg

*ADULT:* 10–20 mg bid PO given morning and evening, or 20 mg PO qd.

### Pharmacokinetics

| Route | Onset | Peak |
|---|---|---|
| Oral | Varies | 4–7 h |

*Metabolism:* Hepatic, $T_{1/2}$: 7–14 d

*Distribution:* Crosses placenta; enters breast milk

*Excretion:* Feces

### Adverse effects

- CNS: Depression, lightheadedness, dizziness, headache, corneal opacity, decreased visual acuity, retinopathy
- GI: *Nausea, vomiting,* food distaste
- **Hematologic**: Hypercalcemia, especially with bone metastases, thrombocytopenia, leukopenia, anemia
- GU: *Vaginal bleeding, vaginal discharge, menstrual irregularities,* pruritus vulvae
- **Dermatologic**: *Hot flashes, skin rash*
- **Other**: Peripheral edema; increased bone and tumor pain and local disease (initially seen with a good tumor response, usually subsides); cancer in animal studies

t

### Clinically important drug-drug interactions
• Increased risk of bleeding with oral anticoagulants • Increased serum levels with bromocriptine

### Drug-lab test interferences
• Possible increase in calcium levels, $T_4$ levels without hyperthyroidism

## ■ Nursing Considerations

### Assessment
- *History:* Allergy to tamoxifen, pregnancy, lactation
- *Physical:* Skin lesions, color, turgor; pelvic exam; orientation, affect, reflexes; ophthalmologic exam; peripheral pulses, edema; liver function tests, CBC and differential, estrogen receptor evaluation of tumor cells

### Implementation
- Administer bid, in the morning and the evening.
- Arrange for periodic blood counts.
- Arrange for initial ophthalmologic exam and periodic exams if visual changes occur.
- Counsel patient to use contraception while taking this drug; inform patient that serious fetal harm could occur.
- Decrease dosage if adverse effects become severe.

### Drug-specific teaching points
- Take the drug twice a day, in the morning and evening.
- The following side effects may occur: bone pain; hot flashes (staying in cool temperatures may help); nausea, vomiting (small, frequent meals may help); weight gain; menstrual irregularities; dizziness, headache, lightheadedness (use caution if driving or performing tasks that require alertness).
- This drug can cause serious fetal harm and must not be taken during pregnancy. Contraceptive measures should be used. If you become pregnant or decide that you would like to become pregnant, consult with your health care provider immediately.
- Report marked weakness, sleepiness, mental confusion, pain or swelling of the legs, shortness of breath, blurred vision.

# tamsulosin hydrochloride

*(tam soo **low'** sin)*

Flomax

**Pregnancy Category B**

### Drug classes
Alpha adrenergic blocker

### Therapeutic actions
Blocks the smooth muscle alpha-1-adrenergic receptors in the prostate, prostatic capsule, prostatic urethra, and bladder neck, leading to relaxation of the bladder and prostate and improving the flow of urine in cases of benign prostatic hypertrophy.

### Indications
- Treatment of the signs and symptoms of benign prostatic hypertrophy

### Contraindications/cautions
- Contraindications: prostatic cancer, pregnancy, lactation.
- Use cautiously with allergy to tamsulosin.

### Dosage
**Available Forms:** Capsules—0.4 mg

*ADULT:* 0.4 mg PO qd 30 min after the same meal each day; if response is not satisfactory in 2–4 wk, dosage may be increased to 0.8 mg PO qd 30 min after the same meal each day.

*PEDIATRIC:* Safety and efficacy not established.

### Pharmacokinetics

| Route | Onset | Peak |
|---|---|---|
| Oral | Varies | 4–6 h |

*Metabolism:* Hepatic; $T_{1/2}$: 9–13 h

*Distribution:* Crosses placenta; passes into breast milk

*Excretion:* Urine and feces

### Adverse effects

- CNS: *Somnolence, insomnia,* amblyopia
- GI: *Nausea,* dyspepsia
- CV: *Orthostatic hypotension,* syncope
- GU: *Abnormal ejaculation, decreased libido,* increased urinary frequency
- Other: Cough, sinusitis, rhinitis

### Clinically important drug-drug interactions

• Increased hypotensive effects with other alpha-adrenergic antagonists • Risk of increased toxic effects of cimetidine, warfarin

## ■ Nursing Considerations

### Assessment

- *History:* Allergy to tamsulosin, pregnancy, lactation, prostatic cancer
- *Physical:* Body weight; skin color, lesions; orientation, affect, reflexes; ophthalmologic exam; P, BP, orthostatic BP; R, adventitious sounds, status of nasal mucous membranes; voiding pattern, normal output, urinalysis

### Implementation

- Ensure that patient does not have prostatic cancer before beginning treatment.
- Administer once a day, 30 min after the same meal each day.
- Resume therapy at 0.4 mg qd if therapy is interrupted for any reason.
- Ensure that patient does not crush, chew, or open capsule. Capsule should be swallowed whole.
- Monitor patient carefully for orthostatic hypotension; chance of orthostatic hypotension, dizziness, and syncope is high with the first dose. Establish safety precautions as appropriate.

### Drug-specific teaching points

- Take this drug exactly as prescribed, once a day. Do not chew, crush, or open capsules; capsules must be swallowed whole. Use care when beginning therapy; the chance of dizziness or syncope is greatest at that time. Change position slowly to avoid increased dizziness. Take the drug 30 min after the same meal each day.
- The following side effects may occur: dizziness, weakness (more likely when you change position, in the early morning, after exercise, in hot weather, and when you have consumed alcohol; some tolerance may occur after you have taken the drug for a while; avoid driving or engaging in tasks that require alertness; change position slowly, use caution in climbing stairs, lie down if dizziness persists); GI upset (eat small, frequent meals); impotence (discuss this with your nurse or physician); stuffy nose. Most of these effects will disappear gradually with continued therapy.
- Report frequent dizziness or fainting, worsening of symptoms.

## temazepam

*(te **maz'** e pam)*

Restoril

**Pregnancy Category X**
**C-IV controlled substance**

### Drug classes

Benzodiazepine
Sedative/hypnotic

### Therapeutic actions

Exact mechanisms of action not understood; acts mainly at subcortical levels of the CNS, leaving the cortex relatively unaffected; main sites of action may be the limbic system and mesencephalic reticular formation; benzodiazepines potentiate the effects of gamma-aminobutyrate (GABA), an inhibitory neurotransmitter.

### Indications

- Insomnia characterized by difficulty falling asleep, frequent nocturnal awakenings, or early morning awakening
- Recurring insomnia or poor sleeping habits
- Acute or chronic medical situations requiring restful sleep

### Contraindications/cautions

- Contraindications: hypersensitivity to benzodiazepines, psychoses, acute narrow-angle glaucoma, shock, coma, acute al-

coholic intoxication with depression of vital signs, pregnancy (risk of congenital malformations, neonatal withdrawal syndrome), labor and delivery ("floppy infant" syndrome), lactation (infants may become lethargic and lose weight).
- Use cautiously with impaired liver or kidney function, debilitation, depression, suicidal tendencies.

### Dosage

**Available Forms:** Capsules—7.5, 15, 30 mg

*ADULT:* 15–30 mg PO before retiring.

*PEDIATRIC:* Not for use in children <18 y.

*GERIATRIC PATIENTS OR THOSE WITH DEBILITATING DISEASE:* Initially 15 mg PO; adjust dosage until individual response is determined.

### Pharmacokinetics

| Route | Onset | Peak |
|---|---|---|
| Oral | Varies | 2–4 h |

*Metabolism:* Hepatic, $T_{1/2}$: 9.5–12.4 h

*Distribution:* Crosses placenta; enters breast milk

*Excretion:* Urine

### Adverse effects

- CNS: *Transient, mild drowsiness initially; sedation, depression, lethargy, apathy, fatigue, lightheadedness, disorientation, restlessness, confusion*, crying, delirium, headache, slurred speech, dysarthria, stupor, rigidity, tremor, dystonia, vertigo, euphoria, nervousness, difficulty concentrating, vivid dreams, psychomotor retardation, extrapyramidal symptoms, *mild paradoxical excitatory reactions during first 2 wk of treatment* (especially in psychiatric patients, aggressive children, and with high dosage), visual and auditory disturbances, diplopia, nystagmus, depressed hearing, nasal congestion
- GI: *Constipation, diarrhea,* dry mouth, salivation, nausea, anorexia, vomiting, difficulty in swallowing, gastric disorders, elevations of blood enzymes: hepatic dysfunction, jaundice
- CV: *Bradycardia, tachycardia*, CV collapse, hypertension and hypotension, palpitations, edema
- Hematologic: Decreased Hct (primarily with long-term therapy), blood dyscrasias
- GU: *Incontinence, urinary retention, changes in libido*, menstrual irregularities
- Dermatologic: Urticaria, pruritus, skin rash, dermatitis
- Dependence: *Drug dependence with withdrawal syndrome* when drug is discontinued
- Other: Hiccups, fever, diaphoresis, paresthesias, muscular disturbances, gynecomastia

### Clinically important drug-drug interactions

- Increased CNS depression with alcohol
- Decreased sedative effects with theophylline, aminophylline, dyphylline, oxitriphylline

## ■ Nursing Considerations

### Assessment

- *History:* Hypersensitivity to benzodiazepines, psychoses, acute narrow-angle glaucoma, shock, coma, acute alcoholic intoxication, pregnancy, lactation, impaired liver or kidney function, debilitation, depression, suicidal tendencies
- *Physical:* Skin color, lesions; T; orientation, reflexes, affect, ophthalmologic exam; P, BP; R, adventitious sounds; liver evaluation, abdominal exam, bowel sounds, normal output; CBC, liver and renal function tests

### Implementation

- Taper dosage gradually after long-term therapy, especially in epileptic patients.

### Drug-specific teaching points

- Take drug exactly as prescribed.
- Do not stop taking this drug (long-term therapy) without consulting your health care provider.
- Avoid pregnancy while taking this drug; use of contraceptive measures is advised; serious fetal harm could occur.

- The following side effects may occur: drowsiness, dizziness (may lessen; avoid driving or engaging in other dangerous activities); GI upset (take drug with water); depression, dreams, emotional upset, crying.
- Nocturnal sleep may be disturbed for several nights after discontinuing the drug.
- Report severe dizziness, weakness, drowsiness that persists, rash or skin lesions, palpitations, swelling of the extremities, visual changes, difficulty voiding.

## teniposide

*(teh **nip'** oh side)*

VM-26

Vumon

**Pregnancy Category D**

### Drug classes

Mitotic inhibitor
Antineoplastic

### Therapeutic actions

Late $S_2$ and early $G_2$ specific cell toxic: lyses cells entering mitosis; inhibits cells from entering prophase; inhibits DNA synthesis, leading to cell death.

### Indications

- In combination with other anticancer drugs for induction therapy with refractory childhood acute lymphoblastic leukemia

### Contraindications/cautions

- Allergy to teniposide, *Cremophor EL*, bone marrow suppression, pregnancy, lactation.

### Dosage

**Available Forms:** Injection—10 mg/ml

Modify dosage based on myelosuppression.

**PEDIATRIC:** 165 $mg/m^2$ teniposide in combination with 300 $mg/m^2$ cytarabine IV twice weekly for eight to nine doses or 250 $mg/m^2$ teniposide in combination with 1.5 $mg/m^2$ vincristine IV weekly for 4–8 wk and prednisone 40 $mg/m^2$ orally for 28 d.

*Renal/hepatic impairment:* Reduced dosage may be necessary.

*Down's syndrome:* Reduce initial dosings; give the first course at half the usual dose.

### Pharmacokinetics

| *Route* | *Onset* | *Peak* |
|---|---|---|
| IV | 30 min | 60 min |

*Metabolism:* Hepatic, $T_{1/2}$: 5 h

*Distribution:* Crosses placenta; enters breast milk

*Excretion:* Urine and bile

### IV facts

**Preparation:** Dilute with 5% Dextrose Injection or 0.9% Sodium Chloride Injection to give a concentration of 0.1, 0.2, 0.4, or 1 mg/ml. Use of glass or polyolefin plastic bags is recommended; PVC containers may crack or break; diluted solutions are stable for 24 h at room temperature.

**Infusion:** Administer slowly over 30–60 min or longer. *Do not give by rapid IV infusion.*

**Compatibilities:** Heparin may cause precipitation; do not mix with other drugs or in other solutions.

### Adverse effects

- CNS: *Somnolence, fatigue,* peripheral neuropathy
- GI: *Nausea, vomiting, anorexia, diarrhea*, stomatitis, aftertaste, liver toxicity
- CV: Hypotension (after rapid IV administration)
- Hematologic: *Myelosuppression*
- Dermatologic: *Alopecia*
- Hypersensitivity: Chills, fever, tachycardia, bronchospasm, dyspnea, anaphylactic-like reaction
- Other: Potentially, carcinogenesis

## ■ Nursing Considerations

### Assessment

- ***History:*** Allergy to teniposide, *Cremophor EL*; bone marrow suppression; pregnancy; lactation
- ***Physical:*** T; weight; hair; orientation, reflexes; BP, P; mucous membranes, abdominal exam; CBC

t

### Implementation

- Do not administer IM or SC because severe local reaction and tissue necrosis occur.
- Avoid skin contact with this drug. The use of rubber gloves is advised; if contact occurs, immediately wash with soap and water.
- Monitor blood pressure during administration; if hypotension occurs, discontinue dose and consult with physician. Fluids and other supportive therapy may be needed.
- Monitor patient before starting therapy and prior to each dose: platelet count, Hgb, WBC count, differential. If severe response occurs, discontinue therapy and consult with physician.

### Drug-specific teaching points

- Prepare a calendar showing return dates for specific treatments and additional courses of therapy.
- The following side effects may occur: loss of appetite, nausea, vomiting, mouth sores (frequent mouth care, small, frequent meals may help; maintain good nutrition; request an antiemetic); loss of hair (obtain a wig or other suitable head covering before the hair loss occurs; keep the head covered in extremes of temperature).
- Have regular blood tests to monitor the drug's effects.
- Report severe GI upset, diarrhea, vomiting, unusual bleeding or bruising, fever, chills, sore throat, difficulty breathing.

## terazosin hydrochloride

*(ter **ay'** zoe sin)*
Hytrin

### Drug classes

Antihypertensive
Alpha adrenergic blocker

### Therapeutic actions

Selectively blocks postsynaptic $alpha_1$-adrenergic receptors, decreasing sympathetic tone on the vasculature, dilating arterioles and veins, and lowering supine and standing BP; unlike conventional alpha-adrenergic blocking agents (eg, phentolamine), it does not also block $alpha_2$ presynaptic receptors, does not cause reflex tachycardia.

### Indications

- Treatment of hypertension
- Treatment of symptomatic benign prostatic hyperplasia (BPH)

### Contraindications/cautions

- Contraindications: hypersensitivity to terazosin, lactation.
- Use cautiously with CHF, renal failure, pregnancy.

### Dosage

**Available Forms:** Capsules—1, 2, 5, 10 mg; tablets (CAN)—1, 2, 5, 10 mg
Adjust dosage at 12- or 24-h intervals.

**ADULT**

- *Hypertension:* 1 mg PO hs. Do not exceed 1 mg; strictly adhere to this regimen to avoid severe hypotensive reactions. Slowly increase dose to achieve desired BP response. Usual range, 1–5 mg PO qd. Up to 20 mg/d has been beneficial. Monitor BP 2–3 h after dosing to determine maximum effect. If response is diminished after 24 h, consider increasing dosage. If drug is not taken for several days, restart with initial 1-mg dose.
- *BPH:* Initial dose, 1 mg PO hs. Increase to 2, 5, or 10 mg PO qd. 10 mg/d for 4–6 wk may be required to assess benefit.

**PEDIATRIC:** Safety and efficacy not established.

### Pharmacokinetics

| Route | Onset | Peak |
|---|---|---|
| Oral | Varies | 1–2 h |

*Metabolism:* Hepatic, $T_{1/2}$: 9–12 h
*Distribution:* Crosses placenta; enters breast milk
*Excretion:* Feces and urine

### Adverse effects

- CNS: *Dizziness, headache, drowsiness, lack of energy, weakness, somnolence,* nervousness, vertigo, depression, paresthesia
- GI: *Nausea,* vomiting, diarrhea, constipation, abdominal discomfort or pain

- **CV**: *Palpitations*, sodium and water retention, increased plasma volume, *edema*, syncope, tachycardia, orthostatic hypotension, angina
- **Respiratory**: *Dyspnea, nasal congestion, sinusitis*
- **GU**: Urinary frequency, incontinence, impotence, priapism
- **EENT**: Blurred vision, reddened sclera, epistaxis, tinnitus, dry mouth, nasal congestion
- **Dermatologic**: Rash, pruritus, alopecia, lichen planus
- **Other**: Diaphoresis, lupus erythematosus

## ■ Nursing Considerations

### Assessment

- ***History:*** Hypersensitivity to terazosin, CHF, renal failure, pregnancy, lactation
- ***Physical:*** Weight; skin color, lesions; orientation, affect, reflexes; ophthalmologic exam; P, BP, orthostatic BP, supine BP, perfusion, edema, auscultation; R, adventitious sounds, status of nasal mucous membranes; bowel sounds, normal output; voiding pattern, urinary output; kidney function tests, urinalysis

### Implementation

- Administer or have patient take first dose just before bedtime to lessen likelihood of first dose effect, syncope, believed due to excessive postural hypotension.
- Have patient lie down, and treat supportively if syncope occurs; condition is self-limiting.
- Monitor patient for orthostatic hypotension, which is most marked in the morning, is accentuated by hot weather, alcohol, exercise.
- Monitor edema, weight in patients with incipient cardiac decompensation, and add a thiazide diuretic to the drug regimen if sodium and fluid retention, signs of impending CHF occur.

### Drug-specific teaching points

- Take this drug exactly as prescribed. Take the first dose just before bedtime. Do not drive or operate machinery for 4 h after the first dose.
- The following side effects may occur: dizziness, weakness (more likely to occur when you change position, in the early morning, after exercise, in hot weather, and when you have consumed alcohol; some tolerance may occur after you have taken the drug for a while, but you should avoid driving or engaging in tasks that require alertness; change position slowly, and use caution when climbing stairs; lie down for a while if dizziness persists); GI upset (frequent, small meals may help); impotence; dry mouth (sucking on sugarless lozenges, ice chips may help); stuffy nose. Most effects will gradually disappear.
- Report frequent dizziness or faintness.

# terbutaline sulfate

*(ter **byoo'** ta leen)*

Brethaire, Brethine, Bricanyl

**Pregnancy Category B**

### Drug classes

Sympathomimetic
Beta-2 selective adrenergic agonist
Bronchodilator
Antiasthmatic agent
Tocolytic agent

### Therapeutic actions

In low doses, acts relatively selectively at $beta_2$-adrenergic receptors to cause bronchodilation and relax the pregnant uterus; at higher doses, $beta_2$ selectivity is lost and the drug acts at $beta_1$ receptors to cause typical sympathomimetic cardiac effects.

### Indications

- Prophylaxis and treatment of bronchial asthma and reversible bronchospasm that may occur with bronchitis and emphysema
- Unlabeled oral and IV use: inhibition of premature labor

### Contraindications/cautions

- Contraindications: hypersensitivity to terbutaline; tachyarrhythmias, tachycardia caused by digitalis intoxication; general anesthesia with halogenated hydrocarbons or cyclopropane, which sensitize the myocardium to catecholamines; unstable vasomotor system disorders; hypertension; pregnancy; labor and delivery (may inhibit labor; parenteral use of beta-adrenergic agonists can accelerate fetal heart beat, cause hypoglycemia, hypokalemia, and pulmonary edema in the mother and hypoglycemia in the neonate); lactation.

- Use cautiously with coronary insufficiency, CAD, history of stroke, COPD patients who have developed degenerative heart disease, hyperthyroidism, history of seizure disorders, psychoneurotic individuals.

### Dosage

**Available Forms:** Tablets—2.5, 5 mg; aerosol—0.2 mg/actuation; injection—1 mg/ml

*ADULT AND PEDIATRIC > 12 Y*

- ***Oral:*** 5 mg at 6-h intervals tid during waking hours. If side effects are pronounced, reduce to 2.5 mg tid. Do not exceed 15 mg/d.
- ***Parenteral***
- *Bronchospasm:* 0.25 mg SC into lateral deltoid area. If no significant improvement in 15 min, give another 0.25-mg dose. Do not exceed 0.5 mg/4 h. If patient fails to respond to second 0.25-mg dose within 15–30 min, other therapeutic measures should be considered.
- *Delay of premature labor:* Initiate IV administration at 10 μg/min. Titrate upward to a maximum of 80 μg/min. Maintain at minimum effective dosage for 4 h. Oral doses of 2.5 mg q4–6h have been used as maintenance therapy until term.
- ***Inhalation (each actuation of aerosol dispenser delivers 0.2 mg terbutaline):*** Two inhalations separated by 60 sec q4–6h. Do not repeat more often than q4–6h.

*PEDIATRIC*

- *<12 Y:* Safety and efficacy not established.

*GERIATRIC:* Patients >60 y are likely to experience adverse effects. Avoid use or use with extreme caution.

### IV facts

**Preparation:** Use of a volume delivery system is suggested; dilute as required in $D_5W$.

**Infusion:** Infuse at rate of up to 80 μg/min for up to 4 h.

### Adverse effects

- CNS: *Restlessness, apprehension, anxiety, fear,* CNS stimulation, hyperkinesia, insomnia, tremor, drowsiness, irritability, weakness, vertigo, headache
- GI: *Nausea,* vomiting, heartburn, unusual or bad taste
- CV: *Cardiac arrhythmias, palpitations,* anginal pain (less likely with bronchodilator doses of this drug than with bronchodilator doses of a nonselective beta-agonist (isoproterenol), changes in BP
- Respiratory: *Respiratory difficulties,* **pulmonary edema,** *coughing,* bronchospasm, paradoxical airway resistance with repeated, excessive use of inhalation preparations
- Other: Sweating, pallor, flushing

### Clinically important drug-drug interactions

- Increased likelihood of cardiac arrhythmias with halogenated hydrocarbon anesthetics (halothane), cyclopropane

## ■ Nursing Considerations

### Assessment

- *History:* Hypersensitivity to terbutaline; tachyarrhythmias; general anesthesia with halogenated hydrocarbons or cyclopropane; unstable vasomotor system disorders; hypertension; CAD; history of stroke; COPD patients who have developed degenerative heart disease; hyperthyroidism; history of seizure disorders; psychoneurotic individuals; pregnancy; labor and delivery; lactation
- *Physical:* Weight; skin color, temperature, turgor; orientation, reflexes; P, BP; R, adventitious sounds; blood and urine

glucose; serum electrolytes; thyroid function tests; ECG

### Implementation

- Use minimal doses for minimal periods of time; drug tolerance can occur with prolonged use.
- Maintain a beta-adrenergic blocker (a cardioselective beta-blocker, such as atenolol, should be used in patients with respiratory distress) on standby in case cardiac arrhythmias occur.
- Do not exceed recommended dosage; administer aerosol during second half of inspiration, because the airways are open wider and distribution is more extensive.

### Drug-specific teaching points

- Do not exceed recommended dosage; adverse effects or loss of effectiveness may result. Read product instructions, and ask your health care provider or pharmacist if you have any questions.
- The following side effects may occur: weakness, dizziness, inability to sleep (use caution when driving or performing activities that require alertness); nausea, vomiting (small, frequent meals may help); fast heart rate, anxiety.
- Report chest pain, dizziness, insomnia, weakness, tremor or irregular heartbeat, failure to respond to usual dosage.

## terpin hydrate

*(ter' pin)*

**Pregnancy Category C**

### Drug classes

Antitussive
Expectorant

### Therapeutic actions

Directly stimulates the respiratory tract secretory glands, increasing the production of respiratory fluids; used mainly as an ingredient in cough medications.

### Indications

- Symptomatic relief of dry, nonproductive cough

### Contraindications/cautions

- Contraindications: diabetes, peptic ulcer, pregnancy, lactation.
- Use cautiously with history of alcohol dependence.

### Dosage

**Available Forms:** Elixir—85 mg/5 ml

*ADULT:* 85–170 mg PO tid–qid.

*PEDIATRIC*

- *1–4 Y:* 20 mg PO tid–qid.
- *5–9 Y:* 40 mg PO tid–qid.
- *10–12 Y:* 85 mg PO tid–qid.

### Pharmacokinetics

Not reported.

### Adverse effects

- CNS: *Drowsiness, dizziness*
- GI: Nausea, vomiting, abdominal pain

## ■ Nursing Considerations

### Assessment

- *History:* Diabetes, peptic ulcer, alcohol abuse, pregnancy, lactation
- *Physical:* R, adventitious sounds; abdominal exam

### Implementation

- Administer with food if severe GI upset occurs.
- Do not give water after administration to make the most of soothing effects.
- Ensure that patient is well hydrated during treatment; humidifier may be helpful in increasing bronchial secretions.

### Drug-specific teaching points

- Take this drug with food if severe GI upset occurs.
- Do not exceed recommended dose.
- The following side effects may occur: drowsiness, dizziness (do not drive or operate dangerous machinery).
- Drink plently of fluids, and consider the use of a humidifier to help facilitate relief of bronchial irritation.
- Report vomiting, worsening of condition being treated, abdominal pain.

# testolactone

*(tess toe **lak'** tone)*

Teslac

**Pregnancy Category C**

## Drug classes

Androgen
Hormone
Antineoplastic

## Therapeutic actions

Synthetic androgen; endogenous androgens are responsible for growth and development of male sex organs and the maintenance of secondary sex characteristics; administration of androgen derivatives increases the retention of nitrogen, sodium, potassium, phosphorus, and decreases urinary excretion of calcium; increases protein anabolism and decreases protein catabolism; stimulates the production of red blood cells; exact mechanism by which antineoplastic effects are exerted is not known.

## Indications

- Palliation of advanced disseminated metastatic breast carcinoma in postmenopausal women when hormonal therapy is indicated
- Disseminated breast carcinoma in premenopausal women in whom ovarian function has been subsequently terminated

## Contraindications/cautions

- Contraindications: known sensitivity to androgens, pregnancy, lactation, carcinoma of the breast in males.
- Use cautiously with liver disease, cardiac disease, nephritis, nephrosis.

## Dosage

**Available Forms:** Tablets—50 mg

*ADULT:* 250 mg PO qid. Continue therapy for a minimum of 3 mo unless there is active disease progression.

*PEDIATRIC:* Safety and efficacy not established.

## Pharmacokinetics

| Route | Onset |
|---|---|
| Oral | Rapid |

*Metabolism:* Hepatic, $T_{1/2}$: unknown
*Distribution:* Crosses placenta; enters breast milk
*Excretion:* Urine

## Adverse effects

- CNS: *Paresthesias*
- GI: *Nausea, vomiting, anorexia, glossitis*, diarrhea, loss appetite, swelling of the tongue
- CV: Hypertension
- **Hematologic**: Hypercalcemia
- **Dermatologic**: Rash, dermatitis, aches of the extremities, edema
- **Virilization**: Hirsutism, hoarseness, deepening of the voice, clitoral enlargement, facial hair growth, affected libido

## ■ Nursing Considerations

### Assessment

- ***History:*** Known sensitivity to androgens, liver or cardiac disease, nephritis, nephrosis, carcinoma of the breast, pregnancy, lactation
- ***Physical:*** Skin color, lesions, texture; hair distribution pattern; P, auscultation; abdominal exam, liver evaluation, mucous membranes; serum electrolytes, liver and renal function tests

### Implementation

- Monitor tumor progression periodically.
- Monitor for occurrence of edema; arrange for diuretic therapy as needed.
- Arrange for periodic monitoring of urine and serum calcium during treatment of disseminated breast carcinoma, and arrange for treatment or discontinuation of the drug if hypercalcemia occurs.

### Drug-specific teaching points

- This drug will need to be taken for long term to evaluate effects.
- The following side effects may occur: body hair growth, baldness, deepening of the voice, loss of appetite, edema or swelling, redness of the tongue.

- This drug is not intended to be taken during pregnancy; serious fetal effects can occur. Use contraceptives during drug treatment.
- Report numbness or tingling of the fingers, toes, face; significant swelling; severe GI upset.

## Testosterone

### testosterone (short-acting)

*(tess **toss'** ter one)*

Histerone, Tesamone

*Transdermal patch:* Testoderm, Andoderm

### testosterone cypionate (long-acting)

dep Andro, Depotest, Depo-Testosterone, Duratest-100

### testosterone enanthate (long-acting)

Andropository, Delatestryl, Durathate-200, Everone

### testosterone propionate (short-acting)

**Pregnancy Category X**

### Drug classes

Androgen
Hormone

### Therapeutic actions

Primary natural androgen; responsible for growth and development of male sex organs and the maintenance of secondary sex characteristics; administration of exogenous testosterone increases the retention of nitrogen, sodium, potassium, phosphorus; decreases urinary excretion of calcium; increases protein anabolism and decreases protein catabolism; stimulates the production of red blood cells.

### Indications

- Replacement therapy in hypogonadism—primary hypogonadism, hypogonadotropic hypogonadism, delayed puberty (men)
- Metastatic cancer, breast cancer in women who are 1–5 y postmenopausal
- Postpartum breast pain/engorgement

### Contraindications/cautions

- Contraindications: known sensitivity to androgens, prostate or breast cancer in males, pregnancy, lactation.
- Use cautiously with MI, liver disease.

### Dosage

**Available Forms:** Short-acting injection—25, 50, 100 mg/ml; long-acting injection—100, 200 mg/ml; transdermal system—2.5, 4, 6 mg/24 h

*Eunuchoidism, eunuchism, postpubertal cryptorchidism for male climateric symptoms, impotence due to:* 25–50 mg IM two to three times per week (testosterone, testosterone propionate).

*Postpartum breast pain/engorgement:* 25–50 mg/d IM for 3–4 d (testosterone propionate).

*Carcinoma of the breast:* 50–100 mg IM three times per week (testosterone, testosterone propionate).

*Male hypogonadism (replacement therapy):* 50–400 mg IM every 2–4 wk (testosterone enanthate, cypionate).

*Males with delayed puberty:* 50–200 mg IM every 2–4 wk for a limited duration (testosterone enanthate, cypionate).

*Primary hypogonadism, hypogonadotropic hypogonadism in males:* Testosterone patch, 4–6 mg/d applied to scrotal skin.

*Palliation of mammary cancer in women:* 200–400 mg IM every 2–4 wk (testosterone enanthate, cypionate).

### Pharmacokinetics

| Route | Onset | Duration |
|---|---|---|
| IM | Slow | 1–3 d |
| IM cypionate | Slow | 2–4 wk |
| IM enanthate | Slow | 2–4 wk |
| IM propionate | Slow | 1–3 d |
| Dermal | Rapid | 2h 4 |

t

*Metabolism:* Hepatic, $T_{1/2}$: 10–100 min; up to 8 d cypionate
*Distribution:* Crosses placenta; enters breast milk
*Excretion:* Urine and feces

### Adverse effects

- CNS: *Dizziness, headache, sleep disorders, fatigue,* tremor, sleeplessness, generalized paresthesia, sleep apnea syndrome, CNS hemorrhage
- GI: *Nausea,* hepatic dysfunction; **hepatocellular carcinoma**
- Hematologic: *Polycythemia, leukopenia,* hypercalcemia, altered serum cholesterol levels, retention of sodium, chloride, water, potassium, phosphates and calcium
- GU: Fluid retention, decreased urinary output
- Dermatologic: *Rash,* dermatitis, anaphylactoid reactions
- Endocrine: *Androgenic effects* (acne, edema, mild hirsutism, decrease in breast size, deepening of the voice, oily skin or hair, weight gain, clitoral hypertrophy or testicular atrophy), *hypoestrogenic effects* (flushing, sweating, vaginitis, nervousness, emotional lability)
- Other: Chills, premature closure of the epiphyses

### Drug-lab test interferences

• Altered glucose tolerance tests • Decrease in thyroid function tests, which may persist for 2–3 wk after therapy • Increased creatinine, creatinine clearance, which may last for 2 wk after therapy

## ■ Nursing Considerations

### Assessment

- ***History:*** Known sensitivity to androgens, prostate or breast cancer in males, MI, liver disease, pregnancy, lactation
- ***Physical:*** Skin color, lesions, texture; hair distribution pattern; injection site; affect, orientation, peripheral sensation; abdominal exam, liver evaluation; serum electrolytes, serum cholesterol levels, liver function tests, glucose tolerance tests, thyroid function tests, long-bone x-ray (in children)

### Implementation

- Apply dermal patch to clean, dry scrotal skin that has been dry shaved. Do not apply elsewhere, and do not use chemical depilatories.
- Inject testosterone deeply into gluteal muscle.
- Shake vials well before use; crystals will redissolve.
- Do not administer frequently; these drugs are absorbed slowly; testosterone enanthate and cypionate are long acting and provide therapeutic effects for about 4 wk.
- Monitor effect on children with long-bone x-rays every 3–6 mo during therapy; discontinue drug well before the bone age reaches the norm for the patient's chronologic age.
- Monitor patient for occurrence of edema; arrange for diuretic therapy as needed.
- Monitor liver function, serum electrolytes periodically during therapy, and consult with physician for corrective measures as needed.
- Periodically measure cholesterol levels in patients who are at high risk for CAD.
- Monitor diabetic patients closely because glucose tolerance may change; adjustments may be needed in insulin, oral hypoglycemic dosage, and diet.
- Periodically monitor urine and serum calcium during treatment of disseminated breast carcinoma, and arrange for appropriate treatment or discontinuation of the drug.
- Monitor geriatric males for prostatic hypertrophy and carcinoma.
- Discontinue drug, and arrange for consultation if abnormal vaginal bleeding occurs.

### Drug-specific teaching points

- This drug can only be given IM. Mark calendar indicating days for injection. Patient receiving the dermal patch must apply the patch to dry, clean scrotal skin that has been dry shaved; do not use chemical depilatories.

- The following side effects may occur: body hair growth, baldness, deepening of the voice, loss of libido, impotence (reversible); excitation, confusion, insomnia (avoid driving or performing tasks that require alertness); swelling of the ankles, fingers (request medication).
- This drug cannot be taken during pregnancy; serious fetal effects could occur. Women should use contraceptive measures.
- Diabetic patients: Monitor urine sugar closely because glucose tolerance may change; report any abnormalities to prescriber, so corrective action can be taken.
- Report ankle swelling; nausea; vomiting; yellowing of skin or eyes; unusual bleeding or bruising; penile swelling or pain; hoarseness, body hair growth, deepening of the voice, acne, menstrual irregularities, pregnancy.

## tetracycline hydrochloride

*(tet ra sye' kleen)*

Cefracycline (CAN), Medicycline (CAN), Neo-Tetrine (CAN), Novotetra (CAN), Panmycin, Sumycin, Tetracap, Tetralean (CAN), Topicycline

**Pregnancy Category D**

### Drug classes
Antibiotic
Tetracycline

### Therapeutic actions
Bacteriostatic: inhibits protein synthesis of susceptible bacteria, preventing cell replication.

### Indications
*Systemic Administration*
- Infections caused by rickettsiae; *Mycoplasma pneumoniae;* agents of psittacosis, ornithosis, lymphogranuloma venereum and granuloma inguinale; *Borrelia recurrentis, Haemophilus ducreyi, Pasteurella pestis, Pasteurella tularensis, Bartonella bacilliformis, Bacteroides, Vibrio comma, Vibrio fetus, Brucella, Escherichia coli, Enterobacter aerogenes, Shigella, Acinetobacter calcoaceticus, Haemophilus influenzae, Klebsiella, Diplococcus pneumoniae, Staphylococcus aureus*
- When penicillin is contraindicated, infections caused by *Neisseria gonorrhoeae, Treponema pallidum, Treponema pertenue, Listeria monocytogenes, Clostridium, Bacillus anthracis, Fusobacterium fusiforme, Actinomyces, Neisseria meningitidis*
- Adjunct to amebicides in acute intestinal amebiasis
- Treatment of acne (oral)
- Uncomplicated urethral, endocervical or rectal infections in adults caused by *Chlamydia trachomatis*
- Instilled in a chest tube, unlabeled use: pleural sclerosing agent in malignant pleural effusions

*Ophthalmic Administration*
- Treatment of superficial ocular infections due to susceptible strains of microorganisms (ophthalmic preparations)
- Prophylaxis of ophthalmia neonatorum due to *N. gonorrrhoeae* or *C. trachomatis* (ophthalmic preparations)

*Topical Administration*
- Treatment of acne vulgaris (topical dermatologic solution)
- Treatment and prophylaxis of minor skin infections due to susceptible organisms (topical dermatologic ointment)

### Contraindications/cautions
- Systemic administration and dermatologic solution: Contraindications: allergy to any of the tetracyclines; allergy to tartrazine (in 250-mg capsules marketed under brand name Panmycin); pregnancy (toxic to the fetus); lactation (causes damage to the teeth of infant).
- Use cautiously with hepatic or renal dysfunction.
- Ophthalmic preparations: Contraindicated in the presence of ocular viral, mycobacterial or fungal infections.

### Dosage
**Available Forms:** Capsules—100, 250, 500 mg; tablets—250, 500 mg; topical so-

lution—2.2 mg/ml; oral suspension—125 mg/5 ml

***Systemic administration***

- *ADULT:* 1–2 g/d PO in two to four equal doses. Up to 500 mg PO qid.
  - *Brucellosis:* 500 mg PO qid for 3 wk with 1 g streptomycin bid IM the first week and qd the second wk.
  - *Syphilis:* 30–40 g PO in divided doses over 10–15 d.
  - *Uncomplicated gonorrhea:* 1.5 g initially, then 500 mg q6h PO to a total of 9 g.
  - *Gonococcal urethritis:* 1.5 g PO initially, then 500 mg q4–6h for 4–6 d.
  - *Severe acne:* 1 g/d PO in divided doses; then 125–500 mg/d.
- *PEDIATRIC*
  - *>8 Y:* 25–50 mg/kg per day PO in four equal doses.

*Topical dermatologic solution:* Apply generously to affected areas bid.

## Pharmacokinetics

| Route | Onset | Peak |
|---|---|---|
| Oral | Varies | 2–4 h |
| Topical: not generally absorbed systemically | | |

*Metabolism:* $T_{1/2}$: 6–12 h

*Distribution:* Crosses placenta; enters breast milk

*Excretion:* Urine

## Adverse effects

*Systemic Administration*

- GI: *Discoloring and inadequate calcification of primary teeth of fetus if used by pregnant women, discoloring and inadequate calcification of permanent teeth if used during period of dental development*, fatty liver, liver failure, *anorexia, nausea, vomiting, diarrhea, glossitis, dysphagia,* enterocolitis, esophageal ulcers
- **Hematologic**: Hemolytic anemia, thrombocytopenia, neutropenia, eosinophilia, leukocytosis, leukopenia
- Dermatologic: *Phototoxic reactions, rash,* exfoliative dermatitis
- Hypersensitivity: Reactions from urticaria to anaphylaxis, including intracranial hypertension
- Other: *Superinfections*, local irritation at parenteral injection sites

*Ophthalmic Preparations*

- Local: *Transient irritation, stinging, itching*, angioneurotic edema, urticaria, dermatitis, superinfections

*Topical Dermatologic Solutions*

- Local: *Stinging, burning during application; skin irritation*; dermatitis; yellowing of areas of application

## Clinically important drug-drug interactions

• Decreased absorption with calcium salts, magnesium salts, zinc salts, aluminum salts, bismuth salts, iron, urinary alkalinizers, food, dairy products, charcoal • Increased digoxin toxicity • Increased nephrotoxicity with methoxyflurane • Decreased effectiveness of oral contraceptives, though rare, has been reported with a risk of breakthrough bleeding or pregnancy • Decreased activity of penicillins

## ■ Nursing Considerations

### Assessment

- *History:* Systemic administration and dermatologic solution: allergy to any of the tetracyclines, tartrazine; hepatic or renal dysfunction, pregnancy, lactation. Ophthalmic preparations: ocular viral, mycobacterial, or fungal infections
- *Physical:* Systemic administration, topical dermatologic solution: site of infection, skin color, lesions; R, adventitious sounds; bowel sounds, output, liver evaluation; urinalysis, BUN, liver and renal function tests. Ophthalmic preparations, dermatologic ointment: site of infection

### Implementation

- Administer oral medication on an empty stomach, 1 h before or 2–3 h after meals. Do not give with antacids. If antacids must be used, give them 3 h after the dose of tetracycline.

- Culture infection before beginning drug therapy.
- Do not use outdated drugs; degraded drug is highly nephrotoxic and should not be used.
- Do not give oral drug with meals, antacids, or food.
- Arrange for regular renal function tests with long-term therapy.
- Use topical preparations of this drug only when clearly indicated. Sensitization from the topical use may preclude its later use in serious infections. Topical preparations containing antibiotics that are not ordinarily given systemically are preferable.

### Drug-specific teaching points

*Oral Preparations*

- Take the drug throughout the day for best results. The drug should be taken on an empty stomach, 1 h before or 2–3 h after meals, with a full glass of water. Do not take the drug with food, dairy products, iron preparations, or antacids.
- Finish your complete prescription; if any is left, discard it immediately. Never take an outdated tetracycline product.
- There have been reports of pregnancy occurring when taking tetracycline with oral contraceptives. To be certain of avoiding pregnancy, use an additional type of contraceptive.
- The following side effects may occur: stomach upset, nausea (reversible); superinfections in the mouth, vagina (frequent washing may help this problem; if severe, request medication); sensitivity of the skin to sunlight (use protective clothing and a sunscreen).
- Report severe cramps, watery diarrhea, rash or itching, difficulty breathing, dark urine or light-colored stools, yellowing of the skin or eyes.

*Topical Dermatologic Solution*

- Apply generously until skin is wet.
- Avoid the eyes, nose, and mouth.
- You may experience transient stinging or burning; this will subside quickly; skin in the treated area may become yellow; this will wash off.
- You may use cosmetics as you usually do.

## tetrahydrozoline hydrochloride

*(tet rah hi **draz'** oh leen)*

Tyzine, Tyzine Pediatric

*OTC ophthalmic preparation:*
Collyrium Fresh Eye Drops, Eyesine, Mallazine Eye Drops, Murine, Optigene 3, Tetrasine, Visine

**Pregnancy Category C**

### Drug classes

Nasal decongestant
Ophthalmic vasoconstrictor/mydriatic

### Therapeutic actions

Acts directly on alpha receptors to produce vasoconstriction of arterioles in nasal passages, which produces a decongestant response; no effect on beta receptors; dilates pupils; increases flow of aqueous humor, vasoconstricts in eyes.

### Indications

- Symptomatic relief of nasal and nasopharyngeal mucosal congestion due to the common cold, hay fever, or other respiratory allergies (topical)
- Relief of redness of eyes due to minor irritations (ophthalmic)
- Temporary relief of burning and irritation due to dryness of the eye or discomfort due to minor irritations or to exposure to wind or sun (ophthalmic)

### Contraindications/cautions

- Contraindications: allergy to tetrahyrozolozine, angle-closure glaucoma, anesthesia with cyclopropane or halothane, thyrotoxicosis, diabetes, hypertension, CV disorders, women in labor whose BP > 130/80.
- Use cautiously with angina, arrhythmias, prostatic hypertrophy, unstable vasomotor syndrome, lactation.

### Dosage

**Available Forms:** Solution—0.05%, 0.1%

ADULT

- ***Nasal:*** 2–4 drops of 0.1% solution in each nostril three to four times a day; 3–4 sprays in each nostril q4h as needed.

- ***Ophthalmic:*** Instill 1–2 drops into eye(s) up to four times a day.

PEDIATRIC

- ***Nasal***
- – *>6 Y:* Adult dosage.
- – *2–6 Y:* 2–3 drops of 0.05% solution in each nostril q4–6h as needed.
- ***Ophthalmic:*** Safety and efficacy not established.

### Pharmacokinetics

| *Route* | *Onset* | *Duration* |
|---|---|---|
| Nasal | 5–10 min | 6–10 h |
| Ophthalmic; not generally absorbed systemically. | | |

*Metabolism:* Hepatic, $T_{1/2}$: unknown

*Distribution:* Crosses placenta; may enter breast milk

*Excretion:* Urine

### Adverse effects

- CNS: *Fear, anxiety, tenseness, restlessness, headache, lightheadedness, dizziness*, drowsiness, tremor, insomnia, hallucinations, psychological disturbances, convulsions, CNS depression, weakness, blurred vision, ocular irritation, tearing, photophobia, symptoms of paranoid schizophrenia
- GI: *Nausea*, vomiting, anorexia
- CV: Arrhythmias, hypertension resulting in intracranial hemorrhage, CV collapse with hypotension, palpitations, tachycardia, precordial pain in patients with ischemic heart disease
- GU: Constriction of renal blood vessels, *dysuria, vesical sphincter spasm,* resulting in difficult and painful urination, urinary retention in males with prostatism
- Local: *Rebound congestion* with topical nasal application
- Other: *Pallor*, respiratory difficulty, orofacial dystonia, sweating

### Clinically important drug-drug interactions

• Severe hypertension when taken with MAOIs, TCAs, furazolidone • Additive effects and increased risk of toxicity with urinary alkalinizers • Decreased vasopressor response with reserpine, methyldopa, urinary acidifiers • Decreased hypotensive action of guanethidine

## ■ Nursing Considerations

### Assessment

- *History:* Allergy to tetrahydrozoline; angle-closure glaucoma; anesthesia with cyclopropane or halothane; thyrotoxicosis, diabetes, hypertension, CV disorders; prostatic hypertrophy, unstable vasomotor syndrome; lactation
- *Physical:* Skin color, temperature; orientation, reflexes, peripheral sensation, vision; P, BP, auscultation, peripheral perfusion; R, adventitious sounds; urinary output pattern, bladder percussion, prostate palpation; nasal mucous membrance evaluation

### Implementation

- Do not administer ophthalmic solution if it is cloudy or changes color.
- Monitor CV effects carefully; patients with hypertension who take this drug may experience changes in BP because of the additional vasoconstriction. If a nasal decongestant is needed, pseudoephedrine is the drug of choice.

### Drug-specific teaching points

- Do not exceed recommended dose. Demonstrate proper administration technique for topical nasal application and administration of eye drops. Avoid prolonged use because underlying medical problems can be disguised.
- The following side effects may occur: dizziness, weakness, restlessness, lightheadedness, tremor (avoid driving or operating dangerous equipment); urinary retention (empty bladder before taking drug).
- Rebound congestion may occur when this drug is stopped; drink plenty of fluids, use a humidifier, avoid smoke-filled areas.
- Report nervousness, palpitations, sleeplessness, sweating.

# Theophylline

## theophylline
*(thee off' i lin)*

*Immediate-release capsules, tablets:* Bronkodyl, Elixophyllin, Quibron-T Dividose, Slo-Phyllin, Theolair

*Timed-release capsules:* Slo-bid Gyrocaps, Slo-Phyllin Gyrocaps, Theo-24, Theobid, Theoclear L.A., Theospan-SR, Theovent

*Timed-release tablets:* Quibron-T/SR Dividose, Respbid, Theochron, Theo-Dur, Theolair-SR, Uniphyl, Uni-Dur

*Liquids:* Aquaphyllin, Asmalix, Elixomin, Elixophyllin, Slo-Phyllin, Theoclear-80, Theolair

## theophylline sodium glycinate

*Elixir:* Acet-Amp (CAN)

**Pregnancy Category C**

### Drug classes
Bronchodilator
Xanthine

### Therapeutic actions
Relaxes bronchial smooth muscle, causing bronchodilation and increasing vital capacity that has been impaired by bronchospasm and air trapping; actions may be mediated by inhibition of phosphodiesterase, which increases the concentration of cyclic adenosine monophosphate; in concentrations that may be higher than those reached clinically, it also inhibits the release of slow-reacting substance of anaphylaxis and histamine.

### Indications
- Symptomatic relief or prevention of bronchial asthma and reversible bronchospasm associated with chronic bronchitis and emphysema
- Unlabeled use of 2 mg/kg per day to maintain serum concentrations between 3 and 5 μg/ml: treatment of apnea and bradycardia of prematurity

### Contraindications/cautions
- Contraindications: hypersensitivity to any xanthines, peptic ulcer, active gastritis, status asthmaticus, pregnancy (neonatal tachycardia, jitteriness, and withdrawal apnea).
- Use cautiously with cardiac arrhythmias, acute myocardial injury, CHF, cor pulmonale, severe hypertension, severe hypoxemia, renal or hepatic disease, hyperthyroidism, alcoholism, labor (may inhibit uterine contractions), lactation.

### Dosage
**Available Forms:** Syrup—80, 150 mg/15 ml; elixir—80 mg/15 ml; solution—80 mg/15 ml; oral solution—150 mg/15 ml; TR capsules—50, 75, 100, 125, 130, 200, 250, 260, 300 mg; TR tablets—100, 200, 250, 300, 400, 500 mg; injection in 5% Dextrose—200, 400, 800 mg/container

Maintain serum levels in the therapeutic range of 10–20 μg/ml; base dosage on lean body mass.

*ADULT*

**Theophylline**

– ***Acute symptoms requiring rapid theophyllinization in patients not receiving theophylline:*** Initial loading dose is required, as indicated below:

| *Patient Group* | *Oral Loading* | *Followed by* | *Maintenance* |
|---|---|---|---|
| Young adult smokers | 6 mg/kg | 3 mg/kg q4h × 3 doses | 3 mg/kg q6h |
| Non-smoking adults, otherwise healthy | 6 mg/kg | 3 mg/kg q6h × 2 doses | 3 mg/kg q8h |

– ***Acute symptoms requiring rapid theophyllinization in patients receiving theophylline:*** A loading dose is required; each 0.5 mg/kg PO administered as a loading dose will result in about a 1 μg/ml increase in serum theophylline. Ideally, defer loading dose until serum theophylline determination is made. Otherwise, base loading dose on clinical judgment and the knowledge that 2.5 mg/kg of a rapidly absorbed preparation will increase serum theophylline levels by about 5 μg/ml and is unlikely to cause dangerous adverse effects if the patient is not experiencing theophylline toxicity before this dose; maintenance doses are as above.

- *Chronic therapy:* Initial dose of 16 mg/kg per 24 h PO or 400 mg/24 h, whichever is less, in divided doses q6–8h for immediate-release preparations or liquids, q8–12 or 24h for timed-release preparations (consult manufacturer's recommendations for specific dosage interval). Increase dosage based on serum theophylline levels, or if these are unavailable, increase in 25%-increments at 2- to 3-d intervals as long as drug is tolerated or until maximum dose of 13 mg/kg per day or 900 mg, whichever is less, is reached.
- ***Dosage adjustment based on serum theophylline levels during chronic therapy***

| Serum Theophylline | Directions |
|---|---|
| Too low | 5–7.5 μg/ml: Increase dose by about 25%, recheck serum level; may need to increase dose.<br>7.5–10 μg/ml: Increase dose by 25%; may need to give total daily dose at more frequent intervals; recheck at 6- to 12-mo intervals. |
| Within normal limits | 10–20 μg/ml: Maintain dosage; recheck level at 6- to 12-mo intervals. |
| Too high | 20–25 μg/ml: Decrease doses by about 10%; recheck level at 6- to 12-mo intervals.<br>25–30 μg/ml: Skip next dose, and decrease subsequent doses by about 25%; recheck levels.<br>>30 μg/ml: Skip next two doses, and decrease subsequent doses by 50%; recheck level. |

Measure serum theophylline in blood sample drawn 1–2 h after administration of immediate-release preparations, 4 h after administration of most sustained-release products.

- ***Rectal:*** 500 mg q6–8h by rectal suppository or retention enema.

**Theophylline sodium glycinate (44.5%–47.3% theophylline):** 330–660 mg PO q6–8h after meals.

PEDIATRIC: Use in children <6 mo not recommended. Use of timed-release products in children <6 y not recommended.

**Theophylline**

- ***Acute symptoms requiring rapid theophyllinization in patients not receiving theophylline;*** An initial loading dose is required, as follows:

| Patient Group | Oral Loading | Followed by | Maintenance |
|---|---|---|---|
| 6 mo–9 y | 6 mg/kg | 4 mg/kg q4h × 3 doses | 4 mg/kg q6h |
| 9–16 y | 6 mg/kg | 3 mg/kg q4h × 3 doses | 3 mg/kg q3h |

- INFANTS PRETERM TO YOUNGER THAN 6 MO: Reduce initial and maintenance doses because elimination of theophylline appears to be delayed in these patients:

| Infant | Loading Dose | Maintenance Dose |
|---|---|---|
| Preterm (≤40 wk postconception) | 1 mg/kg for each 2 μg/ml serum concentration desired | 1 mg/kg q12h |
| Term (birth or 40 wk postconception) | | |
| Up to 4 wk postnatal | | 1–2 mg/kg q12h |
| 4–8 wk | | 1–2 mg/kg q8h |
| >8 wk | | 1–3 mg/kg q6h |

- *Chronic therapy:* Initial dose of 16 mg/kg per 24 h PO or 400 mg/24 h, whichever is less, in divided doses q6–8h for immediate-release preparations or liquids, q8–12 or 24h for timed-release preparations in children <6 y (consult manufacturer's recommendations for specific dosage interval). Increase dosage based on serum theophylline levels, or if these are unavailable, increase in 25%-increments at 2- to 3-d intervals as long as drug is tolerated or until maximum dose given below is reached:

| *Age* | *Maximum Daily Dose* |
|---|---|
| <9 y | 24 mg/kg/d |
| 9–12 y | 20 mg/kg/d |
| 12–16 y | 18 mg/kg/d |
| >16 y | 13 mg/kg/d |

### Theophylline sodium glycinate

- *6–12 Y:* 220–330 mg q6–8h PO after meals.
- *3–6 Y:* 110–165 mg q6–8h PO after meals.
- *1–3 Y:* 55–110 mg q6–8h PO after meals.

*GERIATRIC OR IMPAIRED ADULT:* Use caution, especially in elderly men, and in patients with cor pulmonale, CHF.

- ***Acute symptoms requiring rapid theophyllinization in patients not receiving theophylline:*** An initial loading dose is required, as follows:

| *Patient Group* | *Oral Loading* | *Followed by* | *Maintenance* |
|---|---|---|---|
| Older patients and patients with cor pulmonale | 6 mg/kg | 2 mg/kg q6h for 2 doses | 2 mg/kg q8h |
| Patients with CHF | 6 mg/kg | 2 mg/kg q8h for 2 doses | 1–2 mg/kg q12h |

## Pharmacokinetics

| *Route* | *Onset* | *Peak* |
|---|---|---|
| Oral | Varies | 2 h |

*Metabolism:* Hepatic, $T_{1/2}$: 3–15 h (nonsmoker) or 4–5 h (smokers)

*Distribution:* Crosses placenta; may enter breast milk

*Excretion:* Urine

## Adverse effects

- **Serum theophylline levels < 20 μg/ml:** Adverse effects uncommon.
- **Serum theophylline levels > 20–25 μg/ml:** *Nausea, vomiting, diarrhea, headache, insomnia, irritability* (75% of patients)
- **Serum theophylline levels > 30–35 μg/ml:** Hyperglycemia, hypotension, cardiac arrhythmias, tachycardia (> 10 μg/ml in premature newborns); seizures, brain damage, death
- CNS: *Irritability (especially children); restlessness,* dizziness, muscle twitching, convulsions, severe depression, stammering speech; abnormal behavior characterized by withdrawal, mutism and unresponsiveness alternating with hyperactive periods
- GI: *Loss of appetite*, hematemesis, epigastric pain, gastroesophageal reflux during sleep
- CV: Palpitations, sinus tachycardia, ventricular tachycardia, **life-threatening ventricular arrhythmias,** circulatory failure
- Respiratory: Tachypnea, **respiratory arrest**
- GU: Proteinuria, increased excretion of renal tubular cells and RBCs; diuresis (dehydration), urinary retention in men with prostate enlargement
- Other: Fever, flushing, hyperglycemia, SIADH, rash, increased SGOT

## Clinically important drug-drug interactions

• Increased effects and toxicity with cimetidine, erythromycin, troleandomycin, ciprofloxacin, norfloxacin, enoxacin, ofloxacin, oral contraceptives, ticlopidine, ranitidine • Possibly increased effects with rifampin • Increased serum levels and risk of toxicity in hypothyroid patients, decreased levels in patients who are hyperthyroid; monitor patients on thioamines, thyroid hormones for changes in serum levels as patients becomes euthyroid • Increased cardiac toxicity with halothane • Decreased effects in patients who are cigarette smokers

t

(1–2 packs/day); theophylline dosage may need to be increased 50%–100% • Decreased effects with barbiturates, charcoal • Decreased effects of phenytoins, benzodiazepines, and theophylline preparations • Decreased effects of nondepolarizing neuromuscular blockers • Mutually antagonistic effects of beta-blockers and theophylline preparations.

### Clinically important drug-food interactions

• Theophylline elimination is increased by a low-carbohydrate, high-protein diet and by charcoal broiled beef • Theophylline elimination is decreased by a high-carbohydrate, low-protein diet • Food may alter bioavailability, absorption of timed-release theophylline preparations; these may rapidly release their contents with food and cause toxicity. Timed-release forms should be taken on an empty stomach

### Drug-lab test interferences

• Interference with spectrophotometric determinations of serum theophylline levels by furosemide, phenylbutazone, probenecid, theobromine; coffee, tea, cola beverages, chocolate, acetaminophen cause falsely high values • Alteration in assays of uric acid, urinary catecholamines, plasma free fatty acids

## ■ Nursing Considerations

### Assessment

- *History:* Hypersensitivity to any xanthines, peptic ulcer, active gastritis, status asthmaticus, cardiac arrhythmias, acute myocardial injury, CHF, cor pulmonale, severe hypertension, severe hypoxemia, renal or hepatic disease, hyperthyroidism, pregnancy, lactation
- *Physical:* Skin color, texture, lesions; reflexes, bilateral grip strength, affect; P, auscultation, BP, perfusion; R, adventitious sounds; bowel sounds, normal output; frequency, voiding pattern, normal urinary output; ECG; EEG; thyroid, liver, kidney function tests

### Implementation

- Caution patient not to chew or crush enteric-coated timed-release preparations.
- Give immediate release, liquid dosage forms with food if GI effects occur.
- Do not give timed-release preparations with food; these should be given on an empty stomach, 1 h before or 2 h after meals.
- Monitor results of serum theophylline level determinations carefully, and reduce dosage if serum levels exceed therapeutic range of 10–20 μg/ml.
- Monitor carefully for clinical signs of adverse effects, particularly if serum theophylline levels are not available.
- Maintain diazepam on standby to treat seizures.

### Drug-specific teaching points

- Take this drug exactly as prescribed. If a timed-release product is prescribed, take it on an empty stomach, 1 h before or 2 h after meals. Do not chew or crush timed-release preparations; it may be necessary for you to take this drug around the clock for adequate control of asthma attacks.
- Avoid excessive intake of coffee, tea, cocoa, cola beverages, chocolate. These contain theophylline-related substances that may increase your side effects.
- Smoking cigarettes or other tobacco products may markedly influence the effects of theophylline. It is preferable not to smoke while you are taking this drug. Notify your health care provider if you change your smoking habits while you are taking this drug; it may be necessary to change your drug dosage.
- Have frequent blood tests to monitor drug effects and ensure safe and effective dosage.
- The following side effects may occur: nausea, loss of appetite (take drug with food; applies only to immediate-release or liquid dosage forms); difficulty sleeping, depression, emotional lability.
- Report nausea, vomiting, severe GI pain, restlessness, convulsions, irregular heartbeat.

## thiabendazole

*(thye a **ben'** da zole)*

Mintezol

**Pregnancy Category C**

### Drug classes

Anthelmintic

## Therapeutic actions

Suppresses egg or larva production of helminths and may inhibit the subsequent development of eggs and larvae that are passed in the feces; inhibits a helminth-specific enzyme.

## Indications

- Treatment of strongyloidiasis (threadworm infection), cutaneous larva migrans (creeping eruption), and visceral larva migrans. Not a primary therapy, but no other agent is usually needed with enterobiasis (pinworm) infection with treatment of one of the above.
- When more specific therapy cannot be used or a second agent is desirable, for the treatment of ascariasis (roundworm infection), uncinariasis (hookworm infection), trichuriasis (whipworm infection)
- Alleviation of symptoms of invasive trichinosis

## Contraindications/cautions

- Contraindications: allergy to thiabendazole, pregnancy.
- Use cautiously with renal or hepatic dysfunction, anemia, malnourishment or dehydration.

## Dosage

**Available Forms:** Chewable tablets—500 mg; oral suspension—500 mg/5 ml

***Adult and Pediatric (> 30 lb)***

- *<150 lb:* 10 mg/lb per dose PO.
- *>150 lb:* 1.5 g/dose PO. Maximum daily dose is 3 g. Clinical experience in children weighing < 30 lb is limited.

| *Indication* | *Regimen* |
|---|---|
| Enterobiasis | 2 doses/d for 1 d; repeat in 7 d to reduce risk of reinfection (or 2 doses/d for 2 successive d) |
| Strongyloidiasis, ascariasis, uncinariasis, trichuriasis | 2 doses/d for 2 successive d (or single dose of 20 mg/lb) |
| Cutaneous larva migrans | 2 doses/d for 2 successive d (repeat treatment if lesions still present 2 d after therapy) |
| Trichinosis | 2 doses/d for 2–4 successive d as needed |

## Pharmacokinetics

| *Route* | *Onset* | *Peak* |
|---|---|---|
| Oral | Rapid | 1–2 h |

*Metabolism:* Hepatic, $T_{1/2}$: unknown
*Distribution:* Crosses placenta; may enter breast milk
*Excretion:* Urine

## Adverse effects

- CNS: *Dizziness, drowsiness, giddiness, weariness, headache*, tinnitus, hyperirritability, numbness, abnormal sensation in eyes, blurred vision, xanthopsia
- GI: *Anorexia, nausea,* vomiting, epigastric distress, diarrhea, perianal rash, jaundice, cholestasis, parenchymal liver damage
- CV: Hypotension, collapse
- Hematologic: Rise in SGOT, hyperglycemia, leukopenia
- GU: Enuresis, *malodor of urine*, crystalluria, hematuria
- Hypersensitivity: Reactions ranging from rash, fever, chills, angioedema, lymphadenopathy, anaphylaxis, **Stevens-Johnson syndrome** (sometimes fatal)

## Clinically important drug-drug interactions

- Risk of increased serum levels and toxicity of xanthines if combined; monitor serum xanthine levels and adjust dosage appropriately

## ■ Nursing Considerations

### Assessment

- *History:* Allergy to thiabendazole, renal or hepatic dysfunction, anemia, malnourishment or dehydration, pregnancy, lactation
- *Physical:* Skin color, lesions, turgor; orientation, affect; bowel sounds, output; liver and renal function tests, urinalysis, CBC

### Implementation

- Culture for ova and parasites.
- Administer drug with food; have patient chew tablets before swallowing them.
- Discontinue drug, and consult with physician if hypersensitivity reactions occur.

t

- Arrange for treatment of all family members (pinworm infestations).
- Arrange for disinfection of toilet facilities after patient use (pinworms).
- Arrange for daily laundry of bed linens, towels, nightclothes, and undergarments (pinworms).

### Drug-specific teaching points

- Take drug with food to decrease GI upset. Chew tablets before swallowing.
- Pinworms are easily transmitted; all family members should be treated for complete eradication.
- Strict handwashing and hygiene measures are important; launder undergarments, bedlinens, nightclothes daily; disinfect toilet facilities daily and bathroom floors periodically (pinworms).
- The following side effects may occur: nausea, abdominal pain, diarrhea (small, frequent meals may help); drowsiness, dizziness, insomnia (avoid driving and using dangerous machinery); strange odor may develop in the urine (reversible).
- Report skin rash, joint pain, severe GI upset, fever, chills, swelling of feet or hands, yellow color to skin or eyes.

## thiethylperazine maleate

*(thye eth il* ***per'*** *a zeen)*

Torecan

**Pregnancy Category X**

### Drug classes

Antiemetic
Antivertigo agent

### Therapeutic actions

Mechanism of action not fully understood: acts directly on the CTZ and the vomiting center to suppress nausea and vomiting.

### Indications

- Relief of nausea and vomiting
- Unlabeled use: treatment of vertigo

### Contraindications/cautions

- Allergy to phenothiazines, comatose or severely depressed states, pregnancy, lactation, intracardiac or intracranial surgery.

### Dosage

**Available Forms:** Tablets—10 mg; suppositories—10 mg; injection—5 mg/ml

**ADULT**

- ***Oral and rectal:*** 10–30 mg/d in divided doses.
- ***IM:*** 2 ml, 1–3×/d.

**PEDIATRIC:** Safety and efficacy not determined for children younger than 12 y.

### Pharmacokinetics

| *Route* | *Onset* | *Duration* |
|---|---|---|
| Oral, PR | 60 min | 4 h |
| IM | 30 min | 4 h |

*Metabolism:* Hepatic, $T_{1/2}$: unknown
*Distribution:* Crosses placenta; enters breast milk
*Excretion:* Urine

### Adverse effects

- CNS: *Drowsiness, insomnia, vertigo,* headache, weakness, tremors, ataxia, slurring, cerebral edema, seizures, exacerbation of psychotic symptoms, *extrapyramidal syndromes*; neuroleptic malignant syndrome
- GI: *Dry mouth, salivation, nausea, vomiting, anorexia, constipation*, paralytic ileus, incontinence
- CV: *Hypotension, otrhostatic hypotension,* hypertension, tachycardia, bradycardia, cardiac arrest, CHF, cardiomegaly, refractory arrhythmias, pulmonary edema
- Respiratory: Bronchospasm, laryngospasm, dyspnea, suppression of cough reflex and potential aspiration
- Hematologic: **Eosinophilia, leukopenia, leukocytosis, *anemia*, aplastic anemia, hemolytic anemia, thrombocytopenic or nonthrombocytopenic purpura, pancytopenia, elevated serum cholesterol**
- GU: *Urinary retention,* polyuria, incontinence

- EENT: Nasal congestion, glaucoma, *photophobia, blurred vision*, miosis, mydriasis, deposits in the cornea and lens, pigmentary retinopathy
- Hypersensitivity: Jaundice, *urticaria*, angioneurotic edema, laryngeal edema, photosensitivity, eczema, asthma, anaphylactoid reactions, exfoliative dermatitis
- Endocrine: Lactation, breast engorgement in females, galactorrhea, SIADH secretion, amenorrhea
- Other: Fever, heatstroke, pallor, flushed facies, sweating, *photosensitivity*

### Clinically important drug-drug interactions

• Additive CNS depression, hypotension if given preoperatively with barbiturate anesthetics, alcohol, meperidine • Additive effects of both drugs with beta-blockers • Increased risk of tachycardia, hypotension with epinephrine, norepinephrine • Increased risk of seizure with metrizamide

### Drug-lab test interferences

• False-positive pregnancy tests (less likely if serum test is used) • Increase in PBI, not attributable to an increase in thyroxine

## ■ Nursing Considerations

### Assessment

- *History:* Allergy to phenothiazines, comatose or severely depressed states, lactation, pregnancy, intracranial or intracardiac surgery
- *Physical:* T, body weight, skin color, turgor; reflexes, orientation; P, BP, orthostatic BP, ECG; R, adventitious sounds; bowel sounds, normal output, liver evaluation; prostate palpation, normal urine output; CBC; urinalysis

### Implementation

- Protect the rectal suppositories from light; refrigerate.
- For use after surgery; give slowly by deep IM injection into upper outer quadrant of buttock at or shortly before the termination of anesthesia.
- Keep the patient recumbent for 1/2 h after injection to avoid orthostatic hypotension.
- Be alert to potential for aspiration because of suppressed cough reflex.

### Drug-specific teaching points

- The following side effects may occur: drowsiness (avoid driving or operating dangerous machinery; avoid alcohol, which will increase the drowsiness); faintness, dizziness (change position slowly, use caution climbing stairs).
- Report sore throat, fever, unusual bleeding or bruising, rash, weakness, tremors, impaired vision, dark urine, pale stools, yellowing of the skin and eyes.

# thioguanine

*(thye oh **gwah'** neen)*

TG, 6-Thioguanine

Lanvis (CAN)

**Pregnancy Category D**

### Drug classes

Antimetabolite

Antineoplastic

### Therapeutic actions

Tumor-inhibiting properties, probably due to interference with a number of steps in the synthesis and use of purine nucleotides, which are normally incorporated into DNA and RNA.

### Indications

- Remission induction, consolidation and maintenance therapy of acute leukemias (lymphatic, myelogenous, and acute myelomonocytic) alone and in combination therapy
- Palliative treatment of chronic myelogenous leukemia

### Contraindications/cautions

- Contraindications: allergy to thioguanine, prior resistance to thioguanine, hematopoietic depression, pregnancy (potential mutagen and teratogen), lactation.
- Use cautiously with impaired hepatic function.

t

### Dosage

**Available Forms:** Tablets—40 mg

**ADULT AND PEDIATRIC:** Initial dosage, 2 mg/kg per day PO daily for 4 wk. If no clinical improvement is seen and there are no toxic effects, increase dose to 3 mg/kg per day. If complete hematologic remission is obtained, institute maintenance therapy. No adjustment of dosage is needed if used as part of combination therapy.

### Pharmacokinetics

| *Route* | *Onset* | *Peak* |
|---|---|---|
| Oral | Slow | 8 h |

*Metabolism:* Hepatic, $T_{1/2}$: 11 h
*Distribution:* Crosses placenta; enters breast milk
*Excretion:* Urine

### Adverse effects

- GI: Hepatotoxicity, *nausea, vomiting, anorexia*, diarrhea, stomatitis
- **Hematologic:** *Bone marrow depression, immunosuppression, hyperuricemia* due to rapid lysis of malignant cells
- **Other:** Fever, weakness, cancer, chromosomal aberrations

## ■ Nursing Considerations

### Assessment

- ***History:*** Allergy to thioguanine, prior resistance to thioguanine, hematopoietic depression, impaired hepatic function, pregnancy, lactation
- ***Physical:*** Skin color; mucous membranes, liver evaluation, abdominal exam; CBC, differential, hemoglobin, platelet counts; liver function tests; serum uric acid

### Implementation

- Evaluate hematopoietic status before and frequently during therapy.
- Discontinue drug therapy if platelet count < 50,000; polymorphonuclear granuloctye count < 1,000; consult physician for dosage adjustment.
- Arrange for discontinuation of this drug at any sign of hematologic or hepatic toxicity; consult physician.
- Ensure that patient is well hydrated before and during therapy to minimize adverse effects of hyperuricemia; allopurinal and drugs to alkalinize the urine are sometimes prescribed.
- Administer as a single daily dose.

### Drug-specific teaching points

- Drink adequate fluids while you are on this drug; drink at least 8–10 glasses of fluid each day.
- The following side effects may occur: mouth sores (use frequent mouth care); nausea, vomiting, loss of appetite (small, freqent meals may help); increased susceptibility to infection (avoid crowds and infections).
- This drug may cause miscarriages and birth defects. Use birth control; men also should use birth control measures while on this drug and for a time afterwards.
- Have frequent, regular medical follow-up, including frequent blood tests to assess drug effects.
- Report fever, chills, sore throat, unusual bleeding or bruising, yellow discoloration of the skin or eyes, abdominal pain, flank pain, joint pain, swelling of the feet or legs.

## thioridazine hydrochloride

*(thye oh **rid'** a zeen)*
Apo-Thioridazine (CAN), Mellaril
**Pregnancy Category C**

### Drug classes

Phenothiazine (piperidine)
Dopaminergic blocking agent
Antipsychotic
Antianxiety agent

### Therapeutic actions

Mechanism of action not fully understood: blocks postsynaptic dopamine receptors in the brain, but this may not be necessary and sufficient for antipsychotic activity; depresses the RAS, including the parts of the brain involved with wakefulness and emesis; anticholinergic, antihistaminic ($H_1$), and alpha-adrenergic blocking activity also may contribute to some of its effects.

## Indications

- Management of manifestations of psychotic disorders and short-term treatment of moderate to marked depression with anxiety in adults
- Treatment of multiple symptoms, such as agitation, anxiety, depressed mood, tension, sleep disturbances, and fears in geriatric patients
- Treatment of severe behavioral problems in children marked by combativeness or by explosive hyperexcitable behavior
- Short-term treatment of hyperactive children with accompanying conduct disorders consisting of some or all of the following symptoms: impulsivity, difficulty sustaining attention, aggressivity, mood lability, poor frustration tolerance

## Contraindications/cautions

- Contraindications: coma or severe CNS depression, bone marrow depression, blood dyscrasia, circulatory collapse, subcortical brain damage, Parkinson's disease, liver damage, cerebral arteriosclerosis, coronary disease, severe hypotension or hypertension.
- Use cautiously with respiratory disorders ("silent pneumonia"); glaucoma, prostatic hypertrophy; epilepsy or history of epilepsy (drug lowers seizure threshold); breast cancer; thyrotoxicosis (severe neurotoxicity); peptic ulcer, decreased renal function; myelography within previous 24 h or scheduled within 48 h; exposure to heat or phosphorous insecticides; pregnancy; lactation; children <12 y, especially those with chickenpox, CNS infections (children are especially susceptible to dystonias that may confound the diagnosis of Reye's syndrome).

## Dosage

**Available Forms:** Tablets—10, 15, 25, 50, 100, 150, 200 mg; concentrate—30, 100 mg/ml; suspension—25, 100 mg/5 ml

Full clinical effects may require 6 wk–6 mo of therapy.

### ADULT

- ***Psychotic manifestations:*** 50–100 mg PO tid. Increase gradually to a maximum of 800 mg/d if necessary to control symptoms and then gradually reduce to minimum effective dose. Total daily dose ranges from 200–800 mg divided into two to four doses.

### PEDIATRIC

- *2–12 Y:* 0.5–3.0 mg/kg per day PO.
- ***Moderate disorders:*** Initially, 10 mg PO bid–tid.
- ***Hospitalized, severely disturbed children:*** Initially, 25 mg PO bid–tid.

### GERIATRIC

- ***Short-term treatment of depression with anxiety in geriatric patients:*** Initially, 25 mg PO tid. Dosage ranges from 10 mg bid–qid in milder cases to 50 mg tid–qid for more severely disturbed patients.

## Pharmacokinetics

| Route | Onset | Peak | Duration |
|---|---|---|---|
| Oral | Varies | 2–4 h | 8–12 h |

*Metabolism:* Hepatic, $T_{1/2}$: 10–20 h
*Distribution:* Crosses placenta; enters breast milk
*Excretion:* Urine

## Adverse effects

*Antipsychotic Drugs*

- CNS: *Drowsiness*, insomnia, vertigo, headache, weakness, tremor, ataxia, slurring, cerebral edema, seizures, exacerbation of psychotic symptoms, extrapyramidal syndromes—*pseudoparkinsonism*; *dystonias; akathisia*, tardive dyskinesias, potentially irreversible **neuroleptic malignant syndrome** (NMS)
- CV: Hypotension, orthostatic hypotension, hypertension, tachycardia, bradycardia, cardiac arrest, CHF, cardiomegaly, **refractory arrhythmias** (some fatal), pulmonary edema
- Respiratory: Bronchospasm, laryngospasm, dyspnea; suppression of cough reflex and potential for aspiration
- Hematologic: Eosinophilia, leukopenia, leukocytosis, anemia; aplastic anemia; he-

t

molytic anemia; thrombocytopenic or nonthrombocytopenic purpura; pancytopenia

- **EENT**: Glaucoma, *photophobia, blurred vision*, miosis, mydriasis, deposits in the cornea and lens (opacities), pigmentary retinopathy
- **Hypersensitivity**: Jaundice, urticaria, angioneurotic edema, laryngeal edema, photosensitivity, eczema, asthma, anaphylactoid reactions, exfoliative dermatitis
- **Endocrine**: Lactation, breast engorgement, galactorrhea; SIADH secretion; amenorrhea, menstrual irregularities; gynecomastia; changes in libido; hyperglycemia or hypoglycemia; glycosuria; hyponatremia; pituitary tumor with hyperprolactinemia; inhibition of ovulation, infertility, pseudopregnancy; reduced urinary levels of gonadotropins, estrogens, progestins
- **Autonomic**: *Dry mouth, salivation, nasal congestion, nausea*, vomiting, anorexia, fever, pallor, flushed facies, sweating, constipation, paralytic ileus, urinary retention, incontinence, polyuria, enuresis, priapism, ejaculation inhibition, male impotence
- **Other**: *Urine discolored pink to red-brown*

### Clinically important drug-drug interactions

• Additive CNS depression with alcohol • Additive anticholinergic effects and possibly decreased antipsychotic efficacy with anticholinergic drugs • Increased likelihood of seizures with metrizamide • Increased effects from both drugs in given in combination with propranolol • Decreased antihypertensive effect of guanethidine

### Drug-lab test interferences

• False-positive pregnancy tests (less likely if serum test is used) • Increase in PBI not attributable to an increase in thyroxine

## ■ Nursing Considerations

### Assessment

- *History:* Coma or severe CNS depression; blood dyscrasia; circulatory collapse; subcortical brain damage; Parkinson's disease; liver damage; cerebral arteriosclerosis; coronary disease; severe hypotension or hypertension; respiratory disorders; glaucoma, prostatic hypertrophy; epilepsy; breast cancer; thyrotoxicosis; peptic ulcer, decreased renal function; myelography within previous 24 h or scheduled within 48 h; exposure to heat or phosphorous insecticides; pregnancy; lactation; chickenpox; CNS infections
- *Physical:* Weight, T; reflexes, orientation, intraocular pressure; P, BP, orthostatic BP; R, adventitious sounds; bowel sounds and normal output, liver evaluation; urinary output, prostate size, CBC, urinalysis, thyroid, liver and kidney function tests

### Implementation

- Arrange for ophthalmologic (slit lamp) examination before and during drug therapy.
- Do not change brand names; bioavailability differences have been documented for different brands.
- Oral concentrate may be administered in distilled or acidified tap water or suitable juices, or use the flavored suspension.
- Do not change dosage in chronic therapy more often than weekly; drug requires 4–7 d to achieve steady-state plasma levels.
- Avoid skin contact with oral solution; contact dermatitis has occurred.
- Discontinue drug if serum creatinine, BUN become abnormal or if WBC count is depressed.
- Monitor elderly patients for dehydration, and institute remedial measures promptly; sedation and decreased sensation of thirst related to CNS effects can lead to severe dehydration.
- Consult physician regarding appropriate warning of patient or patient's guardian about tardive dyskinesias.
- Consult physician about dosage reduction, use of anticholinergic antiparkinsonian drugs (controversial) if extrapyramidal effects occur.

### Drug-specific teaching points

- Take drug exactly as prescribed.
- Avoid skin contact with drug solutions.

- Avoid driving or engaging in other dangerous activities if CNS, vision changes occur.
- Avoid prolonged exposure to sun, or use a sunscreen or covering garments.
- Maintain fluid intake and use precautions against heatstroke in hot weather.
- Arrange for ophthalmologic exams periodically during therapy.
- Report sore throat, fever, unusual bleeding or bruising, rash, weakness, tremors, impaired vision, dark urine (pink or reddish brown urine is expected), pale stools, yellowing of the skin or eyes.

## thiotepa

*(thye oh **tep'** ah)*

triethylenethiophosphoramide, TESPA, TSPA

Thioplex

**Pregnancy Category D**

### Drug classes
Alkylating agent
Antineoplastic

### Therapeutic actions
Cytotoxic: disrupts the bonds of DNA, causing cell death; cell cycle nonspecific.

### Indications
- Treatment of adenocarcinoma of the breast, ovary
- Superficial papillary carcinoma of the urinary bladder
- Controlling intracavity effusions secondary to diffuse or localized neoplastic disease of various serosal cavities
- Treatment of lymphoma, including Hodgkin's disease; no longer a drug of choice

### Contraindications/cautions
- Contraindications: allergy to thiotepa, hematopoietic depression, pregnancy, lactation.
- Use cautiously with impaired hepatic or renal function, concomitant therapy with other alkylating agents or irradiation.

### Dosage
**Available Forms:** Powder for injection—15 mg

*Adult*
- ***IV administration:*** 0.3–0.4 mg/kg at 1- to 4-wk intervals.
- ***Intratumor administration:*** Drug is diluted in sterile water to a concentration of 10 mg/ml, then 0.6–0.8 mg/kg is injected directly into the tumor after a local anesthetic is injected through the same needle. Maintainance doses of 0.07–0.8 mg/kg every 1–4 wk depending on patient's condition.
- ***Intracavity administration:*** 0.6–0.8 mg/kg through the same tube that is used to remove fluid from the cavity.
- ***Intravesical administration:*** Dehydrate patient with papillary carcinoma of the bladder for 8–12 h prior to treatment. Then instill 60 mg in 30–60 ml of distilled water into the bladder by catheter. Retain for 2 h. If patient is unable to retain 60 ml, give the dose in 30 ml. Repeat once a week for 4 wk.

### Pharmacokinetics

| Route | Onset |
|---|---|
| IV | Gradual |

*Metabolism:* Hepatic, $T_{1/2}$: unknown
*Distribution:* Crosses placenta; enters breast milk
*Excretion:* Urine

### IV facts
**Preparation:** Reconstitute powder with Sterile Water for Injection. 1.5 ml of diluent gives a drug concentration of 5 mg/0.5 ml of solution. May be further diluted with Sodium Chloride Injection, Dextrose Injection, Dextrose and Sodium Chloride Injection, Ringer's Injection, Lactated Ringer's Injection. Store powder in the refrigerator, reconstituted solution is stable for 5 d if refrigerated. Sterile Water for Injection produces an isotonic solution, other diluents may produce a hypertonic solution that may cause mild to moderate discomfort on injection. Check solution before use; solution should be clear to slightly opaque; grossly opaque solutions or solutions with precipitates should not be used.

t

**Infusion:** Administer IV dose directly and rapidly, 60 mg over 1 min. There is no need for slow IV drip or the use of large volumes of fluid.

### Adverse effects

- CNS: *Dizziness*, headache, blurred vision
- GI: *Nausea, vomiting,* anorexia
- Hematologic: *Hematopoietic toxicity*
- GU: *Amenorrhea, interference with spermatogenesis*, dysuria, urinary retention
- Dermatologic: Hives, skin rash, weeping from subcutaneous lesions, contact dermatitis at injection site
- Other: Febrile reactions, cancer

## ■ Nursing Considerations

### Assessment

- *History:* Allergy to thiotepa, hematopoietic depression, impaired renal or hepatic function, concomitant therapy with other alkylating agents or irradiation, pregnancy, lactation
- *Physical:* Weight; skin color, lesions; T; orientation, reflexes; CBC, differential; urinalysis; liver and renal function tests

### Implementation

- Arrange for blood tests to evaluate bone marrow function before therapy, weekly during therapy and for at least 3 wk after therapy.
- Mix solution with 2% procaine HCl, 1:1,000 epinephrine HCl, or both for local use into single or multiple sites.
- Reduce dosage with renal or hepatic impairment and for bone marrow depression.

### Drug-specific teaching points

- This drug can be given only parenterally. Prepare a calendar of treatment days.
- The following side effects may occur: nausea, vomiting, loss of appetite (request an antiemetic; small frequent meals also may help); dizziness, headache (use special safety precautions to prevent falls or injury); amenorrhea in women, change in sperm production.
- This drug should not be taken during pregnancy; use birth control while you are on this drug. If you become pregnant, consult with your health care provider.
- Have regular medical follow-up, including blood tests, to assess drug effects.
- Report unusual bleeding or bruising, fever, chills, sore throat, stomach or flank pain, severe nausea and vomiting, skin rash or hives.

## thiothixene

*(thye oh **thix'** een)*

thiothixene hydrochloride

Navane

**Pregnancy Category C**

### Drug classes

Dopaminergic blocking agent
Antipsychotic
Thioxanthene, not a phenothiazine

### Therapeutic actions

Mechanism of action not fully understood: blocks postsynaptic dopamine receptors in the brain, but this may not be necessary and sufficient for antipsychotic activity.

### Indications

- Management of manifestations of psychotic disorders

### Contraindications/cautions

- Contraindications: coma or severe CNS depression, blood dyscrasia, circulatory collapse, subcortical brain damage, Parkinson's disease, liver damage, cerebral arteriosclerosis, coronary disease, severe hypotension or hypertension, pregnancy, lactation.
- Use cautiously with respiratory disorders ("silent pneumonia"); glaucoma, prostatic hypertrophy; epilepsy or history of epilepsy (drug lowers seizure threshold); breast cancer; thyrotoxicosis (severe neurotoxicity); peptic ulcer, decreased renal function; myelography within previous 24 h or scheduled within 48 h; exposure to heat or phosphorous insecticides; children <12 y, especially those with chickenpox, CNS infections (children are es-

pecially susceptible to dystonias that may confound the diagnosis of Reye's syndrome).

## Dosage

**Available Forms:** Capsules—1, 2, 5, 10, 20 mg; concentrate—5 mg/ml

Full clinical effects may require 6 wk–6 mo of therapy.

*ADULT*

- ***Oral:*** Initially 2 mg tid (mild conditions) or 5 mg bid (more severe conditions). Increase dose as needed; the usual optimum dose is 20–30 mg/d. May increase to 60 mg/d, but further increases rarely increase beneficial response.
- ***IM (for more rapid control and when oral dosage is not feasible):*** Usual dose is 4 mg bid–qid. Most patients are controlled on 16–20 mg/d. Maximum dosage is 30 mg/d. Institute oral medication as soon as feasible; dosage adjustment may be necessary when changing to oral forms.

*PEDIATRIC:* Not recommended for children <12 y.

*GERIATRIC AND DEBILITATED PATIENTS:* Use lower doses and increase more gradually.

## Pharmacokinetics

| Route | Onset | Duration |
|---|---|---|
| Oral | Slow | 12 h |
| IM | 1–6 h | 12 h |

*Metabolism:* Hepatic, $T_{1/2}$: 34 h

*Distribution:* Crosses placenta; enters breast milk

*Excretion:* Bile and feces

## Adverse effects

*Antipsychotic Drugs*

- CNS: *Drowsiness*, insomnia, vertigo, headache, weakness, tremor, ataxia, slurring, cerebral edema, seizures, exacerbation of psychotic symptoms, extrapyramidal syndromes—*pseudoparkinsonism; dystonias; akathisia*, tardive dyskinesias, potentially irreversible NMS; extrapyramidal symptoms, hyperthermia, **autonomic disturbances** (rare, but 20% fatal)
- CV: Hypotension, orthostatic hypotension, hypertension, tachycardia, bradycardia, cardiac arrest, CHF, cardiomegaly, **refractory arrhythmias** (some fatal), pulmonary edema
- Respiratory: Bronchospasm, laryngospasm, dyspnea, suppression of cough reflex and potential for aspiration
- Hematologic: Eosinophilia, leukopenia, leukocytosis, anemia; aplastic anemia; hemolytic anemia; thrombocytopenic or nonthrombocytopenic purpura; pancytopenia
- EENT: Glaucoma, *photophobia, blurred vision*, miosis, mydriasis, deposits in the cornea and lens (opacities), pigmentary retinopathy
- Hypersensitivity: Jaundice, urticaria, angioneurotic edema, laryngeal edema, photosensitivity, eczema, asthma, anaphylactoid reactions, exfoliative dermatitis
- Endocrine: Lactation, breast engorgement, galactorrhea; SIADH secretion; amenorrhea, menstrual irregularities; gynecomastia; changes in libido; hyperglycemia or hypoglycemia; glycosuria; hyponatremia; pituitary tumor with hyperprolactinemia; inhibition of ovulation, infertility, pseudopregnancy; reduced urinary levels of gonadotropins, estrogens, progestins
- Autonomic: *Dry mouth, salivation, nasal congestion, nausea*, vomiting, anorexia, fever, pallor, flushed facies, sweating, constipation, paralytic ileus, urinary retention, incontinence, polyuria, enuresis, priapism, ejaculation inhibition, male impotence
- Other: *Urine discolored pink to red-brown*

## Drug-lab test interferences

• False-positive pregnancy tests (less likely if serum test is used) • Increase in PBI not attributable to an increase in thyroxine

## ■ Nursing Considerations

### Assessment

- *History:* Severe CNS depression; blood dyscrasia; circulatory collapse; subcortical

brain damage; Parkinson's disease; liver damage; cerebral arteriosclerosis; coronary disease; severe hypotension or hypertension; respiratory disorders; glaucoma, prostatic hypertrophy; epilepsy; breast cancer; thyrotoxicosis; peptic ulcer, decreased renal function; myelography within previous 24 h or scheduled within 48 h; exposure to heat or phosphorous insecticides; pregnancy; lactation; chickenpox; CNS infections
- *Physical:* Weight, T; reflexes, orientation, intraocular pressure; P, BP, orthostatic BP; R, adventitious sounds; bowel sounds and normal output, liver evaluation; urinary output, prostate size. Arrange for CBC, urinalysis, thyroid, liver and kidney function tests.

### Implementation

- Reconstitute the powder for injection with 2.2 ml of Sterile Water for Injection. Store at room temperature for up to 48 h and then discard any unused solution.
- Avoid skin contact with oral solution; contact dermatitis has occurred.
- Discontinue drug if serum creatinine, BUN become abnormal or if WBC count is depressed.
- Monitor elderly patients for dehydration, and institute remedial measures promptly; sedation and decreased sensation of thirst related to CNS effects can lead to severe dehydration.
- Consult physician regarding appropriate warning of patient or patient's guardian about tardive dyskinesias.
- Consult physician about dosage reduction, use of anticholinergic antiparkinsonian drugs (controversial) if extrapyramidal effects occur.

### Drug-specific teaching points

- Take drug exactly as prescribed.
- Avoid skin contact with drug solutions.
- Avoid driving or engaging in other dangerous activities if CNS, vision changes occur.
- Avoid prolonged exposure to sun or use a sunscreen or covering garments.
- Maintain fluid intake, and use precautions against heatstroke in hot weather.
- Report sore throat, fever, unusual bleeding or bruising, rash, weakness, tremors, impaired vision, dark urine (pink or reddish brown urine is to be expected), pale stools, yellowing of the skin or eyes.

## thyroid desiccated

*(thye' roid)*

Armour Thyroid, S-P-T, Thyrar, Thyroid Strong

**Pregnancy Category A**

### Drug classes

Thyroid hormone preparation(contains T3 and T4 in their natural state and ratio)

### Therapeutic actions

Increases the metabolic rate of body tissues, increasing oxygen consumption, respiratory and heart rate; rate of fat, protein, and carbohydrate metabolism; and growth and maturation; exact mechanism of action is not known.

### Indications

- Replacement therapy in hypothyroidism
- Pituitary TSH suppression, in the treatment and prevention of euthyroid goiters and management of thyroid cancer
- Thyrotoxicosis in conjunction with antithyroid drugs and prevention of goitrogenesis, hypothyroidism, and thyrotoxicosis during pregnancy

### Contraindications/cautions

- Contraindications: allergy to active or extraneous constituents of drug (preparations marketed as *Thyrar* are derived from bovine thyroids; preparations marketed as *S-P-T* are derived from porcine thyroids); thyrotoxicosis and acute MI uncomplicated by hypothyroidism.
- Use cautiously with Addison's disease (treatment of hypoadrenalism with corticosteroids should precede thyroid therapy), pregnancy.

### Dosage

**Available Forms:** Tablets—30, 60, 120, 150, 180, 240, 300 mg; capsules—60, 120, 180, 300 mg

**ADULT**

- *Myxedema:* Initial dosage, 16 mg/d PO for 2 wk, followed by 32 mg/d PO for 2 or more wk, then 65 mg/d. Assess after 1 and 2 mo of therapy with the 65-mg dose, and increase dosage if needed up to 130 mg/d for 2 mo. Reassess, and increase to 195 mg/d if needed; make further increases, if needed, in 32- or 65-mg/d increments. Maintenance, 65–195 mg/d.
- *Hypothyroidism without myxedema:* Initial dosage, 65 mg/d PO, increased by 65 mg q30 d PO until desired result is obtained. Maintenance, same as above.

**PEDIATRIC:** Initial dosage, 16 mg/d PO for 2 wk, followed by 32 mg/d PO for 2 or more wk, then 65 mg/d. Assess in 2 mo, and increase dosage if needed up to 130 mg/d for 2 mo. Maintenance, 65–195 mg/d. Actually, dosage may be greater during periods of growth; monitor clinical condition and laboratory tests to determine correct dose (sleeping pulse and basal morning temperature are guides to treatment).

### Pharmacokinetics

| Route | Onset | Peak |
|---|---|---|
| Oral | Varies | 4 h |

*Metabolism:* Liver, kidney, and tissue, $T_{1/2}$: 1–2 d ($T_3$), 6–7 d ($T_4$)
*Distribution:* Crosses placenta; enters breast milk
*Excretion:* Urine and feces

### Adverse effects

All rare at therapeutic doses.

- **Dermatologic**: Partial loss of hair in first few months of therapy in children
- **Endocrine**: Hyperthyroidism (palpitations, elevated pulse pressure, tachycardia, arrhythmias, angina pectoris, cardiac arrest; tremors, headache, nervousness, insomnia; nausea, diarrhea, changes in appetite; weight loss, menstrual irregularities, sweating, heat intolerance, fever)
- **Hypersensitivity**: Allergic skin reactions

### Clinically important drug-drug interactions

• Decreased absorption with cholestyramine • Increased risk of bleeding with warfarin, dicumarol • Decreased effectiveness of digitalis glycosides with thyroid replacement • Alterations in theophylline clearance occur in hypothyroid patients; if thyroid state changes during therapy, monitor patient carefully

## ■ Nursing Considerations

### Assessment

- *History:* Allergy to active or extraneous constituents of drug, bovine, or porcine products; thyrotoxicosis; acute MI uncomplicated by hypothyroidism; Addison's disease; lactation
- *Physical:* Skin lesions, color, temperature, texture; T; muscle tone, orientation, reflexes; P, auscultation, baseline ECG, BP; R, adventitious sounds; thyroid function tests

### Implementation

- Monitor response carefully when beginning therapy, and adjust dosage accordingly.
- Administer as a single daily dose before breakfast.
- Arrange for regular, periodic blood tests of thyroid function.
- Monitor cardiac response throughout therapy.

### Drug-specific teaching points

- Take as a single dose before breakfast.
- This drug replaces a very important hormone and will need to be taken for life. Do not discontinue this drug without consulting your nurse or physician; serious problems can occur.
- Wear or carry a medical alert tag to alert emergency medical personnel that you are on this drug.
- Nausea and diarrhea may occur (dividing the dose may help).
- Have periodic blood tests and medical evaluations while you are on this drug. Keep your scheduled appointments.

- Report headache, chest pain, palpitations, fever, weight loss, sleeplessness, nervousness, irritability, unusual sweating, intolerance to heat, diarrhea.

## thyrotropin

*(thye roe **troe'** pin)*

thyroid-stimulating hormone, TSH

Thytropar

**Pregnancy Category C**

### Drug classes

Hormone
Diagnostic agent

### Therapeutic actions

Produces increased uptake of iodine by the thyroid, increased formation of thyroid hormone, increased release of thyroid hormone, and cellular hyperplasia of the thyroid on prolonged stimulation.

### Indications

- Diagnostic agent to differentiate thyroid failure and to establish a diagnosis of decreased thyroid reserve
- Used for PBI and $I^{131}$ uptake determinations

### Contraindications/cautions

- Contraindications: allergy to thyrotrophin, beef products, coronary thrombosis, untreated Addison's disease.
- Use cautiously with cardiac disease, pregnancy.

### Dosage

**Available Forms:** Powder for injection—10 IU/vial

*ADULT:* 10 IU IM or SC for 1–3 d. Follow by a radioiodine study 24 h after the last injection. No response occurs with thyroid failure; substantial response will occur in pituitary failure.

*PEDIATRIC:* Safety and efficacy not established.

### Pharmacokinetics

| Route | Onset |
|---|---|
| SC, IM | Days |

*Metabolism:* $T_{1/2}$: 30–35 min
*Distribution:* Crosses placenta; enters breast milk
*Excretion:* Urine

### Adverse effects

- CNS: *Headache*
- GI: *Nausea, vomiting*
- CV: Transitory hypotension, tachycardia
- **Hypersensitivity**: Reactions including anaphylaxis
- **Other**: Thyroid gland swelling, *urticaria*

### ■ Nursing Considerations

#### Assessment

- ***History:*** Allergy to thyrotropin, beef products, untreated Addison's disease, cardiac disease, pregnancy
- ***Physical:*** Skin color, lesions; thyroid gland exam; BP, P; R, adventitious sounds; thyroid function tests

#### Implementation

- Store reconstituted solution in refrigerator; do not store >2 wk.
- Administer by IM or SC routes only.

#### Drug-specific teaching points

- Injections will be made on 3 consecutive d. 24 h following the last injection, a radioiodine study will be performed to determine the drug's effects on your thyroid gland.
- The following side effects may occur: nausea, vomiting, rash, swelling on the thyroid gland.
- Report dizziness, palpitations, difficulty breathing.

## tiagabine hydrochloride

*(tye **ag'** ah bine)*

Gabitril

**Pregnancy Category C**

**Drug classes**
Antiepileptic agent

**Therapeutic actions**
Increases GABA levels in the brain, which may result in antiseizure effects. GABA is the major inhibitory neurotransmitter in the CNS; tiagabine binds to GABA reuptake sites, preventing its reuptake, and increases levels in the presynaptic neurons and the glia.

**Indications**
- Adjunctive therapy in patients with partial seizures

**Contraindications/cautions**
- Contraindications: hypersensitivity to tiagabine, hepatic disease or significant hepatic dysfunction.
- Use cautiously with pregnancy, lactation, and the elderly.

**Dosage**
**Available Forms:** Tablets—4, 12, 16, 20 mg
*ADULT:* 4 mg PO qd for 1 wk; may be increased by 4–8 mg/wk until desired response is seen; maximum dose 56 mg/d in 2–4 divided doses.
*PEDIATRIC 12–18 Y:* 4 mg PO qd for 1 wk; may be increased to 8 mg/d in 2 divided doses for 1 wk; then increased by 4–8 mg/wk up to a maximum of 32 mg/d in 2–4 divided doses.
*PEDIATRIC < 12 Y:* Not recommended.

**Pharmacokinetics**

| *Route* | *Onset* | *Peak* |
|---|---|---|
| Oral | Rapid | 1/2–1 h |

*Metabolism:* Hepatic; $T_{1/2}$: 4.5–13.4 h
*Distribution:* Crosses placenta; enters breast milk
*Excretion:* Feces and urine

**Adverse effects**
- CNS: *Dizziness, asthenia, somnolence,* nervousness, tremor, concentration difficulties
- GI: *GI upset, pain*
- GU: Irregular menses, secondary amenorrhea
- EENT: Possible long-term ophthalmic effects
- Dermatologic: **Serious skin rash**

**Clinically important drug-drug interactions**
• Decreased serum levels with carbamazepine, phenytoin, primidone; adjustment in tiagabine dosage may be necessary • Possible interaction with valproate; monitor patient closely

## ■ Nursing Considerations

### Assessment
- ***History:*** Hypersensitivity to tiagabine, hepatic disease or significant hepatic dysfunction, pregnancy, lactation
- ***Physical:*** Body weight; skin color, lesions; orientation, eye exam, affect, reflexes; hepatic function tests

### Implementation
- Give drug with food.
- Reduce dosage and titrate more slowly if patient is not on comcomitant phenytoin, phenobarbital, carbamazepine.
- Provide frequent skin care if dermatologic effects occur.
- Avoid abrupt discontinuation; serious side effects could occur.
- Establish safety precautions (siderails, accompanying patient, etc.) if CNS changes occur.
- Arrange for appropriate counseling for women of childbearing age who wish to become pregnant.

### Drug-specific teaching points
- Take this drug exactly as prescribed.
- Do not discontinue this drug abruptly or change dosage, except on the advice of your physician.
- Avoid the use of alcohol and sleep-inducing or OTC drugs while you are on this drug; these could cause dangerous effects. If you feel that you need one of these preparations, consult your nurse or physician.
- Use contraceptive techniques at all times. If you wish to become pregnant while you are taking this drug, consult your physician.

- The following side effects may occur: drowsiness (avoid driving or performing other tasks requiring alertness); GI upset (take the drug with food or milk; eat small, frequent meals).
- Wear a Medic-Alert bracelet at all times so that any emergency medical personnel will know that you are an epileptic taking antiepileptic medication.
- Report bruising, yellowing of the skin or eyes, pale-colored feces, skin rash, pregnancy, vision changes.

## ticarcillin disodium

*(tye kar **sill'** in)*
Ticar
**Pregnancy Category B**

### Drug classes
Antibiotic
Penicillin with extended spectrum

### Therapeutic actions
Bactericidal: inhibits synthesis of cell wall of action-sensitive organisms, causing cell death.

### Indications
- Severe infections caused by sensitive organisms, particularly *Pseudomonas aeruginosa, Proteus, E. coli*
- Infections caused by anaerobic bacteria
- GU infections caused by the above or *Enterobacter, Streptococcus faecalis*

### Contraindications/cautions
- Contraindications: allergies to penicillins, cephalosporins or other allergens.
- Use cautiously with renal disorders, pregnancy, lactation (may cause diarrhea or candidiasis in the infant).

### Dosage
**Available Forms:** Powder for injection—1, 3, 6, 20, 30 g
Maximum recommended dosage, 24 g/d. Maximum dose of single IM injection, 2 g.

**ADULT**
- *UTIs:* 1 g IM *or* direct IV q6h, up to 150–200 mg/kg per day IV in divided doses q4–6h in severe cases.
- *Other infections:* 200–300 mg/kg per day IV in divided doses q3, 4, or 6h.

**PEDIATRIC**
- *UTIs (< 40 kg):* 50–100 mg/kg per day IM *or* direct IV in divided doses q6–8h up to 150–200 mg/kg per day in divided doses q4–6h IV.
- *Other infections (< 40 kg):* 200–300 mg/kg per day q4–6h IV.

**NEONATES:** May be given IM or over 10–20 min IV.
- *< 2 KG, 0–7 D:* 75 mg/kg q12h initially; after 7 d old, 75 mg/kg q8h.
- *> 2 KG, 0–7 D:* 75 mg/kg q8h; after 7 d old, 100 mg/kg q8h.

**GERIATRIC OR RENAL INSUFFICIENCY:** Initial dose of 3 g IV followed by the following doses:

| *Creatinine Clearance (ml/min)* | *Dosage* |
|---|---|
| >60 | 3 g q4h IV |
| 30–60 | 2 g q4h IV |
| 10–30 | 2 g q8h IV |
| <10 | 2 g q12h IV or 1 g q6h IM |
| <10 with hepatic dysfunction | 2 g qd or 1 g q12h IM |
| Patients on peritoneal dialysis | 3 g q12h IV |
| Patients on hemodialysis | 2 g q12h with 3 g after each dialysis |

### Pharmacokinetics

| *Route* | *Onset* | *Peak* |
|---|---|---|
| IM | Rapid | 30–75 min |
| IV | Rapid | End of infusion |

*Metabolism:* Hepatic, $T_{1/2}$: 0.8–1.4 h
*Distribution:* Crosses placenta; enters breast milk
*Excretion:* Urine

### IV facts
**Preparation:** Reconstitute each gm of ticarcillin for IV use with 4 ml of Sodium Chloride Injection, 5% Dextrose Injection, or Lactate Ringer's Injection. Each 1 ml of solution will contain approximately 200 mg. Date reconstituted solution. Reconstituted solution (10–50 mg/ml) is stable for 72 h at room temperature if diluted with Sodium Chloride or 5% Dex-

trose; 48 h if diluted with Lactated Ringer's; 14 d if refrigerated. Do not store for >72 h if for multidose purposes.
**Infusion:** Direct injection: administer as slowly as possible to avoid vein irritation—over 30 min preferred. Infusion should be run by continuous drip or intermittently from 30 min to 2 h.
**Compatibilities:** Do not mix with solution of gentamicin, tobramycin, amikacin.

### Adverse effects

- CNS: Lethargy, hallucinations, seizures
- GI: *Glossitis, stomatitis, gastritis, sore mouth*, furry tongue, black "hairy" tongue, *nausea, vomiting, diarrhea*, abdominal pain, bloody diarrhea, enterocolitis, pseudomembranous colitis, nonspecific hepatitis
- **Hematologic**: Anemia, thrombocytopenia, leukopenia, neutropenia, prolonged bleeding time
- GU: Nephritis—oliguria, proteinuria, hematuria, casts, azotemia, pyuria
- **Hypersensitivity reactions**: *Rash, fever, wheezing*, anaphylaxis
- Local: *Pain, phlebitis*, thrombosis at injection site
- Other: *Superinfections*—oral and rectal moniliasis, vaginitis, sodium overload

### Clinically important drug-drug interactions

- Decreased effectiveness with tetracyclines
- Inactivation of parenteral aminoglycosides (amikacin, gentamicin, kanamycin, neomycin, metilmicin, streptomycin, tobramycin)

### Drug-lab test interferences

- False-positive Coombs' test with IV use

## ■ Nursing Considerations

### Assessment

- *History:* Allergies to penicillins, cephalosporins, other allergens; renal disorders; pregnancy; lactation
- *Physical:* Culture infection; skin color, lesion; R, adventitious sounds; bowel sounds; CBC, liver and renal function tests, serum electrolytes, Hct, urinalysis

### Implementation

- Culture infection before beginning treatment; reculture if response is not as expected.
- Continue therapy for at least 2 d after signs of infection have disappeared, usually 7–10 d.
- Administer by IM or IV routes only.
- Reconstitute each gram for IM use with 2 ml Sodium Chloride Injection, 5% Dextrose Injection, Lactated Ringer's Injection, or 1% lidocaine HCl without epinephrine. Each 2.6 ml will contain 1 g ticarcillin. Inject deep into a large muscle.
- Maintain epinephrine, IV fluids, vasopressors, bronchodilators, oxygen, and emergency equipment on standby in case of serious hypersensitivity reaction.

### Drug-specific teaching points

- This drug is given by injection.
- The following side effects may occur: upset stomach, nausea, diarrhea (small, frequent meals may help); mouth sores (frequent mouth care may help); pain or discomfort at injection sites.
- Report difficulty breathing, rashes, severe diarrhea, severe pain at injection site, mouth sores.

## ticlopidine hydrochloride

(tye **kloh'** pih deen)

Ticlid

**Pregnancy Category B**

### Drug classes

Antiplatelet agent

### Therapeutic actions

Interferes with platelet membrane function by inhibiting fibrinogen binding and platelet-platelet interactions; inhibits platelet aggregation and prolongs bleeding time; effect is irreversible for life of the platelet.

### Indications

- Reduces risk of thrombotic stroke in patients who have experienced stroke pre-

t

cursors and in patients who have had a completed thrombotic stroke; reserve use for patients who are intolerant to aspirin therapy because side effects may be life-threatening
- Unlabeled uses: intermittent claudication, chronic arterial occlusion, subarachnoid hemmorhage, uremic patients with AV shunts or fistulas, open heart surgery, coronary artery bypass grafts, primary glomerulonephritis, sickle cell disease

### Contraindications/cautions
- Contraindications: allergy to ticlopidine, neutropenia, thrombocytopenia, hemostatic disorders, bleeding ulcer, intracranial bleeding, severe liver disease, lactation.
- Use cautiously with renal disorders, pregnancy, elevated cholesterol, recent trauma.

### Dosage
**Available Forms:** Tablets—250 mg

*ADULT:* 250 mg PO bid with food.

*PEDIATRIC:* Safety and efficacy not established for children younger than 18 y.

### Pharmacokinetics

| *Route* | *Onset* | *Peak* |
|---|---|---|
| Oral | Rapid | 2 h |

*Metabolism:* Hepatic, $T_{1/2}$: 12.6 h, then 4–5 d

*Distribution:* Crosses placenta; enters breast milk

*Excretion:* Urine and feces

### Adverse effects
- CNS: Dizziness
- GI: *Diarrhea, nausea, vomiting, abdominal pain*, flatulence, dyspepsia, anorexia
- Hematologic: *Neutropenia*, bleeding
- Local: *Pain, phlebitis*, thrombosis at injection site
- Other: Rash, purpura

### Clinically important drug-drug interactions
• Decreased effectiveness of digoxin • Increased serum levels and effects of theophylline, aspirin • Increased effects with cimetidine • Decreased absorption with antacids

### Clinically important drug-food interactions
- Increased availability with food

## ■ Nursing Considerations

### Assessment
- ***History:*** Allergy to ticlopidine, neutropenia, thrombocytopenia, hemostatic disorders, bleeding ulcer, intracranial bleeding, severe liver disease, lactation, renal disorders, pregnancy, elevated cholesterol, recent trauma
- ***Physical:*** Skin color, lesions; orientation; bowel sounds, normal output; CBC, liver and renal function tests, serum cholesterol

### Implementation
- Monitor WBC count before use and frequently while initiating therapy; if neutropenia is present or occurs, discontinue drug immediately.
- Administer with food or just after eating to minimize GI irritation and increase absorption.
- Maintain IV methylprednisolone (20 mg) on standby in case excessive bleeding occurs.
- Monitor patient for any sign of excessive bleeding (eg, bruises, dark stools), and monitor bleeding times.
- Provide increased precautions against bleeding during invasive procedures; bleeding will be prolonged.
- Mark patient's chart receiving drug to alert medical personnel of increased risk of bleeding in cases of surgery or dental surgery.

### Drug-specific teaching points
- Take drug with meals or just after eating.
- You will require regular blood tests to monitor your response to this drug.
- It may take longer than normal to stop bleeding; avoid contact sports, use electrical razors; apply pressure for extended periods to bleeding sites.

- The following side effects may occur: upset stomach, nausea, diarrhea, loss of appetite (small, frequent meals may help).
- Notify dentist or surgeon that you are on this drug before invasive procedures.
- Report fever, chills, sore throat, skin rash, bruising, bleeding, dark stools or urine.

## tiludronate sodium

*(tah **loo'** dro nate)*

Skelid

**Pregnancy Category C**

### Drug classes

Biophosphonate

### Therapeutic actions

Affects osteoclast activity by reducing the enzymatic and transport processes that lead to resorption of the bone and by inhibiting the osteoclast protein pump, leading to a rate of bone turnover near normal in patients with Paget's disease.

### Indications

- Treatment of Paget's disease in patients with alkaline phosphatase at least 2 times the upper limit of normal, in those who are symptomatic, and in those at risk for future complications

### Contraindications/cautions

- Contraindications: allergy to biphosphonates, severe renal disease, pregnancy, lactation.
- Use cautiously with hypocalcemia, upper GI disease.

### Dosage

**Available Forms:** Tablets—200 mg tiludronate (as 250-mg tablets)

***Adult:*** 400 mg PO qd for 3 mo taken with 6–8 oz. of plain water at least 2 h before or after any other beverage or food; may retreat after a 3-mo post-treatment period if indicated.

***Pediatric:*** Safety and efficacy not established.

***Renal Impairment:*** Not recommended if Ccr <30 ml/min.

### Pharmacokinetics

| *Route* | *Onset* | *Peak* |
|---|---|---|
| PO | Rapid | 2 h |

*Metabolism:* Not metabolized

*Distribution:* Crosses placenta; may enter breast milk

*Excretion:* Urine

### Adverse effects

- CNS: *Headache,* paresthesia
- GI: *Nausea, diarrhea, dyspepsia*
- CV: Chest pain, edema
- EENT: Glaucoma, conjunctivitis, cataract
- Skeletal: *Increased or recurrent bone pain,* focal osteomalacia
- Other: Hyperparathyroidism, arthrosis, sinusitis

### Clinically important drug-drug interactions

• Absorption decreased by calcium, aspirin, aluminum, magnesium; avoid these drugs for 2 h before to 2 h after taking tulodronate • Effects may be potentiated by indomethacin

## ■ Nursing Considerations

### Assessment

- ***History:*** Allergy to biphosphonates, renal failure, upper GI disease, hypocalcemia, pregnancy, lactation
- ***Physical:*** Muscle tone, bone pain; bowel sounds; eye exam; urinalysis, serum calcium

### Implementation

- Administer with a full glass of plain (not mineral) water, at least 2 h before or after any other beverage, food, or medication.
- Monitor serum calcium levels before, during, and after therapy.
- Ensure a 3-mo rest period after a 3-mo course of treatment if retreatment is required.
- Ensure adequate vitamin D and calcium intake.
- Provide comfort measures if bone pain returns.

### Drug-specific teaching points

- Take this drug with a full glass of plain (not mineral) water, at least 2 hours be-

t

fore or after any other beverage, food, or medication.

- Maintain adequate vitamin D and calcium intake while you are on this drug.
- The following side effects may occur: nausea, diarrhea; bone pain, headache (analgesics may be available to help); visual changes (notify your health care provider and take appropriate safety precautions).
- Report twitching, muscle spasms, dark-colored urine, edema, changes in vision or eye inflammation.

## timolol maleate

*(tye **moe'** lole)*

Blocadren, Timoptic, Timoptic-XE, Betimol

**Pregnancy Category C**

### Drug classes

Beta adrenergic blocker
Antihypertensive
Antiglaucoma agent

### Therapeutic actions

Competitively blocks beta-adrenergic receptors in the heart and juxtaglomerular apparatus, decreasing the influence of the sympathetic nervous system on these tissues and decreasing the excitability of the heart, decreasing cardiac output and oxygen consumption, decreasing the release of renin, and lowering BP; reduces intraocular pressure by decreasing the production of aqueous humor and possibly by increasing aqueous humor outflow.

### Indications

- Hypertension, used alone or in combination with other antihypertensives, especially thiazide-type diuretics
- Prevention of reinfarction in MI patients who are hemodynamically stable
- Prophylaxis of migraine
- Reduction of intraocular pressure in chronic open-angle glaucoma, some patients with secondary glaucoma, aphakic patients with glaucoma (ophthalmic solution)

### Contraindications/cautions

- Contraindications: sinus bradycardia (HR $< 45$ beats/min), second- or third-degree heart block (PR interval $> 0.24$ sec), cardiogenic shock, CHF, asthma, COPD, pregnancy, lactation.
- Use cautiously with diabetes or thyrotoxicosis (timolol can mask the usual cardiac signs of hypoglycemia and thyrotoxicosis).

### Dosage

**Available Forms:** Tablets—5, 10, 20 mg; ophthalmic solution, gel—0.25%, 0.50%

**ADULT**

- ***Oral***
  - *Hypertension:* Initially, 10 mg bid. Increase dosage at 1-wk intervals to a maximum of 60 mg/d divided into two doses, as necessary. Usual maintenance dose is 20–40 mg/d.
  - ***Prevention of reinfarction in MI (long-term prophylaxis in patients who survived the acute phase):*** 10 mg bid PO.
  - *Migraine:* 10 mg PO bid; during maintenance, the 20 mg/d may be given as a single dose. May be increased to a maximum of 30 mg/d in divided doses or decreased to 10 mg/d. Discontinue if satisfactory response is not obtained after 6–8 wk.
- ***Ophthalmic administration:*** Initially 1 drop of 0.25% solution bid into the affected eye(s). Adjust dosage on basis of resonse to 1 drop of 0.5% solution bid or 1 drop of 0.25% solution qd. When replacing other agents, make change gradually and individualize dosage.

**PEDIATRIC:** Safety and efficacy not established.

### Pharmacokinetics

| Route | Onset | Peak |
|---|---|---|
| Oral | Varies | 1–2 h |
| Ophthalmologic | Rapid | 1–5 h |

*Metabolism:* Hepatic, $T_{1/2}$: 3–4 h
*Distribution:* Crosses placenta; enters breast milk
*Excretion:* Urine

### Adverse effects

*Oral*

- CNS: Dizziness, vertigo, tinnitus, fatigue, emotional depression, paresthesias, sleep disturbances, hallucinations, disorientation, memory loss, slurred speech
- GI: *Gastric pain, flatulence, constipation, diarrhea, nausea, vomiting,* anorexia, ischemic colitis, renal and mesenteric arterial thrombosis, retroperitoneal fibrosis, hepatomegaly, acute pancreatitis
- CV: *CHF, cardiac arrhythmias, sinoartial or AV nodal block,* peripheral vascular insufficiency, claudication, CVA, pulmonary edema, hypotension
- **Respiratory**: Bronchospasm, dyspnea, cough, bronchial obstruction, nasal stuffiness, rhinitis, pharyngitis (less likely than with propranolol)
- GU: *Impotence, decreased libido*, Peyronie's disease, dysuria, nocturia, frequent urination
- **MS**: Joint pain, arthralgia, muscle cramp
- **EENT**: Eye irritation, dry eyes, conjunctivitis, blurred vision
- **Dermatologic**: Rash, pruritus, sweating, dry skin
- **Allergic reactions**: Pharyngitis, erythematous rash, fever, sore throat, laryngospasm, respiratory distress
- **Other**: *Decreased exercise tolerance, development of antinuclear antibodies* (ANA), hyperglycemia or hypoglycemia, elevated serum transaminase, alkaline

*Ophthalmic*

- **Local**: Ocular irritation, decreased corneal sensitivity, visual refractive changes, diplopia, ptosis

### Clinically important drug-drug interactions

• Increased effects with verapamil • Increased risk of postural hypotension with prazosin • Decreased antihypertensive effects with NSAIDs, clonidine • Decreased elimination of theophyllines with resultant decrease in expected actions of both drugs when taken concurrently • Peripheral ischemia and possible gangrene with ergotamine, methysergide, dihydroergotamine • Increased risk of hypoglycemia and masked signs of hypoglycemia with insulin • Hypertension followed by severe bradycardia with epinephrine • All of the above may occur with ophthalmic timolol; in addition, additive effects are possible with oral beta-blockers.

### Drug-lab test interferences

• Possible false results with glucose or insulin tolerance tests (oral)

## ■ Nursing Considerations

### Assessment

- ***History:*** Sinus bradycardia, second- or third-degree heart block, cardiogenic shock, CHF, asthma, COPD, pregnancy, lactation, diabetes or thyrotoxicosis
- ***Physical:*** Weight, skin condition, neurologic status, P, BP, ECG, respiratory status, kidney and thyroid function, blood and urine glucose

### Implementation

- Do not discontinue drug abruptly after chronic therapy (hypersensitivity to catecholamines may have developed, causing exacerbation of angina, MI, and ventricular dysrhythmias). Taper drug gradually over 2 wk with monitoring.
- Consult with physician about withdrawal if patient is to undergo surgery (withdrawal is controversial).

### Drug-specific teaching points

- Do not stop taking this drug unless instructed to do so by a health care provider.
- Avoid driving or dangerous activities if CNS effects occur.
- Report difficulty breathing, night cough, swelling of extremities, slow pulse, confusion, depression, rash, fever, sore throat.
- Ophthalmic: Administer eye drops properly to minimize systemic absorption.

## tiopronin

*(tye oh **pro'** nin)*

Thiola

**Pregnancy Category C**

### Drug classes

Thiol compound

### Therapeutic actions

Active reducing and complexing compound, which undergoes thiol-disulfide exchange with cystine during urine formation to form a water-soluble mixed disulfide, reducing cystine and leading to a reduction in the formation of cystine (kidney) stone formation.

### Indications

- Prevention of cystine (kidney) stone formation in patients with severe homozygous cystinuria with urinary cystine greater than 500 mg/d and who are resistant to treatment with conservative measures

### Contraindications/cautions

- Contraindications: hypersensitivity to tiopronin; history of agranulocytosis, aplastic anemia, thrombocytopenia; pregnancy; lactation.
- Use cautiously with history of severe reaction to penicillamine.

### Dosage

**Available Forms:** Tablets—100 mg

Use only after more conservative measures have been tried and failed.

**ADULT:** Initially 800 mg/d PO. Average dose is 1,000 mg/d. Give in divided doses 3×/d at least 1 h before or 2 h after meals. Measure urinary cystine 1 mo after treatment and every 3 mo thereafter. Readjust dosage depending on urinary cystine levels.

**PEDIATRIC:** Safety and efficacy in children <9 y not established.

- *>9 Y:* Initial dosage based on 15 mg/kg per day PO with adjustments based on patient response.

### Pharmacokinetics

| *Route* | *Onset* | *Peak* | *Duration* |
|---|---|---|---|
| Oral | Varies | 4 h | 72 h |

*Metabolism:* Renal, $T_{1/2}$: unknown

*Distribution:* Crosses placenta; enters breast milk

*Excretion:* Urine

### Adverse effects

- **Hematologic:** Leukopenia, eosinophilia, thrombocytopenia
- **GU:** Proteinuria
- **Dermatologic:** *Erythematous, maculopapular* or *morbilliform rash*, lupus erythematous-like reaction, wrinkling and friability of skin
- **General:** *Fever*

## ■ Nursing Considerations

### Assessment

- ***History:*** Hypersensitivity to tiopronin, agranulocytosis, aplastic anemia, thrombocytopenia, severe reaction to penicillamine, pregnancy, lactation
- ***Physical:*** T; skin color, lesions; urinary output; urinalysis, urinary cystine levels, 24 h urinary protein, liver function tests, CBC, Hct, electrolytes

### Implementation

- Attempt conservative measures to decrease stone formation before beginning therapy: Provide at least 3 L of fluid, including two glasses with each meal and hs. Advise patient to get up at night to void and to drink two more glasses of fluid before returning to bed. Additional fluids should be added if sweating, diarrhea occur. A minimum urinary output of 2 L/d should be maintained. Alkali therapy may be used to keep urinary pH in a range of 6.5–7. If cystine stones continue to be formed, tiopronin therapy can be used.
- Initiate therapy at a lower than normal dose in patients with a history of severe penicillamine reaction.
- Administer in divided doses, tid at least 1 h before or 2 h after meals.
- Measure urinary cystine levels 1 mo after treatment and every 3 mo thereafter. Adjust dosage based on amount needed to keep cystine concentration below its solubility limit (generally <250 mg/L).
- Monitor blood counts before and during therapy.
- Monitor patient for abnormal urinary findings. Discontinue if abnormalities occur.

- Discontinue drug if fever occurs; reinstate at a smaller dose, gradually increasing dosage until desired effect is achieved.

### Drug-specific teaching points

- Take this drug three times a day, 1 h before or 2 h after meals. Arrange for periodic blood and urine tests to determine drug's effects on your blood count and urine and to determine the appropriate dosage needed. Keep appointments for these tests.
- Continue to drink at least 3 L of fluid each day. Get up to void during the night, and drink more fluid before returning to bed.
- The following side effects may occur: skin rash, easy breaking of skin (proper skin care is important).
- Report fever, sore throat, chills, bleeding, easy bruising.
- Continue dietary and other treatments prescribed for chronic kidney stone condition.

## tizanidine

*(tis **an'** i deen)*

Zanaflex

**Pregnancy Category C**

### Drug classes

Antispasmodic

Sympatholytic, centrally acting

### Therapeutic actions

Centrally acting alpha-2 agonist; antispasmodic effect thought to be a result of indirect depression of polysynaptic reflexes by blocking the excitatory actions of spinal interneurons.

### Indications

- Acute and intermittent management of of spasticity caused by MS, spinal cord injury, cerebral trauma

### Contraindications/cautions

- Contraindications: hypersensitivity to tizanidine, clonidine
- Use cautiously with hepatic or renal impairment, hypotension, pregnancy, lactation

### Dosage

**Available Forms:** Tablets—4 mg

*ADULT:* 8 mg PO initial dose; repeat as needed q6–8h; maximum dose 36 mg/d.

*PEDIATRIC:* Safety and efficacy not established.

*RENAL IMPAIRMENT:* Use lower doses, monitor response.

### Pharmacokinetics

| Route | Onset | Peak | Duration |
|---|---|---|---|
| Oral | 30–60 min | 1–2 h | 3–4 h |

*Metabolism:* Heptic; $T_{1/2}$: 2.7–4.2 h

*Distribution:* Crosses placenta; may pass into breast milk

*Excretion:* Urine

### Adverse effects

- CNS: *Drowsiness, sedation, dizziness, asthenia,* headache, hallucinations
- GI: *Dry mouth, constipation,* anorexia, malaise, nausea, vomiting, parotid pain, parotitis, mild transient abnormalities in liver function tests
- CV: *Hypotension, orthostatic hypotension,* bradycardia

### Clinically important drug-drug interactions

- Potential risk of increased depression with alcohol, baclofen, other CNS depressants
- Possible increased effects with oral contraceptives; monitor patient and decrease tizanidine dose

## ■ Nursing Considerations

### Assessment

- *History:* Hypersensitivity to tizanidine, clonidine; hepatic or renal impairment, hypotension; pregnancy, lactation
- *Physical:* Mucous membranes—color, lesions; orientation, affect; P, BP, orthostatic BP; perfusion; liver evaluation; liver and renal function tests

### Implementation

- Administer drug q6–8h around the clock for best effects.

t

- Titrate drug dosage slowly, which helps to decrease side effects.
- Continue all supportive measures used for spinal cord–injured or neurologically damaged patients.
- Provide sugarless lozenges or ice chips, as appropriate, if dry mouth or altered taste occur.
- Establish safety precautions if CNS, hypotensive changes occur (siderails, accompany patient when ambulating, etc.).
- Attempt to lower dose if side effects become severe or intolerable.

### Drug-specific teaching points

- Take this drug exactly as prescribed. It is important that you not miss doses. Consult your health care provider to determine a schedule that will not interfere with rest.
- Continue all other supportive measures used for your condition.
- The following side effects may occur: drowsiness, dizziness, lightheadedness, headache, weakness (use caution while driving or performing tasks that require alertness or physical dexterity); dry mouth (such on sugarless lozenges or ice chips); GI upset (eat small, frequent meals); dizziness, lightheadedness when changing position (rise slowly, use caution when transferring).
- Report changes in urine or stool, severe dizziness or passing out, changes in vision, difficulty swallowing.

## tobramycin sulfate

*(toe bra **mye'** sin)*

*Parenteral:* Nebcin

*Ophthalmic:* Tobrex Ophthalmic

**Pregnancy Category B**

### Drug classes

Aminoglycoside antibiotic

### Therapeutic actions

Bactericidal: inhibits protein synthesis in susceptible strains of gram-negative bacteria; mechanism of lethal action is not fully understood, but functional integrity of bacterial cell membrane appears to be disrupted.

### Indications

- Serious infections caused by susceptible strains of *P. aeruginosa, E. coli,* indole-positive *Proteus* species, *Providencia* species, *Klebsiella-Enterobacter-Serratia* group, *Citrobacter* species, and staphylococci (including *S. aureus*; parenteral)
- Staphylococcal infections when penicillin is contraindicated or when the bacteria are not susceptible
- Serious, life-threatening gram-negative infections when susceptibility studies have not been completed (sometimes concurrent penicillin or cephalosporin therapy)
- Treatment of superficial ocular infections due to susceptible strains of organisms (ophthalmic solution)

### Contraindications/cautions

- Contraindications: allergy to aminoglycosides; pregnancy, lactation.
- Use cautiously with elderly or patients with diminished hearing, decreased renal function, dehydration, neuromuscular disorders (myasthenia gravis, parkinsonism, infant botulism); herpes, vaccinia, varicella, mycobacterial infections, fungal infections (ophthalmic solutions).

### Dosage

**Available Forms:** Injection—10, 40 mg/ml; powder for injection—30 mg/ml; ophthalmic solution—0.3%; ophthalmic ointment—3 mg/g

***IM OR IV***

- *ADULT:* 3 mg/kg/d in 3 equal doses q8h. Up to 5 mg/kg/d in 3–4 equal doses can be used in life-threatening infections, but reduce to 3 mg/kg/d as soon as possible. Do not exceed 5 mg/kg/d unless serum levels are monitored.
- *PEDIATRIC:* 6–7.5 mg/kg/d divided into 3–4 equal doses q6–8h.
  – *PREMATURES OR NEONATES* $<1$ *WK:* Up to 4 mg/kg/d in 2 equal doses q12h.
- *GERIATRIC OR RENAL FAILURE PATIENTS:* Reduce dosage, and carefully monitor serum drug levels and renal function tests throughout treatment. Reduced dosage nomogram is available; consult manufacturer's information.

***Eye solution***

- *Mild to moderate disease:* 1–2 drops into conjunctival sac of affected eye(s) q4h.
- *Severe disease:* 2 drops into conjunctival sac of affected eye(s) hourly until improvement occurs.

***Ophthalmic ointment:*** 1/2-in ribbon bid–tid. Severe infection, 1/2-in q3–4h.

## Pharmacokinetics

| *Route* | *Onset* | *Peak* |
|---|---|---|
| IM/IV | Rapid | 30–90 min |
| Ophthalmologic | Rapid | |

*Metabolism:* Minimal hepatic, $T_{1/2}$: 2–3 h
*Distribution:* Crosses placenta; enters breast milk
*Excretion:* Urine

## IV facts

*Preparation:* Dilute vials of solution for injection. Usual volume of diluent is 50–100 ml of 9% Sodium Chloride Injection or 5% Dextrose Injection (less for children). Reconstitute powder for injection with Sterile Water for Injection according to manufacturer's instructions.
*Infusion:* Infuse over 20–60 min.
*Compatibilities:* Do not premix with other drugs; administer other drugs separately.

## Adverse effects

- CNS: Ototoxicity, vestibular paralysis, confusion, disorientation, depression, lethargy, nystagmus, visual disturbances, headache, *numbness, tingling*, tremor, paresthesias, muscle twitching, convulsions, muscular weakness, neuromuscular blockade
- GI: Hepatic toxicity, *nausea, vomiting, anorexia,* weight loss, stomatitis, increased salivation
- CV: Palpitations, hypotension, hypertension
- **Hematologic**: *Leukemoid reaction,* agranulocytosis, granulocytosis, leukopenia, leukocytosis, thrombocytopenia, eosinophilia, pancytopenia, anemia, hemolytic anemia, increased or decreased reticulocyte count, electrolyte disturbances
- GU: *Nephrotoxicity*
- EENT: Localized ocular toxicity and hypersensitivity reactions; *lid itching, swelling;* conjunctival erythema; punctate keratitis
- **Hypersensitivity**: Hypersensitivity reactions: *purpura, rash*, urticaria, exfoliative dermatitis, itching
- **Local**: *Pain, irritation, arachnoiditis at IM injection sites*
- **Other**: Fever, apnea, splenomegaly, joint pain, *superinfections*

## Clinically important drug-drug interactions

• Increased ototoxic, nephrotoxic, neurotoxic effects with other aminoglycosides, cephalothin, potent diuretics • Increased neuromuscular blockade and muscular paralysis with anesthetics, nondepolarizing neuromuscular blocking drugs, succinylcholine • Potential inactivation of both drugs if mixed with beta-lactam-type antibiotics • Increased bactericidal effect with penicillins, cephalopsorins, carbenicillin, ticarcillin

## ■ Nursing Considerations

### Assessment

- ***History:*** Allergy to aminoglycosides; diminished hearing, decreased renal function, dehydration, neuromuscular disorders, lactation, pregnancy; infections (ophthalmic solutions)
- ***Physical:*** Weight; renal function, eighth cranial nerve function; state of hydration; hepatic function, CBC; skin color and lesions; orientation and affect; reflexes; bilateral grip strength; bowel sounds

### Implementation

- Arrange culture and sensitivity tests of infection before beginning therapy.
- Limit duration of treatment to short term to reduce the risk of toxicity; usual duration of treatment is 7–14 d.
- Use ophthalmologic tobramycin only when indicated by sensitivity tests; use of opthalmologic tobramycin may cause

sensitization that will contraindicate the systemic use of tobramycin or other aminoglycosides in serious infections.

- Monitor total serum concentration of tobramycin if ophthalmologic solution is used concurrently with parenteral aminoglycosides.
- Administer IM dose by deep IM injection.
- Ensure that patient is well hydrated before and during therapy.

### Drug-specific teaching points

*Parenteral*

- Report hearing changes, dizziness, pain at injection site.

*Ophthalmic Solution*

- Tilt head back; place medication into conjunctival sac, and close eye; apply light finger pressure on lacrimal sac for 1 min.
- Solution may cause blurring of vision or stinging on administration.
- Report severe stinging, itching, or burning.

## tocainide hydrochloride

*(toe **kay'** nide)*

Tonocard

**Pregnancy Category C**

### Drug classes

Antiarrhythmic

### Therapeutic actions

Type 1B antiarrhythmic: decreases the excitability of myocardial cells by a dose-dependent decrease in $Na^+$ and $K^+$ conductance.

### Indications

- Treatment of life-threatening ventricular arrhythmias
- Unlabeled uses: treatment of myotonic dystrophy, trigeminal neuralgia

### Contraindications/cautions

- Contraindications:allergy to tocainide or amide-type local anesthetics, cardiac conduction abnormalities (heart block in the absence of an artificial ventricular pacemaker), pregnancy (abortions and stillbirths have occurred), lactation.
- Use cautiously with CHF, atrial fibrillation or atrial flutter, renal or hepatic disease, potassium imbalance, bone marrow failure, cytopenia.

### Dosage

**Available Forms:** Tablets—400, 600 mg

Careful patient assessment and evaluation with close monitoring of cardiac response are necessary for determining the correct dosage for each patient.

*ADULT:* 400 mg PO q8h. 1,200–1,800 mg/d in 3 divided doses is the suggested therapeutic range.

*PEDIATRIC:* Safety and efficacy not established.

*GERIATRIC OR RENAL/HEPATIC IMPAIRMENT:* Lower doses required; <1,200 mg/d may suffice.

### Pharmacokinetics

| *Route* | *Onset* | *Peak* |
|---|---|---|
| Oral | Varies | 30–120 min |

*Metabolism:* Hepatic, $T_{1/2}$: 15 h

*Distribution:* Crosses placenta; enters breast milk

*Excretion:* Urine

### Adverse effects

- CNS: *Lightheadedness, dizziness*, fatigue, drowsiness, disorientation, hallucinations, *numbness, paresthesias*, visual disturbances, *tremor*
- GI: *Nausea*, vomiting, abdominal pain, diarrhea
- CV: CHF, cardiac arrhythmias
- **Respiratory**: Pulmonary fibrosis, **pneumonitis**
- **Hematologic**: Leukopenia, agranulocytosis, hypoplastic anemia, thrombocytopenia
- **Dermatologic**: Sweating, hot flashes, night sweats

### Clinically important drug-drug interactions

- Decreased pharmacologic effects with rifampin

## ■ Nursing Considerations

### Assessment

- *History:* Allergy to tocainide or amide-type local anesthetics, CHF, cardiac conduction abnormalities, atrial fibrillation or atrial flutter, hepatic or renal disease, potassium imbalance, pregnancy, lactation
- *Physical:* Weight; orientation, reflexes; P, BP, auscultation, ECG, edema; R, adventitious sounds; bowel sounds, liver evaluation; urinalysis, CBC, serum electrolytes, renal and liver function tests

### Implementation

- Carefully monitor patient response, especially when beginning therapy.
- Reduce dosage in patients with renal or hepatic disease.
- Check serum $K^+$ levels before administration.
- Carefully monitor cardiac rhythm.
- Arrange for regular follow-up of blood counts.
- Evaluate for safe and effective serum levels (4–10 $\mu$g/ml).

### Drug-specific teaching points

- You will require frequent monitoring of cardiac rhythm.
- The following side effects may occur: drowsiness, dizziness, numbness (avoid driving or working with dangerous machinery); nausea, vomiting, diarrhea (small, frequent meals may help); sweating, night sweats, hot flashes.
- Do not stop taking this drug for any reason without checking with your health care provider.
- Have regular follow-up visits to check heart rhythm and blood cell counts.
- Report cough, wheezing, difficulty breathing, unusual bleeding or bruising, fever, chills, sore throat, tremors, visual changes, palpitations.

## tolazamide

*(tole **az'** a mide)*

Tolinase

**Pregnancy Category C**

### Drug classes

Antidiabetic agent
Sulfonylurea, first generation

### Therapeutic actions

Stimulates insulin release from functioning beta cells in the pancreas; may improve binding between insulin and insulin receptors or increase the number of insulin receptors; has significant uricosuric activity.

### Indications

- Adjunct to diet to lower blood glucose in patients with non–insulin-dependent diabetes mellitus (type II)
- Adjunct to insulin therapy in the stabilization of certain cases of insulin-dependent maturity-onset diabetes, reducing the insulin requirement and decreasing the chance of hypoglycemic reactions

### Contraindications/cautions

- Contraindications: allergy to sulfonylureas; diabetes complicated by fever, severe infections, severe trauma, major surgery, ketosis, acidosis, coma (insulin is indicated in these conditions); type I or juvenile diabetes; serious hepatic or renal impairment; pregnancy.
- Use cautiously with uremia, thyroid or endocrine impairment, glycosuria, hyperglycemia associated with primary renal disease, lactation.

### Dosage

**Available Forms:** Tablets—100, 250, 500 mg

*ADULT:* 100 mg/d PO if fasting blood sugar (FBS) is $<$ 200 mg%, or 250 mg/d if FBS is $>$ 200 mg%. Adjust dose accordingly. If dose is larger than 500 mg/d, give in divided doses bid. Dosage greater than 1 g/d not recommended.

*PEDIATRIC:* Safety and efficacy not established.

*GERIATRIC:* Geriatric patients tend to be more sensitive to the drug. Start with a lower initial dose; monitor for 24 h, and gradually increase dose as needed.

### Pharmacokinetics

| *Route* | *Onset* | *Peak* | *Duration* |
|---|---|---|---|
| Oral | Varies | 4–6 h | 12–24 h |

t

*Metabolism:* Hepatic, $T_{1/2}$: 7 h
*Distribution:* Crosses placenta; enters breast milk
*Excretion:* Urine

### Adverse effects

- GI: *Anorexia, nausea, vomiting, epigastric discomfort, heartburn*
- Hematologic: *Hypoglycemia*, leukopenia, thrombocytopenia, anemia
- Dermatologic: Allergic skin reactions, eczema, pruritus, erythema, urticaria, photosensitivity
- Hypersensitivity: Fever, eosinophilia, jaundice
- Other: **Increased risk of CV mortality**

### Clinically important drug-drug interactions

• Increased risk of hypoglycemia with insulin, sulfonamides, chloramphenicol, fenfluramine, oxyphenbutazone, phenylbutazone, salicylates, clofibrate, monoamine oxidase inhibitors • Decreased effectiveness of both tolazamide and diazoxide if taken concurrently • Increased risk of hyperglycemia with thiazides, other diuretics • Risk of hypoglycemia and hyperglycemia with ethanol; "disulfiram reaction" also has been reported.

## ■ Nursing Considerations

### Assessment

- *History:* Allergy to sulfonylureas; diabetes complicated by fever, severe infections, severe trauma, major surgery, ketosis, acidosis, coma; type I or juvenile diabetes; serious hepatic or renal impairment; uremia; thyroid or endocrine impairment; glycosuria; hyperglycemia associated with primary renal disease; pregnancy; lactation
- *Physical:* Skin color, lesions; T; orientation, reflexes, peripheral sensation; R, adventitious sounds; liver evaluation, bowel sounds; urinalysis, BUN, serum creatinine, liver function tests, blood glucose, CBC

### Implementation

- Administer drug in the morning before breakfast. If severe GI upset occurs or if dosage is >500 g/d, dose may be divided with one dose before breakfast and one before the evening meal.
- Monitor urine and serum glucose levels frequently to determine effectiveness of drug and dosage.
- Transfer to insulin therapy during periods of high stress, infections, surgery, trauma, and so forth.
- Use IV glucose if severe hypoglycemia occurs due to overdose.

### Drug-specific teaching points

- Do not discontinue this medication without consulting physician.
- Monitor urine or blood for glucose and ketones as prescribed,
- This drug is not to be used during pregnancy.
- Avoid alcohol while on this drug.
- Report fever, sore throat, unusual bleeding or bruising, skin rash, dark urine, light-colored stools, hypoglycemic or hyperglycemic reactions.

# tolazoline hydrochloride

*(toe **laz'** a leen)*
Priscoline
**Pregnancy Category C**

### Drug classes

Vasodilator
Antihypertensive

### Therapeutic actions

Weak alpha-adrenergic blocker; increases cardiac output and heart rate, increases GI motility, stimulates GI secretions, and causes peripheral vasodilation.

### Indications

- Persistent pulmonary hypertension of the newborn when systemic arterial oxygenation cannot be maintained by the usual methods

### Contraindications/cautions

- Contraindications: allergy to tolazoline.
- Use cautiously with stress ulcers, hypotension, mitral stenosis, pregnancy, lactation.

### Dosage

**Available Forms:** Injection—25 mg/ml

*PEDIATRIC:* 1–2 mg/kg IV through scalp needle over 10 min; follow with an infusion of 1–2 mg/kg per hour for no longer than 36–48 h.

### Pharmacokinetics

| *Route* | *Onset* | *Peak* | *Duration* |
|---|---|---|---|
| IV | Varies | 30–60 min | 3–4 h |

*Metabolism:* Hepatic, $T_{1/2}$: 3–10 h
*Distribution:* May cross placenta or enter breast milk
*Excretion:* Urine

#### IV facts

**Preparation:** No further preparation is required.
**Infusion:** Initial injection over 10 min; then use metered delivery system to deliver 1–2 mg/kg/h and dilute into an infusion of dextrose, saline, Lactated Ringer's or combination of these.
**Compatiblities:** Do not mix with other drugs.

### Adverse effects

- GI: Nausea, vomiting, diarrhea, hepatitis, **GI hemorrhage**
- CV: Hypotension, tachycardia, arrhythmias, hypertension, **pulmonary hemmorhage**
- Hematologic: Leukopenia, thrombocytopenia
- Dermatologic: Flushing, pilomotor acitivity, rash
- Renal: Edema, oliguria, hematuria

### Clinically important drug-drug interactions

- Risk of severe hypotension with epinephrine

## ■ Nursing Considerations

### Assessment

- *History:* Allergy to tolazoline, hypotension, stress ulcers, mitral stenosis, pregnancy, lactation
- *Physical:* Skin color, lesions; T; orientation, reflexes, peripheral sensation; R, adventitious sounds; BP, P, peripheral perfusion; renal and liver function tests

### Implementation

- Store in refrigerator and protect from light.
- Monitor BP closely during administration; arrange for supportive therapy as needed.
- Monitor acid–base balance, oxygenation, vital signs, and electrolytes carefully during administration.
- Assess patients for signs of bleeding: bruising, dark stools, petechiae, vomiting.

### Drug-specific teaching points

- Incorporate teaching about this drug into the overall teaching plan for the parents of the affected newborn.

## tolbutamide

*(tole **byoo'** ta mide)*

Mobenol (CAN), Novobutamide (CAN), Orinase

**Pregnancy Category C**

### Drug classes

Antidiabetic agent
Sulfonylurea, first generation

### Therapeutic actions

Stimulates insulin release from functioning beta cells in the pancreas; may improve binding between insulin and insulin receptors or increase the number of insulin receptors.

### Indications

- Adjunct to diet to lower blood glucose in patients with non–insulin-dependent diabetes mellitus (Type II)

t

- Adjunct to insulin therapy in the stabilization of certain cases of insulin-dependent maturity-onset diabetes, reducing the insulin requirement and decreasing the chance of hypoglycemic reactions

### Contraindications/cautions

- Contraindications: allergy to sulfonylureas; diabetes complicated by fever, severe infections, severe trauma, major surgery, ketosis, acidosis, coma (insulin is indicated in these conditions); Type I or juvenile diabetes; serious hepatic or renal impairment, uremia; thyroid or endocrine impairment; glycosuria, hyperglycemia associated with primary renal disease, pregnancy, lactation.

### Dosage

**Available Forms:** Tablets—500 mg

*ADULT:* 0.25–3 g/d PO in single morning or divided doses. Maintenance dosage, > 2 g/d is seldom required.

*PEDIATRIC:* Safety and efficacy not established.

*GERIATRIC:* Geriatric patients tend to be more sensitive to the drug. Start with a lower initial dose, monitor for 24 h, and gradually increase dose as needed.

### Pharmacokinetics

| Route | Onset | Peak | Duration |
|---|---|---|---|
| Oral | 1 h | 4–6 h | 6–12 h |

*Metabolism:* Hepatic, $T_{1/2}$: 7 h

*Distribution:* Crosses placenta; enters breast milk

*Excretion:* Urine

### Adverse effects

- GI: *Anorexia, nausea, vomiting, epigastric discomfort, heartburn*
- Hematologic: *Hypoglycemia*, leukopenia, thrombocytopenia, anemia
- Dermatologic: Allergic skin reactions, eczema, pruritus, erythema, urticaria, photosensitivity
- Hypersensitivity: Fever, eosinophilia, jaundice
- Other: **Increased risk of CV mortality**

### Clinically important drug-drug interactions

• Increased risk of hypoglycemia with insulin, sulfonamides, chloramphenicol, fenfluramine, oxyphenbutazone, phenylbutazone, salicylates, clofibrate, MAOIs, dicumarol, rifampin • Decreased effectiveness of both tolbutamide and diazoxide if taken concurrently • Increased risk of hyperglycemia with thiazides, other diuretics • Risk of hypoglycemia and hyperglycemia with ethanol

### Drug-lab test interferences

• False-positive reaction for urine albumin if measured with acidification-after-boiling-test; no interference has been reported using sulfosalicylic acid test

## ■ Nursing Considerations

### Assessment

- *History:* Allergy to sulfonylureas; diabetes complicated by fever, severe infections, severe trauma, major surgery, ketosis, acidosis, coma; type I or juvenile diabetes; serious hepatic or renal impairment, uremia; thyroid or endocrine impairment; glycosuria, hyperglycemia associated with primary renal disease; pregnancy; lactation
- *Physical:* Skin color, lesions; T; orientation, reflexes, peripheral sensation; R, adventitious sounds; liver evaluation, bowel sounds; urinalysis, BUN, serum creatinine, liver function tests, blood glucose, CBC

### Implementation

- Administer drug in the morning before breakfast; if severe GI upset occurs, divide dose.
- Monitor urine and serum glucose levels frequently to determine effectiveness of drug and dosage.
- Transfer patients from one oral hypoglycemic agent to another with no transitional period or priming dose.
- Transfer to insulin therapy during periods of high stress (eg, infections, surgery, trauma).

- Use IV glucose if severe hypoglycemia occurs due to overdose.

### Drug-specific teaching points

- Take this drug early in the morning before breakfast. If GI upset occurs, drug may be taken with food or in divided doses. Do not discontinue this medication without consulting your health care provider.
- The following side effects may occur: nausea, GI upset, vomiting (take drug with food); diarrhea; rash, delays in healing (use good skin care; avoid injury).
- This drug is not to be used during pregnancy. If you become pregnant or want to become pregnant, consult your prescriber.
- Avoid alcohol while on this drug; serious reactions can occur.
- Report fever, sore throat, unusual bleeding or bruising, skin rash, dark urine, light-colored stools, hypoglycemic or hyperglycemic reactions.

## tolmetin sodium

***(tole' met in)***

Tolectin, Tolectin DS

**Pregnancy Category C**

### Drug classes

Nonsteroidal anti-inflammatory drug (NSAID)

### Therapeutic actions

Anti-inflammatory, analgesic, and antipyretic activities largely related to inhibition of prostaglandin synthesis; exact mechanisms of action are not known.

### Indications

- Treatment of acute flares and long-term management of rheumatoid arthritis
- Treatment of juvenile rheumatoid arthritis

### Contraindications/cautions

- Contraindications: pregnancy, lactation.
- Use cautiously with allergies, renal, hepatic, CV, and GI conditions.

### Dosage

**Available Forms:** Tablets—200, 600 mg; capsules—400 mg

Do not exceed 2000 mg/d (rheumatoid arthritis) or 1600 mg/d (osteoarthritis).

**ADULT**

- ***Rheumatoid arthritis/osteoarthritis:*** Initial dose, 400 mg PO tid (1200 mg/d) preferably including doses on arising and hs. Maintenance dose, 600–1800 mg/d in 3–4 divided doses for rheumatoid arthritis, 600–1600 mg/d in 3–4 divided doses for osteoarthritis.

***PEDIATRIC (>2 Y):*** 20 mg/kg/d PO in 3–4 divided doses; when control has been achieved, the usual dose is 15–30 mg/kg/d. Do not exceed 30 mg/kg/d.

### Pharmacokinetics

| *Route* | *Onset* | *Peak* |
|---|---|---|
| Oral | Varies | 30–60 min |

*Metabolism:* Hepatic, $T_{1/2}$: 1–1.5 h

*Distribution:* Crosses placenta; enters breast milk

*Excretion:* Urine

### Adverse effects

- CNS: *Headache, dizziness, somnolence, insomnia*, fatigue, tiredness, dizziness, tinnitus, ophthalmologic effects
- GI: *Nausea, dyspepsia, GI pain, diarrhea*, vomiting, constipation, flatulence
- **Respiratory**: Dyspnea, hemoptysis, pharyngitis, bronchospasm, rhinitis
- **Hematologic**: Bleeding, platelet inhibition with higher doses, neutropenia, eosinophilia, leukopenia, pancytopenia, thrombocytopenia, agranulocytosis, granulocytopenia, aplastic anemia, decreased Hgb or Hct, bone marrow depression, mennorhagia
- GU: Dysuria, renal impairment, including renal failure, interstitial nephritis, hematuria
- **Dermatologic**: *Rash*, pruritus, sweating, dry mucous membranes, stomatitis
- **Other**: Peripheral edema, anaphylactoid reactions to fatal anaphylactic shock

### Drug-lab test interferences
- False-positive tests for proteinuria using acid precipitation tests; no interference has been reported with dye-impregnated reagent strips.

## ■ Nursing Considerations
### Assessment
- ***History:*** Allergies, renal, hepatic, CV, and GI conditions; pregnancy, lactation
- ***Physical:*** Skin color, lesions; orientation, reflexes, ophthalmologic and audiometric evaluation, peripheral sensation; P, edema; R, adventitious sounds; liver evaluation; CBC, clotting times, renal and liver function tests; serum electrolytes, stool guaiac

### Implementation
- Administer with milk or food; bioavailability is decreased by up to 16%.
- Use antacids other than sodium bicarbonate if GI upset occurs.
- Arrange for periodic ophthalmologic examination during long-term therapy.
- Institute emergency procedures if overdose occurs—gastric lavage, induction of emesis, supportive therapy.

### Drug-specific teaching points
- Take drug with food.
- Take only the prescribed dosage.
- The following side effects may occur: dizziness, drowsiness can occur (avoid driving or using dangerous machinery).
- Report sore throat, fever, rash, itching, weight gain, swelling in ankles or fingers; changes in vision; black, tarry stools.

## topiramate

*(toe **pie'** rah mate)*

Topamax

**Pregnancy Category C**

### Drug classes
Antiepileptic agent

### Therapeutic actions
Mechanism of action not understood; antiepileptic effects may be due to the actions of blocking sodium channels in neurons with sustained depolarization; increasing GABA activity at receptors, thus potentiating the effects of this inhibitory neurotransmitter; and blocking excitatory neurotransmitters at neuron receptor sites.

### Indications
- Adjunctive therapy for partial-onset seizure treatment in adults

### Contraindications/cautions
- Contraindications: hypersensitivity to any component of the drug.
- Use cautiously with pregnancy (use only if benefits outweigh potential risks to fetus), lactation, renal or hepatic impairment, renal stones.

### Dosage
**Available Forms:** Tablets—25, 100, 200 mg

***Adult:*** 400 mg PO qd in 2 divided doses; begin titration of dose at 50 mg/d in the evening for wk 1; 50 mg AM and PM for wk 2; 50 mg AM and 100 mg PM for wk 3; 100 mg AM and PM for wk 4; 100 mg AM and 150 mg PM for wk 5; 150 mg AM and PM for wk 6; 150 mg AM and 200 mg PM for wk 7; and 200 mg AM and PM for wk 8 and beyond.

***Pediatric:*** Safety and efficacy not established.

***Renal Impairment:*** Ccr <70 ml/min: use 1/2 the usual dose; allow increased time to reach desired level.

### Pharmacokinetics

| *Route* | *Onset* | *Peak* |
|---|---|---|
| Oral | Rapid | 2 h |

*Metabolism:* Hepatic; $T_{1/2}$: 21 h

*Distribution:* Crosses placenta; enters breast milk

*Excretion:* Urine

### Adverse effects
- CNS: *Ataxia, somnolence, dizziness, nystagmus,* nervousness, anxiety, tremor, speech impairment, paresthesias, confusion
- GI: *Nausea, dyspepsia,* anorexia, vomiting

- GU: Dysmenorrhea
- Respiratory: *Upper respiratory infection,* pharyngitis, sinusitis
- Hematologic: Leukopenia
- Other: *Fatigue,* rash

**Clinically important drug-drug interactions**

• Increased CNS depression if taken with alcohol or CNS depresssants; use extreme caution • Increased risk of renal stone development with carbonic anhydrase inhibitors • Decreased effects of oral contraceptives with topiramate; suggest use of barrier contraceptives instead

## ■ Nursing Considerations

### Assessment

- *History:* Hypersensitivity to any component of the drug, pregnancy, lactation, renal or hepatic impairment, renal stones
- *Physical:* Skin color, lesions; orientation, affect, reflexes, vision exam; R, adventitious sounds; liver and renal function tests

### Implementation

- Reduce dosage, discontinue or substitute other antiepileptic medication gradually; abrupt discontinuation may precipitate status epilepticus.
- Administer with food if GI upset occurs.
- Caution patient not to chew or break tablets because of bitter taste.
- Encourage patients with a history of renal stone development to maintain adequate fluid intake while on this drug.
- Suggest the use of barrier contraceptives to patients using this drug.
- Arrange for consultation with appropriate epilepsy support groups as needed.

### Drug-specific teaching points

- Take this drug exactly as prescribed. Do not break or chew tablets; they have a very bitter taste.
- Do not discontinue this drug abruptly or change dosage except on the advice of your heatlh care provider.
- Arrange for frequent check-ups to monitor your response to this drug. It is very important that you keep all appointments for check-ups.
- The following side effects may occur: drowsiness, dizziness, sleepiness (avoid driving or performing other tasks that require alertness; symptoms may occur initially but usually disappear with continued therapy); vision changes (avoid performing tasks that require visual acuity); GI upset (take drug with food; eat small, frequent meals).
- Wear a Medic-Alert bracelet at all times so that any emergency medical personnel will know that you are an epileptic taking antiepileptic medication.
- Avoid using alcohol while you are on this drug; serious sedation could occur.
- Report fatigue, vision changes, speech problems, personality changes.

# topotecan hydrochloride

*(toe **poh'** te kan)*

Hycamtin

**Pregnancy Category C**

**Drug classes**

Antineoplastic

**Therapeutic actions**

Cytotoxic; causes the death of cells during cell division by causing damage to the DNA strand during DNA synthesis.

**Indications**

- Treatment of patients with metastatic ovarian cancer after failure of traditional chemotherapy

**Contraindications/cautions**

- Contraindications: allergy to topotecan; severe bone marrow depression; pregnancy, lactation
- Use cautiously with any bone marrow depression

### Dosage

**Available Forms:** Powder for injection—4 mg

t

*ADULT:* 1.5 $mg/m^2$ IV over 30 min qd for 5 consecutive d; minimum of 4 courses is recommended.
*PEDIATRIC:* Not recommended.
*RENAL IMPAIRMENT:* 0.75 $mg/m^2$ IV over 30 min qd for 5 d is recommended if Ccr is 20–39 ml/min; there is no experience with severe renal dysfunction.

### Pharmacokinetics

| *Route* | *Onset* | *Peak* |
|---|---|---|
| IV | Varies | 1–2 h |

*Metabolism:* Hepatic; $T_{1/2}$: 2–3 h
*Distribution:* Crosses placenta; may pass into breast milk
*Excretion:* Urine

#### IV facts

**Preparation:** Reconstitute each 4-mg vial with 4 ml of Sterile Water for Injection; dilute the appropriate volume of reconstituted topotecan with either 0.9% Sodium Chloride IV infusion or 5% Dextrose IV infusion. Store unreconstituted drug protected from light; reconstituted drug is stable at room light for up to 24 h.
**Infusion:** Infuse total dose over 30 min.

### Adverse effects

- CNS: *Headache, paresthesias,* asthenia, myalgia
- GI: *Nausea, vomiting, diarrhea,* constipation
- Respiratory: *Dyspnea*
- Hematologic: **Neutropenia, leukopenia, thrombocytopenia, anemia**
- Dermatologic: *Total alopecia*
- Other: Fatigue, malaise, pain, myalgia

### Clinically important drug-drug interactions

- Increased myelosuppression with cisplatin; no safe and effective dosage adjustment is available—avoid this combination
- Prolonged neutropenia with filgrastim; avoid this combination until day 6 of the course of therapy, 24 h after completion of treatment with topotecan

## ■ Nursing Considerations

### Assessment

- *History:* Allergy to topotecan, hepatic or renal dysfunction, pregnancy, lactation, bone marrow depression
- *Physical:* Skin lesions, color, turgor; orientation, affect, reflexes; R; liver and renal function tests; CBC with differential

### Implementation

- Obtain CBC before each infusion; do not give to patients with a baseline neutrophil count of <1500 cells/$mm^2$; consult physician for reduction in dose or withholding of drug if bone marrow depression becomes evident.
- Protect patient from exposure to infection.
- Arrange for appropriate analgesic measures if pain and discomfort become severe.
- Arrange for wig or other appropriate head covering when alopecia occurs.

### Drug-specific teaching points

- This drug can only be given by IV infusion, which will run over 30 min. Mark calendar with days to return for infusion. A blood test will be required before each dose is given.
- The following side effects may occur: increased susceptibility to infection (avoid crowds or people with known infections; report any injury); nausea, vomiting (eat small, frequent meals; medication may be ordered); headache; loss of hair (arrange for wig or other head covering; it is important to protect the head from extremes of temperature).
- Report pain at injection site, any injury or illness, fatigue, severe nausea or vomiting.

## toremifene

*(tore **em'** ah feen)*
Fareston
**Pregnancy Category D**

**Drug classes**
Estrogen receptor modulator
Antineoplastic

**Therapeutic actions**
Binds to estrogen receptors, has anti-estrogen effects, and inhibits growth of estrogen receptor–positive and estrogen receptor–negative breast cancer cell lines.

**Indications**
- Treatment of advanced breast cancer in post-menopausal women with estrogen receptor–positive disease

**Contraindications/cautions**
- Contraindications: allergy to toremifene, pregnancy, lactation.
- Use cautiously with history of hypercalcemia, liver dysfunction.

**Dosage**
**Available Forms:** Tablets—60 mg
*ADULT:* 60 mg PO qd.

**Pharmacokinetics**

| *Route* | *Onset* | *Peak* |
|---|---|---|
| Oral | Rapid | 1–6 h |

*Metabolism:* Hepatic; $T_{1/2}$: 5–6 d
*Distribution:* Crosses placenta; enters breast milk
*Excretion:* Feces

**Adverse effects**
- CNS: Depression, lightheadedness, *dizziness,* headache, hallucinations, vertigo
- GI: *Nausea, vomiting,* food distaste
- GU: Vaginal bleeding, vaginal discharge
- Dermatologic: *Hot flashes, skin rash*
- Other: Peripheral edema, hypercalcemia

**Clinically important drug-drug interactions**
- Increased risk of bleeding if taken with oral anticoagulants

## ■ Nursing Considerations

**Assessment**
- *History:* Allergy to toremifene, pregnancy, lactation, hypercalcemia, liver dysfunction
- *Physical:* skin lesions, color, turgor; pelvic exam; orientation, affect, reflexes; BP, peripheral pulses, edema; liver function tests, serum electrolytes

**Implementation**
- Administer qd without regard to food.
- Counsel patient about the need to use contraceptive measures while taking this drug; inform patient that serious fetal harm could occur.
- Provide comfort measures to help patient deal with drug effects: hot flashes (environmental temperature control); headache, depression (monitoring of light and noise); vaginal bleeding (hygiene measures).

**Drug-specific teaching points**
- Take this drug as prescribed.
- The following side effects may occur: hot flashes (stay in cool temperatures); nausea, vomiting (eat small, frequent meals); weight gain; dizziness, headache, lightheadedness (use caution if driving or performing tasks that require alertness).
- This drug can cause serious fetal harm and must not be taken during pregnancy. Contraceptive measures should be used while you are taking this drug. If you become pregnant or decide that you would like to become pregnant, consult with your physician immediately.
- Report marked weakness, sleepiness, mental confusion, changes in color of urine or stool, rash.

## torsemide

*(tor' seh myde)*
Demadex
**Pregnancy Category B**

**Drug classes**
Loop (high-ceiling) diuretic

**Therapeutic actions**
Inhibits the reabsorption of sodium and chloride from the proximal and distal renal tubules and the loop of Henle, leading to a natriuretic diuresis.

## Indications

- Treatment of hypertension and edema associated with CHF, hepatic disease, renal disease

## Contraindications/cautions

- Allergy to torsemide; electrolyte depletion; anuria, severe renal failure; hepatic coma; SLE; gout; diabetes mellitus; lactation

## Dosage

**Available Forms:** Tablets—5, 10, 20, 100 mg; injection—10 mg/ml

Do not exceed 200 mg/d.

*ADULT*

- *CHF:* 10–20 mg PO or IV qd. Dose may be titrated upward until desired results are seen.
- *Chronic renal failure:* 20 mg PO or IV qd. Dose may be titrated upward until desired results are seen.
- *Hepatic failure:* 5–10 mg PO or IV qd. Do not exceed 40 mg/d.
- *Hypertension:* 5 mg PO qd. May be increased to 10 mg if response is not sufficient.

*PEDIATRIC:* Safety and efficacy not established.

## Pharmacokinetics

| *Route* | *Onset* | *Peak* | *Duration* |
|---|---|---|---|
| Oral | 60 min | 60–120 min | 6–8 h |
| IV | 10 min | 60 min | 6–8 h |

*Metabolism:* $T_{1/2}$: 210 min

*Distribution:* Crosses placenta; may enter breast milk

*Excretion:* Unchanged in the urine

### IV facts

**Preparation:** May be given direct IV or diluted in solution with 5% Dextrose in Water, 0.9% Sodium Chloride, Lactated Ringer's Solution. Discard unused solution after 24 h.

**Infusion:** Give by direct injection slowly, over 1–2 min. Further diluted in solution, give slowly, each 200 mg over 2 min.

## Adverse effects

- CNS: *Asterixis, dizziness,* vertigo, paresthesias, confusion, fatigue, nystagmus, *weakness, headache, drowsiness,* fatigue, blurred vision, tinnitus, irreversible hearing loss
- GI: *Nausea, anorexia, vomiting, diarrhea,* gastric irritation and pain, dry mouth, acute pancreatitis, jaundice
- CV: *Orthostatic hypotension,* volume depletion, cardiac arrhythmias, thrombophlebitis
- GU: *Polyuria, nocturia,* glycosuria, renal failure
- **Hematologic:** *Hypokalemia,* leukopenia, anemia, thrombocytopenia
- **Local:** *Pain, phlebitis at injection site*
- **Other:** Muscle cramps and muscle spasms, weakness, arthritic pain, fatigue, hives, photosensitivity, rash, pruritus, sweating, nipple tendernes

## Clinically important drug-drug interactions

• Decreased diuresis and natriuresis with NSAIDs • Increased risk of cardiac glycoside toxicity (secondary to hypokalemia) • Increased risk of ototoxicity with aminoglycoside antibiotics, cisplatin

## ■ Nursing Considerations

### Assessment

- *History:* Allergy to torsemide, electrolyte depletion, anuria, severe renal failure, hepatic coma, SLE, gout, diabetes mellitus, lactation
- *Physical:* Skin color, lesions; edema; orientation, reflexes, hearing; pulses, baseline ECG, BP, orthostatic BP, perfusion; R, pattern, adventitious sounds; liver evaluation, bowel sounds; urinary output patterns; CBC, serum electrolytes, blood sugar, liver and renal function tests, uric acid, urinalysis

### Implementation

- Administer with food or milk to prevent GI upset.
- Mark calendars or other reminders of drug days if intermittent therapy is optimal for treating edema.

- Administer single daily doses early in the day so increased urination will not disturb sleep.
- Avoid IV use if oral use is at all possible.
- Measure and record regular weights to monitor fluid changes.
- Monitor serum electrolytes, hydration, liver function during long-term therapy.
- Provide diet rich in potassium or supplemental potassium.

### Drug-specific teaching points

- Record alternate-day or intermittent therapy on a calendar or dated envelopes.
- Take the drug early in the day so increased urination will not disturb sleep.
- Take the drug with food or meals to prevent GI upset.
- Weigh yourself on a regular basis, at the same time and in the same clothing, and record the weight on your calendar.
- The following side effects may occur: increased volume and frequency of urination; dizziness, feeling faint on arising, drowsiness (avoid rapid position changes, hazardous activities [eg, driving a car] and alcohol consumption); sensitivity to sunlight (use sunglasses or sunscreen, wear protective clothing when outdoors); increased thirst (sucking on sugarless lozenges, frequent mouth care may help); loss of body potassium (a potassium-rich diet, or even a potassium supplement, will be necessary).
- Report weight change of more than 3 lb in one day; swelling in ankles or fingers; unusual bleeding or bruising; nausea, dizziness, trembling, numbness, fatigue; muscle weakness or cramps.

## tramadol hydrochloride

***(tram' ah doll)***
Ultram
**Pregnancy Category C**

### Drug classes

Centrally acting analgesic

### Therapeutic actions

Binds to $\mu$-opioid receptors and inhibits the reuptake of norepinephrine and serotonin; causes many effects similar to the opioids—dizziness, somnolence, nausea, constipation—but does not have the respiratory depressant effects.

### Indications

- Relief of moderate to moderately severe pain

### Contraindications/cautions

- Contraindications: pregnancy; allergy to tramadol; acute intoxication with alcohol, opioids, psychotropic drugs or other centrally acting analgesics; lactation.
- Use cautiously with seizures, concomitant use of CNS depressants or MAOIs, renal or hepatic impairment.

### Dosage

**Available Forms:** Tablets—50 mg

*ADULT:* 50–100 mg PO q4–6 h; do not exceed 400 mg/d.

*PEDIATRIC:* Safety and efficacy not established.

*GERIATRIC, RENAL OR HEPATIC IMPAIRED:* 50 mg PO q12h.

### Pharmacokinetics

| *Route* | *Onset* | *Peak* |
|---|---|---|
| Oral | 1 h | 2 h |

*Metabolism:* Hepatic, $T_{1/2}$: 6–7 h
*Distribution:* Crosses placenta; enters breast milk
*Excretion:* Urine

### Adverse effects

- CNS: *Sedation, dizziness/vertigo, headache,* confusion, dreaming, sweating, anxiety, **seizures**
- GI: *Nausea, vomiting,* dry mouth, constipation, flatulence
- CV: *Hypotension,* tachycardia, bradycardia
- Dermatologic: *Sweating,* pruritus, rash, pallor, urticaria
- Other: **Potential for abuse, anaphylactoid reactions**

t

### Clinically important drug-drug interactions

• Decreased effectiveness with carbamazepine • Increased risk of tramadol toxicity with MAOIs

## ■ Nursing Considerations

### Assessment

- *History:* Hypersensitivity to tramadol; pregnancy; acute intoxication with alcohol, opioids, psychotropic drugs or other centrally acting analgesics; lactation; seizures; concomitant use of CNS depressants or MAOIs; renal or hepatic impairment; past or present history of opioid addiction
- *Physical:* Skin color, texture, lesions; orientation, reflexes, bilateral grip strength, affect; P, auscultation, BP; bowel sounds, normal output; liver and kidney function tests

### Implementation

- Provide environmental control (temperature, lighting) if sweating, CNS effects occur.

### Drug-specific teaching points

- Limit use in patients with past or present history of addiction to or dependence on opioids.
- The following side effects may occur: dizziness, sedation, drowsiness, impaired visual acuity (avoid driving or performing tasks that require alertness); nausea, loss of appetite (lie quietly, eat small frequent meals).
- Report severe nausea, dizziness, severe constipation.

## trandolapril

*(tran* ***dole'*** *ah pril)*

Mavik

**Pregnancy Category C (first trimester)**

**Pregnancy Category D (second and third trimesters)**

### Drug classes

Antihypertensive

Angiotensin converting enzyme inhibitor (ACE inhibitor)

### Therapeutic actions

Blocks ACE from converting angiotensin I to angiotensin II, a powerful vasoconstrictor, leading to decreased blood pressure, decreased aldosterone secretion, a small increase in serum potassium levels, and sodium and fluid loss; increased prostaglandin synthesis may also be involved in the antihypertensive action.

### Indications

- Treatment of hypertension, alone or in combination with other antihypertensives

### Contraindications/cautions

- Contraindications: allergy to ACE inhibitors, history of ACE-associated angioedema
- Use cautiously with impaired renal function, CHF, CAD, salt/volume depletion, surgery, pregnancy, lactation

### Dosage

**Available Forms:** Tablets—1, 2, 4 mg

*ADULT:* African-American patients: 2 mg PO qd. Non–African-American patients: 1 mg PO qd. Maintenance: 2–4 mg/d.

- *Patients on diuretics:* Stop diuretic 2–3 d before beginning trandolapril. Resume diuretic only if BP is not controlled; start at 0.5 mg PO qd and titrate upward as needed.

*PEDIATRIC:* Safety and efficacy not established.

*RENAL OR HEPTIC IMPAIRMENT:* 0.5 mg PO qd, adjust at 1-wk intervals to control BP; usual range is 2–4 mg PO qd.

### Pharmacokinetics

| *Route* | *Onset* | *Peak* |
|---|---|---|
| Oral | 15 min | 2–3 h |

*Metabolism:* $T_{1/2}$: 6–10 h

*Distribution:* Crosses placenta; passes into breast milk

*Excretion:* Urine and feces

### Adverse effects

- GI: *Diarrhea,* GI upset
- CV: *Tachycardia,* angina pectoris, **MI,** Raynaud's syndrome, CHF. hypotension in salt- or volume-depleted patients
- GU: Renal insufficiency, renal failure, polyuria, oliguria, urinary frequency
- Dermatologic: *Rash*
- Other: *Cough, dizziness,* malaise, dry mouth

**Clinically important drug-drug interactions**

• Excessive hypotension may occur with diuretics; monitor closely • Hyperkalemia may occur with potassium supplements, potassium-sparing diuretics, salt substitutes; monitor serum potassium levels • Potential increase in lithium levels if taken concurrently; decreased lithium dose may be needed

## ■ Nursing Considerations

### Assessment

- *History:* Allergy to ACE inhibitors; impaired renal or hepatic function; CAD; CHF; salt/volume depletion; surgery; pregnancy, lactation
- *Physical:* Skin color, lesions, turgor; T; P, BP, peripheral perfusion; mucous membranes, bowel sounds, liver evaluation; urinalysis, renal and liver function tests, CBC and differential

### Implementation

- Administer once a day at same time each day.
- Alert surgeon and mark patient's chart with notice that trandolapril is being taken; angiotensin II formation subsequent to compensatory renin release during surgery will need to be blocked; hypotension may be reversed with volume expansion.
- Monitor patient closely in any situation that may lead to fall in BP secondary to reduction in fluid volume—excessive perspiration and dehydration, vomiting, diarrhea—as excessive hypotension may occur.
- Reduce dosage in patients with impaired renal or hepatic function.
- Discontinue immediately if laryngeal edema, angioedema, or jaundice occurs.

### Drug-specific teaching points

- Take drug once a day at the same general time each day. Do not stop taking this medication without consulting your health care provider.
- The following side effects may occur: GI upset, diarrhea (limited effects that will pass); dizziness, lightheadedness (usually passes after first few days; change position slowly and limit your activities to those that do not require alertness and precision); cough (can be very irritating and does not respond to cough suppressants; notify health care provider if very uncomfortable).
- Be careful in any situation that may lead to a drop in BP (diarrhea, sweating, vomiting, dehydration); if lightheadedness or dizziness occur, consult your health care provider.
- Avoid use of OTC medications while on this drug, especially cough, cold, allergy medications; they may contain ingredients that will interact with this drug. If you feel that you need one of these preparations, consult your nurse or physician.
- Report sore throat, fever, chills; swelling of the hands or feet; irregular heartbeat, chest pains; swelling of the face, eyes, lips, tongue; difficulty breathing; yellowing of skin.

# tranylcypromine sulfate

*(tran ill **sip'** roe meen)*

Parnate

**Pregnancy Category C**

**Drug classes**

Antidepressant

MAOI, hydrazine derivative

**Therapeutic actions**

Irreversibly inhibits MAO, an enzyme that breaks down biogenic amines, such as epinephrine, norepinephrine, and serotonin, allowing these biogenic amines to accumulate in neuronal storage sites; according to the "biogenic amine hypothesis," this accumulation of amines is responsible for the clinical efficacy of MAOIs as antidepressants.

**Indications**

- Treatment of adult outpatients with reactive depression; efficacy in endogenous depression has not been established
- Unlabeled use: treatment of bulimia having characteristics of atypical depression

t

## Contraindications/cautions

- Contraindications: hypersensitivity to any MAOI; pheochromocytoma, CHF; history of liver disease or abnormal liver function tests; severe renal impairment; confirmed or suspected cerebrovascular defect; CV disease, hypertension; history of headache (headache is an indicator of hypertensive reaction to drug); myelography within previous 24 h or scheduled within 48 h; lactation.
- Use cautiously with seizure disorders; hyperthyroidism; impaired hepatic, renal function; psychiatric patients (agitated or schizophrenic patients may show excessive stimulation; manic-depressive patients may shift to hypomanic or manic phase); patients scheduled for elective surgery (MAOIs should be discontinued 10 d before surgery); pregnancy or in women of childbearing age.

## Dosage

**Available Forms:** Tablets—10 mg

Improvement should be seen within 48 h to 3 wk.

*ADULT:* Usual effective dose is 30 mg/d PO in divided doses. If no improvement is seen within 2 wk, increase dosage in 10 mg/d in increments of 1 to 3 wk. May be increased to a maximum of 60 mg/d.

*PEDIATRIC:* Not recommended for children <16 y.

*GERIATRIC:* Patients >60 y are more prone to develop adverse effects; use with caution.

## Pharmacokinetics

| *Route* | *Onset* | *Duration* |
|---|---|---|
| Oral | Rapid | 10 d |

*Metabolism:* Hepatic, $T_{1/2}$: unkown
*Distribution:* Crosses placenta; enters breast milk
*Excretion:* Urine

## Adverse effects

- CNS: *Dizziness, vertigo, headache, overactivity, hyperreflexia, tremors, muscle twitching, mania, hypomania, jitteriness, confusion, memory impairment, insomnia, weakness, fatigue, drowsiness, restlessness, overstimulation, increased anxiety, agitation, blurred vision, sweating,* akathisa, ataxia, coma, euphoria, neuritis, repetitious babbling, chills, glaucoma, nystagmus
- GI: *Constipation, diarrhea, nausea, abdominal pain, edema, dry mouth, anorexia, weight changes*
- CV: **Hypertensive crises, sometimes fatal,** sometimes with intracranial bleeding, usually attributable to tyramine ingestion (see "Drug–Food Interactions" below); symptoms include occipital headache, which may radiate frontally; palpitations; neck stiffness or soreness; nausea; vomiting; sweating (sometimes with fever, cold and clammy skin); dilated pupils; photophobia; tachycardia or bradycardia; chest pain; *orthostatic hypotension, sometimes associated with falling; disturbed cardiac rate and rhythm,* palpitations, tachycardia
- GU: Dysuria, incontinence, urinary retention, sexual disturbances
- Dermatologic: Minor skin reactions, spider telangiectases, photosensitivity
- Other: Hematologic changes, black tongue, hypernatremia

## Clinically important drug-drug interactions

• Increased sympathomimetic effects (hypertensive crisis) with sympathomimetic drugs (norepinephrine, epinephrine, dopamine, dobutamine, levodopa, ephedrine), amphetamines, other anorexiants, local anesthetic solutions containing sympathomimetics • Hypertensive crisis, coma, severe convulsions with TCAs (eg, imipramine, desipramine) • Additive hypoglycemic effect with insulin, oral sulfonylureas (eg, tolbutamide) • Increased risk of adverse interactive actions with meperidine

## Clinically important drug-food interactions

• Tyramine (and other pressor amines) contained in foods are normally broken down by MAO enzymes in the GI tract; in the presence of MAOIs, these vasopressors may be absorbed in high concentrations; in addition, tyramine releases accumulated norepinephrine from nerve terminals; thus, hypertensive crisis may occur when the following foods that contain tyramine or other vasopressors are ingested by a patient on an MAOI: dairy products (blue, camembert, cheddar, mozzarella, parmesan, romano, roquefort, Stilton chesses; sour cream; yogurt); meats, fish (liver, pickled herring, fermented sausages [bologna, pepperoni, salami], caviar, dried fish, other fermented or spoiled meat or fish); unidstilled beverages (imported beer, ale; red wine, especially Chianti; sherry; coffee, tea, colas containing caffeine; chocolate drinks); fruit/vegetables (avocado, fava beans, figs, raisins, bananas, yeast extracts, soy sauce, chocolate)

## ■ Nursing Considerations

### Assessment

- *History:* Hypersensitivity to any MAOI; pheochromocytoma, CHF; abnormal liver function tests; severe renal impairment; confirmed or suspected cerebrovascular defect; CV disease, hypertension; history of headache, myelography within previous 24 h or scheduled within 48 h; lactation; seizure disorders; hyperthyroidism; impaired hepatic, renal function; psychiatric patients; patients scheduled for elective surgery; pregnancy
- *Physical:* Weight; T; skin color, lesions; orientation, affect, reflexes, vision; P, BP, orthostatic BP, perfusion; bowel sounds, normal output, liver evaluation; urine flow, normal output; liver, kidney function tests, urinalysis, CBC, ECG, EEG

### Implementation

- Limit amount of drug that is available to suicidal patients.
- Monitor BP and orthostatic BP carefully; arrange for more gradual increase in dosage initially in patients who show tendency for hypotension.
- Arrange for periodic liver function tests during therapy; discontinue drug at first sign of hepatic dysfunction or jaundice.
- Monitor BP carefully (and if appropriate, discontinue drug) if patient reports unusual or severe headache.
- Provide phentolamine or another alpha-adrenergic blocking drug on standby in case of hypertensive crisis.

### Drug-specific teaching points

- Take drug exactly as prescribed.
- Do not stop taking drug abruptly or without consulting health care provider.
- Avoid ingesting tyramine-containing foods or beverages while on this drug and for 10 d afterward (patient and significant other should receive a list of such foods and beverages).
- The following side effects may occur: dizziness, weakness or fainting when arising from a horizontal or sitting position (transient; change position slowly); drowsiness, blurred vision (reversible; safety measures may need to be taken if severe; avoid driving or performing tasks that require alertness); nausea, vomiting, loss of appetite (small, frequent meals, frequent mouth care may help); nightmares, confusion, inability to concentrate, emotional changes; changes in sexual function.
- Report headache, skin rash, darkening of the urine, pale stools, yellowing of the eyes or skin, fever, chills, sore throat, or any other unusual symptoms.

# trazodone hydrochloride

*(traz' oh done)*
Desyrel
**Pregnancy Category C**

t

### Drug classes

Antidepressant
Selective serotinin reuptake inhibitor (SSRI)

### Therapeutic actions

Mechanism of action unknown; differs from other antidepressants in that it is a triazolopyridine compound, not a TCA, an amphetamine-like CNS stimulant, or an MAOI;

inhibits the presynaptic reuptake of the neurotransmitter serotonin and potentiates the behavioral effects of the serotonin precursor; the relation of these effects to clinical efficacy is unknown.

### Indications

- Treatment of depression in inpatient and outpatient settings and for depressed patients with and without anxiety
- Unlabeled uses: treatment of aggressive behavior, cocaine withdrawal

### Contraindications/cautions

- Contraindications: hypersensitivity to trazodone, EST, recent MI, pregnancy (congenital abnormalities reported).
- Use cautiously with preexisting cardiac disease (arrhythmias, including ventricular tachycardia, may be more likely), lactation.

### Dosage

**Available Forms:** Tablets—50, 100, 150, 300 mg

*ADULT:* Initially 150 mg/d PO. May be increased by 50 mg/d every 3–4 d. Maximum dose for outpatients should not exceed 400 mg/d in divided doses. Maximum dose for inpatients or those severely depressed should not exceed 600 mg/d in divided doses. Use lowest effective dosage for maintenance.

*PEDIATRIC:* Safety and efficacy not established for children <18 y.

### Pharmacokinetics

| *Route* | *Onset* | *Peak* |
|---|---|---|
| Oral | Varies | 1–2 h |

*Metabolism:* Hepatic, $T_{1/2}$: 3–6 h and then 5–9 h

*Distribution:* Crosses placenta; may enter breast milk

*Excretion:* Urine and feces

### Adverse effects

- CNS: *Anger, hostility, agitation, nightmares/vivid dreams, hallucinations, delusions, hypomania, confusion, disorientation, decreased concentration, impaired memory, impaired speech, dizziness, incoordination, drowsiness, fatigue,* excitement, insomnia, nervousness, paresthesia, tremors, akathisia, headache, grand mal seizures, tinnitus, blurred vision, red eyes, nasal/sinus congestion, *malaise*
- GI: *Abdominal/gastric disorder, decreased/increased appetite, bad taste in mouth, dry mouth, hypersalivation, nausea, vomiting, diarrhea, flatulence, constipation*
- CV: *Hypertension, hypotension, shortness of breath, syncope, tachycardia, palpitations,* chest pain, MI, ventricular ectopic activity, occasional sinus bradycardia with long-term use
- **Hematologic**: Anemia, neutropenia, leukopenia, liver enzyme alterations
- GU: *Decreased libido*, impotence, priapism, retrograde ejaculation, early menses, missed periods, hematuria, delayed urine flow, increased urinary frequency
- **MS**: Musculoskeletal aches and pains, muscle twitches
- **Hypersensitivity**: *Allergic skin conditions, edema*, rash
- **Other**: Sweating, clamminess

## ■ Nursing Considerations

### Assessment

- ***History:*** Hypersensitivity to trazodone, EST, recent MI, preexisting cardiac disease, pregnancy, lactation
- ***Physical:*** Skin color, lesions; orientation, affect, reflexes, vision and hearing; P, BP, orthostatic BP, perfusion; bowel sounds, normal output, liver evaluation; urine flow, normal output; usual sexual function, frequency of menses; liver function tests, urinalysis, CBC, ECG

### Implementation

- Ensure that depressed and potentially suicidal patients have access to only limited quantities of drug.
- Administer shortly after a meal or light snack to enhance absorption.
- Administer major portion of dose hs if drowsiness occurs.
- Anticipate symptomatic relief during the first week of therapy with optimal effects

within 2 wk (some patients require 2–4 wk to respond).
- Monitor patient for orthostatic hypotension during therapy.
- Discontinue therapy immediately if priapism occurs.
- Arrange for CBC if patient develops fever, sore throat, or other signs of infection.

### Drug-specific teaching points
- Take drug with food or a snack to enhance absorption and decrease likelihood of dizziness.
- Avoid alcohol, sleep-inducing drugs, and OTC drugs.
- The following side effects may occur: ringing in the ears, headache, dizziness, drowsiness, weakness (reversible; safety measures may need to be taken if severe; avoid driving or performing tasks that require alertness); nausea, vomiting, loss of appetite (small, frequent meals, frequent mouth care may help); dry mouth (sucking sugarless candies may help); changes in sexual function and abilities; nightmares, dreams, confusion, inability to concentrate (may lessen).
- Report dizziness, lightheadedness, faintness, blood in urine, fever, chills, sore throat, skin rash, prolonged or inappropriate penile erection (discontinue immediately).

## tretinoin

***(tret' i noyn)***
retinoic acid
Vesanoid
**Pregnancy Category D**

### Drug classes
Antineoplastic
Retinoid (topical form, see Appendix A)

### Therapeutic actions
Induces cell differentiation and decreases proliferation of acute promyelocytic leukemia (APL) cells, leading to an initial maturation of the primitive promyelocytes, followed by a repopulation of the bone marrow and peripheral blood by normal hematopoietic cells in patients achieving complete remission; exact mechanism of action is not understood.

### Indications
- Induction of remission in APL
- Topical treatment of acne vulgaris

### Contraindications/cautions
- Contraindications: allergy to retinoids or parabens, pregnancy, lactation.
- Use cautiously with liver disease, hypercholesterolemia, hypertriglyceridemia.

### Dosage
*ADULT:* 45 mg/m$^2$/d PO administered in 2 evenly divided doses until complete remission is documented; discontinue therapy 30 d after complete remission is obtained or after 90 d, whichever comes first.
*PEDIATRIC:* Not recommended.

### Pharmacokinetics

| *Route* | *Onset* | *Peak* |
|---|---|---|
| Oral | Slow | 1–2 h |

*Metabolism:* Hepatic; $T_{1/2}$: 0.5–2 h
*Distribution:* Crosses placenta; may enter breast milk
*Excretion:* Urine and feces

### Adverse effects
- CNS: *Fever, headache,* **pseudotumor cerebri** (papilledema, headache, nausea, vomiting, visual disturbances), *earache, visual disturbances, malaise, sweating*
- GI: *Hemorrhage, nausea, vomiting, abdominal pain,* anorexia, inflammatory bowel disease
- CV: Arrhythmias, flushing, hypotension, CHF, **MI, cardiac arrest**
- Respiratory: **RA-APL syndrome** (fever, dyspnea, weight gain, pulmonary infiltrates, pleural and/or pericardial effusion, hypotension may progess to death)
- Hematologic: **Rapid and evolving leukocytosis,** *liver function, elevated lipids, elevated liver enzymes*
- GU: Renal insufficiency, dysuria, frequency, enlarged prostate

- **MS**: Skeletal hyperostosis, arthralgia, *bone and joint pain* and stiffness
- **Dermatologic**: *Skin fragility, dry skin, pruritus, rash,* thinning hair, peeling of palms and soles, skin infections, photosensitivity, nail brittleness, petechiae

### Clinically important drug-drug interactions

- Increased risk of high serum levels and toxicity with ketoconazole

## ■ Nursing Considerations

### Assessment

- *History:* Allergy to retinoids or parabens, pregnancy, lactation, liver disease, hypercholesterolemia, hypertriglyceridemia
- *Physical:* Skin color, lesions, turgor, texture; joints—range of motion; orientation, reflexes, affect, ophthalmologic exam; mucous membranes, bowel sounds; R, adventitious sounds, auscultation; serum triglycerides, HDL, sedimentation rate, CBC and differential, urinalysis, pregnancy test, chest x-ray

### Implementation

- Ensure that patient is not pregnant before administering; arrange for a pregnancy test within 2 wk of beginning therapy. Advise patient to use contraceptives during treatment and for 1 mo after treatment is discontinued.
- Tretinoin is for induction of remission only; arrange for consolidation or maintenance chemotherapy for APL after induction therapy.
- Arrange for baseline recording of serum lipids and triglyceride levels, liver function tests, chest x-ray, CBC with differential and coagulation profile; monitor for changes frequently.
- Discontinue drug and notify physician if liver function tests are >5× upper range of normal, pulmonary infiltrates appear, or patient has difficulty breathing.
- Discontinue drug if signs of papilledema occur; consult with a neurologist for further care.
- Discontinue drug if visual disturbances occur, and arrange for an ophthalmologic exam.
- Discontinue drug if abdominal pain, rectal bleeding, or severe diarrhea occurs, and consult with physician.
- Monitor triglycerides during therapy; if elevations occur, institute other measures to lower serum triglycerides: weight reduction, reduction in dietary fat, exercise, increased intake of insoluble fiber, decreased alcohol consumption.
- Maintain high-dose steroids on standby in case of severe leukocytosis or liver damage.
- Administer drug with meals; do not crush capsules.
- Do not administer vitamin supplements that contain vitamin A.
- Maintain supportive care appropriate for APL patients: monitor for and treat infections, prophylaxis for bleeding, etc.

### Drug-specific teaching points

- Take this drug with meals; do not crush capsules.
- Frequent blood tests will be necessary to evaluate the drug's effects on your body.
- This drug has been associated with severe birth defects and miscarriages; it is contraindicated for pregnant women. Use contraceptives during treatment and for 1 mo after treatment is discontinued. If you think that you are pregnant, consult with your physician immediately.
- You will not be permitted to donate blood while on this drug because of its possible effects on the fetus of a blood recipient.
- The following side effects may occur: dizziness, lethargy, headache, visual changes (avoid driving or performing tasks that require alertness); sensitivity to the sun (avoid sunlamps, exposure to the sun; use sunscreens and protective clothing); diarrhea, abdominal pain, loss of appetite (take drug with meals); dry mouth (sucking sugarless lozenges may help); eye irritation and redness, inability to wear contact lenses; dry skin, itching, redness.
- Avoid the use of vitamin supplements containing vitamin A; serious toxic effects may occur. Limit alcohol consumption. You may also need to limit your intake

of fats and increase exercise to limit the drug's effects on blood triglyceride levels.
- Report headache with nausea and vomiting, difficulty breathing, severe diarrhea or rectal bleeding, visual difficulties.

## Triamcinolone

### triamcinolone
*(trye am **sin'** oh lone)*

*Oral:* Kenacort

### triamcinolone acetonide

*IM, intra-articular, or soft-tissue injection; respiratory inhalant; dermatologic ointment, cream, lotion, aerosol:* Aristocort, Azmacort, Flutex, Kenaject, Kenalog, Triacet, Triamonide, Triderm

### triamcinolone diacetate

*IM, intra-articular, intrasynovial, intralesional injection:* Amcort, Aristocort Intralesional, Articulose, Triam Forte, Triamolone 40, Trilone, Tristoject

### triamcinolone hexacetonide

*Intra-articular, intralesional injection:* Aristospan Intra-articular, Aristospan Intralesional

**Pregnancy Category C**

### Drug classes
Corticosteroid (intermediate acting)
Glucocorticoid
Hormone

### Therapeutic actions
Enters target cells and binds to cytoplasmic receptors, thereby initiating many complex reactions that are responsible for its anti-inflammatory and immunosuppressive effects.

### Indications
- Hypercalcemia associated with cancer (systemic)
- Short-term management of various inflammatory and allergic disorders, such as rheumatoid arthritis, collagen diseases (eg, SLE), dermatologic diseases (eg, pemphigus), status asthmaticus, and autoimmune disorders
- Hematologic disorders: thrombocytopenia purpura, erythroblastopenia
- Ulcerative colitis, acute exacerbations of mutiple sclerosis, and palliation in some leukemias and lymphomas
- Trichinosis with neurologic or myocardial involvement
- Pulmonary emphysema with bronchial spasm or edema; diffuse interstitial pulmonary fibrosis; with diuretics in CHF with refractory edema and in cirrhosis with refractory ascites
- Postoperative dental inflammatory reactions
- Arthritis, psoriatic plaques, and so forth (intra-articular, soft-tissue administration)
- Control of bronchial asthma requiring corticosteroids in conjunction with other therapy (respiratory inhalant)
- Prophylactic therapy in the maintenance treatment of asthma (bid use)
- To relieve inflammatory and pruritic manifestations of dermatoses that are steroid responsive (dermatologic preparations)

### Contraindications/cautions
- Contraindications: infections, especially tuberculosis, fungal infectons, amebiasis, vaccinia and varicella, and antibiotic-resistant infections; lactation; allergy to tartrazine in 8-mg oral tablets marketed under the brand name Kenacort.
- Use cautiously with pregnancy (teratogenic in preclinical studies); kidney or liver disease, hypothyroidism, ulcerative colitis with impending perforation, diverticulitis, active or latent peptic ulcer, inflammatory bowel disease, CHF, hypertension, thromboembolic disorders, osteoporosis, convulsive disorders, diabetes mellitus.

## Dosage
**Available Forms:** Tablets—1, 2, 4, 8 mg; syrup—4 mg/5 ml; injection—5, 20, 25,

40 mg/ml; aerosol—100 μg/actuation; topical ointment—0.25, 0.1, 0.5%; cream—0.25, 0.1, 0.5%; lotion—0.025, 0.1%

***Systemic***

- ADULT: Individualize dosage, depending on the severity of the condition and the patient's response. Administer daily dose before 9 AM to minimize adrenal suppression. If long-term therapy is needed, consider alternate-day therapy. After long-term therapy, withdraw drug slowly to avoid adrenal insufficiency. For maintenance therapy, reduce initial dose in small increments at intervals until the lowest effective dose is reached.
- PEDIATRIC: Individualize dosage, depending on the severity of the condition and the patient's response rather than by formulae that correct adult doses for age or body weight. Carefully observe growth and development in infants and children on prolonged therapy.

***Oral (triamcinolone)***

- *Adrenal insufficiency:* 4–12 mg/d, plus a mineralocorticoid.
- *Rheumatic, dermatologic, allergic, ophthalmologic, hematologic disorders and asthma:* 8–60 mg/d.
- *TB meningitis:* 32–48 mg/d.
- *Acute leukemia: Adult:* 16–40 mg up to 100 mg/d. *Pediatric:* 1–2 mg/kg per day.

***IM (triamcinolone acetonide):*** 2.5–60.0 mg/d.

***IM (triamcinolone diacetate):*** 40 mg/wk. A single parenteral dose 4–7× oral daily dose provides control for 4 d–4 wk.

***Intra-articular, intralesional (dose will vary with joint or soft tissue site to be injected)***

- **Triamcinolone acetonide:** 2.5–15.0 mg.
- **Triamcinolone diacetate:** 5–40 mg.
- **Triamcinolone hexacetonide:** 2–20 mg.

***Respiratory inhalant (triamcinolone acetonide):*** 200 μg released with each actuation delivers about 100 μg to the patient.

- ADULT: 2 inhalations tid–qid, not to exceed 16 inhalations/d.
- PEDIATRIC (6–12 Y): 1–2 inhalations tid–qid, not to exceed 12 inhalations/d.

***Topical dermatologic preparations:*** Apply sparingly to affected area bid–qid.

## Pharmacokinetics

| Route | Onset | Peak | Duration |
|---|---|---|---|
| Oral | 24–48 h | 1–2 h | 2.25 d |
| IM | 24–48 h | 8–10 h | 1–6 wk |

*Metabolism:* Hepatic, $T_{1/2}$: 2–5 h
*Distribution:* Crosses placenta; enters breast milk
*Excretion:* Urine

## Adverse effects

Effects depend on dose, route, and duration of therapy.

- CNS: *Vertigo, headache*, paresthesias, insomnia, convulsions, psychosis, cataracts, increased intraocular pressure, glaucoma (long-term therapy)
- GI: Peptic or esophageal ulcer, pancreatitis, abdominal distention, nausea, vomiting, *increased appetite, weight gain* (long-term therapy)
- CV: Hypotension, shock, hypertension and CHF secondary to fluid retention, thromboembolism, thrombophlebitis, fat embolism, cardiac arrhythmias
- MS: Muscle weakness, steroid myopathy, loss of muscle mass, osteoporosis, spontaneous fractures (long-term therapy)
- Hypersensitivity: Hypersensitivity or anaphylactoid reactions
- Endocrine: Amenorrhea, irregular menses, growth retardation, decreased carbohydrate tolerance, diabetes mellitus, cushingoid state (long-term effect), increased blood sugar, increased serum cholesterol, decreased $T_3$ and $T_4$ levels, hypothalamic-pituitary-adrenal (HPA) suppression with systemic therapy longer than 5 d
- Electrolyte imbalance: *$Na^+$ and fluid retention*, hypokalemia, hypocalcemia
- Other: *Immunosuppression, aggravation, or masking of infections; impaired*

*wound healing*; thin, fragile skin; petechiae, ecchymoses, purpura, striae; subcutaneous fat atrophy

*Intra-articular*

- **Local**: Osteonecrosis, tendon, rupture, infection

*Intralesional (face and head)*

- **Local**: Blindness (rare)

*Respiratory Inhalants*

- **Local**: Oral, laryngeal, and pharyngeal irritation; fungal infections

*Topical Dermatologic Ointments, Creams, Sprays*

- **Local**: Local burning, irritation, acneiform lesions, striae, skin atrophy

### Clinically important drug-drug interactions

• Increased therapeutic and toxic effects with troleandomycin • Risk of severe deterioration of muscle strength when given to myasthenia gravis patients who are also receiving ambenonium, edrophonium, neostigmine, pyridostigmine • Decreased steroid blood levels with barbiturates, phenytoin, rifampin • Decreased effectiveness of salicylates

### Drug-lab test interferences

• False-negative nitroblue-tetrazolium test for bacterial infection • Suppression of skin test reactions

## ■ Nursing Considerations

### Assessment

- *History:* Infections; kidney or liver disease; hypothyroidism; ulcerative colitis with impending perforation; diverticulitis; active or latent peptic ulcer; inflammatory bowel disease; CHF; hypertension; thromboembolic disorders; osteoporosis; convulsive disorders; diabetes mellitus; pregnancy; lactation; allergy to tartrazine
- *Physical:* Weight, T, reflexes and grip strength, affect and orientation, P, BP, peripheral perfusion, prominence of superficial veins, R, adventitious sounds, serum electrolytes, blood glucose.

### Implementation

- Administer once-a-day doses before 9 AM to mimic normal peak corticosteroid blood levels.
- Increase dosage when patient is subject to stress.
- Taper doses when discontinuing high-dose or long-term therapy.
- Do not give live virus vaccines with immunosuppressive doses of corticosteroids.
- Taper systemic steroids carefully during transfer to inhalational steroids; deaths caused by adrenal insufficiency have occurred.
- Use caution when occlusive dressings, tight diapers, and so forth cover affected area; these can increase systemic absorption when using topical preparations.
- Avoid prolonged use of topical preparations near the eyes, in genital and rectal areas, and in skin creases.

### Drug-specific teaching points

- Do not stop taking the drug without consulting your health care provider.
- Avoid exposure to infections.
- Report unusual weight gain, swelling of the extremities, muscle weakness, black or tarry stools, fever, prolonged sore throat, colds or other infections, worsening of your disorder.

*Intra-articular Administration*

- Do not overuse joint after therapy, even if pain is gone.

*Respiratory Inhalant*

- Do not use during an acute asthmatic attack or to manage status asthmaticus.
- Do not use with systemic fungal infections.
- Do not use more often than prescribed.
- Do not stop using this drug without consulting your health care provider.
- Administer inhalational bronchodilator drug first, if receiving concomitant bronchodilator therapy.

*Topical Dermatologic Preparations*

- Apply drug sparingly, avoid contact with eyes.

- Report irritation or infection at the site of application.

## triamterene

*(trye **am'** ter een)*

Dyrenium

**Pregnancy Category B**

### Drug classes

Potassium-sparing diuretic

### Therapeutic actions

Inhibits sodium reabsorption in the renal distal tubule, causing loss of sodium and water and retention of potassium.

### Indications

- Edema associated with CHF, nephrotic syndrome, hepatic cirrhosis; steroid-induced edema, edema from secondary hyperaldosteronism (alone or with other diuretics for added diuretic or antikaliuretic effects)

### Contraindications/cautions

- Contraindications: allergy to triamterene, hyperkalemia, renal disease (except nephrosis), liver disease, lactation.
- Use cautiously with diabetes mellitus, pregnancy.

### Dosage

**Available Forms:** Capsules—50, 100 mg

*ADULT:* 100 mg bid PO if used alone. Reduce dosage if added to other diuretic therapy. Maintenance dosage should be individualized, may be as low as 100 mg every other day. Do not exceed 300 mg/d.

*PEDIATRIC:* Safety and efficacy not established.

### Pharmacokinetics

| *Route* | *Onset* | *Peak* | *Duration* |
|---|---|---|---|
| Oral | 2–4 h | 6–8 h | 12–16 h |

*Metabolism:* Hepatic, $T_{1/2}$: 3 h

*Distribution:* Crosses placenta; enters breast milk

*Excretion:* Urine

### Adverse effects

- CNS: *Headache*, drowsiness, fatigue, *weakness*
- GI: *Nausea, anorexia, vomiting, dry mouth*, diarrhea
- **Hematologic**: Hyperkalemia, blood dyscrasias
- GU: Renal stones, intersititial nephritis
- Dermatologic: Rash, photosensitivity

### Clinically important drug-drug interactions

• Increased hyperkalemia with potassium supplements, diets rich in potassium, ACE inhibitors • Increased serum levels and possible toxicity with cimetidine, indomethacin • Increased risk of amantadine toxicity

### Drug-lab test interferences

- Interference with fluorescent measurement of serum quinidine levels

## ■ Nursing Considerations

### Assessment

- ***History:*** Allergy to triamterene, hyperkalemia, renal or liver disease, diabetes mellitus, pregnancy, lactation
- ***Physical:*** Skin color, lesions, edema; orientation, reflexes, muscle strength; pulses, baseline ECG, BP; R, pattern, adventitious sounds; liver evaluation, bowel sounds; urinary output patterns; CBC, serum electrolytes, blood sugar, liver and renal function tests, urinalysis

### Implementation

- Administer with food or milk if GI upset occurs.
- Mark calendars or provide other reminders of drug days for outpatients if alternate-day or 3- to 5-d/wk therapy is optimal for treating edema.
- Administer early in the day so that increased urination does not disturb sleep.
- Measure and record regular weights to monitor mobilization of edema fluid.
- Arrange for regular evaluation of serum electrolytes, BUN.

### Drug-specific teaching points

- Record alternate-day therapy on a calendar, or make dated envelopes. Take the

drug early in the day as increased urination will occur. The drug may be taken with food or meals if GI upset occurs.
- Weigh yourself on a regular basis, at the same time and in the same clothing, and record the weight on your calendar.
- The following side effects may occur: increased volume and frequency of urination; drowsiness (avoid rapid position changes; do not engage in hazardous activities [eg, driving a car]; this problem is often made worse by the use of alcohol); avoid foods that are rich in potassium (eg, fruits, Sanka); sensitivity to sunlight and bright lights (wear sunglasses, use sunscreens and protective clothing).
- Report weight change of more than 3 lb in one day, swelling in ankles or fingers, fever, sore throat, mouth sores, unusual bleeding or bruising, dizziness, trembling, numbness, fatigue.

## triazolam

*(trye ay' zoe lam)*
Halcion
**Pregnancy Category X**
**C-IV controlled substance**

### Drug classes
Benzodiazepine
Sedative/hypnotic

### Therapeutic actions
Exact mechanisms of action not understood; acts mainly at subcortical levels of the CNS, leaving the cortex relatively unaffected; main sites of action may be the limbic system and mesencephalic reticular formation; benzodiazepines potentiate the effects of GABA, an inhibitory neurotransmitter.

### Indications
- Insomnia characterized by difficulty falling asleep, frequent nocturnal awakenings, or early morning awakening
- Recurring insomnia or poor sleeping habits
- Acute or chronic medical situations requiring restful sleep

### Contraindications/cautions
- Contraindications: hypersensitivity to benzodiazepines; pregnancy (risk of congenital malformations, neonatal withdrawal syndrome); labor and delivery ("floppy infant" syndrome); lactation (infants may become lethargic and lose weight).
- Use cautiously with impaired liver or kidney function, debilitation, depression, suicidal tendencies.

## Dosage
**Available Forms:** Tablets—0.125, 0.25 mg
*ADULT:* 0.125–0.5 mg PO before retiring.
*PEDIATRIC:* Not for use in children <18 y.
*GERIATRIC PATIENTS OR THOSE WITH DEBILITATING DISEASE:* Initially, 0.125–0.25 mg PO. Adjust as needed and tolerated.

### Pharmacokinetics

| *Route* | *Onset* | *Peak* |
|---|---|---|
| Oral | Varies | 1/2–2 h |

*Metabolism:* Hepatic, $T_{1/2}$: 1.5–5.5 h
*Distribution:* Crosses placenta; enters breast milk
*Excretion:* Urine

### Adverse effects
- CNS: *Transient, mild drowsiness initially; sedation, depression, lethargy,* apathy, fatigue, *lightheadedness, disorientation, restlessness, confusion*, crying, delirium, headache, slurred speech, dysarthria, stupor, rigidity, tremor, dystonia, vertigo, euphoria, nervousness, difficulty in concentration, vivid dreams, psychomotor retardation, extrapyramidal symptoms; *mild paradoxical excitatory reactions, during first 2 wk of treatment* (especially in psychiatric patients, aggressive children, and with high dosage), visual and auditory disturbances, diplopia, nystagmus, depressed hearing, nasal congestion, retrograde amnesia, "traveler's amnesia"
- GI: *Constipation, diarrhea,* dry mouth, salivation, nausea, anorexia, vomiting,

t

difficulty in swallowing, gastric disorders, elevations of blood enzymes: hepatic dysfunction, jaundice

- CV: *Bradycardia, tachycardia*, CV collapse, hypertension and hypotension, palpitations, edema
- **Hematologic**: Decreased Hct, blood dyscrasias
- GU: *Incontinence, urinary retention, changes in libido*, menstrual irregularities
- **Dermatologic**: Urticaria, pruritus, skin rash, dermatitis
- **Dependence**: *Drug dependence with withdrawal syndrome* when drug is discontinued (more common with abrupt discontinuation of higher dosage used for longer than 4 mo)
- **Other**: Hiccups, fever, diaphoresis, paresthesias, muscular disturbances, gynecomastia

### Clinically important drug-drug interactions

• Increased CNS depression and sedation with alcohol, cimetidine, omeprazole, disulfiram, oral contraceptives • Decreased sedative effects with theophylline, aminophylline, dyphylline, oxitriphylline • Potentially serious to fatal reactions with ketoconazole, itraconazole; avoid this combination

## ■ Nursing Considerations

### Assessment

- *History:* Hypersensitivity to benzodiazepines, pregnancy, lactation, impaired liver or kidney function, debilitation, depression, suicidal tendencies
- *Physical:* Skin color, lesions; T; orientation, reflexes, affect, ophthalmologic exam; P, BP; R, adventitious sounds; liver evaluation, abdominal exam, bowel sounds, normal output; CBC, liver and renal function tests

### Implementation

- Arrange for periodic blood counts, urinalyses, and blood chemistry analyses with protracted treatment.
- Taper dosage gradually after long-term therapy, especially in epileptic patients.

### Drug-specific teaching points

- Take drug exactly as prescribed.
- Do not stop taking this drug (long-term therapy) without consulting your health care provider.
- Avoid alcohol, sleep-inducing, or OTC drugs.
- Avoid pregnancy while taking this drug; use of contraceptives is advised; serious fetal harm could occur.
- The following side effects may occur: drowsiness, dizziness (may lessen; avoid driving or engaging in hazardous activities); GI upset (take drug with food); depression, dreams, emotional upset, crying; disturbance of nocturnal sleep for several nights after discontinuing the drug.
- Report severe dizziness, weakness, drowsiness that persists, rash or skin lesions, palpitations, swelling of the extremities, visual changes, difficulty voiding.

## trichlormethiazide

*(trye klor meth **eye'** a zide)*

Diurese, Metahydrin, Naqua

**Pregnancy Category C**

### Drug classes

Thiazide diuretic

### Therapeutic actions

Inhibits reabsorption of sodium and chloride in distal renal tubule, thereby increasing excretion of sodium, chloride, and water by the kidney.

### Indications

- Adjunctive therapy in edema associated with CHF, cirrhosis, corticosteroid and estrogen therapy, renal dysfunction
- Hypertension, as sole therapy or in combination with other antihypertensives
- Unlabeled uses: calcium nephrolithiasis alone or with amiloride or allopurinol to prevent recurrences in hypercalciuric or

normal calciuric patients, diabetes insipidus, especially nephrogenic diabetes insipidus

## Contraindications/cautions

- Contraindications: fluid or electrolyte imbalances, pregnancy, lactation, allergy to tartrazine or aspirin (tartrazine contained in tablets marketed under the name Metahydrin).
- Use cautiously with renal or liver disease, gout, SLE, glucose tolerance abnormalities, hyperparathyroidism, manic-depressive disorders.

## Dosage

**Available Forms:** Tablets—2, 4 mg

*ADULT*

- ***Edema, hypertension:*** 2–4 mg PO qd.
- ***Calcium nephrolithiasis:*** 4 mg/d PO.

*PEDIATRIC:* Safety and efficacy not established.

## Pharmacokinetics

| *Route* | *Onset* | *Peak* | *Duration* |
|---|---|---|---|
| Oral | 2 h | 6 h | 24 h |

*Metabolism:* Hepatic, $T_{1/2}$: 2.3–7.3 h

*Distribution:* Crosses placenta; enters breast milk

*Excretion:* Urine

## Adverse effects

- CNS: *Dizziness, vertigo,* paresthesias, weakness, headache, drowsiness, fatigue, leukopenia, thrombocytopenia, agranulocytosis, aplastic anemia, neutropenia
- GI: *Nausea, anorexia, vomiting, dry mouth,* diarrhea, constipation, jaundice, hepatitis, pancreatitis
- CV: Orthostatic hypotension, venous thrombosis, volume depletion, cardiac arrhythmias, chest pain
- GU: *Polyuria, nocturia,* impotence, loss of libido
- Dermatologic: Photosensitivity, rash, purpura, exfoliative dermatitis, hives
- Other: Muscle cramps and muscle spasms, fever, gouty attacks, flushing, weight loss, rhinorrhea

## Clinically important drug-drug interactions

• Risk of hyperglycemia with diazoxide • Decreased absorption with cholestyramine, colestipol • Increased risk of digitalis glycoside toxicity if hypokalemia occurs • Increased risk of lithium toxicity with thiazides • Increased fasting blood glucose leading to need to adjust dosage of antidiabetic agents

## Drug-lab test interferences

• Decreased PBI levels without clinical signs of thyroid disturbances

## ■ Nursing Considerations

### Assessment

- ***History:*** Fluid or electrolyte imbalances, renal or liver disease, gout, SLE, glucose tolerance abnormalities, hyperparathyroidism, manic-depressive disorders, pregnancy, lactation, allergy to tartrazine or aspirin
- ***Physical:*** Skin color and lesions; orientation, reflexes, muscle strength; P, BP, orthostatic BP, perfusion, edema, baseline ECG; R, adventitious sounds; liver evaluation, bowel sounds; CBC, serum electrolytes, blood glucose, liver and renal function tests, serum uric acid, urinalysis

### Implementation

- Administer with food or milk if GI upset occurs.
- Mark calendars or provide other reminders of drug days for outpatients on alternate-day or 3- to 5-d/wk therapy.
- Administer early in the day so increased urination will not disturb sleep.

### Drug-specific teaching points

- Take drug early in the day so sleep will not be disturbed by increased urination.
- Weigh yourself daily, and record weights on your calendar.
- Protect skin from exposure to sun or bright lights.
- Increased urination will occur.
- Use caution if dizziness, drowsiness, feeling faint occur.

t

- Report rapid weight change, swelling in ankles or fingers, unusual bleeding or bruising, muscle cramps.

## trientine hydrochloride

***(trye' en teen)***

Syprine

**Pregnancy Category C**

### Drug classes

Chelating agent for removal of copper from the body

### Therapeutic actions

Chelating agent that combines with copper in the body, making it a more soluble compound that is excreted in the urine.

### Indications

- Treatment of patients with Wilson's disease who are intolerant of penicillamine

### Contraindications/cautions

- Allergy to trientine, pregnancy, lactation.

### Dosage

**Available Forms:** Capsules—250 mg

*Warning:* Interruptions of daily therapy for even a few days have been followed by sensitivity reactions when the drug is reinstituted.

**ADULT:** Initially, 750–1250 mg/d PO in divided doses bid, tid, or qid. May increase to a maximum of 2 g/d. Must be given on an empty stomach.

**PEDIATRIC**

- *<12 Y:* Initially, 500–750 mg/d PO in divided doses bid, tid, qid. May increase to a maximum of 1500 mg/d.

### Pharmacokinetics

| *Route* | *Onset* | *Peak* |
|---|---|---|
| Oral | Varies | 60 min |

*Metabolism:* Hepatic, $T_{1/2}$: unknown

*Distribution:* Crosses placenta; enters breast milk

*Excretion:* Urine

### Adverse effects

- General: *Iron deficiency*, SLE
- Hypersensitivity: Reactions such as asthma, bronchitis, *dermatitis*

## ■ Nursing Considerations

### Assessment

- *History:* Allergy to trientine, pregnancy, lactation
- *Physical:* Skin color, lesions; T; R, adventitious sounds (to detect hypersensitivity reactions); CBC, Hgb levels, titer for ANA, serum and 24-h urine copper levels

### Implementation

- Monitor CBC, Hgb, and serum and 24-h urinary copper levels before and periodically (every 6–12 mo) during therapy.
- Administer drug on an empty stomach, 1 h before or 2 h after meals and at least 1 h apart from any other drug, food, or milk.
- Ensure that patient swallows capsules whole with water; do not open or chew.
- Wash any area that comes in contact with the capsule contents carefully because of the risk of contact dermatitis.
- Monitor T nightly during first month of treatment.
- Arrange for nutritional consultation; if iron supplements are needed, ensure that they are given at least 2 h apart from trientine.
- Evaluate for 24-h urinary copper levels of 0.5–1 mg.

### Drug-specific teaching points

- Do not open or chew capsules. Take on an empty stomach, 1 h before or 2 h after meals and at least 1 h apart from any other drug, food, or milk.
- The following side effects may occur: iron deficiency (periodic blood tests will be needed; iron supplements may be used).
- This drug is not to be used during pregnancy. If you become pregnant or want to become pregnant, consult your prescriber.
- Report skin rash, difficulty breathing, cough or wheezing, fever, chills.

# trifluoperazine hydrochloride

*(trye floo oh **per'** a zeen)*

Apo-Trifluoperazine (CAN), Stelazine

**Pregnancy Category C**

## Drug classes

Phenothiazine (piperazine)
Dopaminergic blocking agent
Antipsychotic
Antianxiety agent

## Therapeutic actions

Mechanism of action not fully understood: antipsychotic drugs block postsynaptic dopamine receptors in the brain, but this may not be necessary and sufficient for antipsychotic activity; depresses the RAS, including the parts of the brain involved with wakefulness and emesis; anticholinergic, antihistaminic ($H_1$), and alpha-adrenergic blocking activity also may contribute to some of its therapeutic (and adverse) actions.

## Indications

- Management of manifestations of psychotic disorders
- Treatment of nonpsychotic anxiety (not drug of choice)

## Contraindications/cautions

- Contraindications: coma or severe CNS depression, bone marrow depression, blood dyscrasia, circulatory collapse, subcortical brain damage, Parkinson's disease, liver damage, cerebral arteriosclerosis, coronary disease, severe hypotension or hypertension.
- Use cautiously with respiratory disorders ("silent pneumonia"); glaucoma, prostatic hypertrophy; epilepsy or history of epilepsy (lowers seizure threshold); breast cancer; thyrotoxicosis (severe neurotoxicity); peptic ulcer, decreased renal function; myelography within previous 24 h or scheduled within 48 h; exposure to heat or phosphorous insecticides; pregnancy; lactation; children <12 y, especially those with chickenpox, CNS infections (children are especially susceptible to dystonias that may confound the diagnosis of Reye's syndrome).

## Dosage

**Available Forms:** Tablets—1, 2, 5, 10 mg; concentrate—10 mg/ml; injection—2 mg/ml

**ADULT**

- *Psychotic disorders*
  - ***Oral:*** 2–5 mg bid. Start small or emaciated patients on the lower dosage. Most patients will show optimum response with 15 or 20 mg/d. Optimum dosage should be reached within 2–3 wk.
  - ***IM:*** For prompt control of severe symptoms, 1–2 mg by deep IM injection q4–6h, as needed. Do not give more often than q4h. More than 6 mg/d is rarely needed. More than 10 mg/d should be given only in exceptional cases.

**PEDIATRIC:** Adjust dosage to weight of child and severity of symptoms. The following dosages are for hospitalized or closely supervised children 6–12 y:

- ***Oral:*** Initially, 1 mg qd–bid. It is usually not necessary to exceed 15 mg/d. Older children with severe symptoms may require higher dosage.
- ***IM:*** For prompt control of severe symptoms, 1 mg qd–bid.

**GERIATRIC:** Use lower doses, and increase dosage more gradually than in younger patients.

- *Nonpsychotic disorders:* Usual dose 1–2 mg bid. Do not administer more than 6 mg/d or for longer than 12 wk.

## Pharmacokinetics

| *Route* | *Onset* | *Peak* | *Duration* |
|---|---|---|---|
| Oral | Varies | 2–4 h | < 12 h |
| IM | Rapid | 1–2 h | < 12 h |

*Metabolism:* Hepatic, $T_{1/2}$: 47–100 h
*Distribution:* Crosses placenta; enters breast milk
*Excretion:* Bile and feces

### Adverse effects

- CNS: *Drowsiness*, insomnia, vertigo, headache, weakness, tremor, ataxia, slurring, cerebral edema, seizures, exacerbation of psychotic symptoms, extrapyramidal syndromes—*pseudoparkinsonism; dystonias; akathisia;* tardive dyskinesias, potentially irreversible (no known treatment), neuroleptic malignant syndrome
- CV: Hypotension, orthostatic hypotension, hypertension, tachycardia, bradycardia, cardiac arrest, CHF, cardiomegaly, **refractory arrhythmias**, pulmonary edema
- Respiratory: Bronchospasm, laryngospasm, dyspnea, suppression of cough reflex and potential for aspiration
- Hematologic: Eosinophilia, leukopenia, leukocytosis, anemia; aplastic anemia; hemolytic anemia; thrombocytopenic or nonthrombocytopenic purpura; pancytopenia
- EENT: Glaucoma, *photophobia, blurred vision*, miosis, mydriasis, deposits in the cornea and lens (opacities), pigmentary retinopathy
- Hypersensitivity: Jaundice, urticaria, angioneurotic edema, laryngeal edema, photosensitivity, eczema, asthma, anaphylactoid reactions, exfoliative dermatitis
- Endocrine: Lactation, breast engorgement, galactorrhea; SIADH; amenorrhea, menstrual irregularities; gynecomastia; changes in libido; hyperglycemia or hypoglycemia; glycosuria; hyponatremia; pituitary tumor with hyperprolactinemia; inhibition of ovulation, infertility, pseudopregnancy; reduced urinary levels of gonadotropins, estrogens, progestins
- Autonomic: *Dry mouth, salivation, nasal congestion, nausea*, vomiting, anorexia, fever, pallor, flushed facies, sweating, constipation, paralytic ileus, urinary retention, incontinence, polyuria, enuresis, priapism, ejaculation inhibition, male impotence
- Other: *Urine discolored pink to red-brown*

### Clinically important drug-drug interactions

• Additive CNS depression with alcohol • Additive anticholinergic effects and possibly decreased antipsychotic efficacy with anticholinergic drugs • Increased likelihood of seizures with metrizamide • Increased frequency and severity of neuromuscular excitation and hypotension in patients who are premedicated with trifluoperazine and are given barbiturate anesthetics (methohexital, thiamylal, phenobarbital, thiopental) • Decreased antihypertensive effect of guanethidine

### Drug-lab test interferences

• False-positive pregnancy tests (less likely if serum test is used) • Increase in PBI, not attributable to an increase in thyroxine

## ■ Nursing Considerations

### Assessment

- *History:* Coma or severe CNS depression; bone marrow depression; blood dyscrasia; circulatory collapse; subcortical brain damage; Parkinson's disease; liver damage; cerebral arteriosclerosis; coronary disease; severe hypotension or hypertension; respiratory disorders; glaucoma, prostatic hypertrophy; epilepsy; breast cancer; thyrotoxicosis; peptic ulcer, decreased renal function; myelography within previous 24 h or scheduled within 48 h; exposure to heat or phosphorous insecticides; pregnancy; lactation; chickenpox; CNS infections
- *Physical:* Weight, T; reflexes, orientation, intraocular pressure; P, BP, orthostatic BP; R, adventitious sounds; bowel sounds and normal output, liver evaluation; urinary output, prostate size; CBC; urinalysis; thyroid, liver, and kidney function tests

### Implementation

- Do not change brand names; bioavailability differences have been documented.
- Dilute oral concentrate (for institutional use only) immediately before use by adding the dose to 60 ml of one of the fol-

lowing: tomato or fruit juice, milk, simple syrup, orange syrup, carbonated beverages, coffee, tea, or water; semisolid foods (soup, pudding) also may be used.
- Avoid skin contact with drug solution; contact dermatitis has occurred.
- Discontinue drug if serum creatinine, BUN become abnormal or WBC count is depressed.
- Monitor elderly patients for dehydration, and institute remedial measures promptly; sedation and decreased sensation of thirst related to CNS effects can lead to severe dehydration.
- Consult physician regarding appropriate warning of patient or patient's guardian about tardive dyskinesias.
- Consult physician about dosage reduction, use of anticholinergic antiparkinsonian drugs (controversial) if extrapyramidal effects occur.

### Drug-specific teaching points

- Take drug exactly as prescribed.
- Avoid skin contact with drug solutions.
- Avoid driving or engaging in other hazardous activities if CNS, vision changes occur.
- Avoid prolonged exposure to sun, or use a sunscreen or covering garments.
- Maintain fluid intake, and use precautions against heatstroke in hot weather.
- Report sore throat, fever, unusual bleeding or bruising, rash, weakness, tremors, impaired vision, dark urine (pink or reddish brown urine is expected), pale stools, yellowing of the skin or eyes.

## triflupromazine hydrochloride

*(trye flu **proe'** ma zeen)*
Vesprin
**Pregnancy Category C**

### Drug classes

Phenothiazine
Dopaminergic blocking agent
Antipsychotic
Antiemetic
Antianxiety agent

### Therapeutic actions

Mechanism of action not fully understood: blocks postsynaptic dopamine receptors in the brain; depresses the parts of the brain involved with wakefulness and emesis; anticholinergic, antihistaminic ($H_1$), and alpha-adrenergic blocking.

### Indications

- Control of severe nausea and vomiting
- Management of manifestations of psychotic disorders

### Contraindications/cautions

- Contraindications: allergy to triflupromazine, comatose or severely depressed states, bone marrow depression, circulatory collapse, subcortical brain damage.
- Use cautiously with Parkinson's disease; liver damage; cerebral or coronary arteriosclerosis; severe hypotension or hypertension; respiratory disorders; glaucoma; epilepsy or history of epilepsy; peptic ulcer or history of peptic ulcer; decreased renal function; prostate hypertrophy; breast cancer; thyrotoxicosis; myelography within 24 h or scheduled within 48 h; lactation; exposure to heat, phosphorous insecticides; children with chickenpox, CNS infections (such children are more susceptible to dystonias, which may confound the diagnosis of Reye's syndrome or other encephalopathy; may mask symptoms of Reye's syndrome, encephalopathies)

### Dosage

**Available Forms:** Injection—10, 20 mg/ml

#### ADULT

- *Nausea and vomiting:* 5–15 mg IM q4h, up to a maximum of 60 mg/d. 1 mg IV up to a maximum of 3 mg/d.
- *Psychotic disorders:* 60 mg IM, up to 150 mg/d.

#### PEDIATRIC (>2 Y)

- *Nausea and vomiting:* 0.2–0.25 mg/kg IM up to a maximum of 10 mg/d. Do not give IV.
- *Psychotic disorders:* 0.2–-0.25 mg/kg IM to a maximum of 10 mg/d.

t

### Pharmacokinetics

| Route | Onset | Peak | Duration |
|---|---|---|---|
| IM | 10–15 min | 15–20 min | 4–6 h |

*Metabolism:* Hepatic, $T_{1/2}$: 10–20 h
*Distribution:* Crosses placenta; enters breast milk
*Excretion:* Urine

### IV facts

**Preparation:** No further preparation required.
**Infusion:** Inject slowly into tubing of actively running IV over 5–10 min.

### Adverse effects

- CNS: *Drowsiness, insomnia, vertigo,* headache, weakness, tremors, ataxia, slurring, cerebral edema, seizures, exacerbation of psychotic symptoms, *extrapyramidal syndromes*; neuroleptic malignant syndrome
- GI: *Dry mouth, salivation, nausea, vomiting, anorexia, constipation*, paralytic ileus, incontinence
- CV: *Hypotension, otrhostatic hypotension,* hypertension, tachycardia, bradycardia, cardiac arrest, CHF, cardiomegaly, refractory arrhythmias, pulmonary edema
- Respiratory: Bronchospasm, laryngospasm, dyspnea, suppression of cough reflex and potential aspiration
- Hematologic: **Eosinophilia, leukopenia, leukocytosis, *anemia*, aplastic anemia, hemolytic anemia, thrombocytopenic or nonthrombocytopenic purpura, pancytopenia, elevated serum cholesterol**
- GU: *Urinary retention,* polyuria, incontinence, priapism, ejaculation inhibition, male impotence, urine discolored pink to red-brown
- EENT: Nasal congestion, glaucoma, *photophobia, blurred vision*, miosis, mydriasis, deposits in the cornea and lens, pigmentary retinopathy
- Hypersensitivity: Jaundice, *urticaria*, angioneurotic edema, laryngeal edema, photosensitivity, eczema, asthma, anaphylactoid reactions, exfoliative dermatitis, contact dermatitis with drug solutions
- Endocrine: Lactation, breast engorgement, galactorrhea, SIADH secretion, amenorrhea, menstrual irregularities; gynecomastia; changes in libido, hyperglycemia, inhibition of ovulation, infertility, pseudopregnancy, reduced urinary levels of gonadotropins, estrogens and progestins
- Other: Fever, heatstroke, pallor, flushed facies, sweating, *photosensitivity*

### Clinically important drug-drug interactions

• Additive anticholinergic effects and possibly decreased antipsychotic efficacy with anticholinergic drugs • Additive CNS depression, hypotension if given preoperatively with barbiturate anesthetics, alcohol, meperidine • Additive effects of both drugs with beta-blockers • Increased risk of tachycardia, hypotension with epinephrine, norepinephrine • Increased risk of seizure with metrizamide • Decreased hypotension effect with guanethidine

### Drug-lab test interferences

• False-positive pregnancy tests (less likely if serum test is used) • Increase in protein-bound iodine, not attributable to an increase in thyroxine

## ■ Nursing Considerations

### Assessment

- *History:* Allergy to triflupromazine; comatose or severely depressed states; bone marrow depression; circulatory collapse; subcortical brain damage, Parkinson's disease; liver damage; cerebral or coronary arteriosclerosis; severe hypotension or hypertension; respiratory disorders; glaucoma; epilepsy; peptic ulcer; decreased renal function; prostate hypertrophy; breast cancer; thyrotoxicosis; myelography within 24 h or scheduled within 48 h; lactation; exposure to heat, phosphorous insecticides; chickenpox, CNS infections
- *Physical:* T; weight, skin color, turgor; reflexes, orientation, intraocular pressure,

ophthalmologic exam; P, BP, orthostatic BP, ECG; R, adventitious sounds; bowel sounds, normal output, liver evaluation; prostate palpation, normal urine output; CBC; urinalysis; thyroid, liver, and kidney function tests; EEG (as appropriate)

### Implementation

- Do not give by SC injection; give slowly by deep IM injection into upper outer quadrant of buttock.
- Reserve IV use for situations when IM use is not possible. Do not use IV in children.
- Keep the patient recumbent for 1/2 h after injection to avoid orthostatic hypotension.
- Avoid skin contact with drug solutions; may cause contact dermatitis.
- Be alert to potential for aspiration because of suppressed cough reflex.
- Monitor renal function tests and discontinue if serum creatinine, BUN become abnormal.
- Monitor CBC and discontinue if WBC count is depressed.
- Withdraw drug gradually after high-dose therapy; gastritis, nausea, dizziness, headache, tachycardia, insomnia have occurred after abrupt withdrawal.
- Monitor elderly patients for dehydration: sedation and decreased sensation of thirst due to CNS effects can lead to dehydration, hemoconcentration, and reduced pulmonary ventilation; promptly institute remedial measures.
- Avoid use of epinephrine as vasopressor if drug-induced hypotension occurs.

### Drug-specific teaching points

- This drug can be given only by injection.
- The following side effects may occur: drowsiness (avoid driving or operating dangerous machinery; avoid alcohol, which will increase the drowsiness); sensitivity to the sun (avoid prolonged sun exposure, and wear protective garments or use a sunscreen); pink or reddish-brown urine (expected effect); faintness, dizziness (transient; change position slowly, use caution climbing stairs).
- Use caution in hot weather; you may be prone to heatstroke; keep up fluid intake, and do not exercise unduly in a hot climate.
- Report sore throat, fever, unusual bleeding or bruising, rash, weakness, tremors, impaired vision, dark urine, pale stools, yellowing of the skin and eyes.

## trihexyphenidyl hydrochloride

*(trye hex ee **fen'** i dill)*

Apo-Trihex (CAN), Artane, Trihexy

**Pregnancy Category C**

### Drug classes

Antiparkinsonism drug (anticholinergic type)

### Therapeutic actions

Has anticholinergic activity in the CNS that is believed to help normalize the hypothesized imbalance of cholinergic/dopaminergic neurotransmission created by the loss of dopaminergic neurons in the basal ganglia of the brain of parkinsonism patients; reduces severity of rigidity and reduces to a lesser extent the akinesia and tremor that characterise parkinsonism; less effective overall than levodopa; peripheral anticholinergic effects suppress secondary symptoms of parkinsonism, such as drooling.

### Indications

- Adjunct in the treatment of parkinsonism (postencephalitic, arteriosclerotic, and idiopathic)
- Adjuvant therapy with levodopa
- Control of drug-induced extrapyramidal disorders

### Contraindications/cautions

- Contraindications: hypersensitivity to trihexyphenidyl; glaucoma, especially angle-closure glaucoma; pyloric or duodenal obstruction, stenosing peptic ulcers, achalasia (megaesophagus); prostatic hypertrophy or bladder neck obstructions; myasthenia gravis; lactation.
- Use cautiously with cardiac arrhythmias, hypertension, hypotension, hepatic or renal dysfunction, alcoholism, chronic illness, people who work in hot environment, pregnancy.

## Dosage

**Available Forms:** Tablets—2, 5 mg; SR capsules—5 mg; elixir—2 mg/5 ml

**ADULT**

- *Parkinsonism:* 1–2 mg PO the first day. Increase by 2-mg increments at 3- to 5-d intervals until a total of 6–10 mg is given daily. Postencephalitic patients may require 12–15 mg/d. Tolerated best if daily dose is divided into three (or four) doses administered at mealtimes (and bedtime).
- *Concomitant use with levodopa:* Usual dose of each may need to be reduced; however, trihexyphenidyl has been shown to decrease bioavailability of levodopa. Adjust dosage on basis of response. 3–6 mg/d PO of trihexyphenidyl is usually adequate.
- *Concomitant use with other anticholinergics:* Gradually substitute trihexyphenidyl for all or part of the other anticholinergic and reduce dosage of the other anticholinergic gradually.
- *Drug-induced extrapyramidal symptoms:* Initially 1 mg PO. If reactions are not controlled in a few hours, progressively increase subsequent doses until control is achieved. Dose of tranquilizer may need to be reduced temporarily to expedite control of extrapyramidal symptoms. Adjust dosage of both drugs subsequently to maintain ataractic effect without extrapyramidal reactions.
- *Sustained-release preparations:* Do not use for initial therapy. Substitute on a milligram for milligram of total daily dose basis after patient is stabilized on conventional dosage forms. A single PO dose after breakfast or two divided doses 12 h apart may be given.

**PEDIATRIC:** Safety and efficacy not established.

**GERIATRIC PATIENTS:** Patients >60 y often develop increased sensitivity to the CNS effects of anticholinergic drugs.

## Pharmacokinetics

| *Route* | *Onset* | *Peak* |
|---|---|---|
| Oral | Varies | 1–1.3 h |

*Metabolism:* Hepatic, $T_{1/2}$: 5.6–10.2 h

*Distribution:* Crosses placenta; enters breast milk

*Excretion:* Urine

## Adverse effects

*Peripheral Anticholinergic Effects*

- CNS (some CNS effects are characteristic of centrally acting anticholinergic drugs): *Disorientation, confusion*, memory loss, hallucinations, psychoses, agitation, nervousness, delusions, delirium, paranoia, euphoria, excitement, *lightheadedness, dizziness*, depression, drowsiness, weakness, giddiness, paresthesia, heaviness of the limbs, numbness of fingers, *blurred vision, mydriasis*, diplopia, increased intraocular tension, angle-closure glaucoma
- GI: *Dry mouth, constipation*, dilation of the colon, paralytic ileus
- CV: Tachycardia, palpitations, hypotension, orthostatic hypotension, acute suppurative parotitis, nausea, vomiting, epigastric distress
- GU: *Urinary retention*, urinary hesitancy, dysuria, difficulty achieving or maintaining an erection
- Dermatologic: Skin rash, urticaria, other dermatoses
- General: *Flushing, decreased sweating*, elevated T
- Other: Muscular weakness, muscular cramping

## Clinically important drug-drug interactions

• Additive adverse CNS effects; toxic psychosis with phenothiazines • Possible masking of the development of persistent extrapyramidal symptoms, tardive dyskinesia, in patients on long-term therapy with antipsychotic drugs, such as phenothiazines, haloperidol • Decreased therapeutic efficacy of antipsychotic drugs (phenothiazines, haloperidol)

## ■ Nursing Considerations

### Assessment

- *History:* Hypersensitivity to trihexyphenidyl, glaucoma, pyloric or duodenal obstruction, stenosing peptic ulcers, achalasia, prostatic hypertrophy or bladder neck obstructions, myasthenia gravis, tachycardia, cardiac arrhythmias, hypertension, hypotension, hepatic or renal dysfunction, alcoholism, chronic illness, people who work in hot environments, pregnancy, lactation

- *Physical:* Weight, T; skin color, lesions; orientation, affect, reflexes, bilateral grip strength, visual exam, including tonometry; P, BP, orthostatic BP, auscultation; bowel sounds, normal output, liver evaluation; urinary output, voiding pattern, prostate palpation; liver and kidney function tests

### Implementation

- Decrease dosage or discontinue drug temporarily if dry mouth is so severe that swallowing or speaking becomes difficult.
- Give with caution and arrange dosage reduction in hot weather; drug interferes with sweating and ability of body to maintain body heat equilibrium; anhidrosis and fatal hyperthermia have occurred.
- Ensure that patient voids before receiving each dose if urinary retention is a problem.

### Drug-specific teaching points

- Take this drug exactly as prescribed.
- The following side effects may occur: drowsiness, dizziness, confusion, blurred vision (avoid driving or engaging in activities that require alertness and visual acuity); nausea (frequent, small meals may help); dry mouth (sucking sugarless lozenges or ice chips may help); painful or difficult urination (emptying the bladder immediately before each dose may help); constipation (if maintaining adequate fluid intake and exercising regularly do not help, consult your health care provider).
- Use caution in hot weather (this drug makes you more susceptible to heat prostration).
- Report difficult or painful urination, constipation, rapid or pounding heartbeat, confusion, eye pain or rash.

## trimethadione

*(trye meth a **dye'** one)*

Tridione

**Pregnancy Category D**

### Drug classes

Anticonvulsant

### Therapeutic actions

Increases seizure threshold; sedative effects that may progress to ataxia.

### Indications

- Control of absence (petit mal) seizures refractory to treatment with other drugs

### Contraindications/cautions

- Contraindications: hypersensitivity to oxazolidinediones; pregnancy, lactation.
- Use cautiously with hepatic, renal abnormalities.

### Dosage

**Available Forms:** Chewable tablets—150 mg; capsules—300 mg

**ADULT:** 300 mg PO tid; may increase by 300 mg/d at weekly intervals; maximum dose, 2.4 g/d.

**PEDIATRIC**

- *>6 Y:* 300–900 mg/d PO in three to four divided doses.

### Pharmacokinetics

| *Route* | *Onset* | *Peak* | *Duration* |
|---|---|---|---|
| Oral | 15–30 min | 1/2–2 h | 5–10 d |

*Metabolism:* Hepatic, $T_{1/2}$: 16–24 h

*Distribution:* Crosses placenta; enters breast milk

*Excretion:* Urine

### Adverse effects

- CNS: *Drowsiness, ataxia, dizziness,* sedation, headache, paresthesias
- GI: GI distress, abnormal liver function tests, hepatitis

- Hematologic: Aplastic anemia
- Dermatologic: *pruritus,* ***exfoliative dermatitis***
- Other: Vaginal bleeding, **lupus-like syndrome**, fetal malformations, *photosensitivity*

## ■ Nursing Considerations

### Assessment

- *History:* Hypersensitivity to oxazolidinediones; hepatic, renal abnormalities; lactation, pregnancy
- *Physical:* Skin color, lesions; orientation, affect, reflexes, bilateral grip strength, vision exam; bowel sounds, normal output, liver evaluation; liver and kidney function tests, urinalysis, CBC with differential, EEG

### Implementation

- Administer with food if GI upset occurs.
- Reduce dosage, discontinue ethosuximide, or substitute other antiepileptic medication gradually; abrupt discontinuation may precipitate absence (petit mal) status.
- Discontinue drug if skin rash, depression of blood count, lupus-like syndrome occur.
- Advise patient to avoid pregnancy; obtain contraceptive counseling.

### Drug-specific teaching points

- Take this drug exactly as prescribed; may be taken with meals if GI upset occurs.
- Do not discontinue this drug abruptly or change dosage, except on the advice of your prescriber.
- Arrange for frequent checkups to monitor your response to this drug.
- The following side effects may occur: drowsiness, dizziness, confusion, blurred vision (avoid driving or performing tasks requiring alertness or visual acuity); GI upset (take drug with food or milk, eat frequent, small meals); sensitivity to sunlight (avoid exposure to sunlight; use a sunscreen and wear protective clothing).
- Wear a medical alert tag at all times so that emergency medical personnel will know that you are an epileptic taking antiepileptic medication.
- This drug has caused serious birth defects; avoid pregnancy.
- Report skin rash, joint pain, unexplained fever, sore throat, unusual bleeding or bruising, drowsiness, dizziness, blurred vision, bruising, pregnancy.

# trimethobenzamide hydrochloride

*(trye meth oh* ***ben'*** *za mide)*

*Oral preparations:* Tigan, Trimazide

*Suppositories:* Tebamide, T-Gen, Tigan, Trimazide

*Parenteral preparations:* Arrestin, Ticon, Tigan

**Pregnancy Category C**

### Drug classes

Antiemetic drug (anticholinergic)

### Therapeutic actions

Mechanism of action not understood; antiemetic action may be mediated through the chemoreceptor trigger zone (CTZ); impulses to the vomiting center do not appear to be affected.

### Indications

- Control of nausea and vomiting

### Contraindications/cautions

- Contraindications: allergy to trimethobenzamide, benzocaine, or similar local anesthetics; uncomplicated vomiting in children (drug may contribute to development of Reye's syndrome or unfavorably influence its outcome; extrapyramidal effects of drugs may obscure diagnosis of Reye's syndrome); pregnancy.
- Use cautiously with lactation; acute febrile illness, encephalitides, gastroenteritis, dehydration, electrolyte imbalance, especially when these occur in children, the elderly, or debilitated; narrow-angle glaucoma; stenosing peptic ulcer; sympto-

matic prostatic hypertrophy; bronchial asthma; bladder neck obstruction; pyloroduodenal obstruction; cardiac arrhythmias.

### Dosage

**Available Forms:** Capsules—100, 200 mg; suppositories—100, 200 mg; injection—100 mg/ml

**ADULT**

- ***Oral:*** 250 mg tid–qid.
- ***Rectal suppositories:*** 200 mg tid–qid.
- ***Parenteral:*** 200 mg IM tid–qid.

**PEDIATRIC:** Do not administer parenterally to children.

- *30–90 lb (13.6–40.9 kg): Oral:* 100–200 mg tid–qid. *Rectal suppositories:* 100–200 mg tid–qid.
- *<30 lb: Rectal suppositories:* 100 mg tid–qid.

**PREMATURE AND NEWBORN:** Not recommended.

**GERIATRIC:** More likely to cause serious adverse reactions in elderly patients; use with caution.

### Pharmacokinetics

| *Route* | *Onset* | *Duration* |
|---|---|---|
| Oral | 10–40 min | 3–4 h |
| IM | 15 min | 2–3 h |

*Metabolism:* Hepatic, $T_{1/2}$: unknown
*Distribution:* Crosses placenta; enters breast milk
*Excretion:* Urine

### Adverse effects

- CNS: Parkinsonlike symptoms, coma, convulsions, opisthotonus, depression, disorientation, *dizziness, drowsiness, headache, blurred vision*
- GI: Diarrhea
- CV: Hypotension
- **Hematologic: Blood dyscrasias, jaundice**
- **Hypersensitivity:** Allergic-type skin reactions
- Local: *Pain following IM injections*

## ■ Nursing Considerations

### Assessment

- *History:* Allergy to trimethobenzamide, benzocaine, or similar local anesthetics; uncomplicated vomiting in children; pregnancy; lactation; acute febrile illness, encephalitides, gastroenteritis, dehydration, electrolyte imbalance; narrow-angle glaucoma; stenosing peptic ulcer; symptomatic prostatic hypertrophy; bronchial asthma; bladder neck obstruction; pyloroduodenal obstruction; cardiac arrhythmias
- *Physical:* Skin color, lesions, texture; T; orientation, reflexes, affect; vision exam; P, BP; R, adventitious sounds; bowel sounds; prostate palpation; CBC, serum electrolytes

### Implementation

- Administer IM injections deep into upper outer quadrant of the gluteal region.
- Teach patient technique of administering rectal suppositories, as appropriate.
- Ensure adequate hydration.

### Drug-specific teaching points

- Take as prescribed. Use proper technique for administering rectal suppositories. Avoid excessive dosage.
- The following side effects may occur: dizziness, sedation, drowsiness (use caution if driving or performing tasks that require alertness); diarrhea; blurred vision (reversible).
- Avoid alcohol while taking this drug; serious sedation could occur.
- Report difficulty breathing, tremors, loss of coordination, sore muscles or muscle spasms, unusual bleeding or bruising, sore throat, visual disturbances, irregular heartbeat, yellowing of the skin or eyes.

t

## trimethoprim

*(trye **meth'** oh prim)*
TMP
Proloprim, Trimpex
**Pregnancy Category C**

### Drug classes

Antibacterial

#### Therapeutic actions

Inhibits the synthesis of nucleic acids and proteins in susceptible bacteria; the bacterial enzyme involved in this reaction is more readily inhibited than the mammalian enzyme.

#### Indications

- Uncomplicated urinary tract infections caused by susceptible strains of *E. coli, Proteus mirabilis, Klebsiella pneumoniae, Enterobacter* species, and coagulase-negative *Staphylococcus* species, including *Staphylococcus saprophyticus*

#### Contraindications/cautions

- Contraindications: allergy to trimethoprim, pregnancy (teratogenic in preclinical studies), megaloblastic anemia due to folate deficiency.
- Use cautiously with hepatic or renal dysfunction, lactation.

#### Dosage

**Available Forms:** Tablets—100, 200 mg

*ADULT:* 100 mg PO q12h *or* 200 mg q24h for 10 d.

*PEDIATRIC:* Effectiveness for children <12 y has not been established.

*GERIATRIC OR RENAL IMPAIRED:* Creatinine clearance of 15–30 ml/min, 50 mg PO q12h; creatinine clearance of < 15 ml/min, not recommended.

#### Pharmacokinetics

| Route | Onset | Peak |
|---|---|---|
| Oral | Varies | 1–4 h |

*Metabolism:* Hepatic, $T_{1/2}$: 8–10 h

*Distribution:* Crosses placenta; enters breast milk

*Excretion:* Urine

#### Adverse effects

- GI: *Epigastric distress*, nausea, vomiting, glossitis
- Hematologic: Thrombocytopenia, leukopenia, neutropenia, megoblastic anemia, methemoglobinemia, elevated serum transaminase and bilirubin, increased BUN and serum creatinine levels
- Dermatologic: *Rash*, pruritus, exfoliative dermatitis
- Other: Fever

### ■ Nursing Considerations

#### Assessment

- *History:* Allergy to trimethoprim, megaloblastic anemia due to folate deficiency, renal or hepatic dysfunction, pregnancy, lactation
- *Physical:* Skin color, lesions; T; status of mucous membranes; CBC; liver and renal function tests

#### Implementation

- Perform culture and sensitivity tests before beginning drug therapy.
- Protect the 200-mg tablets from exposure to light.
- Arrange for regular, periodic blood counts during therapy.
- Discontinue drug, consult with physician if any significant reduction in any formed blood element occurs.

#### Drug-specific teaching points

- Take the full course of the drug; take all the tablets prescibed.
- The following side effects may occur: epigastric distress, nausea, vomiting (small, frequent meals may help); skin rash (consult with your nurse or physician for appropriate skin care).
- Have periodic medical checkups, including blood tests.
- Report fever, sore throat, unusual bleeding or bruising, dizziness, headaches, skin rash.

## trimetrexate glucuronate

*(tri me* ***trex'*** *ate)*

Neutrexin

**Pregnancy Category D**

#### Drug classes

Antineoplastic

Folic acid antagonist

### Therapeutic actions
Inhibits the enzyme responsible for folate activity and DNA, RNA, and protein production, leading to cell death.

### Indications
- Alternate therapy with leucovorin for the treatment of moderate-to-severe *Pneumocystis carinii* pneumonia in immunocompromised patients, including patients with AIDS, who are intolerant to or refractory to trimethoprim-sulfamethoxazole therapy
- Unlabeled use: treatment of non–small cell lung, prostate, and colorectal cancer; metastatic cancer of the head and neck; pancreatic adenocarcinoma

### Contraindications/cautions
- Contraindications: allergy to trimetrexate, leucovorin, or methotrexate; pregnancy (teratogenic in preclinical studies); lactation.
- Use cautiously with hepatic or renal dysfunction, myelosuppression.

### Dosage
**Available Forms:** Powder for injection—25 mg

**ADULT:** 45 mg/m$^2$ IV once a day over 60–90 min with leucovorin IV at a dose of 20 mg/m$^2$ over 5–10 min q6h or orally as four doses of 20 mg/m$^2$. Treatment course is 21 d of trimetrexate and 24 d of leucovorin.

**PEDIATRIC:** Effectiveness for children <18 y has not been established.

**GERIATRIC, RENAL/HEPATIC, OR HEMATOLOGICALLY IMPAIRED:** Reduce dosage, and monitor blood tests before proceeding to next dose.

### Pharmacokinetics

| Route | Onset |
|---|---|
| IV | Rapid |

*Metabolism:* Hepatic, $T_{1/2}$: 7–15 h
*Distribution:* Crosses placenta; enters breast milk
*Excretion:* Urine

### IV facts
**Preparation:** Reconstitute with 2 ml of 5% Dextrose Injection or Sterile Saline for a concentration of 12.5 mg/ml; solution should be pale greenish-yellow with no particulates; may be further diluted with 5% Dextrose to a concentration of 0.25–2 mg/ml; store at room temperature, protect from light; stable for up to 24 h; discard after that time.

**Infusion:** Flush IV line with 10 ml of 5% Dextrose Injection before and after infusing trimetrexate; infuse diluted solution over 60 min; give leucovorin seperately.

### Adverse effects
- CNS: Confusion
- GI: Nausea, vomiting
- **Hematologic**: Hyponatremia, hypocalcemia; increased AST, ALT, alkaline phosphatase, bilirubin, serum creatinine, *neutropenia, thrombocytopenia*, anemia
- **Other**: *Fever*, rash, fatigue

## ■ Nursing Considerations

### Assessment
- *History:* Allergy to trimetrexate, leucovorin, or methotrexate; pregnancy, lactation; use caution in the presence of hepatic or renal dysfunction, myelosuppression
- *Physical:* Skin color, lesions; T; CBC; liver and renal function tests; serum electrolytes

### Implementation
- Avoid contact with solution; if drug contacts skin, flush with soap and water.
- Arrange for proper disposal of drug, using disposal techniques for cytotoxic drugs.
- Ensure that leucovorin is administered as scheduled while on this drug; it is essential for safe use of trimetrexate.
- Arrange for regular, periodic blood counts and liver function tests.
- Protect patient from exposure to infection.
- Consult with physician for changes in drug dose or timing if significant reduction in formed blood elements occurs.

- Monitor for signs of electrolyte disturbances, and arrange for replacement therapy.

### Drug-specific teaching points

- This drug must be given IV in conjunction with another drug, leucovorin. The treatment will last for 21 and 24 d.
- The following side effects may occur: nausea, vomiting (small, frequent meals may help); skin rash.
- You will need regular blood tests during the drug treatment.
- Avoid exposure to infections; you may be more susceptible to infections.
- Report fever, sore throat, unusual bleeding or bruising, extreme fatigue.

## trimipramine maleate

*(trye* ***mi'*** *pra meen)*

Surmontil

**Pregnancy Category C**

### Drug classes

Tricyclic antidepressant (TCA) (tertiary amine)

### Therapeutic actions

Mechanism of action unknown; the TCAs are structurally related to the phenothiazine antipsychotic drugs (eg, chlorpromazine); TCAs inhibit the presynaptic reuptake of the neurotransmitters norepinephrine and serotonin; anticholinergic at CNS and peripheral receptors; the relation of these effects to clinical efficacy is unknown.

### Indications

- Relief of symptoms of depression (endogenous depression most responsive); sedative effects of tertiary amine TCAs may be helpful in patients whose depression is associated with anxiety and sleep disturbance
- Unlabeled uses: treatment of peptic ulcer disease, dermatologic disorders

### Contraindications/cautions

- Contraindications: hypersensitivity to any tricyclic drug, concomitant therapy with an MAOI, recent MI, myelography within previous 24 h or scheduled within 48 h, pregnancy (limb reduction abnormalities may occur), lactation.
- Use cautiously with EST; preexisting CV disorders (eg, severe CAD, progressive CHF, angina pectoris, paroxysmal tachycardia); angle-closure glaucoma, increased intraocular pressure; urinary retention, ureteral or urethral spasm (anticholinergic effects of TCAs may exacerbate these conditions); seizure disorders (TCAs lower the seizure threshold); hyperthyroidism (predisposes to CVS toxicity, including cardiac arrhythmias); impaired hepatic, renal function; psychiatric patients (schizophrenic or paranoid patients may exhibit a worsening of psychosis); manic-depressive patients (may shift to hypomanic or manic phase); elective surgery (TCAs should be discontinued as long as possible before surgery).

### Dosage

**Available Forms:** Capsules—25, 50, 100 mg

**ADULT**

- *Hospitalized patients:* Initially, 100 mg/d PO in divided doses. Gradually increase to 200 mg/d as required. If no improvement in 2–3 wk, increase to a maximum dose of 250–300 mg/d.
- *Outpatients:* Initially 75 mg/d PO in divided doses. May increase to 150 mg/d. Do not exceed 200 mg/d. Total daily dosage may be administered hs. Maintenance dose is 50–150 mg/d given as a single hs dose. After satisfactory response, reduce to lowest effective dosage. Continue therapy for 3 mo or longer to lessen possibility of relapse.

**PEDIATRIC (ADOLESCENT):** 50 mg/d PO with gradual increases up to 100 mg/d. Not recommended for use if <12 y.

**GERIATRIC:** 50 mg/d PO with gradual increases up to 100 mg/d PO.

### Pharmacokinetics

| Route | Onset | Peak |
| --- | --- | --- |
| Oral | Varies | 2 h |

*Metabolism:* Hepatic, $T_{1/2}$: 7–30 h

*Distribution:* Crosses placenta; enters breast milk

*Excretion:* Urine and feces

### Adverse effects

- CNS: *Sedation and anticholinergic (atropine-like) effects; confusion* (especially in elderly), *disturbed concentration,* hallucinations, disorientation, decreased memory, feelings of unreality, delusions, anxiety, nervousness, restlessness, agitation, panic, insomnia, nightmares, hypomania, mania, exacerbation of psychosis, drowsiness, weakness, fatigue, headache, numbness, tingling, paresthesias of extremities, incoordination, motor hyperactivity, akathisia, ataxia, tremors, peripheral neuropathy, extrapyramidal symptoms, *seizures*, speech blockage, dysarthria, tinnitus, altered EEG
- GI: *Dry mouth, constipation*, paralytic ileus, *nausea*, vomiting, anorexia, epigastric distress, diarrhea, flatulence, dysphagia, peculiar taste, increased salivation, stomatitis, glossitis, parotid swelling, abdominal cramps, black tongue, hepatitis, jaundice (rare), elevated transaminase, altered alkaline phosphatase
- CV: *Orthostatic hypotension*, hypertension, syncope, tachycardia, palpitations, MI, arrhythmias, heart block, precipitation of CHF, stroke
- **Hematologic**: Bone marrow depression including agranulocytosis; eosinophila, purpura, thrombocytopenia, leukopenia
- GU: Urinary retention, delayed micturition, dilation of the urinary tract, gynecomastia, testicular swelling; breast enlargement, menstrual irregularity and galactorrhea; increased or decreased libido; impotence
- **Hypersensitivity**: Skin rash, pruritus, vasculitis, petechiae, photosensitization, edema (generalized, facial, tongue), drug fever
- **Endocrine**: Elevated or depressed blood sugar, elevated prolactin levels, SIADH secretion
- **Withdrawal**: Symptoms with abrupt discontinuation of prolonged therapy: nausea, headache, vertigo, nightmares, malaise
- Other: Nasal congestion, excessive appetite, weight gain or loss, sweating, alopecia, lacrimation, hyperthermia, flushing, chills

### Clinically important drug-drug interactions

• Increased TCA levels and pharmacologic (especially anticholinergic) effects with cimetidine, fluoxetine, ranitidine • Increased bleeding effects with dicumarol • Risk of dysrhythmias and hypertension with sympathomimetics • Risk of severe hypertension with clonidine • Hyperpyretic crises, severe convulsions, hypertensive episodes and deaths with MAOIs • Decreased hypotensive activity of guanethidine • *Note:* MAOIs and TCAs have been used successfully in some patients resistant to therapy with single agents; however, case reports indicate that the combination can cause serious and potentially fatal adverse effects.

## ■ Nursing Considerations

### Assessment

- *History:* Hypersensitivity to any tricyclic drug; concomitant therapy with an MAOI; recent MI; myelography within previous 24 h or scheduled within 48 h; pregnancy; lactation; EST; preexisting CV disorders; angle-closure glaucoma, increased intraocular pressure; urinary retention, ureteral or urethral spasm; seizure disorders; hyperthyroidism; impaired hepatic, renal function; psychiatric patients; manic-depressive patients; elective surgery
- *Physical:* Weight; T; skin color, lesions; orientation, affect, reflexes, vision and hearing; P, BP, orthostatic BP, perfusion; bowel sounds, normal output, liver evaluation; urine flow, normal output; usual sexual function, frequency of menses, breast and scrotal examination; liver function tests, urinalysis; CBC, ECG.

### Implementation

- Ensure that depressed and potentially suicidal patients have access to limited quantities of the drug.

t

- Administer major portion of dose at bedtime if drowsiness, severe anticholinergic effects occur.
- Reduce dosage if minor side effects develop; discontinue if serious side effects occur.
- Arrange for CBC if patient develops fever, sore throat, or other sign of infection.

### Drug-specific teaching points

- Take drug exactly as prescribed.
- Do not stop taking this drug abruptly or without consulting your health care provider.
- Avoid alcohol, other sleep-inducing drugs, and OTC drugs.
- Avoid prolonged exposure to sunlight or sunlamps; use a sunscreen or protective garments.
- The following side effects may occur: headache, dizziness, drowsiness, weakness, blurred vision (reversible; safety measures may need to be taken if severe; avoid driving or performing tasks that require alertness); nausea, vomiting, loss of appetite, dry mouth (small, frequent meals, frequent mouth care, sucking sugarless candies may help); nightmares, inability to concentrate, confusion; changes in sexual function.
- Report dry mouth, difficulty in urination, excessive sedation.

## tripelennamine hydrochloride

*(tri pel* ***enn'*** *a meen)*

PBZ, PBZ-SR

**Pregnancy Category C**

### Drug classes

Antihistamine (ethylenediamine type)

### Therapeutic actions

Competitively blocks the effects of histamine at $H_1$ receptor sites; has anticholinergic (atropine-like), antipruritic, and sedative effects.

### Indications

- Symptomatic relief of perennial and seasonal allergic rhinitis, vasomotor rhinitis, allergic conjunctivitis, mild, uncomplicated urticaria and angioedema
- Amelioraton of allergic reactions to blood or plasma
- Dermatographism
- Adjunctive therapy in anaphylactic reactions

### Contraindications/cautions

- Contraindications: allergy to any antihistamines, pregnancy, lactation.
- Use cautiously with narrow-angle glaucoma, stenosing peptic ulcer, symptomatic prostatic hypertrophy, asthmatic attack, bladder neck obstruction, pyloroduodenal obstruction.

### Dosage

**Available Forms:** Tablets—25, 50 mg; ER tablets—100 mg

***Adult:*** 25–50 mg PO q4–6h. Up to 600 mg/d has been used. Sustained-release preparation: 100 mg PO in the morning and the evening; 100 mg q8h may be needed.

***Pediatric:*** 5 mg/kg/d PO or 150 mg/m²/d PO divided into 4–6 doses. Maximum total dose of 300 mg/d. Do not use sustained-release preparations with children.

***Geriatric:*** More likely to cause dizziness, sedation, syncope, toxic confusional states and hypotension in elderly patients; use with caution.

### Pharmacokinetics

| *Route* | *Onset* | *Peak* | *Duration* |
|---|---|---|---|
| Oral | 15–30 min | 1–2 h | 4–6 h |

*Metabolism:* Hepatic, $T_{1/2}$: unknown

*Distribution:* Crosses placenta; enters breast milk

*Excretion:* Urine

### Adverse effects

- CNS: *Drowsiness, sedation, dizziness, disturbed coordination,* fatigue, confusion, restlessness, excitation, nervousness, tremor, headache, blurred vision, diplopia, vertigo, tinnitus, acute labryinthitis, hysteria, tingling, heaviness and weakness of the hands
- GI: *Epigastric distress*, anorexia, increased appetite and weight gain, nausea, vomiting, diarrhea or constipation

- **CV**: Hypotension, palpitations, bradycardia, tachycardia, extrasystoles
- **Respiratory**: *Thickening of bronchial secretions*, chest tightness, wheezing, nasal stuffiness, dry mouth, dry nose, dry throat, sore throat
- **Hematologic**: Hemolytic anemia, hypoplastic anemia, thrombocytopenia, leukopenia, agranulocytosis, pancytopenia
- **GU**: Urinary frequency, dysuria, urinary retention, early menses, decreased libido, impotence
- **Dermatologic**: Urticaria, rash, anaphylactic shock, photosensitivity, excessive perspiration, chills
- **Other**: Drug abuse when used with pentazocine ("Ts and Blues") as a heroin substitute

## ■ Nursing Considerations

### Assessment

- ***History:*** Allergy to any antihistamines, narrow-angle glaucoma, stenosing peptic ulcer, symptomatic prostatic hypertrophy, asthmatic attack, bladder neck obstruction, pyloroduodenal obstruction, pregnancy, lactation
- ***Physical:*** Skin color, lesions, texture; orientation, reflexes, affect; vision exam; P, BP; R, adventitious sounds; bowel sounds; prostate palpation; CBC with differential

### Implementation

- Administer with food if GI upset occurs.
- Administer elixir form if patient is unable to take tablets.
- Caution patient not to crush or chew sustained-release tablets.

### Drug-specific teaching points

- Avoid excessive dosage.
- Take with food if GI upset occurs.
- Do not crush or chew sustained-release tablets.
- The following side effects may occur: dizziness, sedation, drowsiness (use caution if driving or performing tasks that require alertness); epigastric distress, diarrhea, or constipation (take drug with meals); dry mouth (frequent mouth care, sucking sugarless lozenges may help); thickening of bronchial secretions, dryness of nasal mucosa (use a humidifier).
- Avoid alcohol; serious sedation could occur.
- Report difficulty breathing, hallucinations, tremors, loss of coordination, unusual bleeding or bruising, visual disturbances, irregular heartbeat.

# troglitazone

Rezulin

**Pregnancy Category B**

### Drug classes

Antidiabetic agent
Insulin sensitizer

### Therapeutic actions

Resensitizes tissues to insulin; stimulates insulin receptor sites to lower blood glucose and improve the action of insulin.

### Indications

- Adjunct to insulin or sulfonylurea therapy in type II diabetics who are not responding well to traditional therapy
- Adjunct to diet and exercise in the treatment of non–insulin-dependent diabetes mellitus (type II) in patients who have responded poorly to conventional treatment
- Unlabeled use: metabolic control with polycystic ovary disease

### Contraindications/cautions

- Contraindications: allergy to troglitazone; Type I or juvenile diabetes
- Use cautiously with advanced heart disease, liver failure, pregnancy, lactation

### Dosage

**Available Forms:** Tablets—200, 300, 400 mg

*ADULT:* 200 mg PO qd with insulin or sulfonylurea, increasing in 2–4 wk if response is not adequate to 400 mg PO qd; maximum dose 600 mg qd. 400–600 mg PO qd as monotherapy.

*PEDIATRIC:* Safety and efficacy not established.

t

### Pharmacokinetics

| Route | Onset | Peak |
|---|---|---|
| Oral | Rapid | 2–3 h |

*Metabolism:* Hepatic; $T_{1/2}$: h
*Distribution:* Crosses placenta; passes into breast milk
*Excretion:* Bile and urine

### Adverse effects
- CNS: *Headache, pain*
- GI: Anorexia, nausea, vomiting, **acute, potentially fatal liver failure**
- Endocrine: *Hypoglycemia*
- Hypersensitivity: Allergic skin reactions
- Other: *Infections*

### Clinically important drug-drug interactions
• Decreased levels with cholestyramine; avoid this combination • Possible decreased effectiveness of oral contraceptives; advise use of barrier contraceptives

## ■ Nursing Considerations

### Assessment
- ***History:*** Allergy to troglitazone, Type I or juvenile diabetes, serious hepatic impairment, advanced heart disease, pregnancy, lactation
- ***Physical:*** Skin color, lesions; T; orientation, reflexes, peripheral sensation; BP, P; liver evaluation; urinalysis, liver function tests, blood glucose, CBC

### Implementation
- Monitor liver enzymes before administration, once a month for the first 6 mo of therapy and every other month for the next 6 mo. Discontinue drug at any sign of liver failure.
- Monitor urine and serum glucose levels frequently to determine effectiveness of drug and dosage being used.
- Arrange for titration of usual insulin dose under strict medical supervision.
- Arrange for consultation with dietician to establish weight-loss program and dietary control as appropriate.
- Arrange for thorough diabetic teaching program to include disease, dietary control, exercise, signs and symptoms of hypoglycemia and hyperglycemia, avoidance of infection, hygiene.

### Drug-specific teaching points
- Do not discontinue this medication without consulting your health care provider; continue with diet and exercise program for diabetes control.
- This drug may change your body's need for insulin, and careful monitoring will be needed while adjusting to this drug; do not change your insulin dosage without consulting your health care provider.
- Monitor urine or blood for glucose and ketones as prescribed, particularly while adjusting to the drug.
- Report fever, sore throat, unusual bleeding or bruising, skin rash, dark urine, light-colored stools, hypoglycemic or hyperglycemic reactions.

# tromethamine

*(troe **meth'** a meen)*

Tham

**Pregnancy Category C**

### Drug classes
Systemic alkalinizer

### Therapeutic actions
Sodium-free organic amine that acts as a buffer, preventing the occurrence of acidosis; acts as a weak osmotic diuretic; may be preferable to sodium bicarbonate in the treatment of metabolic acidosis when sodium restriction is important.

### Indications
- Prevention or correction of systemic acidosis; metabolic acidosis associated with coronary artery bypass surgery; correction of acidity of acid dextrose blood in cardiac bypass surgery; cardiac arrest

### Contraindications/cautions
- Contraindications: anuria, uremia, pregnancy.
- Use cautiously with respiratory depression, impaired renal function.

### Dosage

**Available Forms:** Injection—18 mg/500 ml

**ADULT AND PEDIATRIC > 12 Y**

- *Acidosis during cardiac bypass surgery:* Single dose of 500 ml IV is usually sufficient; 9 ml/kg IV; do not exceed 500 mg/kg/h.
- *Acidity of ACD blood:* 0.5–2.5 g (15–77 ml) IV added to each 500 ml of ACD blood.
- *Acidosis of cardiac arrest:* Inject 2–6 g directly into ventricular cavity if chest is open; Inject 3.6–10.8 g IV into a large peripheral vein if chest is not open.

### Pharmacokinetics

| *Route* | *Onset* | *Duration* |
|---|---|---|
| IV | Rapid | 8 h |

*Metabolism:* $T_{1/2}$: unknown
*Distribution:* Crosses placenta; enters breast milk
*Excretion:* Urine

### IV facts

**Preparation:** Use as provided by manufacturer.
**Infusion:** Infuse slowly, 5 ml over 1 min, into pump oxygenator, ACD blood, priming fluid or ventricular cavity; infuse slowly into peripheral vein.

### Adverse effects

- GI: Hemorrhagic hepatic necrosis
- Respiratory: Respiratory depression
- Hematologic: Decreased blood glucose
- Local: Phlebitis, infection of injection site

## ■ Nursing Considerations

### Assessment

- *History:* Anuria, uremia, pregnancy, respiratory depression, impaired renal function.
- *Physical:* P, BP; R, adventitious sounds; CBC, blood gases, electrolytes, glucose

### Implementation

- Monitor blood pH, $pCO_2$, bicarbonate, glucose, electrolytes before and during administration.
- Provide supportive or replacement therapy as needed for hematologic changes.
- Use a large needle in the biggest vein available for peripheral use; alkalinity is very irritating to tissues.

### Drug-specific teaching points

- Patients receiving this drug will be unconscious and unaware of its use. If local irritation occurs after use, incorporate some information about the drug into the wound care of the injection site.

# Trovafloxacin

## trovafloxacin

*(troh va* ***flox'*** *a sin)*

Trovan

## alatrofloxacin mesylate

Trovan IV

**Pregnancy Category C**

### Drug classes

Fluoroquinolone-like antibiotic

### Therapeutic actions

Bactericidal; interferes with DNA replication in susceptible gram-negative and gram-positive aerobic and anaerobic bacteria, preventing cell reproduction.

### Indications

- Nosocomial pneumona caused by *E. coli, Pseudomonas aeruginosa, Haemophilus influenzae, Staphylococcus aureus*
- Treatment of adults with community-acquired pneumonia caused by *Streptococcus pneumoniae, H. influenzae, Klebsiella pneumonia, S. aureus, Mycoplasma pneumoniae, Moraxella catarrhalis, Legionella pneumophila, Chlamydia pneumoniae*
- Treatment of acute exacerbation of chronic bronchitis caused by *H. influenzae, M. catarrhalis, Streptococcus pneumoniae, S. aureus, Haemophilus parainfluenzae*

t

- Treatment of acute sinusitis caused by *H. influenzae, M. catarrhalis, S. pneumoniae*
- Treatment of complicated intra-abdominal infections, including postoperative infections caused by susceptible bacteria
- Treatment of gynecologic and pelvic infections including endomyometritis, parametritis, cervicitis, septic abortion, and postpartum infections caused by susceptible bacteria
- Prophylaxis of infection associated with elective colorectal surgery, vaginal and abdominal hysterectomy
- Uncomplicated skin and skin structure infections caused by susceptible bacteria
- Complicated skin and skin structure infections, including diabetic foot infections caused by *S. aureus, Steptococcus agalactiae, P. aeruginosa, E. foecalis, E. coli, Proteus mirabilis*
- Treatment of uncomplicated UTI caused by *E. coli*
- Treatment of chronic bacterial prostatitis caused by *E. coli, E. faecalis, Staphylococcus epidermidis*
- Treatment of urethral gonorrhea in males, endocervical and rectal gonorrhea in females

## Contraindications/cautions

- Contraindications: allergy to any fluoroquinolones, pregnancy, lactation.
- Use cautiously with renal or hepatic dysfunction, seizures.

**Available Forms:** Tablets—100, 200 mg; IV solution—40, 60 ml as single-dose vials of 5 mg/ml

## Dosage

### Adult

- ***Nosocomial pneumonia:*** 300 mg IV followed by 200 mg PO qd for 10–14 d.
- ***Community-acquired pneumonia:*** 200 mg PO or IV followed by 200 mg PO qd for 7–14 d.
- ***Acute sinusitis:*** 200 mg PO qd for 10 d.
- ***Acute bronchitis:*** 100 mg PO for 7–10 d.
- ***Complicated intra-abdominal infections:*** 300 mg IV followed by 200 mg PO qd for 7–10 d.
- ***Gynecologic and pelvic infections:*** 300 mg IV followed by 200 mg PO qd for 7–14 d.
- ***Surgical prophylaxis (colorectal, abdominal, vaginal surgery):*** 200 mg IV or PO as a single dose 30 min–4 h before surgery.
- ***Skin infection, uncomplicated:*** 100 mg PO qd for 7–10 d.
- ***Skin infection, complicated:*** 200 mg PO or IV followed by 200 mg PO qd for 10–14 d.
- ***UTIs:*** 100 mg PO qd for 3 d.
- ***Chronic bacterial prostatitis:*** 200 mg PO qd for 28 d.
- ***Uncomplicated gonorrhea:*** 100 mg PO as a single dose.
- ***Cervicitis:*** 200 mg PO qd for 5 d.
- ***PID (mild):*** 200 mg PO qd for 14 d.

**Pediatric:** Not recommended in children <18 y.

**Hepatic Impairment:** For normal recommended dose of 300 mg IV, use 200 mg IV; for 200 mg IV or PO, use 100 mg IV or PO; for 100 mg PO, use 100 mg PO.

## Pharmacokinetics

| *Route* | *Onset* | *Peak* |
|---|---|---|
| Oral | Varies | 0.5–1 h |
| IV | Rapid | 1 h |

*Metabolism:* Hepatic; $T_{1/2}$: 9–11 h
*Distribution:* Crosses placenta; passes into breast milk
*Excretion:* Bile

## IV facts

**Preparation:** Inspect vial for any discoloration or particulate matter; aseptic technique must be used in preparation of the final solution. Dilute with appropriate amount of 5% Dextrose Injection, 0.45% Sodium Chloride Injection, 5% Dextrose and 0.45% Sodium Chloride Injection, 5% Dextrose and 0.2% Sodium Chloride Injection, or Lactated Ringer's and 5% Dextrose Injection to reach a final concentration of 1–2 mg/ml. Discard any unused portion of the vial. Diluted solution is stable for up to 7 d if refrigerated, for 3 d at room temperature.
**Infusion:** Administer slowly over at least 60 min; avoid rapid or bolus injections.

**Compatibility:** Do not administer in solution with or in the same line with any other drug. If other drugs are given through the same line, the line should be flushed between drugs.

### Adverse effects

- CNS: *Lightheadedness, dizziness, insomnia,* fatigue, somnolence, depression, headache
- GI: *Nausea,* vomiting, dry mouth, *diarrhea,* abdominal pain
- CV: Chest pain, peripheral edema
- Other: Fever, rash, *pruritus,* photosensitivity (low potential for this effect compared with other fluoroquinolones), pain and sensitivity at injection site

### Clinically important drug-drug interactions

• Decreased therapeutic effect with iron salts, sucralfate, antacids, zinc, magnesium; separate by at least 2 h • Decreased absorption of oral trovafloxacin with IV morphine; give IV morphine at least 2 h after oral trovafloxacin given on an empty stomach or 4 h after trovafloxacin given with food

## ■ Nursing Considerations

### Assessment

- *History:* Allergy to fluoroquinolones, hepatic dysfunction, seizures, lactation
- *Physical:* Skin color, lesions; T; orientation, reflexes, affect; mucous membranes, bowel sounds; liver function tests

### Implementation

- Arrange for culture and sensitivity tests before beginning therapy.
- Continue therapy as indicated for condition being treated.
- Separate oral drug from other cation administration, including antacids, by at least 2 h.
- Ensure that patient is well hydrated during course of drug therapy.
- Discontinue drug at any sign of hypersensitivity (rash, photophobia) or at complaint of tendon pain, inflammation, or rupture.
- Monitor clinical response; if no improvement is seen or a relapse occurs, repeat culture and sensitivity.

### Drug-specific teaching points

- Take oral drug without regard to meals. If an antacid is needed, do not take it within 2 hours of trovafloxacin dose.
- Drink plenty of fluids while you are on this drug.
- The following side effects may occur: nausea, vomiting, abdominal pain (eat small, frequent meals); diarrhea or constipation (consult nurse or physician); drowsiness, blurring of vision, dizziness (use caution if driving or operating dangerous equipment); sensitivity to the sun (avoid exposure; use a sunscreen if necessary).
- Report rash, visual changes, severe GI problems, weakness, tremors, sensitivity to light, tendon pain.

## urea

*(yoor ee' a)*

Ureaphil

**Pregnancy Category C**

### Drug classes

Osmotic diuretic

### Therapeutic actions

Elevates the osmolarity of the glomerular filtrate, hindering the reabsorption of water and leading to a loss of water, sodium, and chloride; creates an osmotic gradient in the eye between plasma and ocular fluids, reducing intraocular pressure.

### Indications

- Reduction of intracranial pressure and treatment of cerebral edema
- Reduction of elevated intraocular pressure
- Unlabeled use: induction of abortion when used by intra-amniotic injection

### Contraindications/cautions

- Active intracranial bleeding (except during craniotomy), marked dehydration, severe renal or hepatic disease, pregnancy, lactation.

### Dosage

**Available Forms:** Injection—40 g/150 ml

*ADULT:* Slow IV infusion of 30% solution only: 1–1.5 g/kg. Do not exceed 120 g/d.

*PEDIATRIC:* 0.5–1.5 g/kg, IV. As little as 0.1 g/kg may be adequate in children <2 y.

### Pharmacokinetics

| *Route* | *Onset* | *Peak* | *Duration* |
|---|---|---|---|
| IV | 30–45 min | 60 min | 5–6 h |

*Metabolism:* $T_{1/2}$: unknown

*Distribution:* Crosses placenta; enters breast milk

*Excretion:* Urine

### IV facts

**Preparation:** For 135 ml of a 30% solution of sterile urea, mix one 40-g vial with 105 ml of 5% or 10% Dextrose Injection or 10% Invert Sugar in Water; each ml of a 30% solution provides 300 mg of urea; use only fresh solution; discard any solution within 24 h after reconstitution.

**Infusion:** Administer 30% solution by slow IV infusion; do not exceed 4 ml/min.

**Compatibilities:** Do not administer urea through the same IV set as blood or blood products.

### Adverse effects

- CNS: *Dizziness, headache*, syncope, disorientation
- GI: *Nausea, vomiting*
- **Hematologic**: Hyponatremia, hypokalemia
- **Local**: Tissue necrosis if extravasation occurs at IV site
- **Other**: Thrombophlebitis, febrile response, hypervolemia if improperly administered

## ■ Nursing Considerations

### Assessment

- *History:* Active intracranial bleeding, marked dehydration, hepatic or renal disease, pregnancy, lactation
- *Physical:* Skin color, edema; orientation, reflexes, muscle strength, pupillary reflexes; pulses, BP, perfusion; R, pattern, adventitious sounds; urinary output patterns; serum electrolytes, urinalysis, renal and liver function tests

### Implementation

- Do not infuse in veins of lower extremities of elderly patients.
- Monitor urinary output carefully.
- Monitor BP regularly and carefully.
- Monitor serum electrolytes periodically.
- Use an indwelling catheter in comatose patients.

### Drug-specific teaching points

- This drug can only be given IV.
- The following side effects may occur: increased urination, GI upset (eat small, frequent meals), dry mouth (sugarless lozenges to suck may help), headache, blurred vision (use caution when moving around; ask for assistance).
- Report pain at the IV site, severe headache, chest pain.

## urofollitropin

*(you' ro fol i tro' pin)*

Fertinex, Metrodin

**Pregnancy Category X**

### Drug classes

Hormone

Fertility drug

### Therapeutic actions

Gonadotropin extracted from the urine of postmenopausal women; stimulates ovarian follicular growth and maturation in women who do not have primary ovarian failure; to cause ovulation, human chorionic gonadotropin (HCG) must be given when the follicles are sufficiently mature.

### Indications

- Urofollitropin and HCG are given sequentially for induction of ovulation in patients with polycystic ovarian disease who have an elevated LH/FSH ratio but who

have failed to respond to clomiphene citrate therapy
- Stimulation of multiple follicle development in ovulatory patients in in vitro fertilization programs.

### Contraindications/cautions

- Contraindications: known sensitivity to urofollitropin; high levels of FSH, LH, indicating primary ovarian failure; overt thyroid or adrenal dysfunction; organic cranial lesion; abnormal uterine bleeding of unknown origin; ovarian cysts or enlargement not due to polycystic ovary syndrome; pregnancy (fetal defects).
- Use cautiously with lactation.

### Dosage

**Available Forms:** Powder for injection—75, 150 IU/ampule

Individualize dose to the smallest, effective dose. Must be given only by physicians who are thoroughly familiar with infertility problems; must be given with great care.

**ADULT:** *Initial dose:* 75 IU/d IM urofollitropin for 7–12 d followed by 5,000–10,000 U of HCG 1 d after the last urofollitropin dose. May be repeated for two more courses before increasing dose to 150 IU of FSH/d for 7–12 d followed by 5,000–10,000 U HCG 1 d after the last urofollitropin dose. If evidence of ovulation is present, but pregnancy does not occur, repeat the same dose for two more courses. For assisted fertilization, 150 IU/d cycle day 2, or 3 until follicles are ready. Therapy should not exceed 10 days.

### Pharmacokinetics

| Route | Onset |
|---|---|
| IM | Slow |

*Metabolism:* Hepatic, $T_{1/2}$: unknown

*Distribution:* Crosses placenta; enters breast milk

*Excretion:* Urine

### Adverse effects

- CNS: Headache
- GI: *Abdominal discomfort*, distention, bloating, nausea, vomiting, diarrhea
- CV: Arterial thromboembolism
- GU: Uterine bleeding, *ovarian enlargement*, breast tenderness, ectopic pregnancy, *ovarian overstimulation* (abdominal distention, pain, accompanied in more serious cases by ascites, pleural effusion), multiple births, birth defects in resulting pregnancies
- Local: *Pain, rash, swelling or irritation at injection site*
- Other: Febrile reaction—fever, chills, musculoskeletal aches or pain, malaise, fatigue

## ■ Nursing Considerations

### Assessment

- *History:* Known sensitivity to urofollitropin; high levels of FSH, LH; overt thyroid or adrenal dysfunction; organic cranial lesion; abnormal uterine bleeding of undetermined origin; ovarian cysts or enlargement not due to polycystic ovary syndrome; pregnancy; lactation
- *Physical:* Skin color, temperature; T; injection site; abdominal exam, pelvic exam; urinary pregnanadiol and gonadotropin levels; abdominal ultrasound

### Implementation

- Arrange for a complete pelvic exam before each treatment to rule out ovarian enlargement, pregnancy, other uterine difficulties.
- Caution patient of the risks of multiple births, drug effects, and need for medical evaluation and follow-up.
- Dissolve contents of 1 ampule in 1–2 ml of Sterile Saline. Administer IM immediately; discard any unused reconstituted material.
- Discontinue drug at any sign of ovarian overstimulation, and arrange to have patient admitted to the hospital for observation and supportive measures.
- Examine patient at least every other day for signs of excessive ovarian stimulation during treatment and during a 2-wk post-treatment period.
- Provide women with calendar of treatment days and explanations about the signs of ovulation. Caution patient that

u

24-h urine collections or abdominal ultrasound will be needed periodically to determine drug effects on the ovaries, that timing of intercourse is important for achieving pregnancy. Patient should engage in intercourse daily beginning on the day prior to HCG administration until ovulation is apparent from determination of progestational activity.

### Drug-specific teaching points

- Prepare a calendar showing the treatment schedule and plotting out ovulation.
- The following side effects may occur: abdominal distention, flushing, breast tenderness, pain, rash, swelling at injection site.
- There is an increased incidence of multiple births with this drug.
- Report bloating, stomach pain, fever, chills, muscle aches or pains, abdominal swelling, back pain, swelling or pain in the legs, pain at injection sites.

## urokinase

*(yoor oh **kin'** ase)*

Abbokinase, Abbokinase Open-Cath

**Pregnancy Category B**

### Drug classes

Thrombolytic agent

### Therapeutic actions

Enzyme isolated from human urine; converts plasminogen to the enzyme plasmin (fibrinolysin), which degrades fibrin clots, fibrinogen, and other plasma proteins; lyses thrombi and emboli.

### Indications

- Pulmonary emboli for lysis
- Coronary artery thrombosis within 6 h of onset of symptoms of coronary occlusion
- IV catheter clearance

### Contraindications/cautions

- Contraindications: hypersensitivity to urokinase, active internal bleeding, recent (within 2 mo) CVA, intracranial or intraspinal surgery, intracranial neoplasm.
- Use cautiously with recent major surgery, obstetric delivery, organ biopsy, or rupture of a noncompressible blood vessel; recent serious GI bleed; recent serious trauma, including CPR; severe hypertension; SBE; hemostatic defects; cerebrovascular disease; diabetic hemorrhagic retinopathy; septic thrombosis; pregnancy; lactation.

### Dosage

**Available Forms:** Powder for injection—250,000 IU/vial; powder for catheter clearance—1, 1.8 ml unidose vials

**ADULT**

- ***Pulmonary embolism:*** *Give through constant infusion pump:* Priming dose of 4,400 U/kg as an admixture with 5% Dextrose Injection or 0.9% Sodium Chloride at a rate of 90 ml/h over 10 min. Then give 4,400 U/kg per hour at a rate of 15 ml/h for 12 h. At end of infusion, flush the tubing with 0.9% Sodium Chloride or 5% Dextrose Injection equal to the volume of the tubing. At the end of the infusion, treat with continuous heparin IV infusion, beginning heparin when the thrombin time has decreased to less than twice the normal control.
- *Lysis of coronary artery thrombi:* Before therapy, administer heparin bolus of 2,500–10,000 U IV; infuse urokinase into occluded artery at rate of 6,000 U/min for up to 2 h. Continue infusion until the artery is maximally opened, usually 15–30 min after initial opening.
- *IV catheter clearance:* For clearing a central venous catheter; have patient exhale and hold his or her breath any time catheter is not connected to IV tubing. Disconnect catheter and after determining amount of occlusion, attach tuberculin syringe with urokinase solution and inject amount equal to volume of catheter. Wait 5 min and aspirate; repeat aspirations every 5 min for up to 1 h. A repeat infusion of urokinase may be necessary in severe cases. When patency is restored, aspirate 4–5 ml of blood to ensure removal of drug and residual clot.

Irrigate gently with 0.9% Sodium Chloride in fresh 10 ml syringe and reconnect IV tubing.

*PEDIATRIC:* Safety and efficacy not established.

### Pharmacokinetics

| *Route* | *Onset* | *Peak* |
|---|---|---|
| IV | Immediate | End of infusion |

*Metabolism:* Plasma, $T_{1/2}$: unknown
*Distribution:* Crosses placenta; enters breast milk
*Excretion:* Unknown

### IV facts

**Preparation:** Reconstitute vial with 5.2 ml of Sterile Water for Injection without preservatives. Avoid shaking during reconstitution; gently roll or tilt vial to reconstitute; consult manufacturer's directions for further dilution. Solution may be filtered through 0.45 or smaller cellulose membrane filter in administration set. Use immediately and discard any unused portion of drug; do not store. Refrigerate vials.

**Infusion:** Maintain infusion via an infusion pump to ensure accurate delivery over 12 h.

**Compatibilities:** Do not add other medications to reconstituted solutions.

### Adverse effects

- CNS: Headache
- CV: Angioneurotic edema, arrhythmias (with intracoronary artery infusion)
- Respiratory: Breathing difficulty, bronchospasm
- Hematologic: *Bleeding* (*minor or surface* to major internal bleeding)
- Dermatologic: Skin rash, urticaria, itching, flushing
- Other: Musculoskeletal pain, *fever*

### Clinically important drug-drug interactions

- Increased risk of hemorrhage if used with heparin or oral anticoagulants, aspirin, indomethacin, phenylbutazone

### Drug-lab test interferences

- Marked decrease in plasminogen, fibrinogen; increases in thrombin time, activated partial thromboplastin (APTT), prothrombin time (PT)

## ■ Nursing Considerations

### Assessment

- ***History:*** Hypersensitivity to urokinase; active internal bleeding; recent CVA, intracranial or intraspinal surgery; intracranial neoplasm; recent major surgery, obstetric delivery, organ biopsy, or rupture of a noncompressible blood vessel; GI bleed; recent serious trauma; severe hypertension; SBE; hemostatic defects; cerebrovascular disease; diabetic hemorrhagic retinopathy; septic thrombosis; pregnancy; lactation
- ***Physical:*** Skin color, temperature, lesions; T; orientation, reflexes; P, BP, peripheral perfusion, baseline ECG; R, adventitous sounds; liver evaluation; Hct, platelet count, thrombin time, APTT, PT

### Implementation

- Discontinue heparin unless ordered specifically for coronary artery infusion.
- Regularly monitor coagulation studies.
- Apply pressure or pressure dressings to control superficial bleeding (at invaded or disturbed areas).
- Avoid any arterial invasive procedures.
- Arrange for typing and cross-matching of blood if serious blood loss occurs and whole blood transfusions are required.
- Institute treatment within 6 h of onset of symptoms for evolving MI and within 7 d of other thrombotic event.
- Monitor cardiac rhythm continually during coronary artery infusion.

### Drug-specific teaching points

- You will require frequent blood tests; this drug can only be given IV.
- Report rash, difficulty breathing, dizziness, disorientation, numbness, tingling.

u

# ursodiol

*(ur soe **dye'** ole)*

ursodeoxycholic acid

Actigall, URSO, Ursofalk (CAN)

**Pregnancy Category B**

## Drug classes

Gallstone solubilizing agent

## Therapeutic actions

A naturally occurring bile acid that suppresses hepatic synthesis of cholesterol and inhibits intestinal absorption of cholesterol, leading to a decreased cholesterol concentration in the bile and a bile that is cholesterol solubilizing and not cholesterol precipitating.

## Indications

- Treatment of selected patients with radiolucent, noncalcified gallstones in gallbladders in whom elective surgery is contraindicated
- Treatment of primary biliary cirrhosis (*URSO*)

## Contraindications/cautions

- Contraindications: allergy to bile salts, hepatic dysfunction, calcified stones, radiopaque stones or radiolucent bile pigment stones, unremitting acute cholecystitis, cholangitis, biliary obstruction, gallstone pancreatitis, biliary-gastrointestinal fistula (cholecystectomy required), pregnancy.
- Use cautiously with lactation.

## Dosage

**Available Forms:** Capsules—300 mg, tablets—250 mg

**ADULT:** 8–10 mg/kg/d PO given in 2 to 3 divided doses. Resolution of the gallstones requires months of therapy; condition needs to be monitored with ultrasound at 6-mo and 1-y intervals. Treatment of biliary cirrhosis: 250 mg PO qd.

**PEDIATRIC:** Safety and efficacy not established.

## Pharmacokinetics

| *Route* | *Onset* | *Peak* |
|---|---|---|
| Oral | Varies | Days |

*Metabolism:* Hepatic, $T_{1/2}$: unknown

*Distribution:* Crosses placenta; may enter breast milk

*Excretion:* Feces

## Adverse effects

- CNS: Headache, fatigue, anxiety, depression, sleep disorder
- GI: *Diarrhea,* cramps, heartburn, constipation, nausea, vomiting, anorexia, epigastric distress, dyspepsia, flatulence, abdominal pain
- Respiratory: Rhinitis, cough
- Dermatologic: Pruritus, rash, urticaria, dry skin, sweating, hair thinning
- Other: Back pain, arthralgia, myalgia

## Clinically important drug-drug interactions

- Absorption decreased if taken with bile acid sequestering agents (cholestyramine, colestipol), aluminum-based antacids

## ■ Nursing Considerations

### Assessment

- ***History:*** Allergy to bile salts, hepatic dysfunction, calcified stones, radiopaque stones or radiolucent bile pigment stones, unremitting acute cholecystitis, cholangitis, biliary obstruction, gallstone pancreatitis, biliary-gastrointestinal fistula, pregnancy, lactation
- ***Physical:*** Liver evaluation, abdominal exam; affect, orientation; skin color, lesions; liver function tests, hepatic and biliary radiological studies, biliary ultrasound

### Implementation

- Assess patient carefully for suitability of ursodiol therapy. Alternative therapy should be reviewed before using ursodiol
- Give drug in 2 to 3 divided doses.
- Do not adminster drug with aluminum-based antacids. If such drugs are needed, administer 2–3 h after ursodiol.
- Schedule patients for periodic oral cholecystograms or ultrasonograms to evaluate drug effectiveness at 6-mo intervals until resolution, then every 3 mo to monitor stone formation. Stones recur within

5 y in more than 50% of patients. If gallstones appear to have dissolved, continue treatment for 3 mo and perform follow-up ultrasound.
- Monitor liver function tests periodically. Carefully assess patient if any change in liver function occurs.

### Drug-specific teaching points
- Take drug 2 to 3 times a day. Take the drug as long as prescribed. It may be needed for a prolonged period.
- This drug may dissolve your gallstones; it does not ''cure'' the problem that caused the stones, and in many cases, the stones can recur; medical follow-up is important.
- Arrange to receive periodic x-rays or ultrasound tests of your gallbladder; you also will need periodic blood tests to evaluate your response to this drug. Keep follow-up appointments.
- The following side effects may occur: diarrhea; skin rash (skin care may help); headache, fatigue (request analgesics).
- Do not take with any aluminum-based antacids.
- Report gallstone attacks (abdominal pain, nausea, vomiting), yellowing of the skin or eyes.

## valacyclovir

*(val ah **sye'** kloe ver)*
Valtrex
**Pregnancy Category B**

### Drug classes
Antiviral

### Therapeutic actions
Antiviral activity; inhibits viral DNA replication and deactivates viral DNA polymerase.

### Indications
- Treatment of herpes zoster (shingles) in immunocompromised adults
- Episodic treatment of first-episode or recurrent genital herpes in immunocompromisd adults
- Suppression of recurrent episodes of genital herpes

### Contraindications/cautions
- Contraindications: allergy to valacyclovir or acyclovir, lactation.
- Use cautiously with pregnancy, renal impairment, thrombotic thrombocytopenic purpura.

### Dosage
**Available Forms:** Tablets—500 mg

***Systemic***

**ADULT**
- ***Herpes zoster:*** 1 g tid PO for 7 days; most effective if started within 48 h of onset of symptoms.
- ***Genital herpes:*** 500 mg PO bid for 5 d.
- ***Suppression of recurrent episodes of genital herpes:*** 1 g PO qd; patients with history of <9 episodes 1y may respond to 500 mg PO qd

**PEDIATRIC:** Safety and efficacy not established.

**GERIATRIC OR RENAL IMPAIRED**

| *Creatinine Clearance (ml/min)* | *Dose* |
|---|---|
| >50 | 1 g q8h |
| 30–49 | 1 g q12h |
| 10–29 | 1 g q24h |
| <10 | 500 mg q24h |

### Pharmacokinetics

| *Route* | *Onset* | *Peak* |
|---|---|---|
| Oral | Rapid | 3 h |

*Metabolism:* $T_{1/2}$: 2.5–3.3 h
*Distribution:* Crosses placenta: passes into breast milk
*Excretion:* Unchanged in the urine and feces

### Adverse effects
- CNS: Headache, dizziness
- GI: *Nausea, vomiting,* diarrhea, anorexia



V

**Clinically important drug-drug interactions**
• Decreased rate of effectiveness with probenecid, cimetidine

## ■ Nursing Considerations

### Assessment
- *History:* Allergy to valacyclovir, acyclovir, renal disease, lactation, thrombotic throbocyopenic purpura
- *Physical:* Orientation; urinary output; abdominal exam, normal output; BUN, creatinine clearance

### Implementation
- Begin treatment within 72 h of onset of symptoms of shingles.
- Administer without regard to meals; administer with meals to decrease GI upset if necessary.
- Provide appropriate analgesics for headache, discomfort of shingles.

### Drug-specific teaching points
- Take this drug without regard to meals; if GI upset is a problem, take with meals.
- Take the full course of therapy as prescribed.
- The following side effects may occur: nausea, vomiting, loss of appetite, diarrhea; headache, dizziness.
- Report severe diarrhea, nausea; headache; worsening of the shingles.

# Valproic acid

## Valproic acid
*(val **proe'** ik)*
*Capsules:* Depakene

## sodium valproate
*Syrup:* Depakene
*Injection:* Depacon

## divalproex sodium
*Tablets, enteric coated:*
Depakote, Epival (CAN)
**Pregnancy Category D**

**Drug classes**
Antiepileptic agent

**Therapeutic actions**
Mechanism of action not understood: antiepileptic activity may be related to the metabolism of the inhibitory neurotransmitter, gamma-aminobutyric acid (GABA); divalproex sodium is a compound containing equal proportions of valproic acid and sodium valproate.

**Indications**
- Sole and adjunctive therapy in simple (petit mal) and complex absence seizures
- Adjunctive therapy with multiple seizure types, including absence seizures
- Treatment of mania (divalproex)
- Prophylaxis of migraine headaches (divalproex-DR tablets)
- Treatment of complex partial seizures as monotherapy or with other antiepilepsy drugs (divalproex, sodium valproate injection)
- Unlabeled uses: sole and adjunctive therapy in atypical absence, myoclonic and grand mal seizures; possibly effective therapy in atonic, elementary partial, and infantile spasm seizures; prophylaxis for recurrent febrile seizures in children

**Contraindications/cautions**
- Contraindications: hypersensitivity to valproic acid, hepatic disease or significant hepatic dysfunction.
- Use cautiously with children <18 mo; children <2 y, especially with multiple antiepileptic drugs, congenital metabolic disorders, severe seizures accompanied by severe mental retardation, organic brain disorders (higher risk of developing fatal hepatotoxicity); pregnancy (fetal neural tube defects; do not discontinue to prevent major seizures; discontinuing such medication is likely to precipitate status epilepticus, hypoxia and risk to both mother and fetus); lactation.

### Dosage
**Available Forms:** Capsules—250 mg; syrup—250 mg/5ml; DR tablets—125, 250, 500 mg; sprinkle capsules—125 mg; injection—5 mg

*ADULT:* Dosage is expressed as valproic acid equivalents. Initial dose is 10–15 mg/kg/d PO, increasing at 1-wk intervals by 5–

10 mg/kg/d until seizures are controlled or side effects preclude further increases. Maximum recommended dosage is 60 mg/kg/d PO. If total dose >250 mg/d, give in divided doses.

- *Mania:* 750 mg PO qd in divided doses; do not exceed 60 mg/kg/d.
- *Migraine:* 250 mg PO bid; up to 1,000 mg/d has been used (divalproex DR tablets)

**PEDIATRIC:** Use extreme caution. Fatal hepatotoxicity has occurred. Children <2 y are especially susceptible. Monitor all children carefully.

## Pharmacokinetics

| *Route* | *Onset* | *Peak* |
|---|---|---|
| Oral | Varies | 1–4 h |
| IV | Rapid | 1 h |

*Metabolism:* Hepatic, $T_{1/2}$: 6–1 6 h
*Distribution:* Crosses placenta; enters breast milk
*Excretion:* Urine

## IV facts

**Preparation:** Dilute vial in 5% dextrose injection, 0.9% sodium chloride injection or lactated ringer's injection. Stable for 24 h at room temperature. Discard unused portions.

**Infusion:** Administer over 60 min, not more than 20 mg/min. Do not use > 14 d; switch to oral products as soon as possible.

## Adverse effects

- CNS: *Sedation*, tremor (may be dose-related), emotional upset, depression, psychosis, aggression, hyperactivity, behavioral deterioration, weakness
- GI: *Nausea, vomiting, indigestion*, diarrhea, abdominal cramps, constipation, anorexia with weight loss, increased appetite with weight gain
- Hematologic: Slight elevations in SGOT, SGPT, LDH; increases in serum bilirubin, abnormal changes in other liver function tests, **hepatic failure,** altered bleeding time; thrombocytopenia; bruising; hematoma formation; frank hemorrhage; relative lymphocytosis; hypofibrinogenemia; leukopenia, eosinophilia, anemia, bone marrow suppression
- GU: Irregular menses, secondary amenorrhea
- Dermatologic: Transient increases in hair loss, skin rash, petechiae

## Clinically important drug-drug interactions

• Increased serum phenobarbital, primidone, ethosuximide, diazepam, zidovudine levels • Complex interactions with phenytoin; breakthrough seizures have occurred with the combination of valproic acid and phenytoin • Increased serum levels and toxicity with salicylates, cimetidine, chlorpromazine, erthromycin, felbamate • Decreased effects with carbamazepine, rifampin, lamotrigine • Decreased serum levels with charcoal

## Drug-lab test interferences

- False interpretation of urine ketone test

## ■ Nursing Considerations

### Assessment

- *History:* Hypersensitivity to valproic acid, hepatic dysfunction, pregnancy, lactation
- *Physical:* Weight; skin color, lesions; orientation, affect, reflexes; bowel sounds, normal output; CBC and differential, bleeding time tests, hepatic function tests, serum ammonia level, exocrine pancreatic function tests, EEG

### Implementation

- Give drug with food if GI upset occurs; substitution of the enteric-coated formulation also may be of benefit.
- Reduce dosage, discontinue, or substitute other antiepileptic medication gradually; abrupt discontinuation of all antiepileptic medication may precipitate absence status.
- Arrange for frequent liver function tests; discontinue drug immediately with significant hepatic dysfunction, suspected or apparent; hepatic dysfunction has progressed in spite of drug discontinuation.
- Arrange for patient to have platelet counts, bleeding time determination be-

V

fore therapy, periodically during therapy, and prior to surgery. Monitor patient carefully for clotting defects (bruising, blood tinged toothbrush). Discontinue if there is evidence of hemorrhage, bruising, or disorder of hemostasis.

- Monitor ammonia levels, and discontinue in the presence of clinically significant elevation in levels.
- Monitor serum levels of valproic acid and other antiepileptic drugs given concomitantly, especially during the first few weeks of therapy. Adjust dosage on the basis of these data and clinical response.
- Arrange for counseling for women of childbearing age who wish to become pregnant.
- Evaluate for therapeutic serum levels—usually 50–100 $\mu$g/ml.

### Drug-specific teaching points

- Take this drug exactly as prescribed. Do not chew tablets or capsules before swallowing them. Swallow them whole to prevent local irritation of mouth and throat.
- Do not discontinue this drug abruptly or change dosage, except on the advice of your physician.
- Avoid alcohol, sleep-inducing or OTC drugs. These could cause dangerous effects.
- Have frequent checkups, including blood tests, to monitor your drug response. Keep all appointments for checkups.
- Use contraceptive techniques at all times. If you wish to become pregnant, you should consult your physician.
- The following side effects may occur: drowsiness (avoid driving or performing other tasks requiring alertness; take at bedtime); GI upset (take with food or milk, eat frequent, small meals; if problem persists, substitute enteric-coated drug); transient increase in hair loss.
- Wear a medical ID tag to alert emergency medical personnel that you are an epileptic taking antiepileptic medication.
- This drug may interfere with urine tests for ketones (diabetic patients).
- Report bruising, pink stain on the toothbrush, yellowing of the skin or eyes, pale feces, skin rash, pregnancy.

## valsartan

*(val **sar'** tan)*

Diovan

**Pregnancy Category D**

### Drug classes

Angiotensin II receptor blocker
Antihypertensive

### Therapeutic actions

Selectively blocks the binding of angiotensin II to specific tissue receptors found in the vascular smooth muscle and adrenal gland; this action blocks the vasoconstricting effect of the renin-angiotensin system as well as the release of aldosterone, leading to decreased BP.

### Indications

- Treatment of hypertension, alone or in combination with other antihypertensive agents

### Contraindications/cautions

- Contraindications: hypersensitivity to valsartan, pregnancy (use during second or third trimester can causy injury or even death to fetus), lactation
- Use cautiously with hepatic or renal dysfunction, hypovolemia

### Dosage

**Available Forms:** Capsules—80, 160 mg

*ADULT:* 80 mg PO qd; range 80–320 mg/d

*PEDIATRIC:* Safety and efficacy not established.

### Pharmacokinetics

| *Route* | *Onset* | *Peak* |
|---|---|---|
| Oral | Varies | 1–3 h |

*Metabolism:* Hepatic; $T_{1/2}$: 2 h, then 6–9 h

*Distribution:* Crosses placenta; passes into breast milk

*Excretion:* Feces and urine

### Adverse effects

- CNS: *Headache, dizziness,* syncope, muscle weakness
- GI: *Diarrhea, abdominal pain, nausea,* constipation, dry mouth, dental pain

- **CV:** Hypotension
- **Respiratory:** *URI symptoms, cough,* sinus disorders
- **Dermatologic:** Rash, inflammation, urticaria, pruritus, alopecia, dry skin
- **Other:** Cancer in preclinical studies, back pain, fever, gout

### Clinically important drug-drug interactions

• Decreased serum levels and effectiveness with phenobarbital

## ■ Nursing Considerations

### Assessment

- *History:* Hypersensitivity to valsartan, pregnancy, lactation, hepatic or renal dysfunction, hypovolemia
- *Physical:* Skin lesions, turgor; T; reflexes, affect; BP; R, respiratory auscultation; liver and renal function tests

### Implementation

- Administer without regard to meals.
- Ensure that patient is not pregnant before beginning therapy; suggest use of barrier birth control while on drug; fetal injury and deaths have been reported.
- Find alternative method of feeding infant if drug is being given to nursing mother. Depression of renin-angiotensin system in infants is potentially very dangerous.
- Alert surgeon and mark patient's chart that valsartan is being given. Blockage of renin-angiotensin system following surgery can produce problems. Hypotension may be reversed with volume expansion.
- Monitor patient closely in any situation that may lead to decrease in BP secondary to reduction in fluid volume—excessive perspiration, dehydration, vomiting, diarrhea—as excessive hypotension can occur.

### Drug-specific teaching points

- Take this drug without regard to meals. Do not stop taking drug without consulting your nurse or physican.
- Use a barrier method of birth control while on this drug; if you become pregnant or desire to become pregnant, consult your physician.
- The following side effects may occur: dizziness (avoid driving or performing hazardous tasks); headache (medications may be available to help); nausea, vomiting, diarrhea (proper nutrition is important; consult your dietician); symptoms of upper respiratory tract infection, cough (do not self-medicate; consult your nurse or physician if this becomes uncomfortable).
- Report fever, chills, dizziness, pregnancy.

# vancomycin hydrochloride

*(van koe **mye'** sin)*

Vancocin, Vancoled

**Pregnancy Category C**

### Drug classes

Antibiotic

### Therapeutic actions

Bactericidal: inhibits cell wall synthesis of susceptible organisms, causing cell death.

### Indications

- Potentially life-threatening infections not treatable with other less toxic antibiotics (parenteral)
- Severe staphylococci infections in patients who cannot receive or have failed to respond to penicillins and cephalosporins
- Prevention of bacterial endocarditis in penicillin-allergic patients undergoing dental, upper respiratory, GI, or GU surgery or invasive procedures
- Staphylococcal enterocolitis and antibiotic-associated pseudomembranous colitis caused by *Clostridium difficile* (oral)

### Contraindications/cautions

- Contraindications: allergy to vancomycin.
- Use cautiously with hearing loss, renal dysfunction, pregnancy, lactation.



### Dosage

**Available Forms:** Pulvules—125, 250 mg; powder for oral solution—1, 10 g; powder for injection—1, 5, 10 g

*ADULT:* 500 mg PO q6h *or* 1 g PO q12h. 500 mg IV q6h *or* 1 g IV q6h.
*PEDIATRIC:* 40 mg/kg/d PO in 4 divided doses. 40 mg/kg/d IV in divided doses added to fluids. Do not exceed 2 g/d.
*NEONATES:* Premature and full-term neonates, use with caution because of incompletely developed renal function. Initial dose of 15 mg/kg q12h PO in first week of life, up to age of 1 mo, then q8h thereafter.
***Pseudomembranous colitis caused by C. difficile***: *Adult:* 500 mg to 2 g/d PO in 3 to 4 divided doses for 7–10 d. *Pediatric:* 40 mg/kg/d in 4 divided doses PO. *Neonates:* 10 mg/kg/d PO in divided doses.
***Prevention of bacterial endocarditis in penicillin-allergic patients undergoing dental or upper respiratory procedures***: *Adult and pediatric > 27 kg:* 1 g IV slowly over 1 h, beginning 1 h before the procedure. May repeat in 8–12 h. *< 27 kg:* 20 mg/kg IV slowly over 1 h beginning 1 h before the procedure. May repeat in 8–12 h.
***Prevention of bacterial endocarditis in patients undergoing GI or GU procedures***: *Adult and pediatric >27 kg:* 1 g IV slowly over 1 h plus 1.5 mg/kg gentamicin IM or IV concurrently 1 h before the procedure. May repeat in 8–12 h. *<27 kg:* 20 mg/kg IV slowly over 1 h and 2 mg/kg gentamicin IM or IV concurrently 1 h before the procedure. May repeat in 8–12 h.
*GERIATRIC OR RENAL FAILURE PATIENTS:* Monitor dosage and serum levels very carefully. Dosage nomogram is available for determining the dose according to creatinine clearance (see manufacturer's insert).

### Pharmacokinetics

| *Route* | *Onset* | *Peak* |
|---|---|---|
| Oral | Varies | |
| IV | Rapid | End of infusion |

*Metabolism:* Hepatic, $T_{1/2}$: 4–6 h
*Distribution:* Crosses placenta; may enter breast milk
*Excretion:* Urine

### IV facts

**Preparation:** *Not* for IM administration. Reconstitute with 10 ml Sterile Water for Injection; 500 mg/ml concentration results. Dilute reconstituted solution with 100–200 ml of 0.9% Sodium Chloride Injection or 5% Dextrose in Water for intermittent infusion. For continuous infusion (use only if intermittent therapy is not possible), add 2–4 (1–2 g) vials reconstituted solution to sufficiently large volume of 0.9% Sodium Chloride Injection or 5% Dextrose in Water to permit slow IV drip of the total daily dose over 24 h. Refrigerate reconstituted solution; stable over 14 d. Further diluted solution is stable for 24 h.
**Infusion:** For intermittent infusion, infuse q6h, over at least 60 min to avoid irritation, hypotension, throbbing back and neck pain. Give continuously slowly over 24 h.

### Adverse effects

- CNS: *Ototoxicity*
- GI: *Nausea*
- CV: Hypotension (IV administration)
- Hematologic: Eosinophilia
- GU: *Nephrotoxicity*
- Dermatologic: *Urticaria*, macular rashes
- Other: Superinfections; "**red neck or red man syndrome**" (sudden and profound fall in BP, fever, chills, paresthesias, erythema of the neck and back)

### Clinically important drug-drug interactions

- Increased neuromuscular blockade with atracurium, galamine triethiodide, metocurine, pancuronium, rucuronium, tubocurarine, vecuronium

## ■ Nursing Considerations

### Assessment

- *History:* Allergy to vancomycin, hearing loss, renal dysfunction, pregnancy, lactation
- *Physical:* Site of infection, skin color, lesions; orientation, reflexes, auditory func-

tion; BP, perfusion; R, adventitious sounds; CBC, renal and liver function tests, auditory tests

### Implementation

- Oral solution: Add 115 ml distilled water to contents of 10-g container. Each 6 ml of solution will contain 500 mg vancomycin. Alternatively, dilute the contents of 500-mg vial for injection in 30 ml of water for oral or nasogastric tube administration.
- Observe the patient very closely when giving parenteral solution, particularly the first doses; "red neck" syndrome can occur (see adverse effects); slow administration decreases the risk of adverse effects.
- Culture site of infection before beginning therapy.
- Monitor renal function tests with prolonged therapy.
- Evaluate for safe serum levels; concentrations of 60–80 $\mu$g/ml are toxic.

### Drug-specific teaching points

- This drug is available only in the IV and oral forms.
- Do not stop taking this drug without notifying your nurse or physician.
- Take the full prescribed course of this drug.
- The following side effects may occur: nausea (small, frequent meals may help); changes in hearing; superinfections in the mouth, vagina (frequent hygiene measures will help).
- Report ringing in the ears, loss of hearing, difficulty voiding, rash, flushing.

## vasopressin

*(vay soe **press'** in)*
8-arginine-vasopressin
Pitressin Synthetic
**Pregnancy Category C**

### Drug classes

Hormone

### Therapeutic actions

Purified form of posterior pituitary having pressor and antidiuretic hormone activities; promotes resorption of water in the renal tubular epithelium, causes contraction of vascular smooth muscle, increases GI motility and tone.

### Indications

- Neurogenic diabetes insipidus
- Prevention and treatment of postoperative abdominal distention
- To dispel gas interfering with abdominal roentgenography

### Contraindications/cautions

- Contraindications: allergy to vasopressin or any components, chronic nephritis.
- Use cautiously with vascular disease (may precipitate angina or MI), epilepsy, migraine, asthma, CHF, pregnancy, lactation.

### Dosage

**Available Forms:** Injection—20 U/ml

ADULT: 5–10 U IM or SC. Repeat at 3- to 4-h intervals as needed.

- *Diabetes insipidus*
  - ***Intranasal:*** Administer on cotton pledgets by nasal spray or dropper *or* 5–10 U bid or tid, IM or SC.
- *Abdominal distention:* 5 U IM initially. Increase to 10 U at subsequent injections given IM at 3- to 4-h intervals.
- *Abdominal roentgenography:* Administer 2 injections of 10 U IM or SC each. Give 2 h and 1/2 h before films are exposed. An enema may be given prior to first dose.

PEDIATRIC: Decrease dose proportionately for children.

V

### Pharmacokinetics

| Route | Onset | Duration |
|---|---|---|
| IM/SC | Varies | 2–6 h |

*Metabolism:* Hepatic, $T_{1/2}$: 10–20 min
*Distribution:* Crosses placenta; enters breast milk
*Excretion:* Urine

**Adverse effects**

- CNS: *Tremor, sweating, vertigo*, circumoral pallor, "pounding" in the head
- GI: Abdominal cramps, passage of gas, nausea, vomiting
- Hypersensitivity: Reactions ranging from urticaria, bronchial constriction to anaphylaxis
- Other: *Water intoxication* (drowsiness, lightheadedness, headache, coma, convulsions), local tissue necrosis

## ■ Nursing Considerations

### Assessment

- *History:* Allergy to vasopressin or any components, vascular disease, chronic nephritis, epilepsy, migraine, asthma, CHF, pregnancy
- *Physical:* Skin color, lesions; nasal mucous membranes (if used intranasally); injection site; orientation, reflexes, affect; P, BP, rhythm, edema, baseline ECG; R, adventitous sounds; bowel sounds, abdominal exam; urinalysis, renal function tests, serum electrolytes

### Implementation

- Administer injection by IM route; SC may be used if necessary.
- Monitor condition of nasal passages during long-term intranasal therapy; inappropriate administration can lead to nasal ulceration.
- Monitor patients with CV diseases very carefully for cardiac reactions.
- Monitor fluid volume for signs of water intoxication and excess fluid load; arrange to decrease dosage if this occurs.

### Drug-specific teaching points

- Give nasally on cotton pledgets, by nasal spray, or dropper. (Watch and review drug administration periodically with patient.) Other routes must be IM or SC.
- The following side effects may occur: GI cramping, passing of gas; anxiety, tinnitus, vision changes (avoid driving or performing tasks that require alertness); nasal irritation (proper administration may decrease problem).
- Report swelling, difficulty breathing, chest tightness or pain, palpitations, running nose, painful nasal passages (intranasal).

# venlafaxine

*(vin lah **facks'** in )*

Effexor, Effexor XR

**Pregnancy Category C**

**Drug classes**

Antidepressant

**Therapeutic actions**

Potentiates the neurotransmitter activity in the CNS; inhibits serontonin, norepinephrine, and dopamine reuptake leading to prolonged stimulation at neuroreceptors.

**Indications**

- Treatment of depression

**Contraindications/cautions**

- Allergy to venlafaxine, use of MAOIs, pregnancy, lactation.

### Dosage

**Available Forms:** Tablets—25, 37.5, 50, 75, 100 mg; ER capsules—37.5, 75, 150 mg

**ADULT:** Starting dose, 75 mg/d PO in 2 to 3 divided doses (or once a day, ER capsule) taken with food. May be increased slowly up to 225 mg/d to achieve desired effect.

- *Transfer to or from MAO inhibitor:* At least 14 d should elapse from the discontinuation of the MAOI and the starting of venlafaxine; allow at least 7 d to elapse from the stopping of venlafaxine to the starting of an MAOI.

**PEDIATRIC:** Safety and efficacy not established.

**GERIATRIC:** No dosage adjustment required.

**HEPATIC/RENAL IMPAIRMENT:** Reduce total daily dose by 50%, and increase very slowly to achieve desired effect.

### Pharmacokinetics

| Route | Onset | Duration |
|---|---|---|
| PO | Slow | 48 h |

*Metabolism:* Hepatic, $T_{1/2}$: 1.3–2 h
*Distribution:* Crosses placenta; may enter breast milk
*Excretion:* Urine

### Adverse effects

- CNS: *Somnolence, dizziness, insomnia, nervousness*, anxiety, tremor, dreams
- GI: *Nausea, constipation, anorexia*, diarrhea, vomiting, dyspepsia, *dry mouth*, flatulence
- CV: Vasodilation, hypertension, tachycardia
- GU: *Abnormal ejaculation,* impotence, urinary frequency
- Dermatologic: *Sweating*, rash, pruritus
- Other: *Headache, asthenia,* infection, chills, chest pain

### Clinically important drug-drug interactions

- Increased serum levels and risk of toxicity with MAOIs, cimetidine

## ■ Nursing Considerations

### Assessment

- *History:* Allergy to venlafaxine, use of MAOIs, pregnancy, lactation
- *Physical:* Skin color, temperature, lesions; reflexes, gait, sensation, cranial nerve evaluation; mucous membranes, abdominal exam, normal output; P, BP, peripheral perfusion

### Implementation

- Give with food to decrease GI effects.
- Advise patient to use contraceptives.

### Drug-specific teaching points

- Take with food to decrease GI upset.
- The following side effects may occur: loss of appetite, nausea, vomiting, dry mouth (frequent mouth care, small, frequent meals, sucking sugarless lozenges may help); constipation (request bowel program); dizziness, drowsiness, tremor (avoid driving or operating dangerous machinery).
- Avoid alcohol while on this drug.
- This drug cannot be taken during pregnancy; use birth control. If you become pregnant, consult with your health care provider.
- Report rash, hives, increased depression, pregnancy.

# verapamil hydrochloride

*(ver **ap'** a mill)*

Calan, Calan SR, Covera HS, Isoptin, Verelan

**Pregnancy Category C**

### Drug classes

Calcium channel blocker
Antianginal agent
Antiarrhythmic
Antihypertensive

### Therapeutic actions

Inhibits the movement of calcium ions across the membranes of cardiac and arterial muscle cells; calcium is involved in the generation of the action potential in specialized automatic and conducting cells in the heart, in arterial smooth muscle, and in excitation-contraction coupling in cardiac muscle cells; inhibition of transmembrane calcium flow results in the depression of impulse formation in specialized cardiac pacemaker cells, slowing of the velocity of conduction of the cardiac impulse, the depression of myocardial contractility, and the dilation of coronary arteries and arterioles and peripheral arterioles; these effects lead to decreased cardiac work, decreased cardiac energy consumption, and in patients with vasospastic (Prinzmetal's) angina, increased delivery of oxygen to myocardial cells.

### Indications

- Angina pectoris due to coronary artery spasm (Prinzmetal's variant angina)
- Effort-associated angina

- Chronic stable angina in patients who cannot tolerate or do not respond to beta-adrenergic blockers or nitrates
- Unstable, crescendo, preinfarction angina
- Essential hypertension (sustained-release oral only)
- Treatment of supraventricular tachyarrhythmias (parenteral)
- Temporary control of rapid ventricular rate in atrial flutter or atrial fibrillation (parenteral)
- Unlabeled oral uses: paroxysmal supraventricular tachycardia, migraine headache, nocturnal leg cramps, hypertrophic cardiomyopathy

## Contraindications/cautions

- Contraindications: allergy to verapamil; sick sinus syndrome, except in presence of ventricular pacemaker; heart block (second or third-degree); hypotension; pregnancy; lactation.
- Use cautiously with idiopathic hypertrophic subaortic stenosis, cardiogenic shock, severe CHF, impaired renal or hepatic function.

## Dosage

**Available Forms:** Tablets—40, 80, 120 mg; SR tablets—120, 180, 240 mg; ER tablets—180, 240 mg; SR capsules—120, 180, 240, 360 mg; injection—5 mg/2ml

ADULT

- ***Oral:*** Initial dose of 80–120 mg tid; increase dose every 1–2 d to achieve optimum therapeutic effects. Usual maintenance dose, 320–480 mg/d.
- – ***Hypertension:*** 240 mg PO qd, sustained-release form in morning. 80 mg tid.
- ***Parenteral:*** IV use only. Initial dose, 5–10 mg over 2 min; may repeat dose of 10 mg 30 min after first dose if initial response is inadequate.

PEDIATRIC

- ***IV***
- – *UP TO 1 Y:* Initial dose, 0.1–0.2 mg/kg over 2 min.
- – *1–15 Y:* Initial dose, 0.1–0.3 mg/kg over 2 min. Do not exceed 5 mg. Repeat above dose 30 min after initial dose if response is not adequate.

***GERIATRIC OR RENAL IMPAIRED:*** Reduce dosage, and monitor patient response carefully. Give IV doses over 3 min to reduce risk of serious side effects. Administer IV doses very slowly, over 2 min.

## Pharmacokinetics

| *Route* | *Onset* | *Peak* | *Duration* |
|---|---|---|---|
| Oral | 30 min | 1–2.2 h | 3–7 h |
| IV | 1–5 min | 3–5 min | 2 h |

*Metabolism:* Hepatic, $T_{1/2}$: 3–7 h
*Distribution:* Crosses placenta; enters breast milk
*Excretion:* Urine

## IV facts

**Preparation:** No further preparation required.
**Infusion:** Infuse very slowly over 2–3 min.

## Adverse effects

- CNS: *Dizziness*, vertigo, emotional depression, sleepiness, *headache*
- GI: *Nausea*, constipation
- CV: *Peripheral edema, hypotension*, arrhythmias, bradycardia; AV heart block
- Other: Muscle fatigue, diaphoresis

## Clinically important drug-drug interactions

• Increased cardiac depression with beta-adrenergic blocking agents • Additive effects of verapamil and digoxin to slow AV conduction • Increased serum levels of digoxin, carbamazepine, prazosin, quinidine • Increased respiratory depression with atracurium, gallamine, metocurine, pancuronium, rucuronium, tubocurarine, vecuronium • Risk of serious cardiac effects with IV beta-adrenergic blocking agents; do not give these drugs within 48 h before or 24 h after IV verapamil • Decreased effects with calcium, rifampin

## ■ Nursing Considerations

### Assessment

- *History:* Allergy to verapamil, sick sinus syndrome, heart block, IHSS, cardiogenic shock, severe CHF, hypotension, impaired hepatic or renal function, pregnancy, lactation

- *Physical:* Skin color, edema; orientation, reflexes; P, BP, baseline ECG, peripheral perfusion, auscultation; R, adventitious sounds; liver evaluation, normal output; liver function tests, renal function tests, urinalysis

### Implementation

- Monitor patient carefully (BP, cardiac rhythm, and output) while drug is being titrated to therapeutic dose. Dosage may be increased more rapidly in hospitalized patients under close supervision.
- Monitor BP very carefully with concurrent doses of antihypertensives.
- Monitor cardiac rhythm regularly during stabilization of dosage and periodically during long-term therapy.
- Administer sustained-release form in the morning with food to decrease GI upset.
- Protect IV solution from light.
- Monitor patients with renal or hepatic impairment carefully for possible drug accumulation and adverse reactions.

### Drug-specific teaching points

- Take sustained-release form in the morning with food.
- The following side effects may occur: nausea, vomiting (eat small, frequent meals); headache (monitor the lighting, noise, and temperature; request medication); dizziness, sleepiness (avoid driving or operating dangerous equipment); emotional depression (reversible); constipation (request aid).
- Report irregular heart beat, shortness of breath, swelling of the hands or feet, pronounced dizziness, constipation.

## vinblastine sulfate

*(vin **blas'** teen)*

VLB

Velban, Velbe (CAN)

**Pregnancy Category D**

### Drug classes

Mitotic inhibitor
Antineoplastic

### Therapeutic actions

Affects cell energy production required for mitosis and interferes with nucleic acid synthesis; has antimitotic effect and causes abnormal mitotic figures.

### Indications

- Palliative treatment for generalized Hodgkin's disease (stages III and IV), lymphocytic lymphoma, histiocytic lymphoma, mycosis fungoides, advance testicular carcinoma, Kaposi's sarcoma, Letterer-Siwe disease
- Palliation of choriocarcinoma, breast cancer unresponsive to other therapies
- Hodgkin's disease (advanced) alone or in combination therapies
- Advanced testicular germinal-cell cancers alone or in combination therapy

### Contraindications/cautions

- Contraindications: allergy to vinblastine, leukopenia, acute infection, pregnancy, lactation.
- Use cautiously with liver disease.

### Dosage

**Available Forms:** Powder for injection—10 mg; injection—1 mg/ml

Do not administer more than once a week because of leukopenic response.

**ADULT/PEDIATRIC:** Initial dose, 3.7 mg/m$^2$ as a single IV dose, followed at weekly intervals by increasing doses; a conservative regimen follows:

| *Dose* | *Adult Dose (mg/m$^2$)* | *Pediatric Dose (mg/m$^2$)* |
|---|---|---|
| First | 3.7 | 2.5 |
| Second | 5.5 | 3.75 |
| Third | 7.4 | 5.0 |
| Fourth | 9.25 | 6.25 |
| Fifth | 11.1 | 7.5 |

Use these increments until a maximum dose of 18.5 mg/m$^2$ for adults or 12.5 mg/m$^2$ for children is reached; do not increase dose after WBC is reduced to 3,000/mm$^3$.

- *Maintenance therapy:* When dose produces WBC of 3000/mm$^3$, use a dose one increment smaller for weekly mainte-

V

nance. Do not give another dose until WBC is 4000/mm$^3$ even if 7 d have passed. Duration of therapy depends on disease and response; up to 2 y may be necessary.

### Pharmacokinetics

| Route | Onset |
|---|---|
| IV | Slow |

*Metabolism:* Hepatic, $T_{1/2}$: 3.7 min, then 1.6 h, then 24.8 h
*Distribution:* Crosses placenta; enters breast milk
*Excretion:* Bile

#### IV facts

**Preparation:** Add 10 ml of Sodium Chloride Injection preserved with phenol or benzyl alcohol to the vial for a concentration of 1 mg/ml. Refrigerate drug; opened vials are stable for 30 d when refrigerated.
**Infusion:** Inject into tubing of a running IV or directly into the vein over 20–30 min or as a prolonged infusion over up to 96 h. Rinse syringe and needle with venous blood prior to withdrawing needle from vein (to minimize extravasation). Do not inject into an extremity with poor circulation or repeatedly into the same vein.

### Adverse effects

- CNS: Numbness, paresthesias, peripheral neuritis, mental depression, loss of deep tendon reflexes, headache, seizures, malaise, weakness, dizziness
- GI: Nausea, vomiting, pharyngitis, vesiculation of the mouth, ileus, diarrhea, constipation, anorexia, abdominal pain, rectal bleeding, hemorrhagic enterocolitis
- **Hematologic**: Leukopenia
- GU: Aspermia
- **Dermatologic**: Topical epilation (loss of hair), vesiculation of the skin
- **Local**: Local cellulitis, phlebitis, sloughing if extravasation occurs
- **Other**: Pain in tumor site

### Clinically important drug-drug interactions

- Decreased serum concentrations of phenytoins

## ■ Nursing Considerations

### Assessment

- ***History:*** Allergy to vinblastine, leukopenia, acute infection, liver disease, pregnancy, lactation
- ***Physical:*** Weight; hair; T; reflexes, gait, sensation, orientation, affect; mucus membranes, abdominal exam, rectal exam; CBC, liver function tests, serum albumin

### Implementation

- Do not administer IM or SC due to severe local reaction and tissue necrosis.
- Avoid extravasation; if it occurs, discontinue injection immediately, and give remainder of dose in another vein. Consult physician to arrange for hyaluronidase injection into local area, after which apply moderate heat to disperse drug and minimize pain.
- Avoid contact with the eyes; if contact occurs, thoroughly wash immediately with water.
- Consult with physician if antiemetic is needed for severe nausea and vomiting.
- Check CBC before each dose.

### Drug-specific teaching points

- Prepare a calendar for dates to return for treatment and drug therapy.
- The following side effects may occur: loss of appetite, nausea, vomiting, mouth sores (frequent mouth care, small, frequent meals may help; maintain nutrition; request an antiemetic); constipation (a bowel program may be ordered); malaise, weakness, dizziness, numbness and tingling (avoid injury); loss of hair, skin rash (obtain a wig; keep the head covered in extremes of temperature).
- This drug should not be used during pregnancy. Use birth control. If you become pregnant, consult your physician.

- Have regular blood tests to monitor the drug's effects.
- Report severe nausea, vomiting, pain or burning at injection site, abdominal pain, rectal bleeding, fever, chills, acute infection.

## vincristine sulfate

*(vin **kris'** teen)*

LCR, VCR

Oncovin, Vincasar PFS

**Pregnancy Category D**

### Drug classes
Mitotic inhibitor
Antineoplastic

### Therapeutic actions
Mitotic inhibitor: arrests mitotic division at the stage of metaphase; exact mechanism of action unknown.

### Indications
- Acute leukemia
- Hodgkin's disease, lymphosarcoma, reticulum cell sarcoma, rhabdomyosarcoma, neuroblastoma, Wilms' tumor as part of combination therapy
- Unlabeled uses: idiopathic thrombocytopenic purpura, Kaposi's sarcoma, breast cancer, and bladder cancer

### Contraindications/cautions
- Contraindications: allergy to vincristine, leukopenia, acute infection, pregnancy, lactation.
- Use cautiously with neuromuscular disease, diabetes insipidus, hepatic dysfunction.

### Dosage
**Available Forms:** Injection—1 mg/ml

*ADULT:* 1.4 mg/m$^2$ IV at weekly intervals.

*PEDIATRIC:* 2.0 mg/m$^2$ IV weekly.

- *<10 kg:* 0.05 mg/kg once a week.

*GERIATRIC OR HEPATIC INSUFFICIENCY:* Serum bilirubin 1.5–3.0, reduce dosage by 50%.

### Pharmacokinetics

| Route | Onset | Peak |
|---|---|---|
| IV | Varies | 15–30 min |

*Metabolism:* Hepatic, $T_{1/2}$: 5 min, then 2.3 h, then 85 h

*Distribution:* Crosses placenta; enters breast milk

*Excretion:* Feces and urine

### IV facts
**Preparation:** No further preparation required; drug should be refrigerated.

**Infusion:** Inject solution directly into vein or into the tubing of a running IV infusion. Infusion may be completed within 1 min.

### Adverse effects
- CNS: *Ataxia, cranial nerve manifestations;* foot drop, headache, convulsions, bladder neuropathy, paresthesias, sensory impairment, *neuritic pain, muscle wasting*, SIADH, optic atrophy, transient cortical blindness, ptosis, diplopia, photophobia
- GI: *Constipation,* oral ulcerations, abdominal cramps, vomiting, diarrhea, intestinal necrosis
- Hematologic: *Leukopenia*
- GU: Acute uric acid nephropathy, polyuria, dysuria
- Local: Local irritation, cellulitis if extravasation occurs
- Other: *Weight loss, loss of hair*, fever, **death** with serious overdosage

### Clinically important drug-drug interactions
- Decreased serum levels and therapeutic effects of digoxin

## ■ Nursing Considerations

### Assessment
- *History:* Allergy to vincristine, leukopenia, acute infection, neuromuscular disease, diabetes insipidus, hepatic dysfunction, pregnancy, lactation
- *Physical:* Weight; hair; T; reflexes, gait, sensation, cranial nerve evaluation, ophthalmic exam; mucous membranes, ab-

V

dominal exam; CBC, serum sodium, liver function tests, urinalysis

### Implementation

- Do not administer IM or SC due to severe local reaction and tissue necrosis.
- Take care to avoid extravasation; if it occurs, discontinue injection immediately and give remainder of dose in another vein. Consult with physician to arrange for hyaluronidase injection into local area, and apply heat to disperse the drug and to minimize pain.
- Arrange for wig or suitable head covering if hair loss occurs; ensure that patient's head is covered in extremes of temperature.
- Monitor urine output and serum sodium; if SIADH occurs, consult with physician, and arrange for fluid restriction and perhaps a potent diuretic.

### Drug-specific teaching points

- Prepare a calendar of dates to return for treatment and additional therapy.
- The following side effects may occur: loss of appetite, nausea, vomiting, mouth sores (frequent mouth care, small frequent meals may help; maintain nutrition; request an antiemetic); constipation (bowel program may be ordered); sensitivity to light (wear sunglasses; avoid bright lights); numbness, tingling, change in style of walking (reversible; may persist for up to 6 wk); hair loss (transient; obtain a wig or other suitable head covering; keep the head covered at extremes of temperature).
- This drug cannot be taken during pregnancy; use birth control. If you become pregnant, consult with your physician.
- Have regular blood tests to monitor the drug's effects.
- Report change in frequency of voiding; swelling of ankle, fingers, and so forth; changes in vision; severe constipation, abdominal pain.

## vinorelbine tartrate

*(vin oh **rel'** been)*

Navelbine

**Pregnancy Category D**

### Drug classes

Mitotic inhibitor
Antineoplastic

### Therapeutic actions

Affects cell energy production required for mitosis and interferes with nucleic acid synthesis; has antimitotic effect, prevents the formation of microtubules and leads to cell death; cell cycle specific.

### Indications

- First line treatment of ambulatory patients with unresectable advanced non-small cell lung cancer
- Treatment of stage IV non-small cell lung cancer alone or with cisplatin
- Treatment of stage III non-small cell lung cancer with cisplatin
- Unlabeled uses: breast cancer, ovarian cancer, Hodgkin's disease

### Contraindications/cautions

- Contraindications: allergy to vinca alkaloids, pretreatment granulocyte counts 1000 cells/mm$^3$, pregnancy, lactation.
- Use cautiously with liver disease.

### Dosage

**Available Forms:** Injection—10 mg/ml

Do not administer more than once a week because of leukopenic response.

*ADULT*

- ***Initial dose:*** 30 mg/m$^2$ as single IV dose; repeat once a week until progression of disease or toxicity limits use.
- ***With cisplatin:*** 120 mg/m$^2$ cisplatin on days 1 and 29 and then every 6 wk.
- ***Hepatic impairment:*** Reduce dose.

### Pharmacokinetics

| Route | Onset |
|---|---|
| IV | Slow |

*Metabolism:* Hepatic metabolism; $T_{1/2}$: 22–66 h

*Distribution* : Crosses placenta; passes into breast milk

*Excretion* : Bile and feces

### IV facts

*Preparation*: Dilute for 50 or 10 mg solution. Supplied as single use vials only. Discard after withdrawing solution.

*Infusion*: Inject into tubing of a running IV or directly into the vein over 6–10 min period. Rinse syringe and needle with venous blood prior to withdrawing needle from vein (to minimize extravasation). Do not inject into an extremity with poor circulation or repeatedly into the same vein.

### Adverse effects

- CNS: Numbness, paresthesias (less common than with other vinca alkaloids); headache, weakness, dizziness
- GI: Nausea, vomiting, pharyngitis, vesiculation of the mouth, ileus, diarrhea, constipation, anorexia, abdominal pain, *increased liver enzymes*
- **Hematologic**: ***Granuloctytopenia***, *leukopenia*
- **Dermatologic**: Topical epilation (loss of hair), vesiculation of the skin
- **Local**: Local cellulitis, phlebitis, sloughing with extravasation
- **Other**: myalgia, arthralgia

### Clinically important drug-drug interactions

• Acute pulmonary reactions with mitomycin • Increased risk of granulocytopenia with cisplatin

## ■ Nursing Considerations

### Assessment

- *History:* Allergy to vinca alkaloids, leukopenia, acute infection, liver disease, pregnancy, lactation
- *Physical:* Weight; hair; T; reflexes, gait, sensation, orientation, affect; mucous membranes, abdominal exam; CBC, liver function tests, serum albumin

### Implementation

- Do not administer IM or SC—severe local reaction and tissue necrosis occur.
- Avoid extravasation; if it should occur, discontinue injection immediately and give remainder of dose in another vein. Consult physician to arrange for hyaluronidase injection into local area, after which apply moderate heat to disperse drug and minimize pain.
- Avoid contact with the eyes; if contact occurs, thoroughly wash immediately with water .
- Consult with physician if antiemetic is needed for severe nausea and vomiting.
- Check CBC before each dose.

### Drug-specific teaching points

- Prepare a calendar for dates to return for treatment and additional therapy.
- The following side effects may occur: loss of appetite, nausea, vomiting, mouth sores (frequent mouth care, small frequent meals may help; maintain nutrition; request an antiemetic); constipation (bowel program may be ordered); malaise, weakness, dizziness, numbness and tingling (avoid injury); loss of hair, skin rash (obtain a wig; keep the head covered in extremes of temperature).
- This drug should not be used during pregnancy. Use birth control. If you become pregnant, consult your physician.
- Have regular blood tests to monitor the drug's effects.
- Report severe nausea, vomiting. pain or burning at injection site, abdominal pain, rectal bleeding, fever, chills, acute infection.

## warfarin sodium

*(war' far in)*

Coumadin, Warfilone (CAN), Warnerin (CAN)

**Pregnancy Category D**

### Drug classes

Oral anticoagulant
Coumarin derivative

### Therapeutic actions

Interferes with the hepatic synthesis of vitamin K-dependent clotting factors (factors II-prothrombin, VII, IX, and X), resulting in their eventual depletion and prolongation of clotting times.

### Indications

- Venous thrombosis and its extension, treatment, and prophylaxis

W

- Treatment of atrial fibrillation with embolization
- Pulmonary embolism, treatment, and prophylaxis
- Prophylaxis of systemic emobolization after acute MI
- Unlabeld uses: prevention of recurrent TIAs, prevention of recurrent MI, adjunct to therapy in small-cell carcinoma of the lung

### Contraindications/cautions

- Contraindications: allergy to warfarin; SBE; hemorrhagic disorders; TB; hepatic diseases; GI ulcers; renal disease; indwelling catheters, spinal puncture; aneurysm; diabetes; visceral carcinoma; uncontrolled hypertension; severe trauma (including recent or contemplated CNS, eye surgery; recent placement of IUD); threatened abortion, menometrorrhagia; pregnancy (fetal damage and death); lactation (suggest using heparin if anticoagulation is required).
- Use cautiously with CHF, diarrhea, fever; thyrotoxicosis; senile, psychotic, or depressed patients.

### Dosage

**Available Forms:** Tablets—1, 2, 2.5, 3, 4, 5, 6, 7.5, 10 mg; powder for injection—2 mg

Adjust dosage according to the one-stage PT to achieve and maintain 1.5–2.5 times the control value or prothrombin activity 20%–30% of normal or a PT/INF ratio of 2–3. IV use is reserved for situations in which oral warfarin is not feasible. Dosages are the same for oral and IV forms.

**ADULT:** *Initially:* 10–15 mg/d PO. Adjust dose according to PT response. *Maintenance:* 2–10 mg/d PO based on PT time.

**GERIATRIC:** Lower doses are usually needed; begin dosage lower than adult recommended and closely monitor PT.

### Pharmacokinetics

| *Route* | *Peak* | *Duration* |
|---|---|---|
| Oral | 1 1/2–3 d | 2–5 d |

*Metabolism:* Hepatic, $T_{1/2}$: 1–2.5 d
*Distribution:* Crosses placenta; enters breast milk
*Excretion:* Feces and urine

### IV facts

**Preparation:** Reconstitute 5-mg vial with 2.7 ml of Sterile Water. Protect from light. Use within 4 h of reconstitution.
**Infusion:** Inject slowly over 1–2 min; switch to oral preparation as soon as possible.

### Adverse effects

- GI: *Nausea*, vomiting, anorexia, abdominal cramping, diarrhea, retroperitoneal hematoma, hepatitis, jaundice, mouth ulcers
- Hematologic: Granulocytosis, leukopenia, eosinophilia
- GU: Priapism, nephropathy, red-orange urine
- Dermatologic: *Alopecia, urticaria, dermatitis*
- Bleeding: *Hemorrhage*; GI or urinary tract bleeding (hematuria, dark stools; paralytic ileus, intestinal obstruction from hemorrhage into GI tract); petechiae and purpura, bleeding from mucous membranes; hemorrhagic infarction, vasculitis, skin necrosis of female breast; adrenal hemorrhage and resultant adrenal insufficiency; compressive neuropathy secondary to hemorrhage near a nerve
- Other: Fever, "purple toes" syndrome

### Clinically important drug-drug interactions

• Increased bleeding tendencies with salicylates, chloral hydrate, phenylbutazone, clofibrate, disulfiram, chloramphenicol, metronidazole, cimetidine, ranitidine, cotrimoxazole, sulfinpyrazone, quinidine, quinine, oxyphenbutazone, thyroid drugs, glucagon, danazol, erythromycin, androgens, amiodarone, cefamandole, cefoperazone, cefotetan, moxalactam, cefazolin, cefoxitin, ceftriaxone, meclofenamate, mefenamic acid, famotidine, nizatidine, nalidixic acid • Decreased anticoagulation effect may occur with barbiturates, griseofulvin, rifampin, phenytoin, glutethimide, carbamazepine, vitamin K, vitamin E, cholestyramine, aminoglutethimide, ethchlorvynol • Altered effects with methimazole, propylthiouracil • Increased activity and toxicity of phenytoin when taken with oral anticoagulants

**Drug-lab test interferences**
• Red-orange discoloration of alkaline urine may interfere with some lab tests

## ■ Nursing Considerations

### Assessment

- *History:* Allergy to warfarin; SBE; hemorrhagic disorders; TB; hepatic diseases; GI ulcers; renal disease; indwelling catheters, spinal puncture; aneurysm; diabetes; visceral carcinoma; uncontrolled hypertension; severe trauma; threatened abortion, menometrorrhagia; pregnancy; lactation; CHF, diarrhea, fever; thyrotoxicosis; senile, psychotic or depressed patients
- *Physical:* Skin lesions, color, temperature; orientation, reflexes, affect; P, BP, peripheral perfusion, baseline ECG; R, adventitious sounds; liver evaluation, bowel sounds, normal output; CBC, urinalysis, guaiac stools, PT, renal and hepatic function tests

### Implementation

- Monitor PT or PT/INF ratio regularly to adjust dosage.
- Administer IV form to patients stabilized on Coumadin who are not able to take oral drug. Dosages are the same. Return to oral form as soon as feasible.
- Do not change brand names once stabilized; bioavailability problems exist.
- Evaluate patient regularly for signs of blood loss (petechiae, bleeding gums, bruises, dark stools, dark urine).
- Do not give patient any IM injections.
- Double check all drugs ordered for potential drug–drug interaction; dosage of both drugs may need to be adjusted.
- Use caution when discontinuing other medications; warfarin dosage may need to be adjusted; carefully monitor PT values.
- Maintain vitamin K on standby in case of overdose.
- Arrange for frequent follow-up, including blood tests to evaluate drug effects.
- Evaluate for therapeutic effects: PT 1 1/2–2 1/2 times the control value; PT/INF ratio of 2–3.

### Drug-specific teaching points

- Many factors may change your body's response to this drug—fever, change of diet, change of environment, other medications. Your dosage may have to be changed repeatedly. Write down changes that are prescribed.
- Do not change any medication that you are taking (adding or stopping another drug) without consulting your health care provider. Other drugs can affect your anticoagulant; starting or stopping another drug can cause excessive bleeding or interfere with the desired drug effects.
- Carry or wear a medical ID tag to alert emergency medical personnel that you are taking this drug.
- Avoid situations in which you could be easily injured (contact sports, shaving with a straight razor).
- The following side effects may occur: stomach bloating, cramps (transient); loss of hair, skin rash; orange-red discoloration to the urine (if upsetting, add vinegar to your urine and the color should disappear).
- Have periodic blood tests to check on the drug action. These tests are important.
- Use contraception; do not become pregnant.
- Report unusual bleeding (from brushing your teeth, excessive bleeding from injuries, excessive bruising), black or bloody stools, cloudy or dark urine, sore throat, fever, chills, severe headaches, dizziness, suspected pregnancy.

# xylometazoline hydrochloride

*(zye low met az' oh leen)*

Otrivin Nasal Drops or Spray, Otrivin Pediatric Nasal Drops, Otrivin with M-D Pump (CAN), Sinutab Sinus Spray (CAN)

**Pregnancy Category C**

### Drug classes
Nasal decongestant

### Therapeutic actions
Acts directly on alpha-receptors to produce vasoconstriction of arterioles in nasal passages, which produces a decongestant response; no effect on beta receptors.

### Indications
- Symptomatic relief of nasal and nasopharyngeal mucosal congestion due to the common cold, hay fever, or other respiratory allergies (topical)

### Contraindications/cautions
- Contraindications: allergy to xylometazolozine, angle-closure glaucoma, anesthesia with cyclopropane or halothane, thyrotoxicosis, diabetes, hypertension, CV disorders, women in labor whose BP > 130/80.
- Use cautiously with angina, arrhythmias, prostatic hypertrophy, unstable vasomotor syndrome, lactation.

**Available Forms:** Nasal solution—0.05%, 0.1%

### Dosage
*ADULT:* 2–3 sprays or 2–3 drops in each nostril q8–10h.

*PEDIATRIC 2–12 Y:* 2–3 drops of 0.05% solution in each nostril q8–12h.

### Pharmacokinetics

| *Route* | *Onset* | *Duration* |
|---|---|---|
| Nasal | 5–10 min | 5–6 h |

*Metabolism:* Hepatic, $T_{1/2}$: unknown
*Distribution:* Crosses placenta; may enter breast milk
*Excretion:* Urine

### Adverse effects
Systemic effects are less likely with topical administration than with systemic administration, but because systemic absorption can take place, the systemic effects should be considered.

- CNS: *Fear, anxiety, tenseness, restlessness, headache, lightheadedness, dizziness*, drowsiness, tremor, insomnia, hallucinations, psychological disturbances, convulsions, CNS depression, weakness, blurred vision, ocular irritation, tearing, photophobia, symptoms of paranoid schizophrenia
- GI: *Nausea*, vomiting, anorexia
- CV: Arrhythmias, hypertension, resulting in intracranial hemorrhage, CV collapse with hypotension, palpitations, tachycardia, precordial pain in patients with ischemic heart disease
- GU: Constriction of renal blood vessels, *dysuria, vesical sphincter spasm,* resulting in difficult and painful urination, urinary retention in males with prostatism
- Local: *Rebound congestion* with topical nasal application
- Other: *Pallor*, respiratory difficulty, orofacial dystonia, sweating

### Clinically important drug-drug interactions
• Severe hypertension with MAOIs, TCAs, furazolidone • Additive effects and increased risk of toxicity with urinary alkalinizers • Decreased vasopressor response with reserpine, methyldopa, urinary acidifiers • Decreased hypotensive action of guanethidine

## ■ Nursing Considerations

### Assessment
- ***History:*** Allergy to xylometazoline; angle-closure glaucoma; anesthesia with cyclopropane or halothane; thyrotoxicosis, diabetes, hypertension, CV disorders; prostatic hypertrophy, unstable vasomotor syndrome; lactation.
- ***Physical:*** Skin color, temperature; orientation, reflexes, peripheral sensation, vision; P, BP, auscultation, peripheral perfusion; R, adventitious sounds; urinary output pattern, bladder percussion, prostate palpation; nasal mucous membrance evaluation

### Implementation
- Monitor CV effects carefully in hypertensive patients; change in BP may be from additional vasoconstriction. If a nasal decongestant is needed, pseudoephedrine is the drug of choice.

### Drug-specific teaching points

- Do not exceed recommended dose. Demonstrate proper administration technique for topical nasal application. Avoid prolonged use because underlying medical problems can be disguised.
- The following side effects may occur: dizziness, weakness, restlessness, lightheadedness, tremor (avoid driving or operating dangerous equipment); urinary retention (empty bladder before taking drug).
- Rebound congestion may occur when this drug is stopped; drink plenty of fluids, use a humidifier, avoid smoke-filled areas.
- Report nervousness, palpitations, sleeplessness, sweating.

## zafirkulast

*(zah **fur'** kuh last)*

Accolate

**Pregnancy Category B**

### Drug classes

Antiasthmatic agent

Leukotriene receptor antagonist

### Therapeutic actions

Selectively and competitively blocks receptor for leukotriene $D_4$ and $E_4$, components of SRS-A, thus blocking airway edema, smooth muscle constriction, and cellular activity associated with inflammatory process that contribute to signs and symptoms of asthma.

### Indications

- Prophylaxis and chronic treatment of bronchial asthma in adults and children >12 y

### Contraindications/cautions

- Contraindications: hypersensitivity to zafirkulast or any of its components; acute asthma attacks; status asthmaticus; pregnancy, lactation
- Use cautiously with hepatic or renal impairment; as oral steroid use is decreased; patients who previously required corticosteroid therapy to control asthma.

### Dosage

**Available Forms:** 20 mg

*ADULT AND CHILDREN >12 Y:* 20 mg PO bid on an empty stomach.

*GERIATRIC AND RENAL/HEPATIC IMPAIRED:* Limited experience with drug does not indicate any need to adjust dosage in these populations.

### Pharmacokinetics

| *Route* | *Onset* | *Peak* |
|---|---|---|
| Oral | Rapid | 3 h |

*Metabolism:* Hepatic; $T_{1/2}$: 10 h

*Distribution:* Crosses placenta; passes into breast milk

*Excretion:* Urine and feces

### Adverse effects

- CNS: *Headache,* dizziness, myalgia
- GI: Nausea, diarrhea, abdominal pain, vomiting, liver enzyme elevation
- Other: Generalized pain, fever, accidental injury, infection; **Churg-Strauss syndrome** (eosinophilia, vasculitic rash, pulmonary and cardiac complications) when oral steroid dose is reduced

### Clinically important drug-drug interactions

• Increased risk of bleeding with warfarin; these patients should have PT done regularly and warfarin dose decreased accordingly • Potential for increased effects and toxicity of calcium channel blockers, cyclosporine • Decreased effectiveness with erythromycin, theophylline, terfenadine • Increased effects with aspirin • Possible severe reaction when oral steroid dose is reduced while on zafirkulast; monitor patients very closely

### Clinically important drug-food interactions

• Bioavailability decreased markedly by presence of food; administer at least 1 h before or 2 h after meals

## ■ Nursing Considerations

### Assessment

- *History:* Hypersensitivity to zafirkulast; impaired renal or heaptic function; preg-

nancy, lactation; acute asthma or bronchospasm
- *Physical:* T; orientation, reflexes; R, adventitious sounds; GI evaluation; renal and liver function tests

### Implementation
- Administer on an empty stomach 1 h before or 2 h after meals.
- Ensure that drug is taken continually for optimal effect.
- Do not administer for acute asthma attack or acute bronchospasm.

### Drug-specific teaching points
- Take this drug on an empty stomach, 1 h before or 2 h after meals.
- Take this drug regularly as prescribed; do not stop taking it during symptom-free periods; do not stop taking it without consulting your health care provider.
- Do not take this drug for acute asthma attack or acute bronchospasm; this drug is not a bronchodilator; routine emergency procedures should be followed during acute attacks.
- The following side effects may occur: dizziness (use caution when driving or performing activities that require alertness); nausea, vomiting (eat small, frequent meals); headache (analgesics may be helpful).
- Avoid use of OTC medications while on this drug; many of them contain products that can interfere with drug or cause serious side effects. If you feel that you need one of these products, consult your nurse or physician.
- Report fever, acute asthma attacks, severe headache.

## zalcitabine

***(zal' cye tay been)***

dideoxycytidine, ddC

Hivid

**Pregnancy Category C**

### Drug classes
Antiviral

### Therapeutic actions
Synthetic purine nucleoside, which is active against HIV, inhibits cell protein synthesis, and leads to cell death without viral replication.

### Indications
- Combination therapy with zidovudine in advanced HIV infection

### Contraindications/cautions
- Contraindications: life-threatening allergy to any component, pregnancy, lactation.
- Use cautiously with compromised bone marrow, impaired renal or hepatic function.

### Dosage
**Available Forms:** Tablets—0.375, 0.75 mg

*ADULT:* 0.75 mg PO q8h or 0.75 PO mg administered with 200 mg zidovudine PO q8h.

*PEDIATRIC:* Safety and efficacy not established for children <13 y.

*GERIATRIC OR RENAL IMPAIRED:* Ccr of 10–40 ml/min, reduce dose to 0.75 mg q12h PO; Ccr < 10, reduce dose to 0.75 mg q24h PO.

### Pharmacokinetics

| *Route* | *Onset* | *Peak* |
|---|---|---|
| Oral | Varies | 0.8–1.6 h |

*Metabolism:* Hepatic, $T_{1/2}$: 1–3 h

*Distribution:* Crosses placenta; may enter breast milk

*Excretion:* Urine and feces

### Adverse effects
- CNS: *Headache*, insomnia, myalgia, *asthenia*, malaise, dizziness, paresthesia, somnolence, **peripheral neuropathy**
- GI: *Nausea, GI pain, diarrhea*, anorexia, vomiting, dyspepsia, oral ulcers
- Hematologic: *Agranulocytopenia*, severe anemia requiring transfusions
- Other: *Fever*, diaphoresis, dyspnea, *rash*, taste perversion

## ■ Nursing Considerations

### Assessment

- *History:* Life-threatening allergy to any component, compromised bone marrow, impaired renal or hepatic function, pregnancy, lactation
- *Physical:* Skin rashes, lesions, texture; T; affect, reflexes, peripheral sensation; bowel sounds, liver evaluation; renal and hepatic function tests; CBC and differential

### Implementation

- Monitor hematologic indices every 2 wk.
- Monitor for signs of peripheral neuropathy (numbness, tingling), and reduce drug dose by 50% until sensation returns; gradually reintroduce drug. Permanently discontinue if patient experiences severe discomfort and loss of sensation.
- Administer the drug every 8 h, around the clock with zidovudine; appropriate rest periods may be needed during the day because of interrupted sleep.

### Drug-specific teaching points

- Take drug every 8 h, around the clock. Use an alarm clock to wake you up at night; rest periods during the day may be necessary. Do not share this drug; take exactly as prescribed.
- Zalcitabine and zidovudine do not cure AIDS or ARC; opportunisitc infections may occur, obtain continuous medical care.
- Arrange for frequent blood tests; results of blood counts may indicate a need for decreased dosage or discontinuation of the drug for a period of time.
- The following side effects may occur: nausea, loss of appetite, change in taste (eat small, frequent meals); dizziness, loss of feeling (use precautions); headache, fever, muscle aches.
- These drugs do not reduce the risk of transmission of HIV to others by sexual contact or blood contamination; use precautions.
- Report extreme fatigue, lethargy, severe headache, severe nausea, vomiting, difficulty breathing, skin rash, numbness, tingling, pain in extremities.

# zidovudine

*(zid o **vew'** den)*

azidothymidine, AZT, Compound S

Retrovir

**Pregnancy Category C**

### Drug classes

Antiviral

### Therapeutic actions

Thymidine analogue isolated from the sperm of herring; drug is activated to a triphosphate form that inhibits replication of some retroviruses, including HIV, HTLV III, LAV, ARV.

### Indications

- Management of certain adult patients with symptomatic HIV infection (AIDS and advanced ARC) who have a history of cytologically confirmed *P. carinii* pneumonia or an absolute CD4 (T4 helper/inducer) lymphocyte count of less than 200/mm$^3$ in the peripheral blood before therapy is begun (parenteral)
- Management of patients with HIV infection who have evidence of impaired immunity ($CD_4$ cell count of $< 500/mm^3$) (oral)
- HIV-infected children $>3$ mo who have HIV-related symptoms or who are asymptomatic with abnormal laboratory values indicating significant HIV-related immunosuppression
- Prevention of maternal–fetal HIV transmission

### Contraindications/cautions

- Contraindications: life-threatening allergy to any component, pregnancy, lactation.
- Use cautiously with compromised bone marrow, impaired renal or hepatic function.

### Dosage

**Available Forms:** Capsules—100 mg; syrup—50 mg/5ml; injection—10 mg/ml

**ADULT**

- *Symptomatic HIV infection: Initially:* 200 mg q4h (2.9 mg/kg q4h) PO, around the clock. Monitor hematologic indices every 2 wk. If significant anemia (Hgb $< 7.5$ g/dl, reduction of $> 25\%$) or reduction of granulocytes $> 50\%$ below baseline occurs, dose interruption is necessary until evidence of bone marrow recovery is seen. If less severe bone marrow depression occurs, a dosage reduction may be adequate; *or* 1–2 mg/kg q4h IV.

- *Asymptomatic HIV infection:* 100 mg q4h PO while awake (500 mg/d).
- *Maternal–fetal transmission:* 100 mg PO 5 $\times$/d from $\leq$14 wk gestation to the start of labor.

*PEDIATRIC*

- *3 Mo–12 y:* Initial dose, 180 $mg/m^2$ q6h PO or IV (720 $mg/m^2$/d, not to exceed 200 mg q6h).
- *INFANT BORN TO HIV MOTHER:* 2 mg/kg q6h starting within 12 h of birth to 6 wk of age.

### Pharmacokinetics

| *Route* | *Onset* | *Peak* |
|---|---|---|
| Oral | Varies | 1/2–1 h1/2 |
| IV | Rapid | End of infusion |

*Metabolism:* Hepatic, $T_{1/2}$: 30–60 min
*Distribution:* Crosses placenta; may enter breast milk
*Excretion:* Urine

### IV facts

**Preparation:** Remove desired dose from vial, and dilute in 5% Dextrose in Water to a concentration no greater than 4 mg/ml.

**Infusion:** Administer over 60 min; avoid rapid infusion.

### Adverse effects

- CNS: *Headache*, insomnia, myalgia, *asthenia*, malaise, dizziness, paresthesia, somnolence
- GI: *Nausea, GI pain, diarrhea*, anorexia, vomiting, dyspepsia
- Hematologic: *Agranulocytopenia*, severe anemia requiring transfusions
- Other: *Fever*, diaphoresis, dyspnea, *rash*, taste perversion

## ■ Nursing Considerations

### Assessment

- ***History:*** Life-threatening allergy to any component, compromised bone marrow, impaired renal or hepatic function, pregnancy, lactation
- ***Physical:*** Skin rashes, lesions, texture; T; affect, reflexes, peripheral sensation; bowel sounds, liver evaluation; renal and hepatic function tests, CBC and differential

### Implementation

- Monitor hematologic indices every 2 wk.
- Give the drug around the clock; rest periods may be needed during the day due to interrupted sleep.

### Drug-specific teaching points

- Take drug every 4 h, around the clock. Use an alarm clock to wake you up at night; rest periods during the day may be necessary. Do not share this drug; take exactly as prescribed.
- Zidovudine is not a cure for AIDS or ARC; opportunisitc infections may occur; obtain continuous medical care.
- Arrange for frequent blood tests; results of blood counts may indicate a need for decreased dosage or discontinuation of the drug for a period of time.
- The following side effects may occur: nausea, loss of appetite, change in taste (eat small, frequent meals); dizziness, loss of feeling (use precautions); headache, fever, muscle aches.
- Zidovudine does not reduce the risk of transmission of HIV to others by sexual contact or blood contamination; use precautions.
- Report extreme fatigue, lethargy, severe headache, severe nausea, vomiting, difficulty breathing, skin rash.

## zileuton

***(zye loot' on)***

Zyflo

**Pregnancy Category C**

### Drug classes

Antiasthmatic agent
Leukotriene receptor antagonist

### Therapeutic actions

Selectively and competitively blocks the receptor that inhibits leukotriene formation, thus blocking many of the signs and symptoms of asthma (neutrophil and eosinophil migration, neutrophil and monocyte aggregation, leukocyte adhesion, increased capillary permeability and smooth muscle contraction). These actions contribute to inflammation, edema, mucus secretion and bronchoconstriction caused by cold air challenge in patients with asthma.

### Indications

- Prophylaxis and chronic treatment of bronchial asthma in adults and children > 12 y

### Contraindications/cautions

- Contraindications: hypersensitivity to zileuton or any of its components; acute asthma attacks; status asthmaticus; pregnancy and lactation, severe hepatic impairment.
- Use cautiously with hepatic impairment.

## Dosage

**Available Forms:** Tablets—600 mg

*ADULT AND CHILDREN > 12 Y:* 600 mg PO qid for a total of 2,400 mg/d.

### Pharmacokinetics

| *Route* | *Onset* | *Peak* |
|---|---|---|
| Oral | Rapid | 1.7 h |

*Metabolism:* Hepatic; $T_{1/2}$: 2.5 h
*Distribution:* Crosses placenta; enters breast milk
*Excretion:* Metabolism

### Adverse effects

- CNS: *Headache,* dizziness, myalgia
- GI: Nausea, diarrhea, abdominal pain, vomiting, **elevation of liver enzymes**
- Other: Generalized pain, fever, myalgia

### Clinically important drug-drug interactions

- Increased effects of propranolol, theophylline, terfenadine, warfarin; monitor patient and decrease dose as appropriate

### Clinically important drug-food interactions

- Bioavailability decreased markedly by the presence of food; administer at least 1 h before or 2 h after meals

## ■ Nursing Considerations

### Assessment

- *History:* Hypersensitivity to zileuton; impaired hepatic function; lactation; pregnancy; acute asthma or bronchospasm
- *Physical:* T; orientation, reflexes; R, adventitious sounds; GI evaluation; liver function tests

### Implementation

- Obtain baseline hepatic function tests before beginning therapy; monitor liver enzymes on a regular basis during therapy; discontinue drug and consult prescriber if enzymes rise more than three times normal.
- Administer without regard to food.
- Ensure that drug is taken continually for optimal effect.
- Do not administer for acute asthma attack or acute bronchospasm.

### Drug-specific teaching points

- Take this drug regularly as prescribed; do not stop taking this drug during symptom-free perods; do not stop taking this drug without consulting your health care provider. Continue taking any other antiasthma drugs that have been prescribed for you.
- Do not take this drug for an acute asthma attack or actue bronchospasm; this drug is not a bronchodilator; routine emergency procedures should be followed during acute attacks.
- The following side effects may occur: dizziness (use caution when driving or performing activities that require alertness); nausea, vomiting (eat small, frequent meals; take drug with food); headache (analgesics may be helpful).
- Avoid the use of OTC drugs while you are on this medication; many of them contain products that can interfere with or cause serious side effects when used with

this drug. If you feel that you need one of these products, consult your nurse or physician.
- Report fever, acute asthma attacks, flulike symptoms, lethargy, pruritus, changes in color of urine or stool.

## Zinc

### zinc acetate
Galzin

### zinc sulfate
*OTC and prescription drug:*
Orazinc, Verazinc, Zincate

### zinc gluconate

**Pregnancy Category C**

**Drug classes**
Mineral

**Therapeutic actions**
Natural element that is essential for growth and tissue repair; acts as an integral part of essential enzymes in protein and carbohydrate metabolism.

**Indications**
- Dietary supplement to treat or prevent zinc deficiencies
- Treatment of Wilson's disease (Galzin)
- Unlabeled uses: acrodermatitis enteropathica and delayed wound healing associated with zinc deficiency; treatment of acne, rheumatoid arthritis; treatment of the common cold

**Contraindications/cautions**
- Contraindications: pregnancy and lactation (recommended dietary allowance is needed, but not supplemental replacement).

**Dosage**
**Available Forms:** Tablets—15, 25, 45, 50 mg zinc; 1.4, 2, 7, 11 mg zinc

ADULT
- ***Recommended dietary allowance (RDA):*** 12–15 mg/d PO; pregnancy RDA, 15 mg/d PO; lactation RDA, 6 mg/d PO for the first 6 mo; then 4 mg/d for the next 6 mo.
- ***Dietary supplement:*** 25–50 mg zinc/d PO.

PEDIATRIC
- *RDA:* 5–10 mg/d PO.

**Pharmacokinetics**

| *Route* | *Onset* | *Peak* |
|---|---|---|
| Oral | Slow | Delayed |

*Metabolism:* Hepatic, $T_{1/2}$: unknown
*Distribution:* Crosses placenta; may enter breast milk
*Excretion:* Feces

**Adverse effects**
- GI: Vomiting, *nausea*

## ■ Nursing Considerations

**Assessment**
- *History:* Lactation, pregnancy
- *Physical:* Bowel sounds, normal output; serum zinc levels

**Implementation**
- Give with food if GI upset occurs; avoid bran and other high-fiber foods, calcium and phosphates that may interfere with absorption.
- Ensure that patient receives only the prescribed dosage. Avoid overdose.

**Drug-specific teaching points**
- Take this drug exactly as prescribed. Do not exceed prescribed dosage.
- Take with food, but avoid taking it with bran and other high-fiber foods, dairy products that may interfere with absorption.
- The following side effects may occur: nausea, vomiting (take drug with food).
- Report severe nausea and vomiting, restlessness, fatigue, lethargy.

## zolmitriptan

*(zohl mah **trip'** tan)*
Zomig

**Pregnancy Category C**

### Drug classes

Antimigraine agent
Serotonin selective agonist

### Therapeutic actions

Binds to serotonin receptors to cause vascular constrictive effects on cranial blood vessels, causing the relief of migraine in selected patients.

### Indications

- Treatment of acute migraine attacks with or without aura

### Contraindications/cautions

- Contraindications: allergy to zolmitriptan, active coronary artery disease, Printzmetal's angina, pregnancy.
- Use cautiously with the elderly and with lactation.

### Dosage

**Available Forms:** Tablets—2.5, 5 mg

*ADULT:* 2.5–25 mg PO at onset of headache or with beginning of aura; may repeat dose if headache persists afer 2 h, do not exceed 10 mg in 24 h.

*PEDIATRIC:* Safety and efficacy not established.

### Pharmacokinetics

| *Route* | *Onset* | *Peak* |
|---|---|---|
| PO | Varies | 2–4 h |

*Metabolism:* Hepatic; $T_{1/2}$: 2.5–3.7 h
*Distribution:* Crosses placenta; may pass into breast milk
*Excretion:* Urine and feces

### Adverse effects

- CNS: *Dizziness, vertigo,* headache, anxiety, malaise/fatigue, *weakness, myalgia*
- GI: Abdominal discomfort, dysphagia
- CV: *Blood pressure alterations, tightness or pressure in chest*
- Other: *Tingling, warm/hot sensations, burning sensation, feeling of heaviness, pressure sensation, numbness, feeling of tightness,* feeling strange, cold sensation

### Clinically important drug-drug interactions

• Prolonged vasoactive reactions with ergot-containing drugs • Risk of severe effects with or within <2 wk of discontinuation of an MAO inhibitor

## ■ Nursing Considerations

### Assessment

- *History:* Allergy to zolmitriptan, active CAD, Printzmetal's angina, pregnancy, lactation
- *Physical:* Skin color and lesions; orientation, reflexes, peripheral sensation; P, BP; renal and liver function tests

### Implementation

- Administer to relieve acute migraine, not as prophylactic measure.
- Establish safety measures if CNS, visual disturbances occur.
- Provide environmental control as appropriate to help relieve migraine (lighting, temperature, etc.).
- Monitor BP of patients with possible CAD; discontinue at any sign of angina, prolonged high blood pressure, etc.

### Drug-specific teaching points

- Take this drug exactly as prescribed, at the onset of headache or aura.
- This drug should not be taken during pregnancy; if you suspect that you are pregnant, contact physician and refrain from using drug.
- The following side effects may occur: dizziness, drowsiness (avoid driving or using dangerous machinery); numbness, tingling, feelings of tightness or pressure.
- Maintain any procedures you usually use during a migraine (controlled lighting, noise, etc.).
- Contact your physician immediately if you experience chest pain or pressure that is severe or does not go away.
- Report feelings of heat, flushing, tiredness, feelings of sickness, swelling of lips or eyelids.

## zolpidem tartrate

*(zol' pih dem)*

Ambien

**Pregnancy Category B**
**C-IV controlled substance**

**Drug classes**
Sedative/hypnotic (nonbarbiturate)

**Therapeutic actions**
Modulates GABA receptors to cause suppression of neurons, leading to sedation, anticonvulsant, anxiolytic, and relaxant properties.

**Indications**
- Short-term treatment of insomnia

**Contraindications/cautions**
- Contraindications: hypersensitivity to zolpidem.
- Use cautiously with acute intermittent porphyria, impaired hepatic or renal function, addiction-prone patients, pregnancy, lactation.

**Dosage**
**Available Forms:** Tablets—5, 10 mg
*ADULT:* 10 mg PO hs.
*PEDIATRIC:* Safety and efficacy not established.
*GERIATRIC:* Increased chance of confusion, acute brain syndrome; initiate treatment with 5 mg PO.

**Pharmacokinetics**

| Route | Onset | Peak |
|---|---|---|
| Oral | 45 min | 1.6 h |

*Metabolism:* Hepatic, $T_{1/2}$: 2.6 h
*Distribution:* Crosses placenta; may enter breast milk
*Excretion:* Urine

**Adverse effects**
- CNS: Convulsions, hallucinations, ataxia, EEG changes, pyrexia, *morning drowsiness, hangover, headache, dizziness,* vertigo, acute brain syndrome and confusion; paradoxical excitation, anxiety, depression, nightmares, dreaming, diplopia, blurred vision, *suppression of REM sleep*; REM rebound when drug is discontinued
- GI: Esophagitis, vomiting, *nausea*, diarrhea, constipation
- **Hypersensitivity**: Generalized allergic reactions; pruritus, rash
- Other: Influenza-like symptoms, dry mouth, infection

## ■ Nursing Considerations

### Assessment
- *History:* Hypersensitivity to zolpidem, acute intermittent porphyria, impaired hepatic or renal function, addiction-prone patients, lactation, pregnancy
- *Physical:* T; skin color, lesions; orientation, affect, reflexes, vision exam; P, BP; bowel sounds, normal output, liver evaluation; CBC with differential; hepatic and renal function tests

### Implementation
- Limit amount of drug dispensed to patients who are depressed or suicidal.
- Withdraw drug gradually if patient has used drug long-term or if patient has developed tolerance. Supportive therapy similar to that for withdrawal from barbiturates may be necessary to prevent dangerous withdrawal symptoms.

### Drug-specific teaching points
- Take this drug exactly as prescribed. Do not exceed prescribed dosage. Long-term use is not recommended.
- The following side effects may occur: drowsiness, dizziness, blurred vision (avoid driving or performing tasks requiring alertness or visual acuity); GI upset (eat frequent, small meals).
- Report skin rash, sore throat, fever, bruising.

# APPENDICES

# APPENDIX A

## Alternative and Complementary Therapies

Many natural substances are used by the public for self-treatment of many complaints. These substances, derived from folklore or various cultures, often have ingredients that have been identified and have known therapeutic activities. Some of these substances have unknown mechanisms of action, but over the years have been reliably used to relieve specific symptoms. There is an element of the placebo effect in using some of these substances. The power of believing that something will work and that there is some control over the problem is often very beneficial in achieving relief from pain or suffering. Some of these substances may contain yet unidentified ingredients, which, when discovered, may prove very useful in the modern field of pharmacology. Because these products are not regulated or monitored, there is always a possibility of toxic effects. Some of these products may contain ingredients that interact with prescription drugs. A history of the use of these alternative therapies may explain unexpected reactives to some drugs.

| *Substance* | *Reported Use* |
|---|---|
| alfalfa | Topical: healing ointment, relief of arthritis pain<br>Oral: arthritis treatment, strength giving |
| aloe leaves | Topical: treatment of burns, healing of wounds<br>Oral: treatment of chronic constipation |
| anise | Oral: relief of dry cough, treatment of flatulence |
| apple | Oral: control of blood glucose, constipation |
| arnica gel | Topical: relieves pain from muscle or soft tissue injury |
| bilberry | Oral: treatment of diabetes; cardiovascular problems; lowers cholesterol and triglycerides; treatment of diabetic retinopathy |
| birch bark | Topical: treatment of infected wounds, cuts<br>Oral: as tea for relief of stomach ache |
| blackberry | Oral: as a tea for generalized healing; treatment of diabetes |
| burdock | Oral: treatment of diabetes; atropine-like side effects, uterine stimulant |
| camomile | Topical: treatment of wounds, ulcer, conjunctivitis<br>Oral: treatment of migraines, gastric cramps, relief of anxiety |
| catnip leaves | Oral: treatment of bronchitis, diarrhea |
| cayenne pepper | Topical: treatment of burns, wounds, relief of toothache pain |
| celery | Oral: lowers blood glucose, acts as a diuretic; may cause potassium depletion |
| chicken soup | Oral: breaks up respiratory secretions, bronchodilator, relieves anxiety |
| chicory | Oral: treatment of digestive tract problems, gout; stimulates bile secretions |
| comfrey | Topical: treatment of wounds, cuts, ulcers<br>Oral: gargle for tonsilitis |

*(continued)*

| *Substance* | *Reported Use* |
|---|---|
| coriander | Oral: weight loss, lowers blood glucose |
| dandelion root | Oral: treatment of liver and kidney problems; decreases lactation (after delivery or with weaning); lowers blood glucose |
| DHEA | Oral: slows aging, improves vigor—"Fountain of Youth"; androgenic side effects |
| Di huang | Oral: treatment of diabetes mellitus |
| dried root bark of lycium Chinese mill | Oral: lowers cholesterol, lowers blood glucose |
| echinacea | Oral: treatment of colds, flu; stimulates the immune system, attacks viruses |
| elder bark and/or flowers | Topical: gargle for tonsillitis, pharyngitis<br>Oral: treatment of fever, chills |
| ephedra | Oral: increases energy, relieves fatigue; *warning:* associated with serious complications, withdrawn in some states |
| ergot | Oral: treatment of migraine headaches, treatment of menstrual problems, hemorrhage |
| eucalyptus | Topical: treatment of wounds<br>Oral: decreases respiratory secretions, suppresses cough |
| fennel | Oral: treatment of colic, gout, flatulence; enhances lactation |
| fenugreek | Oral: lowers cholesterol levels; reduces blood glucose; aids in healing |
| fish oil | Oral: treatment of coronary diseases, arthritis, colitis, depression, aggression, attention deficit disorder |
| garlic | Oral: treatment of colds, diuretic; prevention of coronary artery disease, intestinal antiseptic; lowers blood glucose, anticoagulant |
| ginger | Oral: treatment of nausea, motion sickness, postoperative nausea (may increase risk of miscarriage) |
| ginkobe | Oral: increases cerebral blood flow, improves concentration and memory |
| ginseng | Oral: aphrodisiac, mood elevator, tonic; antihypertensive; decreases cholesterol levels; lowers blood glucose |
| goldenrod leaves | Oral: treatment of renal disease, rheumatism, sore throat, eczema |
| goldenseal | Oral: lowers blood glucose, aids healing |
| guayusa | Oral: lowers blood glucose; weight loss |
| hop | Oral: sedative; aids healing; alters blood glucose |
| horehound | Oral: expectorant; treatment of respiratory problems, GI disorders |
| Java plum | Oral: treatment of diabetes mellitus |
| juniper berries | Oral: increases appetite, aids digestion, diuretic, urinary tract disinfectant; lowers blood glucose |
| kava | Oral: treatment of nervous anxiety, stress, restlessness; tranquilizer |
| kudzu | Oral: reduces cravings for alcohol; being researched for use with alcoholics |
| ledum tincture | Topical: treatment of insect bites, puncture wounds; dissolves some blood clots and bruises |

*(continued)*

| *Substance* | *Reported Use* |
|---|---|
| licorice | Oral: prevents thirst, soothes coughs; treats "incurable" chronic fatigue syndrome |
| mandrake root | Oral: treatment of fertility problems |
| marigold leaves/flowers | Oral: relief of muscle tension, increases wound healing |
| melatonin | Oral: relief of jet lag, treatment of insomnia |
| milk thistle | Oral: treatment of hepatitis, cirrhosis, fatty liver due to alcohol or drugs |
| mistletoe leaves | Oral: weight loss; relief of signs and symptoms of diabetes |
| momordica charantia (Karela) | Oral: blocks intestinal absorption of glucose; lowers blood glucose; weight loss |
| nightshade leaves/roots | Oral: stimulates circulatory system; treatment of eye disorders |
| parsley seeds/leaves | Oral: treatment of jaundice, asthma, menstrual difficulties, conjunctivitis |
| peppermint leaves | Oral: treatment of nervousness, insomnia, dizziness, cramps, coughs<br>Topical: rubbed on forehead to relieve tension headaches |
| raspberry | Oral: healing of minor wounds; control and treatment of diabetes |
| rosemary | Topical: relief of rheumatism, sprains, wounds, bruises, eczema<br>Oral: gastric stimulation, relief of flatulence, stimulation of bile release, relief of colic |
| Rue extract | Topical: relief of pain associated with sprains, groin pulls, whiplash |
| saffron | Oral: treatment of menstrual problems, abortifacient |
| sage | Oral: lowers blood pressure; lowers blood glucose |
| sarsaparilla | Oral: treatment of skin disorders, rheumatism |
| saw palmetto | Oral: treatment of benign prostatic hyperplasia |
| St. John's wort | Oral: treatment of depression<br>Topical: treatment of puncture wounds, insect bites, crushed fingers or toes |
| sweet violet flowers | Oral: treatment of respiratory disorders, emetic |
| tarragon | Oral: weight loss; prevents cancer; lowers blood glucose |
| thyme | Topical: liniment, treatment of wounds, gargle<br>Oral: antidiarrhetic, relief of bronchitis and laryngitis |
| valerian | Oral: sedative/hypnotic; reduces anxiety, relaxes muscles |
| white willow bark | Oral: treatment of fevers |
| xuan seng | Oral: lowers blood glucose; slows heart rate; treatment of congestive heart failure |

# APPENDIX B

## Anesthetics

## *General Anesthetics*

General anesthetics are central nervous system depressants that depress the reticular activating system and cerebral cortex, and can produce sedation, hypnosis, anesthesia, and deep coma; these drugs should *only* be given by medical personnel (*eg,* anesthesiologists) trained in resuscitative techniques, including the establishment of an airway. Nursing care related to these drugs involves patient support, teaching, and evaluation.

### Pregnancy Category C

*Contraindicated* in cases of status asthmaticus; absence of suitable veins for IV administration. Caution should be used in cases of severe cardiovascular disease, hypotension or shock, conditions in which hypnotic effects may be prolonged or potentiated, increased intracranial pressure, myasthenia gravis, asthma.

### Adverse Effects

*Circulatory depression,* thrombophlebitis, myocardial depression, cardiac arrhythmias; *respiratory depression including apnea, laryngospasm, bronchospasm,* hiccups, sneezing, coughing; *emergence delirium, headache,* prolonged somnolence and recovery; *nausea,* emesis, salivation.

Patients receiving these drugs will need to be intubated or have immediate access to ventilation to assure adequate ventilation.

### Drug-Specific Teaching Points

What to expect (rapid onset of sleep), what they will feel (with rectal, IV administration), and how they will feel when they wake up.

## *Adjuncts to Anesthetics*

Neuromuscular junction (NMJ) blocking agents (nondepolarizing type) and depolarizing agents are used as adjuncts to general anesthetics to produce paralysis.

### Therapeutic actions

NMJ blockers interfere with neuromuscular transmission and cause flaccid paralysis by blocking acetylcholine receptors at the skeletal neuromuscular junction; succinylcholine is a depolarizing agent that blocks the cholinergic receptors of the motor endplate and causes paralysis of short duration.

### Indications

These drugs are used as adjuncts to general anesthetics, to facilitate endotracheal intubation and relax skeletal muscle and to relax skeletal muscle in order to facilitate mechanical ventilation.

| Drug | Brand Names | Dosage | Special Considerations | Onset/Recovery | Postanesthesia Concerns |
|---|---|---|---|---|---|
| ***Barbiturates*** | | | | | |
| thiopental sodium | *Pentothal* | Test dose: 50–75 mg IV 50–75 mg IV q20–40 sec. Maintenance: 25–50 mg IV | Do not administer in concentrations less than 2% in Sterile Water. C-III controlled substance. | Rapid/ultrashort | Not analgesic, post-op pain common. |
| methohexital sodium | *Brevital* | 5–12 ml of 1% solution. Maintenance; 2–4 ml of 1% solution q4–7 min. | Short acting. do not mix with bacteriostatic water or acid solutions. Should not come in contact with silicone. Avoid contact with rubber stoppers or disposable syringes with silicone. | Rapid/ultra, ultrashort | Respiratory depression and apnea; not analgesic, post-op pain common. |
| ***Gases*** | | | | | |
| nitrous oxide | | | Frequently causes nausea. Nonexplosive gas. Malignant hypothermia can occur. Monitor. Supplied in blue cylinders. | 1–2 min/rapid | Hypoxia; monitor for chest pain, hypertension, stroke. |
| cyclopropane | | | Rapid onset. Malignant hypothermia may occur. Very explosive. Supplied in orange cylinders. | 1–2 min/rapid | Headache, nausea and vomiting; delirium during recovery. |
| ethylene | | | Rapid onset and recovery. Nontoxic. Very explosive. Supplied in red cylinders. | Rapid/rapid | Unpleasant taste, headache. |

| | | | | | |
|---|---|---|---|---|---|
| ***Volatile Liquids*** | | | | | |
| desflurane | *Suprane* | 3%–1% concentrations, inhaled | Not recommended for induction of pediatric patients. May be used as adjunct for maintenance. Can cause respiratory irritation. | Rapid/rapid | Coughing, laryngospasm, increased secretions. |
| enflurane | *Ethrane* | 2%–4.5% produces anesthesia in 7–10 min. | Causes muscle relaxation. May cause renal toxicity. | Rapid/rapid | Cardiac arrhythmias, respiratory depression. |
| halothane | *Fluothane* | Administered by nonrebreathing technique, partial rebreathing or closed technique. | Associated with hepatic toxicity. Monitor for malignant hypothermia. | Rapid/rapid | Hypotension, cardiac arrhythmias. |
| isoflurane | | Inspired 1.5%–3% concentration causes anesthesia in 7–10 min. Maintenance with 1%–2% with nitrous oxide. | Rapid onset and recovery. Causes muscle relaxation. Monitor for hypotension, hypercapnia. | Rapid/rapid | Muscle soreness, bad taste, hypotension |
| methoxyflurane | *Penthrane* | 0.3%–0.8% for anesthesia 0.1%–2% for maintenance | May cause renal toxicity. Used with oxygen or nitrous oxide. | Slow/prolonged | Respiratory depression; hypotension |
| sevoflurane | *Ultane* | 0.5%–3% for anesthesia and maintenance with nitrous oxide | | Rapid/rapid | Coughing, laryngospasm; side effects minimal because of rapid action and excretion |

*(continued)*

| Drug | Brand Names | Dosage | Special Considerations | Onset/Recovery | Postanesthesia Concerns |
|---|---|---|---|---|---|
| *Other* | | | | | |
| droperidol | *Inapsine* | 2.5–10 mg IM or IV | Use caution with renal or hepatic failure. Monitor for hypotension. | 3–10 min/2–4 h | Drowsiness, chills, hypotension, hallucinations during recovery |
| etomidate | *Amidate* | 0.2–0.6 mg/kg IV over 30–60 sec. | Not recommended in children <10 y. Used for sedation for ventilator patients. | 1 min/3–5 min | Myoclonic, tonic movements, nausea and vomiting. |
| ketamine | *Ketalar* | 1–4.5 mg/kg for 5–10 min of anesthesia | Administer slowly over 60 sec. Monitor for severe emergence reactions: dreams, hallucinations, etc. Manage with small dose of hypnotic. | Rapid/45 min | Dissociation, hallucinations; hypertension, increased heart rate |
| midazolam hydrochloride | *Versed* | 0.07–0.06 mg/kg | Onset in 15 min, peaks in 30–60 min. Administer slowly. Monitor for respiratory depression. | Rapid/rapid | Respiratory depression, cough, hiccoughs, nausea and vomiting |
| propofol | *Diprivan* | 100 mcg/kg–2.5 mg/kg | Short-acting. Local burning on injury. Monitor for sedation before discharge; monitor for pulmonary edema. | Rapid/rapid | Hypotension, bradycardia, movement |

## Contraindications/Cautions: Pregnancy Category C

These drugs are contraindicated in the presence of allergy to NMJ drug; myasthenia gravis; Eaton-Lambert syndrome; labor and delivery (drug has been used safely during cesarean section, but the dose may need to be lowered in patients receiving magnesium sulfate to manage pre-eclampsia). Caution should be used in the presence of carcinoma, renal or hepatic disease, respiratory depression, or altered fluid/electrolyte balance.

## Dosage

Primarily administered by anesthesiologists who are skilled in administering artificial respiration and oxygen under positive pressure; facilities for these procedures must be on standby.

## Adverse Effects

**Depressed respiration,** *apnea, histamine release causing wheezing,* bronchospasm; *increased or decreased P, hypotension, vasodilatation—flushing;* profound and prolonged muscle paralysis.

## Important Drug-Drug Interactions

- Increased intensity and duration of neuromuscular block with some anesthetics (isoflurane, enflurane, halothane, diethyl ether, methoxyflurane), some parenteral antibiotics (aminoglycosides, clindamycin, capreomycin, vancomycin, lincomycin, bacitracin, polymyxin B, and sodium colistimethate), ketamine, quinine, quinidine, trimethaphan, carbamazepine, diazepam, azathioprine, mercaptopurine, calcium channel-blocking drugs (verapamil, etc.), $Mg^{2+}$ salts, and in hypokalemia (produced by $K^+$ depleting diuretics).
- Decreased intensity of block with acetylcholine, cholinesterase inhibitors, $K^+$ salts., phenytoin
- Reversal of neuromuscular blockage if taken with aminophylline, dyphylline, oxtriphylline, theophylline

## Implementation

- Have on standby, neostigmine, pyridostigmine, or edrophonium (cholinesterase inhibitors) to overcome excessive neuromuscular block; atropine or glycopyrrolate, to prevent parasympathomimetic effects of cholinesterase inhibitors.
- Change patient's position frequently and provide skin care to prevent decubitus ulcer formation when drug is used for other than brief periods.
- Monitor conscious patient for pain, distress that patient may not be able to communicate, and frequently reassure patient.

## Drug Specific Teaching Points

When a patient is conscious during the use of this drug (ventilator, etc.) include the following points:

- Tell patient drug is being used to paralyze muscles to facilitate treatment.
- Carefully explain all procedures; remember that the patient is not capable of verbal communication but can hear and see.

| Drug | Brand Name | Type | Special Considerations |
|---|---|---|---|
| atracurium besylate | *Tracrium* | NMJ blocker | Has no effect on pain threshold or consciousness; do not use before induction of unconsciousness; bradycardia during anesthesia is more common with this drug. |
| cisatracurium besylate | *Nimbex* | NMJ blocker | Intermediate action/intermediate onset; used for short procedures. |
| doxacurium chloride | *Nuromax* | NMJ blocker | Contains benzyl alcohol and should not be used with premature infants; monitor patient for recovery, prolongation of blockade may occur requiring supportive care. |
| metocurine iodide | *Metubine* | NMJ blocker | Do not give IM; used as adjunct to electroshock therapy. |
| mivacurium chloride | *Mivacron* | NMJ blocker | Has no effect on pain threshold or consciousness; do not use before unconsciousness has been induced. |
| pancuronium bromide | *Pavulon* | NMJ blocker | Used long-term to manage patients on mechanical ventilators; monitor patients for prolongation of neuromuscular effects beyond the time needed or anticipated by drug use; supportive care may be needed. |
| pipercuronium bromide | *Arduan* | NMJ blocker | Recommended only for procedures anticipated to last ≤90 min. Monitor patient for prolongation of neuromuscular blockade; provide supportive care. |
| rocuronium bromide | *Zemuron* | NMJ blocker | 1–2 min onset; short-acting; relatively new drug. |
| succinylcholine chloride | *Anectine, Quelicin* | Depolarizer | Used as adjunct to ECT and for prolonged use on mechanical ventilators; monitor patient for histamine release and resulting hypotension and flushing; monitor patient during recovery for prolonged paralysis and provide supportive care. |
| tubocurarine chloride | | NMJ blocker | Used for diagnosis of myasthenia gravis and for electroshock therapy. Do not use any solution that has developed a faint color. |
| vecuronium bromide | *Norcuron* | NMJ blocker | Has no effect on pain threshold or consciousness; do not use before unconsciousness has been induced. Prolongation of neuromuscular blockade has been reported; monitor patient during recovery and provide supportive care. |

## *Local Anesthetics*

Local anesthetics prevent the conduction of sensory (pain) impulses. Progression of nerve function loss is pain, temperature, touch, proprioception, skeletal muscle tone.

### Indications

Infiltration anesthesia, peripheral nerve block, spinal anesthesia, relief of local pain.

### Pregnancy Category C

*Contraindicated* in cases of hypersensitivity to local anesthetics, para-aminobenzoic acid (PABA), to parabens, heart block, shock, septicemia, reduced levels of plasma esterases.

### Adverse Effects

(Occurrence varies with route of administration): *Headache, backache,* septic meningitis, *restlessness, anxiety, dizziness, tinnitus, blurred vision,* pupil constriction, tremors, nausea, vomiting, *peripheral vasodilation,* myocardial depression, hypotension or hypertension, arrhythmias, **cardiac arrest,** fetal bradycardia, **respiratory arrest,** *sympathetic block and hypotension.*

### Clinically Important Interactions

Increased and prolonged neuromuscular blockade produced by succinylcholine if given concurrently.

### Important Interventions

Ensure that resuscitative equipment is on standby, that drugs for managing seizures, hypotension, cardiac arrest are on standby; ensure that patients receiving spinal anesthetics are well hydrated and remain lying down for up to 12 h after the anesthetic to minimize likelihood of "spinal headache," establish appropriate safety precautions to prevent injury during the time patient has lost sensation.

### Drug-Specific Teaching Points

Incorporate into teaching protocol what feelings to anticipate and what will be experienced; the need to remain lying down after spinal anesthesia; to report burning, pain, headache, difficulty breathing, lack of function in anticipated time frame.

| Drug | Brand-Names | Pharmacokinetics | Uses | Special Considerations |
|---|---|---|---|---|
| benzocaine | *Dermoplast*<br>*Foille*<br>*Lanacane*<br>*Unguentine* | Onset: 1 min<br>Duration: 30–60 min | Skin<br>Mucous membrane | Protect patient from injury; alert patient using skin prep to avoid tight bandages |
| bupivacaine | *Marcaine*<br>*Sensorcaine* | Onset: 5–20 min<br>Duration: 2–7 h | Local<br>Epidural<br>Subarachnoid<br>Caudal<br>Retrobulbar<br>Sympathetic<br>Dental | Do not use for Bier Block—deaths have occurred; do not use .75% solution for obstetric anesthesia |
| butamben picrate | *Butesin Picrate* | Onset: slow<br>Duration: 30–60 min | Skin<br>Mucous membr. | Protect patient from injury; advise patient that swallowing may be difficult with throat use |
| chloroprocaine | *Nesacaine* | Onset: 6–15 min<br>Duration: 15–75 min | Nerve block<br>Caudal<br>Epidural | Do not use with subarachnoid administration |
| dibucaine | *Nupercainal* | Onset: <15 min<br>Duration: 3–4 h | Skin disorders<br>Mucous membranes | Monitor for local reaction; advise patient to use care not to injure themselves |
| dyclonine | *Dyclone* | Onset: <10 min<br>Duration: <60 min | Mucous membranes | Used for preparation for examinations and medical procedures |
| etidocaine | *Duranest HCl* | Onset: 3–15 min<br>Duration: 2–5 h | Peripheral block OB, pelvic, abd. surgery; alveolar block | Monitor for skin breakdown; offer support for lower limb paralysis |
| lidocaine | *Dilocaine*<br>*Nervocaine*<br>*Octocaine*<br>*Solarcaine*<br>*Xylocaine* | Onset: 5–15 min<br>Duration .5–1.5 h | Caudal<br>Epidural<br>Dental<br>Spinal<br>Cervical | Caution patient to avoid injury; shorter acting than many other anesthetics |

| | | | | |
|---|---|---|---|---|
| | | | Peripheral<br>Skin<br>Mucous membranes | |
| mepivacaine | *Carbocaine*<br>*Isocaine*<br>*Polocaine* | Onset: 3–15 min<br>Duration: .75–1.5 h | Nerve block<br>OB use<br>Caudal<br>Epidural<br>Dental<br>Local infiltrate | Use caution in patients with renal impairment |
| pramoxine | *Tronothone*<br>*PrameGel*<br>*Prax*<br>*Itch-X* | Onset: 3–5 min<br>Duration: <60 min | Skin<br>Mucous membr. | Protect patient from injury; advise patient to limit use; do not cover with tight bandages |
| prilocaine | *Citanest* | Onset: 1–15 min<br>Duration: .5–3 h | Nerve block<br>Dental | Advise dental patients not to bite themselves |
| procaine | *Novocain* | Onset: 2–25 min<br>Duration: 15–75 min | Infiltration<br>Peripheral<br>Spinal | Assure patient that feeling will return; monitor skin condition; keep patient supine to avoid headache |
| ropivacaine | *Naropin* | Onset: 1–5 min<br>Duration: 2–6 h | Nerve block<br>Epidural<br>Caudal | Avoid rapid administration; offers postoperative pain management and for obsetrical procedures |
| tetracaine | *Pontocaine* | Onset: 15–30 min<br>Duration: 2–2.5 h | Spinal<br>Prolonged spinal<br>Skin | Protect patient from skin breakdown; offer reassurance with long periods of lower limb paralysis; keep patient supine to avoid headache |

# APPENDIX C

## Anorexiants

The anorexiants are primarily phenethylamines, similar to amphetamine. They act in the CNS to release norepinephrine from nerve terminals. The mechanism of action that leads to appetite-suppression is not known; they may directly stimulate the satiety center in the hypothalamus. The drugs are of limited usefulness and this fact should be weighed against the risks involved in their use.

### Indications

Exogenous obesity as short-term (8–12 week) adjunct to caloric restriction in a weight-reduction program.

### Controlled substances; Pregnancy Category C

*Contraindicated* in cases of allergy to these drugs, cardiovascular disease, hypertension, hyperthyroidism, glaucoma, history of drug abuse, diabetes mellitus, epilepsy, nursing a baby. Not recommended for children <12 yr of age.

### Adverse Effects

*Palpitations, tachycardia,* arrhythmias, dyspnea, **pulmonary hypertension,** hypertension, *overstimulation, restlessness, dizziness, insomnia, weakness, fatigue, drowsiness,* malaise, euphoria, *dry mouth, unpleasant taste, nausea,* vomiting, diarrhea, rash, menstrual irregularities, dependence.

### Clinically Important Interactions

Do not give to patients who have recently (14 days) or are now taking MAO inhibitors; use caution with anyone on antihypertensives, the effect may be blocked.

### Drug-Specific Teaching Points

Take this drug on an empty stomach, 1 h before meals; the drug can only be used for a short time and then it loses its effectiveness; take the drug early in the day to avoid interference with sleep; drug must be used in conjunction with a caloric reduction, weight loss program; avoid driving a car or operating dangerous machinery when on this drug, drug causes drowsiness; do not become pregnant while taking this drug, drug can harm the fetus; report nervousness, palpitations, chest pain, dizziness, bruising, sore throat.

| Drug | Brand Names | Dosage | Special Considerations |
|---|---|---|---|
| benzphetamine hydrochloride | Didrex | 25–50 mg PO qd | C-III controlled substance |
| diethylpropion hydrochloride | *Nobesin* (CAN)<br>*Propiont* (CAN)<br>*Regibon* (CAN)<br>*Tenuate* | 25 mg PO tid; sustained capsules—75 mg qd PO in AM | Do not chew or crush sustained release tablets. Eye pain is common, advise the use of sunglasses in bright light. C-IV controlled substance |
| mazindol | *Mazanor*<br>*Sanorex* | 1 mg PO tid 1 h before meals or 2 mg PO qd, 1 h before lunch | Eye pain common—advise the use of sunglasses in bright light. Headache—analgesics may help. C-IV controlled substance |

*(continued)*

| Drug | Brand Names | Dosage | Special Considerations |
|---|---|---|---|
| phendimetrazine titrate | *Adipost*<br>*Bontril*<br>*Dital*<br>*Melfiat-105*<br>*Dyrexan-OD*<br>*Plegine*<br>*Pre-lu 2*<br>*Rexigen Forte* | 35 mg PO tid; sustained release—105 mg PO qd in AM | Eye pain common—advise the use of sunglasses in bright light; headache—analgesics may help. C-III controlled substance |
| phentermine hydrochloride | *Adipex-P*<br>*Fastin*<br>*Ionamin*<br>*Obe-Nix*<br>*Obephen* | 8 mg PO tid, ½ h before meals; or 15–37.5 mg PO qd as a single daily dose in the AM | Drug is most effective ½ h before meals; eye pain common—advise the use of sunglasses in bright light; headache—analgesics may be helpful. C-IV controlled substance |

# APPENDIX D

## Chemotherapeutic Regimens

Combinations of therapeutic agents are preferable to single agents in the management of many diseases, leading to higher response rates and increased duration of remissions. Common combinations are based on drug action, cell site specificity, responsiveness, and toxic effects.

| *Regimen* | *Use* | *Drugs used* |
|---|---|---|
| ABV | Kaposi's sarcoma | doxorubicin, 40 mg/m$^2$/day IV, day 1<br>bleomycin, 15 units/m$^2$/day IV, day 1 & 15<br>vinblastine, 6 mg/m$^2$/day IV, day 1<br>Repeat every 28 days |
| ABVD | Hodgkin's disease | doxorubicin 25 mg/m$^2$/day IV days 1 and 15<br>bleomycin 10 units/m$^2$/day IV days 1 and 15<br>vinblastine a6 mg/m$^2$/day IV days 1 and 15 with<br>dacarbazine 350–375 mg/m$^2$/day IV days 1 and 15 *or*<br>dacarbazine 150 mg/m$^2$/day IV, days 1–5 |
| AC | Breast cancer | doxorubicin, 75–90 mg/m$^2$ IV, day 1<br>cyclophosphamide, 400–600 mg/m$^2$ IV, day 1<br>Repeat every 21 days. |
| | Sarcoma | doxorubicin, 75–90 mg/m$^2$ IV total infusion over 96 h<br>cisplatin, 90–120 mg/m$^2$ IV, day 6<br>Repeat every 28 days |
| ACe | Breast cancer, metastatic or recurrent disease | cyclophosphamide 200 mg/m$^2$/day PO days 1–3 or 3–6<br>doxorubicin 40 mg/m$^2$ IV day 1<br>Repeat every 21 or 28 days |
| ADIC | Sarcoma | doxorubicin, 45–60 mg/m$^2$ IV, day 1<br>dacarbaazine, 200–250 mg/m$^2$ IV, days 1–15<br>Repeat every 21 days |
| AP | Ovarion, endometrial cancer | doxorubicin, 50–60 mg/m$^2$ IV, day 1<br>cisplatin, 50–60 mg/m$^2$ IV, day 1<br>Repeat every 21 days |
| BCVPP | Hodgkin's disease induction | carmustine 100 mg/m$^2$ IV day 1<br>cyclophosphamide 600 mg/m$^2$ IV day 1<br>vinblastine 5 mg/m$^2$ IV day 1<br>procarbazine 50 mg/m$^2$/day PO day 1<br>procarbazine 100 mg/m$^2$/day PO days 2–10<br>prednisone 60 mg/m$^2$/day PO days 1–10<br>Repeat every 28 days |

*(continued)*

| Regimen | Use | Drugs used |
|---|---|---|
| BEP | Testicular cancer | bleomycin, 30 units IV, days 2, 9, 18<br>etoposide, 100 mg/m$^2$ IV, days 1–15<br>cisplatin, 20 mg/m$^2$ IV, days 1–5<br>Repeat every 21 days |
| BIP | Cervical cancer | bleomycin, 30 units Cl, day 1<br>ifosfamide, 5 g/m$^2$ Cl, day 2<br>cisplatin, 50 mg/m$^2$ IV, day 2<br>mesna 8 g/m$^2$ over 36 h with ifosfamide, day 2<br>Repeat every 21 days |
| BOMP | Cervical cancer | bleomycin, 10 units IM weekly<br>vincristine, 1 mg/m$^2$ IV, days 1, 8, 22, 29<br>cisplatin, 50 mg/m$^2$ IV, days 1 and 22<br>mitomycin, 10 mg/m$^2$ IV day 1<br>Cycle every 6 weeks |
| CAE | Lung cancer | cyclophosphamide 1 g/m$^2$ IV, day 1<br>doxorubicin, 45 mg/m$^2$ IV, day 1<br>etoposide, 50 mg/m$^2$ IV, days 1–5<br>Repeat every 21 days |
| CAF | Breast cancer, metastatic disease | cyclophosphamide 100 mg/m$^2$/day PO days 1–14<br>*or* cylcophosphamide 400–600 mg/m$^2$ IV, day 1<br>doxorubicin 40–60 mg/m$^2$ IV, day 1<br>fluorouracil 400–600 mg/m$^2$ IV, day 1<br>Repeat every 21 days |
| CAL-G | Acute lymphocytic leukemia | cylophosphamide 1.2 g IV, day 1<br>daunorubicin, 45 mg/m$^2$ IV, days 1–3<br>vincristine, 2 mg IV, days 1, 8, 15, 22<br>prednisone 60 mg/m$^2$/d PO days 1–21<br>with asparaginase 6000 units/m$^2$/IV days 5, 8, 11, 15, 21 *or* pegaspargase 2500 units/m$^2$ IM or IV every other week |
| CAMP | Lung cancer | cyclophosphamide 300 mg/m$^2$/day IV days 1 and 8<br>doxorubicin 20 mg/m$^2$/day IV days 1 and 8<br>methotrexate 15 mg/m$^2$/day IV days 1 and 8<br>Procarbazine 100 mg/m$^2$/day PO days 1–10<br>Repeat every 28 days |
| CAP | Non-small cell carcinoma of the lung | cyclophosphamide 400 mg/m$^2$ IV day 1<br>doxorubicin 40 mg/m$^2$ IV, day 1<br>cisplatin 60 mg/m$^2$ IV, day 1<br>Repeat every 28 days |
| CAV | Small cell lung cancer | cyclophosphamide, 750–1000 mg/m$^2$ IV day 1<br>doxorubicin 40–50 mg/m$^2$ IV day 1<br>vincristine 1.4 mg/m$^2$ IV day 1<br>Repeat every 28 days |

*(continued)*

| *Regimen* | *Use* | *Drugs used* |
|---|---|---|
| CAVE | Small cell lung cancer | Add to CAV regimen:<br>etoposide 60–100 mg/m$^2$ IV, days 1–5 |
| CC | Ovarian cancer | cisplatin 300–350 mg/m$^2$ IV, day 1<br>cyclophosphamide 600 mg/m$^2$ IV, day 1<br>Repeat every 28 days |
| CDDP/VP | Pediatric brain tumors | cisplatin 90 mg/m$^2$ IV, day 1<br>etoposide 150 mg/m$^2$ IV, days 2 and 3 |
| CEV | Small cell lung cancer | cyclophosphamide 1 g/m$^2$ IV, day 1<br>etoposide 50 mg/m$^2$ IV, day 1<br>etoposide 100 mg/m$^2$/d PO, days 2–5<br>vincristine 1.4 mg/m$^2$ IV, day 1<br>Repeat every 21 to 28 days |
| CF | Adenocarcinoma, head and neck cancer | cisplatin 100 mg/m$^2$ IV, day 1<br>fluouracil 1 g/m$^2$/d Cl, days 1 through 4 or 5<br>Repeat every 21 to 28 days |
| CF | Head and neck cancer | carboplatin 400 mg/m$^2$ IV, day 1<br>fluouracil 1 g/m$^2$/d Cl, days 1 through 4 or 5<br>Repeat every 21 to 28 days |
| CFM (CNF/FNC) | Breast cancer | cyclophosphamide 500 mg/m$^2$ IV, day 1<br>fluouracil 500 mg/m$^2$ IV, day 1<br>mitoxantrone 10 mg/m$^2$ IV, day 1<br>Repeat every 21 days |
| CHAP | Ovarian cancer | cyclophosphamide 150 mg/m$^2$/d PO days 2–8<br>*or*<br>cyclophosphamide 300–500 mg/m$^2$/d PO day 1 with<br>altretamine 150 mg/m$^2$/d PO days 2–8<br>doxorubicin 30 mg/m$^2$ IV, day 1<br>cisplatin 50–60 mg/m$^2$ IV, day 1 |
| ChiVPP | Hodgkin's lymphoma | chlorambucil 6 mg/m$^2$/d PO days 1–14<br>vinblastine 6 mg/m$^2$ IV, days 1 and 8<br>procarbazine 100 mg/m$^2$/d PO days 1–14<br>prednison 40 mg/m2/d PO days 1–14<br>Repeat every 28 days |
| ChiVPP/EVA | Hodgkin's lymphoma | Use ChiVPP: chlorambucil, procarbazine and prednisone days 1–7 only; vinblastine day 1 only<br>etoposide 200 mg/m$^2$ IV, day 8<br>vincristine 2 mg IV, day 8<br>doxorubicin 50 mg/m$^2$ IV, day 8<br>Repeat every 21 to 28 days |
| CHOP | Non-Hodgkin's lymphoma | cyclophosphamide 750 mg/m$^2$ IV, day 1<br>doxorubicin 50 mg/m$^2$ IV, day 1<br>vincristine 1.4 mg/m$^2$ IV, day 1<br>prednisone 100 mg/day PO, days 1–5<br>Repeat every 21 days |
| CHOP-BLEO | Non-Hodgkin's lymphoma | Add to CHOP: bleomycin, 15 units/day IV, days 1–5 |

*(continued)*

| *Regimen* | *Use* | *Drugs used* |
|---|---|---|
| CISCA | Bladder cancer | cyclophosphamide 650 mg/m$^2$ IV day 1<br>doxorubicin 50 mg/m$^2$ IV day 1<br>cisplatin 70–100 mg/m$^2$ IV, day 2<br>Repeat every 21 to 28 days |
| CISCA/VBiv | Germ cell tumors, advanced | cyclophosphamide 1 g/m$^2$ IV days 1 and 2<br>doxorubicin 80–90 mg/m$^2$ IV days 1 and 2<br>cisplatin 100–120 mg/m$^2$ IV day 3<br>alternating with vinblastine 3 mg/m$^2$ Cl days 1–5<br>bleomycin 30 units/day Cl, days 1–5 |
| CMF | Breast cancer, metastatic or recurrent disease | cyclophosphamide 100 mg/m$^2$/day PO days 1–14<br>*or* cyclophosphamide 400–600 mg/m$^2$ IV, day 1 with:<br>methotrexate 40–60 mg/m$^2$/day IV, day 1<br>fluorouracil 400–600 mg/m$^2$/day IV, day 1<br>Repeat every 21 to 28 days |
| CMFP | Breast cancer, metastatic disease | cyclophosphamide 100 mg/m$^2$/day PO days 1–14<br>methotrexate 30–60 mg/m$^2$/day IV days 1 and 8<br>fluououracil 400–700 mg/m$^2$/day IV days 1 and 8<br>prednisone 40 mg/m$^2$/day PO days 1–14<br>Repeat every 28 days |
| CMFVP | Breast cancer, metastatic or recurrent disease | Add to CMF:<br>vincristine 1 mg IV days 1 and 8<br>prednisone 20–40 mg/d PO days 1–7 or 14<br>Repeat every 21 to 28 days |
| CMV | Bladder cancer | cisplatin 100 mg/m$^2$ IV, day 1<br>methotrexate 30 mg/m$^2$ IV, days 1 and 8<br>vinblastine 4 mg/m$^2$ IV, days 1 and 8 |
| COB | Head and neck cancer | cisplatin 100 mg/m$^2$ IV, day 1<br>vincristine 1 mg IV, days 2 and 5<br>bleomycin 30 units/day Cl, days 2–5<br>Repeat every 21 days |
| CODE | Small cell lung cancer | cisplatin 25 mg/m$^2$ IV q wk for 9 weeks<br>vincristine 1 mg/m$^2$ IV weeks 1, 2, 4, 6, 8<br>doxorubicin 25 mg/m$^2$ IV weeks 1, 3, 5, 7, 9<br>etoposide 80 mg/m$^2$ IV, weeks 1, 3, 5, 7, 9 |
| COMLA | Non-Hodgkin's lymphoma | cyclophosphamide 1.5 mg/m$^2$ IV day 1<br>vincristine 1.4 mg/m$^2$ IV days 1, 8, 15<br>cytarabine 300 mg/m$^2$ IV days 22, 29, 36, 43, 50, 57, 64 and 71<br>methotrexate 120 mg/m$^2$ IV days 22, 29, 36, 43, 50, 57, 64 and 71<br>leucovorin 25 mg/m$^2$ PO q6h ×4 beginning 24h after methotrexate<br>Cycle every 13 weeks |

*(continued)*

| *Regimen* | *Use* | *Drugs used* |
|---|---|---|
| COMP | Pediatric Hodgkin's lymphoma | cyclophosphamide 500 mg/m$^2$ IV days 1 and 15<br>vincristine 1.4 mg/m$^2$ IV days 1 and 3<br>methotrexate 40 mg/m$^2$ IV days 1 and 2<br>prednisone 40 mg/m$^2$/d PO days 1–15 |
| COP | Non-Hodgkin's lymphoma with favorable histology | cyclophosphamide 400–1000 mg/m$^2$ IV day 1<br>vincristine 1.4 mg/m$^2$ IV day 1<br>prednisone 60 mg/m$^2$/day PO days 1–5<br>Repeat every 21 days |
| COPE | Small cell lung cancer | cyclophosphamide 750 mg/m$^2$ IV, day 1<br>vincristine 1.4 mg/m$^2$ IV, day 3<br>cisplatin 20 mg/m$^2$ IV days 1–3<br>etoposide 100 mg/m$^2$ IV, days 1–3<br>Repeat every 21 days |
| COPP or "C" MOPP | Non-Hodgkin's lymphoma, lymphomas with unfavorable histology, Hodgkin's disease | cyclophosphamide 500–650 mg/m$^2$/day IV days 1 and 8<br>vincristine 1.4 mg/m$^2$/day IV days 1 and 8<br>procarbazine 100 mg/m$^2$/day PO days 1–14<br>prednisone 40 mg/m$^2$/day PO days 1–14<br>Repeat every 28 days |
| CP | Chronic lymphocytic leukemia | chlorambucil 0.4 mg/kg/d PO day 1<br>prednisone 100 mg/d PO days 1 and 7 |
| | Ovarian cancer | cyclophosphamide 600–1000 mg/m$^2$ IV, day 1<br>cisplatin 50–100 mg/m$^2$ IV, day 1<br>Repeat every 28 days |
| CT | Ovarian cancer | cisplatin 75 mg/m$^2$ IV, day 1<br>paclitaxel 135 mg/m$^2$ IV, day 1<br>Repeat every 21 days |
| CVD | Malignant melanoma | cisplatin 20 mg/m$^2$ IV, days 1–5<br>vinblastine 1.6 mg/m$^2$ IV days 1–3<br>dacarbazine 800 mg/m$^2$ IV, day 1<br>Repeat every 21 days |
| CVI (VIC) | Lung cancer | carboplatin 300 mg/m$^2$ IV, day 1<br>etoposide 60–100 mg/m$^2$ IV, days 1, 3, 5<br>ifosfamide 1.5 g/m$^2$ IV, days 1, 3, 5<br>mesna 400 mg IV bolus, then 1600 mg over 24h, days 1, 3, 5<br>Repeat every 28 days |
| CVP | Non-Hodgkin's lymphoma, lymphomas with favorable histology | cyclophosphamide 400 mg/m$^2$/day PO days 1–5<br>vincristine 1.4 mg/m$^2$ IV day 1<br>prednisone 100 mg/m$^2$/day PO days 1–6<br>Repeat every 21 days |
| CVPP | Hodgkin's lymphoma | lomustine 75 mg/m$^2$ PO day 1<br>vinblastine 4 mg/m$^2$ IV, days 1 and 8<br>procarbazine 100 mg/m$^2$/d PO days 1–14<br>prednisone 30 mg/m$^2$/d PO days 1–14<br>Repeat every 21 days |

*(continued)*

| Regimen | Use | Drugs used |
|---|---|---|
| CY-VA-DIC | Soft tissue sarcomas, adult sarcomas | cyclophosphamide 400–600 $mg/m^2$ IV day 1<br>vincristine 1.4 $mg/m^2$/day IV days 1 and 5<br>doxorubicin 40–50 $mg/m^2$ IV day 1<br>dacarbazine 200–250 $mg/m^2$ IV, days 1–5<br>Repeat every 21 days |
| DA | AML, pediatric induction | daunorubicin 45–60 $mg/m^2$ IV Cl, days 1–3<br>cytarabine 100 $mg/m^2$ IV q12h for 5–7 days |
| DAL | AML pediatric induction | cytarabine 3 $gm/m^2$ IV q12h days 1–3<br>daunorubicin 45 $mg/m^2$ IV days 1 and 2<br>asparaginase 6000 units/$m^2$ IV day 3 |
| DAT | AML pediatric induction | daunorubicin 45 $mg/m^2$ Cl days 1–3<br>cytarabine 100 $mg/m^2$ Cl days 1–7<br>thioguanine 100 $mg/m^2$ Cl days 1–7 |
| DAV | AML pediatric induction | daunorubicin 60 $mg/m^2$ IV days 1–3<br>cytarabine 200 $mg/m^2$ Cl, days 1–5<br>etoposide 200 $mg/m^2$ Cl, days 5–7 |
| DCT (DAT, TAD) | Adult AML induction | daunorubicin 60 $mg/m^2$ IV, days 1–3<br>cytarabine 200 $mg/m^2$/d Cl days 1–5<br>thioguanine 100 $mg/m^2$ PO q12 h days 1–5 |
| DHAP | Non-Hodgkin's lymphoma | cisplatin 100 $mg/m^2$ Cl over 24 on day 1<br>cytarabine 2 $g/m^2$ IN q12h for 2 doses, day 2<br>dexamethasone 40 mg/d PO or IV days 1–4<br>Repeat every 21 to 28 days |
| DI | Soft tissue sarcoma | doxorubicin 50 $mg/m^2$ IV Cl, day 1<br>ifosfamide 5 $g/m^2$ Cl, day 1<br>mesna 600 $mg/m^2$ bolus, then 2.5 $g/m^2$/d Cl<br>Repeat every 21 days |
| DVP | ALL adult induction | daunorubicin 45 $mg/m^2$ IV, days 1–3 and 14<br>vincristine 2 mg IV weekly for 4 wk<br>prednisone 45 $mg/m^2$/d PO for 28–35 days |
| | ALL pediatric induction | daunorubicin 25 $mg/m^2$ IV days 1 and 8<br>vincristine 1.5 $mg/m^2$ IV, days 1, 8, 15, 22<br>prednisone 40 mg/m2 PO days 1–29 |
| EAP | Gastric, small bowel cancer | etoposide 120 $mg/m^2$ IV, days 4–6<br>doxorubicin 20 $mg/m^2$ IV, days 1 and 7<br>cisplatin 40 $mg/m^2$ IV, days 2 and 8<br>Repeat every 21 to 28 days |
| EC | Small cell lung cancer | etoposide 60–100 $mg/m^2$ IV, days 1–3<br>with carboplatin 400 $mg/m^2$ IV, day 1<br>*or* carboplatin 100–125 $mg/m^2$ IV days 1–3<br>Repeat every 28 days |
| EFP | Gastric, small bowel cancer | etoposide 90 $mg/m^2$ IV, days 1, 3, 5<br>fluouracil 900 $mg/m^2$/d Cl, days 1–5<br>cisplatin 20 $mg/m^2$ IV, days 1–5 |

*(continued)*

| *Regimen* | *Use* | *Drugs used* |
|---|---|---|
| ELF | Gastric cancer | etoposide 120 mg/m$^2$ IV, days 1–3<br>leucovorin 150–300 mg/m$^2$ IV, days 1–3<br>fluouracil 500 mg/m$^2$ IV, days 1–3<br>Repeat every 21 to 28 days |
| EMA 86 | AML adult induction | mitoxatrone 12 mg/m$^2$ IV, days 1–3<br>etoposide 200 mg/m$^2$/d Cl days 8–10<br>cytarabine 500 mg/m$^2$/d Cl, days 1–3 and 8–10 |
| EP | Adenocarcinoma | etoposide 75–100 mg/m$^2$ IV, days 1–3<br>cisplatin 75–100 mg/m$^2$ IV, day 1<br>Repeat every 21 days |
| ESHAP | Non-Hodgkin's lymphoma | methylprednisolone 500 mg/d IV, days 1–4<br>etoposide 40–60 mg/m$^2$ IV, days 1–4<br>cytarabine 2 g/m$^2$ IV, day 5<br>cisplatin 25 mg/m$^2$/d Cl, days 1–4<br>Repeat every 21–28 days |
| EVA | Hodgkin's lymphoma | etoposide 100 mg/m$^2$ IV, days 1–3<br>vinblastine 6 mg/m$^2$ IV, day 1<br>doxorubicin 50 mg/m$^2$ IV, day 1<br>Repeat every 28 days |
| FAC | Breast cancer, metastatic disease | fluorouracil 500 mg/m$^2$/day IV day 1 and bolus on days 4, 5, 8<br>doxorubicin 50 mg/m$^2$ Cl over 48–96 h starting on day 1<br>cyclophosphamide 500 mg/m$^2$ IV, day 1<br>Repeat every 21 days |
| FAM | Gastric carcinoma, adenocarcinoma | fluorouracil 600 mg/m$^2$/day IV days 1, 8, 29, 36<br>doxorubicin 30 mg/m$^2$/day IV days 1 and 29<br>mitomycin 10 mg/m$^2$ IV day 1<br>Repeat every 8 weeks |
| FAMe | Gastric cancer | fluouracil 350 mg/m$^2$ IV, days 1–5, 36–40<br>doxorubicin 40 mg/m$^2$ IV, days 1 and 36<br>semustine 150 mg/m$^2$/d PO day 1<br>Repeat every 10 weeks |
| FAMTX | Gastric cancer | fluouracil 1.5 mg/m$^2$ IV, day 1<br>doxorubicin 30 mg/m$^2$ IV, day 15<br>methotrexate, 1.5 g/m$^2$, IV day 1<br>leucovorin 20–25 mg PO q6h for 8 doses, 24 h after MTX<br>Repeat every 28 days |
| FAP | Gastric cancer | fluouracil 300 mg/m$^2$ IV, days 1–5<br>doxorubicin 40 mg/m$^2$ IV, day 1<br>cisplatin 60 mg/m$^2$ IV, day 1 |
| F-CL(FU/LV) | Colorectal cancer | fluouracil 600 mg/m$^2$ IV, weekly for 6 wk<br>leucovorin 500 mg/m$^2$ IV weekly for 6 wk<br>*or*<br>fluouracil 370–600 mg/m$^2$ IV, or Cl, days 1–5<br>leucovorin 20 mg/m$^2$ IV or Cl, days 1–5<br>Repeat every 6–8 weeks |

*(continued)*

| *Regimen* | *Use* | *Drugs used* |
|---|---|---|
| FED | Lung cancer | fluouracil 960 mg/m$^2$ Cl, days 2–4<br>etoposide 80 mg/m$^2$ IV, days 2–4<br>cisplatin 100 mg/m$^2$ IV, day 1<br>Repeat every 21 days |
| FL | Prostate cancer | flutamide 250 mg PO q8h<br>with leuprolide acetate 1 mg SC daily<br>*or* leuprolide depot 7.5 mg IM q 28 d<br>Repeat every 28 days |
| Fle | Colorectal cancer | fluouracil 450 mg/m$^2$ IV, days 1–5 and 28, weekly thereafter<br>levamisole 50 mg PO q8h days 1–3 and q2wk for 1 y |
| FZ | Prostate cancer | flutamide 250 mg PO q8h<br>goserelin acetate 3.6 mg implant SC q28 days |
| HDMTX | Sarcoma | methotrexate 8–12 g/m$^2$ IV, day 1<br>leucovorin 15 mg/m$^2$ IV PO or IV q6h for 10 doses 30 h after beginning of methotrexate infusion<br>Repeat every 2–4 weeks |
| IE | Sarcoma | ifosfamide 1.8 g/m$^2$ IV, days 1–5<br>etoposide 100 mg/m$^2$ IV, days 1–5<br>mesna 20% of ifosfamide dose, prior to and then 4 and 8 h after ifosfamide<br>Repeat every 21 days |
| IfoVP | Sarcoma, pediatric | ifosfamide 2 g/m$^2$ IV days 1–3<br>etoposide 100 mg/m$^2$ IV, days 1–3<br>mesna 2 g/m$^2$ IV days 1–3 |
| M-2 | Multiple myeloma | vincristine 0.03 mg/kg IV day 1<br>carmustine 0.5–1 mg/kg IV, day 1<br>cyclophosphamide 10 mg/kg IV day 1<br>melphalan 0.25 mg/kg/d PO, days 1–4<br>prednisone 1 mg/kg/d PO days 1–7, tapered over next 14 days<br>Repeat every 5 weeks |
| MACOP-8 | Lymphoma | methotrexate 400 mg/m$^2$ IV, week 2, 6, 10<br>leucovorin 15 mg PO q6h for 6 doses, 24 h after methotrexate<br>doxorubicin 50 mg/m$^2$ IV weeks 1, 3, 5, 7, 9, 11<br>cyclophosphamide 350 mg/m$^2$ IV weeks 1, 3, 5, 7, 9, 11<br>vincristine 1.4 mg/m$^2$ IV, weeks 2, 4, 6, 8, 10, 12<br>bleomycin 10 units/m$^2$ IV weeks 4, 8, 12<br>prednisone 75 mg/d PO for 12 wks tapered over last 2 wk |
| MAID | Sarcoma | mesna 1.5–2.5 mg/m$^2$ IV, days 1–4<br>doxorubicin 15–20 mg/m$^2$/d Cl days 1–3<br>ifosfamide 1.5–2.5 g/m$^2$/d Cl, days 1–3<br>dacarbazine 250–300 mg/m$^2$/d Cl days 1–3<br>Repeat every 21 to 28 days |

*(continued)*

| *Regimen* | *Use* | *Drugs used* |
|---|---|---|
| m-BACOD | Non-Hodgkin's lymphoma | methotrexate 200 mg/m² IV, days 8 and 15<br>leucovorin 10 mg/m² PO q6h for 8 doses starting 24h after methorexate<br>bleomycin 4 units/m² IV, day 1<br>cyclophsphamide 600 mg/m² IV, day 1<br>vincristine 1 mg/m² IV, day 1<br>dexamethasone 6 mg/m²/d PO days 1–15<br>Repeat every 27 days |
| M-BACOD | Non-Hodgkin's lymphoma | See m-BACOD, except:<br>methotrexate 3 g/m² IV, day 14 |
| MBC | Head and neck cancer | methotrexate 40 mg/m² IV, days 1 and 15<br>bleomycin 10 units/m² IM or IV, days 1, 8, 15<br>cisplatin 50 mg/m² IV, day 4<br>Repeat every 21 days |
| MC | AML, adult induction | mitoxantrone 12 mg/m² IV, days 1–3<br>cytarabine 100–200 mg/m²/d Cl, days 1–7 |
| MF | Breast cancer | methotrexate 100 mg/m² IV, days 1 and 8<br>fluouracil 600 mg/m² IV days 1 and 8, given 1 h after methotrexate<br>leucovorin 10 mg/m² IV or PO q6h for 6 doses 24h after methotrexate |
| MICE (ICE) | Sarcoma, lung cancer | mesna 20% ifosfamide dose IV before and every 4 and 8 h after ifosfamide<br>ifosfamide 2 g/m² IV, days 1–3<br>carboplatin 300–600 mg/m² IV, day 1 or 3<br>etoposide 80–100 mg/m² IV, days 1–3<br>Repeat every 28 days |
| MINE-ESHAP | Hodgkin's lymphoma | mesna 1.33 g/m² IV, days 1–3<br>mesna 500 mg PO 4h after ifosfamide<br>ifosfamide 1.33 g/m² IV, days 1–3<br>mitoxantrone 8 mg/m² IV, day 1<br>etoposide 65 mg/m² IV, days 1–3<br>Repeat for 6 cycles, then give ESHAP for 3–6 cycles |
| mini-BEAM | Hodgkin's lymphoma | carmustine 60 mg/m² IV, day 1<br>etoposide 75 mg/m² IV days 2–5<br>cytarabine 100 mg/m² IV q12h days 2–5<br>melphalan 30 mg/m² IV, day 6<br>Repeat every 4–7 weeks |
| MIV | Non-Hodgkin's lymphoma | mitoxantrone 10 mg/m² IV, day 1<br>ifosfamide 1.5 g/m² IV, days 1–3 with mesna<br>etoposide 150 mg/m² IV, days 1–3<br>Repeat every 21 days |
| MOP | Pediatric brain tumors | See MOPP, without prednisone |
| MOPP | Hodgkin's disease, induction | mechlorethamine 6 mg/m² IV days 1 and 8<br>vincristine 1.4 mg/m²/IV days 1 and 8<br>procarbazine 100 mg/m²/day PO days 1–14<br>prednisone 40 mg/m²/day PO days 1–14<br>Repeat every 28 days |

*(continued)*

| *Regimen* | *Use* | *Drugs used* |
|---|---|---|
| MOPP/ABV | Hodgkin's disease advanced | mechlorethamine 6 mg/m$^2$ IV, day 1<br>vincristine 1.4 mg/m$^2$ IV, day 1<br>procarbazine 100 mg/m$^2$/day PO days 1–7<br>prednisone 40 mg/m$^2$/day PO days 1–14<br>alternating every other month with:<br>bleomycin 10 mg/m$^2$ IV day 8<br>vinblastine 6 mg/m$^2$ IV day 8<br>doxorubicin 35 mg/m$^2$ IV, day 8<br>Repeat every 28 days |
| MOPP/ABVD | Hodgkin's lymphoma | Alternate MOPP and ABDV regimens every month |
| MP | Multiple myeloma | melphalan 8–10 mg/m$^2$/d PO days 1–4<br>prednisone 40–60 mg/m$^2$/d, days 1–7<br>Repeat every 28 days |
| MTXCP-PDAdr | Osteosarcoma, pediatric | methotrexate 12 g/m$^2$ IV, days 1 and 8<br>leucovorin 15 mg/m$^2$ PO or IV q6h for 10 doses, 30 h after beginning of methotrexate infusion<br>cisplatin 100 mg/m$^2$ IV, day 1<br>doxorubicin 37.5 mg/m$^2$ IV, days 2 and 3 |
| MV | Breast cancer | mitomycin 20 mg/m$^2$ IV, day 1<br>vinblastine 0.15 mg/m$^2$ IV, days 1 and 21<br>Repeat every 6–8 weeks |
| M-VAC | Transitional cell carcinoma of the bladder | methotrexate 30 mg/m$^2$ IV days 1, 15, 22<br>vinblastine 3 mg/m$^2$ IV days 2, 15, 22<br>doxorubicin 30 mg/m$^2$ IV day 2<br>cisplatin 70 mg/m$^2$ IV day 2<br>Repeat every 28 days |
| MVP | Lung cancer | mitomycin 8 mg/m$^2$ IV, days 1, 29, 71<br>vinblastine 4.5 mg/m$^2$ IV, days 15, 22, 29, then every 2 wk<br>cisplatin 70 mg/m$^2$ IV, day 2<br>Repeat every 28 days |
| MVPP | Hodgkin's lymphoma | mechlorethamine 6 mg/m$^2$ IV, days 1 and 8<br>vinblastine 6 mg/m$^2$ IV, days 1 and 8<br>procarbazine 100 mg/m$^2$/d PO days 1–14<br>prednisone 40 mg/m$^2$/d PO days 1–14<br>Repeat every 4–6 weeks |
| NFL | Breast cancer | mitoxantrone 12 mg/m$^2$ IV, day 1<br>fluouracil 350 mg/m$^2$ IV, days 1–3 after leucovorin<br>leucovorin 300 mg IV days 1–3<br>*or*<br>mitoxantrone 10 mg/m$^2$ IV, day 1<br>fluouracil 1 g/m$^2$/d Cl, days 1–3<br>leucovorin 100 mg/m$^2$ IV, days 1–3<br>Repeat every 21 days |
| NOVP | Hodgkin's lymphoma | mitoxantrone 10 mg/m$^2$ IV, day 1<br>vincristine 2 mg IV, day 8<br>vinblastine 6 mg/m$^2$ IV, day 1<br>prednisone 100 mg/d PO, days 1–5<br>Repeat every 21 days |

*(continued)*

| *Regimen* | *Use* | *Drugs used* |
|---|---|---|
| OPA | Hodgkin's lymphoma, ped. | vincristine 1.5 mg/m$^2$ IV, days 1, 8, 15<br>prednisone 60 mg/m$^2$ IV, days 1–15<br>doxorubicin 40 mg/m$^2$ IV, days 1 and 15 |
| OPPA | Hodgkin's lymphoma | Add to OPA:<br>procarbazine 100 mg/m$^2$/d PO, days 1–15 |
| PAC | Ovarian, endometrial cancer | cisplatin 50–60 mg/m$^2$ IV, day 1<br>doxorubicin 45–50 mg/m$^2$ IV, day 1<br>cyclophosphamide 600 mg/m$^2$ IV, day 1<br>Repeat every 21 to 28 days |
| PC | Lung cancer | paclitaxel 135 mg/m$^2$/d Cl, day 1<br>carboplatin dose by Calvert equation to AUC 7.5, day 1<br>Repeat every 21 days |
| PCV | Brain tumor | lomustine 110 mg/m$^2$/d PO, day 1<br>procarbazine 60 mg/m$^2$/d PO, days 8–21<br>vincristine 1.4 mg/m$^2$ IV, days 8 and 28<br>Repeat every 6–8 weeks |
| PFL | Head and neck, gastric cancer | cisplatin 25 mg/m$^2$/d Cl, days 1–5<br>fluouracil 800 mg/m$^2$/d Cl, days 2–5 or 6<br>leucovorin 500 mg/m$^2$/d Cl, days 1–5 or 6<br>Repeat every 28 days |
| POC | Pediatric brain tumors | prednisone 40 mg/m$^2$/d PO, days 1–14<br>methyl-CCNU 100 mg/m$^2$/d PO, day 2<br>vincristine 1.5 mg/m$^2$ IV, days 1, 8, 15<br>Repeat every 6 weeks |
| ProMACE/cytaBOM | Non-Hodgkin's lymphoma | prednisone 60 mg/m$^2$ PO, days 1–14<br>doxorubicin 25 mg/m$^2$ IV, day 1<br>cyclophosphamide 650 mg/m$^2$ IV, day 1<br>etoposide 120 mg/m$^2$ IV, day 1<br>cytarabine 300 mg/m$^2$ IV, day 8<br>bleomycin 5 units/m$^2$ IV, day 8<br>vincristine 1.4 mg/m$^2$ IV, day 8<br>mitoxantrone 120 mg/m$^2$ IV, day 8<br>leucovorin 25 mg/m$^2$ PO q6h for 6 doses, 24 h after methotrexate |
| ProMACE | Hodgkin's lymphoma | prednisone 60 mg/m$^2$/d PO, days 1–14<br>methotrexate 1.5 mg/m$^2$ IV, day 14<br>leucovorin 50 mg/m$^2$ IV, q6h for 6 doses, 24 hours after methotrexate<br>doxorubicin 25 mg/m$^2$ IV, days 1 and 8<br>cyclophosphamide 650 mg/m$^2$ IV, days 1 and 8<br>etoposide 120 mg/m$^2$ IV, days 1 and 8 |
| ProMACE/MOPP | Hodgkin's lymphoma | Repeat ProMACE for prescribed cycles, then begin MOPP |
| PVB | Testicular carcinoma, adenocarcinoma | cisplatin 20 mg/m$^2$/day IV, days 1–5<br>vinblastine 0.15–0.4 mg/kg IV day 1± day 20<br>bleomycin 30 units IV day 1 or day 2 weekly<br>Repeat every 21 to 28 days |

*(continued)*

| Regimen | Use | Drugs used |
|---|---|---|
| PVDA | ALL, pediatric induction | Add to VDA: prednisone 40 mg/m²/d PO days 1–29 |
| PVP-16 | Lung cancer | cisplatin 60–120 mg/m² IV, day 1<br>etoposide 50–120 mg/m² IV, days 1–3<br>Repeat every 21 to 28 days |
| Stanford V | Hodgkin's lymphoma | mechlorethamine 6 mg/m² IV, weeks 1, 5, 9<br>doxorubicin 25 mg/m² IV, weeks 1, 3, 5, 7, 9, 11<br>vinblastine 6 mg/m2 IV, weeks 1, 3, 5, 7, 9, 11<br>vincristine 1.4 mg/m2 IV, weeks 2, 4, 6, 8, 10, 12<br>bleomycin 5 units/m² IV weeks 2, 4, 6, 8, 10, 12<br>etoposide 60 mg/m² IV, days 1 and 2 in weeks 3, 7<br>prednisone 40 mg/m²/d PO qod, taper last 15 days |
| VAC Pulse | Soft tissue sarcomas | vincristine 2 mg/m²/week IV for 12 weeks<br>dactinomycin 0.015 mg/kg/day IV days 1–5, week 1 and 13<br>cyclophosphamide 10 mg/kg/day IV or PO for 7 days<br>Repeat every 6 weeks |
| VAC Standard | Soft tissue sarcomas | vincristine 2 mg/m²/week IV, weeks 1–12<br>dactinomycin 0.015 mg/kg/day IV days 1–5, every 3 months<br>cyclophosphamide 2.5 mg/kg/day PO for 2 years |
| VACAdr-IfoVP | Sarcoma, pediatric | vincristine 1.5 mg/m² IV days 1, 8, 15<br>dactinomycin 1.5 mg/m² IV every other week<br>doxorubicin 60 mg/m² Cl, day 1<br>cyclophosphamide 1–1.5 m/m² IV, day 1<br>ifosfamide 1.6–2 g/m² IV, days 1–5<br>etoposide 150 mg/m² IV, days 1–5 |
| VAdrC | Pediatric sarcoma | vincristine 1.5 mg/m² IV weekly for 10 wk<br>doxorubicin 35–60 mg/m² IV, day 1<br>cyclophosphamide 500–1500 mg/m² IV, day 1 |
| VAD | Refractory multiple myeloma | vincristine 0.4 mg/day Cl days 1–4<br>doxorubicin 9–12 mg/m²/day Cl days 1–4<br>dexamethasone 20 mg/d PO days 1–4, 9–12, 17–20 |
| | Wilms' tumor | vincristine 1.5 mg/m² IV weekly for 10 wk with dactinomycin 0.45 mg/kg every 3 weeks alternating with doxorubicin 30 mg/m² every 3 weeks |
| VATH | Breast cancer | vinblastine 4.5 mg/m² IV, day 1<br>doxorubicin 45 mg/m² IV, day 1<br>thiotepa 12 mg/m² IV, day 1<br>fluoxymesterone 30 mg/d PO<br>Repeat every 21 days |

*(continued)*

| *Regimen* | *Use* | *Drugs used* |
|---|---|---|
| VBAP | Multiple myeloma | vincristine 1 $mg/m^2$ IV, day 1<br>carmustine 30 $mg/m^2$ IV, day 1<br>doxorubicin 30 $mg/m^2$ IV, day 1<br>prednisone 60 $mg/m^2/d$ PO, days 1–4<br>Repeat every 21 days |
| VC | Lung cancer | vinorelbine 30 $mg/m^2$ IV, weekly<br>cisplatin 120 $mg/m^2$ IV, days 1 and 29<br>Repeat every 6 weeks |
| VCAP | Multiple myeloma | vincristine 1 $mg/m^2$ IV, day 1<br>cyclophosphamide 100–125 $mg/m^2/d$ PO, days 1–4<br>doxorubicin 25–30 $mg/m^2$ IV, day 2<br>prednisone 60 $mg/m^2/d$ PO, days 1–4 |
| VDA | ALL, pediatric induction | vincristine 1.5 $mg/m^2$ IV, days 1, 8, 15, 22<br>daunorubicin 25 $mg/m^2$ IV, days 1 and 8<br>asparaginase 10,000 $units/m^2$ IM, days 2, 4, 6, 8, 10, 12, 15, 17, 19 |
| VDP | Malignant melanoma | vinblastine 5 $mg/m^2$ IV, days 1 and 2<br>dacarbazine 150 $mg/m^2$ IV, days 1–5<br>cisplatin 75 $mg/m^2$ IV, day 5<br>Repeat every 21 to 28 days |
| VIP | Testicular cancer | vinblastine 0.11 mg/kg IV, days 1–2<br>*or* etoposide 75 $mg/m^2$ IV, days 1–5<br>ifosfamide 1.2 $g/m^2/d$ Cl, days 1–5<br>cisplatin 20 $mg/m^2$ IV, days 1–5<br>mesna 400 $mg/m^2$ IV, 15 min pre-ifosfamide infusion on day 1<br>mesna 1.2 $g/m^2/d$ Cl days 1–5<br>Repeat every 21 days |
| VIP-1 | Lung cancer | ifosfamide 1.3 $g/m^2$ IV, days 1–4 with mesna<br>cisplatin 100 $mg/m^2$ IV, days 1 and 8<br>etoposide 60–75 mg/m2 IV, days 1 and 3<br>Repeat every 28 days |
| VIP-2 | Lung cancer | ifosfamide 1–1.2 g $m^2$ IV, day 1 with mesna<br>cisplatin 100 $mg/m^2$ IV, days 1 and 8<br>etoposide 60–75 $mg/m^2$ IV days 1–3<br>Repeat every 28 days |
| VMI | Breast cancer | mitomycin 10 $mg/m^2$ IV, days 1 and 28 for 2 cycles, then 1 only<br>vinblastine 5 $mg/m^2$ IV days 1, 14, 28, 42 for 2 cycles, then days 1 and 21 only<br>Repeat every 6–8 weeks |
| V-TAD | AML induction | etoposide 50 $mg/m^2$ IV, days 1–3<br>thioguanine 75 $mg/m^2$ PO q12h, days 1–5<br>duanorubicin 20 $mg/m^2$ IV, days 1 and 2<br>cytarabine 75 $mg/m^2/d$ Cl, days 1–5 |
| 5 + 2 | AML reinduction | cytarabine 100–200 $mg/m^2/d$ Cl days 1–5 with daunorubicin 45 $mg/m^2$ IV, days 1 and 2<br>*or* mitoxantrone 12 $mg/m^2$ IV days 1 and 2 |

*(continued)*

| *Regimen* | *Use* | *Drugs used* |
|---|---|---|
| 7 + 3 | AML induction | cytarabine 100–200 mg/m²/d Cl days 1–7 with daunorubicin 30–45 mg/m² IV, days 1–3<br>*or* mitoxantrone 12 mg/m² IV days 1–3<br>*or* idarubicin 12 mg/m² IV days 1–3 |
| 8 in 1 | Pediatric brain tumors | methylprednisolone 200 mg/m², day 1<br>vincristine 1.5 mg/m² IV day 1<br>methyl-CCNU 75 mg/m²/d PO, day 1<br>procarbazine 75 mg/m²/d PO, day 1<br>hydroxyurea 1.5–3 mg/m²/d PO, day 1<br>cisplatin 60–90 mg/m² IV, day 1<br>cyclophosphamide 300 mg/m² IV, day 1<br>*or* dacarbazine 150 mg/m² IV, day 1 |

# APPENDIX E

## Commonly Used Biologicals

### diphtheria and tetanus toxoids, combined, absorbed (DT, Td) (available in adult and pediatric preparations)

**Therapeutic Actions**

Contains reduced dose of inactivated diphtheria toxin and full dose of inactivated tetanus toxin to provide adequate immunization in adults without the severe sensitivity reactions caused when full pediatric doses of diphtheria toxoid are given to adults.

**Indications**

Active immunization of adults and children ≥7 y against diphtheria and tetanus.

**Adverse Effects**

Fretfulness; drowsiness; anorexia; vomiting; transient fever; malaise; generalized aches and pains; edema of injection area with redness, swelling, induration, pain (may persist for a few days); hypersensitivity reactions.

**Dosage**

2 primary IM doses of 0.5 ml each given at 4–8 wk intervals, followed by a third 0.5 ml IM dose given in 6–12 mo. Routine booster of 0.5 ml IM every 10 y for maintenance of immunity.

**Nursing Considerations**

- Use caution in pregnant women—**Pregnancy Category C,** safety not established.
- Defer administration of routine immunizing or booster doses in case of acute infection.
- Arrange to interrupt immunosuppressive therapy if emergency booster doses of Td are required due to injury.
- **Not** for treatment of acute tetanus or diphtheria infections.
- Administer by IM injection only, avoid SC or IV injection; deltoid muscle is the preferred site. Do not administer into the same site more than once.
- Arrange for epinephrine 1:1000 to be immediately available at time of injection because of hypersensitivity reactions.
- Provide comfort measures to help the patient cope with the discomforts of the injection: analgesics, warm soaks for injection site, small meals, environmental control—temperature, stimuli.
- Provide patient with written record of immunization and reminder of when booster injection is needed.

### diphtheria and tetanus toxoids and whole cell pertussis vaccine, adsorbed (DTwP)

Tri-Immunol

**Therapeutic Actions**

Provides detoxified diphtheria and tetanus toxins and pertussis vaccine to stimulate an immunologic response in children leading to an active immunity against these diseases.

### Indications

Active immunization of infants and children through 6 y of age (between 6 wk and 7 y) against diphtheria, tetanus, pertussis—for primary immunization and routine recall; start immunization at once if whooping cough is present in the community.

### Adverse Effects

Hypersensitivity reactions; erythema, induration, redness, pain, swelling of the injection area; nodule at the injection site which may persist for several weeks; temperature elevations, malaise, chills, irritability, fretfulness, drowsiness, anorexia, vomiting, persistent crying; rarely—fatal reactions.

### Dosage

- Primary immunization: For children 6 wk to 6 y (ideally, beginning at age 2–3 mo or at the 6 wk check up): 0.5 ml IM on 3 occasions at 4–8 wk intervals with a reinforcing dose administered 1 y after the third injection.
- Booster doses: 0.5 ml IM when the child is 4–6 y old (preferably before beginning kindergarten or elementary school). If 4th dose was given after the 4 y birthday, however, the preschool dose may be omitted. Booster injections every 10 y should be given after this using the adult diphtheria and tetanus toxoids combination; do not give pertussis vaccine to person ≥7 y.

### Nursing Considerations

- Do not use for treatment of acute tetanus, diphtheria or whooping cough infections.
- Do not administer to children >7 y or to adults.
- Do not attempt routine immunization with DTP if the child has a personal history of CNS disease or convulsions.
- Do not administer DTP after recent blood transfusions or immune globulin, in immunodeficiency disorders or with immunosuppressive therapy, or to patients with malignancy.
- Question the parent concerning occurrence of any symptoms or signs of adverse reactions after previous dose before administering repeat dose of the vaccine—if fever >39°C (103°F), convulsions with or without fever, alterations of consciousness, focal neurologic signs, screaming episodes, shock, collapse, somnolence, or encephalopathy have occurred, DTP is contraindicated and diphtheria and tetanus toxoids without pertussis should be used for immunization.
- Administer by IM injection only; avoid SC or IV injection. Midlateral muscle of the thigh is preferred site for infants, deltoid muscle is the preferred site for older children. Do not administer into the same site more than once.
- Arrange for epinephrine 1:1000 to be immediately available at time of injection because of risk of hypersensitivity reactions.
- Provide comfort measures and teach parents to provide comfort measures to help the patient cope with the discomforts of the injection: analgesics, warm soaks for injection site, small meals, environmental control—temperature, stimuli.
- Provide patient with written record of immunization and reminder of when booster injection is needed.

## diphtheria and tetanus toxoids and acellular pertussis vaccine, adsorbed (DTaP)

Acel-Imune, Infanrix, Tripedia

### Therapeutic Actions

Provides detoxified diphtheria and tetanus toxins and acellular pertussis vaccine to stimulate an immunologic response in children leading to an active immunity against these diseases in children who have received 3–4 doses of DTwP vaccine. Use as the 4th or 5th doses only (*Acel-Immune, Tripedia*). For active immunization of children 6 wk–7 y (*Infaurix*).

## Indications

Induction of immunity against diphthera, tetanus, and pertussis as the fourth and fifth dose in children from ages 15 mo (*Tripedia*) or 17 mo (*Acel-Immune*) through the 7th birthday). Children must have been previously immunized with 3 or 4 doses of whole cell DTP. Use in children as young as 15 mo if the child is not expected to return at 18 mo for the fourth dose. Being considered for immunization of adults against pertussis. (*Acel-Immune, Tripedia*). For active immunization of children 6 wk–7 y, acellular pertussis provides superior safety profile to whole cell vaccines (*Infaurix*).

## Adverse Effects

Hypersensitivity reactions; erythema, induration, redness, pain, swelling of the injection area; nodule at the injection site which may persist for several weeks; temperature elevations, malaise, chills, irritability, fretfulness, drowsiness, anorexia, vomiting, persistent crying; rarely—fatal reactions.

## Dosage

- Fourth dose: 0.5 ml IM at 18 mo of age, at least 6 mo after last dose of DTwP.
- Fifth dose: 0.5 ml IM at 4–6 years of age or preferably before entry into school. If 4th dose was given after the 4 y birthday, however, the preschool dose may be omitted. Booster injections every 10 y should be given after this using the adult diphtheria and tetanus toxoids combination; do not give pertussis vaccine to person ≥7 y.

## Nursing Considerations

- Do not use for treatment of acute tetanus, diphtheria, or whooping cough infections.
- Do not administer to children >7 y or to adults (*Acel-Immune, Tripedia*).
- Do not attempt routine immunization with DTaP if the child has a personal history of CNS disease or convulsions.
- Administer only if patient has already received at least 3 doses of DTwP (*Acel-Immune, Tripedia*).
- Do not administer DTaP after recent blood transfusions or immune globulin, in immunodeficiency disorders or with immunosuppressive therapy, or to patients with malignancy.
- Question the parent concerning occurrence of any symptoms or signs of adverse reactions after the previous dose before administering a repeat dose of the vaccine—if fever >39°C (103°F), convulsions with or without fever, alterations of consciousness, focal neurologic signs, screaming episodes, shock, collapse, somnolence, or encephalopathy have occurred, DTP is contraindicated and diphtheria and tetanus toxoids without pertussis should be used for immunization.
- Administer by IM injection only; avoid SC or IV injection. Midlateral muscle of the thigh is preferred site for infants, deltoid muscle is the preferred site for older children. Do not administer into the same site more than once.
- Arrange for epinephrine 1:1000 to be immediately available at time of injection because of risk of hypersensitivity reactions.
- Provide comfort measures and teach parents to provide comfort measures to help the patient cope with the discomforts of the injection: analgesics, warm soaks for injection site, small meals, environmental control—temperature, stimuli.
- Provide parent with written record of immunization and reminder of when booster injection is needed.

## diphtheria and tetanus toxoids and whole cell pertussis vaccine with haemophilus influenzae b conjugates vaccine (DTwP-HIB)

Tetramune

### Therapeutic Actions
Provides detoxified diphtheria and tetanus toxins and whole cell pertussis vaccine and *Haemophilus influenzae* b conjugate vaccine to stimulate an immunologic response in children leading to an active immunity against these diseases.

### Indications
Active immunization of infants and children (2 mo—5 y) against diphtheria, tetanus, pertussis, and *Haemophilus influenzae* b for primary immunization and routine recall. (Not recommended for children who experienced active *Haemophilus influenzae* b infection ≥24 mo.)

### Adverse Effects
Hypersensitivity reactions; erythema, induration, redness, pain, swelling of the injection area; nodule at the injection site which may persist for several weeks; temperature elevations, malaise, chills, irritability, fretfulness, drowsiness, anorexia, vomiting, persistent crying; rarely—fatal reactions.

### Dosage
- Primary immunization: For children 2 mo: three doses of 0.5 ml IM at 2 mo intervals with a fourth dose at 15 mo of age.
- Booster dose: Subsequent DTP or DTaP vaccination is needed at 4–6 y.

### Nursing Considerations
- Do not use for treatment of acute tetanus, diphtheria, whooping cough, or *H. flu* b infections.
- Do not administer to children >5 y or to adults.
- Do not attempt routine immunization if the child has a personal history of CNS disease or convulsions.
- Do not administer after recent blood transfusions or immune globulin, in immunodeficiency disorders or with immunosuppressive therapy, or to patients with malignancy.
- Question the parent concerning occurrence of any symptoms or signs of adverse reactions after the previous dose before administering a repeat dose of the vaccine—if fever >39°C (103°F), convulsions with or without fever, alterations of consciousness, focal neurologic signs, screaming episodes, shock, collapse, somnolence, or encephalopathy have occurred, DTP is contraindicated and diphtheria and tetanus toxoids without pertussis should be used for immunization.
- Administer by IM injection only; avoid SC or IV injection. Midlateral muscle of the thigh is preferred site for infants, deltoid muscle is the preferred site for older children. Do not administer into the same site more than once.
- Arrange for epinephrine 1:1000 to be immediately available at time of injection because of risk of hypersensitivity reactions.
- Provide comfort measures and teach parents to provide comfort measures to help the patient cope with the discomforts of the injection: analgesics, warm soaks for injection site, small meals, environmental control—temperature, stimuli.
- Provide parent with written record of immunization and reminder of when booster injection is needed.

## haemophilus b conjugate vaccine

HibTITTER, PedvaxHIB, ProHIBiT

### Therapeutic Actions

Vaccine prepared from the purified capsular polysaccharide of the *Haemophilus influenzae* type b (Hib) bacterium bound to an inactive noninfective diphtheria toxoid; stimulates long-lived, non-boostable antibody response that prevents Hib diseases.

### Indications

Immunization of children 2 mo–5 y (*Hib TITER*), 18 mo–5 y (*PedvaxHIB* and *ProHIBit*) against diseases caused by *H influenzae* type b.

### Adverse Reactions

Erythema and induration at the injection site, fever, acute febrile reactions.

### Dosage

*PedvaxHIB, ProHIBIT:* 0.5 ml IM
*HibTITER:*

- 2–6 mo old: three separate IM injections of 0.5 ml each given at approximately 2 mo intervals.
- 7–11 mo old: two separate IM injections of 0.5 ml each given at approximately 2 mo intervals.
- 12–14 mo old: one IM injection of 0.5 ml.

All vaccinated children receive a single booster dose at ≥15 mo of age, but not less than 2 mo after the previous dose. Previously unvaccinated children 15–60 mo of age receive a single 0.5 ml IM injection.

### Nursing Considerations

- Do not administer to patient with any history of hypersensitivity to any component of the vaccine.
- Do not administer to any patient with febrile illness or active infection; delay vaccine until patient has recovered.
- Have epinephrine 1:1000 immediately available at time of injection in case of severe anaphylactoid reaction.
- Provide comfort measures—analgesics, antipyretics—or instruct parent to provide comfort measures to help the patient cope with any discomfort from the injection.
- Provide parent with a written record of immunization; identify the particular vaccine that is being used; *HibTITER* requires repeat injections, *PedvaxHIB* and *ProHIBit* require no repeat injections.

## haemophilus b conjugated vaccine and hepatitis B surface antigen (recombinant)

Comvax

### Therapeutic actions

Provides antigenic combination of *Haemophilus* b conjugate vaccine and hepatitis B recombinant vaccine to stimulate an immunologic response in children, leading to an active immunity against these diseases.

### Indications

Active immunization of infants and children (6 wk–15 mo) against *Haemophilus influenzae* b and hepatitis B, for primary immunization and routine recall.

### Adverse effects
Hypersensitivity reactions; erythema, induration, redness, pain, swelling of the injection area; nodule at the injection site, which may persist for several weeks; temperature elevations, malaise, chills, irritability, fretfulness, drowsiness, anorexia, vomiting, persistent crying; rarely—fatal reactions.

### Dosage
- Immunization: 0.5 ml IM at 2, 4, and 12–15 mo.

### Nursing Considerations
- Administer only to children of HBSAG-negative mothers.
- Do not administer to children with immunodeficiency/suppression or malignancy.
- Do not administer to adults.
- Do not administer in the presence of febrile illness.
- Administer by IM injection only; avoid SC or IV injection. Midlateral muscle of the thigh is preferred site for infants; deltoid muscle is preferred site for older children. Do not administer into the same site more than once.
- Arrange for epinephrine 1:1000 to be immediately available at time of injection because of risk of hypersensitivity reactions.
- Provide comfort measures and teach parents to provide comfort measures to help the patient cope with the discomforts of the injection: analgesics, warm soaks for injection site, small meals, environmental control—temperature, stimuli.
- Provide parents with written record of immunization and reminder of when booster injection is needed.

## haemophilus b conjugated vaccine with tetanus toxoid

*ActHIB* (provided with *Tripedia* for 4th dose immunization), *OmniHIB*

### Therapeutic actions
Provides detoxified tetanus toxins and *Haemophilus influenzae* b conjugate vaccine to stimulate an immunologic response in children leading to an active immunity against these diseases.

### Indications
Active immunization of infants and children (2 mo–5 y) against tetanus and *Haemophilus influenzae* b for primary immunization and routine recall.

### Adverse effects
Hypersensitivity reactions; erythema, induration, redness, pain, swelling of the injection area; nodule at the injection site, which may persist for several weeks; temperature elevations, malaise, chills, irritability, fretfulness, drowsiness, anorexia, vomiting, persistent crying; rarely—fatal reactions.

### Dosage
- Primary immunization: For children 2 mo to 5 y, 0.5 ml IM ideally, beginning at age 2 mo; then repeat dose at 4 mo, 6 mo, and 15–18 mo.
- Booster dose: Subsequent DTP or DTaP vaccination is needed at 4–6 y.

### Nursing Considerations
- Do not use for treatment of acute tetanus *H. influenzae* b infections.
- Do not administer to children over the age of 5 y or to adults.

- Do not attempt routine immunization if the child has a personal history of CNS disease or convulsions.
- Do not administer after recent blood transfusions or immune globulin, in immunodeficiency disorders or with immunosuppressive therapy, or to patients with malignancy.
- Administer by IM injection only; avoid SC or IV injection. Midlateral muscle of the thigh is preferred site for infants; deltoid muscle is preferred site for older children. Do not administer into the same site more than once.
- Arrange for epinephrine 1:1000 to be immediately available at time of injection because of risk of hypersensitivity reactions.
- Provide comfort measures and teach parents to provide comfort measures to help the patient cope with the discomforts of the injection: analgesics, warm soaks for injection site, small meals, environmental control—temperature, stimuli.
- Provide parents with written record of immunization and reminder of when booster injection is needed.

## hepatitis A vaccine

*Vaqta*

### Therapeutic effects

Contains hepatitis A antigen that stimulates the production of specific antibodies against HAV, which protects against HAV infection. The immunity does not protect against hepatitis caused by other agents.

### Indications

Active immunization of adults and children $\geq$ 2 mo against disease caused by HAV in situations that warrant immunization (travel, institutionalization, etc); used with IG for immediate and long-term protection against hepatitis A.

### Adverse effects

Transient fever; edema of injection area with redness, swelling, induration, pain (may persist for a few days); upper respiratory illness, headache, rash.

### Dosage

- Adult: 5 U/ml IM as a single dose.
- Pediatric (2 mo–17 y): 25 U/0.5 ml IM with a repeat dose in 6–18 mo.

### Nursing Considerations

- Use caution in pregnancy—**Pregnancy Category C;** safety not established.
- Defer administration in case of acute infection.
- Administer by IM injection only; deltoid muscle is the preferred site, do not give in the gluteal site.
- Arrange for epinephrine 1:1000 to be immediately available at time of injection because of risk of hypersensitivity reactions.
- Provide comfort measures to help the patient cope with the discomforts of the injection: analgesics, warm soaks for injection site, small meals, environmental control—temperature, stimuli.
- Provide patient with written record of immunization and timing for booster immunization.

## hepatitis A vaccine inactivated

Havrix

### Therapeutic Actions

Contains inactivated hepatitis A virus (HAV) that stimulates the production of specific antibodies against HAV, which protect against HAV infection. The immunity does not protect against hepatitis caused by other agents.

### Indications

Active immunization of adults and children ≥ 2 y against disease caused by HAV in situations that warrant immunization (travel, institutionalization, etc.).

### Adverse Effects

Transient fever; edema of injection area with redness, swelling, induration, pain (may persist for a few days); upper respiratory illness, headache, rash.

### Dosage

- Adult: A single dose of 1440 EL U IM.
- Pediatric (2–18 y): 2 doses containing 360 EL U IM.
- Booster dose: A booster dose is recommended 6–12 mo after initial therapy to ensure a sufficient titer of antibodies.

### Nursing Considerations

- Use caution in pregnancy—**Pregnancy Category C;** safety not established.
- Defer administration in case of acute infection.
- Administer by IM injection only; deltoid muscle is the preferred site; do not give in the gluteal site.
- Arrange for epinephrine 1:1000 to be immediately available at time of injection because of risk of hypersensitivity reactions.
- Provide comfort measures to help the patient cope with the discomforts of the injection: analgesics, warm soaks for injection site, small meals, environmental control—temperature, stimuli.
- Provide patient with written record of immunization and timing for booster immunization.

## hepatitis B immune globulin (HBIG)

H-BIG, H-BIGIV, HyperHep

### Therapeutic Actions

Globulin contains a high titer of antibody to hepatitis B surface (HBsAg), providing a passive immunity to hepatitis B surface antigen.

### Indications

- Postexposure prophylaxis following parental exposure (accidental "needle-stick"), direct mucous membrane contact (accidental splash), or oral ingestion (pipetting accident) involving HBsAg-positive materials such as blood, plasma, serum.
- Prophylaxis of infants born to HBsAG-positive mothers.
- Adjunct to hepatitis B vaccine when rapid achievement of protective levels of antibodies is desirable.

### Adverse Effects

Hypersensitivity reactions; tenderness, muscle stiffness at the injection site; urticaria, angioedema; fever, chills, nausea, vomiting, chest tightness.

### Dosage

- Perinatal exposure: 0.5 ml, IM within 12 h of birth; repeat dose at 3 mo and 6 mo after initial dose.
- Percutaneous exposure: 0.06 ml/kg IM, immediately (within 7 d) and repeat 28–30 d after exposure.
- Individuals at high risk of infection: 0.06 ml/kg IM at same time (but at a different site) as hepatitis B vaccine is given.
- IV use approved for prophylaxis against hepatitis B virus reinfection in liver transplant patients.

### Nursing Considerations

- Do not administer to patients with history of allergic response to gamma globulin or with anti-immunoglobulin A antibodies.
- Use caution in pregnant women, **Pregnancy Category C;** safety not established, use only if benefits outweigh potential unknown risks to the fetus.
- HBIG may be administered at the same time or up to 1 mo preceding hepatitis B vaccination without impairing the active immune response from the vaccination.
- Administer IM in the gluteal or deltoid region; do not administer IV.
- Administer the appropriate dose as soon after exposure as possible (within 7 days is preferable); and repeat 28–30 days after exposure.
- Have epinephrine 1:1000 immediately available at time of injection in case of anaphylactic reaction.
- Provide comfort measures to help patient to deal with discomfort of drug therapy—analgesics, antipyretics, environmental control, etc.

## hepatitis B vaccine

Engerix-B, Recombivax-HB

### Therapeutic Actions

Provides inactivated human hepatitis B surface antigen particles to stimulate active immunity and production of antibodies against hepatitis B surface antigens using surface antigen produced by yeast.

### Indications

- Immunization against infection caused by all known subtypes of hepatitis B virus, especially those at high risk for infection—health care personnel, military personnel identified to be at risk, prisoners, users of illicit drugs, populations with high incidence (Eskimos, Indochinese refugees, Haitian refugees), morticians and embalmers, persons at increased risk because of their sexual practices (repeated sexually transmitted diseases, homosexually active males, prostitutes), patients in hemodialysis units, patients requiring frequent blood transfusions, residents of mental institutions, household contacts of people with persistent hepatitis B antigenemia.
- Treatment of choice for infants born to HBsAG-positive mothers.

### Adverse Effects

Soreness, swelling, erythema, warmth, induration at injection site; malaise, fatigue, headache, nausea, vomiting, dizziness, myalgia, arthralgia, rash, low grade fever, pharyngitis, rhinitis, cough, lymphadenopathy, hypotension, dysuria.

### Dosage

- Pediatric (birth–10 y): Initial dose–0.5 ml, IM; followed by 0.5 ml IM at 1 mo and 6 mo after initial dose (*Engerix B*); 0.25 ml IM, followed by 0.25 ml IM at 1 mo and 6 mo after initial dose (*Recombivax–HB*).

- Older children (11–19 y): Initial dose–1 ml, IM; followed by 1 ml IM at 1 mo and 6 mo after initial dose (*Engerix B*); 0.5 ml, IM; followed by 0.5 ml IM at 1 mo and 6 mo after initial dose (*Recombivax–HB*).
- Adults: Initial dose–1 ml, IM; followed by 1 ml IM at 1 mo and 6 mo after initial dose, all types.
- Dialysis or immunocompromised patients: Initial dose—two 1 ml injections at different sites, IM; followed by two 1 ml injections, IM at 1 mo and at 6 mo after initial dose (*Engerix B*).
- Revaccination (a booster dose should be considered if anti-HBs levels $< 10$ mIU/ml 1–2 mo after third dose): Children $\leq 10$ y of age: 10 mcg. Adults and children $> 10$ y: 20 mcg. Hemodialysis patients (when antibody testing indicates need): give two 20 mcg doses.

### Nursing Considerations

- Do not administer to any patient with known hypersensitivity to any component of the vaccine; allergy to yeast.
- Use caution in pregnant or nursing women—**Pregnancy Category C;** safety not established; use only if clearly needed and benefits outweigh potential unknown effects.
- Use caution with any patient with active infection; delay use of vaccine if at all possible; use with caution in any patient with compromised cardiopulmonary status or patients in whom a febrile or systemic reaction could present a significant risk.
- Administer IM, preferably in the deltoid muscle in adults, the anterolateral thigh muscle in infants and small children. Do not administer IV or intradermally; SC route may be used in patients who are at high risk for hemorrhage following IM injection, but increased incidence of local effects has been noted.
- Shake vaccine container well before withdrawing solution; no dilution is needed, use vaccine as supplied. Vaccine will appear as a slightly opaque, white suspension. Refrigerate vials, do not freeze.
- Have epinephrine 1:1000 immediately available at time of injection in case of severe anaphylactic reaction.
- Provide comfort measures—analgesics, antipyretics, care of injection site—to help patient to cope with the effects of the drug.
- Provide patient or parent with a written record of the immunization and dates that repeat injections and antibody tests are needed.

## immunue globulin intramuscular (IG; Gamma Globulin; ISG)

## immune globulin intravenous (IGIV)

Gamimune N, Gammagard S/D, Gammar-P IV, Iveegam, Polygam S/D, Sandoglobulin, Venoglubulin-I, Venoglobulin-S

### Therapeutic Actions

Contains human globulin (16.5% IM, 5% IV) which provides passive immunity through the presence of injected antibodies; IM gamma globulin involves a 2–5 day delay before adequate serum levels are obtained, IV gamma globulin provides immediate antibody levels; mechanism of action in idiopathic thrombocytopenic purpura not determined.

### Indications

- Prophylaxis after exposure to hepatitis A, measles (rubeola), varicella, rubella—IM route preferred.

- Prophylaxis for patients with immunoglobulin deficiency—IM, IV if immediate increase in antibodies is necessary.
- Idiopathic thrombocytopenic purpura—IV route has produced temporary increase in platelets in emergency situations.
- B-cell chronic lymphocytic leukemia (CLL) (*Gammagard, Polygam S/D*)
- Kawasaki syndrome (*Iveegam* only).
- Bone marrow transplant (*Gamimune N* only).
- Pediatric HIV infection (*Gamimune N* only).

## Adverse Effects

Tenderness, muscle stiffness at injection site; urticaria, angioedema, nausea, vomiting, chills, fever, chest tightness; anaphylactic reactions, precipitous fall in blood pressure—more likely with IV administration.

## Dosage

- Hepatitis A: 0.02 ml/kg, IM for household and institutional contacts; persons traveling to areas where hepatitis A is common—0.02 ml/kg IM if staying <2 mo, 0.06 ml/kg IM repeated every 5 mo for prolonged stay.
- Measles (rubeola): 0.2 ml/kg IM if exposed <6 days previously; immunocompromised child exposed to measles—0.5 ml/kg to a maximum of 15 ml IM given immediately.
- Varicella: 0.6–1.2 ml/kg IM given promptly if zoster immune globulin is unavailable.
- Rubella: 0.55 ml/kg IM given to those pregnant women who have been exposed to rubella and will not consider a therapeutic abortion may decrease likelihood of infection and fetal damage.
- Immunoglobulin deficiency: Initial dosage of 1.3 ml/kg IM followed in 3–4 wk by 0.66 ml/kg IM every 3–4 wk; some patients may require more frequent injections.
- *Sandoglobulin:* 200 mg/kg IV, once a month by IV infusion; if insufficient response, increase dose to 300 mg/kg by IV infusion or repeat more frequently. Idiopathic thrombocytopenic purpura—400 mg/kg IV for 5 consecutive days.
- *Gamimune N:* 100 mg/kg IV once a month by IV infusion. May be increased to 200 mg/kg IV or infusion may be repeated more frequently.
- *Gammagard S/D:* 200–400 mg/kg IV, monthly doses of at least 100 mg/kg are recommended. B-cell CLL: 400 mg/kg IV every 3–4 wk. Idiopathic thrombocytopenic purpura: 1000 mg/kg IV, base dose on clinical response. Give up to 3 doses on alternate days if required.
- *Gammar-P IV:* 100–200 mg/kg IV every 3–4 wk.
- *Venoglobulin-I:* 200 mg/kg IV administered monthly. Idiopathic thrombocytopenic purpura: 500 mg/kg/day for 2–7 consecutive days.
- *Iveegam:* 200 mg/kg IV per mo.

## Nursing Considerations

- Do not administer to patients with history of allergy to gamma globulin or anti-immunoglobulin A antibodies.
- Use IM gamma globulin with caution in patients with thrombocytopenia or any coagulation disorder that would contraindicate IM injections—use only if benefits outweigh risks.
- Use with caution in pregnant women—**Pregnancy Category C;** safety not established.
- Administer 2 wk before or 3 mo after immune globulin administration because antibodies in the globulin preparation may interfere with the immune response to the vaccination.
- Have epinephrine 1:1000 immediately available at time of injection in case of anaphylactic reaction, more likely with IV immune globulin, large IM doses, and repeated injections.
- Refrigerate drug, do not freeze, discard partially used vials.

- Administer IM preparation by IM injection only, do not administer SC or intradermally.
- Administer IV preparation with extreme caution as follows:

  *Sandoglobulin:* Give the first infusion as a 3% solution (reconstitute by inverting the 2 bottles so that solvent flows into the IV bottle). Start with a flow rate of 0.5–1 ml/min; after 15–30 min increase infusion rate to 1.5–2.5 ml/min. Administer subsequent infusions at a rate of 2–2.5 ml/min; if high doses must be administered repeatedly after the first infusion of 3% solution, use a 6% solution (reconstitute 1 g vial with 16.5 ml diluent, 3 g vial with 50 ml diluent, 6 g vial with 100 ml diluent) with an initial infusion rate of 1–1.5 ml/min, increased after 15–30 min to a maximum of 2.5 ml/min.

  *Gamimune N:* May be diluted with 5% dextrose, infusion rate of 0.01–0.02 ml/kg/min for 30 min. If patient does not experience any discomfort, the rate may be increased to 0.02–0.04 ml/kg/min. If side effects occur, reduce the rate or interrupt the infusion until the symptoms subside and resume at a rate tolerable to the patient.

  *Gammagard S/D:* Initially administer at a rate of 0.5 ml/kg/h. If rate causes no distress, may be gradually increased, not to exceed 4 ml/kg/h.

  *Gammar-P IV:* Administer at 0.01 ml/kg/min, increasing to 0.02 ml/kg/min after 15–30 min. If adverse reactions occur, slow the infusion rate.

  *Venoglobulin-I:* Infuse at a rate of 0.01–0.02 ml/kg/min for the first 30 min. If patient experiences no distress, may be increased to 0.04 ml/kg/min.

  *Iveegam:* Infuse at rate of 1 ml/min up to a maximum of 2 ml/min of the 5% solution. Drug may be further diluted with 5% dextrose or saline.
- Do not mix immune globulin with any other medications.
- Monitor the patient's vital signs continuously and observe for any symptoms during IV administration—adverse effects appear to be related to the rate of infusion.
- Provide comfort measures or teach patient to provide comfort measures—analgesics, antipyretics, warm soaks to injection site—to help patient to cope with the discomforts of drug therapy.
- Provide patient with written record of injection and dates for follow-up injections as needed.

## influenza virus vaccine

Fluzone, Flu-Shield, Fluvirin

### Therapeutic Effects

Inactivated influenza virus antigens stimulate an active immunity through the production of antibodies specific to the antigens used; the antigens used vary from year to year depending on which influenza virus strains are anticipated to be prevalent.

### Indications

Prophylaxis for people at high risk of developing complications from infection with influenza virus—adults and children with chronic cardiovascular or pulmonary disorders, chronic metabolic disorders, renal dysfunction, anemia, immunosuppression, asthma; residents of chronic care facilities; medical personnel with extensive contact with high-risk patients, to prevent their transmitting the virus to these patients; children on chronic aspirin therapy who are at high risk of developing Reye's syndrome; people who provide essential community services (to decrease the risk of disruption of services).

### Adverse Effects

Tenderness, redness and induration at the injection site; fever, malaise, myalgia; allergic responses—flare, wheal, respiratory symptoms; Guillain-Barré syndrome.

### Dosage

- 6–35 mo—split virus or purified surface antigen only—0.25 ml IM repeated in 4 wk.
- 3–6 y—split virus or purified surface antigen only—0.5 ml IM repeated in 4 wk.
- 9–12 y—split virus or purified surface antigen—0.5 ml IM.
- >12 y—whole or split virus or purified surface antigen—0.5 ml.

### Nursing Considerations

- Do not administer to patients with sensitivities to eggs, chicken, chicken feathers, or chicken dander. If an allergic condition is suspected, administer a scratch test or an intradermal injection (0.05–0.1 ml) of vaccine diluted 1:100 in sterile saline—a wheal greater than 5 mm justifies withholding immunization.
- Do not administer to patient with a hypersensitivity to any component of the vaccine; history of Guillain-Barré syndrome.
- Do not administer to infants and children at the same time as diphtheria, tetanus toxoid, and pertussis vaccine (DTP) or within 14 days after Measles Virus Vaccine.
- Delay administration in the presence of acute respiratory disease or other active infection or acute febrile illness.
- Use caution in pregnant women; **Pregnancy Category C;** safety not established, delay use until the second or third trimester to minimize concern over possible teratogenicity.
- Monitor patient for enhanced drug effects and possible toxicity of *theophylline, warfarin sodium* for as long as 3 wk after vaccine injection.
- Administer IM only; the deltoid muscle is preferred for adults and older children, the anterolateral aspect of the thigh for infants and younger children.
- Consider the possible need for amantadine for therapeutic use for patients in high risk groups who develop illness compatible with influenza during a period of known influenza A activity in the community.
- Have epinephrine 1:1000 immediately available at time of injection in case of anaphylactic reaction.
- Provide comfort measures or teach patient to provide comfort measures—analgesics, antipyretics, warm soaks to injection site—to help patient cope with effects of the drug.
- Provide patient with written record of vaccination and dates of second injection as appropriate.

## measles (rubeola) virus vaccine, live, attenuated

Attenuvax

### Therapeutic Actions

Attenuated measles virus produces a modified measles infection and stimulates an active immune reaction with antibodies to the measles virus.

### Indications

- Immunization against measles (rubeola) immediately after exposure to natural measles, more effective if given before exposure—children ≥ 15 mo (immunization with trivalent MMR vaccine is the preferred product for routine vaccinations).
- Revaccination for children immunized before the age of 12 mo or vaccinated with inactivated vaccine alone.
- Prophylaxis for high school or college age persons in epidemic situations or for adults in isolated communities where measles is not endemic.

### Adverse Effects

Moderate fever, rash; high fever—less common; febrile convulsions, Guillain-Barré syndrome, ocular palsies—less common; burning or stinging wheal or flare at injection site.

### Dosage

Inject the total volume of the reconstituted vaccine or 0.5 ml of multi-dose vial SC into the outer aspect of the upper arm; the dosage is the same for all patients.

### Nursing Considerations

- Do not administer to patients with a history of anaphylactic hypersensitivity to neomycin (contained in injection), to patients with immune deficiency conditions (immunosuppressive therapy with corticosteroids, antineoplastics; neoplasms; immunodeficiency states), to patients receiving immune serum globulin.
- Do not administer to pregnant women, **Pregnancy Category C;** advise patients to avoid pregnancy for 3 mo following vaccination. If measles exposure occurs during pregnancy, provide passive immunity with immune serum globulin.
- Use caution if administering to children with history of febrile convulsions, cerebral injury, or other conditions in which stress due to fever should be avoided.
- Use caution if administering to patient with a history of sensitivity to eggs, chicken, chicken feathers.
- Do not administer within one mo of immunization with other *live virus vaccines;* may be administered concurrently with *monovalent or trivalent polio vaccine, rubella vaccine, mumps vaccine.*
- Do not administer for at least 3 mo following blood or plasma transfusions or administration of serum immune globulin.
- Monitor for possible depression of *tuberculin skin sensitivity;* administer the test before or simultaneously with the vaccine.
- Administer with a sterile syringe free of preservatives, antiseptics, and detergents for each injection (these may inactivate the live virus vaccine); use a 23 gauge, $\frac{5}{8}$″ needle.
- Refrigerate unreconstituted vial; protect from exposure to light. Use only the diluent supplied with the vaccine and reconstitute just before using; discard reconstituted vaccine if not used within 8 h.
- Have epinephrine 1:1000 immediately available at time of injection in case of anaphylactic reaction.
- Provide comfort measures or teach patient or parent to provide comfort measures to help patient to cope with the discomforts of drug therapy—analgesics, antipyretics, warm soaks to injection site, etc.
- Provide patient or parent with a written record of immunization.

## measles, mumps, rubella vaccine, live

MMR-II

### Therapeutic Actions

Attenuated measles, mumps, and rubella viruses produce a modified infection and stimulate an active immune reaction with antibodies to these virus.

### Indications

Immunization against measles, mumps, rubella in children $>15$ mo and adults.

### Adverse Effects

Moderate fever, rash; high fever—less common; febrile convulsions, Guillain-Barré syndrome, ocular palsies—less common; burning or stinging wheal or flare at injection site.

### Dosage

0.5 ml reconstituted vaccine SC into the outer aspect of the upper arm; the dosage is the same for all patients. Booster dose is recommended on entry into school and again at entry into junior high school.

## Nursing Considerations

- Do not administer to patients with a history of anaphylactic hypersensitivity to neomycin (contained in injection), to patients with immune deficiency conditions (immunosuppressive therapy with corticosteroids, antineoplastics; neoplasms; immunodeficiency states), to patients receiving immune serum globulin.
- Do not administer to pregnant women, **Pregnancy Category C;** advice patients to avoid pregnancy for 3 mo following vaccination. If measles exposure occurs during pregnancy, provide passive immunity with immune serum globulin.
- Use caution if administering to children with history of febrile convulsions, cerebral injury, or other conditions in which stress due to fever should be avoided.
- Use caution if administering to patient with a history of sensitivity to eggs, chicken, chicken feathers.
- Do not administer within one mo of immunization with other *live virus vaccines;* may be administered concurrently with *monovalent or trivalent polio vaccine, rubella vaccine, mumps vaccine.*
- Do not administer for at least 3 mo following blood or plasma transfusions or administration of serum immune globulin.
- Monitor for possible depression of *tuberculin skin sensitivity;* administer the test before or simultaneously with the vaccine.
- Administer with a sterile syringe free of preservatives, antiseptics, and detergents for each injection (these may inactivate the live virus vaccine); use a 25-gauge, ⅝″ needle.
- Refrigerate unreconstituted vial; protect from exposure to light. Use only the diluent supplied with the vaccine and reconstitute just before using; discard reconstituted vaccine if not used within 8 h.
- Have epinephrine 1:1000 immediately available at time of injection in case of anaphylactic reaction.
- Provide comfort measures or teach patient or parent to provide comfort measures to help patient to cope with the discomforts of drug therapy—analgesics, antipyretics, warm soaks to injection site, etc.
- Provide patient or parent with a written record of immunization.
- MMR is the vaccination of choice for routine vaccinations. Other combinations that are available—rubella and mumps vaccine (*Biavax II*), and measles and rubella (*MR Vax-II*)—are used for specific situations.

## mumps virus vaccine, live

Mumpsvax

### Therapeutic Actions

Viral antigen stimulates active immunity through production of antibodies to the mumps virus.

### Indications

Immunization against mumps in children >12 mo and adults. (Trivalent MMR vaccine is the drug of choice for routine vaccinations.)

### Adverse Effects

Fever, parotitis, orchitis; purpura and allergic reactions such as wheal and flare at injection site; febrile seizures, unilateral nerve deafness, encephalitis—rare; anaphylactic reactions.

### Dosage

Inject total volume (0.5 ml) of reconstituted vaccine SC into the outer aspect of the upper arm; each dose contains not less than 5000 $TCID_{50}$ (Tissue Culture Infectious Doses) of mumps virus vaccine (vaccine is available only in single dose vials of diluent).

### Nursing Considerations

- Do not administer to patients with history of hypersensitivity to neomycin (each single dose vial of vaccine contains 25 mcg neomycin); immune deficiency conditions; **Pregnancy Category C**—advise patient to avoid pregnancy for 3 mo after vaccination.
- Use caution if administering to patient with history of allergy to eggs, chicken, chicken feathers.
- Delay administration in the presence of active infection.
- Do not administer within one month of immunization with other *live virus vaccines* except may be administered concurrently with *live monovalent or trivalent polio vaccine, live rubella vaccine, live measles vaccine.*
- Do not administer for at least 3 mo following blood or plasma transfusions or administration of serum immune globulin.
- Monitor for possible depression of *tuberculin skin sensitivity;* administer the test before or simultaneously with the vaccine.
- Administer with a sterile syringe free of preservatives, antiseptics, and detergents for each injection (these may inactivate the live virus vaccine); use a 25 gauge, ⅝" needle.
- Refrigerate unreconstituted vial; protect from exposure to light. Use only the diluent supplied with the vaccine and reconstitute just before using; discard reconstituted vaccine if not used within 8 h.
- Have epinephrine 1:1000 immediately available at time of injection in case of anaphylactic reaction.
- Provide comfort measures or teach patient or parent to provide comfort measures to help patient to cope with the discomforts of drug therapy—analgesics, antipyretics, warm soaks to injection site, etc.
- Provide patient or parent with a written record of vaccination.

## pneumococcal vaccine, polyvalent

Pneumovax 23, Pnu-Imune 23

### Therapeutic Actions

Polysaccharide capsules of the 23 most prevalent or invasive pneumococcal types stimulate active immunity through antipneumococcal antibody production against the capsule types contained in the vaccine.

### Indications

- Immunization against pneumococcal pneumonia and bacteremia caused by the types of pneumococci included in the vaccine—specifically in children over 2 y and adults with chronic illnesses or who are immunocompromised and at increased risk for pneumococcal infections.
- Prophylaxis in children ≥2 y with asymptomatic or symptomatic HIV infections.
- Prevention of pneumococcal otitis media in children >2 y.
- Prophylaxis in community groups at high risk for pneumococcal infections—institutionalized persons, groups in an area of outbreak, patients at high risk of influenza complications including pneumococcal infection.

### Adverse Effects

Erythema, induration, soreness at injection site; fever, myalgia; acute febrile reactions, rash, arthralgia—less common; paresthesias, acute radiculoneuropathy—rare; anaphylactic reaction.

### Dosage

One 0.5 ml dose SC or IM. Not recommended for children <2 y.

### Nursing Considerations

- Do not administer to patients with hypersensitivity to any component of the vaccine or with previous immunization with any polyvalent pneumococcal vaccine.
- Do not administer less than 10 days prior to or during treatment for Hodgkin's disease.
- Use caution if administering to patients who are pregnant—**Pregnancy Category C,** safety not established; or patients who are nursing—safety not established.
- Use caution if administering to patients with cardiac, pulmonary disorders—systemic reaction could pose a significant risk.
- May be administered concomitantly with influenza virus vaccine.
- Administer SC or IM only, preferably in the deltoid muscle or lateral mid-thigh; do not give IV.
- Refrigerate vials. Use directly as supplied, do not dilute (reconstitution is not necessary).
- Have epinephrine 1:1000 immediately available at time of injection in case of anaphylactic reaction.
- Provide or teach patient to provide appropriate comfort measures—analgesics, antipyretics, warm soaks to injection site—to help patient to cope with effects of the drug therapy.
- Provide patient with written record of immunization and caution patient not to have another polyvalent pneumococcal vaccine injection.

## poliovirus vaccine, live, oral, trivalent (OPV, TOPV; Sabin)

Orimune

### Therapeutic Actions

Live, attenuated virus stimulates active immunity by simulating the natural infection without producing symptoms of the disease.

### Indications

Prevention of poliomyelitis caused by Poliovirus Types 1, 2, and 3—routine immunization of infants and children through the age of 18 y.

### Adverse Effects

Paralytic diseases in vaccine recipients and their close contacts (risk extremely small).

### Dosage

- Infants: 0.5 ml PO at 2 mo, 4 mo, and 18 mo; an optional dose may be given at 6 mo in areas where polio is endemic. A booster dose is recommended at time of entry into elementary school.
- Older children through 18 yrs: 2 doses of 0.5 ml PO 8 wk apart and a third dose 6–12 mo later.
- Adults: Not usually needed in adults in this country; if unimmunized adult is exposed, is traveling to a high risk area, or is a household contact of children receiving TOPV, IPV (inactivated polio virus vaccine; Salk vaccine) is recommended or immunization using the same schedule as older children.

### Nursing Considerations

- Do not administer to patients with known hypersensitivity to streptomycin or neomycin (each dose contains <25 mcg of each).
- Defer administration in the presence of persistent vomiting or diarrhea and in patients with acute illness or any advanced debilitating condition.

- Do not administer to any patient with immune deficiency conditions; do not administer shortly after immune serum globulin unless absolutely necessary because of travel or exposure; if given with or shortly after ISG, dose should be repeated after 3 mo.
- Use caution if administering to pregnant patients, **Pregnancy Category C,** safety not established, use only if clearly needed and benefits outweigh unknown effects on the fetus; if immediate protection is needed, TOPV is the recommended therapy.
- Do not administer parenterally; administer directly PO or mix with distilled water, tap water free of chlorine, simple syrup or milk; alternately, it may be adsorbed on bread, cake, or cube sugar.
- Store vaccine frozen or refrigerated; thaw before use; vaccine may go through 10 freeze-thaw cycles if temperature does not exceed 46°F and cumulative thaw does not exceed 24h; if it does, vaccine must be refrigerated and used within 30 days.
- Caution unimmunized adults or adults whose immunological status is not known about the risk of paralytic diseases and polio when they are household contacts of children receiving TOPV; risk can be minimized by giving them 3 doses of IPV a month apart before the children receive TOPV.
- Provide patient or parent with a written record of the vaccination and information on when additional doses are needed.

## poliovirus vaccine, inactivated (IPV, Salk)

IPOL

### Therapeutic Actions
Inactivated, attenuated sterile suspension of three types of polio virus used to produce antibody response against poliomyelitis infection.

### Indications
Prevention of poliomyelitis caused by Poliovirus Types 1, 2, and 3 in adults and children who refuse TOPV or in whom TOPV is contraindicated.

### Adverse Effects
Paralytic diseases in vaccine recipients and their close contacts (risk extremely small).

### Dosage
- Children: 0.5 ml SC at 2 mo, 4 mo, and 18 mo. A booster dose is needed at time of entry into elementary school.
- Adults: Not usually needed in adults in this country; if unimmunized adult is exposed, is traveling to a high risk area, or is a household contact of children receiving TOPV, IPV (inactivated polio virus vaccine; Salk vaccine) immunization is recommended. 0.5 ml SC—two doses given at 1–2 mo interval and a third dose given 6–12 mo later. Previously vaccinated adults at risk for exposure should receive a 0.5 ml dose of this drug or TOPV.

### Nursing Considerations
- Do not administer to patients with known hypersensitivity to streptomycin or neomycin (each dose contains <25 mcg of each).
- Defer administration in the presence of persistent vomiting or diarrhea and in patients with acute illness or any advanced debilitating condition.
- Do not administer to any patient with immune deficiency conditions; do not administer shortly after immune serum globulin unless necessary because of travel or exposure; if given with or shortly after ISG, dose should be repeated after 3 mo.

- Use caution if administering to pregnant patients, **Pregnancy Category C,** safety not established, use only if clearly needed and benefits outweigh potential unknown effects on the fetus; if immediate protection is needed, TOPV is the recommended therapy.
- Refrigerate vaccine. Do not freeze.
- Provide patient or parent with a written record of the vaccination and information on when additional doses are needed.

## $RH_o$ (D) immune globulin

Gamulin Rh, HypRho-D, RhoGAM

## $RH_o$ (D) immune globulin IV

WinRHO SD

## $RH_o$ (D) immune globulin micro-dose

HypRho-D Mini-Dose, MICRhoGAM, Mini-Gamulin Rh

### Therapeutic Actions

Suppresses the immune response of nonsensitized $Rh_o$-negative individuals who receive $Rh_o$-positive blood as the result of a fetomaternal hemorrhage or a transfusion accident; each vial of $Rh_o$-immune globulin completely suppresses immunity to 15 ml of Rh-positive packed RBCs (about 30 ml whole blood); each vial $Rh_o$ immune globulin micro-dose suppresses immunity to 2.5 ml Rh-positive packed RBCs.

### Indications

- Prevention of sensitization to the $Rh_o$ factor.
- To prevent hemolytic disease of the newborn (erythroblastosis fetalis) in a subsequent pregnancy—mother must be $Rh_o$ negative, mother must not be previously sensitized to $Rh_o$ factor, infant must be $Rh_o$ positive and direct antiglobulin negative—used at full term delivery, for incomplete pregnancy, for antepartum prophylaxis in case of abortion or ectopic pregnancy.
- To prevent $Rh_o$ sensitization in $Rh_o$-negative patients accidentally transfused with $Rh_o$-positive blood.
- Immune thrombocytopenic purpura (ITP) (IV)

### Adverse Effects

Pain and soreness at injection site.

### Dosage

- Postpartum prophylaxis: 1 vial, IM or IV within 72 h of delivery.
- Antepartum prophylaxis: 1 vial, IM or IV at 28 wk gestation and one vial within 72 h after an Rh-incompatible delivery to prevent Rh isoimmunization during pregnancy.
- Following amniocentesis, miscarriage, abortion, ectopic pregnancy at or beyond 13 wk gestation: 1 vial, IM or IV.
- Transfusion accidents: Multiply the volume in ml of Rh-positive whole blood administered by the hematocrit of the donor unit and divide this volume (in ml) by 15 to obtain the number of vials to be administered. If results of calculation are a fraction, administer the next whole number of vials.
- ITP: 250 IU/kg IV; base therapy on response.

- Spontaneous abortion or induced abortion or termination of ectopic pregnancy up to and including 12 wk gestation (unless the father is Rh negative): 1 vial micro-dose IM given as soon as possible after termination of pregnancy.

### Nursing Considerations

- $Rh_0$ globulin is not needed in $Rh_0$-negative mothers if the father can be determined to be $Rh_0$ negative.
- Do not administer to the $Rh_0$-positive postpartum infant, to a $Rh_0$-positive individual, to a $Rh_0$-negative individual previously sensitized to the $Rh_0$ antigen (if it is not known if a woman is $Rh_0$ sensitized, administer the $Rh_0$ globulin).
- Before administration, determine the infant's blood type and arrange for a direct antiglobulin test using umbilical cord, venous, or capillary blood; confirm that the mother is $Rh_0$ negative.
- Do not administer IV; administer IM within 72 h after $Rh_0$-incompatible delivery, miscarriage, abortion or transfusion.
- Prepare one vial dose by withdrawing entire contents of vial; inject entire contents IM.
- Prepare two or more vial dose using 5–10 ml syringes—withdraw contents from the vials to be administered at one time and inject IM; contents of the total number of vials may be injected as a divided dose at different injection sites at the same time, or the total dosage may be divided and injected at intervals, provided the total dose is administered with 72 h postpartum or after a transfusion accident.
- Refrigerate vials; do not freeze.
- Provide appropriate comfort measures if injection sites are painful.
- Reassure patient and explain what has been given and why; the patient will need to know what was given in the event of future pregnancies.

## rubella virus vaccine, live

Meruvax II

### Therapeutic Actions

Live virus stimulates active immunity through development of antibodies against the rubella virus.

### Indications

- Immunization against rubella—children 12 mo of age to puberty, adolescent and adult males, nonpregnant adolescent and adult females, rubella-susceptible women in the postpartum period, leukemia patients in remission whose chemotherapy has been terminated for at least 3 mo, susceptible persons traveling abroad.
- Revaccination of children vaccinated when <12 mo.

### Adverse Effects

Burning, stinging at injection site; regional lymphadenopathy, urticaria, rash, malaise, sore throat, fever, headache, polyneuritis—symptoms similar to natural rubella; arthritis, arthralgia—often 2–4 wk after receiving the vaccine.

### Dosage

Inject total volume of reconstituted vaccine SC, into the outer aspect of the upper arm; each dose contains not less than 1000 $TCID_{50}$ of rubella.

### Nursing Considerations

- Do not administer to patients with a history of anaphylactic hypersensitivity to neomycin (each dose contains 25 mcg neomycin), to patients with immune deficiency conditions, to patients receiving immune serum globulin or blood transfusions.

- Do not administer to pregnant women, **Pregnancy Category C;** advise patients to avoid pregnancy for 3 mo following vaccination.
- Defer administration in the presence of acute respiratory or other active infections; susceptible children with mild illnesses may be vaccinated.
- Do not administer within one mo of immunization with other *live virus vaccines,* except that rubella vaccine may be administered concurrently with *live monovalent or trivalent polio vaccine live measles virus vaccine, live mumps vaccine.*
- Do not administer for at least 3 mo following blood or plasma transfusions or administration of serum immune globulin.
- Monitor for possible depression of *tuberculin skin sensitivity;* administer the test before or simultaneously with the vaccine.
- Refrigerate vials and protect from light. Reconstitute using only the diluent supplied with the vial, use as soon as possible after reconstitution; discard reconstituted vaccine if not used within 8 h.
- Provide or instruct patient to provide appropriate comfort measures to help patient to cope with the adverse effects of the drug—analgesics, antipyretics, fluids, rest, etc.
- Provide patient or parent with a written record of immunization, inform that revaccination is not necessary.

## typhoid vaccine

Vivotif Berna Vaccine

### Therapeutic Actions

Contains live attenuated strains of typhoid bacteria; produces a humoral antibody response against the causative agent of typhoid fever. Precise mechanism of action is not understood.

### Indications

- Active immunization against typhoid fever (parenteral)
- Immunization of adults and children against disease caused by *Salmonella typhi* (routine immunization is not recommended in the United States but is recommended for travelers, workers in microbiology fields, or those who may come into household contact with typhoid fever)

### Adverse Effects

Transient fever; edema of injection area with redness, swelling, induration, pain (may persist for a few days); headache, malaise.

### Dosage

- Parenteral: Adult and children $\geq$10 y: 2 doses of 0.5 ml each SC at intervals of $\geq$4 wk; children $<$10 y: 2 doses of 0.25 ml each SC at intervals of $\geq$4 wk.
- Booster dose (given every 3 y in cases of continued exposure): Adult and children $\geq$10 y: 0.5 ml SC or 0.1 ml intradermally; children $<$ 10 y: 0.25 ml SC or 0.1 ml intradermally.
- Oral ($>$6 y): One capsule on days 1, 3, 5 and 7 taken 1 h before a meal with a cold or lukewarm drink. There are no data on the need for a booster dose at this time.

### Nursing Considerations

- Use caution with pregnancy—**Pregnancy Category C;** safety not established.
- Defer administration in case of acute infection, GI illness, nausea, vomiting.
- Have patient swallow capsules whole; do not chew. All 4 doses must be taken to ensure antibody response.

- Administer parenteral doses by SC injection; deltoid muscle is the preferred site.
- Arrange for epinephrine 1:1000 to be immediately available at time of injection because of risk of hypersensitivity reactions.
- Provide comfort measures to help the patient cope with the discomforts of the injection: analgesics, warm soaks for injection site, small meals, environmental control—temperature, stimuli.
- Provide patient with written record of immunization and information on booster immunization if appropriate.

## varicella virus vaccine live

Varivax

### Therapeutic Actions

Contains live attenuated varicella virus obtained from human or guinea pig cell cultures. Varicella virus causes chickenpox in children and adults. Vaccine produces an active immunity to the virus; the longevity of immunity is not known.

### Indications

Active immunization of adults and children ≥ 12 mo against chickenpox.

### Adverse Effects

Transient fever; edema of injection area with redness, swelling, induration, pain (may persist for a few days); upper respiratory illness, cough, rash.

### Dosage

- Adult and children ≥ 13 y: 0.5 ml SC in the deltoid area followed by 0.5 ml 4–8 wk later.
- Children 1–12 y: Single 0.5 ml dose SC.

### Nursing Considerations

- Use caution with allergy to neomycin or gelatin, pregnancy—**Pregnancy Category C;** safety not established.
- Defer administration in case of acute infection and for at least 5 mo after plasma transfusion, immune globulin, other immunizations.
- Do not administer salicylates for up to 6 wk after immunization; cases of Reye's syndrome have been reported.
- Administer by SC injection; deltoid muscle is the preferred site.
- Arrange for epinephrine 1:1000 to be immediately available at time of injection because of risk of hypersensitivity reactions.
- Provide comfort measures to help the patient cope with the discomforts of the injection: analgesics, warm soaks for injection site, small meals, environmental control—temperature, stimuli.
- Provide patient with written record of immunization. It is not known at this time if booster immunization will be needed.

## Other Biologicals

| Name | Brand Names | Indications | Dosage | Special Considerations |
|---|---|---|---|---|
| ***Immunoglobulins*** | | | | |
| lymphocyte, immune globulin, anti-thymocyte globulin | *Atgam* | Management of allograft rejection in renal transplants; treatment of aplastic anemia | 10–30 mg/kg/day IV adult transplant; 5–25 mg/kg/day IV pediatric transplant, 10–20 mg/kg/day IV for 8–14 days for aplastic anemia | Possibly useful for other transplants; refrigerate, stable for up to 12 h after reconstitution. |
| rabies immune globulin | *Hyperab*<br>*Imogam* | Passive protection against rabies in nonimmunized patients with exposure to rabies. | 20 IU/kg IM | Refrigerate vial. Infuse wound area if possible. Give in conjunction with rabies vaccine. |
| respiratory syncytial virus immune globulin (human) (RSV-IGIV) | *RespiGam* | Prevention of serious lower respiratory tract infection caused by RSV in children <24 mo with bronchopulmonary dysplasia or history of premature birth. | 1.5 ml/kg/h for 15 min; may increase to 3 ml/kg/h if needed for 15 min; may then increase to 6 ml/kg/h to a total monthly infusion of 750 mg/kg | Administer using infusion pump; use at start of RSV season. Increase rate of infusion only if clinical condition is stable; critically ill children may require a slower rate. |
| tetanus immune globulin | *Hyper-Tet* | Passive immunization against tetanus, useful at time of injury. | 250 units IM | Do not give IV. Arrange proper medical care of wound. Reduce pediatric dosage based on weight. |

*(continued)*

| Name | Brand Names | Indications | Dosage | Special Considerations |
|---|---|---|---|---|
| varicella-zoster immune globulin | *Varicella-Zoster Immune Globulin* | Passive immunity for immunosuppressed patients with significant exposure to varicella. | 125 units/10 kg IM to a max. of 625 units | Administer within 96 h of exposure to chicken pox. Not for use in non-immunosuppressed individuals. |
| ***Antitoxins and antivenins*** | | | | |
| diphtheria antitoxin | | Prevention or treatment of diphtheria. | 20,000–120,000 units IM or by slow IV infusion | Warm before use. Give immediately at first sign of symptoms. |
| antivenin (crotalidae) polyvalent | | Neutralize the venom of pit vipers; inc. rattlesnakes, copperheads, etc. | 20–40 ml IV; up to 100–150 ml IV in severe cases | Removal of venom should be done at once; antivenin to rare breeds of snake may be available from the CDC. |
| antivenin (micrurus fulvius) | | Neutralize the venom of coral snakes in the US | 30–50 ml by slow IV injection | Flush with IV fluids after antivenin has been infused. May require up to 100 ml. |
| Black Widow spider species antivenin | *Antivenin (Latrodectus mactans)* | Treatment of symptoms of Black Widow spider bites. | 2.5 ml IM; may be given IV in 10–50 ml saline over 15 min | Assure supportive therapy and use of muscle relaxants. |
| ***Bacterial vaccines*** | | | | |
| BCG | *TICE BCG* | Exposure to TB of skin-test negative infants and children; treatment of groups with high rates or TB; travel to areas with high rates of endemic TB. | 0.2–0.3 ml percutaneous | Refrigerate, protect from light; keep the vaccination site clean until reaction disappears. |

| | | | | |
|---|---|---|---|---|
| meningococcal polysaccharide vaccine | *Menomune-A/C/Y/W-135* | Prevention of meningitis in patients at risk in epidemic or highly endemic areas. | 0.5 ml SC | Reconstitute with diluent provided. |
| cholera vaccine | | Immunization against cholera for travelers to areas endemic or epidemic in cholera. | 0.2–0.3 ml SC, IM with a booster of 0.5 ml at 10 y | Do not give within 3 wk of yellow fever vaccine. |
| plague vaccine | | Immunization of persons at risk for exposure to plague. | 3 doses IM—1 ml followed by 0.2 ml 4 wk later; and 0.2 ml 5 mo later | Use of vaccine increases chances of recovery in epidemic situations. |
| ***Viral vaccines*** | | | | |
| Japanese encephalitis vaccine | *JE-VAX* | Active immunization in persons >1 y who will reside or travel in areas where it is endemic or epidemic. | 3 SC doses of 1 ml given at days 0, 7, and 30 | Refrigerate vial; do not remove rubber stopper; do not travel within 10 days of vaccination. |
| rabies vaccine | *Imovax Rabies* | Preexposure rabies immunization for patients in high risk area; postexposure antirabies regimen in conjunction with rabies immunoglobulin. | Preexposure; 1 ml IM on days 0, 7, 21, and 28. Postexposure: 1 ml IM on days 0, 3, 7, 21, and 28 | Refrigerate. If titers are low, booster may be needed. |
| yellow fever vaccine | *YF-Vax* | Immunization of travelers to endemic areas. | 0.5 ml SC; booster dose suggested q10 yr | Caution with allergy to chicken or egg products. |

## Recommended Immunization Schedules

| *Immunization* | *Birth* | *2 mo* | *4 mo* | *6 mo* | *12–15 mo* | *18 mo* | *4–6 y* | *11–12 y* | *14–16 y* |
|---|---|---|---|---|---|---|---|---|---|
| Hepatitis B | X | X | | | X | | | | |
| DPT | | X | X | X | X | | | | |
| Tetanus/diphtheria booster | | | | | | | X | X | |
| *H. influenzae* b | | X | X | X | X | | | | |
| Measles, mumps, rubella | | | | | X | | X | | |
| Poliovirus | | X | X | | X | | X | | |

Suggested by the American Academy of Pediatrics, 1995.

# APPENDIX F

## Fixed-Combination Drugs

### *Commonly Prescribed Fixed-Combination Drugs: Dosages*

**Amphetamines**

#### dextroamphetamine with amphetamine

**C II Controlled Substance**
Adderall

Tablets: 2.5 (10 mg tablet) mg or 5 each of (20 mg tablet) dextroamphetamine sulfate and saccharate, amphetamine asparate and sulfate
**Usual adult dosage:** 10–60 mg/d to control symptoms

**Analgesics**

#### acetaminophen with codeine

**C III Controlled Substance**
Tylenol with Codeine

Solution: 12 mg codeine; 120 mg acetaminophen
Tablets No. 2: 15 mg codeine, 300 mg acetaminophen
Tablets No. 3: 30 mg codeine, 300 mg acetaminophen
Tablets No. 4: 60 mg codeine, 300 mg acetaminophen
**Usual adult dosage:** 1–2 tablets q 4–6 h as needed for pain; or 15 ml q 4–6 h.

#### aspirin with codeine

**C-III Controlled Substance**
Empirin with Codeine

Tablets No. 3: 30 mg codeine, 325 mg aspirin
Tablets No. 4: 60 mg codeine, 325 mg aspirin
**Usual adult dosage:** 1–2 tablets q 4–6 h as needed for pain.

Fiorinal with Codeine

Capsules: 30 mg codeine, 325 mg aspirin, 40 mg caffeine, 50 mg butabarbital
**Usual adult dosage:** 1–2 capsules as needed for pain; up to 6/day

## diclofenac sodium and misoprostol

**Pregnancy Category X**

Arthrotec

Tablets
'50': 5 mg diclofenac, 200 mg misoprostol
'75': 75 mg declofenac, 200 mg misoprostol

**Usual adult dosage:**
Osteoarthritis: Arthrotec 50 PO tid or Arthrotec 50 or 75: PO bid
Rheumatoid arthritis: Arthrotec 50 PO tid or qid; or Arthrotec 50 or 75, PO bid.

## hydrocodone with acetaminophen

**C-III Controlled Substance**

Anexsia, Co-Gesic, Duocet, Margesic H, Norco, Panacet 5/500, Vicodin, Zydone

Capsules/tablets: 5 mg hydrocodone, 500 mg acetaminophen
Norco tablets: 10 mg hydrocodone, 325 mg acetaminophen
**Usual adult dosage:** 1–2 tablets/capsules q4h–6 h; up to 8/day.

## hydrocodone with ibuprofen

Vicoprofen

Tablets: 7.5 mg hydrocodone, 200 mg ibuprofen
**Usual adult dosage:** one tablet q 4–6 h as needed for pain

## oxycodone with acetaminophen

**C-II Controlled Substance**

Percocet, Roxicet, Tylox, Roxilox

Tylox capsules: 5 mg oxycodone, 500 mg acetaminophen
Tablets: 5 mg oxycodone, 325 mg acetaminophen
**Usual adult dosage:** 1–2 tablets q 4–6 h as needed for pain.

## oxycodone with aspirin

**C-II Controlled Substance**

Percodan, Roxiprin

Tablets: 4.5 mg oxycodone, 325 mg aspirin
**Usual adult dosage:** 1–2 tablets q6h as needed for pain.

### Antiacne drugs

Ortho Tri-Cyclen tablets

Tablets
0.18 mg norgestimate
35 mcg ethinyl estradiol

**Usual adult dosage:** for women >15 y: 1 tablet PO qd.
Birth control agent used cyclically.
See also **estradiol.**

### Antibacterials

#### Augmentin

Tablets
'250'—250 mg amoxicillin, 125 mg clavulanic acid
'500'—500 mg amoxicillin, 125 mg clavulanic acid
Powder for oral suspension
'125' powder—125 mg amoxicillin, 31.25 mg clavulanic acid
'250' powder—250 mg amoxicillin, 62.5 mg clavulanic acid
Chewable tablets
'125'—125 mg amoxicillin, 31.25 mg clavulanic acid
'250'—250 mg amoxicillin, 62.5 mg clavulanic acid
**Usual adult dosage:** 1 '250' to 1 '500' tablet q8h.
**Usual pediatric dosage:** <40 kg: 20–40 mg amoxicillin/kg/d in divided doses q8h (pediatric dosage is based on amoxicillin content).

Also see **amoxicillin;** clavulanic acid protects amoxicillin from breakdown by bacterial β-lactamase enzymes and is given only in combination with certain antibodies that are broken down by β-lactamase.

### carbapenem

#### Primaxin

Powder for injection
250 mg imipenem and 250 mg cilastatin
500 mg imipenem and 500 mg cilastatin

- Follow manufacturer's instructions for reconstituting and diluting the drug.
- Administer each 250–500 mg dose by IV infusion over 20–30 min; infuse each 1 g dose over 40–60 min.
- Dosage recommendations represent the amount of imipenem to be given. Initial dosage should be individualized on the basis of the type and severity of infection. Subsequent dosage is individualized on the basis of the severity of the patient's illness, the degree of susceptibility of the pathogen(s), the patient's age, weight, and creatinine clearance; dosage for adults with normal renal function ranges from 250 mg 1 g q 6–8 h. Dosage should not exceed 50 mg/kg/d or 4 g/d, whichever is less.
- Dosage for patients with **renal impairment:**

| | *Type of Infection* | |
|---|---|---|
| *CCr (ml/min)* | *Less Severe* | *Life-threatening* |
| 30–70 | 500 mg q8h | 500 mg q6h |
| 20–30 | 500 mg q12h | 500 mg q8h |
| 5–20 | 250 mg q12h | 500 mg q12h |
| or 0–5 with hemodialysis | 250 mg q12h | 500 mg q12h |

- Imipenem is an antibiotic that inhibits cell wall synthesis in susceptible bacteria; cilastatin inhibits the renal enzyme that metabolizes imipenem; these drugs are commercially available only in the combined formulation.

## co-trimoxazole

TMP-SMZ; *Bactrim, Cotrim, Septra, Sulfatrim*

Tablets
80 mg trimethoprim (TMP) and 400 mg sulfamethoxazole (SMZ)
160 mg trimethoprim and 800 mg sulfamethoxazole
Oral suspension
40 mg trimethoprim and 200 mg sulfamethoxazole per 5 ml
IV infusion
84 mg trimethoprim and 400 mg sulfamethoxazole per 5 ml

***Usual adult dosage***

- Urinary tract infections, shigellosis and acute otitis media: 160 mg TMP/800 mg sulfamethoxazole, PO q12h; 8–10 mg/kg/d (based on TMP component) in 2–4 divided doses of q6, 8, or 12h, IV. Treat for up to 14 days (UTIs) or for 5 days (shigellosis).
- Acute exacerbations of chronic bronchitis: 160 mg TMP/800 mg SMZ PO q12h for 14 days.
- *Pneumocystis carinii* pneumonitis: 20 mg/kg TMP and 100 mg/kg SMZ q24h PO in divided doses q6h; 15–20 mg/kg/d (based on TMP component) in 3–4 divided doses q6–8h, IV. Treat for 14 days.

***Usual pediatric dose***

- Urinary tract infections, shigellosis, acute otitis media: 8 mg/kg/d TMP and 40 mg/kg/d SMZ PO in 2 divided doses q12h; 8–10 mg/kg/d (based on TMP component) in 2–4 divided doses q6, 8, or 12h, IV. Treat for 10–14 days (UTIs and acute otitis media) or for 5 days (shigellosis).
- *Pneumocystis carinii* pneumonitis: 20 mg/kg TMP and 100 mg/kg SMZ q24h PO in divided doses q6h; 15–20 mg/kg/d (based on TMP component) in 3–4 divided doses q6–8h, IV. Treat for 14 days.

*IMPAIRED RENAL FUNCTION*

| *Creatinine Clearance (ml/min)* | *Dosage* |
|---|---|
| >30 ml/min | Use standard dosage. |
| 15–30 ml/min | Use ½ standard dosage. |
| <15 ml/min | Not recommended. |

- Administer IV over 60–90 min. Thoroughly flush IV line after each use, do not refrigerate. IV solution must be diluted before use—see manufacturer's instructions. Do *not* give IM.
- Also see **trimethoprim** and **sulfamethoxazole.**

## erythromycin with sulfisoxazole

Eryzole, Pediazole

Granules for oral suspension: erythromycin ethylsuccinate (equivalent of 200 mg erythromycin activity) and 600 mg sulfisoxazole per 5 ml when reconstituted according to manufacturer's directions.

- Usual dosage for acute otitis media: 50 mg/kg/d erythromycin and 150 mg/kg/d sulfisoxazole in divided doses qid for 10 days.
- Administer without regard to meals.
- Refrigerate after reconstitution; use within 14 days.
- Also see **erythromycin** and **sulfisoxazole.**

## piperacillin sodium and tazobactam sodium

Zosyn

Tazobactam is a beta-lactamase inhibitor used in combination with the broad-spectrum penicillin.

- Recommended for appendicitis, peritonitis, postpartum endometritis and PID, community-acquired pneumonia, nosocomial pneumonia if agent is responsive in sensitivity testing.
- Usual daily adult dose: 12 mg/1.5g IV given as 3.375 g q6h.
- Reduced dosage required for renal impairment or dialysis.
- Administer by IV infusion over 30 min. Reconstitute with 5 ml of suitable diluent per 1g piperacillin. Discard after 24h.

See also **piperacillin.**

## ticarcillin with clavulanic acid

Timentin

Powder for injection
  3.1 g vial—3 g ticarcillin, 0.1 g clavulanic acid
  3.2 g vial—3 g ticarcillin, 0.2 g clavulanic acid

- Administer by IV infusion over 30 min.
- Dosage for 60 kg adults: 3.1 g (3 g ticarcillin and 0.1 g clavulanic acid) q4–6h. <60 kg adults: 200–300 mg ticarcillin/kg/d in divided doses q4–6h.
- Urinary tract infections: 3.2 g (3g ticarcillin and 0.2 g clavulanic acid) q8h.
- Pediatric dosage (children <12y): Not established.
- Geriatric or renal failure patients: Initial loading dose of 3.1 g, then as follows:

| *Creatinine Clearance* | *Dosage* |
|---|---|
| >60 | 3.1 g q4h |
| 30–60 | 2 g q4h |
| 10–30 | 2 g q8h |
| <10 | 2 g q12h |
| <10 with hepatic disease | 3.1 g q12h |
| On hemodialysis | 2 g q12h, supplemented with 3.1 g after each dialysis. |

- Continue treatment for 2 days after signs and symptoms of infection have disappeared. (Usual duration of therapy: 10–14 days).

Also see **ticarcillin;** clavulanic acid protects ticarcillin from breakdown by bacterial $\beta$-lactamase enzymes and is given only in combination with certain antibiotics that are broken down by $\beta$-lactamase.

## ampicillin with sulbactam

Unasyn

Powder for injection
  1.5-g vial: 1 g ampicillin, 0.5 g sulbactam
  3-g vial: 2 g ampicillin, 1 g sulbactam

**Usual adult dosage:** 0.5–1 g sulbactam with 1–2 g ampicillin IM or IV q 6–8 h.

Also see **ampicillin;** sulbactam inhibits many bacterial penicillinase enzymes, thus broadening the spectrum of ampicillin; sulbactam is also weakly antibacterial alone.

### Antidepressants

#### Etrafon, Triavil

Tablets
- 2 mg perphenazine, 10 mg amitriptyline
- 2 mg perphenazine, 25 mg amitriptyline
- 4 mg perphenazine, 25 mg amitriptyline
- 4 mg perphenazine, 50 mg amitriptyline (*Triavil* only)

**Usual adult dosage:** 2–4 mg perphenazine with 10–50 mg amitriptyline tid–qid. Reduce dosage after initial response.
Also see **amitriptyline** and **perphenazine.**

#### Limbitrol

Tablets
- 5 mg chlordiazepoxide, 12.5 mg amitriptyline
- 10 mg chlordiazepoxide, 25 mg amitriptyline

**Usual adult dosage:** 10 mg chlordiazepoxide with 25 mg amitriptyline tid–qid up to 6 times daily. 5 mg chlordiazepoxide with 12.5 mg amitriptyline tid–qid for patients who do not tolerate the higher doses. Reduce dosage after initial response.
Also see **amitriptyline** and **chlordiazepoxide.**

### Antidiarrheal drug

## diphenoxylate HCl with atropine sulfate

**C-V Controlled Substance**

Logen, Lomanate, Lomotil, Lonox

Tablets: 2.5 mg diphenoxylate HCl, 0.025 mg atropine sulfate
Liquid: 2.5 mg diphenoxylate HCl, 0.025 mg atropine sulfate/5 ml

- Individualized dosage; usual adult dosage; 5 mg qid.
- Pediatric initial dosage (use only liquid in children 2–12 y of age): 0.3 mg/kg daily in 4 divided doses.

| *Age (years)* | *Weight (kg)* | *Dose* | *Frequency* |
|---|---|---|---|
| 2–5 | 13–20 | 2 mg, 4 ml | 3 times daily |
| 5–8 | 20–27 | 2 mg, 4 ml | 4 times daily |
| 8–12 | 27–36 | 2 mg, 4 ml | 5 times daily |

- Reduce dosage as soon as initial control of symptoms is achieved. Maintenance dosage may be as low as ¼ of the initial dosage.

Also see **atropine sulfate** and **meperidine;** diphenoxylate is chemically and pharmacologically related to meperidine, but lacks analgesic activity.

## Antihypertensive

### Capozide

Tablets
- 25 mg hydrochlorothiazide and 50 or 25 mg captopril
- 15 mg hydrochlorothiazide and 50 or 25 mg captopril

**Usual adult dosage:** 1–2 tablet qd PO taken in the morning.
Dosage should be titrated with the individual products, switching to this combination product when patient is stabilized on the dosage of each drug that is available in this combination.
See also **hydrochlorothiazide, captopril.**

### Combipres

Tablets: 15 mg chlorthalidone with 0.1, 0.2, or 0.3 mg clonidine HCl

**Usual adult dosage:** 1–2 tablet qd PO taken in the morning.
Dosage should be titrated with the individual products, switching to this combination product when patient is stabilized on the dosage of each drug that is available in this combination.
See also **chlorthalidone, clonidine.**

### Hyzaar

Tablets: 50 mg losartan, 12.5 mg hydrochlorothiazide

**Usual adult dosage:** 1 tablet PO qd in the morning.
Not for initial therapy; start using each component and if desired effects are obtained, Hyzaar may be used.
See also **losartan, hydrochlorothiazide.**

### Inderide

Tablets
- 50 mg hydrochlorothiazide with 160, 120, or 80 mg propranolol HCl
- 25 mg hydrochlorothiazide with 80 or 40 mg propranolol HCl

**Usual adult dosage:** 1–2 tablet qd PO taken in the morning.
Dosage should be titrated with the individual products, switching to this combination product when patient is stabilized on the dosage of each drug that is available in this combination.
See also **hydrochlorothiazide, propranolol.**

### Lexxel

Tablets
- 5 mg eualapril, 5 mg felodipine; extended release

**Usual adult dosage:** 1 tablet PO qd.
Dosage should be titrated with the individual products, switching to the combination product when the patient is stabilized on the dosage of each drug that is available in this combination.
See also **eualapril, felodipine.**

## Lotensin HCT

Tablets

25 mg hydrochlorothiazide, 20 mg benazepril
12.5 mg hydrochlorothiazide, 20 mg benazepril
12.5 mg hydrochlorothiazide, 10 mg benazepril
6.25 mg hydrochlorothiazide, 5 mg benazepril

**Usual adult dosage:** 1 tablet qd PO in the morning.
Dosage should be titrated with the individual products, switching to this combination once patient is stabilized.
See also **hydrochlorothiazide, benazepril.**

## Lotrel

Capsule

2.5 mg amlodipine, 10 mg benazepril
5 mg amlodipine, 10 mg benazepril
5 mg amlodipine, 20 mg benazepril

**Usual adult dosage:** 1 tablet qd PO taken in the morning.
Monitor patient for hypertension and adverse effects closely over first 2 wk and regularly thereafter.
See also **amlodipine, benazepril.**

## Teczem

Tablets

enalapril maleate
diltiazem maleate

**Usual adult dosage:** 1–2 tablet qd PO taken in the morning.
Dosage should be titrated with the individual products, switching to this combination product when the patient is stabilized on the dosage of each drug that is available in this combination.
See also **enalapril, diltiazem.**

## Tarka

Tablets

1 mg trandolapril, 240 mg verapamil
2 mg trandolapril, 180 mg verapamil
2 mg trandolapril, 240 mg verapamil
4 mg trandolapril, 240 mg verapamil

**Usual adult dosage:** 1 tablet PO qd.
Take with food.
Dosage should be titrated with the individual products, switching to this combination product when the patient is stabilized on the dosage of each drug that is available in combination.
See also **trandolapril, verapamil.**

### Uniretic

Tablets
15 mg moexipril, 25 mg hydrochlorothiazide
**Usual adult dosage:** 1–2 tablets/d with a meal
Not for initial therapy.
Titrate dose to maintain appropriate BP.
See also **moexipril, hydrochlorothiazide**

### Vaseretic

Tablets
10 mg enalapril maleate and 25 mg hydrochlorothiazide
5 mg enalapril maleate and 12.5 mg hydrochlorothiazide
**Usual adult dosage:** 1–2 tablet qd PO taken in the morning.
Dosage should be titrated with the individual products, switching to this combination product once patient is stabilized on the dosage of each drug that is available in this combination.
See also **enalapril maleate** and **hydrochlorothiazide.**

### Zestoretic, Prinzide

Tablets
12.5 mg lisinopril, 10 mg hydrochlorothiazide
20 mg lisinopril, 12.5 mg hydrochlorothiazide
20 mg lisinopril, 25 mg hydrochlorothiazide
**Usual adult dosage:** 1 tablet qd PO taken in the morning.
Dosage should be titrated with individual products, switching to combination once patient is stabilized.
See also **lisinopril, hydrochlorothiazide.**

### Ziac

Tablets: 2.5, 6.25 or 10 mg bisoprolol and 6.25 mg hydrochlorothiazide
**Usual adult dosage:** 1 tablet/day PO taken in the morning.
Dosage should be titrated within 1 wk, optimal antihypertensive effect may require 2–3 wk.
See also **bisoprolol** and **hydrochlorothiazide.**

## Antimalarials

### Fansidar

Tablets: 500 mg sulfadoxine and 25 mg pyrimethamine
**Usual adult dosage:** Prophylaxis: 1 tablet, PO once/wk.
Presumptive treatment: 3 tablets, PO as a single dose.
**Usual pediatric dosage.**

| *Prophylaxis* | *Presumptive Treatment* |
|---|---|
| 2–11 months: 1/8 tablet PO, once/wk | 2–11 months: 1/4 tablet PO as a single dose |
| 1–3 yrs: 1/4 tablet PO, once/wk | 1–3 yrs: 1/2 tablet PO as a single dose |
| 4–8 yrs: 1/2 tablet PO, once/wk | 4–8 yrs: 1 tablet PO as a single dose |
| 9–14 yrs: 3/4 tablet PO, once/wk | 9–14 yrs: 2 tablets PO as a single dose |
| >14 yrs: 1 tablet/wk | >14 yrs: 3 tablets PO as a single dose |

*Note: Fatalities* have occurred in association with this drug, due to Stevens-Johnson syndrome and toxic epidermal necrolysis; drug should be discontinued at first sign of skin rash, depressed blood count, or active bacterial or fungal infection.
See also **pyrimethamine.**

## Antimigraine drugs

### Cafergot, Ercaf, Wigraine

Tablets: 1 mg ergotamine tartrate, 100 mg caffeine
**Usual adult dosage:** 2 tablets at first sign of attack. Follow with 1 tablet q½h, if needed. Maximum dose is 6 tablets/attack. Do not exceed 10 tablets/wk.

Suppositories: 2 mg ergotamine tartrate, 100 mg caffeine
**Usual adult dosage:** 1 at first sign of attack; follow with second dose after 1h, if needed. Maximum dose is 2/attack. Do not exceed 5/wk.
Also see **ergotamine.**

## Antiparkinsonism drugs

### Sinemet, Sinemet CR

Tablets
- 10 mg carbidopa, 100 mg levodopa
- 25 mg carbidopa, 100 mg levodopa
- 25 mg carbidopa, 250 mg levodopa

Controlled release
- 25 mg carbidopa, 100 mg levodopa
- 50 mg carbidopa, 200 mg levodopa

**Usual adult dosage:** Starting dose for patients not presently receiving levodopa: one tablet of 10 mg carbidopa/100 mg levodopa or 25 mg carbidopa/100 mg levodopa tid. For patients receiving levodopa: start combination therapy with the morning dose, at least 8 h after the last dose of levodopa, and choose a daily dosage of carbidopa/levodopa that will provide 25% of the previous levodopa daily dosage. Dosage must be titrated for each individual, based on the patient's clinical response. See manufacturer's directions for titrating the combination and single agent drugs.
See also **levodopa;** carbidopa is available alone only by a specific request to the manufacturer from physicians who have a patient who needs a different dosage of carbidopa than is provided by the fixed combination drug; carbidopa is a peripheral inhibitor of dopa decarboxylase, an enzyme that converts dopa to dopamine, which cannot penetrate the CNS; the addition of carbidopa to the levodopa regimen reduces the dose of levodopa needed and decreases the incidence of certain adverse reactions to levodopa.

## Antiulcer drugs

### Helidac

Tablets: 524.8 mg bismuth subsalicylate, 250 mg metronidazole, 500 mg tetracycline HCl

**Usual adult dosage:** 1 tablet PO qid for 14 d along with a prescribed $H_2$ antagonist. Indicated for the treatment of active duodenal ulcers associated with *Helicobacter pylori* infection.
See also **bismuth subsalicylate, metronidazole, tetracycline.**

### Tritec (ranitidine bismuth citrate)

Tablets: 162 mg ranitidine, 128 mg trivalent bismuth, 110 mg citrate

**Usual adult dosage:** 400 mg PO bid for 4 wk in combination with clarithromycin, 500 mg PO tid for the first 2 wk.
Indicated for the treatment of active duodenal ulcers associated with *Helicobacter pylori* infection.
See also **ranitidine.**

## Antiviral drugs

### Combivir

Tablets: 150 mg lamivudine, 300 mg zidovudine
**Usual adult dose:** 1 tablet twice daily.
Not recommended for children, adults <50 kg.
May be taken with food.
Does not decrease risk of spreading infections; use caution.
See also **lamivudine, zidovudine.**

## Diuretics

### Aldactazide

Tablets: 25 mg spironolactone, 25 mg hydrochlorothiazide
**Usual adult dosage:** 1–8 tablets daily.
Tablets: 50 mg spironolactone, 50 mg hydrochlorothiazide
**Usual adult dosage:** 1–4 tablets daily.
Also see **hydrochlorothiazide** and **spironolactone.**

### Dyazide

Capsules: 50 mg triamterene, 25 mg hydrochlorothiazide
**Usual adult dosage:** 1 tablet qd or bid after meals.
Also see **hydrochlorothiazide** and **triamterene.**

### Maxzide

Tablets: 75 mg triamterene, 50 mg hydrochlorothiazide
**Usual adult dosage:** 1 tablet qd.
Also see **hydrochlorothiazide** and **triamterene.**

### Moduretic

Tablets: 5 mg amiloride, 50 mg hydrochlorothiazide
**Usual adult dosage:** 1–2 tablets/d with meals.
Also see **amiloride** and **hydrochlorothiazide.**

## Menopause drugs

### Premphase

Tablets: 0.625 mg conjugated estrogens, 5 mg medroxyprogesterone
**Usual adult dosage:** 1 tablet qd PO.

Treatment of moderate to severe symptoms of osteoporosis and prevention of osteoporosis in women with intact uterus.
Also see **estrogen, medroxyprogesterone.**

### Prempro

Tablets: 0.625 mg estrogen, 2.5 mg medroxyprogesterone; 0.625 mg conjugated estrogen; 5 mg medroxyprogesterone
**Usual adult dosage:** 1 tablet qd PO.
For relief of symptoms of menopause and prevention of osteoporosis in women with intact uterus.
See also **estrogen, medroxyprogesterone.**

**Oral contraceptives**

Usual dosage: Take 1 tablet PO daily for 21 d, beginning on day 5 of the cycle (day 1 of the cycle is the first day of menstrual bleeding). Inert tablets or no tablets are taken for the next 7 d. Then start a new course of 21 d.
Suggested measures for missed doses:

One tablet missed—take it as soon as possible, or take 2 tablets the next day.
Two consecutive tablets missed—take 2 tablets daily for the next 2 d, then resume the regular schedule.
Three consecutive tablets missed—begin a new cycle of tablets 7 d after the last tablet was taken; use an additional method of birth control until the start of the next menstrual period.

Postcoital contraception (''morning after'' pills). Safe and effective for emergency contraception. Dosing regimen starts with 72 h of unprotected intercourse with a follow-up dose of the same number of pills 12 h after the first dose.

Ovral: 2 white tablets
Nordette: 4 light orange tablets
Lolouvral: 4 white tablets
Triphasil: 4 yellow tablets
Levlen: 4 light orange tablets
Tri-Levlin: 4 yellow tablets

| *Brand Name* | *Combination* |
|---|---|
| ***Monophasic*** | |
| Alesse | 20 mcg estradiol, 0.10 mg levonorgestrol |
| Brevicon, Modicon, Genora 0.5/35, Nelova 0.5/35 | 35 mcg ethinyl estradiol (estrogen) and 0.5 mg norethindrone (progestin) |
| Demulen 1/50 | 50 mcg ethinyl estradiol (estrogen) and 1 mg ethynodiol diacetate (progestin) |
| Demulen 1/35 | 35 mcg ethinyl estradiol (estrogen) and 1 mg ethynodiol diacetate (progestin) |
| Desogen, Ortho-Cept | 30 mcg ethinyl estradiol and 0.15 mg desogestrel |
| Levlen, Levora, Nordette | 30 mcg ethinyl estradiol (estrogen) and 0.15 mg levonorgestrel (progestin) |
| Loestrin 21 1.5/30 | 30 mcg ethinyl estradiol (estrogen) and 1.5 mg norethindrone acetate (progestin) |
| Loestrin 21 1/20 | 20 mcg ethinyl estradiol (estrogen) and 1 mg norethindrone (progestin) |
| Lo/Ovral | 30 mcg ethinyl estadiol (estrogen) and 0.3 mg norgestrel |
| Norinyl 1 + 50, Genora 1/50, Norethrin 1/50, Nelova 1/50M | 50 mcg mestranol (estrogen) and 1 mg norethindrone (progestin) |

*(continued)*

| *Brand Name* | *Combination* |
|---|---|
| Norinyl 1 + 35, Genora 1/35, N.E.E. 1/35, Nelova 1/35, Norethin 1/35E | 35 mcg ethinyl estradiol (estrogen) and 1 mg norethindrone (progestin) |
| Ortho-Novum 1/50 | 50 mcg ethinyl estradiol (estrogen) and 1 mg norethindrone acetate (progestin) |
| Ovcon-35 | 35 mcg ethinyl estradiol (estrogen) and 1 mg ethynodiol diacetate (progestin) |
| Ovral | 50 mcg ethinyl estradiol (estrogen) and 0.5 mg norgestrel (progestin) course of 21 days |
| ***Biphasic*** | |
| Jenest-28, Ortho-Novum 10/11 | phase 1–10 tablets, 0.5 mg norethindrone (progestin), and 35 mcg ethinyl estradiol (estrogen);<br>phase 2–11 tablets, 1 mg norethindrone (progestin), and 35 mcg ethinyl estradiol (estrogen). |
| ***Tri-phasic*** | |
| Estrostep 21 | phase 1—5 tablets, 1 mg norethindrone and 20 mcg ethinyl estradiol<br>phase 2—7 tablets, 1 mg norethindrone and 30 mcg ethinyl estradiol<br>phase 3—9 tablets, 1 mg norethindrone and 35 mcg ethinyl estradiol |
| Ortho Novum 7/7/7 | phase 1–7 tablets, 0.5 mg norethindrone (progestin), and 35 mcg ethinyl estradiol (estrogen)<br>phase 2—7 tablets, 0.75 mg norethindrone (progestin), and 35 mcg ethinyl estradiol (estrogen)<br>phase 3—7 tablets, 1 mg norethindrone (progestin), and 35 mcg ethinyl estradiol (estrogen) |
| Ortho Tri-cyclen | phase 1—7 tablets, 0.18 mg norgestimate, 35 mcg ethinyl estradiol<br>phase 2—7 tablets, 0.215 mg norgestimate, 35 mcg ethinyl estradiol<br>phase 3—0.25 mg norgestimate, 35 mcg ethinyl estradiol |
| Tri-Levlen | phase 1—6 tablets, 0.05 mg levonorgestrel (progestin), and 30 mcg ethinyl estradiol (estrogen)<br>phase 2—5 tablets, 0.075 mg levonorgestrel (progestin), and 40 mcg ethinyl estradiol (estrogen)<br>phase 3—10 tablets, 0.125 mg levonorgestrel (progestin), and 30 mcg ethinyl estradiol (estrogen) |
| Tri-Norinyl | phase 1—7 tablets, 0.5 mg norethindrone (progestin), and 35 mcg ethinyl estradiol (estrogen)<br>phase 2—9 tablets, 1 mg norethindrone (progestin), and 35 mcg ethinyl estradiol (estrogen)<br>phase 3—5 tablets, 0.5 mg norethindrone (progestin), and 35 mcg ethinyl estradiol (estrogen) |

*(continued)*

| *Brand Name* | *Combination* |
|---|---|
| Triphasil | phase 1—6 tablets, 0.05 mg levonorgestrel (progestin), and 30 mcg ethinyl estradiol (estrogen)<br>phase 2—5 tablets, 0.075 mg levonorgestrel (progestin), and 40 mcg ethinyl estradiol (estrogen)<br>phase 3—10 tablets, 0.125 mg levonorgestrel (progestin), and 30 mg ethinyl estradiol (estrogen) |

## Respiratory Drugs

### Claritin-D 12 Hour

ER Tablets: 5 mg loratidine, 120 mg pseudoephedrine
**Usual adult dosage:** 1 tablet q 12 h.
See also **loratidine, pseudoephedrine**.

### Claritin-D 24 Hour

ER Tablets: 10 mg loratidine, 240 mg pseudoephedrine
**Usual adult dosage:** 1 tablet qd.
See also **loratidine, pseudoephedrine**.

### Combivent

Metered dose inhaler: 18 mcg ipratropium bromide, 90 mcg albuterol
**Usual adult dosage:** 2 inhalations 4 × 1d.
Not for use during acute attack.
Use caution with known sensitivity to atropine, soy beans, joya lecithin, peanuts.
Treatment of bronchospasm with COPD in patients who require more than a single bronchodilator.
See also **ipratropium, albuterol.**

### Tavist-D

Tablets: 75 mg phenylpropanolamine HCl and 1.34 mg clemastine fumarate
**Usual adult dosage:** 1 tablet q12h.
See also **clemastine.**

### Trinalin Repetabs

Tablets: 1 mg azatidine maleate and 120 mg pseudoephedrine sulfate
**Usual adult dosage:** 1 tablet q 12 h for relief of upper respiratory symptoms of colds, allergies, etc.
See also **pseudoephedrine;** azatidine is an antihistamine.

# *Frequently Used Combination Products*

Many products are available on the market in combination form. Many of these are OTC preparations used frequently by consumers, It is helpful to have a guide to the ingredients of these products when instructing patients or assessing for drug interactions. The following is a list of brand names, active ingredients, and common usage. Nursing process information can be checked by looking up the active ingredient.

| *Brand Name* | *Active Ingredients* | *Common Usage* |
|---|---|---|
| *Actifed* | pseudoephedrine, tripolidine | Decongestant |
| *Actified Allergy* | pseudoephedrine, diphenhydramine | Decongestant |
| *Actifed Sinus Daytime* | pseudoephedrine, acetaminophen | Decongestant |
| *Actifed Sinus Nighttime* | pseudoephedrine, diphenhydramine, acetaminophen | Decongestant |
| *Adderall* | dextroamphetamin sulfate and sachavate, amphetamine asperate and sulfate | Amphetamine |
| *Advil Cold and Sinus* | ibuprofen, pseudoephedrine | Decongestant |
| *Aldactazide* | spironolactone, hydrochlorothiazide | Diuretic |
| *Aldoclor* | methyldopa, chlorothiazide | Antihypertensive |
| *Aldoril* | methyldopa, hydrochlorothiazide | Antihypertensive |
| *Alka Seltzer Advanced Formula* | sodium, calcium and potassium bicarbonate; acetaminophen; citric acid | Analgesis, antacid |
| *Alka-Seltzer Cold Medicine* | phenylpropanolamine, chlorpheniramine, dextromethorphan, aspirin | Decongestant, analgesic |
| *Alka-Seltzer Plus Allergy* | pseudoephedrine, chlorpheniramine, acetominephen | Decongestant, antihistamine, analgesic |
| *Alka-Seltzer Plus Cold and Cough* | phenylpropridamine, chlorpheniramine dextromethorphan, aspirin, phenylaline | Decongestants, antihistamine, antitussive |
| *Allerest* | phenylpropanolamine, chlorpheniramine | Decongestant, antihistamine |
| *Amaphen* | acetaminophen, butabarbital, caffeine codeine | Narcotic agonist analgesic |
| *Ambenyl Cough Syrup* | bromodiphenhydramine, codeine, alcohol | Antitussive |
| *Anacin* | aspirin, caffeine | Analgesic |
| *Anacin PM* | diphenhydramine, acetaminophen | Analgesic |
| *Anatuss Syrup* | phenylpropanolamine, dextromethorphan guaifenesin | Antitussive |
| *Anatuss Tablets* | phenylpropanolamine, dextromethorphan guaifenesin, acetaminophen | Antitussive |
| *Anexsia* | hydrocodone, acetaminophen | Analgesic |
| *Antrocol* | atropine, phenobarbital | Sedative, GI anticholinergic |
| *Apresazide* | hydralazine, hydrochlorothiazide | Antihypertensive |
| *Augmentin* | amoxicillin, clavulanic acid | antibiotic |

*(continued)*

| Brand Name | Active Ingredients | Common Usage |
|---|---|---|
| *Bactrim* | trimethoprim, sulfamethoxazole | Antibiotic |
| *Bayer Select Maximum Strength Headache* | acetaminophen, caffeine | Analgesic |
| *Bayer Select Maximum Strength Menstrual* | acetaminophen, pamabrom | Analgesic |
| *Bayer Select Maximum Strength Night Time Pain Relief* | acetaminophen, diphenhydramine | Analgesic |
| *Bayer Select Maximum Strength Sinus Pain Relief* | acetaminophen, pseudoephedrine | Analgesic decongestant |
| *Bellergal-S* | belladonna, phenobarbital, ergotamine | GI anticholinergic, sedative |
| *Benadryl Decongestant* | diphenhydramine, pseudoephedrine | Decongestant |
| *Benylin Decongestant* | diphenhydramine, pseudoephedrine | Decongestant |
| *Bromfed* | brompheniramine, pseudoephedrine | Decongestant, antihistamine |
| *BromoSeltzer* | acetaminophen, sodium bicarbonate, citric acid | Analgesic, antacid |
| *Bronkaid Tablets* | theophylline, ephedrine, guaifensein | Antiasthmatic |
| *Bufferin* | aspirin, magnesium carbonate, aluminum glycinate | Analgesic, antacid |
| *Bufferin AF Nite Time* | diphenhydramine, acetaminophen | Decongestant, analgesic |
| *Cafergot* | ergotamine, caffeine | Antimigraine |
| *Calcidrine Syrup* | codeine, calcium iodide, alcohol | Antitussive |
| *Capozide* | captopril hydrochlorothiazide | Antihypertensive |
| *Cheracol Syrup* | codeine, guaifenesin, alcohol | Antitussive, expectorant |
| *Claritin-D 12 Hour*<br>*Claritin-D 24 Hour* | | |
| *Clindex* | clidinium, chlordiazepoxide | Antispasmodic |
| *Co-Apap* | pseudoephedrine, chlorpheniramine dextromethorphan, acetaminophen | Antihistamine, decongestant |
| *Codimal DH* | phenylephrine, pyrilamine, hydrocodone | Antitussive |
| *Codimal LA* | pseudoephedrine, chlorpheniramine | Antihistamine, decongestant |
| Co-Gesic | hydrocodone, acetaminophen | Analgesic |
| *Col-Probenecid* | probenecid, colchicine | Antigout |
| *Combipres* | Chlorthalidone, clonidine | Antihypertensive |
| *Combivent* | ipratropium, albuterol | Asthma drug |
| *Combivir* | Lamivudine, zidovudine | Antiviral |
| *Comtrex* | pseudoephedrine, chlorpheniramine, dextromethorphan, acetaminophen | Antihistamine, decongestant |
| *Comtrex cough* | pseudoephedrine, dextromethophan, guaifenesin | Decongestant, antitussive, expectorant |

*(continued)*

| Brand Name | Active Ingredients | Common Usage |
|---|---|---|
| *Contac 12 Hour* | phenylpropanolamine, chlorpheniramine | Decongestant, antihistamine |
| *Contac Severe Cold* | pseudoephedrine, chlorpheniramine, dextromethorphan, acetaminophen | Antihistamine, decongestant |
| *COPE* | aspirin, caffeine, magnesium hydroxide, aluminum hydroxide | Analgesis, antacid |
| *Coricidin* | chlorpheniramine, acetaminophen | Antihistamine |
| *Coricidin D* | phenylpropanolamine, chlorpheniramine, acetaminophen | Decongestant, antihistamine, analgesic |
| *Corzide* | nadolol, bendroflumethiazide | Antihypertensive |
| *Cotrim* | trimethoprim, sulfamethoxazide | Anitbiotic |
| *Cyclomydril* | dopentolate, phenylephrine | Ophthalmic |
| *Cylex* | methenamine, sodium salicylate, benzoic acid | Urinary antiinfective |
| *Damason-P* | hydrocodone, aspirin, caffeine | Analgesic |
| *Deconamine* | pseudoephedrine, chlorpheniramine | Antihistamine, decongestant |
| *Deprol* | meprobamate, boractyzine | Anitdepressants |
| *Dermoplast* | benzocaine, menthol, methylparaben | Local anesthetic |
| *Di Gel* | magnesium hydroxide, aluminum hydroxide, magnesium carbonate, simethicone | Local anesthetic Antacid |
| *Dilaudid Cough Syrup* | hydromorphone, guaifenesin | Antitussive |
| *Dimetane Decongestant* | phenylephrine, brompheniramine | Decongestant |
| *Dimetapp* | brompheniramine, phenylpropanolamine | Antihistamine, decongestant |
| *Dimetapp Cold and Flu* | phenylpropanolamine, brompheniramine acetaminophen | Antihistamine, decongestant |
| *Donnagel* | kaolin, pectin, hyoscyamine, atropine, scopalamine | Antidiarrheal |
| *Donnatal* | atropine, scopalamine, hyoscyamine, phenobarbital | Anticholinergic, sedative |
| *Doxidan* | docusate, phenolphthalein | Laxative |
| *Dristan* | phenylephrine, chlorpheniramine, acetaminophen | Antihistamine, decongestant |
| *Dristan Cold* | pseudoephedrine, acetaminophen | Decongestant, analgesic |
| *Drixoral* | pseudoephedrine, dexbrompheniramine, acetaminophen | Antihistamine, decongestant |
| *Duocet* | hydrocodone, acetaminophen | Analgesic |
| *Duo-Medihaler* | isoproterenol, phenylephrine | Bronchodilater |
| *Dyazide* | triamterene, hydrochlorothiazide | Diuretic |
| *Elixophyllin GG* | guaifenesin, theophylline | Antiasthmatic |
| *Empirin with codeine* | aspirin, codeine | Analgesic |
| *Enduronyl* | methycholothiazide, desperidine | Antihypertensive |
| *E-Pilo* (various concentrations) | pilocapine, epinephrine | Antiglaucoma |

*(continued)*

| Brand Name | Active Ingredients | Common Usage |
|---|---|---|
| *Equagesic* | aspirin, meprobamate | Analgesic |
| *Ercaf* | ergotamine, caffeine | Antimigraine |
| *Eryzole* | erythromycin, sulfisoxazole | Anitbiotic |
| *Esimil* | guanethidine, hydrochlorothiazide | Antihypertensive |
| *Etrafon* | perpheruzine, amitriptyline | Anitdepressant |
| *Excedrin Extra Strength* | aspirin, acetaminophen, caffeine | Analgesic |
| *Excedrin P.M.* | acetaminophen, dimenhydramine | Analgesic |
| *Fansidar* | sulfadoxine, pyrimethamine | Antimalarial |
| *Fedahist* | pseudoephedring, chlorpheniramine | Antihistamine, decongestant |
| *Fioricet* | acetaminophen, butalbital, caffeine | Analgesic |
| *Fiorinal* | aspirin, butalbital, caffeine | Analgesic |
| *Fiorinal with Codeine* | aspirin, butalbital, caffeine, codeine | Analgesic |
| *Gaviscon* | aluminum hydroxide, magnesium carbonate | Antacid |
| *Gelusil* | aluminum hydroxide, magnesium hydroxide, simethicone | Antacid |
| *Granulex* | trypsin, Balsam Peru, castor oil | Topical enzyme |
| *Haley's MO* | mineral oil, magnesium hydroxide | Laxative |
| *Halotussin-DM* | guaifenesin, dextromethorphan | Antitussive |
| *Helidac* | bismuth subsalicyate, metronidazole, tetracycline | Anitulcer |
| *Hycomine* | phenylephrine, chlorpheniramine, hydrocodone, acetaminophen, caffeine | Antitussive |
| *Hyzaar* | losartan, hydrochlorothiazide | Anithypertensive |
| *Inderide* | hydrochlorothiazide, propranolol | Anithypertensive |
| *Kapectolin PG* | kaolin, pectin, atropine, hyoscyamine, hyoscine, opium, alcohol | Antidiarrheal |
| *Kondremul with Phenophthalein* | mineral oil, phenolphthalein, Irish moss | Laxative |
| *Lexxel* | enalapril, felodipine | Anithypertensive |
| *Librax* | chlordiazepoxide, clidinium | Anticholinergic |
| *Limbitrol* | chlordiazepoxide, amitriptylene | Antidepressant |
| *Logen* | diphenxylate, atropine | Antidiarrheal |
| *Lomanate* | diphenoxylate, atropine | Antidiarrheal |
| *Lomotil* | diphenoxylate, atropine | Antidiarrheal |
| *Lonox* | diphenoxylate, atropine | Antidiarrheal |
| *Lopressor HCT* | metoprolol, hydrochlorothiazide | Antihypertensive |
| *Lotensin HCT* | hydrochlorothiazide, benazepril | Antihypentensive |
| *Lotrel* | amlodopine, benazepril | Antihypertensive |
| *Lufyllin* | dyphylline, ephedrine, guaifenesin, phenobarbital | Bronchodilator |
| *Lufyllin GG* | theophylline, guaifenesin | Bronchodilator, expectorant |
| *Maalox Plus* | aluminum hydroxide, magnesium hydroxide, simethicone | Antacid |

*(continued)*

| *Brand Name* | *Active Ingredients* | *Common Usage* |
|---|---|---|
| *Maalox Tablets* | aluminum hydroxide, magnesium hydroxide | Antacid |
| *Marax* | theophylline, ephedrine, hydroxyzine | Antiasthmatic |
| *Margesic H* | hydrocodone, acetaminophen | Analgesic |
| *Maxitrol* | dexamethasone, neomycin, polymyxin B | Ophthalmic |
| *Maxzide* | triamterene, hydrochlorothiazide | Diuretic |
| *Menrium* | estrogens, chlordiazepoxide | Antipsychotic |
| *Mepergan* | meperidine, promethazine | Analgesic |
| *Micrainin* | meprobamabate, aspirin | Analgesic |
| *Midol* | cinnamedrine, aspirin, caffeine | Analgesic |
| *Midol PMS* | acetaminophen, pamabrom, pyrilamine | Analgesic |
| *Minizide* | prazosin, polythiazide | Antihypertensive |
| *Modane Plus* | docusate, phenolphthalein | Laxative |
| *Moduretic* | amiloride, hydrochlorothiazide | Diuretic |
| *Mycitracine* | polymyxin B, neomycin, bacitracin | Ophthalmic, antiinfective |
| *Mycolog II* | triamcinolone, nystatin | Antifungal |
| *Mylagen* | calcium carbonate, magnesium carbonate | Antacid |
| *Mylanta* | aluminum hydroxide, magnesium hydroxide simethicone, sorbitol | Antacid |
| *Mylanta II* | aluminum hydroxide, magnesium hydroxide simethicone | Antacid |
| *Mylanta Gekaps* | calcium carbonate, magnesium carbonate | Antacid |
| *Naldecon* | phenylpropanolamine, phenylephrine, chlorpheniramine, phenyltoloxamine | Antihistamine, decongestant |
| *Neo Decadron* | neomycin, dexamethasone | Antibiotic, steroid |
| *Neosporin* | polymyxin B, neomycin, bacitracin | Antibiotic |
| *Nolamine* | phenylpropanolamine, chlorpheniramine, phenindamine | Antihistamine, decongestant |
| *Norco* | hydrocodone, acetaminophen | Analgesic |
| *Norgesic* | orphenadrine, aspirin, caffeine | Skeletal muscle relaxant |
| *Novafed A* | chlorpheniramine, pseudoephedrine | |
| *Nyquil Hot Therapy* | pseudoephedrine, acetaminophen, dextromethorphan, doxylamine | Antihistamine, decongestant |
| *Nyquil Nighttime* | pseudoephedrine, doxylamine, dextromethorphan | Antihistamine, decongestant |
| *Ornade Spanules* | phenylpropanolamine, chlorpheniramine | Antihistamine, decongestant |
| *Ornex* | phenylpropanolamine, acetaminophen | Analgesic, decongestant |
| *Ortho Tri-Cyclen* | norgestimate, ethinylestradiol | Antiacue |

*(continued)*

| Brand Name | Active Ingredients | Common Usage |
|---|---|---|
| *Otocort* | hydrocortisone, neomycin, polymyxin B | Antibiotic, steroid |
| *Pamprin* | acetaminophen, pamabrom, pyrilamine | Analgesic |
| *Panacet 5/500* | hydrocodone, acetaminophen | Analgesic |
| *Pediazole* | erythromycin, sulfisoxazole | Antibiotic |
| *Percocet* | oxycodone, acetaminophen | Analgesic |
| *Percodan* | oxycodone, aspirin | Analgesic |
| *Peri-Colace* | docusate, casanthranol | Laxative |
| *Phenergan/Codeine* | promethazine, codeine | Antitussive |
| *Phrenilin* | acetaminophen, butalbital | Analgesic |
| *Polaramine* | guaifenesin, dexchlorpheniramine, pseudoephedrine | Antihistamine, decongestant, expectorant |
| *Poly-Histine* | pheniramine, pyrilamine, phenytoloxamine | Antihistamine, decongestant |
| *Polysporin* | polymyxin B, bacitracin | Antibiotic |
| *Premphase* | estrogen, medroxyprogesterone | Menopause drug |
| *Prempro* | estrogen, medroxyprogesterone | Menopause drug |
| *Premsyn PMS* | acetaminophen, pamabrom, pyrilamine | Analgesic |
| *Primatene* | theophylline, ephedrine | Antiasthma |
| *Primaxin* | imipenem, cilastin | Antibiotic |
| *Priuzide* | lisinopril, hydrochlorothiazide | Antihypertensive |
| *Probampacin* | ampicillin, probenecid | Antibiotic |
| *Quadrinal* | ephedrine, theophylline, potassium iodide, phenobarbital | Bronchodilator |
| *Quibron* | theophylline, guaifenesin | Antiasthma, expectorant |
| *R&C Shampoo* | pyrethins, piperonyl butoxide | Pediculocide |
| *Regulace* | docusate, casanthranol | Laxative |
| *Repan* | acetaminophen, caffeine, butalbital | Analgesic |
| *RID* | pyrethins, piperonyl butoxide | Pediculocide |
| *Rifamate* | isoniazid, rifampin | Antituberculosis |
| *Riopan Plus* | magaldrate, simethicone | Antacid |
| *Robaxisal* | methocarbamol, aspirin | Skeletal muscle relaxant |
| *Robitussin AC* | codeine, guaifenesin, alcohol | Antitussive, expectorant |
| *Robitussin CF* | phenylpropanolamine, guaifenesin, alcohol, dextromethorphan | Antitussive, expectorant |
| *Robitussin DAC* | codeine, guaifenesin, alcohol pseudoephedrine | Antitussive, expectorant |
| *Robitussin DM* | guaifenesin, dextromethorphan, alcohol | Antitussive, expectorant |
| *Robitussin PE* | pseudoephedrine, guaifenesin, alcohol | Antitussive, expectorant |
| *Rondec* | pseudophedrine, carbinoxamine | Antihistamine, decongestant |
| *Roxilox* | oxycodone, acetaminophen | Analgesic |
| *Roxiprin* | oxycodone, aspirin | Analgesic |

*(continued)*

| Brand Name | Active Ingredients | Common Usage |
|---|---|---|
| *Rulox* | aluminum hydroxide, magnesium hydroxide, simethicone | Antacid |
| *Ru-Tuss* | phenylepinephrine, propanolamine, chlorpheniramine, hysocyamine, propanolamine, alcohol | Decongestant, antihistamine |
| *Ryna* | pseudoephedrine, chlorpheniramine | Antihistamine, decongestant |
| *Ryna-C* | codeine, pseudoephedrine, chlorpheniramine | Antihistamine, decongestant |
| *Sedapap* | acetaminophen, butabital | Analgesic |
| *Seldane-D* | terfenadine, pseudoephedrine | Antihistamine, decongestant |
| *Senokot-S* | senna, docusate | Laxative |
| *Septra* | trimethoprim, sulfamethoxazole | Antibiotic |
| *Sine-Aid IB* | pseudoephedrine, ibuprofen | Decongestant |
| *Sinemet* | carbidopa, levodopa | Antiparkinsonism drug |
| *Sinemet-CR* | carbidopa, levodopa | Antiparkinsonism drug |
| *Sine-Off No Drowsiness* | pseudoephedrine, acetaminophen | Decongestant |
| *Sinutab* | pseudoephedrine, chlorpheniramine, acetaminophen | Decongestant |
| *Soma Compound* | aspirin, carisoprodol | Skeletal Muscle relaxant |
| *Sudafed Plus* | pseudoephedrine, chlorpheniramine | Antihistamine, decongestant |
| *Sulfatrim* | trimethoprim, sulfamethoxazole | Antibiotic |
| *Sultrin Triple* | sulfathiazole, sulfacetamide, sulfamenzamide, urea | Antibiotic |
| *Synalgos DC* | aspirin, caffeine, dihydrocodeine | Analgesic |
| *Talacen* | pentazocine, acetaminophen | Analgesic |
| *Talwin Compound* | aspirin, pentazocine | Analgesic |
| *Talwin NX* | pentazocine, naloxone | Analgesic |
| *Tarka* | trandolapril, verapamil | Antihypertensive |
| *Tavist-D* | phenylpropanolamine, clemastine | Antihistamine |
| *Teczem* | enalapril, diltiazem | Antihypertensive |
| *Theodrine* | ephedrine, theophylline, phenobarbital | Antiasthma |
| *TheraFlu Flu and Cold* | pseudoephedrine, chlorpheniramine, acetaminophen | Antihistamine, decongestant |
| *TheraFlu Flu, Cold & Cough* | pseudoephedrine, chlorpheniramine, dextromethorphan, acetaminophen | Antihistamine, decongestant, antitussive |
| *Timolide* | hydrochlorthaizide, timolol | Antihypertensive |
| *TMP-SMZ* | trimethoprim, sulfamethoxasole | Antidepressant |
| *Triacin C* | pseudoephedrine, tripolidine, codeine | Antitussive |
| *Triad* | acetaminophen, caffeine, butabital | Analgesic |
| *Triaminic* | pyrilamine, pheniramine, phenylpropanolamine | Antihistamine, decongestant |
| *Triaminic Allergy* | chlorpheniramine, phenylpropanolamine | Antihistamine, decongestant |

*(continued)*

| Brand Name | Active Ingredients | Common Usage |
|---|---|---|
| *Triaminic-DM* | dextramethorphan, phenylpropanolamine | Antihistamine, decongestant |
| *Triaminic-TR* | pyrilamine, pheniramine, phenylpropanolamine | Antihistamine, decongestant |
| *Triaminicol* | phenylpropanolamine, chlorpheniramine, dextromethorphan | Antihistamine, decongestant |
| *Triavil* | perphoriazine, amitriptyline | Antidepressant |
| *Trinalin Repetabs* | azatidine, pseudoephedrine | Antihistamine |
| *Tritec* | ranitidine, trivalent bismuth, citrate | Antiulcer |
| *Tylenol Cold & Flu* | acetaminophen, chlorpheniramine, pseudoephedrine, dextromethorphan | Antihistamine, decongestant |
| *Tylenol PM* | acetaminophen, diphenhydramine | Antihistamine, decongestant |
| *Tylenol with codeine* | tylenol, codeine | Analgesic |
| *Tylox* | oxycodone, acetaminophen | Analgesic |
| *Unasyn* | ampicillin, sulbactam | Antibiotic |
| *Uniretic* | moexipril, hydrochlorothiazide | Antihypertensive |
| *Vanex* | chlorpheniramine, hydrocodone, phenylephrine | Antihistamine, decongestant |
| *Vaseretic* | enalapril, hydrochlorothiazide | Antihypertensive |
| *Vicks DayQuil* | dextromethorphan, pseudoephedrine, acetaminophen, guaifenesin | Antihistamine, decongestant |
| *Vicks Formula 44* | dextromethorphan, chlorpheniramine, alcohol | Antihistamine, decongestant |
| *Vicks Nyquil* | dextromethorphan, doxylamine, pseudoephedrine, acetaminphen | Antihistamine, antitussive, decongestant |
| *Vicoden* | hydrocodone, acetaminophen | Analgesic |
| *Vicoprofen* | hydrocodone, ibuprofen | Analgesic |
| *Wigraine* | caffeine, ergotamine | Antimigraine |
| *Zestoretic* | lisinopril, hydrochlorothiazide | Antihypertensive |
| *Ziac* | bisopropol, hydrochlorothiazide | Antihypertensive |
| *Zosyn* | piperacillin, tazobactam | Antibiotic |
| *Zydone* | hydrocodone, acetaminophen | Analgesic |

# APPENDIX G

## Laxatives

Laxative use has been replaced by the use of proper diet and exercise in many clinical situations. Most laxatives are available as OTC preparations and are often abused by people who become dependent on them for GI movement.

### Indications

Short-term relief of constipation; to prevent straining; to evacuate the bowel for diagnostic procedures; to remove ingested poisons from the lower GI tract; as adjunct in anthelmintic therapy.

### Pregnancy Category C

*Contraindicated* in cases of allergy to these drugs, third trimester of pregnancy, acute abdomen.

### Adverse Effects

*Excessive bowel activity, perianal irritation, abdominal cramps,* weakness, dizziness, *cathartic dependence.*

### Drug-Specific Teaching Points

Use as a temporary measure; swallow tablets whole; do not take this drug within 1 h of any other drugs; report sweating, flushing, muscle cramps, excessive thirst.

Adverse effects in *Italics* are most common; those in **Bold** are life-threatening.

| Drug | Brand Names | Dosage | Type | Onset | Special Considerations |
|---|---|---|---|---|---|
| bisacodyl | *Dulcolax*<br>*Fleet lax.*<br>*Dulcagen*<br>*Bisco-Lax* | 10–15 mg PO<br>2.5 g in water via enema | Stimulant | 6–10 h<br>Rapid | Allergy to tartrazine in *Dulcolax* tablets; may discolor urine. |
| cascara | | 325–650 mg PO | Stimulant | 6–10 h | |
| castor oil | *Neolid*<br>*Purge*<br>*Fleet-Flavored Castor*<br>*Emulosil* | 15–30 ml | Stimulant | 2–6 h | May be very vigorous; abdominal cramping. |
| docusate | *Regutol*<br>*Colace*<br>*Disonate*<br>*DOK*<br>*DOS Softgel*<br>*D-S-S*<br>*Modane Soft*<br>*Diocto C* | 50–240 mg | Detergent<br>Softener | 24–72 h | Gentle; beneficial with anorectal conditions that are painful and with dry or hard feces |
| glycerin | *Sani-Supp*<br>*Fleet Babylex* | Suppository; 4 ml liquid | Hyperosmolar | 15–30 min | Insert suppository high into rectum, retain 15 min; insert liquid dispenser and apply gentle, steady pressure until all liquid is gone, then remove. |

*(continued)*

| *Drug* | *Brand Names* | *Dosage* | *Type* | *Onset* | *Special Considerations* |
|---|---|---|---|---|---|
| lactulose | *Cephulac*<br>*Cholac*<br>*Chronulac*<br>*Constilac*<br>*Constulose*<br>*Duphalac*<br>*Enulose* | 51–30 ml PO | Hyperosmolar | 24–48 h | Also used for treatment of portal-system encephalopathy. May be more palatable mixed with fruit juice, water, or milk. |
| magnesium citrate | *Citrate of Magnesia* | 1 glassful | Saline | 0.5–3 h | Reduce pediatric dosage by $^1/_2$. |
| magnesium hydroxide | *Milk of Magnesia,*<br>*MOM*<br>*Philip's MOM* | 15–30 ml | Saline | 0.5–3 h | Take with liquids; flavored varieties available. |
| magnesium sulfate | *Epsom Salts* | 10–25 g | Saline | 0.5–3 h | Take mixed with glass of water; reduce pediatric dose to 5–10 g in glass of water. |
| mineral oil | *Kondremul Plain*<br>*Milkinol*<br>*Neo-Cultol* | 5–45 ml PO | Emollient | 6–8 h | Reduce pediatric dose to 5–20 ml. May decrease absorption of fat-soluble vitamins.<br>Use caution to avoid lipid pneumonia with aspiration. |
| phenolphthalein | *Alophen Pills*<br>*Ex-Lax*<br>*Lax Pills*<br>*Espotabs*<br>*Feen-a-mint* | 60–194 mg PO at bedtime | Stimulant | 6–10 h | Yellow phenolphthalein is 2–3 times more potent than phenolphthalein; keep away from pets, may be neurotoxic. |

| | | | | | |
|---|---|---|---|---|---|
| | *Modane*<br>*Evac-U-Gen*<br>*Medilax* | | | | |
| polycarbophil | *FiberCon*<br>*Equalactin*<br>*Mitrolan*<br>*Fiber-Lax*<br>*Fiberall* | 1 g PO<br>1–4 times/d as needed; do not exceed 6 g/d in adults or 3 g/d in children | Bulk | 12–24 h | Good with irritable bowel syndrome, diverticulitis. Abdominal fullness may occur. Smaller doses more frequently may alleviate discomfort. |
| psyllium | *Fiberall Natural*<br>*Hydrocil Instant*<br>*Konsyl*<br>*Metamucil* | 1 tsp or packet in cool water or juice, 1–3 times/d in children | Bulk | 12–24 h | Safest and most physiological. Assure that patient has sufficient water to completely swallow dose. |
| senna | *Senokot*<br>*Senna-Gen*<br>*Senokotxtra*<br>*Black-Draught*<br>*Gentlax*<br>*Fletcher's Castoria*<br>*Dr. Caldwell Senna* | 1–8 tablets/d at bedtime; suppository; syrup—10–25 ml | Stimulant | 6–10 h | May be very aggressive; abdominal cramps and discomfort may occur. |

# APPENDIX H

## Ophthalmic Agents

Ophthalmic agents are drugs that are intended for direct administration into the conjunctiva of the eye. These drugs are used to treat glaucoma (miotics constrict the pupil and decrease the resistance to aqueous flow), to aid in diagnosis of eye problems (mydriatics—dilate the pupil for examination of the retina; cyclopegics paralyze the muscles that control the lens to aid refraction), or treat local ophthalmic infections or inflammation; and to provide relief from the signs and symptoms of allergic reactions.

### Pregnancy Category C

*Contraindicated* in cases of allergy to these drugs. These drugs are seldom absorbed systemically, but caution should be taken with any patient who would have problems with the systemic effects of the drug if it were absorbed systemically.

### Adverse Effects

*Local irritation,* stinging, burning, blurring of vision (prolonged when using ointment), tearing; headache.

### Dosage

1–2 drops to each eye bid to qid or .25–.5 in of ointment to each eye is the usual dosage.

***Solution/drops***

Wash hands thoroughly before administering; do not touch dropper to eye or to any other surface; have patient tilt head backward or lie down, stare upward; gently grasp lower eyelid and pull the eyelid away from the eyeball; instill drop(s) into pouch formed by eyelid; release lid slowly; have patient close eye and look downward; apply gentle pressure to the inside corner of the eye for 3–5 min to retard drainage; do not rub eyes; do not rinse eyedropper. Do not use eyedrops that have changed color; if more than one type of eyedrop is used, wait 5 min before administration.

***Ointment***

Wash hands thoroughly before administering; hold tube between hands for several minutes to warm the ointment; discard the first cm of ointment when opening the tube for the first time; tilt head backward or lie down and stare upward; gently pull out lower lid to form pouch; place 0.25–0.5 in of ointment inside the lower lid; have patient close eyes for 1–2 min and roll eyeball in all directions; remove any excess ointment from around eye. If using more than one kind of ointment, wait 10 min between administration.

### Drug Specific Teaching Points

Teach patient the proper administration technique for the ophthalmic agent ordered; caution patients that transient stinging or burning may occur and that blurring vision may also occur—appropriate safety measures should be taken; sensitivity to sun will occur with mydriatic agents which cause pupils to dilate, sunglasses may be needed; report severe eye discomfort, palpitations, nausea, headache.

| Drug | Brand Names | Usage | Special Considerations |
|---|---|---|---|
| apraclonidine | *Iopidine* | To control or prevent postsurgical elevations of IOP in patients after argon-laser eye surgery | Monitor for the possibility of vasovagal attack; do not give to patients with allergy to clonidine. |
| brimonidine tartrate | *Alphagan* | Treatment of open-angle glaucoma and ocular hypertension; selective alpha-2 antagonist. | Selective alpha-2 antagonist; minimal effects on CV and pulmonary systems. Do not use with MAOIs. 1 gt tid. |
| carbachol | *Miostat*<br>*Isopto Carbachol* | Direct acting miotic; for treatment of glaucoma; for miosis during surgery | Surgical dose a one-use only portion; 1–2 gt up to tid as needed for glaucoma. |
| cyclopentolate | *Cyclogyl* | Mydriasis/cycloplegia in diagnostic procedures | Individuals with dark pigmented irides may require higher doses; compress lacrimal sac for 1–2 min after admin. to decrease any systemic absorption. |
| dapiprazole | *Rev-Eyes* | Miotic: iatrogenically induced mydriasis produced by adrenergic or parasympathetic agents | Not for use to reduce IOP; do not use if constriction is undesirable. Do not use more than once a week. |
| demecarium | *Humorsol* | Treatment of glaucoma and strabismus; cholinesterase inhibitor | If response is not adequate in first 24h, consider another drug. Do not use more often than necessary—1–2 gt/wk up to 1–2 gt/d have been used. |
| diclofenac sodium | *Voltaren Ophthalmic* | Photophobia; for use in patients undergoing incisional refractive surgery. | Apply 1 gt qid beginning 24-h after cataract surgery; continue through the first 2 wk postoperatively. |
| dorzolamide | *Trusopt* | Treatment of elevated IOP in patients with ocular hypertension or open-angle glaucoma. | A sulfonamide; monitor patients on parenteral sulfonamides for possible additive effects. |
| echothiopate | *Phospholine lodide* | Treatment of glaucoma; irreversible cholinesterase inhibitor; long-acting. Accommodative esotropia | Given only once a day because of long action; tolerance may develop with prolonged use, usually responds to a rest period. |

*(continued)*

| *Drug* | *Brand Names* | *Usage* | *Special Considerations* |
|---|---|---|---|
| fluorometholone | *Fluor-Op, FML* | Topical corticosteroid used for treatment of inflammatory conditions of the eye | Improvement should occur within several days, discontinue if no improvement is seen. Discontinue if swelling of the eye occurs. |
| homatropine | *Isopto-Homatropine Homatropine HBr* | Long-acting mydriatic and cycloplegic used for refraction and treatment of inflammatory conditions of the uveal tract. | Individuals with dark pigmented irides may require larger doses; 5–10 min is usually required for refraction. |
| idoxuridine (IDU) | *Herplex* | Antiviral; used to treat herpes simplex keratitis | Transient burning and stinging may occur; reconsider drug if improvement is not seen within 7–8 d. Do not administer for longer than 21 d at a time. Protect drug from light; do not mix with other medications. |
| latanoprost | *Xalatan* | Treatment of open-angle glaucoma or ocular hypertension in patients intolerant or nonresponsive to other agents | Remove contact lenses before use and for 15 min after use; allow at least 5 min between this and the use of any other agents; expect burning, blurred vision. |
| levocabastine | *Livostin* | Relief of allergic conjunctivitis | Treatment may be needed for up to 2 wk. Do not wear soft contact lenses during use of this drug. Shake well before use and do not use any discolored solution. |
| Iodoxamide | *Alomide* | Treatment of vernal conjunctivitis and keratitis | Patients should not wear contact lenses while using this drug; discontinue if stinging and burning persist after instillation. |
| metipropranolol | *OptiPranolol* | Beta blocker; used in treating chronic open-angle glaucoma and ocular hypertension | Concomitant therapy may be needed; caution patient about possible vision changes. |
| natamycin | *Natacyn* | Antibiotic used to treat fungal blepharitis, conjunctivitis and keratitis; drug of choice for *Fusarium sotani* keratitis | Shake well before each use; store at room temp.; failure to improve in 7–10 d suggests a nonsusceptible organism, re-evaluate. |

*(continued)*

| Drug | Brand Names | Usage | Special Considerations |
|---|---|---|---|
| olopatadine hydrochloride | *Patanol* | Mast cell stabilizer and antihistamine; provides fast onset of relief of itching due to conjunctivitis with prolonged action | Not for use with contact lenses; headache is common side effect. |
| physostigmine | *Eserine* | Miotic, cholinesterase inhibitor; used only for reduction of IOP in primary glaucoma | Headache may occur and may be unresponsive to analgesics; avoid night driving or performing tasks in low light. |
| pilocarpine | *Pilocar*<br>*Piloptic*<br>*Pilostat*<br>*Akarpine* | Chronic and acute glaucoma; treatment of mydriasis caused by drugs; direct acting miotic agent | Can be stored at room temp. for up to 8 wk, then discard. 1–2 gt up to 6 times/d may be needed, based on patient response. |
| polydimethylsiloxane | *AdatoSil* | Treatment of retinal detachments where other therapy is not effective or is inappropriate; primary choice for retinal detachment due to AIDS-related CMV retinitis or viral infection | Monitor for cataracts; must be injected into aqueous humor. |
| rimexolone | *Vexol* | Corticosteroid; postop ocular surgery and for treatment of anterior uveitis | Monitor for signs of steroid absorption. |
| suprofen | *Profenal* | NSAID; used to inhibit intraoperative miosis | Local burning may occur; monitor patient for any cross sensitivities to other NSAIDs. |
| trifluridine | *Viroptic* | Antiviral; used to treat primary keratoconjunctivitis and recurrent epithelial keratitis due to herpes simplex virus types 1 & 2 | Transient burning and stinging may occur; reconsider drug if improvement is not seen within 7 d. Do not administer for longer than 21 d at a time. |
| vidarabine | *Vira-A* | Acute keratoconjunctivitis and recurrent epithelial keratitis due to herpes simplex 1 and 2; superficial keratitis caused by herpes simplex virus and not responding to idoxuridine | Treat an additional 7 d after repithelialization has occurred; if no improvement in 21 d, consider other therapy. |

# APPENDIX I

## Peripheral Vasodilators

The peripheral vasodilators are direct-acting, vascular smooth muscle relaxants with no adrenergic stimulating or blocking actions. They are labeled as *"Possibly effective"* for adjunctive treatment of intermittent claudication, arteriosclerosis obliterans, thrombophlebitis, nocturnal leg cramps, Raynaud's phenomenon, and selected cases of ischemic cerebral vascular disease. Although many other drugs that have proven efficacy and therapeutic value are now available for these conditions, these drugs are still available and may be used in some situations.

### Pregnancy Category C

*Contraindicated* in cases of allergy to the drug, severe obliterative coronary artery disease, severe obliterative cerebral vascular disease, glaucoma, active bleeding, bleeding tendency.

### Adverse Effects

Heartburn, abdominal pain, eructation; *flushing, headache,* feeling of weakness; *tachycardia;* orthostatic hypotension, dizziness.

### Drug-Specific Teaching Points

Take drug with meals or antacids (if prescribed) if GI upset occurs. Report severe headache, chest pain, shortness of breath, loss of consciousness, numbess, tingling in the extremities.

| *Drug* | *Brand Name* | *Dosage* | *Special Considerations* |
|---|---|---|---|
| cyclandelate | | 1.2–1.6 g/d PO in divided doses after meals and at bedtime. With improvement, decrease in 200 mg intervals. Maintenance: 400–800 mg/d PO in 2–4 divided doses. | Short-term use is rarely beneficial. |
| isoxsuprine hydrochloride | *Vasodilan*<br>*Voxsuprine* | 10–20 mg PO 3–4 times/d | Has been used to inhibit premature labor. Can cause serious problems. Not recommended. Rash may occur. Stop drug if rash appears. |
| papaverine hydrochloride | *Pavabid*<br>*Pavagen TD* | 100–300 mg PO 3–5 times/d<br>150 mg q12h PO timed release | Long-term use is needed. |

# APPENDIX J

## Prophylaxis for the Prevention of Bacterial Endocarditis

### Conditions Considered at Risk for Endocarditis—Prophylaxis Recommended

High risk

- Prosthetic cardiac valves
- Previous endocarditis
- Complex cyanotic congenital heart disease (single ventricles, transposition of the great vessels, tetralogy of Fallot)
- Surgically constructed systemic pulmonary shunts or conduits

Moderate risk

- Most other congenital cardiac malformations
- Acquired valvular dysfunction (rheumatic heart disease)
- Hypertrophic cardiomyopathy
- Mitral valve prolapse with regurgitation and/or thickened valves

### Conditions Considered at Negligible Risk—Prophylaxis Not Recommended

- Isolated secundum atrial septal defect
- Surgical repair or atrial septal defect, ventricular septal defect, PDA
- Previous coronary artery bypass graft surgery
- Mitral valve prolapse without valvular regurgitation
- Physiologic, functional or innocent heart murmurs
- Previous Kawasaki disease without valvular dysfunction
- Previous rheumatic fever without valvular dysfunction
- Cardiac pacemakers and implanted defibrillators

### Procedures for Which Endocarditis Prophylaxis Is Recommended

Dental

- Dental extractions
- Periodontal procedures
- Dental implant placement and reimplantation of avulsed teeth
- Endodontic (root canal) instrumentation or surgery
- Subgingival placement of antibiotic fibers or strings
- Initial placement of orthodontic bands but not braces
- Intraligamentary local anesthetic injections
- Prophylactic cleaning of teeth or implants where bleeding is anticipated

Respiratory Tract

- Tonsillectomy and/or adenoidectomy
- Surgical operations that involve respiratory mucosa
- Bronchoscopy with a rigid bronchoscope

GI tract

- Sclerotherapy for esophageal varices
- Esophageal structure dilation
- Endoscopic retrograde cholangiography with biliary obstruction
- Biliary tract surgery
- Surgical operations that involve intestinal mucosa

GU tract
- Prostatic surgery
- Cystoscopy
- Urethral dilation

## Procedures for Which Endocarditis Prophylaxis Is Not Recommended

Dental
- Restorative dentistry
- Local anesthetic injections
- Intracanal endodontic treatment and post placement and buildup
- Placement of rubber dams
- Postoperative suture removal
- Placement of removable prosthodontic or orthodontic appliances
- Taking of oral impressions
- Fluoride treatments
- Taking of oral radiographs
- Orthodontic appliance adjustment
- Shedding of primary teeth

Respiratory Tract
- Endotracheal intubation
- Bronchoscopy with a flexible bronchoscope
- Tympanostomy tube insertion

GI Tract
- Transesophageal echocardiography
- Endoscopy with or without gastrointestinal biopsy

GU Tract
- Vaginal hysterectomy
- Vaginal delivery
- Cesarean section
- In uninfected tissues: urethral catheterization, uterine dilation and curettage, therapeutic abortion, sterilization procedures, insertion or removal of intrauterine devices

Other
- Cardiac catheterization
- Balloon angioplasty
- Implanted cardiac pacemakers, defibrillators, stents
- Incision, biopsy, or surgically scrubbed skin
- Circumcision

## Prophylaxis Regimens for Dental, Oral, Respiratory or Esophageal Procedures

| *Situation* | *Agent* | *Regimen* |
|---|---|---|
| Standard prophylaxis | amoxicillin | Adults: 2.0 g PO, children 50 mg/kg PO 1 h before procedure |
| Unable to take oral meds | ampicillin | Adults: 2.0 g IM or IV, children 50 mg/kg IM or IV within 30 min before procedure |
| Allergic to penicillins | clindamycin *or* | Adults: 600 mg PO, children 20 mg/kg PO 1 h before procedure |
| | cephalexin or cefadroxil | Adults: 2.0 g PO, children 50 mg/kg PO 1 h before procedure |
| | azithromycin or clarithromycin | Adults: 500 mg PO, children 15 mg/kg PO 1 h before procedure |

*(continued)*

| Situation | Agent | Regimen |
|---|---|---|
| Allergic to penicillins and unable to take oral meds | clindamycin *or* cefazolin | Adults 600 mg IV, children 20 mg/kg IV within 30 min of procedure<br>Adults: 1.0 g IM or IV, children 25 mg/kg IM or IV within 30 before procedure |

## Prophylaxis Regimens for Genitourinary, Gastrointestinal (Excluding Esophageal) Procedures

| Situation | Agent | Regimen |
|---|---|---|
| High-risk patients | ampicillin plus gentamicin | Adults: ampicillin 2.0 g IM or IV plus gentamicin 1.5 mg/kg IM or IV within 30 min before procedure; 6 h later, ampicillin 1 g, IM or IV or amoxicillin 1 g PO<br>Children: ampicillin 50 mg/kg IM or IV plus gentamicin 1.5 mg/kg within 30 min of procedure; 6 h later, ampicillin 25 mg/kg IM or IV, or amoxicillin 25 mg/kg PO |
| High-risk patients allergic to penicillins | vancomycin plus gentamicin | Adults: vancomycin 1.0 g IV over 1–2 h plus gentamicin, 1.5 mg/kg; complete dose within 30 before procedure<br>Children: vancomycin 20 mg/kg IV over 1–2 h plus gentamicin 1.5 mg/kg IV or IM; complete dose within 30 min before procedure |
| Moderate-risk patients | amoxacillin or ampicillin | Adults: amoxicillin 2.0 g PO 1 h before procedure or ampicillin 2.0 g IM or IV within 30 min before starting procedure<br>Children: amoxicillin 50 mg/kg PO 1 h before procedure, or ampicillin 50 mg/kg IM or IV within 30 min before procedure |
| Moderate-risk patients allergic to penicillins | vancomycin | Adults: vancomycin 1.0 g IV over 1–2 h; complete within 30 before procedure<br>Children: vancomycin 20 mg/kg IV over 1–2 h complete within 30 min before procedure |

(From the American Heart Association, June 1997.)

# APPENDIX K

## Topical Agents

Topical agents are drugs that are intended for surface use, not ingestion or injection. They may be very toxic if absorbed into the system, but serve several purposes when used topically.

### Pregnancy Category C

*Contraindicated* in cases of allergy to these drugs, open wounds or abrasions.

### Adverse Effects

*Local irritation,* stinging, burning, dermatitis, toxic effects if absorbed systemically.

### Drug-Specific Teaching Points

Apply sparingly as directed. Do not use with open wounds or broken skin. Avoid contact with eyes. Report any local irritation, allergic reaction, worsening of condition being treated.

| *Drug* | *Brand Names* | *Dosage* | *Special Considerations* |
|---|---|---|---|
| *Emollients* | | | |
| boric acid ointment | *Borofax* | Apply as needed | Relieves burns, itching, irritation. |
| dexpanthenol | *Panthoderm* | Apply qd-bid. | Relieves itching and aids in healing for mild skin irritations. |
| glycerin | | Combined with other ingredients—rose water | Moisturing effect |
| lanolin | | Ointment base, applied generously | Allergy to sheep or sheep products—use caution; base for many ointments |

*(continued)*

| Drug | Brand Names | Dosage | Special Considerations |
|---|---|---|---|
| urea | *Aquacare*<br>*Carmol*<br>*Gordon's Urea*<br>*Gormel*<br>*Lanaphilic*<br>*Nutraplus*<br>*Ureacin* | 2–4 times/d to area affected | Rub in completely. Used to restore nails—cover with plastic wrap; keep dry and remove in 3, 7, 10, or 14 d. |
| vitamin A and D | | Apply locally with gentle massage bid-qid. | Relieves minor burns, chafing skin irritations. Consult physician if not improved within 7 d. |
| zinc oxide | | Apply as needed. | Relieves burns, abrasion, diaper rash. |
| ***Growth Factor*** | | | |
| becaplermin | *Regranax Gel* | Apply to diabetic foot ulcers bid–qid | Increases the incidence of healing of diabetic foot ulcers as adjunctive therapy; must have an adequate blood supply. |
| ***Lotions and Solutions*** | | | |
| Burow's solution aluminum acetate | *Bluboro Powder*<br>*Boropak Powder*<br>*Domeboro Powder*<br>*Pedi-Boro Soak Paks* | Dissolve one packet in a pint of water, apply q15–30 min for 4–8h | Astringent wet dressing for relief of inflammatory conditions, insect bites, athlete's foot, bruise, etc; do not use occlusive dressing. |
| calamine lotion | *Calamatum*<br>*Calamox*<br>*Resinol* | Apply to affected area tid-qid. | Relieves itching, pain of poison ivy, poison sumac and oak, insect bites, and minor skin irritations. |
| hamamelis water | *A-E-R*<br>*Tucks*<br>*Witch Hazel* | Apply locally up to 6 times/d. | Relieves itching and irritation of vaginal infection, hemorrhoids, postepisotomy discomfort, post hemorrhoidectomy care. |
| quaternium-18 bentonite | *Ivy Block* | Apply at least 15 min before exposure to poison ivy and every 4 h for continued protection. | Barrier lotion to prevent poison ivy/oak/sumac reactions. |

| | | | |
|---|---|---|---|
| ***Antiseptics*** | | | |
| Benzalkonium chloride | *BAC*<br>*Benza*<br>*Zephiran* | Mix in solution as needed; spray for preoperative use; storage of instruments in solution | Thoroughly rinse detergents and soaps from skin before use; add anti-rust tablets for instruments stored in solution; dilute solution as indicated for use. |
| chlorhexidine gluconate | *Dyna-Hex*<br>*Exidine*<br>*Hibiciens*<br>*Hibistat* | Scrub or rinse; leave on for 15 seconds, for surgical scrub—3 min. | Use for surgical scrub, preoperative skin prep., wound cleansing; preop bathing and showering. |
| hexachlorophene | *pHisoHex*<br>*Septisol* | Apply as wash. | Surgical wash, scrub; do not use with burns or on mucous membranes; rinse thoroughly. |
| iodine | | Wash affected area with solution. | Highly toxic; avoid occlusive dressings; stains skin and clothing. |
| povidone iodine | *ACU-dyne*<br>*Aerodine*<br>*Betadine*<br>*Betagen*<br>*Iodex* | Apply as needed. | Treated areas may be bandaged. HIV is inactivated in this solution; causes less irritation than iodine; less toxic. |
| sodium hypochlorite | *Dakin's* | Apply as antiseptic. | Caution—chemical burns can occur. |
| thimersol | *Aeroaid*<br>*Mersol* | Apply qd-tid. | Contains mercury compound; used preop and as first aid for abrasions, wounds. |
| ***Antibiotics*** | | | |
| mupirocin | *Bactroban* | Apply small amt. to affected area tid. May be covered with a gauze dsg. | Use to treat impetigo caused by *Staph. aureus, Streptococcus* and *S. pyogens.* Monitor for signs of superinfection; reevaluate if not clinical response in 3–5 d. |
| ***Antivirals*** | | | |
| imiquimod | *Aldara* | Apply a thin layer to warts and rub in 3×/wk at bedtime for 16 wks. | Remove with soap and water after 6–10 h; for treatment of external genital warts and perianal warts. |

*(continued)*

| Drug | Brand Names | Dosage | Special Considerations |
|---|---|---|---|
| penciclovir | *Denavir* | Apply thin layer to affected area q2h while awake for 4 d. Use at first sign of cold sore. | Treatment of cold scores in healthy patients. Reserve use for herpes labialis on lips and face—avoid mucous membranes. |
| ***Antipsoriatics*** | | | |
| Ammoniated mercury | *Emersal* | Apply qd-bid. | Protect from light; potential sensitizer provoking severe allergic reactions. |
| anthralin | *Anthra-Derm*<br>*Drithocreme* | Apply qd only to psoriatic lesions | May stain fabrics, skin, hair, fingernails; use protective dressing. |
| calcipotriene | *Dovonex* | Apply thin layer twice a day | Monitor serum calcium levels with extended use; use only for disorder prescribed; may cause local irritation; is a synthetic vitamin $D_2$. |
| ***Antiseborrheics*** | | | |
| selenium sulfide | *Selsun Blue* | Massage 5–10 ml into scalp; rest 2–3 min., rinse | May damage jewelry, remove before use; discontinue if local irritation occurs |
| chloroxine | *Capitrol* | Massage into wet scalp; leave lather on for 3 min | May discolor blond, gray, bleached hair. Do not use on active lesions. |
| ***Antifungals*** | | | |
| butenafine HCl | *Mentax* | Apply to affected area only once a day for 4 wk. | Treatment of intradigital pedia (athlete's foot), tinea corporis, ringworm, tinea cruris. |
| clotrimazole | *Lotrimin*<br>*Mycelex* | Gently massage into affected area bid. | Cleanse area before applying; use for up to 4 wk. Discontinue if irritation, worsening of condition occurs. |
| econzole nitrate | *Spectazole* | Apply locally qd-bid. | Cleanse area before applying; treat for 2–4 wk. Discontinue if irritation, burning or worsening of condition occurs. For athlete's foot, change socks and shoes at least once a day. |
| gentian violet | | Apply locally bid. | May stain skin and clothing; do not apply to active lesions. |
| naftitine HCl | *Naftin* | Gently massage into affected area bid. | Avoid occlusive dressings; wash hands thoroughly after application. Do not use longer than 4 wk. |

| | | | |
|---|---|---|---|
| oxiconazole | *Oxistat* | Apply qd-bid. | May be needed for up to 1 mo. |
| terbinafine | *Lamisil* | Apply to area bid until clinical signs are improved; 1–4 wk | Do not use occlusive dressings; report local irritation; discontinue if local irritation occurs. |
| tolnaftate | *Aftate*<br>*Genaspor*<br>*Tinactin*<br>*Ting* | Apply small amount bid for 2–3 wk; 4–6 wk may be needed if skin is very thick | Cleanse skin with soap and water before applying drug, dry thoroughly, wear loose, well-fitting shoes, change socks at least qid. |
| ***Pediculocides/scabicides*** | | | |
| lindane | *G-Well*<br>*Scabene* | Apply thin layer to entire body, leave on 8–12h, then wash thoroughly. Shampoo 1–2 oz. into dry hair and leave in place 4 min. | For external use only. Single application is usually sufficient, reapply after 7 d at signs of live lice. Teach hygiene and prevention; treat all contacts. Assure parents this is a readily communicable disease. |
| crotamiton | *Eurax* | Thoroughly massage into skin of entire body; repeat in 24h. Take a cleansing bath or shower 48h after last application. | For external use only. Change bed linens and clothing the next day. Contaminated clothing can be dry cleaned or washed on hot cycle. Shake well before using. |
| permethrin | *Elimite, Nix* | Thoroughly massage into all skin areas (30g/adult); wash off after 8–14h. Shampoo into freshly washed, rinsed and towel dried hair. Leave on for 10 min.; rinse. | For external use only. Single application is usually curative. Notify health care provider if rash, itching become worse. Approved for prophylactic use during head lice epidemics. |
| ***Keratolytics*** | | | |
| cantharidin | | Apply to lesion; cover with tape; remove in 24h | Replace tape with loose bandage; may cause itching and burning, may be tender for 2–6 d; if spilled on skin, wipe off with acetone or tape remover; if contacts eyes, flush immediately and contact physician. |
| podophyllium resin | *Pod-Ben-25*<br>*Podocon-25*<br>*Podofin* | Applied only by physician. | Do not use if wart is inflamed or irritated. Very toxic, minimum amount possible is used to avoid absorption. |
| podofilox | *Condylox* | Apply q12h for 3 consecutive d. | Allow to dry before using area; dispose of used applicator; may cause burning and discomfort. |

*(continued)*

| Drug | Brand Names | Dosage | Special Considerations |
|---|---|---|---|
| ***Topical hemostatics*** | | | |
| absorbable gelatin | *Gelfoam* | Smear or press paste to cut surface; when bleeding stops, remove excess. Apply sponge and allow to remain in place, will be absorbed. | Prepare paste by adding 3–4 ml sterile saline to contents of jar. Apply sponge dry or saturated with saline. Assess continually for any sign of infection, agent may act as site of infection or abscess formation. Do not use in presence of infection. |
| microfibrillar collagen | *Avitene* | Use dry. Apply directly to the source of bleeding; apply pressure, time will vary from 3–5 min depending on the site. Discard any unused product. | Monitor for infection; do not use in the presence of infection. Remove any excess material once bleeding has been controlled. |
| thrombin | *Thrombinar, Thrombostat* | Prepare in Sterile Distilled Water of Isotonic Saline; 100–1000 units/ml. Mix freely with blood on the surface of injury. | Contraindicated in presence of any bovine allergies. Watch for any sign of severe allergic reaction in sensitive individuals. |
| ***Pain Relief*** | | | |
| capsaicin | *Zostrix* | Apply not more than 3–4 times/day. | Applied locally, provides temporary relief from the pain of osteoarthritis, rheumatoid arthritis, neuralgias. Do not bandage tightly; stop use and seek health care if condition worsens or persists after 14–28 d. |
| ***Burn Preparations*** | | | |
| mafenide | *Sulfamylon* | Apply to a clean, debrided wound, 1–2 times/d with a gloved hand. Cover burn at all times with drug, reapply as needed. | Bathe patient in a whirlpool daily to aid debridement. Continue until healing occurs; monitor for infection and toxicity—acidosis. May cause marked discomfort on application. |
| nitrofurazone | *Furacin* | Apply directly to burn or place on gauze; reapply qd. | Flushing the dressing with sterile saline will facilitate removal. Monitor for signs of superinfections; treat supportively. Rash frequently occurs. |

| | | | |
|---|---|---|---|
| silver sulfadiazine | *Silvadene, Thermazene SSF Cream* | Apply qd-bid to a clean, debrided wound; use a $^{1}/_{16}$ in thickness. | Bathe patient in a whirlpool to aid debridement. Dressings are not necessary but may be used; reapply whenever necessary. Monitor for fungal superinfections. |
| ***Acne Product*** | | | |
| adapalene | *Differin* | Apply a thin film to affected area after washing. | Do not use on cuts or any open area. Avoid use on sunburned skin in combination with other products, or exposure to sun. Less drying than other products. |
| azelaic acid | *Azelex* | Wash and dry skin, massage a thin layer into affected area bid. | Wash hands thoroughly after application. Improvement usually occurs within 4 wk. Initial irritation usually occurs but will pass with time. |
| sodium sulfacetamide | *Klaron* | Apply a thin film bid to affected areas. | Wash affected area with mild soap and water; pat dry. Avoid use in denuded or abraded areas. |
| tazarotene | *Tazorac* | Apply thin film, once daily in the evening. | Avoid use in pregnancy. Drying, causes photosensitivity; Do not use with irritants or products with high alcohol. |
| tretinoin, 0.025% cream | *Avita* | Apply thin layer once/d. | Discomfort, peeling redness may occur for the first 2–4 wk. Worsened acne may occur in first few wk. |
| tretinoin, gel | *Retin-A* micro* | Apply to cover, once/d after cleansing | Exacerbation of inflammation may occur at first. Therapeutic effects usually seen in first 2 wk. |
| ***Oral Preparations*** | | | |
| amlexanox | *Aphthasol* | Apply to aphthous ulcers qid: after meals and hs, following oral hygiene; 4×/d for 10 d. | Consult with dentist if ulcers are not healed within 10 d. May cause local pain. |
| ***Antiadhesion agent*** | | | |
| sodium hyaluronate and carboxymethylcellulose | *Seprafilm* | Placed during open abdominal or pelvic surgery to reduce the occurrence and extent of postoperative adhesions. | Turns into gel within 24–48 h; resorbed within 1 wk, excreted within 28 d. Monitor for abscess and pulmonary embolus. |

# Corticosteroids

## Drug Classes

Hormonal agents
Corticosteroids
Glucocorticoids/mineralcorticoids

## Therapeutic Actions

Enter cells and bind cytoplasmic receptors, thereby initiating complex reactions that are responsible for the anti-inflammatory, antipruritic, and anti-proliferative effects.

## Indications

- Relief of inflammatory and pruritic manifestations of corticosteroid-sensitive dermatoses
- Temporary relief of minor skin irritations, itching and rashes—nonprescription products

## Adverse Effects

- Local: Burning, irritation, acneiform lesions, striae, skin atrophy, secondary infection
- CNS: Glaucoma, cataracts after prolonged periorbital use that allows the drug to enter the eyes
- Systemic: Systemic absorption can occur, leading to the adverse effects experienced with systemic use; growth retardation and suppression of the HPA (more likely to occur with occlusive dressings, in patients with liver failure, and with children who have a larger skin surface–to–body weight ratio)

## Dosage

Apply sparingly to affected area bid–tid.

## Drug-Specific Teaching Points

- Apply sparingly in a light film, rub in gently. Washing the area before application may increase drug penetration.
- Do not use occlusive dressings, tight-fitting diapers or plastic pants unless otherwise indicated. This may increase systemic absorption (except with aclometasone used to treat psoriasis).
- Avoid prolonged use, especially near the eyes, in genital or rectal areas, on the face, and in skin creases. Avoid any direct contact with eyes.
- Use this drug only for the purpose indicated. Do not apply to open lesions.
- Notify nurse or physician if condition becomes worse or persists, if burning or irritation occurs, or if infection occurs in the area.

| *Drug* | *Brand Name* | *Preparations* |
|---|---|---|
| alclometasone dipropionate | *Aclovate* | Ointment, cream: 0.05% concentration |
| amcinonide | *Cyclocort* | Ointment, cream, lotion: 0.1% concentration |
| betamethasone dipropionate | *Diprosone, Maxivate, Rhoprosone* (CAN), *Taro-Stone* (CAN), *Teledar* | Ointment, cream, lotion, aerosol: 0.05% concentration |
| betamethasone dipropionate augmented | *Diprolene* | Ointment, cream, lotion: 0.05% concentration |
| betamethasone valerate | *Betacort* (CAN), *Betaderm* (CAN), *Betatrex, Beta-Val, Betnovate* (CAN), *Celestroderm* (CAN), *Prevex, B*(CAN), *Rholosone* (CAN), *Valisone* | Ointment, cream, lotion: 0.1% concentration |

*(continued)*

| Drug | Brand Name | Preparations |
|---|---|---|
| clobetasol propionate | *Dermovate* (CAN), *Temovate* | Ointment, cream: 0.05% concentration |
| clocortolone pivalate | *Cloderm* | Cream: 0.1% concentration |
| desonide | *DesOwen, Tridesiolon* | Ointment, cream: 0.05% concentration |
| desoximetasone | *Topicort* | Ointment, cream: 0.25% concentration<br>Gel: 0.05% concentration |
| dexamethasone | *Aeroseb-Dex* | Aerosol: 0.01% concentration |
| dexamethasone sodium phosphate | *Decadron Phosphate* | Cream: 0.1% concentration |
| diflorasone diacetate | *Florone, Maxiflor, Psorcon* | Ointment, cream: 0.05% concentration |
| | *Florone E* | Cream: 0.5% concentration |
| fluocinolone acetonide | *Flurosyn, Synalar* | Ointment: 0.025% concentration<br>Cream: 0.01% concentration |
| | *Flurosyn, Synalar, Synemol* | Cream: 0.025% concentration |
| | *Fluonid, Flurosyn, Synalar* | Solution: 0.01% concentration |
| fluocinonide | *Lidex* | Ointment: 0.05% concentration |
| | *Fluonex, Lidex, Lyderm Cream* (CAN) | Cream: 0.05% concentration |
| | *Lidex, Topsyn Gel* (CAN) | Solution, gel: 0.05% concentration |
| flurandrenolide | *Cordran* | Ointment, cream: 0.025% concentration<br>Ointment, cream, lotion: 0.05% concentration<br>Tape: 4 mcg/cm$^2$ |
| fluticasone propionate | *Cutivate* | Cream: 0.05% concentration<br>Ointment: 0.05% concentration |
| halcinonide | *Halog* | Ointment, cream, solution: 0.1% concentration<br>Cream: 0.025% concentration |
| halobetasol propionate | *Ultravate* | Ointment, cream: 0.05% concentration |
| hydrocortisone | *Cortizone 5, Bactine Hydrocortisone, Cort-Dome, Dermolate, Dermtex HC, HydroTEX* | Lotion: 0.25% |
| | *Cortizone 10, Hycort, Tegrin-HC* | Cream, lotion, ointment, aerosol: 0.5% |
| | *Hytone* | Cream, lotion, ointment, solution: 1% |

*(continued)*

| Drug | Brand Name | Preparations |
|---|---|---|
| hydrocortisone acetate | *Cortaid, Lanacort-5* | Ointment: 0.5% concentration |
| | *Corticaine* ($R_x$), *FoilleCort, Gyne-cort, Lanacort 5* | Cream: 0.5% concentration |
| | *Anusol-HC, U-Cort* | Cream: 1% concentration |
| | *Caldecort, Cortaid with Aloe* | Cream: 0.5% concentration |
| | *CortaGel* | Gel: 0.5% concentration |
| hydrocortisone buteprate | *Pandel* | Cream: 0.1% |
| hydrocortisone butyrate | *Locoid* | Ointment, cream: 0.1% concentration |
| hydrocortisone valerate | *Westcort* | Ointment, cream: 0.2% concentration |
| mometasone furoate | *Elocon* | Ointment, cream, lotion: 0.1% concentration |
| | *Nasonex* | Nasal Spray: 0.2% |
| prednicarbate | *Dermatop* | Cream: 0.1% concentration: preservative free |
| triamcinolone acetonide | *Flutex, Kenalog* | Ointment: 0.025% concentration |
| | *Aristocort* | Ointment: 0.1% concentration and 0.5% concentration<br>Cream: 0.025% concentration and 0.5% concentration |
| | *Triacet, Triderm* | Cream: 0.1% concentration |
| | | Lotion: 0.025% and 0.1% concentration |

# APPENDIX L

## Vitamins

Vitamins are substances that the body requires for carrying out essential metabolic reactions. The body cannot synthesize enough of these components to meet all of its needs; therefore, they must be obtained from animal and vegetable tissues taken as food. Vitamins are needed only in small amounts because they function as coenzymes that activate the protein portion of enzymes; which catalyze a great deal of biochemical activity. Vitamins are either water soluble and excreted in the urine, or fat soluble and capable of being stored in adipose tissue.

### Indications

- Treatment of vitamin deficiency
- Dietary supplement when needed
- Specific therapeutic uses related to vitamin activity

### Pregnancy Category C

*Contraindicated* in cases of allergy to these drugs, colorants, additives, or preservatives.

### Drug-Drug Interactions

Pyrodoxine interferes with effectiveness of levodopa; fat-soluble vitamins may not be absorbed if given concurrently with mineral oil, cholestyramine, colestipol.

| Vitamin | Brand Names | Type | RDA (PO) | Therapeutic Uses/Special Consideration |
|---|---|---|---|---|
| A | *Aquasol A*<br>*Del-vi-A* | Fat soluble | 1000 mcg (males)<br>800 mcg (females)<br>1300 mcg (nursing)<br>375–700 mcg (ped.) | Severe deficiency—500,000 IU/d–3 days; then 50,000 IU/d for 2 wk PO or IM. Protect IM vial from light. Hypervitaminosis A can occur—cirrhotic-like liver syndrome with CNS effects, GI drying, rash, liver changes. Treat by discontinuing vitamin; saline, prednisone, calcitonin IV. Liver damage may be permanent. |
| ascorbic acid (C) | *Cebid*<br>*Cevalin*<br>*Cevi-Bid*<br>*Dull-C*<br>*Flavorcee*<br>*N'Ice Vitamin C drops*<br>*Vita-C* | Water soluble | 50–60 mg (males)<br>50–60 mg (females)<br>70–90 mg (nursing)<br>70 mg (pregnancy)<br>30–45 mg (ped.) | May be given PO, IM, IV (slowly), SC. Treatment of scurvy—300 mg–1 g daily; enhanced wound healing—300–500 mg/d for 7–10 d; burns—1–2 g/d. Also being studied for treatment of common cold, asthma, CAD, wound healing, cancer, schizophrenia. |
| calcifediol ($D_3$) | | Fat soluble | | Management of metabolic bone disease or hypocalcemia in patients on chronic renal dialysis: 300–350 mcg/wk given daily or on alternate days. Discontinue if hypercalcemia occurs. |
| calcitriol ($D_3$) | *Calcijex*<br>*Rocaltrol* | Fat soluble | | Management of hypocalcemia in patients on renal dialysis: 0.25 mcg/d. Reduction of elevated parathyroid hormone: 0.25 mcg/d in the morning as an initial dose then 0.5–2 mcg/d. May be effective in the treatment of psoriasis. |
| cholecalciferol ($D_3$) | *Delta-D* | Fat soluble | 200–400 IU (males)<br>200–400 IU (females)<br>400 IU (nursing)<br>400 IU (pregnancy)<br>300–400 IU (ped.) | Vitamin D deficiency—400–1000 IU/d. May be useful for treatment of hypocalcemic tetany and hypoparathyroidism. |

| | | | | |
|---|---|---|---|---|
| cyanocobalamin ($B_{12}$) | *Ener-B* | Water soluble | 2 mcg (males)<br>2 mcg (females)<br>2.6 mcg (nursing)<br>2.2 mcg (pregnancy)<br>0.3–1.4 mcg (ped.) | Deficiency—25–250 mcg/d. Note: not for the treatment of pernicious anemia. |
| D | | Fat soluble | 200–400 IU (males)<br>200–400 IU (females)<br>400 IU (nursing)<br>400 IU (pregnancy)<br>300–400 IU (ped.) | Vitamin D deficiency—400–1000 IU/d. May be useful for treatment of hypocalcemic tetany and hypoparathyroidism. Encourage balanced diet and exposure to sunlight. Do not use with mineral oil. |
| dihydrotachysterol (DHT; $D_2$) | *DHT*<br>*Hytakerol* | Fat soluble | | Treatment of postoperative tetany, idiopathic tetany, hypoparathyroidism: Initial dose 0.8–2.4 mg/d for several days, then 0.2–1 mg/d to achieve normal serum calcium. May supplement with oral calcium. |
| E | *Aquasol E*<br>*Vita-Plus E Softgels*<br>*E Complex*<br>*Amino-Opti E* | Fat soluble | 15 IU (males)<br>12 IU (females)<br>16–18 IU (nursing)<br>15 IU (pregnancy)<br>4–10 IU (ped.) | Used in certain premature infants to reduce the toxic effects of oxygen on the lung and retina; do not give IV; report—fatigue, weakness, nausea, headache, blurred vision, diarrhea. |
| ergocalciferol ($D_2$) | *Drisdol drops* | Fat soluble | 200–400 IU (males)<br>200–400 IU (females)<br>400 IU (nursing)<br>400 IU (pregnancy)<br>300–400 IU (ped.) | Give IM in GI, biliary, liver disease. Refractory rickets—12,000–500,000 IU/d Hypoparathyroidism—50,000–200,000 IU/d Familial hypophosphatemia—10,000–80,000 IU/d plus 1–2 g phosphorus. |

(continued)

| *Vitamin* | *Brand Names* | *Type* | *RDA (PO)* | *Therapeutic Uses/Special Consideration* |
|---|---|---|---|---|
| menadiol sodium diphosphate ($K_4$) | | Fat soluble | 45–80 mcg (males)<br>45–65 mcg (females)<br>65 mcg (nursing)<br>65 mcg (pregnancy)<br>5–50 mcg (ped.) | Hypoprothrombinemia due to obstructive jaundice—5 mg/d PO, IM, SC, IV, Hypoprothrombinemia due to antibiotics or salicylates—5–10 mg/d. |
| niacin ($B_3$) | *Niacor*<br>*Nicolar*<br>*Nicotinic acid* | Water soluble | 15–20 mg (males)<br>13–15 mg (females)<br>20 mg (nursing)<br>17 mg (pregnancy)<br>5–13 mg (ped.) | Prevention and treatment of pellagra: up to 500 mg/d; niacin deficiency: up to 100 mg/d, also used for treatment of hyperlipidemia in patients who do not respond to diet and exercise—1–2 g tid. Do not exceed 6 g/d. Feelings of warmth, flushing may occur with administration but usually pass within 2h. |
| nicotinamide ($B_3$) | | Water soluble | 15–20 mg (males)<br>13–15 mg (females)<br>20 mg (nursing)<br>17 mg (pregnancy)<br>5–13 mg (ped.) | Prevention and treatment of pellagra: up to 50 mg 3–10 times/d. |
| P (Bioflavonoids) | *Amino-Opti-C*<br>*Bio Acerola C*<br>*Citro-Flav 2000*<br>*Flavons-500*<br>*Pan C-500*<br>*Peridin C*<br>*Span C* | Water soluble | None known | Used to treat bleeding, abortion, poliomyelitis, arthritis, diabetes, etc. There is little evidence that these uses have any clinical efficacy. |

| | | | | |
|---|---|---|---|---|
| phytonadione (K) | *Mephyton* | Fat soluble | 45–80 mcg (males)<br>45–65 mcg (females)<br>65 mcg (nursing)<br>65 mcg (pregnancy)<br>5–30 mcg (ped.) | Hypoprothrombinemia due to anticoagulants—2.5–10 mg PO, IM. Hemorrhagic disease of the newborn: 0.5–1 mg IM within 1h of birth, 1–5 mg IM may be given to the mother before delivery; hypoprothrombinemia in adults 2.5–25 mg PO or IM. |
| pyridoxine HCl ($B_6$) | *Nestrex* | Water soluble | 1.7–2 mg (males)<br>1.4–1.6 mg (females)<br>2.1 mg (nursing)<br>2.2 mg (pregnancy)<br>0.3–1.4 mg (ped.) | Deficiency: 10–20 mg/d PO or IM for 3 wk. Vitamin $B_6$ deficiency syndrome: up to 600 mg/day for life. INH poisoning–give an equal amount of pyridoxine: 4 g IV followed by Ig IM q30min. Reduces effectiveness of *levodopa* and leads to serious toxic effects—avoid this combination. |
| riboflavin ($B_2$) | | Water soluble | 1.4–1.8 mg (males)<br>1.2–1.3 mg (females)<br>1.7–1.8 mg (nursing)<br>1.6 mg (pregnancy)<br>0.4–1.2 mg (ped.) | Treatment of deficiency; 5–15 mg/day. May cause a yellow/orange discoloring of the urine. |
| thiamine HCl ($B_1$) | | Water soluble | 1.2–1.5 mg (males)<br>1–1.1 mg (females)<br>1.6 mg (nursing)<br>1.5 mg (pregnancy)<br>0.3–1 mg (ped.) | Treatment of wet beriberi: 10–30 mg IV tid; treatment of beriberi: 10–20 mg IM tid for 2 wk with an oral multivitamin containing 5–10 mg/d for 1 mo. Do not mix in alkaline solutions. Used orally as a mosquito repellant, alters body sweat composition. Feeling of warmth and flushing may occur with administration. |

# Part II
# Administration-Related Content

# APPENDIX M

## Formulae for Calculating Dosages

### *Pediatric Dosages*

Children often require different doses of drugs than adults because children's bodies often handle drugs very differently from adults' bodies. The "standard" drug dosages listed in package inserts and references such as the PDR refer to the adult dosage. In some cases, a pediatric dosage is suggested, but in many cases it will need to be calculated based on the child's age, weight, or body surface. The following are some standard formulae for calculating the pediatric dose.

**Fried's rule**

$$\text{infant's dose } (<1 \text{ y}) = \frac{\text{infant's age (in mo)}}{150 \text{ mo}} \times \text{average adult dose}$$

**Young's rule**

$$\text{child's dose } (1\text{–}12 \text{ y}) = \frac{\text{child's age (in yrs)}}{\text{child's age (in yrs)} + 12} \times \text{average adult dose}$$

**Clark's rule**

$$\text{child's dose} = \frac{\text{weight of child (lb)}}{150 \text{ lb}} \times \text{average adult dose}$$

**Surface area rule**

$$\text{child's dose} = \frac{\text{surface area of child (in square meters)}}{1.73} \times \text{average adult dose}$$

The surface area of a child is determined using a nomogram which determines surface area based on height and weight measurements.

Pediatric dosage calculations should be checked by two persons. Many institutions have procedures for double checking the dosage calculation of those drugs (eg, digoxin) used most frequently in the pediatric area.

## Commonly Used Calculations

In many situations, the nurse needs to calculate the correct dosage of a prescribed drug from the drug form or concentration that is available.

**Prescribed versus available quantity or concentration**

A common situation occurs when the amount of a drug prescribed is not the same as the standard form that is available. To determine the correct amount to give, the prescribed units need to be converted to the available units.

$$\frac{\text{dose ordered}}{\text{dose available}} \times \text{volume available} = \text{volume to administer}$$

For example: the order reads 0.125 mg digoxin, the drug is available in 0.25-mg tablets.

$$\frac{0.125 \text{ mg}}{0.250 \text{ mg}} \times 1 \text{ tablet} = \tfrac{1}{2} \text{ tablet to be administered}$$

Or, using a ratio, or cross-multiplying calculation such as:

$$\frac{\text{Ordered amount}}{\text{Amount to give } (x)} = \frac{\text{Available unit}}{1}$$

For example: the order reads 0.125 mg digoxin, the drug is available in 0.25-mg tablets. Use a simple algebra, cross multiplying to determine the correct amount needed:

$$\frac{0.125 \text{ mg}}{x} = \frac{0.25 \text{ mg}}{1 \text{ tablet}}$$

$$1 \text{ tablet } (0.125 \text{ mg}) = 0.25 \text{ mg } x$$

$$x = \frac{0.125 \text{ mg (tablet)}}{0.25 \text{ mg}}$$

$$x = 0.5 \text{ tablets}$$

**Parenteral**

Using the same basic concept to determine how much of a liquid to give in injection, determine the amount of solution that will contain the prescribed dose:

$$\frac{\text{dose ordered}}{\text{dose available}} \times \text{volume on hand} = \text{volume to give}$$

For example: the order is for 0.4 mg atropine IM; the atropine available comes in 0.3-mg/ml vials.

$$\frac{0.4 \text{ mg}}{0.3 \text{ mg}} \times 1 \text{ ml} = \text{volume to give}$$

$$\tfrac{4}{3} \times 1 \text{ ml} = 4/3 \text{ or } 1.3 \text{ ml to give}$$

### IV Flow Rates

IV flow rate is determined by rate of infusion and the number of drops/ml of the fluid being given. This ranges from 10 (maxi) to 15 (micro) drops/ml, depending on the infusion set being used.

$$\text{drops/ml} \times \text{ml/min} = \text{IV flow rate (drops/min)}$$

For example: the antibiotic ordered to be given IV is 60 ml being given through a maxi-drip set and is to be given over 30 min.

$$\frac{10 \text{ drops}}{1 \text{ ml}} \times \frac{60 \text{ ml}}{30 \text{ min}} = 20 \text{ drops/min}$$

$$\frac{\text{total fluid to be infused}}{\text{total time of infusion}} \times \text{drops/min} = \text{IV flow rate (drops/min)}$$

For example: the order reads 500 ml D5W to be infused over 5 hours; the infusion unit uses a microdrip drip set of 15 drops/ml.

$$\frac{500 \text{ ml}}{5 \text{ h } (\times 60 \text{ min/h})} \times \frac{15 \text{ drops}}{\text{ml}} = \text{IV flow rate}$$

$$\frac{500 \text{ ml}}{300 \text{ min}} \times \frac{15 \text{ drops}}{\text{ml}} = 25 \text{ drops/min}$$

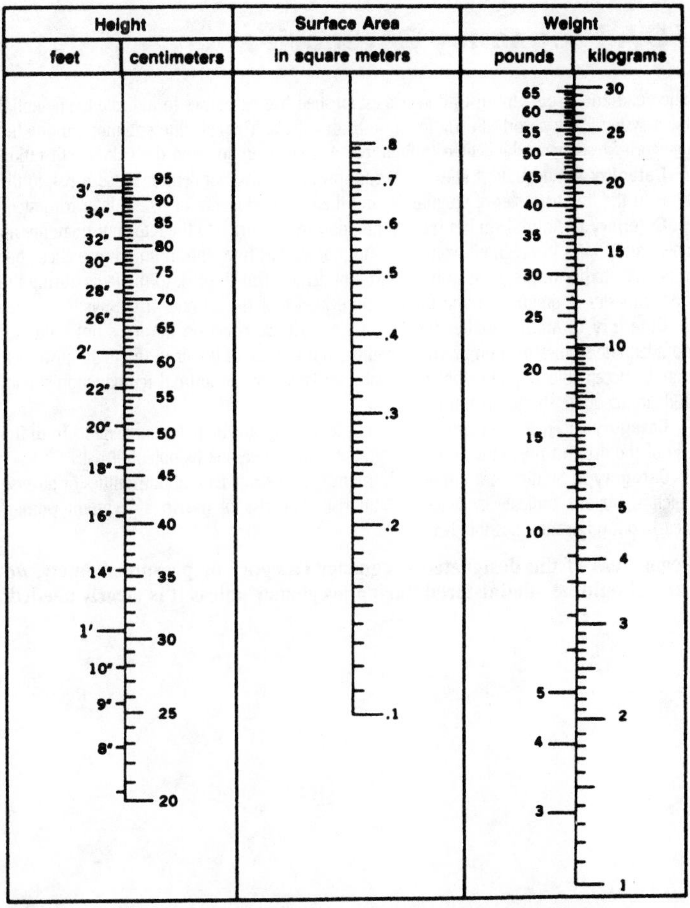


Nomogram for estimating surface area of infants and young children. To determine the surface area of the patient, draw a straight line between the point representing the height on the left vertical scale and the point representing the weight on the right vertical scale. The point at which this line intersects the middle vertical scale represents the patient's surface area in square meters. (Courtesy of Abbott Laboratories.)

# APPENDIX N

## FDA Pregnancy Categories

The Food and Drug Administration has established five categories to indicate the potential for a systemically absorbed drug to cause birth defects. The key differentiation among the categories rests upon the degree (reliability) of documentation and the risk-benefit ratio.

**Category A:** Adequate studies in pregnant women have not demonstrated a risk to the fetus in the first trimester of pregnancy, and there is no evidence of risk in later trimesters.

**Category B:** Animal studies have not demonstrated a risk to the fetus but there are no adequate studies in pregnant women. *or* Animal studies have shown an adverse effect, but adequate studies in pregnant women have not demonstrated a risk to the fetus during the first trimester of pregnancy, and there is no evidence of risk in later trimesters.

**Category C:** Animal studies have shown an adverse effect on the fetus but there are no adequate studies in humans; the benefits from the use of the drug in pregnant women may be acceptable despite its potential risks. *or* There are no animal reproduction studies and no adequate studies in humans.

**Category D:** There is evidence of human fetal risk, but the potential benefits from the use of the drug in pregnant women may be acceptable despite its potential risks.

**Category X:** Studies in animals or humans demonstrate fetal abnormalities or adverse reaction; reports indicate evidence of fetal risk. The risk of use in a pregnant woman clearly outweighs any possible benefit.

**Regardless of the designated Pregnancy Category or presumed safety, *no* drug should be administered during pregnancy unless it is clearly needed.**

# Appendix O

## Drugs Withdrawn or Discontinued Since the Last Edition

*Achromycin* (tetracycline)
*Agoral Plain* (mineral oil)
*AK-Dex Ophthalmic* (dexamethasone)
*AminFreAmine* (amino acids)
*Apo*-Allopurinol (CAN) (allupurinal)
*Aralen Phosphate with Primaquine Phosphate* (combination)
*Atesol* (CAN) (acetaminophen)
*Bretylol* (bretylium)
*Buffaprin* (aspirin)
*Campain* (acetaminophen)
*Ceclor Pulvules* (cefaclor)
**chloramphenicol palmitate**
*Chloromycetin Kapseals* (chloramphenicol)
**codeine sulfate**
*Corticosporin* (combination)
*Cyclan* (cyclandelate)
*Cyclospasmol* (cyclandelate)
*D-Amp* (ampicillin)
*Dapex* (phentermine)
*Decaderm* (dexamethasone)
*Decadrol* (dexamethasone)
*Decameth* (dexamethasone)
*Decaspray* (dexamethasone)
*Depitol* (carbamazepine)
*Deprol* (meprobamate, bractyzine)
*Dexasen-4* (dexamethasone)
**dexfenfluramine**
**diphenidol**
*Dispos-a-Med Isoproterenol Hcl* (isoproterenol)
*Dolanex* (acetaminophen)
*Eldepryl* (selegiline)
*Endep* (amitriptyline)
*Enovid* (combination)
*Enovid E 21* (combination)
*Enovil* (amitriptyline)
**ethaverine**
*Exdol* (acetaminophen)
*Femcare* (clotrimazole)
**fenfluramine hydrochloride**
*Fertux* (urofollitropin)
*Fluogen* (influenza virus vaccine)
*Gamastan* (immune globulin IM)
*Gammar* (immune globulin IM)
*Genabid* (papaverine)
*Gen-Salbutamol* (CAN) (albuterol)
*Geridium* (phenazophyridine)
*Humulin R U-500* (insulin)
*L-Deprenyl* (selegiline)
*Ledercillin-VK* (penicillin V)
*Liquaemin Sodium* (heparin)
*Lorcet* (hydrocodone, acetaminophen)
*Medrol Acetate* (methylpredisolone)
*Meprospan* (meprobamate)
*Monitan* (CAN) (acebutolol)
*Myidil* (tripolidine)
*Neo Cortef* (combination)
*Neothylline* (dyphylline)
*Nevlova 10/11* (combination)
*Novahistine DH* (combination)
*Novahistine DMX* (combination)
*Novahistine Expectorant* (combination)
*Obermine* (phentermine)
*Obestine* (phentermine)
*Pamprin-IB* (ibuprofen)
*Panasol* (prednisone)
*Panex* (acetaminophen)
*Parmine* (phentermine)
*Pavadine* (papaverine)
*Pfizerpen-AS* (penicillin G procaine)
**phenacemide**
*Phentrol* (phentermine)
*Phenetron* (chlorphemiramine)
*Phenolax* (phenolphthaline)
*Phenuron* (phenacemide)
*Platinol* (cisplatin)
*Ponderal* (CAN) (fenfluramine)
*Pondimin* (fenfluramine)
*Proben C* (combination)
*Profilate-HP* (antihemophilic factor)
*Pyronium* (CAN) (phenazophyridine)
*Reactine* (cetrizine)
*Redux* (dexfenfluramine)
*Rhotral* (CAN) (acebutolol)
*Robitet* (tetracycline)
*Rufen* (ibuprofen)
*Seldane* (terfenadine)
**selegiline hydrochloride**
*St. Joseph's Aspirin Free* (acetaminophen)

**streptomycin sulfate**
*Suppap* (acetaminophen)
*Surital* (thiamylal)
**terfenadine**
*Tetralan* (tetracycline)
**thiamylal sodium**
*Trendar* (ibuprofen)
*Tricosal* (choline magnesium salicylate)
*Tylenol with Codeine #1* (acetaminophen, codeine)
*Ultraject* (morphine)
*Ultralente U* (insulin)
**uracil mustard**
*Uri-tet* (oxytetracycline)
*Urobak* (sulfamethoxazole)
*Urodine* (phenazophyridine)
*Verr-Canth* (cantharidin)
*Vontrol* (diphenidol)
*Zartman* (cephalexin)

# APPENDIX P

## DEA Schedules of Controlled Substances

The Controlled Substances Act of 1970 regulates the manufacturing, distribution, and dispensing of drugs which are known to have abuse potential. The Drug Enforcement Agency (DEA) is responsible for the enforcement of these regulations. The controlled drugs are divided into five DEA schedules based on their potential for abuse and physical and psychological dependence.

**Schedule I** ***(C-I):*** High abuse potential and no accepted medical use (heroin, marijuana, LSD)

**Schedule II** ***(C-II):*** High abuse potential with severe dependence liability (narcotics, amphetamines, and barbiturates)

**Schedule III** ***(C-III):*** Less abuse potential than Schedule II drugs and moderate dependence liability (nonbarbiturate sedatives, nonamphetamine stimulants, limited amounts of certain narcotics)

**Schedule IV** ***(C-IV):*** Less abuse potential than Schedule III and limited dependence liability (some sedatives, antianxiety agents, and nonnarcotic analgesics)

**Schedule V** ***(C-V):*** Limited abuse potential. Primarily small amounts of narcotics (codeine) used as antitussives or antidiarrheals. Under federal law, limited quantities of certain Schedule V drugs may be purchased without a prescription directly from a pharmacist. The purchaser must be at least 18 years of age and must furnish suitable identification. All such transactions must be recorded by the dispensing pharmacist.

Prescribing physicians and dispensing pharmacists must be registered with the DEA, which also provides forms for the transfer of Schedule I and II substances and establishes criteria for the inventory and prescribing of controlled substances. State and local laws are often more stringent than federal law. In any given situation, the more stringent law applies.

# APPENDIX Q

## Injections Information

| Type | Needle Gauge | Needle Length | Syringe | Comments |
|---|---|---|---|---|
| Intradermal | 26 | ⅜ in | Tuberculin | Area must be marked or mapped if repeated tests done. |
| Subcutaneous | 25 | ½ in | Tuberculin, insulin | Rotate sites. |
| Intramuscular | 20–23 | 1–3 in | 2–3 ml | Rapid insertion and slow injection help to decrease pain. |
| Intravenous | 20, 21 | | Bag with tubing. | Monitor site and needle-placement. |
| Blood | 16, 18 | | Bag with tubing. | Check equipment, needle placement, and injection site regularly. |

**Injection Procedures**

**Intradermal injection:** Inject directly below the surface of the skin. The injection should produce a wheal or fluid-filled bump that can be seen beneath the skin at the injection site. Skin on the back of the forearm is the usual site for these injections. The area should be marked or mapped for reading tests in 24–48h.

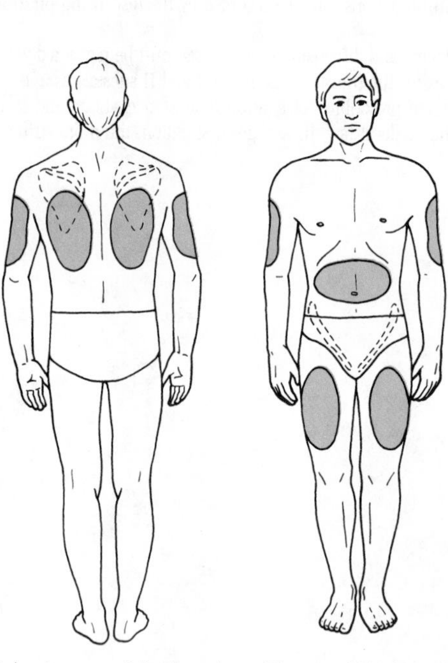

Subcutaneous injection sites. (Earnest, V.V. [1992]. *Clinical skills in nursing practice,* [2nd ed., p. 864]. Philadelphia: J.B. Lippincott.)

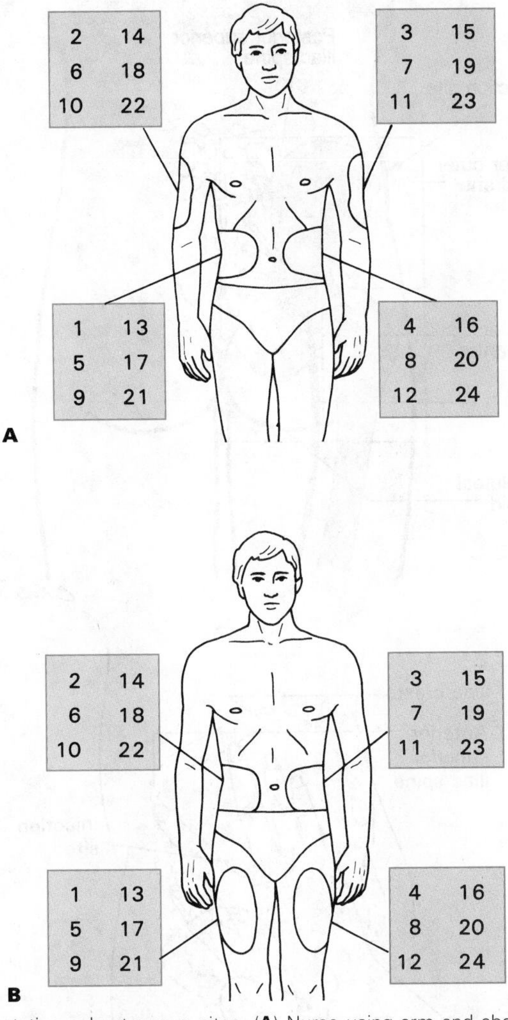


Chart for rotating subcutaneous sites. (**A**) Nurse using arm and abdomen. (**B**) Client using abdomen and thighs. (Earnest, V.V. [1992]. *Clinical skills in nursing practice,* [2nd ed., p. 864]. Philadelphia: J.B. Lippincott.)

**Subcutaneous injection:** Inject into the loose connective tissue underneath the skin; do not inject more than 2 ml at a time. Areas of the body that can be "pinched up" are best suited—abdomen, upper thigh, upper arm. The needle is inserted at 45 degrees; the plunger is pulled back to assure that no blood returns and the needle is not in a vein; if no blood returns, inject solution. Subcutaneous sites should be rotated for frequent injections. Monitor sites for signs of abscess or necrotic tissue. Do not use this method for patients in shock, and monitor patients with poor perfusion or low blood pressure, as the drug may not be absorbed or may be absorbed very slowly.

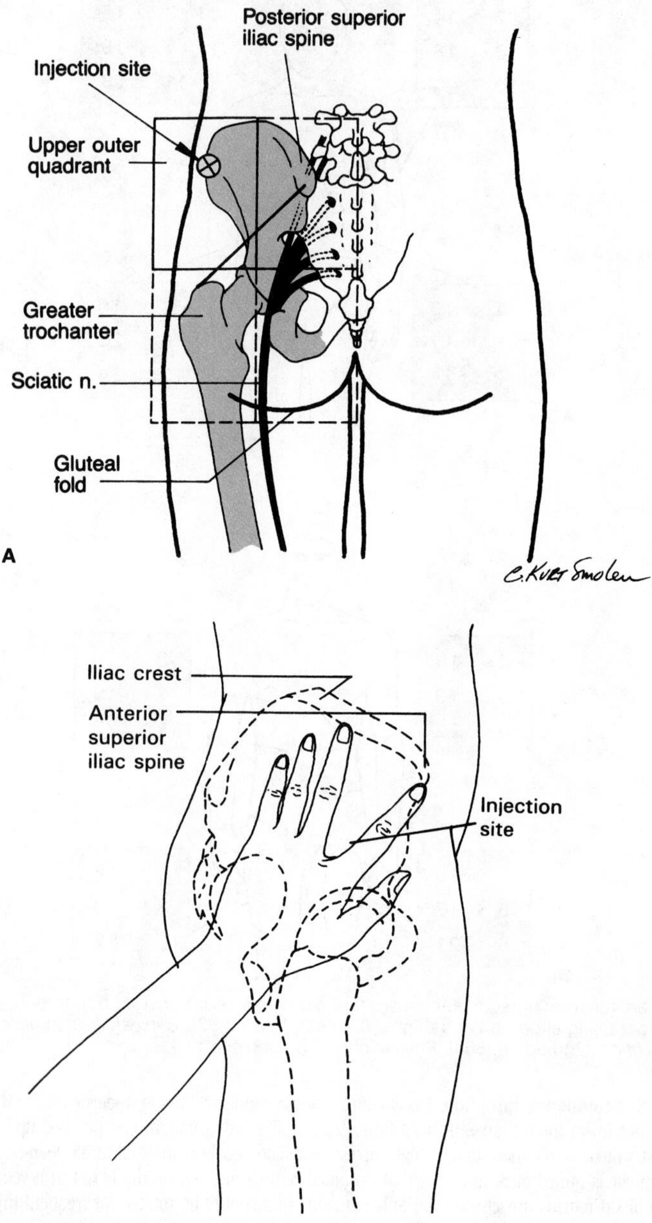


Intramuscular injection sites. (**A**) Landmarks for the dorsogluteal injection site. (**B**) Landmarks for the ventrogluteal injection site. *(continued)*

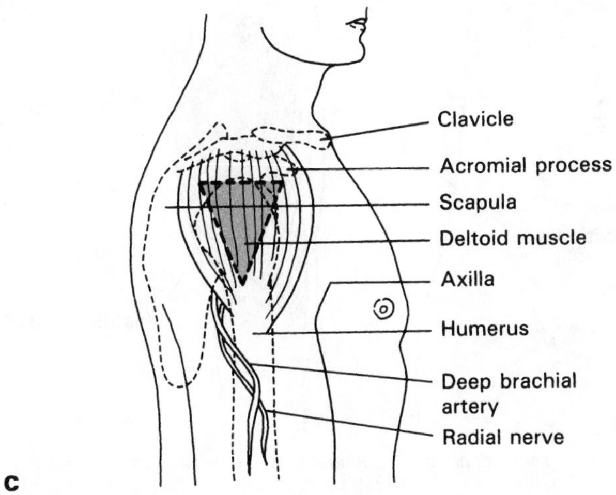


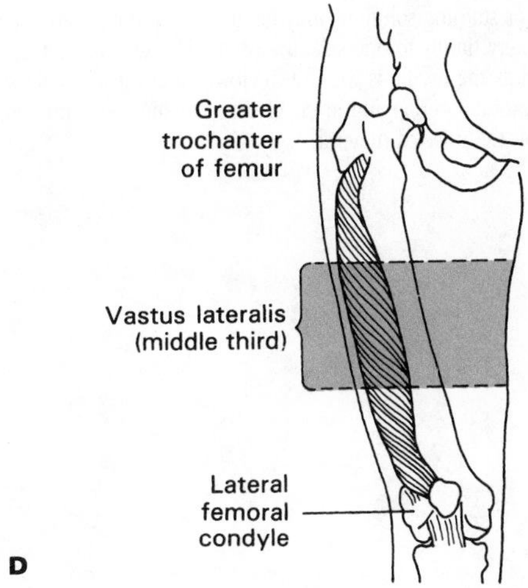


Intramuscular injection sites *(continued)*. (**C**) Landmarks for the deltoid injection site. (**D**) Landmarks for the vastus lateralis injection site. *(continued)*

**Intramuscular injection:** Insert needle quickly into big muscle; pull the plunger back to assure that no blood returns and the needle is not in a vein; if no blood returns, inject slowly. Position the patient to relax the muscle, which will increase blood flow, aid absorption, and decrease pain. Vastus lateralis muscle of the thigh is site of choice for children up to 3 y; ventrogluteal muscle is the site of choice for older children and adults; deltoid muscle and gluteus maximus are other possible sites in special situations.

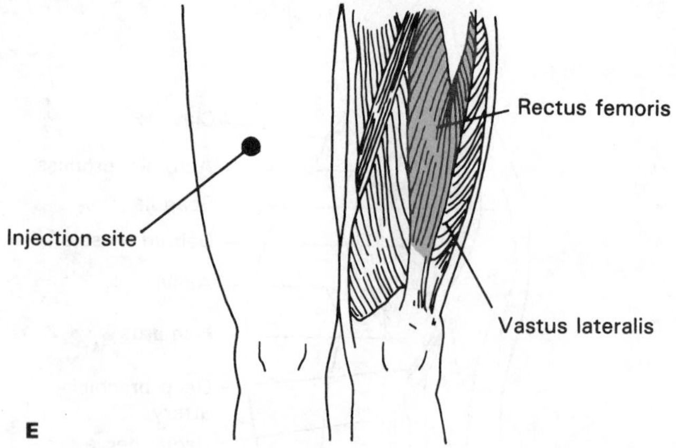


Intramuscular injection sites *(continued)*. (**E**) Landmarks for the rectus femoris injection site. (Earnest, V.V. [1992]. *Clinical skills in nursing practice* [2nd ed., pp. 865–866]. Philadelphia: JB Lippincott.)

**Z-Track:** Very irritating or staining solutions may be given by Z-track technique. The skin is prepped and pulled very tightly to one side; the needle is inserted into the muscle; the drug is injected as the needle is withdrawn slowly, and the skin released. This procedure allows the various overlapping layers of tissue to slide back into position in a Z formation, sealing off the injected material.

# APPENDIX R

## Narcotic Equianalgesic Dosages

The following are dosages for equal relief of pain when used in the acute care setting for the narcotic drugs below. Chronic administration or abuse of these drugs may alter the pharmacokinetics of the drugs, resulting in varying equivalents.

| *Drug* | *Duration* | *Half-life* | *Route* | *Equianalgesic Dosage* |
|---|---|---|---|---|
| Alfentanil | NA | 1–2 h | IM | 0.4–0.8 mg |
| Codeine | 4–6 h | 3 h | IM | 120 mg |
| | | | PO | 200 mg |
| Fentanyl | 1–2 h | 1.5–6 h | IM | 0.1 mg |
| | | | PO | NA |
| Hydrocodone | 4–8 h | 3.3–4.5 h | NA | NA |
| | | | PO | 5–10 mg |
| Hydromorphone | 4–5 h | 2–3 h | IM | 1.3–1.5 mg |
| | | | PO | 7.5 mg |
| Levorphanol | 6–8 h | 12–16 h | IM | 2 mg |
| | | | PO | 4 mg |
| Meperidine | 2–4 h | 3–4 h | IM | 75 mg |
| | | | PO | 300 mg |
| Methadone | 4–6 h | 15–30 h | IM | 10 mg |
| | | | PO | 10–20 mg |
| Morphine | 3–7 h | 1.5–2 h | IM | 10 mg |
| | | | PO | 30–60 mg |
| Oxycodone | 4–6 h | NA | PO | 30 mg |
| | | | IM | 10–15 mg |
| Oxymorphone | 3–6 h | NA | IM | 1 mg |
| | | | PR | 10 mg |
| Propoxyphene | 4–6 h | 6–12 h | PO | 130/200 mg |
| Sufentanil | NA | 2.5 h | IM | 0.02 mg |

# APPENDIX S

## Patient Teaching Guide

Patient's name ______________________________

Prescriber's name ______________________________

Phone number ______________________________

Instructions:

1. The name of your drug is ____________________ ; it is used for ____________________
2. The dose of the drug that is ordered for you is ______________________________.
3. Special storage instruction for your drug:
4. The drug should be taken ________ times a day. The best time to take your drug is ____________ , ____________ , etc.
5. The drug should (not) be taken with meals, because food will affect the way the drug is absorbed.
6. Special activities that should be considered when taking this drug:
7. Be aware that the following side effects may occur:
8. Do not take this drug with other drugs, including over-the-counter medications without first checking with your health care provider.
9. Tell any nurse, physician, or dentist who is taking care of you that you are taking this drug.
10. Keep this and all medications out of the reach of children.

*Notify your nurse or physician if any of the following occur:*

1. Report: (specific signs or symptoms associated with drug toxicity)
2. Abrupt stoppage of the drug. Abrupt stoppage of this drug can cause ____________________.

Whenever a patient is given the responsibility for drug administration, there are certain facts to which the patient should have ready access. Some states require that patients be given written information about their drugs. Nursing care always includes patient teaching activities. This teaching guide is designed to be copied for distribution to the patient, and the specific information about each drug—which is found in the patient teaching section of each drug monograph—can be added for a quick, precise teaching aid. The patient needs to know what the drug is and the dosage prescribed, especially if he or she sees more than one physician or travels; special storage information; how many times a day and *when* the drug should be taken; how to take the drug in relation to meals; specific adverse effects that are expected with this drug; special precautions or activities that are related to the use of this drug, including follow-up visits or tests; signs and symptoms to report to his or her health care provider; and dangers of abrupt stoppage of the drug. Good practice also requires reminding the patient to avoid all other medications (including OTC drugs) without checking first, keeping drugs away from children, and reporting to any other health care provider that he or she is taking this drug.

# APPENDIX T

## Important Dietary Guidelines for Patient Teaching

*Tyramine-Rich foods* (important to avoid with MAO inhibitors, some antihypertensives)

| | | | | |
|---|---|---|---|---|
| Aged cheeses | Avocados | Bananas | Beer | Bologna |
| Caffeine beverages | Chocolate | Liver | Over-ripe fruit | Pepperoni |
| Pickled fish | Red wine (Chianti) | Salami | Smoked fish | Yeast |
| Yogurt | | | | |

*Potassium-Rich Foods* (important to eat with potassium wasting diuretics)

| | | | | |
|---|---|---|---|---|
| Avocados | Bananas | Broccoli | Cantaloupe | Dried fruits |
| Grapefruit | Lima Beans | Nuts | Navy beans | Oranges |
| Peaches | Potatoes | Prunes | Rhubarb | Sanka coffee |
| Sunflower seeds | Spinach | Tomatoes | | |

*Calcium-Rich Foods* (important after menopause, in children, in hypocalcemic states)

| | | | | |
|---|---|---|---|---|
| Bok choy | Broccoli | Canned salmon | Canned sardines | Clams |
| Cream soups (made with milk) | Spinach | Dairy products | Milk | Molasses |
| | | Tofu | | |
| Oysters | | | | |

*Urine Acidifiers* (important in maintaining excretion of some drugs)

| | | | | | |
|---|---|---|---|---|---|
| Cheese | Cranberries | Eggs | Fish | Grains | Plums |
| Poultry | Prunes | Red meats | | | |

*Urine alkalinizer* (important in maintaining excretion of some drugs)

| | | | | |
|---|---|---|---|---|
| Apples | Berries | Citrus fruit | Milk | Vegetables |

*Iron-Rich Foods* (important in maintaining RBC)

| | | | | |
|---|---|---|---|---|
| Beets | Cereals | Dried beans/peas | Dried fruit | Enriched grains |
| Leafy-green vegetables | | Organ meats (liver, heart, kidney) | | |

*Low-Sodium Foods* (important in CHF, hypertension, fluid overload, etc.)

| | | | | | |
|---|---|---|---|---|---|
| Egg yolk | Fresh vegetables | Fresh fruit | Grits | Honey | Jam/jellies |
| Lean meats | Lima beans | Macaroons | Potatoes | Poultry | Pumpkin |
| Puffed rice | Puffed wheat | Red kidney beans | | Sherbet | Unsalted nuts |

*High-Sodium Foods* (important in CHF, hypertension, fluid overload, etc.)

| | | | | |
|---|---|---|---|---|
| BBQ | Beer | Buttermilk | Butter | Canned soups |
| Canned seafood | Canned spaghetti sauce | Pre-packaged dinners, cookies, mixes | Cured meats | "Fast foods" |
| Microwave dinners | Pickles | Snack foods | Tomato ketchup | TV dinners |
| Pretzels | Sauerkraut | | | |

# Appendix U

## NANDA-APPROVED NURSING DIAGNOSES

This list represents the NANDA-approved nursing diagnoses for clinical use and testing (1994)

PATTERN 1: EXCHANGING

| | |
|---|---|
| 1.1.2.1 | Altered Nutrition: More than Body Requirements |
| 1.1.2.2 | Altered Nutrition: Less than Body Requirements |
| 1.1.2.3 | Altered Nutrition: Risk for More Than Body Requirements |
| 1.2.1.1 | Risk for Infection |
| 1.2.2.1 | Risk for Altered Body Temperature |
| 1.2.2.2 | Hypothermia |
| 1.2.2.3 | Hyperthermia |
| 1.2.2.4 | Ineffective Thermoregulation |
| 1.2.3.1 | Dysreflexia |
| 1.3.1.1 | Constipation |
| 1.3.1.1.1 | Perceived Constipation |
| 1.3.1.1.2 | Colonic Constipation |
| 1.3.1.2 | Diarrhea |
| 1.3.1.3 | Bowel Incontinence |
| 1.3.2 | Altered Urinary Elimination |
| 1.3.2.1.1 | Stress Incontinence |
| 1.3.2.1.2 | Reflex Incontinence |
| 1.3.2.1.3 | Urge Incontinence |
| 1.3.2.1.4 | Functional Incontinence |
| 1.3.2.1.5 | Total Incontinence |
| 1.3.2.2 | Urinary Retention |
| 1.4.1.1 | Altered (Specify Type) Tissue Perfusion (Renal, cerebral, cardiopulmonary, gastrointestinal, peripheral) |
| * 1.4.1.2.1 | Fluid Volume Excess |
| * 1.4.1.2.2.1 | Fluid Volume Deficit |
| 1.4.1.2.2.2 | Risk for Fluid Volume Deficit |
| * 1.4.2.1 | Decreased Cardiac Output |
| 1.5.1.1 | Impaired Gas Exchange |
| 1.5.1.2 | Ineffective Airway Clearance |
| * 1.5.1.3 | Ineffective Breathing Pattern |
| 1.5.1.3.1 | Inability to Sustain Spontaneous Ventilation |
| 1.5.1.3.2 | Dysfunctional Ventilatory Weaning Response (DVWR) |
| 1.6.1 | Risk for Injury |
| 1.6.1.1 | Risk for Suffocation |
| 1.6.1.2 | Risk for Poisoning |
| 1.6.1.3 | Risk for Trauma |
| 1.6.1.4 | Risk for Aspiration |
| 1.6.1.5 | Risk for Disuse Syndrome |
| 1.6.2 | Altered Protection |
| 1.6.2.1 | Impaired Tissue Integrity |
| 1.6.2.1.1 | Altered Oral Mucous Membrane |
| 1.6.2.1.2.1 | Impaired Skin Integrity |

| | |
|---|---|
| 1.6.2.1.2.2 | Risk for Impaired Skin Integrity |
| 1.7.1 | Decreased Adaptive Capacity: Intracranial |
| 1.8 | Energy Field Disturbance |

PATTERN 2: COMMUNICATING

| | |
|---|---|
| 2.1.1.1 | Impaired Verbal Communication |

PATTERN 3: RELATING

| | |
|---|---|
| 3.1.1 | Impaired Social Interaction |
| 3.1.2 | Social Isolation |
| 3.1.3 | Risk for Loneliness |
| 3.2.1 | Altered Role Performance |
| 3.2.1.1.1 | Altered Parenting |
| 3.2.1.1.2 | Risk for Altered Parenting |
| 3.2.1.1.2.1 | Risk for Altered Parent/Infant/Child Attachment |
| 3.2.1.2.1 | Sexual Dysfunction |
| 3.2.2 | Altered Family Processes |
| 3.2.2.1 | Caregiver Role Strain |
| 3.2.2.2 | Risk for Caregiver Role Strain |
| 3.2.2.3.1 | Altered Family Process: Alcoholism |
| 3.2.3.1 | Parental Role Conflict |
| 3.3 | Altered Sexuality Patterns |

PATTERN 4: VALUING

| | |
|---|---|
| 4.1.1 | Spiritual Distress (Distress of the Human Spirit) |
| 4.2 | Potential for Enhanced Spiritual Well-Being |

PATTERN 5: CHOOSING

| | |
|---|---|
| * 5.1.1.1 | Ineffective Individual Coping |
| 5.1.1.1.1 | Impaired Adjustment |
| 5.1.1.1.2 | Defensive Coping |
| 5.1.1.1.3 | Ineffective Denial |
| * 5.1.2.1.1 | Ineffective Family Coping: Disabling |
| * 5.1.2.1.2 | Ineffective Family Coping: Compromised |
| 5.1.2.2 | Family Coping: Potential for Growth |
| 5.1.3.1 | Potential for Enhanced Community Coping |
| 5.1.3.2 | Ineffective Community Coping |
| 5.2.1 | Ineffective Management of Therapeutic Regimen (Individuals) |
| 5.2.1.1 | Noncompliance (Specify) |
| 5.2.2 | Ineffective Management of Therapeutic Regimen: Families |
| 5.2.3 | Ineffective Management of Therapeutic Regimen: Community |
| 5.2.4 | Effective Management of Therapeutic Regimen: Individual |
| 5.3.1.1 | Decisional Conflict (Specify) |
| 5.4 | Health Seeking Behaviors (Specify) |

PATTERN 6: MOVING

| | |
|---|---|
| 6.1.1.1 | Impaired Physical Mobility |
| 6.1.1.1.1 | Risk for Peripheral Neurovascular Dysfunction |
| 6.1.1.1.2 | Risk for Perioperative Positioning Injury |
| 6.1.1.2 | Activity Intolerance |

| | | |
|---|---|---|
| | 6.1.1.2.1 | Fatigue |
| | 6.1.1.3 | Risk for Activity Intolerance |
| | 6.2.1 | Sleep Pattern Disturbance |
| | 6.3.1.1 | Diversional Activity Deficit |
| | 6.4.1.1 | Impaired Home Maintenance Management |
| | 6.4.2 | Altered Health Maintenance |
| | 6.5.1 | Feeding Self Care Deficit |
| | 6.5.1.1 | Impaired Swallowing |
| | 6.5.1.2 | Ineffective Breastfeeding |
| | 6.5.1.2.1 | Interrupted Breastfeeding |
| | 6.5.1.3 | Effective Breastfeeding |
| | 6.5.1.4 | Ineffective Infant Feeding Pattern |
| | 6.5.2 | Bathing/Hygiene Self Care Deficit |
| | 6.5.3 | Dressing/Grooming Self Care Deficit |
| | 6.5.4 | Toileting Self Care Deficit |
| | 6.6 | Altered Growth and Development |
| | 6.7 | Relocation Stress Syndrome |
| | 6.8.1 | Risk for Disorganized Infant Behavior |
| | 6.8.2 | Disorganized Infant Behavior |
| | 6.8.3 | Potential for Enhanced Organized Infant Behavior |

PATTERN 7: PERCEIVING

| | | |
|---|---|---|
| | 7.1.1 | Body Image Disturbance |
| * | 7.1.2 | Self Esteem Disturbance |
| * | 7.1.2.1 | Chronic Low Self Esteem |
| * | 7.1.2.2 | Situational Low Self Esteem |
| | 7.1.3 | Personal Identity Disturbance |
| | 7.2 | Sensory/Perceptual Alterations (Specify) (Visual, Auditory, Kinesthetic, Gustatory, Tactile, Olfactory) |
| | 7.2.1.1 | Unilateral Neglect |
| | 7.3.1 | Hopelessness |
| | 7.3.2 | Powerlessness |

PATTERN 8: KNOWING

| | | |
|---|---|---|
| * | 8.1.1 | Knowledge Deficit (Specify) |
| | 8.2.1 | Impaired Environmental Interpretation Syndrome |
| | 8.2.2 | Acute Confusion |
| | 8.2.3 | Chronic Confusion |
| | 8.3 | Altered Thought Processes |
| | 8.3.1 | Impaired Memory |

PATTERN 9: FEELING

| | | |
|---|---|---|
| * | 9.1.1 | Pain |
| * | 9.1.1.1 | Chronic Pain |
| * | 9.2.1.1 | Dysfunctional Grieving |
| * | 9.2.1.2 | Anticipatory Grieving |
| * | 9.2.2 | Risk for Violence: Self-Directed or Directed at Others |
| | 9.2.2.1 | Risk for Self-Mutilation |
| | 9.2.3 | Post-Trauma Response |

| | |
|---|---|
| 9.2.3.1 | Rape-Trauma Syndrome |
| 9.2.3.1.1 | Rape-Trauma Syndrome: Compound Reaction |
| 9.2.3.1.2 | Rape-Trauma Syndrome: Silent Reaction |
| 9.3.1 | Anxiety |
| 9.3.2 | Fear |

*Diagnoses revised by small work groups at the 1994 Biennial Conference on the Classification of Nursing Diagnoses; changes approved and added in 1996.

## Information About Nursing Diagnoses

The diagnoses are in taxonomic order, including definition, defining characteristics, risk factors and related factors. Because the process of developing and reviewing diagnoses has evolved, not all components are available for all diagnoses. For diagnoses approved in the early stages, critical defining characteristics were identified. This is denoted by an asterisk. Later, critical and supporting components were replaced by major and minor defining characteristics. The date next to the diagnostic title represents the conference year in which the general assembly accepted the diagnosis. Revised lists appear in subsequent proceedings. Those diagnoses accepted prior to 1986 do not have defining characteristics differentiated as major or minor. The diagnoses accepted in 1986 have identified defining characteristics as major (critical indicators) and minor (supporting indicators). Major defining characteristics are present in 80 to 100% of the clients experiencing the diagnosis and minor as present in 50 to 79% of the clients experiencing the diagnosis.

# APPENDIX V: **Drug Compatibility Guide**

| | aminophylline | amphotericin B | ampicillin | atropine | calcium gluconate | carbenicillin | cefazolin | cimetidine | clindamycin | diazepam | dopamine | epinephrine | erythromycin | fentanyl | furosemide | gentamicin |
|---|---|---|---|---|---|---|---|---|---|---|---|---|---|---|---|---|
| aminophylline | * | | Y | | Y | N | N | | N | Y | Y | N | N | | | |
| amphotericin B | | * | N | | N | N | | N | | | N | | | | | N |
| ampicillin | Y | N | * | N | N | Y | Y | | N | | N | | N | | | N |
| atropine | | | N | * | | | | Y | | N | | N | | Y | | |
| calcium gluconate | Y | N | N | | * | | N | | N | | Y | N | Y | | | |
| carbenicillin | N | N | Y | | | * | | Y | Y | | Y | N | N | | | N |
| cefazolin | N | | Y | | N | | * | N | | Y | | | N | | | N |
| cimetidine | | N | | Y | | Y | N | * | Y | | | Y | Y | | Y | Y |
| clindamycin | N | | N | | N | Y | | Y | * | | | | | | | Y |
| diazepam | Y | | | N | | | Y | | | * | | N | | | N | |
| dopamine | Y | N | N | | Y | Y | | | | | * | | | | | N |
| epinephrine | N | | | N | N | N | | Y | | N | | * | N | | N | |
| erythromycin | N | | N | | Y | N | N | Y | | | | N | * | | | |
| fentanyl | | | | Y | | | | | | | | | | * | | |

| | glycopyrrolate | heparin sodium | hydrocortisone | hydroxyzine | levarterenol | lidocaine | meperidine | morphine | nitroglycerin | pentobarbital | potassium choride | sodium bicarbonate | tetracycline | vancomycin | verapamil | viatmin B & C complex |
|---|---|---|---|---|---|---|---|---|---|---|---|---|---|---|---|---|
| aminophylline | | Y | Y | N | N | Y | N | N | Y | Y | Y | Y | N | N | Y | N |
| amphotericin B | | Y | Y | | | N | | | | | N | Y | N | | N | |
| ampicillin | | Y | N | | | Y | | | | | Y | | N | | Y | Y |
| atropine | Y | N | | Y | N | | Y | Y | | N | Y | N | | | Y | Y |
| calcium gluconate | | Y | Y | | Y | Y | | | | | Y | N | N | Y | Y | Y |
| carbenicillin | | | Y | | N | Y | | | | | Y | | N | | Y | N |
| cefazolin | | | Y | | N | N | | | | N | Y | | N | | Y | Y |
| cimetidine | | Y | | | Y | Y | | | | N | Y | | Y | Y | Y | Y |
| clindamycin | | Y | Y | | | | | | | N | Y | Y | | | Y | Y |
| diazepam | N | N | | N | N | N | N | N | | N | N | N | | | Y | N |
| dopamine | | Y | Y | | | Y | | | Y | | Y | | Y | | Y | Y |
| epinephrine | | Y | | | N | N | Y | | | | N | N | | | Y | Y |
| erythromycin | | N | Y | | | Y | | | | N | Y | Y | N | Y | Y | N |
| fentanyl | | | | Y | | | Y | Y | | N | | | | | | |

| | | | | | | | | | | | | | | | | | | | | | | | | | | | | | | | | |
|---|---|---|---|---|---|---|---|---|---|---|---|---|---|---|---|---|---|---|---|---|---|---|---|---|---|---|---|---|---|---|---|---|
| furosemide | | | | | | | | Y | | N | | N | | | * | N | | Y | | | N | | | | Y | | Y | | N | | Y | Y |
| gentamicin | | N | N | | | N | N | | Y | | Y | | | | N | * | | N | | | | | | | | | | | | | Y | Y |
| glycopyrrolate | | | | Y | | | | | | N | | | | | | | * | | | Y | | Y | Y | Y | | N | | N | | | | |
| heparin sodium | Y | Y | Y | N | Y | | | Y | Y | N | Y | Y | N | | Y | N | | * | N | N | Y | Y | N | N | | | Y | Y | N | N | Y | Y |
| hydrocortisone | Y | Y | N | | Y | Y | Y | | Y | | Y | | Y | | | | | N | * | | Y | Y | | | | N | Y | Y | N | Y | Y | Y |
| hydroxyzine | N | | | Y | | | | | | N | | | | Y | | | Y | N | | * | | Y | Y | Y | | N | | | | | | N |
| levarterenol | N | | | N | Y | N | N | Y | | N | | N | | | N | | | Y | Y | | * | | | | | N | Y | | Y | | Y | Y |
| lidocaine | Y | N | Y | | Y | Y | N | Y | | N | Y | N | Y | | | | Y | Y | Y | Y | | * | | | Y | Y | Y | Y | Y | | Y | Y |
| meperidine | N | | | Y | | | | | | N | | Y | | Y | | | Y | N | | Y | | | * | N | | N | | N | | | Y | |
| morphine | N | | | Y | | | | | | N | | | | Y | | | Y | N | | Y | | | N | * | | N | Y | N | | | Y | Y |
| nitroglycerin | Y | | | | | | | | | | Y | | | | Y | | | | | | | Y | | | * | | | | | | Y | |
| pentobarbital | Y | | | N | | | N | N | N | N | | | N | N | | | N | | N | N | N | Y | N | N | | * | | N | N | N | Y | |
| potassium chloride | Y | N | Y | Y | Y | Y | Y | Y | Y | N | Y | N | Y | | Y | | | Y | Y | | Y | Y | | Y | | | * | Y | Y | Y | Y | |
| sodium bicarbonate | Y | Y | | N | N | | | | Y | N | | N | Y | | | | N | Y | Y | | | Y | N | N | | N | Y | * | N | N | Y | N |
| tetracycline | N | N | N | | N | N | N | Y | | | Y | | N | | N | | | N | N | | Y | Y | | | | N | Y | N | * | | | Y |
| vancomycin | N | | | | Y | | | Y | | | | | Y | | | | | N | Y | | | | | | | N | Y | N | | * | Y | Y |
| verapamil | Y | N | Y | Y | Y | Y | Y | Y | Y | Y | Y | Y | Y | | Y | Y | | Y | Y | | Y | Y | Y | Y | Y | Y | Y | Y | | Y | * | Y |
| vitamin B & C complex | N | | Y | Y | Y | N | Y | Y | Y | N | Y | Y | N | | Y | Y | | Y | Y | N | Y | Y | | Y | | | | N | Y | Y | Y | * |

KEY:
Y = Compatible
N = Incompatible
Blank space = Information about compatibility was not available

NOTE: Because the compatibility of two or more drugs in solution depends on several variables such as the solution itself, drug concentration and the method of mixing (bottle, syringe, or Y-site), this table is intended to be used solely as a guide to general drug compatibilities. Before mixing any drugs, the health-care professional should ascertain if a potential incompatibility exists by referring to an appropriate information source.

(Reprinted from Malseed, R.T., Goldstein, F.J. & Balkon, N. (1995). *Phamacology: Drug therapy and nursing management* (4th ed) Philadelphia: JB Lippincott Co. Used with permission.)

# APPENDIX W: Quick Check: Compatibility of Drugs in Syringe

| | atropine | butorphanol | chlorpromazine | cimetidine | dimenhydrinate | dimenhydramine | fentanyl | glycopyrrolate | heparin | hydroxyzine | meperidine | metoclopramide | midazolam | morphine | nalbuphine | pentazocine | pentobarbital | prochlorperazine | promethazine | ranitidine | secobarbital | thiopental |
|---|---|---|---|---|---|---|---|---|---|---|---|---|---|---|---|---|---|---|---|---|---|---|
| atropine | Y | Y | Y | Y | M | M | M | Y | M | Y | Y | M | Y | M | Y | M | M | M | M | Y | | |
| butorphanol | Y | Y | Y | Y | N | Y | Y | | | Y | M | | Y | Y | | Y | N | Y | Y | | | |
| chlorpromazine | Y | Y | Y | N | N | M | M | Y | N | M | M | M | Y | M | | M | N | Y | M | Y | | N |
| cimetidine | Y | Y | N | Y | | Y | Y | Y | Y | Y | Y | | Y | Y | Y | Y | N | Y | Y | | N | |
| dimenhydrinate | M | N | N | | Y | M | M | N | M | N | M | M | N | M | | M | N | N | N | Y | | N |
| dimenhydramine | M | Y | | Y | M | Y | | Y | | M | M | Y | Y | M | | M | N | M | M | Y | | N |
| fentanyl | M | Y | M | | M | M | Y | | M | Y | M | M | Y | M | | M | N | M | M | Y | | |
| glycopyrrolate | Y | | Y | Y | N | Y | | Y | | Y | Y | | Y | Y | | N | N | Y | Y | Y | N | N |
| heparin | M | | N | | M | | M | | Y | | N | M | | N | | N | | | N | | | |

| | | | | | | | | | | | | | | | | | | | | | | |
|---|---|---|---|---|---|---|---|---|---|---|---|---|---|---|---|---|---|---|---|---|---|---|
| hydroxyzine | Y | Y | M | Y | N | M | Y | Y | | Y | M | M | Y | Y | Y | Y | N | M | M | N | | |
| meperidine | Y | M | M | Y | M | M | M | Y | N | M | Y | M | Y | N | | M | N | M | Y | Y | | N |
| metoclopramide | M | | M | | M | Y | M | | M | M | M | Y | Y | M | | M | | M | M | Y | | |
| midazolam | Y | Y | Y | Y | N | Y | Y | Y | | Y | Y | Y | Y | Y | Y | | N | N | Y | N | | |
| morphine | M | Y | M | Y | M | M | M | Y | N | Y | N | M | Y | Y | | M | N | M | M | Y | | N |
| nalbuphine | Y | | | Y | | | | | | Y | | | Y | | Y | | N | Y | Y | Y | | |
| pentazocine | M | Y | M | Y | M | M | M | N | N | Y | M | M | | M | | Y | N | M | Y | Y | | |
| pentobarbital | M | N | N | N | N | N | N | N | | N | N | N | N | N | N | N | Y | N | N | | | Y |
| prochlorperazine | M | Y | Y | Y | N | M | M | Y | | M | M | M | N | M | Y | M | N | Y | M | Y | | N |
| promethazine | M | Y | M | Y | N | M | M | Y | N | M | Y | M | Y | M | Y | Y | N | M | Y | Y | | N |
| ranitidine | Y | | Y | | Y | Y | Y | Y | | N | Y | Y | N | Y | Y | Y | | Y | Y | Y | | |
| secobarbital | | | | N | | | | N | | | | | | | | | | | | | Y | |
| thiopental | | | N | | N | N | | N | | | N | | | N | | | Y | N | N | | | Y |

KEY:
Y = Compatible in syringe
M = Moderately compatible, inject immediately after combining
N = Incompatible, do not mix in syringe
Blank space = Information about compatibility is not currently available

# Bibliography

*Drug evaluations subscription* (1998). Chicago: American Medical Association.

Carpenito, L.J. (1995). *Nursing diagnosis* (6th ed.). Philadelphia: J.B. Lippincott Company.

*Drug facts and comparisons* (1998). St. Louis, MO: J.B. Lippincott-Raven.

*Drug Facts Update: Physicians On-Line.* Multimedia, 1998.

Tatro, D.S. (Ed.). (1998). *Drug interaction facts.* St. Louis, MO: J.B. Lippincott-Raven.

Gilman, A.G., Goodman, L.S., Rall, T.W., and Murad, F. (Eds.). (1993) *Goodman and Gilman's the pharmacological basis of therapeutics* (8th ed.) New York: Macmillan.

*Handbook of adverse drug interactions.* (1998). New Rochelle, NY: The Medical Letter.

Katzung, B.G. (1987). *Basic and clinical pharmacology* (3rd ed.). Norwalk, Connecticut: Appleton and Lange.

Levine, R.R. (1993). *Pharmacology: Drug actions and reactions (3rd ed.). Boston: Little, Brown.*

Lindberg, J. et al. (1998). *Introduction to nursing (2nd ed.).* Philadelphia: J.B. Lippincott-Raven.

Malseed, R. (1995). *Textbook of pharmacology and nursing care.* Philadelphia: J.B. Lippincott Company.

*PDR for nonprescription drugs.* (1998). Oradell, NJ: Medical Economics Company.

*PDR for ophthalmology.* (1998). Oradell, NJ: Medical Economics Company.

*Physicians' desk reference* (44th ed.) (1998). Oradell, NJ: Medical Economics Company.

*Professionals guide to patient drug facts.* (1998). St. Louis, MO: J.B. Lippincott-Raven.

Rodman, M.J., Karch, A.M., Boyd, E.H., and Smith, D.W. (1985). *Pharmacology and drug therapy in nursing* (3rd ed.). Philadelphia: J.B. Lippincott Company.

Smeltzer, S.C., & Bare, B.G. (1996). *Brunner and Suddarth's textbook of medical-surgical nursing* (8th ed.). Philadelphia: J.B. Lippincott-Raven.

Spencer, Nichols, Waterhouse, et al. (1993). *Clinical pharmacology and nursing management.* Philadelphia: J.B. Lippincott Company.

*The medical letter on drugs and therapeutics* (1998). New Rochelle, NY: Medical Letter.

Griffiths, M.C. (Ed.). (1987) *USAN 1987 and the USP dictionary of drug names.* Rockville, MD: United States Pharmacopeial Convention.

# Index

Official generic names are shown in **bold face**. Brand names of drugs are shown in *italics* followed by the generic name in parentheses. Brand names of Canadian drugs are indicated by (CAN). Chemical or nonofficial names appear in plain print. Drug classes appear in **BOLD CAPITAL LETTERS** with the drugs that fall in that class listed as official names under the class heading.

## A

## B

## C

## D

## E

## F

## G

## H

## I

## J



## K

## N

## O

## P

## Q



## R

## S

## T

## U



## V

## Example of a Drug Monograph that can be printed directly from the enclosed disk

*captopril*

***(kap' toe pril)***

Apo-Capto (CAN), Capoten, Novo-Captopril (CAN), Nu-Capto (CAN), Syn-Captopril (CAN)

**Pregnancy Category C**

### Drug classes

Antihypertensive

Angiotensin-converting enzyme (ACE) inhibitor

### Therapeutic actions

Blocks ACE from converting angiotensin I to angiotensin II, a powerful vasoconstrictor, leading to decreased blood pressure, decreased aldosterone secretion, a small increase in serum potassium levels, and sodium and fluid loss; increased prostaglandin synthesis also may be involved in the antihypertensive action.

### Indications

- Hypertension alone or in combination with thiazide-type diuretics
- CHF in patients unresponsive to conventional therapy; used with diuretics and digitalis
- Diabetic nephropathy
- Left ventricular dysfunction after MI
- Unlabeled uses: management of hypertensive crises; treatment of rheumatoid arthritis; diabetic nephropathy, diagnosis of anatomic renal artery stenosis, hypertension related to scleroderma; renal crisis; diagnosis of primary aldosteronism, idiopathic edema; Bartter's syndrome; Raynaud's syndrome; hypertension of Takayasu's disease

### Contraindications/cautions

- Allergy to captopril; impaired renal function; CHF; salt/volume depletion, lactation.

### Dosage

ADULT

- *Hypertension:* 25 mg PO bid or tid; if satisfactory response is not noted within 1–2 wk, increase dosage to 50 mg bid–tid; usual range is 25–150 mg bid–tid PO with a mild thiazide diuretic. Do not exceed 450 mg/d.
- *Congestive heart failure:* 6.25–12.5 mg PO tid in patients who may be salt/volume depleted. Usual initial dose is 25 mg PO tid; maintenance dose of 50–100 mg PO tid. Do not exceed 450 mg/d. Use in conjunction with diuretic and digitalis therapy.
- *Left ventricular dysfunction after MI:* 50 mg PO tid, starting as early as 3 days post MI. Initial dose of 6.25 mg, then 12.5 mg tid, increasing slowly to 50 mg tid.
- *Diabetic nephropathy:* 25 mg PO tid.

PEDIATRIC: Safety and efficacy not established.

GERIATRIC AND RENAL IMPAIRED: Excretion is reduced in renal failure; use smaller initial dose; titrate at smaller doses with 1- to 2-wk intervals between increases; slowly titrate to smallest effective dose. Use a loop diuretic with renal dysfunction.

### Pharmacokinetics

| Route | Onset | Peak |
|---|---|---|
| Oral | 15 min | ½–1½ h |

*Metabolism:* $T_{1/2}$: 2 h

*Distribution:* Crosses placenta; passes into breast milk

*Excretion:* Urine

### Adverse effects

- CV: *Tachycardia,* angina pectoris, **MI,** Raynaud's syndrome, CHF, hypotension in salt/volume depleted patients
- GI: *Gastric irritation, aphthous ulcers, peptic ulcers, dysgeusia,* cholestatic jaundice, hepatocellular injury, anorexia, constipation
- Hematologic: Neutropenia, agranulocytosis, thrombocytopenia, hemolytic anemia, **fatal pancytopenia**

Adverse effects in *Italics* are most common; those in **Bold** are life-threatening.

- GU: *Proteinuria,* renal insufficiency, renal failure, polyuria, oliguria, urinary frequency
- **Dermatologic:** *Rash, pruritus,* pemphigoid-like reaction, scalded mouth sensation, exfoliative dermatitis, photosensitivity, alopecia
- **Other:** Cough, malaise, dry mouth, lymphadenopathy

### Clinically important drug-drug interactions

• Increased risk of hypersensitivity reactions with allopurinol • Decreased antihypertensive effects with indomethacin

### Clinically important drug-food interactions

• Decreased absorption of captopril with food

### Drug-lab test interferences

• False-positive test for urine acetone

## ■ Nursing Considerations

### Assessment

- *History:* Allergy to captopril, impaired renal function, CHF, salt/volume depletion, pregnancy, lactation
- *Physical:* Skin color, lesions, turgor; T; P, BP, peripheral perfusion; mucous membranes, bowel sounds, liver evaluation; urinalysis, renal and liver function tests, CBC and differential

### Implementation

- Administer 1 h before or 2 h after meals.
- Alert surgeon and mark patient's chart with notice that captopril is being taken; the angiotensin II formation subsequent to compensatory renin release during surgery will be blocked; hypotension may be reversed with volume expansion.
- Monitor patient closely for fall in BP secondary to reduction in fluid volume (excessive perspiration and dehydration, vomiting, diarrhea); excessive hypotension may occur.
- Reduce dosage in patients with impaired renal function.

### Drug-specific teaching points

- Take drug 1 h before or 2 h after meals; do not take with food.
- Do not stop without consulting your physician.
- The following side effects may occur: GI upset, loss of appetite, change in taste perception (limited effects, will pass); mouth sores (frequent mouth care may help); skin rash; fast heart rate; dizziness, lightheadedness (usually passes after the first few days; change position slowly, and limit your activities to those that do not require alertness and precision).
- Be careful of drop in blood pressure (occurs most often with diarrhea, sweating, vomiting, dehydration); if lightheadedness or dizziness occurs, consult your care provider.
- Avoid OTC medications, especially cough, cold, allergy medications that may contain ingredients that will interact with it.
- Report mouth sores; sore throat, fever, chills; swelling of the hands, feet; irregular heartbeat, chest pains; swelling of the face, eyes, lips, tongue, difficulty breathing.

## Example of a Patient Teaching Printout that can be formulated using your own word processing software

Patient's Name: ______________________________

*You should know the following information about the drug that has been prescribed for you:*

**Drug Name: captopril**

How to pronounce: ***kap' toe pril***

Other names that this drug is known by: Capoten: this drug is used to treat your hypertension.

## Instructions to follow for your safety:

- Take drug 1 hour before or 2 hours after meals; do not take with food.
- Do not stop without consulting your physician.
- The following side effects may occur: gastrointestinal upset, loss of appetite, change in taste perception (these effects will pass); mouth sores (frequent mouth care may help); skin rash; fast heart rate; dizziness, lightheadedness (usually passes after the first few days; change position slowly, and limit your activities to those that do not require alertness and precision).
- Be careful of drop in blood pressure (diarrhea, sweating, vomiting, dehydration); if lightheadedness or dizziness occurs, consult your care provider.
- Avoid taking over-the-counter medications, especially cough, cold and allergy medications that may contain ingredients that will interact with it.
- Report mouth sores; sore throat, fever, chills; swelling of the hands, feet; irregular heartbeat, chest pains; swelling of the face, eyes, lips, tongue; difficulty breathing.
- Keep this and all medications out of the reach of children.
- Tell any doctor, dentist, or nurse who is taking care of you that you are on this drug.

A: Louis

# 1999 Lippincott's Quick-Access Drug Disk

This software program has been designed to be used with an IBM or IBM-compatible computer and Microsoft Windows. This program enables you to access information on more than 140 generic drugs and more than 500 trade name drugs, using either a generic or trade name. Once you have selected a drug, you can view the complete drug monograph, print the drug monograph, make an ASCII file, make your own drug cards, or create patient teaching printouts. If you choose to make an ASCII file, you will then be able to edit the drug information, using your own word processing program; change the information in any way that suits your needs; and print out edited information.

## YOU CAN CHOOSE EITHER PRINT OPTION TO CREATE YOUR OWN DRUG CARDS!!!!

**To start the program:**

- insert the diskette into the floppy drive
- choose the Run command from the Windows Program Manager
- type A:QUIKDRUG and click OK. (or B:QUIKDRUG if your diskette drive is :>B:)
- view the Disk Title/Copyright Screen introducing *1999 Lippincott's Quick-Access Drug Disk* and the drug disclaimer
- proceed by clicking OK

**The generic drug name list will appear on your computer screen. You will now have seven (7) options:**

- scroll through the list of drug names, using the mouse or UP and DOWN arrow keys
- view a monograph for a highlighted drug name
- switch from the generic drug name list to the trade drug name list
- search for a specific drug name
- print a drug monograph
- create an ASCII file
- exit the program

**If you have selected to view a drug monograph, the monograph will appear on your computer screen. You now have four (4) options:**

- scroll forward or backward through the monograph listing, using the mouse or the UP and DOWN arrow keys
- print the monograph
- create an ASCII file
- close the monograph and return to the drug name list

**If you have selected to create an ASCII file:**

- select and type in the drug file name using up to eight (8) characters
- click OK
- exit this program to use the file in your word-processing program; if prompted for convert file format, choose ASCII (DOS) Text

**To exit the program:**

- click Exit

**Refer to the previous three pages for an EXAMPLE OF A PATIENT TEACHING HANDOUT THAT YOU CAN CREATE and a SAMPLE DRUG MONOGRAPH PRINTOUT.**